Harrell

August's Consultations in
FELINE INTERNAL
MEDICINE
VOLUME 7

About The Cover

The handsome feline on the cover is the late Tuxedo Stan. Stanley, one of four boys born to a homeless mother, rose from his humble beginnings to international stardom when he ran for mayor of Halifax, Nova Scotia, Canada in October, 2012. His campaign helped raise awareness of the plight of neglected and homeless cats in Halifax and around the world. Tuxedo Stan's election slogan, "Because neglect isn't working," has been adopted by many feline rescue groups. The newly elected Halifax municipal government donated $40,000.00 to the local SPCA to help build a low-cost spay and neuter clinic as a direct result of the *Tuxedo Stan for Mayor* campaign. Sadly, Tuxedo Stan succumbed to aggressive renal lymphosarcoma 8 months after the election, at just 3-1/2 years of age. Stan's brother, Earl Grey, continues his work as leader of The Tuxedo Party of Canada. You can follow Earl Grey and the Tuxedo Party at www.earlgreycat.com or at www.facebook.com.

Dr. Hugh Chisholm, Tuxedo Stan's manager

August's Consultations in
FELINE INTERNAL MEDICINE

VOLUME 7

Edited by

Susan E. Little
DVM, DABVP (Feline)
Owner, Bytown Cat Hospital
Ottawa, Ontario, Canada

ELSEVIER

ELSEVIER

3251 Riverport Lane
St. Louis, MO 63043

AUGUST'S CONSULTATIONS IN FELINE INTERNAL MEDICINE   ISBN: 978-0-323-22652-3
VOLUME 7

International Standard Book Number: 978-0-323-22652-3

Vice President and Publisher: Loren Wilson
Content Strategy Director: Penny Rudolph
Content Development Manager: Jolynn Gower
Content Development Specialist: Brandi Graham
Publishing Services Manager: Julie Eddy
Design Direction: Amy Buxton
Cover photo: Dr. Hugh Chisholm

Printed in the United States of America

Last digit in the print number: 9 8 7 6 5 4 3 2 1

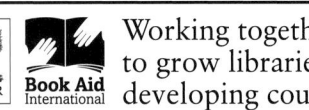

Working together
to grow libraries in
developing countries

www.elsevier.com • www.bookaid.org

It is a daunting task to take over the editorial duties for this volume of Consultations in Feline Internal Medicine *from the esteemed Dr. John R. August. The first volume in this series was published in 1991, and here we are, almost 25 years later, with the publication of volume 7. My career as a feline specialist was shaped and enriched by these volumes and I never dreamt that one day I'd have the honor of becoming editor. I hope this volume continues the tradition of excellence in cutting-edge feline medicine encompassed in the previous six volumes. It is only fitting that this volume is dedicated to the person whose vision is responsible for this body of work. Here's to you,*
Dr. August!

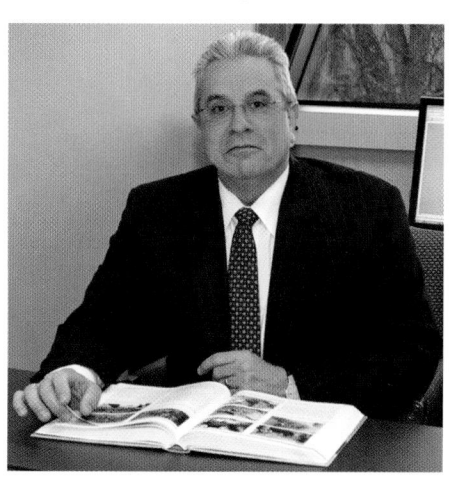

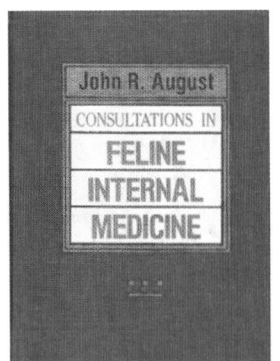
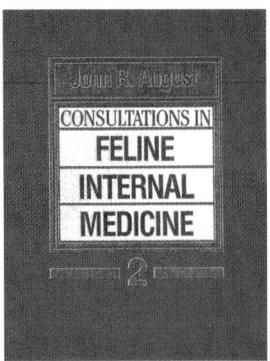
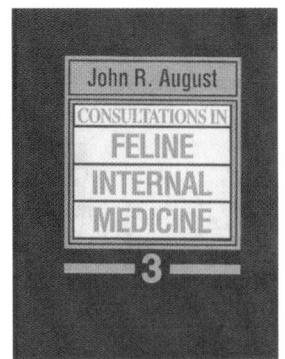
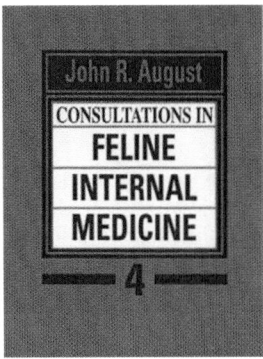
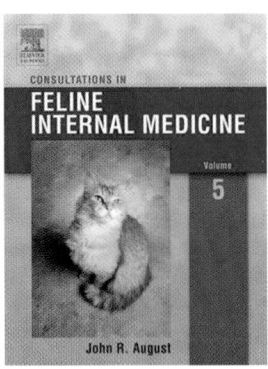
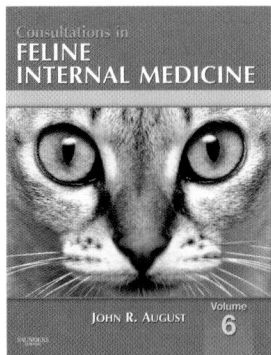

Preface

"Eeyore was saying to himself, 'This writing business. Pencils and what-not. Over-rated, if you ask me. Silly stuff. Nothing in it.'"—A.A. Milne, *Winnie-the-Pooh*

In the preface to the first volume of this series in 1991, Dr. John August wrote, "I wanted to develop a book that addressed key issues in feline medicine that were topical, practical, and controversial." He noted that the section editors for that first volume, and for every succeeding volume, were tasked with identifying hot topics and recruiting the very best authors. I have taken those words to heart and attempted to continue the tradition of publishing the best current topics in feline medicine in this volume. Such an important task was not possible without the expert assistance of the 17 section editors to identify and recruit an outstanding panel of more than 100 international authors who are experts in their fields.

The first volume in this series contained nine sections: Special Problems, Dermatology, Cardiology and Respiratory Disorders, Endocrine and Metabolic Disorders, Urinary Tract, Hematopoietic System, Gastrointestinal System, Neurology, and Infectious Diseases. Throughout the years, in keeping with the changing face of feline medicine, the sections have occasionally changed. This volume of *Consultations in Feline Internal Medicine* contains 12 sections, covering Infectious Diseases (8 chapters), Gastrointestinal Diseases (8 chapters), Endocrine and Metabolic Diseases (9 chapters), Dermatology (8 chapters), Cardiology and Respiratory Medicine (13 chapters), Upper and Lower Urinary Tract Diseases (7 chapters), Oncology (7 chapters), Nutrition (6 chapters), Population Medicine (9 chapters), as well as three new sections.

A section on Emergency and Critical Care Medicine appears for the first time in this volume. This new section, designed by editors Dr. Tony Johnson and Dr. Gretchen Statz, contains 13 chapters on diverse topics such as the new evidence-based guidelines for cardiopulmonary resuscitation in cats, treatment of hypertensive crises, and cutting-edge endourology procedures (urinary diversion techniques). Also new in this volume is a section on Behavioral Medicine with 6 chapters, edited by Dr. Debra Horwitz. The inclusion of this section reflects the growing body of research that helps us understand both normal behavior and behavior problems in cats. Behavior problems are some of the most common concerns that cat owners bring to veterinarians, so it is a delight to see the excellent content designed by Dr. Horwitz and her authors covering subjects such as anxiety disorders, intercat aggression, and house soiling. Finally, 10 chapters on Pediatric and Geriatric Medicine were separated from Population Medicine and organized into their own section by Dr. Margie Scherk. A growing body of work is illuminating the special physiology and needs of cats at either end of the life span. Chapters on anesthesia and sarcopenia in senior cats will be of special interest to clinicians, and the chapter on neonatal resuscitation covers information that is difficult to find in other sources.

In addition to the new sections, there are some new and exciting topics in the traditional sections. These include chapters on the gut microbiome, complementary and alternative therapies for inflammatory bowel disease, continuous glucose monitoring for diabetic patients, stem cell therapy for chronic kidney disease, emerging dermatoses, cardiorespiratory disease in the shelter setting, electrochemotherapy, management of large-scale cruelty cases, and controversies in feline nutrition. As always, the chapters in this book provide a mix of practical information and new ideas, even controversial topics. They contain things you will put into everyday use and material that will be thought-provoking.

Writing is essentially a lonely business, as many of the authors included in this book will tell you, but I will have to disagree with Winnie the Pooh as it is clearly not "silly stuff." The fruits of the labors of many experts are now shared with you and the feline medicine community. Cats do not give up their secrets easily, but this volume contains many important pieces of the puzzle.

ACKNOWLEDGMENTS

Putting together a textbook of this magnitude is not possible without an excellent publishing team and my thanks go to my colleagues at Elsevier, including Brandi Graham, Penny Rudolph, and others for their support and advice. Textbooks depend on the willingness of experts to share and teach, so I would like to express my gratitude to the section editors and authors who gave freely of their time and expertise in what I know are already busy professional schedules. The real reason I love to work on textbooks is how much I learn from my wonderful colleagues in the process! Finally, I want to thank the excellent veterinarians and team members I work with every day at Bytown Cat Hospital in Ottawa, Ontario for their support and understanding of the seemingly endless work of editing a textbook.

Section Editors

P. Jane Armstrong, DVM, MS, MBA
Professor of Small Animal Internal Medicine
Department of Veterinary Clinical Sciences
University of Minnesota
St. Paul, Minnesota
Nutrition

Joseph W. Bartges, DVM, PhD
Staff Internist and Academic Director
Cornell University Veterinary Specialists
Stamford, Connecticut
Adjunct Clinical Professor
Small Animal Clinical Sciences
Cornell University
Ithaca, New York
Upper and Lower Urinary Tract Diseases

Christine L. Cain, DVM, DACVD
Assistant Professor of Dermatology
Department of Clinical Studies
University of Pennsylvania
School of Veterinary Medicine
Philadelphia, Pennsylvania
Dermatology

Craig A. Datz, DVM, MS, DABVP, DACVN
Adjunct Associate Professor
College of Veterinary Medicine
University of Missouri
Columbia, Missouri
Senior Scientific Affairs Manager
Royal Canin USA
St. Charles, Missouri
Infectious Diseases

Brian A. DiGangi, DVM, MS, DABVP
Clinical Assistant Professor
Department of Small Animal Clinical Sciences
University of Florida
Gainesville, Florida
Population Medicine

Brenda Griffin, DVM, MS, DACVIM
Adjunct Associate Professor of Shelter Medicine
Department of Small Animal Clinical Sciences
College of Veterinary Medicine
University of Florida
Gainesville, Florida
Population Medicine

Debra F. Horwitz, DVM, DACVB
Veterinary Behaviorist
Veterinary Behavior Consultations
St. Louis, Missouri
Behavioral Medicine

Albert E. Jergens, DVM, PhD, DACVIM
Professor and Associate Chair for Research and Graduate
    Studies
Department of Veterinary Clinical Sciences
College of Veterinary Medicine
Iowa State University
Ames, Iowa
Gastrointestinal System

Tony Johnson, DVM, DACVECC
Medical Director
Veterinary Information Network
Davis, California
Emergency and Critical Care Medicine

Antony S. Moore, BVSc, MVSc
Veterinary Oncology Consults
Wauchope, New South Wales, Australia
Oncology

Mark E. Peterson, DVM, DACVIM
Department of Endocrinology and Nuclear Medicine
Animal Endocrine Clinic
New York, New York
Adjunct Professor of Medicine
Department of Clinical Sciences
New York State College of Veterinary Medicine
Cornell University
Ithaca, New York
Endocrine and Metabolic Diseases

Elizabeth Rozanski, DVM
Associate Professor
Department of Clinical Sciences
Tufts Cummings School of Veterinary Medicine
North Grafton, Massachusetts
Cardiology and Respiratory Medicine

John Rush, DVM, MS, DACVIM (Cardiology), DACVECC
Professor
Department of Clinical Sciences
Tufts Cummings School of Veterinary Medicine
North Grafton, Massachusetts
Cardiology and Respiratory Medicine

Margie Scherk, DVM, Dip ABVP (Feline Practice)
catsINK
Vancouver, British Columbia, Canada
Pediatric and Geriatric Medicine

Gretchen Statz, DVM, DACVECC
Staff Criticalist
Department of Internal Medicine and Critical Care
Veterinary Specialty and Emergency Care
Indianapolis, Indiana
Internal Medicine Consultant
Antech Diagnostics
Irvine, California
Emergency and Critical Care Medicine

Séverine Tasker, BSc, BVSc (Hons), PhD, DSAM, DipECVIM-CA, FHEA, MRCVS
Reader in Feline Medicine
The Feline Centre
Langford Veterinary Services & School of Veterinary
   Sciences
University of Bristol
Langford, Bristol, United Kingdom
Infectious Diseases

Angela Witzel, DVM, PhD
Assistant Clinical Professor of Nutrition
Small Animal Clinical Sciences
University of Tennessee
Knoxville, Tennessee
Nutrition

Contributors

Jill L. Abraham, VMD, DACVD
Dermatologist
Department of Dermatology
BluePearl Veterinary Partners
New York, New York
Feline Food Allergy

Karin Allenspach, DMV, ECVIM-CA, FVH, PhD, FHEA
Professor in Small Animal Internal Medicine
Department of Veterinary Clinical Sciences
Royal Veterinary College
London, Hertfordshire, Great Britain
Feline Inflammatory Gastrointestinal Disease

Jennifer Baez, VMD, DACVIM (Internal Medicine, Oncology)
Veterinary Medical Oncologist
Department of Oncology
Center for Animal Referral and Emergency Services (CARES)
Langhorne, Pennsylvania
Feline Mammary Carcinoma

Melissa Bain, DVM, DACVB, MS, DACAW
Associate Professor of Clinical Animal Behavior
Veterinary Medicine and Epidemiology
UC Davis School of Veterinary Medicine
Davis, California
Update on Feline Housesoiling and Urine Marking

Joseph W. Bartges, DVM, PhD
Staff Internist and Academic Director
Cornell University Veterinary Specialists
Stamford, Connecticut
Adjunct Clinical Professor
Small Animal Clinical Sciences
Cornell University
Ithaca, New York
Update on Feline Urolithiasis
Urinary Tract Infection

Marie C. Bélanger, DVM, MSc, ACVIM
Professor of Small Animal Internal Medicine and Cardiology
Department of Clinical Sciences
University of Montreal
St-Hyacinthe, Quebec, Canada
Cardiorenal Syndrome

David Bennett, BSc, BVetMed, PhD, DVM, DSAO, FHEA, MRCVS
Professor
School of Veterinary Medicine
University of Glasgow
Glasgow, Great Britain
Osteoarthritis in the Aging Cat

Allyson Berent, DVM, DACVIM
Staff Veterinarian, Director of Interventional Endoscopy Services
Department of Interventional Radiology / Endoscopy
The Animal Medical Center
New York, New York
Endourology in the Feline Patient: Urinary Diversion Techniques

Darren Berger, DVM, DACVD
Assistant Professor of Dermatology
Department of Veterinary Clinical Sciences
College of Veterinary Medicine
Iowa State University
Ames, Iowa
Malassezia spp. in Feline Dermatology

Jeannine M. Berger, DVM, DACVB, DACAW, CAWA
Director of Behavior Resources
Department of Behavior
San Francisco SPCA
San Francisco, California
Feline Aggression Toward People

April E. Blong, DVM, DACVECC
Post-Doctoral Associate
Cornell Clinical Fellow
Small Animal Nutrition Resident
Cornell University
College of Veterinary Medicine
Ithaca, New York
Feline Cardiopulmonary Resuscitation: Current Evidence-Based Guidelines

Manuel Boller, Dr. Med. Vet., MTR, DACVECC
Senior Lecturer Emergency and Critical Care
Faculty of Veterinary and Agricultural Sciences
University of Melbourne
Werribee, Victoria, Australia
Feline Cardiopulmonary Resuscitation: Current Evidence-Based Guidelines

Dawn Merton Boothe, DVM, MS, PhD, DACVIM, DACVCP
Professor, Director Clinical Pharmacology
Anatomy Physiology and Pharmacology; Clinical Sciences
Auburn University
Auburn, Alabama
Medicating the Very Young and the Very Old Cat

Allison Bradley, BA, DVM, DACVIM
VCA Veterinary Specialists of Northern Colorado
Loveland, Colorado
Feline Extrahepatic Bile Duct Obstruction: Medical versus Surgical Management

Benjamin Brainard, VMD, DACVAA, DACVECC
Associate Professor, Critical Care
Department of Small Animal Medicine and Surgery
College of Veterinary Medicine, University of Georgia
Athens, Georgia
Current Diagnostics and Therapeutics in Feline Hypercoagulability

Jennifer Broadhurst, DVM
Division Director
Clay County Animal Care & Control
Clay County, Florida
Kitten Nurseries: A Practical Guide

Michael R. Broome, DVM, MS, DABVP
Advanced Veterinary Medical Imaging
Tustin, California
Treatment of Severe, Unresponsive, or Recurrent Hyperthyroidism
Treatment of Hyperthyroidism and Concurrent Renal Disease

Scott A. Brown, VMD, PhD
Josiah Meigs Distinguished Teaching Professor
Department of Physiology & Pharmacology
University of Georgia
Edward Gunst Professor of Small Animal Medicine
Department of Small Animal Medicine & Surgery
UGA College of Veterinary Medicine
Athens, Georgia
Chronic Kidney Disease: An Update

C.A. Tony Buffington, DVM, PhD
Professor
Veterinary Clinical Sciences
The Ohio State University
Columbus, Ohio
Feline Idiopathic Cystitis
Environmental Strategies to Promote Health and Wellness

Christopher G. Byers, DVM, DACVECC, DACVIM (SAIM), CVJ
Medical Doctor
VCA Midwest Veterinary Specialists of Omaha
Omaha, Nebraska
Adjunct Associate Professor of Emergency & Critical Care
Kansas State University College of Veterinary Medicine
Manhattan, Kansas
Acute Hemolytic Disorders in Cats

Alane Kosanovich Cahalane, DVM, MA, DACVS-SA
CEO and Co-Founder
VSH Hong Kong
Hong Kong, SAR China
Vascular Access Ports in Cats

Christine L. Cain, DVM, DACVD
Assistant Professor of Dermatology
Department of Clinical Studies
University of Pennsylvania
School of Veterinary Medicine
Philadelphia, Pennsylvania
Diagnostically Challenging Dermatoses of Cats

Amanda Callens, BS, LVMT
Veterinary Technician
Update on Feline Urolithiasis

Daniel L. Chan, DVM, DACVECC, DACVN, DECVECC, FHEA, MRCVS
Professor of Emergency and Critical Care Medicine and Clinical Nutrition
Section of Emergency and Critical Care
Department of Clinical Science and Services
The Royal Veterinary College
University of London
Critical Care Nutrition

Dennis J. Chew, DVM, DACVIM (Internal Medicine)
Professor Emeritus
Department of Veterinary Clinical Sciences
The Ohio State University College of Veterinary Medicine
Columbus, Ohio
Management of Idiopathic Hypercalcemia

Martha G. Cline, DVM, DACVN
Clinical Veterinary Nutritionist
Department of Clinical Nutrition
Red Bank Veterinary Hospital
Tinton Falls, New Jersey
Current Feeding Practices of Cat Owners

Rachel Dean, BVMS, PhD, DSAM(fel), MRCVS
Director of the Centre for Evidence-Based Veterinary
    Medicine
Clinical Associate Professor in Feline Medicine
School of Veterinary Medicine and Science
University of Nottingham, Sutton Bonington Campus
Loughborough, Great Britain
Evidence-Based Feline Medicine: Principles and Practicalities

Joao Felipe de Brito Galvao, MV, MS, DACVIM (SAIM)
Internal Medicine Specialist and Medical Director
Department of Internal Medicine
VCA Arboretum View Animal Hospital
Downers Grove, Illinois
Management of Idiopathic Hypercalcemia

Amy DeClue, DVM, MS, DACVIM
Associate Professor of Small Animal Internal Medicine
Department of Veterinary Medicine and Surgery
University of Missouri
Columbia, Missouri
Continuous Glucose Monitoring in Cats with Diabetes

Alison Diesel, DVM, DACVD
Clinical Assistant Professor
Department of Small Animal Clinical Sciences
College of Veterinary Medicine and Biomedical Sciences
Texas A&M University
College Station, Texas
*Recognition of and Approach to Feline Cutaneous Reaction
    Patterns*

**Brian A. DiGangi, DVM, MS, DABVP (Canine & Feline
Practice)**
Clinical Assistant Professor
Department of Small Animal Clinical Sciences
University of Florida
Gainesville, Florida
Strategies for Infectious Disease Management in Shelter Cats

Ray Dillon, DVM, MS, MBA, DACVIM (IM)
Jack Rash Professor of Medicine
Department of Clinical Sciences
College of Veterinary Medicine
Auburn University
Auburn, Alabama
Feline Heartworm Disease

Adam Eatroff, DVM, DACVIM (SAIM)
Department of Internal Medicine / Hemodialysis Unit
BluePearl Veterinary Partners
New York, New York
Acute Kidney Injury

Amy K. Farcas, DVM, MS, DACVN
Owner, Clinical Nutritionist
Veterinary Nutrition Care
Belmont, California
Feeding the Senior and Geriatric Cat

Daniel J. Fletcher, PhD, DVM
Associate Professor, Section of Emergency and Critical Care
Associate Chair, Department of Clinical Sciences
Cornell University
College of Veterinary Medicine
Ithaca, New York
*Feline Cardiopulmonary Resuscitation: Current Evidence-
    Based Guidelines*

J.D. Foster, VMD, DACVIM
Staff Veterinarian
Department of Small Animal Internal Medicine
University of Pennsylvania, School of Veterinary Medicine
Philadelphia, Pennsylvania
Cutaneous Manifestations of Internal Disease

Susan Foster, BVSc, MVetClinStud, FANZCVS
Small Animal Medicine Consultant
Vetnostics
North Ryde, New South Wales, Australia
Adjunct Senior Lecturer in Small Animal Medicine
School of Veterinary and Life Sciences
Murdoch University
Murdoch, Western Australia
*Dealing with Toxoplasmosis: Clinical Presentation, Diagnosis,
    Treatment and Prevention*

Diane Frank, DVM, DACVB
Professor
Department of Clinical Sciences
Université de Montréal
St-Hyacinthe, Quebec, Canada
Intercat Aggression

Lisa M. Freeman, DVM, PhD, DACVN
Professor
Department of Clinical Sciences
Cummings School of Veterinary Medicine at Tufts
    University
North Grafton, Massachusetts
Nutritional Management of Heart Disease

Frédéric Gaschen, Dr. Med. Vet., Dr. Habil.
Professor and Chief
Companion Animal Medicine Service
Louisiana State University School of Veterinary Medicine
Baton Rouge, Louisiana
*Disorders of Esophageal, Gastric, and Intestinal Motility in
    Cats*

Lorrie Gaschen, DVM, PhD, Dr. Med. Vet., Dipl. DECVDI
Associate Dean for Diversity and Faculty Affairs
Blanche Donaldson Professor
Professor of Diagnostic Imaging
Department of Veterinary Clinical Sciences
Louisiana State University
Baton Rouge, Louisiana
*Diagnostic Imaging of the Gastrointestinal Tract and Tissue
    Sampling*

Sonya G. Gordon, DVM, DVSc, DACVIM-CA
Associate Professor
Department of Small Animal Clinical Science
Texas A&M University
College Station, Texas
Update on the Management of Feline Cardiomyopathy

Brenda Griffin, DVM, MS, DACVIM
Adjunct Associate Professor of Shelter Medicine
Department of Small Animal Clinical Sciences
College of Veterinary Medicine
University of Florida
Gainesville, Florida
Lost Cats: Epidemiology and Best Practices for Identification and Recovery

Tamara Grubb, DVM, PhD, DACVAA
Assistant Professor of Anesthesia & Analgesia
Department of Veterinary Clinical Sciences
College of Veterinary Medicine, Washington State University
Pullman, Washington
Anesthesia for the Aging Cat

Danièlle Gunn-Moore, BSc(Hon), BVM&S, PhD, FHEA, MANZCVS, MRCVS
Professor of Feline Medicine, RCVS Specialist in Feline Medicine, Division of Veterinary Clinical Sciences
Royal (Dick) School of Veterinary Studies and the Roslin Institute,
University of Edinburgh
Edinburgh, Scotland
Cognitive Dysfunction in the Cat

Beth Hamper, DVM, PhD, DACVN
Small Animal Nutritionist
Hamper Veterinary Nutritional Consulting
Indianapolis, Indiana
The Unique Metabolic Adaptations and Nutrient Requirements of the Cat

Katrin Hartmann, Dr. Med. Vet., Dr. Habil., ECVIM-CA (Internal Medicine)
Professor and Department Head
Center of Clinical Veterinary Sciences
Clinic of Small Animal Medicine
Munich, Germany
Update on Antiviral Therapies

Andrea Harvey, BVSc, DSAM(Feline), DipECVIM-CA, MRCVS, MANZCVS (Associate)
RCVS Recognised & Registered (NSW) Specialist in Feline Medicine
Small Animal Specialist Hospital
Sydney, Australia
Feline Laryngeal Disease

Daniel F. Hogan, DVM
Professor and Chief
Comparative Cardiovascular Medicine and Interventional Cardiology
College of Veterinary Medicine
Veterinary Clinical Sciences
Purdue University
West Lafayette, Indiana
Treatment and Prevention of Feline Arterial Thromboembolism

Katherine Irwin, DVM, DACVD
Dermatologist
Dermatology for Animals
Omaha and Lincoln, Nebraska
Cyclosporine in Feline Dermatology

Stephanie Janeczko, DVM, MS, DABVP (Canine & Feline Practice), CAWA
Senior Director, Shelter Medicine Programs
Department of Research & Development
American Society for the Prevention of Cruelty to Animals
New York, New York
Foster Care Programs in Animal Shelters

Rosanne E. Jepson, BVSc, MVetMed, PhD, DipACVIM, DipECVIM
Lecturer in Small Animal Internal Medicine
Department of Clinical Sciences and Services
Royal Veterinary College
London, Great Britain
Phosphate and the Kidney

Albert E. Jergens, DVM, PhD, DACVIM
Professor and Associate Chair for Research and Graduate Studies
Department of Veterinary Clinical Sciences
College of Veterinary Medicine
Iowa State University
Ames, Iowa
Feline Inflammatory Gastrointestinal Disease

Tony Johnson, DVM, DACVECC
Medical Director
Veterinary Information Network
Davis, California
Fibrosing Pleuritis

SeungWoo Jung, DVM, MS, PhD, DACVIM (Cardiology)
Assistant Professor of Cardiology
Department of Clinical Sciences
Auburn University
Auburn, Alabama
Feline Heartworm Disease

Rebecca Kirby, DVM, DACVIM, DACVECC
Gainesville, Florida
Feline Circulatory Shock

Claudia A. Kirk, DVM, PhD, DACVN, DACVIM
Professor and Associate Dean
Office of the Associate Dean for Academic Affairs and
 Student Services
College of Veterinary Medicine
University of Tennessee
Knoxville, Tennessee
Cats and Carbohydrates: How Much Should We Feed?

Erika L. Krick, VMD
Assistant Professor of Oncology
Department of Clinical Studies
University of Pennsylvania School of Veterinary Medicine
Philadelphia, Pennsylvania
A Review and Update on Gastrointestinal Lymphoma in Cats

Darcie Kunder, VMD
Resident
Department of Dermatology and Allergy
Matthew J Ryan Veterinary Hospital, University of
 Pennsylvania
Philadelphia, Pennsylvania
Cutaneous Manifestations of Internal Disease

Michelle Kutzler, DVM, PhD, DACT
Associate Professor of Companion Animal Industries
Department of Animal and Rangeland Sciences
Oregon State University
Corvallis, Oregon
Neonatal Resuscitation and Supportive Care in Cats

D. P. Laflamme, DVM, PhD, Dipl. ACVN
Veterinary Nutritionist
Department of Basic Research
Nestle Purina PetCare Research
St. Louis, Missouri
Sarcopenia and Weight Loss in the Geriatric Cat

Selena Lane, DVM
Critical Care Resident
Department of Small Animal Medicine and Surgery
University of Georgia
Athens, Georgia
*Current Diagnostics and Therapeutics in Feline
 Hypercoagulability*

Cathy Langston, DVM, DACVIM
Associate Professor
Department of Small Animal Internal Medicine
The Ohio State University
Columbus, Ohio
Acute Kidney Injury

**Jacqui Ley, BVSc(hons), PhD(Psychology),
FANZCVS(Veterinary Behaviour), DECAWBM**
Registered Specialist in Veterinary Behaviour
Animal Behaviour Consultations
Melbourne Veterinary Specialist Centre
Melbourne, Victoria, Australia
Feline Social Behavior and Personality

Susan E. Little, DVM, DABVP (Feline)
Owner, Bytown Cat Hospital
Ottawa, Ontario, Canada
Emerging Aspects of Streptococcal Infections in Cats

Andrew Lowe, DVM, MSc, DACVD
Dermatologist
Department of Dermatology
Alta Vista Animal Hospital
Ottawa, Ontario, Canada
Glucocorticoids in Feline Dermatology

**Virginia Luis Fuentes, MA, VetMB, PhD, DACVIM,
DECVIM-CA (Cardiology)**
Professor of Veterinary Cardiology
Department of Clinical Science and Services
Royal Veterinary College
Hatfield, Hertfordshire, Great Britain
*Ultrasound Imaging for Diagnosis and Staging of Feline
 Cardiomyopathy*

Leslie A. Lyons, BS, MS, PhD
Gilbreath McLorn Professor of Comparative Medicine
Department of Veterinary Medicine & Surgery
College of Veterinary Medicine
University of Missouri
Columbia, Missouri
Population Structure and Genetic Testing in Cats

Caroline Mansfield, BSc, BVMS, MVM, PhD, DECVIM-CA
Associate Professor in Small Animal Medicine
Faculty of Veterinary and Agricultural Science
University of Melbourne
Werribee, Victoria, Australia
*The Challenges of Pancreatitis in Cats: A Diagnostic and
 Therapeutic Conundrum*

**Stanley L. Marks, BVSc, PhD, DACVIM (Internal
Medicine, Oncology), DACVN**
Professor
Department of Medicine and Epidemiology
University of California, Davis, School of Veterinary
 Medicine
Davis, California
*Rational Approach to Diagnosing and Managing Infectious
 Causes of Diarrhea in Kittens*

Elizabeth A. Mauldin, DVM, DACVP, DACVD
Associate Professor
Department of Pathobiology
School of Veterinary Medicine
University of Pennsylvania
Philadelphia, Pennsylvania
Diagnostically Challenging Dermatoses of Cats

Elisa Mazzaferro, MS, DVM, PhD, DACVECC
Staff Criticalist
Cornell University Veterinary Specialists
Stamford, Connecticut
Emergency Approach to Respiratory Distress: Heart Versus Lung

Paul Mellor, BSc, BVM&S, CSAM, DECVIM
Pinnacle Specialists
Maidstone, Kent, Great Britain
Plasma Cell Disorders

Melinda D. Merck, DVM
Owner
Veterinary Forensics Consulting, LLC
Austin, Texas
Clinical Management of Large-Scale Cruelty Cases

Kathryn M. Meurs, DVM, PhD
Professor
Department of Clinical Sciences
North Carolina State University College of Veterinary Medicine
Raleigh, North Carolina
Genetics of Feline Heart Disease

Kathryn E. Michel, DVM, MS, MSED, DACVN
Professor of Nutrition
Department of Clinical Studies
School of Veterinary Medicine, University of Pennsylvania
Philadelphia, Pennsylvania
Feeding the Senior and Geriatric Cat

Kristina Miles, DVM, MS
Assistant Professor & Section Head, Radiology
Department of Veterinary Clinical Sciences
College of Veterinary Medicine
Iowa State University
Ames, Iowa
Diagnostic Imaging of the Gastrointestinal Tract and Tissue Sampling

Carmel T. Mooney, MVB, MPhil, PhD, DECVIM-CA
Associate Professor
Small Animal Clinical Studies
School of Veterinary Medicine
University College Dublin
Belfield, Dublin, Ireland
Diagnostic Testing for Hyperthyroidism in Cats

Karen A. Moriello, DVM, Diplomate American College of Veterinary Dermatology
Clinical Professor of Dermatology
Department of Medical Sciences
School of Veterinary Medicine
University of Wisconsin-Madison
Madison, Wisconsin
Dermatophytosis: Decontamination Recommendations

Suzanne Murphy, BVM&S, MSc (Clin. Onc.), DECVIM-CA (Onc.), MRCVS
RCVS Specialist in Veterinary Oncology
Head of Clinics
Centre for Small Animal Studies
Animal Health Trust
Newmarket, Suffolk, Great Britain
Squamous Cell Carcinoma in Cats

Stijn Niessen, DVM, PhD, DECVIM, FHEA, MRCVS
Senior Lecturer and Co-Head of Internal Medicine
Department of Clinical Science and Services
Royal Veterinary College
London, Great Britain
Research Associate
Diabetes Research Group
Newcastle Medical School
Newcastle-upon-Tyne, Tyne and Wear, Great Britain
The Diabetic Cat: Insulin Resistance and Brittle Diabetes

Shila Nordone, MS, PhD
Research Assistant Professor
Department of Molecular Biomedical Sciences
North Carolina State University College of Veterinary Medicine
Raleigh, North Carolina
Proactive Maintenance of the Aging Feline Immune System

Carolyn O'Brien, BVSc, MVetClinStud, FANZCVS
PhD Candidate
Faculty of Veterinary and Agricultural Sciences
University of Melbourne
Parkville, Victoria, Australia
Specialist in Feline Medicine
Melbourne Cat Vets
Fitzroy, Victoria, Australia
Update on Mycobacterial Infections: Diagnosis, Management, Zoonotic Considerations

Robert T. O'Brien, DVM, MS
Specialist in Veterinary Radiology
Director of Imaging
Epica Medical Innovations
Staff Radiologist
Oncura Partners Diagnostics, LLC
Nobleboro, Maine
Radiographic and Computed Tomography Imaging of the Feline Thorax

edan

Adesola Odunayo, DVM, MS, DACVECC
Clinical Assistant Professor
Department of Small Animal Clinical Sciences
University of Tennessee
Knoxville, Tennessee
Traumatic Brain Injury
Pyothorax

Shelly Olin, DVM, DACVIM (SAIM)
Clinical Assistant Professor
Department of Small Animal Clinical Sciences
University of Tennessee
Knoxville, Tennessee
Urinary Tract Infection

Beth Overley-Adamson, VMD, DACVIM (Oncology)
Veterinary Medical Oncologist
Department of Oncology
Center for Animal Referral and Emergency Services
   (CARES)
Langhorne, Pennsylvania
Feline Mammary Carcinoma

Mark A. Oyama, DVM, DACVIM-Cardiology
Professor
Department of Clinical Studies—Philadelphia
University of Pennsylvania
Philadelphia, Pennsylvania
Cardiac Blood Tests

Valerie J. Parker, DVM, DACVIM, DACVN
Assistant Professor
Department of Veterinary Clinical Sciences
The Ohio State University
Columbus, Ohio
Management of Idiopathic Hypercalcemia

Adam P. Patterson, DVM, DACVD
Clinical Assistant Professor
Department of Small Animal Clinical Sciences
Texas A&M University
College Station, Texas
Recognition of and Approach to Feline Cutaneous Reaction
   Patterns

Mark E. Peterson, DVM, DACVIM
Department of Endocrinology and Nuclear Medicine
Animal Endocrine Clinic
New York, New York
Adjunct Professor of Medicine
Department of Clinical Sciences
New York State College of Veterinary Medicine
Cornell University
Ithaca, New York
Treatment of Severe, Unresponsive, or Recurrent
   Hyperthyroidism
Diagnosis and Management of Iatrogenic Hypothyroidism

Jessica M. Quimby, DVM, PhD, DACVIM
Assistant Professor
Department of Clinical Sciences
Colorado State University
Fort Collins, Colorado
Chronic Kidney Disease: Stem Cell Therapy

Nicki Reed, BVM&S, Cert VR, DSAM (Feline) DECVIM-CA, MRCVS
European Veterinary Specialist in Internal Medicine
RCVS Specialist in Feline Medicine
Lumbry Park Veterinary Specialists
Alton, Hampshire, Great Britain
Respiratory and Ocular Mycoplasmal Infections: Significance,
   Diagnosis, and Management

Alexander M. Reiter, Dipl. Tzt., Dr. Med. Vet., Dipl. AVDC, Dipl. EVDC
Associate Professor of Dentistry and Oral Surgery
Department of Clinical Studies
University of Pennsylvania School of Veterinary Medicine
Philadelphia, Pennsylvania
Update on Oral Inflammation in the Cat

Sheilah A. Robertson, BVMS (Hons), PhD, DACVAA, DECVAA, DACAW, DECAWBM (WSEL), MRCVS
Associate Professor
Department of Small Animal Clinical Sciences
College of Veterinary Medicine
Michigan State University
East Lansing, Michigan
Anesthetic-Related Morbidity and Mortality in Cats

Judy Rochette, DVM, FAVD, DAVDC
Referral Specialist
West Coast Veterinary Dental Services
Vancouver, British Columbia, Canada
Consultant
VIN
Disorders and Normal Variations of the Oral Cavity of Kittens
   and Senior Cats

Elizabeth Rozanski, DVM
Associate Professor
Department of Clinical Sciences
Tufts Cummings School of Veterinary Medicine
North Grafton, Massachusetts
Feline Lower Airway Disease

Elke Rudloff, DVM, DACVECC
Residency Training Supervisor
Lakeshore Veterinary Specialists
Glendale, Wisconsin
Feline Circulatory Shock

Nancy A. Sanders, DVM, DACVIM (SAIM), DACVECC
Internal Medicine Consultant
IDEXX Laboratories, Inc.
Westbrook, Maine
Recognition and Treatment of Hypertensive Crises

Brian A. Scansen, DVM, MS, DACVIM (Cardiology)
Associate Professor of Cardiology
Department of Veterinary Clinical Sciences
Colorado State University
Fort Collins, Colorado
Feline Hypertension

Kenneth W. Simpson, BVM&S, PhD, DACVIM, DECVIM-CA
Professor of Small Animal Medicine
Department of Clinical Sciences
Cornell University
Ithaca, New York
The Role of the Microbiota in Feline Inflammatory Bowel Disease

Carlo Siracusa, DVM, MS, PhD, DACVB, DECAWBM
Clinical Assistant Professor of Animal Behavior
Department of Clinical Studies
School of Veterinary Medicine
University of Pennsylvania
Philadelphia, Pennsylvania
Creating Harmony in Multiple Cat Households

Katherine A. Skorupski, DVM, DACVIM (Oncology)
Associate Professor of Clinical Medical Oncology
Department of Veterinary Surgical and Radiological Sciences
University of California, Davis
Davis, California
Feline Soft Tissue Sarcomas

Dan D. Smeak, BS, DVM, DACVS
Professor, Chief of Surgery
Department of Veterinary Clinical Sciences
Colorado State University
Fort Collins, Colorado
Feline Extrahepatic Bile Duct Obstruction: Medical versus Surgical Management

Martha Smith-Blackmore, DVM
Clinical Assistant Professor and Fellow
Center for Animals and Public Policy
Tufts Cummings School of Veterinary Medicine
North Grafton, Massachusetts
Executive Board Member
American Heartworm Society
Wilmington, Delaware
Approach to Feline Cardiorespiratory Disease in Shelter Medicine

Maria Soltero-Rivera, DVM, DAVDC
VCA San Francisco Veterinary Specialists
San Francisco, CA
Update on Oral Inflammation in the Cat

Karin U. Sorenmo, DVM, Dipl ACVIM (Oncology), ECVIM-CA
Professor of Oncology
Department of Clinical Studies
School of Veterinary Medicine
University of Pennsylvania
Philadelphia, Pennsylvania
A Review and Update on Gastrointestinal Lymphoma in Cats

Enrico P. Spugnini, DVM, PhD, DACVIM (Oncology), DECVIM-CA (Oncology)
Biopulse S.r.l.
Naples, Italy
Electrochemotherapy in Feline Oncology

Gretchen Statz, DVM, DACVECC
Staff Criticalist
Department of Internal Medicine and Critical Care
Veterinary Specialty and Emergency Care
Indianapolis, Indiana
Internal Medicine Consultant
Antech Diagnostics
Irvine, California
Feline Diabetic Ketoacidosis

Judith L. Stella, PhD
USDA-APHIS Science Fellow
Department of Comparative Pathobiology
Purdue University
West Lafayette, Indiana
Environmental Strategies to Promote Health and Wellness

Meredith E. Stepita, DVM, DACVB
Owner
Veterinary Behavior Specialists
Dublin, California
Feline Anxiety and Fear-Related Disorders

Harriet M. Syme, BSc, BVetMed, PhD, FHEA, Dipl. ACVIM, Dipl. ECVIM-CA
Professor of Small Animal Internal Medicine
Department of Clinical Science and Services
Royal Veterinary College
North Mymms, Hatfield, Hertfordshire, Great Britain
Are Methimazole Trials Really Necessary?

Viktor Szatmári, DVM, PhD, Dipl. ECVIM-CA (Cardiology)
Assistant Professor
Department of Clinical Sciences of Companion Animals
Faculty of Veterinary Medicine
Utrecht University
Utrecht, Netherlands
Feline Lungworm Infection

Samantha Taylor, BVetMed (Hons), CertSAM, DipECVIM-CA, MRCVS
European Veterinary Specialist in Internal Medicine
RCVS Specialist in Feline Medicine
Distance Education Coordinator
International Cat Care
Wiltshire, Great Britain
Feline Laryngeal Disease

Elizabeth Thomovsky, DVM, MS, DACVECC
Clinical Assistant Professor
Department of Small Animal Emergency and Critical Care
Purdue University
West Lafayette, Indiana
Selection and Use of Blood Products in the Feline Patient

Katrina R. Viviano, DVM, PhD, DACVIM, DACVCP
Clinical Associate Professor
Department of Medical Sciences
University of Wisconsin
Madison, Wisconsin
Practical Antimicrobial Therapy

Craig B. Webb, PhD, DVM, DACVIM
Professor
Department of Clinical Sciences
Colorado State University
Fort Collins, Colorado
Complementary and Alternative Medicine Therapies for Inflammatory Bowel Disease

Tracy L. Webb, DVM, PhD
Research Scientist
Department of Clinical Sciences
Colorado State University
Fort Collins, Colorado
Complementary and Alternative Medicine Therapies for Inflammatory Bowel Disease

J. Scott Weese, DVM, DVSc, DACVIM
Professor of Pathobiology
Professor, Centre for Public Health and Zoonoses
University of Guelph
Guelph, Ontario, Canada
The Gut Microbiome

Jodi L. Westropp, DVM, PhD, DACVIM
Associate Professor
Department of Veterinary Medicine and Epidemiology
University Of California Davis
Davis, California
Feline Idiopathic Cystitis

Charles E. Wiedmeyer, DVM, PhD, DACVP
Associate Professor
Veterinary Medical Diagnostic Laboratory
College of Veterinary Medicine
University of Missouri
Columbia, Missouri
Continuous Glucose Monitoring in Cats with Diabetes

Rebecca P. Wilkes, DVM, PhD, DACVM
Assistant Professor
Department of Infectious Diseases
College of Veterinary Medicine
University of Georgia
Tifton, Georgia
Update on Antiviral Therapies

Tina Wismer, DVM, DABVT, DABT
Medical Director
ASPCA Animal Poison Control Center
Urbana, Illinois
Feline Toxins: Recognition, Diagnosis, Treatment

Angela Witzel, ACVN, DVM, PhD
Assistant Clinical Professor of Nutrition
Department of Small Animal Clinical Sciences
University of Tennessee
Knoxville, Tennessee
Current Concepts in Preventing and Managing Obesity

Eric Zini, PD, PhD, Dipl. ECVIM-CA (Internal Medicine)
Clinic for Small Animal Internal Medicine
University of Zurich
Zurich, Switzerland
Department of Animal Medicine, Production and Health
University of Padova
Legnaro, Padova, Italy
Department of Small Animal Internal Medicine
Istituto Veterinario di Novara
Granozzo con Monticello
Novara, Italy
Clinical Remission and Survival in Diabetic Cats: What Has Changed Over the Last Decade

Contents

SECTION 11
Behavioral Medicine

SECTION 12
Pediatric and Geriatric Medicine

Craig A. Datz, DVM and Séverine Tasker, PhD

CHAPTER

1

Rational Approach to Diagnosing and Managing Infectious Causes of Diarrhea in Kittens

Stanley L. Marks

Diarrhea in kittens is a frequent disorder facing veterinarians and managers of feline shelters and catteries;[1] however, there is scant literature providing specific information on causes and management of this problem. An innumerable number of kittens are abandoned or relinquished shortly after birth to be fostered by 4,000 to 6,000 American animal shelters (Humane Society of the United States report, www.humanesociety.org), and a recent survey of the Association of Shelter Veterinarians identified kitten diarrhea as one of the top two concerns of veterinarians treating shelter cats, second only to upper respiratory infections (K. Hurley, personal communication). Infectious disease was reported by Cave et al. to be the most common cause (55%) of kitten mortality identified from the necropsy findings of 274 kittens from private homes and rescue centers within the United Kingdom, with 25% of kitten mortality being attributed specifically to feline parvovirus (FPV).[2]

Knowledge of the most common causes of diarrhea in kittens is integral to formulating appropriate diagnostic and therapeutic plans, as well as guiding the veterinarian when standard therapeutic recommendations fail (Table 1-1). *Diarrhea in kittens is often associated with the effects of stress,[3] dietary intolerance, primary intestinal disease (congenital short colon, intussusception,[4] or inflammatory bowel disease [IBD]), and infections with enteropathogenic bacteria, viruses,[5] parasites, and protozoa.[6]* Although bacterial enteropathogens have been associated with diarrhea in kittens, identifying a causal relationship is difficult because potentially pathogenic enteric organisms can frequently be isolated in clinically healthy kittens. Routine bacterial examination of 57 clinically healthy kittens presented for initial vaccination revealed bacterial enteropathogens and intestinal parasites in 45% of the kittens.[7] These findings were substantiated by a study that documented a significantly higher incidence of *Campylobacter* spp. in 28% of 54 nondiarrheic cats compared to 10% of 219 diarrheic cats.[8] In addition, this study demonstrated that

there was no significant difference in the prevalence of intestinal parasites between diarrheic and nondiarrheic cats.[8] Determination of the frequency of enteropathogens in 100 cats entering an animal shelter in Florida confirmed that cats with diarrhea were no more likely to be infected with one or more (84%) enteropathogen than were cats with normal feces (84%).[9] Only feline coronavirus (FCoV) was significantly more prevalent in cats with diarrhea (58%) compared with cats with normal feces (36%).[9]

The high prevalence of enteropathogens in healthy feline populations underscores the challenges faced by veterinarians when trying to attribute causality in diarrheic kittens infected with the same enteropathogens. These studies highlight the importance of establishing practical guidelines for the treatment of the most common and important enteropathogens, as it is challenging and cost-prohibitive to test all shelter cats for all possible infections.

PARASITIC CAUSES OF DIARRHEA

Trichomoniasis

Over the past 15 years the protozoan parasite *Tritrichomonas blagburni* (formerly known as *Tritrichomonas foetus*) has emerged as an important cause of feline diarrhea worldwide (Figure 1-1).[10,11] Experimental cross-infection studies between cats and cattle using both feline and bovine isolates of the parasite, the differences in pathogenicity between *T. foetus* in cattle and *T. blagburni* in domestic cats, and molecular gene sequencing differences between parasites obtained from domestic cats and parasites obtained from cattle have resulted in characterization and differentiation of this new species of *Tritrichomonas* infecting cats.[12] Infected cats are generally young, but have ranged in age from 3 months to 13 years (median 9 months). The pathogenicity

Text continued on page 6

Table 1-1   Parasitic, Bacterial, and Viral Causes of Diarrhea in Kittens

Disease	Clinical Signs	Diagnostic Test(s)	Infectious Agent	Comments	Treatment
Parasitic Causes of Diarrhea in Kittens					
Trichomoniasis	Large bowel diarrhea Subclinical infection is common	1. Direct fecal smear 2. InPouch fecal culture 3. Fecal PCR	*Tritrichomonas blagburni* trophozoites identified on fecal smear and culture DNA detected via PCR	Fecal PCR testing is the most sensitive method. Fecal InPouch culture can take up to 10 days to yield a positive result	Ronidazole 30 mg/kg PO every 24 h for 14 days. Isolate infected cats. Retest.
Cryptosporidiosis	Subclinical infection is common Small bowel or mixed-bowel diarrhea	1. Acid-fast stain on fecal cytology 2. DFA testing 3. Fecal PCR	*Cryptosporidium felis* oocysts	More common in kittens and immunocompromised cats. Infection can be self-limiting.	Treatment can be challenging. No drug is FDA approved. Azithromycin (7-10 mg/kg PO every 12 h for 10 days) is recommended.
Giardiasis	Small bowel diarrhea Subclinical infection is common	1. Direct fecal smear 2. Fecal flotation (centrifugation) 3. Fecal ELISA 4. Fecal DFA 5. Fecal PCR (recommended for determination of *Giardia* assemblages if warranted)	*Giardia intestinalis* (has 8 assemblages [A-H] that determine its zoonotic potential) Flotation and DFA detect cysts via microscopy and ELISA detects soluble antigen	Fecal flotation combined with fecal ELISA has a combined sensitivity of > 97% PCR testing has a lower sensitivity than ELISA and flotation ELISA testing should be used for baseline screening only	None of the treatments are FDA approved. Metronidazole 25 mg/kg PO every 12 h for 7 days or Fenbendazole 50 mg/kg PO every 24 h for 5 days. Environmental control is important.
Coccidiosis	Subclinical infection is common Large bowel to mixed-bowel diarrhea	Fecal flotation (centrifugation)	*Cystoisospora felis* oocysts *Cystoisospora rivolta* oocysts	Coccidiosis is typically a disease of kittens, and diarrhea can be self-limiting.	Sulfadimethoxine is approved but is coccidiostatic, label dose is 55 mg/kg PO initial dose followed by 27.5 mg/kg every 24 h for up to 14 days. Ponazuril 50 mg/kg PO every 24 h for 4 days. Environmental control.
Whipworms	Large bowel diarrhea	Fecal flotation (centrifugation)	*Trichuris serrata*	Rare in domestic cats.	Fenbendazole 50 mg/kg PO every 24 h for 5 days (not FDA approved).
Roundworms	Small bowel diarrhea, failure to thrive, "pot-bellied" appearance	Fecal flotation (centrifugation)	*Toxocara cati* *Tocascaris leonina*	Common in kittens < 6 months old.	Pyrantel pamoate 20 mg/kg PO beginning at 2 wks of age, or Fenbendazole 50 mg/kg PO every 24 h for 5 days.

Hookworms	Small bowel diarrhea, melena, iron-deficiency anemia, failure to thrive	Fecal flotation (centrifugation)	Ancylostoma tubaeforme, Ancylostoma braziliense, Uncinaria stenocephala Ancylostoma caninum	Relatively uncommon in cats.	Selamectin, moxidectin, milbemycin oxime, emodepside. Fenbendazole and pyrantel pamoate are not FDA approved but are used off-label.

Bacterial Causes of Diarrhea in Kittens

Clostridium perfringens	Subclinical infection is occasionally seen. Diarrhea can be small bowel, large bowel, or mixed in nature	1. ELISA test for C. perfringens enterotoxin 2. Fecal PCR for enterotoxin gene (should not be used alone to make a diagnosis)	C. perfringens enterotoxin	The pathogenicity of C. perfringens is unclear in cats, and detection of the enterotoxin via ELISA in diarrheic kittens and cats is far less common compared with dogs. A stained fecal smear for detecting endospores is highly insensitive and is not recommended. Fecal culture alone is of no diagnostic utility.	Supportive treatment is sufficient in most cases. In cats with systemic illness, metronidazole (10 mg/kg PO every 12 h for 5-7 days), amoxicillin (22 mg/kg PO every 12 h for 5-7 days), or tylosin (10 mg/kg PO every 24 h for 5-7 days) is recommended.
Clostridium difficile	Subclinical infection is occasionally seen. Diarrhea can be small bowel, large bowel, or mixed in nature	1. Fecal culture (negative culture rules out infection) 2. ELISA test for C. difficile toxins A&B	C. difficile toxins A&B	Detection of C. difficile toxins A&B in asymptomatic kittens is not uncommon.	Supportive treatment is sufficient in most cases. In cats with systemic illness, metronidazole (10 mg/kg PO every 12 h for 5-7 days) is the drug of choice.
Campylo-bacteriosis	Subclinical infection is commonly seen with nonpathogenic species. C. jejuni can cause large bowel diarrhea	1. Fecal culture 2. Fecal PCR 3. Stained fecal smear is extremely unreliable and insensitive	Over 14 species described in dogs and cats. C. jejuni is pathogenic and zoonotic	Most Campylobacter spp. are non-pathogenic. Prevalence rates of Campylobacter spp. are higher in non-diarrheic cats vs. diarrheic cats. PCR is helpful to differentiate Campylobacter species.	Avoid injudicious antimicrobial therapy. Supportive treatment and appropriate barrier control is optimal. Azithromycin (5-10 mg/kg PO every 24 h for 5-21 days) is warranted in immunocompromised cats or cats with systemic illness.

Continued

Table 1-1   Parasitic, Bacterial, and Viral Causes of Diarrhea in Kittens—cont'd

Disease	Clinical Signs	Diagnostic Test(s)	Infectious Agent	Comments	Treatment
Salmonellosis	Subclinical infection is uncommonly seen Diarrhea is typically small bowel Other clinical signs include fever, lethargy, anorexia, vomiting	1. Fecal culture 2. Fecal PCR	Two main species, *Salmonella enterica* and *Salmonella bongori*, each of which contains multiple serotypes	Infection of cats with *Salmonella* has been associated with feeding of raw meats. Outbreaks of *S. enterica serovar* Typhimurium infection in cats have been associated with seasonal song bird migrations ("songbird fever").	Avoid injudicious antimicrobial therapy. Supportive treatment and appropriate barrier control is optimal. Amoxicillin (22 mg/kg PO every 12 h for 7 days with enrofloxacin 5 mg/kg PO every 24 h for 7 days) is warranted in immunocompromised cats or cats with systemic illness.
Anaerobiospirillum infection	Large bowel diarrhea	1. Histopathology of colon with special stains	*A. succuniciproducens*	Infection is relatively rarely documented in cats.	Amoxicillin-clavulanic acid 15 mg/kg PO every 12 h for 14 days.
Gastric and intestinal *Helicobacter* infections	Subclinical infection is very common Clinical signs can range from vomiting to anorexia to diarrhea and lethargy depending on which species and organ system are involved	1. PCR of gastric biopsies (helpful for determination of species) 2. Serology (only determines exposure) 3. Cytology of impression smears or biopsies 4. Rapid urease testing of gastric biopsies 5. Culture is of low sensitivity	Over 15 species of *Helicobacter* described in dogs and cats	Majority of cats show no clinical signs.	Treatment is not routinely administered in infected cats. A 2-3 wk course of omeprazole with metronidazole and clarithromycin PO has been used with varying success in eradicating the infection.
Tyzzer's disease	Small and large bowel diarrhea, hepatic disease	1. PCR of affected intestinal or liver biopsies 2. Histopathology and special stains of intestine and liver	*Clostridium piliforme*	Infection can be rapidly fatal.	Amoxicillin 22 mg/kg PO every 12 h for 10 days.

Viral Causes of Diarrhea in Kittens

Disease	Clinical Signs	Diagnostic Test(s)	Infectious Agent	Comments	Treatment
Feline Panleukopenia Virus	Fever, lethargy, inappetence, vomiting, diarrhea, sudden death Cerebellar signs can also occur	1. Canine parvovirus fecal antigen (ELISA) 2. Histopathology (usually necropsy) 3. PCR of feces, tissue samples 4. Fecal electron microscopy 5. Virus isolation (feces, tissues)	FPV, occasionally infection with related mink enteritis virus, CPV-2a, CPV-2b, or CPV-2c	Pathogenesis of FPV is similar to that of CPV infection. Subclinical infection is probably widespread. Marked variation in the sensitivity and specificity of fecal ELISA tests. Disinfection of the environment with bleach or potassium peroxymonosulfate is important.	Supportive care, IV crystalloids and parenteral antimicrobials (ampicillin and fluoroquinolone), antiemetics, dextrose, colloids, antacids (H₂-blockers or proton pump inhibitors).

Organism	Clinical Signs	Abbreviation/Agent	Diagnostics	Comments/Treatment
Feline Coronavirus	Enteric FCoV subclinical infection is common or may result in diarrhea. If FIP develops, may see fever, lethargy, inappetence, vomiting, diarrhea, icterus, uveitis, neurologic signs, abdominal distension (effusion)	FCoV	1. RT-PCR for detection of FCoV in feces (enteric FCoV) 2. Serology for detection of antibodies to FCoV indicates exposure only 3. For FIP, immunohistochemical staining for coronavirus antigen within lesions characterized by pygranulomatous or granulomatous vasculitis 4. Diagnosis also supported by analysis of abdominal effusion (high protein exudate that contains low numbers of nucleated cells [<5000 cells/μL] 5. RT-PCR for detection of FCoV in effusion or tissue samples	FCoV is commonly detected in healthy and diarrheic cats with a prevalence ranging from 36-75%. Interpretation of positive FCoV serological or PCR-based tests must be made cautiously. / No cure exists for FIP. Prednisolone therapy with or without chlorambucil has been associated with prolongation of life span and improved quality of life. Several immunomodulators and antiviral drugs have been tried, but none has shown convincing benefit *in vivo*.
Feline Leukemia Virus	Extremely variable and depends on the strain involved, challenge dose, host immune function, age, and coinfections. Uncommonly, FeLV causes enteritis that clinically and histologically resembles that caused by FPV, except that lymphoid depletion is absent	FeLV-A (present in all cats with FeLV) FeLV-B FeLV-C	1. Screening via ELISA or related immunochromatographic in-house assays for free FeLV antigen (targets FeLV p27 antigen in serum or blood) 2. IFA on serum or bone marrow targets FeLV antigen in blood cells 3. PCR on blood, bone marrow, or tissue targets FeLV RNA or proviral DNA	The use of tears or saliva is suboptimal compared to serum for ELISA testing. Infected cats should be housed indoors to prevent spread of infection to other cats. Avoid feeding raw-food diets to infected cats. / Supportive care with management of opportunistic infections when warranted. Antiviral agents and immunomodulators are of limited benefit for treatment of cats with FeLV infections.

CPV, Canine parvovirus; DFA, direct fluorescent antibody; ELISA, Enzyme-linked immunosorbent assay; FCoV, feline coronavirus; FDA, U.S. Food and Drug Administration; FeLV, feline leukemia virus; FIP, feline infectious peritonitis; FPV, feline panleukopenia virus; IFA, indirect immunofluorescent antibody assay; IV, intravenous; PCR, polymerase chain reaction; RT-PCR, reverse transcriptase-polymerase chain reaction

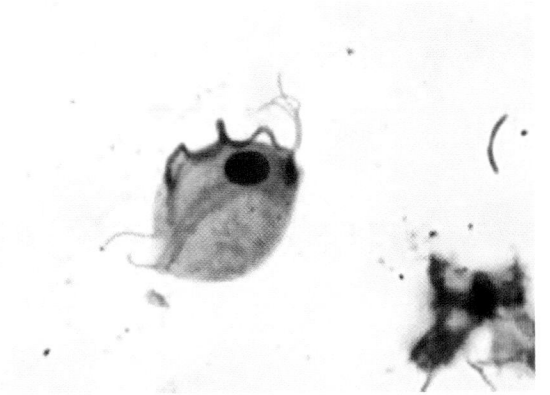

Figure 1-1: Giemsa-stained fecal smear showing characteristic appearance of *Tritrichomonas foetus* with its three anterior flagellae and long undulating membrane (magnification ×1000).

of *T. blagburni* for cats was demonstrated when eight cats were experimentally infected with a *T. blagburni* strain isolated from a diarrheic kitten.[13] Trophozoites were cultured from the feces of all eight cats within 1 week following oral inoculation, with infection persisting throughout the entire 203 days of the study, even when stools became normal.

Prevalence of *Tritrichomonas blagburni*

Natural *T. blagburni*-associated intestinal disease has been described mainly in younger cats (<2 years old) from multi-cat environments such as catteries, shelters, or cat shows.[14-16] The prevalence of *T. blagburni* infection at an international cat show was found to be 31% (36 out of 117 cats), with 28 out of 89 catteries affected.[11] Coinfection by *T. blagburni* and *Giardia* spp. was common and was documented in 12% of cats.[11] Xenoulis and colleagues documented coinfections with *T. blagburni* and *Giardia* in 22% of 104 cats, underscoring the importance of differentiating these enteropathogens.[16] Improper treatment of *T. blagburni* infection with metronidazole is common in cats because the trophozoites can be confused with those of *Giardia* spp. Risk factors for protozoal shedding and exacerbation of diarrhea included concurrent infection with *Cryptosporidium* spp. and cats living in close proximity with one another.[11] The predominance of infection in young cats from dense housing conditions may reflect an increased opportunity for exposure, or enhanced susceptibility to infection because of environmental stress or immunologic immaturity.

Clinical Signs

T. blagburni infection in cats can be associated with a chronic or recurrent large intestinal diarrhea characterized by increased mucus, tenesmus, occasional hematochezia, and increased frequency.[16] The median duration of diarrhea was 135 days, with a range of 1 day to 7.9 years.[16] The anus frequently is red, swollen, and painful, and fecal incontinence is not uncommon. Most cats usually are bright, alert, and responsive, and in good body condition with a normal appetite. *T. blagburni* can be isolated from the feces of asymptomatic cats, many of whom will not develop diarrhea.

Diagnosis

Multiple Direct Fecal Smears on Diarrheic Fecal Specimens. Direct fecal smears are indicated for the recovery of motile trophozoites of *Giardia* spp. and trichomonads such as *T. blagburni*. The procedure should be performed with saline (0.9%) on fresh feces (body temperature, <2 hours old). Trophozoites in older specimens lose their motility, degenerate, and become unrecognizable. The survival of trichomonads can be prolonged by adding 3 mL of 0.9% saline to 2 g of feces. A small amount of feces (size of a match head) is placed on a warm slide and a drop of 0.9% saline is mixed with the feces. Alternatively, a miniscule amount of fresh feces can be collected by insertion of a cotton-tipped swab into the rectum. The smear must not be too thick because trophozoites will be missed easily. A simple rule of thumb is that the observer should be able to read the fine newsprint of a newspaper through the smear.

After application of a coverslip, the smear is evaluated for motile organisms by examining at 100× magnification, with confirmation at 400× magnification. After the wet preparation has been checked thoroughly for motile trophozoites, a drop of D'Antoni's iodine can be placed at the edge of the coverslip, or a new wet mount can be prepared with iodine alone for morphological identification of the organism. A weak iodine solution that resembles "strong tea" is recommended.

The main limitation of direct fecal smears is sample size, with the result that negative smears are not uncommon with low fecal parasite burdens. The sensitivity of direct fecal smear examination for diagnosis of *T. blagburni* is relatively low in cats with spontaneous disease (14%).[17] In addition, the trophozoites of *T. blagburni* can be very difficult to distinguish from those of nonpathogenic intestinal trichomonads such as *Pentatrichomonas hominis* in the absence of fixation and staining. *T. blagburni* should also be distinguished from *Giardia* spp. *Giardia* trophozoites have a concave ventral disc and motility that mimics a falling leaf. In contrast, trichomonads are spindle shaped, have an undulating membrane that courses the entire length of the body, and move in a more irregular and jerky fashion. In contrast to *Giardia* spp., trichomonads do not have a cyst stage, which underscores the limitations of the fecal flotation technique for diagnosis of trichomoniasis. Trichomonads will not survive refrigeration and are rarely found in formed fecal specimens.

Fecal Cultures Performed with an InPouch TF Feline Test Kit. A commercially available system marketed for diagnosis of *T. blagburni* infection in cats (InPouch TF Feline, Biomed Diagnostics, White City, Oregon) should be considered if multiple direct fecal smears are negative for trophozoites.[17] Approximately 0.05 g (match head size) of freshly voided feces can be placed in the InPouch for culture, or alternatively, a saline-moistened cotton-tipped swab can be placed in the rectum and then gently agitated in the InPouch for culture. The InPouch should be incubated at room temperature in an upright position in the dark and examined every 48 hours for up to 10 days for motile trophozoites with use of a 20× or 40× objective (Figure 1-2). Incubation of the InPouch at

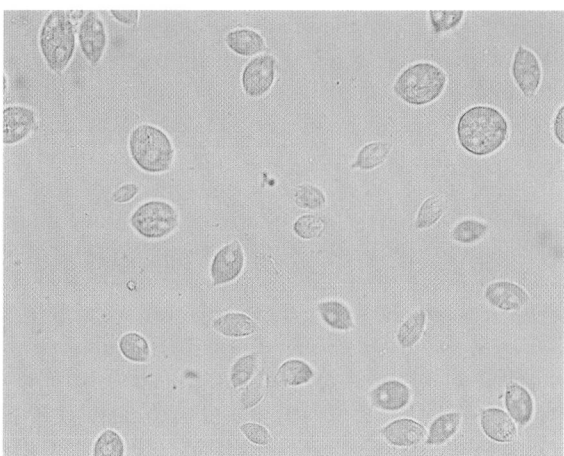

Figure 1-2: *Tritrichomonas* trophozoites in culture medium (InPouch Feline TF) isolated from a diarrheic cat (magnification ×400).

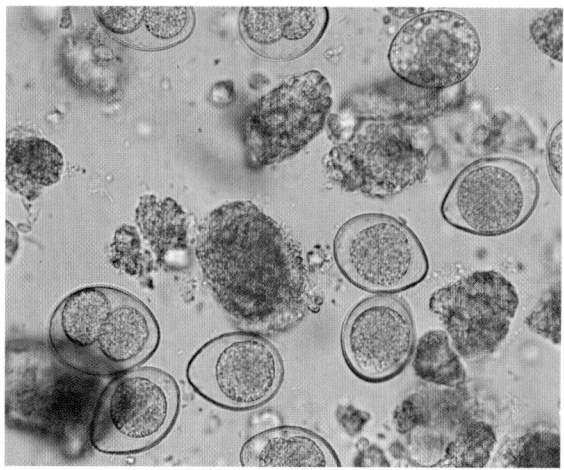

Figure 1-3: Zinc sulfate fecal flotation showing *Cystoisospora* spp. oocysts recovered from a diarrheic kitten (magnification ×400).

37°C (98.6°F) for 24 hours before incubation at room temperature can facilitate an earlier diagnosis because the warmer temperature is more conducive to replication of the trophozoites. Before microscopic evaluation, it is easiest to place the pouch in a plastic clamp provided by the manufacturer that facilitates mounting the pouch onto the stage of a light microscope. Possible reasons for negative fecal culture results include the use of old, desiccated, nondiarrheic, or refrigerated feces in which trophozoites are unlikely to survive; the use of bacteriostatic lubricant to collect the feces; or the placement of excessive feces in the InPouch resulting in overgrowth of bacteria or yeast in the culture medium.

Polymerase Chain Reaction (PCR). PCR is the most sensitive test for detecting *T. blagburni* in cats, but also the most expensive of the three options.[18] The PCR test is more sensitive than fecal culture and resulted in positive tests in 55% of cultures that were negative for *T. blagburni*, even when feces were normal. Fresh viable fecal specimens should be used for PCR testing whenever feasible.

Treatment

A nitroimidazole drug, ronidazole, is the drug of choice for the treatment of *T. blagburni* in cats.[19] The dosage is 30 mg/kg orally (PO) once a day for 14 consecutive days. In a retrospective study of 104 cats infected with *T. blagburni*, 64% of cats treated with ronidazole had a good response to treatment, while about 36% of cats had an inadequate response or a relapse shortly after treatment.[16] It is important that the amount of ronidazole be accurately calculated for each cat on the basis of its body weight. There is no evidence that higher doses of ronidazole are more effective, and they could increase the risk of neurotoxicity.[20] Clinical signs of neurotoxicity include lethargy, inappetence, ataxia, and seizures. These signs generally resolve upon cessation of drug therapy, but can last for 1 to 2 weeks. The drug must be immediately discontinued if signs of neurotoxicity are observed.

Cats that have persistent diarrhea despite ronidazole administration should be further evaluated for other enteropathogens or a persistent *T. blagburni* infection. Additional

considerations for a suboptimal response to ronidazole therapy include quality control problems at the compounding pharmacy or inadequate dosing of the ronidazole. Consider repeating the treatment regime with an appropriate dose and formulation of ronidazole only if the cat is not exhibiting any signs of neurotoxicity.

Ronidazole is not approved by the United States Food and Drug Administration (FDA) for use in companion animals, and veterinarians are advised to obtain informed consent before using this drug. The drug is obtained from compounding pharmacies and is best compounded into capsules because of the drug's bitter taste. In light of the poor host specificity of *T. blagburni* and the intimate association between infected cats and their human companions, the potential for zoonotic transmission should be considered. A single case of human infection with *T. blagburni* has been documented in the literature to date. In that case, the infection presented as epididymitis and meningoencephalitis following immunosuppression and peripheral blood stem cell transplantation.[21]

Environmental Control of *Tritrichomonas blagburni*

T. blagburni is extremely fragile because of its inability to form a cyst. Desiccation, refrigeration, exposure to temperatures above 40.6°C (105°F), and prolonged exposure to oxygen will kill the organism. Litter should be replaced and boxes disinfected to prevent cats from getting reinfected with *T. blagburni* during the treatment period.

Coccidia Species

Coccidia are obligate, intracellular protozoan parasites commonly found in the gastrointestinal tract of dogs and cats. They include the *Cryptosporidium* spp. described later. The most commonly diagnosed coccidial infections in cats are *Cystoisospora felis* and *Cystoisospora rivolta* (Figure 1-3).[22] Coccidiosis is typically a disease of puppies and kittens less than 6 months old; parasite recurrence is rare in animals greater than 1 year of age. In most cases, diarrhea, if present, is self-limiting or rapidly responsive to treatment for coccidiosis.

The presence of enteric protozoans in diarrheic stool does not denote a causal association, and reinfection with *Cystoisospora* spp. is common. Immunity in kittens to *C. rivolta* is not complete, and some oocysts are shed after challenge.[23] Four-week-old kittens are most susceptible to infection with *C. felis*. Enteritis, emaciation, and death can occur after inoculation of 10^5 oocysts,[24] although older kittens can exhibit large- or mixed-bowel diarrhea and abdominal discomfort.

Diagnosis

Fecal flotation with zinc sulfate is the recommended method for diagnosis. Examination of stools for infectious agents that cause disease in these animals is important because coccidiosis usually is asymptomatic. Cats can have oocysts in their fecal specimens from ingestion of prey. These should be recognized as pseudoparasites. The most common of these are *Eimeria* species from ruminants, rabbits, or rodents. These oocysts will not be in the two-celled stage as is common for *Cystoisospora* species. They often will have ornamentations such as micropyle caps or dark thick walls that are not found on *Cystoisospora* oocysts.

Treatment

Sulfadimethoxine is the only drug that has been approved for the treatment of coccidiosis in dogs and cats, but because sulfonamides are coccidiostatic, a low level of persistent infection is possible after treatment. Sulfadimethoxine given at 50 mg/kg PO every 24 hours for 10 to 14 days eliminates oocyst excretion in most animals,[26] but doses and duration of treatment do vary; the label dose of sulfadimethoxine specifies 55 mg/kg PO as an initial dose followed by 27.5 mg/kg PO thereafter, for up to 14 days. Trimethoprim and sulfonamide, furazolidone, and amprolium are also commonly used drugs. Cats do not like the taste of trimethoprim sulfa and will drool profusely. Providing the drug as a capsule or some other compounded dosage form may facilitate ease of administration.

Ponazuril is currently the treatment of choice for many clinicians and shelter managers for eradication of *Cystoisospora* spp. infections in dogs and cats. It is available in the United States in paste form (Marquis paste, Bayer Animal Health; ponazuril 150 mg/g concentration) as a treatment for *Sarcocystis neurona* infection in horses. The drug appears to be well tolerated even in very young kittens and puppies; the dosage is 30 to 50 mg/kg PO every 24 hours for 3 consecutive days. A study in shelter-housed cats and dogs revealed that a dose of 50 mg/kg every 24 hours for 3 consecutive days was not always effective at reducing fecal oocyst counts to levels below the detection limit by 3 to 4 days after the initiation of treatment.[27] Single doses of less than 50 mg/kg do not appear efficacious. Future studies should evaluate increasing the dose rate or continuing treatment for a longer period. Toltrazuril (Baycox, Bayer Animal Health) has been used successfully for the management of kittens infected with *Cystoisospora* spp. in Canada, Australia, and the United Kingdom. The drug is not available in the United States. In addition, environmental oocyst contamination should be reduced by cleaning contaminated surfaces thoroughly, preferably with 10% ammonia with 10 minutes contact time, and by bathing infected animals.

Cryptosporidium Species

Coccidia of the genus *Cryptosporidium* are small, obligate intracellular protozoan parasites that replicate in the microvillous borders of the intestinal and respiratory epithelium of many vertebrates, including birds, mammals, reptiles, and fish.[28] The *Cryptosporidium* genus currently contains at least 20 species and over 40 genotypes, most of which are host adapted and have a narrow host range (e.g., *Cystoisospora canis* in dogs, *C. felis* in cats, and *Cystoisospora hominis* in human beings).[29] The zoonotic risk of feline cryptosporidiosis is relatively low, as most human cases of cryptosporidiosis are associated with *C. hominis* and *Cystoisospora parvum*.[30]

Clinical Signs

Infection with *Cryptosporidium* spp. in kittens and immunosuppressed cats causes a spectrum of disease ranging from an asymptomatic carrier state to mild, transient diarrhea, cholera-like illness, or prolonged and severe life-threatening malabsorption syndrome.[31] The organism has also been associated with diarrhea in adult cats without obvious evidence of immunosuppression. In addition, *Cryptosporidium* spp. infection has been diagnosed in association with intestinal cellular infiltrates indistinguishable from those seen with IBD in cats.[32] Caution should be taken against overinterpretation of the presence of the organism with these infiltrates, because other co-factors, including diet, might be associated with these cellular infiltrates. *Cryptosporidium* spp. was identified in 10 of 50 nondiarrheic cats entering an animal shelter (20%) and in 5 of 50 diarrheic cats (10%), illustrating the fact that many cats can be subclinically infected with *Cryptosporidium* spp.[9]

Diagnosis

Despite the relatively high seroprevalence rates of *C. parvum*-specific immunoglobulin G (IgG) in cats (8.3% to 87%),[33-35] the laboratory detection of this ubiquitous protozoan parasite in spontaneously infected diarrheic cats is difficult, predominantly because the organism is so small (average 4.6×4.0 µm), is difficult to find in fecal specimens via light microscopy,[36] and because fecal shedding may be intermittent. Current laboratory protocols for detection of *Cryptosporidium* oocysts in fecal specimens include microscopic examination of smears stained with Giemsa stain, the modified Ziehl-Neelson (ZN) technique (Figure 1-4), the modified Kinyoun acid-fast technique, or an immunofluorescent detection procedure (Figure 1-5).[37,38] Immunofluorescent detection procedures are more sensitive and specific than acid-fast stains and are generally the method of choice for morphological diagnosis in human beings.[39] Microscopic techniques work well when clinical signs are present and oocyst numbers are relatively high; however, once clinical signs abate and oocyst numbers are greatly decreased, the sensitivity of tests relying

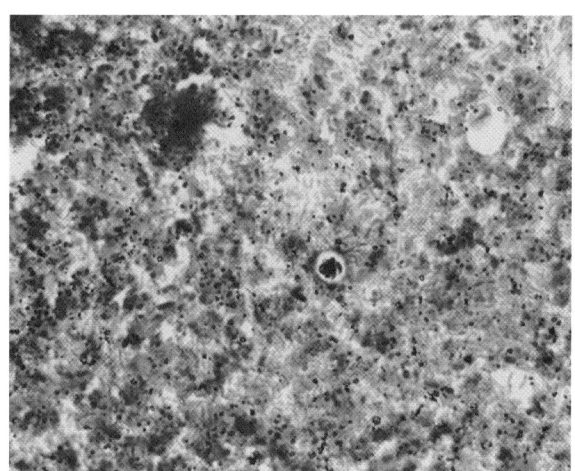

Figure 1-4: Fecal smear showing a single acid-fast (modified Ziehl-Neelson) staining *Cryptosporidium* oocyst from a diarrheic cat (magnification ×1000).

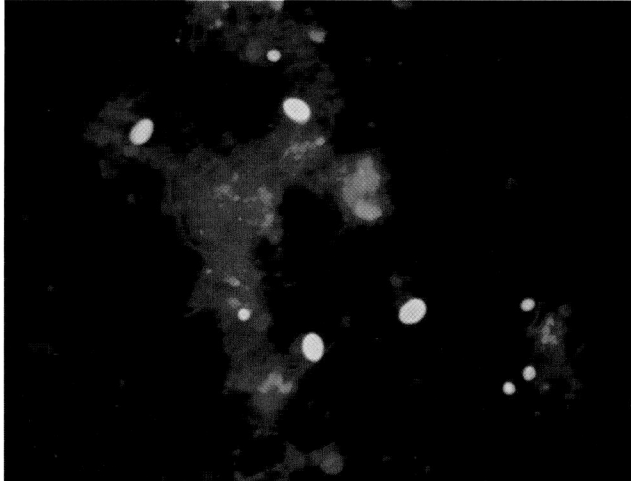

Figure 1-5: Direct immunofluorescent assay (Merifluor *Cryptosporidium/Giardia* direct Immunofluorescent kit, Meridian Diagnostics Inc, Cincinnati, Ohio) showing fluorescent *Giardia* cysts (*larger, oval*) and *Cryptosporidium* oocysts (*smaller, round*) (magnification ×400).

on morphological identification is reduced and diagnosis often requires examination of multiple fecal specimens. In these cases, the newer enzyme immunoassays designed to detect *Cryptosporidium* antigens in feces have proven more sensitive.[40] Difficulties in detection and enumeration of oocysts in fecal specimens are compounded by variation in consistency among individual fecal specimens, the amount of specimen used, and oocyst losses incurred during recovery processes. Real-time PCR for diagnosis of *Cryptosporidium* spp. infection is readily available in large reference laboratories, and studies utilizing this diagnostic modality have demonstrated a significantly higher prevalence of *Cryptosporidium* spp. in infected cats compared with microscopic evaluation and immunoassay methods.[6]

A study compared the performance characteristics of a ZN stain, direct fluorescent antibody technique, and three enzyme-linked immunosorbent assay (ELISA) tests (Table 1-2).[21] It revealed that the Remel ProSpecT Microplate ELISA (Thermo Fisher Scientific, Lenexa, Kansas) was the most sensitive diagnostic test for *Cryptosporidium* spp. on a single day, whereas the ProSpecT Rapid ELISA was highly insensitive and should not be utilized by veterinary diagnostic laboratories.

Treatment

Eradication of this parasite has proven difficult, and many putatively effective drugs are either toxic or ineffective in cats. The aminoglycoside paromomycin is potentially nephrotoxic[41] and ototoxic in cats, and preferably should not be used. Although the benzamide antimicrobial nitazoxanide has been shown to eradicate *Cryptosporidium* spp. in humans and cats, its use in cats is associated with unacceptable adverse effects (i.e., vomiting and anorexia). One report stated that tylosin was effective in eradicating *Cryptosporidium* infection in a cat[32]; however, this drug failed to eradicate infection in a prospective double-blind study conducted by the author in naturally infected cats. Azithromycin is used in humans for management of cryptosporidiosis, and the author has used this drug successfully in cats, administered at a dosage of 7 to 10 mg/kg PO every 12 hours for 7 days. Veterinarians should make every effort to identify and treat underlying causes of immunosuppression and/or concurrent disorders in

Table 1-2	Cumulative Sensitivities of Five Methods of Detection of *Cryptosporidium* Species in Fecal Specimens Collected Once Daily over 4 Consecutive Days from 104 Naturally Exposed Kittens			
Detection Method		**Day 1 (%)**	**Day 3 (%)**	**Day 4 (%)**
Ziehl-Neelson technique		72	91	94
Direct immunofluorescence detection		50	83	84
Premier ELISA* (Meridian Bioscience, Inc., Cincinnati, Ohio)		80	93	93
Remel ProSpecT Microplate ELISA (Thermo Fisher Scientific, Lenexa, Kansas)		89	94	95
Remel ProSpecT Rapid ELISA (Thermo Fisher Scientific, Lenexa, Kansas)		15	43	49

*Enzyme-linked immunosorbent assay

infected kittens because infection with the parasite is often self-limiting.

Giardia Species

Giardia spp. are an important cause of outbreaks of water-borne infection resulting from contamination of raw municipal water, backcountry streams, and lakes with human effluent or infected animal feces.[42] The overall prevalence of *Giardia* in cats in North America has been reported at about 4%, with much higher levels in kittens and in cats housed in shelters.[43] Fourteen percent of cats entering an animal shelter in Florida tested positive for *Giardia* spp.[9] Interestingly, adult cats with diarrhea were significantly more likely (odds ratio [OR] 5.00) to be infected with *Giardia* spp. (10/15 [67%]) than were juveniles with diarrhea (10/35 [29%]).[9]

Epidemiological studies have focused on the transmission route of *Giardia* spp. and have sought to determine their zoonotic potential. *Giardia intestinalis* assemblages A-H have been defined by DNA sequence analysis so far, of which assemblages A and B are mainly virulent for humans and are often referred to as "zoonotic assemblages."[44] A study comparing mammalian *G. intestinalis* assemblages studied 13 feline isolates, of which seven were assemblage F, two were assemblage D, three were assemblage A, and one contained both assemblages C and D.[45] These results support the notion that *Giardia* spp. isolated from infected cats can be zoonotic, although transmission from cats to humans appears to be rare.

Clinical Signs

Giardia infections in adult cats are often subclinical or associated with a transient softening of the stool early in the infection; however, acute diarrhea tends to occur in kittens shortly after infection. Feces are often malodorous and pale, and may contain mucus.

Diagnosis

Giardiasis is commonly misdiagnosed or underdiagnosed because of intermittent shedding and difficulty identifying cysts and trophozoites. The Companion Animal Parasite Council (CAPC; http://www.capcvet.org/) recommends testing symptomatic cats with a combination of direct smear, fecal flotation via centrifugation, and a sensitive, specific ELISA optimized for use in companion animals. A commercially available dual (*Cryptosporidium* spp. and *Giardia* spp.) direct fluorescent antibody (DFA) assay is available and is more sensitive than fecal flotation for detection of *Giardia* spp.; however, the procedure requires a fluorescent microscope to evaluate the fecal specimen. Fecal PCR is commonly performed at reference laboratories, although the author recommends the use of conventional testing (i.e., fecal flotation via centrifugation, ELISA testing, and DFA) whenever feasible. The author combines the use of the dual DFA test with a fecal flotation and wet mount preparation in dogs and cats with diarrhea.

Fecal PCR for *Giardia* should not be used in lieu of fecal flotation or other tests because the sensitivity of the currently available PCR assays is low. *Giardia* PCR fails to amplify DNA from approximately 20% of samples that are positive for *Giardia* cysts or antigens in other assays.[46] This finding likely results from the presence of PCR inhibitors in feces. PCR should only be used for *Giardia* if genotyping of the previously detected *Giardia* spp. is desired to determine the *Giardia* assemblage. The latter assay can be performed at the Veterinary Diagnostic Laboratory at Colorado State University (http://dLab.colostate.edu/).

The diagnosis of *Giardia* spp. infection traditionally has depended on microscopic identification of trophozoites (Figure 1-6) or cysts (Figure 1-7) in feces from affected animals. However, microscopic diagnosis of giardiasis can be difficult, because cysts may be shed intermittently and the cysts are so delicate. Many artifacts (e.g., grass pollen, yeast) mimic the morphology of *Giardia* cysts to varying degrees, and care must be exercised in differentiating these from *Giardia* spp. A survey evaluated the sensitivity of fecal

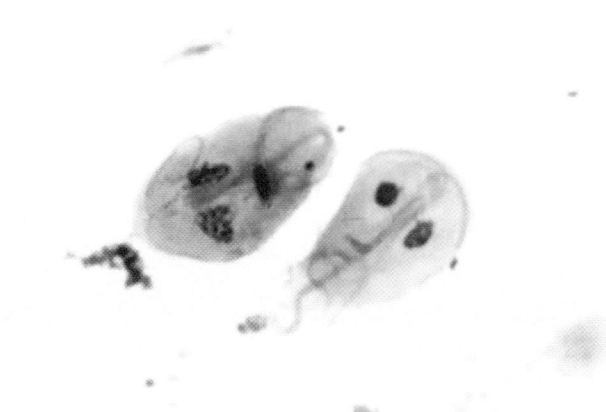

Figure 1-6: Giemsa-stained fecal smear showing two *Giardia* trophozoites exhibiting the characteristic pear, or tear-drop, shape with bilateral symmetry when viewed from the top, two nuclei, and fibrils running the length of the parasite (magnification ×400).

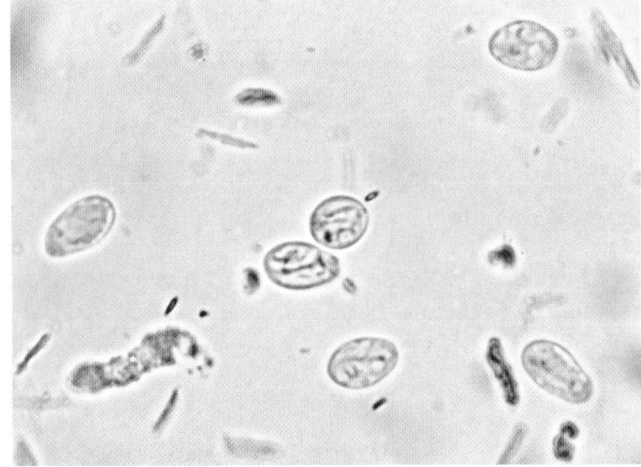

Figure 1-7: Zinc sulfate fecal flotation showing *Giardia* cysts with distinctive fibrils (axonemes) coursing the length of the cyst (magnification ×400).

flotation for detection of *Giardia* spp. in dogs and confirmed the poor performance of current in-house microscopy testing for *Giardia* spp. compared with microplate ELISA. In that study, microscopy following fecal flotation identified only half of the infected dogs and falsely diagnosed up to 25% of uninfected animals.[47]

Many veterinarians and reference laboratories have resorted to using ELISA tests that rely upon detection of *Giardia* cyst wall protein 1 (GCWP 1).[48] The ELISA tests are advantageous because they are generally easy to perform and results are easy to interpret. In addition, the test does not rely upon morphological identification of cysts via microscopy, which saves technician time and potentially avoids false-negative interpretations. The ELISA tests also can detect GCWP 1 in the absence of detectable cysts.[48] However, the SNAP *Giardia* Test (IDEXX Laboratories, Westbrook, Maine) is the only commercially available *Giardia* ELISA assay approved for patient-side testing of giardiasis in dogs and cats. The SNAP *Giardia* Test is a rapid in-house enzyme immunoassay that can be performed on fresh feces, previously frozen feces, or feces stored at 2° to 7°C (35.6 to 44.6°F) for up to 7 days. The test has the added advantages of simplicity, rapid availability of results (8 minutes after mixing of the conjugate solution with feces), and low cost. However, such *Giardia* antigen assays should be supplemental tests because they only detect *Giardia* spp. and should not replace fecal flotation and wet mount examination to detect a wide variety of intestinal parasites, including *Giardia* spp. In addition, the *Giardia* antigen test is best used as a baseline supplemental test to diagnose new infections in animals and should not be used to assess efficacy of therapy because antigen can persist for up to 4 weeks or longer in the absence of *Giardia* cysts.

The performance characteristics of the SNAP *Giardia* test were evaluated in 304 diarrheic and nondiarrheic shelter cats that had also undergone fecal testing via direct immunofluorescence, fecal flotation via centrifugation, and four other human-based immunoassays.[49] Both the sensitivity and specificity of the SNAP Giardia test were 85.3%. When the SNAP *Giardia* test was used in parallel with fecal flotation, the sensitivity of the combined tests increased to 97.8% for detection of *Giardia* spp.[49]

Treatment

In the United States, there is no drug that is FDA approved for treating giardiasis in dogs and cats, and the use of different drugs has been extrapolated from use in humans. The majority opinion of the CAPC is that *asymptomatic* cats may not require treatment. A cat without clinical signs found to be infected with *Giardia* may be treated with a single course of antigiardial therapy. If other cats or dogs live with an infected kitten, all those of the same species may also be treated with a single course of antigiardial therapy. *Repeated courses of treatment are not indicated in dogs and cats without clinical signs.*

Metronidazole was shown to be highly effective and safe when given at 25 mg/kg PO every 12 hours for 7 days to cats with experimental infections.[50] Albendazole also is relatively

effective when dosed at 25 mg/kg PO every 12 hours for 5 days; however, the drug has been associated with pancytopenia and is teratogenic. A trial evaluating the efficacy of fenbendazole (50 mg/kg PO every 24 hours for 5 days) in cats coinfected with *C. parvum* revealed that the drug was safe; however, it was relatively ineffective (50%).[51] Fenbendazole may be administered in combination with metronidazole in refractory cases, and the combination may result in better resolution of clinical disease and cyst shedding. A combination of febantel, pyrantel, and praziquantel (Drontal Plus, Bayer HealthCare LLC, Animal Health Division, Shawnee Mission, Kansas) was shown to be relatively safe and effective in experimentally infected kittens when given at twice the dose recommended for dogs. The dose of febantel used was 56.5 mg/kg PO every 24 hours for 5 days.[52] If treatment combined with bathing (see Control of *Giardia* Infection) does not eliminate infection, as evidenced by testing feces for persistence of cysts in a diarrheic kitten, treatment with either fenbendazole alone or in combination with metronidazole may be extended for another 10 days.

Control of *Giardia* Infection

The following four fundamental steps should be taken to control *Giardia* infection and minimize reinfection of treated animals:

1. The environment is decontaminated. Simultaneous treatment of animals with medication and decontamination of the environment with quaternary ammonium-based (QUAT) disinfectant such as Roccal-D Plus (Zoetis, Florham Park, New Jersey), Quatsyl 256 (Lehn & Fink Products, Montvale, New Jersey), or Aqua Quat 400 (Arysta LifeScience, South Africa) should improve effectiveness of treatment and maximize the possibility of eliminating *Giardia* spp. from the cattery or shelter. Specifically, gross fecal contamination should be removed as much as possible on a daily basis. Runs should be rinsed with water, after which a layer of disinfectant foam (e.g., Roccal-D Plus) should be applied. After 10 to 20 minutes, the foam should be rinsed away with fresh water. Cages should be sponged clean on a daily basis with a dilute disinfectant or mix of bleach (e.g., Clorox, The Clorox Company, Oakland, California) diluted at 1:32 and Quatsyl 256 at 1:256.
2. The animal is treated with effective drugs.
3. The animal is bathed to clean cysts from the coat.
4. Reintroduction of infection is prevented.

Unfortunately, the last three recommendations have limitations and inherent challenges in a cattery or shelter environment. There are no consistently effective antigiardial drugs, and it is difficult to bathe cats. Reinfection is common, so decontamination of the environment in shelters is paramount.

Whipworms

Domestic cats rarely acquire whipworm infections in North America, although they are a possibility in animals with

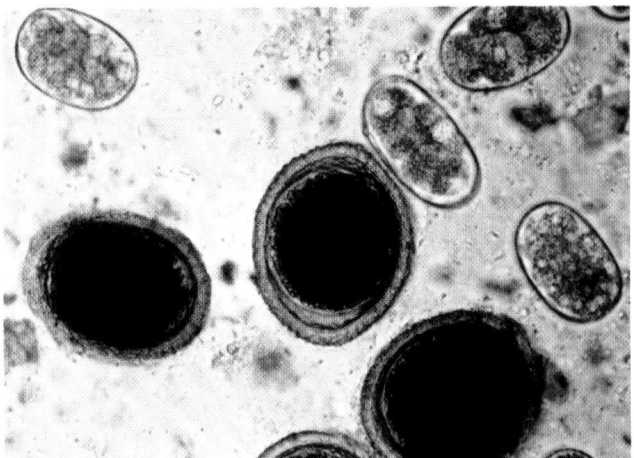

Figure 1-8: Fecal flotation showing large, thick-walled ova of *Toxocara cati* and *Ancylostoma caninum* ova (magnification ×400).

clinical signs of colitis. The adult worms burrow into the colonic and cecal mucosa and may cause inflammation, hematochezia, and intestinal protein loss.

Diagnosis. *Trichuris serrata* should be considered in cats with evidence of colonic disease. A fecal flotation by centrifugation test should allow recognition of the bioperculate ova. However, intermittent shedding of *Trichuris vulpis* and *Trichuris campanula* has been well documented in dogs; therefore cats with a negative fecal flotation should be dewormed empirically.

Treatment. Fenbendazole is a safe broad-spectrum anthelminthic. The drug is administered at 50 mg/kg PO every 24 hours for 5 consecutive days, and the regime is repeated at 3 weeks and 3 months after initiation of therapy. Despite its reported safety in cats even when administered at 5 times the recommended dosage and 3 times the duration approved for use in dogs, fenbendazole is not approved for use in cats in the United States (although it is in other countries), so the drug is typically prescribed off-label to treat cats.

Roundworms

Roundworms (*Toxocara cati* and *Toxascaris leonina*) are particularly common in kittens <6 months old and can cause diarrhea, failure to thrive, a poor quality coat, and a "potbellied" appearance. Vomiting is observed occasionally when the roundworms gain access to the stomach.

Diagnosis. The large ova (approximately 80 μm) with a characteristic thick wall are easy to recognize on fecal flotation (Figure 1-8).

Treatment. Pyrantel pamoate at 20 mg/kg PO is safe in kittens over 2 weeks of age. The treatment should be repeated at approximately 2 weeks. Fenbendazole also is an effective anthelminthic and can be administered to kittens from 4 weeks of age at 50 mg/kg PO for 5 days to kill more than 90% of prenatal larvae. Because the prepatent period of *T. cati* is 8 weeks, kittens do not need to be treated for roundworms until 6 weeks of age. However, given the concern

about hookworm infection, all kittens should be routinely dewormed with pyrantel pamoate beginning at 2 weeks of age and then placed on a monthly heartworm preventative with efficacy against *Toxocara* spp.

Hookworms

Cats can be infected with *Ancylostoma tubaeforme*, *Ancylostoma braziliense*, *Uncinaria stenocephala*, and less commonly, the canine hookworm *Ancylostoma caninum*. The worms are voracious blood suckers and attach to the mucosa of the small intestine. Hookworm infections in cats are relatively uncommon with reported prevalences of 0.9% and 1.1%.[53] Kittens are infected by ingestion of larvae from a contaminated environment, larval skin penetration, or ingestion of larvae in the tissues of vertebrate hosts (usually rodents). Infected kittens occasionally can have life-threatening blood loss or iron-deficiency anemia, melena, hematochezia, and failure to thrive.

Diagnosis. Fecal flotation should be positive because the worms produce a large amount of eggs.

Treatment. Effective drugs that are FDA approved in the United States include selamectin (Revolution, Zoetis, Florham Park, New Jersey), moxidectin (Advantage Multi, Bayer Animal Health Division, Germany), milbemycin oxime (Milbemax, Novartis Animal Health, New York, New York), and emodepside (Profender Bayer Animal Health Division, Germany). Fenbendazole and pyrantel are not FDA approved, but are frequently used off-label in cats at the same doses as those used for treatment of roundworms.

BACTERIAL CAUSES OF DIARRHEA

Diagnosis of bacterial-associated diarrhea in kittens is challenging for two reasons: (1) the isolation rates for putative bacterial enteropathogens often are similar in diarrheic and nondiarrheic animals and (2) the incidence of bacterial-associated diarrhea is extremely variable. Caution should be heeded in interpretation of the results of fecal ELISAs for *Clostridium perfringens* enterotoxin (CPE) and *Clostridium difficile* toxin A and/or B in neonatal kittens because of the high incidence of positive ELISAs (up to 40%) observed in apparently healthy kittens by the author. Although testing of human infants is not recommended, data have shown that 26% of children hospitalized with *C. difficile* infections (CDIs) were younger than 1 year, and 5% were neonates.[54] What cannot be determined from these data are whether the rates of hospitalization for CDIs represent true disease or asymptomatic carriage. *C. difficile* carriage rates average 37% for infants 0 to 1 month of age and 30% between 1 and 6 months of age.[55] The rate of carriage is similar to that of nonhospitalized adults (0% to 3%) by 3 years of age. It is plausible that neonates and infants may lack the cellular machinery to bind and process the toxins of *Clostridium* species. This phenomenon is underscored in neonatal puppies that have been shown to have a high incidence of carriage of toxigenic

C. difficile (up to 58% of puppies) with no demonstration of pathogenicity.[56] These findings highlight the potential concerns with overinterpreting fecal PCR panels that detect the genes for the CPE or *C. difficile* toxins A and B.

The indications for performance of fecal enteric panels on diarrheic kittens are poorly defined, which results in indiscriminate testing and misinterpretation of results. Fecal PCR and toxin analysis for specific bacteria should be reserved for (1) kittens that develop diarrhea after kenneling or show attendance once parasitic and viral (feline panleukopenia virus [FPV]) causes for diarrhea have been ruled out, (2) kittens with an acute onset of bloody diarrhea in association with evidence of sepsis, (3) outbreaks of diarrhea occurring in more than one household pet, and (4) screening for enteropathogens (*Campylobacter jejuni* or *Salmonella* spp.) when zoonotic concerns are present. The prevalence of five groups of potentially zoonotic enteric infections (*Salmonella* spp., *Campylobacter* spp., *Cryptosporidium* spp., *Giardia* spp., and *T. cati*) in fecal samples from cats under 1 year of age that were either housed in humane shelters or presented to primary-care veterinarians in central New York State was studied.[57] Possible associations of these organisms with the cat's source or with the presence of diarrhea were evaluated. The presence of diarrhea was not significantly associated with the number of organisms identified. Of the 74 cats with diarrhea, 35% (26/74) had one or more types of organisms identified, but of the 189 without diarrhea, 43% (81/189) had one or more types of organisms identified. The proportion of fecal samples with one or more zoonotic organisms was 35.1% among client-owned cats and 44.2% among shelter cats. The prevalence of *Salmonella* spp. was 0.8%, which is similar to the reported prevalence of *Salmonella* spp. in cats in Colorado[58] and in kittens from shelters in Japan (1.1%).[59]

Campylobacter spp. was isolated from significantly fewer diarrheic (21 of 219 or 9.6%) versus nondiarrheic cats (15 of 54 or 27.8%) in a study evaluating the prevalence of bacterial and parasitic agents in feces from diarrheic and healthy cats from northern California.[8] Caution should be heeded in overinterpreting the isolation of *Campylobacter* spp. from diarrheic kittens, because many species are nonpathogenic. In addition, fecal cultures are relatively insensitive for isolation of *Campylobacter* spp. compared with PCR-based testing. In the study by Queen and colleagues[8] only 13.2% of cats were positive for *Campylobacter* spp. via fecal culture versus 56.5% via PCR. It has been well documented that biochemical and phenotypical characterization of *Campylobacter* spp. in cat feces is insufficient to characterize the infection. Molecular-based testing allows differentiation of enteric *Campylobacter* spp. from *Helicobacter* spp., and also allows identification of multiple *Campylobacter* spp. in individual animals.[60] Molecular-based testing allows the clinician to detect zoonotic enteropathogens such as *Campylobacter jejuni* and avoid injudicious antimicrobial therapy for kittens infected with *Campylobacter helveticus*, an organism of questionable pathogenicity given its high prevalence in healthy cats.

Wright- or Gram-stained fecal smears have been suggested as a tool to diagnose enterotoxigenic *C. perfringens*-

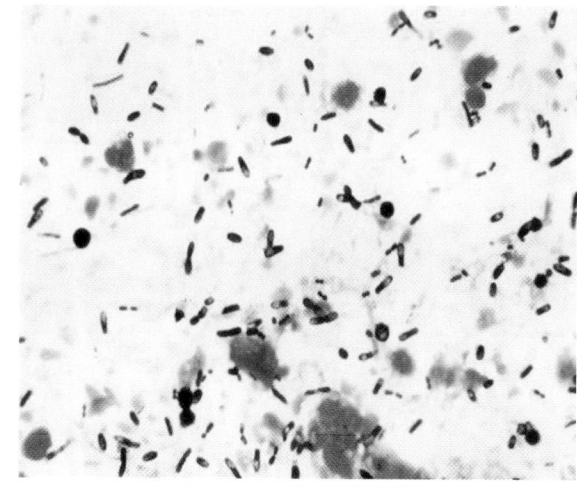

Figure 1-9: Stained fecal smear (modified Wright's stain) from a healthy, nondiarrheic cat showing numerous endospores of *Clostridium perfringens* (magnification ×1000).

associated disease as well as infection with *Campylobacter* spp. (Figure 1-9). Several studies in dogs have reported no association between fecal endospore counts and the presence of diarrhea, or between spore counts and the detection of the CPE in fecal specimens.[61,62] In addition, the identification of spiral-shaped bacteria on fecal smears is suboptimal for diagnosis of *Campylobacter* spp. infection for two reasons: (1) most *Campylobacter* spp. infections in cats are nonpathogenic and observation of stained fecal smears does not allow differentiation of pathogenic versus nonpathogenic species and (2) *Campylobacter* spp. cannot be differentiated from other spiral-shaped bacteria such as *Arcobacter* spp., *Anaerobiospirillum* spp., and *Helicobacter* spp. PCR testing of oral swabs collected from 85 cats in Southern Italy documented carriage of *Arcobacter* spp. in 78.8% of the cats,[63] highlighting the limitations of stained fecal smears for identifying spiral-shaped bacteria.

A recent study demonstrated an association between mortality in kittens and a shift in ileum mucosa-associated enterococci from *Enterococcus hirae* to *Enterococcus faecalis* and adherent *Escherichia coli*.[64] In addition, the *E. faecalis* isolates obtained from these kittens were characterized as carrying multiple genotypic and phenotypic attributes of virulence. However, whether the colonization of ileum-mucosa-associated microbiota by *E. faecalis* was a contributing cause or consequence of gastrointestinal disease and terminal illness in the sick kittens is unknown.

Miscellaneous Bacterial Causes of Diarrhea

Anaerobiospirillum Species

Anaerobiospirillum spp. are motile, spiral-shaped, anaerobic gram-negative rods that were first identified by Malnick and colleagues in 1983 in two human patients with diarrhea.[64] Since then, *Anaerobiospirillum succiniciproducens* and *Anaerobiospirillum thomasii* have been recognized as causes of septicemia, particularly in immunocompromised humans, and have been isolated from the throat and feces of healthy dogs

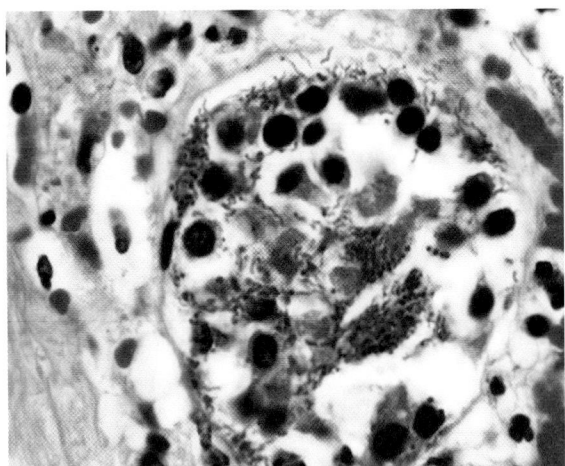

Figure 1-10: Light photomicrograph of colon obtained from a cat, showing spiral-shaped *Anaerobiospirillum* bacteria inside the lumen of a dilated crypt (Steiner stain) (magnification ×1200).

and cats.[65,66] The author has identified three cats (one of which was a 6-month-old kitten) with clinical signs of either acute onset of vomiting, diarrhea, or abdominal pain that progressed rapidly to systemic disease characterized by lethargy and collapse. On necropsy, an acute to subacute ileocolitis was found in association with abundant spiral-shaped organisms confirmed as *Anaerobiospirillum* spp.[67] (Figure 1-10). *Anaerobiospirillum* spp. and *Campylobacter* spp. are morphologically similar and can be confused. *Anaerobiospirillum* spp. are oxidase- and catalase-negative, whereas *Campylobacter* spp. usually are oxidase- and catalase-positive. *Anaerobiospirillum* demonstrate corkscrew motility, whereas *Campylobacter* display darting motility. *Anaerobiospirillum* has bipolar tufts of flagella, whereas *Campylobacter* has a single flagellum on one or both poles. Although the organisms have been isolated from the rectal swabs of asymptomatic dogs and cats, they have not been isolated from the feces of asymptomatic human beings. Most human patients infected with *Anaerobiospirillum* spp. are immunocompromised, and the organism is a rare cause of bacteremia in people. According to the National Committee for Clinical Laboratory Standards breakpoints for anaerobes, the isolates are susceptible to amoxicillin-clavulanic acid, cefoxitin, imipenem, and penicillin, intermediately susceptible to metronidazole, and resistant to clindamycin.

Helicobacter Species

Helicobacter spp. are gram-negative, microaerophilic spiral-shaped, motile bacteria that colonize the gastrointestinal tract of several mammalian and avian hosts. Although *Helicobacter* spp. are better known as gastric pathogens, accumulating reports describe enteric pathogenic helicobacters in dogs, humans, and birds. *Helicobacter canis* was isolated from two adult Bengal cats and two 8-month-old Bengal kittens with and without chronic diarrhea.[68] Because the cats were coinfected with other potential pathogens, including *C. helveticus*,

and because *H. canis* was isolated from nondiarrheic cats, the causal role of *H. canis* in production of the diarrhea could not be proven.[69] Histologically, the colons of the four affected cats were characterized by mild to moderate neutrophilic, plasmacytic, and histiocytic infiltrates in the lamina propria, with crypt abscesses.

A 4-month-old male British Blue cat with catarrhal to hemorrhagic enteritis showed massive colonization of the stomach, small intestine, and cecum with spiral-shaped bacilli that strongly resembled *Flexispira rappini*, a spiral-shaped *Helicobacter* species known as a normal intestinal colonizer in dogs and mice.[70] Inflammatory infiltration was moderate and dominated by T cells. In the intestine, bacilli were found in the gut lumen, between villi, in crypt lumina, and within epithelial cells. Degeneration of crypt epithelial cells was observed, in addition to crypt dilation and moderate to massive macrophage-dominated infiltration of the mucosa and submucosa.

A morphologically, ecologically, and genetically unique helicobacter was recovered from an 8-week-old domestic shorthaired stray kitten with severe diarrhea.[69] A Gram stain of the fecal smear showed large numbers of *Helicobacter*-like curved, gram-negative rods. The kitten was ultimately euthanized and necropsied. Histopathologic assessment of the intestine revealed a thick layer of densely packed bacteria that covered the mucosal surface of the cecum and colon. The bacteria stained strongly with Warthin-Starry stain. The appearance of the duodenum, jejunum, and ileum were within normal limits. The organism could not be cultured but was described on the basis of the 16S ribosomal ribonucleic acid gene sequence analysis and morphology, and appeared to be a new species, with *H. canis* being the most genetically similar species. The new helicobacter organism was proposed as a candidate species, with the specific designation *Helicobacter colefelis*.[69] It is unclear how pathogenic *H. colefelis* is, and attempts to transfect other cats did not induce diarrhea after inoculation, despite the cats becoming PCR-positive.

There are a plethora of protocols that have been utilized in an effort to eradicate *Helicobacter* spp. from infected cats, and most protocols incorporate a gastric protectant agent in combination with one or two antimicrobials. Only a few controlled, randomized, blind therapeutic studies in cats have been published. Twenty-three cats naturally infected with *Helicobacter heilmannii* were randomized to four treatment groups to receive a placebo (group 1); azithromycin, tinidazole, ranitidine, and bismuth once daily for 4 days (group 2); clarithromycin, metronidazole, ranitidine, and bismuth twice daily for 4 days (group 3); or clarithromycin, metronidazole, ranitidine, and bismuth twice daily for 7 days (group 4).[71] Ten days after treatment, all of the cats in the placebo group were infected with *H. heilmannii* following testing utilizing a urea breath test. The urea breath test is the most reliable noninvasive test for *Helicobacter pylori* infection in humans and has been used in natural and experimental animal *Helicobacter* infections.[72] Four of 6 cats in group 2 and all the cats in groups 3 and 4 had a negative result for the urea breath test. Forty-two days after treatment, 0 of 4, 3 of 6, 7 of 11, and 4 of 8 cats in groups 1 to 4, respectively, still had a negative result, underscoring the challenges of maintaining a definitive long-term cure in cats naturally infected with *Helicobacter* spp. A recent study in 13 asymptomatic cats with naturally acquired *Helicobacter* spp. infection evaluated the efficacy of a quadruple therapy protocol utilizing a regime of omeprazole, amoxicillin, metronidazole, and clarithromycin for 14 days.[73] Molecular analysis of gastric biopsies revealed persistence of *Helicobater* spp. DNA in four cats that were negative on quantitative urease testing in biopsies, cytology, and histopathology. These results suggest that antibiotic regimes that are effective against *H. pylori* in people are less effective at eradicating *Helicobacter* spp. in cats with naturally acquired infection.

Clostridium piliforme

Tyzzer's disease caused by *C. piliforme* infection has been reported in immunocompromised kittens with feline infectious peritonitis (FIP),[74] feline leukemia virus infection (FeLV),[75] or FPV infection.[76] Histopathologic lesions caused by *C. piliforme* are characterized by necrotizing enteritis or multifocal hepatic necrosis, and special stains (toluidine blue, Giemsa, periodic acid-Shiff, and Warthin-Starry methods) reveal large filamentous bacilli in bundles or crisscross patterns in the cytoplasm of the epithelial cells. PCR of affected intestinal biopsies can be used to detect the 196-bp bands specific to 16S rDNA of *C. piliforme.*

Although the liver is the most commonly involved organ, necrotizing enterocolitis has been well documented in infected kittens. *C. piliforme* has been reported to be susceptible to penicillin, tetracycline, and erythromycin in studies using infected embryonated eggs; however, the author is unaware of any studies evaluating the efficacy of antimicrobial therapy in infected cats. Avoiding contact with environments contaminated by rodents is important to minimize transmission of the organism.

Treatment of Enteropathogenic Bacteria in Kittens

The lack of well-scrutinized therapeutic guidelines for veterinarians that provide objective recommendations for implementing fecal bacterial testing, combined with the clinical documentation of enteropathogenic bacteria in diarrheic and healthy kittens, has resulted in indiscriminate testing and misinterpretation of results. In addition, antimicrobial therapy is commonly administered injudiciously to diarrheic kittens, with cessation of diarrhea erroneously equated with eradication of the putative enteropathogen. Veterinarians should be cognizant of the fact that most bacterial enteropathogens are associated with self-limiting diarrhea, and the injudicious administration of antimicrobials could be more harmful than beneficial. Supportive therapy and appropriate hygiene control should be considered in all kittens with suspected or confirmed bacterial-associated diarrhea, and antimicrobials should only be administered to immunocompromised kittens or kittens manifesting systemic signs of illness.

Management of *Clostridium perfringens*-Associated Diarrhea

Kittens that are systemically ill (e.g., fever, hemorrhagic gastroenteritis, inflammatory or toxic leukogram) merit appropriate antimicrobial therapy. There is no documented evidence for the benefits of antimicrobial therapy in dogs or cats with uncomplicated diarrhea associated with *C. perfringens*. Antibiotics that have been recommended for the treatment of canine *C. perfringens*-associated diarrhea include ampicillin (22 mg/kg PO every 12 hours for 5 to 7 days), erythromycin (10 to 15 mg/kg PO every 8 hours for 5 to 7 days), metronidazole (10 to 15 mg/kg PO every 12 hours for 5 to 7 days), and tylosin (10 mg/kg PO every 24 hours for 5 to 7 days). Tylosin is an extremely bitter-tasting powder that should be compounded into empty gelatin capsules or into a palatable suspension before administration to cats.

Management of *Clostridium difficile*-Associated Diarrhea

In general, CDI is treated like any other diarrheal disease. Supportive therapy should be administered. If CDI is suspected to be antimicrobial associated, antimicrobial therapy should be discontinued if possible. Metronidazole (10 to 15 mg/kg PO every 12 hours for 5 to 7 days) is commonly used, although it is unclear whether it is needed in all cases. Other treatment options that have been used with a lack of objective scrutiny in kittens include intestinal adsorbents such as di-tri-octahedral smectite (Bio-Sponge, Platinum Performance, Buellton, California), probiotics, and dietary modification with increased soluble fiber.

Management of *Salmonella*-Associated Diarrhea

It is widely accepted (although supportive scientific evidence is lacking) that the administration of antimicrobials is not warranted for uncomplicated episodes of *Salmonella* infection, and only supportive therapy is recommended. In the event of systemic disease or an immunocompromised patient, antimicrobials may be necessary and a combination of ampicillin and a fluoroquinolone for 5 to 7 days is advocated as empirical therapy. If culture results are available, antimicrobial susceptibility testing should be performed to optimize antimicrobial therapy.

Management of *Campylobacter*-Associated Diarrhea

The majority of cases are uncomplicated, self-limiting, and will resolve with supportive therapy alone. Because isolation of *Campylobacter* does not necessarily imply causation of clinical signs, treatment may not be warranted and may further disrupt the intestinal microbiota. However, in immunocompromised or febrile kittens, or in kittens with evidence of hemorrhagic diarrhea, antimicrobial treatment may be indicated. Macrolides and fluoroquinolones are most commonly used to treat *Campylobacter* infections, although the macrolides are the drugs of choice in light of the increasing resistance to fluoroquinolones observed in people and dogs. Erythromycin administered at 10 to 15 mg/kg PO every 8 hours or azithromycin at 5 to 10 mg/kg PO every 24 hours can be given for 5 to 21 days as treatment. Azithromycin is better tolerated, but to the author's knowledge, no published studies regarding efficacy of azithromycin for treatment of campylobacteriosis in cats or its comparison with other macrolides or fluoroquinolones are available.

Enteropathogenic Bacteria Zoonotic Considerations

All kittens with idiopathic diarrhea or a diagnosis of infection with any of the bacteria described here should be considered potentially contagious. Salmonellosis and campylobacteriosis are diseases of major zoonotic importance, and contact with diarrheic animals has been identified as a risk factor for diarrhea in humans. Nosocomial transmission of *C. difficile* and *Salmonella* has been identified in small animal clinics and outbreaks of human salmonellosis in clinic personnel have been documented. The risk of nosocomial and zoonotic transmission of *C. perfringens* probably is minimal, but cannot be dismissed.

Basic practices such as isolation, use of appropriate personal protective equipment, and proper cleaning and disinfection practices are the main control measures. Handwashing is preferred over alcohol-based hand sanitizers because spores of *C. difficile* and *C. perfringens* are alcohol resistant. Litter boxes should be cleaned and disinfected regularly. Gloves should be worn when handling litter boxes and hands washed after glove removal. *C. difficile* and *C. perfringens* spores are highly resistant to most disinfectants but susceptible to bleach (1:10 to 1:20 dilution of regular household bleach) and some oxidizing agents such as accelerated hydrogen peroxide.

VIRAL CAUSES OF DIARRHEA

Feline viral enteritis is usually diagnosed in younger unvaccinated animals. The animal's signalment, history, clinical signs, and hematologic findings are important in ranking a viral etiology as a likely cause of the animal's diarrhea. The two most common viral enteropathogens in cats are FPV and FCoV.

Feline Panleukopenia Virus

Feline panleukopenia is the prototype parvovirus of carnivores and is environmentally stable, highly contagious and spread by direct contact with the feces, urine, and blood of infected cats. Without thorough disinfection with an appropriate disinfectant suitable for nonenveloped viruses such as bleach, potassium peroxymonosulfate (Trifectant, Tomlyn Products, Division of Vétoquinol, USA, Buena, New Jersey) or Virkon-S (DuPont Animal Health Solutions), environmental contamination can remain infectious for many months. Bleach must be applied to a clean surface to be effective. Five percent household bleach should be freshly diluted 1:32 (½ cup per gallon). Correct dilution is very important for maximizing effectiveness. Historically, feline panleukopenia was caused exclusively by FPV; however, it has now been confirmed that feline panleukopenia can be caused by canine parvovirus (CPV) 2a, 2b, and 2c.[77] Because of the widespread use of highly effective vaccines against FPV, the disease has become much less prevalent over the last 20 years, particularly in private practice.[78] The disease seems more prevalent in animal shelters which are home to a continual influx of cats of unknown vaccination status, particularly during the summer and fall when large numbers of kittens with waning maternal immunity are admitted.[79] Because the incubation period is 2 to 14 days, exposed cats that are clinically healthy but incubating the infection might not show clinical signs until days after they have arrived at a shelter or an adoptive home.

Clinical Signs

The hallmark of FPV is diarrhea caused by marked shortening of the intestinal villi with impaired regeneration of the enterocytes. In the peracute form, kittens can die within 12 hours due to septic shock, dehydration, and hypothermia, and clinical signs can be minimal or absent. The more common acute form is characterized by fever for 3 to 4 days, lethargy, anorexia, vomiting, and diarrhea. The disease has an acute self-limiting course and cats that survive infection for longer than 5 days usually recover over the course of several weeks.[78] Intrauterine or perinatal infection may affect the central nervous system of the fetus, leading to cerebellar ataxia and intention tremor in affected kittens.

Diagnosis

Diagnosis is supported on the basis of the cat's history, physical examination findings, and results of a hemogram (neutropenia and lymphopenia). In clinical practice, virus isolation from blood and feces is impractical, and most veterinarians rely upon detection of FPV in feces using either ELISA or immunochromatographic technology. The ELISA tests marketed for detection of CPV-2 antigen can be used for detection of FPV antigen due to cross-reactivity between the two viruses. *FPV infection should never be ruled out on the basis of a negative fecal ELISA.* Reference laboratories offer PCR-based testing of whole blood or feces, facilitating the diagnosis of FPV in those cats that are ELISA negative. In-house parvovirus antigen tests may be positive up to 2 weeks after administration of modified live vaccines; therefore, in recently vaccinated cats, positive results do not necessarily equate with infection.[80]

Management

A cat diagnosed with FPV should be kept in isolation. Treatment is supportive and virtually identical to that described for the dog with parvovirus. Restoration of fluid, electrolyte, and acid-base balance with intravenous (IV) fluid and electrolyte therapy is indicated, with particular attention given to potassium repletion. The intraosseous route can be utilized in kittens, because the subcutaneous route is likely to be inadequate. Enteral administration of dextrose solution (2.5% to 5%) is recommended if the kitten is hypoglycemic. Parenteral administration of dextrose should be reserved for kittens with intractable vomiting. Plasma or colloids (hetastarch) are indicated if the serum albumin concentration drops below 2.0 g/dL (20 g/L), and whole blood transfusions can be used if the cat is anemic with concurrent severe hypoalbuminemia.

The compromised intestinal mucosal barrier facilitates bacterial translocation, and the presence of bacteremia in combination with neutropenia may lead to sepsis in these immunocompromised patients. Prevention of sepsis is important and a broad-spectrum parenterally administered antibiotic with efficacy against gram-negative and anaerobic bacteria is recommended. Examples include ampicillin (20 mg/kg IV every 8 hours) or piperacillin in combination with aminoglycosides, fluoroquinolones (despite not being FDA-approved for parenteral administration in cats in the United States), or cephalosporins. Human granulocyte colony-stimulating factor at 5 µg/kg every 24 hours subcutaneously (SC) will increase neutrophil numbers, but may not influence outcome. Antiemetics such as prochlorperazine, metoclopramide, ondansetron, dolasetron, or maropitant are indicated if the kitten is vomiting. Maropitant is FDA approved for parenteral (SC) administration in kittens older than 16 weeks of age at a dose of 1 mg/kg administered once daily for up to 5 consecutive days. Use of refrigerated product may reduce the pain response associated with the injection. Metoclopramide is a less effective centrally acting antiemetic in cats compared to dogs because chemoreceptor trigger zone D_2-dopamine receptors may not be as important in mediating humoral emesis in the cat. In addition, the drug has an extremely short half-life (90 minutes in dogs) necessitating administration via a constant rate infusion at a dose of 1 mg/kg every 24 hours to maximize its efficacy.

Gastric protectants including the H2-receptor antagonists famotidine at 0.5 to 1 mg/kg PO every 12 to 24 hours (Pepcid, Alchemy Importers, Inc.); ranitidine at 1 to 2 mg/kg PO, IV, SC every 12 hours (Zantac, SmithKline Beecham); sucralfate at 0.25 to 0.3 g PO every 6 to 8 hours (Carafate, Nostrum Laboratories, Inc.); and proton pump inhibitors such as omeprazole at 0.7 to 1 mg/kg PO every 12 to 24 hours (Prilosec, AstraZeneca) are indicated if there is evidence of secondary esophagitis or gastrointestinal bleeding. Broad-spectrum anthelminthics to treat concurrent intestinal parasites should be administered when the cat is no longer vomiting. Oral intake of water and food should be restricted only if vomiting persists, and enteral feeding should be restarted as soon as possible. Beneficial effects of early enteral nutrition have been documented in dogs with CPV.[81] Cats with persistent vomiting, diarrhea, or anorexia will require parenteral nutrition, preferably via a central venous catheter in the jugular or the saphenous vein depending on the size of the cat.

Feline recombinant interferon-omega (Virbagen Omega, Virbac) is effective in the treatment of CPV and also inhibits replication of FPV in cell culture.[82] Interferon-omega was administered to cats in a cattery at the onset of an outbreak of FPV infection.[83] A dose of 1 MU/kg SC once daily for 3 days was given to some of the cats, whereas the remaining control cats were untreated. Although clinical signs and survival were similar for both cat groups, treated cats had lower levels of α-1 globulins and higher mean levels of γ-globulins. Following recovery and subsequent modified live virus vaccination, treated cats had higher levels of γ-globulin and anti-FPV–specific IgG as compared to untreated control cats.

In a disease outbreak, passive immunization can be used to protect susceptible young kittens with an incomplete vaccination history or unvaccinated adult cats. Homologous antisera from cats with a high titer to infection can be used to provide immunity. The recommended dose is 2 mL per kitten given SC or intraperitoneally. Because administered immunoglobulins persist for up to 2 to 4 weeks, the neonatal vaccination series must be delayed. Passive administration of antisera is recommended for use only in exposed susceptible (unvaccinated) cats that require immediate protection or in colostrum-deprived kittens.

Feline Enteric Coronavirus

Feline coronavirus is an enveloped single-stranded RNA virus that occurs as two pathotypes: feline enteric coronavirus (FECV), defined as the "ubiquitous enteric biotype," and feline infectious peritonitis virus (FIPV), the "virulent biotype" that causes FIP in individual cats.[84] Feline coronavirus is transmitted via the fecal-oral route and primarily infects enterocytes. Cats can become persistently infected and continuously or intermittently shed virus with the feces. They generally remain healthy despite systemic infection, indicating that healthy FECV carriers play a key role in the epidemiology of FIP. Feline enteric coronavirus is generally regarded as the avirulent pathotype of FCoV and in older cats oral FECV infection only leads to mild, nonspecific clinical signs such as transient anorexia. However, in young kittens after waning of maternal antibodies, oral FECV infection can induce severe enteritis. There have also been reports of fatal coronavirus enteritis in naturally infected juvenile and adult cats. Affected cats presented with catarrhal to hemorrhagic enteritis, and immunohistopathology confirmed that the virus infected the fully differentiated villous epithelial cells.[85] Infected cats can seroconvert and test positive on FCoV serological testing. Feline coronavirus is commonly detected in healthy and diarrheic cats with a prevalence ranging from 36% to 75%.[6,7] Interpretation of positive FCoV serological or PCR-based test results must be made cautiously because most cats that are infected with FECV have mild clinical signs, unless the animal is coinfected with other enteropathogens. There is no specific treatment for coronaviral enteritis in cats; treatment is symptomatic and supportive. Please refer to Table 1-1 for a summary of the parasitic, bacterial, and viral infections of kittens.

DIAGNOSTIC APPROACH TO THE KITTEN WITH SUSPECTED INFECTIOUS DIARRHEA

The widening array of recognized enteropathogens in kittens and the increasing demand for cost-containment in the face of a need for rapid turnaround of results increases the need for judicious implementation of fecal testing. Thorough clinical and epidemiological evaluation must define the severity and type of illness (e.g., febrile, hemorrhagic diarrhea, nosocomial infection, inflammatory leukogram), exposure (travel history, ingestion of raw or undercooked meat products, contacts that are ill, recent antibiotic use), and determination of whether the animal or owner is immunocompromised to facilitate fecal testing and optimization of antimicrobial therapy.

A rational understanding of the indications and limitations of different fecal examination techniques is of paramount importance for optimizing the diagnosis of infectious diarrhea in the kitten. Specific fecal examination techniques for the diagnosis of intestinal parasites that should be considered in all diarrheic kittens include the fecal wet mount (direct smear) for motile protozoan trophozoites of *Giardia* spp. and *T. blagburni*; fecal flotation via centrifugation for parasitic oocysts, cysts, and ova; acid-fast staining of a fecal smear to assess for the presence of *Cryptosporidium* spp. oocysts; fecal ELISA for *Giardia* spp.; and fecal DFA for *Giardia* spp. and *Cryptosporidium* spp. Stained fecal smears using Wright-Giemsa or Diff-Quik to assess feces for endospores, Campylobacter-like organisms, and white blood cells are of limited diagnostic utility. A rectal scraping to evaluate the colorectal mucosa for inflammatory cells, neoplastic cells, or infectious agents can be performed in cats with clinical signs of colitis or dyschezia. Fecal culture for *T. blagburni* is somewhat time-consuming to perform and is less sensitive than the commercially available fecal PCR. A detailed overview of fecal flotation via centrifugation, fecal culture for enteropathogenic bacteria, fecal immunoassays, and fecal PCR is provided later. The author does not advocate fecal fat assessment with Sudan IV stain because the test is highly insensitive and nonspecific.

Fecal Flotation via Centrifugation

Fecal flotations are indicated to find cysts, oocysts, and ova in feces. Different flotation procedures have been described but not all provide optimal conditions for parasite identification. For example, the duration and speed of centrifugation together with the amount of time the coverslip sits on the tube after centrifugation are important.

Fresh feces should be examined whenever possible, or a fresh specimen can be refrigerated for up to 72 hours for detection of cysts, oocysts, or ova via a concentration technique. Fresh feces also can be placed in 10% buffered formalin if evaluation will be delayed more than 72 hours. Specimens fixed in formalin are suitable for concentration techniques, acid-fast stains, and immunoassays. Although standing (gravitational) flotation methods are easier and quicker to perform than centrifugation flotation (Figure 1-11), the latter clearly has superior sensitivity (up to eight times).[86] Animals with low parasite burdens in feces could have a false-negative result if the gravitational method is utilized. Fecal flotations have limitations and should not be used to detect heavy ova that do not float (*Paragonimus* spp.) or larvae (*Aelurostrongylus* spp.).

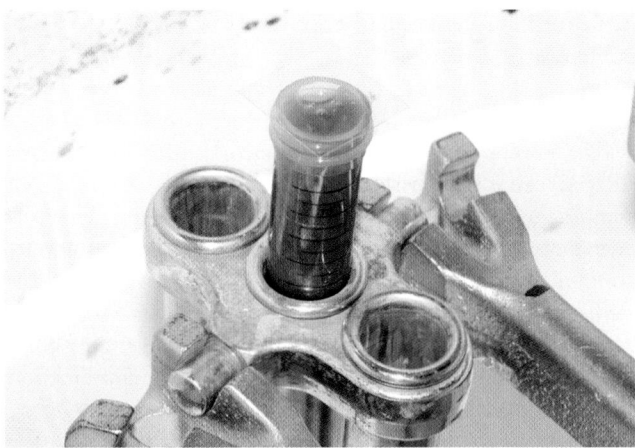

Figure 1-11: Centrifuge with free swinging buckets showing a coverslip in place before centrifugation.

The type of flotation solution used and its specific gravity are important considerations. The author recommends zinc sulfate with a specific gravity of 1.18 or 1.20 for flotations. This solution and specific gravity are optimal for flotation of ova and *Giardia* cysts, while the structural detail of the *Giardia* cyst is maintained.

Procedure for Centrifugal Flotation

1. A fecal emulsion is prepared with use of 2 to 5 g of feces and 5 to 10 mL of flotation solution.
2. The emulsion is strained through a tea strainer or cheesecloth with 10- to 15-mL flotation solution into a 15- to 20-mL conical centrifuge tube.
3. The tube is filled with flotation medium to create a positive meniscus.
4. A coverslip is placed on top of the tube.
5. The tube is balanced in the centrifuge.
6. The tubes are centrifuged for 5 minutes at 1200 rpm (280 × g).
7. Remove the tube and let it stand with the coverslip for 10 minutes.
8. The coverslips are removed carefully from the tubes by lifting straight up; they are placed on a clean slide.
9. Systematically examine the entire area under the coverslip at 100 diameters (i.e., 10× magnification). The 40× objective lens can be used to confirm the diagnosis and make measurements.

Modification

With a centrifuge that is fixed-angle and does not have free-swinging buckets, the above procedure should be followed but the centrifuge tube is filled to within an inch or so from the top, and a coverslip is not added for the final spin. When the final centrifugation step is complete, the tube is set upright carefully in a test tube rack. A pipette is used to gently run additional flotation solution down the side of the tube while disturbing the contents as little as possible. A positive meniscus is created and a coverslip set on top. This preparation should be allowed to stand for 10 minutes only.

The coverslip is removed to a slide and examined as described in step 8.

Fecal Culture for Enteropathogenic Bacteria

The indications for performing fecal enteric panels on diarrheic dogs and cats are poorly defined, resulting in indiscriminate testing and misinterpretation of results. Fecal cultures for *C. difficile*, *C. perfringens*, *Campylobacter* spp., and *Salmonella* spp. can be time-consuming and insensitive. In addition, isolation of a putative bacterial enteropathogen does not denote causation. The author discourages the use of bacterial culture for isolation of *C. perfringens* and *C. difficile* in cats in the clinical setting, as both enteropathogens are infrequently associated with disease based upon detection of enterotoxins and toxins, respectively, the organisms are of dubious pathogenicity, and isolation can take up to 72 hours. Most clinicians prefer real-time PCR for detection of *Salmonella* spp. and *Campylobacter* spp. and for differentiation of pathogenic from nonpathogenic *Campylobacter* spp. Most regional veterinary reference laboratories are able to use molecular-based methods to differentiate *Campylobacter* spp.

Fecal Immunoassays for Parasitic, Viral, and Bacterial Enteropathogens

A DFA has been validated for concurrent detection of *Giardia* spp. cysts and *Cryptosporidium* spp. oocysts in dog and cat feces. This assay requires a fluorescent microscope and is available at commercial reference laboratories or universities. A variety of highly sensitive and specific CPV antigen tests are commercially available for the detection of FPV; however, antigen shedding can be intermittent thus limiting the sensitivity of the test as a screening tool. Animal shelter veterinarians should select fecal tests for FPV detection that have high sensitivity for FPV and low frequency of vaccine-related test interference. The SNAP Parvo test (IDEXX Laboratories, Westbook, Maine) had the lowest incidence of positive results in sixty-four 8- to 10-week-old specific-pathogen-free kittens inoculated with a modified-live (MLV) or inactivated FPV vaccine. The AGEN CPV (AGEN Biomedical Ltd, Brisbane, Queensland, Australia) and in particular the WITNESS CPV (Synbiotics Corp, San Diego, California) have a much higher frequency of vaccine-related interference.[74] Detection of FeLV antigen is warranted in kittens failing to respond to conventional therapy, although detection of the antigen denotes exposure of the kitten to the virus, but does not prove that clinical disease is due to the virus. The *Giardia* ELISA test has been validated in both dogs and cats, and is an excellent in-house immunoassay that should be used in conjunction with fecal flotation and wet mounts to increase the diagnostic yield for *Giardia* spp. Commercially available enterotoxin and toxin ELISAs are available for diagnosis of *C. perfringens* and *C. difficile* infections; however, none of the immunoassays have been validated in cats or dogs to date, and caution should be heeded in interpreting these results as these organisms are of dubious pathogenicity.

Polymerase Chain Reaction for Parasitic, Viral, and Bacterial Enteropathogens

Diagnosis of *Giardia* spp. infection is generally made with the combination of fecal flotation technique, wet mount, and fecal antigen tests (ELISA or DFA). Fecal PCR assays for *Giardia* can have false-negative results because of PCR inhibitors in feces, and PCR should not be used as a screening procedure for this organism. Large commercial reference laboratories that routinely perform PCR have incorporated a number of controls to ensure quality at each step in the process: quantitative DNA/RNA controls to assess the quality of each clinical sample; extraction controls for every DNA/RNA extraction cycle to ensure the absence of contamination; and internal positive and negative controls to verify each real-time PCR test for optimal performance and the absence of contamination. The primary indication for *Giardia* spp. PCR is for determining whether the infective species is a zoonotic assemblage. The latter assay can be performed at the Veterinary Diagnostic Laboratory, Colorado State University (http://dLab.colostate.edu/). This PCR test is different from the RealPCR Feline Diarrhea Panel (IDEXX Laboratories, Westbrook, Maine) or the FastPanel PCR Feline GI Profile Panel (Antech Diagnostics, Irvine, California) performed at commercial reference laboratories. PCR can be used to diagnose *Cryptosporidium* spp. in kittens; however, the author prefers using a DFA test that allows direct visualization of oocysts under a fluorescent microscope. Detection of *C. felis* and *C. canis* do not always prove that the agent is the cause of the clinical disease. Fecal PCR testing is recommended for the diagnosis of *T. blagburni* infection in cats; however, DNA of *T. blagburni* can be detected in healthy carrier cats and so positive results must be interpreted in the context of the animal's history, physical examination findings, and environment. Polymerase chain reaction is a sensitive method for detecting DNA of *Salmonella* spp. and *Campylobacter* spp., but positive results do not inherently necessitate antimicrobial therapy as discussed previously. In cats, the positive predictive value of *Clostridium* spp. PCR assays on feces is low, and should best be combined with toxin immunoassays to increase the diagnostic yield. Reverse transcriptase–PCR is used to detect coronavirus RNA in feces; however, positive test results do not differentiate FIP-inducing strains from FECV, and the prevalence of coronavirus in healthy, nondiarrheic cats is high.

It is incumbent upon the clinician to be aware of the limitations and benefits of each of the fecal diagnostic tests, and to recognize that the mere detection of DNA from a putative enteropathogen or the detection of *Giardia* spp. cysts or *Cryptosporidium* spp. oocysts in a fecal specimen do not denote a cause-and-effect phenomenon. It should be recognized that a kitten demonstrating signs of colitis (tenesmus, hematochezia, increased fecal mucus, scant fecal volume with a marked increase in frequency) with evidence of *Giardia* spp. on fecal flotation or ELISA has another cause for the colitis signs, because *Giardia* is a small bowel pathogen. Further investigation for known causes of colitis in kittens (e.g.,

T. blagburni, Cystoisospora spp., *Campylobacter* spp., *C. perfringens, C. difficile*, food intolerance) should be undertaken.

EMPIRICAL THERAPY FOR KITTENS WITH DIARRHEA OF UNKNOWN CAUSE

The most common causes of diarrhea in neonatal and juvenile kittens are the rapid introduction of milk replacer or rapid transition from formula to commercial diets (weaning period) and infectious causes of diarrhea, specifically parasites (e.g., *Cystoisospora* spp., *Giardia* spp.) and viral enteropathogens (e.g, FCoV). The stress of changing the kitten's environment can exacerbate the diarrhea. The author deworms kittens with simple diarrhea routinely using a broad-spectrum anthelminthic (e.g., fenbendazole) even in the face of a negative fecal flotation or negative *Giardia* ELISA. Metronidazole administration at 10 to 15 mg/kg PO every 12 hours for 5 to 7 days often is associated with partial to complete amelioration of diarrhea, possibly because of altering the intestinal microbiota, dampening cell-mediated immunity, or activity against a specific pathogen such as *C. difficile* or *C. perfringens*. Dietary modification should be considered in kittens that fail to respond to empirical antiparasitic therapy and metronidazole administration. One can temporarily dilute the milk replacer with an oral electrolyte solution such as Pedialyte (Abbott Laboratories, Abbott Park, Illinois) to facilitate acclimation to the formula. One can also feed a highly digestible therapeutic intestinal diet for kittens that have been weaned, and there is compelling evidence documenting the benefits of canned therapeutic diets for the management of adult cats with naturally occurring chronic diarrhea.[87]

Dietary fat restriction does not appear to be of benefit in adult cats with chronic diarrhea, according to a study that compared the effects of a high-fat (45.1% of calories from fat) versus a low-fat (23.8% of the calories from fat), highly digestible diet.[88] Caution should be heeded in extrapolating the results of these studies in adult cats to kittens, because similar studies have not been undertaken to date. Kittens that fail to improve on a commercial diet can be fed a cooked turkey or chicken diet (without carbohydrates) for 5 to 10 days to provide a highly digestible meal containing moderate amounts of fat. Home-cooked diets are not complete and balanced, and should not be fed to kittens for more than 10 days. Probiotics containing *Enterococcus faecium, Lactobacillus* spp., or *Bifidobacterium bifidum* can be used in kittens with simple diarrhea, and several studies have shown benefit for the use of these nutraceuticals.[89] Kittens that have failed to respond adequately to administration of fenbendazole, metronidazole, and dietary therapy are given a 3-day course of ponazuril at 50 mg/kg PO. The author has observed many diarrheic neonatal kittens diagnosed with *Cystoisospora* spp. on fecal flotation at 6 weeks of age that had negative fecal flotations at 2 to 3 weeks of age, due to the long incubation period, and intermittent shedding of the parasite is also well documented. Ronidazole is only administered for the treatment of *T. blagburni* infection.

Kittens with complicated diarrhea characterized by worsening of clinical signs in the face of hematochezia or melena should undergo fecal testing (PCR or ELISA) for FPV and PCR testing for enteropathogenic bacteria, in particular *C. jejuni* and *Salmonella* spp. A complete blood cell count should be done, and the kitten should undergo serological screening for FeLV and feline immunodeficiency virus if this has not been done before. Metronidazole administered for 5 to 7 days should effectively treat *C. perfringens* and *C. difficile*, and kittens infected with *C. jejuni* and showing evidence of systemic clinical signs should be managed with a macrolide antibiotic such as azithromycin at 7 to 10 mg/kg PO every 12 hours for 10 days. Fecal PCR testing can also detect DNA of *C. felis*, and kittens infected with this protozoan can be treated with azithromycin at the same dose.

Inflammatory bowel disease primarily is a disease of middle-aged to older cats, and kittens are more likely to have diarrhea resulting from an infectious cause. The author discourages the administration of prednisolone to diarrheic kittens unless a comprehensive work-up, including intestinal biopsies, warrants this therapy. Kittens with chronic ileitis could have secondary deficiencies of vitamin B_{12} (cobalamin), an important micronutrient for DNA replication in the intestinal crypts. Vitamin B_{12} can be administered empirically to kittens at 100 μg per kitten, given SC once weekly for 6 weeks. Repeat injections should be based on determination of serum cobalamin concentrations. Cobalamin is safe, easy to administer, and inexpensive.

CONCLUSION

Comprehensive fecal exams are important in the diagnostic evaluation of kittens with diarrhea. The diagnostic yield will be markedly increased with the examination of fresh fecal specimens, the use of a centrifugation technique with zinc sulfate solution, and the timely incorporation of immunoassays for diagnosing *Giardia* and *Cryptosporidium* spp. Diagnosis of *T. blagburni* is enhanced with the utilization of PCR, although InPouch culture kits facilitate the growth and direct visualization of motile trophozoites. The author recommends using PCR over InPouch cultures because of the PCR test's increased sensitivity over culture and rapid turnaround.

The clinical documentation of enteropathogenic bacteria that cause diarrhea in kittens is clouded by the presence of many of these organisms existing as normal constituents of the indigenous intestinal microbiota. Attributing disease to a putative bacterial enteropathogen(s) in kittens should be made only after considering the animal's signalment, predisposing factors, clinical signs, fecal assays for toxins, fecal culture, and/or PCR. Relying on results of fecal culture alone is discouraged, because *C. perfringens, C. difficile, Campylobacter* spp., and pathogenic and nonpathogenic *E. coli* are commonly isolated from apparently healthy kittens.

Accurate diagnosis of infections may require diagnostic laboratories to incorporate PCR-based assays using genus- and species-specific primers to facilitate detection of toxin genes and differentiation of species that appear phenotypically and biochemically similar. In assessment of a diarrheic kitten not responding to therapy and for which a diagnosis has not been made, repeating previously negative diagnostic tests frequently is more helpful than performing endoscopy and biopsy.

References

1. Swihart EV: Chronic diarrhea in kittens: ending the never ending story. *Vet Forum* June:52–61, 1997.
2. Cave TA, Thompson H, Reid SWJ, et al: Kitten mortality in the United Kingdom: a retrospective analysis of 274 histopathological examinations (1986-2000). *Vet Rec* 151:497–501, 2002.
3. Buffington CA: External and internal influences on disease risk in cats. *J Am Vet Med Assoc* 220:994–1002, 2002.
4. Burkitt JM, Drobatz KJ, Saunders HM, et al: Signalment, history, and outcome of cats with gastrointestinal tract intussusception: 20 cases (1986-2000). *J Am Vet Med Assoc* 234:771–776, 2009.
5. Litster A, Benjanirut C: Case series of feline panleukopenia virus in an animal shelter. *J Feline Med Surg* 16:346–353, 2014.
6. Paris JK, Wills S, Balzer HJ, et al: Enteropathogen co-infection in UK cats with diarrhea. *BMC Vet Res* 10:13, 2014.
7. Gow AG, Gow DJ, Hall EJ, et al: Prevalence of potentially pathogenic enteric organisms in clinically healthy kittens in the UK. *J Feline Med Surg* 11:655–662, 2009.
8. Queen EV, Marks SL, Farver TB: Prevalence of selected bacterial and parasitic agents in feces from diarrheic and healthy control cats from northern California. *J Vet Int Med* 26:54–60, 2012.
9. Sabshin SJ, Levy JK, Tupler T, et al: Enteropathogens identified in cats entering a Florida animal shelter with normal feces or diarrhea. *J Am Vet Med Assoc* 241:331–337, 2012.
10. Gookin JL, Breitschwerdt EB, Levy MG, et al: Diarrhea associated with trichomonosis in cats. *J Am Vet Med Assoc* 215(10):1450–1454, 1999.
11. Gookin JL, Stebbins ME, Hunt E, et al: Prevalence of and risk factors for feline *Tritrichomonas foetus* and *Giardia* infection. *J Clin Microbiol* 42(6):2707–2710, 2004.
12. Walden HS, Dykstra C, Dillon A, et al: A new species of *Tritrichomonas* (Sacrcomastigophora: Trichomonida) from the domestic cat (*Felis catus*). *Parasitol Res* 112:2227–2235, 2013.
13. Gookin JL, Levy MG, Law JM, et al: Experimental infection of cats with *Tritrichomonas foetus*. *Am J Vet Res* 62:1690–1697, 2001.
14. Kuehner KA, Marks SL, Kass PH, et al: *Tritrichomonas foetus* infection in purebred cats in Germany: prevalence of clinical signs and the role of co-infection with other enteroparasites. *J Feline Med Surg* 13:251–258, 2011.
15. Kingsbury DD, Marks SL, Cave NJ, et al: Identification of *Tritrichomonas foetus* and *Giardia* spp. infection in pedigree show cats in New Zealand. *N Z Vet J* 58:6–10, 2010.
16. Xenoulis PG, Lopinski DJ, Read SA, et al: Intestinal *Tritrichomonas foetus* infection in cats: a retrospective study of 104 cases. *J Feline Med Surg* 15:1098–1103, 2013.
17. Gookin JL, Foster DM, Poore MF, et al: Use of a commercially available culture system for diagnosis of *Tritrichomonas foetus* infection in cats. *J Am Vet Med Assoc* 222:1376–1379, 2003.
18. Gookin JL, Birkenheuer AJ, Breitschwerdt EB, et al: Single-tube nested PCR for detection of *Tritrichomonas foetus* in feline feces. *J Clin Microbiol* 40(11):4126–4130, 2002.
19. Gookin JL, Copple CN, Papich MG, et al: Efficacy of ronidazole for treatment of feline *Tritrichomonas foetus* infection. *J Vet Int Med* 20:536–543, 2006.
20. Rosado TW, Specht A, Marks SL: Neurotoxicosis in 4 cats receiving ronidazole. *J Vet Int Med* 21:328–331, 2007.
21. Okamoto S, Wakui M, Kobayashi H, et al: *Trichomonas foetus* meningoencephalitis after allogeneic peripheral blood stem cell transplantation. *Bone Marrow Transplant* 21(1):89–91, 1998.
22. Gates MC, Nolan TJ: Endoparasite prevalence and recurrence across different age groups of dogs and cats. *Vet Parasitol* 166:153–158, 2009.
23. Dubey JP: Life cycle of *Isospora rivolta* in cats and mice. *J Protozool* 26:433–443, 1979.
24. Andrews JM: Coccidiosis in mammals. *Am J Hyg* 6:784–794, 1926.
25. Lindsay DS, Blagburn BL: Practical treatment and control of infections caused by canine gastrointestinal parasites. *Vet Med* 89:441–455, 1995.
26. Litster AL, Nichols J, Hall K, et al: Use of ponazuril to treat coccidiosis in shelter-housed cats and dogs. *Vet Parasitol* 2014 [ahead of print].
27. Fayer R, Speer CA, Dubey JR: General biology of *Cryptosporidium*. In Dubey JR, Speer CA, Fayer R, editors: *Cryptosporidiosis of man and animals*, Boca Raton, 1990, CRC Press, pp 1–29.
28. Xiao L, Fayer R: Molecular characterization of species and genotypes of *Cryptosporidium* and *Giardia* and assessment of zoonotic transmission. *Int J Parasitol* 38:1239–1255, 2008.
29. Xiao L, Feng Y: Zoonotic cryptosporidiosis. *FEMS Immunol Med Microbiol* 52:309–323, 2008.
30. Current WL: Cryptosporidiosis. *J Am Vet Med Assoc* 187:1334–1338, 1985.
31. Lappin MR, Dowers K, Taton-Allen G, et al: Cryptosporidiosis and inflammatory bowel disease in a cat. *Feline Pract* 25:10–13, 1997.
32. McReynolds CA, Lappin MR, Ungar B, et al: Regional seroprevalence of *Cryptosporidium parvum* specific IgG of cats in the United States. *Vet Parasitol* 80:187–195, 1999.
33. Mtambo MMA, Nash AS, Wright SE, et al: Prevalence of specific anti-*Cryptosporidium* IgG, IgM, and IgA in cat sera using an indirect immunofluorescence antibody test. *Vet Rec* 60:37–43, 1995.
34. Tzipori S, Campbell I: Prevalence of *Cryptosporidium* antibodies in 10 animal species. *J Clin Microbiol* 14:455–456, 1981.
35. Sargent KD, Morgan UM, Elliot A, et al: Morphological and genetic characterization of *Cryptosporidium* oocysts from domestic cats. *Vet Parasitol* 77:221–227, 1998.
36. Garcia LS, Brewer TC, Bruckner DA: Fluorescence detection of *Cryptosporidium* oocysts in human fecal specimens by using monoclonal antibodies. *J Clin Microbiol* 25:119–121, 1987.
37. Marks SL, Hanson TE, Melli AC: Comparison of direct immunofluorescence, modified acid-fast staining, and enzyme immunoassay techniques for detection of *Cryptosporidium* spp. in naturally exposed kittens. *J Am Vet Med Assoc* 225:1549–1553, 2004.
38. Arrowood MJ, Sterling CR: Comparison of conventional staining methods and monoclonal antibody-based methods for *Cryptosporidium* oocyst detection. *J Clin Microbiol* 27:1490–1495, 1989.
39. Garcia LS, Shimizu RY: Evaluation of nine immunoassay kits (enzyme immunoassay and direct fluorescence) for detection of *Giardia lamblia* and *Cryptosporidium parvum* in human fecal specimens. *J Clin Microbiol* 35(6):1526–1529, 1997.
40. Gookin JL, Riviere JE, Gilger BC, et al: Acute renal failure in four cats treated with paromomycin. *J Am Vet Med Assoc* 215(12):1821–1823, 1999.
41. Marshall MM, Naumovitz D, Ortega Y, et al: Waterborne protozoan pathogens. *Clin Microbiol Rev* 10:67–85, 1997.
42. Kirkpatrick CE: Enteric protozoal infections. In Greene CE, editor: *Infectious diseases of the dog and cat*, Philadelphia, 1990, Saunders, pp 804–814.
43. Plutzer J, Ongerth J, Karanis P: Giardia taxonomy, phylogeny and epidemiology: Facts and open questions. *Int J Hyg Environ Health* 213:321–333, 2010.
44. Scorza AV, Ballweber LR, Tangtrongsup S, et al: Comparison of mammalian Giardia assemblages based on β-giardin, glutamate dehydrogenase, and triose phosphate isomerase genes. *Vet Parasitol* 189(2–4):182–188, 2012.
45. Tangtrongsup S, Scorza V: Update on the diagnosis and management of *Giardia* spp. infections in dogs and cats. *Topics Comp Anim Med* 25:155–162, 2010.

46. Groat R, Monn M, Flynn L, et al Survey of clinic practices and testing for diagnosis of Giardia infections in dogs and cats. Abstract, IDEXX Laboratories, Information brochure, 2004.

47. Boone JH, Wilkins TD, Nash TE: Techlab and Alexon *Giardia* enzyme-linked immunosorbent assay kits detect cyst wall protein 1. *J Clin Microbiol* 37:611–614, 1999.

48. Mekaru SR, Marks SL, Felley AJ, et al: Comparison of direct immunofluorescence, immunoassays, and fecal flotation for detection of *Cryptosporidium* spp. and *Giardia* spp. in naturally exposed cats in 4 Northern California animal shelters. *J Vet Intern Med* 21:959–965, 2007.

49. Kirkpatrick CE: Epizootiology of endoparasitic infections in pet dogs and cats presented to a veterinary teaching hospital. *Vet Parasitol* 30(2):113–124, 1988.

50. Scorza AV, Lappin MR: Metronidazole for the treatment of feline giardiasis. *J Feline Med Surg* 6(3):157–160, 2004.

51. Scorza AV, Radecki SV, Lappin MR: Efficacy of febantel/pyrantel/praziquantel for the treatment of *Giardia* infection in cats. *J Vet Int Med* 18(3):388, 2004. (Abstract).

52. Zimmer JF, Miller JJ, Lindmark DG: Evaluation of the efficacy of selected commercial disinfectants in inactivating *Giardia muris* cysts. *J Am Anim Hosp Assoc* 24:379–385, 1988.

53. Kim J, Smathers SA, Prasad P, et al: Epidemiological features of *Clostridium difficile*-associated disease among inpatients at children's hospitals in the United States, 2001-2006. *Pediatrics* 122:1266–1270, 2008.

54. Jangi S, Lamont JT: Asymptomatic colonization by Clostridium difficile in infants: implications for disease in later life. *J Pediatr Gastroenterol Nutr* 51:2–7, 2010.

55. Perrin J, Buogo C, Gallusser A, et al: Intestinal carriage of *Clostridium difficile* in neonate dogs. *Zentralbl Veterinarmed B* 40:222–226, 1993.

56. Spain CV, Scarlett JM, Wade SE, et al: Prevalence of enteric zoonotic agents in cats less than 1 year old in central New York State. *J Vet Intern Med* 15(1):33–38, 2001.

57. Hill SL, Cheney JM, Taton-Allen GF, et al: Prevalence of enteric zoonotic organisms in cats. *J Am Vet Med Assoc* 216:687–692, 2000.

58. Kaneuchi C, Shishido K, Shibuya M, et al: Prevalences of Campylobacter, Yersinia, and Salmonella in cats housed in an animal protection center. *Jpn J Vet Sci* 49:499–506, 1987.

59. Koene MGJ, Houwers DJ, Dijkstra JR, et al: Strain variation within *Camylobacter* species in fecal samples from dogs and cats. *Vet Micro* 133:199–205, 2009.

60. Weese JS, Staempfli H, Prescott JF, et al: The roles of *Clostridium difficile* and enterotoxigenic *Clostridium perfringens* in diarrhea in dogs. *J Vet Intern Med* 15:374–378, 2001.

61. Marks SL, Kather EJ, Kass PH, et al: Genotypic and phenotypic characterization of *Clostridium perfringens* and *Clostridium difficile* in diarrheic and healthy dogs. *J Vet Intern Med* 16:533–540, 2002.

62. Fera MT, La Camera E, Carbone M, et al: Pet cats as carriers of *Arcobacter* spp. in Southern Italy. *J Appl Microbiol* 106:1661–1666, 2009.

63. Ghosh A, Borst L, Stauffer SH, et al: Mortality in kittens is associated with a shift in ileum mucosa-associated enterococci from *Enterococcus hirae* to biofilm-forming *Enterococcus faecalis* and adherent *Escherichia coli. J Clin Micro* 51:3567–3578, 2013.

64. Malnick H, Thomas M, Lotay H, et al: *Anaerobiospirillum* species isolated from humans with diarrhoea. *J Clin Path* 36:1097–1101, 1983.

65. Malnick H: *Anaerobiospirillum thomasii* sp. nov., an anaerobic spiral bacterium isolated from the feces of cats and dogs and from diarrheal feces of humans, and emendation of the genus *Anaerobiospirillum. Int J Syst Bacteriol* 47:381–384, 1997.

66. Malnick H, Williams K, Phil-Ebosie J, et al: Description of a medium for isolating *Anaerobiospirillum* spp., a possible cause of zoonotic disease, from diarrheal feces and blood of humans and use of the medium in a survey of human, canine, and feline feces. *J Clin Microbiol* 28:1380–1384, 1990.

67. DeCock HE, Marks SL, Stacy BA, et al: Ileocolitis associated with Anaerobiospirillum in cats. *J Clin Microbiol* 42(6):2752–2758, 2004.

68. Foley JE, Solnick JV, Lapointe J, et al: Identification of a novel enteric *Helicobacter* species in a kitten with severe diarrhea. *J Clin Micro* 36:908–912, 1998.

69. Kipar A, Weber M, Menger S, et al: Fatal gastrointestinal infection with 'Flexispira rappini'-like organisms in a cat. *J Vet Med B Infect Dis Vet Public Health* 48(5):357–365, 2001.

70. Neiger R, Seiler G, Schmassmann A: Use of a urea breath test to evaluate short-term treatments for cats naturally infected with *Helicobacter heilmannii. Am J Vet Res* 60:880–883, 1999.

71. Glauser M, Michetti P, Blum AL, et al: Carbon-14-urea breath test as a noninvasive method to monitor *Helicobacter felis* colonization in mice. *Digestion* 57:30–34, 1996.

72. Khoshnegah J, Jamshidi S, Mohammadi M, et al: The efficacy and safety of long-term Helicobacter species quadruple therapy in asymptomatic cats with naturally acquired infection. *J Feline Med Surg* 13(2):88–93, 2011.

73. Kubokawa K, Kubo M, Takasaki Y, et al: Two cases of feline Tyzzer's disease. *Jpn J Exp Med* 43:413–421, 1973.

74. Bennett AM, Huxtable CR, Love DN: Tyzzer's disease in cats experimentally infected with feline leukemia virus. *Vet Microbiol* 2:49–56, 1977.

75. Ikegami T, Shirota K, Goto K, et al: Enterocolitis associated with dual infection by *Clostridium piliforme* and feline panleukopenia virus in three kittens. *Vet Pathol* 36:613–615, 1999.

76. Nakamura K, Sakamoto M, Ikeda Y, et al: Pathogenic potential of canine parvovirus types 2a and 2c in domestic cats. *Clin Diag Lab Immunol* 8:663–668, 2001.

77. Greene CE: Feline parvovirus infection. In Greene CE, editor: *Infectious diseases of the dog and cat*, ed 4, St Louis, 2012, Elsevier/Saunders, pp 80–88.

78. Patterson EV, Reese MJ, Tucker SJ, et al: Effect of vaccination on parvovirus antigen testing in kittens. *J Am Vet Med Assoc* 230:359–363, 2007.

79. Neuerer FF, Horlacher K, Truyen U, et al: Comparison of different in-house test systems to detect parvovirus in faeces of cats. *J Fel Med Surg* 10:247–251, 2008.

80. Mohr AJ, Leisewitz AL, Jacobson LS, et al: Effect of early enteral nutrition on intestinal permeability, intestinal protein loss and outcome in dogs with severe parvoviral enteritis. *J Vet Intern Med* 17:791–798, 2003.

81. Martin V, Najbar W, Gueguen S, et al: Treatment of canine parvoviral enteritis with interferon-omega in a placebo-controlled challenge trial. *Vet Microbiol* 89:115–127, 2002.

82. Paltrinieri S, Crippa A, Comerio T, et al: Evaluation of inflammation and immunity in cats with spontaneous parvoviral infection: consequences of recombinant feline interferon-omega administration. *Vet Immnol Immunopathol* 118(1–2):68–74, 2007.

83. Pedersen NC: A review of feline infectious peritonitis virus infection: 1963-2008. *J Feline Med Surg* 11:225–258, 2009.

84. Kipar A, Kremendahl J, Addie DD, et al: Fatal enteritis associated with coronavirus infection in cats. *J Comp Pathol* 119:1–14, 1998.

85. Alcaino HA, Baker NF: Comparison of two flotation methods for detection of parasite eggs in feces. *J Am Vet Med Assoc* 164(6):620–622, 1974.

86. Laflamme DP, Xu H, Cupp CJ, et al: Evaluation of canned therapeutic diets for the management of cats with naturally occurring chronic diarrhea. *J Fel Med Surg* 14:669–677, 2012.

87. Laflamme DP, Xu H, Long GM: Effect of diets differing in fat content on chronic diarrhea in cats. *J Vet Int Med* 25:230–235, 2011.

88. Bybee SN, Scorza AV, Lappin MR: Effect of the probiotic *Enterococcus faecium* SF68 on the presence of diarrhea in cats and dogs housed in an animal shelter. *J Vet Intern Med* 25:856–860, 2011.

89. Hart ML, Suchodolski JS, Steiner JM, et al: Open-label trial of a multi-strain synbiotic in cats with chronic diarrhea. *J Fel Med Surg* 14:240–245, 2012.

Respiratory and Ocular Mycoplasmal Infections: Significance, Diagnosis, and Management

Nicki Reed

ETIOLOGY

Mycoplasma spp. are acellular, prokaryotic organisms within the class Mollicutes.[1] The absence of a cell wall, small genome, and restricted metabolic capacity compromise their ability to survive outside a host environment.[1] There are numerous publications about the feline hemotropic *Mycoplasma* spp., which survive attached to red blood cells; however, this chapter will focus on the nonhemotropic strains, which favor attachment to mucous membranes, such as those lining the conjunctiva, respiratory tract, synovial joints, and mammary glands.

EPIDEMIOLOGY

Mycoplasma spp. are generally considered to be host-specific, although some species may be found in different hosts; for example, *Mycoplasma gateae* is found in both cats and dogs. Several different species of *Mycoplasma* have been isolated from healthy domestic felines, including *M. gateae*, *Mycoplasma felis*, *Mycoplasma feliminutum*, *Mycoplasma arginini*, *Mycoplasma pulmonis*, *Mycoplasma arthritidis*, and *Mycoplasma gallisepticum*. Early studies[2-5] suggested that *Mycoplasma* spp. were normal commensal flora of the upper respiratory tract but not the lower respiratory tract in cats. Of these species, *M. gateae* is the most commonly isolated, being identified in up to 93% of throat swabs[2] followed by *M. felis* in up to 15% of throat swabs.[3] Such commensal organisms were considered to be transmitted from cat to cat by close contact.[5] Attempts to establish mycoplasmal infections by direct inoculation of experimental kittens with *M. felis*, *M. gateae*, and *M. arginini* in early studies suggested that although colonization occurred, development of clinical signs or pathologic lesions did not.[6,7] It also proved difficult to establish colonization with species that did not originate from domestic cats[6]; this supports host specificity.

The role of *Mycoplasma* spp. in respiratory infections was thus considered of minimal significance for several years, comprising mainly solitary case reports of cats with pneumo-

nia or pyothorax.[8-11] The finding of organisms in tracheobronchial lavages in cats with respiratory disease but not healthy cats[12,13] again raised the question of whether *Mycoplasma* spp. are primary pathogens or merely opportunistic invaders.

The confinement of multiple cats together provides an ideal environment for spread of respiratory pathogens. The role of *Mycoplasma* spp. in upper respiratory tract disease in shelters has also been evaluated, and prevalence rates of up to 65% have been documented in cats with upper respiratory tract disease.[14-17] The presence of *Mycoplasma* spp. was significantly associated with signs of upper respiratory tract infection in one study[17] but not in a study in which *M. felis* was isolated more frequently from asymptomatic than symptomatic cats.[16]

Although there appears to be an association between infection with *Mycoplasma* spp. and signs of respiratory tract disease, they have not been definitively identified as primary pathogens in respiratory disease.[14] *Mycoplasma* spp. are currently considered to be a "suspected" primary pathogen in respiratory tract disease. However, *M. felis* is now considered to be a primary pathogen in conjunctivitis because the ability to induce disease in experimentally inoculated kittens was demonstrated in a study.[18]

Potential reasons as to why the role of *Mycoplasma* spp. in respiratory disease is unclear may include variation in the pathogenicity of individual *Mycoplasma* spp. and the role of host defenses in the establishment of disease. One study demonstrated that *M. felis* was only identified from multicat households in which upper respiratory tract disease was present and not from control households that were disease free.[19] In this study *M. felis* was present in cats with and without clinical signs, suggesting that some cats had immunity to the infection whereas others did not.[19]

PATHOGENESIS

Although direct comparisons with other species cannot be made, studies into the pathogenicity of *M. pneumoniae* in humans, *M. bovis* in cattle, *M. hyopneumoniae* in pigs, and

M. pulmonis in mice offer some interesting insights into how *Mycoplasma* spp. may play a role in feline respiratory disease.

Virulence typically involves adhesion of the bacterium to the host cell by an attachment organelle and other adhesin proteins and lipoproteins.[20,21] Cytotoxicity may then occur through the release of inflammatory cytokines and generation of hydrogen peroxide and superoxide radicals, which lead to loss of respiratory cilia and interleukin (IL)-5-induced wheezing.[20-22] Ineffective humoral immunity may lead to the development of chronic disease states with establishment of intracellular infections that evade the immune response[21] (Figure 2-1).

The nature of the immune response mounted by the host may also play a role in disease pathogenesis. A mouse model of mycoplasmal infection has shown that interferon-gamma (IFN-γ)-driven, type 1 helper T cell (Th1) responses appear to be associated with improved resistance to infection, whereas IL-4-driven type 2 (Th2) responses are associated with pulmonary pathology.[23] An association between mycoplasmal infection and asthma has been recognized in humans, with increased recovery of *M. pneumoniae* in asthmatics compared with nonasthmatics[24] and an association with acute exacerbation of asthma.[25] The effect that mycoplasmal infection has on the development of asthma may depend on the timing of infection. A study in mice demonstrated that airway responsiveness was reduced by prior infection with *M. pneumoniae*, accompanied by increased IFN-γ production (Th1 response).[26] However, if the infection occurred after allergen sensitization, the airway hyperresponsiveness was increased, accompanied by increased production of IL-4 (Th2 response) (Figure 2-2).

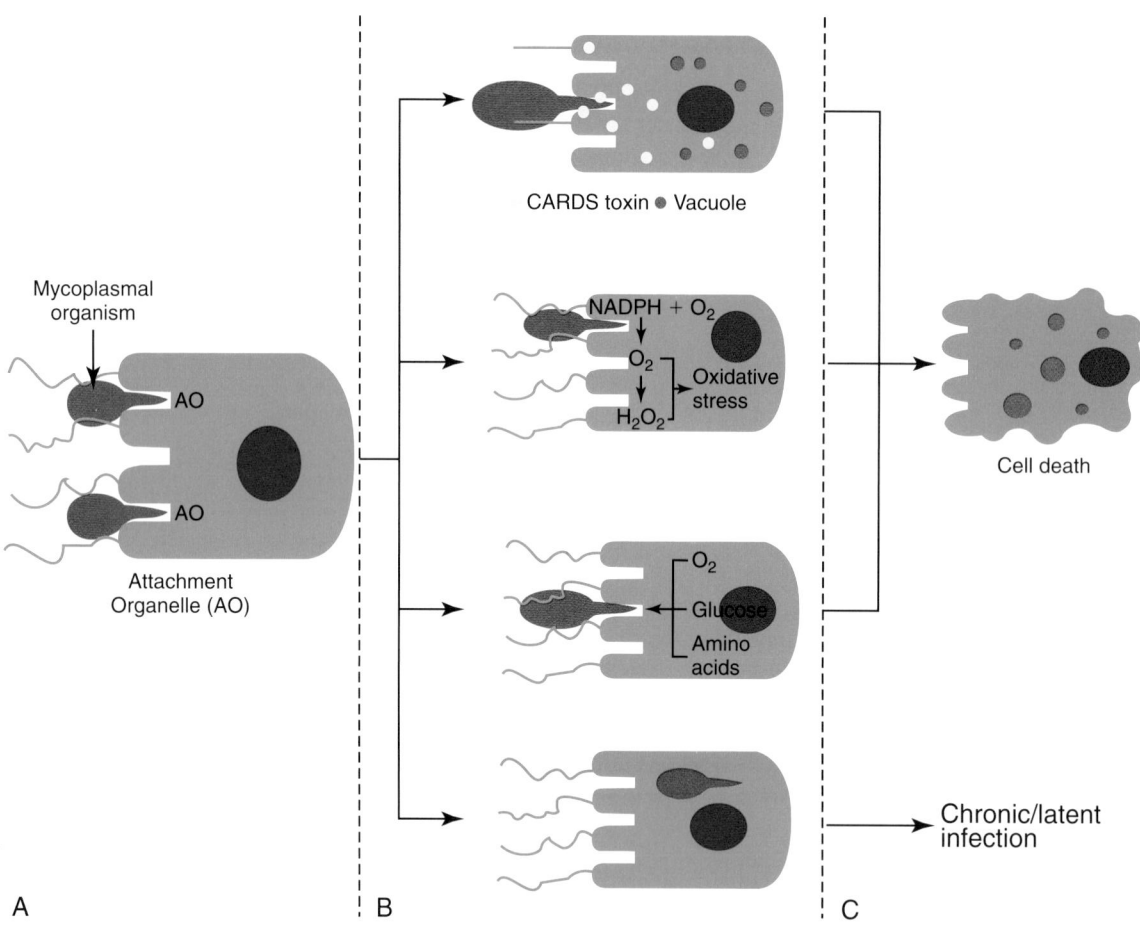

Figure 2-1: Potential Pathogenic Mechanisms of *Mycoplasma* spp. A, Attachment of mycoplasmal organisms to respiratory epithelial cells is facilitated by the attachment organelle (AO), which contains cytoadhesin proteins, such as P_1. Variations in P_1 may be involved in immunity to subtypes. **B,** Mycoplasmal organisms may then (from top to bottom): (1) produce community-acquired respiratory distress syndrome (CARDS) toxin, which causes ciliostasis and vacuolation; (2) produce superoxide and hydrogen peroxide, which cause oxidative stress; (3) utilize nutrients, such as oxygen, glucose, and amino acids, normally required by the epithelial cell; and (4) move intracellularly. **C,** *Top:* Loss of ciliary function, oxidative stress, and lack of nutrients cause cell death and exfoliation, which can contribute to the inflammation seen with mycoplasmal infection. *Bottom:* Mycoplasmal organisms residing intracellularly avoid immune surveillance and contribute to chronic or latent infections.

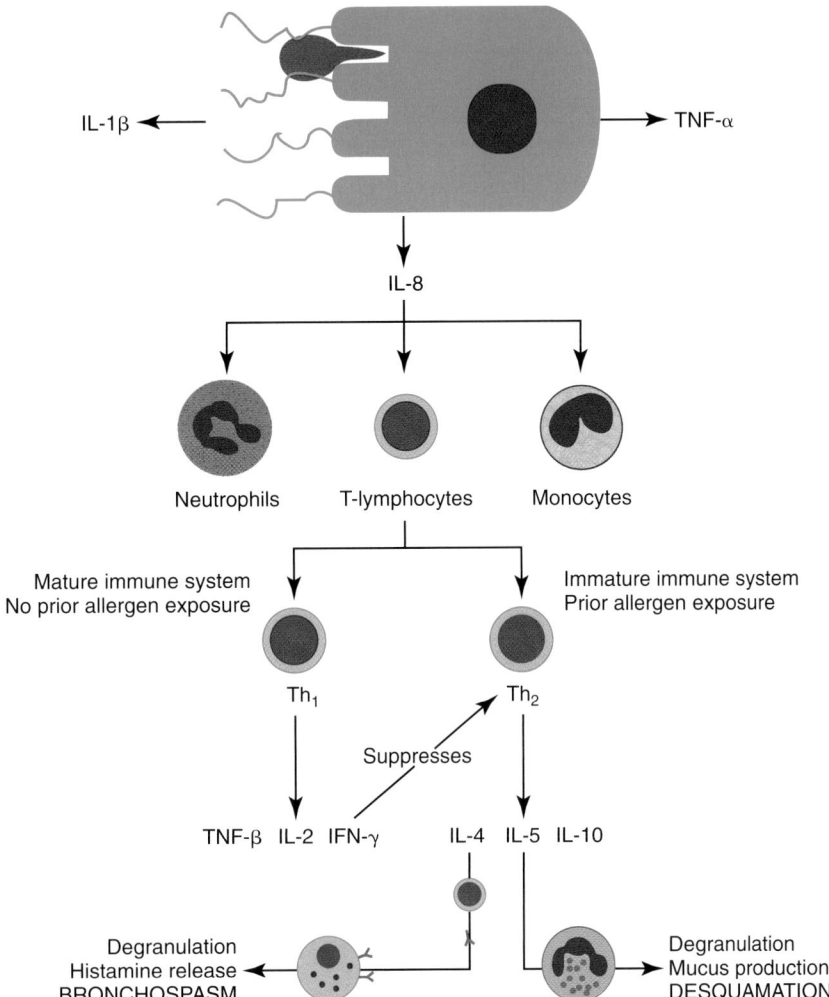

Figure 2-2: Proposed effect of immune response to mycoplasmal infection and the development or exacerbation of asthma. Attachment of mycoplasmal organisms to respiratory epithelium stimulates release of inflammatory cytokines (interleukin [IL]-1β, IL-8, and tumor necrosis factor-α [TNF-α]). IL-8 attracts inflammatory cells, including lymphocytes. Patients with a mature, functional immune system and no previous history of allergen exposure develop a Th1-mediated response and produce interferon-γ (IFN-γ), which suppresses the Th2 response. Development of a Th2-mediated response to mycoplasmal infection occurs in patients with an immature immune system and/or prior allergen exposure. It results in increased IL-4 and IL-5 production. IL-4 stimulates B cells to produce immunoglobulin E (IgE), resulting in degranulation and histamine release from mast cells and bronchospasm. IL-5 stimulates migration of eosinophils. Degranulation of eosinophils increases mucus production and desquamation. Mycoplasmal infection may therefore potentially result in development of asthma, a Th2-mediated disease, in immature patients and cause exacerbation of clinical signs in those already diagnosed (prior allergen exposure).

CLINICAL DISEASE AND DIFFERENTIAL DIAGNOSES

Ocular Disease

Signs of conjunctivitis in cats include serous, mucoid, or purulent ocular discharge, conjunctival hyperemia, blepharospasm, and chemosis (Figure 2-3). Infectious agents most commonly associated with feline conjunctivitis are feline herpesvirus type 1 (FHV-1), *Chlamydophila felis*, and feline calicivirus (FCV).[27] However, *Mycoplasma* spp. have been reported to be present in 16% to 25% of cases of feline conjunctivitis.[28,29] One study[30] reported a prevalence of up to 49%

in cats with conjunctivitis and upper respiratory tract disease, although this included cocarriage with other infectious agents. A further study[31] identified *Mycoplasma* spp. more commonly than either FHV-1 or *C. felis* and significantly more frequently in cats with conjunctivitis than in healthy cats. Conjunctivitis in cats with concurrent upper respiratory tract signs in which the presence of *Mycoplasma* spp. are identified may be associated with more severe clinical signs.[17,32]

M. felis and *M. gateae* have also been reported to be associated with ulcerative keratitis,[33] although the role of mycoplasmas in initiating this disease process is uncertain because all cases reported had received previous treatment for FHV-1 or corticosteroids.

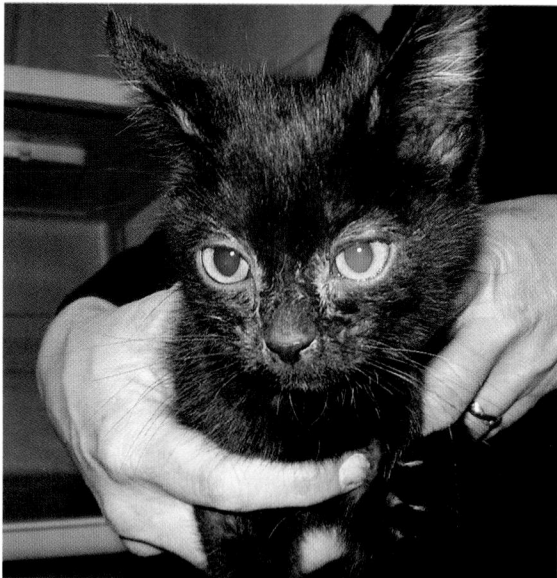

Figure 2-3: Bilateral serous ocular and nasal discharges in a young cat with respiratory mycoplasmal infection.

Upper Respiratory Tract Disease

Nasal discharge and sneezing are common conditions affecting cats, and *Mycoplasma* spp. have been associated with acute upper respiratory tract infections.[17,19,32,34] Other infectious agents that may cause signs consistent with cat "flu" include FHV-1, FCV, *C. felis,* and *Bordetella bronchiseptica*; therefore diagnostic tests are required to differentiate the causal agent and hence identify the most appropriate treatment.

Mycoplasma spp. have also been identified in cats with chronic rhinosinusitis but not in healthy control cats.[35] However, the numbers were too small to be statistically significant and thus confirm an association between *Mycoplasma* spp. and chronic rhinosinusitis. Imaging findings from radiography, computed tomography (CT), and endoscopy are not specific for mycoplasmal infections, although they may help to exclude neoplasia, foreign bodies, nasopharyngeal polyps, or nasopharyngeal stenosis as a cause for chronic rhinitis (Figure 2-4).

An initial study evaluating formalin-fixed tissues by polymerase chain reaction (PCR) for FHV-1, *Bartonella,* and *Mycoplasma* spp. DNA had suggested an association between mycoplasmal infection and the formation of nasopharyngeal polyps.[36] However, this was not substantiated when fresh tissue samples were analyzed and compared with healthy control cats.[37]

Lower Respiratory Tract Disease

Lower respiratory tract disease may manifest as coughing, tachypnea, or respiratory distress. Several studies have documented *Mycoplasma* spp. infection in association with lower respiratory tract disease in cats,[13,38,39] with up to 22% of cases having positive culture results. It is of note that a number of the cases in these studies had concurrent upper airway signs or conjunctivitis, as was also identified in the smaller case

series and case reports of *Mycoplasma*-associated pneumonia.[10,11,40-42] The frequency of this association suggests that lower respiratory tract disease may result from aspiration of pharyngeal organisms associated with upper respiratory tract disease.

Clinical signs reported in cats affected by *Mycoplasma* pneumonia have included nasal discharge, sneezing, ocular discharge, coughing, wheezing, tachypnea, dyspnea, pyrexia, hypothermia, cyanosis, and acute respiratory distress.[11,41,43,44] In addition to pneumonia, lower respiratory tract infection with *Mycoplasma* spp. has been associated with pulmonary abscessation and pyothorax.[9,10,45] One study suggested that mycoplasmal infections should be suspected as a cause of pyothorax when the pleural effusion is nonodorous and bacteria cannot be detected by Gram-stained smears of the fluid; however, this theory has not been validated.[10]

Imaging studies have identified bronchointerstitial and alveolar lung patterns, lung lobe consolidation, and pleural effusions (Figure 2-5). Spontaneous pneumomediastinum and subcutaneous emphysema have been described in one severe case of *Mycoplasma* pneumonia.[43] Computed tomography findings have been reported in two cases[43,44] and have comprised patchy, multifocal consolidation, areas of ground-glass attenuation, and nodular and reticular markings. Residual fibrosis may occur, but this has not been documented histopathologically.[44]

DIAGNOSIS

Collection of Diagnostic Samples

Samples may be obtained for diagnosis from several areas, depending on clinical signs. Conjunctival swabs may be obtained by rolling a sterile culture swab along the conjunctival mucosa of the lower eyelid. Samples for ocular cytology may also be obtained using a brush technique.[46] Nasal swabs are best obtained with fine-tipped sterile bacteriology swabs following removal of any gross discharges. Oropharyngeal swabs can be obtained by rolling a sterile bacterial swab against the surface of the pharyngeal mucosa. Oropharyngeal swabs may yield a higher level of recovery than nasal swabs and are easier to perform; however, there may only be moderate agreement between the two sites.[14]

Samples that may be obtained under general anesthesia include nasal flush fluid, nasal biopsies, and bronchoalveolar lavage fluid. Discordance has been reported between samples of nasal flush fluid and nasal biopsies submitted for culture, and due to the potential for *Mycoplasma* spp. to attach to epithelial cells, some flush samples may not reflect true mycoplasmal infection status.[47]

Cytology
Detection of Organisms

Cytologic detection of *Mycoplasma* organisms (small, lightly basophilic structures of 0.2 to 0.8 μm diameter, in clusters adherent to the cell surface) on Romanowsky-stained smears

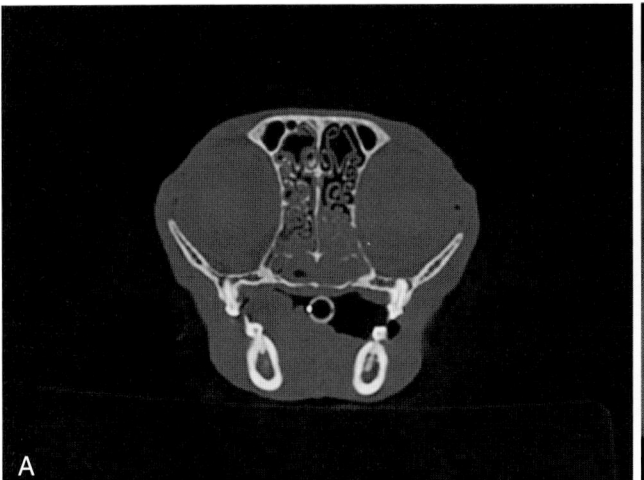
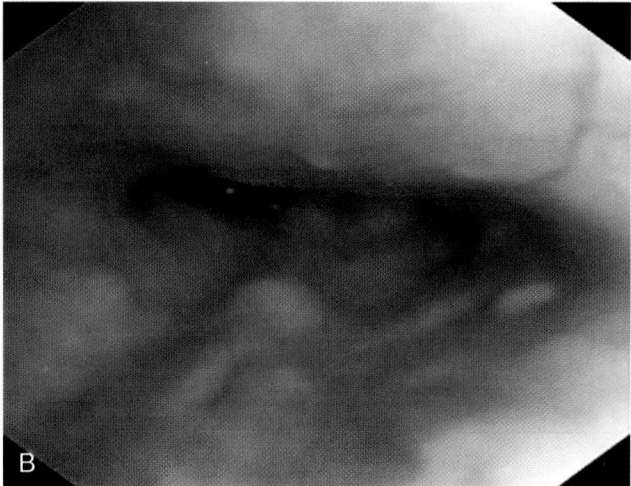

Figure 2-4: Investigations in a Cat with Chronic Rhinitis. A 9½-year-old male neutered cat was investigated for sneezing and nasal discharge of 4 months duration. The cat had been acquired from a rescue center at 8 weeks of age, was fully vaccinated, and led an indoor/outdoor lifestyle. The cat was reported to sneeze up to 20 times per day and had shown some improvement to long-acting cefovecin injections, although the sneezing had not completely resolved. The nasal discharge was reported to have initially been localized to the right side and was purulent in nature, but at time of presentation it was bilateral and serous. The cat was also reported to have a chronic, left-sided, ocular serous discharge, which had been present since acquisition and had increased respiratory noise when sleeping. No dyspnea or tachypnea was reported, and the cat was otherwise well. Physical examination was unremarkable with the exception of a serous discharge present at the left nostril. There was no evidence of facial asymmetry or pain, and normal airflow was present bilaterally. No ocular discharge was detected on this occasion. Blood tests comprising hematology, biochemistry, and assessment of clotting were all unremarkable. An oral examination under general anesthesia did not identify any abnormalities. **A,** The computed tomography scan shows evidence of fluid accumulation in the nasal passages, with no nasal deformity or turbinate destruction. *(Right is on the left side of the image.)* **B,** Retroflexed view of the nasopharynx of the case shown in Figure 2-4A. There is lymphoid hyperplasia with mucus accumulation in the right nasal passage, causing partial occlusion of the choana. *(Right is on the right side of the image.)* The findings are nonspecific and could be attributed to feline herpesvirus type 1 (FHV-1) infection (with or without other bacterial infections), lymphocytic-plasmacytic rhinitis, fungal rhinitis, or allergic rhinitis. Pinch biopsies were obtained from the nasal passages and submitted for bacterial culture and histopathology. Histopathology identified a neutrophilic infiltrate. An oropharyngeal swab was obtained and tested for *Mycoplasma felis*, FHV-1, feline calicivirus, *Bordetella bronchiseptica*, and *Chlamydophila felis* by polymerase chain reaction (PCR). *M. felis* was diagnosed by PCR at high levels. In the absence of any other respiratory pathogens, treatment was commenced with oral doxycycline (10 mg/kg by mouth every 24 hours), and the cat was reported to have shown a marked improvement after 1 week of therapy. The cat was treated for 6 weeks but showed a relapse when off antibiotics.

has been reported for conjunctival samples,[46] but detection of organisms is known to be insensitive and nonspecific. Identification is not improved by Gram-staining due to the absence of a cell wall.

Inflammatory Cells Detected on Cytology

Inflammation associated with *Mycoplasma* spp. infection appears to be predominantly neutrophilic in a study of conjunctivitis cases.[46] Cytology of bronchoalveolar lavage samples typically also demonstrates a predominantly neutrophilic population.

Bacterial Culture

Due to their lack of cell wall, *Mycoplasma* spp. are delicate organisms with special culture requirements. Transport media, such as Amies charcoal, may be recommended,[14] although

one study[39] found no benefit to using a specific mycoplasma transport medium when rapid culture was available. Prior to obtaining samples, clarification should be sought from the laboratory to which the samples will be submitted for their preferred method of transportation. Biphasic culture is typically performed, comprising inoculation onto a solid agar overlain with a liquid broth, such as modified Hayflick's or Friis. Then aerobic incubation in a carbon dioxide-enriched (5% to 10%) environment is performed. Colonies have a classic "fried egg" appearance, enabling their identification (Figure 2-6). *Mycoplasma* spp. are slow-growing organisms; therefore culture for 10 to 14 days is usually required before a definitive negative result can be given.

The *Mycoplasma* spp. cultured may be presumptively identified based on their ability to ferment different sugars, utilize arginine, reduce methylene blue, and their hemolytic ability.[2,48] Additionally, serologic methods, such as metabolic

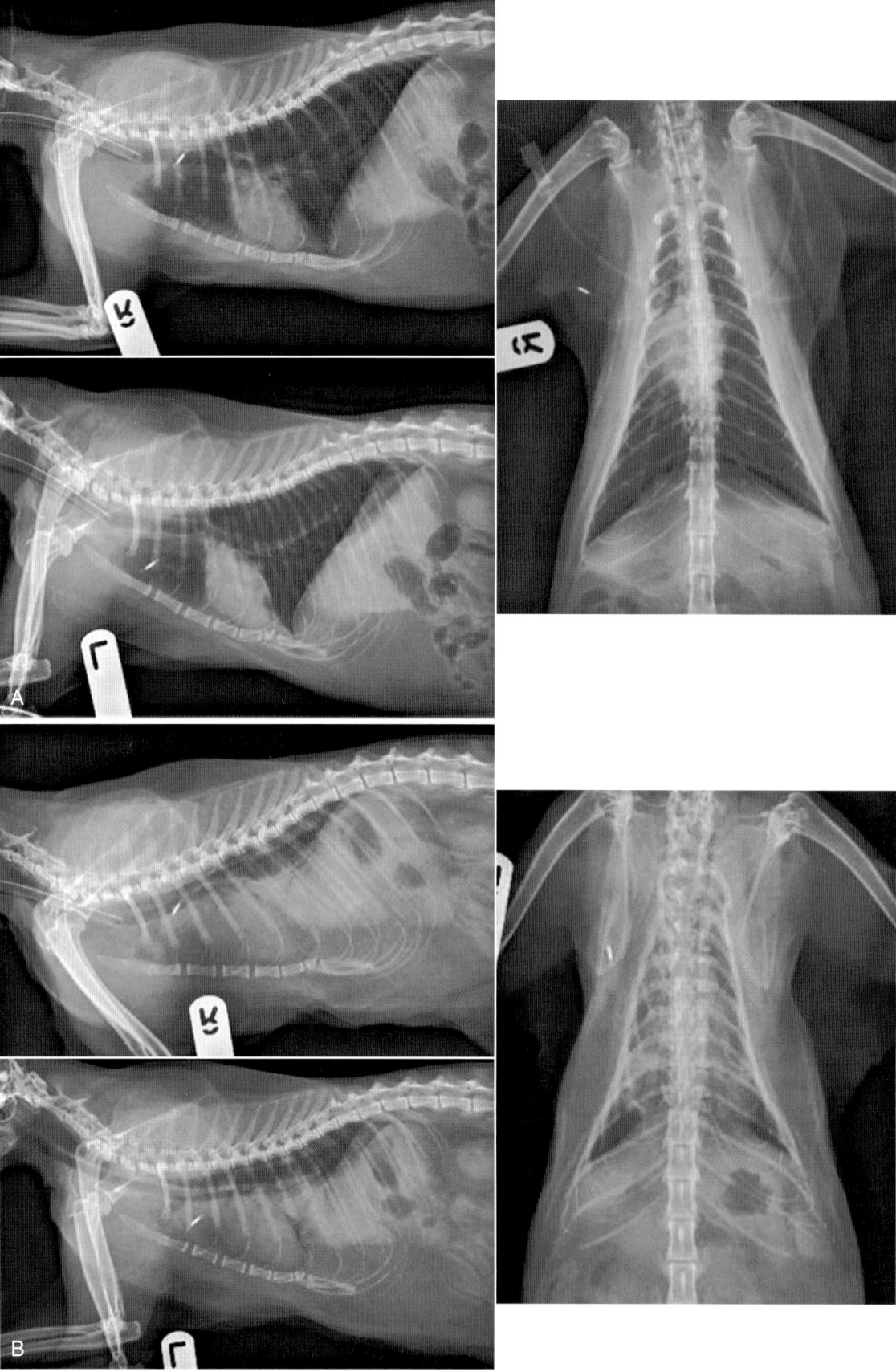

Figure 2-5: Thoracic radiographs before and after bronchoalveolar lavage in a cat with *Mycoplasma felis* pneumonia. **A,** Right lateral, left lateral, and dorsoventral views of the thorax of a cat prior to bronchoalveolar lavage. The cat is intubated and inflated views have been obtained. There is a diffuse bronchointerstitial pattern present. **B,** Right lateral, left lateral, and dorsoventral views of the same cat following bronchoalveolar lavage with two 3 mL aliquots of warm saline. There is evidence of pneumothorax, pneumomediastinum, and lung lobe atelectasis. The cat recovered with oxygen supplementation, inhaled salbutamol (albuterol), and intravenous dexamethasone. *M. felis* was identified in the bronchoalveolar lavage fluid. Pneumothorax is a recognized risk of bronchoalveolar lavage but has also been reported to occur spontaneously in a cat with mycoplasmal pneumonia.[43]

inhibition, growth inhibition, immunofluorescence, and immunobinding, have also been used to more definitively identify the species of *Mycoplasma* cultured.[49] However, these methods are not generally available commercially, with most laboratories simply stating that *Mycoplasma* spp. has been cultured.

Polymerase Chain Reaction

Due to the difficulties associated with *Mycoplasma* spp. culture, PCR assays are being used more routinely to identify *Mycoplasma* organisms. Special transport media are not required because DNA is stable, results can be obtained more rapidly, noncultivable species may be identified, and speciation is more accurate.[50] Both conventional and real-time (quantitative) *M. felis*-specific PCR tests have been developed[51,52] and are now becoming widely available commercially. Although this may enable more frequent detection of *M. felis* infection in respiratory disease, other species of *Mycoplasma* may be overlooked in clinical cases because PCR is species-specific. In contrast, use of a generic *Mycoplasma* genus-specific PCR followed by DNA sequencing of any resulting PCR product may allow identification of the *Mycoplasma* species involved.[53] Alternatively, a more generic bacterial 16S rDNA PCR and denaturing gradient gel electrophoresis allows detection of individual species but is not so widely available.[54] Although PCR may be more sensitive than culture, a positive result theoretically reflects only the presence of *Mycoplasma* DNA, not viable organisms.[14,39] However, because dead organisms are generally considered to be rapidly cleared, positive PCR results are usually given credence.

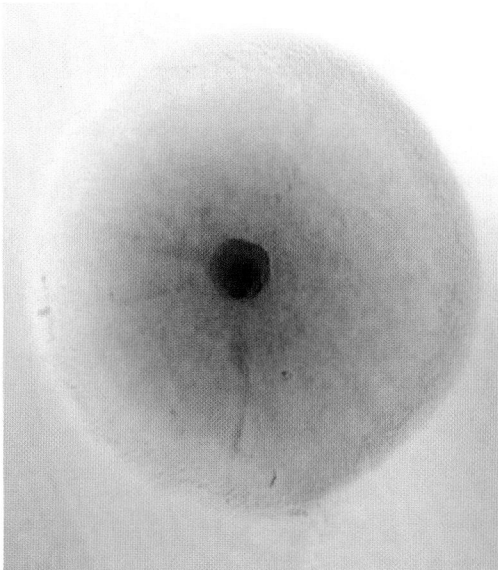

Figure 2-6: Classic "fried egg" appearance of *Mycoplasma* colonies. (Courtesy V. Bermudez, Ontario Veterinary College, Guelph, Ontario, Canada. In Greene CE: Infectious diseases of the dog and cat, 4th edition, St Louis, 2012, Saunders.)

Serology

Although serology may be used to diagnose mycoplasmal infections, particularly with regard to demonstrating rising titres, this has not been used clinically in feline medicine. In human medicine, detection of respiratory mycoplasmal infections by serology has been superseded by PCR assays, due to low sensitivity of serology in the acute phase of the disease.[55]

TREATMENT

Conjunctivitis

When *M. felis* is the sole infectious agent isolated and there are no associated upper respiratory tract disease signs, topical treatment with an ophthalmic ointment containing oxytetracycline, chloramphenicol, or a fluoroquinolone may be appropriate. If conjunctivitis is seen in association with systemic signs, then use of systemic antibacterial therapy combined with an ocular lubricant may be more appropriate.

Systemic Antibacterial Therapy

Due to the difficult culture requirements of *Mycoplasma* spp., determination of antibacterial sensitivity is rarely carried out, although guidelines for minimal inhibitory testing in *Mycoplasma* spp. have been published.[56] *Mycoplasma* spp. are generally reported to be sensitive to tetracyclines, fluoroquinolones, macrolides, azalides, lincosamides, and chloramphenicol, although it is the first three of these antibacterial groups that are most commonly used in clinical practice (Table 2-1).

Tetracyclines

Doxycycline is the preferred tetracycline due to its increased intracellular concentration and once-daily administration

Table 2-1	Oral Antibacterial Therapy for Respiratory Mycoplasmal Infections in Cats*
Antibacterial	**Dosage**
Doxycycline[†]	10 mg/kg every 24 h[59] 5 mg/kg every 12 h[58]
Marbofloxacin	2 mg/kg every 24 h
Pradofloxacin[‡]	5 mg/kg every 24 h[34,58] 10 mg/kg every 24 h[34]
Azithromycin	5-10 mg/kg every 24 h for 5 days, then every 48 h[§]

*See text for discussion on duration of treatment
[†]Use of twice daily dosing may be associated with less vomiting
[‡]Both doses appear well-tolerated. In a study of multi-etiology feline rhinitis, 10 mg/kg resolved 92% of cases and 5 mg/kg resolved 85% of cases (i.e., there was no significant difference in outcome). The label dose (Veraflox, Bayer) is 7.5 mg/kg every 24 hours.
[§]Plumb DC: *Plumb's veterinary drug handbook,* ed 8, Malden, MA, 2015, Wiley-Blackwell.

compared with other tetracyclines. In addition it is speculated that it may have anti-inflammatory effects due to its ability to inhibit matrix metalloproteinases, although this has yet to be demonstrated in feline disease.[57] Care has to be taken with the potential for esophageal ulceration and stricture formation, especially with tablets or capsules containing the hyclate and hydrochloride salt formulations. The use of doxycycline has been investigated in a number of studies of upper respiratory tract infections in shelter cats in which *Mycoplasma* spp. were implicated; clinical efficacy was demonstrated within 14 days of treatment.[15,58,59]

Fluoroquinolones

The response to fluoroquinolones appears to be variable. No improvement was seen when enrofloxacin was administered to a kitten with mycoplasmal pneumonia in one report.[44] A lower airway disease case excluded from a study by this author[39] because it had received marbofloxacin prior to investigation was culture positive for *Mycoplasma* spp. However, pradofloxacin is reported to have an enhanced spectrum against *Mycoplasma* spp. compared with other fluoroquinolones, as well as decreased resistance.[34] *Mycoplasma* spp. could, however, still be recovered in cats following 7-day courses of oral pradofloxacin at 5 mg/kg/day and even at 10 mg/kg/day[34]; however, when administered at 5 mg/kg/day for 42 days, *Mycoplasma* spp. were no longer identified by PCR.[58] Pradofloxacin is secreted into tears and saliva, which may provide a theoretical advantage of pradofloxacin over doxycycline in treatment of upper respiratory tract infection.[60] However, whether pradofloxacin is taken into cells is unclear at this time.[58]

Macrolides

Azithromycin has been recommended because it is reported to be very effective against mycoplasmas.[11] Other features of azithromycin that may be beneficial include the dosing regimen allowing administration every 72 hours and its ability to accumulate inside phagocytes.[61] One study of upper respiratory tract infections in shelter cats did not show azithromycin to be any more efficacious than amoxicillin (which is not effective for *Mycoplasma* spp., which are cell wall free). However, these cats had multiple infectious agents present, which may have affected responses.[62] Macrolides may have an immunomodulatory effect as well as an antibacterial effect. One study looking at the effect of clarithromycin on *M. pneumoniae* infection in mice revealed that the improvement appeared to be due to its antibacterial effect.[63] Macrolide resistance has been documented in human *Mycoplasma* spp.,[21] although other sources suggest they are the antibacterial agent of choice for *M. pneumoniae*.[64]

Duration of Treatment

The duration of treatment required is unclear. Clinical signs may often resolve within 7 days[59]; however, chronic intracellular infections may prevent complete elimination. One study demonstrated a mean time to elimination of *Mycoplasma* spp. of 20 days for treatment with pradofloxacin and 19 days

for treatment with doxycycline, as assessed by PCR.[58] A minimum treatment period of 42 days was advised, however, due to some cats being PCR-positive at 28 days. The author of this chapter also currently recommends a 6-week treatment period. One case was treated with doxycycline for a total of 65 days, having previously failed to improve with initial therapy of ticarcillin-clavulanate and enrofloxacin.[44]

Fluoroquinolones are bactericidal, whereas tetracyclines and macrolides are bacteriostatic. This may be of significance if treating immunocompromised patients. Due to the finding of *M. felis* in asymptomatic cats in households where upper respiratory tract disease has been identified, treatment of in-contact cats has been suggested,[19] although there is a lack of evidence to support this indiscriminate use of antibacterials.

Although azithromycin may facilitate compliance, the author of this chapter will generally use doxycycline for 6 weeks as first-line therapy, preferring to use fluoroquinolones for cats that do not respond to doxycycline or that relapse. Failure to respond seems more common with azithromycin than doxycycline in this author's experience. Despite recommending prolonged courses of treatment, recrudescence of disease is not unusual once antibacterial therapy has stopped. This may reflect underlying deficits within the respiratory immune system that make cats prone to mycoplasmal infections; therefore trying to address underlying pathology, such as feline asthma, and improve airway hygiene are also important.

Supportive Treatments

Supportive treatments include removal of ocular and nasal discharges and use of saline nebulization therapy for cats affected by upper respiratory tract signs. Bronchodilators, such as oral theophylline or inhaled salbutamol (albuterol) or salmeterol, may be beneficial in cats coughing or showing signs of lower airway disease. Ensuring adequate hydration and nutrition is also of importance and may necessitate intravenous fluid therapy and placement of feeding tubes.

Corticosteroids

Although corticosteroids may be beneficial in reducing the inflammation associated with the Th2 response potentially induced by *Mycoplasma* spp., they may also allow bacterial proliferation and recrudescence of chronic infection. If *Mycoplasma* spp. infection is diagnosed in a cat with signs consistent with feline asthma, the author will defer use of corticosteroids until a 4- to 6-week course of antibacterial therapy has been provided (where possible) or use both concurrently if the severity of signs warrants it.

Monitoring of Therapy

Response to therapy is often used to support the role that *Mycoplasma* spp. play in respiratory disease, but ideally repeat sampling following a course of treatment should be performed to demonstrate clearance of the infection. This may be relatively easily accomplished with ocular or oropharyngeal swabs for conjunctivitis or upper respiratory tract disease. However, owners may be less willing to have repeated bronchoalveolar lavage performed for evaluation of lower respiratory tract disease. Although radiography may be less invasive, it is an insensitive technique to assess response to therapy for mycoplasmal infection. In addition, it would be extremely useful to have studies documenting response to therapy so that the most appropriate antibacterial drugs can be identified, the ideal duration of therapy can be determined, and differences in antibacterial susceptibility among the different strains or species of *Mycoplasma* can be detected.

PREVENTION

Vaccination

No feline vaccines are currently available to prevent infection with *Mycoplasma* organisms. The absence of a vaccine may reflect the difficulty in knowing the significance of *Mycoplasma* spp. as primary pathogens versus commensal flora of the respiratory tract. It is of note, however, that in some host species in which *Mycoplasma* spp. are recognized to be a primary respiratory pathogen, vaccine development has been hampered by lack of efficacy or unacceptable side effects, and recombinant vaccines or stimulation of mucosal immunity may be vaccine targets for the future.[65]

ZOONOTIC POTENTIAL

The majority of *Mycoplasma* spp. are considered host specific, although some species have been documented to move between species.[66] Although *M. felis* may cause respiratory tract disease in horses,[66] neither it nor any of the other species commonly isolated from the feline oropharynx (*M. gateae*, *M. feliminutum*, and *M. arginini*) have been reported to cause respiratory disease in humans. There are two reported cases of potential zoonotic infection from cats to humans.[67,68] One case of *M. felis* septic arthritis has been reported in a patient with hypogammaglobulinemia and on prednisolone therapy—both predisposing factors for mycoplasmal infections in humans.[67] The patient owned a cat and had been bitten on the hand 6 months previously by a different cat; therefore the definitive source was not confirmed because neither cat was sampled. A second case of mycoplasmal infection of suspected feline origin was identified in a veterinarian who sustained a cat scratch injury on the hand and developed subsequent cellulitis.[68] Serology performed on the veterinarian demonstrated similar inhibiting antibodies as in a second cat that the veterinarian had treated for a purulent cat-bite wound on its leg but not with the cat that inflicted the scratch. The actual species of *Mycoplasma* was not confirmed. The high prevalence of *Mycoplasma* spp. within the oropharyngeal cavity of cats makes it somewhat surprising that these organisms are not more commonly identified in cat-bite injuries. This may reflect the difficulties with isolation of *Mycoplasma* spp. or that increased awareness by physicians of *Bartonella* spp. infections from cat bites may result in antibiotics to which *Mycoplasma* spp. are also susceptible being prescribed more frequently. Alternatively, host specificity may make it genuinely difficult for the feline mycoplasmas to establish infections in people.

SUMMARY

For a simple organism, there is still much to be learned about the pathogenicity of *Mycoplasma* spp., and the role that they play in respiratory disease actually appears to be very complex. Improved detection through the use of PCR and recognition of the potential for the immune system to play a role in establishment of disease will hopefully lead to a better understanding not only of the disease process but also of its management.

References

1. Greene CE, Chalker VJ: Nonhemotropic mycoplasmal, ureaplasmal, and L-form infections. In Greene CE, editor: *Infectious diseases of the dog and cat*, ed 4, St Louis, 2012, Elsevier/Saunders, pp 319–325.
2. Heyward J, Sabry M, Dowdle W: Characterization of *Mycoplasma* species of feline origin. *Am J Vet Res* 30:615–622, 1967.
3. Tan R, Wang Lim E, Ishak B: Ecology of *Mycoplasmas* in clinically healthy cats. *Aust Vet J* 53:515–518, 1977.
4. Spradbrow PB, Marley J, Portas B, et al: The isolation of *Mycoplasmas* from cats with respiratory disease. *Aust Vet J* 46:109–110, 1970.
5. Blackmore D, Hill A, Jackson O: The incidence of *Mycoplasma* in pet and colony maintained cats. *J Small Anim Pract* 12:207–216, 1971.
6. Blackmore D, Hill A: The experimental transmission of various *Mycoplasmas* of feline origin to domestic cats (*Felis catus*). *J Small Anim Pract* 14:7–13, 1973.
7. Tan RJ, Wang Lim E, Ishak B: Significance and pathogenic role of *Mycoplasma arginini* in cat diseases. *Can J Comp Med* 41:349–354, 1977.
8. Wong W, Noor F: Pyothorax in the cat—a report of two cases. *Kajian Veterinar Malaysia* 16:15–17, 1984.
9. Crisp M, Birchard S, Lawrence AE, et al: Pulmonary abscess caused by a *Mycoplasma* species in a cat. *J Am Vet Med Assoc* 191:340–342, 1987.
10. Malik R, Love D, Hunt G, et al: Pyothorax associated with a *Mycoplasma* species in a kitten. *J Small Anim Pract* 32:31–34, 1991.
11. Foster S, Barrs V, Martin P, et al: Pneumonia associated with *Mycoplasma* spp in three cats. *Aust Vet J* 76:460–464, 1998.
12. Moise N, Wiedenkeller D, Yeager A, et al: Clinical, radiographic and bronchial cytologic features of cats with bronchial disease: 65 cases (1980-1986). *J Am Vet Med Assoc* 194:1467–1473, 1989.
13. Randolph J, Moise N, Scarlett J, et al: Prevalence of mycoplasmal and ureaplasmal recovery from tracheobronchial lavages and of mycoplasmal recovery from pharyngeal swab specimens in cats with or without pulmonary disease. *Am J Vet Res* 54:897–900, 1993.
14. Veir J, Ruch-Gallie R, Spindel M, et al: Prevalence of selected infectious organisms and comparison of two anatomic sampling sites in

shelter cats with upper respiratory tract disease. *J Feline Med Surg* 10:551–557, 2008.

15. Litster AW: Comparison of the efficacy of amoxicillin-clavulanic acid, cefovecin and doxycycline in the treatment of upper respiratory tract disease in cats housed in animal shelters. *J Am Vet Med Assoc* 241:218–226, 2012.

16. Gourkow N, Lawson J, Hamon S, et al: Descriptive epidemiology of upper respiratory disease and associated risk factors in cats in an animal shelter in coastal western Canada. *Can Vet J* 54:132–138, 2013.

17. Bannasch M, Foley J: Epidemiologic evaluation of multiple respiratory pathogens in cats in animal shelters. *J Feline Med Surg* 7:109–119, 2005.

18. Tan R: Susceptibility of kittens to *Mycoplasma felis* infection. *Jpn J Exp Med* 44:235–240, 1974.

19. Holst B, Hanas S, Berndtsson L, et al: Infectious causes for feline upper respiratory tract disease—a case-control study. *J Feline Med Surg* 12:783–789, 2010.

20. Caswell J, Archambault M: *Mycoplasma bovis* pneumonia in cattle. *Anim Health Res Rev* 8:161–186, 2008.

21. Waites K, Balish M, Atkinson T: New insights into the pathogenesis and detection of *Mycoplasma pneumoniae* infections. *Future Microbiol* 3:635–648, 2008.

22. Waites K, Talkington D: *Mycoplasma pneumonia* and its role as a human pathogen. *Clin Microbiol Rev* 17:697–728, 2004.

23. Bodhanker S, Sun X, Woolard M, et al: Interferon gamma and interleukin 4 have contrasting effects on immunopathology and the development of protective adaptive immunity against *Mycoplasma* respiratory disease. *J Infect Dis* 202:39–51, 2010.

24. Kraft M, Cassell G, Henson J, et al: Detection of *Mycoplasma pneumoniae* in the airways of adults with chronic asthma. *Am J Resp Crit Care Med* 158:998–1001, 1998.

25. Lieberman D, Lieberman D, Printz S, et al: Atypical pathogen infection in adults with acute exacerbation of bronchial asthma. *Am J Resp Crit Care Med* 167:406–410, 2003.

26. Chu H, Honour J, Rawlinson C, et al: Effects of respiratory *Mycoplasma pneumoniae* infection on allergen-induced bronchial hyperresponsiveness and lung inflammation in mice. *Infect Immun* 71:1520–1526, 2003.

27. Gerriets W, Joy N, Huebner-Guthardt J, et al: Feline calicivirus: a neglected cause of feline ocular surface infections. *Vet Ophthalmol* 15:172–179, 2012.

28. Shewen P, Povey R, Wilson M: A survey of the conjunctival flora of clinically normal cats and cats with conjunctivitis. *Can Vet J* 21:231–233, 1980.

29. Haesebrouck F, Devriese L, van Rijssen B, et al: Incidence and significance of isolation of *Mycoplasma felis* from conjunctival swabs of cats. *Vet Microbiol* 26:95–101, 1991.

30. Hartmann A, Hawley J, Werkenthin C, et al: Detection of bacterial and viral organisms from the conjunctiva of cats with conjunctivitis and upper respiratory tract disease. *J Feline Med Surg* 12:775–782, 2010.

31. Low HC, Powell CC, Veir JK, et al: Prevalence of feline herpesvirus 1, *Chlamydophila felis,* and *Mycoplasma* spp DNA in conjunctival cells collected from cats with and without conjunctivitis. *Am J Vet Res* 68:643–648, 2007.

32. Burns R, Wagner DC, Leutenegger CM, et al: Histologic and molecular correlation in shelter cats with acute upper respiratory infection. *J Clin Microbiol* 49:2454–2460, 2011.

33. Gray L, Ketring KT: Clinical use of 16S rRNA gene sequencing to identify *Mycoplasma felis* and *Mycoplasma gateae* associated with feline ulcerative keratitis. *J Clin Microbiol* 43:3431–3434, 2005.

34. Spindel MV: Evaluation of pradofloxacin for the treatment of feline rhinitis. *J Feline Med Surg* 10:472–479, 2008.

35. Johnson L, Foley JE, de Cock HE, et al: Assessment of infectious organisms associated with chronic rhinosinusitis in cats. *J Am Vet Med Assoc* 227:579–585, 2005.

36. Klose T, Rosychuk R, MacPhail C, et al: Association between upper respiratory tract infections and inflammatory aural and nasopharyngeal polyps in cats. *J Vet Int Med* 21:628, 2007.

37. Klose T, MacPhail C, Schultheiss P, et al: Prevalence of select infectious agents in inflammatory aural and nasopharyngeal polyps from client-owned cats. *J Feline Med Surg* 12:769–774, 2010.

38. Foster S, Martin P, Braddock J, et al: A retrospective analysis of feline bronchoalveolar lavage cytology and microbiology (1995-2000). *J Feline Med Surg* 6:189–198, 2004.

39. Reed N, Simpson KE, Ayling R, et al: *Mycoplasma* species in cats with lower airway disease: improved detection and species identification using a polymerase chain reaction assay. *J Feline Med Surg* 14:833–840, 2012.

40. Chandler J, Lappin M: Mycoplasmal respiratory infections in small animals: 17 cases (1988-1999). *J Am Anim Hosp Assoc* 38:111–119, 2002.

41. Foster S, Martin P, Allan G, et al: Lower respiratory tract infections in cats: 21 cases (1995-2000). *J Feline Med Surg* 6:167–180, 2004.

42. Barrs V, Allan G, Beatty J, et al: Feline pyothorax: a retrospective study of 27 cases in Australia. *J Feline Med Surg* 7:211–222, 2005.

43. Trow A, Rozanski E, Tidwell A: Primary *Mycoplasma* pneumonia associated with reversible respiratory failure in a cat. *J Feline Med Surg* 10:398–402, 2008.

44. Bongrand Y, Blais M, Alexander K: Atypical pneumonia associated with a *Mycoplasma* isolate in a kitten. *Can Vet J* 53:1109–1113, 2012.

45. Gulbahar M, Gurturk K: Pyothorax associated with a *Mycoplasma* sp and *Arcanobacterium pyogenes* in a kitten. *Aust Vet J* 80:344–345, 2002.

46. Hillstrom A, Tvedten H, Kallberg M, et al: Evaluation of cytologic findings in feline conjunctivitis. *Vet Clin Pathol* 41:283–290, 2012.

47. Johnson L, Kass P: Effect of sample collection methodology on nasal culture results in cats. *J Feline Med Surg* 11:645–649, 2009.

48. Cole BC, Golightly L, Ward JR: Characterization of *Mycoplasma* strains from cats. *J Bacteriol* 94:1451–1458, 1967.

49. Brown M, Gionet P, Senior D: Identification of *Mycoplasma felis* and *Mycoplasma gateae* by an immunobinding assay. *J Clin Microbiol* 28:1870–1873, 1990.

50. Brown DR, McLaughlan GS, Brown MB: Taxonomy of the feline *Mycoplasmas Mycoplasma felifaucium, Mycoplasma feliminutum, Mycoplasma felis, Mycoplasma gateae, Mycoplasma leocaptivus, Mycoplasma leopharyngis,* and *Mycoplasma simbae* by 16S rRNA gene sequence comparisons. *Int J Syst Bacteriol* 45:560–564, 1995.

51. Chalker VJ, Owen WMA, Paterson CJI, et al: Development of a polymerase chain reaction for the detection of *Mycoplasma felis* in domestic cats. *Vet Microbiol* 100:77–82, 2004.

52. Söderlund R, Bölske G, Ström Holst B, et al: Development and evaluation of a real-time polymerase chain reaction method for the detection of *Mycoplasma felis. J Vet Diagn Invest* 23:890–893, 2011.

53. Johnson L, Drazenovich N, Foley J: A comparison of routine culture with polymerase chain reaction technology for the detection of *Mycoplasma* species in feline nasal samples. *J Vet Diagn Invest* 16:347–351, 2004.

54. McAuliffe L, Ellis R, Lawes J, et al: 16S rDNA PCR and denaturing gradient gel electrophoresis; a single generic test for detecting and differentiating *Mycoplasma* species. *J Med Microbiol* 54:731–739, 2005.

55. Templeton K, Scheltinga S, Graffelmann A, et al: Comparison and evaluation of real-time PCR, real-time nucleic acid sequence-based amplification, conventional PCR and serology for diagnosis of *Mycoplasma pneumoniae. J Clin Microbiol* 41:4366–4371, 2003.

56. Hannan P: Guidelines and recommendations for antimicrobial minimum inhibitory concentration (MIC) testing against veterinary *Mycoplasma* species. *Vet Res* 31:373–395, 2000.

57. Leemans J, Kirschvink N, Bernaerts F, et al: Salmeterol or doxycycline do not inhibit acute bronchospasm and airway inflammation in cats with experimentally-induced asthma. *Vet J* 192:49–56, 2012.

58. Hartmann AH: Efficacy of pradofloxacin in cats with feline upper respiratory tract disease due to *Chlamydophila felis* or *Mycoplasma* infections. *J Vet Int Med* 22:44–52, 2008.

59. Kompare B, Litster AL, Leutenegger CM, et al: Randomised, masked controlled clinical trial to compare 7-day and 14-day course length of doxycycline in the treatment of *Mycoplasma felis* infection in shelter cats. *Comp Immunol Microbiol Inf Dis* 36:129–135, 2013.

60. Hartmann AK: Pharmacokinetics of pradofloxacin and doxycycline in serum, saliva and tear fluid of cats after oral administration. *J Vet Pharmacol Ther* 31:87–94, 2008.

61. Hunter RP, Lynch MJ, Ericson JF, et al: Pharmacokinetics, oral bioavailability and tissue distribution of azithromycin in cats. *J Vet Pharmacol Ther* 18:38–46, 1995.

62. Ruch-Gallie R, Veir J, Spindel M, et al: Efficacy of amoxycillin and azithromycin for the empirical treatment of shelter cats in suspected bacterial upper respiratory tract infections. *J Feline Med Surg* 10:542–550, 2008.

63. Hardy R, Rios A, Chavez-Bueno S, et al: Antimicrobial and immunologic activities of clarithromycin in a murine model of *Mycoplasma pneumoniae*-induced pneumonia. *Antimicrob Agents Chemother* 47:1614–1620, 2003.

64. Blasi F: Atypical pathogens and respiratory tract infection. *Eur Respir J* 24:171–181, 2004.

65. Nicholas R, Ayling R, McAuliffe L: Vaccines for *Mycoplasma* diseases in animals and man. *J Comp Pathol* 140:85–96, 2009.

66. Pitcher D, Nicholas R: *Mycoplasma* host specificity: fact or fiction. *Vet J* 170:300–306, 2005.

67. Bonillo H, Chenoweth C, Tully J, et al: *Mycoplasma felis* septic arthritis in a patient with hypogammaglobulinemia. *Clin Infect Dis* 24:222–225, 1997.

68. McCabe S, Murray J, Ruhnke H, et al: *Mycoplasma* infection of the hand acquired from a cat. *J Hand Surg* 12A:1085–1088, 1987.

Update on Mycobacterial Infections: Diagnosis, Management, and Zoonotic Considerations

Carolyn O'Brien

Mycobacteria cause a variety of clinical syndromes in the cat, ranging from localized skin disease to disseminated and potentially fatal infections. Cutaneous disease is the most common manifestation; however, the respiratory, skeletal, and nervous systems, abdominal organs, peripheral and internal lymph nodes, and eye may be involved.

Mycobacteria are gram-positive, aerobic, non–spore forming, nonmotile, rod-shaped bacteria. Identification of the causative agent either via culture or genetic testing is important for treatment, prognostic and epidemiologic reasons, and especially for assessing the potential for zoonotic transmission. Conceptually, mycobacteria can be divided into three main groups (Box 3-1):

1. Obligate pathogens that require a mammalian host such as the tuberculous mycobacteria, also known as members of the *Mycobacterium tuberculosis* (MTB) complex. Species in this category reported to cause disease in cats include *M. tuberculosis sensu stricto, Mycobacterium bovis,* and *Mycobacterium microti.*
2. Species that have pathogenic potential but are generally considered opportunistic saprophytes, variably distributed in the environment. This group can be subdivided into (1) slowly growing mycobacteria (e.g., *Mycobacterium avium* complex [MAC]) and (2) rapidly growing mycobacteria, previously known as Runyon group IV or "atypical" mycobacteria.
3. Species that cause cutaneous leproid/tuberculous granulomata, with or without systemic involvement, which cannot be cultured by routine laboratory methods and have an enigmatic ecologic niche. These are known as the "lepromatous" mycobacteria.

ETIOLOGY AND EPIDEMIOLOGY

Feline mycobacterial infections have been documented since the late 1880s; however, there is much yet to be learned about the ecology and transmission of these organisms. Relatively few studies have examined large cohorts of cats with mycobacteriosis.[1-5] These studies are generally restricted to animals in a particular country or region, and therefore may not be representative of the condition in cats in other parts of the world, particularly with regard to causative species. In some studies, only a small number of cases definitively identify the mycobacteria species via culture and/or genetic analysis.

Most cats with mycobacterial infections do not appear to have underlying immunosuppressive conditions, except for some cats with "tuberculoid" leprosy.[6] Moreover, no particular association has been made with mycobacteriosis and positive retroviral status, unlike people with human immunodeficiency virus (HIV)/acquired immunodeficiency syndrome (AIDS) and MAC infections. Regardless of causative species, most cases of mycobacteriosis occur in adult cats with outdoor access, although infections have also been reported in indoor cats.

Tuberculous Mycobacteria

The vast majority of human tuberculosis (TB) around the world is caused by *M. tuberculosis.* Cats are naturally resistant to this organism, but occasional infections have been documented[7] (Box 3-2).

M. bovis and *M. microti* are the main MTB complex species associated with disease in cats, especially in the United Kingdom and some parts of Western Continental Europe.[2,10] *M. microti* was first recognized in voles in the 1930s and was previously termed "*microti*-like" or "*M. tuberculosis-M. bovis* variant" in some publications. In a study reporting cases of feline mycobacteriosis in Great Britain, of 159 samples that yielded a positive culture result, 40% were *M. microti,* and 33% were *M. bovis.*[2] In the study, when comparisons were made between these two cohorts, it was found that those cats with *M. bovis* were likely to be younger, with a mean age of 3 years, whereas the *M. microti*-infected cats had a mean age of 8 years.[2]

M. bovis has worldwide endemicity, although some areas are virtually free of the disease, such as most of Continental Europe and parts of the Caribbean and Australia. In developed nations, the incidence of bovine TB has been greatly reduced via widespread surveillance, slaughter of test-positive cattle, and the pasteurization of milk. *M. microti* is found in

BOX 3-1 Mycobacteria Causing Feline Infections

Mycobacteria that cause feline infections can be grouped into tuberculous, slowly growing and rapidly growing opportunistic saprophytic, and lepromatous species.

BOX 3-2 Tuberculosis

Tuberculosis has plagued mankind for millennia. In fact, whole genome analysis suggests that the major *Mycobacterium tuberculosis* (MTB) complex strains have been co-evolving with humans for around 70,000 years, starting prior to the Neolithic Demographic Transition from Africa.[8] It was previously thought that *Mycobacterium bovis* was the precursor to MTB; however, genetic studies suggest that the opposite is more likely to be true.[9]

Western Europe, the United Kingdom, South Africa, and South America. Its main reservoir appears to be voles (also known as field mice in North America), shrews, wood mice, and other small rodents found in woodland areas.[11]

Cats are generally considered incidental or spillover hosts for the tuberculous mycobacteria, but it is unknown whether they are involved in the transmission of the infection to other species. Direct cat-to-cat transmission was documented in an outbreak of *M. bovis* infection in a group of research cats,[12] but the likelihood for this to occur in the field setting is not clear.

Cats rarely acquire *M. tuberculosis*, but they can become exposed by humans infected with this organism, likely by inhalation of infective droplets. However, there are relatively few completely documented cases of anthropozoonotic infection in the literature. Cats are more commonly infected with *M. bovis*, albeit at a greatly reduced rate in most of the developed world because of intensive bovine TB eradication and control programs. Direct exposure to *M. bovis*-infected humans may also be a source of the disease in cats, although it is more likely via ingestion of unpasteurized milk, uncooked meat, or offal from infected cattle. This may especially be a problem in *M. bovis*-endemic countries such as Argentina, where it is customary to feed pet and stray cats raw bovine lung.[13] It is not known to what extent these types of practices contribute to infection in cats domiciled in the rest of Latin America, Eastern Europe, Asia, Africa, and the Indian subcontinent. Feral cats have been observed to scavenge the carcasses of two *M. bovis*-reservoir species in New Zealand, the Australian common brushtail opossum and the domestic ferret.[14] It is conceivable that pet cats may also participate in this practice. The European badger is also a potential source of *M. bovis* infection in cats in the United Kingdom and the Irish Republic. The exact route of transmission from this species is not clear, but it may involve fomites, direct interspecies aggression, and/or consumption of infected carrion by

cats, although the latter two scenarios seem unlikely.[2,15] In a recent necropsy survey of wild mammals collected from "bovine TB hot-spots" of southwest England, numerous potential feline prey species, including mice, grey squirrels, a vole, and a shrew, were found to be infected with *M. bovis*.[16] It has also been proposed that cutaneous wounds could become secondarily contaminated with *M. bovis* from the environment. However, it is perhaps more conceivable that the organism is directly inoculated via bites or scratches obtained in altercations with, or ingestion of, infected prey. Investigators in the United States have postulated that wild deer carcasses infected with *M. bovis* provide a potential source of infection for cats in that country.[17] Suspected nosocomial contamination of surgical wounds has been reported.[18]

Feline *M. microti* infections are likely acquired by ingestion of, or being bitten by, infected prey species. These infections tend to occur in southeastern England, northern England, and southern Scotland, where infection is found in the resident wild vole populations.[19] These "*M. microti* areas" in the United Kingdom may be relatively geographically distinct from those in which *M. bovis* infection is common.[2] That being said, cases of *M. bovis* can and do occur in some of these areas, and *vice versa* for *M. microti*, although the exception to this may be southern Scotland, where cats do not appear likely to be infected with locally acquired *M. bovis*.[2] As is the case for *M. bovis*, genotyping of *M. microti* isolates divides this species into a number of different genotypes that tend to be distinctly geographically clustered.[19,20] Serum hydroxyvitamin D levels of cats with active TB are lower than those of healthy controls (as is the case in humans)[21]; however, the significance of this finding is not known.

Mycobacterium avium Complex and Other Slowly Growing Saprophytes

Numerous saprophytic slowly growing mycobacterial species have been known to cause disease in cats. The most common of these are members of the MAC; however, infections caused by numerous other mycobacterial species have been documented (Table 3-1). Very little is known about the prevalence of cats with slowly growing saprophytic mycobacteriosis. Approximately 16% of cats with culture-positive mycobacteriosis in Great Britain were infected with an MAC organism, and many were domiciled in a geographical cluster in the eastern counties of England.[2]

These slow-growing saprophytes are found worldwide in natural and municipal water sources and soil that is rich in organic matter. In addition, they are associated with certain plant species, especially sphagnum moss. Many of these organisms are ubiquitous; however, some have a higher environmental presence in certain geographical areas or environmental niches; for example, *M. malmoense* or biofilms with *M. intracellulare* in the United Kingdom and Sweden. Some environmental mycobacteria have highly restricted, focal areas of endemicity, as is the case for *M. ulcerans* infection, where the only nonhuman cases have been reported in a

Table 3-1 **Characteristics of Mycobacterial Species Known to Cause Infections in Cats**

Mycobacterial Species	Suspected Transmission*	Clinical Features	Public health Risk	Recommended Treatment[†,‡,§]
Tuberculous Mycobacteria				
Mycobacterium bovis	Ingestion of infected unpasteurized cow's milk, offal, or wildlife prey species. Cutaneous inoculation directly from infected wildlife or from contaminated environmental material.	Cutaneous nodules or fistulae most common. Regional peripheral lymphadenopathy. Internal organ, particularly abdominal, involvement, including regional lymphadenopathy (especially mesenteric). Any anatomical site may be involved.	Likely to be low in developed countries and unknown in developing countries. Precautionary measures such as PPE should be used when handling animals, especially with discharging wounds or during surgery or necropsy exam, because of the known pathogenicity of this organism in humans.	Medical treatment is instituted with two or three of the following drugs: clarithromycin (or azithromycin), rifampicin, pradofloxacin (or moxifloxacin) or clofazimine, depending on availability and/or owner finances. Modifications to the drug regimen are then made depending on susceptibility data, response to therapy, or the development of side effects necessitating drug cessation (e.g., hepatotoxicity). If drug resistance develops, treatment may include ethambutol, dihydrostreptomycin, isoniazid, or pyrazinamide.[ǁ] Surgical excision of cutaneous nodules is advised if practicable.
Mycobacterium microti	Ingestion of infected wildlife prey species. Cutaneous inoculation directly from infected wildlife or from contaminated environmental material.		Unknown, but likely to be very low, given apparently low pathogenicity of *M. microti* in immunocompetent humans.	
Mycobacterium tuberculosis	Inhalation of infective respiratory secretions from humans.	Internal organ involvement, including lymphadenopathy. Any anatomical site may be involved. (Few cases are reported in the literature.)	Low in developed countries and unknown in developing countries. Precautionary measures such as PPE should be used when handling animals, especially with discharging wounds or during surgery or necropsy exam, because of the known pathogenicity of this organism in humans.	The treatment of *M. tuberculosis* in pet animals is not generally advised.

Table 3-1   Characteristics of Mycobacterial Species Known to Cause Infections in Cats—cont'd

Mycobacterial Species	Suspected Transmission*	Clinical Features	Public health Risk	Recommended Treatment[†,‡,§]
Slowly Growing Saprophytes				
Most commonly: *Mycobacterium avium* complex: *M. avium* subsp. *avium*, *M. avium* subsp. *hominissuis*, and *M. intracellulare* Rarely: *M. genavense*, *M. malmoense*, *M. celatum*, *M. terrae* complex, *M. simiae*, *M. xenopi*, *M. ulcerans*, and *M. heckeshornense*	Cutaneous inoculation with contaminated environmental material via cat fights or other breaches of the integument. Ingestion of contaminated municipal or environmental water sources or infected wildlife prey species.	Internal organ, particularly abdominal, involvement, including regional lymphadenopathy (especially mesenteric). Pulmonary involvement (with or without accompanying clinical signs) common with *M. avium* infections. Any anatomical site may be involved. Cutaneous nodules or fistulae (uncommon). Regional peripheral lymphadenopathy (uncommon).	Unknown, but likely to be low, given the low pathogenicity of saprophytic mycobacteria in immunocompetent humans.	Medical treatment is instituted with clarithromycin (or azithromycin) and one or two of the following: rifampin, pradofloxacin (or moxifloxacin)[¶] or clofazimine, depending on availability and/or owner finances. Modifications to the drug regimen are then made depending on species identification, susceptibility data, response to therapy, or the development of side effects necessitating drug cessation (e.g., hepatotoxicity). Surgical excision of cutaneous nodules is advised if practicable.
Rapidly Growing Saprophytes				
Mycobacterium fortuitum group: *M. fortuitum sensu stricto*, *M. porcinum*, and *M. alvei* *M. smegmatis* group: *M. smegmatis sensu stricto*, *M. goodii*, and *M. wolinskyi* *M. chelonae-abscessus* group: *M. chelonae sensu stricto* and *M. abscessus* subsp. *bolletti* (formerly *M. massiliense*) Rarely: *M. mageritense* group, *M. mucogenicum* group, *M. falvenscens*, *M. phlei*, and *M. thermoresistible*	Cutaneous inoculation with contaminated environmental material via cat fights or other breaches of the integument. Inhalation in the case of pneumonia (rare).	Dermatitis/panniculitis of the caudoventral abdominal (most common), lateral thoracic or flank skin and subcutis, particularly in overweight cats. Pneumonia (rare).	Unknown, but likely to be low, given the low pathogenicity of saprophytic mycobacteria in immunocompetent humans.	Medical treatment is instituted with two of the following drugs: ideally, pradofloxacin (or moxifloxacin) depending on availability and/or owner finances, plus doxycycline (if in a country with a high proportion of *M. smegmatis* group infections, e.g., Australia) or clarithromycin (if in the United States). Modifications to the drug regimen are then made depending on drug susceptibility data and/or response to therapy. Wide surgical excision of granulomatous tissue is recommended if lesions are no longer improving with medical therapy.

Continued

Mycobacterial Species	Suspected Transmission*	Clinical Features	Public health Risk	Recommended Treatment†,‡,§
Lepromatous Mycobacteria				
Mycobacterium lepraemurium	Cutaneous inoculation from altercations with infected rodents.	Single or multiple cutaneous nodules, may be ulcerated. Regional peripheral lymphadenopathy (common).	Unknown, but likely to be negligible.	Medical treatment is instituted with two of the following drugs: rifampin, clofazimine, clarithromycin, or pradofloxacin-moxifloxacin, (or a second-generation fluoroquinolone if identified as the novel Australia-New Zealand species). Surgical excision of nodules is recommended as an adjunct to medical therapy if practicable.
Mycobacterium sp. "Tarwin"	Cutaneous inoculation with contaminated environmental material via cat fights or other breaches of the integument.	Single or multiple cutaneous nodules, may be ulcerated, typically on the head or forelimbs. Ocular involvement (cornea, conjunctiva, and eyelid margins) is common. Regional peripheral lymphadenopathy (uncommon).	Unknown, but likely to be low.	
Novel Australia-New Zealand species	Cutaneous inoculation with contaminated environmental material via cat fights or other breaches of the integument.	Single or multiple cutaneous nodules, may be ulcerated. Regional peripheral lymphadenopathy (common). Some have aggressive clinical course with regional subcutaneous edema and internal organ involvement.	Unknown, but likely to be low.	
Mycobacterium visibile	Unknown.	Aggressive clinical course with widespread dermal and internal organ involvement.	Unknown.	No treatment attempts have been documented for this organism, but medical therapy as per the other lepromatous organisms would be appropriate.

PPE, Personal protective equipment (e.g., gloves, gown, face mask, and glasses or goggles).

*No routes of transmission have been definitively proven for *M. microti,* the slowly and rapidly growing saprophytic or lepromatous mycobacteria.

†Infections with *M. bovis* and *M. tuberculosis* are notifiable in many countries. Please check local legislation regarding compulsory euthanasia in microbiologically confirmed cases in some regions.

‡For all mycobacterial species, treatment is continued for 2 months after all lesions have resolved clinically or via imaging studies. If recurrence is documented, some cats may require lifelong therapy with at least one drug (e.g., clarithromycin), especially if there are immunosuppressive comorbidities.

§See Table 3-2 for information on drug doses, potential side effects, and recommended monitoring of therapy.

‖Not *M. bovis.*

¶With some slowly growing mycobacteria, pradofloxacin-moxifloxacin may be substituted with a second-generation fluoroquinolone such as orbifloxacin or marbofloxacin, according to published empiric drug susceptibility, once the species has been identified (e.g., *M. ulcerans*).

narrow region along the southern and southeastern coast of Victoria, Australia.

M. avium subsp. *avium* is the causative agent of classic avian TB. This subspecies only occasionally causes disease in humans. The majority of human *M. avium* infections, particularly cervical lymphadenitis in children, disseminated infection in the setting of AIDS, and lung disease in humans with cystic fibrosis or bronchiectasis, are caused by *M. avium* subsp. *hominissuis,* which also causes disease in pigs. Both of these *M. avium* subspecies have been documented to cause clinical disease in cats (as well as one report of a variant MAC "X"); however, most of the cases of feline MAC infection discussed in the literature have not been typed to the subspecies level. *M. intracellulare* infection in cats appears to be less common than *M. avium.*

As with the tuberculous mycobacteria, the route of infection determines the clinical picture. It is assumed that cats acquire infection via ingestion of contaminated or infected prey (possibly birds in the case of *M. avium* subsp. *avium* or *Mycobacterium genavense* infection) or via oral or transcutaneous inoculation of contaminated environmental material. Inhalation of organisms is another possible route; however, this seems less likely given that most cases with pulmonary disease appear to have disseminated infection seemingly arising from primary gastrointestinal or cutaneous infections. Most cats with slow-growing mycobacterial infections have outdoor access. Occasional cases have been reported in strictly indoor animals, or in those with only limited, supervised outdoor access.

In humans, disseminated infection with slowly growing saprophytic mycobacteria is more frequently observed in individuals with disturbances of cell-mediated immunity; for example, patients with HIV/AIDS, where the CD4+ T cell count has fallen below 50/μL. Indeed, there are numerous reports of cats with disseminated mycobacteriosis caused by slowly growing saprophytes with acquired defects of immunity, such as cyclosporine treatment in the context of renal transplantation, retroviral infection (plus lymphoma in one case), idiopathic CD4+ lymphopenia, systemic glucocorticoid administration, or comorbidities such as advanced chronic kidney disease and cryptococcosis. The suspected predisposition of young Abyssinian, Somali, and possibly Siamese cats to *M. avium* infection gives rise to the speculation that there may be an inherited defect of cell-mediated immunity in these breeds. The vast majority of the reported cases of disseminated disease has no apparent predisposing conditions and is mostly negative for retroviruses, although almost none have undergone laboratory evaluation of humoral and cell-mediated immunity. That being said, the rarity of disease compared to the likely high incidence of exposure to these organisms suggests that most cats are innately resistant to infection.

The slowly growing saprophytic organisms may also cause localized cutaneous disease with or without involvement of local lymph nodes. These infections presumably arise because of the introduction of organisms via a breach in the integument. In almost all of these localized cases, the cat had no overt predisposing conditions, although one case was concurrently being treated with a multidrug chemotherapy protocol for lymphoma.

Rapidly-Growing Saprophytes

The causative agents of rapidly growing mycobacterial infections are ubiquitous saprophytes that are able to grow on synthetic culture media within 7 days at 75° to 113°F (24° to 45°C). Cases have been reported from tropical (Brazil), subtropical (the Southeastern and Southwestern United States), and temperate regions of the world (Australia, New Zealand, Canada, Finland, Germany, the Netherlands, and the United Kingdom). Individual species reported to have caused disease in cats are recorded in Table 3-1. Geographical differences exist with respect to the incidence of particular causative organisms. The *M. smegmatis* group, followed by *Mycobacterium fortuitum*, cause most infections in cats domiciled in eastern Australia. In the Southwestern United States, *M. fortuitum* group infections, followed by *M. chelonae,* appear to be more common.

It is thought that lesions acquired via environmentally contaminated cat fight injuries account for the typically observed initial anatomical sites of the inguinal region, and less commonly, the axillae, flanks, or dorsum. Likewise, other breaches to the integument, such as bite wounds, penetrating foreign bodies, injections, or surgery may also allow rapidly growing mycobacteria to overcome normal host defenses. It appears that cats with a tendency toward adiposity, especially spayed females with a prominent ventral abdominal fat pad, have a predisposition toward these infections, likely because of the preference of rapidly growing mycobacteria for tissues rich in lipids. It is thought that the adipose tissue may provide triglycerides for growth of organisms and/or protection from the immune responses of the host. Indeed, experimental infections cannot be induced in cats that do not have a significant amount of subcutaneous fat.

Pneumonia caused by *M. fortuitum* infection has been reported in two cats, and *M. thermoresistibile* was confirmed as the causative agent in one instance. One of the *M. fortuitum* infections was thought possibly to be associated with a lipoid pneumonia secondary to aspiration of orally administered lactulose, and the cat with *M. thermoresistibile* pneumonia acquired the infection following a bath, which had presumably resulted in aspiration of contaminated water.

Lepromatous Mycobacteria

Feline leprosy was first described in 1962. Found in an urban-dwelling cat from Auckland, New Zealand, it presented with subcutaneous nodules containing many acid-fast bacilli (AFB). Under the assumption that the index case was infected with a tuberculous mycobacterium, the cat was euthanized, and its body submitted for necropsy. When no evidence of systemic disease could be found, and the inoculation of the organism failed to produce disease in a guinea pig, nor any growth on mycobacterial media—nor did clinical material from two further cases—the authors concluded that this was likely to be a new disease entity. They compared the condition to human and rat leprosy with respect to the microbiologic, clinical, and histopathologic picture. In the subsequent decades, the condition was reported in eastern Australia, Western Canada, the United Kingdom, Southwestern United States, and the Netherlands. Later, cases were identified in France, New Caledonia, Italy, the Greek islands, and Japan. Historically, New Zealand and Australia have reported the highest incidence of cases worldwide, which the author subjectively believes to be the case as of 2014.

Based on rodent inoculation studies, and concordant delayed-type hypersensitivity skin reactions between cell homogenates made from the causative agent of feline leprosy (lepromin) and *Mycobacterium lepraemurium* in sensitized guinea pigs, early researchers concluded that *M. lepraemurium* was the likely causative agent of the disease in cats. In the absence of evidence to the contrary, it was assumed for decades that this organism was the sole causative agent of the condition. However, publication of the work of Hughes and colleagues[22] in the late 1990s showed that despite similar clinical and histologic patterns, the etiology of feline leprosy was heterogeneous according to genetic analysis, and could not be solely ascribed to *M. lepraemurium*. That analysis, as well as subsequent studies, identified the involvement of at least two other "non-culturable" species of mycobacteria. One is related to the *M. simiae* group, provisionally known as *Mycobacterium* sp. "Tarwin,"[23] with cases geographically restricted to approximately 9000 km^2 east of Melbourne, Australia (C. O'Brien, unpublished data), and the other, a novel, genetically heterogeneous mycobacterial species related to *M. leprae,* is found along the eastern coast of Australia and both islands of New Zealand.[6]

Epidemiologic data suggest that many cats with feline leprosy are young males, although females and cats of any age may be affected. The disease occurs mostly in animals with outdoor access. It is supposed that young male cats are more likely to fight and hunt and thus face greater potential to be exposed to the organisms via inoculation by contaminated teeth or claws of other cats or prey species.

A mycobacterial disease characterized by diffuse cutaneous infection and widespread systemic dissemination has been documented in cats from Western Canada and the states of Idaho and Oregon in the United States, caused by the apparently non-culturable *Mycobacterium visibile.*[24] This organism is phylogenetically similar to the species novel to the eastern coast of Australia and New Zealand.

CLINICAL FEATURES

It is often difficult, if not impossible, to differentiate the causative mycobacterial species based on clinical presentation alone; however, the main findings are summarized in Table 3-1. The majority of cats with mycobacteriosis have skin lesions, especially located in anatomical areas associated with wounds acquired via altercations with prey species or other cats,[25] with many having multiple cutaneous sites affected. Peripheral lymphadenopathy, especially of the head and/or neck, may accompany the skin lesions or may be the primary presenting sign. If internal involvement is detected, the most common causative agents are either the tuberculous mycobacteria (especially in the United Kingdom and New Zealand) or members of the MAC. Rarely, systemic infections caused by other mycobacterial species, including other slowly growing saprophytes, rapidly growing mycobacteria, and the novel Australia and New Zealand lepromatous organism have been documented.

Tuberculous Mycobacteria

It is possible that, like humans, many cats exposed to tuberculous mycobacteria are asymptomatic. Indeed, a necropsy study of feral cats from an *M. bovis*-endemic area of New Zealand found that of the six cats from which *M. bovis* was isolated, only two had gross lesions.

Independent of the causative species, signs of disease are generally clinically similar and are typically referable to the route of infection. Ingestion tends to result in alimentary infection, typically manifesting as submandibular or mesenteric lymphadenopathy. Inhalation may result in pneumonia, although respiratory involvement is likely to be due to hematogenous spread from the skin or abdomen. Cutaneous lesions are thought to be due to local inoculation, but in some cases may also be the manifestation of disseminated disease. That being said, any anatomical site can theoretically be affected via hematogenous and/or lymphatic spread of organisms. Most cats with localized cutaneous lesions or superficial regional lymphadenopathy are constitutionally well, but systemically infected individuals often display signs of weight loss, lethargy, and inappetence, particularly if the intestinal tract is involved.

Cats with *M. microti* or *M. bovis* infection mostly present with solitary or multiple cutaneous nodules, typically located on the face or gingiva, limbs, lateral thorax, tail base, or perineum, and they may have mandibular, or less commonly, superficial cervical lymphadenopathy.[2,10] The cutaneous lesions and skin overlying affected lymph nodes may ulcerate or fistulate, and sometimes infection involves contiguous muscle and bone, especially where nodules are adherent to the underlying structures.

Cats may also have evidence of internal disease, such as pulmonary, liver, spleen, and/or mesenteric lymph node involvement, with or without concurrent cutaneous or superficial lymph node disease. Uncommonly, ocular involvement (e.g., chorioretinitis and conjunctivitis) and tuberculous arthritis or osteomyelitis have been reported.

Mycobacterium avium Complex and Other Slowly Growing Saprophytes

Most cases reported in the literature have involved animals with systemic disease, and findings of weight loss, inappetence, and lethargy are commonly reported. Many

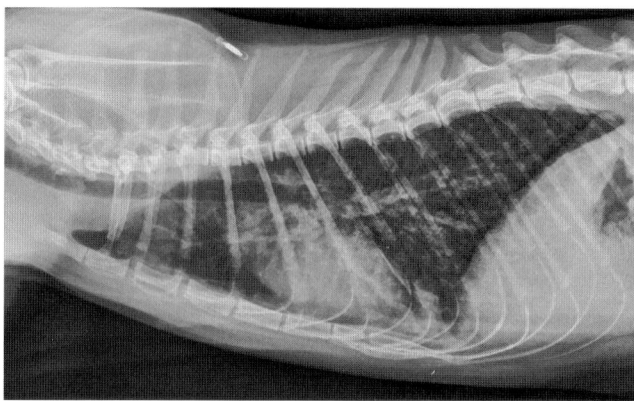

Figure 3-1: Lateral thoracic radiograph of a cat with disseminated *Mycobacterium avium* infection demonstrating a diffuse bronchointerstitial pattern. The cat presented for vomiting and inappetence. The main clinical finding was palpable mesenteric lymphadenopathy. Respiratory signs were absent. (Courtesy of Amanda Nott.)

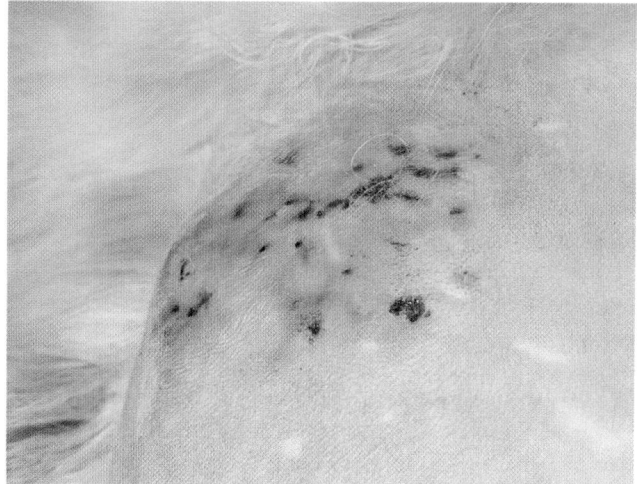

Figure 3-2: The typical pepper pot appearance of a cutaneous infection caused by a rapidly growing mycobacterial species on the ventrolateral thorax of a cat. (Courtesy of Gregory Raspbury and Janet Newell.)

systemically affected cats have mild to moderate fever and localized or generalized peripheral or abdominal, particularly mesenteric, lymphadenopathy. The latter finding may be accompanied by mild to moderate abdominal discomfort. Cranial organomegaly related to hepatic and/or splenic involvement, and thickening of the intestines may be appreciated on abdominal palpation and/or imaging. Some animals with abdominal organ involvement may also have peritoneal effusion, though this is usually not marked. Many cats have a history of localized skin lesions on the face or limbs, with or without lymphadenopathy, prior to the disease becoming generalized. Systemic spread is occasionally documented in the literature following a course of empirical therapy involving inappropriate antibiotics or glucocorticoids. Pulmonary involvement manifesting as respiratory distress and/or cough may also be apparent, and is typically accompanied by evidence of disease elsewhere in the body, particularly the abdomen and/or cutaneous sites. Even in the absence of clinical signs referable to the lower respiratory system, many cats with systemic MAC infection have radiographic evidence of respiratory involvement (Figure 3-1). As with the tuberculous mycobacteria, it appears that any anatomical site can be affected. Less common manifestations of systemic involvement discussed in the literature include chorioretinitis in a cat with *M. simiae,* pyelonephritis and pancreatitis in a cat with *M. xenopi,* and vulvitis, pyelonephritis, and central nervous system involvement in cats with *M. avium.*

Localized, predominantly cutaneous disease without evidence of systemic involvement has been reported with *M. avium, M. malmoense, M. terrae* complex, and *M. ulcerans.* A MAC infection was the causative agent in a case of granulomatous otitis causing vestibular dysfunction, facial nerve paralysis, and invasion into the oral cavity, and *M. intracellulare* has been reported as a cause of corneal infection.

pneumonia in cats. Animals with mycobacterial panniculitis typically present with a localized plaque or nodule of the skin and subcutis at a site of confirmed or presumed injury on the ventral abdomen, especially the inguinal area, lateral thorax, or flank. Diagnostic clues to the possibility of an unusual infectious etiology in these cases, as opposed to the usual microbes associated with a cat fight abscess, are absence of the typically malodorous pus, less localized swelling and pain, absence of systemic signs of illness, and the lack of response to surgical drainage and antibiotics typically utilized for this condition (e.g., amoxicillin/clavulanate).

As the condition progresses, the subcutaneous tissue develops a so-called pepper pot appearance (Figure 3-2), thin alopecic areas of epidermis overlying and adherent to thickened subcutaneous tissue. The collections of pus within the subcutis lead to characteristic focal purple depressions in the skin, eventually breaking down to become fistulae, exuding a watery discharge. The condition tends to be chronically progressive in both depth and width, and may eventually involve the entire ventral abdomen, flanks, perineum, and occasionally, limbs. Fortunately, spread to internal organs or lymph nodes is very unusual, although adjacent structures such as the abdominal wall can be involved. Affected cats have few signs of systemic illness, even in cases where skin involvement is extensive. Occasionally, cats may develop constitutional signs of malaise, fever, inappetence, weight loss, and reluctance to move, particularly if skin lesions become secondarily infected with *Staphylococcus* and *Streptococcus* spp. Lower respiratory tract infection caused by rapidly growing mycobacteria typically causes coughing, respiratory distress, fever, malaise, and weight loss.

Rapidly-Growing Saprophytes

Rapidly growing mycobacteria typically cause a distinctive mycobacterial panniculitis[5,26,27] and rarely pyogranulomatous

Lepromatous Mycobacteria

Feline leprosy is characterized by the finding of a single or multiple cutaneous and/or subcutaneous nodules often located on the head, limbs, or trunk.[6] The nodules are typically not painful, well circumscribed, and not adherent to underlying tissues. The overlying skin tends to be intact; however, it may be alopecic or ulcerated, particularly if the lesion is large, and local lymph nodes may also be involved.

There are a number of reports of feline leprosy in the veterinary literature; however, before the use of molecular methods of species identification, it is unclear which species of mycobacteria was actually involved. Some publications describe clinical data from patients where the etiologic agent has been confirmed by polymerase chain reaction (PCR) analysis, and in some reports, only scant information on disease presentation is provided.

Lesions caused by *M. lepraemurium* and the novel Australia-New Zealand species tend to be found on the head, limbs, and trunk (although anywhere on the integument can theoretically be involved), or may be widespread, involving many cutaneous sites (Figure 3-3). Intriguingly, lesions caused by *Mycobacterium* sp. "Tarwin" are mostly found on the head, particularly the eyes (Figures 3-4A and B), muzzle and lips (Figure 3-4C), mouth (Figure 3-4D), and front limbs. The author does not believe this species has been documented to cause widespread cutaneous or systemic disease.

The clinical course of feline leprosy infection may range from indolent to aggressive. Cases often have a tendency toward local spread, ulceration, and development of widespread lesions over several weeks to months. The nature of the disease may be influenced by host factors (e.g., age, concurrent illness, and immunologic status) or the causal species or route and size of the inoculum. Some of these factors are the subject of ongoing investigation by the author and colleagues. Cases of *M. visibile* infection (and at least one case of the novel Australia-New Zealand species [C. O'Brien, unpublished observations]) have been documented to have widespread cutaneous lesions and systemic involvement confirmed at necropsy.

DIAGNOSIS

Differential diagnoses of nodular lesions of the skin and subcutis include infections caused by other saprophytic bacterial species (especially *Nocardia* and *Rhodococcus*, which may also be acid-fast), fungi, and algae, or primary or metastatic neoplasia. No pathognomonic clinical, clinicopathologic, radiographic, or ultrasonographic findings differentiate systemic mycobacterial infections from the aforementioned etiologies. Animals with extensive cutaneous or systemic involvement may have hypercalcemia that is due to granulomatous disease. The slowly growing saprophytic mycobacteria (and on rare occasions, the rapidly growing species) can produce disease that is clinically indistinguishable from those that cause feline leprosy and feline TB caused by the MTB complex.

Collection of representative tissue and/or fluid samples for cytology or histopathology and microbiology is necessary for the diagnosis of feline mycobacterial disease. Occasionally, organisms may be visualized microscopically in circulating leukocytes, bone marrow aspirates, or urine sediment.

It is important that in areas endemic for the MTB complex, the diagnosis of TB is not based simply on the cytologic or histopathologic finding of AFB and/or pyogranulomatous inflammation in clinical samples, especially where mandatory reporting of such cases may result in compulsory euthanasia. Every effort should be made to identify the causative agent either via mycobacterial culture and/or molecular methodologies, and it is recommended that clinicians and/or pathologists involved in these cases endeavor to contact a relevant mycobacterium reference laboratory, or equivalent, for further processing of these samples if necessary.

Cytologic and Histopathologic Samples

The diagnosis of cutaneous infections caused by tuberculous (MTB complex) organisms, slow-growing saprophytes and the causative agents of feline leprosy is often relatively simple, provided the clinician has a high index of suspicion. The key to diagnosis is the collection of adequate samples for cytology, histopathology, and microbiology. In areas where members of the MTB complex are endemic, precautions such as wearing appropriate personal protective equipment (PPE), such as gloves, gowns, surgical masks, and protective eyewear should be taken during any procedure in which discharging or ulcerated lesions, and/or surgical or necropsy tissues are handled. Techniques for obtaining fine-needle aspirate and biopsy material are described in Box 3-3.

Cytology

Romanowski-stained cytologic smears obtained by fine-needle aspiration will demonstrate granulomatous to pyogranulomatous inflammation with mycobacterial rods recognized by their characteristic negatively staining

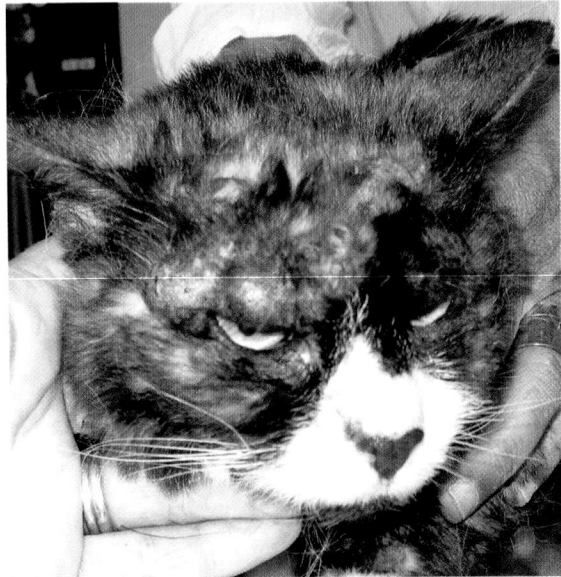

Figure 3-3: A cat with feline leprosy caused by the novel Australia-New Zealand *Mycobacterium*. This cat had widespread cutaneous lesions, and evidence of systemic disease was found at necropsy. (Courtesy of Anna Day.)

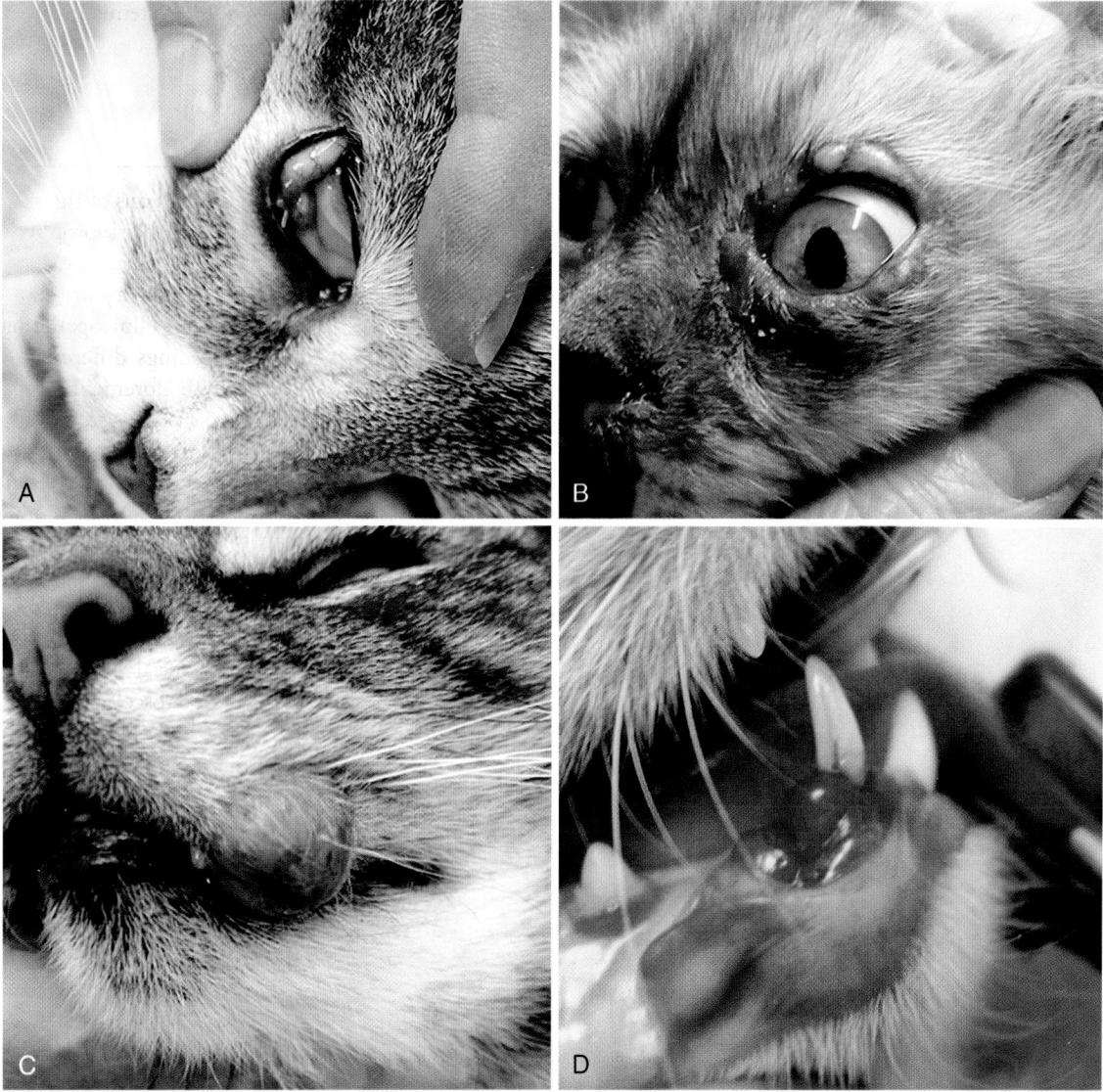

Figure 3-4: Feline leprosy lesions caused by *Mycobacterium* species "Tarwin" involving the conjunctiva **(A)**, eyelids **(B)**, muzzle **(C)**, and gingiva **(D)**. **(A,** Courtesy of Andrew Tresize. **C,** Courtesy of Stacie Lethlean. **D,** Courtesy of Juliet Mills.)

BOX 3-3 Collection of Fine-Needle Aspirate and Biopsy Material

Cutaneous Nodules and Peripheral Lymph Nodes
Aspiration of the nodule should always be performed prior to surgical excision to try to establish a presumptive diagnosis and aid in surgical planning. Intact cutaneous nodules should be excised with an elliptical pattern with at least a 5-mm margin (ideally in all dimensions, although it is not necessary to include underlying musculoskeletal structures if a 5-mm deep margin cannot be obtained). Aspiration and/or excisional or wedge biopsy of peripheral lymph nodes using standard techniques may also be necessary to differentiate the disease from other causes of lymphadenopathy in the cat (e.g., lymphoma or deep fungal infections).

Subcutaneous Panniculitis
Fine-needle aspiration and cytology may establish the presence of pyogranulomatous inflammation, but may not allow

visualization of acid-fast bacteria. Enough subcutaneous pus may be obtained from this technique to allow culture of the organism, thus establishing the diagnosis (see the Mycobacterial Culture section). Punch biopsies are also usually inadequate for obtaining representative tissue samples for the diagnosis of rapidly growing mycobacterial infection. For optimal histopathologic samples, a deep wedge subcutaneous tissue biopsy should be obtained from the margin of the lesion.

Internal Organs and Lymph Nodes
Standard techniques for obtaining ultrasound-guided fine-needle aspirates and surgical tissue biopsies should be followed to obtain adequate clinical material for cytological, histopathologic, and microbiological investigation.

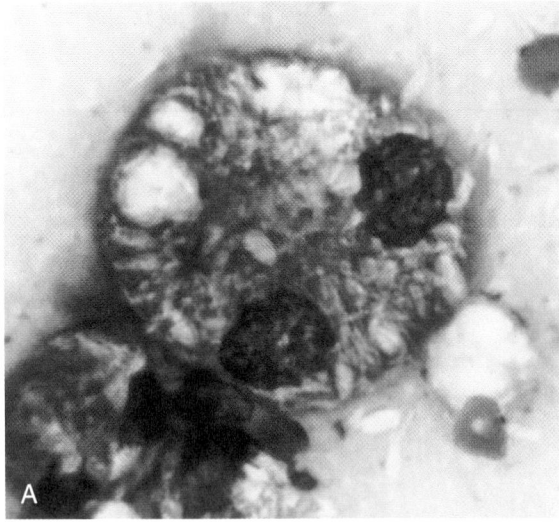

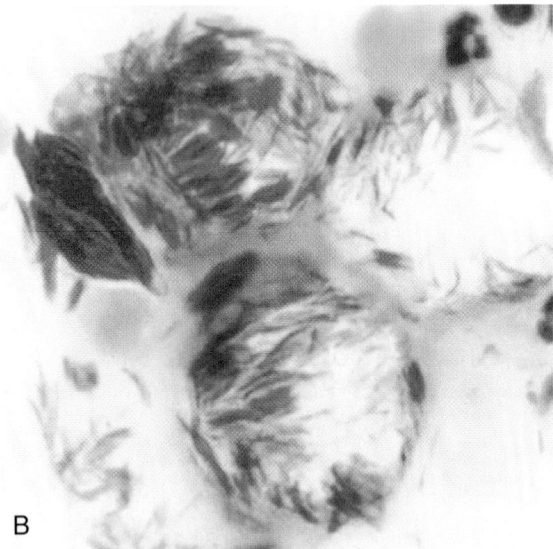

Figures 3-5: **A,** Photomicrograph of a Diff Quik–stained fine-needle aspirate of a nodular skin lesion from a cat with leprosy caused by the novel Australia-New Zealand species (1000×). Note the large number of "negatively" staining bacteria within the multinucleate macrophage. **B,** A Ziehl-Neelson–stained slide from the same cat demonstrating large numbers of mycobacteria that stain as pink rods (1000×). (Courtesy of George Reppas.)

appearance, usually located within macrophages (Figure 3-5A). Typically, mycobacteria are not visible on hematoxylin and eosin (H&E)–stained histopathology sections of biopsy samples, except *M. visibile* and the novel mycobacterial species that causes feline leprosy in Australia and New Zealand. Instead, they must be visualized using acid-fast staining techniques, such as Ziehl-Neelson (ZN) (see Figure 3-5B) or similar (e.g., Fite's), although bacterial numbers may be variable, depending on mycobacterial species and host immune response. A modified ZN-staining procedure may be needed to visualize rapidly growing mycobacteria, as they are not as acid-fast as other species are. Unlike MAC infections and feline leprosy, some tuberculous (especially *M. microti*) and rapidly growing mycobacteria may be much fewer in number and harder to visualize in diagnostic material. A thorough search of several smears is sometimes

required to identify organisms, and the diagnosis should not be ruled out if no organisms are found. The tendency for rapidly growing mycobacteria to accumulate extracellularly in fat vacuoles in tissues may contribute to the difficulty in finding these organisms because of loss during regular processing of cytologic and histopathologic samples, which typically involves lipid solvents. For optimal visualization of mycobacteria in these instances, fluorescent Auramine O staining or frozen tissue processing may provide superior sensitivity. On occasion, samples that are AFB-negative will be positive on mycobacterial culture or molecular methods such as PCR (although culture is typically more sensitive in these instances).

Histopathology

Tuberculous Mycobacteria. All of the members of the MTB complex produce histopathologically similar lesions, with characteristic solitary to coalescing granulomas (tubercles). Granulation tissue surrounds a mixed layer of inflammatory cells, consisting of macrophages, neutrophils, lymphocytes, and plasma cells. Within the center of the granuloma resides a collection of epithelioid macrophages and some neutrophils. This central area contains variable, but usually low numbers of AFB and may or may not contain necrotic tissue. In some species, this necrotic material may become mineralized, but this appears to be rare in the cat.

Mycobacterium avium *Complex and Other Slowly Growing Saprophytic Mycobacteria.* Cutaneous MAC infections are usually characterized histopathologically by the finding of pyogranulomatous or granulomatous inflammation admixed with a variable fibroblastic response. Rarely, the fibroblastic reaction may be so pronounced as to make it difficult for a pathologist to differentiate the lesion from an inflamed fibrosarcoma (mycobacterial pseudotumor). In these cases, numerous AFB are typically found within both macrophages and spindle cells. Lesions without a prominent fibroblastic response can mimic lepromatous leprosy histopathologically.

Rapidly-Growing Saprophytes. The histopathologic characteristics of rapidly growing mycobacterial dermatitis and panniculitis include an ulcerated or acanthotic dermis and overlying multifocal to diffuse pyogranulomatous inflammation, typically extending to the deep subcutis. Within discrete pyogranulomata, a thin rim of neutrophils usually surrounds a clear, inner zone, caused by degenerate adipocytes, which may contain scant, faintly H&E staining or acid-fast mycobacteria, with an outer collection of epithelioid macrophages. Sometimes the pyogranulomatous areas lack these clear zones. In between each pyogranuloma tends to be a mixed inflammatory response, predominantly neutrophils and macrophages, but also containing lymphocytes and plasma cells. AFB may also occasionally be visualized within macrophages, but often mycobacteria can be frustratingly difficult to find within tissue sections.

Lepromatous Mycobacteria. The pathologic picture of feline leprosy is subdivided into (1) lepromatous and (2) tuberculoid. The types are thought to correspond to the host immunologic response. The lepromatous, or multibacillary, form is thought to correspond with a poor cell-mediated immune response, characterized by infiltration of tissue with many foamy or multinucleate macrophages containing huge numbers of mycobacteria, no necrosis, and virtually no lymphocytes and plasma cells. Tuberculoid, or pauci-bacillary, feline leprosy is thought to occur when the patient exhibits a more effective cell-mediated immune response, and it is characterized by pyogranulomatous inflammation dominated by epithelioid histiocytes, with moderate numbers of lymphocytes and plasma cells, and moderate to few observable AFB often in areas of multifocal to coalescing necrosis. It has been postulated in cats that the predominant histopathologic picture may be influenced by the causative agent,[6] although the validity of this assumption has been questioned by other investigators.[28] Invasion of peripheral nerves, which is a feature of human leprosy, is not typically observed in cats. That being said, mycobacterial sciatic neuritis has been described in a cat; however, unfortunately the causative species was not able to be determined in this case, despite the use of molecular methods.[29]

Collection of Samples for Culture

Ideally, all tissue samples collected for biopsy—not just in cases of suspected mycobacterial disease—should be divided into formalin-fixed and fresh aliquots in case microbiologic processing is required. The fresh tissue samples should be wrapped in sterile gauze swabs moistened with saline then placed in a sterile container for submission to the pathology laboratory. Concerning culture of rapidly growing mycobacterial species from panniculitis lesions, material swabbed from cutaneous draining sinus tracts is usually unsuitable because of high numbers of contaminating secondary bacteria; thus, fine-needle samples obtained through intact skin decontaminated with 70% ethanol or surgically collected tissue biopsies are preferred.

As mycobacterial culture and identification, especially of the tuberculous and slowly growing saprophytes, requires specialized expertise, and thus the pathology laboratory should ideally be contacted before submission if a mycobacterial infection is suspected. Fresh samples collected for culture do not require specialized handling or storage.

Mycobacterial Culture

The culture of viable mycobacterial organisms from clinical specimens is considered the gold standard for the diagnosis of infection caused by the tuberculous and saprophytic mycobacteria. Broth systems have the advantage of more rapid growth and the ability for automation compared to solid media; however, they do not supersede the requirement for the latter. Indeed, there are occasions where isolates grow preferentially on a surface rather than in liquid, or growth-positive broth tubes have been observed that do not flag as positive in an automated system, such as BACTEC MGIT (Mycobacterial Growth Indicator Tube, Becton Dickinson Microbiology Systems, Sparks, Maryland) (Box 3-4).

BOX 3-4 Normal Procedures for Mycobacterial Culture Carried Out in the Mycobacterium Reference Laboratory Known to the Author

If samples are procured from sites normally considered sterile (e.g., tissue biopsies, cerebrospinal fluid, or effusion fluid), no decontamination is performed before inoculation. For other samples (e.g., bronchial washes, fresh skin or gut biopsies, swabs, pus, or postmortem specimens), half of the specimen is generally inoculated directly onto media and the other half undergoes decontamination; for example, using 2% to 4% sodium hydroxide (modified Petroff's method). Samples are then neutralized prior to inoculation onto several suitable media, usually a combination of a broth (e.g., Middlebrook 7H12 or Mycobacterial Growth Indicator Tube [MGIT], Becton Dickinson Microbiology Systems, Sparks, Maryland), and solid egg-based (e.g., Lowenstein Jensen [LJ]) or non-egg-based media (e.g., Middlebrook 7H10 or 7H11). Glycerol-free media (e.g., pyruvate-containing LJ or Stonebrink) must be used if *M. bovis* is to be cultured. Primary cultures are then incubated at 82° to 88°F (28° to 31°C) and 95° to 99°F (35° to 37°C) for up to 12 weeks. Although most slowly growing mycobacteria will be detected in less than 6 to 8 weeks (and typically much sooner with broth culture), some strains of *M. microti*, *M. ulcerans*, and *M. genavense* may take up to 12 weeks to show detectable growth. Typically, *M. genavense* is fastidious and will only grow in broth media.

The BACTEC MGIT system is perhaps the most widely used liquid broth system for the recovery of viable mycobacteria from clinical samples, except urine and blood or bone marrow cultures, which tend to utilize the BacT/Alert system (Biomeriux, Craponne, France) or BACTEC Myco/F Lytic medium placed in a BACTEC 9050 instrument, and it has mostly superseded radiometric culture systems. The MGITs contain Middlebrook 7H9 broth, supplemented with antibiotic and enrichment mixtures. The inoculated tube is then incubated at 97°F (36°C) and monitored continuously by a BACTEC 960 instrument for 42 days. The MGIT system allows rapid and automated detection of mycobacterial growth using a fluorescent indicator embedded in silicone at the bottom of the tube that is quenched while there is oxygen dissolved in the broth. Once the oxygen in the tube is utilized by growing organisms, the unmasked fluorescence is detected by the system and flagged as positive. In laboratories that do not have a BACTEC 960 machine, or for tubes incubated at 88°F (31°C) (e.g., for *M. ulcerans*), the tubes can be monitored manually with the use of a Wood's lamp or other fluorescence reader. Positive tubes that are determined to contain AFB (by examination of a ZN-stained smear prepared from the culture) are then subcultured onto solid media and incubated at 88°F (31°C) and/or 97°F (36°C) for up to 12 weeks.

Although much slower in terms of turnaround time, use of solid media allows for the examination of colony morphology, which may assist with species identification, and allows for the detection of mixed growth.

It should be noted that culture attempts for the lepromatous organisms are usually unsuccessful. However, the clinician should still consider collecting fresh tissue samples in each presumptive case, in case the etiologic agent actually turns out to be a culturable organism.

Methods for Differentiating Mycobacterial Species

If a presumptive MTB complex organism is identified from the primary culture (based on colony and organism morphology), the isolates often undergo further confirmatory testing, such as antigen testing (e.g., SD BIOLINE MPT64 Ag Rapid ITC kit, Alere, Waltham, Massachusetts) or nucleic acid hybridization (DNA probe) testing (e.g., AccuProbe MTB Complex Culture Identification Test, Hologic Gen-Probe, San Diego, California).

MPT64 is a protein secreted by some MTB complex cells, including *M. tuberculosis*, *M. bovis*, and *M. microti*, which can be identified via a benchtop immunochromatography kit. Nucleic acid hybridization testing assesses the ability of rRNA derived from the mycobacterial isolate to specifically align and bind with a complimentary DNA probe bound to a chemiluminescent label. The resulting RNA/DNA hybrid can be detected with a specific luminometer supplied by the manufacturer. Further biochemical testing and/or PCR-based genetic fingerprinting are required for identification to the species and/or strain level.

If the results of initial tests demonstrate a presumptive MAC organism, a nucleic acid hybridization test (AccuProbe Mycobacterium Avium Complex Culture Identification Test, Hologic Gen-Probe, San Diego, California) or similar may be used for confirmation. Further biochemical testing and PCR-based genetic fingerprinting allow identification to the species and/or strain level.

For mycobacteria other than MTB complex or MAC, a suite of other tests such as biochemical, and assessment of growth conditions (e.g., duration to detection of positive growth on primary culture [rapid or slow growing]), preferred temperature, colony pigment production (nonchromogenic, photochromogenic, or scotochromogenic), and growth on different media (e.g., blood and/or MacConkey's agar plates at 86° F [30° C] for rapid growers) are traditionally carried out, although these are often replaced with molecular methods of identification.

The Inno-LiPA Mycobacteria v2 line probe assay (Fujirebio Diagnostics, Malvern, Pennsylvania) detects the presence of any mycobacteria, and is able to identify the presence of up to 16 different mycobacterial species simultaneously, including MTB complex, MAC, and a variety of slowly and rapidly growing organisms, based on genetic differences in the 16S-23S rRNA internal transcribed spacer (ITS) region. A similar assay, the GenoType Mycobacterium assay (Hain

Lifescience, Nehren, Germany), tests for MTB complex and 40 other mycobacterial species. It should be noted, however, that with the AccuProbe, InnoLiPa, and GenoType assays, errors of identification, especially with MAC and other slowly growing mycobacteria, might occur.[30] The emerging methodology, matrix-assisted laser desorption ionization-time of flight (MALDI-tof) mass spectrometry, has been validated for identification of a number of mycobacterial species.[31] It can provide results in as little as 2 hours. The MALDI-tof method, however, cannot differentiate between some species of clinically significant mycobacteria; therefore, superior accuracy means that the gold standard for mycobacterial species identification remains DNA gene sequencing.[30]

PCR has the advantage of providing a rapid and highly accurate diagnosis, except in instances where the sample has become contaminated with environmental mycobacteria. Fresh or frozen tissue, Romanowsky-stained cytology slides, and formalin-fixed paraffin-embedded tissue sections can all be used to potentially amplify and identify mycobacterial genetic material at diagnostic laboratories with mycobacterial expertise and suitable PCR facilities. The use of cytology slides for PCR is particularly appealing in feline practice because it may circumvent the need for invasive biopsy procedures.[32] It should be remembered that for AFB-negative samples, mycobacterial infections cannot be ruled out based on a negative PCR result.

Real-time PCR is an increasingly used method to identify the presence of mycobacterial DNA in human and animal clinical samples. Assays targeting the IS*6110* element for MTB complex, IS*2404* for *M. ulcerans*, multiplex IS*901*, and IS*1245* for differentiation of *M. avium* subsp. *avium* and *M. avium* subsp. *hominissuis*, have been developed and have shown to be useful in the diagnosis of feline infections.[33,34] As of 2014, real-time PCR assays specific for the causative agents of feline leprosy are in development (C. O'Brien and J. Fyfe, unpublished data).

The members of the MTB complex can be difficult to differentiate using routine molecular tests, because all have identical sequences at the 16S rRNA gene and the 16S-23S rRNA gene ITS region. In addition, all tuberculous mycobacteria contain IS*6110*, the most commonly used genetic target for real-time PCR diagnosis of human TB infections. Other molecular methods to differentiate and phylogenetically analyze the members of the MTB complex include genomic deletion analysis, spoligotyping, and mycobacterium interspersed repetitive unit and variable number of tandem repeats (MIRU-VNTR) analysis.

PCR-restriction fragment analysis (PRA) via amplification of particular genes, subsequent restriction enzyme digestion, and then analysis via gel electrophoresis is a commonly used DNA profiling technique for identification of nontuberculous mycobacteria, (Figure 3-6) although the popularity of this methodology is waning because of the increased availability of competitively priced genetic sequencing.

Amplification and sequencing of 16S rRNA, *hsp*65, or *rpoB* genes and/or the 16S-23S rRNA ITS region, or in some cases multigene analysis, are now considered the most

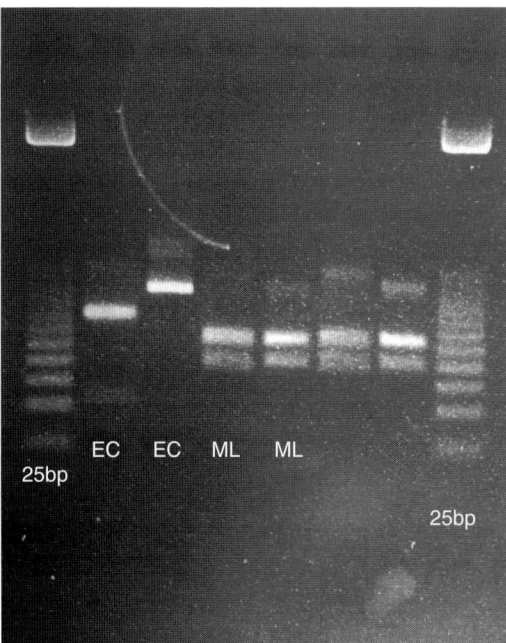

Figure 3-6: Restriction-fragment-length-polymorphism analysis of the 16S-23S ribosomal ribonucleic acid internal transcribed spacer region of an organism causing leprosy in a New Zealand cat. The DNA fragments from the case *(lanes 6 and 7, the unlabeled lanes)* are compared to those from known *Mycobacterium lepraemurium (ML)* and the novel Australia-New Zealand species *(EC)* cases. Molecular weight markers are found at either side of the gel *(25 bp)* to allow sizing of the bands found.

accurate and practical ways to identify most mycobacterial species, although these methods cannot differentiate members of the MTB complex. Draft- and full-genome sequencing of mycobacteria of medical and veterinary importance is also becoming increasingly common, although mostly in a research setting. It is hoped that these data will shed light on the ecology, and possibly transmission, of many of these enigmatic species, especially those that have an undefined ecologic niche such as the lepromatous mycobacteria.

Immunologic Tests

The purified protein derivative (PPD) intradermal test, or Mantoux test, developed in the early 1900s, is still widely used around the world, mainly in humans and cattle, to detect the presence of a delayed-type hypersensitivity response to "tuberculin" extracts of *M. tuberculosis* or *M. bovis*, as an indication of exposure to any member of the MTB complex. Intradermal testing of cats has been shown to be insensitive. Snider and colleagues found that none of 49 cats domiciled on *M. bovis*-endemic farms reacted to intradermal tuberculin testing, despite histopathologic changes suggestive of TB at necropsy in 21 of these animals, and culture-confirmed *M. bovis* infection in 12 cats.[35]

In vitro testing of humans for exposure to *M. tuberculosis-M. bovis* and cattle for exposure to *M. bovis* via interferon-gamma (IFN-γ) release assay (e.g., QuantiFERON-TB,

Cellestis, Valencia, California, or T-SPOT.*TB*, Oxford Immunotech, Abingdon, United Kingdom) has been utilized for a number of years. These assays work by testing whether an individual's T lymphocytes release IFN-γ in response to specific antigens (specifically, ESAT-6 and CFP-10), which are present in *M. tuberculosis* and *M. bovis* but absent in *M. bovis* bacille Calmette-Guérin (BCG) vaccine, *M. microti*, and other environmental mycobacteria. These tests were primarily developed to try to avoid the cross-reactivity seen with the PPD test in BCG-vaccinated humans. Interferon-γ release assays utilize either enzyme-linked immunosorbent assay (ELISA) or enzyme-linked immunospot (ELISPOT) technology. Peripheral blood mononuclear cells are separated from whole blood samples and mixed with an appropriate mycobacterial antigen. The IFN-γ released from stimulated T lymphocytes is captured by anti-IFN-γ antibodies bound to the ELISPOT plates. Spots of IFN-γ are then identified by a second antibody, which has been conjugated to a fluorochrome. A feline IFN-γ ELISPOT test utilizing both bovine tuberculin and ESTAT6/CFP10 for the identification of cats infected with either *M. bovis* or *M. microti*, with the ability to differentiate the two, has been developed in the United Kingdom,[36] and is currently commercially available via Biobest Laboratories. The test is reported as having a sensitivity of 90% for detecting feline *M. bovis* infections, 83.3% sensitivity for detecting feline *M. microti* infections, and 100% specificity for both.[37] The IFN-γ response of one cat undergoing treatment for suspected *M. bovis* infection showed a significant decline—almost to baseline levels—at the cessation of treatment and at 6-month follow-up when compared to pretreatment values.[37]

Serum antibody tests have also been evaluated for use in the diagnosis of clinical feline TB. Multiantigen print immunoassay (MAPIA) strips, the TB STAT-PAK test, and the Rapid DPP VetTB kit results were evaluated for cats with culture-confirmed *M. bovis* and *M. microti* infections and compared with negative controls and cats with non-MTB complex mycobacterial infections.[37] Overall sensitivity was 90% for the detection of *M. bovis* infection and greater than 40% for *M. microti*, with a specificity of 100%.

An important point to emphasize is that, like the situation in humans, these tests do not specifically differentiate active and latent infection or previous exposure, and the gold standard for the diagnosis of active TB remains culture of viable organisms from clinical samples obtained from cats with signs and cytologic and/or histopathologic findings consistent with mycobacterial infection.

TREATMENT

Because most nontuberculous mycobacteria are ubiquitous in the environment, the clinician should work with both a microbiologist and, if necessary, a companion animal infectious disease expert, to assess the clinical significance of any cultured or molecularly detected unusual isolates before a decision is made to treat the animal, especially if the clinical picture is not consistent with the diagnosis. The nature of the disease presentation, cytologic or histopathologic findings, anatomical site of specimen collection, and the established or assumed immunologic status of the patient are all considered.

There are no published prospective controlled studies regarding treatment of any of the feline mycobacterioses, and the existing literature consists of single case reports or a few retrospective, observational case series. Treatment recommendations for cats are typically based on extrapolation from human data or from the respective author's experience. The recommendations are summarized in Table 3-1. The drugs and their recommended doses typically chosen to treat feline mycobacterial infections in cats are listed in Table 3-2. Drug side effects, American trade names and formulations, and other pertinent information are also presented in Table 3-2.

Empirical Therapy

Because identification of the causative organism may take weeks to months, or may not be available at all, the clinician will need to start empirical treatment in almost all cases of feline mycobacteriosis (Box 3-5). The choice and number of initial drugs used in a particular case depends on various factors including:

- The most likely or suspected etiologic agent, based on the clinical presentation and geographical location
- The breed of the cat
- Owner finances and/or ability to potentially medicate the cat for an extended duration (months to years) with multiple drugs (up to twice a day)
- The existence of any comorbidities (for example, hepatic disease that may limit the tolerance of certain drugs)

As a general guide, initial empirical therapy—especially where the tuberculous mycobacteria are endemic—should include at least two, and ideally three, of the following drugs: rifampin, clarithromycin (or azithromycin), and pradofloxacin (or moxifloxacin). In areas where feline leprosy is more common, clofazimine would also be a reasonable choice as a substitution for one of the drugs in the treatment of nodular cutaneous mycobacteriosis, depending on availability. In non-TB-endemic areas, systemic mycobacteriosis is likely to be caused by a MAC organism, and clarithromycin or azithromycin should always be included in the initial treatment regimen. Cutaneous panniculitis is usually caused by a rapidly growing mycobacterial species, and initial treatment choices of doxycycline (in Australia) or clarithromycin (in the United States) and pradofloxacin or moxifloxacin—or less ideally a second-generation fluoroquinolone (see Table 3-2)—are appropriate for empirical therapy. Once the organism has been identified, treatment can be modified as per the guidelines in Table 3-1 or depending on response to treatment and/or the results of drug susceptibility testing, if available. Treatment in all cases should continue for at least 2 months past resolution of signs as assessed via clinical examination and/or diagnostic imaging. It has been suggested that esophagostomy tube placement be considered in some cases to

facilitate the administration of multidrug therapy over the extended periods required to treat most mycobacterial infections.[38] In most cases, it is not necessary to quarantine the animal, unless it has been diagnosed with a tuberculous mycobacterial infection. As some of the anti-mycobacterial drugs induce photosensitivity, it is recommended that owners try to keep the cat indoors during therapy, especially in the summer months.

BOX 3-5 Examples of Factors Influencing Clinical Decision Making with Regard to Empirical Therapy in Cats with Mycobacteriosis

Clinical Presentation
- Disseminated mycobacterial diseases are most likely due to tuberculous or MAC organisms
- Panniculitis is most likely due to rapidly growing saprophytic organisms

Geographical Location
- Infection with tuberculous organisms is very unlikely in nonendemic countries
- Infection with the lepromatous organisms is particularly common in Australia and New Zealand
- Certain drugs may not be available for use in certain countries (e.g., pradofloxacin is not available as of 2014 in Australia and New Zealand)

Breed Susceptibility
- Abyssinian and Somali cats are possibly predisposed to MAC infections

Owner Finances
- Older generic drugs are the most cost effective, whereas newer human drugs, especially those that need to be compounded for veterinary use, usually are much more expensive

Case Examples
Scenario 1: A young Abyssinian cat with systemic mycobacteriosis domiciled in Australia is most likely to have a MAC infection. Therefore, initial therapy should include clarithromycin (plus at least one other drug, but this should not be a second-generation fluoroquinolone).

Scenario 2: A cat with inguinal panniculitis domiciled in the United States is most likely to have an infection caused by a rapidly growing organism (either *M. fortuitum* or *M. chelonae*), and although the ideal empirical drug choices in this case are the new 8-cyano-fluoroquinolone, pradofloxacin, and twice-daily clarithromycin, in a situation where the owner has limited funds and the cat is difficult to medicate, a combination of a second-generation fluoroquinolone (e.g., marbofloxacin or orbifloxacin) plus once daily azithromycin may be a better initial choice.

MAC, Mycobacterium avium complex.

Table 3-2	Drugs Typically Chosen to Treat Feline Mycobacterial Infections		
Drug	**Dosage**	**Side Effects/Comments**	**American Proprietary Name(s)/ Comments**
Clofazimine	25 mg total dose by mouth (PO) every 24 h or 50 mg total dose every 48 h	Pitting corneal lesions. Skin and body fluid discoloration (pink-brown), photosensitization. Nausea, vomiting, and abdominal pain caused by crystalline drug deposits in abdominal viscera. Possible hepatotoxicity. Administration with food improves absorption. Restricted access in some parts of the world (through compounding pharmacists only). Monitor serum hepatic enzymes. Reduce dose or discontinue drug if clinical signs appear.	Lamprene, Novartis (Human); 50 mg and 100 mg capsules. Not registered for use in cats. Due to limited availability, may be restricted by the FDA for treating human disease only, contact the FDA Center for Veterinary Medicine for further information.
Clarithromycin	62.5 mg/cat PO every 12 h	Cutaneous erythema and edema, hepatotoxicity, diarrhea and/or vomiting, neutropenia, thrombocytopenia. Can be given with food. Reduce dose in cats with renal or severe hepatic failure. Monitor hepatic enzymes* during treatment. Elevation of enzymes or the development of GI signs may require dose reduction. If cytopenias or allergic skin reactions develop, discontinue drug. Interacts with metabolism of drugs by cytochrome P450 system.	Biaxin, Abbott (Human); 250 mg and 500 mg tablets; 125 mg/5 mL and 250 mg/5 mL suspension. Shake suspension before use. Develops a bitter taste if stored in the refrigerator.
Azithromycin	5-15 mg/kg PO every 24 h	Vomiting, diarrhea, abdominal pain, and hepatotoxicity. Monitor hepatic enzymes* during treatment. Pre-existing hepatic disease or elevation of enzymes or the development of GI signs during treatment may require dose reduction. Do not mix with food.	Numerous generic brands; 250 mg, 500 mg, and 600 mg tablets; 100 mg/5 mL and 200 mg/5 mL oral suspension.
Rifampin (Rifampicin)	10 mg/kg PO every 24 h	Not registered for use in cats. Hepatotoxicity and/or inappetence necessitating dose reduction or cessation of drug. Cutaneous erythema-pruritus may occur, necessitating pretreatment with antihistamine and dose reduction. If animal displays signs of anaphylaxis, discontinue drug immediately and administer epinephrine and glucocorticoids. May need to be compounded into suitably sized doses. Monitor hepatic enzymes* during treatment; every 2 weeks initially, then monthly.	Rifadin, Sanofi-Aventis; 150 mg and 300 mg oral capsules. May be split and placed into gelatin capsules (wear gloves). Generic formulation available.

Continued

Table 3-2 **Drugs Typically Chosen to Treat Feline Mycobacterial Infections—cont'd**

Drug	Dosage	Side Effects/Comments	American Proprietary Name(s)/ Comments
Doxycycline	5-10 mg/kg PO every 12 h	Hydrochloride or hyclate tablet and capsule formulations may cause esophageal irritation and possibly stricture. Give with food or oral fluids to ensure that tablet/capsule does not irritate the esophagus. Alternatively, tablets may be crushed and mixed with food.	Vibra-Tabs, Vibramycin, Pfizer (Human); 50 mg and 100 mg oral tablets; 50 mg/5 mL oral syrup; 25 mg or 50 mg/5 mL oral suspension.
Enrofloxacin	5 mg/kg PO every 24 h	Enrofloxacin has the potential to cause retinal toxicity in cats.	Enrofloxacin: Baytril, Bayer (Veterinary); 22.7 mg, 68 mg, and 136 mg oral tablets; 22.7 mg/mL parenteral injection (IM).
Marbofloxacin	2.75-5.5 mg/kg PO every 24 h	Marbofloxacin or orbifloxacin are preferred for use in cats.	Marbofloxacin: Marbocyl, Vetoquinol (Veterinary); 5 mg, 20 mg, and 80 mg oral tablets. Zeniquin, Zoetis Animal Health (Veterinary); 25 mg, 50 mg, 100 mg, and 200 mg oral tablets.
Orbifloxacin	7.5 mg/kg PO every 24 h	Most *M. avium* complex organisms are resistant to second-generation fluoroquinolones.	
All second-generation fluoroquinolones			Orbifloxacin: Orbax, Merck Animal Health (Veterinary); 5.7 mg, 22.7 mg, 68 mg oral tablets, 30 mg/mL oral suspension.
Pradofloxacin Third-generation fluoroquinolone	7.5 mg/kg PO every 24 h	Give without food unless GI side effects occur.	Veraflox, Bayer (Veterinary); 15 mg, 60 mg, and 120 mg tablets; 25 mg/mL suspension. Only approved for use in the cat for 7 days; off-label for extended periods of treatment, although appears to be safe.
Moxifloxacin Fourth-generation fluoroquinolone	10 mg/kg PO every 24 h	Vomiting and anorexia. Possible tendon inflammation and rupture (not reported in cats). Not registered for use in cats. May need to be compounded into suitable-sized doses. The dose can be divided 12 hourly and/or administered with food if GI side effects are observed.	Avelox, Bayer (Human); 400 mg film-coated tablets.
Gentamicin	2 mg/kg SC, IM, IV every 24 h	Can be nephrotoxic and ototoxic. Monitor renal function and ensure adequate hydration.	Gentamicin: Gentocin, Garasol, Merck Animal Health (Veterinary); 50 mg/mL injectable solution.
Amikacin	10 mg/kg SC, IM, IV every 24 h	Generally used perioperatively for durations of less than 7-10 days before and after surgical resection of lesions caused by rapidly growing mycobacteria.	Amikacin: Amiglyde-V, Zoetis Animal Health (Veterinary); 50 mg/mL and 250 mg/mL injectable solution.

FDA, U.S. Food and Drug Administration; *GI*, gastrointestinal; *IM*, intramuscularly; *IV*, intravenously; *PO, per os* (by mouth); *SC*, subcutaneously.
*Hepatic enzymes that warrant monitoring are alanine aminotransferase (ALT) and alkaline phosphatase (ALP).

Antimicrobial Susceptibility Testing

An attempt should be made to obtain drug susceptibility data if the isolate is able to be cultured. This is especially important for organisms that may have variable drug susceptibility, such as the rapidly growing species *Mycobacterium fortuitum,* or for recurrent mycobacterial infections where the animal has previously undergone antibiotic treatment and may have acquired drug resistance. Because extended incubation is required for *M. genavense* and *M. ulcerans,* antimicrobial susceptibility testing is not routinely performed on these species. Drug susceptibility testing is not carried out on the lepromatous mycobacterial species, because they cannot be grown in the laboratory using standard methods.

The Clinical and Laboratory Standards Institute (CLSI) criteria for the antimicrobial susceptibility testing of mycobacteria recommend broth microdilution as the gold standard, preferably performed by a mycobacterium reference laboratory (MRL), or similarly experienced facility.[39] Most published drug susceptibility data apply to members of the TB complex, MAC, and some slowly and rapidly growing mycobacterial species isolated from human infections, although some data exist for species isolated from cats, especially the rapidly growing mycobacteria.[40,41]

Many MRLs deal almost exclusively with organisms isolated from human cases, and, in many countries, laboratories with specialized expertise in veterinary mycobacteriology do not exist. Many MRLs use standardized minimum inhibitory concentration (MIC) microbroth plates (Box 3-6) or automated systems such as the BACTEC MGIT 960 for drug susceptibility testing. With the latter system, the emphasis is usually on the rapid detection of strains of *M. tuberculosis* that are resistant to isoniazid and rifampin, and additionally fluo-roquinolones and aminoglycosides, known as multidrug- and extensive drug-resistant TB respectively. These strains are of grave public health concern, but are not generally of veterinary relevance. As per the CLSI guidelines, many MRLs only test MAC organisms for clarithromycin susceptibility, as the *in vitro* susceptibility to other antituberculous agents does not always predict clinical response in human patients.[39] Manual microbroth dilution testing may be available against drugs that are not included on the standardized plates, including clofazimine and other trimethoprim and sulfonamide drugs, but the opportunity to have isolates tested against some drugs used in feline patients, especially those licensed only for animal use (e.g., pradofloxacin) may be limited. Ideally, the spectrum of drugs that can be incorporated into an isolate's susceptibility testing should be discussed with the individual laboratory involved in each case.

Tuberculous Mycobacteria

Cats with *M. microti* infection have been treated successfully using combinations of rifampin, enrofloxacin or marbofloxacin, and clarithromycin or azithromycin. It is recommended that cats infected with MTB complex organisms receive a combination of rifampin, a fluoroquinolone (pradofloxacin or moxifloxacin, or a second-generation agent) and a macrolide (clarithromycin or azithromycin) for the first 2 months, followed by consolidation therapy with a macrolide and fluoroquinolone for at least 4 months.[42] Occasionally, other agents such as ethambutol and isoniazid have been used in the treatment of feline TB, although the toxicity of these agents tends to limit their use in cats, and they are typically only utilized in the setting of drug resistance to one of the more commonly utilized agents.[43]

Mycobacterium avium Complex and Other Slowly Growing Saprophytes

The British and the American Thoracic Societies have both published guidelines that recommend humans with slowly growing mycobacterial infections be treated with clarithromycin-based multidrug regimens.[44,45] There are no published guidelines on the duration of management of feline infections caused by the slowly growing saprophytes. However, multidrug regimens of durations similar to those for the tuberculous mycobacteria, that is for a duration of at least 2 months past resolution of disease signs—likely for at least 6 to 7 months in the case of systemic infection—would be appropriate.

Treatment of *Mycobacterium avium* Complex Infections

Although there are some reports of clarithromycin resistance in wild strains of *M. avium* and *M. intracellulare,* the vast majority of isolates are highly susceptible to this drug, with MICs of 4 to 8 mg/L.[46]

Systemic feline *M. avium* infections have been successfully treated with clarithromycin and clofazimine,[47] or a variable combination of clarithromycin plus ethambutol, rifampin,

---

BOX 3-6 Examples of Standardized Minimum Inhibitory Concentration Microliter Plates

Some examples of standardized minimum inhibitory concentration microliter plates used in some laboratories for drug susceptibility testing of mycobacteria are as follows:
- Sensititre MYCOTB (Thermo Scientific) tests isolates against ethambutol, isoniazid, rifampicin, amikacin, cycloserine, ethionamide, kanamycin, moxifloxacin, ofloxacin, *p*-aminosalicylic acid, rifabutin, and streptomycin.
- Sensititre SLOMYCO (Thermo Scientific) tests isolates against clarithromycin, rifampin, ethambutol, isoniazid, moxifloxacin, ciprofloxacin, rifabutin, trimethoprim-sulfamethoxazole (SXT), amikacin, linezolid, streptomycin, doxycycline, and ethionamide.
- Sensititre RAPMYCO (Thermo Scientific) tests isolates against SXT, ciprofloxacin, moxifloxacin, cefoxitin, amikacin, doxycycline, tigecycline, clarithromycin, linezolid, imipenem, cefepime, amoxicillin/clavulanic acid, ceftriaxone, minocycline, and tobramycin.

and enrofloxacin, in one instance.[48] The combination of clarithromycin and rifampin may be effective; however, the success of therapy is less clear, with relapses reported.[47] The author also is aware of a systemically *M. avium*-infected Abyssinian cat that responded promptly and completely to a regimen of clarithromycin, rifampin, and moxifloxacin. MAC organisms tend to be resistant to the second-generation fluoroquinolones, for example ciprofloxacin. However, better susceptibility is observed to the fourth-generation drugs such as moxifloxacin,[46] and likely the veterinary third-generation drug, pradofloxacin, although the latter has not been validated via susceptibility testing against these bacteria. The use of doxycycline for feline MAC infections has also been reported, but the contribution of doxycycline to apparently successful treatment of local and disseminated MAC-infected cats is difficult to interpret, because these cats were usually also concurrently treated with drugs known to be effective against these species (clarithromycin and/or clofazimine). Even though doxycycline is effective against some species of rapidly growing mycobacteria, *M. avium* appears to have generally poor *in vivo* susceptibility to this drug.[49,50] If feasible, surgical excision of granulomatous tissue may be beneficial in addition to medical therapy, especially if the infection is restricted to a localized cutaneous site. Subjectively, wound breakdown in these cases appears to be less likely than with infections caused by the rapidly growing mycobacteria, especially if surgical margins of 0.5 to 1.0 cm can be obtained; however, owners should still be advised of this possibility. Cutaneous lesions treated with surgical excision alone tend to be locally recurrent, and in many cases the infection may have already spread to local lymph nodes or beyond, thus adjunctive medical therapy is always advised for at least 2 months after surgical resection.

Treatment of Other Slowly-Growing Saprophytes

The treatments of other agents that cause sporadic disease in cats (e.g., *M. terrae* complex) have not been extensively studied, even in the setting of human disease. Susceptibility data obtained from isolates causing human tenosynovitis and pulmonary disease suggest that the majority of these organisms are susceptible to clarithromycin or azithromycin, but are variably susceptible to amikacin, rifampin, clofazimine, and ciprofloxacin.[51] An otherwise healthy young cat with localized *M. terrae* complex infection of the hind paw was successfully treated empirically with enrofloxacin, rifampin, and clarithromycin.[52]

M. ulcerans isolates are not routinely subjected to antibiotic susceptibility testing because of their extremely slow growth, but fortunately, they have a relatively predictable antibiogram. A combination of surgical débridement and rifampin plus a fluoroquinolone or clarithromycin is the recommended treatment in humans. Dogs with ulcerative skin disease responded successfully to an 8 to 10 week course of rifampin plus a fluoroquinolone (with or without minimal surgical intervention),[53] and a cat with a preulcerative nodule on the bridge of the nose was successfully treated with surgical debulking and a course of clarithromycin.[34] A paradoxical

worsening of clinical lesions can occur with successful treatment of *M. ulcerans* infection in humans, presumably because of resolution of the local immunosuppressive effects of the toxin mycolactone secreted by the organism, and these are managed with anti-inflammatory doses of systemic glucocorticoids. This phenomenon has not yet been documented in animals.

Clarithromycin-based protocols appear to produce the most favorable outcomes in human *M. simiae* infections, and the organism may be susceptible to moxifloxacin, even when resistance to the second-generation fluoroquinolones has been demonstrated *in vitro*. Disseminated *M. simiae* infection was successfully treated in an otherwise healthy 8-year-old cat with empirically prescribed enrofloxacin, rifampin, and clarithromycin.[54]

Disseminated *M. xenopi*, involving the kidneys, pancreas, abdominal lymph nodes, and bone marrow was diagnosed in a young cat with idiopathic CD4+ lymphocytopenia.[55] Treatment with rifampin and ciprofloxacin was continued until the cat died of malignant melanoma 7 years later. Necropsy examination showed persistence of disseminated rifampin and ciprofloxacin-resistant mycobacteriosis, despite susceptibility data demonstrating sensitivity to both of these drugs in the initial period of treatment.

Rapidly-Growing Saprophytes

The medical and surgical management of mycobacterial panniculitis in cats is well described.[56,57] Even though some cases (particularly those caused by strains of *M. fortuitum* found in the United States) can be difficult to treat, most cats can be successfully managed by the use of lipophilic antimicrobial agents directed by susceptibility data and, where appropriate, radical surgical resection and reconstructive techniques.

Members of the *M. smegmatis* complex are usually susceptible to doxycycline and fluoroquinolones but are often resistant to clarithromycin. *M. fortuitum* tends to show higher levels of resistance to antimicrobials in general, although it tends to be susceptible to fluoroquinolones and clarithromycin, and *M. chelonae* tends to be resistant to all commonly used drugs except clarithromycin and linezolid. MICs for ciprofloxacin, enrofloxacin, moxifloxacin, and pradofloxacin using the broth microdilution method have been reported for feline *M. fortuitum*, *Mycobacterium goodii*, and *M. smegmatis sensu stricto* isolates.[40,58]

In geographical areas where *M. smegmatis* and *M. fortuitum* complex infections predominate (e.g., Australia), treatment should begin empirically with doxycycline and pradofloxacin or moxifloxacin. However, in the United States, where significant numbers of *M. chelonae* infections are recorded, the drugs of choice would be clarithromycin with pradofloxacin. Multidrug therapy reduces the induction of resistant clones, and ideally, therapy should be adjusted based on *in vitro* susceptibility data. In refractory cases, clofazimine, cefoxitin, linezolid, or amikacin may be used, if indicated by drug susceptibility data.

Because there may be issues with drug penetration into the granulomatous subcutaneous tissue, drugs should be administered at the high end of the dose ranges. Cases should be monitored via clinical examination every few weeks for evidence of clinical response. In some cases, a cure may be achieved with medical therapy alone. However, it appears that some infections eventually become refractory to treatment (i.e., the lesions no longer appear to be reducing in size), requiring wide *en bloc* surgical resection of residual foci of infection, along with perioperative administration of an aminoglycoside for a few days, if indicated by susceptibility data, and then continuation of appropriate antibiotics for several more months. Numerous techniques, such as skin fold advancement flaps, have been published with regard to reconstruction of large cutaneous deficits in the cat. If the area to be resected is particularly large, or in an awkward anatomical location, consultation with an experienced soft tissue surgeon is strongly encouraged. Anecdotally, some cases have benefited from the use of vacuum-assisted closure of resultant surgical wounds.

The total duration of therapy for mycobacterial panniculitis caused by rapidly growing mycobacteria is usually 3 to 12 months. Ideally, treatment should be continued for 2 months past clinical resolution of signs, which should be ascertained by thorough palpation of the previously affected area, rather than just visual inspection.

With regard to pneumonia caused by rapidly growing mycobacteria, empiric treatment with pradofloxacin or moxifloxacin and clarithromycin should be started immediately and then adjusted if necessary based on susceptibility data. Treatment should always consist of using two or three suitable drugs and should be continued for 2 months past resolution of clinical and/or radiographic signs. Discrete pulmonary lesions that do not respond completely to appropriate medical therapy may need to be surgically resected, with antibiotic therapy continued after surgery for at least 2 months.

Lepromatous Mycobacteria

Although there have been rare instances of spontaneous resolution of feline leprosy infection,[59] the vast majority of cases require treatment to effect a cure. Definitive treatment guidelines for each of the causative agents are yet to be established, because the antibiotic susceptibility of these organisms is largely unknown and because of the paucity of data from any large-scale case series. Work on *M. lepraemurium* grown in viability assays within cell culture suggests that the organism is highly susceptible to rifampin and clofazimine.[60] Even though this organism appears to be somewhat susceptible to dapsone, a drug used to treat leprosy in humans, the potential side effects of this drug (e.g., hepatotoxicity, neurotoxicity, and blood dyscrasias) limit its use in cats.

A combination of two to three of the following drugs; rifampin, clofazimine, clarithromycin, or pradofloxacin or moxifloxacin, ideally with surgical resection of lesions, appears to be the most efficacious treatment regimen[6,61] (C. O'Brien,

personal observations). Subjectively, some cases of feline leprosy caused by the novel Australia–New Zealand organism appear to respond favorably to a second-generation fluoroquinolone, so one could be substituted for pradofloxacin or moxifloxacin.

As with other mycobacterial infections, it is recommended that medical therapy be continued for 2 months past resolution of clinical signs, and in most cases, 4 to 6 months or more of therapy is required. Even if all visible cutaneous lesions have been removed surgically, it is recommended that medical therapy be continued for 2 months because recurrence at the same or distant anatomical sites is relatively common.

PREVENTION OF INFECTION

Because it is assumed that most cases of feline mycobacteriosis are acquired via either inoculation or ingestion of organisms from the environment or infected prey species, the most prudent intervention owners can implement to reduce the chance of infection is to keep cats indoors. Avoiding the feeding of unpasteurized milk or offal (in areas of *M. bovis* endemicity) is also recommended.

PROGNOSIS

The prognosis depends on a number of factors, including the causative agent and the extent of the infection, with systemic disease holding a guarded prognosis. The commitment of the owner to the implementation of a potentially expensive and time-consuming schedule of multidrug therapy for many months also influences the outcome, with many treatment failures resulting from lack of compliance. Generally, localized infections caused by all species have a relatively favorable prognosis if treated with an appropriate combination of drugs and surgery, if necessary.

PUBLIC HEALTH RISKS

Although *M. bovis* remains an important cause of TB in humans living in developing nations, this organism causes a very small proportion of the disease in humans in industrialized countries. Interestingly, although the incidence of TB in the United Kingdom in cattle has been increasing since the start of the 1990s, no coincident increase in the incidence of locally acquired *M. bovis* infection in humans has been observed. The risk of cat-to-human transfer of *M. bovis* appears to be low[62]; however, a recent news report from the United Kingdom details the infection in four people (two clinically and two subclinically affected) associated with an infected pet cat.[63] There is a case in the literature of human *M. bovis* infection supposedly acquired by a cat bite,[64] and a laboratory worker was observed to have seroconverted after exposure to an accidentally infected research cat colony.[12]

Humans seem relatively resistant to infection with *M. microti*—indeed, for a period in the 1940s and 1950s it was touted as an alternative agent to *M. bovis* BCG as an anti-TB vaccine—although infections have been documented in both immunodeficient and immunocompetent individuals. Currently, there have been no confirmed cases of cat-to-human transmission of *M. microti* infection.

Slowly growing saprophytic mycobacterial infections, particularly caused by MAC organisms, may cause considerable morbidity and mortality in humans with inherited or acquired immunologic defects. Healthy humans can acquire these infections, although they tend to be localized. It is likely that almost all of these infections are derived from environmental sources; however, potential zoonotic transfer from infected pets cannot be completely discounted. That being said, there are no confirmed cases of cat-to-human transmission of slowly growing mycobacteria, apart from one report of a person contracting *Mycobacterium marinum* secondary to a cat scratch.[65] This scenario likely represented the mechanical inoculation of an environmentally acquired contaminant, rather than a true zoonotic transfer.

As with the slowly growing saprophytes, zoonotic transmission of rapidly growing mycobacteria organisms from infected animals to humans is unlikely, but there has been a report of *M. fortuitum* infection secondary to a cat bite to the forearm of an otherwise healthy middle-aged woman.[66]

There appears to be little to no risk of humans acquiring *M. lepraemurium* from cats. The ecology and transmission of other etiologic agents of feline leprosy syndrome are still poorly characterized and it is difficult to ascertain their potential for zoonotic transfer, but it appears to be low.

The zoonotic potential of any mycobacterial infection must be carefully considered before an attempt is made to treat infected animals. Indeed, some authors recommend against treatment of confirmed cases of *M. bovis* and *M. tuberculosis* infection.[67] Published guidelines from feline practitioner groups, such as the European Advisory Board on Cat Diseases, recommend that all owners, regardless of immunologic status, but especially if any member of the household is immunocompromised, should be made aware of the low but potential risk of zoonotic transfer of feline mycobacterial diseases, particularly those caused by *M. bovis*, *M. microti*, and the MAC complex[42] (perhaps especially, but not exclusively, *M. avium* subsp. *hominissuis*). The use of gloves is recommended when treating these animals. Veterinary personnel in areas endemic for *M. bovis* or with high rates of human TB (*M. tuberculosis*, that may be passed on to pets) should be cognizant of any potential zoonotic risk and utilize PPE, such as gloves, masks, and protective clothing, especially when handling cats with cutaneous lesions, collecting biopsies, or performing necropsy studies. Because most humans acquire TB via inhalation, the highest risk of zoonotic transmission is likely to be during procedures that may produce infectious aerosols, especially bronchoscopy, and surgery or necropsy on patients with high numbers of AFB. If bronchoscopy or surgery is deemed beneficial to the management of cats with *M. bovis*, ideally the procedure should be postponed until after the onset of medical therapy (approximately 1 to 2 weeks) (although bronchoscopy may have been done diagnostically for collection of samples before confirming the diagnosis). Occupational health and safety recommendations for the management of potentially contagious human TB patients undergoing bronchoscopy, surgery, or autopsy include the use of operating or autopsy rooms maintained at negative atmospheric pressure with respect to surrounding areas that exhaust via a high-efficiency particulate air (HEPA) filter directly to the outside, or less ideally, utilize a portable HEPA unit in the procedure room. Additionally, respiratory protection, ideally via an individually fitted N95 respirator mask, is recommended for all personnel who may be exposed to infectious aerosols. These measures have been established to protect workers from the much higher risk of disease transmission from *M. tuberculosis*-infected human patients. Moreover, it is likely that the risk of transmission of *M. bovis* from infected cats is quite low in comparison; however, the aforementioned measures could be used to reduce the risk further if desired. It would also seem prudent to ensure that the remains of any deceased cat with a mycobacterial infection be cremated rather than buried, to reduce the risk of environmental contamination.

References

1. De Lisle G, Collins D, Loveday A, et al: A report of tuberculosis in cats in New Zealand, and the examination of strains of *Mycobacterium bovis* by DNA restriction endonuclease analysis. *N Z Vet J* 38(1):10–13, 1990.
2. Gunn-Moore DA, McFarland SE, Brewer JI, et al: Mycobacterial disease in cats in Great Britain: I. Culture results, geographical distribution and clinical presentation of 339 cases. *J Feline Med Surg* 13:934–944, 2011.
3. Gunn-Moore DA, McFarland SE, Schock A, et al: Mycobacterial disease in a population of 339 cats in Great Britain: II. Histopathology of 225 cases, and treatment and outcome of 184 cases. *J Feline Med Surg* 13:945–952, 2011.
4. Thompson EJ, Little PB, Cordes DO: Observations of cat leprosy. *N Z Vet J* 27:233–235, 1979.
5. Malik R, Wigney DI, Dawson D, et al: Infection of the subcutis and skin of cats with rapidly growing mycobacteria: a review of microbiological and clinical findings. *J Feline Med Surg* 2:35–48, 2000.
6. Malik R, Hughes MS, James G, et al: Feline leprosy: two different clinical syndromes. *J Feline Med Surg* 4:43–59, 2002.
7. Haligur M, Vural SA, Sahal M, et al: Generalised tuberculosis in a cat. *Bull Vet Inst Pulawy* 51:531–534, 2007.
8. Comas I, Coscolla M, Luo T, et al: Out-of-Africa migration and Neolithic coexpansion of *Mycobacterium tuberculosis* with modern humans. *Nat Genet* 45:1176–1182, 2013.
9. Mostowy S, Cousins D, Brinkman J, et al: Genomic deletions suggest a phylogeny for the *Mycobacterium tuberculosis* complex. *J Infect Dis* 186:74–80, 2002.
10. Rufenacht S, Bogli-Stuber K, Bodmer T, et al: *Mycobacterium microti* infection in the cat: a

case report, literature review and recent clinical experience. *J Feline Med Surg* 13:195–204, 2011.

11. Cavanagh R, Begon M, Bennett M, et al: *Mycobacterium microti* infection (vole tuberculosis) in wild rodent populations. *J Clin Microbiol* 40:3281–3285, 2002.

12. Isaac J, Whitehead J, Adams JW, et al: An outbreak of *Mycobacterium bovis* infection in cats in an animal house. *Aust Vet J* 60:243–245, 1983.

13. Zumarraga MJ, Martinez Vivot M, Marticorena D, et al: *Mycobacterium bovis* in Argentina: isolates from cats typified by spoligotyping. *Rev Argent Microbiol* 41:215–217, 2009.

14. Ragg JR, Mackintosh CG, Moller H: The scavenging behaviour of ferrets (*Mustela furo*), feral cats (*Felis domesticus*), possums (*Trichosurus vulpecula*), hedgehogs (*Erinaceus europaeus*) and harrier hawks (*Circus approximans*) on pastoral farmland in New Zealand: implications for bovine tuberculosis transmission. *NZ Vet J* 48:166–175, 2000.

15. Monies RJ, Cranwell MP, Palmer N, et al: Bovine tuberculosis in domestic cats. *Vet Rec* 146:407–408, 2000.

16. Delahay RJ, Smith GC, Barlow AM, et al: Bovine tuberculosis infection in wild mammals in the South-West region of England: a survey of prevalence and a semi-quantitative assessment of the relative risks to cattle. *Vet J* 173:287–301, 2007.

17. Kaneene JB, Bruning-Fann CS, Dunn J, et al: Epidemiologic investigation of *Mycobacterium bovis* in a population of cats. *Am J Vet Res* 63:1507–1511, 2002.

18. Murray A, Dineen A, Kelly P, et al: Nosocomial spread of *Mycobacterium bovis* in domestic cats. *J Feline Med Surg* 17:173–180, 2015.

19. Smith NH, Crawshaw T, Parry J, et al: *Mycobacterium microti*: more diverse than previously thought. *J Clin Microbiol* 47:2551–2559, 2009.

20. Emmanuel FX, Seagar AL, Doig C, et al: Human and animal infections with *Mycobacterium microti*, Scotland. *Emerg Infect Dis* 13:1924–1927, 2007.

21. Lalor SM, Mellanby RJ, Friend EJ, et al: Domesticated cats with active mycobacteria infections have low serum vitamin D (25(OH) D) concentrations. *Transbound Emerg Dis* 59:279–281, 2012.

22. Hughes MS, Ball NW, Beck LA, et al: Determination of the etiology of presumptive feline leprosy by 16S rRNA gene analysis. *J Clin Microbiol* 35:2464–2471, 1997.

23. Fyfe JA, McCowan C, O'Brien CR, et al: Molecular characterization of a novel fastidious mycobacterium causing lepromatous lesions of the skin, subcutis, cornea, and conjunctiva of cats living in Victoria, Australia. *J Clin Microbiol* 46:618–626, 2008.

24. Appleyard GD, Clark EG: Histologic and genotypic characterization of a novel *Mycobacterium* species found in three cats. *J Clin Microbiol* 40:2425–2430, 2002.

25. Malik R, Norris J, White J, et al: Wound cat. *J Feline Med Surg* 8:135–140, 2006.

26. Horne KS, Kunkle GA: Clinical outcome of cutaneous rapidly growing mycobacterial

infections in cats in the Southeastern United States: a review of 10 cases (1996-2006). *J Feline Med Surg* 11:627–632, 2009.

27. Jassies-van der Lee A, Houwers DJ, Meertens N, et al: Localised pyogranulomatous dermatitis due to *Mycobacterium abscessus* in a cat: a case report. *Vet J* 179:304–306, 2009.

28. Davies JL, Sibley JA, Myers S, et al: Histological and genotypical characterization of feline cutaneous mycobacteriosis: a retrospective study of formalin-fixed paraffin-embedded tissues. *Vet Dermatol* 17:155–162, 2006.

29. Paulsen DB, Kern MR, Weigand CM: Mycobacterial neuritis in a cat. *J Am Vet Med Assoc* 216:1589–1591, 2000.

30. Brown-Elliott BA, Wallace RJ: Enhancement of conventional phenotypic methods with molecular-based methods for the more definitive identification of nontuberculous mycobacteria. *Clin Microbiol Newslett* 34:109–115, 2012.

31. Saleeb PG, Drake SK, Murray PR, et al: Identification of mycobacteria in solid-culture media by matrix-assisted laser desorption ionization-time of flight mass spectrometry. *J Clin Microbiol* 49:1790–1794, 2011.

32. Reppas G, Fyfe J, Foster S, et al: Detection and identification of mycobacteria in fixed stained smears and formalin-fixed paraffin-embedded tissues using PCR. *J Small Anim Pract* 54:638–646, 2013.

33. Kriz P, Novakova B, Nagl I, et al: *Mycobacterium avium* subsp. *hominissuis*: generalized infection of cats. *Veterinarstvi* 62:680–684, 2012.

34. Elsner L, Wayne J, O'Brien CR, et al: Localised *Mycobacterium ulcerans* infection in a cat in Australia. *J Feline Med Surg* 10:407–412, 2008.

35. Snider WR, Cohen D, Reif JS, et al: Tuberculosis in canine and feline populations. Study of high-risk populations in Pennsylvania, 1966-1968. *Am Rev Respir Dis* 104:866–876, 1971.

36. Rhodes SG, Gruffydd-Jones T, Gunn-Moore D, et al: Adaptation of IFN-gamma ELISA and ELISPOT tests for feline tuberculosis. *Vet Immunol Immunopathol* 124:379–384, 2008.

37. Rhodes SG, Gunn-Moore D, Boschiroli ML, et al: Comparative study of IFN-gamma and antibody tests for feline tuberculosis. *Vet Immunol Immunopathol* 144:129–134, 2011.

38. Sykes JE, Gunn-Moore DA: Mycobacterial infections. In Sykes JE, editor: *Canine and feline infectious diseases*, St Louis, 2013, Elsevier.

39. CLSI: *Susceptibility testing of mycobacteria, nocardiae, and other aerobic actinomycetes: approved standard*, Wayne, 2011, Clinical and Laboratory Standards Institute.

40. Govendir M, Hansen T, Kimble B, et al: Susceptibility of rapidly growing mycobacteria isolated from cats and dogs, to ciprofloxacin, enrofloxacin and moxifloxacin. *Vet Microbiol* 147(1/2):113–118, 2011.

41. Govendir M, Hansen T, Kimble B, et al: Clinical efficacy of moxifloxacin for treating rapidly growing mycobacteria (RGM) infections in cats. *J Vet Pharmacol Ther* 32(S1):71, 2009.

42. Lloret A, Hartmann K, Pennisi MG, et al: Mycobacterioses in cats: ABCD guidelines on

prevention and management. *J Feline Med Surg* 15:591–597, 2013.

43. Gunn-Moore D, Dean R, Shaw S: Mycobacterial infections in cats and dogs. *In Pract* 32:444–452, 2010.

44. Griffith DE, Aksamit T, Brown-Elliott BA, et al: American Thoracic Society Documents. *Am J Respir Crit Care Med* 175:367–416, 2007.

45. Campbell I, Drobniewski F, Novelli V, et al: Management of opportunist mycobacterial infections: Joint Tuberculosis Committee guidelines 1999. *Thorax* 55:210–218, 2000.

46. Hombach M, Somoskovi A, Homke R, et al: Drug susceptibility distributions in slowly growing non-tuberculous mycobacteria using MGIT 960 TB eXiST. *Int J Med Microbiol* 303:270–276, 2013.

47. Baral RM, Metcalfe SS, Krockenberger MB, et al: Disseminated *Mycobacterium avium* infection in young cats: overrepresentation of Abyssinian cats. *J Feline Med Surg* 8:23–44, 2006.

48. de Groot PHS, van Ingen J, de Zwaan R, et al: Disseminated *Mycobacterium avium* subsp *avium* infection in a cat, the Netherlands. *Vet Microbiol* 144:527–529, 2010.

49. Collins L, Franzblau SG: Microplate alamar blue assay versus BACTEC 460 system for high-throughput screening of compounds against *Mycobacterium tuberculosis* and *Mycobacterium avium*. *Antimicrob Agents Chemother* 41:1004–1009, 1997.

50. Maugein J, Fourche J, Mormede M, et al: *In vitro* sensitivity of *Mycobacterium avium* and *Mycobacterium xenopi* to erythromycin, roxithromycin and doxycycline. *Pathol Biol* 37:565, 1989.

51. Smith DS, Lindholm-Levy P, Huitt GA, et al: *Mycobacterium terrae*: case reports, literature review, and *in vitro* antibiotic susceptibility testing. *Clin Infect Dis* 30:444–453, 2000.

52. Henderson SM, Baker J, Williams R, et al: Opportunistic mycobacterial granuloma in a cat associated with a member of the *Mycobacterium terrae* complex. *J Feline Med Surg* 5:37–41, 2003.

53. O'Brien CR, McMillan E, Harris O, et al: Localised *Mycobacterium ulcerans* infection in four dogs. *Aust Vet J* 89:506–510, 2011.

54. Dietrich U, Arnold P, Guscetti F, et al: Ocular manifestation of disseminated *Mycobacterium simiae* infection in a cat. *J Small Anim Pract* 44:121–123, 2003.

55. Meeks C, Levy J, Crawford P, et al: Chronic disseminated *Mycobacterium xenopi* infection in a cat with idiopathic CD4+ T lymphocytopenia. *J Vet Int Med* 22:1043–1047, 2008.

56. Malik R, Hunt GB, Goldsmid SE, et al: Diagnosis and treatment of pyogranulomatous panniculitis due to *Mycobacterium smegmatis* in cats. *J Small Anim Pract* 35:524–530, 1994.

57. O'Brien CR, Fyfe J, Malik R: Infections caused by rapidly growing mycobacteria. In Greene CE, editor: *Infectious diseases of the dog and cat*, ed 4, St Louis, 2012, Elsevier, pp 515–521.

58. Govendir M, Norris JM, Hansen T, et al: Susceptibility of rapidly growing mycobacteria and *Nocardia* isolates from cats and dogs to

pradofloxacin. *Vet Microbiol* 153:240–245, 2011.

59. Roccabianca P, Caniatti M, Scanziani E, et al: Feline leprosy: spontaneous remission in a cat. *J Am Anim Hosp Assoc* 32:189–193, 1996.

60. Mendoza-Aguilar M, Almaguer-Villagrán L, Jiménez-Arellanes A, et al: The use of the microplate alamar blue assay (MABA) to assess the susceptibility of *Mycobacterium lepraemurium* to anti-leprosy and other drugs. *J Infect Chemother* 18:652–661, 2012.

61. Malik R, Smits B, Reppas G, et al: Ulcerated and nonulcerated nontuberculous cutaneous mycobacterial granulomas in cats and dogs. *Vet Dermatol* 24:146–153, e32–e33, 2013.

62. Human Animal Infections and Risk Surveillance (HAIRS): qualitative assessment of the risk that cats infected with *Mycobacterium bovis* present to human health, www.hpa.org.uk/webc/HPAwebFile/HPAweb_C/1317140243205. Accessed April 28, 2014.

63. PubMed Health Web site. http://www.ncbi.nlm.nih.gov/pubmedhealth/behindthehead lines/news/2014-03-28-first-cat-to-human-tb-infections-reported/. Accessed March 28, 2015.

64. Lewis-Jonsson J: The transmission of tuberculosis from cats to human beings. *Acta Tuberc Pneum Sc* 20:102–105, 1946.

65. Phan TA, Relic J: Sporotrichoid *Mycobacterium marinum* infection of the face following a cat scratch. *Aust J Dermatol* 51:45–48, 2010.

66. Ngan N, Morris A, de Chalain T: *Mycobacterium fortuitum* infection caused by a cat bite. *N Z Med J* 118:U1354, 2005.

67. Greene CE, Gunn-Mooore D: Infections caused by slow-growing mycobacteria. In Greene CE, editor: *Infectious diseases of the dog and cat*, ed 4, St Louis, 2012, Elsevier, pp 495–510.

Practical Antimicrobial Therapy

Katrina R. Viviano

Despite being one of the greatest medical discoveries of the twentieth century, antimicrobials also contribute to the continued evolution of bacteria and the emergence of bacterial antimicrobial resistance.[1,2] In human medicine, studies have estimated that 25% to 50% of antimicrobial use is unnecessary or inappropriate,[3-5] with similar reports from veterinary medicine.[6-10] These data highlight the importance of approaching every antimicrobial prescription using a rational clinical strategy to optimize success, minimize adverse outcomes, and avoid unnecessary prescriptions. This chapter reviews some of the common challenges associated with antimicrobial therapy with a focus on the more recently approved antimicrobials and their feline-specific adverse effects, as well as guidelines to optimize antimicrobial use in an era of increasing antimicrobial resistance.

CEPHALOSPORINS

A third-generation cephalosporin, cefovecin, has been recently approved for use in cats as a single subcutaneous injection for the treatment of skin infections including wounds and abscesses.[11,12] Other reported uses include the treatment of bacteriuria associated with feline urinary tract infections.[13] Compared to other third-generation cephalosporins, cefovecin's spectrum of activity *(Escherichia coli, Staphylococcus pseudintermedius,* and *Pasteurella multocida)* and clinical use more closely parallels that of a first-generation cephalosporin. Cefovecin has no activity against *Pasteurella aeruginosa* or *Enterococcus* spp.[14] The most commonly reported adverse reactions include vomiting, diarrhea, anorexia, and lethargy.

In cats, cefovecin is highly protein bound (≈99%) with an extended elimination half-life of 6.9 days and therapeutic serum concentrations against *P. multocida* for 7 days.[15] Cefovecin's extended exposure time following a single subcutaneous injection prohibits drug withdrawal once administered, leading to potentially higher risks of adverse effects including the development of bacterial antimicrobial resistance.[16]

Judging by published reports in companion animal medicine journals, the use of cefovecin in cats is relatively common; it is reported as one of the top three systemic antimicrobials used in feline patients.[17,18] In a review of antimicrobial use in companion animal practice in Ontario, cefovecin use was reported in 38 of the 219 feline cases evaluated.[18] Six of these 38 cefovecin prescriptions were for the treatment of

conditions with a low bacterial risk (e.g., lower urinary tract disease or acute feline upper respiratory tract disease), suggesting that cefovecin may be overprescribed in cats. In a randomized prospective clinical trial, amoxicillin-clavulanic acid or doxycycline was reported to be more efficacious than cefovecin in shelter cats with clinical signs consistent with upper respiratory disease.[19] These findings are reflective of the common bacterial isolates (i.e., *Mycoplasma* spp., *Chlamydophila felis,* or *Bordetella bronchiseptica*) linked to complicated upper respiratory infections in cats and kittens for which doxycycline has the most appropriate spectrum.

The extended duration of antimicrobial coverage offered by cefovecin in cats is attractive, as daily oral therapy can be a challenge in some cats. However, cefovecin should be treated as a second-line antimicrobial that is prescribed when a first-line antimicrobial is not an option or organism susceptibility supports its use based on *in vitro* testing. The use of third-generation cephalosporins in human medicine is reserved for the treatment of serious bacterial infections with limited antimicrobial alternatives. Cefovecin has a role in treating bacterial infections in cats, but its use needs to be judicious and limited to clinical situations in which alternative antimicrobials are inappropriate because of spectrum of activity, susceptibility data, or patient compliance.

FLUOROQUINOLONES

Fluoroquinolones have evolved over time with the goal of improved oral bioavailability and a broader spectrum of activity. Veterinary-approved fluoroquinolones licensed for the cat include second-generation fluoroquinolones (e.g., enrofloxacin, marbofloxacin, and orbifloxacin) and the third-generation fluoroquinolone pradofloxacin. Retinal toxicity in cats has been reported for enrofloxacin and orbifloxacin (Table 4-1), but all fluoroquinolones have the potential to cause retinal toxicity and blindness in cats and should be used with caution.

Fluoroquinolone-associated retinal degeneration in cats is dose dependent and species specific. Cats are deficient in the ATP-binding cassette subfamily G member 2 (ABCG2) protein encoded by the *ABCG2* gene. The ABCG2 protein functions as part of the blood-retinal barrier, preventing xenobiotics, including the photosensitive fluoroquinolones, from entering the retina.[20] Cats treated with high doses or moderate overdoses of a fluoroquinolone are at risk for retinal degeneration and blindness. To minimize retinal toxicity in

Table 4-1 — Summary of Postapproval Studies That Have Evaluated the Dosage of the Veterinary-Approved Fluoroquinolones Associated with Retinal Degeneration in Young Healthy Cats

Fluoroquinolone	Label Dose (mg/kg/day)	No Retinal Lesions (mg/kg/day)	Multiple of Minimum Label Dose	Retinal Degeneration (mg/kg/day)	Multiple of Label Dose
Enrofloxacin[21,43]	5	5	1×	≥20	4×
Orbifloxacin[21]	2.5-7.5	15	6×	≥45	18×
Marbofloxacin[21]	2.75-5.5	55	20×	N/R	N/A
Pradofloxacin[44]	7.5	50	6×	N/R	N/A

N/A, Not applicable; *N/R*, none reported.

cats, clinicians may preferentially use marbofloxacin or pradofloxacin instead of enrofloxacin. In addition, when prescribing any fluoroquinolone for a cat the recommended label dose should not be exceeded, extra-label intravenous use or prolonged treatment durations should be avoided, and empirical dosage adjustments should be considered in cats with underlying kidney disease.[21] For example, fluoroquinolones are primarily excreted in the urine and are considered concentration-dependent antibiotics; therefore extending the dosing interval to every other day versus once a day may be an empirical dosage adjustment in a cat with kidney disease and a serum creatinine concentration of 2 mg/dL (177 mmol/L).

Pradofloxacin is a third-generation fluoroquinolone available in Europe for the treatment of bacterial infections in cats and approved in the United States as an oral suspension for feline skin infections.[22] The antimicrobial spectrum of pradofloxacin provides a broader gram-positive spectrum relative to other fluoroquinolones and is effective against some anaerobes, while maintaining susceptibility in gram-negative, *Mycoplasma*, *Bartonella*, and intracellular bacteria (e.g., *Rickettsia*, *Mycobacterium*) species.[23-26] Compared with other fluoroquinolones, pradofloxacin has a comparatively low minimum inhibitory concentration (MIC) against susceptible bacterial pathogens (e.g., *S. pseudintermedius*, *E. coli*, beta-hemolytic streptococci, *P. multocida*, and *B. bronchiseptica*), which supports inhibition of microorganism growth at lower antibiotic dilutions.[27]

Reported indications for pradofloxacin use in cats include wound infections and abscesses, hemoplasma infections, bacterial urinary tract infections, upper respiratory infections, and infections associated with mycobacteria.[28-30] Saliva and tear concentrations of pradofloxacin exceed serum concentrations in healthy cats.[31] However, in one study of cats with upper respiratory infections due to *Mycoplasma* spp. and *C. felis*, *C. felis* DNA persisted in some cats treated with pradofloxacin while all doxycycline-treated cats had negative results when tested with a polymerase chain reaction (PCR) assay.[32] The use of pradofloxacin in the treatment of upper respiratory and lower urinary tract infections in cats should be based on organism isolation and susceptibility data to avoid overuse of this antibiotic, as both of these diseases are not commonly of bacterial origin. Rational use of pradofloxacin should focus

on the treatment of serious bacterial infections (e.g., mixed bacterial infections including pyothorax, cholangitis, or peritonitis) or when supported by bacterial culture and antimicrobial susceptibility testing.

TETRACYCLINES

Minocycline is a lipophilic semisynthetic tetracycline with a spectrum of activity similar to doxycycline. Susceptible organisms encompass some gram-positive species (e.g., *Staphylococcus* and *Streptococcus*), gram-negative species (e.g., *Bordetella*, *Brucella*, *Bartonella*, and *Pasteurella* spp.), as well as other species including *Rickettsiae*, *Leptospira*, *Chlamydophila*, *Borrelia*, *Mycoplasma*, and *Wolbachia* spp. Common resistant species include *E. coli*, *Klebsiella*, *Bacteroides*, *Enterobacter*, *Proteus*, and *Pseudomonas* spp.

Routine antimicrobial susceptibility testing uses tetracyclines as the representative for this class of antimicrobials; however, some bacterial isolates reported to be tetracycline-resistant may still be sensitive to doxycycline or minocycline. For example, many methicillin-resistant *Staphylococcus pseudintermedius* (MRSP(I)) isolates remain sensitive to minocycline despite reported resistance to tetracycline and doxycycline.[33] Antimicrobial susceptibility testing of MRSP(I) isolates for doxycycline and minocycline requires a special induction susceptibility assay to identify the presence of inducible resistance gene(s). Not all microbiology laboratories have a validated induction susceptibility assay available for minocycline.

Compared with doxycycline, minocycline has not been widely used in veterinary medicine in part due to the limited availability of routine susceptibility testing of minocycline versus doxycycline and the fact that doxycycline is well tolerated. With the recent decreased availability and increased cost of doxycycline in some geographic regions, the use of minocycline as an alternative tetracycline may increase in veterinary medicine. For example, doxycycline has been in short supply in the United States over the past few years and the cost has significantly increased. Limited clinical experience and lack of published studies on the use of minocycline in cats make evidence-based recommendations difficult. In addition, no minocycline pharmacokinetic data have been published for cats. However, a pharmacokinetic study was recently presented as an abstract suggesting a feline minocycline dosage of 8.8 mg/kg (or 50 mg/cat) by mouth every 24 hours[34] for susceptible bacterial species versus the previously extrapolated dosage of 5 to 10 mg/kg by mouth every 12 hours.[35]

The formation of focal esophageal strictures in cats administered oral capsules or tablets of doxycycline salts (hyclate or hydrochloride forms more so than monohydrate forms) has been reported.[36,37] The likely mechanism for stricture formation is the retention of the capsule or tablet in the esophagus as it dissolves, leading to a caustic burn associated with the acidity of doxycycline and subsequent fibrosis and stricture formation. Treatment requires endoscopic-guided esophageal dilation. The risk of forming an esophageal stricture can be avoided by administering doxycycline as an oral suspension in cats rather than as capsules or tablets or by following capsule or tablet administration with water or food. The risk of esophageal strictures in cats administered oral minocycline is unknown. Following minocycline capsule administration with water or food or the use of an oral suspension would likely minimize the risk of stricture formation.

PRINCIPLES TO OPTIMIZE THE CLINICAL USE OF ANTIMICROBIALS

To minimize unnecessary antimicrobial administration and optimize the use of the currently available antimicrobials, each antimicrobial prescription needs to be preceded by a careful clinical patient evaluation and investigation in order to:

- Identify the site of a documented or suspected infection
- Provide a rational approach for the selection of empirical antimicrobial therapy
- Collect appropriate biologic sample(s) for bacterial culture and antimicrobial susceptibility testing to optimize definitive antimicrobial therapy

Patient Evaluation

The cat's history, clinical signs, physical examination findings, and diagnostic investigation should be used to define or localize the site of a suspected or confirmed bacterial infection, to assist in determining if an appropriate sample is needed for bacterial culture, and to generate a rational empirical antimicrobial therapeutic plan. The decision to prescribe antimicrobials should be limited to those clinical indications known to be associated with a bacterial infection in cats. Common errors that can lead to an inappropriate antimicrobial prescription in cats include the presence of a fever, which alone should not be an indication for antimicrobial use.

For example, feline upper respiratory infections are often triggered by stress and associated with a fever but more commonly have a viral origin (90% of cases are due to herpesvirus and/or calicivirus infections) rather than a primary bacterial etiology. In addition, feline lower urinary tract disease and pancreatitis have an inflammatory etiology despite the onset of acute clinical signs including fever; the presence of an underlying bacterial pathogen is uncommon. In most feline patients these conditions are self-limiting, responsive to supportive care, and do not require antimicrobial therapy.

Bacterial Culture and Antimicrobial Susceptibility

Appropriate biologic sample(s) for bacterial culture and antimicrobial susceptibility should be acquired prior to the initiation of antimicrobial therapy. Ideally, sample collection should be from the site of infection, but in some cases indirect sampling may be necessary. For example, urine collected from the bladder versus the kidney is used for culture in most cats diagnosed with pyelonephritis. In a few clinical situations in which the common bacterial pathogens are predictable and unlikely to carry antimicrobial resistance, an initial bacterial culture may not be required (e.g., the treatment of a lanced, uncomplicated cat bite abscess).

For some bacterial diseases, establishing a diagnosis is best accomplished using alternative diagnostic tools rather than a bacterial culture; for example, using PCR to diagnose *Mycoplasma haemofelis* (formerly *Hemobartonella felis*) in a cat being investigated for anemia. When serologic antibody testing is used (e.g., for *Toxoplasma gondii*), convalescent titers may be required to establish a diagnosis; in the absence of clinical disease, positive titers may only represent exposure, not active infection.

Empirical Antimicrobial Therapy

The goal of empirical antimicrobial therapy is to begin effective treatment for the most likely bacterial pathogen(s) while minimizing adverse effects including the development of antimicrobial resistance. In less severe or self-limiting infections, antimicrobial administration may be delayed until a bacterial pathogen is isolated and antimicrobial susceptibility data are available. In some cases antimicrobial administration alone is likely to be unsuccessful without additional interventions, such as the removal of cystoliths in a patient with bacterial cystitis, abscess drainage to overcome the low surface area to volume ratio, or chest tube placement and/or thoracotomy in cases of pyothorax.

The rational selection of empirical antimicrobial therapy requires knowledge about the antimicrobial, including spectrum of antimicrobial activity, ability to penetrate site of infection, and common adverse effects or drug interactions. Antimicrobial susceptibility patterns of bacterial isolates can vary among geographic regions and over time within a geographic region. Just as previous antimicrobial use in an individual cat can lead to the development of a more resistant bacterial infection, local community or hospital antimicrobial use patterns influence regional bacterial resistance. Therefore, knowledge of the local resistance patterns of the common bacterial pathogens encountered in feline medicine can be

Table 4-2 Clinical Conditions in Cats Associated with Bacterial Infections and the Most Common Bacterial Isolates to Guide Empirical Antimicrobial Therapy

Clinical Condition	Bacterial Isolates
Abscess (cat bite)	*Pasteurella* spp.
Cholangitis/Hepatitis	*Escherichia coli, Enterococcus* spp., anaerobes
Neutropenia	*E. coli, Enterococcus* spp., anaerobes
Pneumonia	*Mycoplasma* spp.
Pyelonephritis	*E. coli, Enterococcus* spp.
Pyothorax	*Pasteurella* spp., anaerobes
Systemic inflammatory response syndrome	*E. coli*

Maddison J, Page S, Church D: *Small animal clinical pharmacology,* Edinburgh, 2008, Saunders.

invaluable to assist with empirical antimicrobial selection. Unfortunately, only limited published data are available for cats.[38]

Of equal importance is knowledge of patient-specific factors including the site of infection and/or source of infection, the most common infecting bacterial pathogens (Table 4-2), the severity of the patient's clinical condition, past medical history including response to previous antimicrobial therapy, and other concurrent problems (e.g., kidney or liver disease; immunosuppression).

A final but important consideration in designing an effective therapeutic plan when prescribing antibiotics is the owner's ability to medicate the cat and be compliant in administering the prescribed antibiotics at the optimal dosing interval and for the intended duration. Pilling cats can be difficult; hiding antibiotics in food is generally not an option and will only lead to food aversion. Often small pills or capsules and stable liquid formulations are more easily administered in cats. However, not all medications are stable or bioavailable in a compounded liquid formulation, so it is important to consult with a licensed pharmacist about stability and efficacy. The owner's input is essential in developing a successful therapeutic plan. Educating the owner on the purpose or rationale for antibiotic therapy and possible or anticipated side effects as well as discussing the importance of compliance will likely go a long way in improving clinical outcomes. In addition, always keep in mind many ill cats may be taking multiple medications, further complicating owner compliance and resulting in drug-drug interactions or undesirable adverse effects.

The more difficult parameters to apply to clinical situations in the design of an antibiotic therapeutic plan are

estimating the antimicrobial's ability to penetrate the site of infection, the need for a bacteriostatic versus a bactericidal antibiotic, and the optimal dose and interval, which may be in part dependent on time-versus concentration-dependent killing.

Antimicrobial Tissue Penetration

Effective antimicrobial therapy requires that the antibiotic reach the site of infection and that a therapeutic concentration of antibiotic is achieved. Antibiotic tissue penetration is an important part of efficacy and is influenced by many factors including the antibiotic's lipid solubility (one of the many physiochemical properties of a drug that enables passive diffusion across the lipid bilayer of cell membranes) and the target tissue's blood supply and presence or absence of inflammation. Tissue and intracellular penetration is critical for obligate intracellular pathogens and infections in protected sites (e.g., central nervous system, prostate, or bronchial secretions; Table 4-3).

Bacteriostatic versus Bactericidal Antimicrobials

The distinction between *in vitro* bacteriostatic and bactericidal antibiotic activity is less clinically important for nonimmunocompromised, uncomplicated cases. However, clinical situations in which bactericidal antibiotics are historically preferred in human medicine include immunocompromised individuals and patients diagnosed with bacterial endocarditis, bacterial meningitis, bacterial osteomyelitis, or neutropenic fevers.[39] In cats, clinical situations in which bactericidal antibiotics are often used or recommended include immunocompromised or retroviral-infected cats. Table 4-3 provides general information on *in vitro* bacteriostatic versus bactericidal information for the common classes of antimicrobials prescribed in cats.

Time-Dependent versus Concentration-Dependent Antimicrobials

A final consideration in optimizing empirical as well as definitive antimicrobial therapy is to ensure that the antimicrobial is prescribed at an appropriate dose and dosing interval. Successful bacterial clearance requires that the antimicrobial concentration at the site of infection is above the MIC of the organism for at least a portion of the dosing interval. The required duration of time above the MIC is antimicrobial dependent and estimated using pharmacokinetic-pharmacodynamic principles.

For some antimicrobials, bacterial killing is optimized by maintaining drug serum concentrations above the MIC for most of the dosing interval (i.e., time-dependent killing) or achieving a targeted maximum serum concentration (Cmax) or area under the curve (AUC), with the serum drug concentration falling below the MIC for a portion of the dosing interval (i.e., concentration-dependent killing). The

| Table 4-3 | The Physicochemical Properties, *In Vitro* Activity (Bactericidal vs Bacteriostatic), Bacterial Kill Kinetics (Time- vs Concentration-Dependent Bacterial Killing), and Sites of Distribution (Extracellular Fluid, Tissue, or Intracellular Penetration) of the Common Antimicrobials Used in Cats |

Antimicrobial	Lipid Solubility*	Distribution	*In Vitro* Activity	Kinetics
Beta-Lactams Penicillins Cephalosporins	Low	Extracellular fluid	Bactericidal[†]	Time-dependent
Aminoglycosides Amikacin Gentamicin	Low	Extracellular fluid	Bactericidal	Concentration-dependent
Lincosamides Clindamycin	Moderate	Tissues: Bone Intracellular: WBC	Bacteriostatic[‡]	Time-dependent
Macrolides Azithromycin Tylosin	Moderate	Intracellular: WBC	Bacteriostatic[§]	Time-dependent[ǁ]
Potentiated Sulfonamides TMS/sulfa	Moderate	Tissues: CNS/CSF, ocular, prostate	Bactericidal	Time-dependent
Tetracyclines Doxycycline Minocycline	High	Tissue: Bronchial secretions Intracellular: WBC	Bacteriostatic	Time-dependent
Chloramphenicol	High	Tissues: CNS/CSF, ocular, bronchial secretions	Bacteriostatic[§]	Time-dependent
Fluoroquinolones Enrofloxacin Marbofloxacin Pradofloxacin	High	Tissues: Prostate, liver, lung, bone, kidney, bronchial secretions Intracellular: WBC	Bactericidal	Concentration-dependent
Metronidazole	High	Tissues: CNS, bronchial secretions, bone	Bactericidal	Concentration-dependent

Maddison J, Page S, Church D: *Small animal clinical pharmacology*, Edinburgh, 2008, Saunders; Bonagura J, Twedt D: *Kirk's current veterinary therapy XV*, St Louis, 2014, Elsevier, pp 1219-1223.
CNS, Central nervous system; *CSF*, cerebrospinal fluid; *TMS/sulfa*, trimethoprim/sulfonamides; *WBC*, white blood cell.
*One of the many physicochemical properties of a drug that enables passive diffusion across the lipid bilayer of cell membranes.
[†]Except *Enterococcus* spp.
[‡]Bactericidal in high concentrations against very susceptible organisms.
[§]Bactericidal against some very sensitive bacteria.
[ǁ]Exception is azithromycin which appears to have concentration-dependent activity.

beta-lactam antimicrobials (e.g., penicillins and cephalosporins) are examples of time-dependent killing antimicrobials (see Table 4-3). For beta-lactam antimicrobials, the serum drug concentration should be above the MIC for at least 50% of the dosing interval, which requires frequent dosing. Beta-lactam dosing intervals range from intermittent dosing every 8 to 12 hours for some of the beta-lactams (e.g., amoxicillin, amoxicillin-clavulanic acid) to the use of constant-rate infusions (e.g., ticarcillin, ceftazidime). Some time-dependent

antimicrobials (e.g., macrolides, lincosamides) require serum drug concentrations above the MIC for the entire dosing interval.

The aminoglycosides and fluoroquinolones are considered concentration-dependent antimicrobials (see Table 4-3) and are the most effective at bacterial killing (i.e., attaining a targeted Cmax or AUC). For most bacteria, concentration-dependent killing is associated with a postantibiotic effect that does not require drug serum concentrations to be above the MIC for the entire dosing interval. A multiple of the serum drug concentration/MIC ratio is used as the serum target concentration to achieve effective tissue concentrations (e.g., for aminoglycosides, Cmax/MIC ratio of 8 to 10; for fluoroquinolones, AUC^{0-24}/MIC ratio of 100 to 125). For these concentration-dependent antimicrobials, once a day dosing is clinically used to maximize efficacy and minimize side effects. For example, animal models have shown more effective killing and less nephrotoxicity when aminoglycosides are administered once daily.[40,41]

Definitive Antimicrobial Therapy

Bacterial culture and antimicrobial susceptibility data provide characterization of the type of bacteria present and *in vitro* antimicrobial susceptibility, enabling prescribers to tailor antimicrobial therapy according to patient-specific data. The interpretation of the clinical significance of these data requires an assessment of the patient, a fundamental working knowledge of the spectrum of action and the tissue penetration of the antimicrobials tested, the number of colony-forming units (CFUs) of the bacteria isolated, as well as the type of sample submitted and collection method used. For example, isolating more than 100,000 CFU/mL of *E. coli* in cat urine collected by cystocentesis in a cat newly diagnosed with renal azotemia would be clinically significant and supportive of a diagnosis of pyelonephritis. However, 1000 CFU/mL of three different bacterial isolates in a urine sample collected off the examination table from a healthy cat would be more suggestive of sample contamination. Important consider-

ations when evaluating the organism's susceptibility pattern include the following: whether the antimicrobial therapy needs to be narrowed, broadened, or discontinued based on *in vitro* susceptibility; the patient's clinical response to empirical therapy; the long term plan for the patient (e.g., duration of therapy, need for follow up culture, etc.).

The next important consideration in determining definitive antimicrobial therapy is the duration of therapy and monitoring. The duration of therapy for most bacterial infections in cats remains empirical as published studies evaluating the most effective durations are limited. Extrapolation from human and a few veterinary studies indicates that a shorter duration of therapy may be effective in some cases.[42,43] For example, the recently published antimicrobial use guidelines for the treatment of urinary tract disease suggest that treatment of uncomplicated urinary tract infections for up to 7 days may be as effective as therapeutic trials of 14 days.[42]

Complicated and Recurrent Infections

A follow-up monitoring plan for bacterial eradication should be considered in all cases in which clinical failure is suspected or in cases of recurrent infections. Follow-up cultures need to be considered; for some cases this may be during antimicrobial therapy and/or following therapy, to determine efficacy by documenting bacterial resolution or recurrence. As bacteria continue to evolve and adapt to antimicrobial exposure, the roles of bacterial cultures and antimicrobial susceptibility are becoming increasingly important.

References

1. Dellit TH, Owens RC, McGowan JE, Jr, et al: Infectious Diseases Society of America and the Society for Healthcare Epidemiology of America guidelines for developing an institutional program to enhance antimicrobial stewardship. *Clin Infect Dis* 44:159–177, 2007.
2. Fishman N: Antimicrobial stewardship. *Am J Med* 119:S53–S61, discussion S62–S70, 2006.
3. Gonzales R, Malone DC, Maselli JH, et al: Excessive antibiotic use for acute respiratory infections in the United States. *Clin Infect Dis* 33:757–762, 2001.
4. Marr JJ, Moffet HL, Kunin CM: Guidelines for improving the use of antimicrobial agents in hospitals: a statement by the Infectious Diseases Society of America. *J Infect Dis* 157:869–876, 1988.
5. Pestotnik SL: Expert clinical decision support systems to enhance antimicrobial stewardship programs: insights from the society of infectious diseases pharmacists. *Pharmacotherapy* 25:1116–1125, 2005.
6. Black DM, Rankin SC, King LG: Antimicrobial therapy and aerobic bacteriologic culture patterns in canine intensive care unit patients:

74 dogs (January-June 2006). *J Vet Emerg Crit Care (San Antonio)* 19:489–495, 2009.
7. Escher M, Vanni M, Intorre L, et al: Use of antimicrobials in companion animal practice: a retrospective study in a veterinary teaching hospital in Italy. *J Antimicrob Chemother* 66:920–927, 2011.
8. Holso K, Rantala M, Lillas A, et al: Prescribing antimicrobial agents for dogs and cats via university pharmacies in Finland—patterns and quality of information. *Acta Vet Scand* 46:87–93, 2005.
9. Rantala M, Holso K, Lillas A, et al: Survey of condition-based prescribing of antimicrobial drugs for dogs at a veterinary teaching hospital. *Vet Rec* 155:259–262, 2004.
10. Wayne A, McCarthy R, Lindenmayer J: Therapeutic antibiotic use patterns in dogs: observations from a veterinary teaching hospital. *J Small Anim Pract* 52:310–318, 2011.
11. Six R, Cleaver DM, Lindeman CJ, et al: Effectiveness and safety of cefovecin sodium, an extended-spectrum injectable cephalosporin, in the treatment of cats with abscesses and infected wounds. *J Am Vet Med Assoc* 234:81–87, 2009.

12. Stegemann MR, Sherington J, Passmore C: The efficacy and safety of cefovecin in the treatment of feline abscesses and infected wounds. *J Small Anim Pract* 48:683–689, 2007.
13. Passmore CA, Sherington J, Stegemann MR: Efficacy and safety of cefovecin for the treatment of urinary tract infections in cats. *J Small Anim Pract* 49:295–301, 2008.
14. Stegemann MR, Passmore CA, Sherington J, et al: Antimicrobial activity and spectrum of cefovecin, a new extended-spectrum cephalosporin, against pathogens collected from dogs and cats in Europe and North America. *Antimicrob Agents Chemother* 50:2286–2292, 2006.
15. Stegemann MR, Sherington J, Coati N, et al: Pharmacokinetics of cefovecin in cats. *J Vet Pharmacol Ther* 29:513–524, 2006.
16. Lawrence M, Kukanich K, Kukanich B, et al: Effect of cefovecin on the fecal flora of healthy dogs. *Vet J* 198:259–266, 2013.
17. Mateus A, Brodbelt DC, Barber N, et al: Antimicrobial usage in dogs and cats in first opinion veterinary practices in the UK. *J Small Anim Pract* 52:515–521, 2011.
18. Murphy CP, Reid-Smith RJ, Boerlin P, et al: Out-patient antimicrobial drug use in

dogs and cats for new disease events from community companion animal practices in Ontario. *Can Vet J* 53:291–298, 2012.

19. Litster AL, Wu CC, Constable PD: Comparison of the efficacy of amoxicillin-clavulanic acid, cefovecin, and doxycycline in the treatment of upper respiratory tract disease in cats housed in an animal shelter. *J Am Vet Med Assoc* 241:218–226, 2012.
20. Ramirez CJ, Minch JD, Gay JM, et al: Molecular genetic basis for fluoroquinolone-induced retinal degeneration in cats. *Pharmacogenet Genomics* 21:66–75, 2011.
21. Wiebe V, Hamilton P: Fluoroquinolone-induced retinal degeneration in cats. *J Am Vet Med Assoc* 221:1568–1571, 2002.
22. Bayer HealthCare LLC AHD: Veraflox Oral Suspension for cats. In *Freedom of information summary, original new animal drug application*, Washington, 2012, FDA.
23. Biswas S, Maggi RG, Papich MG, et al: Comparative activity of pradofloxacin, enrofloxacin, and azithromycin against Bartonella henselae isolates collected from cats and a human. *J Clin Microbiol* 48:617–618, 2010.
24. Dowers KL, Tasker S, Radecki SV, et al: Use of pradofloxacin to treat experimentally induced *Mycoplasma hemofelis* infection in cats. *Am J Vet Res* 70:105–111, 2009.
25. Silley P, Stephan B, Greife HA, et al: Comparative activity of pradofloxacin against anaerobic bacteria isolated from dogs and cats. *J Antimicrob Chemother* 60:999–1003, 2007.
26. Silley P, Stephan B, Greife HA, et al: Bactericidal properties of pradofloxacin against veterinary pathogens. *Vet Microbiol* 157:106–111, 2012.
27. Schink AK, Kadlec K, Hauschild T, et al: Susceptibility of canine and feline bacterial pathogens to pradofloxacin and comparison with other fluoroquinolones approved for companion animals. *Vet Microbiol* 162:119–126, 2013.

28. Litster A, Moss S, Honnery M, et al: Clinical efficacy and palatability of pradofloxacin 2.5% oral suspension for the treatment of bacterial lower urinary tract infections in cats. *J Vet Intern Med* 21:990–995, 2007.
29. Malik R, Smits B, Reppas G, et al: Ulcerated and nonulcerated nontuberculous cutaneous mycobacterial granulomas in cats and dogs. *Vet Dermatol* 24:146–153, e32–e33, 2013.
30. Spindel ME, Veir JK, Radecki SV, et al: Evaluation of pradofloxacin for the treatment of feline rhinitis. *J Feline Med Surg* 10:472–479, 2008.
31. Hartmann A, Krebber R, Daube G, et al: Pharmacokinetics of pradofloxacin and doxycycline in serum, saliva, and tear fluid of cats after oral administration. *J Vet Pharmacol Ther* 31:87–94, 2008.
32. Hartmann AD, Helps CR, Lappin MR, et al: Efficacy of pradofloxacin in cats with feline upper respiratory tract disease due to *Chlamydophila felis* or *Mycoplasma* infections. *J Vet Intern Med* 22:44–52, 2008.
33. Weese JS, Sweetman K, Edson H, et al: Evaluation of minocycline susceptibility of methicillin-resistant *Staphylococcus pseudintermedius*. *Vet Microbiol* 162:968–971, 2013.
34. Tynan BE, Cohn LA, Kerl ME, et al: Pharmacokinetics of minocycline in domestic cats [abstract]. *J Vet Intern Med* 28:1097, 2014.
35. Papich MG: Antibiotic treatment of resistant infections in small animals. *Vet Clin North Am Small Anim Pract* 43:1091–1107, 2013.
36. German AJ, Cannon MJ, Dye C, et al: Oesophageal strictures in cats associated with doxycycline therapy. *J Feline Med Surg* 7:33–41, 2005.
37. Trumble C: Oesophageal stricture in cats associated with use of the hyclate (hydrochloride) salt of doxycycline. *J Feline Med Surg* 7:241–242, 2005.

38. Authier S, Paquette D, Labrecque O, et al: Comparison of susceptibility to antimicrobials of bacterial isolates from companion animals in a veterinary diagnostic laboratory in Canada between 2 time points 10 years apart. *Can Vet J* 47:774–778, 2006.
39. Pankey GA, Sabath LD: Clinical relevance of bacteriostatic versus bactericidal mechanisms of action in the treatment of gram-positive bacterial infections. *Clin Infect Dis* 38:864–870, 2004.
40. Drusano GL, Ambrose PG, Bhavnani SM, et al: Back to the future: using aminoglycosides again and how to dose them optimally. *Clin Infect Dis* 45:753–760, 2007.
41. Nordstrom L, Lerner SA: Single daily dose therapy with aminoglycosides. *J Hosp Infect* 18(Suppl A):117–129, 1991.
42. Weese JS, Blondeau JM, Boothe D, et al: Antimicrobial use guidelines for treatment of urinary tract disease in dogs and cats: antimicrobial guidelines working group of the international society for companion animal infectious diseases. *Vet Med Int* 2011:263768, 2011.
43. Westropp JL, Sykes JE, Irom S, et al: Evaluation of the efficacy and safety of high dose short duration enrofloxacin treatment regimen for uncomplicated urinary tract infections in dogs. *J Vet Intern Med* 26:506–512, 2012.
44. Gelatt KN, van der Woerdt A, Ketring KL, et al: Enrofloxacin-associated retinal degeneration in cats. *Vet Ophthalmol* 4:99–106, 2001.
45. Messias A, Gekeler F, Wegener A, et al: Retinal safety of a new fluoroquinolone, pradofloxacin, in cats: assessment with electroretinography. *Doc Ophthalmol* 116:177–191, 2008.

Emerging Aspects of Streptococcal Infections in Cats

Susan E. Little

Streptococci are gram-positive, facultative anaerobic cocci known to cause both local and generalized pyogenic infections in humans and animals. Many streptococcal species are pathogenic, but others are commensal flora of the oral cavity, nasopharynx, skin, urogenital, and gastrointestinal tracts. Opportunistic infections occur when the host defenses are breached, leading to a variety of clinical manifestations. Rarely, invasive and life-threatening infections occur, including necrotizing fasciitis (NF) and streptococcal toxic shock syndrome (STSS). The Lancefield classification system based on cell wall antigens (groups A through W) and hemolytic activity (nonhemolytic, alpha-hemolytic, and beta-hemolytic) is commonly used to group species of streptococci. Streptococcal species in group A,[1,2] group B,[3] and group D[4,5] are rarely reported to cause clinical disease in cats; most infections belong to groups C and G (Table 5-1). This chapter focuses on the traditional and emerging clinical syndromes associated with *Streptococcus canis* and *Streptococcus equi* subspecies *zooepidemicus* (SEZ) in cats.

STREPTOCOCCUS CANIS

Pathogenicity and Epidemiology

The most commonly reported streptococcal pathogen in cats is *S. canis* (beta-hemolytic, Lancefield group G). *S. canis* is a commensal of the skin, oropharynx, and urogenital tract of cats. Isolation rates for *S. canis* vary depending on the population studied and the anatomic location cultured. When cultures from various anatomic sites in 71 cats were reviewed, 12.7% of cats were positive for *S. canis*, with the oropharynx and rectum being the most commonly colonized sites.[6] An earlier study of 66 cats found 19% had oropharyngeal and 30% had rectal carriage of *S. canis*.[7] Two retrospective studies evaluated infectious agents in a total of 85 cats with chronic rhinitis/rhinosinusitis and 10 healthy control cats without finding evidence of *S. canis*.[8,9] In one study of the bacterial populations of the vagina in 66 female cats and the prepuce of 29 male cats undergoing surgical sterilization, *S. canis* was cultured from 15% of the female and 17% of the male cats.[10] Another study of vaginal and uterine swabs from 53 healthy female cats (13 breeding queens, 10 kittens, and 30 cats undergoing ovariohysterectomy) isolated *S. canis* from 43% of the cats.[11]

Clinical Manifestations

Reports of various types of clinical disease due to *S. canis* in cats appear in the literature (see Table 5-1). Case reports and case series include urogenital infections,[12-14] skin wounds and abscesses,[15] vegetative endocarditis,[16] myocarditis,[17] lymphadenitis,[18,19] otitis media and leptomeningitis,[20] and discospondylitis.[21] Outbreaks of disease in closed research colonies have been reported, including abscesses[22]; fever, depression, lymphadenopathy, pharyngitis, and submandibular edema;[23] pyothorax;[24] and arthritis.[25]

Sepsis due to *S. canis* is a common cause of morbidity and mortality in neonatal kittens. The infection is acquired from the vagina and oropharynx of the queen, and the bacteria gain entrance through the umbilical vein after the umbilical cord is severed, causing omphalophlebitis, peritonitis, and sepsis. Kittens born to queens less than 2 years of age are most at risk, because young queens maintain a high vaginal population of *S. canis*. More than one kitten in a litter may be affected, and mortality rates in the first 2 weeks of life may be high, especially when the organism is first introduced into a naïve population, such as a pedigreed cattery. Affected kittens fail to thrive and may have omphalophlebitis. They may also be found dead with minimal antemortem clinical signs (Figure 5-1). Diagnosis is made by culture of umbilical exudates or at necropsy, when *S. canis* can be cultured from several locations, including the liver, lung, umbilicus, pericardial cavity (Figure 5-2), and peritoneal cavity. Kittens with omphalophlebitis or lymphadenitis should be treated with appropriate antibiotics (typically beta-lactams in this age group) and drainage of abscesses.

Streptococcal Toxic Shock Syndrome and Necrotizing Fasciitis

Streptococcal Toxic Shock Syndrome and Necrotizing Fasciitis in Humans. STSS is a multisystem syndrome characterized by the sudden onset of shock and organ failure that was first recognized in humans in 1978. In humans, STSS is typically caused by group A streptococci (especially *Streptococcus pyogenes*); about half of patients have concurrent NF. The portal of entry is often the site of a minor local trauma, but in at least 50% of cases, the route of acquisition is unknown. Streptococcal superantigens are thought to be key virulence factors that result in the sudden massive release of

Table 5-1	Streptococcal Species Associated with Clinical Disease in Cats		
Species	**Lancefield Group**	**Disease Syndromes**	**References**
S. pneumoniae	A	Polyarthritis, bacteremia, necrotizing fasciitis	1, 2
S. agalactiae	B	Peritonitis, septicemia, placentitis	3
S. equi ssp. *zooepidemicus*	C	Upper respiratory tract disease, meningoencephalitis	54, 62-65
S. suis	D	Dermatitis, fibrinonecrotic pleuropneumonia, meningoencephalitis	4, 5
S. canis	G	Abscesses, neonatal sepsis, umbilical infections, pyelonephritis, rhinitis, sinusitis, pharyngitis, otitis media, lymphadenopathy, pyothorax, meningitis, discospondylitis, necrotizing fasciitis, toxic shock, skin ulceration, endocarditis, myocarditis	11-16, 22-25, 39, 42

S., Streptococcus; ssp., subspecies.

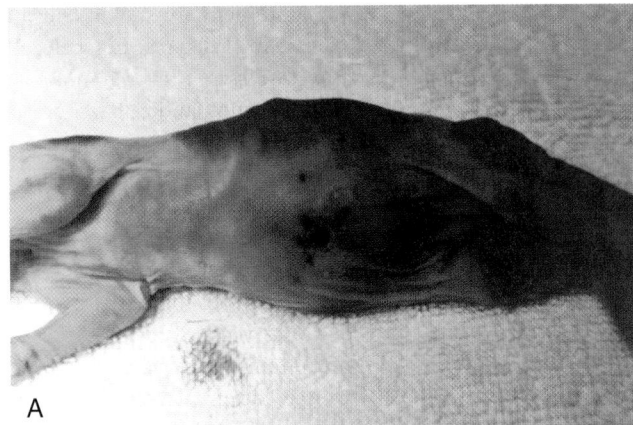

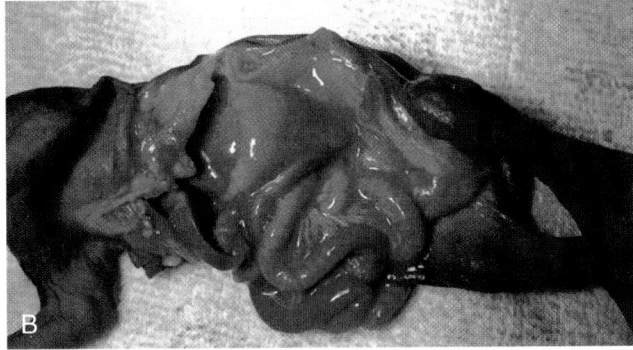

Figure 5-1: A, This Sphynx kitten was found suddenly dead. The only evidence of omphalophlebitis was discoloration around the umbilicus. **B,** On postmortem examination, septic peritonitis was found, and *S. canis* was cultured from the abdominal effusion.

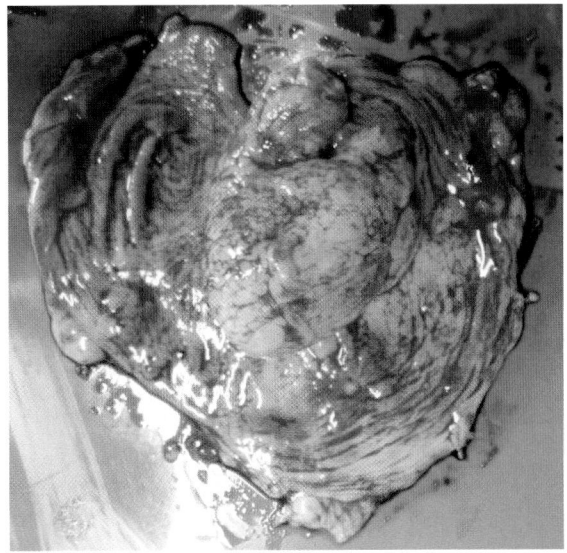

Figure 5-2: Pyopericardium in a Persian kitten that died from bronchopneumonia. *S. canis* was cultured from the lungs and pericardial fluid.

cytokines leading to fever, vomiting, hypotension, tissue damage, respiratory failure, vascular leakage, disseminated intravascular coagulation, and shock.[26] Death can occur within 48 hours of onset of clinical signs. Mortality rates for STSS in humans remain at about 50% despite advances in understanding the immunopathogenesis.[27] NF is an invasive bacterial infection ("flesh-eating bacteria") of deep subcutaneous tissues and fascia with necrosis and gangrene that may be caused by pathogens such as *S. pyogenes, Staphylococcus aureus,* and *Clostridium* spp. NF may begin as an insignificant wound and, like STSS, can progress rapidly. Risk factors for NF in humans include diabetes mellitus, intravenous drug use, hypertension, malnutrition, and obesity.[28]

Streptococcal Toxic Shock Syndrome and Necrotizing Fasciitis in Cats. Feline and canine cases of STSS and NF (Figure 5-3) bear striking similarity to human cases although not enough cases have been studied to determine predisposing factors. Suggested diagnostic criteria for STSS in dogs and cats have been adapted from criteria used in humans (Box 5-1).[29] The Laboratory Risk Indicator for Necrotizing Fasciitis score (Table 5-2) was developed to help physicians distinguish early NF lesions from other soft tissue infections,

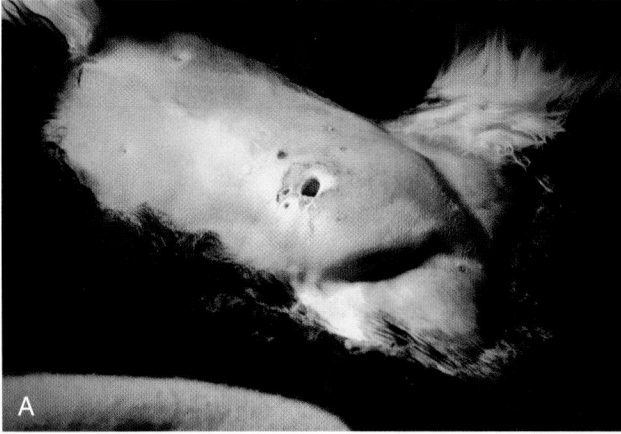

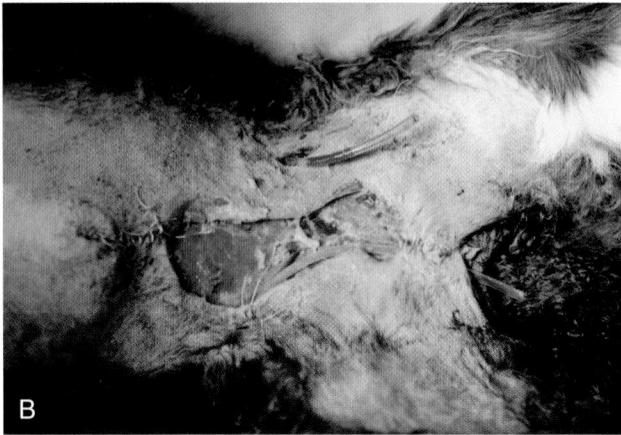

Figure 5-3: Necrotizing fasciitis often begins with a small skin wound. **A,** The small wound in this cat was surgically explored and discovered to be more extensive than originally expected. **B,** *S. canis* was cultured from the purulent material in the wound, which progressed rapidly to involve large areas of skin, subcutaneous fat, and fascia.

<table>
<tr><td colspan="2">

BOX 5-1   Proposed Criteria for the Diagnosis of Streptococcal Toxic Shock Syndrome in Dogs and Cats

</td></tr>
</table>

 I. Isolation of group G streptococci *(Streptococcus canis)*
   A. From a normally sterile site
   B. From a nonsterile site
 II. Clinical signs
   A. Hypotension
     1. Systolic blood pressure less than 90 mm Hg in dogs
     2. Systolic blood pressure less than 80 mm Hg in cats
   and
   B. Two or more of the following signs
     1. Renal impairment: serum creatinine above the reference range
     2. Coagulopathy: thrombocytopenia or disseminated intravascular coagulation (prolonged clotting times, decreased serum fibrinogen, and increased fibrin degradation products)
     3. Liver involvement: serum AST, ALT, or total bilirubin at least twice the upper limit of the reference range
     4. Acute respiratory distress syndrome: acute onset of diffuse pulmonary infiltrates and hypoxemia in the absence of cardiac failure, or evidence of diffuse capillary leakage manifested as acute onset of pulmonary edema, or pleural or peritoneal effusions with hypoalbuminemia
     5. Generalized erythematous macular rash that may desquamate
     6. Soft tissue necrosis, including NF or myositis, or gangrene

Adapted from Sykes JE: Streptococcal and enterococcal infections. In *Canine and feline infectious diseases,* St Louis, 2013, Elsevier/Saunders, pp 334–346.
ALT, Alanine aminotransferase; *AST,* aspartate aminotransferase, *NF,* necrotizing fasciitis.
Note: Cases that fulfill criteria IA and II are definite cases; cases that fulfill criteria IB and II are probable cases if no other cause is identified.

such as cellulitis and abscesses, and is based on changes associated with systemic inflammatory response syndrome and sepsis.[30] No similar scoring system has been proposed for veterinary patients. Therefore, NF in veterinary patients is initially suspected based on the physical findings (e.g., local erythema, edema, and severe pain, sometimes with signs of shock) and surgical findings (e.g., easy separation of fascia from other tissues and copious exudate that is thin and malodorous).[31] Tissue for culture and histopathology should be taken from the leading edge of the lesion.

Most cases of STSS/NF documented in the veterinary literature involve canine patients. Canine STSS cases caused by *S. canis* were first identified in Ontario, Canada, in 1995.[32-34] Diagnosis of STSS was established if the animal had evidence of hypotensive shock and involvement of at least one organ or system in association with isolation of *S. canis* from a normally sterile site. Many cases had both STSS and NF, which appears to increase mortality as it does in humans. NF lesions often involve limbs and are characterized by intense pain with localized swelling that requires extensive drainage and débridement. Also similar to human cases, onset of

clinical signs is sudden, disease progression is rapid, and the mortality rate is high.

Toxic shock-like syndrome associated with septicemia caused by group G *Streptococcus* spp. was reported in three related kittens that presented with depression, pyrexia, respiratory signs, and limb swelling (although findings were not compatible with NF).[35] Two of the three kittens died. Sporadic case reports of NF in cats appear in the literature associated with various pathogens, including *Prevotella bivia,*[36] *Acinetobacter baumannii,*[37] and Fournier's gangrene.[38,39] A few reported cases involved *S. canis,* including one fatal case of NF and necrotizing myositis with pneumonia[40] and another case that survived after extensive débridement and negative pressure wound management.[41]

In contrast to individual case reports, reports of invasive streptococcal disease resembling STSS/NF affecting large

Table 5-2	Laboratory Criteria for the Diagnosis of Necrotizing Fasciitis in Humans	
Test		**Score***
C-reactive protein (mg/L)		
<150		0
≥150		4
Total white blood cell count (mm³)		
<15		0
15-25		1
>25		2
Hemoglobin (g/dL)		
>13.5		0
11-13.5		1
<11		2
Sodium (mmol/L)		
≥135		0
<135		2
Creatinine (μmol/L)		
≤141		0
>141		2
Glucose (mmol/L)		
≤10		0
>10		1

Adapted from Wong CH, Khin LW, Heng KS, et al: The LRINEC (Laboratory Risk Indicator for Necrotizing Fasciitis) score: a tool for distinguishing necrotizing fasciitis from other soft tissue infections. *Crit Care Med* 32(7):1535-1541, 2004.
*A score ≥6 is suspicious of necrotizing fasciitis; a score ≥8 is strongly predictive.

numbers of intensively housed shelter cats have been reported in the United States with mortality rates up to 30%.[42] Two distinct presentations have been noted.[42] In two shelter outbreaks, skin ulceration and chronic respiratory infection progressed to necrotizing rhinitis/sinusitis and suppurative meningitis (Figure 5-4). Skin ulceration was most often found on distal limbs, and two or more limbs could be affected. Necrosis and perforation of the nasal bone overlying the frontal sinus were seen with subsequent cellulitis and edema of subcutaneous tissues causing the nasal bridge area to swell. In another shelter, rapid progression from NF with skin ulceration (Figure 5-5) to toxic shock-like syndrome, sepsis, and death occurred.

These shelter outbreaks share some common and alarming characteristics. Although upper respiratory tract disease (URTD) was endemic in both shelters, *S. canis* was typically the sole pathogen reported in these cases. Despite the fact the cultured *S. canis* was sensitive to multiple antibiotics *in vitro*, treatment of patients was not always successful. Also, extensive environmental cleaning was often unable to prevent persistence of the bacteria in the environment. In an older report of an outbreak in a closed specific pathogen-free

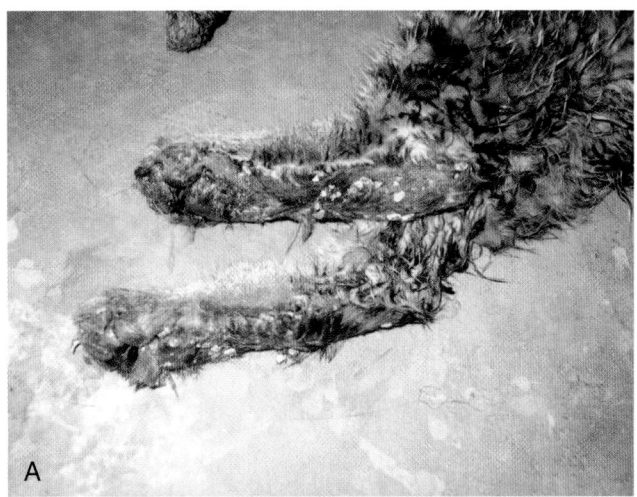
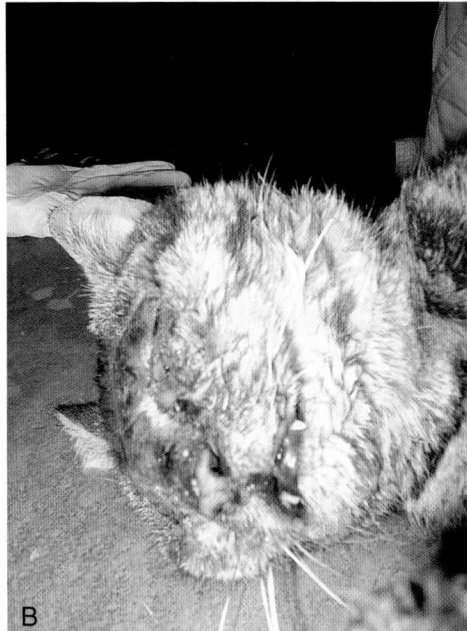

Figure 5-4: Ulcerated foot pads (**A**) and necrotizing rhinitis/sinusitis (**B**) due to *S. canis* in cats involved in a shelter outbreak with high mortality. (Copyright Dr. Kate Hurley.)

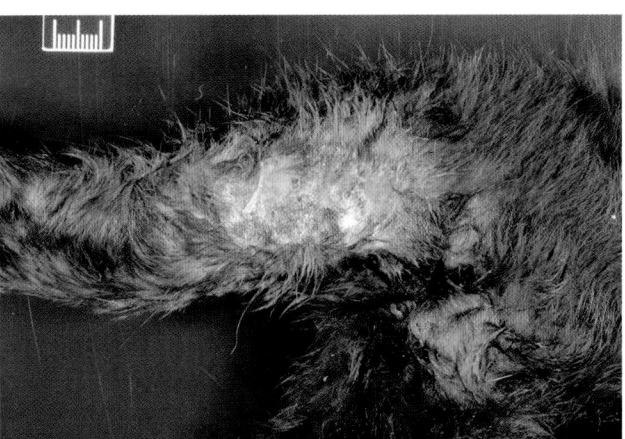

Figure 5-5: Necrotizing fasciitis with skin ulceration in a cat involved in a shelter outbreak of streptococcal disease. (From Pesavento PA, Bannasch J, Bachmann R, et al: Fatal Streptococcus canine infections in intensively housed shelter cats, *Vet Path* 44: 218-221, 2007.)

Table 5-3	Drug Therapy for Streptococcal Infections in Cats
Drug	**Dosage***
Amoxicillin/clavulanate	62.5 mg/cat, PO, every 12 h
Cephalexin	22-30 mg/kg, PO, every 12 h
Chloramphenicol	10-20 mg/kg, PO/IV/SC, every 12 h
Clindamycin	10 mg/kg, PO/IV, every 12 h
Erythromycin	20 mg/kg, PO, every 8 h
Penicillin G (procaine)	10,000-20,000 IU/kg, IM or SC, every 12-24 h
Pradofloxacin	7.5 mg/kg, PO, every 24 h
Trimethoprim/ sulfonamide	15-30 mg/kg, PO, every 12 h

IM, Intramuscularly; *IU*, international unit; *IV*, intravenously; *PO, per os* (by mouth); *SC*, subcutaneously.
*Duration of treatment is dictated by the clinical presentation; a minimum of 2 weeks is suggested.

colony, only depopulating the affected building stopped the outbreak.[23] The factors that allow a typically commensal organism to cause invasive life-threatening disease are not well understood. Little is known about *S. canis* virulence factors in severe disease. All affected cats in one study carried almost identical isolates based on molecular typing, suggesting a clonal origin and spread of a virulent strain.[43] Other factors could include shelter management practices, stress, and antibiotic therapy for other conditions. Control measures for shelter outbreaks are discussed later.

Treatment

Group G isolates are generally susceptible to erythromycin, clindamycin, and beta-lactam antibiotics (Table 5-3). In the study of cultures from 71 cats mentioned earlier, all streptococcal isolates were susceptible to penicillin G and ampicillin; the least effective antimicrobial was tetracycline.[6] Aminoglycoside susceptibility is reported to be variable. In a study of 500 *Streptococcus* isolates from swine, horses, cats, and dogs, the most commonly detected resistances were against sulfamethoxazole (20% to 78%), tetracycline (17% to 93%), and gentamicin (14% to 79%), regardless of species of origin.[44] Resistance to penicillins or cephalosporins was rarely detected. Choices for central nervous system infections include high-dose intravenous penicillin, trimethoprim sulfonamide, clindamycin, or intravenous third-generation cephalosporins.[45] Prevention of neonatal infection in endemic environments has been described by treating the queen with 1.0 mL/cat subcutaneous (SC) injection of a combined benzathine/procaine penicillin (300,000 International Unit/mL) at the time of delivery.[46] Newborn kittens are treated

with the same product (diluted 1:6 with sterile 0.9% saline, 0.25 mL/kitten, SC).

Successful treatment of NF and/or STSS in veterinary patients parallels recommendations for humans. The life of the patient depends on prompt initiation of aggressive therapy that is based on a presumptive diagnosis before test results are available. Treatment includes complete surgical débridement of necrotic tissue (often requiring multiple procedures or limb amputation), hemodynamic support, nutritional support, and analgesia. Antibiotic therapy is based on culture results, but broad-spectrum treatment is begun in the interim. Recommended drug regimens based on experience with human cases include a combination of penicillin, an aminoglycoside, and clindamycin.[31] Fluoroquinolones are not recommended despite *in vitro* bacterial sensitivity. In fact, the use of enrofloxacin in dogs with *S. canis* infections is suspected to have contributed to the emergence of canine STSS/NF because fluoroquinolones may induce bacteriophages encoding superantigen genes and enhance virulence.[33,34,47] Wound management techniques such as active closed-suction drainage[48] and negative pressure wound therapy[41,49] have been associated with success in veterinary patients.

Zoonotic Potential

Humans have only rarely been reported to be infected by *S. canis,* and there is no evidence that cats or dogs represent a significant source of infection. Regardless, it would be prudent for veterinarians to take precautions against inadvertent infection of skin breaks or cuts when treating animals with STSS/NF by wearing latex gloves and protective clothing. Although most cases of STSS/NF in humans are caused by group A organisms, there is at least one case report of group G streptococcal myositis and STSS resulting in a patient's death.[50]

STREPTOCOCCUS EQUI SUBSPECIES *ZOOEPIDEMICUS*

S. equi ssp. *equi* (beta-hemolytic, Lancefield group C), commonly known as *S. equi*, is well known as the cause of strangles in horses and donkeys. SEZ is an opportunistic commensal organism in horses but is a zoonotic pathogen for humans, causing septicemia, pneumonia, arthritis, and meningitis.[51] SEZ has not historically been known as a commensal of dogs or cats, and not all infected animals have a history of exposure to farm animals or horses.

Streptococcus Equi Subspecies *Zooepidemicus* in Dogs

Reports of acute, fatal necrohemorrhagic pneumonia and septicemia due to SEZ first appeared in racing kennels in the United Kingdom and in research colony dogs more than 30 years ago.[52,53] More recently, the pathogen has become known as a cause of contagious canine infectious respiratory disease complex. Reports have described large-scale outbreaks in intensively housed shelter and kennel dogs in different countries, with high morbidity (up to 90%) and mortality (up to 50%).[54-58] The disease is highly contagious and is characterized by sudden onset of pyrexia, cough, dyspnea, lethargy, and hemorrhagic nasal discharge. Initially, affected animals may appear to have typical "kennel cough" but the disease progresses rapidly; death often occurs within 24 to 48 hours of the first clinical signs.[57] On histopathology, most cases have fibrinosuppurative, necrotizing, and hemorrhagic pneumonia.[57] It is possible that coinfection with an organism such as *Bordetella bronchiseptica*, *Mycoplasma* spp., canine influenza virus, or canine herpesvirus may be necessary for maximum virulence.[57,59] However, outbreaks may also be due to the introduction of either a high pathogen load or a virulent SEZ clone in a densely populated environment with susceptible dogs.[56]

Diagnosis of SEZ infection in dogs has been made by culturing lung samples, nasal swabs, transtracheal lavage fluid, or throat swabs. A polymerase chain reaction (PCR) assay is also commercially available. Animals that die or are euthanized should undergo necropsy with bacterial culture to confirm the diagnosis. Isolates of SEZ from dogs have been reported to be susceptible to penicillin, ampicillin, amoxicillin, and enrofloxacin.[54] Some isolates have been reported to be resistant to tetracycline and doxycycline.[54,56,60] Despite appropriate antibiotic therapy, mortality rates in densely housed animals are high, at least in part due to the rapid progression of the disease. Virulence factors (such as superantigens or bacterial toxins) and management factors (e.g., close confinement, transport stress, social stress, etc.) that may contribute to disease severity have not been well explored.

Sporadic cases of nonfatal chronic rhinitis and pneumonia due to SEZ have been reported in pet dogs living on horse farms.[61-63] One in-contact dog was positive on oropharyngeal culture but had no clinical signs despite being infected with the known virulent SEZ strain ST173,[63] suggesting that infection may arise from exposure to horses but factors other than bacterial strain alone play a role in the severity of disease.

Streptococcus Equi Subspecies Zooepidemicus in Cats

Streptococcus equi subspecies *zooepidemicus* has not previously been known as a pathogen causing lower respiratory tract disease in cats based on published retrospective studies and case series, although *S. canis* is sometimes isolated.[64-66] Recently, however, SEZ has been identified as an important emerging feline pathogen in shelters and large-scale hoarding situations. SEZ infection in cats is clinically different from that in dogs, because it lacks the hemorrhagic component. Disease in cats is associated with purulent nasal discharge (Figure 5-6), cough, rhinitis/sinusitis, respiratory distress, pneumonia, meningoencephalitis, and death.[67-69] The first report of an outbreak of disease due to SEZ in cats was

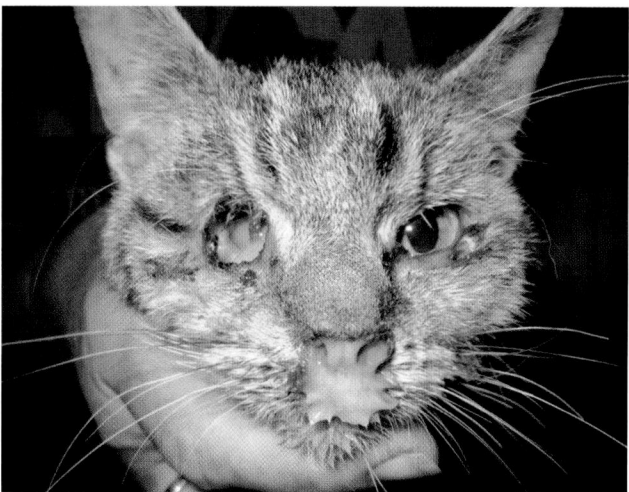

Figure 5-6: Purulent nasal and ocular disease with severe rhinitis/sinusitis in a cat with *S. equi* ssp. *zooepidemicus*. (Copyright Dr. Julie Levy.)

published in 2010 when 78 cats in a large shelter in Israel died.[67] On postmortem examination of 39 cats, most had severe acute diffuse bronchopneumonia and some had pleuritis, peritonitis, or pyogranulomatous meningoencephalitis. Diagnosis was made by culture of nasal and pharyngeal swabs, bronchoalveolar lavage fluid, and various tissue samples (primarily lung). Although other pathogens were also isolated (e.g., *Pasteurella multocida* and *Chlamydophila* spp.), SEZ was the predominant organism. SEZ was also isolated from cats with mild signs of URTD, suggesting that the pathogen may have become persistent in the shelter through cats that were shedding the organism before being detected and treated.

In a report of four large seizures of cats from failed sanctuaries in the United States (2009 to 2012), 55% of 81 cats with URTD tested positive for SEZ.[59] Infection was detected by real-time PCR performed on conjunctival and oropharyngeal swabs, and coinfection with other pathogens (e.g., feline calicivirus, feline herpesvirus, *B. bronchiseptica*, *Mycoplasma felis*, and *Chlamydophila felis*) was common. The authors speculate that SEZ coinfection may account for the severity of URTD in large cat-dense populations in contrast to the milder, self-limiting form of URTD commonly seen in traditional shelters where SEZ is uncommon. Because cats with URTD entering shelters may represent the point of introduction for SEZ, it is important that all cats have a thorough physical examination upon admission and that URTD is promptly and appropriately treated.

SEZ is capable of causing rapid disease progression in cats as well as dogs. In two cats from separate shelters in British Columbia, Canada, acute onset of URTD progressed to death in less than 24 hours.[68] On postmortem examination, rhinitis and meningitis (Figure 5-7) were found, and SEZ was isolated from the nasal cavity and brain.

A case report of SEZ causing meningoencephalitis via extension of otitis media/otitis interna in a 5-year-old

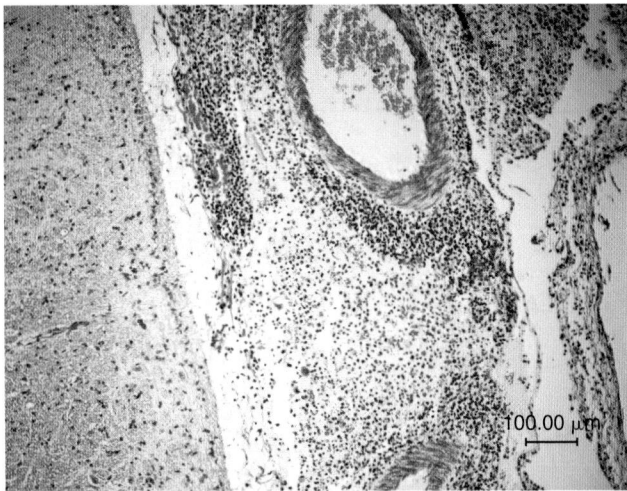

Figure 5-7: Brain and leptomeninges from a cat that died of *S. equi* ssp. *zooepidemicus* infection. Lymphoplasmacytic perivascular cuffing with expansion of the leptomeninges by neutrophils, macrophages and red blood cells. Hematoxylin and eosin (H&E) stain. (Copyright Dr. Ann Britton.)

castrated male cat living exclusively indoors with no known route of exposure has been published.[69] The cat was referred for evaluation of neurologic signs (dull mentation, head tilt, and vestibular ataxia). SEZ was isolated in high numbers from cerebrospinal fluid. The cat was initially treated with ampicillin/sulbactam and enrofloxacin. After the culture results were received, treatment was changed to trimethoprim/sulfamethoxazole and amoxicillin/clavulanic acid. Treatment was continued for 8 weeks, and the cat gradually made a full recovery.

The first report of SEZ infection in an exotic felid was published in 2012. A 16-year-old male snow leopard *(Panthera uncia)* died from meningoventriculitis due to SEZ within 1 month of the onset of neurologic signs.[70] This animal had been fed horse meat, which may have been the source of infection. Another possible route of SEZ exposure for both cats and humans is guinea pigs. In 2013, a small cluster of SEZ cases in humans was linked epidemiologically and genetically to infected guinea pigs.[71]

As in canine outbreaks of disease due to SEZ, contributing factors in feline outbreaks are not well understood. Although there is evidence that some canine outbreaks may be due to virulent SEZ strains, molecular analysis of feline isolates has not been reported. Environmental and management factors, as well as coinfections, may also play a role in feline disease outbreaks due to the majority of cases being reported in intensively housed populations. Unfortunately, there is a lack of knowledge about the incubation period and ease of transmission outside of the shelter environment, as well as the frequency and manner of shedding after recovery for highly pathogenic *S. canis* and SEZ infections in dogs and cats.

Control of SEZ and *S. canis* shelter outbreaks involves isolation of infected cats as the bacteria are shed in respiratory secretions.[56] Clinically affected, as well as exposed,

individuals should be treated with an appropriate antibiotic as early as possible; duration of treatment is suggested to be 2 weeks.[72] If humane care and adequate housing cannot be provided (e.g., for feral cats), euthanasia is recommended. Recovered cats should be quarantined for 2 weeks following complete resolution of clinical signs.[72] Steps should be taken to prevent fomite transmission; environmental cleaning and disinfection are very important. Streptococcal species are inactivated by commonly used quaternary ammonium compounds and oxidizing agents. They are also susceptible to phenol-based compounds, but these should not be used because they are known to be toxic to cats. Although antibiotic choices for treatment of *S. canis* are predictable, little has been published about antimicrobial sensitivities for SEZ in cats. In general, group C isolates would be expected to be susceptible to penicillin, erythromycin, chloramphenicol, and cephalosporins.[46]

Zoonotic Potential of *Streptococcus Equi*

Human infection with *S. equi* is rare but can be fatal. Septicemia, meningitis, pneumonia, arthritis, nephritis, and toxic shock cases have been reported in the literature. The first report of zoonotic transmission of SEZ from a dog occurred in 2010.[63] The dog in this report had chronic (rather than acute) respiratory tract disease. Genetic analysis of the SEZ isolate confirmed an identical organism in the dog and the person. To date, no reports have documented transmission from an infected cat to a human. Nevertheless, it is prudent to take measures to protect veterinary staff and owners when dealing with cats or dogs where SEZ infection is possible.

SEZ is likely to be an under-recognized cause of severe respiratory disease in cats because testing is not routinely part of URTD screening panels and the disease presents differently from the hemorrhagic form seen in dogs. Clinicians should be alert to the possibility of SEZ infection in cats with compatible clinical signs that come from high-density populations.

SUMMARY

Although streptococcal disease is common in animals, emerging clinical syndromes associated with *S. canis* and SEZ have been reported in cats in recent years. Clinical disease associated with *S. canis* is highly variable and most often involves individual cats—although shelter outbreaks of unusually severe, invasive disease have been reported. Clinicians should be aware of the clinical signs of STSS/NF as a high index of suspicion and prompt aggressive treatment is necessary. Disease associated with SEZ has not historically been documented in cats. Reports involving this emerging pathogen have primarily involved high-density populations but rarely may involve individual pet cats. Work remains to be done to further the understanding of risk factors, disease transmission, optimal treatment, and disease prevention for both pathogens.

References

1. Stallings B, Ling GV, Lagenaur LA, et al: Septicemia and septic arthritis caused by Streptococcus pneumoniae in a cat: possible transmission from a child. *J Am Vet Med Assoc* 191(6):703–704, 1987.

2. Zhang S, Wilson F, Pace L: Streptococcus pneumoniae-associated cellulitis in a two-month-old domestic shorthair kitten. *J Vet Diagn Invest* 18(2):221–224, 2006.

3. Dow SW, Jones RL, Thomas TN, et al: Group B streptococcal infection in two cats. *J Am Vet Med Assoc* 190(1):71–72, 1987.

4. Roels S, Devroye O, Buys H, et al: Isolation of Streptococcus suis from a cat with meningo-encephalitis. *Vet Microbiol* 136(1–2):206–207, 2009.

5. Devriese LA, Haesebrouck F: Streptococcus suis infections in horses and cats. *Vet Rec* 130(17):380, 1992.

6. Lysková P, Vydržalová M, Královcová D, et al: Prevalence and characteristics of Streptococcus canis strains isolated from dogs and cats. *Acta Vet Brno* 76(4):619–625, 2007.

7. Devriese LA, Cruz Colque JI, De Herdt P, et al: Identification and composition of the tonsillar and anal enterococcal and streptococcal flora of dogs and cats. *J Appl Bacteriol* 73(5):421–425, 1992.

8. Demko JL, Cohn LA: Chronic nasal discharge in cats: 75 cases (1993-2004). *J Am Vet Med Assoc* 230(7):1032–1037, 2007.

9. Johnson LR, Foley JE, De Cock HE, et al: Assessment of infectious organisms associated with chronic rhinosinusitis in cats. *J Am Vet Med Assoc* 227(4):579–585, 2005.

10. Strom Holst B, Bergstrom A, Lagerstedt AS, et al: Characterization of the bacterial population of the genital tract of adult cats. *Am J Vet Res* 64(8):963–968, 2003.

11. Clemetson LL, Ward ACS: Bacterial flora of the vagina and uterus of healthy cats. *J Am Vet Med Assoc* 196(6):902–905, 1990.

12. Lawler DF, Evans RH, Reimers TJ, et al: Histopathologic features, environmental factors, and serum estrogen, progesterone, and prolactin values associated with ovarian phase and inflammatory uterine disease in cats. *Am J Vet Res* 52(10):1747–1753, 1991.

13. Kenney KJ, Matthiesen DT, Brown NO, et al: Pyometra in cats: 183 cases (1979-1984). *J Am Vet Med Assoc* 191(9):1130–1132, 1987.

14. Axnér E, Ågren E, Båverud V, et al: Infertility in the cycling queen: seven cases. *J Feline Med Surg* 10(6):566–576, 2008.

15. Roy J, Messier S, Labrecque O, et al: Clinical and in vitro efficacy of amoxicillin against bacteria associated with feline skin wounds and abscesses. *Can Vet J* 48(6):607–611, 2007.

16. Malik R, Barrs VR, Church DB, et al: Vegetative endocarditis in six cats. *J Feline Med Surg* 1(3):171, 1999.

17. Matsuu A, Kanda T, Sugiyama A, et al: Mitral stenosis with bacterial myocarditis in a cat. *J Vet Med Sci* 69(11):1171–1174, 2007.

18. Bedford SW: Streptococcal suppurative lymphadenitis in a cat. *Vet Rec* 144(1):28, 1999.

19. Swindle MM, Narayan O, Luzarraga M, et al: Contagious streptococcal lymphadenitis in cats. *J Am Vet Med Assoc* 177(9):829–830, 1980.

20. Van der Heyden S, Butaye P, Roels S: Cholesterol granuloma associated with otitis media and leptomeningitis in a cat due to Streptococcus canis infection. *Can Vet J* 154(1):72–73, 2013.

21. Malik R, Latter M, Love DN: Bacterial discospondylitis in a cat. *J Small Anim Pract* 31(8):404–406, 1990.

22. Goldman PM, Moore TD: Spontaneous Lancefield group G streptococcal infection in a random source cat colony. *Lab Anim Sci* 23(4):565–566, 1973.

23. Tillman PC, Dodson ND, Indiveri M: Group G streptococcal epizootic in a closed cat colony. *J Clin Microbiol* 16(6):1057–1060, 1982.

24. Wu CC, Kiupel M, Raymond JT, et al: Group G streptococcal infection in a cat colony. *J Vet Diagn Invest* 11(2):174–177, 1999.

25. Iglauer F, Kunstýr I, Mörstedt R, et al: Streptococcus canis arthritis in a cat breeding colony. *J Exp Anim Sci* 34(2):59–65, 1991.

26. Commons RJ, Smeesters PR, Proft T, et al: Streptococcal superantigens: categorization and clinical associations. *Trends Mol Med* 20(1):48–62, 2014.

27. Low DE: Toxic shock syndrome: major advances in pathogenesis, but not treatment. *Crit Care Clin* 29(3):651–675, 2013.

28. Francis KR, Lamaute HR, Davis JM, et al: Implications of risk factors in necrotizing fasciitis. *Am Surg* 59(5):304–308, 1993.

29. Sykes JE: Streptococcal and enterococcal infections. In *Canine and feline infectious diseases*, St Louis, 2013, Elsevier/Saunders, pp 334–346.

30. Wong CH, Khin LW, Heng KS, et al: The LRINEC (Laboratory Risk Indicator for Necrotizing Fasciitis) score: a tool for distinguishing necrotizing fasciitis from other soft tissue infections. *Crit Care Med* 32(7):1535–1541, 2004.

31. Naidoo SL, Campbell DL, Miller LM, et al: Necrotizing fasciitis: a review. *J Am Anim Hosp Assoc* 41:104–109, 2005.

32. Prescott JF, Miller CW, Mathews KA, et al: Update on canine streptococcal toxic shock syndrome and necrotizing fasciitis. *Can Vet J* 38(4):241–242, 1997.

33. Prescott JF, Mathews K, Gyles CL, et al: Canine streptococcal toxic shock syndrome in Ontario: an emerging disease? *Can Vet J* 36(8):486–487, 1995.

34. Miller CW, Prescott JF, Mathews KA, et al: Streptococcal toxic shock syndrome in dogs. *J Am Vet Med Assoc* 209(8):1421–1426, 1996.

35. Taillefer M, Dunn M: Group G streptococcal toxic shock-like syndrome in three cats. *J Am Anim Hosp Assoc* 40:418–422, 2004.

36. Hess MO: Necrotising fasciitis due to Prevotella bivia in a cat. *J Small Anim Pract* 50(10):558–560, 2009.

37. Brachelente C, Wiener D, Malik Y, et al: A case of necrotizing fasciitis with septic shock in a cat caused by Acinetobacter baumannii. *Vet Dermatol* 18(6):432–438, 2007.

38. Berube DE, Whelan MF, Tater KC, et al: Fournier's gangrene in a cat. *J Vet Emerg Crit Care (San Antonio)* 20(1):148–154, 2010.

39. Vaske H, Ragan I, Harkin K, et al: Successful conservative management of suspected Fournier's gangrene in cats: 3 cases. *J Feline Med Surg Open Reports* 1(1):2055116915589837, 2015.

40. Sura R, Hinckley LS, Risatti GR, et al: Fatal necrotising fasciitis and myositis in a cat associated with Streptococcus canis. *Vet Rec* 162(14):450–453, 2008.

41. Nolff MC, Meyer-Lindenberg A: Necrotising fasciitis in a domestic shorthair cat—negative pressure wound therapy assisted débridement and reconstruction. *J Small Anim Pract* 56(4):218–284, 2015.

42. Pesavento PA, Bannasch MJ, Bachmann R, et al: Fatal *Streptococcus canis* infections in intensively housed shelter cats. *Vet Pathol* 44(2):218–221, 2007.

43. Kruger EF, Byrne BA, Pesavento P, et al: Relationship between clinical manifestations and pulsed-field gel profiles of *Streptococcus canis* isolates from dogs and cats. *Vet Microbiol* 146(1–2):167–171, 2010.

44. Schwarz S, Alesík E, Grobbel M, et al: Antimicrobial susceptibility of streptococci from various indications of swine, horses, dogs and cats as determined in the BfT-GermVet monitoring program 2004-2006. *Berl Munch Tierarztl Wochenschr* 120(9–10):380–390, 2007.

45. Greene CE, Prescott JF: Streptococcal infections. In Greene CE, editor: *Infectious diseases of the dog and cat*, ed 4, St Louis, 2012, Elsevier/Saunders, pp 325–332.

46. Blanchard P, Wilson D: Group G streptococcal infections in kittens. In Kirk RW, editor: *Current veterinary therapy X: Small animal practice*, Philadelphia, 1989, Saunders, pp 1091–1093.

47. Ingrey KT, Ren J, Prescott JF: A fluoroquinolone induces a novel mitogen-encoding bacteriophage in Streptococcus canis. *Infect Immun* 71(6):3028–3033, 2003.

48. Csiszer AB, Towle HA, Daly CM: Successful treatment of necrotizing fasciitis in the hind limb of a great dane. *J Am Anim Hosp Assoc* 46(6):433–438, 2010.

49. Maguire P, Azagrar J, Carb A: The successful use of negative-pressure wound therapy in two cases of canine necrotizing fasciitis. *J Am Anim Hosp Assoc* 51(1):43–48, 2015.

50. Wagner JG, Schlievert PM, Assimacopoulos AP, et al: Acute group G streptococcal myositis associated with streptococcal toxic shock syndrome: case report and review. *Clin Infect Dis* 23(5):1159–1161, 1996.

51. Pelkonen S, Lindahl SB, Suomala P, et al: Transmission of Streptococcus equi subspecies zooepidemicus infection from horses to

humans. *Emerg Infect Dis* 19(7):1041–1048, 2014.

52. Sundberg JP, Hill D, Wyand DS, et al: Streptococcus zooepidemicus as the cause of septicemia in racing greyhounds. *Vet Med Small Anim Clin* 76(6):839–842, 1981.

53. Garnett NL, Eydelloth RS, Swindle MM, et al: Hemorrhagic streptococcal pneumonia in newly procured research dogs. *J Am Vet Med Assoc* 181(11):1371–1374, 1982.

54. Byun JW, Yoon SS, Woo GH, et al: An outbreak of fatal hemorrhagic pneumonia caused by Streptococcus equi subsp. zooepidemicus in shelter dogs. *J Vet Sci* 10(3):269–271, 2009.

55. Kim MK, Jee H, Shin SW, et al: Outbreak and control of haemorrhagic pneumonia due to Streptococcus equi subspecies zooepidemicus in dogs. *Vet Rec* 161(15):528–530, 2007.

56. Pesavento PA, Hurley KF, Bannasch MJ, et al: A clonal outbreak of acute fatal hemorrhagic pneumonia in intensively housed (shelter) dogs caused by Streptococcus equi subsp. zooepidemicus. *Vet Pathol* 45(1):51–53, 2008.

57. Priestnall S, Erles K: Streptococcus zooepidemicus: an emerging canine pathogen. *Vet J* 188(2):142–148, 2011.

58. Chalker VJ, Brooks HW, Brownlie J: The association of Streptococcus equi subsp. zooepidemicus with canine infectious respiratory disease. *Vet Microbiol* 95(1–2):149–156, 2003.

59. Polak KC, Levy JK, Crawford PC, et al: Infectious diseases in large-scale cat hoarding investigations. *Vet J* 201(2):189–195, 2014.

60. Chalker VJ, Waller A, Webb K, et al: Genetic diversity of Streptococcus equi subsp. zooepidemicus and doxycycline resistance in kennelled dogs. *J Clin Microbiol* 50(6):2134–2136, 2012.

61. Acke E, Abbott Y, Pinilla M, et al: Isolation of Streptococcus zooepidemicus from three dogs in close contact with horses. *Vet Rec* 167(3):102–103, 2010.

62. Piva S, Zanoni RG, Specchi S, et al: Chronic rhinitis due to Streptococcus equi subspecies zooepidemicus in a dog. *Vet Rec* 167(5):177–178, 2010.

63. Abbott Y, Acke E, Khan S, et al: Zoonotic transmission of Streptococcus equi subsp. zooepidemicus from a dog to a handler. *J Med Microbiol* 59(1):120–123, 2010.

64. Macdonald ES, Norris CR, Berghaus RB, et al: Clinicopathologic and radiographic features and etiologic agents in cats with histologically confirmed infectious pneumonia: 39 cases (1991-2000). *J Am Vet Med Assoc* 223(8):1142–1150, 2003.

65. Foster SF, Martin P, Allan GS, et al: Lower respiratory tract infections in cats: 21 cases (1995-2000). *J Feline Med Surg* 6(3):167–180, 2004.

66. Bart M, Guscetti F, Zurbriggen A, et al: Feline infectious pneumonia: a short literature review and a retrospective immunohistological study on the involvement of Chlamydia spp. and distemper virus. *Vet J* 159(3):220–230, 2000.

67. Blum S, Elad D, Zukin N, et al: Outbreak of Streptococcus equi subsp. zooepidemicus infections in cats. *Vet Microbiol* 144(1–2):236–239, 2010.

68. Britton AP, Davies JL: Rhinitis and meningitis in two shelter cats caused by Streptococcus equi subspecies zooepidemicus. *J Comp Pathol* 143(1):70–74, 2010.

69. Martin-Vaquero P, da Costa RC, Daniels JB: Presumptive meningoencephalitis secondary to extension of otitis media/interna caused by Streptococcus equi subspecies zooepidemicus in a cat. *J Feline Med Surg* 13(8):606–609, 2011.

70. Yamaguchi R, Nakamura S, Hori H, et al: Purulent meningoventriculitis caused by Streptococcus equi subspecies zooepidemicus in a snow leopard (Panthera uncia). *J Comp Pathol* 147(2–3):397–400, 2012.

71. Gruszynski K, Young A, Levine SJ, et al: Streptococcus equi subsp. zooepidemicus infections associated with guinea pigs. *Emerg Infect Dis* 21(1):2015.

72. Hurley KF, Pesavento PA: Emerging streptococcal diseases of dogs and cats. ACVIM Forum/Canadian VMA Convention. Montreal, QC, 2009, pp 512–514.

Dealing with Toxoplasmosis: Clinical Presentation, Diagnosis, Treatment, and Prevention

Susan Foster

Toxoplasma gondii is an obligate, intracellular Apicomplexan parasite. The Apicomplexa is a large, diverse group of eukaryocytes, most of which possess a unique organelle called an apicoplast (a vestigial plastid that is the site of manufacture and storage of a range of important chemical compounds) and an apical complex structure (involved in penetrating a host's cell).

T. gondii infects virtually all species of mammals. Domestic cats and other Felidae are the definitive hosts that excrete oocysts. Both Felidae and non-Felidae can act as intermediate hosts that harbor tissue cysts. There are three infectious stages: sporozoites in oocysts, tachyzoites (actively multiplying stage), and bradyzoites enclosed in tissue cysts (slowly multiplying stage). Transmission is usually by ingestion of infected tissues or oocyst-contaminated food or water, but congenital infection also occurs.

T. gondii was initially described as being highly clonal and exhibiting a low genetic diversity because in North America and Europe, isolates were predominantly from three *T. gondii* clonal lineages designated as types I, II, and III.[1-3] Studies of genetic polymorphism revealed that at each gene locus there were only two alleles, indicating that these three lineages arose from a common source and that they have since undergone limited genetic exchange.[4,5] However, in regions of the world other than North America and Europe and in select niches within Europe and North America, types I, II, and III do not predominate.[1] Some isolates have mixtures of the two-allele patterns seen in the type strains, indicating that they are natural recombinants. Less common are exotic strains which have many unique polymorphisms, indicating they have a more ancient origin.[5] South America has the greatest diversity of strains of any region yet examined,[1,2] suggesting that South America may have been the birthplace of *Toxoplasma*.[1]

The clonal types of *T. gondii* show different virulence in mice: type I always causes lethal infection whereas types II and III are far less virulent. Less is known about genotype and virulence in feline toxoplasmosis. In experimental infection of immunocompetent cats, parenteral infection with type I *T. gondii* (RH strain) resulted in severe to fatal disease.[6] Parenteral infection with type II (ME49 strain) has usually led to mild transient signs of which chorioretinitis has been

the most specific,[7] although the ME49 strain has caused death (or resulted in euthanasia) in experimentally infected cats.[8-11] A type II (Apico I) *T. gondii* also led to fatal systemic toxoplasmosis in a naturally infected, apparently immunocompetent cat.[3] Natural infection with *T. gondii* of the type 12 lineage (a fourth clonal lineage recognized in North American wildlife) has caused disease in a North American domestic cat.[12] Further genotype information in clinical cases will be required to assess clinical relevance of clonal lineage in cats.

CLINICAL PRESENTATION

Clinical signs may have a sudden onset, and disease can be rapidly fatal in some cats. In other cats there may be a slower onset and progression. It is yet to be determined whether the type and severity of clinical illness depends on the strain of *T. gondii*, host genotype, or both. However, for practical purposes, type and severity can be related to the degree of tissue injury and location. Tachyzoites are the invasive asexual forms of the parasite that require intracellular existence for replication and survival. Cell necrosis is caused by the intracellular growth of *T. gondii*.

Cats ingesting sporulated oocysts or tissue bradyzoites have necrosis of the intestine and associated lymphoid organs and can develop self-limiting, small bowel diarrhea lasting up to 10 days. However, it is more usual that this phase of illness is subclinical.[13] Clinical signs in cats can occur after acute exposure or reactivation of tissue cysts, with release of bradyzoites, following immunosuppression. Clinical toxoplasmosis from systemic spread is most severe in transplacentally or lactationally infected kittens because tachyzoite replication can be overwhelming.[13,14]

In 100 cats with histologically confirmed systemic toxoplasmosis, lesions in the available tissues were most commonly found in lungs (97.7%), central nervous system (CNS) (96.4%), liver (93.3%), pancreas (84.4%), heart (86.4%), and eyes (81.8%).[15] The lung appears to be a common target organ in both primary and reactivated toxoplasmosis in cats.[16]

Kittens with toxoplasmosis may be stillborn or die before weaning. Clinical signs pertain to involvement of the liver, lungs, and CNS. Lethargy, depression, hypothermia, and sudden death can occur, with some kittens suckling until death.[13] Kittens may have abdominal distension due to an enlarged liver and ascites. Encephalitic kittens may sleep most of the time or cry continuously.[13] It is not known how frequently kittens develop toxoplasmosis as many kitten deaths and illnesses are not investigated or reported. It is also not known whether the genotype of *T. gondii* is important. Kittens born to queens experimentally infected with Mozart, Maggie, or ME49 strains of *T. gondii* develop chorioretinitis (some with transient concurrent anterior uveitis), sometimes in absence of other illness.[8] Lesion differences were found in kittens from queens infected with the Mozart strain of *T. gondii* compared with kittens from queens infected with ME49 or Maggie strains; however, other experimental factors may have been responsible.[8]

In older cats, anorexia, lethargy, and dyspnea are commonly recognized features of clinical toxoplasmosis[13]; coughing, although less common, has also been reported.[17] Persistent or intermittent fever is a frequent finding[13,15] with some cats paradoxically eating well despite a high fever.[15] Weight loss and wasting are commonly reported in case reports and series.[18-27] Icterus caused by liver or pancreatic involvement was recorded in 24% of 100 fatal feline cases.[15] Abdominal pain or discomfort, likely attributable to hepatitis, pancreatitis, or discomfort from interference with respiration in cats with pneumonia, is a frequent finding,[15] and abdominal effusion may be present.[13,15] Eosinophilic fibrosing gastritis has been reported in one cat with confirmed toxoplasmosis.[28]

Anterior or posterior uveitis in one or both eyes is common. Iritis, iridocyclitis, or chorioretinitis can occur alone or concomitantly.[13] Ocular toxoplasmosis occurs in some cats without systemic clinical signs of disease.[13] Both ocular and neurologic manifestations in the absence of other systemic signs are reportedly more common with reactivated infection than acute infection.[13]

Signs attributable to CNS involvement have been variable and include hypothermia, blindness, increased affectionate behavior, stupor, inability to stand, extensor rigidity, hind limb paralysis and inability to urinate, incoordination, atypical cry, ear twitch, circling, torticollis, head bobbing, anisocoria and seizures.[15,18,20,24,27,29]

Other reported findings include vomiting, diarrhea, cardiac arrhythmias, splenomegaly, lymphadenomegaly, muscle hyperesthesia, muscle atrophy, lower motor neuron deficits, stiffness of gait, lameness, joint pain, cutaneous nodules and sudden death.[13,15,19,20,30] Abdominal mass lesions have been recorded in naturally occurring cases of toxoplasmosis.[25,26]

Risk of clinical toxoplasmosis is increased with immunocompromise caused by infection (e.g., feline immunodeficiency virus [FIV], feline leukemia virus, feline infectious peritonitis, hemoplasmosis) or drug therapy.* There are an increasing number of reports of toxoplasmosis in cats that have been treated with cyclosporine.[16,32-34,36,37] Clinical cases of toxoplasmosis in immunosuppressed cats often feature respiratory signs and pulmonary pathology.[16]

DIAGNOSIS

Hematology

Hematology findings are nonspecific. There may be anemia, leukocytosis, or leukopenia. In severely affected cats, leukopenia can persist until death. Experimentally, leukocytosis has been associated with the recovery phase,[13] although neutrophilic leukocytosis also occurs in fatal clinical cases.[23,26,38] A left shift,[22,23,26,32,39] sometimes degenerative,[3,17] has been reported in a number of cases. Lymphopenia,[17,23,32,35,38-40] likely stress related, is often present. Eosinophilia is listed as a common finding.[13] However, although two cases in one case series were reported to have eosinophilia,[20] eosinophilia seems to be rarely reported in published clinical cases* and was not present in a cat with eosinophilic lesions.[28]

Serum Biochemistry and Urinalysis

The most common serum biochemical abnormalities would appear to be increased bilirubin, alanine aminotransferase (ALT), and aspartate aminotransferase (AST).† Increases in AST or ALT activity may reflect liver or muscle necrosis.[13] Creatine kinase can be increased if there is muscle necrosis.[13] Hyperproteinemia due to hyperalbuminemia[20] or hyperglobulinemia[19,20,41] may be noted, although hypoproteinemia and hypoalbuminemia can occur during acute illness.[13,26,32,33] Although serum amylase is not commonly increased in cats with pancreatitis, when pancreatitis occurs due to toxoplasmosis, increased serum amylase may be present.[15,23] It is not known whether feline pancreatic lipase immunoreactivity (fPLI) is a more sensitive marker of pancreatitis in cats with toxoplasmosis because the majority of the clinical literature on toxoplasmosis preceded the development of this assay. Bilirubinuria and proteinuria may be present on urinalysis.[15]

Cytology and Histopathology

Tachyzoites can be detected in various tissues and body fluids by cytology during acute illness but are rarely found in blood or cerebrospinal fluid (CSF). More commonly, they are detected in peritoneal or thoracic effusions.[13] Although it is reported that tachyzoites are rarely found in transtracheal aspirate (TTA) or bronchoalveolar lavage (BAL) samples,[13,42] BAL/TTA has enabled a definitive diagnosis of toxoplasmosis in a number of cats.[16] An experimental study also demonstrated BAL cytology to be useful in the diagnosis of toxoplasmosis in cats and more sensitive than histologic examination of tissues for identification of tachyzoites.[11]

---

*References 7,18,22,24,26,31-37.

*References 3,17,22,23,26,35,38-40.
†References 3,10,15,17,20,22,23,26,28,33.

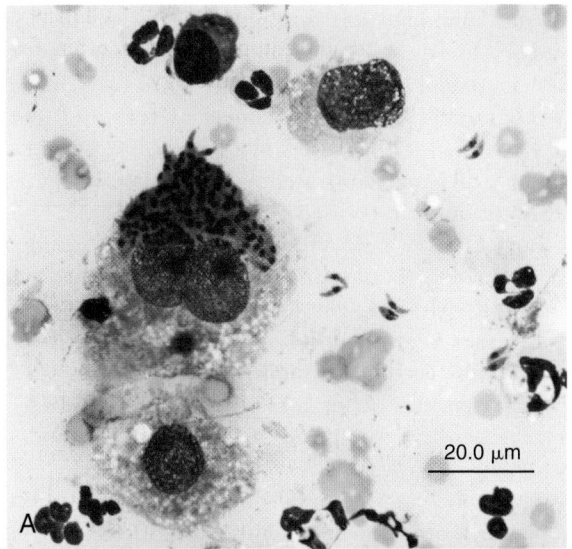

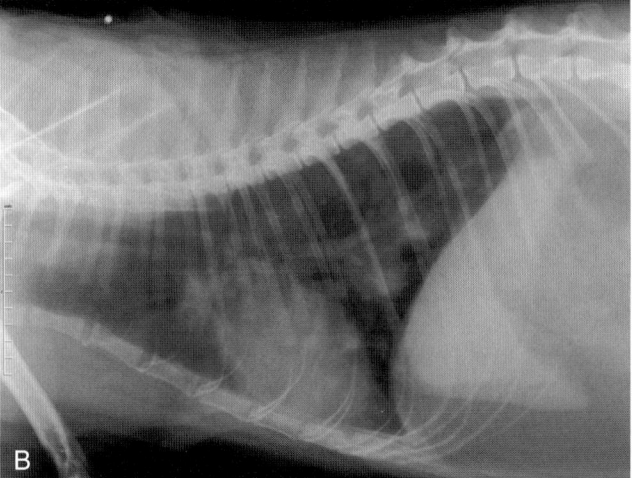

Figure 6-1: A, Diff Quick-stained smear of a fine-needle lung aspirate obtained under ultrasound guidance from one of the pulmonary nodules in the cat shown in part B. Note the individual tachyzoites and an aggregate of tachyzoites within a macrophage. The cat was successfully treated with clindamycin and pyrimethamine.[16] **B,** Left lateral radiograph of a 7-year-old, castrated, male Devon Rex, which had been treated with cyclosporine and developed toxoplasmosis. Throughout all lung lobes are multiple, rounded, variably sized nodules. Although there are a number of differential diagnoses (including abscesses, granulomas, and hematomas), this nodular pattern could have resulted in a misdiagnosis of pulmonary neoplasia. (**A,** Case details courtesy of Dr. Katherine Briscoe. In Foster SF, Martin P: Lower respiratory tract infections in cats. Reaching beyond empirical therapy. *J Feline Med Surg* 13:313-332, 2011.)

Lung fine-needle aspiration (FNA) cytology has enabled the diagnosis of *T. gondii* infection[16,37] (Figure 6-1A); however, FNA cytology and lung biopsy evaluation sometimes fail to identify *T. gondii*.[16,18,19] In addition, with organisms not always evident and cellular features sometimes consistent with neoplasia, FNA cytology can be misleading.[18,19] Detection of *T. gondii* by polymerase chain reaction (PCR) is considered more sensitive and specific than cytologic or histopathologic detection of the organism, so PCR should be considered if toxoplasmosis is suspected but not demonstrated cytologically.[14]

Cerebrospinal Fluid Analysis

Published CSF abnormalities vary. Protein is reportedly increased[41,43] or normal to increased.[13] Gunn-Moore and Reed[43] described a mildly increased number of lymphocytes (and occasionally neutrophils) which would be in agreement with Lappin.[14] However, one reported case had a mild suppurative inflammation[41] with neutrophils comprising more than 50% of the nucleated cells.

Radiology

Thoracic radiographic findings, especially in cats with acute disease, usually consist of a diffuse interstitial to alveolar pattern with a patchy distribution[13,17,22,33,39]; mild to marked pleural effusion can be present.[3,13,32]

However, radiographic signs are variable, and symmetrical alveolar coalescence has been noted in some severely affected animals[13] and asymmetric lung lobe consolidation in others.[22] Of particular concern are radiographs demonstrating a discrete mass[19] or a nodular pattern.[18] Nodules may be ill-defined[33] and appear to adjoin bronchi[18,44] or well-defined (see Figure 6-1B). The combination of a nodular pattern of radiographic change and cytology suggestive of neoplasia has resulted in misdiagnosis of pulmonary carcinoma in cats with toxoplasmosis.[16,18,19] It is prudent to assume any cyclosporine-treated cat with a nodular pulmonary pattern has clinical toxoplasmosis until proven otherwise. In addition, the possibility of other opportunistic infections, such as mycobacteriosis, is worth considering.[45]

Abdominal radiographic findings may consist of masses in intestines or mesenteric lymph nodes or a homogeneous increase in density due to effusion. Loss of contrast in the right abdominal quadrant can indicate pancreatitis. Organ pathology may also be present on ultrasonographic examination.

Fecal Oocysts

There is a high prevalence of feline exposure to *T. gondii* worldwide with, for example, 9% to 87% seroprevalence in North, Central, and South America and the Caribbean.[46] However, the prevalence of oocysts in feces is low (<1%) in most feline populations[46] because shedding usually occurs for only 1 to 2 weeks postexposure.[13] Some cats experimentally reinfected with a different strain of *T. gondii* from that used in initial challenge (or challenges) 6 years prior have been shown to reshed oocysts.[10]

Oocysts are only rarely found in cats ill with systemic toxoplasmosis. In a study of 100 cats with clinical toxoplasmosis in 1993 by Dubey and Carpenter,[15] only two cats had *T. gondii*-like oocysts.[15] Presumably, these were both young cats because it was stated in 1995 by Dubey[10] that there was only one report, unrelated to the 1993 study,[15] of oocyst shedding occurring in a naturally infected adult cat with clinical toxoplasmosis.[10] Experimental immunosuppression with doses of corticosteroids that would exceed those used clinically has resulted in re-excretion of oocysts, but commonly used anti-inflammatory or immunosuppressive doses of glucocorticoids do not appear to predispose to reactivated toxoplasmosis.[13,14] It should be noted that it is not possible to distinguish *T. gondii* oocysts from oocysts of *Hammondia* or *Besnoitia* species on routine microscopy; thus mouse bioassay is the usual method of differentiation in experimental studies.[46] In an individual cat, performing *T. gondii* serology and documenting seroconversion within 3 weeks of oocyst detection is more practical.

Serum Antibody Tests

Serologic tests for detection of *T. gondii*-specific antibodies do not provide a definitive diagnosis. Following initial exposure, immunoglobulin M (IgM) increases first, and this is followed by increased immunoglobulin G (IgG). Once infected, animals have *Toxoplasma* tissue cysts for life, and this stimulates a long-term humoral immune response in infected cats. Prevalence of seropositivity increases with age because of increased chance of exposure with time rather than increased susceptibility.[13]

Theoretically a high IgM titer with negative IgG titer indicates a recent exposure. Documentation of an increasing IgG titer (fourfold or greater) can also verify recent infection but not necessarily oocyst shedding or clinical disease.[13] A high IgG titer with a negative IgM titer indicates chronic infection.

However, there are numerous confounding possibilities with serologic testing. After experimental inoculation, most cats are positive for *T. gondii*-specific IgM within 2 weeks.[47] However, some cats do not have increased IgM until 4 to 10 weeks postinfection despite having detectable IgG titers after 3 to 6 weeks, depending on the assay used.[47] In addition, approximately 20% of cats do not develop IgM titers, and the antibody class shift from IgM to IgG may not occur in FIV-infected cats or cats treated with glucocorticoids.[13] IgM is also occasionally detected in the serum of cats with chronic or reactivated infection, and IgM may persist in some cats for months to years after infection.[13,47]

IgG testing is also problematic. In most cats, there is a narrow window for documentation of a rising titer with maximal titers being reached in 2 to 3 weeks, although some cats may not develop IgG titers for 4 to 6 weeks[13,48] and some will die before IgG titers are increased.[15] IgG in chronically affected queens is transferred in colostrum to kittens, and these maternal antibodies persist for 8 to 12 weeks after birth.[49] High IgG titers do not prove recent or active infection. Chronic persistence of high IgG titers merely reflects continued presence of *Toxoplasma* antigen after infection[13] and does not preclude the possibility of reshedding oocysts.[10]

Thus antibody class does not accurately predict the oocyst-shedding period, likelihood of oocyst shedding, or stage of infection. Magnitude of titer is also not helpful, with some healthy cats having extremely high titers and some clinically ill cats having low titers.[14] There is no clinical value in repeat-ing serum antibody titers to monitor resolution of clinical disease because animals are antibody-positive for life.[14]

Test methodology must be known when assessing antibody test results. There are a number of tests available for detection of *T. gondii*-specific antibodies. Indirect fluorescent antibody (IFA) and enzyme-linked immunosorbent assay (ELISA) testing can be used for detection of IgM, IgG, or immunoglobulin A (IgA). The indirect hemagglutination test (IHA) primarily measures IgG as does the modified agglutination test (MAT).[13] The latex agglutination test (LAT) cannot be used to distinguish immunoglobulin class. In comparing sensitivities, ELISA methods are as sensitive as IFA and more sensitive than LAT or IHA.[13] The MAT is extremely sensitive compared to the other methods for detecting IgG. With the MAT, antibodies to acetone-fixed (AF) tachyzoites are increased only during acute infection (less than 3 months), whereas antibodies to formalin-fixed (FF) tachyzoites can remain high for years.[13] This phenomenon has been attributed to the variation in IgG profiles in response to shifting *Toxoplasma* surface antigens as the infection progresses from an acute to a more chronic stage. The acetone preparation contains stage-specific antigens, which are recognized by IgG antibodies formed against *Toxoplasma* tachyzoites early in infection. These antibodies have different specificities from those formed later in infection.[50] The differential agglutination test, which compares AF titers with FF titers, has been used in human medicine to help differentiate acute and chronic infections in immunocompromised individuals and pregnant women. However, the absence of knowledge about the exact time of infection in humans has made it difficult to provide an accurate time of conversion of the acute to nonacute pattern in the differential agglutination test.[50] The differential agglutination test has now been further tested experimentally in mice in combination with ELISA IgG and IgM testing to differentiate between acute and late experimental toxoplasmosis in this species.[50] The potential usefulness for such testing in cats is unknown.

Polymerase Chain Reaction

T. gondii DNA can be detected in the blood of healthy cats so that positive PCR results do not necessarily indicate clinical disease.[14,51] The source of the organism in these cats could be bradyzoites from tissue cysts or tachyzoites in subclinically affected cats.[14,51] The main roles for PCR in veterinary medicine are confirming toxoplasmosis when *T. gondii*-like organisms are seen cytologically or histologically, demonstrating the presence of *T. gondii* when there is a high likelihood of toxoplasmosis clinically or histologically but no organisms found in the sample, or diagnosing ocular or CNS toxoplasmosis when used in conjunction with antibody testing on aqueous humor or CSF (see later). PCR assays may also be used more in the future to determine which strains of *T. gondii* are responsible for infection in clinical cases.[1]

For routine PCR analysis, fresh samples can be submitted. Tissues, fluids, or aspirates for *T. gondii* PCR testing can also be maintained frozen until assayed because DNA is very stable.[14] PCR assays are reportedly less sensitive on FF samples; however, immunohistochemistry can be performed on these samples.[14]

Aqueous Humor and Cerebrospinal Fluid Antibody and Antigen Testing

Testing for antibodies and antigen in aqueous humor and CSF may be more useful than serologic tests. *T. gondii*-specific IgA, IgG, and DNA can be detected in aqueous humor and CSF of both normal and clinically ill cats. When assessing specific antibodies in aqueous humor or CSF, those produced locally must be differentiated from those passively diffusing across a damaged vascular barrier. This can be done by calculating the Goldmann-Witmer coefficient (GWC). For *T. gondii* the coefficient is defined as GWC = X/Y, in which X is *T. gondii*-specific antibody in aqueous or CSF sample divided by total IgG in sample, and Y is *T. gondii*-specific antibody in serum divided by total IgG in serum. Alternatively, an antibody coefficient can be calculated by measuring a specific antibody for a nonocular infectious agent, such as feline calicivirus, for comparison instead of total IgG.[13] Coefficients of 1 to 8 are suggestive of local production of antibody, and coefficients greater than 8 provide definitive evidence for local production of antibody.[13,52] However, unpublished data indicate that *T. gondii*-specific IgM has only been detected in the aqueous humor or CSF of clinically ill cats; this may be the best indicator of clinical disease.[14]

The presence of *T. gondii* in aqueous humor as detected by PCR may correlate to clinical disease in some but not all cats.[53] Some ophthalmoscopically normal cats have *T. gondii* detected in aqueous humor by PCR. Conversely, cats with posterior segment disease may have the organism localized in vitreous rather than aqueous humor, resulting in false negative tests.[53] In humans, ocular toxoplasmosis is diagnosed by ophthalmic examination but in cats, ophthalmic findings are not pathognomonic; thus calculation of sensitivity, specificity, and predictive values for PCR testing on aqueous humor samples in cats is not possible.[53]

The combination of *T. gondii*-specific IgM antibody detection in aqueous humor or CSF and organism DNA amplification by PCR is reportedly the most accurate way to diagnose ocular or CNS toxoplasmosis in cats,[14] but comprehensive data on sensitivity and specificity are lacking. In addition, assessment of commercially available PCR assays is often difficult as few, if any, technical details are routinely provided.

Summary

Definitive diagnosis of clinical toxoplasmosis requires demonstration of *T. gondii* tachyzoites in tissues or fluids by cytology, histopathology, or immunohistochemistry. Ocular or CNS toxoplasmosis may be diagnosed with a combination of PCR and IgM testing on aqueous humor or CSF, respectively. Because a definitive diagnosis is not always possible

antemortem, a provisional diagnosis may be made when there is a combination of serologic evidence of recent or active infection (high IgM titer or fourfold or greater increase in IgG titer), exclusion of other causes of clinical signs, and beneficial clinical response to appropriate therapy.

TREATMENT

Drug therapy for toxoplasmosis in humans has long centered on inhibitors of parasite nucleotide metabolisms, specifically pyrimethamine (inhibiting dihydrofolate reductase) and sulfa-based compounds (inhibiting dihydropteroate synthase). Clindamycin, an antibiotic that inhibits prokaryotic translation machinery, has proven effective as a second-line drug.[1]

In cats, clindamycin is routinely recommended as a first-line drug for treatment of toxoplasmosis, with concurrent topical, oral, or injectable corticosteroids if there is anterior uveitis.[13] Trimethoprim sulfonamide has also been recommended.[14] However, it is important to note that there has been no published work comparing the relative clinical efficacy of drugs used to treat feline toxoplasmosis. In addition, as there has been little genotyping in clinical cases of feline toxoplasmosis to determine the virulence and drug susceptibility of different strains, it is difficult to assess drug efficacy in reported cases.

Clindamycin

Clindamycin is the most commonly used first-line drug for feline toxoplasmosis. Clindamycin targets ribosomes in the plastid (apicoplast),[54,55] but the effect of the drug is delayed because complete loss of plastid DNA is required. Given the relatively high copy number of DNA in each plastid, this could take several parasite divisions to occur.[54] Thus the antimicrobial effect of clindamycin is delayed *in vitro* for 1 to 3 days.[56]

The recommended dose of clindamycin is 10 to 12.5 mg/kg every 12 hours by mouth (PO) for 4 weeks[14,42] with each oral dose followed by a food or water swallow to prevent possible esophagitis.[57] If oral dosing is not possible, clindamycin can be given subcutaneously at the same dose. It is reported that clinical signs of systemic illness, including inappetence, fever, and hyperesthesia, usually begin to resolve within 24 to 48 hours of clindamycin therapy, and active chorioretinitis generally subsides within 1 week.[13] Lower motor neuron deficits and muscle atrophy may take longer (e.g., weeks) to resolve in animals with polymyositis, and neurologic deficits may not totally resolve because of permanent damage.[13] It is recommended that cats with anterior uveitis should be treated with clindamycin and concurrent topical, oral, or injectable corticosteroids to avoid potential adverse sequelae, such as lens luxation and glaucoma. Although anti-inflammatory doses of glucocorticoids are not likely to exacerbate systemic disease, topical glucocorticoid therapy is still preferable.[13]

Despite being widely accepted, these recommendations warrant further analysis. A study of clindamycin efficacy in an experimental model of acute feline toxoplasmosis with the ME49 strain demonstrated that there was increased morbidity and mortality from hepatitis and interstitial pneumonia in both clindamycin treatment groups (12.5 mg/kg every 12 hours PO or 11 mg/kg every 24 hours PO) compared with both control groups (placebo once or twice daily PO).[9] Possible causes for this were discussed, including the potential for clindamycin to inhibit phagocyte action.[9] In addition, the report noted that clindamycin is more suppressive than curative for *T. gondii*, concentrations found to be inhibitory *in vitro* may not be achieved *in vivo*, and the antimicrobial effect of clindamycin is delayed.[9] It is also reported that clindamycin is not effective against extracellular tachyzoites.[58]

Although it has been stated that disease-enhancing effects of clindamycin have not been substantiated in naturally infected cats,[13] a number of cats in the literature have died (or been euthanized due to clinical deterioration) despite clindamycin treatment.[16,28,36,40] Assessment of the efficacy of clindamycin in clinical cases is thus difficult, especially without strain and virulence data. Clindamycin was reported to be efficacious in one North American case study[20]; however, the selection criteria for that study included response to appropriate treatment or histopathologic confirmation, and the only case with definite histologic confirmation died without treatment; another cat with possible tachyzoites on histopathology responded poorly to clindamycin treatment. Davidson and colleagues[9] specifically commented that any clinical improvement in chorioretinitis in pet cats treated with clindamycin should be interpreted cautiously and not used as *de facto* evidence of toxoplasmosis. However, cats with uveitis and either *T. gondii*-specific antibodies (IgG, IgM, or both) in aqueous humor (GWC greater than 1) or serum were shown to be statistically more likely to have a positive therapeutic response if treated with clindamycin and glucocorticoids than if treated with glucocorticoids alone.[52,53]

A review of 10 cases of pulmonary toxoplasmosis revealed that only one cat survived long-term with sole clindamycin therapy, and no cats survived with clindamycin and sulfonamide treatment with or without trimethoprim.[16] The only clindamycin combination therapy that was successful was clindamycin and pyrimethamine.[16] The two cats that received this combination had both been receiving cyclosporine. One cat was treated with clindamycin and pyrimethamine for 16 days followed by trimethoprim sulfonamide and pyrimethamine for 26 days[32] and the other with clindamycin for 10 weeks (2 weeks past radiographic resolution) and pyrimethamine for 4 weeks (K. Briscoe, personal communication); the latter cat was still alive at the time of writing, 3.5 years after successful treatment (see Figure 6-1). One cannot draw any real conclusions from such a limited number of cases. It may be that cats with pulmonary toxoplasmosis and critical presentation have a very poor prognosis regardless of which antimicrobial agent is used, or that the cats which survived had a less virulent strain or more chronic disease course.

However, it could also be that clindamycin alone is poorly efficacious and possibly even detrimental in these situations as was demonstrated in the experimental study.[9] As such, based on the clinical cases reported and the experimental and theoretical data regarding clindamycin, it is difficult to recommend clindamycin alone in critical cases of pulmonary toxoplasmosis or acute disseminated toxoplasmosis. Clindamycin and pyrimethamine may be a better option, especially in cats immunosuppressed with cyclosporine.

Pyrimethamine, Trimethoprim, and Sulfonamides

Treatment of systemic toxoplasmosis with sulfonamides at a dosage of 60 mg/kg every 12 hours PO for 4 weeks if used as sole therapy, or 30 mg/kg every 12 hours PO for 4 weeks if used in combination with trimethoprim (15 mg/kg every 12 hours PO) or pyrimethamine (0.25 to 0.5 mg/kg every 12 hours PO), has been reported.[13] Parenteral administration of trimethoprim sulfonamide could also be considered if oral medication is not appropriate. However, sulfonamides, like clindamycin, have also been ineffective in clinical cases. Dubey and Carpenter[15] reported that treatment of 17 cats with sulfonamides failed to prevent death: 12 died or were euthanized within 30 hours, and the other five lived from 2 to 13 days. Eight of these cats were treated concurrently with pyrimethamine.

Pyrimethamine alone has marked *in vitro* activity against *T. gondii* whereas sulfadiazine (a sulfonamide) has not, but pyrimethamine and sulfadiazine have synergistic activity.[59] Pyrimethamine has greater efficacy than trimethoprim when used in combination with a sulfonamide but can cause bone marrow suppression in cats.[13] Regardless, it is probably worth considering pyrimethamine (dosed at 0.25 to 0.5 mg/kg every 12 hours PO) in the initial acute phases of disease. If bone marrow suppression occurs, it can often be corrected with the addition of folinic acid (5 mg per cat every 24 hours PO) or brewer's yeast (100 mg/kg every 24 hours PO) to the cat's diet.[13] Supplementation is not advisable prophylactically because there will be some decrease in drug efficacy against the parasite; it should only be used if documented bone marrow suppression has occurred.

Triazines

It is perhaps also worth considering the use of triazines, such as diclazuril and toltrazuril, because these have reasonable clinical efficacy (60% to 70%) for equine protozoal myeloencephalitis.[60] Diclazuril, especially when combined with pyrimethamine, was also efficacious in mice with experimentally induced acute toxoplasmosis,[61] and toltrazuril has been shown to be effective against the intestinal developmental stages of *T. gondii* and reasonably effective against extraintestinal stages of *T. gondii* in cats.[62] The dose of toltrazuril in cats reported for treatment of the enteroepithelial cycle is 5 to 10 mg/kg every 24 hours PO for 2 weeks;[13] the dose for systemic toxoplasmosis is unknown.

Fluconazole and Fluconazole-Combination Protocols

One of the latest treatments being investigated is fluconazole with or without pyrimethamine and sulfonamides. A 10-day treatment with fluconazole had a significant effect on survival in mice experimentally infected with the ME49 strain of *T. gondii*.[63] The combination of fluconazole, sulfadiazine, and pyrimethamine was also very effective, resulting in 93% survival in mice infected with the highly virulent *T. gondii* RH strain compared with 36% survival when treated with sulfadiazine and pyrimethamine alone.[64] The combination of fluconazole plus pyrimethamine with no sulfadiazine was also efficient in reducing mortality compared with treatment without fluconazole.[64] These results may be due to an additive effect, *in vivo* synergistic effect, or pharmacokinetic changes. Fluconazole is a strong competitive inhibitor of cytochrome P450 isoform 2C9, which metabolizes sulfadiazine, but its effect on pyrimethamine metabolism is unknown.[64] The method of action of the azoles has yet to be elucidated, but it is likely that there is a specific molecular target in *T. gondii*.[64] Interestingly, itraconazole did not improve survival in experimentally-infected mice despite reducing brain cyst burden.[63]

Other Drugs

Doxycycline, minocycline, clarithromycin, and various combinations with pyrimethamine and sulfonamides are also outlined as possible treatment protocols.[13,14] Azithromycin, despite having a delayed onset of action similar to clindamycin,[58] has been used successfully at 7.5 mg/kg every 12 hours PO.[14] That this drug may not be uniformly useful is demonstrated by the report of a case of azithromycin-resistant, clindamycin-responsive pulmonary toxoplasmosis in a dog.[14]

PREVENTION

Cats

The only way to prevent toxoplasmosis in cats is to keep cats indoors, ensuring no access to rodents or mechanical vectors of oocysts, and feed them appropriately cooked or commercially processed food. If raw meat and bones are fed to cats, freezing any such products at −12° C (10° F) or lower for at least 3 days before feeding should kill tissue cysts.[2] Care would still be required as cysts can remain viable for more than 11 days at −7° C (19° F)[2]; if freezer temperature were insufficient, cysts could remain viable.

Cyclosporine-Treated Cats

With increased use of cyclosporine in feline medicine and both anecdotal and published[16,32-34,36,37] reports of toxoplasmosis in cyclosporine-treated cats, this population of cats requires separate consideration. Although it could be argued that there are many immunosuppressive therapies that could predispose to acute or reactivated clinical toxoplasmosis, many of these therapies are used in life-threatening illnesses, such as chemotherapy for neoplasia or immunosuppression for immune-mediated hemolytic anemia. Cyclosporine, however, although it can be used as an adjunct in general immunosuppressive therapy for critical diseases and renal transplants, is increasingly being used to treat relatively benign diseases, such as atopic dermatitis and other dermatologic conditions. The possibility of inducing a life-threatening infection in such a situation is one that requires serious consideration.

One published case treated with cyclosporine alone for atopy died from acute systemic toxoplasmosis,[34] and it has been suggested anecdotally that most toxoplasmosis in cats treated with cyclosporine for atopy is due to acute infection rather than reactivation. However, there is supportive evidence from published cases[32,33] that toxoplasmosis in cats treated with cyclosporine, as sole therapy or in combination with prednisolone, can also be due to reactivated infection.

There are no published studies to indicate whether cyclosporine concentration plays a role in individual cats. Trough cyclosporine concentrations are variable in cats on similar doses of cyclosporine, and cats with reactivated toxoplasmosis after cyclosporine have reportedly had extremely high blood concentrations of the drug.[42] It has been suggested that cats with trough concentrations of >1000 ng/mL may be at increased risk.[65] It has also been suggested that concurrent prednisolone may enhance the risk (V. Barrs, personal communication), although cyclosporine has resulted in systemic toxoplasmosis when used as sole therapy.[32,34]

Until such time as a large case series is available, the risk factors will remain subjective and accurate advice difficult to formulate. It is not known whether testing patients for *T. gondii* antibody prior to cyclosporine therapy and then treating positive animals with a drug with activity against *T. gondii* would be of benefit.[42] It would be prudent to reduce chance of acute infection in cyclosporine-treated cats by keeping them indoors and feeding commercial food. It is probably worthwhile measuring trough cyclosporine concentrations approximately 2 weeks after initiating therapy[42] with the aim of keeping them ≤1000 ng/mL but remembering there will be differences in concentrations between different assays. Avoiding concurrent prednisolone may also be worthwhile if possible.

Both prevention and detection of recrudescent infection are challenging. Antibody titers in previously infected cats are unlikely to be of assistance, apart from identifying a potential risk factor for recrudescent toxoplasmosis. The best advice in a cat with evidence of *T. gondii* exposure prior to cyclosporine therapy may be to watch carefully for any signs of illness and seek veterinary attention immediately.

With respect to oocyst shedding in cyclosporine-treated cats, it has been demonstrated experimentally that cyclosporine dosed at 7.5 mg/kg every 24 hours PO prior to *T. gondii* infection actually lessened oocyst shedding and that cyclosporine did not induce repeat shedding. Thus, this protocol is unlikely to increase risk of *T. gondii* oocyst shedding in client-owned cats.[66]

Public Health

T. gondii is an important zoonotic agent. Acquired infection in immunocompetent humans is relatively innocuous and results in self-limiting fever, malaise, and lymphadenopathy. However, *T. gondii* can have serious adverse effects on human fetuses (e.g., stillbirth, CNS disease, and ocular disease) and immunocompromised patients.[14] Reactivated toxoplasmosis resulting in encephalitis in patients with acquired immuno-deficiency syndrome (AIDS) has been a very significant issue but one that has all but disappeared in patients treated with highly active antiretroviral therapy.[1]

The possibility that infection with *T. gondii* changes the behavior of its host to increase transmission has long been recognized.[67,68] More recently, laboratory experiments have shown that rats chronically infected with *T. gondii* lose their innate fear of cats, making them more likely to become prey.[69,70] In humans, reports of correlations between *T. gondii* seropositivity and schizophrenia date as far back as 1966.[1] There have also been reported associations between *T. gondii* and behavior changes (e.g., risk of being in a car accident), cognition, and suicide.[71,72] A comprehensive review of *T. gondii* and schizophrenia[71] assessed evidence for and against a causal association. Interestingly, although seroprevalence of toxoplasmosis has decreased in the United States and Europe, there has been no concomitant decrease in the prevalence of schizophrenia.[71] In addition, countries and regions (rural) with a high prevalence of antibodies to *T. gondii* have not demonstrated an unusually high prevalence of schizophrenia.[71] Thus a definitive causal link has not been proven, and much work remains to clarify the association between toxoplasmosis and schizophrenia. Similarly, toxoplasmosis does not necessarily cause increased suicide risk despite an epidemiologic association in some studies.[72] Individuals with an increased suicide risk may just lead lifestyles that predispose them to infection with *T. gondii*.[72]

The majority of cases of horizontal transmission to humans are caused by ingestion of tissue cysts in infected meat or by the ingestion of soil, water, or food contaminated with sporulated oocysts derived from the environment.[2] Until recently, only risk factor studies gave an indication of the predominant route of transmission in a given population. The relative importance of transmission via tissue cysts versus oocysts in any given population is often unknown except in case of outbreaks with a well-defined source. However, the discovery of a sporozoite-specific protein, which elicited antibody production and differentiated oocyst-infected pigs and mice from tissue-cyst infected animals, may help clarify the method of transmission in future studies.[73]

Infection from tissue cysts occurs with eating or preparing undercooked or raw meat, such as pork, goat, and lamb.[13,46] Ingestion of such meat, failing to wash hands thoroughly after handling raw meat, and contamination of other uncooked foods, such as salads, by utensils used to prepare raw meat are all possible mechanisms of infection. Ingestion of raw goat's milk may be an additional source of human toxoplasmosis.[13] Another risk factor is consumption of raw oysters, clams, or mussels, which presumably filter *T. gondii* from seawater.[74]

The prevalence of *T. gondii* infection in human populations that do not consume meat or eat it well-cooked suggests that infection from the environment via oocysts in soil, water, or on uncooked vegetables is also important.[46] When cats become infected with *T. gondii* they pass unsporulated (non-infectious) oocysts in feces for 1 to 2 weeks. After exposure to moisture and air, these oocysts mature in 1 to 5 days to become infectious (sporulated oocysts), and the sporulated oocysts survive for months to years. Thus frequent gardening and occupations that involve regular soil contact, such as farming, are risks.[46]

Increased risk of acquired toxoplasmosis was not associated with cat ownership in studies of veterinary health care providers or humans with AIDS,[14] and risk of acquiring *T. gondii* from cat feces collected in litter boxes is negligible when appropriate measures are used[46] because oocysts require at least 24 hours for sporulation and unsporulated oocysts are more susceptible to disinfection and environmental destruction.[13] Touching cats is probably not a common way to acquire toxoplasmosis because of the short oocyst shedding period, rarity of repeat shedding, and cats' fastidious grooming habits which result in removal of feces and thus oocysts.[14]

It is possible that with their habits of both eating and rolling in feces, dogs are likely to act as mechanical vectors for oocysts. Viable sporulated oocysts were present in dog feces for up to 2 days after feeding sporulated oocysts.[75] Nonsporulated oocysts did not sporulate on dog fur,[75] but there is still a possibility that dogs may act as a vector for sporulated oocysts. Some studies have identified dog ownership as a risk factor for human exposure to *T. gondii*[76,77]; thus hand washing after contact with dogs[77] and avoidance of dog contact have been suggested as precautions against infection.[78] It is worth noting that earthworms, houseflies, cockroaches, and snails can also act as mechanical vectors.[13]

Prevention of toxoplasmosis in humans involves avoiding exposure of susceptible hosts. Risk of exposure by ingesting tissue cysts in meat can be avoided by cooking all meat to an internal temperature greater than 67° C (153° F). Freezing of meat in home freezers (−12° C [10° F]) for at least 24 hours is also an effective method for killing organisms if meat is to be consumed rare.[2] Hands should be thoroughly washed after handling raw meat and care should be taken with chopping boards and utensils, ideally having a dedicated board for meat preparation. Gloves should be worn when gardening, and hands should be washed thoroughly when finished. Hands should also be washed after handling dogs. Care should be taken when cleaning litter trays. Sporulated oocysts resist most disinfectants, and immersing litter pans in boiling or scalding water is usually the easiest means of disinfection. However, there is little likelihood of sporulation if litter boxes are changed daily.

Advice given to pregnant women often includes the erroneous suggestion that seropositive cats should be removed from the household. An IgG-seropositive cat is probably not shedding oocysts and is less likely to shed oocysts if re-exposed or immunosuppressed.[13] Seronegative cats are in fact the greatest public health risk because, although they are not likely to be shedding, they will shed oocysts if exposed. Thus advice should really be concentrated on reducing risk of infection from soil (wearing gloves when gardening), water (filtering or boiling water), meat (appropriate food hygiene and cooking), and litter trays (see earlier). Although it is often recommended to only feed cats cooked or commercially processed food[14], and this may be valid during a human pregnancy, this recommendation would seem unnecessary for routine human prophylaxis if the precautions with respect to litter trays are taken.

Environmental Contamination

The issue of how to dispose of cat feces is challenging. Human infection is one important factor, but clinical toxoplasmosis in wildlife is also a concern. For example, toxoplasmosis resulting in death has been demonstrated in sea otters in California.[79] Experimental evidence shows that T. gondii oocysts survive chemical and physical inactivation treatments at levels four to six times higher than those used to treat raw sewage.[46] Thus, in California, a bill was passed that required manufacturers of cat litter to label their packaging with an advisory cautioning against cat litter disposal in toilets.[46] The recommendation is that feces should be bagged in plastic[42] and disposed of in garbage destined for landfill specifically designed to prevent waste materials leaking into groundwater.[46] This may be valid in situations in which particular wildlife populations have been shown to be at risk. However, most cats probably shed oocysts for no more than 21 days of their life,[46] if they get infected with toxoplasmosis at all. Regardless of whether litter from owned cats (especially low-risk cats, such as indoor cats on commercial diets) is diverted from sewage to landfill, outdoor and feral cats will still be defecating outdoors. In addition, dogs may be acting as mechanical vectors, potentially contaminating water sources by feces or swimming. Thus, a recommendation to contaminate landfill (that may or may not leak into groundwater) with at least one plastic bag daily for the life of an owned cat (potentially up to 17 years or more) to prevent, for example, 7 to 21 days of possible contamination with oocysts, would appear to be an inappropriate environmental recommendation in most situations, in this author's opinion.

CONCLUSION

T. gondii has been the subject of a very large volume of clinical and research data in multiple species, but there is still much to be learned about this parasite, its detection, most likely mode of transmission for different species and locations, strain and virulence variations, most effective treatment, and mitigation of factors that predispose to clinical disease.

References

1. Boothroyd JC: *Toxoplasma gondii*: 25 years and 25 major advances for the field. *Int J Parasitol* 39:935–946, 2009.
2. Robert-Gangneux F, Dardé M-L: Epidemiology of and diagnostic strategies for toxoplasmosis. *Clin Microbial Rev* 25:264–296, 2012.
3. Spycher A, Geiby C, Howard J, et al: Isolation and genotyping of *Toxoplasma gondii* causing fatal systemic toxoplasmosis in an immunocompetent 10-year-old cat. *J Vet Diagn Invest* 23:104–108, 2011.
4. Grigg ME, Bonnefoy S, Hehl AB, et al: Success and virulence in *Toxoplasma* as the result of sexual recombination between two distinct ancestries. *Science* 294:161–165, 2001.
5. Khan A, Su C, German M, et al: Genotyping of *Toxoplasma gondii* strains from immunocompromised patients reveals high prevalence of type I strains. *J Clin Microbiol* 43:5881–5887, 2005.
6. Parker GA, Langloss JM, Dubey JP, et al: Pathogenesis of acute toxoplasmosis in specific-pathogen-free cats. *Vet Pathol* 18:786–803, 1981.
7. Davidson MG, Rottman JB, English RV, et al: Feline immunodeficiency virus predisposes cats to acute generalized toxoplasmosis. *Am J Pathol* 143:1486–1497, 1993.
8. Powell CC, Lappin MR: Clinical ocular toxoplasmosis in neonatal kittens. *Vet Ophthalmol* 4:87–92, 2001.
9. Davidson MG, Lappin MR, Rottman JR, et al: Paradoxical effect of clindamycin in experimental, acute toxoplasmosis in cats. *Antimicrob Agents Chemother* 40:1352–1359, 1996.
10. Dubey JP: Duration of immunity to shedding of *Toxoplasma gondii* oocysts by cats. *J Parasitol* 81:410–415, 1995.
11. Hawkins EC, Davidson MG, Meuten DJ, et al: Cytologic identification of *Toxolasma gondii* in bronchoalveolar lavage fluid of experimentally infected cats. *J Am Vet Med Assoc* 210:648–650, 1997.
12. Dubey JP, Prowell M: Ante-mortem diagnosis, diarrhea, oocyst shedding, treatment, isolation, and genetic typing of *Toxoplasma gondii* associated with clinical toxoplasmosis in a naturally infected cat. *J Parasitol* 99:158–160, 2013.
13. Dubey JP, Lappin MR: Toxoplasmosis and neosporosis. In Greene CE, editor: *Infectious diseases of the dog and cat*, 3rd ed, St Louis, 2006, Elsevier/Saunders, pp 754–775.
14. Lappin MR: Toxoplasmosis. In Bonagura JD, Twedt DC, editors: *Kirk's current veterinary therapy XIV*, ed 14, St Louis, 2009, Saunders/Elsevier, pp 1254–1258.
15. Dubey JP, Carpenter JL: Histologically confirmed clinical toxoplasmosis in cats: 100 cases (1952-1990). *J Am Vet Med Assoc* 203:1556–1566, 1993.
16. Foster SF, Martin P: Lower respiratory tract infections in cats. Reaching beyond empirical therapy. *J Feline Med Surg* 13:313–332, 2011.
17. Feeney DA, Sautter JH, Lees GE: An unusual case of acute disseminated toxoplasmosis in a cat. *J Am Anim Hosp Assoc* 17:311–314, 1981.
18. Foster SF, Charles JA, Canfield PJ, et al: Reactivated toxoplasmosis in a FIV-positive cat. *Aust Vet Practit* 28:159–163, 1998.
19. Litster AL, Mitchell G, Menrath V: Pulmonary toxoplasmosis in a FIV-negative cat. *Aust Vet Pract* 29:154–158, 1999.
20. Lappin MR, Greene CE, Winston S, et al: Clinical feline toxoplasmosis. Serologic diagnosis and therapeutic management of 15 cases. *J Vet Intern Med* 3:139–143, 1989.
21. Sardinas JC, Chastain CB, Collins BK, et al: Toxoplasma pneumonia in a cat with incongruous serological test results. *J Small Anim Pract* 35:104–107, 1994.

22. Eddlestone SM, Hoskins JD, Hosgood G, et al: Take the Compendium challenge [Concurrent *Haemobartonella felis* and *Toxoplasma gondii* infection in a cat]. *Compendium* 18:774–779, 1996.

23. Poitout F, Weiss DJ, Dubey JP: Lung aspirate from a cat with respiratory distress. *Vet Clin Path* 27:10, 21–22, 1998.

24. Heidel JR, Dubey JP, Blythe LL, et al: Myelitis in a cat infected with *Toxoplasma gondii* and feline immunodeficiency virus. *J Am Vet Med Assoc* 196:316–318, 1990.

25. Reppas GP, Dockett AG, Burrell DH: Anorexia and an abdominal mass in a cat. *Aust Vet J* 77:784, 789–790, 1999.

26. Duncan RB, Lindsay D, Chickering WR, et al: Acute primary toxoplasmic pancreatitis in a cat. *Feline Pract* 28:6–8, 2000.

27. Holzworth J: Encephalitic toxoplasmosis in a cat. *J Am Vet Med Assoc* 313–316, 1954.

28. McConnell JF, Sparkes AH, Blunden AS, et al: Eosinophilic fibrosing gastritis and toxoplasmosis in a cat. *J Feline Med Surg* 9:82–88, 2007.

29. Henriksen P, Dietz HH, Henriksen SA: Fatal toxoplasmosis in five cats. *Vet Parasitol* 55:15–20, 1994.

30. Anfray P, Bonetti C, Fabbrini F, et al: Feline cutaneous toxoplasmosis: a case report. *Vet Dermatol* 16:131–136, 2005.

31. Peterson JL, Willard MD, Lees GE, et al: Toxoplasmosis in two cats with inflammatory intestinal disease. *J Am Vet Med Assoc* 199:473–476, 1991.

32. Barrs VR, Martin P: Beatty JA: Antemortem diagnosis and treatment of toxoplasmosis in two cats on cyclosporin therapy. *Aust Vet J* 84:30–35, 2006.

33. Bernsteen L, Gregory CR, Aronson LR, et al: Acute toxoplasmosis following renal transplantation in three cats and a dog. *J Am Vet Med Assoc* 215:1123–1126, 1999.

34. Last RD, Suzuki Y, Manning T, et al: A case of fatal systemic toxoplasmosis in a cat being treated with cyclosporin A for feline atopy. *Vet Dermatol* 15:194–198, 2004.

35. Toomey JM, Carlisle-Nowak MM, Barr SC, et al: Concurrent toxoplasmosis and feline infectious peritonitis in a cat. *J Am Anim Hosp Assoc* 31:425–428, 1995.

36. Nordquist BC, Aronson LR: Pyogranulomatous cystitis associated with *Toxoplasma gondii* infection in a cat after renal transplantation. *J Am Vet Med Assoc* 232:1010–1012, 2008.

37. Ploeg R: Pulmonary toxoplasmosis in a cat. *Aust Vet Practit* 37:118, 2007.

38. Spada E, Proverbio D, Giudice C, et al: Pituitary-dependent hyperadrenocorticism and generalised toxoplasmosis in a cat with neurological signs. *J Feline Med Surg* 12:654–658, 2010.

39. Brownlee L, Sellon RK: Diagnosis of naturally occurring toxoplasmosis by bronchoalveolar lavage in a cat. *J Am Anim Hosp Assoc* 37:251–255, 2001.

40. Lindsay SA, Barrs VR, Child G, et al: Myelitis due to reactivated spinal toxoplasmosis in a cat. *J Feline Med Surg* 12:818–821, 2010.

41. Singh M, Foster DJ, Child G, et al: Inflammatory cerebrospinal fluid analysis in cats: clinical diagnosis and outcome. *J Feline Med Surg* 7:77–93, 2005.

42. Dubey JP, Lindsay DS, Lappin MR: Toxoplasmosis and other intestinal coccidial infections in cats and dogs. *Vet Clin North Am Small Anim Pract* 39:1009–1034, 2009.

43. Gunn-Moore DA, Reed N: CNS disease in the cat. Current knowledge of infectious causes. *J Feline Med Surg* 13:824–836, 2011.

44. Bartels JE: Toxoplasma pneumonia in the cat. *Feline Pract* 2:11–13, 1972.

45. Griffin A, Newton AL, Aronson LR, et al: Disseminated *Mycobacterium avium* complex infection following renal transplantation in a cat. *J Am Vet Med Assoc* 222:1097–1101, 2003.

46. Dabritz HA, Conrad PA: Cats and *Toxoplasma*: implications for public health. *Zoonoses Public Health* 57:34–52, 2010.

47. Lappin MR, Greene CE, Prestwood AK, et al: Diagnosis of recent *Toxoplasma gondii* infection in cats by use of an enzyme-linked immunosorbent assay for immunoglobulin M. *Am J Vet Res* 50:1580–1585, 1989.

48. Lappin MR, Greene CE, Prestwood AK, et al: Enzyme-linked immunosorbent assay for the detection of circulating antigens of *Toxoplasma gondii* in the serum of cats. *Am J Vet Res* 50:1586–1590, 1989.

49. Omata Y, Oikawa H, Kanda M, et al: Transfer of antibodies to kittens from mother cats chronically infected with *Toxoplasma gondii*. *Vet Parasitol* 52:211–218, 1994.

50. Ali NM, Habib KSM: Kinetics and time dependence of the differential agglutination of acetone [AC]- and formalin [HS]-fixed *Toxoplasma* tachyzoites by serum of mice with experimental toxoplasmosis. *J Parasit Dis* 36:112–119, 2012.

51. Burney DP, Lappin MR, Spilker M, et al: Detection of *Toxoplasma gondii* parasitemia in experimentally inoculated cats. *J Parasitol* 85:947–951, 1999.

52. Lappin MR, Roberts SM, Davidson MG, et al: Enzyme-linked immunosorbent assays for the detection of *Toxoplasma gondii*-specific antibodies and antigens in the aqueous humor of cats. *J Am Vet Med Assoc* 201:1010–1016, 1992.

53. Lappin MR, Burney DP, Dow SW, et al: Polymerase chain reaction for the detection of *Toxoplasma gondii* in aqueous humor of cats. *Am J Vet Res* 57:1589–1593, 1996.

54. Fichera ME, Roos DS: A plastid organelle as a drug target in apicomplexan parasites. *Nature* 390:407–409, 1997.

55. Camps M, Arrizabalaga G, Boothroyd J: An rRNA mutation identifies the apicoplast as the target for clindamycin in *Toxoplasma gondii*. *Mol Microbiol* 43:1309–1318, 2002.

56. Pfefferkorn ER, Nothnagel RF, Borotz SE: Parasiticidal effect of clindamycin on *Toxoplasma gondii* grown in cultured cells and selection of a drug-resistant mutant. *Antimicrob Agents Chemother* 36:1091–1096, 1992.

57. Beatty JA, Swift N, Foster DJ, et al: Suspected clindamycin-associated oesophageal injury in cats: five cases. *J Feline Med Surg* 8:412–419, 2006.

58. Fichera ME, Bhopale MK, Roos DS: In vitro assays elucidate peculiar kinetics of clindamycin action against *Toxoplasma gondii*. *Antimicrob Agents Chemother* 39:1530–1537, 1995.

59. Harris C, Salgo MP, Tanowitz HB, et al: In vitro assessment of antimicrobial agents against *Toxoplasma gondii*. *J Infect Dis* 157:14–22, 1988.

60. Dirikolu L, Foreman JH, Tobin T: Current therapeutic approaches to equine protozoal myeloencephalitis. *J Am Vet Med Assoc* 242:482–491, 2013.

61. Lindsay DS, Rippey NS, Blagburn BL: Treatment of acute *Toxoplasma gondii* infections in mice with diclazuril or a combination of diclazuril and pyrimethamine. *J Parasitol* 81:315–318, 1995.

62. Haberkorn A: Chemotherapy of human and animal coccidioses: state and perspectives. *Parasitol Res* 82:193–199, 1996.

63. Martins-Duarte ÉS, Lemgruber L, de Souza W, et al: *Toxoplasma gondii*: fluconazole and itraconazole activity against toxoplasmosis in a murine model. *Exp Parasitol* 124:466–469, 2010.

64. Martins-Duarte ÉS, de Souza W, Vommaro RC: *Toxoplasma gondii*: the effect of fluconazole combined with sulfadiazine and pyrimethamine against acute toxoplasmosis in murine model. *Exp Parasitol* 133:294–299, 2013.

65. Jeromin AM: Cyclosporine in veterinary dermatology. In *Proceedings*, 84th Annual Western Veterinary Conference, Nevada, 2012.

66. Lappin MR, Scorza V: *Toxoplasma gondii* oocyst shedding in normal cats and cats treated with cyclosporine. *J Vet Intern Med* 25:709, 2011 (Abstract).

67. Hay J, Aitken PP, Hair DM, et al: The effect of congenital *Toxoplasma* infection on mouse activity and relative preference for exposed areas over a series of trials. *Ann Trop Med Parasitol* 78:611–618, 1984.

68. Webster JP, Brunton CF, MacDonald DW: Effect of *Toxoplasma gondii* upon neophobic behaviour in wild brown rats, *Rattus norvegicus*. *Parasitology* 109:37–43, 1994.

69. Berdoy M, Webster JP, MacDonald DW: Fatal attraction in rats infected with *Toxoplasma gondii*. *Proc Biol Sci* 267:1591–1594, 2000.

70. Vyas A, Kim SK, Giacomini N, et al: Behavioral changes induced by *Toxoplasma* infection of rodents are highly specific to aversion of cat odors. *Proc Natl Acad Sci USA* 104:6442–6447, 2007.

71. Yolken RH, Dickerson FB, Fuller Torrey E: Toxoplasma and schizophrenia. *Parasite Immunol* 31:706–715, 2009.

72. Sparkes A: Elevated suicide risks, cats and toxoplasmosis. *Vet Rec* 171:303, 2012.

73. Hill D, Coss C, Dubey JP, et al: Identification of a sporozoite-specific antigen from

Toxoplasma gondii. J Parasitol 97:328–337, 2011.

74. Jones JL, Dargelas V, Roberts J, et al: Risk factors for *Toxoplasma gondii* infection in the United States. *Clin Infect Dis* 49:878–884, 2009.

75. Lindsay DS, Dubey JP, Butler JM, et al: Mechanical transmission of *Toxoplasma gondii* oocysts by dogs. *Vet Parasitol* 73:27–33, 1997.

76. Sroka S, Bartelheimer N, Winter A, et al: Prevalence and risk factors of toxoplasmosis among pregnant women in Fortaleza, Northeastern Brazil. *Am J Trop Med Hyg* 83:528–533, 2010.

77. Frenkel JK, Parker BB: An apparent role of dogs in the transmission of *Toxoplasma gondii.* The probable importance of xenosmophilia. *Ann N Y Acad Sci* 791:402–407, 1996.

78. Frenkel JK, Lindsay DS, Parker BB, et al: Dogs as possible mechanical carriers of *Toxoplasma,* and their fur as a source of infection of young children. *Int J Infect Dis* 7:292–293, 2003.

79. Shapiro K, Miller M, Mazet J: Temporal association between land-based runoff events and California sea otter (*Enhydra lutris nereis*) protozoal mortalities. *J Wildl Dis* 48:394–404, 2012.

Update on Antiviral Therapies

Rebecca P. Wilkes and Katrin Hartmann

Antiviral chemotherapy use is still relatively uncommon in veterinary medicine. Controlled studies evaluating the efficacy of antiviral drugs in cats are lacking, or, if studies have been done, in many cases, the data are insufficient to determine effective dosing for these drugs. With the exception of the recombinant feline interferon (rFeIFN)-omega, so far no antiviral drugs are specifically licensed for veterinary medicine, which leaves the veterinary community with the option to use off-label antivirals made for humans to combat viral diseases in feline patients.

The goal of research in antiviral chemotherapy is the discovery of antiviral agents that are specific for the inhibition of viral multiplication without affecting normal cell division; however, because viruses are dependent on host cell machinery for replication, drug targets are often nonspecific. This makes antivirals inherently more toxic than antimicrobials are because the antiviral drugs are damaging to not only the virus but also the host cells as well. In addition, agents considered safe for human use are not always safe when administered to cats.[1] Antivirals made for systemic use often require host and/or viral metabolism to be active. Therefore, agents designed for use in humans are neither reliably nor predictably metabolized by cats or their viruses. Thus antiviral agents should always be tested first *in vitro* for efficacy and safety, and then followed by pharmacokinetic studies in cats.[1] Systemic antivirals often have a relatively narrow safety margin, and special considerations should always be given to patients with reduced hepatic or renal function. Well-designed blinded, placebo-controlled studies in client-owned animals should follow studies in laboratory-bred, experimentally infected cats to confirm results in genetically diverse cats.[1]

Most of the human antivirals are specifically intended for treatment of human immunodeficiency virus (HIV) or human herpesvirus infections. Therefore, feline immunodeficiency virus (FIV) and feline herpesvirus type 1 (FHV-1) infections have been the most important indications for antiviral chemotherapy in veterinary medicine. Topical antiviral therapy has been mainly used for herpetic ocular disease, but studies have evaluated a systemic antiviral compound (famciclovir) for treatment of multiple clinical syndromes associated with FHV-1 infections. Even though combination antiviral therapy has been successful in slowing disease progression in people with HIV, similar therapy has not been thoroughly evaluated in cats.[2] Recent studies have focused on combination therapy and evaluation of additional HIV drugs that have not been previously evaluated in feline

cells. It is hoped that expanding the number of drugs that are shown to be effective for FIV will lead to effective combination therapy for feline patients.

Some additional feline infections that have been the focus of current antiviral studies are feline leukemia virus (FeLV) infection and feline infectious peritonitis (FIP). Some of the HIV antivirals, such as raltegravir, are nonspecific, and they display activity against additional retroviruses, including FeLV, in *in vitro* studies. Identification of the human coronavirus that causes severe acute respiratory syndrome (SARS) has led to evaluation of antivirals for treatment of various coronaviruses, including the feline coronaviruses (FCoVs) that cause FIP, although testing is mainly in *in vitro* stages. Several studies have also evaluated the use of rFeIFN-omega for treatment of multiple feline viruses. A review of the literature for antiviral treatment in cats, including current recommendations for drug dosages and use, is given in Table 7-1.

FELINE IMMUNODEFICIENCY VIRUS

Feline immunodeficiency virus infects lymphocytes, cells of the monocyte-macrophage lineage, and cells of the central nervous system causing a variety of clinical signs (Figure 7-1). The viral replication cycle of FIV is highly similar to HIV. Feline immunodeficiency virus binds to host cells by an initial interaction of the FIV envelope (Env) glycoprotein with the CD134 molecule on the host cell, resulting in subsequent interaction with the co-receptor CXCR4 on the host cell, followed by viral envelope fusion with the host cell membrane. This allows entry of the viral nucleocapsid into the cytoplasm. The viral RNA is released into the cytoplasm and transcribed to complementary DNA (cDNA) by the reverse transcriptase (RT) enzyme, which is specific to retroviruses. The cDNA is subsequently synthesized to double-stranded DNA, transported to the nucleus, and integrated into the host genome by another virus-specific enzyme, the integrase. Viral messenger ribonucleic acid (mRNA) and genomic RNA are then transcribed and transported to the cytoplasm. Viral proteins are translated and processed by a third virus-specific enzyme, the protease. The immature virion moves to the cell membrane and acquires the viral envelope and glycoproteins and then is finally released from the cells.[2]

Antiretroviral drugs studied extensively in HIV infection have targeted the three virus-specific enzymes (protease, RT,

Table 7-1	Some Current Recommendations for Antiviral Administration in Cats	
Drug	**Dose**	**Indication**
Zidovudine (AZT)	5-10 mg/kg every 12 h PO or SC (the higher dose may cause nonregenerative anemia)	FIV or FeLV
rHIFN-α*	10^4 to 10^6 IU per kg SC every 24 h (associated with development of neutralizing antibodies within 3 wks with the higher dose) Oral application of low-dose (1 to 50 IU per kg every 24 h)—no antibody development	FIV, FeLV, FCV (oral dose), or ±FHV-1
rFeIFN-omega†	Licensed protocol: 3 cycles of injections at day zero, day 14, and day 60; each treatment cycle consists of 10^6 IU/kg/day SC for 5 consecutive days Recently used oral protocol: 10^5 IU/cat PO every 24 h for 90 consecutive days	FIV, FeLV, panleukopenia (parvovirus), ±FCV (oral protocol), ±FCoV, or ±FHV-1
L-lysine	500 mg every 12 h PO (twice daily important to maintain efficacy); must be given as a bolus and not in food; only an adjunctive therapy	FHV-1, long-term (likely lifelong) treatment in cats with recurring clinical signs to prevent reactivation of latent infection
Famciclovir	40 mg/kg PO 3 times daily (most recent recommendation; definitive dose and rate have not been established)[19]	FHV-1-associated clinical disease

*Recombinant human interferon alpha.
†Recombinant feline interferon omega.
FCoV, feline coronavirus; *FCV*, feline calicivirus; *FeLV*, feline leukemia virus; *FHV-1*, feline herpesvirus type 1; *FIV*, feline immunodeficiency virus; *IU*, international unit; *PO*, orally; *SC*, subcutaneous(ly) .

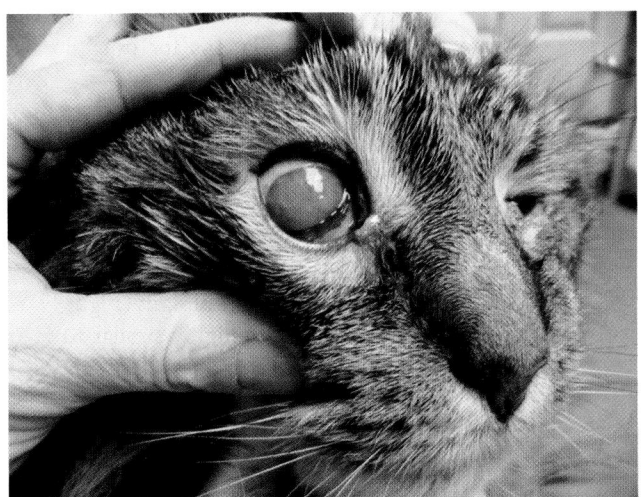

Figure 7-1: Severe anterior uveitis in a cat diagnosed with feline immunodeficiency virus infection. Photo courtesy of Dr. Susan Little.

and integrase), as well as some additional targets, interfering with different steps of the virus replication cycle.[3] As of 2014, approximately 30 compounds are approved by the U.S. Food and Drug Administration (FDA) for treatment of different stages of HIV infection.[2] Some of these drugs can also be used for FIV, and steps that can be inhibited include: (1) virus entry into susceptible cells by blocking attachment to the host cell co-receptor CXCR4; (2) reverse transcription of viral genomic RNA; (3) viral DNA integration into host genomes; and (4) proteolytic processing of precursor viral proteins into mature viral proteins (Figure 7-2).[2,3]

Reverse Transcriptase Inhibitors

Close similarities exist between the RT of HIV and FIV, and it has been shown that several RT-targeted antiviral compounds active against HIV are also effective in inhibiting FIV replication *in vitro*.[4] The RT of HIV is actually the target for three classes of inhibitors: nucleoside RT inhibitors (NRTI), nucleotide RT inhibitors (NtRTI), and nonnucleoside RT inhibitors (NNRTI). Nucleoside RT inhibitors and NtRTI interact with the catalytic site (the substrate-binding site) of the RT enzyme, whereas NNRTI interact with an allosteric site located at a short distance from the catalytic site. For the NRTI and NtRTI to interact with the substrate-binding site, they need to be phosphorylated.[3]

All of the NRTI (zidovudine [AZT], didanosine [ddI], zalcitabine [ddC], stavudine [d4T], lamivudine [3TC], abacavir [ABC], and emtricitabine) can be considered as nucleoside analogues, and they act in a similar fashion. After they have been taken up by the cells, they are phosphorylated three times to the active triphosphate form, and they act as competitive inhibitors of the normal deoxynucleoside triphosphate (dNTP) substrates, which are used by the cell to make DNA. Unlike dNTP substrates, NRTI lack a 3′-hydroxyl group on the deoxyribose moiety. Once incorporated into the DNA chain, the absence of a 3′-hydroxyl group, which normally forms the 5′- to 3′-phosphoester bond with the next nucleic acid, blocks further extension of the DNA by RT, resulting in DNA chain termination. The analogues cannot be cleaved from the active center and thus block the RT enzyme.[3] Nucleoside analogues are not only accepted as false substrates by viral enzymes, but also by cellular enzymes, and

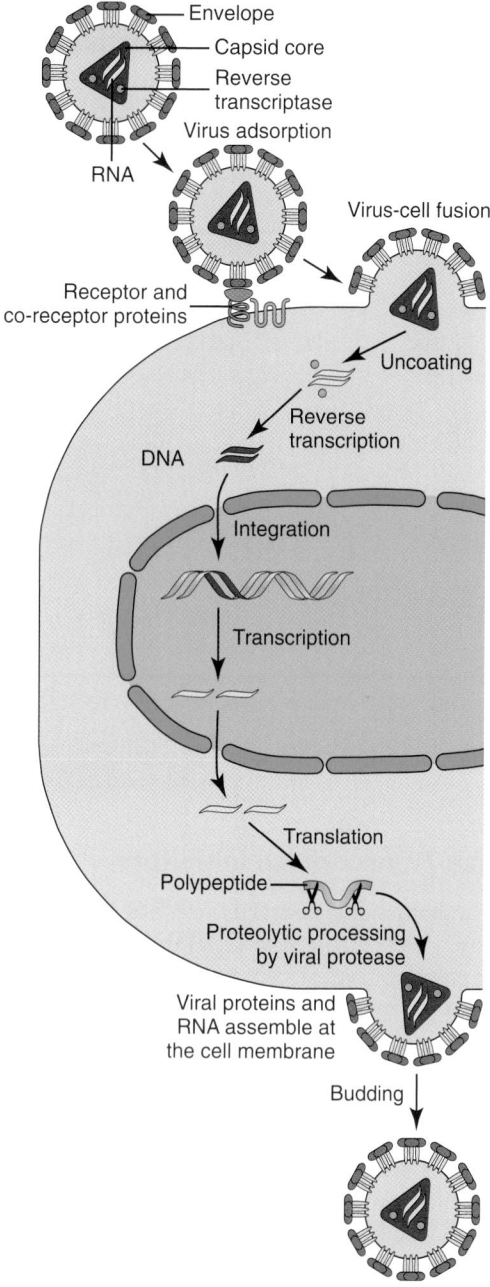

Figure 7-2: Replicative cycle of feline immunodeficiency virus and human immunodeficiency virus, demonstrating targets for therapeutic intervention, including co-receptor interaction, reverse transcription (by reverse transcriptase), integration, and proteolytic processing (by viral protease).

this is the major cause of their toxicity. Zidovudine is the NRTI most studied in cats, including *in vivo* studies evaluating the clinical response of experimentally and naturally FIV-infected cats treated with the drug. Zidovudine can increase the CD4+/CD8+ ratio and improve clinical condition scores in FIV-infected cats; however, it can result in adverse effects, such as dose-dependent nonregenerative anemia and neutropenia.[4,5] In addition, mutations producing resistance against the drug can develop.[4,5] Therefore, a study evaluated nine NRTI to inhibit FIV replication in feline peripheral blood

mononuclear cells.[4] Six of these drugs (ABC, ddI, emtricitabine, 3TC, d4T, and AZT) had been previously evaluated in feline cells, and three (amdoxovir, racivir, and dexelvucitabine) had not. Significant differences among the drugs were not found, but based on the data obtained, amdoxovir, dexelvucitabine, and racivir appear to be options for future studies investigating their potential use in FIV-infected cats. Though pharmacological data for cats are not available for these drugs, cytotoxic properties of these compounds suggest they could likely be used *in vivo* at dosages comparable to that for AZT.[4]

Nucleotide RT inhibitors are distinguished from NRTI as they are nucleotide analogues (not nucleoside analogues), which means that they only need two (not three) phosphorylation steps to be converted to their active form. Most importantly, they contain a phosphonate group that cannot be cleaved by hydrolases (esterases), which would make it more difficult to cleave off these compounds, once incorporated at the 3′-terminal end, compared with their regular nucleotide counterparts. Use of these compounds also results in DNA chain termination. One of these drugs, cidofovir, is active against virtually all DNA viruses, including polyoma-, papilloma-, adeno-, herpes-, and poxviruses. Cidofovir has been used for treatment of FHV-1 (see Feline Herpesvirus Type 1). Adefovir (9-(2-phosphonylmethoxyethyl)adenine [PMEA]) has a spectrum of activity that partially overlaps with cidofovir, in that both are active against herpesviruses, but adefovir is also active against hepadnaviruses (hepatitis B) and retroviruses, including FIV and FeLV. The antiviral activity spectrum of tenofovir (PMPA) is narrower than that of PMEA, in that it no longer extends to herpesviruses but is confined to hepadna- and retroviruses.[6] This drug has been tested *in vitro* against FeLV (see Feline Leukemia Virus).

Adefovir has been tested in FIV-infected cats in a 6-week placebo-controlled, double-blinded, clinical trial; 10 cats received adefovir (10 mg/kg subcutaneously [SC] twice weekly) and 10 cats received a placebo.[7] There was no decrease in the proviral or viral loads in treated cats, and the cats developed a progressive, life-threatening anemia. This is a common adverse effect of some nucleotide analogues.[7] Adefovir was also tested in combination with the co-receptor inhibitor plerixafor (see Co-receptor Inhibitors) in the same study, producing the same outcome as seen with use of the adefovir alone.[7]

A related drug, (*R*)-9-(2-phosphonylmethoxypropyl)-2,6-diaminopurine (PMPDAP), has been shown previously to be a potent inhibitor of FIV replication in cell culture and has reduced the viral load in three of four cats experimentally infected with FIV when treated at 20 mg/kg SC three times per week for 6 weeks. There were no changes in the red blood cell counts or hemoglobin values with treatment.[8] A recent study evaluated the efficacy of this drug in a placebo-controlled, double-blind study with a population of 20 cats naturally infected with FIV.[8] No significant differences were found between PMPDAP-treated (25 mg/kg SC twice weekly for 6 weeks) and placebo-treated cats, although cats treated with PMPDAP showed a tendency for improvement in their clinical signs and CD4+/CD8+ ratios. Mild hematological side effects (slight decline in packed cell volume and hemoglobin values) were seen in the treatment group. Compared with other NtRTI, PMPDAP seems to be slightly less toxic.[8]

Unlike the NRTI and NtRTI, NNRTI are an active form, with no dependence on intracellular metabolic pathways. NNRTI inhibit the RT by binding to the enzyme in a hydrophobic pocket that is located away from its catalytic site. The interaction of the compounds with the RT induces conformational changes that affect the catalytic activities of the enzyme.[9] Nonnucleoside RT inhibitors are considered highly specific inhibitors of HIV-1, and thus not active against other retroviruses, including FIV.[9] This is due to differences in the structure and/or flexibility of FIV RT that prevent NNRTI from interacting with the FIV RT.[10]

Protease Inhibitors

Protease inhibitors are based on the "peptidomimetic" principle, that is, they contain a hydroxyethylene scaffold that mimics the normal peptide linkage (cleaved by the HIV protease) but which itself cannot be cleaved. They thus prevent the HIV protease from carrying out its normal function, which is the proteolytic processing of precursor viral proteins into mature viral proteins.[3] Despite similarities between the HIV and FIV proteases, all but one of the currently available HIV protease inhibitors have failed to inhibit the protease of FIV. The one compound of interest, tipranavir, has only been tested against FIV *in vitro* so far.[4] However, studies have demonstrated that these compounds can be used to inhibit FCoV replication (see Feline Coronavirus).

Co-Receptor Inhibitors

Co-receptor inhibitors block viral attachment by binding to receptors on the host cell membrane to obscure the site of interaction of Env with the receptor.[2] Most of the receptor homologues or antagonists are highly selective for HIV and not useful for veterinary medicine. One exception can be used in cats with FIV infection, the class of bicyclams (e.g., plerixafor). Plerixafor (1,1′-[1,4-phenylenebismethylene]-bis(1,4,8,11-tetraazacyclotetradecane)-octachloride dehydrate, [AMD3100], [JM3100]), is the prototype compound among the bicyclams. Bicyclams are dimeric low-molecular weight nonpeptidic compounds that bind selectively to the chemokine receptor CXCR4. This is the cell surface co-receptor used by both HIV and FIV for attachment and infection of susceptible CD4+ lymphocytes, and the amino acid sequences of human and feline CXCR4 are highly similar. Drug binding inhibits attachment of the viral envelope to the host cell. The efficacy of plerixafor against FIV was recently investigated in naturally FIV-infected cats that were treated in a placebo-controlled, double-blind clinical trial.[7] Plerixafor was administered at 0.5 mg/kg SC every 12 hours. Treatment of FIV-infected cats with plerixafor caused

a significant decrease in the provirus load but did not lead to improvement of clinical or immunological variables. A statistical decrease in serum magnesium levels was observed in the treatment group, without clinical consequences. No development of resistance of FIV isolates to plerixafor was found during the treatment period, making it a potential treatment for FIV-infected cats.[7] Limited oral bioavailability and short half-life preclude clinical use of plerixafor in HIV infection,[2,7] but additional CXCR4 antagonists are under development and should be tested for efficacy against FIV when available.

Integrase Inhibitors

Integrase catalyzes strand transfer (3′-end joining), which inserts both viral DNA ends into a host cell chromosome.[3] Integrase inhibitors are used to treat HIV infection. One of the integrase inhibitors (raltegravir) has been shown to be effective for inhibition of FeLV (see Feline Leukemia Virus).

Highly Active Antiretroviral Therapy

Administration of a combination of drugs from different classes, termed highly active antiretroviral therapy (HAART), to HIV-infected patients has turned an invariably fatal disease into a chronic but manageable condition.[2,3] The goals associated with the use of combinations of three (or more) anti-HIV compounds are: (1) to obtain synergism among different compounds acting at different molecular targets; (2) to lower the individual drug dosages to reduce their adverse side effects; and (3) to diminish the likelihood of development of drug resistance.[3] Combination therapy has not been thoroughly investigated for treatment of FIV infection in cats,[2] and use of multiple classes of drugs is more difficult in cats because some of the drug classes that are effective for HIV do not work for FIV.[2,4] However, the need for combination antiretroviral therapy for feline patients has been the focus of recent studies.

The goal of antiviral therapy should be improvement of the cat's clinical status. This is not always correlated with virus replication, as measured by a plasma viral load.[9] It has been suggested that antiretroviral therapy should be administered to FIV-infected cats in the later stages of the asymptomatic phase of infection, during which the cat does not show clinical signs and the immune system is relatively normal and more likely to respond to treatment.[5] After experimental infection, when the CD4+/CD8+ ratio decreases, viral load increases markedly, and clinical signs of immunosuppression begin to appear. However, the situation in naturally infected cats is different, and the quality of life is not associated with the viral load.[11] Therefore, it is debated at which time point antiviral therapy should be started and whether it should be administered to asymptomatic cats. In a recent study, antiretroviral therapy was initiated during the later stages of the asymptomatic phase of infection in naturally infected cats. The cats were defined as being in the later stages of the asymptomatic phase of infection when the CD4+/CD8+ ratio reached 0.9, because at this stage of infection, the viral load increased markedly, and clinical signs of immunosuppression began to appear. The ratios were calculated every 4 months for 2 to 5 years prior to initiation of the antiviral therapy, and viral loads of all cats were quantified once a year. The cats were randomly assigned to treatment groups of eight cats each. Treatment included combination therapy, but no placebo group was used, and the study was not blinded.[5] The follow-up was performed over 1 year, through clinical evaluation and the determination of viral loads and CD4+/CD8+ ratios. Comparisons of pretreatment and post-treatment values from the cats were performed, as well as comparison of values between treatment groups. A combination of two NRTI (AZT + 3TC, 25 mg/kg every 12 hours orally [PO]) was compared to treatment with AZT alone (5 mg/kg every 12 hours PO). The combination of AZT and 3TC is often used in HIV-infected patients, given that both drugs show a synergistic effect. Treatment with AZT alone or in combination with 3TC induced a significant increase in the CD4+/CD8+ ratio and a significant decrease in viral load within and among groups, with an even greater reduction with combination therapy than with AZT alone. Only mild side effects, including vomiting in one of eight cats, anorexia in two of eight cats, and anemia in one of eight cats, were seen with this treatment combination, but therapeutic interventions resolved the problems, and treatment did not have to be stopped.[5] However, the lack of a control group and lack of blinding make the results of the study very difficult to interpret. Therefore, treatment of asymptomatic FIV-infected cats with antivirals cannot be generally recommended based on the currently available data. An earlier *in vivo* study was performed in experimentally FIV-infected cats that were treated with a high-dose AZT and 3TC combination (100 or 150 mg/kg/day PO for each drug). The combination had no anti-FIV activity in these chronically infected cats. Severe side effects, which included fever, anorexia, and marked hematologic changes, were observed in some of the cats with such high-dose dual-drug treatment, but the toxic effects were reversed when the dose was lowered to 20 mg/kg every 24 hours.[12]

Ideally, combination therapy for feline patients will contain at least two to three drugs from at least two different classes, as recommended for human patients.[9] As previously mentioned, PMEA (an NtRTI) was tested in combination with the co-receptor inhibitor plerixafor; however, because of the toxicity associated with the PMEA, this combination cannot be recommended.[7] Therefore, use of plerixafor in combination with other NtRTI that are less toxic than PMEA or compounds of other drug classes are should be further investigated in the future.

Immunomodulator

Lymphocyte T-cell immunomodulator (LTCI), a protein produced by a bovine-derived thymic stromal epithelial cell line, is conditionally licensed by the United States Department of Agriculture (USDA) as a treatment aid for cats infected with FIV or FeLV. The primary therapeutic effect is activation of progenitor CD4 T-cells to mature cells, which then produce cytokines, including interleukin (IL)-2 and interferon (IFN). A few studies performed by the manufacturer are highlighted in a review article.[13] The studies suggest reduced virus load, improved clinical signs, and improved hematological parameters with treatment. However, the data for placebo-controlled studies were not shown, and a field study with naturally infected cats lacked a control group. Independent placebo-controlled, blinded studies are warranted. Additional information about immunomodulators and immunostimulants is provided in the feline herpesvirus type 1 and feline coronavirus sections.

FELINE LEUKEMIA VIRUS

Feline leukemia virus, like FIV, is a member of the family *Retroviridae*, but unlike FIV, FeLV is a gammaretrovirus and not a lentivirus. Feline leukemia virus causes a wide variety of clinical signs in infected cats (Figure 7-3). Structural differences affect the susceptibility of gammaretroviruses to anti-HIV drugs, but the similarities in mechanism of replication suggest that some of these drugs can also inhibit FeLV. This is true of most NRTI.[14] Zidovudine effectively inhibits FeLV replication *in vitro*, and *in vivo* in experimental infections. However, in naturally FeLV-infected cats, it did not reduce plasma virus load, improve immunological and clinical status, increase quality of life, nor prolong life expectancy.[15] Its bone marrow toxicity can also cause adverse side effects (e.g., nonregenerative anemia) that are more pronounced in FeLV-infected cats than in FIV-infected cats. Therefore, it is not recommended as a first line of therapy for FeLV infection.[16]

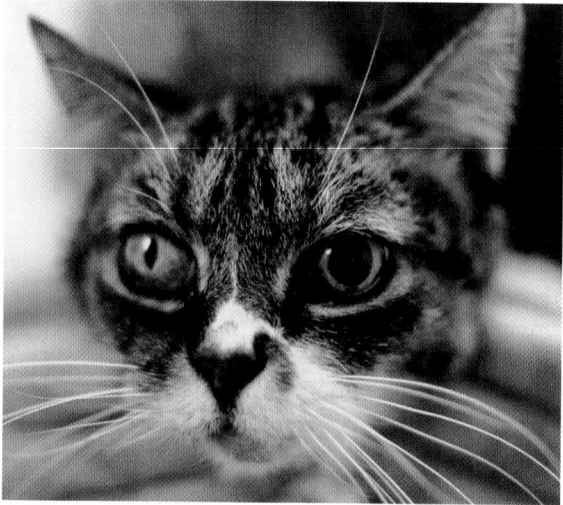

Figure 7-3: Anisocoria in a Cat Infected with FeLV. (Photo courtesy of Dr. Susan Little.)

Tenofovir, an NtRTI used for treatment of HIV, has been shown to be effective against FeLV *in vitro*.[14] The anti-FeLV mechanism of tenofovir is probably similar to what has been described for HIV-1. Tenofovir is given in the form of a prodrug, which is converted to an acyclic nucleoside phosphate. Once converted to the active diphosphate form, tenofovir is incorporated by RT into viral DNA, where it acts as a chain terminator to inhibit further elongation of the viral DNA.[14] However, *in vivo* studies in FeLV-infected cats are lacking.

Raltegravir

Another compound currently used for human HIV therapy, raltegravir, could be considered for the treatment of FeLV-infected cats.[14] The high degree of conservation across lentiviruses, betaretroviruses, gammaretroviruses, and alpharetroviruses of integrase active sites suggests that FeLV might be highly sensitive to integrase inhibitors.[16] The mechanism of action against FeLV is the same as for FIV, inhibition of integration of the viral dsDNA that is produced by reverse transcription of the viral RNA genome.[14]

An *in vitro* study evaluated the effective 50% inhibitory concentration (EC_{50}) for FeLV inhibition of raltegravir in several feline cell lines and found these values are in the range of that observed for HIV and a related gammaretrovirus, xenotropic murine leukemia virus, and are well below the minimal plasma concentrations found in humans.[16] The effective concentration of raltegravir had no appreciable effect on cell viability nor induced apoptosis, suggesting that this could be an effective and safe drug also *in vivo*.[16] However, raltegravir is partly eliminated as glucuronide, a metabolic pathway that is not very efficient in cats, and it would increase the risk of toxicity resulting from drug accumulation.[16] As of 2014, no *in vivo* studies have been published.

FELINE HERPESVIRUS TYPE 1

Feline herpesvirus type 1 is a member of the subfamily *Alphaherpesvirinae*, order *Herpesvirales*. Herpes simplex viruses 1 and 2 and varicella zoster virus are also members of this subfamily, and antivirals developed for the treatment of these human viruses have been used for treatment of FHV-1 in cats. Feline herpesvirus type 1 typically infects epithelial and mucosal surfaces and travels retrograde along sensory axons to establish latency in the trigeminal ganglia. Reactivated virus travels down those same axons to infect similar tissues to those that were originally infected, potentially resulting in recurrent or chronic sequelae, including keratitis, conjunctivitis, rhinosinusitis, dermatitis (Figure 7-4), and potentially blindness.[17] Whereas drug combinations have become standard procedure for the treatment of HIV infections, the treatment of other virus infections, including herpesviruses, is routinely based on the use of a single antiviral drug.[18]

A group of antiviral drugs known as acyclic nucleoside analogues are used for the systemic treatment of human

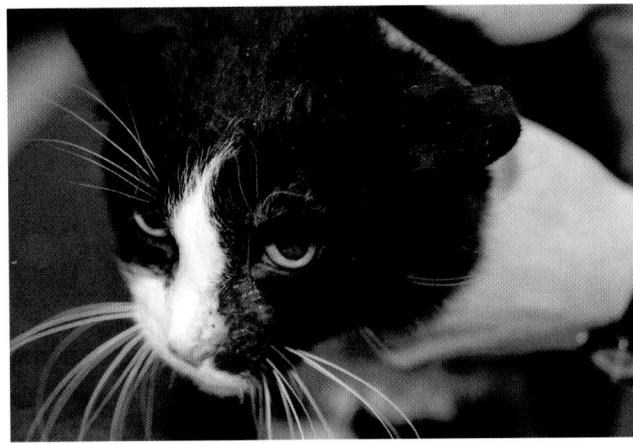

Figure 7-4: Herpetic dermatitis. (Photo courtesy of Dr. Elizabeth May, University of Tennessee College of Veterinary Medicine.)

alphaherpesviruses, such as herpes simplex virus 1 (HSV-1). They have been investigated for treatment of FHV-1. Members of this group of antiviral agents include acyclovir (and its prodrug, valacyclovir), ganciclovir, and penciclovir (and its prodrug, famciclovir). All require three phosphorylation steps for activation. The first of these steps must be catalyzed by the FHV-1 viral enzyme, thymidine kinase. This makes the drugs less toxic *in vivo* compared to many of the other antiviral drugs. However, the activity of the thymidine kinase in FHV-1 is not equivalent to the enzyme of human herpesviruses. The second and third phosphorylation steps must be performed by host enzymes, which are not as effective in cats as they are in humans. This knowledge helps explain why the acyclic nucleoside antiviral agents developed for humans infected with HSV-1 are not predictably effective when administered to cats infected with FHV-1 and why pharmacokinetic and efficacy studies are always needed to establish appropriate dosing in cats.[1]

Acyclovir has been adequately tested in cats for the treatment of FHV-1, but it has a relatively low antiviral potency and poor bioavailability. A very high dose is required for effective treatment, which is associated with unacceptable toxicity, with signs related to bone marrow suppression and nephrotoxicity.[1] A prodrug of acyclovir, valacyclovir, was developed for increased bioavailability in humans, but use for FHV-1 treatment in experimentally infected cats induced fatal renal and hepatic necrosis and bone marrow suppression, and did not reduce viral shedding or clinical disease severity.[1,19] Therefore, despite its superior pharmacokinetics, valacyclovir should not be used in cats.[1]

Ganciclovir

Ganciclovir appears to be at least 10-fold more effective against FHV-1 than acyclovir *in vitro*. Ganciclovir is available for systemic as well as topical use in the form of a 0.15% ophthalmic gel formulation in humans. Ganciclovir holds promise for feline FHV-1 infection and currently available formulations warrant safety and efficacy studies in cats.[1]

Famciclovir

The most promising systemic drug for the treatment of FHV-1 is famciclovir, a prodrug of the active compound penciclovir, which has been shown to be highly efficacious in inhibiting FHV-1 replication *in vitro*. Penciclovir is absorbed poorly when given orally, so the oral form famciclovir was developed with increased bioavailability and uptake from the intestinal tract.[1] Famciclovir requires di-deacetylation, mainly in the blood, and oxidation by a hepatic aldehyde oxidase for conversion to the active compound penciclovir. Unfortunately, hepatic aldehyde oxidase activity is basically absent in cats, which makes the pharmacokinetics of this drug complex and results in lower than expected plasma penciclovir concentrations despite administration of relatively high doses of famciclovir.[20,21] Despite this, studies evaluating famciclovir *in vivo* have shown it to be safe and efficacious for use in feline patients.[20,22] Cats experimentally infected with FHV-1 and receiving famciclovir 90 mg/kg PO three times daily for 21 days had significantly improved outcomes for systemic, ophthalmic, clinicopathologic, virologic, serologic, and histologic variables when compared with placebo-treated cats. Treatment was initiated on day zero, the same day the cats were infected.[20] Even though this study did not mimic how cats with natural infection would be treated, results from a clinical case study suggested this drug is likely effective for treatment of clinical cases, though it was not blinded and placebo controlled.[22] Clinical cases with primary ocular disease, rhinosinusitis, and dermatitis each attributed to FHV-1 (though not definitively diagnosed), were treated with famciclovir at doses of 62.5 mg PO once or twice daily for ocular herpetic disease or rhinosinusitis or up to 125 mg PO three times daily for dermatitis. Famciclovir was well tolerated with each dose and had a positive effect on each clinical condition.[22]

A definitive dose rate has not been established for famciclovir. However, penciclovir has no appreciable *in vitro* effect if present for 24 hours prior to infection, suggesting that famciclovir should be administered more frequently than once every 24 hours to ensure exposure to penciclovir as additional epithelial cells become exposed to viral infection.[21] Current pharmacokinetic data suggest that dosing three times daily is required,[21] and 40 mg/kg PO three times daily has been suggested for treatment of cats infected with FHV-1, based on effective concentrations obtained in *in vivo* studies[20,22] and determination of new *in vitro* 50%-inhibitory concentrations.[21] The most commonly reported adverse effects of famciclovir treatment in humans include urticaria, hallucinations, headaches, and confusion (especially in elderly humans), which would likely be more difficult to detect in animals. For these reasons, judicious use of this drug is recommended in client-owned cats, especially those with pre-existing hepatic or renal insufficiency.[21]

Pharmacokinetic studies have also evaluated the concentration of penciclovir in tears, and treatment with an oral dose of 40 mg of famciclovir/kg three times daily achieves a penciclovir concentration at the ocular surface likely to be effective against FHV-1.[23] This is potentially an alternative therapy to the use of topical drugs, the majority of which require multiple daily applications.[23] However, an implantable silicone polymer device impregnated with penciclovir has been developed that holds promise for long-term, steady-state subconjunctival delivery of the drug for the treatment of ocular herpetic disease.[17]

Cidofovir

Although herpetic ocular disease is commonly treated with topical antiviral ophthalmic solutions or ointments (including idoxuridine, vidarabine, or trifluridine),[1] these antivirals do not require a virus-specific phosphorylation step for activation. Moreover, they damage host cells, specifically resulting in bone marrow suppression. Therefore, they should not be used systemically.[1] For good reviews of these topical drugs, see the reports of Maggs[1] and Gould.[24] Cidofovir, a member of the NtRTI class of drugs, has been tested for topical treatment of FHV-1 ocular disease but not for systemic use. It appears to be efficacious topically and is a newer drug (therefore it is included in this section). Cidofovir requires the typical two host-mediated phosphorylation steps without virally mediated phosphorylation.[1] Its safety when given topically arises from its relatively high affinity for HSV DNA polymerase compared with human DNA polymerase. It is commercially available only in injectable form in the United States for treatment of a human betaherpesvirus. When applied topically as a 0.5% solution twice daily to cats experimentally infected with FHV-1, it led to reduced viral shedding and improvement of clinical disease compared to the placebo group.[25] Its efficacy with only twice daily administration (despite being virostatic) is believed to be due to the long tissue half-lives of the metabolites of this drug. There are reports of its experimental topical use in humans and rabbits being associated with stenosis of the nasolacrimal duct, but this has not been shown in cats. The fact that a twice-daily topical treatment is sufficient, whereas all other topical antivirals require application every 3 to 4 hours, makes cidofovir a useful alternative for ocular topical treatment.[1,24,25]

Small Interfering RNA

Small interfering RNAs (siRNAs) designed to target the FHV-1 DNA polymerase[26] and glycoprotein D[27] have been used *in vitro* to induce RNA interference in an immortalized cell line and in primary feline corneal epithelial cells to inhibit FHV-1 replication. RNA interference is a post-transcriptional, RNA-guided gene-silencing mechanism present in eukaryotes.[28] Interference of the FHV-1 essential genes resulted in reduction of virus replication up to 98 ± 1%. This type of therapy is intended for topical treatment of chronic herpetic disease. However, a preliminary *in vivo* study evaluating topical delivery of siRNAs to feline corneas was unsuccessful.[29] The lack of delivery was likely the result of siRNA dilution and rapid removal by tear film and blinking. Studies are ongoing to identify a means of increasing contact time between the corneal cells and siRNAs to allow delivery.

Lysine

Twice-daily oral L-lysine bolus administration, initiated prior to experimental infection, reduced the severity of conjunctivitis in cats undergoing primary infection. L-lysine bolus administration also reduced viral shedding in latently infected cats experimentally infected with FHV-1, following changes in husbandry and housing but not following corticosteroid administration. *In vitro*, lysine supplementation led to reduction of FHV-1 replication.[1] Arginine exerts a substantial growth-promoting effect on FHV-1 and is an essential amino acid for viral protein synthesis, and lysine antagonizes this effect. Lysine and arginine competitively inhibit transport of each other by using a common transport system, and lysine induces arginase, an enzyme that causes the degradation of arginine. Arginine deficiency inhibits synthesis of infectious viral particles and downregulates synthesis of viral proteins. However, unlike the protocol for HSV-1-infected humans, owners of cats receiving lysine for FHV-1 should not be advised to restrict their cat's arginine intake[1] because feeding a diet lacking L-arginine is associated with a severe risk of hyperammonemia and encephalopathy.[30]

It has been suggested that the ratio of L-lysine to L-arginine, rather than the concentration of each amino acid, is critical in achieving an inhibitory effect on viral replication. Dietary supplementation increases mean plasma concentrations of L-lysine without reducing L-arginine concentrations and has been shown to be safe for use in cats, up to 86 g/kg of diet. Supplementation with higher doses has been shown to result in reduced food intake.[30,31]

Despite promising initial *in vitro* data and *in vivo* results from experimental studies, current studies question whether viral inhibition with increased lysine concentrations, in the absence of decreased arginine concentrations, can be biologically important. A new study evaluating the effect of various ratios of L-lysine and L-arginine on FHV-1 DNA replication *in vitro* demonstrated only a modest reduction in viral DNA (less than 1 log) at ratios considered difficult to obtain *in vivo* in healthy cats.[31]

A lack of efficacy of L-lysine supplementation has also been demonstrated *in vivo* in shelter settings.[1,32] Dietary supplementation was unsuccessful, likely because the cats were anorexic during peak disease and were not ingesting the lysine when they needed it the most. Bolus administration was also unsuccessful, likely because of stress associated with the lysine administration.[1,32] The stress of bolus administration in shelter situations could negate its effects and even cause transfer of pathogens among cats by shelter workers administering the lysine. However, data do not support dietary supplementation.[1,32]

Unfortunately, no studies to date have been conducted on client-owned cats; however, anecdotal evidence suggests that there is a benefit from administration of lysine in individuals. Dosing is 500 mg PO twice daily, which should be given as a bolus and not added to food. Any benefit from lysine therapy is likely only possible with daily, lifelong treatment of cats with chronic herpetic disease, rather than use of lysine as a treatment during acute or recrudescent episodes. Potentially, daily therapy would reduce episodes of viral recrudescence. However, clinical studies in pet cats are lacking. The cost of this therapy should be weighed against the potential benefits. Owners should be made aware that this is only an adjunctive therapy and that administration of antiviral drugs might be necessary to gain better control of signs.

Polyprenyl Immunostimulant

Polyprenyl immunostimulant (PI) is an immunomodulator that has a conditional license in the United States for treatment of FHV-1 infection. In blinded, placebo-controlled, experimental challenge studies, PI started on the day of virus exposure significantly reduced the severity and duration of rhinitis and conjunctivitis associated with acute FHV-1 disease (Legendre and Kuritz, manuscript in preparation). According to the manufacturer, PI upregulates the innate immune system and modulates the immune response toward a cellular response. This activity was attributed to positive effects associated with treatment of FHV-1, which requires a cell-mediated immune response for control. Viral titers were not compared between treatment and control groups in the studies, but based on the reduced signs associated with treatment, clinical studies are warranted.

FELINE CORONAVIRUS AND FELINE INFECTIOUS PERITONITIS

Feline infectious peritonitis is associated with clinical signs that can affect almost any body system (Figure 7-5). Currently, there is no effective treatment for FIP despite its importance as the leading infectious cause of death in young cats.[33] Following the discovery that SARS is caused by a coronavirus (SARS-CoV), efforts to find an antiviral drug for coronaviruses increased. A few antiviral agents that target different steps in the replication cycle have been tested against feline FCoV. Coronavirus spike proteins on the viral envelope initially bind to receptors on the host cell membrane.[33] The spike protein mediates fusion of the viral envelope with host cell membranes. During this process, heptad repeats 1 and 2 (HR1 and HR2) of the spike protein assemble to form a complex, resulting in a conformational change that is necessary for fusion.[34] Peptides have been used as antivirals by inhibiting the HR1-HR2 interaction, thus preventing membrane fusion.[34] The spike protein must be cleaved for entry of the virus into the cytoplasm. Feline coronavirus infection is dependent on cathepsin B, a host cysteine protease found within the cell, making this the likely protease responsible for spike protein cleavage. Therefore, cathepsin B can serve as a potential target for the development of therapeutic drugs against FCoV. Following entry into the cell, FCoV produce viral polyproteins that are processed into

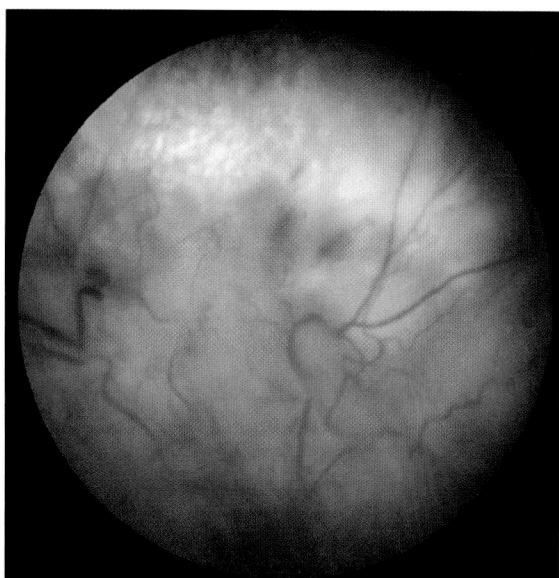

Figure 7-5: Chorioretinitis in a cat diagnosed with feline infectious peritonitis. (Photo courtesy of Drs. Dan Ward and Diane Hendrix, University of Tennessee College of Veterinary Medicine.)

mature proteins by viral-specific proteases, the main protease (3C-like [3CL] protease) and the papain-like protease. Because the cleavages of viral polyproteins are an essential step for virus replication, blockage of viral protease is also an attractive target for therapeutic intervention.[33]

Protease and Cathepsin Inhibitors

In an *in vitro* experiment in Crandell-Rees feline kidney cells, 3CL protease inhibitors and cathepsin inhibitors were tested for their ability to inhibit FCoV replication.[33] Both types of drugs produced effective inhibition with EC_{50} values in the nanomolar range and each drug tested was nontoxic to the cells at effective concentrations. The 3CL protease inhibitors were more effective than the cathepsin inhibitors and when used in combination, these drugs had strong synergic effects. There have not been any *in vivo* studies with these drugs in cats to date. In one *in vitro* study, 16 antiviral compounds, including nucleoside analogues used to treat herpesviruses, NRTI used for HIV, and protease inhibitors also used for HIV, were tested for their ability to inhibit FCoV in cell culture.[35] Among the 16 drugs tested, two showed significant inhibition of FCoV when compared to the untreated cells. These were nelfinavir and *Galanthus nivalis* agglutinin (GNA). Nelfinavir is a HIV protease inhibitor that has been shown to target the 3CL protease of SARS-CoV by interacting with 18 residues of the protease. The drug was slightly less effective against FCoV than against SARS-CoV, likely because only seven of the corresponding residues of the 3CL protease of FCoV are identical to the SARS-CoV protease.[35] GNA, a carbohydrate-binding agent, exhibits its antiviral effect by binding to coronavirus glycosylated envelope glycoproteins, thereby inhibiting viral attach-

ment to the host cell. The antiviral effects were concentration dependent, and nelfinavir displayed cellular toxicity at higher doses. GNA was a better inhibitor of FCoV, and when the two agents were added together, a synergistic antiviral effect was produced. The results suggest that the combined use of GNA and nelfinavir could have therapeutic potential in the treatment of cats with FIP.[35]

Fusion Inhibitors

Viral fusion has also been targeted effectively with a synthetic peptide based on the putative HR2 sequence of FCoV. Virus replication was significantly inhibited *in vitro* compared to controls, and the peptide was nontoxic.[34] This peptide was also used in combination with human IFN-alpha. The two displayed a synergistic effect, but the cells were pretreated with IFN prior to infection by the virus.[34] See the section on interferon for further information about interferon treatment for FIP.

Polyprenyl Immunostimulant

Immunomodulators have been considered because FIP is an immune-mediated disease.[35]

A drug that has shown promise for immunomodulation is PI.[36] This drug has a conditional license in the United States for treatment of FHV-1 infection. In a case series of three cats, PI was associated with prolonged survival in cats with noneffusive FIP.[36] No placebo group was included for comparison, so definitive conclusions about the effectiveness of this drug for treatment of FIP cannot be drawn.

Additional immunostimulants such as ImmunoRegulin (*Propionibacterium acnes*), an inactivated bacterin, and a T-cell receptor peptide (manufactured by Imulan Biotherapeutics), have been suggested for treatment of FIP. These are not antiviral drugs; instead, each of these products is reported to stimulate the immune response toward a cell-mediated response or to reduce an overactive type 2 helper T-cell (Th2) response. An imbalance in T-cell versus B-cell immune response has been suggested to contribute to the development of FIP. It has been proposed that a strong cell-mediated immune response protects a cat from the development of FIP, whereas the production of antibodies is counterproductive, enhancing the uptake and replication of feline infectious peritonitis virus (FIPV) in macrophages and contributing to the pathology by producing a type III hypersensitivity vasculitis. However, this hypothesis has been questioned.[37] Therefore, even though the use of these types of drugs for stimulation of a cell-mediated response might seem a logical approach for the treatment of FIP, there is currently no data to support their use.

An additional non-antiviral drug that has been evaluated for treatment of FIP is propentofylline. This drug appears to downregulate proinflammatory cytokines, which in turn can reduce vasculitis. Vasculitis, as stated earlier, is responsible for pathology associated with FIP. However, in a placebo-controlled, double-blind study in cats with late stage FIP, there was no statistically significant difference in the survival time, the quality of life, or any clinical or laboratory parameter in cats treated with this drug versus cats receiving a placebo.[38] Of the cats in the study, 21 of 23 cats displayed effusion at the start of the study. The drug might be more useful in cats without effusion because it may have a chance to prevent vasculitis and therefore effusions, but studies are lacking.

INTERFERON

Interferons are molecules produced by vertebrate cells in response to viral infections or certain inert substances, such as double-stranded RNA, and other microbial agents. There are three types of IFNs. Type I IFNs comprise the largest subfamily and include IFN-α, IFN-β, and IFN-omega. Type I IFNs are produced by various cell types, such as leukocytes and fibroblasts, in direct response to virus infection.[39] There is only one member of the type II IFN subfamily, IFN-γ, that is an immunomodulatory cytokine, produced in response to recognition of infected cells by T lymphocytes and natural killer cells of the host's immune system.[39] Type III IFNs, which contain three ILs, (IL-28A, IL-28B, and IL-29), are identified. This subfamily also has the ability to interfere with virus replication and has been suggested to be the ancestral antiviral system of vertebrates.[39] Interferons are not virucidal; rather, they trigger expression of various antiviral proteins and thus induce an antiviral state within the host cell to limit replication and spread of viruses. Further, type I IFNs have been shown to potently enhance innate and adaptive immune responses *in vivo*, through various immunomodulatory effects, such as activation of dendritic cells (DCs), amplification of antibody response, and enhancement of T-cell and natural killer cell cytotoxicity.[40] Viruses causing lysis of their target cell are most effectively inhibited by IFN through their antiviral activity in noninfected cells. Therefore, IFNs have their highest utility in the prophylaxis or early postexposure management for virus infections. Given that IFNs are not specific for a particular virus, they have been tested for the treatment of multiple feline viruses, including FHV-1, FIV, FeLV, feline calicivirus (FCV), and FCoV.[40]

Two molecules of type I IFNs are currently being used for therapy in cats: human recombinant interferon alpha (rHuIFN-α), and rFeIFN-omega, which is licensed for use in cats and dogs in Europe, Australia, and some Asian countries. IFNs are not strictly species-specific in their effects; however, their biologic activity and toleration are greater in cells of genetically related species. *In vitro* results suggest that rFeIFN-omega would likely be more effective than rHuIFN-α *in vivo*, although both IFNs have been shown to have therapeutic value in cats.[40]

There are two common treatment regimens for use of rHuIFN-α in cats: injection of a high dose (10^4 to 10^6 International Unit per kg SC every 24 hours) or oral application of a low dose (1 to 50 International Unit [IU] per kg every 24 h). When given parenterally to cats, rHuIFN-α becomes ineffective within a few weeks because of the development of neutralizing antibodies that limit its activity.[40,41] rHuIFN-α can be given orally for a longer period because no antibodies will develop during oral treatment. Unlike rHuIFN, rFeIFN-omega, being a feline recombinant product does not induce neutralizing antibodies when administered SC. This means that the high-dose parenteral protocol can be used safely and efficiently even if repeat administration is required. This is an important factor to consider in a condition where management needs to be lifelong.[42]

Given PO, IFNs are inactivated by gastric acid and destroyed by trypsin and other proteolytic enzymes in the duodenum and therefore are not absorbed and cannot be detected in the blood after oral administration. Direct antiviral effects are unlikely after oral application; however, IFN still seem to have immunomodulatory activity. Type I IFNs likely bind to mucosal receptors in the oral cavity, stimulating the local lymphoid tissue, leading to cytokine release from lymphatic cells in the oropharyngeal lymphoid tissues, triggering a cascade of immunologic responses that act systemically.[43]

Feline Retroviruses

Interferons have been used for the treatment of feline retrovirus infections. Treatment with IFN improved the clinical condition scores of cats infected with FeLV and FIV, but not because of a reduction in viral load. This suggests that the improved clinical condition seen with treatment is not specific to an antiviral effect, at least not for FIV and FeLV, but instead is a result of immunomodulation, potentially associated with the innate immune response.[40,42,44]

Some clinical signs in FIV-infected cats are caused by immunopathological reactions, such as gingivostomatitis and uveitis. Immunomodulation might be the cause of improvement of some clinical signs associated with IFN treatment, probably the result of an effective control over inflammatory cytokines in diseased organs.[44] It has been suggested that a nonspecific stimulation of the immune system with IFN therapy might be contraindicated in FIV-infected cats because it could lead to a rise in viral replication produced by the activation of lymphocytes and macrophages harboring latent infections and therefore accelerate disease progression in these cats, and the use of IFN in HIV-infected humans is controversial.[5] However, use of low-dose oral HuIFN (natural, not recombinant in this study) in ill FIV-infected cats (50 IU per kg on the oral mucosa daily for 7 days on alternating weeks for 6 months, followed by a 2-month break, and then repetition of the 6-month treatment) resulted in improvement of clinical signs in a placebo-controlled, double-blind study.[44] Parenteral rFeIFN-omega used according to the licensed protocol (Table 7-1) resulted in decreased mortality rates in FeLV-infected cats, compared with the control group in another placebo-controlled study.[40,45] In another study evaluating FIV- and/or FeLV-infected cats housed in a shelter, hematologic values remained within reference ranges, and there were no biochemical abnormalities associated with rFeIFN-omega treatment used according to the licensed protocol.[41] These findings suggest that IFN treatment is safe for treatment of FIV- and FeLV-infected cats,[40,41,44,45] but further studies are required to clearly demonstrate its efficacy against FIV and FeLV *in vivo*.

A recent study evaluated the use of oral administration of rFeIFN-omega for the treatment of symptomatic naturally infected, client-owned FIV-infected cats.[42] The treatment protocol was 10^5 IU/cat PO every 24 hours for 90 consecutive days, administered by the cats' owners. A historical group that was treated SC with the licensed protocol[41] was used as a control for comparison, but no placebo group was included. Treatment resulted in significant improvement of clinical scores between pretreatment and post-treatment values, and there was no significant difference between the SC historical control group and the PO group, suggesting that PO administration of rFeIFN-omega could be used effectively as an alternative to the licensed protocol, at a significantly reduced cost.[42]

An additional benefit of using IFN therapy for FIV and FeLV treatment could be the effect of IFN on opportunistic infections by other viruses, including FHV-1 and FCV.[41] In fact, the effect of IFN on these additional viral infections might be the cause of the improved clinical scores associated with IFN treatment.[40,41] Both FIV and FeLV replicate in lymphoid and monocytoid cell subsets and cause immunosuppression. In FIV-infected cats, most of the clinical signs are not directly caused by the FIV itself but are the result of secondary infections, as well as neoplasia.[40,46] Although FeLV causes more severe clinical syndromes than FIV does, diseases secondary to immunosuppression account for a large portion of the syndromes seen in FeLV-infected cats as well.[11] Considering that IFN therapy seems to have no effect on FIV and FeLV virus load but it is immunomodulatory, it would seem advisable to treat retrovirus-infected cats with IFN when they have clinical signs, as they would benefit from its effects in improving their clinical condition.[40]

Feline Herpesvirus Type I and Feline Calicivirus

A recent study attempted to evaluate the hypothesis that improvement in clinical scores with IFN treatment in FIV- and FeLV-infected cats might be a reflection of reduction in viral shedding of secondary viruses in these cats.[41] Sixteen naturally infected FIV- and/or FeLV-infected cats (seven FIV, six FeLV, and three coinfected) were followed during rFeIFN-omega therapy (used according to the licensed protocol) to monitor clinical signs and to correlate them with excretion of concomitant viruses (FCV, FHV-1, FCoV, and feline parvovirus [FPV]). Shedding of these viruses was evaluated by real-time quantitative polymerase chain reaction (PCR) (FHV-1 and FCoV) or conventional PCR (FCV and FPV). Pretreatment and post-treatment samples were compared. Feline calicivirus shedding was detected in 13 of 16 cats on day 0 and not detected on day 65. The amount of FHV-1 shedding was significantly reduced in the cats at the end of the study (day 65), compared with the beginning.

Feline coronavirus shedding was reduced but not significantly, and there was not enough FPV detected in the population to draw any significant conclusions.[41] However, there was no placebo group used for this study, and without a placebo group, it is difficult to determine definitively if the results are due to antiviral effects of IFN or are just consistent with the natural resolution of viral shedding.

In a separate study, 36 cats with naturally acquired upper respiratory tract disease housed in a humane society facility were treated with one drop of rFeIFN-omega solution (10^6 unit/mL), rHuIFN-α solution (10^6 IU/mL), or saline (0.9% NaCl) solution (12 cats/group) in each eye twice daily for 14 days for the treatment of keratoconjunctivitis.[46] There was no statistical difference between the treatment groups and the placebo group with regard to clinical scores or viral shedding (FHV-1 and FCV), determined by real-time quantitative PCR from oropharyngeal and conjunctival swabs. Feline herpesvirus type 1 shedding was lower, though not statistically significant, on day 14 compared with day 0 for all groups (including the placebo group), and clinical scores were significantly decreased on day 14 compared to day 0, again for all groups including the placebo group.[46] Therefore, comparing results between days 0 and 14 in the treated cats without the inclusion of the placebo group would have resulted in a different conclusion for this study. These cats were not infected with FeLV, and even though the FIV status was unknown for all the cats, the ones that were tested were negative. However, this study highlights the need for a placebo group for accurate evaluation of the effect of IFN therapy on FHV-1 and FCV shedding and associated disease.

Oral and SC IFN therapy has been associated with an improvement in oral ulcers and gingivitis and gingivostomatitis in cats infected with FIV,[40,41] a condition that is common in cats with FCV infections.[41] Feline calicivirus is also associated with chronic gingivostomatitis in cats not infected with FIV or FeLV,[43] and a study evaluated the efficacy of rFeIFN-omega (10^5 IU/day for 90 days by topical oromucosal administration) for the treatment of FCV-associated feline chronic gingivostomatitis (FCGS) and caudal stomatitis in FIV-/FeLV-negative cats.[43] Cats were included in the study if they continued to show persistence of clinical signs of FCGS at least 2 months after periodontal treatment (scaling, subgingival débridement, and polishing), tooth extraction, and 3 weeks of antibiotics with analgesic and anti-inflammatory drugs as needed. Twenty-four cats were treated with the IFN, and the effect was compared with a positive control group that received a standard corticosteroid therapy. The results suggested that the IFN therapy was as effective as the corticosteroid treatment for this condition for improvement in clinical signs.[43] Feline calicivirus viral loads were not evaluated in this study, and there was no placebo group used for comparison. However, assuming the IFN therapy was the cause of the improvement seen in these cats, the results add to the hypothesis that improvement in oral lesions in FIV- and/or FeLV-infected cats likely is associated with the effect of IFN on opportunistic viral infections. Differences in the outcome of the different studies could be due to different application methods (e.g., ocular versus oral); however, definitive conclusions cannot be drawn without additional studies that also evaluate viral load in naturally infected cats that are randomized, placebo-controlled, and double-blinded.

Feline Coronavirus and Feline Infectious Peritonitis

IFN has also been evaluated for treatment of FIP. In a randomized placebo-controlled, double-blinded treatment trial, 37 cats with FIP were treated with rFeIFN-omega or placebo.[47] In all cats, FIP was confirmed by histology and/or immunohistochemical or immunofluorescence staining of FCoV antigen in effusion or tissue macrophages. All cats received glucocorticoids, either as dexamethasone in case of effusion (1 mg/kg intrathoracic or intraperitoneal injection every 24 hours) or prednisolone (2 mg/kg PO every 24 hours). Cats also received either a placebo or rFeIFN-omega at 10^6 IU/kg SC every 24 hours for 8 days and subsequently once a week. There was no statistically significant difference in the mean survival time of cats treated with rFeIFN-omega versus the placebo. Cats survived for a period of 3 to 200 days before euthanasia with a mean survival time of 18 days. There was only one long-term survivor (>3 months) in the rFeIFN-omega group. Interferon treatment might be more effective if started earlier, but this is not of relevance in the treatment of cats with FIP in the field.[47] However, IFN therapy might be useful for treatment of cats with chronic FCoV shedding, but further studies are required. As previously mentioned, treatment with rFeIFN-omega (licensed SC protocol) was associated with a decrease in FCoV shedding in FIV- and/or FeLV-infected cats; however, the results were not compared with a placebo group.[41]

SUMMARY

In conclusion, antivirals are still in their infancy for the treatment of feline diseases. However, as new drugs are produced for human viral diseases that can be used for feline patients, and testing of currently available drugs continues, it is hoped that determination of effective protocols for treatment of feline viral diseases will be possible in the future.

References

1. Maggs DJ: Antiviral therapy for feline herpesvirus infections. Vet Clin Small Anim 40:1055–1062, 2010.
2. Mohammadi H, Bienzle D: Pharmacological inhibition of feline immunodeficiency virus (FIV). Viruses 4:708–724, 2012.
3. De Clercq E: Anti-HIV drugs: 25 compounds approved within 25 years after the discovery of HIV. Int J Antimicrob Agents 33:307–320, 2009.
4. Schwartz AM, McCrackin MA, Schinazi RF, et al: Antiviral efficacy of nine nucleoside reverse transcriptase inhibitors against feline immunodeficiency virus in feline peripheral blood mononuclear cells. Am J Vet Res 75:273–281, 2014.
5. Gómez NV, Fontanals A, Castillo V, et al: Evaluation of different antiretroviral drug protocols on naturally infected feline immunodeficiency virus (FIV) cats in the late phase of the asymptomatic stage of infection. Viruses 4:924–939, 2012.
6. De Clercq E: Acyclic nucleoside phosphonates: past, present and future bridging chemistry to HIV, HBV, HCV, HPV, adeno-, herpes-, and poxvirus infections: the phosphonate bridge. Biochem Pharmacol 73:911–922, 2007.
7. Hartmann K, Stengel C, Klein D, et al: Efficacy and adverse effects of the antiviral compound plerixafor in feline immunodeficiency virus-infected cats. J Vet Intern Med 26:483–490, 2012.
8. Hartmann AD, Wilhelm N, Balzarini J, et al: Clinical efficacy of the acyclic nucleoside phosphonate 9-(2-phosphonylmethoxypropyl) -2,6-diaminopurine (PMPDAP) in the treatment of feline immunodeficiency virus-infected cats. J Feline Med Surg 14:107–112, 2011.
9. De Bethune MP: Non-nucleoside reverse transcriptase inhibitors (NNRTIs), their discovery, development, and use in the treatment of HIV-1 infection: A review of the last 20 years (1989-2009). Antiviral Res 85:75–90, 2010.
10. Auwerx J, Esnouf R, De Clercq E, et al: Susceptibility of feline immunodeficiency virus/human immunodeficiency virus type 1 reverse transcriptase chimeras to non-nucleoside RT inhibitors. Molec Pharmacol 65:244–251, 2004.
11. Hartmann K: Clinical aspects of feline immunodeficiency and feline leukemia virus infection. Vet Immunol Immunopathol 143:190–201, 2011.
12. Arai M, Earl DD, Yamamoto JK: Is AZT/3TC therapy effective against FIV infection or immunopathogenesis? Vet Immunol Immunopathol 85:189–204, 2002.
13. Gingerich DA: Lymphocyte-cell immunomodulator (LTCI): review of the immunopharmacology of a new veterinary biologic. Intern J Appl Res Vet Med 6:61–68, 2008.
14. Greggs WM, III, Clouser CL, Patterson SE, et al: Discovery of drugs that possess activity against feline leukemia virus. J Gen Virol 93:900–905, 2012.
15. Stuetzer B, Brunner K, Lutz H, et al: A trial with 3′-azido-2′,3′-dideoxythymidine and human interferon-a in cats naturally infected with feline leukaemia virus. J Feline Med Surg 5:667–671, 2013.
16. Cattori V, Weibel B, Lutz H: Inhibition of feline leukemia virus replication by the integrase inhibitor Raltegravir. Vet Microbiol 152:165–168, 2011.
17. Semenkow SL, Johnson NM, Maggs DJ, et al: Controlled release delivery of penciclovir via a silicone (MED-4750) polymer: kinetics of drug delivery and efficacy in preventing primary feline herpesvirus infection in culture. Virol J 11:34, 2014.
18. De Clercq E: A 40-year journey in search of selective antiviral chemotherapy. Annu Rev Pharmacol and Toxicol 51:1–24, 2011.
19. Nasisse MP, Dorman DC, Jamison KC, et al: Effects of valacyclovir in cats infected with feline herpesvirus 1. Am J Vet Res 58:1141–1144, 1997.
20. Thomasy SM, Lim CC, Reilly CM, et al: Evaluation of orally administered famciclovir in cats experimentally infected with feline herpesvirus type-1. Am J Vet Res 72:85–95, 2011.
21. Groth AD, Contreras MT, Kado HK, et al: In vitro cytotoxicity and antiviral efficacy against feline herpesvirus type 1 of famciclovir and its metabolites. Vet Ophthalmol 1–7, 2013.
22. Malik R, Lessels NS, Webb S, et al: Treatment of feline herpesvirus-1 associated disease in cats with famciclovir and related drugs. J Feline Med Surg 11:40–48, 2009.
23. Thomasy SM, Covert JC, Stanley SD, et al: Pharmacokinetics of famciclovir and penciclovir in tears following oral administration of famciclovir to cats: a pilot study. Vet Ophthalmol 15:299–306, 2012.

24. Gould D: Feline herpesvirus-1: ocular manifestations, diagnosis and treatment options. *J Feline Med Surg* 13:333–346, 2011.

25. Fontenelle JP, Powell CC, Veir JK, et al: Effect of topical ophthalmic application of cidofovir on experimentally induced primary ocular feline herpesvirus-1 infection in cats. *Am J Vet Res* 69:289–293, 2008.

26. Wilkes RP, Kania SA: Evaluation of the effects of small interfering RNAs on in vitro replication of feline herpesvirus-1. *Am J Vet Res* 71:655–663, 2010.

27. Wilkes RP, Kania SA: Use of interfering RNAs targeted against feline herpesvirus 1 glycoprotein D for inhibition of feline herpesvirus 1 infection of feline kidney cells. *Am J Vet Res* 70:1018–1025, 2009.

28. Gavrilov K, Saltzman WM: Therapeutic siRNA: principles, challenges, and strategies. *Yale J Biol Med* 85:187–200, 2012.

29. Wilkes RP, Ward D, Newkirk KM, et al: Evaluation of delivery agents used for introduction of small interfering RNAs into feline corneal cells. *Am J Vet Res* 74:243–247, 2013.

30. Fascetti AJ, Maggs DJ, Kanchuk ML, et al: Excess dietary lysine does not cause lysine-arginine antagonism in adult cats. *J Nutrition* 134(8 Suppl):2042S–2045S, 2004.

31. Cave NJ, Dennis K, Gopakumar G, et al: Effects of physiologic concentrations of L-lysine on in vitro replication of feline herpesvirus 1. *Am J Vet Res* 75:572–580, 2014.

32. Rees TM, Lubinski JL: Oral supplementation with L-lysine did not prevent upper respiratory infection in a shelter population of cats. *J Feline Med Surg* 10:510–513, 2008.

33. Kim Y, Mandadapu SR, Groutas WC, et al: Potent inhibition of feline coronaviruses with peptidyl compounds targeting coronavirus 3C-like protease. *Antiviral Res* 97:161–168, 2013.

34. Liu I, Tsai W, Hsieh L, et al: Peptides corresponding to the predicted heptad repeat 2 domain of the feline coronavirus spike protein are potent inhibitors of viral infection. *PLoS ONE* 8:e82081, 2013.

35. Hsieh L, Lin C, Su B, et al: Synergistic antiviral effect of *Galanthus nivalis* agglutinin and nelfinavir against feline coronavirus. *Antiviral Res* 88:25–30, 2010.

36. Legendre AM, Bartges JW: Effect of Polyprenyl Immunostimulant on the survival times of three cats with the dry form of feline infectious peritonitis. *J Feline Med Surg* 11:624–626, 2009.

37. Pedersen NC: An update on feline infectious peritonitis: virology and immunopathogenesis. *Vet J* 2014, doi: 10.1016/j.tvjl.2014.04.017.

38. Fischer R, Ritz K, Webber C, et al: Randomized, placebo controlled study of the effect of propentofylline on survival time and quality of life of cats with feline infectious peritonitis. *J Vet Intern Med* 25:1270–1276, 2011.

39. Bonjardim CA, Ferreira PCP, Kroon EG: Interferons: signaling, antiviral and viral evasion. *Immunol Lett* 122:1–11, 2009.

40. Domenech A, Miro G, Collado VM, et al: Use of recombinant interferon omega in feline retrovirosis: from theory to practice. *Vet Immunol Immunopathol* 143:301–306, 2011.

41. Gil S, Leal RO, Duarte A, et al: Relevance of feline interferon omega for clinical improvement and reduction of concurrent viral excretion in retrovirus infected cats from a rescue shelter. *Res Vet Sci* 94:753–763, 2013.

42. Gil S, Leal RO, McGahie N, et al: Oral recombinant feline interferon-omega as an alternative immune modulation therapy in FIV positive cats: clinical and laboratory evaluation. *Res Vet Sci* 96:79–85, 2014.

43. Hennet PR, Camy GAL, McGahie DM, et al: Comparative efficacy of a recombinant feline interferon omega in refractory cases of calicivirus-positive cats with caudal stomatitis: a randomised, multi-centre, controlled, double-blind study in 39 cats. *J Feline Med Surg* 13:577–587, 2011.

44. Pedretti E, Paseri B, Amadori M, et al: Low-dose interferon-treatment for feline immunodeficiency virus infection. *Vet Immunol Immunopathol* 109:245–254, 2006.

45. de Mari K, Maynard L, Sanquer A, et al: Therapeutic effects of recombinant feline interferon-omega on feline leukemia virus (FeLV)-infected and FeLV/feline immunodeficiency virus (FIV)-coinfected symptomatic cats. *J Vet Intern Med* 18:477–482, 2004.

46. Slack JM, Stiles J, Leutenegger CM, et al: Effects of topical ocular administration of high doses of human recombinant interferon alpha-2b and feline recombinant interferon omega on naturally occurring viral keratoconjunctivitis in cats. *Am J Vet Res* 74:281–289, 2013.

47. Ritz S, Egberink H, Hartmann K: Effect of feline interferon-omega on the survival time and quality of life of cats with feline infectious peritonitis. *J Vet Intern Med* 21:1193–1197, 2007.

The Gut Microbiome

J. Scott Weese

The intestinal tract houses one of the most abundant microbial populations on the planet. It is estimated that the microbial population of an individual (the microbiota) contains 10 times more cells than the host. When the sum of the genetic makeup of the microbiota (the microbiome) is considered, microbial dominance increases to approximately 100 to 1000 times that of the host. Much of the microbiota has likely evolved with its particular host species, and it should come as no surprise that there is an intimate relationship between the animal host and its microbial residents.

The role of the intestinal microbiota in intestinal health and digestion has been recognized (or appreciated) for many years. It is clear that the intestinal microbiota performs many important functions to maintain health and prevent disease, and that alterations in the microbiota can be associated with various disease processes. The gastrointestinal microbiota aids in digestion, helps exclude ingested pathogens, interacts with the local and systemic immune systems, and performs a wide array of other activities, most of which are poorly understood. Many potential impacts of the microbiota on disease, particularly extraintestinal disease, are probably not even realized.

As research advances, it becomes abundantly clear that the microbiota interacts closely with the body in diverse and complicated ways and well beyond the intestinal tract. The body is constantly encountering bacterial metabolites, in the gut and beyond, and it is estimated that up to one third of small molecules circulating in the human bloodstream originate from the gut microbiota.[1] These can have complex and wide-ranging effects, and there is increasing information about potential roles of the microbiota in a wide range of conditions, including infectious, allergic, metabolic, and neoplastic diseases, as well as obesity. In humans, data suggest that the intestinal microbiota may even be involved in diseases that have not traditionally had any clear connection to the intestinal tract, such as neurocognitive disorders and autism.

ASSESSMENT OF THE GUT MICROBIOTA

Early study of the feline gut microbiota involved the use of bacterial culture and resulted in what we now know to be a tremendous underestimation of the composition and structure of the microbiota. As limitations of culture were recognized and new technologies were developed, broader insight was gained using culture-independent methods. The development of next generation sequencing, which allows for analysis of thousands to millions of DNA sequences, has revolutionized the study of complex bacterial populations. Combined with parallel advances in bioinformatics, it is now possible to identify thousands of bacteria in a sample and to get a better understanding of the microbiota. This approach has been used extensively in humans and some other animal species, with studies providing unprecedented information about the intestinal microbiota in health and various disease states. While powerful, there are still limitations, such as an inability to provide absolute (as opposed to relative) quantification and an inability to evaluate spatial distribution. These are strengths of another currently used method, fluorescence *in situ* hybridization (FISH), a method that allows for objective quantification of bacterial groups, as well as spatial distribution within tissue or samples. However, FISH is labor intensive, not amenable to high throughput, and focused on specific known bacterial groups; it is best used for evaluation of the presence and distribution of selected bacterial groups in biopsy samples. An ideal (but rarely applied) approach is to use a combination of methods (Table 8-1).

Normal Feline Fecal Microbiota

Comparison of results from earlier culture-dependent studies with recent FISH and DNA sequence–based studies shows the remarkable evolution in our understanding of the feline microbiota. A 1971 study reported isolation of only a small number of different genera (maximum six per cat) and a dominance of enterococci, streptococci, coliforms, and lactobacilli.[2] Clostridia were found in a minority of cats. In hindsight, these findings clearly provide a superficial, if not potentially misleading, assessment of the gut microbiota. However, that was inevitable because of the limitations of available technology combined with the highly complex microbiota and presence of a large number of organisms that are not able to be cultured using standard methods. It is likely that tens of thousands of different bacterial species can be found in the intestinal tract of an individual animal, with an overall bacterial abundance estimated to be in the range of 10^{10} to 10^{11} (10 to 100 billion) bacteria per gram of feces.[3] Further, the bacterial genera that dominated early culture-based studies are now known to comprise a minority of the microbiota, whereas anaerobes such as clostridia were underestimated.

Table 8-1	Summary of Different Methods of Evaluating Gastrointestinal Microbiota		
Method	**Description**	**Advantages**	**Disadvantages**
Culture	Inoculation onto nonselective or selective culture media, with subsequent biochemical or molecular identification of individual bacteria	• Can obtain isolates for definitive identification, susceptibility testing, and typing • Inexpensive • Limited need for specialized equipment • Quantitative	• Cannot grow a large percentage of the microbiota • Profound culture bias because some bacteria grow much better than others • Cannot properly evaluate an environment with thousands of different species
Fluorescence *in situ* hybridization (FISH)	Use of fluorescent probes that bind to specific bacteria/genes, with visualization via fluorescence microscopy	• Semiquantitative • Can evaluate distribution of bacteria within tissue • Can be highly specific, identifying selected species (or genes) • No bias from differences in amplification efficiency (PCR bias)	• Limited throughput • Dependent on known gene sequences; unable to identify unknown organisms • Unable to characterize vast numbers of different microorganisms in a sample
16S rRNA gene cloning	Use of broad range (eubacterial) PCR followed by cloning of PCR products into plasmids, then sequencing the plasmids	• Culture-independent: Can identify unknown and unculturable organisms	• Limited throughput • Labor intensive and expensive • PCR and cloning bias • May have limited species resolution (i.e., good for identifying bacteria to the genus level but not necessarily species level)
Next generation sequencing of PCR products	Use of broad range (eubacterial) PCR and subsequent direct sequencing of PCR products	• Culture-independent: Can identify unknown and unculturable organisms • Now amenable to high throughput approaches • Can identify thousands of different bacteria in a single sample • Allows for assessment of microbial community composition and structure	• PCR bias • Does not quantify total bacterial numbers • Indicates microbial composition but not function • May have limited species resolution
Shotgun next generation sequencing	Direct sequencing of DNA from samples	• Can identify unknown and unculturable organisms • No PCR bias • Can also provide information about nonbacterial components (e.g., Archaea, fungi, viruses) • Massive amount of data • Can evaluate functional characteristics of the microbiota, not just phylogeny	• Expensive • Database limitations hamper classification of a large percentage of non–16S rRNA gene sequences • May have limited species resolution • Requires advanced computational resources

PCR, Polymerase chain reaction; *rRNA,* ribosomal ribonucleic acid.

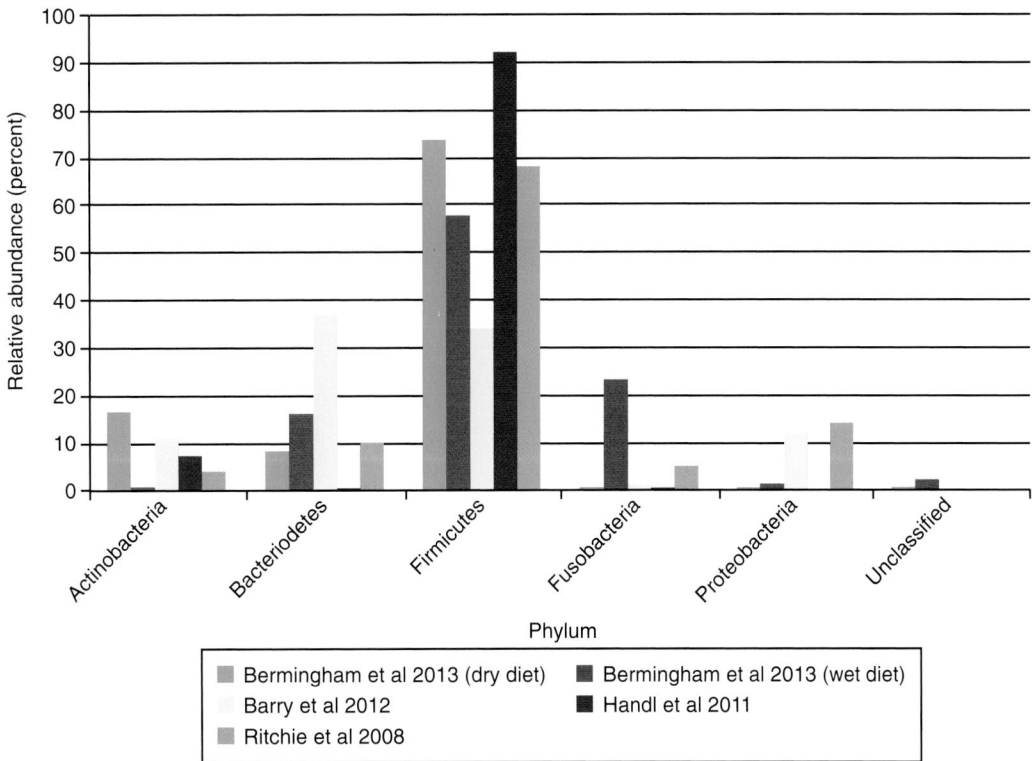

Figure 8-1: Relative abundances of different bacterial phyla from 16S ribosomal ribonucleic acid gene sequence–based studies evaluating the fecal microbiome in cats.

Whereas care should be taken in directly comparing results from different studies, a crude representation of the phylum-level distribution of the fecal microbiome from some recent culture-independent feline studies is illustrated in Figure 8-1. Studies have reported variable results, even at the phylum level. For context, the difference between a cat and a tapeworm is at the phylum level, so it can reasonably be assumed that phylum-level changes in the gut microbiota could result in marked functional changes. Whether this is because of small study size, differences in methodology, differences in cat populations (e.g., research colony versus household pets, indoor versus outdoor cats), geographic variation, bioinformatics approaches, or spurious results is unknown.

The normal or optimal intestinal microbiome in healthy cats is currently unknown, if one even exists. It likely varies with age, diet, and management (e.g., outdoor environment) among other factors, playing a role in its development and maintenance.[3-5] There can be remarkable variation among healthy cats and indeed, what is optimal for one cat may be suboptimal for another. Further, in humans, the concept of *enterotypes* has been put forth. Although not universally accepted, it has been postulated that there are a few main types of microbiota distribution (enterotypes) among healthy individuals in the same population, each of which seems entirely appropriate for the given host. Whether this means that some individuals are better suited for different enterotypes or whether any of these types are equally suitable for all individuals is unknown. There has been no investigation of this in cats.

Despite the wide variations reported in limited feline studies, five main phyla tend to predominate: Firmicutes, Bacteroidetes, Proteobacteria, Actinobacteria, and Fusobacteria. Within the typically dominant Firmicutes phylum, members of the Clostridia class and Clostridiales order usually account for the highest percentage of sequences in feline fecal samples.[6] The high prevalence of *Clostridium* spp. in healthy animals is noteworthy because of the widespread notion that clostridia are bad bacteria. This raises questions about the frequent use of empirical antimicrobial therapy directed against clostridia (e.g., metronidazole, tylosin) for the treatment of idiopathic diarrhea, because of the broad efficacy of those drugs against clostridia. Rather than being a bad group of bacteria, many (if not most) *Clostridium* spp., and in particular other genera from the Clostridiales order, such as *Roseburia, Lachnospira, Ruminococcus, Faecalibacterium,* and *Eubacterium,* may be critical components of gut health, and treatments that would also kill these beneficial clostridiales may not be optimal. Another main bacterial class within the Firmicutes phylum is Bacilli, which includes the *Lactobacillus, Streptococcus, Enterococcus,* and *Staphylococcus* genera. Many of these are typically considered "good" bacteria, and they may play important roles in gut health, although clear data are lacking.

The Bacteriodetes phylum is often reported as the second-most abundant phylum after Firmicutes and consists of various gram-negative species. This phylum tends to receive less attention because its members are less often implicated as pathogens or considered high-profile members of the microbiota. However, there have been some reports of overrepresentation of this phylum in some diseases in certain species (e.g., Crohn's disease in humans). Further, as this is a relatively common component of the microbiota in healthy cats, it is reasonable to assume that Bacteroidetes do have an important role in the normal microbiota. Recently, attention has been paid to the potential role of Bacteroidetes in prevention of obesity or in weight loss in humans and laboratory species.[7,8] Feline studies are lacking, but the role of Bacteroidetes in obesity management in cats requires evaluation.

The Proteobacteria phylum includes various clinically relevant genera such as *Salmonella, Escherichia, Shigella, Campylobacter,* and *Pasteurella.* This phylum tends to be less common in healthy cats, with higher levels found in some disease states, such as inflammatory bowel disease (IBD).[9,10] It is possible that an increase in Proteobacteria is an indicator of dysbiosis rather than an implication of these bacteria as a cause of IBD, since profound increases in Proteobacteria can be found in some diseases that are clearly not initiated by this bacterial group, such as *Clostridium difficile* diarrhea (or enteritis) in humans.[11]

Variable relative amounts of the Actinobacteria phylum have been reported, which may in part be a result of decreased efficiency of some universal bacterial primers for some members of this phylum.[12] A study using *cpn*60 instead of 16S ribosomal ribonucleic acid (rRNA) gene primers reported a relatively high prevalence of this phylum in dogs.[13] Similarly, polymerase chain reaction (PCR) assays specifically targeting *Bifidobacterium* (a member of this group that is available in some commercial probiotics) can find that genus much more commonly than typical 16S rRNA gene studies. It has been reported that Actinobacteria were more prevalent in obese dogs.[14] This should not be taken as implying that bifidobacteria supplementation should be avoided, but that investigation of this phylum (among others) in obesity in cats is necessary before drawing conclusions.

With any study of microbiome composition, care must also be taken to remember that phylogeny and function are not necessarily the same thing. Although it is reasonable to assume that bacteria of different taxonomic levels, particularly higher levels such as phylum or order, have different functions, there can be a remarkable degree of functional redundancy (at least in humans), whereby diverse microorganisms can perform the same core functions, and phylogeny is only one piece of the puzzle that is the feline intestinal microbiota.

Assessing the Microbiota: From Individuals to Populations

Traditionally, the focus of microbiota assessment has been on individual microorganisms, mainly the number present (abundance) or their percentage of the total population (relative abundance). Relative abundance is still widely used for microbiota assessment, but it is clear that the microbiota is a functioning population that is not simply the sum of all its microbial parts. Rather, it is a community that interacts with itself and the body, and so measures typically applied to ecologic studies are now used to assess the intestinal microbiota. Among the more common are diversity, evenness, and richness, presumably important descriptors of the microbiota but also ones where an optimal state is unknown (and perhaps variable among cats). Mathematical methods can also be used to compare bacterial community membership (bacterial groups that are present) and structure (groups that are present along with their relative abundance). Each of these can be calculated in different ways, usually with complex mathematical formulae, but the general principles of each are relatively straightforward and applicable to various studies. At this time, with advances in methodologies, it is becoming easy to produce abundant data describing the fecal microbiota of an individual animal. Yet, determining the clinical relevance to an individual animal is difficult because of deficiencies in understanding the "normal" microbiota and its variations, as well as the biologic relevance of any observed changes. Whereas microbiota assessment will likely be used as a tool for diagnosis of disease in individual animals in the future, much more study is required to get to this point.

What Does Fecal Analysis Indicate?

Disease does not occur in feces. Rather, it occurs in the tissues of the intestinal tract. It is important to remember that the gut is composed of many distinct ecologic niches. The environments in the stomach, small intestine, and large intestine are distinct, and are therefore quite different microbial habitats. It should not be surprising that there can be striking differences in the microbial compositions of those sites in other animal species.[15] Feline data are limited, but a culture-based study identified significant differences among intestinal locations.[2] While acknowledging the variability of the gastrointestinal tract, most research involves assessment of feces because of the ease and minimally invasive nature of sampling. It is reasonable to assume that significant variation exists, with feces more accurately representing distal intestinal locations. That does not mean that fecal analysis is not useful. Rather, it should serve as a reminder that feces only provide a partial reflection of the state of the microbiota elsewhere in the gastrointestinal tract. Better study of the composition of different intestinal tract locations and the correlation between changes in feces and other intestinal samples is required.

Cause versus Effect

One major challenge for studies of the gut microbiota is differentiating cause and effect. Cross-sectional studies are a mainstay of veterinary research and provide important information but rarely have any ability to demonstrate causation. Therefore, finding a difference in gut microbiota composition between two groups simply means that there was a difference. It could have occurred because the altered microbiota resulted in development of disease, but alteration of the microbiota as a result of disease is equally likely in many situations, or it could have occurred from some unrelated and irrelevant event. For example, the gut microbiota and its relation to obesity is an area of active research in humans, and something that may be relevant in cats. It is clear that obesity can be associated with a different gut microbiota, as was shown in people in a study comparing the fecal microbiota of lean and obese twins.[7] But, does that mean that different gut microbiota resulted in a development of obesity in those individuals, or were microbiota differences simply a result of different dietary intake by lean versus obese individuals? Further studies in laboratory animals have supported the hypothesis that obesity may indeed have an infectious component, with transfer of selected microbial components or the whole microbiota from an obese mouse being able to cause weight gain in a lean mouse.[8] A definitive answer to the question of the gut microbiota and obesity is still lacking, and this example shows the need for further studies to address the issue.

THERAPEUTIC MANIPULATION OF THE MICROBIOME

As it becomes clear that alterations in the gut microbiome can be associated with disease, measures to stabilize or restore the microbiome become more appealing. Yet, this is a complicated area because of our limited understanding of how (and why) the microbiome changes in different disease states, difficulties differentiating cause from effect, interindividual variation that might preclude a one-size-fits-all approach, and limited evidence of therapeutic effects on this complex microbial population. There are few feline studies and those that are available are often small, with limited statistical power or with design concerns.

Antimicrobial therapy is widely used to treat some gastrointestinal disorders, with anecdotal success. However, clear efficacy data are lacking; anecdotal response to therapy could indicate clinical efficacy, but it may also be a result of self-limiting disease or non-antimicrobial (e.g., anti-inflammatory) effects of administered drugs. It is likely that antimicrobials have a profound impact on the gut microbiome, and that this can result in clinical cure in many animals. However, it is a nonspecific, and in many ways crude, approach that carries some risk of further microbiome disruption, adverse effects, and antimicrobial resistance selection pressure.

Diet can play a role in microbiome development in other species, and unsurprisingly, there are data indicating that dietary changes can modify the feline fecal microbiome. Cats fed a dry diet had differences in the abundances of several phyla, with more Actinobacteria and fewer Fusobacteria and Proteobacteria.[16] Presumably, those changes were the result of different dietary compositions, such as differences in dietary protein to carbohydrate ratios,[17] not simply whether the diet was in a kibble or wet form. However, it indicated that relatively major fecal microbiome shifts can occur in clinically normal animals through dietary change. Dietary supplementation with fructooligosaccharide (FOS),

cellulose, or pectin can also modify the fecal microbiome,[18] something that is not surprising because these are nutritional substrates for some components of the intestinal microbiota. Extrapolating these data into clinical use is challenging, as the clinical relevance of these changes is largely unknown. Diverse therapeutic commercial diets are available, with anecdotal success but limited objective information. It is logical that modifying the nutritional source of the gut microbiome could alter its composition, but diets specifically targeting a desired microbiota modification (or specific microbiota effects) are lacking.

Probiotic therapy is also commonly used for various gastrointestinal disorders. In humans, probiotic therapy has received much attention, with highly mixed results. Interestingly, much of the strongest probiotic data from humans and other species involve efficacy against extraintestinal disease (e.g., allergy, vaginitis), not enteric disease, perhaps indicative of both the difficulty in manipulating the intestinal microbiota in enteric disease and the role of the microbiota in extraintestinal disease. Convincing feline data for efficacy of probiotics are currently lacking. No change in the microbiota was noted in a study of healthy cats,[19] although subtle (yet potentially relevant) changes may be difficult to identify. An impact of *Enterococcus faecium* (SF68) on feline herpesvirus type 1 (FHV-1)–associated morbidity was suggested in one study,[20] although the data were not particularly convincing. There is evidence from humans that the microbiota composition is strongly influenced early in life, with relative stability thereafter. This might suggest that it is difficult to modify the microbiota in healthy animals once they are adults.

Recently, there has been tremendous interest in fecal transplantation in humans, particularly as a treatment for refractory and recurrent *Clostridium difficile* infection (CDI). Also referred to as stool transplantation, transfaunation, or human biotherapy, this rather crude but potentially effective treatment is based on the concept that because the ideal components of a probiotic cocktail are not known, the entire fecal population from a healthy individual should be administered. This has been shown to have high cure rates in humans with CDI, with a parallel restoration of the microbiota of the recipient to a normal state, much more similar to the donor's than the patient's pretreatment microbiota.[11] Preliminary data from cats in a small, uncontrolled trial suggests that this might be an effective approach for chronic diarrhea,[21] although further study is required.

BEYOND BACTERIA

While bacteria make up the most abundant and probably most important components of the intestinal microbiota, there are also populations of Archaea,[22] fungi,[22,23] viruses,[22] and parasites that likely play some role in health and certainly in disease. These have received limited attention, in part because of the perceived importance of bacteria and because of the greater difficulty in assessing these groups. One study of healthy cats reported that bacteria accounted for 97.8% of the microbial DNA, with Archaea at 0.9%, viruses at 0.09%, and Eukaryota (e.g., fungi, protozoa) accounting for 1.2%.[22] While these groups make up minor components of the intestinal microbial community, they should not be ignored, and further study of their roles in health and disease, both independently and through interactions with other microbes, is required.

One closing point must be considered. The profound differences in culture-dependent and DNA sequence–based studies should perhaps serve as a reminder that we presumably have not yet reached the pinnacle of microbiota assessment. It is possible (if not likely) that in future years, reviews similar to this will point out the profound deficiencies in the methods of the early twenty-first century. Regardless, currently available technologies have revolutionized research, and few would deny that remarkable, important information is now being obtained and that the role of the microbiota in feline health and disease is profound.

References

1. Wikoff WR, Anfora AT, Liu J, et al: Metabolomics analysis reveals large effects of gut microflora on mammalian blood metabolites. *Proc Natl Acad Sci U S A* 106:3698–3703, 2009.
2. Osbaldiston GW, Stowe EC: Microflora of alimentary tract of cats. *Am J Vet Res* 32:1399–1405, 1971.
3. Jia J, Frantz N, Khoo C, et al: Investigation of the faecal microbiota of kittens: monitoring bacterial succession and effect of diet. *FEMS Microbiol Ecol* 78:395–404, 2011.
4. Jia J, Frantz N, Khoo C, et al: Investigation of the faecal microbiota of geriatric cats. *Lett Appl Microbiol* 53:288–293, 2011.
5. Desai A, Musil K, Carr A, et al: Characterization and quantification of feline fecal microbiota using *cpn*60 sequence-based methods and investigation of animal-to-animal variation in microbial population structure. *Vet Microbiol* 137:120–128, 2009.
6. Ritchie L, Steiner JM, Suchodolski JS: Assessment of microbial diversity along the feline intestinal tract using 16S rRNA gene analysis. *FEMS Microbiol Ecol* 66:590–598, 2008.
7. Turnbaugh PJ, Hamady M, Yatsunenko T, et al: A core gut microbiome in obese and lean twins. *Nature* 457:480–484, 2009.
8. Turnbaugh PJ, Ley RE, Mahowald MA, et al: An obesity-associated gut microbiome with increased capacity for energy harvest. *Nature* 444:1027–1031, 2006.
9. Inness VL, McCartney AL, Khoo C, et al: Molecular characterisation of the gut microflora of healthy and inflammatory bowel disease cats using fluorescence in situ hybridisation with special reference to *Desulfovibrio* spp. *J Anim Physiol Anim Nutr* 91:48–53, 2007.
10. Janeczko S, Atwater D, Bogel E, et al: The relationship of mucosal bacteria to duodenal histopathology, cytokine mRNA, and clinical disease activity in cats with inflammatory bowel disease. *Vet Microbiol* 128:178–193, 2008.
11. Shahinas D, Silverman M, Sittler T, et al: Toward an understanding of changes in diversity associated with fecal microbiome transplantation based on 16S rRNA gene deep sequencing. *MBio* 3:e338–e412, 2012.
12. Krogius-Kurikka L, Kassinen A, Paulin L, et al: Sequence analysis of percent G+C fraction libraries of human faecal bacterial DNA reveals a high number of Actinobacteria. *BMC Microbiol* 9:68, 2009.
13. Chaban B, Links MG, Hill JE: A molecular enrichment strategy based on *cpn*60 for detection of epsilon-proteobacteria in the dog fecal microbiome. *Microbiol Ecol* 63:348–357, 2012.
14. Handl S, German A, Holden S, et al: Fecal microbiota in lean and obese dogs. *FEMS Microbiol Ecol* 84:332–343, 2013.
15. Suchodolski JS, Camacho J, Steiner JM: Analysis of bacterial diversity in the canine duodenum, jejunum, ileum, and colon by comparative 16S rRNA gene analysis. *FEMS Microbiol Ecol* 66:567–578, 2008.
16. Bermingham EN, Young W, Kittelmann S, et al: Dietary format alters fecal bacterial populations in the domestic cat *(Felis catus)*. *MicrobiologyOpen* 2:173–181, 2013.
17. Hooda S, Vester Boler BM, Kerr KR, et al: The gut microbiome of kittens is affected by dietary protein:carbohydrate ratio and associated with blood metabolite and hormone concentrations. *Br J Nutr* 109:1637–1646, 2013.
18. Barry KA, Middelbos IS, Vester Boler BM, et al: Effects of dietary fiber on the feline gastrointestinal metagenome. *J Proteome Res* 11:5924–5933, 2012.
19. Garcia-Mazcorro JF, Lanerie DJ, Dowd SE, et al: Effect of a multi-species synbiotic formulation on fecal bacterial microbiota of healthy cats and dogs as evaluated by pyrosequencing. *FEMS Microbiol Ecol* 78:542–554, 2011.
20. Veir JK, Knorr R, Cavadini C, et al: Effect of supplementation with *Enterococcus faecium* (SF68) on immune functions in cats. *Vet Ther* 8:229–238, 2008.
21. Weese JS, Webb JA, Abrams-Ogg A, et al: Preliminary clinical and microbiome assessment of fecal transplantation in dogs and cats. *J Vet Intern Med* 27:651, 2013. (Abstract).
22. Tun HM, Brar MS, Khin N, et al: Gene-centric metagenomics analysis of feline intestinal microbiome using 454 junior pyrosequencing. *J Microbiol Methods* 88:369–376, 2012.
23. Handl S, Dowd SE, Garcia-Mazcorro JF, et al: Massive parallel 16S rRNA gene pyrosequencing reveals highly diverse fecal bacterial and fungal communities in healthy dogs and cats. *FEMS Microbiol Ecol* 76:301–310, 2011.

Complementary and Alternative Medicine Therapies for Inflammatory Bowel Disease

Craig B. Webb and Tracy L. Webb

CURRENT THERAPEUTIC STRATEGY

Diet, corticosteroids, and antibiotics are the mainstays of therapy for cats diagnosed with inflammatory bowel disease (IBD).[1,2] The goals of therapy are to reduce or eliminate the patient's clinical signs (e.g., decreased appetite, nausea, vomiting, diarrhea, and weight loss) and to reverse, repair, and normalize the gastrointestinal (GI) pathophysiology responsible for intestinal inflammation. The current therapeutic strategy for feline IBD is designed, in general, to limit the antigenic stimulation and dampen the inflammatory response of the GI immune system. Treatments are also used to address specific GI signs: an antiemetic for vomiting, an appetite stimulant for anorexia, and cobalamin supplementation as needed.

Dietary intervention in the treatment of feline IBD usually involves the use of a single-protein, single-carbohydrate source hypoallergenic diet or a hydrolyzed protein diet.[3] Guilford and colleagues[4] showed that 50% of cats with clinical signs consistent with an idiopathic chronic enteropathy improved significantly following several weeks of hypoallergenic dietary therapy. Although dietary intervention is an essential and often the first component of the sequential treatment plan for any cat with a chronic enteropathy, Guilford's data mean that at least 50% of these cases are not diet responsive; the designation of idiopathic IBD includes a failure to respond adequately to a dietary change alone.

Corticosteroids form the foundation of therapy in the majority of feline IBD cases. Prednisolone is commonly started at 5 mg/cat given once or twice daily so that the patient is initially receiving an immunosuppressive dose (1 to 2 mg/kg daily). Other immunosuppressive drugs are used in addition to or instead of prednisolone if the clinical response is unsatisfactory or prednisolone side effects are unacceptable (Table 9-1). These include dexamethasone or methylprednisolone acetate injections at the prednisolone dosage equivalent, budesonide, or cyclosporine.[2] Chlorambucil, considered a chemotherapeutic drug, was originally used in conjunction with prednisolone for treating cats with GI lymphoma,[5] but anecdotally is apparently becoming more popular as a second immunosuppressive drug in cats with IBD refractory to prednisolone treatment. The side effects associated with these drugs may include polyuria and polydipsia, and diabetes mellitus; however, many cats appear to tolerate corticosteroids well especially when used conservatively for the shortest duration possible.[6]

A course of antibiotics is frequently added to the diet change and immunosuppressive treatment for cats with IBD. Although tylosin is the antibiotic featured in recent research on canine antibiotic-responsive diarrhea, it is likely that metronidazole continues to be the most frequently prescribed antibiotic for cats with IBD. The motivation for adding antibiotics to the treatment protocol likely includes the belief that this will result in a beneficial change in the intestinal microbiota, may reduce the dosage of glucocorticoids when both drugs are used concurrently, or, in the case of metronidazole, may add an additional immunomodulatory agent.

The resolution of clinical signs in cats with IBD treated with diet, antibiotics, and/or immunosuppressive drugs is variable as to the degree and duration of clinical improvement. The reasons for seeking additional, alternative, or complementary therapies for feline IBD range from an inadequate clinical response to traditional therapy, frequent relapses, severity of medication side effects, difficulty administering medications, and/or the desire to use a more specific, targeted, or "natural" treatment for the disease.

Table 9-1	Drugs Commonly Used in the Treatment of Feline Inflammatory Bowel Disease
Drug	**Dosage**
Prednisolone	Starting dose 5 mg/cat PO, once or twice daily
Budesonide	0.5-1.0 mg/cat/day PO
Cyclosporine	5 mg/kg PO, once or twice daily
Chlorambucil	2 mg/cat PO, every 48-72 hours
Cobalamin	250 µg/cat SC; 1 injection weekly for 6 weeks, then 1 injection 30 days later, then retest 30 days after the last dose

PO, per os (orally); *SC,* subcutaneously.

COBALAMIN

Cobalamin refers to vitamin B_{12}, for which there are a number of chemical forms. Cyanocobalamin is the most common manufactured form of vitamin B_{12} for supplementation. In 1967 Gazet and McColl[7] compared the absorption of cobalamin across the small intestine of the cat to that of dogs, monkeys, and humans. Almost 10 years later Okuda and colleagues again looked at this absorptive process in the cat.[8] In 1992 Vaden and colleagues[9] presented a case study of a cat suffering from methylmalonic acidemia secondary to a putative defect in cobalamin absorption across the GI tract. In 1999 the Texas A&M GI Laboratory took note of cobalamin deficiency in cats with exocrine pancreatic insufficiency, finding serum levels to be severely decreased and recommending parenteral cobalamin supplementation.[10] Then in 2001 Simpson and colleagues[11] confirmed that a significant number of cats with GI, hepatic, and/or pancreatic disease had subnormal serum cobalamin concentrations. In 2005, Ruaux and colleagues[12] showed that cobalamin supplementation in cats with signs of GI disease (e.g., IBD) improved their biochemical abnormalities, and most importantly, led to decreased vomiting and diarrhea in a majority of cases when combined with other treatments. Thus cobalamin supplementation quickly went from a novel therapy to an accepted practice in many cases of feline GI disease. In fact, Reed and colleagues[13] suggest that we should consider supplementing cobalamin in a greater number and more varied distribution of feline illness cases.

Cobalamin is now well established as a complementary treatment for cats with IBD[14] (see Table 9-1). In fact, many cats with chronic GI signs receive cobalamin supplementation regardless of their endogenous level and so that level is often left unmeasured. But research suggests that the lowest cobalamin levels may be found in cats with GI lymphoma, and gastroenterologists are forever struggling with the important distinction between IBD and GI lymphoma. Of course cats with IBD can also have very low cobalamin levels, and cats with GI lymphoma can have normal cobalamin levels, but the initial cobalamin concentration could be an important piece of the overall diagnostic picture when attempting

to distinguish between these two diseases in cats.[15] Hypocobalaminemia strongly indicates the need for collection of ileal biopsies that aid in the diagnosis of feline alimentary lymphoma.[16]

PROBIOTICS

There are, of course, normal microbial inhabitants of the feline GI tract, such as *Firmicutes, Bacteroidetes,* and *Fusobacteria.* The commensal GI microbiota help to regulate innate and adaptive immunity.[17] Other bacteria are considered pathogens in the feline GI tract, such as select *Clostridium* spp., *Campylobacter, Salmonella,* and certain *Escherichia* spp. Dysbiosis is a common finding associated with IBD in dogs.[18] Accordingly, there is interest in microbiota as a potential therapeutic target in cats with chronic enteropathies and an interest in probiotics as one of those targeted therapies. Although that interest has translated into hundreds of studies and publications on the effects of probiotics in humans with GI disease, the number of articles in the feline veterinary literature is not nearly so extensive. As demonstrated in Table 9-2, our knowledge of the feline GI microbiota and the impact of probiotics on feline acute and chronic enteropathies is quite limited.

Probiotics are "Living organisms, which upon ingestion in a certain number exert health benefits beyond inherent basic nutrition."[19] The individual components of this definition are important considerations for veterinarians contemplating the use of probiotics in the therapy of feline GI diseases. The organisms in the intended product must be living, and their concentrations should be abundant. In addition, the organisms must be resistant to the acidic conditions of the stomach and the bile encountered in the proximal duodenum as well as metabolically active in the lumen of the GI tract where they would ideally adhere to the mucosa and persist during their administration period. Finding a commercial product that meets these requirements can be challenging at best. Weese and Martin[20] assessed 25 probiotics for label claims and bacterial content, finding significant deficiencies and inaccuracies in the majority of products. In only 4 of 15 products did the contents meet or exceed label claims, and only two of these provided labels with a proper description of the contents of the product. ConsumerLab.com is one low-cost, user-friendly source of information on product claims and quality that may help in evaluating the myriad of probiotics used by veterinary clients. But even starting with the assumption that a clinician is able to obtain a probiotic organism(s) as advertised, which ones should be prescribed?

There is, as of now, no evidence to support the claim that probiotics must be species-specific, as cross-species organisms have proven beneficial. There is, however, clear variability in the response, or lack of response, when administering probiotics to human patients with different GI diseases. It is clear that different probiotic strains of bacteria have different effects in different hosts. Two studies in cats found benefit in the administration of a single-organism product to shelter cats with acute diarrhea or use of a multi-organism product

Table 9-2 Feline Probiotic Literature: Citations of Probiotic Use in Cats with Enteropathies

Citation	Population (Number)	Key*	Reported Effect
Marshall-Jones, et al.[33]	Healthy adult cats (12)	1	Increased *Lactobacillus,* decreased *Clostridium* and *Enterococcus*
Veir, et al.[34]	Kittens (9)	2	Increased CD4+ cells
Lappin, et al.[35]	Chronic feline herpesvirus type 1 cats (12)	2	Lessened morbidity
Rishniw and Wynn[36]	Chronic kidney disease cats (10)	3	Failed to reduce azotemia when sprinkled on food
Garcia-Mazcorro, et al.[37]	Healthy cats (12) and dogs (12)	4	Increased abundance of probiotic bacteria in feces
Bybee, et al.[21]	Shelter cats (217)	2	Significantly fewer episodes of upper respiratory tract disease lasting 2 days or longer
Hart, et al.[22]	Feline chronic diarrhea (53)	4	70% of owners perceived improvement in diarrhea
Lalor and Gunn-Moore[23]	*Tritrichomonas foetus* (26)	2	Decreased risk of relapse

*1, Lactobacillus acidophilus (noncommercial source); 2, Enterococcus faecium SF68 (FortiFlora, Purina); 3, Azodyl (Vetoquinol); 4, Proviable-DC (Nutramax).

BOX 9-1 Feline Conditions That Can Be Considered for Probiotic Supplementation

- Acute onset idiopathic diarrhea
- Diarrhea associated with overcrowding, shelter environment, young cats
- Chronic diarrhea where response to traditional therapy is less than satisfactory
- In anticipation of stress, diet change, medication, travel
- Antibiotic-associated diarrhea (consider concurrent use as it appears that the probiotics used in veterinary products are resistant to the antibiotics used in veterinary patients, allowing for concurrent administration)
- Diarrhea associated with gastrointestinal parasites (consider as adjunctive therapy)

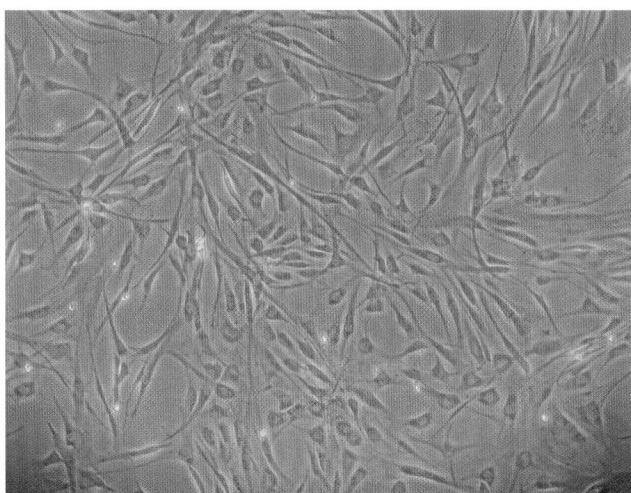

Figure 9-1: Adipose-derived feline mesenchymal stem cells in culture.

in client-owned cats with chronic enteropathy, respectively.[21,22] It would appear that the effect a probiotic has on the qualitative make-up of the recipient's microbiota is dependent on the continual use of the product during the treatment period. Box 9-1 lists feline GI conditions where probiotic supplementation may potentially play a beneficial role. The clinician is warned that the entries in this table are loosely based on theory, extrapolation from the human model, and anecdotal reports or experience. However, one of the more exciting recent findings is the positive effect on *Tritrichomonas foetus* diarrhea relapse in cats supplemented with a probiotic product.[23]

STEM CELLS

Stem cells were discovered approximately 50 years ago, and the field has rapidly expanded in the last decade. In general, stem cells are defined by the following three characteristics: capability of dividing and renewing through cell division for long periods of time, lack of specialization, and capability of giving rise to specialized cell types. Stem cells are divided into two main categories: embryonic (or pluripotent cells to include induced pluripotent stem cells) and adult (or somatic cells, which have more limited *in vitro* self-renewal capabilities). Adult stem cells can be divided into hematopoietic and mesenchymal types. Mesenchymal stem cells (MSC), also referred to as *multipotent stromal cells,* are identified mainly by their ability to differentiate into multiple mesenchymal tissues: chondrocytes, osteoblasts, and adipocytes. In fact, trilineage differentiation is one of three defining characteristics of MSC in addition to plastic adherence and self-renewal.[24] Mesenchymal stem cells can be derived from a multitude of adult tissues. Two of the most common tissues used for MSC generation are bone marrow and adipose tissue (Figure 9-1). Mesenchymal stem cells have been generated from many species, including recently from the domestic cat. Mesenchymal stem cells are considered important for both their potential regenerative capabilities as well as their immunomodulatory properties. Mesenchymal stem cells appear to avoid allogenic recognition and to target areas of inflammation, and therefore represent an interesting potential therapy for several disease processes affecting both human and veterinary patients.

There is currently very little published on feline MSC (fMSC).[25,26] However, the available research shows that fMSC are similar to MSC from other species. Feline MSC harvested from a variety of tissues show appropriate stem cell morphology and plastic adherence as well as the ability to propagate for several passages *in vitro*. All of the tested tissue types have also shown multilineage differentiation potential when cultured in the appropriate induction medium. Direct comparisons of the potential tissues of origin of fMSC are limited. One study found that, consistent with studies in other species, feline adipose tissue generates significantly more MSC in a shorter time period than does bone marrow.[27] Clinically useful numbers of early passage, culture-expanded adipose-derived fMSC can be generated in 7 to 10 days. Adipose tissue is collagenase-digested, the stromal vascular fraction (SVF) is isolated, and the cells are then cultured in a flask to allow isolation of the MSC and cell growth.

The majority of the available fMSC literature has been descriptive, and functional data for fMSC are lacking. Mesenchymal stem cells from other species are known to suppress T-cell function *in vitro*. Culture-expanded adipose-derived fMSC are similarly capable of suppressing mitogen-induced T-cell proliferation (T. Webb, unpublished data). Of additional importance, adipose-derived fMSC can be safely administered to allogeneic recipients without generating a clinically apparent immune response.[28,29] Culture-expanded allogeneic adipose-derived fMSC are currently being used in clinical trials to evaluate their therapeutic effects on several feline diseases including chronic kidney disease, asthma, and IBD.[28,29,30] Data from these various pilot studies suggest that when harvested, prepared, and handled appropriately, fMSCs can be safely administered to cats with a variety of chronic diseases. The presence and prevalence of long-term side effects occurring greater than 2 years following treatment have not yet been determined and are important areas of future research.

Of clinical significance, information concerning the ideal treatment parameters for fMSC is lacking. The ideal donor (e.g., autologous versus allogeneic, donor age, sex), tissue of origin, number of cells, method of cell preparation, site or route of injection, number of treatments, among other variables, remain unknown. These parameters may be dependent on multiple factors including the specific disease process being treated. Significant additional research is needed to further investigate the therapeutic potential of fMSC for cats.

There is significant immune dysregulation in feline IBD, and although the cytokine profile is complex and incompletely understood, limited data suggest that cytokine expression is a mixed response with select type 1 helper T cell (Th1) cytokines being differentially expressed, similar to humans with Crohn's disease.[31] The trophic properties along with the anti-inflammatory and immunomodulatory effects of MSC administration make it a theoretically beneficial treatment modality for feline IBD. The early success reported in animal models and clinical trials in humans with Crohn's disease further suggest that the use of MSC therapy in IBD warrants further consideration for use in cats. But at what point should the feline practitioner consider the leap from consideration to recommendation?

Adipose-derived fMSC are not embryonic stem cells, and so a significant barrier to their use (e.g., those based on philosophical, religious, and ethical beliefs) has been removed. Any client with a keyboard can quickly immerse themselves in the internet enthusiasm for the "silver bullet" potential of stem cell therapy—and then make an appointment with their veterinarian. As summed up by Dr. Dori Borjesson, many veterinarians offer stem cell therapies to satisfy demanding customers, so "Clinicians are sucked into giving treatment" even in the absence of research to support such treatment.[32]

Currently there are no U.S. Food and Drug Administration (FDA)-approved veterinary stem cell products. Several veterinary companies are providing commercially-available stem cell products, two of which advertise feline products: Vet-Stem (www.vet-stem.com), which offers Vet-Stem Regenerative Cell Therapy, and MediVet America, LLC (www.medivet-america.com), which offers an in-house kit. In both cases, the majority of these commercial treatments involve patients with orthopedic and musculoskeletal problems (e.g., chronic osteoarthritis, soft tissue injuries of the joints, tendons and ligaments, and fractures). However, feline gingivitis, kidney disease, IBD, and pulmonary fibrosis are also reported as targets. Neither website provides any references or cites any research on the use of their product in cats with chronic enteropathies including IBD.

For both of these companies, the process of stem cell therapy for feline IBD begins with the harvesting of adipose tissue from the patient to be treated (i.e., autologous treatment). In the case of Vet-Stem, the adipose tissue is shipped to their facility for processing, and the company returns the injection-ready product within 24 hours for an approximate cost of U.S. $2000 to $3500. Veterinarians are required to complete the company's accreditation course. MediVet America provides a kit for the in-house processing of adipose tissue, producing an injection-ready product in approximately 4 hours, at a cost of about $1800. Both companies claim to have serviced thousands of pets, although neither provides a specific number for the cats that have received treatment.

MediVet America states that:

- "Adult stem cells are highly concentrated in the fat tissue. … At this concentration, it is no longer necessary to culture the stem cells to acquire the necessary cell numbers to make a healing impact."
- "The stem cells are contained within a pool of cells in the fat termed the Stromal Vascular Fraction (SVF). The SVF may impart anti-inflammatory effects, add bioactive peptides, and contribute to reformation and architectural organization. These are benefits lost once stem cells are cultured."

The company provides an enzyme system to break down the adipose tissue and a filter and antibiotic wash for sterility of the resultant SVF. A key step appears to be the light-emitting diode (LED) activation of proliferation, differentiation, and induction prior to the reintroduction into the patient. MediVet claims that "we have seen positive clinical improvement in 95% of the arthritic cases performed nationwide".

The Vet-Stem website states "Regenerative cells 'communicate' with the cells of their local environment through paracrine and autocrine modalities, creating the optimal environment for natural healing" (http://www.vet-stem.com/science.php). Bob Harman, CEO of Vet-Stem, Inc., is quoted as saying there is "an 80% success rate in improvement of quality of life" (http://www.vet-stem.com/pdfs/6110 -0007-002%20Quality%20of%20Life%20Handout.pdf). Again, there are no references or cited research on the use of this therapy in cats with chronic enteropathies including IBD. The website states that Vet-Stem is currently evaluating the use of stem cells for the treatment of IBD, feline chronic kidney disease, liver disease, immune-mediated diseases, and heart disease. Their website states that cancer, systemic infection, neurologic disorders (including spinal cord injuries), uncontrolled diabetes mellitus, and any organ disease disqualifies a pet for Vet-Stem therapy.

Box 9-2 summarizes important parameters to consider prior to any recommendations for the use of stem cell therapy in cats, including those with IBD. Perhaps the first entry on that list should actually be the reminder: "At first, do no harm." Keeping this cautionary note in mind, at Colorado State University (CSU), a blinded, placebo-controlled clinical trial using allogeneic fMSCs harvested, processed, culture-expanded, and administered at CSU yielded promising results in cats with chronic enteropathies that have failed other therapies.[30]

Feline MSC research has been in progress for just over a decade but is currently expanding significantly as human and rodent studies have suggested several potential clinical applications of MSC for disease processes. Although fMSC thus far appear similar to MSC from other species, little published data are currently available. There is a significant lack of information on optimal details for fMSC use and function at this time. Current clinical trials have demonstrated safety and feasibility of administration of autologous and allogeneic adipose-derived fMSC, and further results from ongoing *in vitro* and *in vivo* studies should provide additional information in the near future.

BOX 9-2 Considerations Regarding Stem Cell Therapy in Cats

1. Stem cell therapy is not currently regulated by the FDA.
2. Stem cell therapy is generally the injection of a heterogenous population of cells, including MSC, endothelial progenitor cells, fibroblasts, hematopoietic and immune cells, and others.
3. A search of PubMed for studies on MSC therapy in clinical cases of feline diseases produces three pilot studies from a single investigator looking at their use in cats with CKD.[28,30,38]
4. Stem cells have become the latest in a long line of therapies in veterinary medicine where our use is fast and far outpacing our understanding.
5. Proceed with optimism and hope, but have significant contemplation and caution.

CKD, chronic kidney disease; *FDA*, U.S. Food and Drug Administration; *MSC*, mesenchymal stem cells.

References

1. de Rezende CE, Al-Ghazlat S: Feline small cell lymphosarcoma versus inflammatory bowel disease: treatment and prognosis. *Compend Contin Educ Vet* 35:E1–E6, 2013.
2. Trepanier L: Idiopathic inflammatory bowel disease in cats—rational treatment selection. *J Feline Med Surg* 11:32–38, 2009.
3. Mandigers PJ, Biourge V, German AJ: Efficacy of a commercial hydrolysate diet in eight cats suffering from inflammatory bowel disease or adverse reaction to food. *Tijdschr Diergeneeskd* 135:668–672, 2010.
4. Guilford WG, Jones BR, Markwell PJ, et al: Food sensitivity in cats with chronic idiopathic gastrointestinal problems. *J Vet Intern Med* 15:7–13, 2001.
5. Lingard AE, Briscoe K, Beatty JA, et al: Low-grade alimentary lymphoma: clinicopathological findings and response to treatment in 17 cases. *J Feline Med Surg* 11:692–700, 2009.
6. Plumb DC: *Veterinary drug handbook*, ed 7, Ames, 2011, Wiley-Blackwell.
7. Gazet JC, McColl I: Absorption of vitamin B-12 from the small intestine. Study in man, monkey, cat and dog. *Br J Surg* 54:128–131, 1967.
8. Okuda K, Kitazaki T, Morokuma M: Intestinal vitamin B12 absorption and gastric juice in the cat. *Digestion* 8:417–428, 1973.
9. Vaden SL, Wood PA, Ledley FD, et al: Cobalamin deficiency associated with methylmalonic academia in a cat. *J Am Vet Med Assoc* 200:1101–1103, 1992.
10. Steiner JM, Williams DA: Feline exocrine pancreatic disorders. *Vet Clin North Am Small Anim Pract* 29:551–575, 1999.
11. Simpson KW, Fyfe J, Cornetta A, et al: Subnormal concentrations of serum cobalamin (vitamin B12) in cats with gastrointestinal disease. *J Vet Intern Med* 15:26–32, 2001.
12. Ruaux CG, Steiner JM, Williams DA: Relationships between low serum cobalamin concentrations and methylmalonic academia in cats. *J Vet Intern Med* 23:472–475, 2009.
13. Reed N, Gunn-Moore D, Simpson K: Cobalamin, folate and inorganic phosphate abnormalities in ill cats. *J Feline Med Surg* 9:278–288, 2007.
14. Ruaux CG, Steiner JM, Williams DA: Early biochemical and clinical responses to cobalamin supplementation in cats with signs of gastrointestinal disease and severe hypocobalaminemia. *J Vet Intern Med* 19:155–160, 2005.
15. Scott KD, Zoran DL, Mansell J, et al: Utility of endoscopic biopsies of the duodenum and ileum for diagnosis of inflammatory bowel disease and small cell lymphoma in cats. *J Vet Intern Med* 25:1253–1257, 2011.
16. Kiselow MA, Rassnick KM, McDonough SP, et al: Outcome of cats with low-grade lympocytic lymphoma: 41 cases (1995-2005). *J Am Vet Med Assoc* 232:405–410, 2008.
17. Purchiaroni F, Tortora A, Gabrielli M, et al: The role of intestinal microbiota and the immune system. *Eur Rev Med Pharmacol Sci* 17:323–333, 2013.
18. Hooda S, Minamoto Y, Suchodolski JS, et al: Current state of knowledge: the canine gastrointestinal microbiome. *Anim Health Res Rev* 13:78–88, 2012.
19. FAO/WHO Expert Consultation: Health and nutritional properties of probiotics in food

including powder milk with live lactic acid bacteria. American Córdoba Park Hotel, Córdoba, Argentina; Oct 2001.

20. Weese JS, Martin H: Assessment of commercial probiotic bacterial contents and label accuracy. *Can Vet J* 52:43–46, 2011.

21. Bybee SN, Scorza AV, Lappin MR: Effect of probiotic Enterococcus faecium SF68 on presence of diarrhea in cats and dogs housed in an animal shelter. *J Vet Intern Med* 25:856–860, 2011.

22. Hart ML, Suchodolski JS, Steiner JM, et al: Open-label trial of a multi-strain symbiotic in cats with chronic diarrhea. *J Feline Med Surg* 14:240–245, 2012.

23. Lalor SM, Gunn-Moore DA: Effects of concurrent ronidazole and probiotic therapy in cats with *Tritrichomonas foetus*-associated diarrhea. *J Feline Med Surg* 14:650–658, 2012.

24. Dominici M, LeBlanc K, Mueller I, et al: Minimal criteria for defining multipotent mesenchymal stromal cells. The International Society for Cellular Therapy position statement. *Cytotherapy* 8:315–317, 2006.

25. Fortier LA, Travis AJ: Stem cells in veterinary medicine. *Stem Cell Res Ther* 2:9, 2011.

26. Gattegno-Ho D, Argyle SA, Argyle DJ: Stem cells and veterinary medicine: tools to understand diseases and enable tissue regeneration and drug discovery. *Vet J* 191:19–27, 2012.

27. Webb TL, Quimby JM, Dow SW: In vitro comparison of feline bone marrow-derived and adipose tissue-derived mesenchymal stem cells. *J Feline Med Surg* 14:165–168, 2012.

28. Quimby JM, Webb TL, Gibbons DS, et al: Evaluation of intrarenal mesenchymal stem cell injection for treatment of chronic kidney disease in cats: a pilot study. *J Feline Med Surg* 13:418–426, 2011.

29. Trzil JE, Chang CH, Webb T, et al: Short term use of mesenchymal stem cells fails to modulate BGA-specific airflow limitation in experimental feline asthma. *Veterinary Comparative Respiratory Society Annual Symposium*, Columbia, MO, 2012.

30. Webb TL, Webb CB: Stem cell therapy in cats with chronic enteropathy: a proof-of-concept study. *J Feline Med Surg* [Epub ahead of print].

31. Waly NE, Peters IR, Day MJ, et al: Measurement of IL-12 (p 40, 35), IL-23p19, and IFN-γ mRNA in duodenal biopsies of cats with inflammatory enteropathy. *J Vet Intern Med* 28:42–47, 2014.

32. Cyranoski D: Stem cells boom in vet clinics. *Nature* 11:96, 2013.

33. Marshall-Jones ZV, Baillon ML, Croft JM, et al: Effects of *Lactobacillus acidophilus* DSM13241 as a probiotic in healthy adult cats. *Am J Vet Res* 67:1005–1012, 2006.

34. Veir JK, Knorr R, Cavadini C, et al: Effect of supplementation with *Enterococcus faecium* (SF68) on immune functions in cats. *Vet Ther* 8:229–238, 2007.

35. Lappin MR, Veir JK, Satyaraj E, et al: Pilot study to evaluate the effect of oral supplementation of *Enterococcus faecium* SF68 on cats with latent feline herpesvirus 1. *J Feline Med Surg* 11:650–654, 2009.

36. Rishniw M, Wynn SG: Azodyl, a synbiotic, fails to alter azotemia in cats with chronic kidney disease when sprinkled onto food. *J Feline Med Surg* 13:405–409, 2011.

37. Garcia-Mazcorro JF, Lanerie DJ, Dowd SE, et al: Effect of a multi-species synbiotic formulation on fecal bacterial microbiota of healthy cats and dogs as evaluated by pyrosequencing. *FEMS Microbiol Ecol* 78:542–554, 2011.

38. Quimby JM, Webb TL, Habenicht LM, et al: Safety and efficacy of intravenous infusion of allogeneic cryopreserved mesenchymal stem cells for treatment of chronic kidney disease in cats: results of three sequential pilot studies. *Stem Cell Res Ther* 4:48, 2013.

The Role of the Microbiota in Feline Inflammatory Bowel Disease

Kenneth W. Simpson

Inflammatory bowel disease (IBD) is the collective term applied to a group of chronic enteropathies characterized by persistent or recurrent gastrointestinal (GI) signs and inflammation of the GI tract. It is widely accepted that IBD involves a complex interplay among host genetics, the intestinal microenvironment (principally bacteria and dietary constituents), the immune system, and environmental "triggers" of intestinal inflammation.[1] However, the specific steps that lead to IBD and the basis for phenotypic variation and unpredictable responses to treatment are not known. Recent advances in microbiology have enabled unforeseen insights into the composition and spatial distribution of intestinal bacteria, fungi, viruses, and protozoa (collectively the microbiota) in health and disease across species.[2-4] This chapter summarizes current knowledge of the role of the microbiota in feline IBD with a focus on bacteria.

WHAT BACTERIA COLONIZE THE HEALTHY FELINE GASTROINTESTINAL TRACT?

Culture-Based Analyses

Until recently, our knowledge of the bacterial composition of the feline GI tract was based on the culture of duodenal/jejunal juice or mucosa, colonic contents, and feces.[5-8] These studies found that *Bacteroides* spp., *Clostridium* spp., *Enterococcus* spp., *Streptococcus* spp., *Fusobacteria* spp., and *Eubacteria* spp. are the most common bacteria cultured from the feline GI tract. In general, the number and type of bacteria vary according to the intestinal region, with the number and proportion of strictly anaerobic bacteria increasing from the duodenum to the colon, peaking at 10^{11} colony-forming unit (CFU)/g of feces. Although the small intestine contains fewer bacteria than the colon or feces, bacterial numbers in the small intestines of healthy cats vary widely, from less than 10^2 to greater than 10^8 CFU/mL, and frequently exceed the 10^5 CFU/mL reported as the upper limit of normal in healthy people.[7] This has important implications for clinicians seeking to make diagnosis of small intestinal bacterial overgrowth (SIBO).[7]

Culture-Independent Analyses

The advent of molecular microbiology has enabled the identification of bacteria using their genetic signatures without the need to grow them. Culture-independent analyses have revealed that culture-based methods dramatically underestimate the diversity of the enteric flora, typically identifying only 20% of the bacteria recognized by their 16S RNA signatures.[9] In other words, culture-based methods only identify bacteria that you know how to grow. The principal culture-independent methods used to identify bacteria are polymerase chain reaction (PCR), 16S ribosomal ribonucleic acid (rRNA) sequencing, and fluorescence *in situ* hybridization (FISH; Box 10-1). The 16S sequencing is frequently employed as a first step to create an inventory of bacteria that are present and their relative proportions.[10-12] Bacteria of interest can then be targeted for precise enumeration by PCR (primers with or without probes against a bacterial target) or FISH with oligonucleotide probes directed against bacterial 16 or 23S rRNA.[13] FISH can also be used to gain insight into the spatial distribution of bacteria in formalin fixed biopsies. For example, are they luminal, adherent, crypt associated, or invasive?[13]

16S-based studies in cats indicate that Firmicutes (most are gram-positive bacteria) is the dominant bacterial phylum throughout the GI tract, with Clostridiales (predominately *Clostridium* cluster XIVA) and Lactobacillales (includes the Enterococcaceae, Lactobacillaceae, and Streptococcaceae families) being the predominant orders.[12,14,15] These findings broadly parallel the results of culture-based studies where *Clostridium* spp. were identified in duodenal aspirates of more than 90% of cats.[6-8] *Enterococcus* spp., *Streptococcus* spp., and *Lactobacillus* spp. were the dominant species from the jejunum,[5] and *Enterococcus* spp. and *Lactobacillus* were the dominant species from the colon and feces.[5] The 16S-based analyses to date have indicated that the microbiota tends to be more similar within an individual than when comparing the same intestinal region among different cats.[15] FISH-based studies of duodenal mucosa-associated bacteria in healthy cats have shown that the majority of bacteria are present in free and adherent mucus, with a median of 48

(0-399) bacteria/mm^2 of mucosa.[13] In healthy cats, the total numbers of bacteria hybridizing to probes against *Clostridium* spp., *Bacteroides* spp., *Streptococcus* spp., and Enterobacteriaceae represented only 6% of bacteria hybridizing to the EUB-338 probe.[13]

BACTERIA AND INFLAMMATORY BOWEL DISEASE/CHRONIC ENTEROPATHIES

When considering the role of bacteria in IBD, it is important to understand that IBD is a term applied to a diverse group of chronic enteropathies that are characterized by persistent or recurrent GI signs and inflammation of the GI tract.[16] IBD is often subcategorized on the basis of clinical signs (e.g., vomiting, diarrhea, and/or weight loss), clinicopathologic abnormalities (e.g., low cobalamin and/or low albumin), ultrasonographic findings (e.g., muscularis hypertrophy and/or regional lymphadenopathy), histopathology (cellular infiltrates and mucosal architecture), the anatomic region(s) involved (e.g., proximal small intestine, ileum, and/or colon), and response to therapy (e.g., diet-responsive, antibiotic-responsive, steroid-responsive, or unresponsive).[13,16-20] Feline IBD is also considered in the context of concurrent inflammation of other organs, such as the liver and pancreas ("triaditis") and kidneys.[21]

The most commonly diagnosed form of feline IBD is lymphocytic-plasmacytic inflammation of the proximal small intestine.[21] Unfortunately, this nomenclature is somewhat misleading as the numbers of lymphocytes and plasma cells in the small intestinal mucosa of cats with and without GI signs are broadly similar.[22] Thus the term *lymphoplasmacytic enteritis* is often more helpful at distinguishing this group of patients from those with neutrophilic, granulomatous, or eosinophilic infiltrates, than identifying cats with increased numbers of lymphocytes and plasma cells. The emergence of low-grade, T-cell, alimentary lymphoma in cats means that careful consideration has to be given to the number and regional distribution of mucosa-associated lymphocytes (e.g., clusters of intraepithelial lymphocytes) to enable distinction between lymphoplasmacytic enteritis and lymphoma.[23,24] It is common practice for pathologists to emphasize mucosal cellularity as the dominant histopathologic feature, with scant information provided about mucosal architecture. However, the finding that abnormalities in mucosal architecture, such as villous atrophy and fusion, correlate with proinflammatory cytokine upregulation and the severity of clinical signs in cats with IBD[13] indicates the importance of reporting architecture and cellularity.

There is a paucity of studies that have evaluated the microbiota in cats with GI disease. Studies to date have included client-owned cats with lymphocytic plasmacytic enteritis, less commonly neutrophilic or granulomatous ileitis or colitis; foster kittens with ill thrift; and colony-housed cats with signs of GI disease.

Intestinal Bacteria in the Duodenum of Cats with Lymphocytic Plasmacytic Enteritis

The only culture-independent study of the duodenal mucosal bacteria in cats to date employed FISH analysis to evaluate the numbers and types of bacteria associated with the duodenal mucosa and their relationship to clinical signs, histopathology, and mucosal cytokines.[13] Cats with signs of GI disease had more mucosal Enterobacteriaceae than healthy cats (Figure 10-1). The total number of mucosal bacteria was strongly associated with changes in mucosal architecture and the density of cellular infiltrates, particularly macrophages and T cells. A subset of bacteria comprising Enterobacteriaceae, *Escherichia coli*, and *Clostridium* spp. correlated with abnormalities in mucosal architecture (principally atrophy and fusion), proinflammatory cytokine upregulation (interleukin [IL]-1, -8, and -12), and the number of clinical signs exhibited by the affected cats (Figure 10-2). This study shows that changes in the number and type of mucosa-associated bacteria are related to the presence and severity of IBD in cats and raises the possibility that abnormal mucosal flora are involved in the etiopathogenesis of feline IBD. These changes in the microbiota closely parallel the microbial shifts, termed *dysbiosis*, observed in people, dogs, and murine models of IBD.[10-12,25] From a comparative standpoint, the histopathologic findings, microbial shifts, and cytokine profiles in cats with moderate to severe lymphoplasmacytic IBD resemble those associated with active celiac disease in people.[26-28] The potential for IBD-associated dysbiosis to effect change outside of the gut is increasingly recognized. Studies in cats with inflammatory liver disease[29] and severe pancreatitis (K.W. Simpson and D.C. Twedt, unpublished observations) have revealed the presence of intrahepatic and intrapancreatic bacteria, notably *E.coli* and *Enterococcus* spp., and raise the possibility that the inflamed, dysbiotic gut may be the source for these bacteria (Figure 10-3).[21,29]

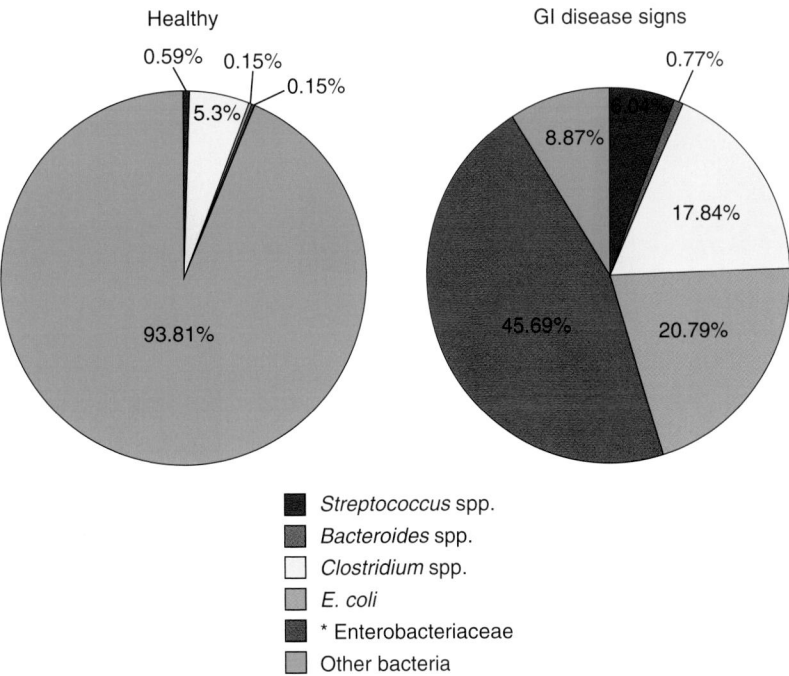

Figure 10-1: Proportion of mucosal *Streptococcus* spp., *Bacteroides* spp., *Clostridium* spp., *E. coli*, and Enterobacteriaceae in healthy cats and cats with signs of gastrointestinal (GI) disease. Numbers indicate the proportion (%) of bacteria recognized by the EUB-338 probe. *Enterobacteriaceae recognized by 1531 minus *E. coli*. (From Janeczko S, Atwater D, Bogel E, et al: The relationship of mucosal bacteria to duodenal histopathology, cytokine mRNA, and clinical disease activity in cats with inflammatory bowel disease. *Vet Microbiol* 128:178-193, 2008.)

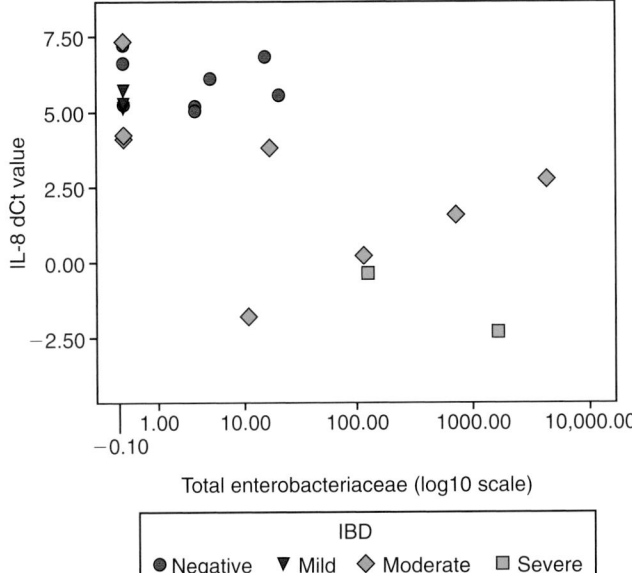

Figure 10-2: Interrelationship of interleukin *(IL)-8* upregulation (lower values for delta cycle threshold (dCT) on the Y axis indicate more upregulation), mucosal Enterobacteriaceae, and histopathologic severity of inflammatory bowel disease *(IBD)*. (From Janeczko S, Atwater D, Bogel E, et al: The relationship of mucosal bacteria to duodenal histopathology, cytokine mRNA, and clinical disease activity in cats with inflammatory bowel disease. *Vet Microbiol* 128:178-193, 2008.)

Bacterial Involvement in Neutrophilic and Granulomatous Ileitis or Colitis

There is growing evidence to implicate bacteria and other infectious agents in the development of granulomatous and neutrophilic intestinal inflammation across species. Nonbacterial infections associated with this type of intestinal inflammation in cats include feline infectious peritonitis, fungi, and *Tritrichomonas fetus*.[30,31] Bacterial pathogens such as *Salmonella*, *Campylobacter*, and *Yersinia* have been associated with neutrophilic enteritis, whereas mycobacteria have been associated with granulomatous inflammation and regional lymphadenopathy.[32] The discovery of invasive *E. coli* in dogs with granulomatous colitis has changed our perception of this disease as an idiopathic immune-mediated condition to a bacterially driven disease in a susceptible host.[10] To date, there is only a single report of granulomatous/histiocytic ulcerative colitis in cats with invasive bacteria that responded to antibiotics.[33] Ileocolitis associated with spiral bacteria identified as an *Anaerobiospirillum* spp. has been described in six cats.[34] Four cats had clinical signs related to the GI tract, whereas two did not. The most significant and consistent histologic change was present in the colon and consisted of marked multifocal to diffuse dilations of the crypt lumina that were filled with large numbers of spiral bacteria, often accompanied by necrotic epithelial cells and degenerate leukocytes or associated with crypt abscesses consisting of

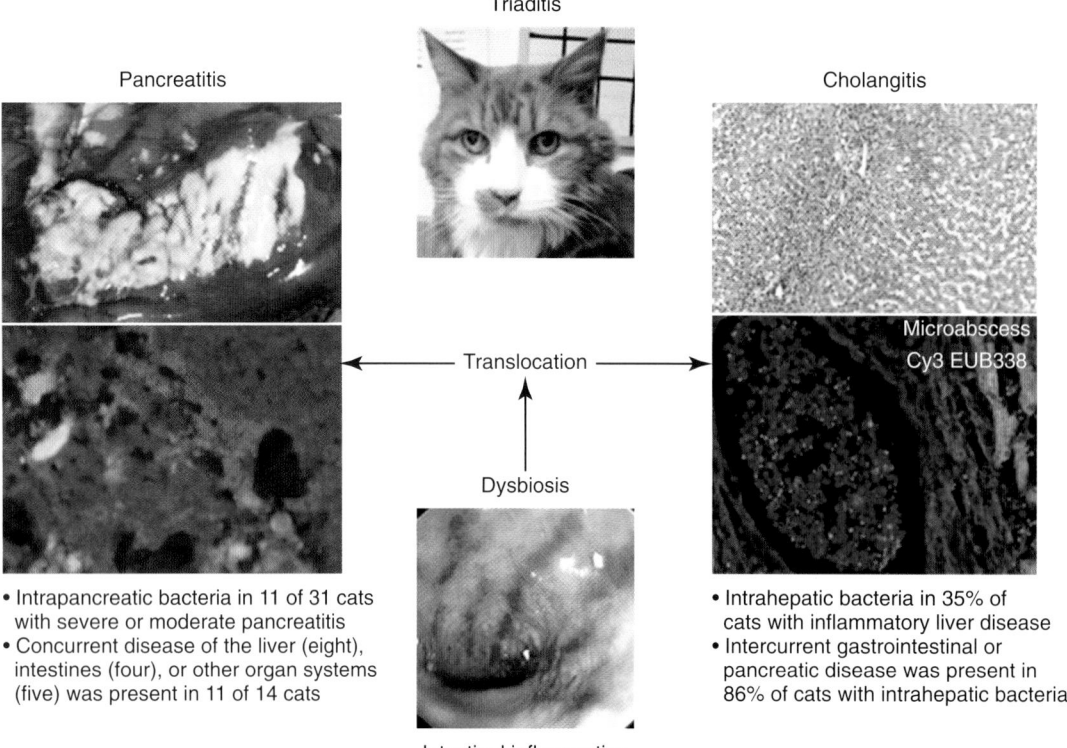

Triaditis

Pancreatitis

Cholangitis

Microabscess
Cy3 EUB338

← Translocation →

↑

Dysbiosis

- Intrapancreatic bacteria in 11 of 31 cats with severe or moderate pancreatitis
- Concurrent disease of the liver (eight), intestines (four), or other organ systems (five) was present in 11 of 14 cats

- Intrahepatic bacteria in 35% of cats with inflammatory liver disease
- Intercurrent gastrointestinal or pancreatic disease was present in 86% of cats with intrahepatic bacteria

Intestinal inflammation

Figure 10-3: Could intestinal dysbiosis promote bacterial translocation to the liver and pancreas? "Intestinal inflammation", most frequently "lymphocytic plasmacytic" or small cell lymphoma, could promote dysbiosis and the translocation of enteric bacteria to the pancreas and liver across the inflamed intestines or pancreatico-biliary papilla. This scenario could lead to the development of triaditis.[21]

necrosis of the crypt epithelium and accumulation of polymorphonuclear neutrophils. Changes in the surface epithelium ranged from focal sloughing to multifocal erosions, particularly over submucosal lymphoid aggregates, to diffuse epithelial necrosis and mucosal ulceration. Inflammatory cells were usually relatively sparse and consisted mainly of lymphocytes, with fewer histiocytes and polymorphonuclear neutrophils. The presence of an *Anaerobiospirillum* spp. was demonstrated by genus-specific 16S PCR and electron microscopy. Nucleotide sequencing of three affected cats showed a close relationship to *Anaerobiospirillum succiniciproducens*. The colons of three clinically healthy cats without lesions and one cat with mild colitis not associated with spiral bacteria were negative for *Anaerobiospirillum* spp. in the same assay. Another study has also correlated the presence of bacteria with spiral morphology with enterocolitis in cats, but the identity of these bacteria was not determined.[35]

It is becoming apparent that routine histopathology is an insensitive means of detecting infectious agents in tissue samples with evidence of neutrophilic and granulomatous inflammation. Although histochemical stains for fungi, argyrophilic and acid-fast bacteria, coronavirus, and culture may improve detection (Figure 10-4A), it is these cases that are likely to benefit most from additional culture-independent evaluation using PCR, 16S sequencing, or FISH analysis.[10,31,34] Eubacterial FISH analysis of formalin-fixed tissues can be performed on the same tissue block used for histopathology. It seems a reasonable first step for screening for the presence of bacteria and their regional distribution within the gut (i.e., luminal, adherent, or invasive).[13] For example, FISH analysis enabled the identification of invasive spiral bacteria in the ileum, colon, and regional lymph nodes of a cat with pyogranulomatous ileocolitis associated with recurrent episodes of fever and leukocytosis whose inflammatory process was considered sterile on the basis of histopathology (see Figure 10-4C). FISH analysis of colonic mucosa from a cat with dilated crypts and neutrophilic infiltrates enabled the detection of bacteria in and around degenerating glands (see Figure 10-4D) that responded to tylosin but not metronidazole or enrofloxacin.

Ileal Biofilm-Forming Bacteria in Foster Kittens

Approximately 15% of foster kittens die before 8 weeks of age, with most of these kittens demonstrating clinical signs or postmortem evidence of enteritis.[36,37] Lesions observed via light microscopy in the GI tract of kittens were largely nonspecific as to etiology and characterized in many cases as

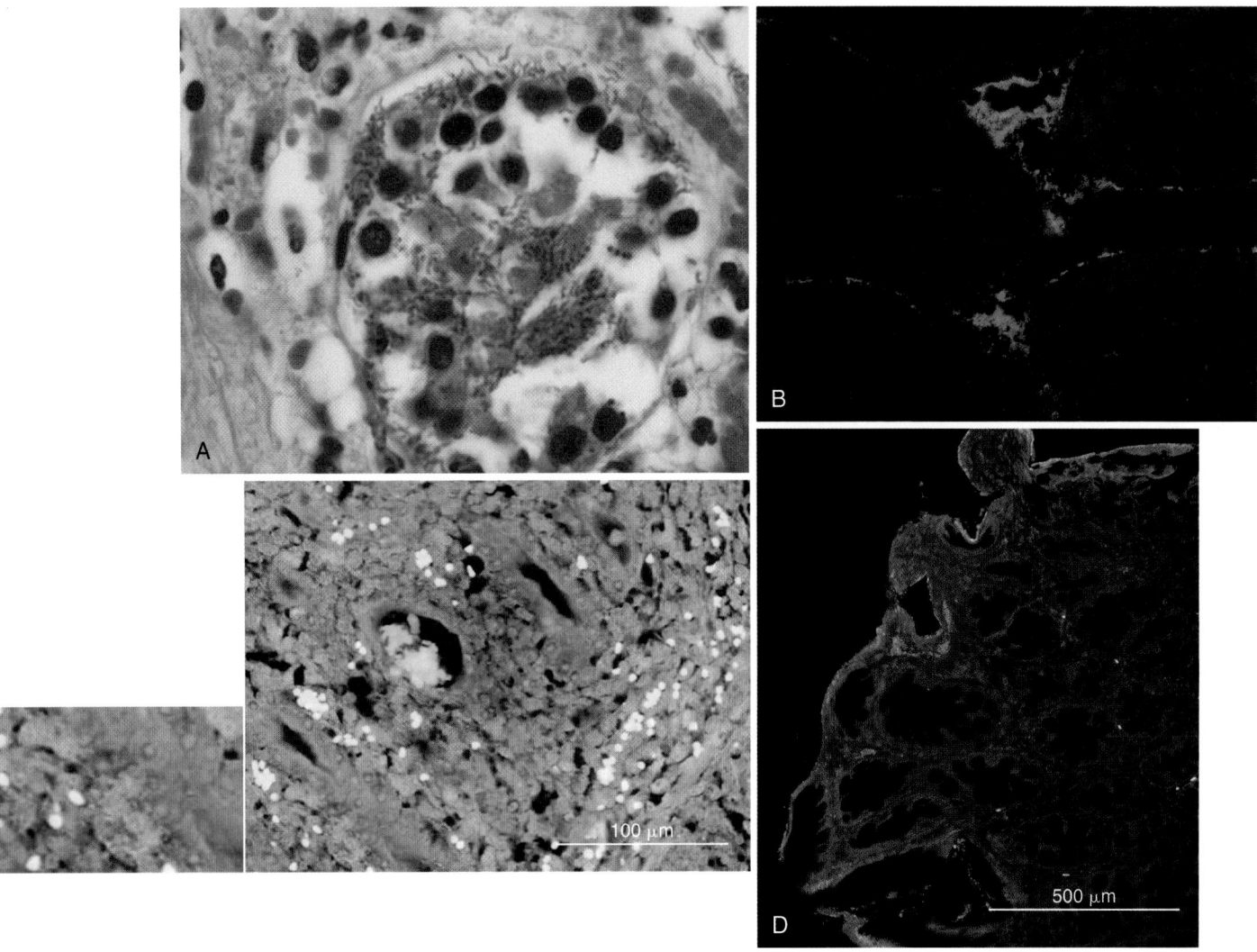

Figure 10-4: Spatial Distribution of Enteric Bacteria. A, Spiral bacteria inside the lumen of a dilated crypt (H&E, magnification, ×120). Histopathology revealed a severe, diffuse lymphoplasmactic, necrotizing enteritis with crypt necrosis and intraluminal spiral bacteria confirmed to be Anaerobiospirillum spp. **B,** Enteroadherent enterococci in the ileum of healthy kittens. Moderate **(C)** to severe **(D)** diffuse bacterial adherence of healthy small intestinal mucosa visualized with fluorescence *in situ* hybridization (FISH) using an oligonucleotide probe specific for eubacteria (Eub-338-FAM) or *Enterococcus* spp. (Enc-221-Cy3). Specimens were nuclear counterstained with 4′,6-diamidino-2-phenylindole (DAPI). **C,** Mucosally invasive spiral bacteria in a cat with pyogranulomatous ileitis visualized with FISH using an oligonucleotide probe specific for eubacteria (bacteria are *red:* Eub-338-Cy3). Specimens were nuclear counterstained with DAPI. Clinical signs resolved in response to doxycycline and enrofloxacin. **D,** Bacteria in and around degenerating crypts in cat with neutrophilic colitis visualized with FISH using an oligonucleotide probe specific for eubacteria (bacteria are *red:* Eub-338-Cy3). Specimens were nuclear counterstained with DAPI. Clinical signs resolved in response to tylosin. (**A,** Image is courtesy of Dr. Stan Marks. **B,** Copyright 2015 Jody Gookin; used with permission.)

consisting of mild inflammatory infiltrates and crypt abscesses. Ghosh and colleagues[37] used culture and FISH analysis to characterize the ileum mucosa-associated enterococcal community of 50 apparently healthy and 50 terminally ill foster kittens. In healthy kittens, *Enterococcus hirae* was the most common species of ileum mucosa-associated enterococci and was often observed to adhere extensively to the small intestinal epithelium (see Figure 10-4B). *E. faecalis*, with numerous virulence traits and multiple antimicrobial resistances, was more commonly isolated from the ileum mucosa of kittens with terminal illness. In addition, attachment of *E. coli* to the intestinal epithelium was significantly associated with terminal illness and was not observed in any kitten with adherent *E. hirae*.

Fecal Bacteria in Colony Cats with Signs of Gastrointestinal Disease

FISH analysis was performed to investigate the microbiota in a colony of cats that developed severe GI disease while undergoing an experimental trial.[38] This colony of cats, which underwent initial clinical investigations at Cornell University, had an ill-defined virus-like enteropathy that was associated with multisystemic and sometimes fatal disease that led to closure of the colony and its relocation to a research facility. These cats are described by Inness and colleagues[38] as having IBD, but they clearly had an unexplained severe enteropathy that is far removed from what is considered IBD in client-owned cats. FISH analysis showed total bacteria, *Bifidobacterium* spp., and *Bacteroides* spp. counts were higher in healthy cats when compared with affected cats, whereas *Desulfovibrio* spp. (producers of toxic sulphides) numbers were found to be significantly higher in affected cats.

The fecal microbiota of 15 colony cats with chronic diarrhea was evaluated using massive parallel 16S sequencing before and after dietary modification to determine the impact of diet change and related improvement in diarrhea.[39] Alterations in the intestinal microbiota were associated with improvement in diarrhea, but their relationship to disease was unclear.

IMPLICATIONS FOR THERAPY

From the limited clinical studies performed to date, it is clear that changes in the microbiota (i.e., dysbiosis) can accompany a variety of GI disorders in cats. It remains to be determined if dysbiosis is a cause or a consequence of GI disease in cats. Recent research indicates that acute, nonspecific intestinal inflammation can induce a consistent shift in the microbiome from Firmicutes to Proteobacteria, accompanied by a reduction in microbial diversity and proliferation of *E. coli* that recapitulates the dysbiosis of IBD.[25] There appears to be an interdependence of inflammation and dysbiosis, with inflammation promoting dysbiosis, and dysbiosis promoting inflammation. Genetic susceptibility may impact the threshold for dysbiosis in response to an external trigger and may also influence the ability of an individual to resolve the self-perpetuating cycle of dysbiosis and inflammation generated by an acute insult.[25]

From a therapeutic standpoint, it is tempting to equate dysbiosis with a need for antimicrobial therapy. However, this may not be required in patients that lack evidence of invasive bacteria (e.g., neutrophilic or granulomatous inflammation, intramucosal bacteria) or enteric translocation (e.g., fever, neutrophilia, regional lymphadenopathy). Because intestinal dysbiosis is an endpoint of many adverse stimuli, simply removing the initiating inflammatory stimulus, without recourse to antimicrobial intervention, may effect clinical resolution. From a mechanistic standpoint, bacteria and diet are frequently separated, but it is important to consider that they are not mutually exclusive, and the ability of diet to alter

microbial populations in healthy cats is well established.[40-43] Changes in the microbiome are present in diet-responsive enteropathies such as celiac disease,[26,28] and responses to diet, without recourse to immunomodulatory drugs, have also been observed in people with Crohn's disease. Clinical signs in dogs with lymphoplasmacytic enteritis and concurrent dysbiosis can also resolve in response to a controlled diet without recourse to antimicrobial therapy.[16] With this in mind, it is noteworthy that 49% of 55 cats with chronic GI disease, which would typically be defined as low-grade lymphoplasmacytic enteritis, responded to an antigen-restricted diet without recourse to antimicrobial or immunosuppressive therapy.[17] Similar responses have also been reported in cats fed hydrolyzed diets.[44] Thus it seems prudent that cats with signs of chronic GI disease (that have undergone a thorough workup to exclude infectious or parasitic agents, non-GI disorders, exocrine pancreatic insufficiency, and intestinal structural abnormalities requiring surgery) with biopsy findings that are considered normal, minimal change, or "lymphoplasmacytic enteritis" are treated in a sequential, stepwise manner with progression to more aggressive therapeutics dictated by a lack of response.

For example, dietary modification (e.g., antigen-restricted or hydrolyzed diet) and cobalamin supplementation[45] for 2 weeks could be followed by the addition of an antimicrobial (e.g., tylosin) for 2 weeks, then by the addition of an immunosuppressive agent (e.g., prednisolone). This stepwise approach, which has been very effective in dogs with chronic enteropathies,[16] will hopefully identify subsets of cats that are diet-responsive, antibiotic-responsive, prednisolone-responsive, or unresponsive, and provide a phenotype that is important in ongoing efforts to inform understanding of the pathogenesis, diagnosis, and treatment of IBD. In cats with more severe lymphoplasmacytic enteritis, simultaneous therapy with diet, vitamins, antibiotics, and immunosuppressive agents may be prescribed, with treatments sequentially withdrawn if remission is achieved. In cats with neutrophilic or granulomatous inflammation, infectious agents must be strongly suspected. An aggressive search for organisms in the intestinal mucosa or regional lymph nodes (culture, histopathology and special stains, PCR, and FISH analysis) and potential systemic dissemination is of paramount importance to enable specific therapy. For proven and suspected bacterial infections, antimicrobials are the mainstay of therapy, and choice of treatment should take into consideration the spatial distribution of bacteria (i.e., antimicrobial sensitivities determined *in vitro* have to be reconciled with the ability of an antimicrobial to penetrate tissues and cells harboring the bacteria). Immunosuppression of these patients should be a last resort. Despite great expectations that probiotic bacteria given alone or in combination with prebiotics will alleviate or prevent the dysbiosis associated with IBD or chronic enteropathies, studies that show a positive effect are lacking. Some formulations have been evaluated in healthy cays and cats with chronic diarrhea,[46,47] but clinical trials in cats with IBD have not been reported to date.

SUMMARY

Recent advances in microbiology provide new insights into the composition and spatial distribution of intestinal bacteria, fungi, viruses, and protozoa in health and disease. A picture is emerging that correlates changes in the relative proportions of resident enteric bacterial populations—"dysbiosis"— with clinical signs and mucosal inflammation. The role of dysbiosis in the disease process remains to be elucidated. Is it a cause or a consequence, or a cause and a consequence, of intestinal disease? From a clinical perspective, it seems wise to adopt a stepwise approach to treating cats with lymphocytic plasma-cytic enteritis with diet, then antimicrobials, and then immunosuppression as the default approach in most cases. In cats with evidence of neutrophilic or granulomatous intestinal inflammation, the onus is very much on the clinician to search aggressively for infectious agents before defaulting to immunosuppression of an idiopathic disease. Much remains to be learned about the complex interplay among host genetics, the intestinal microenvironment (principally bacteria and dietary constituents), the immune system, and environmental triggers of intestinal inflammation that lead to the development of IBD in cats.

References

1. Jergens AE, Simpson KW: Inflammatory bowel disease in veterinary medicine. *Front Biosci (Elite Ed)* 4:1404–1419, 2012.
2. Barry KA, Wojcicki BJ, Middelbos IS, et al: Dietary cellulose, fructooligosaccharides, and pectin modify fecal protein catabolites and microbial populations in adult cats. *J Anim Sci* 88:2978–2987, 2010.
3. Handl S, Dowd SE, Garcia-Mazcorro JF, et al: Massive parallel 16S rRNA gene pyrosequencing reveals highly diverse fecal bacterial and fungal communities in healthy dogs and cats. *FEMS Microbiol Ecol* 76(2):301–310, 2011.
4. Tun HM, Brar MS, Khin N, et al: Gene-centric metagenomics analysis of feline intestinal microbiome using 454 junior pyrosequencing. *J Microb Meth* 88:369–376, 2012.
5. Osbaldiston GW, Stowe EC: Microflora of alimentary tract of cats. *Am J Vet Res* 32:1399–1405, 1971.
6. Papasouliotis K, Sparkes AH, Werrett G, et al: Assessment of the bacterial flora of the proximal part of the small intestine in healthy cats, and the effect of sample collection method. *Am J Vet Res* 59(1):48–51, 1998.
7. Johnston KL: Small intestinal bacterial overgrowth. *Vet Clin North Am Small Anim Pract* 29(2):523–550, vii, 1999.
8. Johnston KL, Swift NC, Forster-van Hijfte M, et al: Comparison of the bacterial flora of the duodenum in healthy cats and cats with signs of gastrointestinal tract disease. *J Am Vet Med Assoc* 218:48–51, 2001.
9. Eckburg PB, Bik EM, Bernstein CN, et al: Diversity of the human intestinal microbial flora. *Science* 308:1635–1638, 2005.
10. Simpson KW, Dogan B, Rishniw M, et al: Adherent and invasive *Escherichia coli* is associated with granulomatous colitis in boxer dogs. *Infect Immun* 74(8):4778–4792, 2006.
11. Suchodolski JS: Intestinal microbiota of dogs and cats: a bigger world than we thought. *Vet Clin North Am Small Anim Pract* 41(2):261–272, 2011.
12. Minamoto Y, Hooda S, Swanson KS, et al: Feline gastrointestinal microbiota. *Anim Health Res Rev* 13(1):64–77, 2012.
13. Janeczko S, Atwater D, Bogel E, et al: The relationship of mucosal bacteria to duodenal histopathology, cytokine mRNA, and clinical disease activity in cats with inflammatory bowel disease. *Vet Microbiol* 128:178–193, 2008.
14. Ritchie LE, Burke KF, Garcia-Mazcorro JF, et al: Characterization of fecal microbiota in cats using universal 16S rRNA gene and group-specific primers for Lactobacillus and Bifidobacterium spp. *Vet Microbiol* 144:140–146, 2010.
15. Ritchie LE, Steiner JM, Suchodolski JS: Assessment of microbial diversity along the feline intestinal tract using 16S rRNA gene analysis. *FEMS Microbiol Ecol* 66(3):590–598, 2008.
16. Simpson KW, Jergens AE: Pitfalls and progress in the diagnosis and management of canine inflammatory bowel disease. *Vet Clin North Am Small Anim Pract* 41(2):381–398, 2011.
17. Guilford WG, Jones BR, Markwell PJ, et al: Food sensitivity in cats with chronic idiopathic gastrointestinal problems. *J Vet Intern Med* 15(1):7–13, 2001.
18. Simpson KW, Fyfe J, Cornetta A, et al: Subnormal concentrations of serum cobalamin (vitamin B$_{12}$) in cats with gastrointestinal disease. *J Vet Intern Med* 15(1):26–32, 2001.
19. Jergens AE: Feline idiopathic inflammatory bowel disease: what we know and what remains to be unraveled. *J Feline Med Surg* 14(7):445–458, 2012.
20. Daniaux LA, Laurenson MP, Marks SL, et al: Ultrasonographic thickening of the muscularis propria in feline small intestinal small cell T-cell lymphoma and inflammatory bowel disease. *J Feline Med Surg* 16(2):89–98, 2014.
21. Simpson KW: Pancreatitis and triaditis in cats: causes and treatment. *J Small Anim Pract* 56(1):40–49, 2015.
22. Waly N, Gruffydd-Jones TJ, Stokes CR, et al: The distribution of leucocyte subsets in the small intestine of healthy cats. *J Comp Pathol* 124(2–3):172–182, 2001.
23. Kiselow MA, Rassnick KM, McDonough SP, et al: Outcome of cats with low-grade lymphocytic lymphoma: 41 cases (1995-2005). *J Am Vet Med Assoc* 232(3):405–410, 2008.
24. Moore PF, Rodriguez-Bertos A, Kass PH: Feline gastrointestinal lymphoma: mucosal architecture, immunophenotype, and molecular clonality. *Vet Pathol* 49(4):658–668, 2012.
25. Craven MD, Egan CE, Dowd SE, et al: Inflammation drives dysbiosis and bacterial invasion in murine models of ileal Crohn's disease. *PLoS ONE* 7(7):e41594, 2012.
26. Sanz Y, De Pama G, Laparra M: Unraveling the ties between celiac disease and intestinal microbiota. *Int Rev Immunol* 30(4):207–218, 2011.
27. Sjöberg V, Sandström O, Hedberg M, et al: Intestinal T-cell responses in celiac disease—impact of celiac disease associated bacteria. *PLoS ONE* 8(1):e53414, 2013.
28. Olivares M, Neef A, Castillejo G, et al: The HLA-DQ2 genotype selects for early intestinal microbiota composition in infants at high risk of developing coeliac disease. *Gut* 64(3):406–417, 2015.
29. Twedt DC, Cullen J, McCord K, et al: Evaluation of fluorescence *in situ* hybridization for the detection of bacteria in feline inflammatory liver disease. *J Feline Med Surg* 16(2):109–117, 2014.
30. Van Kruiningen HJ, Ryan MJ, Shindel NM: The classification of feline colitis. *J Comp Pathol* 93(2):275–294, 1983.
31. Gookin JL, Stone MR, Yaeger MJ, et al: Fluorescence in situ hybridization for identification of Tritrichomonas foetus in formalin-fixed and paraffin-embedded histological specimens of intestinal trichomoniasis. *Vet Parasitol* 172(1–2):139–143, 2010.
32. Elze J, Grammel L, Richter E, et al: First description of Mycobacterium heckeshornense infection in a feline immunodeficiency virus-positive cat. *J Feline Med Surg* 15(12):1141–1144, 2013.
33. Van Kruiningen HJ, Dobbins WO: Feline histiocytic colitis: a case report with electron microscopy. *Vet Pathol* 16(2):215–222, 1979.
34. De Cock HE, Marks SL, Stacy BA, et al: Ileocolitis associated with Anaerobiospirillum in cats. *J Clin Microbiol* 42(6):2752–2758, 2004.
35. Feinstein RE, Olsson E: Chronic gastroenterocolitis in nine cats. *J Vet Diagn Invest* 4(3):293–298, 1992.
36. Nicklas JL, Moisan P, Stone MR, et al: *In situ* molecular diagnosis and histopathological characterization of enteroadherent

Enterococcus hirae infection in pre-weaning-age kittens. *J Clin Microbiol* 48(8):2814–2820, 2010.

37. Ghosh A, Borst L, Stauffer SH, et al: Mortality in kittens is associated with a shift in ileum mucosa-associated enterococci from Enterococcus hirae to biofilm-forming Enterococcus faecalis and adherent Escherichia coli. *J Clin Microbiol* 51(11):3567–3578, 2013.

38. Inness VL, McCartney AL, Khoo C, et al: Molecular characterisation of the gut microflora of healthy and inflammatory bowel disease cats using fluorescence in situ hybridisation with special reference to Desulfovibrio spp. *J Anim Physiol Anim Nutr (Berl)* 91(1–2): 48–53, 2007.

39. Ramadan Z, Xu H, Laflamme D, et al: Fecal microbiota of cats with naturally occurring chronic diarrhea assessed using 16S rRNA gene 454-pyrosequencing before and after dietary treatment. *J Vet Intern Med* 28(1):59–65, 2014.

40. Sparkes AH, Papasouliotis K, Sunvold G, et al: Bacterial flora in the duodenum of healthy cats, and effect of dietary supplementation with fructo-oligosaccharides. *Am J Vet Res* 59:431–435, 1998.

41. Lubbs DC, Vester BM, Fastinger ND, et al: Dietary protein concentration affects intestinal microbiota of adult cats: a study using DGGE and qPCR to evaluate differences in microbial populations in the feline gastrointestinal tract. *J Anim Physiol Anim Nutr (Berl)* 93(1):113–121, 2009.

42. Barry KA, Middelbos IS, Vester Boler BM, et al: Effects of dietary fiber on the feline gastrointestinal metagenome. *J Proteome Res* 11(12):5924–5933, 2012.

43. Hooda S, Vester Boler BM, Kerr KR, et al: The gut microbiome of kittens is affected by dietary protein:carbohydrate ratio and associated with blood metabolite and hormone concentrations. *Br J Nutr* 109(9):1637–1646, 2013.

44. Mandigers PJ, Biourge V, German AJ: Efficacy of a commercial hydrolysate diet in eight cats suffering from inflammatory bowel disease or adverse reaction to food. *Tijdschr Diergeneeskd* 135(18):668–672, 2010.

45. Worhunsky P, Toulza O, Rishniw M, et al: The relationship of serum cobalamin to methylmalonic acid concentrations and clinical variables in cats. *J Vet Intern Med* 27(5):1056–1063, 2013.

46. Hart ML, Suchodolski JS, Steiner JM, et al: Open-label trial of a multi-strain synbiotic in cats with chronic diarrhea. *J Feline Med Surg* 14(4):240–245, 2012.

47. Biagi G, Cipollini I, Bonaldo A, et al: Effect of feeding a selected combination of galacto-oligosaccharides and a strain of Bifidobacterium pseudocatenulatum on the intestinal microbiota of cats. *Am J Vet Res* 74(1):90–95, 2013.

Disorders of Esophageal, Gastric, and Intestinal Motility in Cats

Frédéric Gaschen

Disorders of digestive motility include esophageal, gastric, small intestinal, and colonic dysmotility. Their prevalence is difficult to establish due to a lack of appropriate epidemiological studies. Motility disorders resulting from obstruction of esophageal, gastric, small intestinal, or colonic transit by foreign bodies or space-occupying lesions are a common occurrence in clinical practice. However, there is little data about nonobstructive digestive motility disorders, and it is thought that they are generally under recognized in feline practice. As well, available diagnostic tools and treatment modalities are limited.

Nonobstructive digestive motility disorders may go unnoticed by the cat's owner because of subtle clinical signs that are difficult to recognize until the problem is severe. They may result from primary segmental or diffuse inflammatory or neoplastic infiltration of the esophageal or gastrointestinal (GI) wall. Gastrointestinal motility also may be influenced by a variety of diseases affecting other organs, such as abdominal inflammation or endocrinopathies, electrolyte abnormalities, and uremic syndrome. Further, diseases affecting the autonomous nervous system, although rare, may have devastating consequences.

The diagnosis and treatment of cats with esophageal and GI obstructions are generally relatively straightforward. Therefore, these diseases will not be further discussed in this chapter.

ESOPHAGUS

Anatomy and Physiology

The upper esophageal sphincter (UES) consists of striated muscle fibers of both cricopharyngeal and esophageal origin. The two spirally arranged muscularis layers of the esophagus wind in opposite directions. They consist of striated muscle fibers in the proximal third of the esophagus (cervical segment), whereas they contain only smooth muscle fibers in the distal two-thirds of the esophagus (thoracic segment).[1] A thickening of the esophageal muscle is noticeable at the gastroesophageal junction and functions as the lower esophageal sphincter (LES).[1] A significant thickening of the muscularis mucosae is observed at the level of the LES, and the circular muscle layer contains annulospiral elastic fibers.[2]

The function of the esophagus is tightly regulated. After the oropharyngeal phase of swallowing, the UES relaxes and a primary esophageal motility wave is triggered, which propels the food bolus aborally toward the LES. Presence of a bolus in the distal esophagus causes relaxation of the LES to allow passage into the stomach. Presence of a bolus remaining in the esophagus after primary peristalsis has occurred triggers secondary peristalsis.[3]

Esophageal motility is under the control of neurons originating in the nucleus ambiguus located in the brain stem (motor) and solitary tract nucleus in the medulla oblongata (sensory), the cervical ganglia, and a complex network of interneurons.[1] The vagus nerve and its various branches, such as the recurrent laryngeal nerves and cranial laryngeal nerves, connect the muscular layers of the esophagus to the higher centers.[4]

Evaluation of Esophageal Motility

Esophageal function is evaluated using survey radiographs looking for abnormalities along the length of the organ, such as megaesophagus, radiopaque foreign body, or esophageal mass. Static or dynamic contrast studies (esophagram) are recommended in the presence of clinical signs of esophageal disease if no abnormality can be identified on survey films. These studies allow identification of radiolucent foreign bodies and esophageal strictures. Fluoroscopy is required for evaluation of esophageal motility.[3] Endoscopic examination of the esophagus may allow visualization of obstructions (e.g., foreign bodies, strictures) or esophagitis. High-resolution manometry is a technique commonly used in humans for thorough evaluation of esophageal function; it has been used successfully in unsedated cats (P. Kook, personal communication, 2014) and may represent a valuable tool to enhance the knowledge of feline esophageal function in health and disease (Figure 11-1).

Motility Disorders

Esophageal diseases are uncommon in cats. Studies from referral institutions reported a prevalence ranging from 0.05% to 1% of all feline patients.[5,6] Median age of affected cats ranges from 3 to 6 years.[5,7] Associated clinical signs

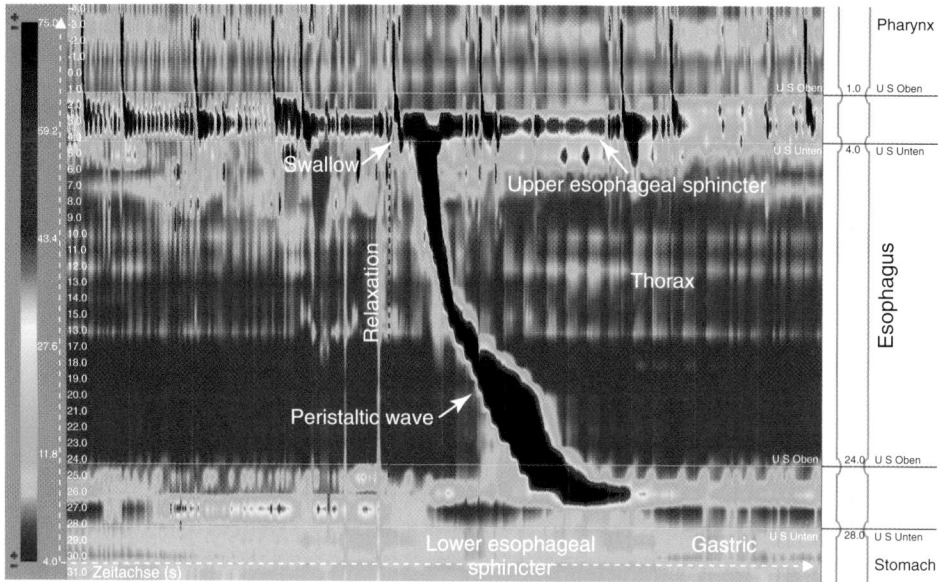

Figure 11-1: Topographic analysis of esophageal peristalsis using a 36-channel, high-resolution manometry system in a healthy unsedated Maine Coon cat. The vertical axis represents the distance in centimeters from the tip of the catheter, which is located in the stomach (see schematic drawing of the esophagus on the right), and the horizontal axis represents time. Pressure magnitude is encoded in color corresponding to the scale shown on the left; high-pressure regions are denoted by the red end of the spectrum and the low-pressure regions by the blue end. (Courtesy Dr. P. Kook, University of Zurich Vetsuisse Faculty.)

include regurgitation and/or vomiting, dysphagia, odynophagia, hypersalivation, anorexia, and weight loss. A retrospective study of 44 cats with esophageal dysmotility reported a high prevalence of respiratory signs, such as coughing, noisy breathing, nasal discharge, dyspnea, or combinations of those signs.[6] These signs may have resulted from effects of gastroesophageal reflux (GER) and esophageal acidification on airways and lungs.[6,8] Interestingly, an association between GER and asthmatic conditions has been well documented in humans.[8] GER was documented in 12% to 22% of young and adult cats undergoing general anesthesia using different protocols. Reflux episodes usually occurred within a few minutes and lasted for 20 minutes or longer.[9,10] In severe cases with significant damage to the esophageal mucosa, postanesthetic esophageal stricture may develop.

Apart from esophageal obstructions (e.g., foreign body, stricture, vascular ring anomaly, luminal mass), GER, megaesophagus, and type I (sliding) hiatal hernia were common causes identified in reported cases.[6,7] Abnormal esophageal motility in cats with GER and/or hiatal hernia is most likely due to secondary esophagitis. A subset of cats had idiopathic esophageal dysmotility.[6,7] Megaesophagus is a rare occurrence in cats; congenital forms have been reported. Acquired megaesophagus is a feature of feline dysautonomia (see Generalized Motility Disorders). Additionally, dysphagia and/or megaesophagus were identified in 15% of cats with myasthenia gravis, a rare disease commonly associated with thymic pathology.[11]

Administration of tablets and capsules to cats often challenges esophageal motility with significant midcervical retention after a dry swallow.[12,13] Tablets and capsules containing substances with irritating properties, such as doxycycline and clindamycin, have been shown to cause esophagitis and esophageal stricture.[14,15]

Prevention and Treatment

Successful prevention of esophageal retention is easy and consists of administering 6 mL water orally (PO) using a syringe immediately after pilling,[12] a one-step pill gun with flavored liquid (Flavo Rx Pill Glide), or a pill delivery treat (Greenies Pill Pockets).[16]

Once esophageal obstruction has been ruled out (via esophagram or esophagoscopy), there is no easy treatment for cats with decreased esophageal motility. Owners need guidance with selecting the optimal food consistency (often a trial and error process) and should be advised to make the best possible use of gravity by keeping the cat upright after each meal. GER can be prevented by administration of prokinetics, which increase LES muscle tone, such as cisapride and erythromycin (see Stomach and Table 11-2).

STOMACH

Anatomy and Physiology

The enteric nervous system is a complex grid that plays an essential role in the multiple functions of the GI tract. The myenteric plexus (Auerbach's plexus) located between the longitudinal and circular muscular layers is for the most part responsible for coordination of intrinsic (entero-enteric) and extrinsic (under the influence of the central nervous system

[CNS]) information and subsequent regulation of GI motility. The interstitial cells of Cajal form a network of cells located in the muscular layers of the gastric and intestinal wall. They have a pacesetter function and generate a slow wave pattern. However, smooth muscle contractions only occur when spike potentials are generated on top of the slow waves and trigger the release of acetylcholine in the synaptic cleft.

When assessing motility in cats, the stomach can be divided into two parts: the gastric reservoir, consisting of the fundus and a large part of the body area, and the gastric pump, consisting of a part of the gastric body and the pyloric antrum.

The role of the gastric reservoir is to store and eventually evacuate ingesta toward the pump. The function of the gastric pump is to mix and grind the gastric content before evacuation into the proximal duodenum. Peristaltic waves originate in the proximal stomach and propagate to the pylorus. When a peristaltic wave propagates to the distal antrum, a small part of the ingesta will pass through the pylorus into the duodenum whereas the largest part will be propelled into the proximal antrum to undergo further grinding (retropulsion).

A feline peculiarity is the absence of the typical pattern of fasting GI motility seen in other small carnivores and humans. In particular, type III migrating motor complexes (MMCs) have a housekeeping function, which allows emptying of large, ingestible particles from the stomach when it is nearly empty and propagates them to the entire small intestine. Instead, cats display spike burst activity followed by migrating spike complexes that are probably responsible for the important housekeeping function.[17]

In healthy animals, the rate of gastric emptying is modulated by the size of the meal and the composition of the diet (e.g., moisture and fat, protein and carbohydrate content) and is under the influence of neural and endocrine factors. Liquid meals are emptied faster than solid meals.[18] The gastric emptying time (GET) is shorter for canned diets than for dry kibbles,[19] with triangular-shaped kibbles emptied slower than round kibbles.[20] Drinking water seems to shorten the GET of cats fed dry food.[19] Age does not appear to significantly slow down gastric motility because there was no significant difference in GET between young and old cats in one study.[21]

Sedation may influence gastric motility. Cats receiving diazepam (0.18 mg/kg intravenously [IV]) were shown to eat larger meals than control cats, and their GET was increased, probably due to the larger meal size. In another study, ketamine and acepromazine administered IV tended to shorten the orocecal transit time (OCTT) of liquid barium in healthy cats, whereas ketamine and valium mixtures did not have any effect.

Diagnostic Approach

A detailed history and physical examination may detect signs suggestive of GI dysmotility (Box 11-1). The initial approach to the cat with a suspected GI motility disorder consists in first ruling out obstructive GI disease and requires abdominal

BOX 11-1 Clinical Signs Associated with Delayed Gastric Emptying

- Nausea with associated signs, such as drooling and lip smacking
- Vomiting
  - May occur long after food intake, when the stomach should be empty (greater than 8 to 10 hours postprandial)
  - Occasionally projectile vomiting (without prodromal signs, such as nausea with salivation)
- Abdominal distension, bloated abdomen
- Cranial abdominal discomfort, colic
- Dysorexia and anorexia
- Weight loss
- Pica and/or polydipsia
- Increased belching

radiographs, possibly followed by ultrasound examination. Presence of food in the stomach after prolonged fasting (i.e., more than 12 hours) suggests delayed gastric emptying. Moreover, abdominal ultrasound may reveal severely decreased or absent gastric and duodenal motility. Once GI obstruction has been ruled out, complete blood count, serum chemistry panel, and urinalysis are necessary to look for underlying disorders that may secondarily influence motility.

Evaluation of Gastric Motility
Several techniques have been used to evaluate GET in the cat. Table 11-1 provides examples of published GET data obtained from measurements with various techniques.

Gastric Radionuclide Scintigraphy. Gastric radionuclide scintigraphy is the gold standard technique. The cat is fed a solid meal mixed with radiolabeled technetium-99m (^{99m}Tc), and postprandial scans are performed at regular intervals with a gamma camera to allow quantification of the radioactivity present in the stomach. A time curve is drawn and $T_{1/2}$ (time at which one-half of the initial radioactivity remains in the stomach) and $T_{50\%}$ (time at 50% of the area under the curve) can be calculated.[18,19] Unfortunately, the method is only available at academic institutions and select referral centers and is used mostly for research purposes. Data from the literature do not provide consistent reference values due to varied meal composition and sizes.

Liquid Barium Sulfate Gastrogram. Liquid barium sulfate gastrogram has been widely used to assess GI transit times. The dose of 36% weight per volume barium suspension in cats is 12 mL/kg and should be administered when the stomach is empty.[22] Liquid barium should be present in the duodenum after 30 minutes and should have moved away from the stomach 3 hours postadministration. However, assessment of gastric emptying of liquids is an insensitive technique, with the exception of mechanical obstructions. Although mixing barium with food may allow better evaluation of the solid phase of gastric emptying, barium can easily

Table 11-1 **Examples of Gastric Emptying Times Obtained in Healthy Cats after Using Various Techniques**

Technique	Measured Parameter	Meal Type and Size	Time (h)	Source
Radionuclide scintigraphy: Ingestion of a meal mixed with technetium-99m (99mTc)	T_{50} and T_{80} (times when 50% and 80%, respectively, of the radioactivity has left the stomach)	25 kcal/kg or approx. one-half of daily caloric requirement (canned)	$T_{50} = 2.7 \pm 0.2$ $T_{80} = 4.9 \pm 0.8$	19
	T_{50} and T_{80}	40 kcal/kg or approx. 80% of daily caloric requirements (dry)	$T_{50} = 3.9 \pm 0.2$ $T_{80} = 10.2 \pm 0.8$	
BIPS: Ingestion of a meal mixed with 1.5- and 5-mm diameter spheres	$GE_{50\%}$ (time when 50% of all spheres have left the stomach) GET (time when 100% of all spheres have left the stomach)	Whiskas Supermeat, Pedigree Pet Foods (canned), approx. one-quarter of daily caloric needs	7.7 (range: 3.5-10.9) 12 (range: 6-14)	23
Sodium acetate breath test: Ingestion of a meal mixed with Na-acetate	$T_{1/2}$ (time when 50% of the meal has left the stomach)	a/d, Hill's Pet Nutrition (canned), unspecified amount	4.5	25
Abdominal ultrasound: Ingestion of a meal and serial measurements of antral pyloric diameter	Time to total emptying	Full daily caloric requirement Half of daily caloric requirement	24 (range: 16-26) 14 (range: 12-14)	26

Data extracted from selected publications.
BIPS, Barium-impregnated polyethylene spheres; *GET,* Gastric emptying time

dissociate from the test meal and empty into the duodenum even though the solid food is still in the stomach, rendering the study unreliable.

Barium-impregnated polyethylene spheres (BIPS, Med ID, Grand Rapids, Michigan) have been used for evaluation of GI transit times in cats. Capsules contain several each of two sphere sizes (1.5- and 5-mm diameter) and can easily be used in practice.[23] However, correlation between gastric emptying of BIPS and scintigraphy has been disappointing in cats,[24] and the clinical utility of these spheres has been questioned.

Breath Tests. Breath tests using markers, such as octanoic acid or sodium acetate radiolabeled with the stable isotope ^{13}C, have been established in cats. The marker is absorbed in the duodenum and processed in the liver with release of ^{13}C, which is ultimately exhaled. Postprandial time plotting of ^{13}C/^{12}C ratios in the breath is used to obtain $T_{1/2}$ values. A fair correlation was observed between the sodium acetate breath test and ^{99m}Tc scintigraphy.[25] Although this technique may be more practical than scintigraphy, availability is still limited to research facilities at this time.

Ultrasound Evaluation. Ultrasound evaluation of GET relies on the postprandial measurement of the cross-sectional area or estimated volume of the relaxed pyloric antrum over time. As the stomach empties, the size of the antrum decreases and ultimately returns to fasted values. GET can be derived from a time plot of the obtained values. Although the technique has only been validated in dogs, it has been used in cats as well (Figure 11-2).[26] Ultrasound also allows the evaluation of amplitude and frequency of antral contractions, two potentially useful parameters of gastric motility based on studies performed in dogs.[27] If the technique proves reliable

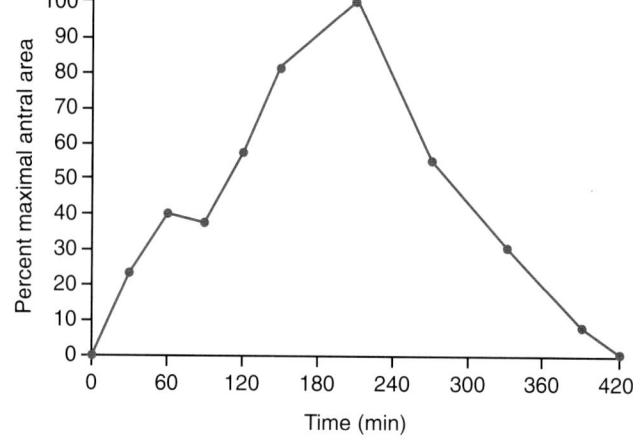

Figure 11-2: Evaluation of gastric emptying by abdominal ultrasonography in a healthy cat after a meal consisting of dry kibbles meeting one-quarter of the daily requirements. The *Y*-axis represents the percentage of the maximal antral area, and the *X*-axis represents time. $GET_{50\%}$ is 276 minutes, and the stomach is 98% empty at 420 minutes. There is a 210-minute latency until the antrum reaches its maximum diameter, which has been reported in another study, and attributed to rehydration of kibbles and slow antral dilation with minimal increase in luminal pressure.[24] $GET_{50\%}$, time when 50% of meal has left the stomach.

in cats as well, the wide availability of ultrasound equipment would render it very applicable in the clinical setting.

Motility Disorders

Generally, there are very little published data on disorders of gastric emptying in cats; much of the data given later is derived from clinical observations.

Primary Disorders of Gastric Motility

Primary functional disorders appear to be rare in cats. Dysautonomia is discussed in detail later. A review of hairballs suggested that peculiarities of feline gastric motility may be involved in their etiopathogenesis, in particular of the apparent lack of organized interdigestive motility.[28] In humans and dogs, type III MMC efficiently eliminates non-digestible content larger than 1 to 2 mm in diameter. Their absence in felines may prevent passage of hair material through the pylorus and promote gastric retention and ultimately formation of a hairball. In particular, in shorthaired cats, frequent vomiting of hairballs may also be an early sign of chronic enteropathies and should prompt clinicians to initiate further diagnostic tests.[28]

Secondary Disorders of Gastric Motility

Gastric, intestinal, and abdominal inflammation are common causes of gastric dysmotility in cats. Examples include intestinal parasitoses, acute gastroenteritis, chronic enteropathies (such as inflammatory bowel disease), alimentary lymphoma, and gastric ulcers. Additionally, inflammatory diseases of abdominal organs have the potential to cause paralytic ileus (see Generalized Motility Disorders) that may result in prolonged anorexia and hospitalization. Interestingly, GET is not prolonged after endoscopic placement of a percutaneous gastrostomy tube.[29]

Diseases affecting multiple organ systems may also impact GI motility. Hyperthyroid cats had a significantly shorter OCTT after receiving a liquid meal with lactulose than healthy cats.[30] Successful treatment with radioactive iodine (^{131}I) at least partially normalized the OCTT.[31] Diabetes mellitus is the most common cause of delayed gastric emptying in humans. However, in spite of the frequent occurrence of feline diabetes mellitus, there are no available data describing delayed GET in cats with spontaneous diabetes to date. Dogs with significant (66%) experimental reduction of renal mass show decreased small intestinal and colonic motility, but gastric motility is preserved. There are no similar data available for cats. It is conceivable that loss of 75% or more of the renal parenchyma, as is common in cats with chronic kidney disease, may have repercussions on gastric motility as well. Finally, electrolyte disorders, such as hypokalemia, hypocalcemia, hypercalcemia, and hypomagnesemia, may negatively impact smooth muscle function and decrease GI motility.

Drugs may also induce delayed gastric emptying; opioids and anticholinergics may cause impaired smooth muscle function. Delayed GI transit times were documented in dogs undergoing general anesthesia; this is likely to occur in cats as well.

Stress and release of sympathetic transmitters may occur in association with trauma, other painful events, or unusual surroundings and has the potential to inhibit gastric motility.

Treatment of Disorders of Gastric Motility

If decreased gastric motility appears to be secondary, treatment aimed at addressing the underlying disorder is an essential premise to ultimate resolution of the dysmotility. Disturbances in GI motility contribute to the perpetuation of anorexia.

Diet. A dietary approach for treatment of delayed gastric motility relies on applied physiology. Small meals consisting of an easily digestible liquid or canned diet of low caloric density and fat content are more likely to be emptied rapidly from the stomach. Unfortunately, such diets may not be appetizing to finicky cats, and a compromise between palatability and optimal meal composition needs to be found in such cases.

Prokinetics. Table 11-2 summarizes site and mechanism of action, dosage recommendation, and side effects of GI prokinetics for clinical use in cats. A discussion of the drugs can be found at the end of this chapter.

SMALL INTESTINE

Anatomy and Physiology

Surprisingly little is known about feline small intestinal motility patterns. As stated earlier, the interdigestive motility is different from that observed in other species. In cats, spike burst electrical activity is followed by migrating spike complexes that generate giant aboral contractions. These contractions are probably responsible for moving large, indigestible particles toward the large intestine.[17,32] The fed motility patterns described in other carnivorous species are presumed to be present in cats as well. They consist of peristaltic waves, or circular contractions propagating aborally, and of stationary (also called phasic or segmenting) contractions that occur at single sites and are responsible for mixing content.

Diagnostic Approach

When abnormal small intestinal transit is suspected, the first step consists of rigorously ruling out obstructive disease, such as foreign bodies and intramural or extramural masses, because these often necessitate a surgical approach. Once an obstruction has been ruled out, evaluation of the small intestinal transit time (SITT) may be useful. Small intestinal transit time can be estimated using the OCTT determined using the hydrogen breath test. This test measures hydrogen production after administration of lactulose, which is only metabolized by the large intestinal microbiota.[33] The OCTT is comprised of both GET and SITT and was reported to be between 30 and 45 minutes in healthy cats after administration of lactulose without solid food.[33] SITT can also be determined using radiopaque spheres administered with a solid meal.[23,34] Published times for SITT in healthy cats ranged from 2.25 to 3.05 hours in one study.[34] However, in most clinical situations, qualitative evaluation of small intestinal motility is more practical. Abdominal radiographs may show dilated and gas-filled intestinal segments (Figure 11-3), and abdominal ultrasonography may reveal large, hypomotile intestinal loops (Figure 11-4).

Table 11-2	Prokinetic Drugs Most Commonly Used in Cats with Delayed Esophageal and Gastrointestinal Motility (in Alphabetical Order)*,†		
Name	**Mechanism and Site of Action**	**Posology**	**Side Effects**
Bethanechol	Parasympathomimetic agent Esophagus, LES, gastric antrum, small intestine, colon	1.25-5 mg/cat PO every 8 h Start at low end of dosing range	Vomiting, diarrhea, salivation, anorexia Cardiovascular and respiratory effects usually only with excessive dose
Cisapride	Serotonin agonist ($5HT_4$ receptors) LES, gastric antrum, duodenum, colon	1 mg/kg PO every 8 h or 1.5 mg/kg PO every 12 h Start at low end of dosing range and titrate to effect	Inhibitor of cytochrome P-450 enzyme, may increase half-life of other drugs eliminated via this pathway
Erythromycin	Motilin agonist Esophagus, LES Unknown in cats: gastric antrum or small intestine	0.5-1 mg/kg IV, PO every 8 h	None described at that dose
Metoclopramide	Dopamine antagonist (D2 receptors), $5HT_3$ antagonist, $5HT_4$ agonist Gastric antrum	0.2-0.4 mg/kg SC every 8 h 1-2 mg/kg/day IV CRI	Excitation, restlessness, muscle tremor after overdosing

*See text for more details and additional drugs for which clinical experience is currently more limited.
†Prokinetic drugs should not be used before obstructive disease has been definitively ruled out. They are also contraindicated in the presence of gastrointenstinal hemorrhage or perforation. These drugs are not approved for use in cats in the United States.
CRI, Constant rate infusion; *IV,* intravenously; *LES,* lower esophageal sphincter; *PO,* per os; *SC,* subcutaneously.

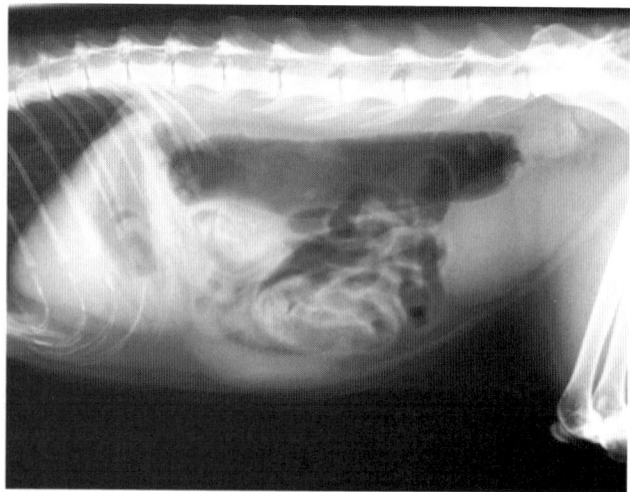

Figure 11-3: Lateral radiograph of the abdomen of a cat with dysautonomia showing gassy distension of the small intestine and colon. There is generalized gas distension of the small intestine and some loops measure more than 1.2 cm. A moderate amount of granular mineral opacity is seen in some loops of small intestine. (From Novellas R, Simpson KE, Gunn-Moore DA, et al: Imaging findings in 11 cats with feline dysautonomia. *J Feline Med Surg* 12:584-591, 2010.)

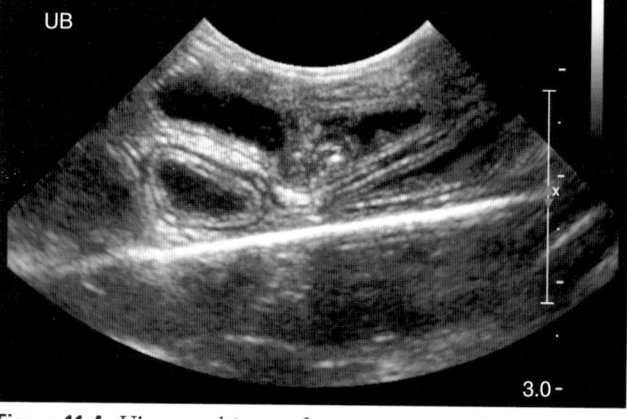

Figure 11-4: Ultrasound image from a 12-year-old male neutered cat with sepsis and acute diarrhea showing multiple jejunal segments that are dilated and fluid filled. The walls are normal in thickness but have an indistinct layering, thin mucosa, and prominent submucosa. Because of their generalized distribution and the mild fluid distention, these findings are characteristic of functional ileus. (Courtesy Dr. Lorrie Gaschen, Louisiana State University.)

Motility Disorders

Enteritis is associated with abnormal intestinal motility patterns that generally result in decreased SITT through a combination of decreased phasic contractions and increased aboral giant contractions. These abnormalities resolve with successful treatment of enteritis. Mechanical ileus is commonly observed and can be caused by intestinal foreign bodies, granulomas, or neoplastic masses (e.g., alimentary lymphoma). Chronic intestinal pseudo-obstruction is a syndrome that generally occurs as a consequence of chronically abnormal intestinal motility in a segment of small intestine. It was reported to be the result of visceral myopathy in a young cat presented for a weeklong history of anorexia, intermittent vomiting, and diarrhea, and also evidence of dilated and hypomotile small bowel loops on imaging. The cat did well after surgical resection of a 20-cm segment of dilated jejunum.[35] Many diseases originating outside the GI tract may have repercussion on small intestinal motility and cause paralytic ileus (see Generalized Motility Disorders). As mentioned earlier, hyperthyroidism shortens the OCTT.[30,31]

Treatment

The principles listed under the approach to gastric motility disorders also apply to small intestinal dysmotility. Any underlying disorder needs to be addressed. Gastrointestinal prokinetics are discussed in detail later and in Table 11-2. Chronic intestinal pseudo-obstruction may require a surgical approach.

COLON

Anatomy and Physiology

In the cat, the colon has two main functions: water absorption, which occurs in the proximal colon, and storage of feces until defecation. Although the physiology of colonic motility has not been studied extensively in the cat, it is likely that principles observed in other species can be applied. Stationary contractions mix the content and indirectly promote water absorption. Peristaltic contractions move the feces aborally over small distances. Finally, giant contractions precede defecation and move feces over longer segments. The gastrocolic reflex is mediated by enteric nerves and enhances colonic motility after a meal, leading to defecation.

Diagnostic Approach

As is the case in other segments of the GI tract, obstructive diseases must first be differentiated from nonobstructive disorders because the approach will be significantly different for each category. Obstruction results in the hypertrophic form of megacolon. If the cause of the obstruction can be addressed in a timely manner, colonic function may be preserved. However, prolonged obstruction is ultimately associated with loss of colonic contractility. Colonic motility can be evaluated qualitatively with radiographs and ultrasound (with enlargement of the colon indicative of dysfunction). Transit of radiopaque spheres can be used to measure the large bowel transit time (LBTT). Large bowel transit time measured at the time of complete evacuation of radiopaque spheres was 40 hours in healthy cats.[36]

Motility Disorders

Colonic inflammation is associated with decreased nonpropulsive motility and excessive propulsive motility, which results in diarrhea with frequent defecation of feces of decreased consistency, and resolves with treatment of colitis. Prolonged LBTT causes constipation.

Constipation, Obstipation, and Megacolon

Definitions. Constipation is characterized by infrequent or difficult evacuation of feces. Obstipation is the result of recurrent, intractable constipation. Constipation and obstipa-

tion may culminate in the syndrome of megacolon.[37] Constipation is a relatively frequent problem in the cat, whereas obstipation and megacolon are less prevalent.

Etiology. Differential diagnoses for constipation in the cat are summarized in Box 11-2.

Clinical Presentation. Obstipation and megacolon are observed in middle-aged cats (mean age: 5.8 years).[38] Typical clinical signs include reduced, absent, or painful defecation, which may be progressive, and are often present for weeks to months before presentation. Dry feces may be seen inside or outside the litter box, and dyschezia may be observed. Chronic constipation and obstipation may have systemic repercussions, such as anorexia, lethargy, weight loss, and vomiting. A thorough physical examination is required in constipated and obstipated cats and may reveal varying degrees of

---

BOX 11-2 Differential Diagnosis of Constipation in the Cat with Prevalence of Most Common Causes of Obstipation (in Parentheses)

Mechanical Obstruction
- Intraluminal—foreign body, neoplasia, stricture, perineal hernia, rectal diverticulum
- Intramural—neoplasia, granuloma
- Extraluminal—pelvic fractures (23%), neoplasia, prostatic disease

Behavioral
- Soiled litter box, change in environment, behavioral issues, inactivity, hospitalization

Inflammation
- Perianal bite wounds, anal sacculitis and abscess, proctitis, anorectal foreign bodies, perineal fistula, arthritis

Metabolic, Endocrine
- Metabolic—obesity, dehydration, hypokalemia, hypercalcemia, chronic kidney disease
- Endocrine—hypothyroidism, hyperparathyroidism

Neuromuscular Dysfunction
- Spinal cord disease—lumbosacral disease, sacral spinal cord deformity, such as in Manx cats (5%)
- Hypogastric or pelvic nerve—injury (6%), malignancy, dysautonomia
- Submucosal or myenteric plexus neuropathy—dysautonomia, aging
- Colonic smooth muscle—idiopathic megacolon (62%), aging

Drugs
- Opiates, anticholinergics, diuretics, phenothiazine, barium sulfate

Washabau RJ, Hasler AH: Constipation, obstipation, and megacolon. In August JR, editor: *Consultations in feline internal medicine*, Philadelphia, 1997, pp 104-112.

dehydration, weight loss, and abdominal pain. Digital rectal palpation should be performed under sedation or anesthesia and may reveal pelvic canal abnormalities or more rarely a rectal foreign body, stricture, or presence of secondary perineal hernia.

Diagnostic Approach. A thorough screening of cats presented with recurrent constipation is recommended to rule out underlying diseases and evaluate the systemic repercussions of the problem. Chronic degenerative conditions, such as chronic kidney disease or arthritis, are commonly associated with constipation episodes. Abdominal radiographs with orthogonal views are recommended. They are useful for assessing the pelvic canal and may be helpful in grading the severity of the fecal impaction. A study established the ratio of maximal colon diameter to the fifth lumbar vertebra (L5) length.[39] A ratio less than 1.28 was indicative of a normal colon, whereas a ratio greater than 1.48 was a good indicator of megacolon.[39] Abdominal ultrasonography may additionally reveal enlarged regional lymph nodes attributable to the presence of chronic inflammation.

Treatment. Identified underlying problems should be treated. The different methods for treatment of constipation include the following options:

- *Oral laxatives* are all administered to effect, starting at the low end of the recommended dose. Bulk laxatives, such as psyllium (1 to 4 teaspoons mixed with food every 12 to 24 hours) or canned pumpkin (1 to 4 teaspoons per day mixed with food), have been used with good success. A specially formulated psyllium-enriched diet is commercially available (Royal Canin Intestinal Fiber Response). In an open trial, the diet was shown to be palatable, improve fecal consistency, and decrease the necessity for other treatments, such as lactulose or cisapride.[40] Dioctyl sodium sulfosuccinate (docusate, DSS) is an emollient agent (50 mg PO every 24 hours), which is commonly used in constipated cats. Mineral oil (10 to 25 mL PO daily) and petrolatum (various specially formulated products) are lubricant laxatives. Hyperosmotic laxatives include lactulose (0.5 mL/kg PO every 8 to 12 hours) and polyethylene glycol 3350 (Miralax, GoLytely), which has been shown to be safe and palatable in cats.[41] Polyethylene glycol 3350 can also be administered through a naso-esophageal tube at rates between 6 to 10 mL/kg/h in constipated and obstipated cats. The mean total dose required was 80 mL/kg (range: 40 to 156), and defecation occurred on average 8 hours after initiation of treatment (range: 5 to 24).[42] The technique has considerably decreased the need for enemas in feline practice (S. Little, personal communication, 2014).
- *Enemas* should be injected slowly. Rapid administration may cause reflex vomiting and rapid, excessive efflux of the liquid and may also increase the risk of colonic perforation. Warm tap water or warm physiologic saline are administered at a dose of 5 to 10 mL/kg. Docusate, mineral oil, or lactulose may also be administered rectally (5 to 10 mL/cat). Avoid combining DSS and mineral oil. Docusate suppositories are available for use at home if the cat tolerates them.

- Prokinetic agents are discussed later. Currently, the most commonly used prokinetic in cats with constipation and obstipation is cisapride.
- A stepwise approach has proven useful in cats with constipation and obstipation. Cats with mild constipation (e.g., first occurrence or recurrence after a long interval with normal defecation) can be treated with oral laxatives and may require an initial enema. Maintaining these cats on a psyllium-enriched diet or continuing supplementation with laxatives may be beneficial. Moderate or recurrent constipation usually benefits from naso-esophageal administration of Polyethylene glycol 3350 (see earlier). Refractory cases may require administration of several enemas and/or manual extraction of feces. Manual extraction is useful when all other options have failed. It is best performed on the anesthetized cat with careful transabdominal colonic massage with simultaneous rectal administration of a combination of warm water or physiologic saline with water-soluble lubricants in an attempt to break down the impacted feces. Instruments, such as sponge forceps, may be useful if used cautiously. In refractory cases, more than one session may be required to evacuate the colon without taking excessive risks. Some authors recommend administering a low dose of metronidazole (7.5 to 15 mg/kg PO every 12 hours) in order to address the risk of bacterial translocation during or after the procedure. Long-term treatment should consist of fiber supplementation with additional lactulose and cisapride. Regular administration of enemas by the owner in the home environment is unlikely to be easy in the majority of cases, and compliance may be low. A surgical approach should be considered for severe cases with obstipation or megacolon that does not respond to the treatments mentioned earlier, and different techniques for colectomy have been successful in these cats.[37] A description of the procedures is best found in surgical texts.

GENERALIZED MOTILITY DISORDERS

Several conditions may cause a generalized impairment of digestive motility. Paralytic ileus is a common occurrence, and feline dysautonomia is a rare disease that may affect all parts of the digestive system and other organ systems as well.

Paralytic Ileus

Etiopathogenesis

Early experimental studies performed on anesthetized cats demonstrated that mechanical stimulation of the small and large intestine, intestinal surgery, and peritoneal inflammation all induce gastric inhibition. Probable pathways included sympathetic nerves, vagus nerve, and spinobulbar ascending pathways as well as local vagovagal reflexes.[43] There is evidence that dogs have decreased gastric emptying after laparotomy.[44,45] Four major pathways have been identified for postobstructive ileus (POI) in animal models and in humans: (1) *neurogenic* with stimulation of inhibitory neural pathways associated with surgical stress, (2) *inflammatory* with stimulation of macrophages and neutrophils upon bowel manipulation and release of proinflammatory mediators that reduce GI motility, and (3) *hormonal* with release of corticotrophin-releasing factor and stimulation of proinflammatory cytokines in the bowel. Finally, POI may be compounded by (4) *pharmacologic* interventions, in particular by the use of exogenous opioids as analgesics and their general inhibitory effect on GI motility. Among opioid analgesics, mu-receptor agonists increase antral contractions but decrease antral propulsion; similarly they increase intestinal tone and segmentation but decrease intestinal propulsion. Finally, they strengthen the activity of the ileocolic and anal sphincters. Mu-receptor agonists, such as loperamide, or those combined with anticholinergics, such as diphenoxylate and atropine, are used in the treatment of acute episodes of diarrhea. They may lead to dysmotility if administered for more than a few days.

Anticholinergics administered alone also have the potential to elicit adynamic ileus. Box 11-3 lists diseases likely to cause adynamic ileus. There is preliminary data suggesting delayed GI transit times can occur in dogs and cats with pyloric diseases, pancreatitis, and uremic syndrome.[44] In cats, acute pancreatitis, cholangitis, peritonitis, and uremic syndrome are common extraintestinal processes that have the potential to decrease GI motility.

Clinical Signs and Diagnosis
Clinical signs include those listed in Box 11-1 in association with signs of the primary underlying disease. Gut sounds are usually absent on abdominal auscultation. Typically, abdominal radiographs show moderately distended bowel loops filled with gas and liquid content (see Figure 11-3), and abdominal ultrasound reveals distended and hypomotile stomach and intestine (see Figure 11-4).

Treatment
Proper management is important because lack of GI motility prevents the use of the GI tract for feeding. Any identifiable cause needs to be treated, and prokinetic agents may be useful. A constant rate infusion (CRI) of lidocaine (initially 0.025 mg/kg/min IV after loading bolus of 0.5 mg/kg IV) during any surgical intervention was thought to decrease the severity of POI through the drug's antinociceptive, antihyperalgesic, and anti-inflammatory properties. However, the current consensus is that lidocaine CRI does not have any direct effect on GI motility.

Feline Dysautonomia

Dysautonomia is a disease of yet unknown origin; it was first described in cats in the early 1980s. It is characterized by generalized and progressive dysfunction of the autonomic nervous system. There is circumstantial evidence from an outbreak in a closed cat colony that dysautonomia may be associated with *Clostridium botulinum* type C toxin.[46] Several hundred cats with dysautonomia have been reported worldwide, with a cluster in the United Kingdom and, to a lesser extent, the European continent. Peak prevalence occurred in the early to mid-1980s, and the disease appears to be less prevalent at this time.[47] In the United States, isolated indigenous cases were also reported from the Midwestern states of Missouri and Kansas.[48]

Clinical Signs and Diagnosis
Cats with dysautonomia display signs of generalized autonomic dysfunction, such as bilateral mydriasis unresponsive to light, prolapse of the third eyelid, dry mucous membranes, dry crusted nasal secretions, bradycardia (heart rate less than 150 or even less than 120 bpm) in spite of apparent nervousness, and/or dehydration. A large, easily expressible urinary bladder may be palpated and associated with urinary incontinence. GI signs include anorexia, constipation, regurgitation or vomiting, and areflexic anus with or without fecal incontinence.[48,49] Megaesophagus may be present, although some cats only show decreased esophageal motility in a fluoroscopic study. Abdominal radiographs may reveal gas-filled, dilated stomach and bowels (see Figure 11-3). Decreased tear production is often present, as assessed with Shirmer tear test. In the presence of the signs mentioned, the diagnosis is confirmed by applying dilute (0.05% to 0.1%) pilocarpine eye drops. This causes rapid development of miosis, demonstrating the presence of autonomic dysfunction and denervation hypersensitivity of the iris muscle.[47-49] The presentation of feline dysautonomia is acute to subacute, and the disease usually progresses over days to weeks.

Treatment
Treatment is aimed at supporting the essential body functions (including IV fluids, urinary bladder expression, feeding in an upright position), and affected cats often require intensive care in the hospital and home environment. Multiple GI prokinetic drugs are often used together in an attempt to support digestive motility. Pilocarpine eye drops are used to prevent photophobia and third eyelid prolapse, and artificial tears are applied. The cautious use of bethanechol may also be beneficial. The posology of GI prokinetic drugs is listed in Table 11-2.

BOX 11-3   Causes of Adynamic Ileus

- Abdominal surgery
- Peritonitis
- Intestinal ischemia
- Sepsis
- Electrolyte imbalance (hypokalemia)
- Uremic syndrome
- Dysautonomia
- Spinal cord injuries
- Lead poisoning
- Anticholinergic drugs

Adapted from Guilford WG: Motility disorders of the bowel. In Guilford WG, Center SA, Strombeck DR, et al, editors: *Strombeck's small animal gastroenterology*, ed 3, Philadelphia, 1996, Saunders, pp 532-539.

Prognosis

The prognosis is poor, with only 25% of cats recovering from the disease over several months, sometimes only partially.[33] Cats showing mild clinical signs appear to have the best chance for clinical recovery.[48,49]

Histopathologic Evaluation

Postganglionic neurons are more commonly affected, although lesions may also be seen in preganglionic neurons. Cranial nerve ganglia and dorsal root ganglia may also be affected. The lesions consist of loss of Nissl substance, pyknotic nuclei, and disappearance of neurons in autonomic ganglia in the absence of marked inflammation. These changes can also be seen in some somatic neurons. Electron microscopy reveals typical ultrastructural lesions of large cisternae and complex membranous stacks.[49]

GASTROINTESTINAL PROKINETIC DRUGS FOR USE IN CATS

Prokinetic drugs should not be administered before a GI obstruction has been definitely ruled out. The available published evidence on the effect of various prokinetic drugs in healthy cats is tenuous, whereas it is almost nonexistent for cats with GI dysmotility. Therefore, collective clinical experience plays an important role in most recommendations for drug usage and dosage (see also Table 11-2).

Cisapride

Cisapride is a serotonergic drug, and its main site of action is the type 4 serotonin ($5HT_4$) receptors located on enteric cholinergic neurons that innervate intestinal smooth muscle. Activation results in release of acetylcholine in the synaptic cleft and excitation of the postsynaptic cell membrane. Cisapride also interacts with $5HT_1$ and $5HT_3$ receptors (antagonist) and $5HT_2$ receptors (agonist) in the enteric nervous system. It is a substrate of CYP3A, a cytochrome P450 enzyme. Cisapride was shown to have effects in the feline LES, gastric antrum, and colon. It stimulates *in vitro* contractions of colon smooth muscle strips collected from healthy cats and from cats with megacolon.[50,51] It is assumed to also have prokinetic properties in the small bowel of cats. Unlike what is observed in humans, cisapride does not cause prolongation of the QT interval and polymorphic ventricular arrhythmia in cats unless administered at doses 20 times higher than currently recommended.[52] It is therefore safe to use in cats. Cisapride is recommended for use in cats with GER, delayed gastric emptying, paralytic ileus, and colonic dysmotility and is widely used clinically for the treatment of feline megacolon.

Prucalopride

Prucalopride is a newer serotonergic compound with high affinity for the $5HT_4$ receptor that is currently available in Europe (Resolor, Shire), Canada (Resotran, Janssen), and Australia (Resotrans, Janssen) but not yet in the United States. In the cat, only very preliminary data is available. Prucalopride was shown to trigger defecation within 1 hour of oral administration to healthy cats at the empiric dose of 0.64 mg/kg, although a dose of 0.32 mg/kg had no effect.[53] Prucalopride has prokinetic properties on the canine gastric antrum, small intestine, and colon, but there is no further published evidence of its effects on the various segments of the feline GI tract. Although the drug holds great promise, no further recommendations can be made at this time for its use in cats.

Mosapride

Mosapride is a selective $5HT_4$ agonist that is approved for use in dogs in Japan (Pronamid, Dainippon Sumitomo Pharma). It lacks cardiotoxicity in cats[52] and was shown to evoke concentration-dependent contractions of feline ileal muscle fibers *in vitro*.[54] A dose of 5 mg/cat PO twice daily was reported to be helpful in constipated cats.[55] This compound may ultimately prove useful for a variety of indications.

Metoclopramide

Metoclopramide has a variety of effects with repercussions on GI motility. It is an antagonist of dopamine type 2 (D_2) receptors, the major mechanism of its antiemetic action in dogs, but not in cats because they lack D_2 receptors in their chemoreceptor trigger zone or emetic center. However, dopamine antagonism may also play a role in the drug's prokinetic properties because D_2 receptors have been shown to impair acetylcholine release in muscarinic endplates located in the stomach. Most of the prokinetic effects are due to the drug's affinity for the $5HT_4$ receptor. Additionally, metoclopramide is also a $5HT_3$ inhibitor. The drug has no significant effect on the LES but was shown to cause antral contractions in cats.

Erythromycin

Erythromycin is a motilin agonist that initiates interdigestive type III MMC and is commonly used in the dog. However, cats do not display a classic type of interdigestive motility pattern. Functional motilin receptors and motilin precursor have been identified in the feline GI tract, with highest concentrations in the duodenum and lowest in the colon. Erythromycin increases muscle tone *in vitro* in the feline LES but not in the colon. There are no studies evaluating the effects of erythromycin on gastric emptying or small intestinal transit in cats, and its benefits as a GI prokinetic in cats are unknown.

Ranitidine and Nizatidine

Ranitidine and nizatidine are antagonists of the histamine type 2 receptors. In addition, they exert acetylcholinesterase-inhibiting properties in the muscarinic cholinergic endplates connecting enteric motoneurons and smooth muscle cells, with GI prokinetic effects. In the cat, the prokinetic properties of ranitidine and nizatidine on colonic muscle cells have been documented *in vitro* only in a preliminary study,[56] and their effect on gastric or small intestinal motility is unknown. The dosage is the same as that recommended when these drugs are used as H_2 antagonists.

Bethanechol

Bethanechol directly stimulates cholinergic receptors. At therapeutic doses, its effects are usually limited to muscarinic receptors; however, nicotinic stimulation may occur with higher doses. Bethanechol is a cholinergic drug with significant stimulating effects on the GI and urinary tracts. However, it is not a recognized prokinetic agent that promotes coordinated GI motility. The only recommended use is in the treatment of feline dysautonomia.[48,49]

Mirtazapine

Mirtazapine is a tetracyclic antidepressant and $5HT_3$ antagonist. It has documented appetite stimulant and antiemetic properties in cats with chronic kidney disease at a dose of 1.88 mg PO every 48 hours (one-quarter of a 7.5 mg tablet).[57] A study performed in dogs documented that high doses of mirtazapine accelerated both gastric emptying of solid food and colonic transit time but had no effect on SITT.[58] Although this has not been studied in cats, it is possible that part of the positive effects of the drug in nauseous patients may be due to improved digestive motility. Further studies about the use of mirtazapine as a GI prokinetic agent in cats are needed before any recommendation for clinical use in cats with disorders of GI motility can be made.

References

1. Venker-van Haagen AJ: Esophagus—structure and function. In Washabau R, Day MJ, editors: *Canine and feline gatroenterology*, St Louis, 2013, Elsevier, pp 570–573.
2. Clerc N: Histological characteristics of the lower oesophageal sphincter in the cat. *Acta Anat (Basel)* 117:201–208, 1983.
3. Gaschen L: The canine and feline esophagus. In Thrall DE, editor: *Textbook of veterinary diagnostic radiology*, St Louis, 2013, Elsevier, pp 500–522.
4. Lang IM, Medda BK, Jadcherla S, et al: The role of the superior laryngeal nerve in esophageal reflexes. *Am J Physiol Gastrointest Liver Physiol* 302:G1445–G1457, 2012.
5. Frowde PE, Battersby IA, Whitley NT, et al: Oesophageal disease in 33 cats. *J Feline Med Surg* 13:564–569, 2011.
6. Moses L, Harpster NK, Beck KA, et al: Esophageal motility dysfunction in cats: a study of 44 cases. *J Am Anim Hosp Assoc* 36:309–312, 2000.
7. Levine JS, Pollard RE, Marks SL: Contrast videofluoroscopic assessment of dysphagic cats. *Vet Radiol Ultrasound* 55:465–471, 2014.
8. Tuchman DN, Boyle JT, Pack AI, et al: Comparison of airway responses following tracheal or esophageal acidification in the cat. *Gastroenterology* 87:872–881, 1984.
9. Galatos AD, Savas I, Prassinos NN, et al: Gastro-oesophageal reflux during thiopentone or propofol anaesthesia in the cat. *J Vet Med A Physiol Pathol Clin Med* 48(5):287–294, 2001.
10. Sideri AI, Galatos AD, Kazakos GM, et al: Gastro-oesophageal reflux during anaesthesia in the kitten: comparison between use of a laryngeal mask airway or an endotracheal tube. *Vet Anaesth Analg* 36:547–554, 2009.
11. Shelton GD, Ho M, Kass PH: Risk factors for acquired myasthenia gravis in cats: 105 cases (1986-1998). *J Am Vet Med Assoc* 216:55–57, 2000.
12. Westfall DS, Twedt DC, Steyn PF, et al: Evaluation of esophageal transit of tablets and capsules in 30 cats. *J Vet Intern Med* 15:467–470, 2001.
13. Graham JP, Lipman AH, Newell SM, et al: Esophageal transit of capsules in clinically normal cats. *Am J Vet Res* 61:655–657, 2000.
14. Beatty JA, Swift N, Foster DJ, et al: Suspected clindamycin-associated oesophageal injury in cats: five cases. *J Feline Med Surg* 8:412–419, 2006.
15. German AJ, Cannon MJ, Dye C, et al: Oesophageal strictures in cats associated with doxycycline therapy. *J Feline Med Surg* 7:33–41, 2005.
16. Bennett AD, MacPhail CM, Gibbons DS, et al: A comparative study evaluating the esophageal transit time of eight healthy cats when pilled with the flavorx pill glide versus pill delivery treats. *J Feline Med Surg* 12:286–290, 2010.
17. De Vos WC: Migrating spike complex in the small intestine of the fasting cat. *Am J Physiol* 265:G619–G627, 1993.
18. Costello M, Papasouliotis K, Barr FJ, et al: Determination of solid- and liquid-phase gastric emptying half times in cats by use of nuclear scintigraphy. *Am J Vet Res* 60:1222–1226, 1999.
19. Goggin JM, Hoskinson JJ, Butine MD, et al: Scintigraphic assessment of gastric emptying of canned and dry diets in healthy cats. *Am J Vet Res* 59:388–392, 1998.
20. Armbrust LJ, Hoskinson JJ, Lora-Michiels M, et al: Gastric emptying in cats using foods varying in fiber content and kibble shapes. *Vet Radiol Ultrasound* 44:339–343, 2003.
21. Peachey SE, Dawson JM, Harper EJ: Gastrointestinal transit times in young and old cats. *Comp Biochem Physiol A Mol Integr Physiol* 126:85–90, 2000.
22. Hogan PM, Aronson E: Effect of sedation on transit time of feline gastrointestinal contrast studies. *Vet Radiol* 29:85–88, 1988.
23. Sparkes AH, Papasouliotis K, Barr FJ, et al: Reference ranges for gastrointestinal transit of barium-impregnated polyethylene spheres in healthy cats. *J Small Anim Pract* 38:340–343, 1997.
24. Goggin JM, Hoskinson JJ, Kirk CA, et al: Comparison of gastric emptying times in healthy cats simultaneously evaluated with radiopaque markers and nuclear scintigraphy. *Vet Radiol Ultrasound* 40:89–95, 1999.
25. Schmitz S, Gotte B, Borsch C, et al: Direct comparison of solid-phase gastric emptying times assessed by means of a carbon isotope-labeled sodium acetate breath test and technetium ^{99m}Tc albumin colloid radioscintigraphy in healthy cats. *Am J Vet Res* 75:648–652, 2014.
26. Coradini M, Rand J, Filippich L, et al: Associations between meal size, gastric emptying and postprandial plasma glucose, insulin and lactate concentrations in meal-fed cats. *J Anim Physiol Anim Nutr (Berl)* 2014. doi: 10.1111/jpn.12280. [Epub ahead of print].
27. Tsukamoto A, Ohno K, Tsukagoshi T, et al: Real-time ultrasonographic evaluation of canine gastric motility in the postprandial state. *J Vet Med Sci* 73:1133–1138, 2011.
28. Cannon M: Hair balls in cats: a normal nuisance or a sign that something is wrong? *J Feline Med Surg* 15:21–29, 2013.
29. Smith SA, Ludlow CL, Hoskinson JJ, et al: Effect of percutaneous endoscopic gastrostomy on gastric emptying in clinically normal cats. *Am J Vet Res* 59:1414–1416, 1998.
30. Papasouliotis K, Muir P, Gruffydd-Jones TJ, et al: Decreased orocaecal transit time, as measured by the exhalation of hydrogen, in hyperthyroid cats. *Res Vet Sci* 55:115–118, 1993.
31. Schlesinger DP, Rubin SI, Papich MG, et al: Use of breath hydrogen measurement to

evaluate orocecal transit time in cats before and after treatment for hyperthyroidism. *Can J Vet Res* 57:89–94, 1993.

32. Weisbrodt NW, Christensen J: Electrical activity of the cat duodenum in fasting and vomiting. *Gastroenterology* 63:1004–1010, 1972.

33. Muir P, Papassouliotis K, Gruffydd-Jones TJ, et al: Evaluation of carbohydrate malassimilation and intestinal transit time in cats by measurement of breath hydrogen excretion. *Am J Vet Res* 52:1104–1109, 1991.

34. Chandler ML, Guilford G, Lawoko CR: Radiopaque markers to evaluate gastric emptying and small intestinal transit time in healthy cats. *J Vet Intern Med* 11:361–364, 1997.

35. Harvey AM, Hall EJ, Day MJ, et al: Chronic intestinal pseudo-obstruction in a cat caused by visceral myopathy. *J Vet Intern Med* 19:111–114, 2005.

36. Fucci V, Pechman RD, Hedlund CS, et al: Large bowel transit times using radiopaque markers in normal cats. *J Am Anim Hosp Assoc* 31:473–477, 1995.

37. Washabau RJ: Colonic dysmotility. In Washabau RJ, Day MJ, editors: *Canine and feline gastroenterology*, St Louis, 2013, Elsevier, pp 757–764.

38. Washabau RJ, Hasler AH: Constipation, obstipation, and megacolon. In August JR, editor: *Consultations in feline internal medicine*, Philadelphia, 1997, Elsevier, pp 104–112.

39. Trevail T, Gunn-Moore D, Carrera I, et al: Radiographic diameter of the colon in normal and constipated cats and in cats with megacolon. *Vet Radiol Ultrasound* 52:516–520, 2011.

40. Freiche V, Houston D, Weese H, et al: Uncontrolled study assessing the impact of a psyllium-enriched extruded dry diet on faecal consistency in cats with constipation. *J Feline Med Surg* 13:903–911, 2011.

41. Tam FM, Carr AP, Myers SL: Safety and palatability of polyethylene glycol 3350 as an oral laxative in cats. *J Vet Intern Med* 24(3):723, 2010.

42. Carr AP, Gaunt MC: Constipation resolution with administration of polyethylene-glycol solution in cats. *J Vet Intern Med* 24(3):723, 2010.

43. Glise H, Abrahamsson H: Reflex vagal inhibition of gastric motility by intestinal nociceptive stimulation in the cat. *Scand J Gastroenterol Suppl* 15:769–774, 1980.

44. Allan FJ, Guilford WG: Radiopaque markers: preliminary clinical observations. *J Vet Intern Med* 8(2):151, 1994.

45. Schmitz S, Jansen N, Failing K, et al: ^{13}C-sodium acetate breath test for evaluation of gastric emptying times in dogs with gastric dilatation-volvulus. *Tierarztl Prax Ausg K Kleintiere Heimtiere* 41:87–92, 2013.

46. Nunn F, Cave TA, Knottenbelt C, et al: Association between key-gaskell syndrome and infection by *Clostridium botulinum* type C/D. *Vet Rec* 155:111–115, 2004.

47. Novellas R, Simpson KE, Gunn-Moore DA, et al: Imaging findings in 11 cats with feline dysautonomia. *J Feline Med Surg* 12:584–591, 2010.

48. Kidder AC, Johannes C, O'Brien DP, et al: Feline dysautonomia in the midwestern United States: a retrospective study of nine cases. *J Feline Med Surg* 10:130–136, 2008.

49. Sharp NJ: Feline dysautonomia. *Semin Vet Med Surg (Small Anim)* 5:67–71, 1990.

50. Washabau RJ, Sammarco J: Effects of cisapride on feline colonic smooth muscle function. *Am J Vet Res* 57:541–546, 1996.

51. Hasler AH, Washabau RJ: Cisapride stimulates contraction of idiopathic megacolonic smooth muscle in cats. *J Vet Intern Med* 11:313–318, 1997.

52. Kii Y, Nakatsuji K, Nose I, et al: Effects of 5-HT(4) receptor agonists, cisapride and mosapride citrate on electrocardiogram in anaesthetized rats and guinea-pigs and conscious cats. *Pharmacol Toxicol* 89:96–103, 2001.

53. Briejer MR, Engelen M, Jacobs J, et al: R093877 enhances defecation frequency in conscious cats. *Gastroenterology* 112:A705, 1997.

54. Wang Y, Park SY, Oh KH, et al: Characteristics of 5-hydroxytryptamine receptors involved in contraction of feline ileal longitudinal smooth muscle. *Korean J Physiol Pharmacol* 15:267–272, 2011.

55. Kang JH, Lee M, Noh S, et al: Use of mosapride citrate in cats with chronic constipation. *Proceedings* World Small Animal Veterinary Congress, Birmingham, 2012.

56. Washabau RJ, Pitts MM, Hasler A: Nizatidine and ranitidine stimulate feline colonic smooth muscle contraction. *J Vet Intern Med* 10:157, 1996.

57. Quimby JM, Lunn KF: Mirtazapine as an appetite stimulant and anti-emetic in cats with chronic kidney disease: a masked placebo-controlled crossover clinical trial. *Vet J* 197:651–655, 2013.

58. Yin J, Song J, Lei Y, et al: Prokinetic effects of mirtazapine on gastrointestinal transit. *Am J Physiol Gastrointest Liver Physiol* 306:G796–G801, 2014.

59. Guilford WG: Motility disorders of the bowel. In Guilford WG, Center SA, Strombeck DR, et al, editors: *Strombeck's small animal gastroenterology*, ed 3, Philadelphia, 1996, Saunders, pp 532–539.

Feline Inflammatory Gastrointestinal Disease

Albert E. Jergens and Karin Allenspach

Feline inflammatory gastrointestinal (GI) disease is a collective term applied to a group of multi-organ inflammatory disorders characterized by persistent or recurrent GI signs with inflammation of the liver, pancreas, and/or small intestine. This ill-defined, but often cited, multi-organ disease entity is also termed *triaditis;* however, there are no peer-reviewed published reports using this definition found in PubMed. Anecdotally, multi-organ GI inflammation in cats would seem to be a clinically prevalent disorder that complicates treatment strategies and impacts outcome for affected cats versus cats having single organ inflammation alone. But is this really the case? This chapter reviews the evidence-based data supporting the presence of simultaneous multi-organ inflammatory disease in cats, as well as how to diagnose and treat these disorders, and whether inflammation in multiple organs affects long-term prognosis.

TRIADITIS: PAST AND PRESENT PERSPECTIVE

The exact origin of the term *triaditis* is unknown. Perhaps the first reference made to feline inflammatory GI disease was made by Zawie and Garvey when they reported a possible association between cholecystitis, duodenitis, and pancreatitis in a series of feline patients with chronic hepatopathy.[1] In the mid-1990s, a series of reports from different investigative groups at different institutions were published evaluating multi-organ inflammation in cats (Table 12-1). The most extensive case series was published by Weiss and colleagues[2], where a potential association between inflammation in the gut, liver, pancreas, and even the kidneys was observed in necropsy specimens. The prevalence of inflammatory bowel disease (IBD; 15/18; 83%) and pancreatitis (9/18; 50%) was greater for cats with cholangiohepatitis, compared with cats without inflammatory hepatic disease. Thirty-nine percent of cats (7/18) with cholangiohepatitis had IBD and pancreatitis. This report was soon followed by observations defining an association between hypocobalaminemia and feline GI disease,[3] acute necrotizing/suppurative pancreatitis in cats,[4] and outcome in cats having acute pancreatitis with and without hepatic lipidosis.[5] Potential limitations of these earlier reports included the retrospective design of most studies, the focus on specific feline subsets with alimentary tract disorders, the use of less-sophisticated diagnostic tests (as compared with present assays), and the inability to

definitively confirm the temporal relationship that multi-organ inflammation occurred simultaneously.

One contemporary investigation (necropsy study) evaluated the histopathologic findings in 44 cats diagnosed with cholangitis based on the World Small Animal Veterinary Association (WSAVA) classification scheme (see later).[6] Results indicated that liver enzyme activity did not predict the degree of parenchymal inflammation. Inflammatory bowel disease (50%), pancreatitis (60%), or both (32%) commonly accompanied cholangitis. Cholangitis appeared to contribute to death in most cats in the study; however, the majority of mortality was associated with concurrent disease. Unfortunately, indices for histopathologic scoring of intestines were not defined, different segments of the GI tract in different cats were sampled, and gut biopsies were not performed in all cats. Still others[2] have utilized big data obtained from veterinary reference laboratories to describe the prevalence of feline multi-organ GI inflammation. In separate searches utilizing various serological markers (including feline trypsin-like immunoreactivity [fTLI], feline pancreas-specific lipase [fPL], cobalamin, folate, alanine aminotransferase [ALT], alkaline phosphatase [ALP]) of GI inflammation from different laboratories, the prevalence of triaditis was similar from two sites (32/1345 cats = 2.4% and 51/3816 cats = 1.3%), whereas the prevalence of both intestinal inflammation and pancreatitis from a third site was 22%.

PROPOSED MECHANISMS FOR MULTI-ORGAN INFLAMMATION

The mechanisms for simultaneous inflammation involving the small intestine, pancreas, and/or liver might be related to the unique pancreaticobiliary anatomy of the cat. Multi-organ inflammation is possible because the feline pancreatic duct enters the common bile duct before it opens into the duodenum. Unlike the anatomy in the dog, the accessory pancreatic duct is small and only present in approximately 20% of cats. Cats also have naturally high numbers of bacteria in their duodenum, which might predispose them to ascending passage of bacteria and/or their products into the pancreatic and biliary system; or alternatively, retrograde ejection of bile up the pancreatic and common bile ducts during vomiting episodes could also increase the risk for pancreatic

Table 12-1   Retrospective Analyses on the Potential Associations among Multi-Organ Gastrointestinal Inflammatory Disorders in Cats

Author	Study Type	Aim	Conclusions
Weiss et al.[2]	Retrospective analysis of 78 cats at necropsy	Assess the association of feline ILD with inflammation in other organs	Inflammation in the liver, pancreas, gut, and/or kidneys was observed; 15 of 18 cats with ILD had IBD; 9 of 18 cats with ILD had pancreatitis; 7 of 18 cats with ILD had IBD and pancreatitis ILD may be associated with IBD or pancreatitis
Simpson et al.[23]	Retrospective analysis of 49 cats with GI disease; 22 of 49 cats had subnormal cobalamin for inclusion	Identify the spectrum of feline GI diseases associated with hypocobalaminemia	Multi-organ inflammation of the liver, pancreas, and/or gut can be seen with hypocobalaminemia
Hill and Van Winkle[5]	Retrospective analysis of 40 cats at necropsy	Characterize the histology of feline pancreatitis	Most cats (32 of 40) had acute necrotizing pancreatitis vs suppurative pancreatitis Nonpancreatic pathology to gut or liver was uncommon
Akol et al.[7]	Retrospective study of 13 cats	Evaluate recovery rate of AP vs AP and HL	AP and HL was observed in 38% of cats Recovery rate for AP plus HL was 20% vs 50% for HL alone Liver and pancreatic pathology may occur together

AP, Acute pancreatitis; *GI*, gastrointestinal; *HL*, hepatic lipidosis; *IBD*, inflammatory bowel disease; *ILD*, inflammatory liver disease.

inflammation and cholangitis.[7] Cats with IBD likely have increases in intestinal permeability associated with mucosal inflammation, which also contributes to bacterial translocation into the portal circulation and endotoxemia. Thus, when inflammatory disease occurs in the small intestine, it may ascend the common bile duct and affect the pancreas and biliary tree or vice versa. The communication between these organs facilitates bidirectional movement of bacteria, inflammatory mediators, bile, and/or pancreatic secretions from one area to another (Figure 12-1).

A critical assessment on the potential role for bacteria causing multi-organ inflammation in cats has been investigated in separate studies. Warren and colleagues[8] first compared the histopathologic features, immunophenotyping, clonality, and *in situ* localization of bacteria in 51 cats diagnosed with lymphocytic cholangitis (LC). Using fluorescence *in situ* hybridization (FISH) for detection of eubacteria in hepatic biopsy specimens, the majority (*n* = 32 of 36; 89%) of tissues examined had no detectable *in situ* bacterial colonization. Inflammation of the liver, pancreas, and GI tract concurrently was reported in 10 out of 31 cholangitis cases (32%) in which histopathology results were available for all three organs. In another report, FISH detected the presence and distribution of intact bacteria in hepatic biopsies

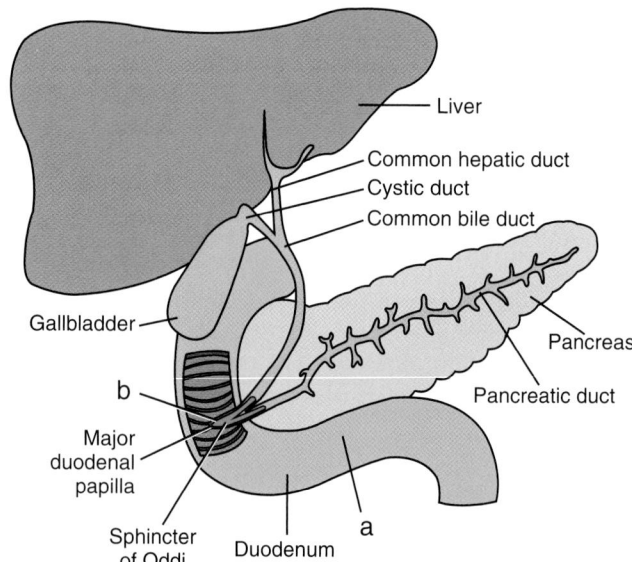

Figure 12-1: Illustration depicting the close proximity and potential anatomic relationship among the liver, pancreas, and duodenum, which may predispose to multi-organ gastrointestinal inflammation. Specifically, microbial imbalances, intestinal inflammation, and increased gut permeability contribute to bacterial translocation. Retrograde passage of luminal contents and biliary secretions may also predispose to pancreatitis and cholangitis. (Image courtesy of Ms. Katy Van Est.)

obtained from 39 cats with inflammatory liver disease (ILD; comprised of a variety of hepatopathies, including neutrophilic cholangitis [NC]) and 19 cats with histologically normal livers (controls).[8] Results indicated that intrahepatic bacteria were observed in 13 out of 39 ILD and 1 out of 19 control cats. Moreover, bacteria in ILD were most frequently localized to portal vessels with bacterial colonization highest in *Escherichia coli*–positive NC cats. Concurrent non-hepatic disease, predominantly pancreatic and intestinal (8/10 cats biopsied), was present in all 13 cats with intrahepatic bacteria. Taken together, these findings support the possibility that intrahepatic bacteria contribute to the pathogenesis of ILD and that hepatic colonization may arise from either enteric translocation and/or hematogenous seeding in affected cats.

RECLASSIFICATION OF FELINE INFLAMMATORY LIVER DISEASE

The WSAVA Liver Standardization Group has revised the histopathologic classification of feline liver disease for consistency of diagnostic interpretation and dissemination of observations among investigators.[9] The term *cholangitis*, rather than *cholangiohepatitis*, is preferred because disruption of the limiting plate to involve hepatic parenchyma is not a consistent feature, and when present, is an extension of primary cholangitis. Using this grading scheme, four distinct forms of feline cholangitis are now recognized, including NC, LC, destructive cholangitis, and cholangitis associated with liver fluke infestation (Table 12-2). Neutrophilic and lymphocytic cholangitis are the most common forms of ILD in cats.[8] Although the causes of most feline ILD have not been determined, it is suspected that infectious agents and/or the immune mechanisms they evoke contribute to the inflammatory process in many cases.

Neutrophilic Cholangitis

In this classification of cholangitis, infiltration of the liver and biliary tree is primarily neutrophilic. The cause is uncertain, but NC may be the result of biliary tract infection ascending from the GI tract.[9,10] This type of cholangitis is composed of both acute and chronic forms, with acute neutrophilic cholangitis (ANC) characterized by neutrophilic inflammation alone within the portal areas, which may extend into the hepatic parenchyma. Chronic neutrophilic cholangitis (CNC) is thought to occur as a progression of ANC and is characterized histologically by variable infiltrates of neutrophils, lymphocytes, and plasma cells. Varying degrees of biliary hyperplasia and fibrosis will be present in biopsy specimens depending on the chronicity of the disease.

Neutrophilic cholangitis is often associated with extrahepatic biliary obstruction (EHBO). In one study,[11] EHBO was identified in 40% of cats with ANC and 76% of cats with CNC, whereas a separate report[12] found that 64% of cats with EHBO had cholangitis. It remains unknown whether infection is the cause or effect of EHBO; however, cholangitis has been implicated as the sole cause of EHBO, resulting from proliferation of mucosa within the common bile duct.

Cats with NC are often young (approximately 3 to 5 years old) and present with an acute illness, which is usually a week or so in duration.[13] Cats often present with nonspecific clinical signs of anorexia, lethargy, vomiting, and weight loss (Figure 12-2). Physical examination findings commonly include icterus and dehydration, with fever, hepatomegaly, and abdominal pain observed in fewer than half of all cases. Hematologic abnormalities are variable but may include a neutrophilia with or without a left shift. Routine biochemical analysis confirms elevation of ALT, aspartate aminotransferase (AST), ALP, and serum total bilirubin ranging in severity from mild to severe. Survey abdominal radiographs are rarely useful for NC. Abdominal ultrasound should be performed to rule out EHBO and to evaluate for abnormalities in gallbladder and hepatic morphology. Both diffuse hypoechoic and hyperechoic changes in the hepatic parenchyma have been reported with NC.[15] Dilation of the common bile duct or gallbladder distension with or without increased bile sediment are the most consistent changes indicative of EHBO (Figure 12-3). Ultrasonography also provides useful information on the presence of multi-organ inflammatory disease involving the pancreas and/or alimentary tract.

Table 12-2	World Small Animal Veterinary Association Histopathologic Classification of Feline Cholangitis by Etiology		
Neutrophilic Cholangitis	**Lymphocytic Cholangitis**	**Destructive Cholangitis**	**Chronic Cholangitis**
Neutrophils in the lumen and/or epithelium of bile ducts	Infiltration of small lymphocytes in and restricted to portal areas	Destruction and loss of bile ducts with inflammation and fibrosis	Dilated larger bile ducts with papillary projections and fibrosis
Chronic stage is characterized by a mixed cellular infiltrate	Variable fibrosis and bile duct proliferation may also be seen	Reported in dogs	Seen in dogs and cats
Etiology: Ascending bacterial infection from GI tract	Etiology: Immune-mediated onset and progression	Etiology: Idiosyncratic reaction to drugs, as well as viral and toxin causes	Etiology: Liver fluke infestation in dogs and cats

Adapted from van den Ingh TS, Cullen JM, Twedt DC, et al: Morphological classification of biliary disorders of canine and feline liver. In Rothuizen J, Bunch SE, Charles JA, et al, editors: *WSAVA standards for clinical and histological diagnosis of canine and feline liver diseases*, Edinburgh, 2006, Saunders/Elsevier.
GI, Gastrointestinal.

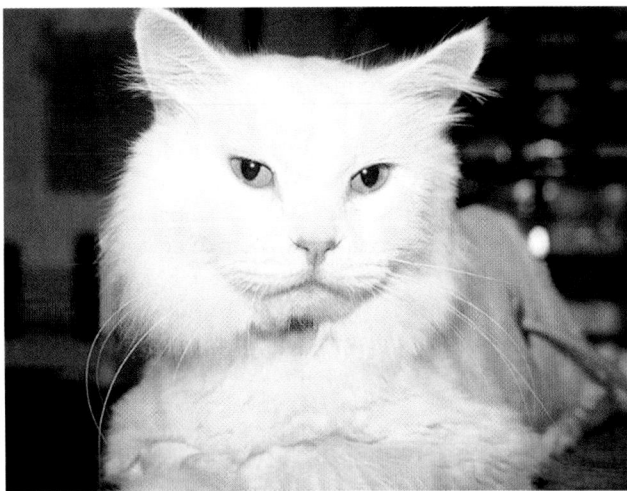

Figure 12-2: General malaise, anorexia, and icterus in a 3-year-old domestic shorthair with neutrophilic cholangitis. A percutaneous endoscopic gastrostomy tube has been placed to provide enteral nutrition support.

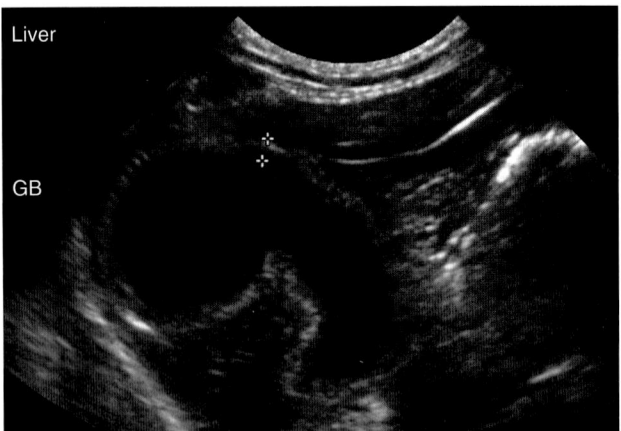

Figure 12-3: Hepatic ultrasonography showing dilatation of the common bile duct and thickening of the gallbladder wall *(asterisks)* in association with feline neutrophilic cholangitis. (Image courtesy of Dr. Kristina Miles, DACVR, Iowa State University.)

Lymphocytic Cholangitis

Lymphocytic cholangitis is characterized by infiltration of lymphocytes and plasma cells confined around portal areas with variable degrees of fibrosis and biliary hyperplasia[9] (Figure 12-4). The nature of the inflammatory infiltrate suggests an underlying immune-mediated pathogenesis for this form of cholangitis. In contrast to NC, LC is uncommonly associated with bacterial colonization with infection documented in less than 20% of cats.[8,14] Lymphocytic cholangitis typically has a chronic progressive clinical course over months or years. Affected cats may be young or old, and Persian cats appear to be overrepresented, suggesting a possible genetic predisposition.[16]

Cats with LC may come to the clinic in chronic progressive hepatic failure with salient clinical signs of anorexia, lethargy, vomiting, and weight loss. The most common physical examination findings include icterus, ascites, and

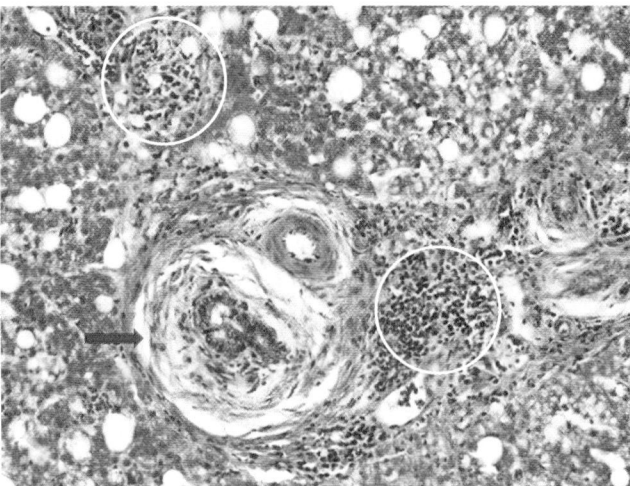

Figure 12-4: Tru-Cut biopsy core showing histologic inflammation of lymphocytic cholangitis in a cat. Note the two focal areas of lymphocytic infiltrates *(white circles)* and the onion skin fibrosis *(red arrow)* surrounding the bile duct. Hematoxylin and eosin (H&E) stain.

hepatomegaly. Signs of hepatic encephalopathy (dullness, ptyalism, and seizures) may develop with severe disease. Typical laboratory abnormalities include elevations in serum ALT, AST, and total bilirubin with hypergammaglobulinemia reported frequently. Abdominal radiography is useful in confirming free abdominal fluid and hepatomegaly. Ultrasonography demonstrates diffuse heterogeneous hepatic echogenicity with segmental dilatations in intrahepatic and extrahepatic bile ducts suggestive of obstructions. It also may aid in the recognition of concurrent disease.

Differentiation of Cholangitis Syndromes

Distinction among the different syndromes of NC and LC is difficult because they share many overlapping features of signalment, clinical presentation, physical examination findings, biochemistry abnormalities, and the potential to be associated with multi-organ inflammation involving the pancreas and/or alimentary tract. Ultimately, hepatic biopsy (methodology does matter; see later) is required for definitive diagnosis and may be aided by FISH for detection of *in situ* bacteria associated with NC. Differentiation between LC and well-differentiated lymphoma is difficult for even the best pathologist and, unfortunately, is not aided by the use of specialized immunohistochemical or molecular (polymerase chain reaction for antigen receptor rearrangement [PARR]) techniques.

Diagnosis of Cholangitis

Accurate diagnosis of the form of cholangitis present requires histopathologic examination of hepatic biopsy specimens coupled with the previously mentioned supportive clinical information. Liver biopsy specimens may be obtained by multiple methods, including laparotomy, laparoscopy, and ultrasound-guided (Tru-Cut needle) techniques. Although these different techniques may have their place in different

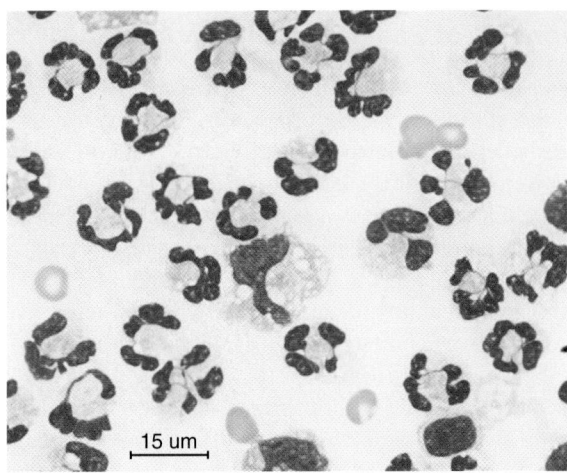

Figure 12-5: Bile collected via ultrasound-guided cholecystocentesis showing marked neutrophilic inflammation in the lumen of the gallbladder as viewed cytologically (using a Cytospin 4 Cytocentrifuge). (Image courtesy of Dr. Shannon Hostetter, DACVP, Iowa State University.)

clinical situations and with clients having varying financial constraints, surgical wedge liver biopsies provide the largest and most diagnostically accurate tissues.[17] Acquisition of forceps biopsy specimens using laparoscopy also provides quality specimens for diagnostic evaluation. Both laparotomy and laparoscopy allow for direct visualization of most hepatobiliary structures and sampling of extrahepatic tissues if needed. Laparotomy is the diagnostic procedure of choice in cats suspicious for EHBO. Although Tru-Cut needle biopsies may be obtained quickly using ultrasound guidance, it is noteworthy that the histopathology of needle biopsy specimens correlates with wedge biopsies in only 50% of cases.[18] Multiple hepatic lobes should always be biopsied, regardless of the biopsy method utilized, because inflammatory lesion severity may vary anatomically. Lastly, fine-needle aspiration (FNA) offers limited sensitivity for diagnosis of cholangitis with liver cytology correlating with biopsy results in only 39% to 60% of cases.[19]

Samples for aerobic and anaerobic bacteriologic culture should be obtained in all cats suspicious for cholangitis (Figure 12-5). Gallbladder bile is preferred over culture of hepatic tissues and may be safely obtained via ultrasound-guided percutaneous cholecystocentesis.[20] In one study of cats with cholangitis, bile cultures were more likely to detect pathogens (75% versus 33%) and less likely to yield contaminants (4% versus 29%) than liver cultures.[11] Moreover, bacterial culture was positive (predominantly *E. coli* and *Enterococcus* spp.) in 11 out of 23 (48%) samples and concurred with FISH in 15 out of 23 cases of cats with ILD.[8] These collective observations in different studies suggest that bacterial culture (and potentially FISH) have an essential role in the accurate diagnosis of bacterial infection in cats with cholangitis.

Treatment Strategies

Treatment of cholangitis is both specific and supportive. Note that treatment strategies for either form of cholangitis are largely empirical, and the optimal protocol is unknown. Antibiotics are the mainstay of therapy in cats with NC and are based on the results of bacterial culture/susceptibility testing. When bacterial culture is unavailable, an antibiotic is used that provides broad-spectrum activity against the most commonly isolated pathogens, including *E. coli*, *Enterococcus* spp., and Clostridia.[8,13,20] First-choice antibiotics include ampicillin/clavulanic acid or a fluoroquinolone with metronidazole for a minimum of 4 to 6 weeks. Clinical signs and serial hepatic enzymes are used to monitor treatment effects.

The primary treatment of cats with LC involves immunosuppressive drug therapy using prednisolone (1 to 2 mg/kg by mouth [PO] every 12 hours) for induction of remission, then slowly tapering over 6 to 8 weeks to the lowest effective dose.[13] It is also recommended to use antibiotics concurrently for 2 to 4 weeks given the possibility of bacterial infection complicating the effects of immunosuppressive therapy.[17] Clinical response and repeat hepatic enzyme concentrations will guide the duration of prednisolone therapy; however, some cats will require continuous drug therapy over 4 to 6 months, whereas others require lifelong therapy.

Other medications and nutritional supplements to consider for use with feline cholangitis are ursodeoxycholic acid (UDCA), S-adenosylmethionine (SAMe), milk thistle, and vitamin E.[13,17] Although the clinical benefit of any of these drugs has not been proven, their use is supported by numerous anecdotal reports. Ursodeoxycholic acid is a nontoxic hydrophilic bile acid that favors a beneficial bile acid milieu when administered.[13] This drug is reported to promote choleresis, reduce inflammation, and alter bile acid composition to less toxic concentrations. Antioxidants (SAMe and milk thistle) are of value in reducing oxidative damage to hepatocytes. Nutritional support for liver disease is crucial and best accomplished using enteral feeding methods. The authors recommend placement of an esophagostomy tube if the cat is stable enough for short-term general anesthesia; otherwise, a nasoesophageal feeding tube can be considered in debilitated cats.

Cats with EHBO are medical emergencies and may require surgical intervention to decompress the obstruction and flush the biliary system (See Chapter 16). Unfortunately, surgery in cats with EHBO is associated with considerable short-term mortality (36% to 57%) due to decreased vascular responsiveness and poor myocardial contractility.[12,21] Therefore, surgical diversion of the biliary system is only indicated as a last resort and when medical therapy alone offers little hope for survival.

Prognosis

The prognosis in cats with NC is generally good with one study reporting median survival times of 29.3 months with no difference found in survival times between ANC and CNC.[22] Some report that LC had a better response when treated with UDCA rather than with corticosteroids.[13] Cats having EHBO warrant a guarded-to-poor prognosis, which improves with time if they survive surgery to discharge from the hospital. Prognostic factors for cats with multi-organ inflammatory GI disease have not been identified.

FELINE PANCREATITIS

Feline pancreatitis has been recognized to occur more commonly than previously thought, which is mainly because the clinical signs associated with this disease are very vague and nonspecific.[24] This is particularly true for chronic pancreatitis and also for the more acute form of the disease. Cats with pancreatitis also commonly present with other diseases concurrently, such as idiopathic IBD of the small intestine, hepatic lipidosis, and cholangitis.[24] Furthermore, pancreatitis is often seen in cats with diabetes mellitus and can be a factor that contributes to deterioration of the disease or leads to the development of diabetic ketoacidosis.[7] Histologically, feline pancreatitis is categorized into acute necrotizing, acute suppurative, and chronic non-suppurative forms of the disease. The latter seems to be more common in cases that show less fulminant clinical signs and is characterized by a mononuclear cell infiltration and various degrees of fibrosis.

Evidence of Concurrent Inflammatory Liver or Intestinal Disease in Cats with Pancreatitis

Few studies have investigated cats with pancreatitis for any concurrent diseases.[3,4,7] There seems to be more evidence for cats with pancreatitis to have concurrent cholangitis than IBD. In one postmortem study identifying pancreatitis, 92% of 62 cats also had LC, hepatic lipidosis, or diabetes mellitus.[4] However, this study only looked at histology of the pancreas at postmortem, and few of the cats in the study actually showed clinical signs attributable to pancreatitis before death. Another early study looked at 40 cats with acute pancreatitis and showed that they frequently had elevations in ALT, ALP, bilirubin, and cholesterol.[5] However, in this study, there were only mild changes detectable on histology of the liver or small intestine, which would not strongly support the presence of triaditis.[5] Evidence for triaditis as defined by significant concurrent inflammation of the pancreas, small intestine, and liver has been documented in several published studies.[3,6] The evidence is relatively strong for a link of pancreatitis and cholangitis: Two studies report that 50%[2] or 65% of cats,[3] respectively, with cholangitis had concurrent histologic evidence of pancreatic inflammation. There is growing substantial evidence that there could be a link between possible bacterial infection of the liver and pancreas, as two studies elegantly showed that bacterial DNA can be found in the liver of up to 33% of cats with cholangitis and up to a third of pancreata of cats with clinically moderate to severe pancreatitis.[8] These studies used FISH to detect bacterial DNA; and therefore, caution must be exercised to extrapolate this finding to an actual bacterial infection of the liver or pancreas. However, it is intriguing to think that an ascending infection from the duodenum could lead to pancreatitis and cholangitis in at least some cats with clinical signs attributable to multi-organ inflammation (i.e., triaditis).

Diagnosis of Pancreatitis in Cats

The diagnosis of pancreatitis in cats is hampered by the fact that the clinical signs are often nonspecific. In one study, anorexia, lethargy, diarrhea, icterus, and an abdominal mass effect were the most common clinical findings. Therefore, the classic clinical signs seen in many dogs with acute pancreatitis, such as vomiting and abdominal pain, may not be appreciated in cats. Chemistry profile and complete blood count (CBC) are also of little diagnostic use, although some studies report that hypercholesterolemia can be found in up to 72% of cats with pancreatitis.[5,9,10] Amylase and lipase are too unspecific for the diagnosis of pancreatitis in cats and are not recommended. Hypocalcemia can be found in up to 65% of pancreatitis cases[4,9] and has been associated with a worse prognosis.[11] Abdominal ultrasound is routinely performed in cats with signs of possible pancreatitis and serves to identify acute pancreatitis as much as eliminating other causes of vague GI signs. If ultrasonographic signs of pancreatitis are found (e.g., an enlarged, hypoechoic or hyperechoic pancreas) surrounded by hyperechoic mesentery, this will be highly specific for acute pancreatitis[12] (Figure 12-6). However, the sensitivity of abdominal ultrasound is affected by the chronicity of the disease—the more chronic the pancreatitis, the less likely it is to be able to detect ultrasonographic changes. Consequently, the sensitivity of the test has been reported to vary from 24% to 67%.[13]

Assays for feline pancreatic lipase immunoreactivity (fPLI) have become widely available. It is produced only in the exocrine pancreas, and therefore has the potential to be a highly specific test. Only one published study to date has evaluated the sensitivity and specificity of this test in feline pancreatitis cases. The sensitivity for fPLI in moderate to severe histologic pancreatitis was 100%, but it dropped to 54% in mild pancreatitis cases.[15] This finding highlights an important aspect of accuracy testing for fPLI, because the

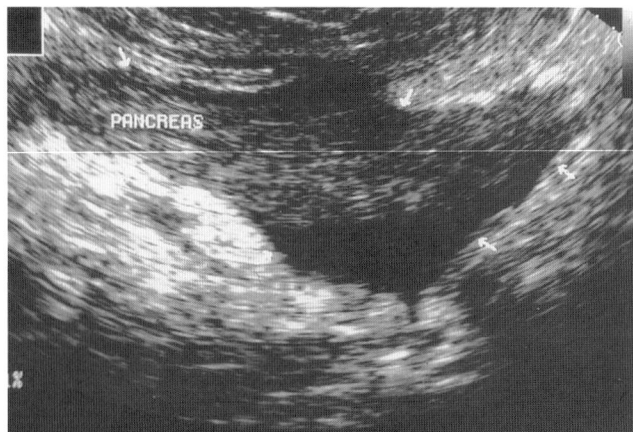

Figure 12-6: Ultrasonographic image of acute pancreatitis in a cat. Note the hypoechoic pancreatic parenchyma surrounded by the hyperechoic mesentery, which is highly specific for acute pancreatic inflammation. (Image courtesy of Dr. Kristina Miles, DACVR, Iowa State University.)

gold standard used in most studies is histological evidence of pancreatitis, which may or may not translate into clinical signs of pancreatitis in the cats. It also points to the fact that the more chronic the pancreatitis is, the less leakage of fPLI is expected, and therefore the sensitivity of the test drops to levels that are clinically useless. In a follow-up study from the same group, 182 cats were included, reporting a sensitivity of 79% and a specificity of 100% for detecting pancreatitis in cats that presented with clinical signs suspicious of pancreatitis.[16] Moreover, fPLI does not seem to be affected by prerenal azotemia and can, therefore, be helpful in the assessment of cats with dehydration or shock that present with signs attributable to possible pancreatitis.[17] In another study, it was also reported that the magnitude of fPLI concentration is correlated with negative outcome in cats with acute pancreatitis.[18]

Treatment of Acute Pancreatitis

Because most cases of acute pancreatitis in cats are idiopathic, supportive treatment is the main means of treatment. Fluid therapy should be initiated without delay and has been shown in human cases to improve microcirculation of the pancreas and to improve outcome.[19] Supportive treatment should include considering colloid or plasma transfusion in case of hypoalbuminemia; however, no studies have been done to show any efficacy for this. Analgesia is another very important aspect of treatment of acute pancreatitis. Buprenorphine or butorphanol have good efficacy, and some cats are visibly a lot more comfortable after having been given analgesia. The authors also have had good success with transdermal fentanyl patches in cats with acute pancreatitis. Furthermore, antiemetics are given to counteract vomiting and nausea, and they are important measures while trying to feed the cats enterally as well. Maropitant citrate (Cerenia) at 1 mg/kg once daily PO or subcutaneously is very effective and is used commonly in the authors' practice. Enteral feeding should be initiated early on in these cats and can be achieved through naso-esophageal tubes or esophageal tubes. It is important to note that it is not necessary to insist on a low-fat diet in cats with pancreatitis; therefore higher calorie diets that can be fed through the tube are acceptable.

Treatment of Chronic Pancreatitis

The treatment of chronic pancreatitis is not straightforward; because many times, there may not be obvious clinical signs, and sometimes the only indication of chronic pancreatitis is an elevated fPLI in a cat with vague GI signs. Serum cobalamin concentrations should always be measured in such cases as well and, if found to be low, should be supplemented. Low cobalamin concentrations can be a sign of pancreatic exocrine disease (because extrinsic factor is produced in the pancreas in cats) and/or indicative of ileal disease, such as IBD or lymphoma. In some cats with chronic relapsing pancreatitis, the exocrine pancreas can get exhausted over time, resulting in clinical signs of exocrine pancreatic insufficiency. Even before obvious clinical signs develop, it is prudent to assess exocrine pancreatic function by measuring fTLI and, if necessary, supplementing pancreatic enzymes as well as cobalamin. Corticosteroids have long been assumed to be contraindicated in pancreatitis; however, current thoughts about the pathogenesis of chronic pancreatitis suggest that there could be a degree of autoimmune inflammation involved, as has been seen in dogs and humans alike. Based on this assumption, the authors have treated several cases of chronic pancreatitis with anti-inflammatory doses of steroids (1 mg/kg PO of prednisolone every 24 hours) for several weeks, with good success of decreasing signs of vague GI upset and decreasing fPLI concentration after treatment. Care must be taken if there is the possibility of subclinical *Toxoplasma* infection in cats, which can flare up when treatment with prednisolone is initiated. In cases where there is evidence or suspicion of concurrent IBD, prednisolone is initiated at an immune-suppressive dose (2 mg/kg PO once a day for 2 weeks) and then tapered slowly over several weeks.

IDIOPATHIC INFLAMMATORY BOWEL DISEASE

Inflammatory bowel disease in cats is an exclusion diagnosis and comprises a phenotype of chronic GI disease, mainly diarrhea, vomiting, and weight loss, with histological evidence of lymphoplasmacytic inflammation in the small and/or large intestine. Other causes of chronic GI signs need to be excluded before the diagnosis of idiopathic IBD is made. Similar to people and dogs, the pathogenesis of IBD in cats is thought to involve the intestinal microbiome, dietary antigens, and the intestinal immune system. The primary cytokine profile that has been identified from biopsies of cats with IBD is of a predominant type 1 helper T cell (Th1)-type, with cytokines such as interleukin (IL)-1, IL-8, and IL-12 elevated when compared with biopsies from healthy cats.[20] A recent publication also suggests the possibility of some IL-17 cytokine messenger ribonucleic acid (mRNA) levels being elevated in biopsies from cats with IBD.[21] This finding still needs to be confirmed at the protein level and does not seem to fit with the histological phenotype of lymphoplasmacellular infiltration, because IL-17 cytokines are normally found to be locally increased in diseases with granulocytic infiltration, such as human Crohn's disease. However, there is clear evidence that the microbiome plays an important role in the development of IBD in cats. One study showed a direct correlation of the numbers of mucosa-associated *Enterobacteriaceae*, as well as *E. coli* and *Clostridium* species, with the amount of Th1-type cytokines found in the same biopsies, as well as clinical severity and histological changes.[20] Importantly, there is growing evidence that relying solely on the number of infiltrating lymphocytes and plasma cells in the lamina propria of cats with IBD may not be as helpful as more subtle, architectural changes of the mucosa for the diagnosis and severity grading of the disease.[20,22]

Evidence for Concurrent Liver or Pancreatic Inflammatory Disease in Cats with Inflammatory Bowel Disease

The evidence of proven concurrent diseases in cats with IBD is sparse. One necropsy study looking at 78 cats with cholangitis identified 83% of cats in that population that also had IBD, and 50% that also had evidence of pancreatitis.[2] In 39% of cats, all three diagnoses were made, making the case for possible triaditis. A study looking at cobalamin serum concentrations in 80 cats with vague GI signs identified 49 cats with cobalamin values below the reference range, with many of these having histological evidence of pancreatitis and cholangitis, as well as IBD.[23] In another study, 23 cats diagnosed with IBD were evaluated for serum fPLI concentrations, regardless of whether there was any clinical suspicion for pancreatitis or not.[25] In this study, 16 out of 23 cats had elevated fPLI. This correlated with hypoalbuminemia and hypocobalaminemia in the same cats; however, the outcome was not affected by fPLI. This study indicates that cats with IBD could have concurrent pancreatitis, although biopsies of the pancreata were not performed in this study.

Diagnosis of Inflammatory Bowel Disease in Cats

Because IBD is an exclusion diagnosis, the usual workup consists of a fecal examination for worms and giardia, blood work (including CBC and biochemistry profile), urinalysis, and abdominal ultrasound examination. In addition, it may be indicated to test for the presence of *Tritrichomonas* in the feces, especially if signs of large bowel diarrhea are predominant and are associated with minimal clinical signs otherwise. Other blood tests to consider are a total thyroxine (T4) and possibly a fTLI; the latter mainly if there are clinical signs suggestive of exocrine pancreatic insufficiency. In addition, many clinicians evaluate serum cobalamin and folate. Low cobalamin could give an indication of diffuse small intestinal, ileal, and/or exocrine pancreatic disease, and a low folate can be seen with either diffuse or proximal small intestinal disease. fPLI can be useful to assess for additional pancreatic inflammation as well and has been shown to be elevated in 70% of cats with IBD in one study.[25] When these tests have been performed and point toward the possibility of a diffuse intestinal disease that is likely to affect the duodenum, ileum, and/or colon, then endoscopy is indicated as a next step. It is important to recognize that many cats with either IBD or intestinal lymphoma will have the ileum affected, so sampling from this site is imperative to make a diagnosis in many cases.[26] There is increasing awareness that intestinal small cell lymphoma in cats can clinically mimic moderate to severe IBD and that tests up to the point of biopsy sampling can yield the exact same results. In some cases, mesenteric lymph nodes will be enlarged and can be sampled by FNA, which can sometimes help in the differentiation of the two diseases. In one study, it was shown that the muscularis propria layer of the mucosa can be thickened and identified by abdominal ultrasound, which can be indicative of small cell lymphoma.[27]

Additional tools to help differentiate between small cell lymphoma and IBD are immunohistochemistry for B and T cells (small cell lymphoma are mostly of T-cell type), and PARR[28] (Figure 12-7). Both of these tests should only be used in conjunction with the aforementioned tests and appropriate clinical signs to diagnose the disease. Finally, it may be of little clinical relevance to make this distinction anyway, as both severe IBD and intestinal small cell lymphoma respond reasonably well to immunosuppressive treatments and are associated with a fairly good prognosis.[29] In most cases, histology for IBD shows a variable degree of infiltration with lymphocytes and plasma cells into the lamina propria, as well as mucosal architectural changes, such as villous atrophy and villous fusion (Figure 12-8). These latter changes

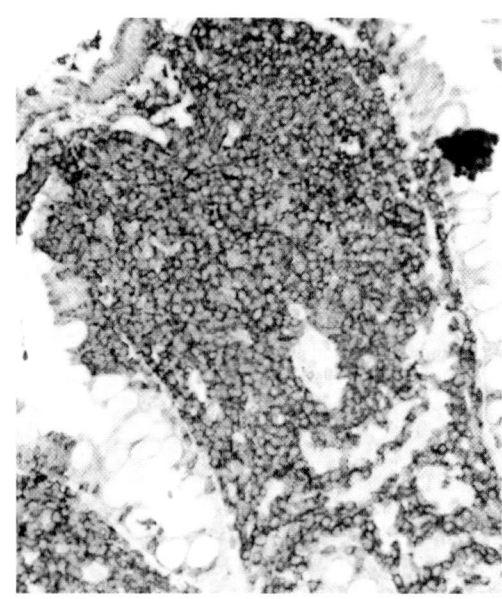

Figure 12-7: Endoscopic ileal biopsy in a cat with chronic diarrhea and weight loss. Immunophenotyping using a CD3+ T-cell antibody shows that more than 95% of the mucosal cellular infiltrates are CD3+ positive lymphocytes. This histopathologic observation is consistent with a diagnosis of feline alimentary lymphoma.

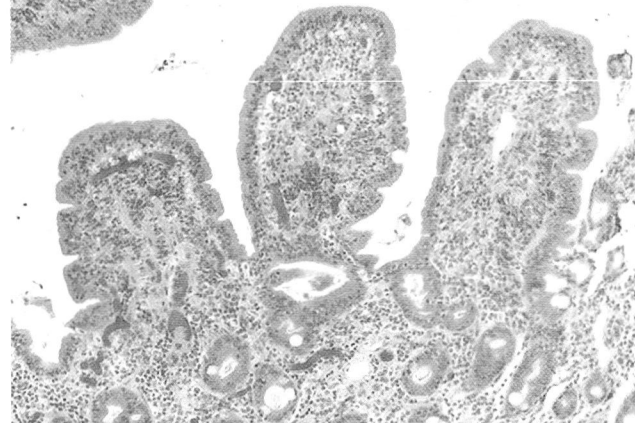

Figure 12-8: Endoscopic duodenal biopsy showing moderate feline lymphocytic-plasmacytic enteritis. Note cellular infiltrates within the lamina propria accompanied by increased numbers of intraepithelial lymphocytes and villus atrophy.

seem to be more important than the inflammatory infiltrate with regards to the severity of disease, as one publication showed.[20]

Treatment of Inflammatory Bowel Disease in Cats

The treatment of IBD in cats should follow a sequential approach. The first treatment to try is an elimination diet or hydrolyzed diet, given exclusively for at least 7 days. It has been shown that up to 50% of cats with IBD respond very quickly, within several days, to this treatment. Hydrolyzed diets seem to work as well as elimination diets,[30] although no direct comparisons of these approaches have been published.

If the cat will not respond to a dietary trial, then corticosteroids at immunosuppressive doses (2 mg/kg PO for 2 weeks, then slow tapering doses over several weeks) are indicated, either alone or in combination with tylosin or metronidazole.[31,32] In cats with incomplete or no response within 2 weeks of starting corticosteroid treatment, chlorambucil can be added in at a dosage of 2 mg/kg PO every 24 to 72 hours or 2 mg/m² every 14 days. A CBC should be performed every 3 to 4 weeks to monitor for myelosuppression; however, this has only rarely been reported in cats. The treatment approach for cats diagnosed with small cell lymphoma is the same as for severe IBD (i.e., a combination protocol of prednisolone and chlorambucil, which has been associated with prolonged survival times).[29]

References

1. Zawie DA, Garvey MC: Feline hepatic disease. *Vet Clin North Am* 2:1201–1230, 1984.
2. Weiss DJ, Gagne JM, Armstrong PJ: Relationship between inflammatory hepatic disease and inflammatory bowel disease, pancreatitis, and nephritis in cats. *J Am Vet Med Assoc* 209:1114–1116, 1996.
3. Callahan Clark JE, Haddad JL, Brown DC, et al: Feline cholangitis: a necropsy study of 44 cats (1986-2008). *J Feline Med Surg* 13:570–576, 2011.
4. Ferreri JA, Hardam E, Kimmel SE, et al: Clinical differentiation of acute necrotizing from chronic nonsuppurative pancreatitis in cats: 63 cases (1996-2001). *J Am Vet Med Assoc* 223:469–474, 2003.
5. Hill RC, Van Winkle TJ: Acute necrotizing pancreatitis and acute suppurative pancreatitis in the cat: A retrospective study of 40 cases (1976-1989). *J Vet Intern Med* 7:25–33, 1993.
6. Marolf AJ, Kraft SL, Dunphy TR, et al: Magnetic resonance (MR) imaging and MR cholangiopancreatography findings in cats with cholangitis and pancreatitis. *J Feline Med Surg* 15:285–294, 2013.
7. Akol KG, Washabau RJ, Saunders HM, et al: Acute pancreatitis in cats with hepatic lipidosis. *J Vet Intern Med* 7:205–209, 1993.
8. Warren A, Center S, McDonough S, et al: Histopathologic features, immunophenotyping, clonality, and eubacterial fluorescence *in situ* hybridization in cats with lymphocytic cholangitis/cholangiohepatitis. *Vet Pathol* 48:627–641, 2011.
9. Swift NC, Marks SL, MacLachlan NJ, et al: Evaluation of serum feline trypsin-like immunoreactivity for the diagnosis of pancreatitis in cats. *J Am Vet Med Assoc* 217:37–42, 2000.
10. Gerhardt A, Steiner JM, Williams DA, et al: Comparison of the sensitivity of different diagnostic tests for pancreatitis in cats. *J Vet Intern Med* 15:329–333, 2001.
11. Kimmel SE, Washabau RJ, Drobatz KJ: Incidence and prognostic value of low plasma ionized calcium concentration in cats with acute pancreatitis: 46 cases (1996-1998). *J Am Vet Med Assoc* 219:1105–1109, 2001.
12. Williams JM, Panciera DL, Larson MM, et al: Ultrasonographic findings of the pancreas in cats with elevated serum pancreatic lipase immunoreactivity. *J Vet Intern Med* 27:913–918, 2013.
13. Saunders HM, VanWinkle TJ, Drobatz K, et al: Ultrasonographic findings in cats with clinical, gross pathologic, and histologic evidence of acute pancreatic necrosis: 20 cases (1994-2001). *J Am Vet Med Assoc* 221:1724–1730, 2002.
14. Twedt DC, Armstrong PJ, Simpson KW: Feline cholangitis. In Bonagura JD, Twedt DC, editors: *Kirk's current veterinary therapy XV*, St Louis, 2014, Elsevier/Saunders.
15. Forman MA, Marks SL, De Cock HE, et al: Evaluation of serum feline pancreatic lipase immunoreactivity and helical computed tomography versus conventional testing for the diagnosis of feline pancreatitis. *J Vet Intern Med* 18:807–815, 2004.
16. Forman MA, Shiroma J, Armstrong PJ, et al: Evaluation of feline pancreas-specific lipase (spec-fPL) for the diagnosis of feline pancreatitis. *J Vet Intern Med* 23:2009. (ACVIM Abstract #250).
17. Jaensch S: The effect of naturally occurring renal insufficiency on serum pancreatic-specific lipase in cats. *Comp Clin Pathol* 22:801–803, 2014.
18. Stockhaus C, Teske E, Schellenberger K, et al: Serial serum feline pancreatic lipase immunoreactivity concentrations and prognostic variables in 33 cats with pancreatitis. *J Am Vet Med Assoc* 243:1713–1718, 2013.
19. Warndorf MG, Kurtzman JT, Bartel MJ, et al: Early fluid resuscitation reduces morbidity among patients with acute pancreatitis. *Clin Gastroenterol Hepatol* 9:705–709, 2011.
20. Janeczko S, Atwater D, Bogel E, et al: The relationship of mucosal bacteria to duodenal histopathology, cytokine mRNA, and clinical disease activity in cats with inflammatory bowel disease. *Vet Microbiol* 128:178–193, 2008.
21. Waly NE, Peters IR, Day MJ, et al: Measurement of IL-12 (p40, p35), IL-23p19, and IFN-gamma mRNA in duodenal biopsies of cats with inflammatory enteropathy. *J Vet Intern Med* 28:42–47, 2014.
22. Washabau RJ, Day MJ, Willard MD, et al: Endoscopic, biopsy, and histopathologic guidelines for the evaluation of gastrointestinal inflammation in companion animals. *J Vet Intern Med* 24:10–26, 2010.
23. Simpson KW, Fyfe J, Cornetta A, et al: Subnormal concentrations of serum cobalamin (vitamin B₁₂) in cats with gastrointestinal disease. *J Vet Intern Med* 15:26–32, 2001.
24. Gagne JM, Weiss DJ, Armstrong PJ: Histopathologic evaluation of feline inflammatory liver disease. *Vet Pathol* 33:521–526, 1996.
25. Bailey S, Benigni L, Eastwood J, et al: Comparisons between cats with normal and increased fPLI concentrations in cats diagnosed with inflammatory bowel disease. *J Small Anim Pract* 51:484–489, 2010.
26. Scott KD, Zoran DL, Mansell J, et al: Utility of endoscopic biopsies of the duodenum and ileum for diagnosis of inflammatory bowel disease and small cell lymphoma in cats. *J Vet Intern Med* 25:1253–1257, 2011.
27. Zwingenberger AL, Marks SL, Baker TW, et al: Ultrasonographic evaluation of the muscularis propria in cats with diffuse small intestinal lymphoma or inflammatory bowel disease. *J Vet Intern Med* 24:289–292, 2010.
28. Moore PF, Woo JC, Vernau W, et al: Characterization of feline T cell receptor gamma (TCRG) variable region genes for the molecular diagnosis of feline intestinal T cell lymphoma. *Vet Immunol Immunopathol* 106:167–178, 2005.
29. Stein TJ, Pellin M, Steinberg H, et al: Treatment of feline gastrointestinal small-cell lymphoma with chlorambucil and glucocorticoids. *J Am Anim Hosp Assoc* 46:413–417, 2010.
30. Mandigers PJ, Biourge V, German AJ: Efficacy of a commercial hydrolysate diet in eight cats suffering from inflammatory bowel disease or adverse reaction to food. *Tijdschr Diergeneeskd* 135:668–672, 2010.
31. Dennis JS, Kruger JM, Mullaney TP: Lymphocytic/plasmacytic colitis in cats: 14 cases (1985-1990). *J Am Vet Med Assoc* 202:313–318, 1993.
32. Jergens AE, Crandell JM, Evans R, et al: A clinical index for disease activity in cats with chronic enteropathy. *J Vet Intern Med* 24:1027–1033, 2010.

Update on Oral Inflammation in the Cat

Maria Soltero-Rivera and Alexander M. Reiter

Oral inflammation can have various presentations depending on the etiology, progressiveness, extent, and location. It can be acute, chronic, or acute-on-chronic. Lesions can be localized, multifocal, or generalized. The margins of the lesions can be well-defined or ill-defined. Additionally, the inflammation can be centered over teeth, or it can be in edentulous areas. Oftentimes the duration of clinical signs along with the distribution of the lesions can aid in determining the etiology of the condition. The location of the lesions in the oral cavity is also important, because certain diseases preferentially target specific structures (Table 13-1).

Histologically, oral inflammation can range in appearance from an ulcerated area to a bullous lesion to proliferation of tissues (through hyperplasia or granulation tissue formation) to areas of necrosis. The main differential diagnoses for oral inflammation include gingivitis, periodontitis, gingivostomatitis, neoplasia, eosinophilic granuloma, foreign body reaction, immune-mediated and autoimmune disease, metabolic disease, and burn injury (i.e., chemical, electric, or thermal). It is important to keep in mind that some of these conditions may be a manifestation of systemic disease. Also, some systemic diseases (such as those that cause immunosuppression) can predispose patients to any form of oral inflammation. It is extremely important to obtain a detailed medical history from cat owners when evaluating each individual case.

This chapter discusses the epidemiology, pathology/pathogenesis, clinical presentation, diagnostic evaluation, treatment options, chronic management, and prognosis of these diseases.

HEALTHY ORAL TISSUES

The factors that play a major role in protecting the oral cavity from insults include the oral epithelium, taste buds, salivary secretions, gingival crevicular fluid, resident microbiota, and the initial inflammatory response by the host.

Masticatory mucosa and lining mucosa are the tissues primarily affected by oral inflammation. The epithelium of masticatory mucosa is moderately thick and frequently orthokeratinized. It is inextensible and well adapted to withstanding abrasion. The epithelium of lining mucosa is thicker than that of masticatory mucosa and is non-keratinized. The surface is flexible, and the submucosa is elastic, allowing it to stretch.[1] Taste buds protect the mucosa via rejection of

potentially toxic materials.[2] Saliva has a diluting and neutralizing function in addition to antimicrobial effects through enzymes and immunoglobulins.[1] The gingival crevicular fluid is believed to cleanse the gingival sulcus, improve adhesion of the epithelium to the tooth via plasma proteins, possess antimicrobial properties, and exert antibody activity to protect the gingiva.[3] The normal bacterial flora of the oral cavity plays a role in innate immunity by preventing colonization and growth of potential pathogens.

The lamina propria contains several different cell types, including macrophages, fibroblasts, mast cells, and inflammatory cells. Inflammatory cells are for the most part found in significant numbers in connective tissue. When these are present as a result of injury or as part of a disease process, the overlying epithelium is affected via cytokine release. As in other parts of the body, the type of inflammatory cell infiltrate depends on disease etiology and duration.[1]

When further characterizing the leukocyte subsets present in the oral mucosa of healthy cats, the normal feline oral mucosa clearly contains a range of immune cell populations. CD3+ intraepithelial lymphocytes and CD8+ T cells are more common than CD4+ T cells. Cells with a characteristic dendritic morphology are present in the intraepithelial and subepithelial compartments. At times, these are associated with clusters of CD3+ T cells comprised of both CD8+ and CD4+ T cells. Mast cells are most commonly found in the lamina propria and submucosal compartments. In these compartments, CD3+ T cells are also observed, and there are similar numbers of CD4+ and CD8+ cells. The few plasma cells that are present are generally either immunoglobulin (Ig) G+ or IgA+ in their immunophenotype.[4]

GINGIVITIS AND PERIODONTITIS

Periodontal disease involves inflammation of the gingiva, periodontal ligament, cementum, and alveolar bone.[5] Ninety-six percent of 109 cats with a mean age of 6.2 ± 5.2 years showed evidence of gingival inflammation in one study[6] (Figure 13-1). Gingivitis may remain stable throughout the life of the animal. However, with the aid of additional factors, it may progress to periodontitis. Periodontitis is inflammation of the periodontal ligament, cementum, and alveolar bone, resulting in pocket formation, gingival recession, and alveolar bone loss (Figure 13-2). A recent study demonstrated

Table 13-1	Nomenclature of Oral and Oropharyngeal Inflammation According to the American Veterinary Dental College	
Location	**Term**	**Definition**
Gingiva	Gingivitis	Inflammation of gingiva
Periodontal ligament, alveolar bone, and cementum	Periodontitis	Inflammation of nongingival periodontal tissues
Bone and bone marrow	Osteomyelitis	Inflammation of the bone and bone marrow
Alveolar mucosa	Alveolar mucositis	Inflammation of alveolar mucosa (i.e., mucosa overlying the alveolar process and extending from the mucogingival junction without obvious demarcation to the vestibular sulcus and to the floor of the mouth)
Sublingual mucosa	Sublingual mucositis	Inflammation of mucosa on the floor of the mouth
Labial/buccal mucosa	Labial/buccal mucositis	Inflammation of the lip/cheek mucosa
Mucosa of the caudal oral cavity	Caudal mucositis	Inflammation of mucosa of the caudal oral cavity, bordered medially by the palatoglossal folds and fauces, dorsally by the hard and soft palate, and rostrally by alveolar and buccal mucosa
Palatal mucosa	Palatitis	Inflammation of mucosa covering the hard and/or soft palate
Lingual mucosa	Glossitis	Inflammation of mucosa of the dorsal, lateral, and/or ventral tongue surface
Lip	Cheilitis	Inflammation of the lip (including the mucocutaneous junction area and skin of the lip)
Mouth	Stomatitis	Inflammation of the mucous lining of any of the structures in the mouth; in clinical use, the term should be reserved to describe widespread oral inflammation (beyond gingivitis and periodontitis) that may also extend into submucosal tissues (e.g., marked caudal mucositis extending into submucosal tissues may be termed caudal stomatitis)
Palatine tonsil	Tonsillitis	Inflammation of the palatine tonsil
Pharynx	Pharyngitis	Inflammation of the pharynx

Data from AVDC Nomenclature Committee; American Veterinary Dental College. (2012, May 1). Retrieved July 1, 2015, from http://www.avdc.org/nomenclature.html.

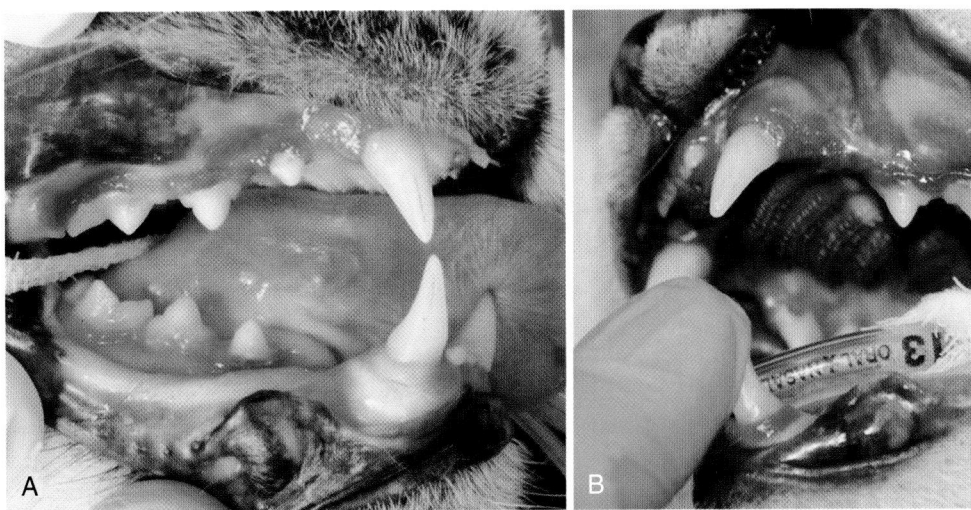

Figure 13-1: Photographs of a 2-year-old Maine Coon **(A)** and 7-year-old domestic shorthair **(B)**, showing gingivitis, early gingival recession, and alveolar mucositis. (Copyright 2014 Alexander M. Reiter; used with permission.)

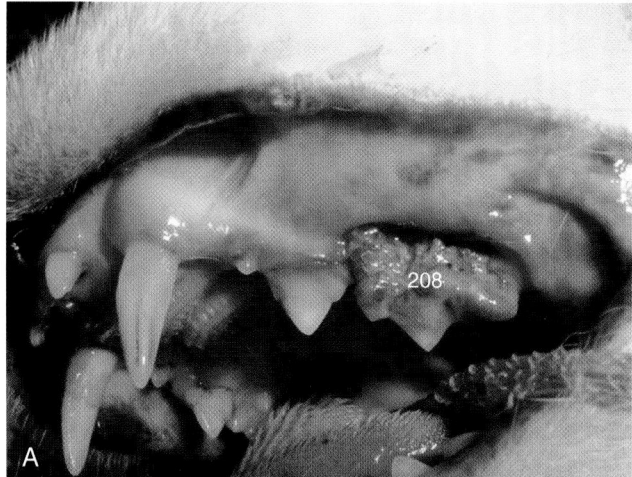

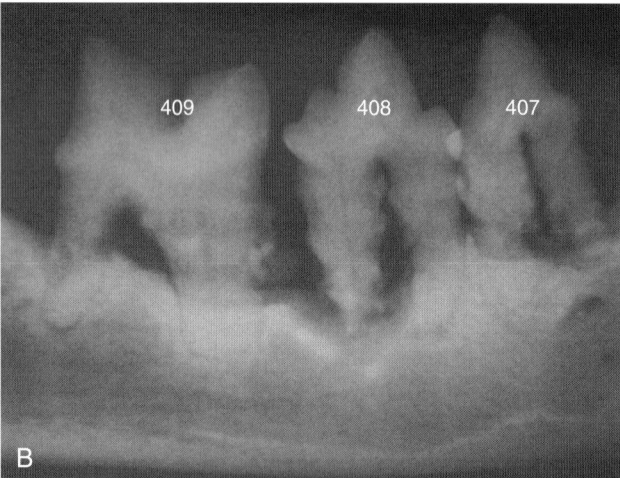

Figure 13-2: Photographs showing localized severe periodontitis at the left maxillary fourth premolar (tooth #*208*) in an 8-year-old domestic shorthair **(A)** and generalized severe periodontitis of the right mandibular third and fourth premolars and first molar (teeth #*407, 408,* and *409*) in a 13-year-old domestic shorthair **(B)**. (Copyright 2014 Alexander M. Reiter; used with permission.)

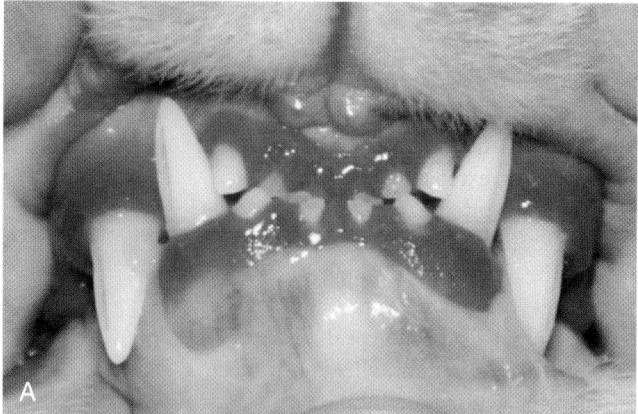

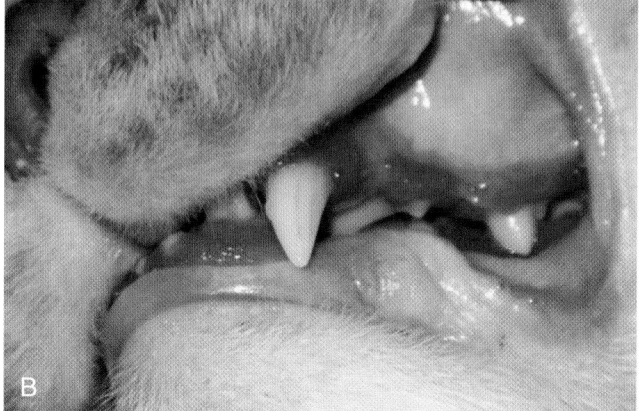

Figure 13-3: Front **(A)** and side **(B)** views of the mouth (lips retracted) of a 6½-month-old Maine Coon with juvenile hyperplastic gingivitis. (Copyright 2014 Alexander M. Reiter; used with permission.)

that 13% of cats suffering from periodontal disease also had evidence of aggressive periodontitis.[6] That same study also found a strong association between periodontal disease and type I tooth resorption. This is similar to another study where 72% of teeth with type I resorption also showed periodontitis as opposed to only 15.6% in teeth with type II resorption.[7]

A strong suspicion for a genetic predisposition exists in cats. Purebred cats are said to develop dental calculus more commonly than domestic cats.[8] Additionally, rapidly progressing and refractory periodontitis have been reported to occur more commonly in young Somali and Abyssinian cats exhibiting gingivostomatitis or with feline immunodeficiency virus (FIV) infection.[9] In humans, periodontitis has been associated with abnormal phagocytic activity as well as immunosuppressive states.[10] Hypoplasia of root cementum has also been implicated as a cause specifically in human cases of juvenile periodontitis.[11] A condition known as *juvenile hyperplastic gingivitis* has been described as occurring in cats

younger than 1 to 2 years of age (Figure 13-3). Periodic professional dental cleanings, careful gingivectomy and gingivoplasty, extraction of teeth with severe attachment loss, and rigorous home oral hygiene are recommended until patients outgrow the potential causes of this disease.[12]

Amoxicillin/clavulanic acid had the highest *in vitro* susceptibility against all isolates and all anaerobes isolated from the subgingival spaces of cats with gingivitis. Additionally, enrofloxacin showed the highest *in vitro* susceptibility for the anaerobes isolated.[13] In cases where professional dental cleaning and extraction of severely affected teeth do not resolve periodontal inflammation, patients should be tested for feline leukemia virus (FeLV) and FIV infection. A greater prevalence and increased severity of oral inflammation was noted in cats infected with FIV. The disease was worse in those with FIV and feline calicivirus (FCV) coinfection, or with FCV and FeLV coinfection.[14]

In dogs, increasing severity of attachment loss was associated with changes in systemic inflammatory variables and renal indices.[15] In cats, the severity of periodontitis has been associated with increases in globulins, alanine aminotransferase, and IgG blood levels, suggesting that periodontal disease is not simply a localized disease but may also evoke systemic host responses.[16]

STOMATITIS

Stomatitis is a complex, chronic, and destructive inflammatory process affecting the epithelium and lamina propria, with frequent extension into the submucosal tissues.[17] This more widespread inflammation of the oral mucosa is estimated to affect 0.7% of cats presented to veterinary practices.[18] The etiology of stomatitis is not fully understood; however, it is suspected to be multifactorial. This is in contrast to the stomatitis or mucosal ulceration that results from contact with an irritant, allergen, or antigen, most often in areas of a heavy plaque burden. This condition is known as *chronic ulcerative paradental stomatitis.* However, the lesions are commonly referred to as "kissing ulcers" or "contact ulcers." A similar type of lesion that is proliferative rather than ulcerative in nature develops in the alveolar or buccal mucosa distobuccal to the mandibular first molar tooth in cats (Figure 13-4). The lesions may result from continued trauma secondary to a tight caudal occlusion between the maxillary fourth premolar and the mandibular first molar, or due to continued trauma from the maxillary fourth premolar on an area of inflammation on the distobuccal aspect of the mandibular first molar. Surgical excision of the mass and blunting or extraction of the involved tooth or teeth has been reported to be 100% effective.[19]

Some of the common bacterial isolates in cats with stomatitis include *Pasteurella pneumotropica, Pasteurella multocida,* and *Capnocytophaga canimorsus.*[20] Prior exposure to viral diseases such as FCV, feline herpesvirus (FHV), FeLV, and FIV is thought to be a risk factor for developing stomatitis.[21] This is likely due to the progressive decline in immune function caused by infection with FIV and FeLV.[8,22] On the other hand, FCV does seem to play a more direct role, as shown by persistent shedding of this virus in all cats with chronic

ulceroproliferative stomatitis as compared to only 20% in normal cats.[23] Ulcers on the tongue, philtrum, and palate can be seen in cases of FHV. However, they are infrequent compared to FCV infection.[8] Infection with FIV, FeLV, and FCV may also influence disease severity.[8] The role of infection with *Bartonella* remains controversial.[24] Infection with feline panleukopenia virus, feline syncytium-forming virus, feline infectious peritonitis, and/or *Candida albicans* have also been implicated as causes of stomatitis.[25,26] During inflammation, the number of CD79a[+] cells, leukocyte antigen 1 (L1)[+] cells, and CD3[+] T cells and the level of major histocompatibility complex (MHC) class II expression tend to correlate with disease severity.[17] Additionally, CD8[+] T cells are more numerous than CD4[+] T cells, and the majority of plasma cells are of the IgG isotype. When compared to oral mucosal samples from healthy cats, the number of cells labeled for CD3, CD4, CD8, CD79a, IgG, IgA, or L1 and the number of mast cells within the lamina propria and submucosa of cats with oral inflammation significantly increase. The epithelial compartment in these cats also has more CD3[+] T cells compared to healthy cats. Mast cell density is also significantly increased in gingival tissues adjacent to areas affected by stomatitis.[27]

Affected animals often show signs of oral discomfort when eating, grooming, or manipulating their mouths. In addition to the often symmetric, bright, ulcerated or proliferative lesions of the gingiva, alveolar mucosa, buccal mucosa (Figure 13-5), and/or the area lateral to the palatoglossal folds (Figure 13-6), physical examination findings may include a poor hair coat and decreased body condition. In some cases, the lateral margins of the tongue and the areas of the hard palate that are in contact with the teeth may also be involved. Of cats with stomatitis, 59% to 61% show radiographic evidence of resorption of multiple teeth,[28] and differentiation into squamous cell carcinoma (SCC) has been reported in some cats.[29,30]

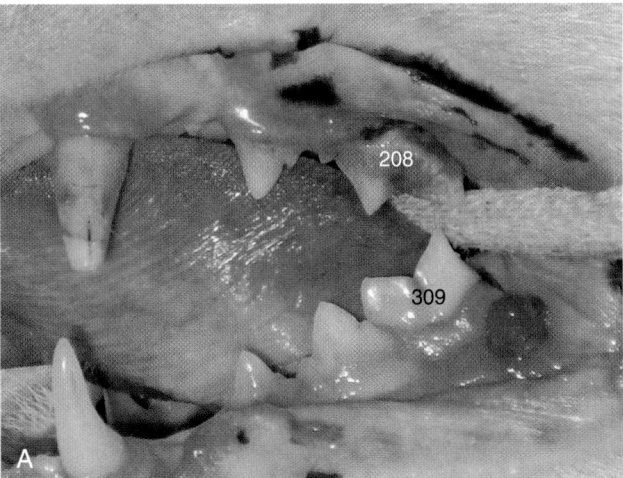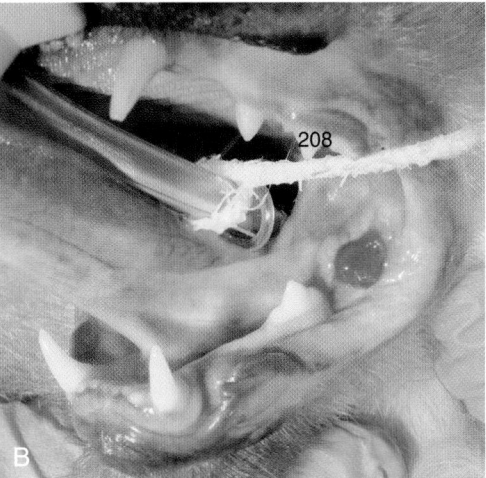

Figure 13-4: A, Photograph of an 8-year-old domestic shorthair with pyogenic granuloma in alveolar and buccal mucosa at the distobuccal aspect of the left mandibular first molar (tooth #*309*). **B,** Note that the lesion continued to proliferate even after extraction of tooth #*309* in a 9-year-old Himalayan, indicating that the true culprit is the left maxillary fourth premolar (tooth #*208*). (Copyright 2014 Alexander M. Reiter; used with permission.)

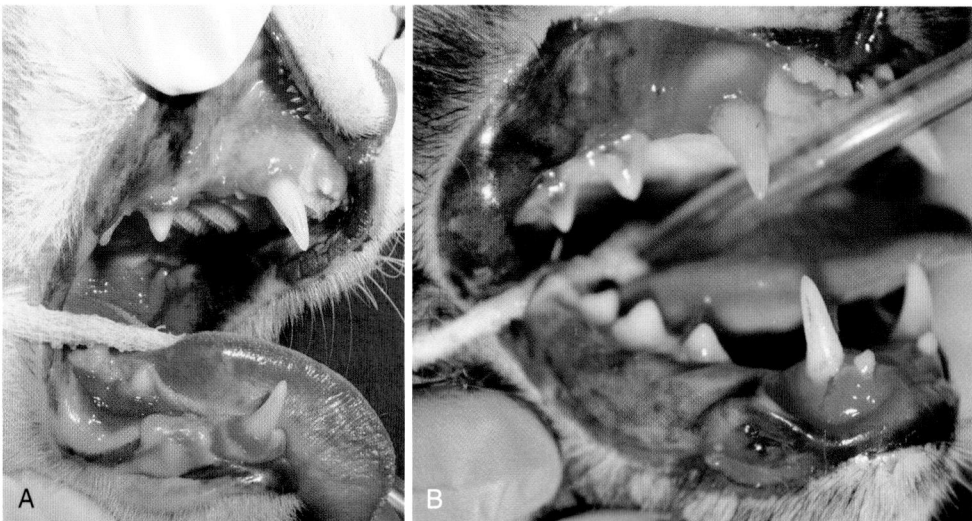

Figure 13-5: Photographs of a 12½-year-old domestic shorthair **(A)** and a 3-year-old domestic shorthair **(B)** with stomatitis, manifesting as gingivitis and inflammation of alveolar, labial, and buccal mucosa; the latter cat **(B)** also shows involvement of the philtrum, lip commissure, and mucocutaneous junction near the lateral frenulum of the left lower lip. (Copyright 2014 Alexander M. Reiter; used with permission.)

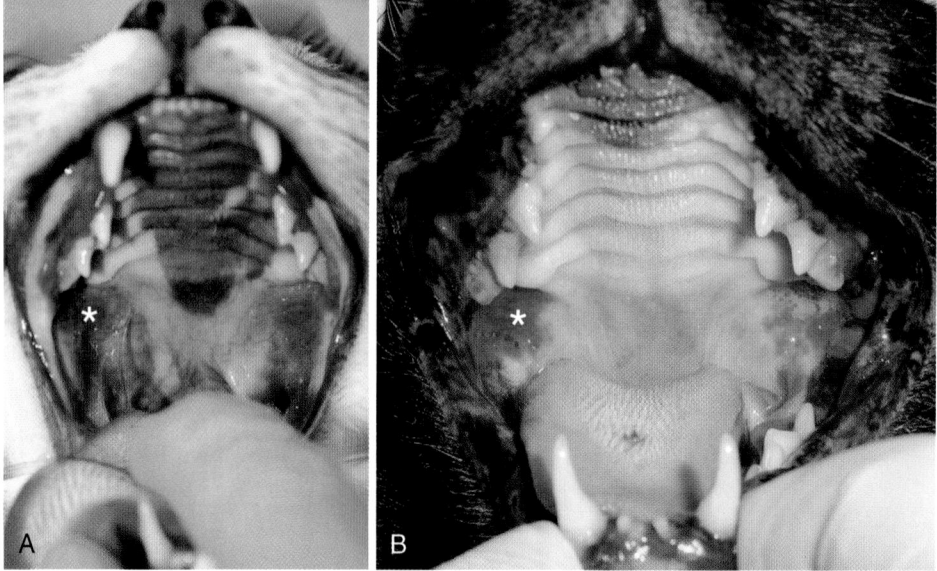

Figure 13-6: Photographs of a 7-year-old domestic shorthair **(A)** and 5-year-old domestic shorthair **(B)** with stomatitis; there is bilateral gingivitis, alveolar and buccal mucositis, and inflammation *(asterisks)* of the caudal aspect of the oral cavity lateral to the palatoglossal folds; the hard and soft palate are usually not involved in this classic type of stomatitis. (Copyright 2014 Alexander M. Reiter; used with permission.)

Acutely, treatment consists of controlling the inflammation via immunosuppression or immune modulation along with symptomatic therapy. Corticosteroids, such as prednisone or prednisolone, are typically used at a dose of 0.5 to 1 mg/kg *per os* (PO) once or twice daily. Corticosteroids can be effective in 73% to 86% of cases.[31] Antibiotics may also be used. However, only 30% of cases respond, and the response is only transient.[31] Amoxicillin/clavulanic acid (13.75 mg/kg every 12 hours PO) or clindamycin (5 to 11 mg/kg every 12 hours PO) are most commonly used. Nutritional support is

sometimes necessary, especially in chronic cases with severe weight loss and evidence of dehydration. Otherwise, the patient should only be offered soft food. If symptoms resolve or the patient improves significantly, plaque control measures, namely daily toothbrushing, should be instituted. However, many cats have too much pain to allow this. Pain control with oral transmucosal buprenorphine (0.01 mg/kg every 8 to 12 hours), sustained release buprenorphine (0.12 mg/kg every 48 to 72 hours subcutaneously [SC]) or a transdermal fentanyl patch should also be considered.

Chronic treatment with corticosteroids is not recommended due to the undesirable long-term side effects that may develop, including diabetes mellitus, polyuria, and polydipsia. Full-mouth extractions are recommended and have achieved a nearly 80% success rate with a complete cure in 60% of cases and a clinical cure in 20% of cases.[30] This supports the theory of stomatitis resulting from a hypersensitivity reaction to plaque. In severe cases, transient treatment with corticosteroids (prednisolone 0.5 to 1 mg/kg every 12 to 24 hours PO) immediately after full-mouth extractions may be necessary.

When cases are refractory, treatment with feline interferon omega (Virbagen Omega) may be considered—although it is currently not available in the United States or Canada. Daily use of this medication (0.1 MU every 24 hours PO) has resulted in significant improvement of clinical lesions as well as a decrease in pain scores up to 90 days post-treatment.[32] Intralesional injections with feline interferon omega can be considered prior to oral administration. A randomized, placebo-controlled, double-blinded clinical trial evaluating the effectiveness of cyclosporine in cats that had undergone partial or full-mouth extractions for treatment of stomatitis found significant improvement in residual oral inflammation in patients with cyclosporine blood levels >300 ng/mL.[33] Finally, ablation of inflamed tissues with carbon dioxide (CO_2) laser has been reported to promote fibrosis after repeated treatments in one refractory case.[34]

Stomatitis can be a frustrating condition for the patient and the owner, as well as the veterinarian. Thirteen percent of cases are only slightly improved with full-mouth extractions and will need further therapy. Additionally, 7% of cases will be unimproved altogether.[30] When treating with feline interferon omega or CO_2 laser, the owners need to understand that repeated treatments are often necessary before even slight improvements are seen. Retroviral status should be assessed prior to therapy, as this may affect prognosis.

SQUAMOUS CELL CARCINOMA

Squamous cell carcinoma is the most common oral tumor in domestic cats.[35] These tumors can vary in appearance and may present as an ulcerated area or a mass. Sometimes the ulcerated area appreciated on oral examination may represent the "tip of the iceberg" (Figure 13-7). Historically, the sublingual/lingual region has been reported to be the most commonly affected site.[36] However, recent reports show the gingiva on the mandible[37] and maxilla[38] to be most often involved. Metastasis to mandibular lymph nodes in these cases, as evaluated by fine-needle aspiration cytology, has been previously documented to be as high as 31% to 36%.[38,39] A significant association between mandibular lymph node metastasis and survival time has not been found.[38] Evidence of pulmonary metastasis, which had been evaluated by three-view thoracic radiography or necropsy, was present in 10% of cases but was not a significant negative prognostic factor. Interestingly, tumor volume appeared not to be a predictor for regional and distant metastasis, because no significant association was seen between tumor size and metastasis.[38]

Despite its historically low metastatic potential, feline oral SCC is generally considered to carry a poor prognosis. Outcome has been largely dependent on the degree of primary tumor invasion at diagnosis,[36] and most cats with oral SCC succumb to the effects of progressive local disease and local treatment failure.[40,41] The prognostic impact of completeness of surgical margins is unclear, and studies evaluating multimodal treatment have shown improved survival times compared to monotherapy.[40,42,43] A study evaluating

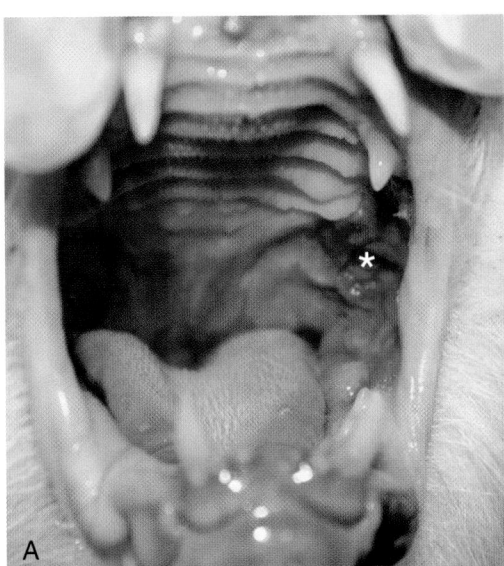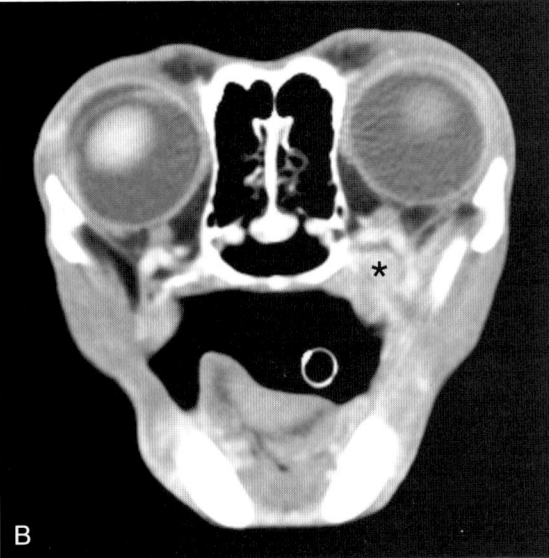

Figure 13-7: Photograph (**A**) and transverse computed tomographic image in soft tissue algorithm obtained after intravenous administration of contrast medium (**B**) of a 12-year-old Persian with squamous cell carcinoma (*asterisks*) of the left caudal upper jaw. Note orbital invasion of the tumor. (Copyright 2014 Maria Soltero-Rivera and Alexander M. Reiter; used with permission.)

multimodal therapy for non-resectable tumors found survival times with complete remission of up to 759 days.[44] Most recently, 21 cats treated with 10 once daily radiation fractions of 4.8 Gy showed a median overall survival of 174 days.[45]

EOSINOPHILIC GRANULOMA

Eosinophilic granuloma is a disease that results from underlying antigenic stimulation. The eosinophil is one of the major sources of the inflammatory mediators associated with type I hypersensitivity reactions. The most commonly identified underlying causes in cats include ectoparasites and other insects, environmental allergens (i.e., atopic dermatitis), or dietary hypersensitivity. Histopathologic examination is useful in order to rule out other differential diagnoses, such as neoplasia or infection. Distinctive histopathologic features of eosinophilic granuloma are small foci of collagen degeneration in which degenerated collagen fibers are surrounded by degranulated eosinophils, resulting in flame figures.[46]

Clinically these lesions are characterized by a proliferative or ulcerative component with yellow pinpoint areas consistent with sulfur granules. The nodular form is commonly found in the oral cavity. Granulomas can be seen in the tongue, palate, and/or glossopharyngeal arches (Figure 13-8). Indolent ulcers, another presentation for this type of inflammatory process, are commonly seen near the midline of the (usually) upper lip and adjacent to the canine tooth; however, these can also be seen on the lower lip.[25,26] The appearance of the lesions that arise on the lip range from a puffy area to

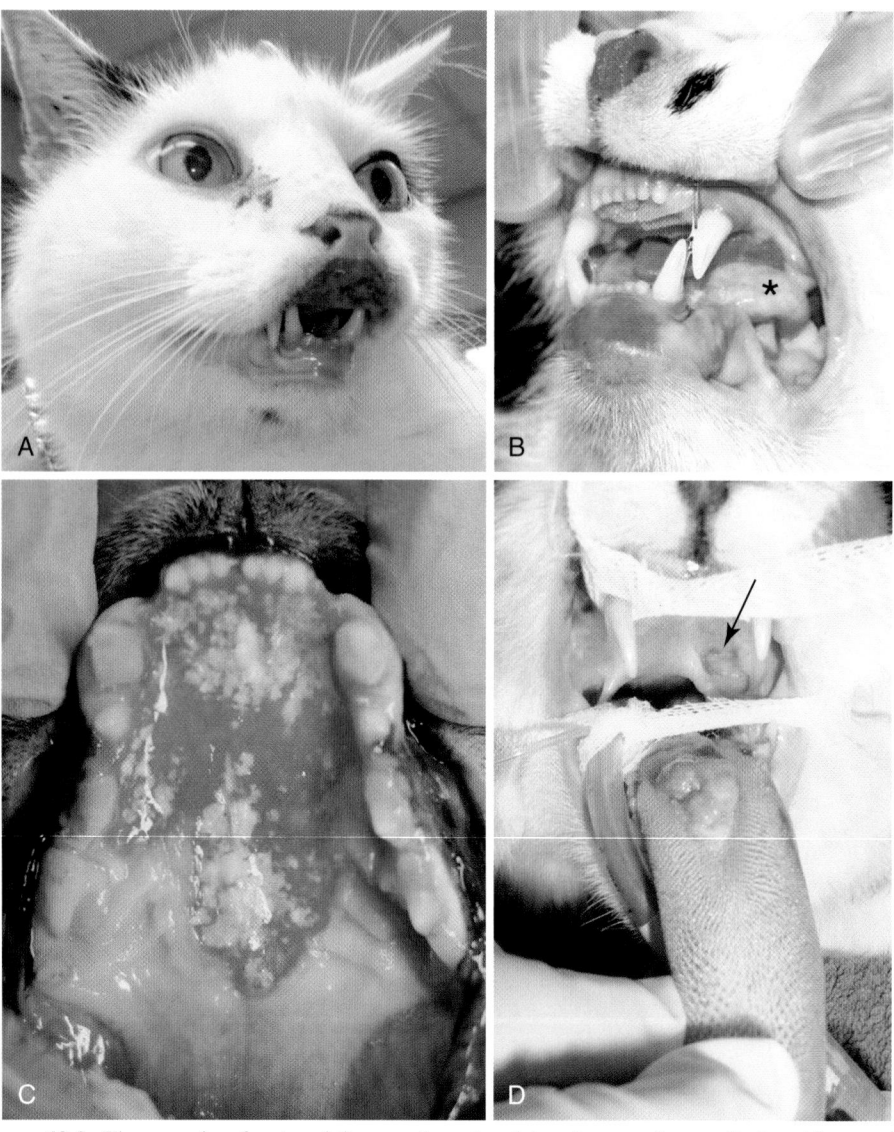

Figure 13-8: Photographs of eosinophilic granuloma involving the rostral upper lip in a 10-year-old domestic shorthair **(A)**, the rostral lower lip in a 5-year-old domestic shorthair that also has severe sublingual edema *(black asterisk)* **(B)**, the hard palate in an 8½-year-old Russian Blue **(C)**, and an area near the soft palate *(black arrow)* and the dorsal aspect of the tongue in a 12-year-old domestic shorthair **(D)**. (Copyright 2014 Alexander M. Reiter; used with permission.)

erosive or ulcerative lesions with raised edges. Some cats are asymptomatic, and in some, lesions resolve with time.

Treatment involves removing the underlying cause by recommending flea prevention and a hypoallergenic diet. Additionally, immunosuppressive therapy with prednisone or prednisolone at 0.5 to 1 mg/kg every 12 to 24 hours PO may be necessary. Recently a study evaluating the efficacy of treatment with amoxicillin/clavulanic acid for 21 days showed a 42.6% reduction in mean lesion size for lip ulcers and a 96.2% reduction in plaque size.[47] If the area shows evidence of chewing trauma or exposure to foreign objects, debulking with the CO_2 laser may be considered as well as intralesional corticosteroid injections (e.g., triamcinolone). Treatment with palmitoylethanolamide, PLR120 (comicronized Palmidrol INN), an endogenous fatty acid amide that downregulates mast cell degranulation, showed clinical improvement in 67% of affected cats.[48] Switching from plastic to stainless steel bowls has anecdotally shown to help.

For cats with severe ulcerative cutaneous or oral lesions that are unresponsive to corticosteroid treatment, FHV type 1 infection should be considered, and the diagnosis can be achieved via immunohistochemistry or polymerase chain reaction testing.[49-51] Eosinophilic vasculitis, which is a rare disease of dogs and cats seen in association with arthropod and insect bite-induced lesions, and occasionally in mast cell tumors, can also be seen along with cutaneous eosinophilic granulomas and plaques in the absence of cutaneous vasculitis.[52]

FOREIGN BODY

A retrospective study evaluating gastrointestinal (GI) foreign bodies in dogs and cats showed that 63% of linear foreign bodies originated from the base of the tongue (Figure 13-9). The most common types of foreign object recovered from cats were string, rope, or fishing lines.[53] Burdock and foxtails can also become entrapped in the oral mucosa, and in dogs they have been reported to elicit a type of granular stomatitis. These oral lesions most often occur on the tip and edges of the tongue and the rostral portions of the upper lip and gingiva. Occasionally the philtrum is involved. Initially they appear as small papules that can then coalesce, and eventually a necrotic center may develop. Removal of the foreign body along with thorough débridement and flushing of the wound is the treatment of choice. Oral antibiotics and soft food should also be considered postextraction.[54]

IMMUNE-MEDIATED AND AUTOIMMUNE DISEASES

Failure of desmosomal adhesion can result from genetic, autoimmune, or infectious causes.[55] The diagnosis of these disorders is based on both morphologic as well as immunologic criteria. Proper site selection, biopsy technique, and sample handling are extremely important in order to reach a

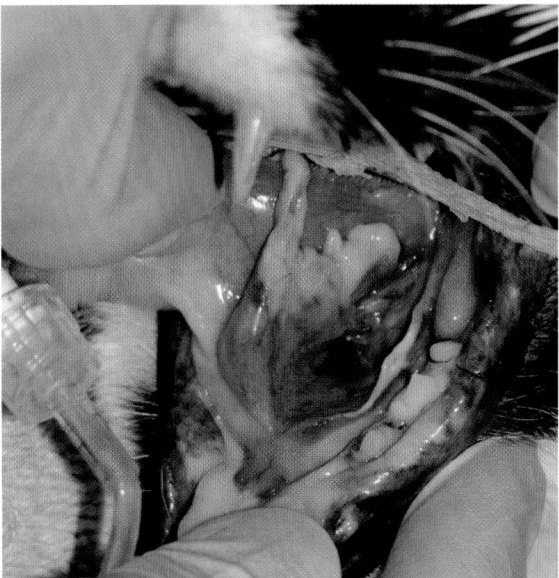

Figure 13-9: Photograph of a 12-year-old domestic shorthair with a non-healing wound in the left sublingual region as a result of foreign body penetration. Note the necrotic tissue margins. (Copyright 2014 Alexander M. Reiter; used with permission.)

definitive diagnosis. Biopsy of the leading edge of a lesion when an intact blister is not found may be sufficient. Preserving the samples in Michel's solution is also preferred by some pathologists, because it preserves tissue antigenicity at ambient temperatures.[56]

Pemphigus represents the most common autoimmune blistering dermatosis in domestic animals. Pemphigus vulgaris is a deep, acantholytic dermatosis. It is rare in feline patients with an estimated incidence of one per 10,000 veterinary dermatology cases per year. It can have mucosal and mucocutaneous manifestations. The presentation can be acute or chronic, and the direct Nikolsky sign (skin fragility) is usually positive.[55] Affected animals are usually mature, and lesions can present as erythema, erosions, ulcerations, scales, and crusts. Erosive lesions are preferentially located in the oral cavity and mucocutaneous junctions.[57] In fact, oral involvement, which may include gingivitis, stomatitis, or glossitis, has been reported to occur in approximately 90% of cases and may be the initial manifestation of the disease in about 50% of cases.[58] Most patients with pemphigus vulgaris show signs of systemic disease, such as anorexia, lethargy, weight loss, and fever. Light microscopy performed on biopsy specimens shows suprabasal acantholysis and cleft formation.[55] Spontaneous resolution of cases has been reported. However, when treatment is necessary, corticosteroids with or without cyclophosphamide are recommended.[57] Side effects seen with cyclophosphamide treatment include hemorrhagic cystitis, bone marrow suppression, GI disturbances, nephrotoxicity, and hepatotoxicity. Cyclophosphamide is also presumed to be carcinogenic.[56]

Of the autoimmune subepidermal blistering dermatoses, 80% of patients with bullous pemphigoid develop oral lesions at the initial onset of disease or later during its course.[58]

Bullous pemphigoid represents 50% of subepidermal autoimmune blistering dermatoses in cats. As opposed to pemphigus vulgaris, this disease can affect animals of any age, even before puberty. Lesions consist primarily of turgid vesicles, erosions, ulcers, and crusts. In cats as opposed to dogs, few lesions are present, and erosions predominate on the face and in the oral cavity. In cats as well as in horses, subepithelial vesicles exhibit fewer inflammatory cells, and special stains are needed to visualize degranulating eosinophils. Long-term remission of bullous pemphigoid has been seen in one cat treated with corticosteroids.[57]

Mucous membrane pemphigoid, although uncommon, has been reported in at least two cats,[57] and the authors have witnessed one additional case. Laminin 5 and 6, collagen XVII, and integrin alpha-6/beta-4 have been implicated as autoantigens in both humans and dogs. However, only laminin 5 has been recognized in the feline homologue of this disease.[59]

Systemic lupus erythematosus has been reported in at least two cats with palatine and glossal ulceration. Behavioral changes, non-erosive polyarthritis, fever, lymphadenomegaly, weight loss, and leukopenia are primarily seen with this condition. The oral ulceration is likely a complication of the systemic vasculitis that occurs.[8,25,26] Erythema multiforme (Figure 13-10) accounted for 0.11% of dermatology cases

seen in the feline population at one academic institution.[60] In this report, only 38% of dogs showed oral lesions, and no oral lesions were reported in the only cat described. In a case report of erythema multiforme, the cat first developed lesions on the face and head, but there were no visible lesions in the oral cavity. This patient did not respond to withdrawal of current medications, but a significant improvement was noted approximately 1 week after treatment with human immunoglobulin.[61] Toxic epidermal necrolysis[62] and idiopathic vasculitis[8] have also been reported to occur in a small number of cats.

Treatment for these conditions should be considered lifelong, and owner commitment for periodic monitoring is imperative. Animals must be routinely monitored with complete blood counts and serum chemistry panels. Although corticosteroids have been reported to be successful in treating most of these conditions, some cases require other forms of immunosuppressive or immunomodulating therapy. Some immune-mediated skin diseases have also been treated with tetracycline, niacinamide, and pentoxifylline, which together can have immunomodulating and anti-inflammatory effects.[63,64] Antibiotics should be prescribed in cases with a secondary infection. Symptomatic treatment is required acutely, including nutritional support and pain control until long-term therapy takes effect.

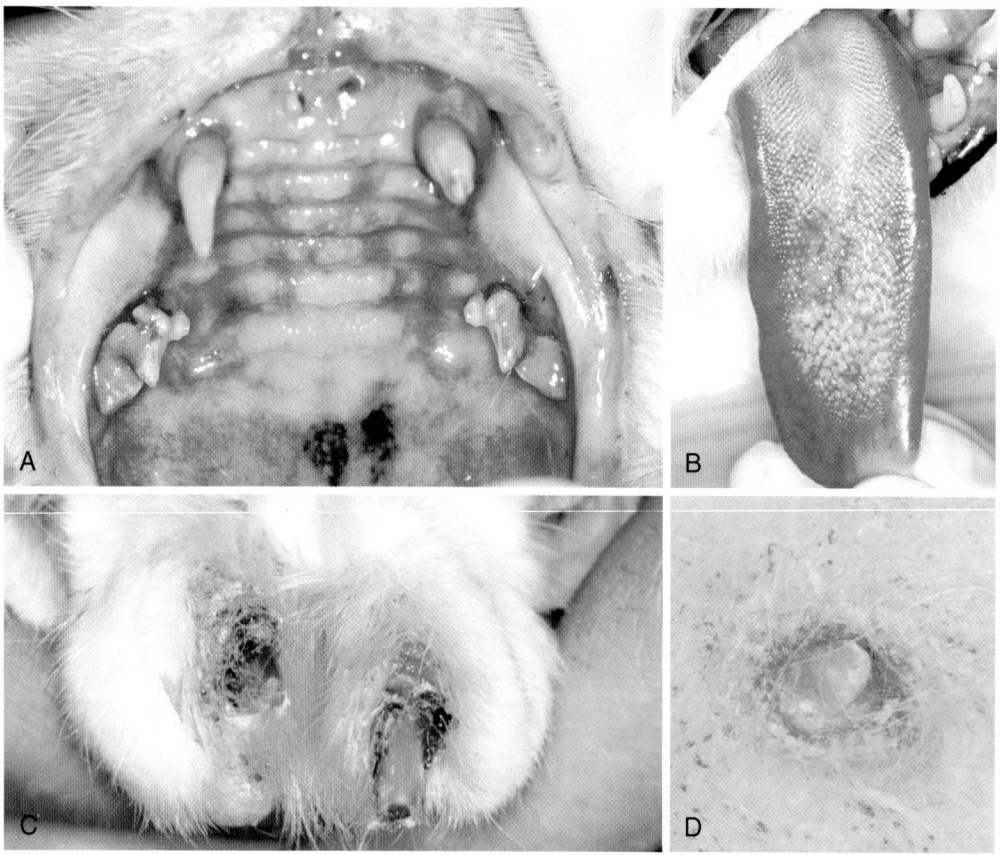

Figure 13-10: Photographs of a 10-year-old domestic shorthair with erythema multiforme manifesting at the hard palate **(A)**, dorsal tongue surface **(B)**, nail beds **(C)**, and nipple **(D)**. (Copyright 2014 Alexander M. Reiter; used with permission.)

METABOLIC DISEASE

Acute uremia is defined as a rapid decline in renal function leading to retention of uremic wastes. The incidence of acute uremia in animals is unknown, but in humans it accounts for 1% of hospital admissions.[26] Uremic halitosis and oral ulcerations are common findings on physical examination of severely affected patients. Ulceration occurs especially at the labial and buccal mucosa, lateral margins of the tongue, lateral lip frenula, and lip commissures (Figure 13-11).

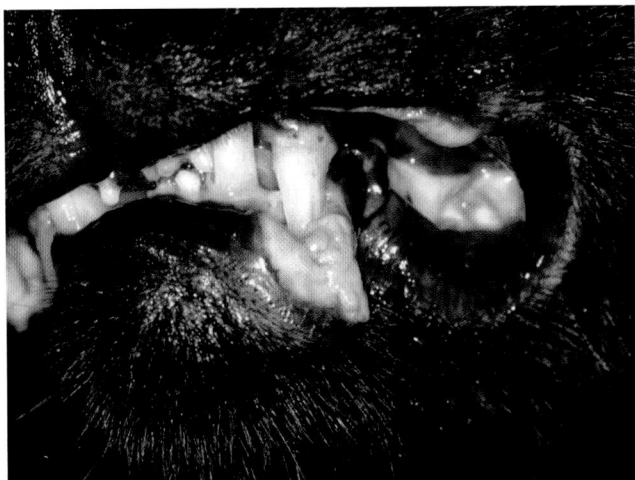

Figure 13-11: Photograph of a 16-year-old domestic shorthair in renal failure, showing uremic ulcerations at the mucosa and mucocutaneous junction areas of the upper and lower lips. (Copyright 2014 Alexander M. Reiter; used with permission.)

Uremic vasculitis and thrombosis lead to necrosis and sloughing of the mucosa. Halitosis is often a feature of this syndrome, because the lesions become secondarily infected with oral bacteria such as *Fusobacterium necrophorum*. In severe cases, there may be extensive subepithelial necrosis and sloughing of the tip of the tongue. The lesions are often very painful and contribute to the anorexia often observed in animals with kidney disease.

Treatment is symptomatic and includes pain management (buprenorphine 0.01 mg/kg every 8 to 12 hours intravenously), bypassing the mouth with supplemental enteral or parenteral nutrition, and use of gastric protectants (sucralfate 0.25 to 0.5 g every 8 to 12 hours PO). Topical mouthwashes such as a mixture of diphenhydramine, sucralfate or aluminum and magnesium hydroxide (Maalox), and lidocaine may provide some local pain control.[25,26] Dilute (0.12%) chlorhexidine rinses also play a role in preventing secondary infection of the necrotic areas. Other metabolic disease such as diabetes mellitus, liver failure, and respiratory disease, as well as immunosuppressive medications, have also been reported to lead to oral ulceration and necrosis.[25,26]

BURNS

Burns can be caused by electricity, chemicals, heat, friction, or radiation (Figure 13-12). Chewing on household power cords is the most common cause of electric burns in dogs and cats, and these are usually low-voltage injuries. The electrical current can cause damage through its direct effect as well as via transformation of electric energy into heat. Ultimately,

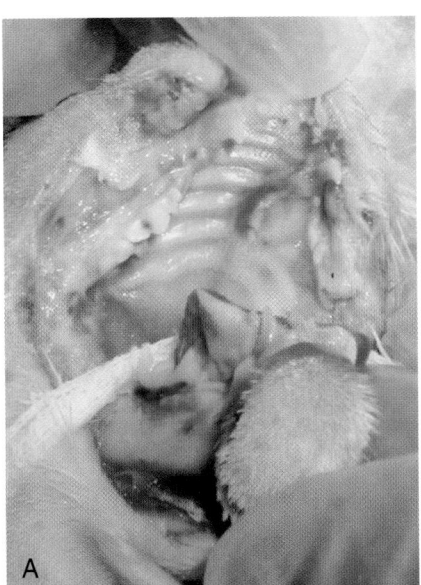 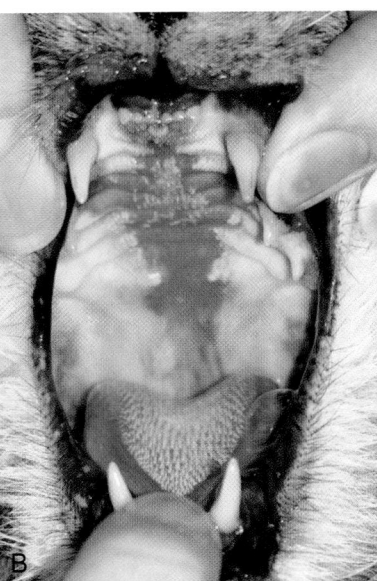 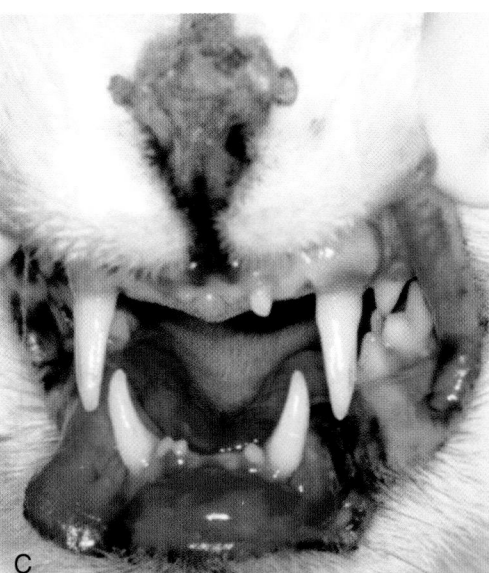

Figure 13-12: Photographs of a 2-month-old domestic shorthair with electric burns and extensive tissue necrosis at the lips, cheeks, tongue, and hard palate **(A),** an 8-year-old domestic shorthair with chemical burns of the hard and soft palate and the tip and lateral aspects of the tongue **(B),** and a 12-year-old domestic shorthair with thermal burns at the nasal plane, lips, and the tip and lateral aspects of the tongue after being offered microwaved milk **(C).** (Copyright 2014 Alexander M. Reiter; used with permission.)

superheated tissues become necrotic, and ischemia results from the vascular insults that occur. Moist mucus membranes are severely affected due to their low electrical resistance. The patient should be evaluated for cardiac arrhythmias and neurogenic pulmonary edema prior to evaluating the oral cavity under sedation or anesthesia.[65] Edema and necrosis are typically seen in the tongue, palate, and lip commissures. Discoloration of adjacent teeth secondary to pulpitis can also be seen. Palatal necrosis can lead to the development of an oronasal fistula, and a portion of the necrotic tongue may be sloughed. Patients should be treated symptomatically for at least 7 to 10 days or until tissues appear healthy. Until definitive surgery can be performed, antibiotics and pain medication should be instituted. Nutritional supplementation should be considered when patients refuse to eat soft food. Definitive therapy consists of débridement of the lesions unless these are superficial enough to heal by contraction and re-epithelialization.[66,67]

Chemical burns can result from exposure to household cleaning products, phenolic compounds, essential oils, heavy metal (thallium), or plant toxins (i.e., *Dieffenbachia*). The rostral and dorsal aspects of the tongue and the palate are usually affected. A poison control center (e.g., American Society for the Prevention of Cruelty to Animals Animal Poison Control—http://www.aspca.org/pet-care/animal-poison-control) should be contacted in these cases for treatment of any ingested substances. Similar to electric cord injuries, treatment should be symptomatic, but débridement is less often necessary. Patients should be evaluated for esophagitis and gastritis and treated accordingly. The hair of affected patients should be clipped or washed if the hair coat is contaminated to prevent contact via grooming. Thermal injuries can be encountered in animals that are fed home-prepared diets or heated milk. Injuries are similar to those seen with chemical burns with the lips and nasal plane also being affected. Similar to chemical and electric burn injuries, symptomatic treatment and client education are necessary.

SUMMARY

The oral tissues can respond to insults in various ways, including vasodilation, hypertrophy or atrophy, capillary rupture, infarction, ulceration, and necrosis.[68] A thorough patient history can provide a definitive diagnosis in cases of foreign body trauma and toxic exposure. Oral inflammation may only be a component of a general malaise. In many cases, a professional dental cleaning, including diagnostic imaging, biopsy and culture, and sensitivity testing may be required in order to reach a definitive diagnosis. Outcome ultimately depends on the cause of the disease with immune-mediated diseases and neoplasia carrying the worst prognosis.

References

1. Squier CA, Finkelstein MW: Oral mucosa. In Nanci A, Ten Cate AR, editors: *Ten Cate's oral histology: development, structure, and function*, ed 6, St Louis, 2003, Mosby, pp 329–375.
2. Gelber HB: Alimentary system and the peritoneum, omentum, mesentery and peritoneal cavity. In Zachary JF, McGavin MD, editors: *Pathologic basis of veterinary disease*, ed 5, Philadelphia, 2012, Elsevier, pp 322–401.
3. Bulkacz J, Carranza FA: Defense mechanisms of the gingiva. In Newman MG, Takei HH, Carranza FA, editors: *Carranza's clinical periodontology*, ed 11, Philadelphia, 2012, Elsevier, pp 66–70.
4. Harley R, Gruffydd-Jones TJ, Day MJ: Characterization of immune cell populations in oral mucosal tissue of healthy adult cats. *J Comp Pathol* 128:146–155, 2003.
5. Lommer MJ, Verstraete FJ: Radiographic patterns of periodontitis in cats: 147 cases (1998-1999). *J Am Vet Med Assoc* 218:230–234, 2001.
6. Girard N, Servet E, Biourge V, et al: Periodontal health status in a colony of 109 cats. *J Vet Dent* 26:147–155, 2009.
7. DuPont GA, DeBowes LJ: Comparison of periodontitis and root replacement in cat teeth with resorptive lesions. *J Vet Dent* 19:71–75, 2002.
8. Pedersen NC: Inflammatory oral cavity diseases of the cat. *Vet Clin North Am Small Anim Pract* 22:1323–1345, 1992.
9. Wiggs RB, Lobprise HB: Domestic feline oral and dental disease. In Wiggs RB, Lobprise

HB, editors: *Veterinary dentistry: principles and practice*, ed 1, Philadelphia, 1997, Lippincott-Raven, pp 482–517.
10. Tapashetti RP, Sharma S, Patil SR, et al: Potential effect of neutrophil functional disorders on pathogenesis of aggressive periodontitis. *J Contemp Dent Pract* 14:387–393, 2013.
11. Lindskog S, Blomlöf L: Cementum hypoplasia in teeth affected by juvenile periodontitis. *J Clin Periodontol* 10:443–451, 1983.
12. Reiter AM: Dental and oral diseases. In Little SE, editor: *The cat: clinical medicine and management*, ed 1, St Louis, 2012, Saunders, pp 329–370.
13. Harvey CE, Thornsberry C, Miller BR, et al: Antimicrobial susceptibility of subgingival bacterial flora in cats with gingivitis. *J Vet Dent* 12:157–160, 1995.
14. Tenorio AP, Franti CE, Madewell BR, et al: Chronic oral infections of cats and their relationship to persistent oral carriage of feline calici-, immunodeficiency, or leukemia viruses. *Vet Immunol Immunopathol* 29:1–14, 1991.
15. Rawlinson JE, Goldstein RE, Reiter AM, et al: Association of periodontal disease with systemic health indices in dogs and the systemic response to treatment of periodontal disease. *J Am Vet Med Assoc* 238:601–609, 2011.
16. Cave NJ, Bridges JP, Thomas DG: Systemic effects of periodontal disease in cats. *Vet Q* 32:131–144, 2012.
17. Harley R, Gruffydd-Jones TJ, Day MJ: Immunohistochemical characterization of oral

mucosal lesions in cats with chronic gingivostomatitis. *J Comp Pathol* 144:239–250, 2011.
18. Healey KAE, Dawson S, Burrow R, et al: Prevalence of feline chronic gingivo-stomatitis in first opinion veterinary practice. *J Feline Med Surg* 9:373–381, 2007.
19. Soukup J: Feline oral pyogenic granuloma: a previously unnamed mucogingival lesion. In *Proceedings 27th Annual Veterinary Dental Forum (New Orleans, LA)*, 2013, p 19.
20. Dolieslager SMJ, Riggio MP, Lennon A, et al: Identification of bacteria associated with feline chronic gingivostomatitis using culture-dependent and culture-independent methods. *Vet Microbiol* 148:93–98, 2011.
21. Knowles JO, Gaskell RM, Gaskell CJ, et al: Prevalence of feline calicivirus, feline leukaemia virus and antibodies to FIV in cats with chronic stomatitis. *Vet Rec* 124:336–338, 1989.
22. Torten M, Franchini M, Barlough JE, et al: Progressive immune dysfunction in cats experimentally infected with feline immunodeficiency virus. *J Virol* 65:2225–2230, 1991.
23. Reubel GH, Hoffmann DE, Pedersen NC: Acute and chronic faucitis of domestic cats: a feline calicivirus-induced disease. *Vet Clin North Am Small Anim Pract* 22:1347–1360, 1992.
24. Dowers KL, Hawley JR, Brewer MM, et al: Association of Bartonella species, feline calicivirus, and feline herpesvirus 1 infection with gingivostomatitis in cats. *J Feline Med Surg* 12:314–321, 2010.

25. Taney K, Smith M: Oral and salivary gland disease. In Ettinger SJ, Feldman EC, editors: *Textbook of veterinary internal medicine: diseases of the dog and the cat,* ed 7, Philadelphia, 2010, Elsevier, pp 1479–1486.

26. DiBartola SP: Clinical approach and laboratory evaluation of renal disease. In Ettinger SJ, Feldman EC, editors: *Textbook of veterinary internal medicine: diseases of the dog and the cat,* ed 7, Philadelphia, 2010, Elsevier, pp 1955–1956.

27. Arzi B, Murphy B, Cox DP, et al: Presence and quantification of mast cells in the gingiva of cats with tooth resorption, periodontitis and chronic stomatitis. *Arch Oral Biol* 55:148–154, 2010.

28. Lommer MJ, Verstraete FJM: Concurrent oral shedding of feline calicivirus and feline herpesvirus 1 in cats with chronic gingivostomatitis. *Oral Microbiol Immunol* 18:131–134, 2003.

29. Signorelli PS, Stefanelle D, Roccabianca P: Differentiation of chronic stomatitis in oral squamous cell carcinoma in three cats. In *Proceedings 15th European Congress of Veterinary Dentistry (Cambridge, UK),* 2006, pp 77–78.

30. Hennet P: Chronic gingivo-stomatitis in cats: long-term follow-up of 30 cases treated by dental extractions. *J Vet Dent* 14:15–21, 1997.

31. White SD, Rosychuk RA, Janik TA, et al: Plasma cell stomatitis-pharyngitis in cats: 40 cases (1973-1991). *J Am Vet Med Assoc* 200:1377–1380, 1992.

32. Hennet PR, Camy GAL, McGahie DM, et al: Comparative efficacy of a recombinant feline interferon omega in refractory cases of calicivirus-positive cats with caudal stomatitis: a randomised, multi-centre, controlled, double-blind study in 39 cats. *J Feline Med Surg* 13:577–587, 2011.

33. Lommer MJ: Efficacy of cyclosporine for chronic, refractory stomatitis in cats: a randomized, placebo-controlled, double blinded clinical study. *J Vet Dent* 30:8–17, 2013.

34. Lewis JR, Tsugawa AJ, Reiter AM: Use of CO_2 laser as an adjunctive treatment for caudal stomatitis in a cat. *J Vet Dent* 24:240–249, 2007.

35. Stebbins KE, Morse CC, Goldschmidt MH: Feline oral neoplasia: a ten-year survey. *Vet Pathol* 26:121–128, 1989.

36. Postorino Reeves NC, Turrel JM, Withrow SJ: Oral squamous cell carcinoma in the cat. *J Am Anim Hosp Assoc* 29:438–441, 1993.

37. Martin CK, Tannehill-Gregg SH, Wolfe TD, et al: Bone-invasive oral squamous cell carcinoma in cats: pathology and expression of parathyroid hormone-related protein. *Vet Pathol* 48:302–312, 2011.

38. Soltero-Rivera MM, Krick EL, Reiter AM, et al: Prevalence of regional and distant metastasis in cats with advanced oral squamous cell carcinoma: 49 cases (2005-2011). *J Feline Med Surg* 16:164–169, 2014.

39. Gendler A, Lewis JR, Reetz JA, et al: Computed tomographic features of oral squamous cell carcinoma in cats. *J Am Vet Med Assoc* 236:319–325, 2010.

40. Hutson C, Willauer C, Walder E, et al: Treatment of mandibular squamous cell carcinoma in cats by use of mandibulectomy and radiotherapy—7 cases (1987-1989). *J Am Vet Med Assoc* 201:777–781, 1992.

41. Northrup NC, Selting KA, Rassnick KM, et al: Outcomes of cats with oral tumors treated with mandibulectomy: 42 cases. *J Am Anim Hosp Assoc* 42:350–360, 2006.

42. Fidel J, Lyons J, Tripp C, et al: Treatment of oral squamous cell carcinoma with accelerated radiation therapy and concomitant carboplatin in cats. *J Vet Intern Med* 25:504–510, 2011.

43. Fidel JL, Sellon RK, Houston RK, et al: A nine-day accelerated radiation protocol for feline squamous cell carcinoma. *Vet Radiol Ultrasound* 48:482–485, 2007.

44. Marconato L, Buchholz J, Keller M, et al: Multimodal therapeutic approach and interdisciplinary challenge for the treatment of unresectable head and neck squamous cell carcinoma in six cats: a pilot study. *Vet Comp Oncol* 11:101–112, 2013.

45. Poirier VJ, Kaser-Hotz B, Vail DM, et al: Efficacy and toxicity of an accelerated hypofractionated radiation therapy protocol in cats with oral squamous cell carcinoma. *Vet Radiol Ultrasound* 54:81–88, 2013.

46. Fondati A, Fondevila D, Ferrer L: Histopathological study of feline eosinophilic dermatoses. *Vet Dermatol* 12:333–338, 2001.

47. Wildermuth BE, Griffin CE, Rosenkrantz WS: Response of feline eosinophilic plaques and lip ulcers to amoxicillin trihydrate-clavulanate potassium therapy: a randomized, double-blind placebo-controlled prospective study. *Vet Dermatol* 23:110–118, e24–e25, 2012.

48. Scarampella F, Abramo F, Noli C: Clinical and histological evaluation of an analogue of palmitoylethanolamide, PLR 120 (comicronized Palmidrol INN) in cats with eosinophilic granuloma and eosinophilic plaque: a pilot study. *Vet Dermatol* 12:29–39, 2001.

49. Lee M, Bosward KL, Norris JM: Immunohistological evaluation of feline herpesvirus-1 infection in feline eosinophilic dermatoses or stomatitis. *J Feline Med Surg* 12:72–79, 2010.

50. Persico P, Roccabianca P, Corona A, et al: Detection of feline herpes virus 1 via polymerase chain reaction and immunohistochemistry in cats with ulcerative facial dermatitis, eosinophilic granuloma complex reaction patterns and mosquito bite hypersensitivity. *Vet Dermatol* 22:521–527, 2011.

51. Malik R, Lessels NS, Webb S, et al: Treatment of feline herpesvirus-1 associated disease in cats with famciclovir and related drugs. *J Feline Med Surg* 11:40–48, 2009.

52. Scott DW: Eosinophils in the walls of large dermal and subcutaneous blood vessels in biopsy specimens from cats with eosinophilic granuloma or eosinophilic plaque. *Vet Dermatol* 10:77–78, 1999.

53. Hayes G: Gastrointestinal foreign bodies in dogs and cats: a retrospective study of 208 cases. *J Small Anim Pract* 50:576–583, 2009.

54. Thiverge G: Granular stomatitis in dogs due to Burdock. *Can Vet J* 14:96–97, 1973.

55. Olivry T, Linder KE: Dermatoses affecting desmosomes in animals: a mechanistic review of acantholytic blistering skin diseases. *Vet Dermatol* 20:313–326, 2009.

56. Ackerman LJ: Pemphigus and pemphigoid in domestic animals: an overview. *Can Vet J* 26:185–189, 1985.

57. Olivry T, Chan LS: Autoimmune blistering dermatoses in domestic animals. *Clin Dermatol* 19:750–760, 2001.

58. Verstraete FJM: *Self-assessment color review of veterinary dentistry,* ed 1, Ames, 1999, Iowa State University Press, p 104.

59. Olivry T, Dunston SM, Zhang G, et al: Laminin-5 is targeted by autoantibodies in feline mucous membrane (cicatricial) pemphigoid. *Vet Immunol Immunopathol* 88:123–129, 2002.

60. Scott DW, Miller WH: Erythema multiforme in dogs and cats: literature review and case material from the Cornell University College of Veterinary Medicine (1988-1996). *Vet Dermatol* 10:297–309, 1999.

61. Byrne KP, Giger U: Use of human immunoglobulin for treatment of severe erythema multiforme in a cat. *J Am Vet Med Assoc* 220:197–201, 2002.

62. Scott DW, Halliwell R, Goldschmidt MH, et al: Toxic epidermal necrolysis in two dogs and one cat. *J Am Anim Hosp Assoc* 15:271–279, 1979.

63. Chaidemenos GC: Tetracycline and niacinamide in the treatment of blistering skin diseases. *Clin Dermatol* 19:781–785, 2001.

64. Marks SL, Merchant S, Foil C: Pentoxifylline: wonder drug? *J Am Anim Hosp Assoc* 37:218–219, 2001.

65. Mann FA: Electrical and lightning injuries. In Silverstein DC, Hopper K, editors: *Small animal critical care medicine,* ed 1, St Louis, 2009, Elsevier, pp 687–690.

66. Kolata R, Burrows C: The clinical features of injury by chewing electrical cords in dogs and cats. *J Am Anim Hosp Assoc* 17:219–222, 1981.

67. Presley R, Macintire D: Electrocution and electrical cord injury. *Stand Care Emer Crit Care Med* 7:7–11, 2005.

68. Anderson J: Approach to diagnosis of canine oral lesions. *Compend Contin Educ Pract Vet* 13:1215–1226, 1991.

Diagnostic Imaging of the Gastrointestinal Tract and Tissue Sampling

Lorrie Gaschen and Kristina Miles

Radiography remains an important imaging modality for screening the feline patient with signs of gastrointestinal (GI) disease such as vomiting, anorexia, icterus, and diarrhea. Abdominal radiography allows the size, shape, and opacity of the liver to be determined. In some instances, it allows an enlarged gallbladder to be diagnosed, as well as gas or mineralization of the hepatic parenchyma or biliary structure such as a cyst to be recognized. Radiographically, the liver may appear normal even if severely diseased.[1] In vomiting or anorectic cats, it is important to identify obstructive ileus, foreign bodies, or abdominal masses radiographically. Ultrasonography is the most frequently used modality for detailed assessment of the hepatobiliary system and intestinal wall in the cat. High-resolution images of the intestinal wall layering, liver, gallbladder, common bile duct, major duodenal papilla, and pancreas can be performed consistently in most cats with both portable and console ultrasound units. High-frequency transducers, either curved-array or linear, are both suitable to assess these structures in cats. Nuclear scintigraphy has the advantage of being able to assess liver function as well as biliary. Endoscopic retrograde cholangiopancreatography (ERCP) is a modality that combines endoscopy with fluoroscopy and allows the common bile duct to be catheterized and visually examined as well as biopsy samples to be obtained. Magnetic resonance imaging (MRI) and computed tomography (CT) are more widely available advanced imaging modalities that can be used to assess the hepatobiliary system, but as with ERCP, they are not yet well established in cats.

HEPATIC PARENCHYMAL DISEASE

Hepatomegaly is one of the hallmark signs of hepatobiliary disease. However, the absence of an enlarged liver does not rule out the existence of disease, and the plan to pursue additional imaging should be based on the clinical findings. Radiography has the immediate benefit of being able to diagnose liver size and opacity. An enlarged liver has contours that extend caudal to the costal arch, and the stomach is usually caudodorsally displaced (Figure 14-1). A large amount of falciform fat can displace the liver dorsally, and it can also

be falsely diagnosed as hepatomegaly (Figure 14-2). An enlarged and fluid-filled stomach can also be misinterpreted as hepatomegaly in the cat (Figure 14-3). The most common change in opacity is the presence of mineralizations. These may appear as multifocal linear or irregularly-shaped mineralizations randomly arranged throughout the hepatic parenchyma or localized to one region, such as the gallbladder (Figure 14-4A and B). Randomly arranged mineralizations, when linear, typically are seen when they are associated with the biliary system. Choledocholithiasis (Figure 14-4C) can be present within the intrahepatic and extrahepatic bile ducts as well as within the common bile or pancreatic ducts. The presence of gas associated with the liver generally indicates the presence of infection, usually ascending from the GI tract via the common bile duct or due to necrosis.

Radiography is insensitive for differentiating diffuse versus multifocal or vascular causes of changes in size and shape of the liver, and ultrasonography is generally required for differentiation.

Diffuse Hepatic Parenchymal Disease

Ultrasonography of the liver is used to further assess size, shape, margination, and opacity changes detected radiographically or prior to advanced cross sectional imaging, such as CT or MRI.

The liver is divided into left, quadrate, right, and caudate lobes, but the separation of lobes is not well seen sonographically unless abdominal fluid is present. The normal hepatic parenchyma has a uniform echogenicity. The echotexture is coarser and more hypoechoic when compared to that of the spleen, and the hepatic and portal veins are distributed evenly throughout the parenchyma (Figure 14-5). Hepatic echogenicity must be evaluated in comparison to neighboring organs at the same depth and preferably within the same image. The liver is hypoechoic to the falciform ligament and the spleen (Figure 14-6). Due to the small size of the feline spleen, it is not always possible to have the spleen and the liver in the same field of view. Portal veins have echogenic walls and can be traced back to the porta hepatis in cases where Doppler ultrasound is not available. Hepatic veins lack these echogenic walls and may be seen entering the caudal

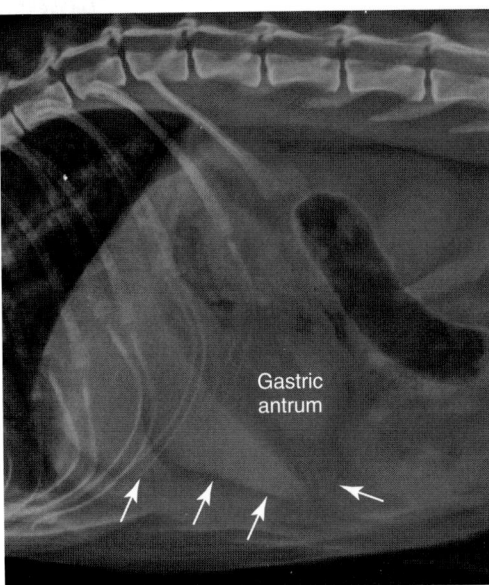

Figure 14-1: Hepatomegaly. The *arrows* mark the ventral contour of the liver, which has rounded borders and extends caudal to the costal arch. The stomach is displaced caudally, another feature of hepatomegaly.

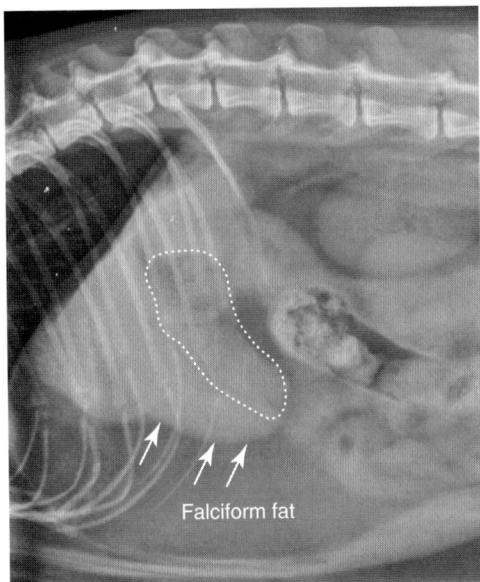

Figure 14-2: This cat has a large amount of falciform fat, which can also create the appearance of hepatomegaly due to displacement of the liver. The liver border is marked by *arrows,* and the gastric antrum is marked by a *dotted line.*

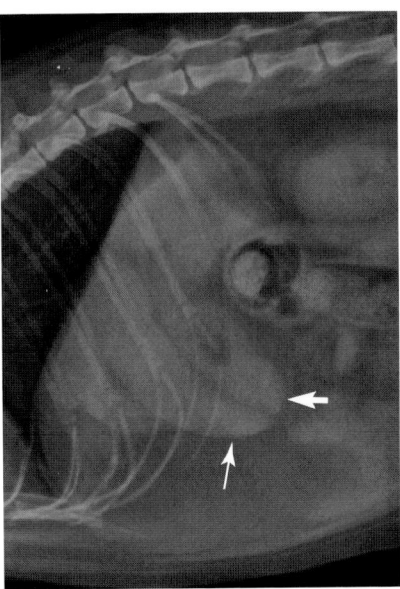

Figure 14-3: The *large arrow* points to the gastric antrum, which is fluid opaque and silhouettes the liver. The silhouetting of the stomach with the liver can create the appearance of a rounded or enlarged liver. The *thin arrow* points to the liver border that is displaced by the large amount of falciform fat, which can make the liver appear larger than it is.

hypoechoic (e.g., due to congestion, suppurative hepatitis, or lymphoma).[1] Diffuse (infiltrative but not nodular) liver diseases (such as inflammation, round-cell neoplasia, non–round-cell infiltrative, prenodular (early) metastatic neoplasia, lipidosis, and vacuolar hepatopathy) cannot be differentiated from one another or from normal liver based on sonographic features.[2] Ultrasonographic diagnosis of diffuse liver disease should be substantiated by biopsy and histopathologic evaluation if suspected clinically (Figure 14-7). It should be noted that clinically normal obese cats may have a liver that is hyperechoic relative to the fat of the falciform ligament.[3]

Multifocal Hepatic Parenchymal Disease

Nodules are most commonly hypoechoic, but hyperechoic, isoechoic, and mixed echogenic nodules also occur. Focal and multifocal nodules are most commonly due to nodular hyperplasia and metastatic disease. The presence of target lesions (hypoechoic nodules with a hyperechoic center) are more commonly malignant than benign but can be due to necrosis from nonneoplastic causes (Figure 14-8). Causes of focal or multifocal nodules in the feline liver include primary or metastatic neoplasia, nodular hyperplasia, pyogranulomas and abscesses, and parasitic infection. Anechoic cavities in the liver are typically the result of cysts in cats (e.g., congenital, biliary pseudocysts, cystadenoma or cystadenocarcinoma, parasitic, or necrosis due to infection or neoplasia). Contrast-enhanced ultrasonography can be used to detect metastatic hepatic nodules and to differentiate them from benign lesions.[4] In particular, the accurate detection and characterization of lesions with acoustic properties similar to those of the surrounding normal parenchyma (i.e., isoechoic lesions)

vena cava. The intrahepatic biliary tree is not seen in normal cats. The size of the liver is subjectively assessed using ultrasonography and should be determined together with the radiographic findings.

Both focal and diffuse disease can be diagnosed sonographically, but sonography is more sensitive for identifying focal lesions, both hypoechoic and hyperechoic. Diffuse liver disease appears ultrasonographically normal or as a change in liver echogenicity from normal and can be characterized as either hyperechoic (e.g., due to fatty change, diabetes mellitus, steroid hepatopathy, chronic hepatitis, or cirrhosis) or

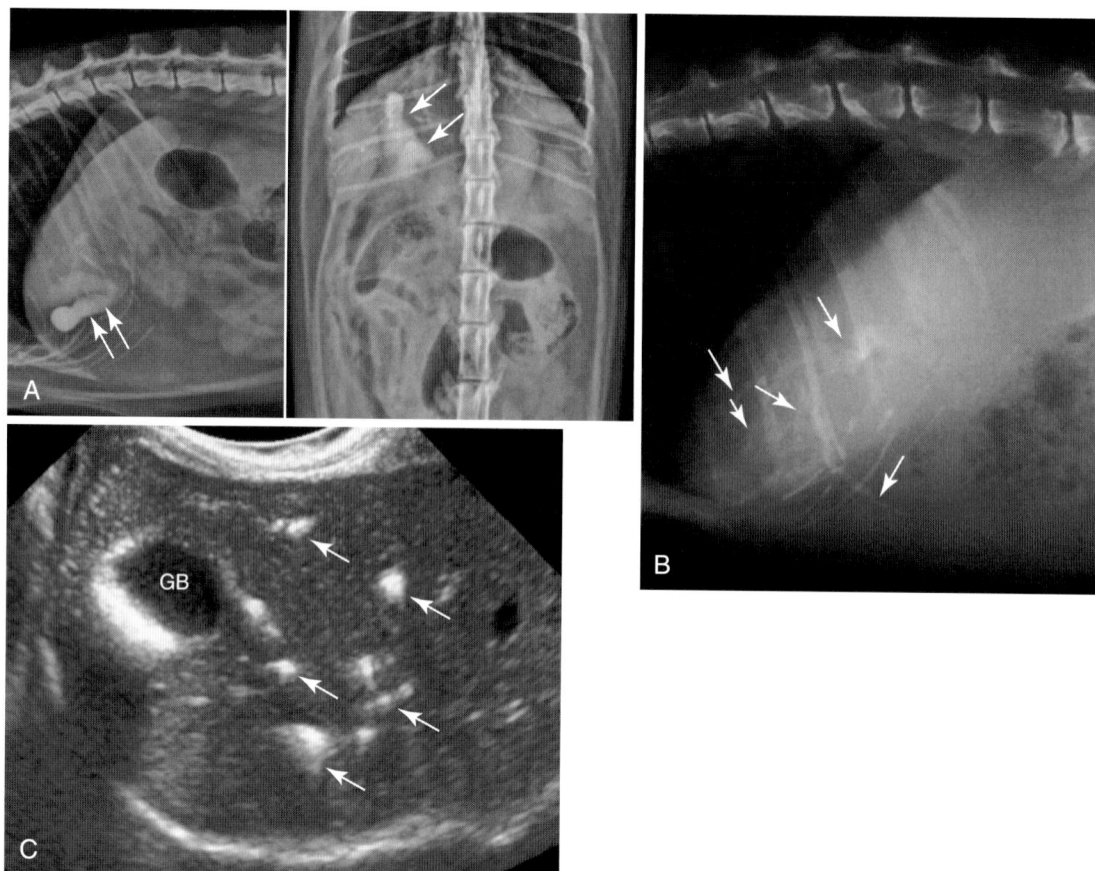

Figure 14-4: **A,** Lateral *(left)* and ventrodorsal *(right)* images of a cat with cholelithiasis *(arrows).* The mineral opacity in the gallbladder marks its location in the right cranioventral part of the abdomen. **B,** The *arrows* mark numerous linear and tortuous mineral opacities in the liver, which are located in the intrahepatic bile ducts representing intrahepatic choledocholithiasis, which is often an incidental finding in cats. **C,** Ultrasound images of intrahepatic biliary mineralizations (choledocholithiasis). There is mineralized dependent content in the gallbladder *(GB)* creating acoustic shadowing (cholecystolithiasis).

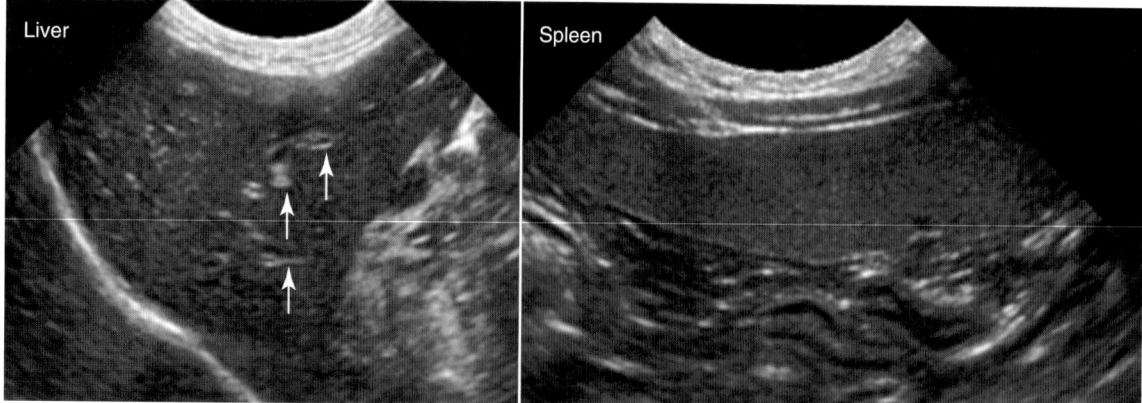

Figure 14-5: Side-by-Side Images of the Normal Feline Liver and Spleen. The liver is hypoechoic compared with the spleen and has a coarser echotexture, which is mainly due to the presence of hyperechoic striations that represent the portal vein walls *(arrows* point to a number of them).

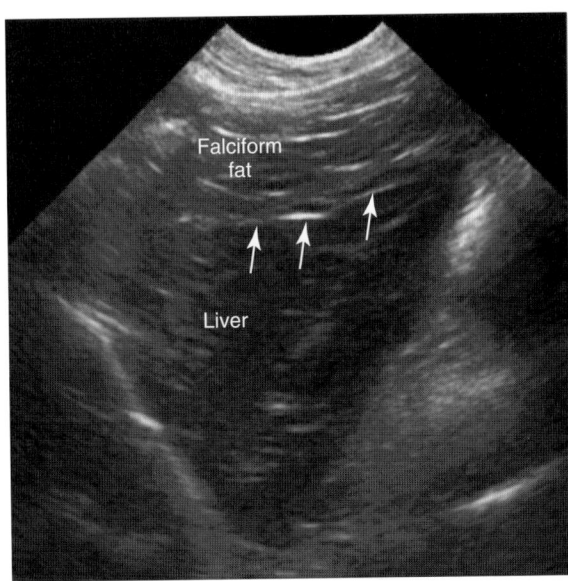

Figure 14-6: Ultrasound Image of a Cat with a Large Amount of Falciform Fat. The *arrows* point to the hyperechoic liver capsule, which helps to differentiate the liver parenchyma from the fat, because the fat can appear very similar to the liver and is often mistaken for the liver in cats. Note that the liver is hypoechoic in comparison to the falciform fat in normal cats.

is a significant limitation of B-mode gray-scale ultrasonography.[5] The use of ultrasonographic contrast media to assist in the characterization of benign and malignant hepatic lesions in humans and the dog has been reported.[6] Its use has been described in one cat that had isoechoic hepatic metastatic nodules due to splenic hemangiosarcoma.[4] Contrast-enhanced ultrasonography of the liver, kidney, pancreas, small intestine, and lymph nodes has been performed in healthy cats.[7] One quantitative study in cats was performed with contrast-enhanced power and color Doppler techniques to assess vascularity and blood flow in the pancreas.[8] Contrast-enhanced ultrasound imaging in the cat is not yet well established, but the obtained baseline data may serve as reference values in the future assessment of cats with kidney, liver, pancreatic, intestinal, or lymph node disease or suspected vascular compromise.[7] However, the only well-established and current clinical indication for use of contrast-enhanced ultrasound in veterinary medicine is detection and characterization of focal lesions in the liver and spleen in dogs.

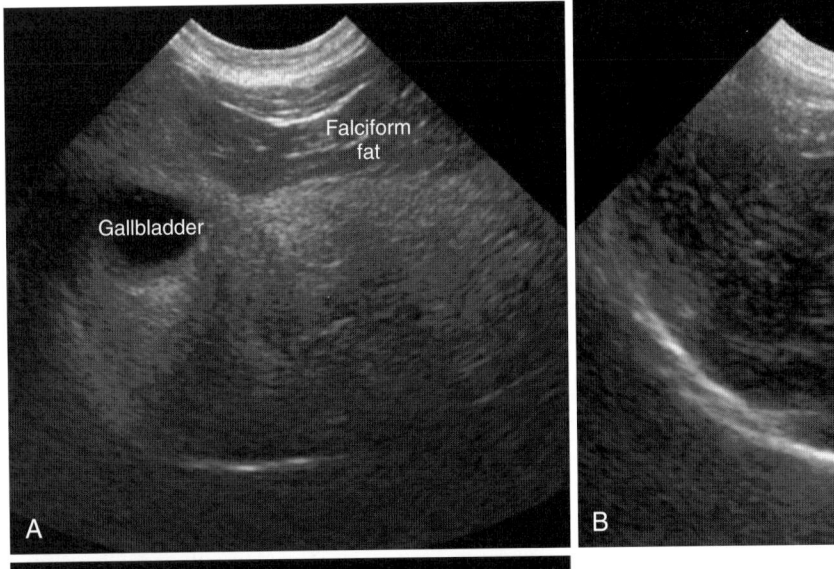

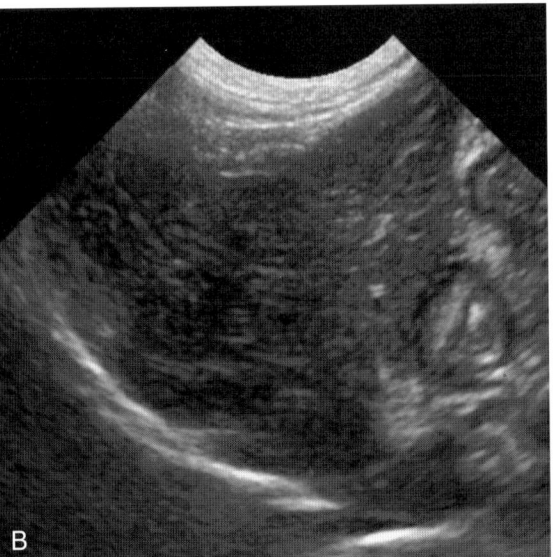

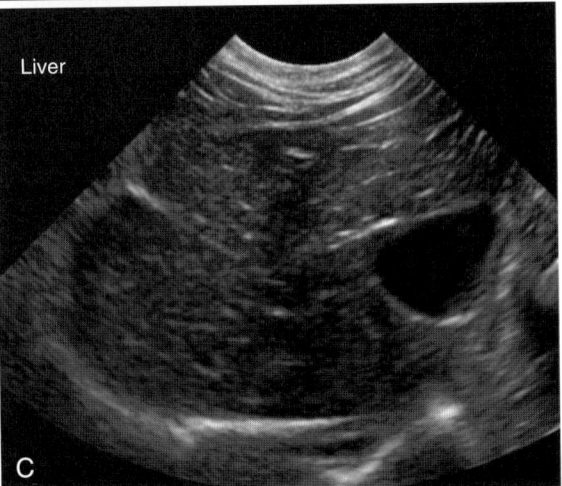

Figure 14-7: A, Transverse ultrasound image of a diffusely hyperechoic liver. Note that the liver is hyperechoic compared to the falciform fat. Also, the liver is diffusely homogenous and the portal vein markings are no longer as evident as in a normal liver. Diagnosis in this cat was hepatic lipidosis. Common differential diagnoses for this appearance are diabetes mellitus, lymphoma, or hepatitis. **B,** Diffusely hypoechoic pancreas in a cat with acute hepatitis. **C,** Diffusely hypoechoic liver in a cat with hepatic lymphoma. Note the similarity with the image in **B.** This underscores the necessity for tissue sampling.

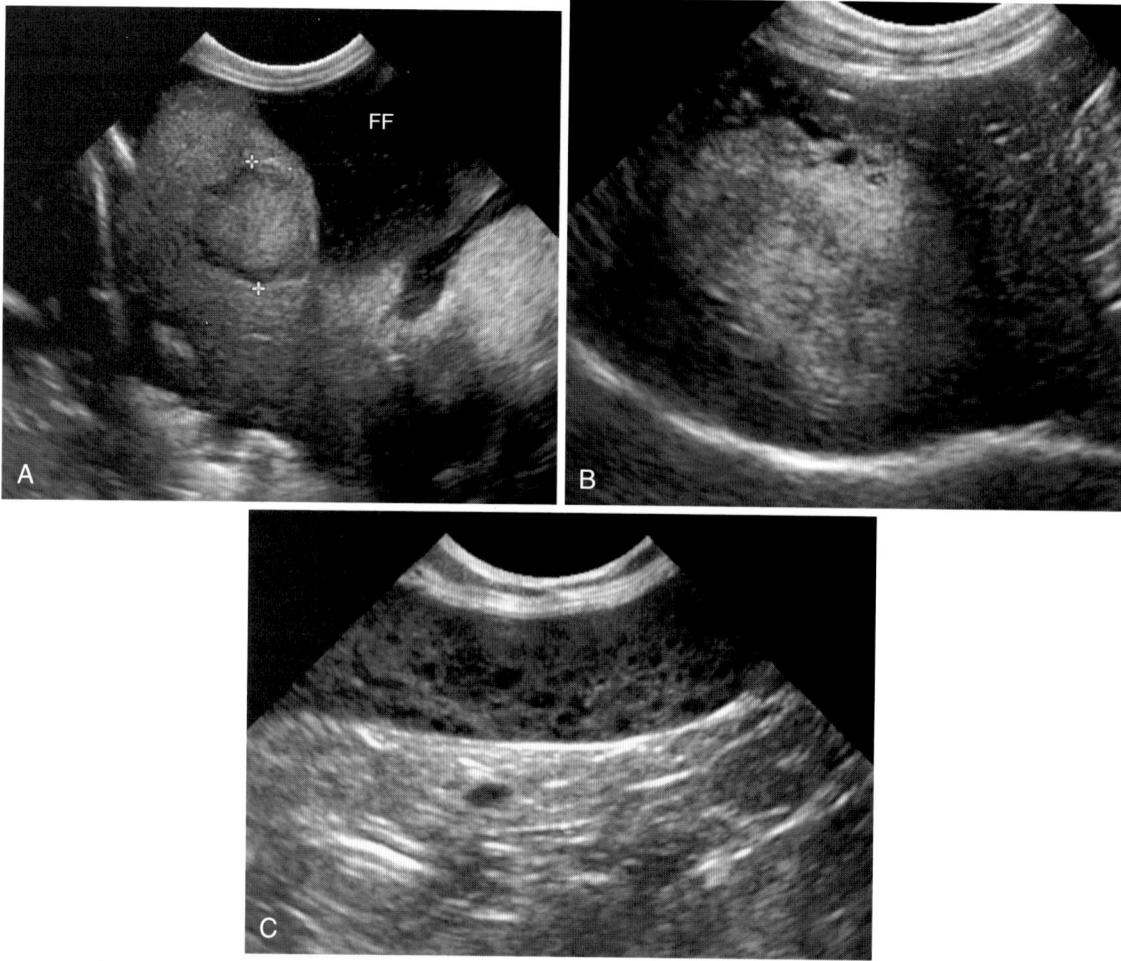

Figure 14-8: A, Cat with hepatic lymphoma. There is a targetoid lesion (+ to +) in the liver, as well as free peritoneal fluid. The focal nodule has an outer hypoechoic rim and a hyperechoic center, the main feature of a targetoid lesion. The presence of a targetoid lesion increases the likelihood of neoplasia, but necrosis due to infection cannot be ruled out. Tissue sampling is indicated to differentiate the two. The targetoid liver lesion was confirmed as lymphoma. **B,** Large irregularly shaped hyperechoic hepatic mass diagnosed as lymphoma. **C,** Spleen in the same cat shown in **B** with lymphoma. The splenic parenchyma has diffuse small and variably-sized hypoechoic foci. The main differential for this finding is lymphoma or extramedullary hematopoiesis.

GALLBLADDER

Radiographically, an enlarged gallbladder typically appears as a focal, well-demarcated, soft tissue mass at the cranioventral aspect of the liver, on the right of midline, adjacent to the thoracic spine (Figure 14-9). It can be mistaken as an enlarged liver lobe because the gallbladder can become enlarged to that extent. The presence of an enlarged gallbladder may be due to fasting or anorexia as well as obstruction, and ultrasonography is generally the next diagnostic test required to confirm and determine the cause of an enlarged gallbladder.

Ultrasonographically, the gallbladder, cystic duct, and common bile duct can be consistently visualized in the cat. The gallbladder may be bilobed as a normal variant in the cat (Figure 14-10). In most cats, the common bile duct can be traced to the major duodenal papilla where it joins with the major pancreatic duct before entering the papilla and duodenum. The gallbladder wall should be barely perceptible as a

thin hyperechoic rim or possibly no rim at all may be visible. The content should be anechoic. This is the same for the cystic and bile ducts. The common bile duct can be identified as a tubular structure coursing ventral to and parallel with the portal vein, most easily recognized at the porta hepatis (Figure 14-11). The gallbladder wall should be less than 1 mm thick and the diameter of the common bile duct less than 4 mm. Gallbladder volume can be calculated with the basic measurements package of most ultrasound units. Fasted mean gallbladder volume has been shown to be 2.42 mL with a range of 0.84 to 4.50 mL in healthy cats.[9] Gallbladder distention is not always present in cats with bile duct obstruction. Gallbladder dilation was seen in less than 50% of cats with bile duct obstruction in one study.[10] Bile duct obstruction can be recognized sonographically as either luminal, mural, or extramural. External compression by regional lymph nodes, the pancreas, or hepatic masses can occur. Duodenal foreign body has also been documented as causing blockage of the bile duct.[11] Mural thickening can lead to stenosis and

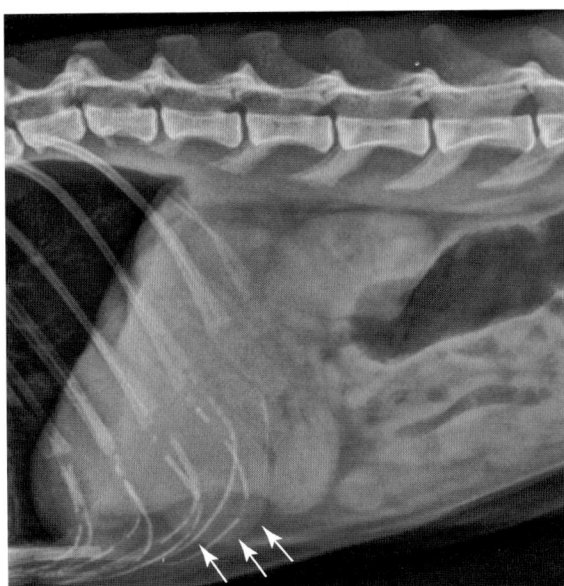

Figure 14-9: Enlarged Gallbladder. The *arrows* mark the ventral borders of an enlarged gallbladder and its typical radiographic location. The gallbladder appears as a focal, soft tissue opaque, rounded, and smoothly-bordered structure at the ventral liver margin.

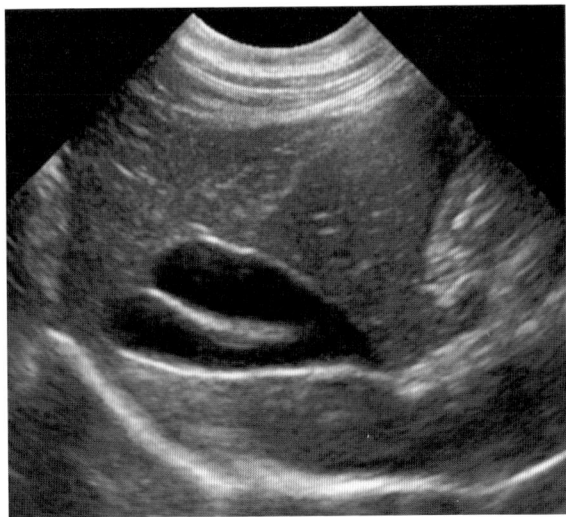

Figure 14-10: Ultrasound Image of a Bilobed Gallbladder. This is a normal finding in the cat.

intraluminal sludge balls, and choledocholiths can similarly cause complete or partial obstruction. Determining if a bile duct obstruction is present in the presence of one of these findings is not necessarily easy. The determination is often a combination of the ultrasound findings, clinical condition, and bilirubin levels. Obstructions can occur at any point along the path of the bile duct, but the papilla is a common site. Extrahepatic biliary obstruction in cats can be due to neoplasia, inflammation, and choleliths (see Chapter 16).[10] A common bile duct diameter over 5 mm has been reported in 97% of cats with extrahepatic biliary obstruction. In that study, ultrasound identified all obstructive choleliths (calculus or plugs) in the common bile duct. Cholestasis due to biliary mucocele has been reported but is extremely rare.[12]

A thickened gallbladder wall is generally seen in cats with cholangitis or cholecystitis. Wall thickness greater than 1 mm

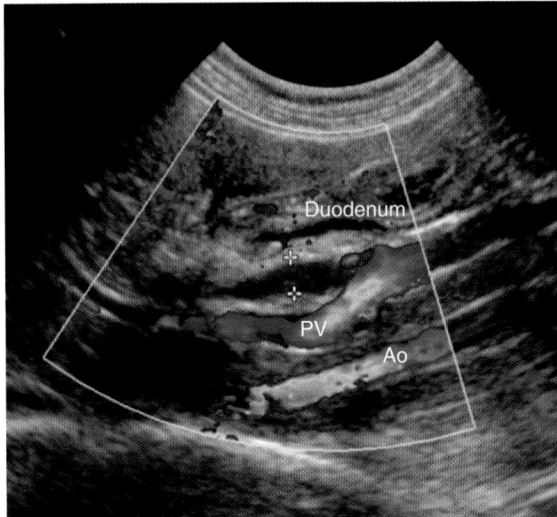

Figure 14-11: Color Doppler ultrasound image showing the normal common bile duct (+ to +) located between the portal vein *(PV)* and duodenum. *Ao,* Aorta.

is accurate in predicting gallbladder disease in cats, although a thickness less than 1 mm cannot rule out mild or chronic inflammation[13] (Figure 14-12). Gallbladder and ductal content that becomes echogenic can be mobile or wall associated. Biliary sludge, sludge balls, and mucosal hyperplasia can be detected. However, Doppler ultrasonography should be utilized in order to assess whether focal accumulation of echogenic material is attached to the wall or not. Wall-associated structures can be due to inflammatory polyps or neoplasia. Similar focal infiltrative nodules can occur at the major duodenal papilla and be either obstructive or nonobstructive. Having fewer mucus glands in the gallbladder may explain why mucoceles do not develop in the cat.[14]

BILE DUCTS

The common bile duct of the cat is long and sinuous compared with the dog. In the cat, the common bile duct fuses in an ampulla with the pancreatic duct just before entering the duodenal papilla about 3 cm caudal to the pylorus.[14] In some cats, the major pancreatic duct opens separately but immediately adjacent to the common bile duct. Approximately 2 cm caudal to the major duodenal papilla, the accessory pancreatic duct enters the duodenum (minor duodenal papilla) in 20% of cats.[14] Although two ducts nearly always drain the pancreas in both species, a great deal of variation exists. Because of the close proximity of the pancreas and common bile duct, pancreatitis commonly influences bile flow through the major bile duct, causing obstruction to flow and jaundice. In the cat, inflammatory, neoplastic, or obstructive disorders involving the distal common bile duct can affect both the biliary tree and pancreas (Figure 14-13). In fact, it is possible that microlithiasis or sludged bile transiently obstructing the distal common bile duct causes intermittent bile duct occlusion and idiopathic pancreatitis in the cat. Blood supply to the intrahepatic bile ducts is provided

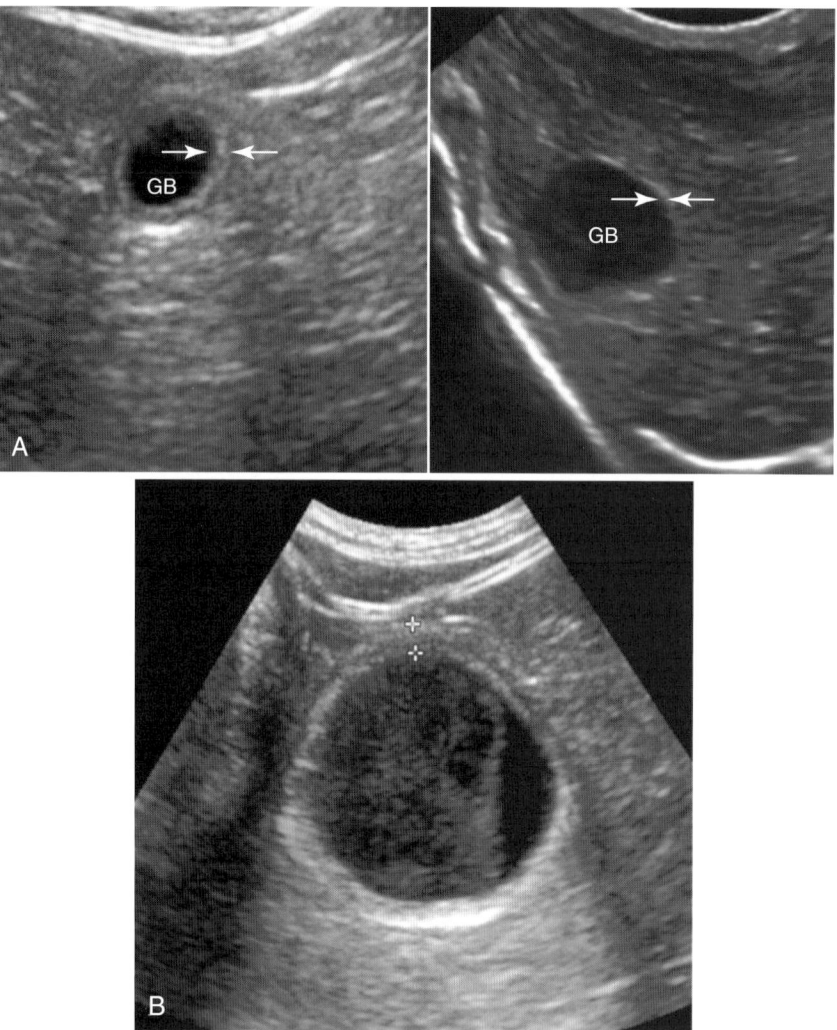

Figure 14-12: **A,** The ultrasound image on the *left* is from a cat with cholecystitis. There is generalized thickening of the gallbladder wall *(between arrows)*. Compare to the normal, thin-walled feline gallbladder on the *right*. **B,** Cat with icterus and cholecystitis. The gallbladder wall is thickened (+ to +), and there is heterogenous echogenic sludge in the bile in the lumen.

GB, gallbladder.

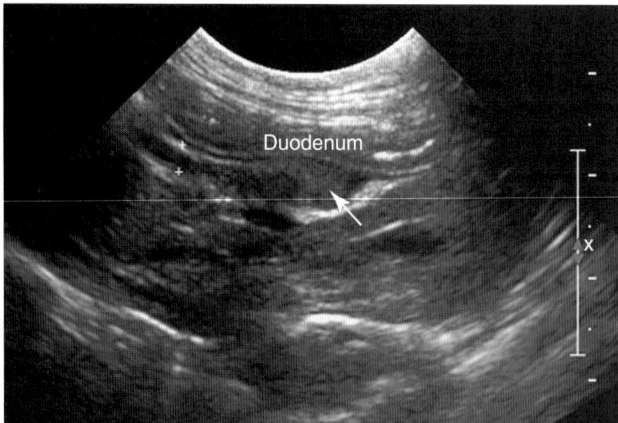

Figure 14-13: Inflammatory polyp of the major duodenal papilla *(arrow)* confirmed at surgery in an icteric cat. Partial obstruction of the common bile duct was occurring (+ to +).

by the hepatic arterial and portal venous circulations. Consequently, hematogenously disseminated infectious agents may involve the intrahepatic biliary tree.[14]

Cholangiohepatitis and cholecystitis can give rise to choleliths in cats or the choleliths can be caused by bile duct obstruction.[15,16] Choleliths in cats are reported as being composed of calcium salts and cholesterol (Figure 14-14). Mixed composition can be a combination of cholesterol with lesser amounts of protein, bilirubin, bile salts, and inorganic minerals.[17] They can also be comprised entirely of bilirubin due to chronic hemolysis in cats with pyruvate kinase deficiency that may be found in Abyssinians and Somalis. They can be incidental findings or associated with extrahepatic bile duct obstruction.

Biliary cystadenomas (Figure 14-4A) can create a large, smoothly marginated mass of soft tissue opacity in the cranioventral abdomen that silhouettes with the liver, but they are more typically identified sonographically.[18] Biliary cystadenomas are usually solitary but can be multiple, and cats

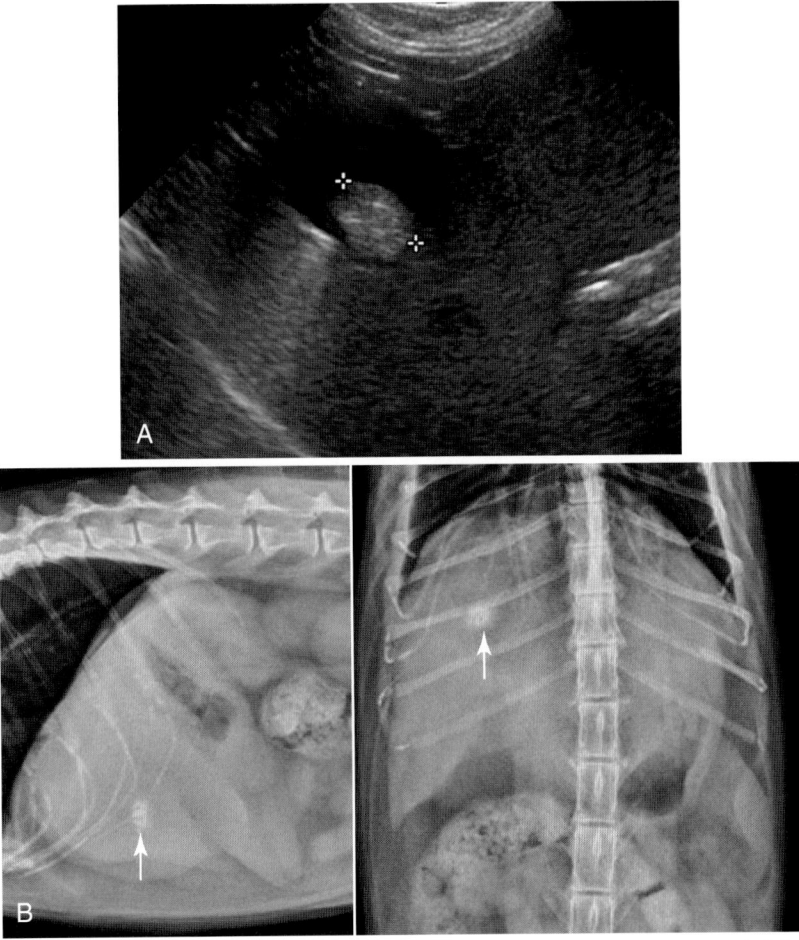

Figure 14-14: **A,** A round hyperechoic structure with distal shadowing represents a cholelith (+ to +). **B,** Radiographs of the same cat as in **A,** showing the cholelith *(arrow).* Note the cranioventral and right-sided location of the gallbladder.

greater than 10 years of age are more commonly affected. They usually do not result in clinical signs unless they become very large and compress adjacent structures, such as the stomach.[18]

Multifocal hypoechoic or anechoic cavities or tubular structures in the liver are commonly associated with dilation of the intrahepatic bile ducts. Causes include cholestasis due to biliary cystadenomas and cystadenocarcinomas, as well as parasitic cysts. Color Doppler ultrasonography is a useful tool for differentiating dilated intrahepatic bile ducts from vascular structures (Figure 14-15B).

Extrahepatic cyst (choledochal cyst) is a rare cause of bile duct obstruction.[19,20] Surgical drainage, subtotal resection, and omentalization of the cyst, along with supportive medical management, has been reported as successful treatment of the clinical signs. A common bile duct cyst was established by ultrasound examination and laparotomy and was ultimately confirmed by histological analysis and removed surgically. Cysts of the common bile duct require treatment because of their common association with cholangitis, pancreatitis, and cystic rupture.[20] Histological examination of cyst tissue is mandatory for a definitive diagnosis and to differentiate it from neoplasia.

Gas can be recognized in the bile duct lumen as hyperechoic foci that have reverberation artifacts. Gas generally originates from the GI tract and can be a source of not only biliary emphysema but also infection.

Cholangitis is a common inflammatory disorder of the biliary system in cats, and ultrasound is a common imaging modality used to screen for it. In a retrospective study evaluating 26 cats with a histologic diagnosis of cholangitis, most had a sonographically normal liver size, echogenicity, and normal biliary system.[21] Statistically significant sonographic changes for cats with cholangitis included hyperechoic liver parenchyma, hyperechoic gallbladder contents, and increased pancreatic size. Cats with the sonographic features of diffuse liver hyperechogenicity, gallbladder contents, and enlarged pancreas may suggest cholangitis.[21]

Hepatobiliary scintigraphy (HBS) can be used to diagnose biliary obstruction. In seven animals with biliary obstruction that had HBS performed, using nonvisualization of the intestine by 180 minutes as the scintigraphic criterion for diagnosis of biliary obstruction, sensitivity was 83%, and specificity was 94% in this series.[22] Hepatobiliary scintigraphy failed to demonstrate radiolabel within either the gallbladder or intestine at any time when obstruction was

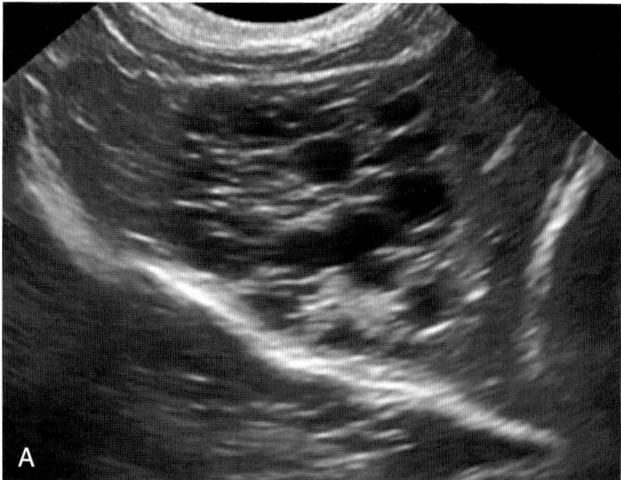

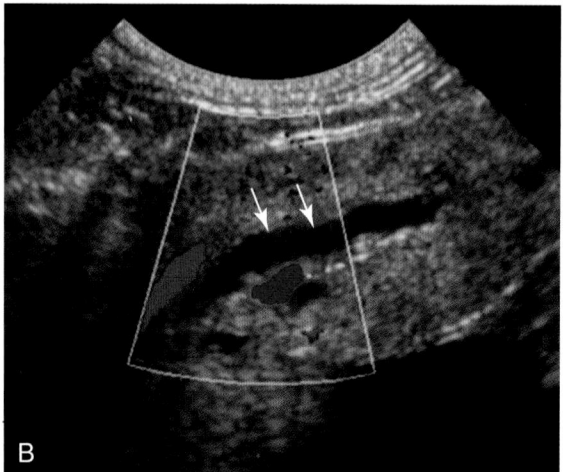

Figure 14-15: A, Multiple hypoechoic cavities throughout the liver parenchyma in a cat with biliary cystadenomas. Differential diagnoses include biliary adenocarcinoma, and parasitic infection. **B,** Intrahepatic bile duct dilation *(arrows)* due to chronic cholangiohepatitis and bile duct obstruction. Doppler ultrasound aids in differentiating dilated blood vessels from bile ducts.

present.[23] Hepatobiliary scintigraphy was concluded to be an accurate indicator of extrahepatic biliary obstruction in this group of animals.[22]

HEPATIC FUNCTION

Hepatobiliary scintigraphy can be useful in cats with hepatobiliary disease, to assess the severity of hepatic dysfunction and to determine if extrahepatic biliary obstruction is present.[24] In a group of 10 cats with histologically documented hepatobiliary disease, the scintigraphic pattern could be correlated to the histological severity. However, correlation between hepatobiliary scintigraphic patterns and specific disease entities (such as hepatic lipidosis or cholangitis-cholangiohepatitis syndrome) could not be made in this study.[24] In another study that assessed hepatic function pre- and post-liver fluke infestation *(Platynosomum concinnum)*, it was shown that despite the presence of severe multifocal histologic abnormalities, minimal clinical, biochemical, and scintigraphic derange-

ments were identified using this model of cholangiohepatitis.[25] Based on this study, HBS appears to be an insensitive test for structural hepatobiliary abnormalities.[25]

PORTOSYSTEMIC VASCULAR DISEASE

Congenital portosystemic shunting is not as common in cats as in dogs, and abdominal ultrasonography is generally the most common imaging modality used for confirmation following clinical pathology and abdominal radiography. Although abdominal radiographs may show a small liver, ultrasonography allows the shunt vessel to be directly visualized (Figure 14-16). However, the lack of identification of a shunting vessel does not rule out its presence, and cross-sectional imaging (such as CT-angiography or portal scintigraphy) may be required.[26,27] Trans-splenic portal scintigraphy using ^{99m}Tc-pertechnetate is a well-established technique in the dog and can also be used in the cat.[27] Extrahepatic portosystemic shunts are the most common and are usually left gastric vein, portoazygous, portocaval, colonic, or gastrosplenic types.[26,28] In one study, 70% of cats with left gastric vein shunts had a shunt that entered the left phrenic vein, and 30% entered the post hepatic caudal vena cava.[29] Both intrahepatic and extrahepatic shunts can be diagnosed with a high level of accuracy using ultrasonography.[28] Acquired shunts are even less common than the congenital type and splenosystemic shunts are described (see Figure 14-16D). Forty-two percent of cats with splenosystemic shunts in a recent study had hepatopathy associated with the presence of a splenosystemic shunt, but no specific diseases were found to be correlated in the remainder.[30]

THE PANCREAS

The diagnosis of feline pancreatitis is complex and should be based on a combination of clinical signs, blood results including feline pancreatic lipase immunoreactivity (fPLI) and ultrasound (see Chapter 15).[31] The sensitivity of ultrasound alone for diagnosing pancreatitis in cats is low, ranging from 11% to 35%. Currently, there are no universally agreed upon guidelines or parameters for diagnosing feline pancreatitis with ultrasound. However, attention to pancreatic size, echotexture and peripancreatic changes, and the presence of multi-organ disease help support the diagnosis.

Ultrasonography is currently one of the most commonly used tools for the diagnosis of pancreatitis in dogs and cats. Ultrasound is widely available today, but the sonographic examination of the pancreas is highly user dependent. An excellent knowledge of anatomy, as well as experience, is required to both locate the pancreas and interpret its appearance.[32]

The normal feline pancreas is best visualized with a high frequency transducer, curved or linear array, at least 7.5 MHz (Figure 14-17). The portal vein is a consistent anatomic landmark for identification of the left lobe and body of the

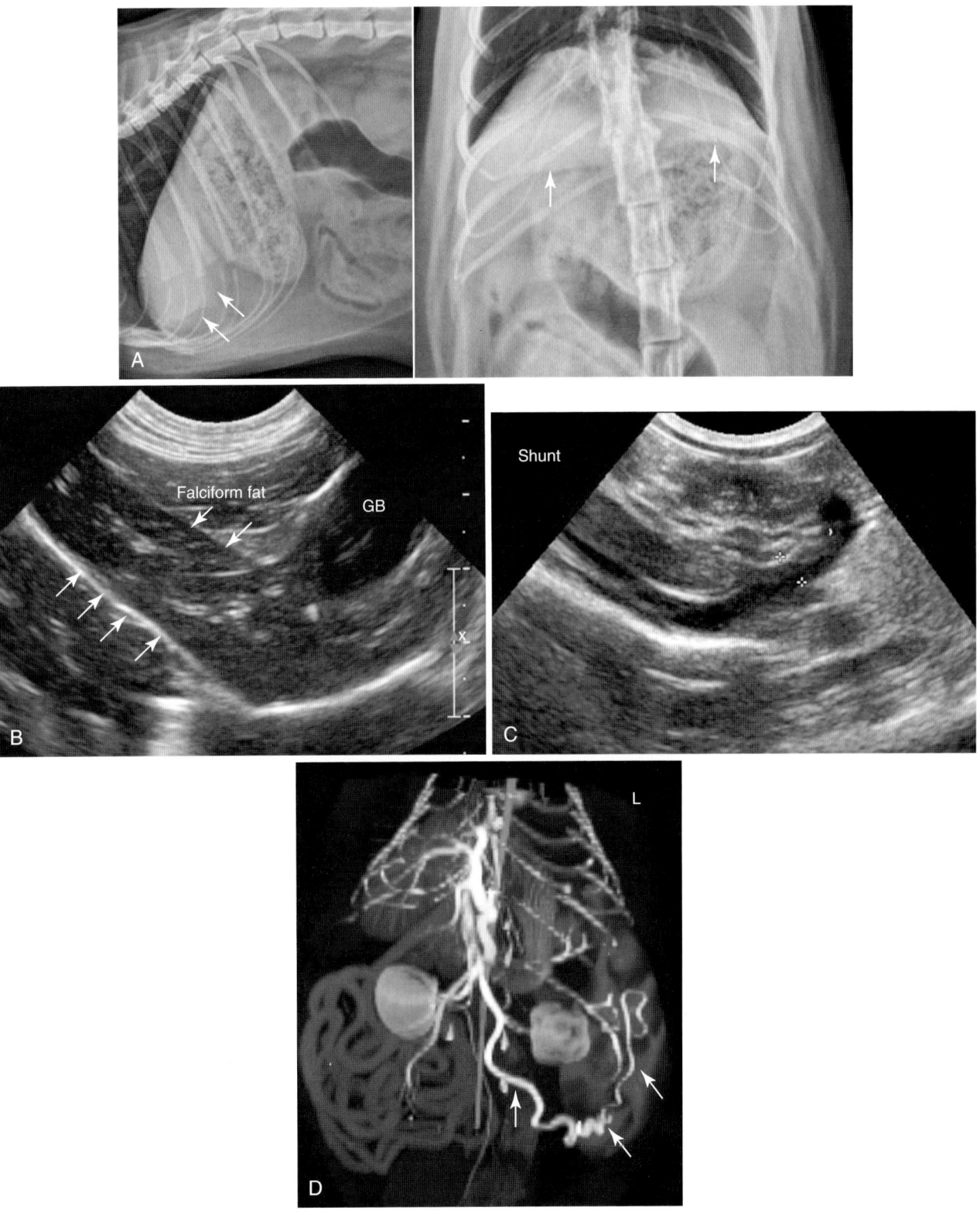

Figure 14-16: A, Lateral *(left)* and ventrodorsal *(right)* radiographs of a cat with an extrahepatic portosystemic shunt. Microhepatia is present. *Arrows* mark the caudal extent of the liver, which is very small. **B,** Small liver *(between arrows)* in the same cat as in **A,** which is due to extrahepatic portosystemic shunt. **C,** Large aberrant extrahepatic shunt vessel in the same cat as in **A** and **B.** **D,** Maximum intensity projection image of a computed tomographic (CT) angiogram in a cat with a splenorenal shunt *(arrows).* The cat was examined for assessment of a soft tissue sarcoma with CT, and this was an incidental finding. The cat had no clinical signs at the time.

GB, gallbladder.

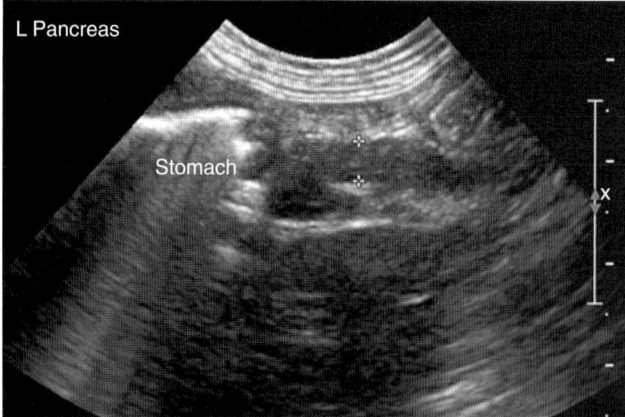

Figure 14-17: Ultrasound of a Normal Feline Left Pancreatic Limb. The left limb is immediately caudal to the gastric body and is smoothly bordered and hypoechoic.

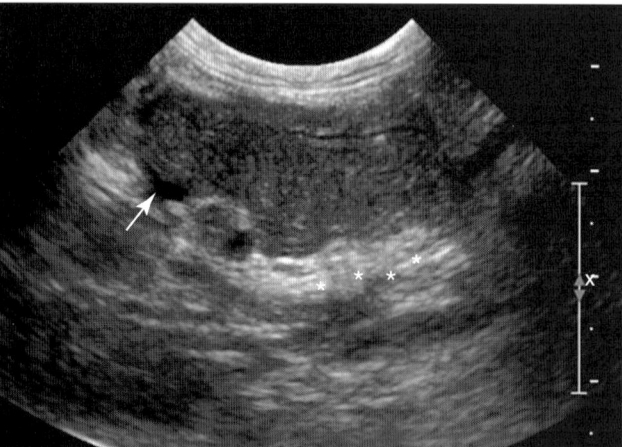

Figure 14-18: Acute Pancreatitis. Enlarged, hypoechoic pancreas with irregular borders and a small amount of peritoneal free fluid *(arrow)* and peripancreatic hyperechoic mesentery *(*).

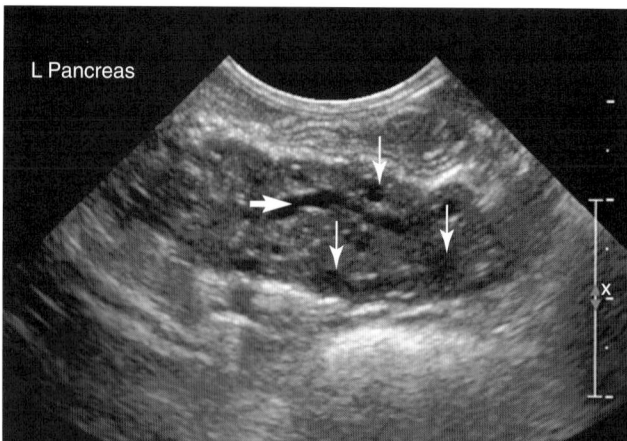

Figure 14-19: Irregularly-Shaped Left Pancreatic Limb. The parenchyma is heterogenous, and there are multiple small, rounded, hypoechoic foci randomly arranged throughout the parenchyma *(small arrows mark some of these).* The *large arrow* points to the tubular pancreatic duct in the center of the pancreas. The hypoechoic foci are commonly associated with hyperplastic nodules. Differentials include retention cysts and neoplasia.

pancreas. The duodenum serves as a landmark for identification of the right pancreatic limb. Once the portal vein is located in the sagittal plane, the left pancreatic limb is located to its left and caudal to the body of the stomach. The left limb is generally much easier to identify due to its size and location compared with the right limb in the cat.

The normal pancreas is homogenous, finely textured, and isoechoic to the surrounding mesentery, hyperechoic to the liver, and hypoechoic to the spleen.[32] The mean thickness measurements for the right pancreatic lobe, body, and left pancreatic lobe were 4.5 mm (range 2.8 to 5.9), 6.6 mm (range 4.7 to 9.4), and 5.4 mm (range 3.4 to 9.0), respectively.[32] The pancreatic duct is consistently visualized in the left pancreatic lobe and has a mean thickness of 0.8 mm (range 0.5 to 1.3).[32]

In acute disease, the pancreas may become enlarged as in dogs (Figure 14-18). However, this finding is much more inconsistent in cats than in dogs. In chronic disease, the pancreas may be of normal size or smaller and may be hypoechoic or hyperechoic, or normal in appearance. Unremarkable findings do not rule out pancreatitis in cats. In cats,

multiple hypoechoic round foci of a few millimeters in diameter may also be recognized. These may represent nodular hyperplasia or dilated pancreatic ducts[33] (Figure 14-19). The main differential diagnosis for an enlarged, irregularly-shaped pancreas with nodules is pancreatic carcinoma (Figure 14-20). Tissue sampling is imperative for diagnosis.

Cavities of the pancreas in cats are typically either due to abscesses or pseudocysts and appear anechoic or hypoechoic, possibly with a thickened wall (Figure 14-21). A number of investigators have attempted to assess the sensitivity and specificity of ultrasound compared to other imaging modalities for diagnosing pancreatitis in cats, however, with greatly varying results.[34]

Magnetic resonance imaging and magnetic resonance cholangiopancreatography (MRCP) have developed into accurate, highly sensitive and specific imaging tools for the diagnosis of biliary and pancreatic duct disorders in humans.[35] Little has been published in veterinary medicine using MRI to diagnose hepatobiliary disease, however. One study in cats showed that MRI could detect pancreatic abnormalities not seen with ultrasonography.[35] These abnormalities consisted of a pancreatic parenchymal T2 hyperintensity and T1 hypointensity in cats suspected of having pancreatitis.[35] The advantages of MRI/MRCP over sonography of these cats included the striking pancreatic signal changes associated with pancreatitis and the ability to comprehensibly assess and measure the pancreas and hepatobiliary structures without operator dependence or interference from bowel gas. MRI/MRCP imaging of the feline abdomen may be beneficial in cases with equivocal ultrasound imaging findings.[35]

INTERVENTIONAL PROCEDURES

Due to the lack of sensitivity and specificity of ultrasonography for liver disease, tissue sampling is necessary in most cats

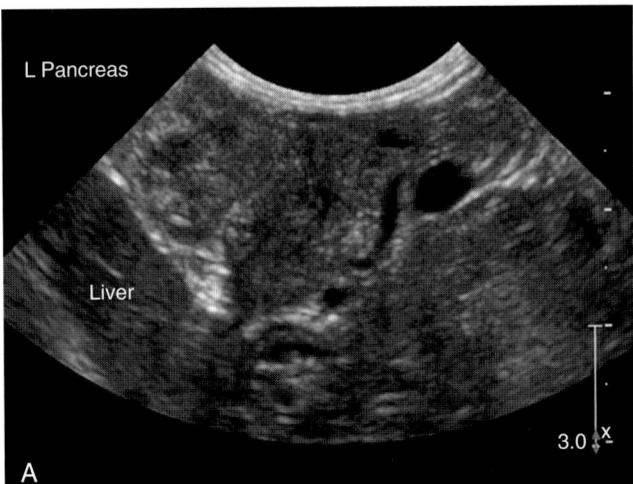

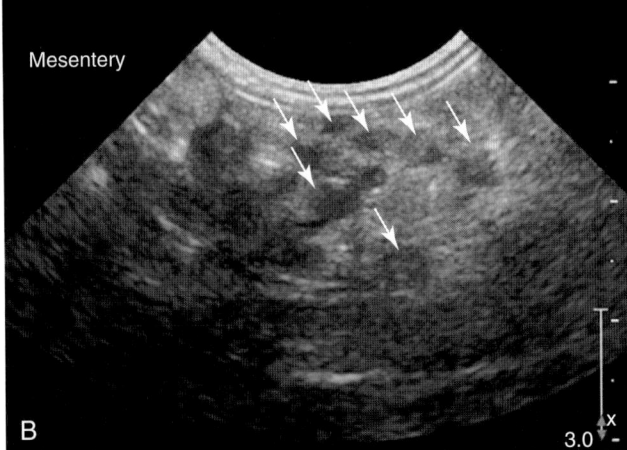

Figure 14-20: A, Large heterogenous pancreas with an irregular shape and nodular architecture in a cat with pancreatic carcinoma. **B,** Carcinomatosis in same cat as in **A.** There are numerous small hypoechoic nodules *(arrows)* throughout the mesentery that were due to carcinomatosis secondary to pancreatic carcinoma.

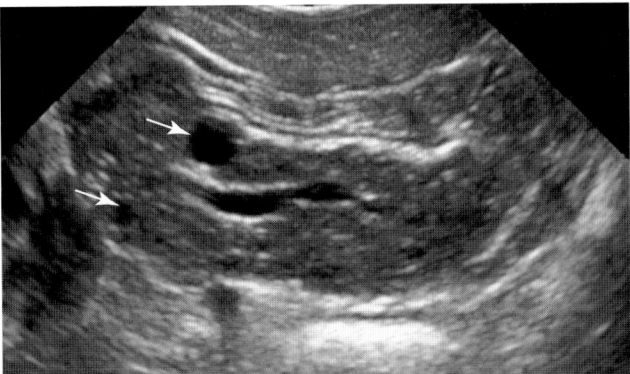

Figure 14-21: Two round anechoic cavities *(arrows)* present in this pancreas are consistent with retention cysts.

with suspected liver disease. If liver disease is suspected and the liver appears normal on ultrasound, tissue sampling should still be performed. Fine-needle aspiration (FNA) of the liver can be performed quickly and relatively inexpensively for cytological analysis of the liver for either diffuse or

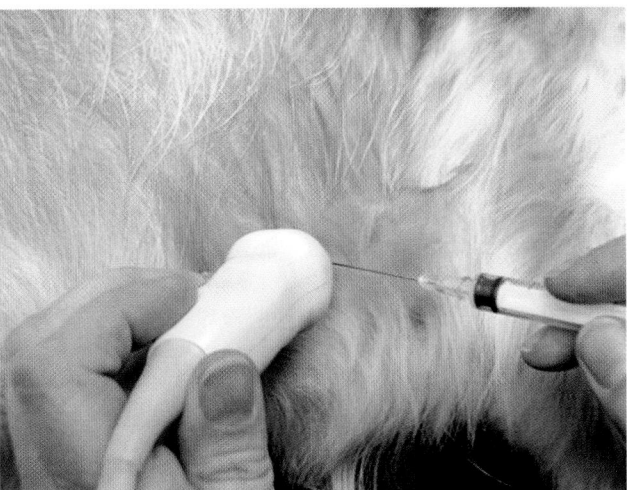

Figure 14-22: Ultrasound-Guided Fine-Needle Aspiration of the Liver. The needle is manually lined up with the center of the probe and angled at 45 degrees so that it is best visible in the center of the ultrasound image.

multifocal disease. Ultrasound-guided Tru-Cut liver biopsies can also be performed. A solitary report emphasized that these can have complications in cats. However, it is a widely used and commonly performed procedure that has been shown to be safe in the cat. Coagulation parameters should be assessed prior to Tru-Cut biopsy but are not necessarily required prior to FNA unless an underlying coagulopathy is suspected.

Ultrasound-guided FNA and Tru-Cut biopsy are commonly used for tissue sampling of the liver in cats because they can be performed in the sedated animal compared with the need for general anesthesia and laparotomy for obtaining larger samples. However, ultrasound-guided FNA for cytologic examination of the liver has limitations when used to identify the primary disease process in dogs and cats compared to histological evaluation.[36] Cytological evaluation of the liver may correlate to histopathological examination in cats only approximately 50% of the time.[36] Vacuolar hepatopathy is one of the most common cytological diagnoses in dogs and cats, being more prevalent in cats.[36] Unfortunately, vacuolar hepatopathy is often present secondary to other primary liver diseases that are better recognized histopathologically. Fine-needle aspiration and cytology may not detect infiltrative lesions, particularly those that are nodular, multifocal, or localized around the portal regions.[37] Fine-needle aspiration cytology is a useful diagnostic procedure with many advantages, but care must be taken to avoid diagnosing hepatic lipidosis as the cause of illness when an infiltrative lesion is responsible.[37]

Fine-Needle Aspiration and Biopsy

Technique for Fine Needle-Aspiration

A 22-gauge, 1.5 inch needle is adequate for obtaining FNA samples for cytology. Free-hand (Figure 14-22) or guided techniques can be used, but free-handed needle insertion is generally used for small animals, such as cats, where the distance to the target organ is small. The plane of needle insertion must be in the midline plane of the transducer, and the needle should pass obliquely across the ultrasound beam to enhance visibility. The sampling technique varies among operators and organs being aspirated. The stab or woodpecker technique involves getting the needle tip to the region of interest and stabbing the needle back and forth a few times and then withdrawing the needle. The suction technique involves three to four gentle suctions when the needle tip is in the area of interest but may result in more blood contamination of the sample.

Technique for Tru-Cut Biopsy

Tru-Cut type tissue biopsy needles are used to obtain samples for histology. Needle size for cats should be 18-gauge for most organs due to their smaller size. Needle guidance systems can be used, but the free-hand method is commonly employed because of the small size of the cat. Both can be performed at the same time in the same cat if desired. Semiautomated or fully automated spring-loaded needles are most commonly used and easiest. The spring loaded device should be checked for needle depth penetration and compared to the region of the liver that is to be sampled. Typical depths are 2 cm for fully automated devices, and the depth of the liver needs to be approximately twice that for safety reasons. The diaphragm and the liver hilus need to be avoided. If the liver is too small, Tru-Cut samples should not be obtained and surgical biopsies should be performed instead.

Automated biopsy gun samples in feline hepatic biopsies have been associated with 19% of cats developing severe shock compared to 0% when using a semiautomated biopsy gun. This is believed to be due to the pressure wave created by the automatic device resulting in intense vagotonia.[38] However, this complication has not been encountered by others.

Cholecystocentesis

Percutaneous ultrasound-guided cholecystocentesis is an effective, minimally-invasive, and safe technique enabling identification of bacterial isolates in cats with inflammatory hepatobiliary disease.[39,40] One study showed that the technique is safe in cats.[40] The procedure is performed with a 22-gauge 1.5-inch (3.81 cm) needle with an attached 12-mL syringe via a right-sided transhepatic approach or, more commonly, into the fundus of the gallbladder via a right ventral abdominal approach. Generally, an attempt is made to completely empty the gallbladder during the procedure. Ultrasonographic complications with the right ventral abdominal technique were not observed.[40] Decreased appetite and evidence of mild abdominal pain were detected in four of 12 cats within 2 days after performing cholecystocentesis, and the mean neutrophil count increased 2 days afterward but remained within the reference range.

Samples for aerobic and anaerobic bacteriologic culture should be obtained in cats with the differential diagnoses of bacterial hepatitis/cholangitis. Gallbladder bile is preferred over culture of hepatic tissues and may be obtained with ultrasound-guided percutaneous cholecystocentesis.[41] Complications of image-guided sampling are uncommon but include hemorrhage, which may be assessed postbiopsy via color Doppler screening. Fine-needle aspiration offers limited sensitivity for diagnosis of cholangitis with liver cytology correlating with biopsy results in only 39% to 60% of cases.[42]

Cholangitis is the most common inflammatory condition involving the feline liver and requires special consideration. Multiple hepatic lobes should be biopsied, regardless of the biopsy method employed, because inflammatory lesion severity may vary within and between lobes. Surgical wedge liver biopsies provide the largest and most diagnostically accurate samples. Acquisition of forceps biopsy specimens using laparoscopy may also provide good quality specimens for diagnostic evaluation. Both laparotomy and laparoscopy allow for direct visualization of most hepatobiliary structures and sampling of extrahepatic tissues, as required.

GASTROINTESTINAL RADIOGRAPHY

Survey abdominal radiographs are commonly obtained for noninvasive screening of feline patients presented with clinical signs of GI disease (e.g., vomiting, diarrhea, inappetence, and/or constipation). As a result, a variety of techniques have been proposed to more objectively differentiate between normal and abnormal small intestinal and colonic total diameter in cats.[43,44] The generally uniform size of feline patients provides consistent osseous structures for use as reference standards in determining maximum small intestinal and colonic diameter ratios. Initially, a feline small intestinal diameter greater than 10 to 12 mm was considered abnormally enlarged.[45] Normal feline colonic diameter was previously described as ranging between 1 and 1.5 times the length of the L7 vertebral body.[46] However, recent studies have advocated alternate methods for identification of normal size of these structures (Table 14-1).

Table 14-1	**Feline Total Diameter Ratios for Small Intestine and Colon**	
	Normal Ratio (Lateral View)	**Abnormal Ratio**
Small intestine*	<2 times cranial end plate of the L2 vertebra	>2 times L2 cranial end plate
Colon†	<1.28 times the length of the L5 vertebral body	>1.48 times L5 length

*Adams WM, Sisterman LA, Klauer JM, et al: Association of intestinal disorders in cats with findings of abdominal radiography. *J Am Vet Med Assoc* 236:880-886, 2010.
†Trevail T, Gunn-Moore D, Carrera I, et al: Radiographic diameter of the colon in normal and constipated cats and in cats with megacolon. *Vet Radiol Ultrasound* 52:516-520, 2011.

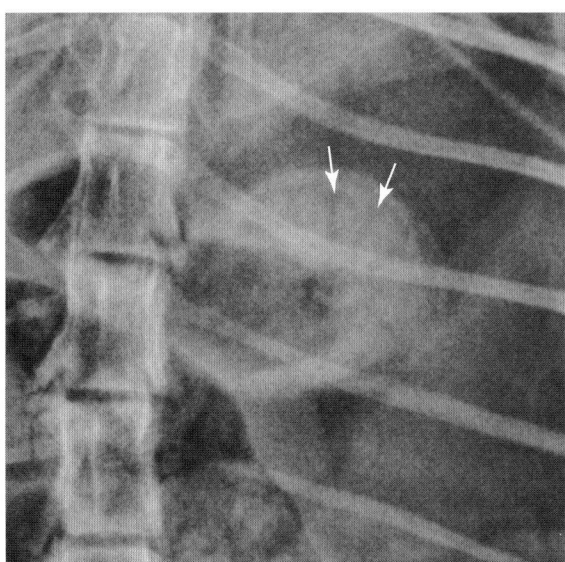

Figure 14-23: Ventrodorsal Radiograph of the Feline Abdomen. The feline stomach has a specific feature where a radiolucent band is interposed between the rugal folds and represents fat *(arrows)* in the submucosa of the gastric wall.

Table 14-2	Feline Positive Contrast Upper Gastrointestinal Study Dose Rates	
Contrast	**Concentration**	**Dose**
Barium sulfate suspension	50% to 60% weight/ volume (liquid)	12-16 mL/kg* or 5 mL/lb
Nonionic iodinated	240 mg Iodine/mL	10 mL/kg (1 : 2 dilution with water)†

*Morgan JP: The upper gastrointestinal examination in the cat: normal radiographic appearance using positive contrast medium. *Vet Radiol* 22:159-169, 1981.
†Williams J, Biller DS, Miyabayashi T, et al: Evaluation of Iohexol as a gastrointestinal contrast medium in normal cats. *Vet Radiol Ultrasound* 34(5):310-314, 1993.

Radiographic variations of the GI tract specific to cats include location of the pylorus at or near midline and fat opacity within the gastric wall, each best seen on the ventrodorsal projection (Figure 14-23). The feline cecum is small, cone-shaped, and not typically air-filled. As a result, visualization of the feline cecum as a specific structure is uncommon, particularly on survey images. The presence of intraluminal GI gas in the cat has been suggested as an unusual finding in earlier investigations.[45,47] However, a more recent study[43] demonstrates that observation of intraluminal gas in the feline GI tract may be more associated with the animal's physical parameters at the time of imaging, such as length of time from most recent meal, administration of enemas, or aerophagia due to stress or pain. A normal intraluminal gas pattern of the small intestine typically consists of linear gas lucencies, which may become round to oval when viewed end-on. Abnormal intraluminal gas patterns include short angular gas lucencies, which are fragmented into irregular segments within tortuous small bowel loops, suggesting a linear foreign body, or disorganized heterogenous gas and soft tissue opacities associated with ingestion of other foreign material.

Survey abdominal radiographs allow for rapid evaluation of the GI tract in cats with suspected mechanical obstruction due to intraluminal, mural, or extrinsic lesions. Addition of a left lateral recumbent view, following a right lateral recumbent projection and prior to the ventrodorsal view, provides an opportunity for gas within the stomach to progress into the proximal duodenum, enhancing duodenal localization and assessing pyloric patency to gas. Survey abdominal radiographs provide a rapid, affordable method for determination of next diagnostic and/or therapeutic steps. Additionally, use of a wooden spoon to gently compress the abdomen may aid in separating bowel loops from one another to better identify abnormal segments (Figure 14-24).[48]

Although less commonly performed in the cat than in the dog, introduction of negative contrast (air) into the stomach or descending colon may provide additional information concerning location of, or communication between, specific anatomic structures (Figure 14-24C). Positive contrast radiography to further assess the feline esophagus or upper gastrointestinal (UGI) tract may be performed with liquid barium.[45] Alternatively, nonionic iodinated contrast agents,[49] such as iohexol, may be administered *per os* if GI perforation is suspected based on survey radiographs (Table 14-2). Images are obtained at 5, 30, and 60 minutes post-contrast administration in the cat. Initiation of gastric emptying during positive contrast UGI studies may be delayed for 20 to 30 minutes due to patient excitement or stress.[44]

GASTROINTESTINAL ULTRASOUND

Abdominal ultrasound plays an integral role in evaluation of feline GI disease through discrimination of mural abnormalities that cannot be differentiated with survey and/or contrast radiographs alone[50,51] (Figure 14-25). Although ultrasound examination of GI wall layers is best performed in cats that have been fasting for 12 hours, ideal patient preparation may not always be obtained. Patient sedation may be required in uncooperative animals or to minimize aerophagia due to vocalization, stress, or discomfort and the resultant increase in gas-soft tissue interface artifacts.

Normal sonographic GI wall layering in cats is well documented.[52-54] A mucosal surface-to-surface hyperechoic interface is present in the empty intestine, surrounded by a distinct hypoechoic mucosal layer (Figure 14-26). The feline GI mucosa is consistently the most prominent layer observed. A thin hyperechoic submucosa, with connective tissue stroma, is fairly consistent in thickness throughout the GI tract. Thickness of the muscularis layer is greatest in the feline ileum, compared with other areas (Figure 14-27). Overall, the hypoechoic muscularis is normally less prominent than the mucosal layer. The feline distal ileum, typically located medial

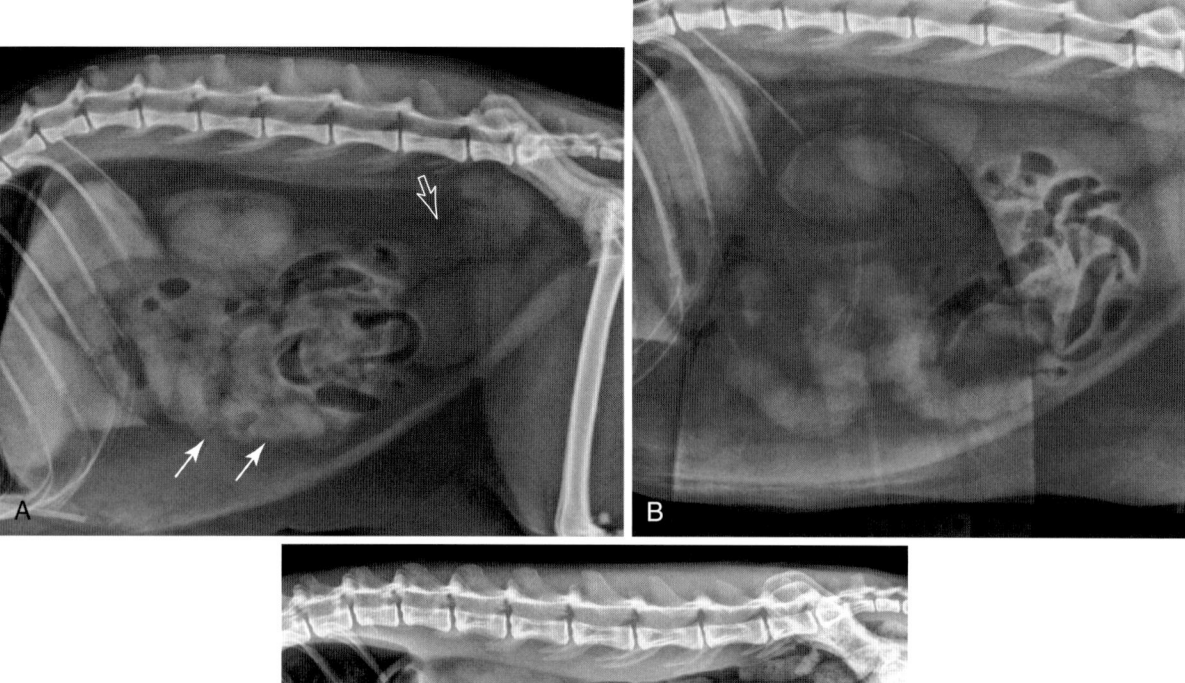

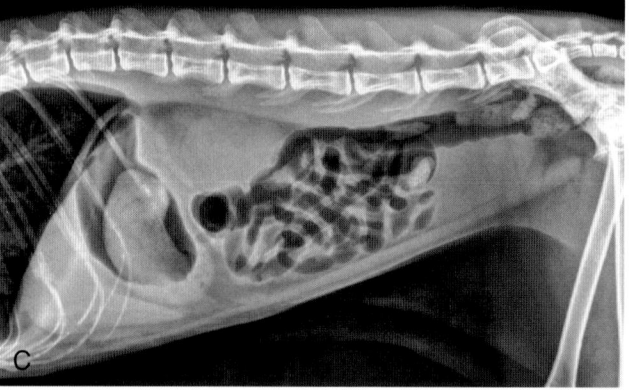

Figure 14-24: A, Lateral abdomen of a vomiting cat. The jejunum in the mid-ventral abdomen is bunched *(arrows),* and there is focal loss of detail. The colon also has an irregular shape *(open arrow).* **B,** Compression of the cranial abdomen with a wooden spoon shows that the bunched jejunal segments in **A** are actually plicated and have a garland-like shape consistent with a linear foreign body, which was confirmed at surgery. **C,** Left lateral recumbent view of an 8-year-old, neutered male domestic longhair cat. The gas-filled stomach highlights the smooth margins of an intraluminal soft tissue/fluid opaque structure. A very large trichobezoar lodged in the pylorus was identified and then removed via endoscopy.

to the right kidney, exhibits a distinctive "wagon wheel" pattern on short-axis images.[55] Finally, the thin, hyperechoic serosa is best seen when oriented as a specular reflector at a 90-degree angle to the transducer. The cecum is infrequently observed, but it can be identified when enlarged or thickened.[56]

Abnormalities of the intestinal wall may be focal, segmental, or diffuse and may obliterate or maintain wall layering. Total thickness (mucosa-to-serosa) of the various portions of the GI tract, as well as thickness of individual layers, should be determined, preferably at multiple sites.[57] A general expectation of a muscularis layer thickness of less than half the submucosal layer thickness has been described.[58] Objective maximum total intestinal wall thickness measurements in cats vary from 0.25 to 0.38 cm.[52,55,57,59,60] Gastric (0.27 to 0.36 cm) and colonic (0.13 to 0.25 cm) maximum total wall thickness ranges have also be described.[53,54] Recently, measurement standardization has been suggested in cats

through determination of ratios between the thickness of the mucosal and muscularis layers and the transverse aortic diameter.[53]

Although considerable overlap between the sonographic appearance of neoplastic disease and nonspecific inflammation of the intestine exists,[57-61] focal loss of wall layering is much more commonly observed with neoplastic conditions or fungal infections. Absence or alteration of normal peristaltic contractions throughout the GI tract should also be noted. Surrounding tissues should be evaluated for abnormally hyperechoic mesenteric fat; pockets of free peritoneal fluid; or enlarged (greater than 0.4 cm),[60] rounded, and/or hypoechoic regional lymph nodes. Identification of changes involving these ancillary structures is critical for prioritizing differentials and next diagnostic steps.

Chronic inflammatory disease may result in mild to moderate increases in total wall thickness or may alter individual layers. Inflammatory bowel disease (IBD) is typically

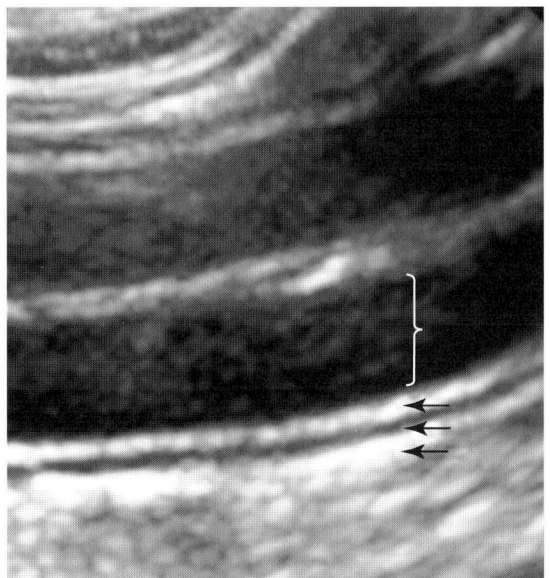

Figure 14-25: Normal longitudinal ultrasound image of the jejunum showing the wall layering. The alternating hyperechoic, hypoechoic, and hyperechoic layers moving from the mucosa to the serosa *(black arrows)* are thin and uniform. *Bracket,* Mucosal layer.

generalized but can be segmental. Distinction between the wall layers is typically preserved in animals with lymphocytic, plasmacytic, and eosinophilic enteritis. However, the muscularis may be thickened in both diffuse IBD as well as diffuse lymphoma[58] (see Figures 14-26 and 14-27; Figure 14-28.)

Sonographic evaluation of the GI tract is also commonly performed to confirm the presence of suspected GI foreign bodies, including linear foreign bodies, prior to surgical removal.[62-67]

ULTRASOUND-GUIDED SAMPLE COLLECTION

Common clinical indications in animals with chronic gastroenteritis include evaluation of enlarged mesenteric lymph nodes, increased intestinal wall thickness, and intestinal masses. For FNA, an 18- to 20-gauge needle is inserted into the selected site with ultrasound-guidance and aspirated, most commonly using a free-hand technique. Specific needle types may vary, including standard hypodermic needles or those containing stylets (Wescott spinal needles) for

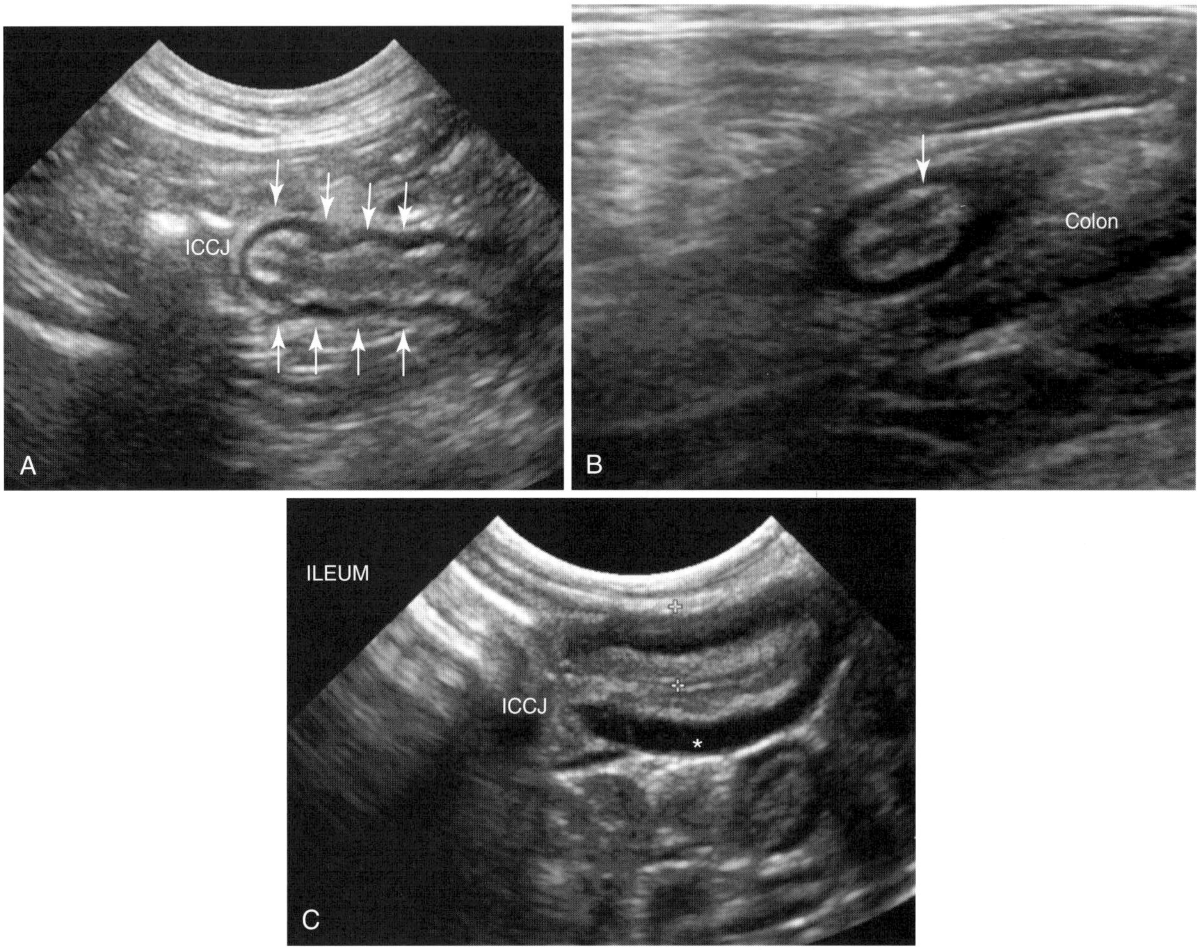

Figure 14-26: **A,** Longitudinal ultrasound image of the feline ileum at the ileocecocolic junction *(ICCJ).* **B,** Normal ileum in the transverse plane has a wagon wheel appearance *(arrow)* adjacent to the ascending colon. **C,** Cat with lymphoma. The ileum is infiltrated, and its wall is 6 mm thick (+ to +) with prominent hypoechoic muscular wall layer *(*).*

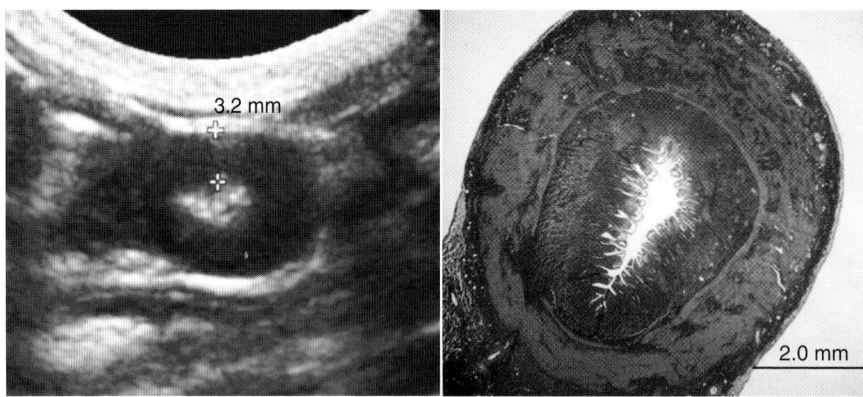

Figure 14-27: Transverse Image of a Jejunal Segment in a Vomiting Cat. The wall is thickened at 3.2 mm (+ to +), and there is transmural hypoechoic loss of wall layering. The corresponding histopathologic image shows a uniform population of round cells stained purple (hematoxylin and eosin stain) throughout all layers of the intestinal wall.

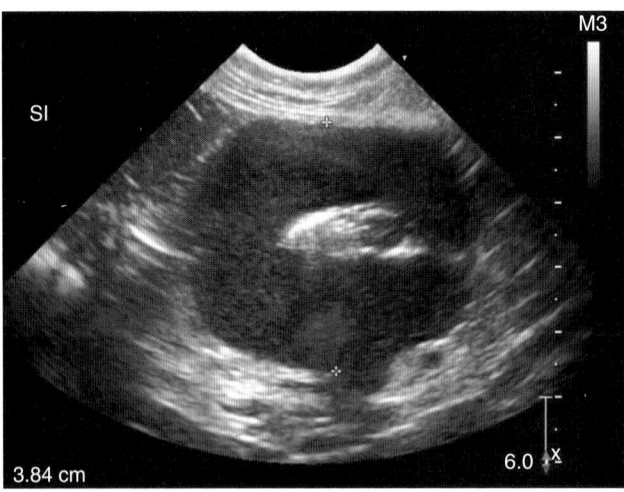

Figure 14-28: Transverse ultrasound images of a cat with chronic vomiting and diarrhea due to lymphocytic, plasmacytic enteritis confirmed by surgical biopsy. The thickening of the muscularis is generalized and cannot be differentiated from diffuse lymphoma, which can also lead to diffuse muscularis thickening. *SI*, small intestine.

microcore samples. Alternatively, the tip of the needle may be repeatedly repositioned within the tissue without aspiration to obtain the cytologic specimen. Gastrointestinal mass lesions and enlarged lymph nodes are more successfully sampled than focal regions of mild intestinal thickening. The FNA specimens may then be submitted as fixed slide smears or needle aspirates intended for rapid cytospin analysis and/or bacteriologic culture.

Tissue core biopsies for histopathology are obtained using a larger needle (Tru-Cut) with or without a semiautomatic biopsy device, which allows the operator to control the depth of needle placement and length of sample obtained. An 18-gauge needle is suggested (with or without a biopsy guide transducer attachment) for feline patients depending on the location and size of the lesion being sampled. Generally, two to three specimens are obtained for histopathologic evaluation.

References

1. Biller DS, Kantrowitz B, Miyabayashi T: Ultrasonography of diffuse liver disease: a review. *J Vet Intern Med* 6:71–76, 1992.
2. Feeney DA, Anderson KL, Ziegler LE, et al: Statistical relevance of ultrasonographic criteria in the assessment of diffuse liver disease in dogs and cats. *Am J Vet Res* 69:212–221, 2008.
3. Nicoll RG, Jackson MW, Knipp BS, et al: Quantitative ultrasonography of the liver in cats during obesity induction and dietary restriction. *Res Vet Sci* 64:1–6, 1998.
4. Webster N, Holloway A: Use of contrast ultrasonography in the diagnosis of metastatic feline visceral haemangiosarcoma. *J Feline Med Surg* 10:388–394, 2008.
5. Nyman HT, Kristensen AT, Flagstad A, et al: A review of the sonographic assessment of tumor metastases in liver and superficial lymph nodes. *Vet Radiol Ultrasound* 45:438–448, 2004.
6. O'Brien RT: Improved detection of metastatic hepatic hemangiosarcoma nodules with contrast ultrasound in three dogs. *Vet Radiol Ultrasound* 48:146–148, 2007.
7. Leinonen MR, Raekallio MR, Vainio OM, et al: Quantitative contrast-enhanced ultrasonographic analysis of perfusion in the kidneys, liver, pancreas, small intestine, and mesenteric lymph nodes in healthy cats. *Am J Vet Res* 71:1305–1311, 2010.
8. Rademacher N, Ohlerth S, Scharf G, et al: Contrast-enhanced power and color Doppler ultrasonography of the pancreas in healthy and diseased cats. *J Vet Intern Med* 22:1310–1316, 2008.
9. Penninck DG, Brisson JO, Webster CR: Sonographic assessment of gallbladder volume in normal cats. *Vet Radiol Ultrasound* 51:665–666, 2010.
10. Gaillot HA, Penninck DG, Webster CR, et al: Ultrasonographic features of extrahepatic biliary obstruction in 30 cats. *Vet Radiol Ultrasound* 48:439–447, 2007.
11. Della Santa D, Schweighauser A, Forterre F, et al: Imaging diagnosis—extrahepatic biliary

tract obstruction secondary to a duodenal foreign body in a cat. *Vet Radiol Ultrasound* 48:448–450, 2007.

12. Woods KS, Brisson BA, Defarges AM, et al: Congenital duplex gallbladder and biliary mucocele associated with partial hepatic cholestasis and cholelithiasis in a cat. *Can Vet J* 53:269–273, 2012.

13. Hittmair KM, Vielgrader HD, Loupal G: Ultrasonographic evaluation of gallbladder wall thickness in cats. *Vet Radiol Ultrasound* 42:149–155, 2001.

14. Center SA: Diseases of the gallbladder and biliary tree. *Vet Clin North Am Small Anim Pract* 39:543–598, 2009.

15. Harvey AM, Holt PE, Barr FJ, et al: Treatment and long-term follow-up of extrahepatic biliary obstruction with bilirubin cholelithiasis in a Somali cat with pyruvate kinase deficiency. *J Feline Med Surg* 9:424–431, 2007.

16. Elwood CM, White RN, Freeman K, et al: Cholelithiasis and hyperthyroidism in a cat. *J Feline Med Surg* 3:247–252, 2001.

17. Morrison WB: Cholangitis, choledocholithiasis, and icterus in a cat. *Vet Pathol* 22:285–286, 1985.

18. Kristick KL, Ranck RS, Fink M: What is your diagnosis? Biliary cystadenoma of the liver causing deviation of the stomach to the left. *J Am Vet Med Assoc* 236:1065–1066, 2010.

19. Best EJ, Bush DJ, Dye C: Suspected choledochal cyst in a domestic shorthair cat. *J Feline Med Surg* 12:814–817, 2010.

20. Grand JG, Doucet M, Albaric O, et al: Cyst of the common bile duct in a cat. *Aust Vet J* 88:268–271, 2010.

21. Marolf AJ, Leach L, Gibbons DS, et al: Ultrasonographic findings of feline cholangitis. *J Am Anim Hosp Assoc* 48:36–42, 2012.

22. Boothe HW, Boothe DM, Komkov A, et al: Use of hepatobiliary scintigraphy in the diagnosis of extrahepatic biliary obstruction in dogs and cats: 25 cases (1982–1989). *J Am Vet Med Assoc* 201:134–141, 1992.

23. Head LL, Daniel GB: Correlation between hepatobiliary scintigraphy and surgery or postmortem examination findings in dogs and cats with extrahepatic biliary obstruction, partial obstruction, or patency of the biliary system: 18 cases (1995–2004). *J Am Vet Med Assoc* 227:1618–1624, 2005.

24. Newell SM, Selcer BA, Roberts RE, et al: Hepatobiliary scintigraphy in the evaluation of feline liver disease. *J Vet Intern Med* 10:308–315, 1996.

25. Newell SM, Graham JP, Roberts GD, et al: Quantitative hepatobiliary scintigraphy in normal cats and in cats with experimental cholangiohepatitis. *Vet Radiol Ultrasound* 42:70–76, 2001.

26. Tivers M, Lipscomb V: Congenital portosystemic shunts in cats: investigation, diagnosis and stabilisation. *J Feline Med Surg* 13:173–184, 2011.

27. Vandermeulen E, Combes A, de Rooster H, et al: Transsplenic portal scintigraphy using ^{99m}Tc-pertechnetate for the diagnosis of portosystemic shunts in cats: a retrospective review of 12 patients. *J Feline Med Surg* 15:1123–1131, 2013.

28. Lamb CR, Forster-van Hijfte MA, White RN, et al: Ultrasonographic diagnosis of congenital portosystemic shunt in 14 cats. *J Small Anim Pract* 37:205–209, 1996.

29. White RN, Parry AT: Morphology of congenital portosystemic shunts emanating from the left gastric vein in dogs and cats. *J Small Anim Pract* 54:459–467, 2013.

30. Palerme JS, Brown JC, Marks SL, et al: Splenosystemic shunts in cats: a retrospective of 33 cases (2004–2011). *J Vet Intern Med* 27:1347–1353, 2013.

31. Xenoulis PG, Steiner JM: Current concepts in feline pancreatitis. *Top Companion Anim Med* 23:185–192, 2008.

32. Etue SM, Penninck DG, Labato MA, et al: Ultrasonography of the normal feline pancreas and associated anatomic landmarks: a prospective study of 20 cats. *Vet Radiol Ultrasound* 42:330–336, 2001.

33. Wall M, Biller DS, Schoning P, et al: Pancreatitis in a cat demonstrating pancreatic duct dilatation ultrasonographically. *J Am Anim Hosp Assoc* 37:49–53, 2001.

34. Saunders HM: Ultrasonography of the pancreas. *Probl Vet Med* 3:583–603, 1991.

35. Marolf AJ, Kraft SL, Dunphy TR, et al: Magnetic resonance (MR) imaging and MR cholangiopancreatography findings in cats with cholangitis and pancreatitis. *J Feline Med Surg* 15:285–294, 2013.

36. Wang KY, Panciera DL, Al-Rukibat RK, et al: Accuracy of ultrasound-guided fine-needle aspiration of the liver and cytologic findings in dogs and cats: 97 cases (1990–2000). *J Am Vet Med Assoc* 224:75–78, 2004.

37. Willard MD, Weeks BR, Johnson M: Fine-needle aspirate cytology suggesting hepatic lipidosis in four cats with infiltrative hepatic disease. *J Feline Med Surg* 1:215–220, 1999.

38. Proot SJ, Rothuizen J: High complication rate of an automatic Tru-Cut biopsy gun device for liver biopsy in cats. *J Vet Intern Med* 20:1327–1333, 2006.

39. Brain PH, Barrs VR, Martin P, et al: Feline cholecystitis and acute neutrophilic cholangitis: clinical findings, bacterial isolates and response to treatment in six cases. *J Feline Med Surg* 8:91–103, 2006.

40. Savary-Bataille KC, Bunch SE, Spaulding KA, et al: Percutaneous ultrasound-guided cholecystocentesis in healthy cats. *J Vet Intern Med* 17:298–303, 2003.

41. Wagner KA, Hartmann FA, Treoanier LA: Bacterial culture results from liver, gall bladder or bile in 248 dogs and cats evaluated for hepatobiliary disease: 1998–2003. *J Vet Intern Med* 21:417–424, 2007.

42. Wang KY, Panciera DL, Al-Rukibat RK, et al: Accuracy of ultrasound-guided fine-needle aspiration of the liver and cytologic findings in dogs and cats: 97 cases (1990–2000). *J Am Vet Med Assoc* 224:75–78, 2004.

43. Adams WM, Sisterman LA, Klauer JM, et al: Association of intestinal disorders in cats with findings of abdominal radiography. *J Am Vet Med Assoc* 236:880–886, 2010.

44. Trevail T, Gunn-Moore D, Carrera I, et al: Radiographic diameter of the colon in normal and constipated cats and in cats with megacolon. *Vet Radiol Ultrasound* 52:516–520, 2011.

45. Morgan JP: The upper gastrointestinal examination in the cat: normal radiographic appearance using positive contrast medium. *Vet Radiol* 22:159–169, 1981.

46. O'Brien TR: Radiographic diagnosis of abdominal disorders in the dog and cat: radiographic interpretation, clinical signs, pathophysiology. *WB Saunders* 141–395, 1981.

47. Weichselbaum RC, Feeney DA, Hayden DW: Comparison of upper gastrointestinal radiographic findings to histopathologic observations: a retrospective study of 41 dogs and cats with suspected small bowel infiltrative disease (1985 to 1990). *Vet Radiol Ultrasound* 35:418–426, 1994.

48. Silva AC, Pimenta M, Guimaraes LS: Small bowel obstruction: what to look for. *Radiographics* 29:423–439, 2009.

49. Williams J, Biller DS, Miyabayashi T, et al: Evaluation of Iohexol as a gastrointestinal contrast medium in normal cats. *Vet Radiol Ultrasound* 34(5):310–314, 1993.

50. Penninck DG, Nyland TG, Kerr LY, et al: Ultrasonographic evaluation of gastrointestinal diseases in small animals. *Vet Radiol Ultrasound* 31:134–141, 1990.

51. Gaschen L: Ultrasonography of small intestinal inflammatory and neoplastic diseases in dogs and cats. *Vet Clin North Am Small Anim Pract* 41:239–244, 2011.

52. Di Donato P, Penninck D, Pietra M, et al: Ultrasonographic measurement of the relative thickness of intestinal wall layers in clinically healthy cats. *J Feline Med Surg* 16:333–339, 2014.

53. Winter MD, Londono L, Berry CR, et al: Ultrasonographic evaluation of relative gastrointestinal layer thickness in cats without clinical evidence of gastrointestinal tract disease. *J Feline Med Surg* 16:118–124, 2014.

54. Newell SM, Graham JP, Roberts GD, et al: Sonography of the normal feline gastrointestinal tract. *Vet Radiol Ultrasound* 40:40–43, 1999.

55. Goggin JM, Biller DS, Debey BM, et al: Ultrasonographic measurement of gastrointestinal wall thickness and the ultrasonographic appearance of the ileocolic region in healthy cats. *J Am Anim Hosp Assoc* 36:224–228, 2000.

56. Taeymans O, Holt N, Penninck DG, et al: Ultrasonographic characterization of feline ileocecolic abnormalities. *Vet Radiol Ultrasound* 52:335–339, 2011.

57. Norsworthy GD, Estep JS, Kiupel M, et al: Diagnosis of chronic small bowel disease in cats: 100 cases (2008–2012). *J Am Vet Med Assoc* 243:1455–1461, 2013.

58. Zwingenberger AL, Marks SL, Baker TW, et al: Ultrasonographic evaluation of the muscularis propria in cats with diffuse small intestinal lymphoma or inflammatory bowel disease. *J Vet Intern Med* 24:289–292, 2010.

59. Daniaux LA, Laurenson MP, Marks SL, et al: Ultrasonographic thickening of the muscularis propria in feline small intestinal small cell

T-cell lymphoma and inflammatory bowel disease. *J Feline Med Surg* 16:89–98, 2014.

60. Tucker S, Penninck DG, Keating JH, et al: The clinicopathological and ultrasonographic features of cats with eosinophilic enteritis. *J Feline Med Surg* 16:943–949, 2014.

61. Baez JL, Hendrick MJ, Walker LM, et al: Radiographic, ultrasonographic, and endoscopic findings in cats with inflammatory bowel disease of the stomach and small intestine: 33 cases (1990–1997). *J Am Vet Med Assoc* 215:349–354, 1999.

62. Garcia DAA, Froes TR, Vilani RGDOC, et al: Ultrasonography of small intestinal obstructions; a contemporary approach. *J Small Animal Practice* 52:484–490, 2011.

63. Tidwell AS, Penninck DG: Ultrasonography of gastrointestinal foreign bodies. *Vet Radiol Ultrasound* 33:160–169, 1992.

64. Tyrrell D, Beck C: Survey of the use of radiography vs. ultrasonography in the investigation of gastrointestinal foreign bodies in small animals. *Vet Radiol Ultrasound* 47:404–408, 2006.

65. Boysen SR, Tidwell AS, Penninck DG: Ultrasonographic findings in dogs and cats with gastrointestinal perforation. *Vet Radiol Ultrasound* 44:556–564, 2003.

66. Grassi R, Romano S, Pinto A, et al: Gastroduodenal perforations: conventional plain film, ultrasonography and CT findings in 166 consecutive patients. *Eur J Radiol* 50:30–36, 2004.

67. Ferrell EA, Graham JP: Ultrasound corner diagnosis of pneumoperitoneum. *Vet Radiol Ultrasound* 44:307–308, 2003.

The Challenges of Pancreatitis in Cats: A Diagnostic and Therapeutic Conundrum

Caroline Mansfield

> *To know that we know what we know, and that we do not know what we do not know, that is true knowledge.*
>
> —*Henry David Thoreau*

The optimal diagnosis and treatment of pancreatitis in cats remains elusive despite a number of advances and increasing awareness of the condition by the veterinary profession. Diagnosis may be confounded by comorbidities, and in most cats, clinical signs of pancreatitis remain vague and nonspecific. In general, acute pancreatitis is easier to diagnose than chronic pancreatitis but presents challenges for optimal management, particularly in the face of serious concurrent disease. Chronic pancreatitis is more difficult to diagnose, and its true clinical significance is not universally accepted. As a result, the treatment recommendations for chronic pancreatitis are highly variable, and there is little evidence to favor one particular approach.

One reason for the high number of comorbidities in cats with pancreatitis is the unique anatomy of the cat. Most cats have only one pancreatic duct that enters the small intestine through the major duodenal papilla, with this opening being contiguous with the bile duct[1,2] (Figure 15-1).

CLASSIFICATION

The classification of pancreatitis is usually based on histology. This classification is sometimes arbitrary, because in many cases a pancreatic biopsy is not obtained.

Chronic non-suppurative pancreatitis is the histologic type that occurs most commonly in cats. This form is defined as a mononuclear (often lymphocytic) inflammation, with disruption of the pancreatic architecture due to concurrent fibrosis.[3,4] The inflammation may be minimal and recurrent at the time of diagnosis. It has been shown that pancreatic inflammation is present variably throughout the pancreas in dogs; single biopsies may miss the true extent of the disease.[5] This has not been evaluated in cats.

Histologically, acute pancreatitis is defined as a neutrophilic inflammation without fibrosis or exocrine atrophy and

is present within the body of the pancreas and/or peripancreatic fat.[6] There also appears to be an acute suppurative form that is unique to cats. This type is uncommon and tends to affect younger cats. A possible autoimmune form with periductular lymphocytic inflammation has also been described.[1]

Clinically, the term *chronic pancreatitis* is given to cases in which there are only mild clinical signs and *acute pancreatitis* when there are severe clinical signs. In cats, it does appear as if there is a reasonable correlation between the clinical and histologic classifications.

INCIDENCE

A survey of 115 feline postmortem examinations at a tertiary referral institution found that there was an overall prevalence of 67% for pancreatitis, with 45% of clinically healthy cats also having pancreatic lesions.[7] This study demonstrates that chronic pancreatitis may be grossly under recognized in cats. However, it also raises the possibility that mild histologic changes in the pancreas may not be clinically important and actually represent a spectrum of normal. Cats have been increasingly reported to develop acute pancreatitis (AP) similar to dogs, with necrosis of the peripancreatic fat region being a predominant feature.

ETIOLOGY

The etiology of chronic pancreatitis is most widely explored and understood in humans and laboratory rodent models. The currently accepted hypothesis in humans is the sentinel acute pancreatitis event (SAPE) hypothesis.[8] In this hypothesis, the pancreatic acinar cells come under oxidative stress (e.g., from fats, alcohol, oxidative products in the bile). There

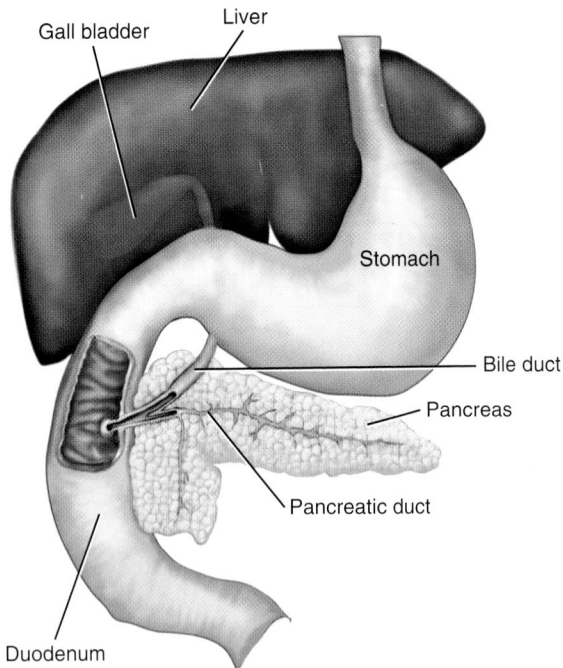

Figure 15-1: Anatomical representation of the relationship between the biliary and pancreatic systems in the cat. (Courtesy of Dr. Kate Patterson, MediPics and Prose.)

is a massive pro-inflammatory response, followed by an influx of stellate cells that are pro-fibrotic. If the oxidative stresses are removed at this point in time, the pancreas heals with no consequences. However, if there is a continued low-grade secretion of cytokines in response to continued oxidative stress or recurrent bouts of inflammation, then the stellate cells respond and cause periacinar fibrosis. It is unknown if this SAPE phenomenon occurs in cats. It could be hypothesized that it does and that initial oxidative stress plays an important role, especially since due to the unique feline anatomy, any abnormality in the bile is also carried to the pancreas (see Figure 15-1).

Triaditis refers to concurrent inflammatory bowel disease (IBD), chronic pancreatitis, and cholangiohepatitis. One postmortem study identified a greater prevalence of pancreatitis (9/18) and intestinal inflammation (15/18) in cats with cholangiohepatitis.[9] However, the concept of "triaditis" is being challenged (see Chapter 12). The association between cholangiohepatitis and pancreatitis appears to be low, whereas the association between IBD and pancreatitis is high. There are two major hypotheses as to why there could be a relationship between IBD and pancreatitis. First, inflammation in the gut may cause distant inflammation in the pancreas, which could occur via upregulation of inflammatory mediators or their receptors. Second, there may be inflammation in response to enteric bacteria, which have been documented in the pancreas of cats via culture-independent means.[10] This latter hypothesis is perhaps even more relevant in the face of concurrent cholangitis, as discussed later. Other possible relationships between pancreatitis and IBD could be due to development of pancreatitis in response to treatment for IBD, changes in cholesterol, or anatomic abnormalities of the duodenum.[11,12]

Autoimmune pancreatitis (AIP) is an uncommon phenomenon in humans but is reported in association with IBD.[11,13] In humans, AIP is categorized as type 1 when the pancreas is involved in a multisystemic fibroinflammatory disease (immunoglobulin (Ig) G4-associated systemic diseases) and as type 2 when associated with IBD.[14] Up to 39% of humans with Crohn's disease have circulating pancreatic autoantibodies, although evidence supporting an association between these antibodies and clinical pancreatitis is lacking.[12] The presence of IgG4 staining cells in the pancreas and incidence of circulating antibodies against the pancreas have not been established in cats.

Enteric bacteria have been identified in the pancreas of some cats via fluorescent *in situ* hybridization (FISH).[10] Bacterial involvement appears to be more common in moderate to severely affected cats with acute pancreatitis and with concurrent hepatic disease than in those with chronic pancreatitis.[10] In one retrospective study, 60% of cats with cholangitis had concurrent pancreatitis, whereas in a case series, 50% of cats with cholecystitis had pancreatic inflammation.[15,16] Pancreatic necrosis has been induced in cats by perfusion of infected bile through the pancreatic duct but not by perfusion of sterile bile or saline.[17] When a solution of bacteria suspended in saline was perfused, only mild edematous pancreatitis developed.[17] This suggests that an inflammatory response severe enough to induce necrosis may require both bile substrate and bacteria. Despite these reports, the exact pathogenic role bacteria may play in naturally occurring pancreatitis is unclear, and whether the bacteria identified in such cases[10] are present due to translocation or are direct contaminants is unknown. Certainly in a feline experimental model and one case report, translocation of *Escherichia coli* from blood into the pancreas has been documented.[18,19]

Pancreatitis in cats has also been associated with toxoplasmosis and feline infectious peritonitis.[20,21] In one postmortem review of cats with toxoplasmosis, over 80% of cats had pancreatic inflammation,[22] and pancreatitis has been reported as being a presentation of acute toxoplasmosis.[23] However, a study based on serologic testing suggested that there was no association between *Toxoplasma gondii* (or *Bartonella* species) and pancreatitis in cats.[24] A proposed association between herpesvirus, parvovirus infection, and pancreatitis has not been supported, but an association between calicivirus infection and severe pancreatitis has.[25,26] Aberrant migration of the liver fluke *Amphimerus pseudofelineus* is a documented but extremely rare cause of pancreatitis.[27]

High dietary fat intake, particularly when there is concurrent low dietary protein, is a frequent cause of pancreatitis in the dog.[28] However, dietary fat intake does not seem to be a cause of pancreatitis in cats.[28,29] In support of this, one experimental study showed that hyperlipidemia did not induce pancreatic histologic change in cats.[30] Toxic causes are also reported in greater frequency in dogs than in cats, but organophosphate toxicity due to application of topical insecticides is certainly a potential cause of pancreatitis in cats.[31]

Trauma, in particular falling from a height, has been associated with the development of pancreatitis in cats.[32] Although

Labels in figure: Gall bladder, Liver, Stomach, Bile duct, Pancreas, Pancreatic duct, Duodenum not quantified, it is likely that other types of trauma, such as motor vehicle accidents, are also likely to cause pancreatitis even if not clinically apparent. There are multiple genetic abnormalities reported in humans that predispose to chronic pancreatitis that include cationic trypsinogen mutations.[8] To date, no such genetic mutation has been identified in cats.

Despite this long list of potential etiologies, in most cats an underlying cause of pancreatitis is never found.

COMORBIDITIES

Concurrent disease has been reported in the majority of cats with chronic pancreatitis, as well as a large number of cats with acute pancreatitis.[7,15,16,33-36] As suggested by the earlier discussion, this comorbidity may have a direct causal relationship. Certainly the most commonly reported organs concurrently involved with pancreatitis are the hepatobiliary and intestinal systems.[31] There does not appear to be a negative prognosis associated with concurrent IBD and pancreatitis.[35] Extrahepatic biliary tract obstruction (see Chapter 16) can occur as a complication of pancreatitis in cats and may require specific intervention.[36] The development of hepatic lipidosis is commonly reported in cats with acute pancreatitis, with or without diabetic ketoacidosis.[33,37,38] The presence of hepatic lipidosis is likely a result of a period of starvation and markedly worsens the prognosis for cats with pancreatitis.[39,40] Renal disease also has a high incidence in pathology-based reports, but this may be related to the fact that the studies assessed older cats that are more likely to have unrelated renal pathology.[9]

Concurrent diabetes mellitus and exocrine pancreatic disease is a challenging issue in feline medicine, due to the difficulties this combination of conditions poses for treatment. A large number of cats with diabetes mellitus were found to have chronic pancreatitis in one postmortem survey (17/37)[41]; however, the presence of pancreatitis was not negatively associated with survival. Two European studies presented as abstracts identified pancreatic abnormalities (via ultrasound and/or increased pancreatic lipase) in 30% to 43% of diabetic cats.[42,43] In the study that documented ultrasonographic changes, there were no clinical signs associated with pancreatitis observed in any of the cats.[42] Similarly, in another study there appeared to be no correlation between glycemic control and feline pancreatic lipase concentration.[44]

One experimental study found that hyperglycemia increased neutrophil numbers within the pancreas,[30] and the authors postulated that diabetes may in fact have caused the pancreatitis rather than the other way around. This is a similar theory to that proposed in human medicine, in which acinar acidosis is thought to predispose to pancreatitis.[45,46] The alternative theory is that a subset of cats develop pancreatitis and have subsequent reduction of pancreatic endocrine function due to fibrosis. It is possible that there are genetic and regional differences in terms of the relationship between pancreatitis and diabetes in cats. However, in terms of feline clinical practice, determining the order of events is often a chicken or egg question ("Which came first—the chicken or the

egg?") that is clinically irrelevant because most cats have both conditions at presentation.

CLINICAL SIGNS

There is no overwhelming age, breed, or sex predisposition for pancreatitis. Due to the high incidence of concurrent morbidities, it is likely that cats will be at least 6 years of age. In contrast with dogs, there is no reported association with obesity.

The clinical signs in cats are much more subtle and easy to miss than in dogs. This is the case even when cats have acute pancreatitis, as summarized in Table 15-1.

DIAGNOSTIC METHODS

Laboratory Testing
Routine
Traditional biochemical methods are notoriously nonspecific and poorly sensitive for diagnosing pancreatic inflammation in the cat, and changes generally reflect concurrent disease and the associated electrolyte/fluid imbalances. However,

Table 15-1 **A Summary of Clinical Signs Reported From Three Different Studies of Cats with Acute Pancreatitis**

Clinical Sign	Hill and Van Winkle[31]	Kimmel, Washabau, and Drobatz[47]	Ferreri, Hardam, Kimmel, et al.[34]
Case numbers	n = 40 (necropsy based)	n = 46	n = 30
Lethargy	100%	83%	50%
Anorexia	97%	96%	63%
Dehydration	92%	NR	33%
Hypothermia	68%	NR	NR
Vomiting	35%	43%	43%
Abdominal pain	25%	17%	10%
Palpable abdominal mass	23%	4%	3%
Diarrhea	15%	11%	NR
Dyspnea	20%	NR	16%
Ataxia	15%	NR	NR
Weight loss	NR	39%	40%
Jaundice	NR	22%	16%
Pallor	NR	NR	30%

NR, Not recorded.

routine biochemistry is important to perform in order to obtain basic information to direct fluid and electrolyte therapy and assess for evidence of concurrent disease. One study showed hypocalcemia to be a poor prognostic indicator in cats, even in the absence of associated clinical signs.[47] However, another study showed no difference in ionized calcium between cats with acute pancreatitis and those with chronic pancreatitis.[34] One interesting observation is that the most common routine biochemical change in cats with pancreatitis is hypercholesterolemia.[33] The exact cause of this is unknown, and it is an interesting phenomenon in light of the fact that excess dietary fat does not seem to predispose cats to the development of pancreatitis. Because there are few differentials for hypercholesterolemia, its presence in a sick cat should alert veterinarians to the possibility of pancreatitis.

Total Lipase, Amylase, and Trypsin-Like Immunoreactivity

The increase in serum lipase and amylase in cats with pancreatitis tends to be less than in the dog, and these values are seldom diagnostic in their own right. However, a study suggests that using an alternative assay type (1,2-*o*-dilaurylrac-glycero-3-glutaric acid-[6′-methylresorufin] ester [DGGR]) to measure lipase activity may have a higher sensitivity, equivalent to pancreatic lipase immunoreactivity (PLI).[48] This is a colorimetric assay, whereas a 1,2-diglyceride assay has traditionally been used. A prospective study showed that the DGGR lipase assay had a sensitivity of 47.8% in 23 cats that had pancreatic histology performed.[48] The sensitivity was higher for the acute form of pancreatitis than chronic and had a similar sensitivity to feline pancreatic lipase immunoreactivity (fPLI) (56.5%). Similarly, another abstract showed that lipase was increased in 80% of cats with an increased PLI; the conclusion was that a combination of pancreatic ultrasound abnormalities and a high total lipase activity (using traditional assay methodology) had a perfect (100%) predictive value for high fPLI.[49] Conversely, the absence of ultrasound abnormalities plus normal lipase activity was perfectly predictive of a normal fPLI. This study did not have histologic confirmation of pancreatitis.

A feline trypsin-like immunoreactivity (fTLI) assay is commercially available, and it is highly sensitive and specific for the diagnosis of exocrine pancreatic insufficiency.[50] Unfortunately fTLI is not very useful clinically, with a reported sensitivity of 8% to 33% in chronic pancreatitis,[51-54] although higher with more severe disease.[53] Concentration of fTLI may also be increased by other diseases, such as chronic kidney disease, IBD, lymphosarcoma, and starvation.[52,54]

Pancreatic Lipase Immunoreactivity

A fPLI radioimmunoassay with a reference interval of 1.2 to 3.8 µg/L was established initially in cats.[55,56] This type of assay was originally developed in dogs and is based on the premise that different isoenzymes of lipase are produced solely by the pancreas.[57] There have been studies that show immunolocalization of canine pancreatic lipase within acinar cells, and dogs without exocrine pancreatic function have no measurable circulating pancreatic lipase.[58,59] These studies have been not performed in cats. However, a similar approach was taken in development of the feline assay by purifying pancreatic lipase from cat pancreata and developing polyclonal antibodies against pancreatic lipase.[56] The PLI radioimmunoassay was then replaced commercially by an enzyme-linked immunosorbent assay (Spec feline pancreas-specific lipase (fPL), IDEXX Laboratories, Westbrook, ME) that used recombinant peptide as the antigen in its development (instead of isolated pancreatic lipase) and monoclonal antibodies, as well as a commercially available semiquantitative in-clinic test (SNAP fPL, IDEXX Laboratories).[55] No validation studies have been published for the new feline assays; however, the manufacturer claims good reproducibility and accuracy. The current reference interval for Spec fPL suggests normal values are <3.5 µg/L, with a value >5.3 µg/L considered consistent with pancreatitis. The SNAP fPL test records a positive when the result is >3.5 µg/L. Again, no studies on correlation between SNAP fPL and Spec fPL have been published, but the manufacturer reports agreement of 82% (for "abnormal" results) and 92% (for "normal" results).

Variable sensitivities have been reported for fPLI and Spec fPL, which probably reflects the lack of a noninvasive, gold-standard diagnosis in cats as well as differences in clinical presentation and study design. In addition, many studies are under powered. One study showed a sensitivity of 100% for fPLI in five cats with AP, but only 54% for 13 cats with chronic pancreatitis.[51] An abstract assessing 31 cats with definite or probable pancreatitis determined a sensitivity for Spec fPL of 79%, whereas another study assessing 35 cats with suspected pancreatitis had a sensitivity of 54%.[60,61]

Specificity of Spec fPL appears to be relatively high, but large studies are lacking. One study comparing 18 cats with pancreatitis (five acute and 13 chronic) to eight healthy cats and three symptomatic cats with normal pancreatic histopathology reported a specificity of 91%.[51] Similarly, a large abstract study of 59 sick cats that were unlikely to have pancreatitis determined a specificity of 82%.[61] There appears to be no statistically significant increase in fPLI or Spec fPL in cats with experimentally induced renal failure.[62] This suggests that there may be minimal effects from other diseases; however, the effect of renal disease in clinical situations requires further evaluation.

All in all, the use of Spec fPL and SNAP fPL is recommended by the author as supportive evidence for pancreatitis, and a diagnosis of pancreatitis should also take into account the clinical presentation and imaging findings.

Novel Laboratory Testing

Unfortunately, there have been no new assays developed for the diagnosis of pancreatitis in cats. Assessment of pancreas-specific markers, such as trypsinogen activation peptide, more than 10 years ago were not helpful.[43] New diagnostic tests that measure markers of inflammation are increasingly being studied in domestic animals. In one study, serum amyloid A (SAA) decreased over time and correlated with clinical improvement in a cat with pancreatitis.[63] It appears that the human SAA assay is valid to use in cats; however, the main clinical utility would be for clinical prognostication and monitoring rather than diagnosis *per se*.[64]

Cytology

Although uncommonly performed, fine-needle biopsy of the pancreas is a relatively safe procedure when ultrasound guided.[65] The author recommends using a 25-gauge needle attached to a 3-mL syringe containing a small amount of air. The needle enters the pancreas and is moved backward and forward along the same line several times. No redirection or aspiration should be used. The clinical usefulness of this test in cats is unknown, but because the changes in other diagnostic modalities (including ultrasound) are nonspecific, this could be considered more frequently to differentiate inflammation from neoplasia, particularly lymphoma.

Diagnostic Imaging

Radiography and Ultrasound

Feline pancreatitis is difficult to assess via diagnostic imaging. Abdominal radiographs tend to be unhelpful, particularly in chronic pancreatitis, although they may be useful to assess for other abdominal disease. Occasionally in obese cats, the left limb of the pancreas is visible on ventrodorsal radiographs (Figure 15-2).

The increased availability of ultrasound has made this a commonly used method of diagnosis for pancreatitis in cats. Despite an increase in operator expertise, some studies have shown a very disappointing sensitivity for the diagnosis of pancreatitis (particularly the chronic form) in cats. Reported sensitivities range from 11% to 84%.[53,60,66,67] However, the sensitivity increases with the severity of disease.[60]

A "normal" pancreas has smooth borders, is not enlarged (left limb <9.5 mm, body <8 mm, and right limb <6 mm), and is isoechoic compared to the liver[60] (Figure 15-3). There should be no fluid around the pancreas, and the lymph nodes should be of normal size. The right limb of the pancreas is the most difficult to locate using ultrasound, and so many studies report solely on the left limb. Nodular changes within the pancreas may be observed as an age-related change, but masses more than 2 cm in diameter are considered consistent with neoplasia.[68] Although it has been shown that the pancreatic duct diameter increases with age, it should not exceed 2.5 mm in diameter at any age.[69,70] Stimulation with secretin does lead to a detectable increase in the diameter of the pancreatic duct, but whether this is useful clinically for diagnosing chronic pancreatitis is unknown.[71]

Classic ultrasonographic findings of AP are reported as being similar to those in dogs (e.g., enlarged hypoechoic pancreas with hyperechoic peripancreatic tissue).[32] The presence of hyperechoic peripancreatic fat is considered the most sensitive ultrasonographic feature of AP in cats[60] (Figure 15-4). Other changes such as severely altered pancreatic margination (roughened appearance) and pancreatic limb thickness are less sensitive.[60] The least specific ultrasound change reported is mildly altered pancreatic margination.[60] The time of onset of clinical signs may precede ultrasonographic changes, further confounding the utility of this diagnostic tool.[32] In cats with suspected acute pancreatitis, it is therefore recommended that repeat ultrasound be performed 36 to 49 hours after the first assessment if there are no supportive changes on initial assessment.

Endosonography is a technique performed under general anesthesia whereby the ultrasound transducer is placed in the stomach and pressed against the pancreas through the

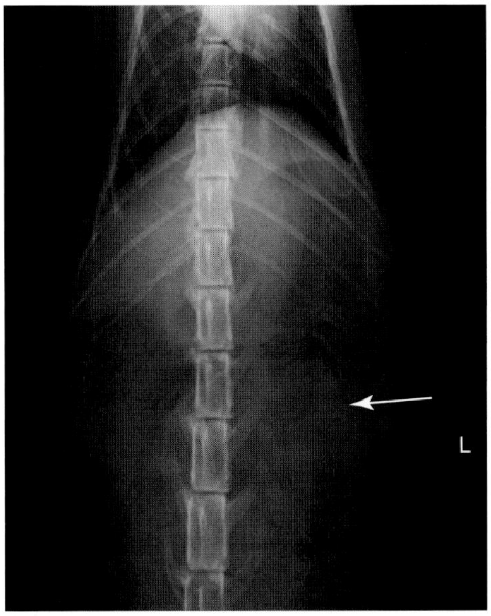

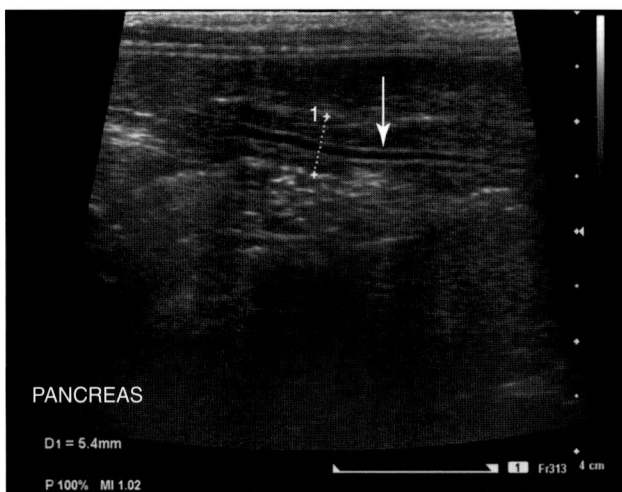

Figure 15-2: A ventrodorsal radiograph of cat (without pancreatitis) that shows the left limb of the pancreas highlighted in the cranial left quadrant of the abdomen *(arrow)*. (Courtesy of Dr. Cathy Beck, University of Melbourne.)

Figure 15-3: Longitudinal ultrasound image of the left limb of a normal pancreas in a cat. The thickness of the pancreas is less than 1 cm (5.4 mm) as shown by the calipers, and the pancreatic duct is seen as a hypoechoic tubular structure *(arrow)*. There is smooth margination of the pancreas with no surrounding hyperechogenicity. (Courtesy of Dr. Cathy Beck, University of Melbourne.)

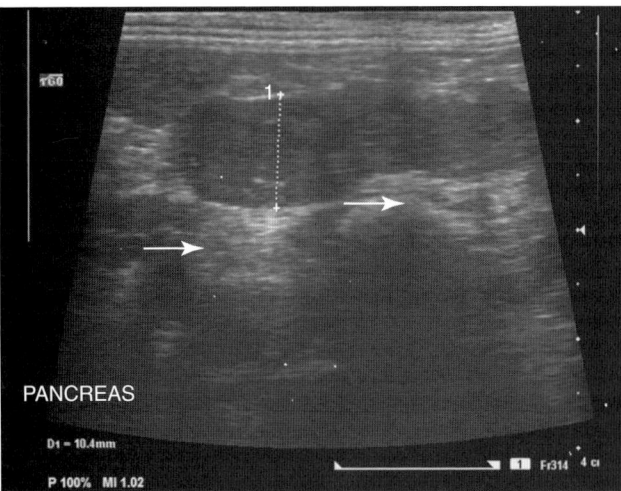

Figure 15-4: Abdominal ultrasound image showing a thickened pancreas (calipers), undulating pancreatic margin, and hyperechoic peripancreatic fat *(arrows)*. (Courtesy of Dr. Cathy Beck, University of Melbourne.)

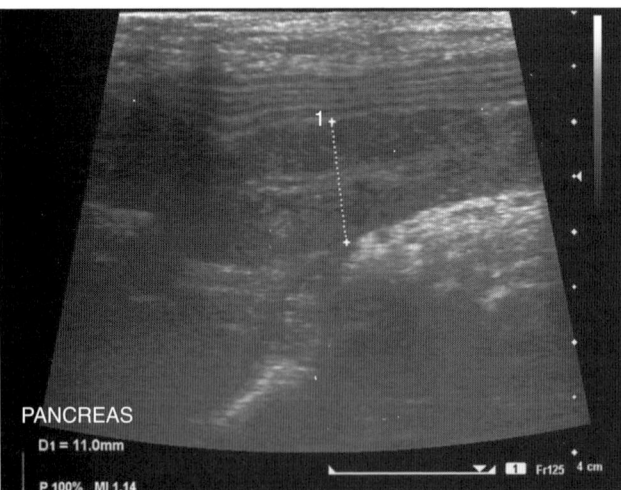

Figure 15-5: Abdominal ultrasound image showing a thickened pancreas (calipers), altered echogenicity of the pancreas, and peripancreatic fat. Fine-needle aspiration was consistent with lymphoma, emphasizing that ultrasound changes are not 100% specific for inflammation. (Courtesy of Dr. Cathy Beck, University of Melbourne.)

stomach wall and theoretically provides a better quality image of the pancreas. However, in initial evaluation, it appears to have no advantage over transabdominal ultrasound, except perhaps in obese cats.[72] Color-flow Doppler ultrasonography has also been evaluated, with the premise that vascularization of the pancreas will be different between malignant and benign processes.[73] Although this is a relatively widely available modality, it has not been assessed in clinical situations.

In effect the appearance of a normal pancreas on ultrasound does not rule out pancreatitis, and changes observed in the pancreas may be due to other diseases, such as neoplasia or nodular hyperplasia (Figure 15-5). More advanced ultrasound techniques require further evaluation for their true clinical utility to be known.

Advanced Imaging Techniques

Unfortunately, despite being considered the gold standard in human medicine, computed tomography (CT) evaluation of the abdomen shows little benefit in cats with acute or chronic pancreatitis.[51,53,74] One prospective study found that magnetic resonance imaging (MRI) was highly sensitive in the diagnosis of pancreatitis.[75] This increased sensitivity of MRI over CT or ultrasound may be due to the increased ability to detect soft tissue abnormalities. Magnetic resonance cholangiopancreatography (MRCP) uses T2-weighted images to highlight pancreatic and biliary ducts following secretin stimulation.[76] Currently, MRI is not routinely available for all feline patients, and the associated costs and anesthesia time required for MRI do not appear to be justified in comparison to conventional ultrasonography. The use of radiolabeled leukocytes and scintigraphy has been evaluated in normal cats and shown to be altered in one cat with pancreatitis.[77,78] However, most practices do not have scintigraphy or radioisotope handling capacity; for the moment, this remains a tertiary referral option.

Surgical Biopsy

Laparotomy. In many cases, a diagnosis can be made only by histologic evaluation of the pancreas. Surgical exploration may be contraindicated in severely ill cats, but full evaluation of the abdomen and sampling from the liver, mesenteric lymph nodes, and intestines may be justified in order to fully evaluate for concurrent disease. Pancreatic biopsies are not necessarily deleterious, but decreased blood flow or hypotension during general anesthesia may worsen or precipitate inflammation of the organ.

Laparoscopy. The increasing use of laparoscopy in veterinary practice makes this modality an increasingly attractive method of confirming the presence of pancreatitis and ruling out other diseases, such as neoplasia or nodular hyperplasia.[79] However, as with exploratory laparotomy, it is important to never evaluate the pancreas in isolation. Assessment and biopsy of other organs, in particular the liver, mesenteric lymph nodes, and intestine, is always advisable.

With adequate skill and training, laparoscopy can be performed quickly and has a reduced morbidity compared to exploratory laparotomy. Careful attention to anesthetic technique is required to maintain blood pressure (as for exploratory laparotomy) to ensure that no episodes of hypovolemia or hypotension occur. Anesthetic risks aside, obtaining biopsies of the pancreas during laparoscopy appears to be safe and effective for diagnosis in cats.[76,80,81] Discussion of the specific technique to perform laparoscopy is beyond the scope of this chapter. Extensive further reading and training is recommended for this procedure to be used safely and effectively.[79]

TREATMENT

Most, if not all, of the treatment options for pancreatitis in the cat are untested and extrapolated either from canine or human medicine, where they tend to be equally untested. Much of the management comes down to common sense; the sicker the cat, the more intensive the treatment that is required. For the purposes of this chapter, treatment has been classified into outpatient and inpatient rather than acute and chronic pancreatitis, because definitive differentiation is not always possible. The outpatient cat with pancreatitis tends to have the chronic disease with waxing and waning clinical signs, whereas the inpatient is generally sicker and shows signs of metabolic derangement.

Both the sick feline inpatient and not-so-sick feline outpatient are likely to benefit from cobalamin supplementation.[82] Cobalamin can be given weekly until there is a documented improvement in serum cobalamin concentrations or empirically (250 µg/cat subcutaneously [SC] once weekly for 4 weeks).

Outpatient

Because there are no specific treatment options for pancreatitis, management of concurrent disease takes precedence. In cats with coexisting IBD, cholangitis, or cholangiohepatitis, an antibiotic (e.g., amoxicillin) that is excreted in the bile should be prescribed. Monitoring of serum cholesterol may be beneficial, and feeding a low-fat diet or supplementing with omega-3 fatty acids could be considered if serum cholesterol is persistently elevated. Extrapolated dosages for omega-3 fatty acids in cats are 17 to 25 mg/kg/day eicosapentaenoic acid (EPA) and 8 to 18 mg/kg/day docosahexaenoic acid (DHA). Care should be taken with introducing EPA/DHA, because they may cause diarrhea or make the food unpalatable to cats.

A certain level of pain should be presumed to be present in cats during bouts of inflammation, even if they do not show typical signs. On an outpatient basis, buprenorphine (Table 15-2) or gabapentin (10 mg/kg *per os* [PO] every 12 hours) are relatively safe and reasonable alternatives for long-term pain relief in cats. Gabapentin is an anticonvulsant that is effective against pain, and one of the mechanisms is via inhibition of substance P.[83] Nonsteroidal anti-inflammatory medication could be considered if the cat has a reasonable appetite, is well hydrated, and has good renal function.

A common clinical dilemma is whether to treat with analgesia alone or with additional anti-inflammatory/immune suppression as well. Ideally, immune suppression should only be used when there is histologic confirmation of lymphocytic inflammation within the pancreas. If the cat is not diabetic, prednisolone is the drug of choice for both immune suppression (2 to 4 mg/kg/day PO) and to treat inflammation/fibrosis (1 to 2 mg/kg/day PO). Prednisolone has been removed from the register of drugs that can potentially cause pancreatitis in humans and so is not contraindicated. If the animal is diabetic, then prednisolone may not be appropriate due to increased insulin resistance.

Management of concurrent diabetes mellitus may be difficult, because the insulin requirement may increase during bouts of active pancreatitis and then decrease during periods of recovery, leading to poorly sustained glycemic control.[41,84] One of the biggest risks associated with this waxing and waning illness is that when the disease is no longer present, the insulin requirements may drop precipitously. Due to this reason, some authors recommend the cautious use of doses of insulin in cats during the bouts of pancreatitis to prevent ketosis and avoid ensuing hypoglycemia when the inflammation resolves.[29] Education of the owner to carefully adjust the insulin dose and to have regular monitoring (at home or in clinic) is also essential. Despite the aversion to using prednisolone in a diabetic cat, a short course of prednisolone at anti-inflammatory doses may be helpful if the endogenous cause of the insulin resistance (pancreatic inflammation) is resolved.

An alternative immune suppressive option for cats is cyclosporine (5 mg/kg/day PO), because it is affordable and

Table 15-2	Dosage Rates for Analgesic Agents Potentially Useful in Treatment of Pancreatitis in Cats		
Drug	**Dosage**	**Duration of Action**	**Comment**
Full mu Agonist			
Methadone	0.1-1.0 mg/kg IV, IM, SC	4-6 h	
Fentanyl	2 µg/kg IV bolus	0.3 h	
	0.2-0.8 µg/kg/min	CRI	
	12.5 or 25 µg/h transdermal patch	Up to 5 days	Inconsistent efficacy Do not cut the patch
Remifentanil	2-4 µg/kg/h	CRI	
Partial mu Agonist			
Buprenorphine	10-40 µg/kg, IV, IM, sublingually	6-8 h	Generally start at a higher dose and frequency, then taper down if possible
Butorphanol	0.2 mg/kg IV, IM, SC	<2 h	Minimal analgesia

CRI, Continuous rate infusion; *IM,* intramuscularly; *IV,* intravenously; *SC,* subcutaneously.

generally well tolerated. However, there is a risk of unmasking latent toxoplasmosis; *Toxoplasma* titers[85] should be measured before and 2 to 4 weeks after starting cyclosporine. Chlorambucil (1 to 2 mg/m^2/day PO) is another immune suppressive drug that could be used in cats with chronic inflammation in the same way as used in IBD. Neither cyclosporine nor chlorambucil have been assessed in feline pancreatitis, and so their use remains speculative.

There is no evidence that dietary changes need to be made in feline pancreatitis, the exceptions being if there is concurrent disease that requires this or there is persistent hyperlipidemia.

INPATIENT

Cats that require hospitalization due to AP are at high risk for the development of concurrent disease, such as hepatic lipidosis or diabetic ketoacidosis. Treatment of these conditions takes priority, and the possibility of hepatic lipidosis must be considered at all times. As for dogs, AP can cause systemic organ complications, such as acute respiratory distress syndrome, cardiac arrhythmias, and disseminated intravascular coagulation, as well as local fluid collections within the pancreas and biliary duct obstruction.[86] The presence of hyperkalemia, dyspnea, and fPLI concentrations more than 20 μg/L appeared to correlate with prognosis in one prospective case series of 33 cats.[66] However, because cats were euthanized, this finding may be biased. In addition, nutritional management of the patients was unclear.

The basic tenets of management of pancreatitis are fluid therapy, pain relief, antiemetic therapy, and nutritional support. No specific fluid therapy protocol has been shown to be particularly advantageous in pancreatitis in cats. Extrapolation of experimental and medical data would suggest that lactated Ringer's solution is superior to normal saline, early fluid resuscitation is essential, and colloid therapy may be necessary.[46,87,88] However, fluid therapy should always be tailored to the individual animal.

Major mediators of pain in pancreatitis appear to be calcitonin gene-related peptide and substance P, acting through the neurokinin-1 (NK1) receptor.[89] Therefore during acute bouts of inflammation, treatment with an NK1-receptor antagonist, such as maropitant (0.5 to 1.0 mg/kg/day SC), may be of benefit in multiple ways: as an antiemetic, reducing pain, and potentially directly attenuating the systemic inflammatory response.[90] Maropitant is not licensed for use in cats in many countries, and so the use should be considered off label. Additional pain relief is often required and generally is based around opioid use. Full mu agonist opioids (e.g., morphine, methadone, hydromorphone, and fentanyl) are usually used to treat moderate to severe pain, whereas the partial mu agonists (e.g., buprenorphine) and the mu antagonist kappa agonists (e.g., butorphanol) are used for milder pain (see Table 15-2).[91] Fentanyl is a potent analgesic agent but does have profound effects on gastrointestinal motility.

Unfortunately the systemic absorption of fentanyl from transdermal patches is erratic; an intravenous (IV) route (2–4 μg/kg/h) may be preferable if methadone or buprenorphine is ineffective. Gabapentin can also be used as an adjunct analgesic agent in the acute setting.

Although many cats do not vomit when they have pancreatitis, there may be nausea that impacts their clinical recovery, and so treatment with at least one antiemetic agent is indicated even in the absence of vomiting. The exact mechanisms by which vomiting and nausea are mediated in pancreatitis are unknown. However, extrapolation would suggest that it is both peripherally and centrally mediated.[89,92] As a result, and due to the potential additional analgesic effects, maropitant is indicated as the first-line therapy. Adjunct antiemetic agents include ondansetron (0.5 mg/kg IV loading dose followed by 0.5 mg/kg/h infusion for 6 hours or 0.5 to 1 mg/kg PO every 12 to 24 hours) and mirtazapine (1.88 mg/cat PO every 48 hours).

Nutritional support is increasingly gaining attention in treatment of feline pancreatitis, similar to trends in human and canine medicine. One retrospective analysis of feline pancreatitis showed the most common complication of parenteral nutrition in cats was hyperglycemia, which is associated with a poor prognosis in humans.[39] The study also found that the presence of hepatic lipidosis and prolonged starvation before institution of parenteral nutrition was negatively associated with survival in cats.[39] As a result, the author recommends early interventional enteral nutrition. If anesthesia is indicated for a medical reason or the cat is clinically stable with no bleeding deficits, an esophagostomy feeding tube can be inserted. Alternatively, a naso-esophageal tube can be placed using only local anesthesia in severely ill cats.[93]

There are no studies that indicate the preferred food to give; it is generally a question of available formulations for the size of feeding tube that is being used. Naso-esophageal tubes are narrow in diameter; in countries where liquid veterinary diets are not available, human enteral formulas can be given. Human enteral formulas tend to be low in protein and lower than the recommended daily intake for cats (7.5 to 12 g/100 kcal). For example, Ensure (Abbott Laboratories), a commonly-available human convalescent diet, contains only 3.2 g protein/100 kcal. In our institution, if this diet is fed to cats for more than 24 hours, whey protein isolate (2.4 g/100 g) is added to the formulation. For this reason, larger gauge tubes inserted into the esophagus or stomach are preferred in order to feed veterinary convalescent diets in our hospital population. There is no evidence that fat restriction is necessary in the acute setting, nor is it established that providing the full caloric requirement is necessary to gain clinical benefit. In fact, cautious increases in the caloric intake may be a better strategy than titrating up to 100% quickly. The potential role of additives, such as omega-3 fatty acids or glutamine, is currently not known.

Although antibiotics are not routinely used in dogs with pancreatitis, there is a possible association with either bacterial translocation or bacterial reflux up the pancreatic duct in cats. Additionally, treatment of concurrent diseases (e.g., infectious cholangitis or hepatic lipidosis) with antibiotics is generally indicated. Therefore, use of an antibiotic that is excreted in the bile and can be given parenterally (e.g., ticarcillin or ampicillin) is advisable. Parenteral vitamin K and multivitamins may also be beneficial, especially if hepatic lipidosis is present.

Surgery is no longer recommended in the treatment of AP in humans,[94,95] with two exceptions. The first being when there is a documented septic process (within the pancreas) or when there is pathology (e.g., duct obstruction) that requires surgical correction. The consensus among human pancreatic surgeons is that even in the face of infection, the prognosis is improved if patients are treated with antibiotics for a period of time prior to surgery.[95] There are no well-powered studies that suggest débridement of pancreatic necrosis is useful in the management of pancreatitis in cats, and these procedures carry a high risk of morbidity. This author feels that percutaneous drainage of pancreatic fluid masses along with supportive care and antimicrobial therapy should be the first line of treatment for cats and may remove the need for surgical intervention. For the presence of pathology within the biliary or intestinal system, surgical intervention may be necessary but ideally in the least invasive manner.

SUMMARY

Pancreatitis in the cat can occur as a mild inflammatory process, associated with concurrent disease or as a severe presentation with systemic complications. Noninvasive diagnosis at the moment appears to rely on a combination of clinical signs, measurement of serum fPLI (or total serum lipase concentration), and abdominal ultrasound. When evaluating cats for intestinal or hepatic disease, pancreatic biopsy is recommended as well, because histopathology is the current gold standard for diagnosis. Laparoscopic techniques provide a less invasive method by which to obtain biopsies. Treatment of concurrent disease takes precedence in the management of cats. Close attention needs to be given to analgesia and nutritional support of severely ill cats. To date, there is no preferred diet to feed in either the acute or chronic setting. Cats with chronic disease, especially if insulin resistance is of concern, may benefit from anti-inflammatory therapy.

References

1. Garvey MS, Zawie DA: Feline pancreatic disease. *Vet Clin North Am Small Anim Pract* 14:1231–1246, 1984.
2. Charles J: Pancreas. In Maxie MG, editor: *Jubb, Kennedy, and Palmer's pathology of domestic animals*, ed 5, Edinburgh, 2007, Saunders/Elsevier, pp 389–423.
3. Watson PJ, Roulois AJ, Scase T, et al: Prevalence and breed distribution of chronic pancreatitis at post-mortem examination in first-opinion dogs. *J Small Anim Pract* 48:609–618, 2007.
4. de Cock HEV, Forman MA, Farver T, et al: Prevalence and histopathologic characteristics of pancreatitis in cats. *Vet Pathol* 44:39–49, 2007.
5. Newman S, Steiner J, Woosley K, et al: Localization of pancreatic inflammation and necrosis in dogs. *J Vet Intern Med* 18:488–493, 2004.
6. Newman SJ, Steiner JM, Woosley K, et al: Histologic assessment and grading of the exocrine pancreas in the dog. *J Vet Diagn Invest* 18:115–118, 2006.
7. De Cock HEV, Forman MA, Farver TB, et al: Prevalence and histopathologic characteristics of pancreatitis in cats. *Vet Pathol* 44:39–49, 2007.
8. Stevens T, Conwell DL, Zuccaro G: Pathogenesis of chronic pancreatitis: an evidence-based review of past theories and recent developments. *Am J Gastroenterol* 99:2256–2270, 2004.
9. Weiss DJ, Gagne JM, Armstrong PJ: Relationship between inflammatory hepatic disease and inflammatory bowel disease, pancreatitis, and nephritis in cats. *J Am Vet Med Assoc* 209:1114–1116, 1996.
10. Simpson KW, Twedt D, McDonough SP, et al: Culture-independent detection of bacteria in feline pancreatitis. *J Vet Intern Med* 25:2011. (Abstract).
11. Navaneethan U, Shen B: Hepatopancreatobiliary manifestations and complications associated with inflammatory bowel disease. *Inflamm Bowel Dis* 16:1598–1619, 2010.
12. Pitchumoni CS, Rubin A, Das K: Pancreatitis in inflammatory bowel diseases. *J Clin Gastroenterol* 44:246–253, 2010.
13. Finkelberg D, Sahani V, Deshpande W, et al: Autoimmune Pancreatitis. *N Engl J Med* 355:2670–2676, 2006.
14. Sugumur AS, Chari ST: Autoimmune pancreatitis. *J Gastroenterol Hepatol* 23:1368–1373, 2011.
15. Brain PH, Barrs VR, Martin P, et al: Feline cholecystitis and acute neutrophilic cholangitis: clinical findings, bacterial isolates and response to treatment in six cases. *J Feline Med Surg* 8:91–103, 2006.
16. Callahan Clark JE, Haddad JL, Brown DC, et al: Feline cholangitis: a necropsy study of 44 cats (1986-2008). *J Feline Med Surg* 13:570–576, 2011.
17. Arendt T: Bile-induced acute-pancreatitis in cats—roles of bile, bacteria, and pancreatic duct pressure. *Dig Dis Sci* 38:39–44, 1993.
18. Widdison AL, Karanjia ND, Reber HA: Routes of spread of pathogens into the pancreas in a feline model of acute-pancreatitis. *Gut* 35:1306–1310, 1994.
19. Son TT, Thompson L, Serrano S, et al: Surgical intervention in the management of severe acute pancreatitis in cats: 8 cases (2003-2007). *J Vet Emerg Crit Care (San Antonio)* 20:426–435, 2010.
20. Smart ME, Downey RS, Stockdale PH: Toxoplasmosis in a cat associated with cholangitis and progressive pancreatitis. *Can Vet J* 14:313–316, 1973.
21. Simpson KW: Current concepts of the pathogenesis and pathophysiology of acute pancreatitis in the dog and cat. *Compend Contin Educ Vet* 15:247–251, 1993.
22. Dubey JP, Carpenter JL: Histologically confirmed clinical toxoplasmosis in cats: 100 cases (1952-1990). *J Am Vet Med Assoc* 203: 1993.
23. Duncan RB, Lindsay D, Chickering WR, et al: Acute primary toxoplasmic pancreatitis in a cat. *Feline Pract* 28:6–8, 2000.
24. Bayliss DB, Steiner JM, Sucholdolski JS, et al: Serum feline pancreatic lipase immunoreactivity concentration and seroprevalences of antibodies against Toxoplasma gondii and Bartonella species in client-owned cats. *J Feline Med Surg* 11:663–667, 2009.
25. Pedersen NC, Elliott JB, Glasgow A, et al: An isolated epizootic of hemorrhagic-like fever in cats caused by a novel and highly virulent strain of feline calicivirus. *Vet Microbiol* 73:281–300, 2000.
26. Pesavento PA, MacLachlan NJ, Dillard-Telm L, et al: Pathologic, immunohistochemical, and electron microscopic findings in naturally occurring virulent systemic feline calicivirus infection in cats. *Vet Pathol* 41:257–263, 2004.
27. Steiner JM, Williams DA: Feline pancreatitis. *Compend Contin Educ Vet* 19:590–603, 1997.
28. Mansfield CS: Acute pancreatitis in dogs: advances in understanding, diagnostics and treatment. *Top Companion Anim Med* 27:123–132, 2012.

29. Caney SM: Pancreatitis and diabetes in cats. *Vet Clin North Am Small Anim Pract* 43:303–317, 2013.

30. Zini E, Osto M, Moretti S, et al: Hyperglycaemia but not hyperlipidaemia decreases serum amylase and increases neutrophils in the exocrine pancreas of cats. *Res Vet Sci* 89:20–26, 2010.

31. Hill RC, Van Winkle TJ: Acute necrotizing pancreatitis and acute suppurative pancreatitis in the cat. A retrospective study of 40 cases (1976-1989). *J Vet Intern Med* 7:25–33, 1993.

32. Zimmermann E, Hittmair KM, Suchodolski JS, et al: Serum feline-specific pancreatic lipase immunoreactivity concentrations and abdominal ultrasonographic findings in cats with trauma resulting from high-rise syndrome. *J Am Vet Med Assoc* 242:1238–1243, 2013.

33. Armstrong PJ, Williams DA: Pancreatitis in cats. *Top Companion Anim Med* 27:140–147, 2012.

34. Ferreri JA, Hardam E, Kimmel SE, et al: Clinical differentiation of acute necrotizing from chronic nonsuppurative pancreatitis in cats: 63 cases (1996-2001). *J Am Vet Med Assoc* 223:469–474, 2003.

35. Bailey S, Benigni L, Eastwood J, et al: Clinical significance of increased serum feline pancreatic lipase immunoreactivity concentrations in cats with inflammatory bowel disease. *J Vet Intern Med* 23:2009. (Abstract).

36. Mayhew PD, Weisse CW: Treatment of pancreatitis-associated extrahepatic biliary tract obstruction by choledochal stenting in seven cats. *J Small Anim Pract* 49:133–138, 2008.

37. Bruskiewicz KA, Nelson RW, Feldman EC, et al: Diabetic ketosis and ketoacidosis in cats: 42 cases (1980-1995). *J Am Vet Med Assoc* 211:188–192, 1997.

38. Dimski DS, Taboada J: Feline idiopathic hepatic lipidosis. *Vet Clin North Am Small Anim Pract* 25:357–373, 1995.

39. Queau Y, Larsen JA, Kass PH, et al: Factors associated with adverse outcomes during parenteral nutrition administration in dogs and cats. *J Vet Intern Med* 25:446–452, 2011.

40. Akol KG, Washabau RJ, Saunders HM, et al: Acute pancreatitis in cats with hepatic lipidosis. *J Vet Intern Med* 7:205–209, 1993.

41. Goossens MMC, Nelson RW, Feldman EC, et al: Response to insulin treatment and survival in 104 cats with diabetes mellitus (1985-1995). *J Vet Intern Med* 12:1–6, 1998.

42. Zini E, Hafner M, Osto M, et al: Pancreatic enzymes activity and ultrasonographic findings in diabetic cats at diagnosis and during follow-up. In *European College of Veterinary Internal Medicine Congress*, Sevilla, Spain, 2011. (Abstract).

43. Schafer S, Kooistra HS, Kunzle A, et al: Evaluation of insulin-like growth factor 1 (IGF-1), total thyroxine (TT4), feline pancreatic lipase immunoreactivity (fPLI) and urinary corticoid creatinine ratio (UCCR) in cats with diabetes mellitus in Switzerland and the Netherlands. In *European College of Veterinary Internal Medicine Congress*, Mainz, Germany, 2013. (Abstract).

44. Forcada Y, German AJ, Noble PJ, et al: Determination of serum fPLI concentrations in cats with diabetes mellitus. *J Feline Med Surg* 10:480–487, 2008.

45. Bhoomagoud M, Jung T, Atladottir J, et al: Reducing extracellular pH sensitizes the acinar cell to secretagogue-induced pancreatitis responses in rats. *Gastoenterol* 137:1083–1092, 2009.

46. Wu BU, Hwang JQ, Gardner TH, et al: Lactated Ringer's solution reduces systemic inflammation compared with saline in patients with acute pancreatitis. *Clin Gastroenterol Hepatol* 9(8):710–717, 2011.

47. Kimmel SE, Washabau RJ, Drobatz KJ: Incidence and prognostic value of low plasma ionized calcium concentration in cats with acute pancreatitis: 46 cases (1996-1998). *J Am Vet Med Assoc* 219:1105–1109, 2001.

48. Oppliger S, Hartnack S, Riond B, et al: Agreement of the serum spec fPL (TM) and 1,2-O-dilauryl-rac-glycero-3-glutaric acid-(6'-methylresorufin) ester lipase assay for the determination of serum lipase in cats with suspicion of pancreatitis. *J Vet Intern Med* 27:1077–1082, 2013.

49. Abrams-Ogg A, Ruotsalo K, Kocmarek H, et al: Total serum lipase activity for the antemortem diagnosis of feline pancreatitis. *J Vet Intern Med* 27:708–708, 2013.

50. Steiner JM, Williams DA: Serum feline trypsin-like immunoreactivity in cats with exocrine pancreatic insufficiency. *J Vet Intern Med* 14:627–629, 2000.

51. Forman MA, Marks SL, De Cock HEV, et al: Evaluation of serum feline pancreatic lipase immunoreactivity and helical computed tomography versus conventional testing for the diagnosis of feline pancreatitis. *J Vet Intern Med* 18:807–815, 2004.

52. Swift NC, Marks SL, MacLachlan NJ, et al: Evaluation of serum feline trypsin-like immunoreactivity for the diagnosis of pancreatitis in cats. *J Am Vet Med Assoc* 217:37–42, 2000.

53. Gerhardt A, Steiner JM, Williams DA, et al: Comparison of the sensitivity of different diagnostic tests for pancreatitis in cats. *J Vet Intern Med* 15:329–333, 2001.

54. Allen HS, Steiner J, Broussard J, et al: Serum and urine concentrations of trypsinogen-activation peptide as markers for acute pancreatitis in cats. *Can J Vet Res* 70:313–316, 2006.

55. Xenoulis PG, Steiner JM: Canine and feline pancreatic lipase immunoreactivity. *Vet Clin Pathol* 41:312–324, 2012.

56. Steiner JM, Wilson BG, Williams DA: Development and analytical validation of a radiommunoassay for the measurement of feline pancreatic lipase immunoreactivity in serum. *Can J Vet Res* 68:309–314, 2004.

57. Steiner JM, Teague SR, Williams DA: Development and analytic validation of an enzyme-linked immunosorbent assay for the measurement of canine pancreatic lipase immunoreactivity in serum. *Can J Vet Res* 67:175–182, 2003.

58. Steiner JM, Berridge BR, Wojcieszyn J, et al: Cellular immunolocalization of gastric and pancreatic lipase in various tissues obtained from dogs. *Am J Vet Res* 63:722–727, 2002.

59. Steiner JM, Rutz GM, Williams DA: Serum lipase activities and pancreatic lipase immunoreactivity concentrations in dogs with exocrine pancreatic insufficiency. *Am J Vet Res* 67:84–87, 2006.

60. Williams JM, Panciera DL, Larson MM, et al: Ultrasonographic findings of the pancreas in cats with elevated serum pancreatic lipase immunoreactivity. *J Vet Intern Med* 27:913–918, 2013.

61. Forman MA, Shiroma JT, Armstrong PJ: Evaluation of feline pancreas-specific lipase (Spec fPL) for the diagnosis of feline pancreatitis. *J Vet Intern Med* 23:733–734, 2009. (Abstract).

62. Xenoulis P, Finco D, Suchodolski J, et al: Serum fPLI and Spec fPL concentrations in cats with experimentally induced chronic renal failure. *J Vet Intern Med* 23:758, 2009. (Abstract).

63. Tamamoto T, Ohno K, Ohmi A, et al: Time-course monitoring of serum amyloid A in a cat with pancreatitis. *Vet Clin Pathol* 38:83–86, 2009.

64. Christensen M, Jacobsen S, Ichiyanagi T, et al: Evaluation of an automated assay based on monoclonal anti-human serum amyloid A (SAA) antibodies for measurement of canine, feline, and equine SAA. *Vet J* 194:332–337, 2012.

65. Bjorneby JM, Kari S: Cytology of the pancreas. *Vet Clin North Am Small Anim Pract* 32:1293–1312, 2002.

66. Stockhaus C, Teske E, Schellenberger K, et al: Serial serum feline pancreatic lipase immunoreactivity concentrations and prognostic variables in 33 cats with pancreatitis. *J Am Vet Med Assoc* 243:1713–1718, 2013.

67. Saunders HM, VanWinkle TJ, Drobatz K, et al: Ultrasonographic findings in cats with clinical, gross pathologic, and histologic evidence of acute pancreatic necrosis: 20 cases (1994-2001). *J Am Vet Med Assoc* 221:1724–1730, 2002.

68. Hecht S, Penninck D, Keating JH: Imaging findins in pancreatic neoplasia and nodular hyperplasia in 19 cats. *Vet Radiol Ultrasound* 48:45–50, 2007.

69. Wall M, Biller DS, Schoning P, et al: Pancreatitis in a cat demonstrating pancreatic duct dilatation ultrasonographically. *J Am Anim Hosp Assoc* 37:49–53, 2001.

70. Larson MM, Panciera DL, Ward DL, et al: Age-related changes in the ultrasound appearance of the normal feline pancreas. *Vet Radiol Ultrasound* 46:238–242, 2005.

71. Baron ML, Hecht S, Matthews AR, et al: Ultrasonographic observation of secretin-induced pancreatic duct dilation in healthy cats. *Vet Radiol Ultrasound* 51:86–89, 2010.

72. Schweighauser A, Gaschen F, Steiner J, et al: Evaluation of endosonography as a new diagnostic tool for feline pancreatitis. *J Feline Med Surg* 11:492–498, 2009.

73. Rademacher N, Ohlerth S, Scharf G, et al: Contrast-enhanced power and color doppler ultrasonography of the pancreas in healthy and diseased cats. *J Vet Intern Med* 22:1310–1316, 2008.

74. Head LL, Daniel GB, Becker TJ, et al: Use of computed tomography and radiolabeled leukocytes in a cat with pancreatitis. *Vet Radiol Ultrasound* 46:263–266, 2005.

75. Marolf AJ, Kraft SL, Dunphy TR, et al: Magnetic resonance (MR) imaging and MR cholangiopancreatography findings in cats with cholangitis and pancreatitis. *J Feline Med Surg* 15:285–294, 2013.

76. Marolf AJ, Stewart JA, Dunphy TR, et al: Hepatic and pancreaticobiliary MRI and MR cholangiopancreatography with and without secretin stimulation in normal cats. *Vet Radiol Ultrasound* 52:415–421, 2011.

77. Head LL, Daniel GB, Becker TJ, et al: Use of computed tomography and radiolabeled leukocytes in a cat with pancreatitis. *Vet Radiol Ultrasound* 46:263–266, 2005.

78. Head LL, Daniel GB, Tobias K, et al: Evaluation of the feline pancreas using computed tomography and radiolabeled leukocytes. *Vet Radiol Ultrasound* 44:420–428, 2003.

79. Robertson E, Twedt D, Webb C: Diagnostic laparoscopy in the cat 1: rationale and equipment. *J Feline Med Surg* 16:5–16, 2014.

80. Webb CB: Feline laparoscopy for gastrointestinal disease. *Top Companion Anim Med* 23:193–199, 2008.

81. Cosford KL, Shmon CL, Myers SL, et al: Prospective evaluation of laparoscopic pancreatic biopsies in 11 healthy cats. *J Vet Intern Med* 24:104–113, 2010.

82. Ruaux CG, Steiner JM, Williams DA: Early biochemical and clinical responses to cobalamin supplementation in cats with signs of gastrointestinal disease and severe hypocobalaminemia. *J Vet Intern Med* 19:155–160, 2005.

83. Lamont LA: Adjunctive analgesic therapy in veterinary medicine. *Vet Clin North Am Small Anim Pract* 38:1187–1203, 2008.

84. Rand JS: Pathogenesis of feline diabetes. *Vet Clin North Am Small Anim Pract* 43:221–231, 2013.

85. Barrs VR, Martin P, Beatty JA: Antemortem diagnosis and treatment of toxoplasmosis in two cats on cyclosporin therapy. *Aust Vet J* 84:30–35, 2006.

86. Mansfield CS: Pathophysiology of acute pancreatitis: potential application from experimental models and human medicine to dogs. *J Vet Intern Med* 26:875–887, 2012.

87. Horton JW, Dunn CW, Burnweit CA, et al: Hypertonic saline-dextran resuscitation of acute canine bile-induced pancreatitis. *Am J Surg* 158:48–56, 1989.

88. Warndorf MG, Kurtzman JT, Bartel MJ, et al: Early fluid resuscitation reduces morbidity among patients with acute pancreatitis. *Clin Gastroenterol Hepatol* 9:705–709, 2011.

89. Frossard JL, Pastor CM: Experimental acute pancreatitis: new insights into the pathophysiology. *Front Biosci* 7:d275–d287, 2002.

90. Bhatia M, Saluja AK, Hofbauer B, et al: Role of substance P and the NK1 receptor in acute pancreatitis and pancreatitis-associated lung injury. *Proc Natl Acad Sci USA* 95:4760–4765, 1998.

91. Lemke KA, Creighton CM: Analgesia for anesthetized patients. *Top Companion Anim Med* 25:70–82, 2010.

92. Elwood C, Devauchelle P, Elliot J, et al: Emesis in dogs: a review. *J Small Anim Pract* 51:4–22, 2010.

93. Klaus JA, Rudloff E, Kirby R: Nasogastric tube feeding in cats with suspected acute pancreatitis: 55 cases (2001-2006). *J Vet Emerg Crit Care* 19:337–346, 2009.

94. Wu BU, Conwell DL: Acute pancreatitis part I: approach to early management. *Clinical Gastroenterol Hepatol* 8:410–416, 2010.

95. Nordback IH, Sand J, Saaristo R, et al: Early treatment with antibiotics reduces the need for surgery in acute necrotizing pancreatitis: a single-center randomized study. *J Gastrointest Surg* 5:113–118, 2001.

Feline Extrahepatic Bile Duct Obstruction: Medical versus Surgical Management

Allison Bradley and Dan D. Smeak

EPIDEMIOLOGY

Extrahepatic bile duct obstruction (EHBDO) is defined as the lack of bile transit into the duodenum due to blockage along the common bile duct (CBD) or at its junction with the duodenum. The pathology may be intraluminal, mural, or extramural (Table 16-1). EHBDO is an uncommon but often life-threatening problem that may require timely surgical intervention. However, in many cases, the indications for medical or surgical management are not straightforward,[1] and the risks and frequently poor prognosis associated with biliary surgery in cats often make this decision difficult.

Extrahepatic bile duct obstruction is less common in cats than dogs,[23] likely due to the higher incidence of acute pancreatitis and gallbladder mucoceles in dogs. Although no true breed predilections have been reported for EHBDO in cats, anecdotally Siamese may be overrepresented, possibly due to their increased incidence of cholangitis and pancreatitis.[24] Cats of any age can be affected by EHBDO, but the majority of them are middle-aged or older. There do not appear to be significant sex predilections for diseases associated with feline EHBDO.

HISTORY AND CLINICAL SIGNS

Although EHBDO can occasionally be an incidental finding, most affected cats present with icterus and nonspecific signs, such as anorexia, lethargy, and vomiting. Diarrhea is less consistently reported, but weight loss is common with chronic disease. Polyphagia—secondary to fat maldigestion—is rarely reported.[16,25] The owner may note pigmenturia or acholic feces, the latter being an insensitive but fairly specific indication of the lack of bilirubin entering the intestinal tract. Abdominal pain, abdominal effusion, and fever are variably present, as are gastrointestinal (GI) bleeding and other evidence of bleeding tendencies. Abdominal palpation may reveal hepatomegaly or a palpable gallbladder.[26,27] Hepatic encephalopathy (HE) is not common in cats with biliary disease; signs include obtundation and ptyalism.[28] Although uncommon, alopecia has been reported in cats with bile duct carcinoma.[29] Signs of EHBDO can be acute (days) or chronic (weeks to months). Acute, obstructive cholelithiasis may be associated with a briefer duration of clinical signs than chronic inflammatory or neoplastic disease.[20,24] History regarding previous bouts of illness that might suggest chronic inflammatory disease, as well as the possibility of trauma or parasite exposure (e.g., travel and hunting behavior) should be elicited.

DIAGNOSTIC WORKUP

Minimum Database

The diagnostic investigation should begin with a serum biochemistry panel, complete blood count (CBC) with slide review, and urinalysis. Cats with EHBDO have an elevated serum bilirubin, and this change is typically quite marked,[26] often with bilirubin increased tenfold or more above the reference range. Mild elevations in bilirubin (e.g., less than 34.2 μmol/L [2 mg/dL]) are common in cats with other systemic illnesses and are unlikely to reflect EHBDO, unless the obstruction has just occurred.[30] The liver enzymes alanine aminotransferase (ALT), aspartate aminotransferase (AST), alkaline phosphatase (ALP), and gamma-glutamyltransferase (GGT) are typically elevated. In contrast to dogs with markedly elevated cholestatic enzymes secondary to EHBDO, in the cat, ALT concentrations often exceed ALP, due to the smaller pool and shorter half-life of feline ALP.[1,24,26,31-33] GGT is typically elevated in EHBDO,[34] and concentrations may also exceed ALP.[35] With chronic obstruction, cholesterol is usually elevated[26]; however, many cats in published case series have normal cholesterol in the face of EHBDO.[1,32,36] Other important findings on the serum biochemistry panel include azotemia (which is often a poor prognostic indicator);[37] hyperglobulinemia (often observed with lymphoma or lymphocytic cholangitis [LC]),[5] and biochemistry tests affected by decreased hepatic function (e.g., hypoglycemia, hypoalbuminemia, hypocholesterolemia, and low blood urea nitrogen). Low ionized calcium should increase the index of suspicion for acute pancreatitis and may be a poor prognostic indicator.[38]

The CBC may reveal an inflammatory leukogram that becomes more severe with increasing chronicity of EHBDO.[26]

Table 16-1	Differential Diagnoses of Feline Extrahepatic Bile Duct Obstruction
Causes of Extrahepatic Bile Duct Obstruction*	**Medical or Surgical[†]**
Inflammatory mural—cholangitis/choledochitis	M: Bacterial or sterile; cholangitis can be the cause or result of EHBDO[1,2]
Inflammatory extramural (e.g., pancreatitis, pancreatolith,[3] lymphadenopathy, duodenal disease)	M: Pancreatitis can be the cause or result of EHBDO[4]
Neoplasia—luminal/mural or extramural (e.g., biliary, duodenal, pancreatic)	S: Unless lymphoma
Obstructive cholelithiasis, biliary sludge, blood clot	S: Biliary sludge/stones can be the cause or result of EHDBO[1,5]
Parasites • Flukes (*Platynosomum* spp. and others) • Ascarids • Other	M and S: Endemic in all tropical and subtropical regions; obstruction may be due to parasites, sludge, or secondary inflammation or fibrosis;[6-11] ascarids and *Echinococcus* spp. are causes of EHBDO in people, not yet reported in cats[12,13]
Diaphragmatic hernia[14]	S
Bile duct stricture	S
Congenital/anatomic abnormalities (e.g., choledochal duct cyst,[15-17] polycystic liver disease,[16] biliary atresia[2])	M or S: If small number of obstructive lesions, surgery can be curative but may not be an option with diffuse disease
Gallbladder mucocele[18-20]	S
Duodenal or biliary foreign body[21,22]	S
Gallbladder torsion	S: Not yet reported in the cat[6]
Any case complicated by bile peritonitis	S: Surgery usually necessary, but some small sterile bile leaks may resolve without complication[18]

EHBDO, Extrahepatic bile duct obstruction.
*In approximate order of frequency.
[†]*M*, Medical; *S*, surgical. Indicates preferred treatment. In all cases, surgery may be required if obstruction does not resolve with medical therapy.

Neutropenia or marked left shift may increase the suspicion of a bacterial etiology. Eosinophilia may be associated with parasitism. Anemia is frequently present and may be nonregenerative due to chronic disease, or it may be regenerative in association with GI bleeding secondary to prolonged EHBDO.[26] If anemia is present, or the packed cell volume or hematocrit have dropped relative to a particular patient's historical values, then it is important to investigate the possibility of a prehepatic cause of hyperbilirubinemia. The blood smear should be reviewed for evidence of hemolytic disease and *Mycoplasma haemofelis* or other parasitic infection, and a saline agglutination test should be performed.

The urinalysis will reveal bilirubinuria; unlike in dogs, any bilirubinuria is significant in the cat and will precede jaundice.[26] Although the lack of urobilinogen may be evidence of complete EHBDO, this test is error-prone and correlates poorly with disease. Although most other changes will be nonspecific relative to EHBDO, it is important to note the cat's baseline urine specific gravity and any proteinuria, because renal complications of EHBDO may occur. Bacteriuria should be evaluated, and a urine culture performed if present, or if sepsis is suspected, because organisms affecting the hepatobiliary system and/or translocated from the GI tract secondary to EHBDO might be identified in this manner.[16]

Imaging

Once hyperbilirubinemia is identified, and hemolysis has been ruled out, the next diagnostic step is abdominal imaging to investigate hepatic versus posthepatic causes of icterus. Although abdominal radiographs are likely to be insensitive for many causes of hepatobiliary disease, routine radiographs should be performed in order to evaluate for diaphragmatic hernia, duodenal foreign body, emphysematous cholecystitis, or mass effects, as well as to assess the size of the liver. They may also identify radiopaque choleliths; however, these can be an incidental finding.[6,23] Evidence of free abdominal fluid or gas within hepatobiliary structures should prompt urgent assessment for septic or bile peritonitis.[16]

Abdominal ultrasound is required to thoroughly evaluate the gallbladder, cystic duct, CBD, and intrahepatic bile ducts for dilation and other abnormalities. Because the biliary tree can be difficult to image, this should be performed by a highly-skilled ultrasonographer, and the patient should be fasted. Often, changing patient positioning is required to visualize the entire biliary system. Color-flow Doppler distinguishes blood vessels from bile ducts.

The normal diameter of the feline CBD is 4 mm or less.[39] Because even an enlarged CBD can be missed on ultrasonographic exam, serial imaging should be performed if clinical suspicion of EHBDO persists. In dogs with experimental CBD ligation, the CBD dilates after 24 to 48 hours.[42] Distended intrahepatic biliary ducts, which occur approximately 4 to 5 days after experimental EHBDO in dogs, are seen as hypoechoic tubular structures adjacent to the intrahepatic portal veins (they are not normally visualized unless distended).[40] Although they provide supportive evidence, dilated intrahepatic ducts do not confirm EHBDO,[20] and normal intrahepatic ducts do not rule it out.[20,39] If biliary dilation is seen, a thorough search for the cause of obstruction (see Table 16-1) should be performed along the length of the CBD to its termination at the duodenal papilla. In a study of 30 cats with EHBDO, the most common site for an obstruction was in the distal CBD or duodenal papilla, and asymmetrical, irregular thickening of the CBD wall was associated with bile duct adenocarcinoma.[20] If a mass is present and accessible, fine-needle aspiration (FNA) and cytology should be performed. In most cases, ultrasonography cannot distinguish between inflammatory and neoplastic masses.[20]

Thickened (1 mm or greater), hyperechoic, and layered gallbladder walls are associated with disease, including EHBDO, but a normal-appearing wall does not rule out pathology.[41] Aberrant gallbladder anatomy (e.g., bilobed or duplex) is relatively common and likely incidental.[16,19] Unlike in dogs, feline gallbladder sludge may not be incidental and has been associated with hepatobiliary disease.[42,43] Obstructive masses in the gallbladder may be benign polyps or malignant neoplasia.[41] The integrity of the gallbladder should be carefully evaluated, because confirmed or impending gallbladder rupture is an indication for prompt surgical intervention. However, ultrasound may be insensitive for gallbladder rupture.[44,45] It is important to note that with acute EHBDO, the gallbladder may not yet be dilated, and serial ultrasound examinations and/or advanced imaging may be required if clinical suspicion persists.[46] However, in some cases of EHBDO, the gallbladder may remain contracted due to inflammation or fibrosis and therefore never becomes dilated.[20,39,47,48]

Examination of the other abdominal organs may provide clues as to the cause of EHBDO. For example, although ultrasound is insensitive for feline pancreatitis, hyperechoic pancreas, dilated pancreatic duct or pancreatic cysts, and increased pancreatic blood flow may suggest pancreatitis.[49,50,51] Thickened or poorly layered loops of bowel may suggest inflammatory bowel disease (IBD) or lymphoma.[43] Lymph node abnormalities may be seen with a variety of infectious, inflammatory, and neoplastic conditions, and cytology of lymph node aspirates may yield a diagnosis. The appearance of the liver is nonspecific for most conditions associated with EHBDO, and it may be normal, hypoechoic, or hyperechoic.[43,50,52,53] Chronic EHBDO results in hepatomegaly.[26,27]

If no obvious cause of obstruction or evidence of bile peritonitis is found, the decision to pursue surgery should be contingent upon progressive worsening of clinical signs, laboratory abnormalities, or bile duct dilation on serial ultrasounds. Biliary dilation alone is not specific for obstruction.[1,54-56] Many cases of nonsurgical diseases, such as cholangitis, will have biliary dilation,[4,52,52,53] and biliary dilation may persist indefinitely after a previous episode of obstruction[16,56] or cholecystectomy, as has been reported in dogs and humans.[45,57] In the authors' experience, it is common to find dilated bile ducts in cats with normal serum bilirubin, indicating patent bile flow (Figure 16-1). In addition, a necropsy study of 44 cats with cholangitis revealed that many cats with dilated CBDs and/or gallbladders were not obstructed.[53]

If clinical suspicion of EHBDO persists but cannot be confirmed with serial ultrasound exams, then other imaging modalities may be considered. Although hepatobiliary scintigraphy may be more accurate than ultrasound for diagnosis

of EHBDO,[55] its utility is restricted by its limited availability and the need to scan patients multiple times over at least 24 hours, during which time the patients are radioactive. Hyperbilirubinemia and sepsis can also confound interpretation of results.[57] Magnetic resonance imaging (MRI) is commonly used in people when ultrasound and computed tomography (CT) fail to reveal the cause of icterus. MRI was utilized in one report of 10 cats with suspected cholangitis and/or pancreatitis and may be of particular use for diagnosing pancreatitis and obtaining complete images of the biliary tract without interference from bowel gas.[50] Computed tomography would seem to offer some of these same advantages, but so far studies have shown little diagnostic value in cats with pancreatitis.[58,59] Endoscopic retrograde cholangiopancreatography combines endoscopy and fluoroscopy for imaging of the biliary and pancreatic ducts and may also facilitate therapeutic interventions, such as sphincterotomy and stent placement. It has been attempted with some success in healthy cats[60] and is under investigation in cats with suspected EHBDO (A. Berent, personal communication, April 1, 2014).

Adjunct Diagnostics

If basic lab work and abdominal imaging do not reveal a definitive cause of EHBDO, then adjunct diagnostics should be pursued. Every effort should be made to obtain a diagnosis before proceeding to surgery, although in some cases exploratory laparotomy with biopsy may be the only way to obtain a definitive diagnosis. Additional tests that should be considered on a case-by-case basis are described later.

Thoracic radiographs are indicated in most cases to screen for metastasis or concurrent disease (e.g., heart failure and aspiration pneumonia) that might alter the prognosis and therapeutic plan. Pleural effusion is commonly seen in cases of acute necrotizing pancreatitis (ANP),[49] and sternal lymphadenopathy is common with feline inflammatory liver disease.[16]

Coagulation status should be assessed in all patients. Prothrombin time (PT) and activated partial thromboplastin time (aPTT) should be measured, because EHBDO and its associated diseases can result in deficiency of vitamin K-dependent clotting factors or other coagulopathies. Although clotting times are poorly correlated with bleeding complications following FNA or biopsy of the liver,[61] we believe their measurement is still prudent, and correction with vitamin K and fresh frozen plasma is indicated if they are significantly (greater than 25%) prolonged prior to any invasive procedures. At the authors' institution, the authors also measure *buccal mucosal bleeding time* prior to liver biopsy, because thrombopathia can be a complication of hepatobiliary disease. Assays supportive of hypercoagulability, which can also occur with EHBDO in dogs and people,[62] such as thromboelastography and platelet function testing, are less widely available and not routinely performed, although they may be helpful in investigation of select cases in which thromboembolic complications are suspected.

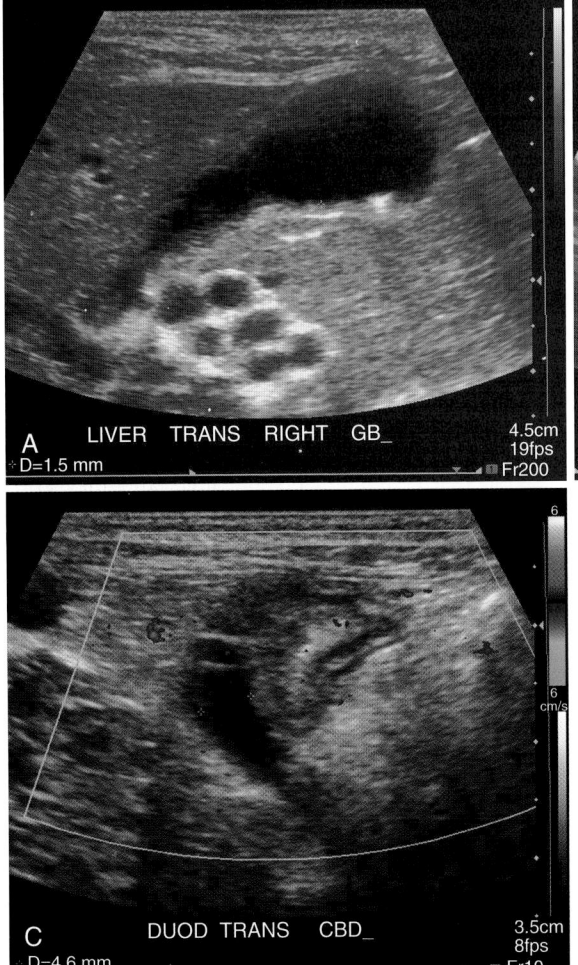

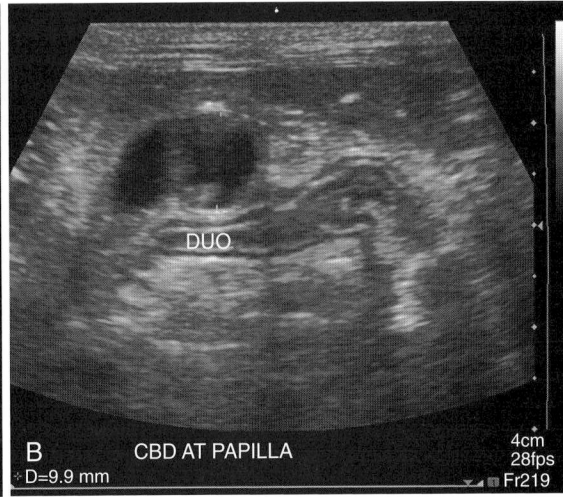

Figure 16-1: Nonobstructive biliary dilation due to chronic pancreatitis in a cat with normal serum bilirubin. **A,** A classic tortuous common bile duct (CBD) is visible adjacent to the gallbladder. **B,** The CBD (denoted by calipers) measures 9.9 mm at the duodenal papilla. **C,** Use of color Doppler to differentiate the large tubular structure as a bile duct rather than a blood vessel (*red and blue* indicate blood flow).

Cytology of Fine-Needle Aspirates of Liver, Pancreas, Masses, and Enlarged Lymph Nodes

Cytology of liver aspirates is fairly sensitive for lymphoma and mast cell tumor, and it can be diagnostic for carcinomas in some cases; however, multiple studies have demonstrated that results should be interpreted with caution.[2,61,63] It is also sensitive for hepatic lipidosis.[2] Although this will not rule out another underlying condition, the presence of hepatic lipidosis may affect prognosis[33] and medical management. Inflammation seen on cytology of fine-needle aspirates may be primary or secondary; however, it may guide medical management. For example, if septic suppurative inflammation is identified, a Gram stain may help with initial antibiotic selection.[16]

Bile cytology and culture (aerobic and anaerobic) should be performed whenever possible in cases not proceeding directly to surgery, especially those of suspected cholangitis.[64] Bile is a more sensitive sample for culture than liver tissue.[2,65] Fluke ova may also be identified on bile cytology.[7] "White bile," which appears grossly more like serum, is a rare finding and almost always indicates complete EHBDO.[6,48]

Percutaneous ultrasound-guided cholecystocentesis has been demonstrated to be safe in healthy cats and is commonly performed at many institutions. A transhepatic approach, rather than direct puncture of the fundus, has been recommended so that the liver tissue can seal off small bile leaks,[16] but in a study of 12 healthy cats, the one cat in which a transhepatic approach was used had a hemorrhagic complication, versus no complications in the 11 cats in which direct puncture was employed (using a 22-gauge 1.5-inch spinal needle with attempted complete drainage from the fundus).[66] Ultrasound-guided cholecystocentesis has also been utilized in cats with neutrophilic cholangitis[67] and dogs with cholecystitis,[68] but a higher complication rate may be seen, and it is not recommended if there is ultrasonographic evidence of severe cholecystitis.[67] The procedure should be done under heavy sedation and can stimulate a lethal vasovagal response, so anticholinergic and ventilatory support should be available.[16]

Abdominal Effusion Analysis

Ascites is uncommon in cats with experimental EHBDO[26] and in cats with cholangitis,[43] although it may be more common with LC.[5,43] The presence of abdominal effusion in the absence of severe hypoalbuminemia should increase the suspicion of bile peritonitis, pancreatitis,[69] and neoplasia, and the fluid should be sampled as close to the biliary structures as possible[16] and submitted for fluid analysis and cytology, as well as culture if indicated. Bile peritonitis may be suspected if the gallbladder appears compromised, or the fluid cytology is consistent with bile peritonitis (e.g., high-protein, suppurative exudate with or without bile crystals). In those cases, the fluid bilirubin concentration should be measured. If it exceeds the serum bilirubin concentration, or a urine dipstick is positive for bilirubin when used to test the fluid,[70] surgical intervention is indicated.

Fecal Examination

Formalin-ether centrifugation is the recommended method for detecting fluke ova[8,71] and will identify most helminth eggs, as well. However, false-negative results may be obtained due to intermittent shedding of ova, or with complete EHBDO, in which fluke ova may not be shed in the feces.[16]

Gastrointestinal Function Panel, Including Feline Pancreatic Lipase Immunoreactivity

In a necropsy study of 44 cats with cholangitis, 50% had concurrent IBD, 60% had concurrent pancreatitis, and 32% had evidence of all three conditions.[53] Accordingly, clinicians should remain vigilant for the possibility of "triaditis" in all cases of feline inflammatory hepatobiliary disease (see Chapter 12). Pancreatitis can be difficult to diagnose in cats,[49,50,69] and the combination of feline pancreatic lipase immunoreactivity (fPLI) with clinical suspicion and ultrasound findings is often necessary (see Chapter 15).[38] Abnormalities in cobalamin and folate levels may point to underlying intestinal disease, as well as the need for cobalamin supplementation. Cobalamin levels can also be decreased with cholangitis and pancreatitis but increased with cholestasis.[72]

Serology for feline leukemia and feline immunodeficiency viruses and *Toxoplasma gondii* should be performed.[8]

Additional Bacterial Culture

If bile cannot be safely obtained, or if bile cytology is nondiagnostic, additional (albeit likely lower yield) samples that may be cultured in patients with suspected sepsis include blood, urine, and aspirates of the liver and pancreas.[5,16,73]

TREATMENT

Surgical versus Medical Therapy— The Decision-Making Process

Conventional wisdom states that permanent and complete biliary obstruction warrants surgical intervention. However, partial obstructions or temporary complete obstructions— such as those seen with cholangitis and acute pancreatitis—may respond favorably to medical management.[23,57] It is important to differentiate permanent versus temporary obstructions during surgical decision making,

because the therapeutic options and expected patient outcomes may differ dramatically. Given the difficulty of diagnosing an EHBDO as complete and ongoing before surgery, as well as the challenge, complications, and poor prognosis often associated with biliary surgery in cats, surgery should only be considered after a methodical diagnostic workup and, when appropriate, a trial of medical therapy, or in cats that cannot be medically stabilized and are strongly suspected of having an EHBDO (Figure 16-2).

To be sure, there are certain causes of EHBDO (i.e., complete and permanent) where surgery is effective at creating a patent avenue for bile transport to the small bowel, and these are clear indications for prompt surgical intervention. These include a lodged, obstructive duodenal foreign body, diaphragmatic hernia, obstructive choleliths, and EHBDO associated with gallbladder mucocele. Additionally, cats with evidence of bile or septic peritonitis or impending gallbladder rupture warrant emergency surgery. Other conditions, such as pancreatitis and cholangitis, that can present clinically and sonographically as apparent EHBDO[23,67,69] are best handled medically and should only be taken to surgery if the patient is not responding well to medical management. In these refractory cases, an exploratory laparotomy may reveal a previously undiagnosed, yet surgically correctable, cause of the EHBDO. For example, although pancreatitis can cause EHBDO, EHBDO due to a choledocholith can cause pancreatitis.[4,16] Alternatively, surgical procedures (e.g., temporary stent placement, procurement of samples for histopathology and culture, and placement of a feeding tube) may aid in both the diagnosis and medical management of the case. It is the third category of EHBDO—cases in which the potential benefits of surgery are not well-defined or cases with temporary partial or complete obstructions that might respond to medical therapy (e.g., firm sludge, inflammatory extramural masses [such as pancreatitis or lymphadenopathy], partial bile duct stenosis from infection or inflammation, incidental cholelithiasis, and cases in which an underlying cause cannot be identified)—that presents the biggest treatment conundrum. When deciding whether or not to intervene surgically in cases that do not have a definitive surgical indication, the following factors come into play:

- Prognosis associated with the underlying disease: Is it reversible with surgery, or would it be readily managed medically postoperatively?
- Is biliary-enteric diversion likely to be necessary?
- What comorbidities or poor prognostic indicators (e.g., hepatic lipidosis,[33] severe hypocalcemia,[38,69] hypotension, sepsis, acute renal failure, coagulopathy)[37] are present?
- Is the patient already failing medical therapy, leaving little choice other than surgical exploration?
- Is surgery the only way to obtain a diagnosis of the underlying disease?
- Are there concomitant intra-abdominal conditions in the patient that need surgical attention?
- Does the patient need a feeding tube, and/or would the patient benefit from biliary stenting to palliate the obstruction or buy time for medical therapy?

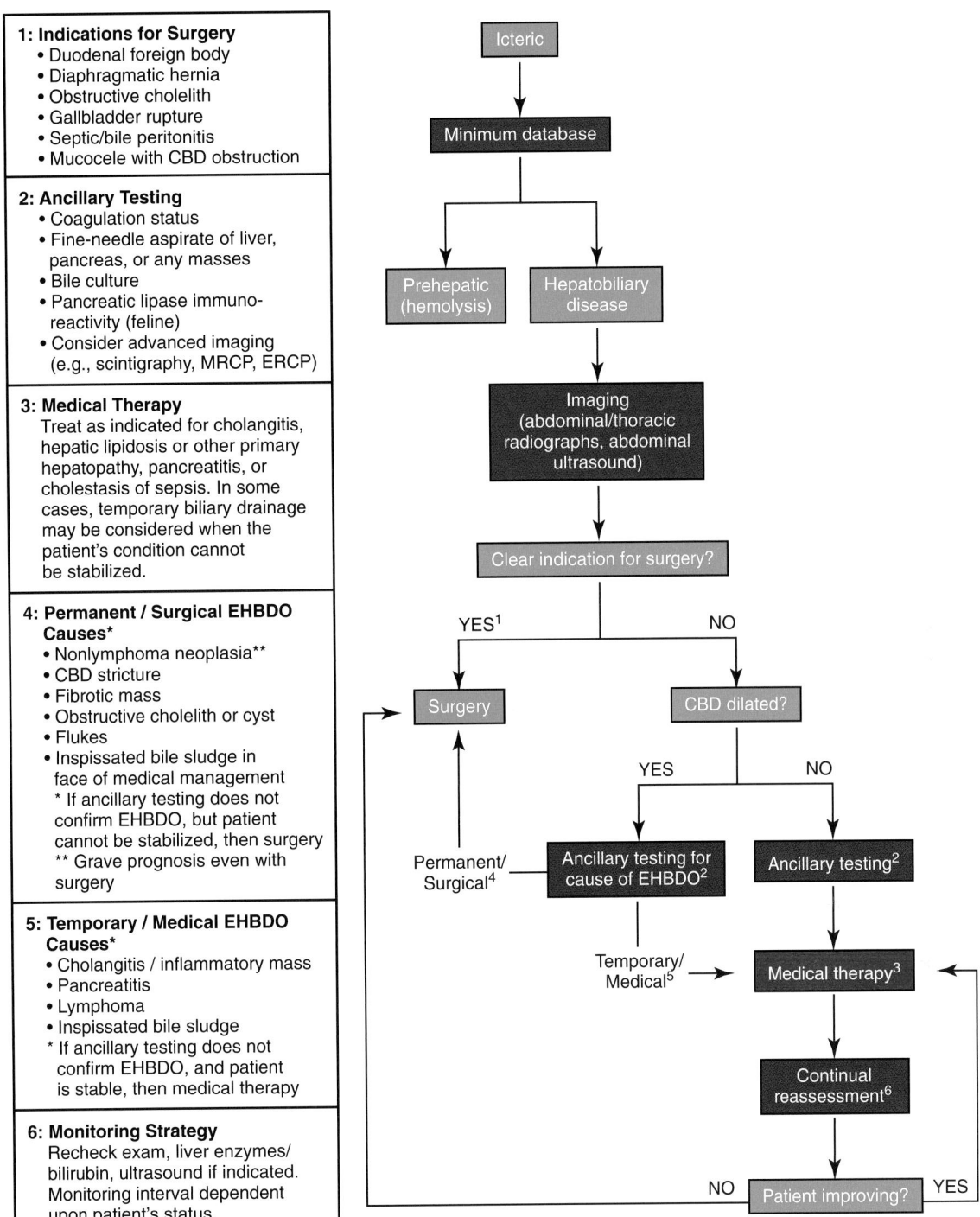

1: Indications for Surgery
- Duodenal foreign body
- Diaphragmatic hernia
- Obstructive cholelith
- Gallbladder rupture
- Septic/bile peritonitis
- Mucocele with CBD obstruction

2: Ancillary Testing
- Coagulation status
- Fine-needle aspirate of liver, pancreas, or any masses
- Bile culture
- Pancreatic lipase immuno-reactivity (feline)
- Consider advanced imaging (e.g., scintigraphy, MRCP, ERCP)

3: Medical Therapy
Treat as indicated for cholangitis, hepatic lipidosis or other primary hepatopathy, pancreatitis, or cholestasis of sepsis. In some cases, temporary biliary drainage may be considered when the patient's condition cannot be stabilized.

4: Permanent / Surgical EHBDO Causes*
- Nonlymphoma neoplasia**
- CBD stricture
- Fibrotic mass
- Obstructive cholelith or cyst
- Flukes
- Inspissated bile sludge in face of medical management
  * If ancillary testing does not confirm EHBDO, but patient cannot be stabilized, then surgery
  ** Grave prognosis even with surgery

5: Temporary / Medical EHBDO Causes*
- Cholangitis / inflammatory mass
- Pancreatitis
- Lymphoma
- Inspissated bile sludge
  * If ancillary testing does not confirm EHBDO, and patient is stable, then medical therapy

6: Monitoring Strategy
Recheck exam, liver enzymes/bilirubin, ultrasound if indicated. Monitoring interval dependent upon patient's status.

Figure 16-2: Algorithm for therapeutic decision making in feline extrahepatic bile duct obstruction *(EHBDO). CBD,* common bile duct; *ERCP,* endoscopic retrograde cholangiopancreatography; *MRCP,* magnetic resonance cholangiopancreatography.

Severity Assessment and Stabilization

Based on history, physical examination, and measurement of systemic blood pressure, cases of possible EHBDO can be divided into three major categories:

1. *Stable outpatient:* These cats are hydrated and euvolemic. They are either eating or can be maintained at home with an appetite stimulant or after placement of an esophagostomy feeding tube. In these cases, if surgery is clearly indicated, it should be performed electively as soon as possible, ideally when the cat is on a solid nutritional plane. If the need for surgery is unclear, repeated assessment of clinicopathologic and ultrasound parameters may be most appropriate in approximately 1 week.

2. *Stable inpatient:* These cats may be dehydrated, severely anemic, in significant pain, and/or have intractable

vomiting and need more supportive care than can be provided at home, but they do not demonstrate signs of sepsis or circulatory shock. If surgery is clearly indicated, it should be performed as soon as any significant dehydration, coagulopathy, or anemia has been corrected. Otherwise, as long as they remain stable, reassessment of the need for surgery may be most appropriate after 1 to 2 days of medical therapy.

3. *Critical:* These patients may be hypotensive or show other evidence of sepsis. Their condition is dynamic, and they may display progressive discomfort or declining neurologic or cardiovascular status. They must be continually reassessed, and if they cannot be stabilized, exploratory surgery may be required in the absence of a definitive diagnosis of EHBDO.

Perioperative stabilization and initial management of a cat with EHBDO should include the following considerations, which are discussed in more detail in the following medical therapy section:

- Correction of dehydration, hypovolemia, and hypotension
- Correction of coagulopathy and anemia
- Correction of electrolyte abnormalities and acid-base derangement
- Antibiotic therapy
- Treatment of fulminant HE
- Provision of analgesia
- Control of vomiting and GI hemorrhage

Because concurrent hepatic lipidosis may be a poor prognostic factor, and a poor nutritional state is associated with decreased immune function, wound healing, and overall prognosis, enteral nutrition should be provided in any patient that can tolerate it (i.e., conscious, not recumbent, and with vomiting controlled).[74] Naso-esophageal feeding tubes can typically be placed quickly with only local anesthesia.[74] A variety of therapies aimed at decreasing endotoxemia secondary to the lack of bile flow to the intestines have demonstrated variable success in people but have not been explored in cats.[1,34,75] Of these, lactulose, early enteral feeding, glutamine supplementation, and internal bile replacement seem the most promising.[75] All cats undergoing surgery should be blood-typed, and the appropriate blood product should be readily available.[34] Crossmatching is required in cases having received a transfusion at least 4 days prior and may be ideal in all cases.[76]

In some cases, biliary decompression may also be considered as a component of presurgical stabilization. The decision to pursue procedures, such as therapeutic cholecystocentesis or temporary diversion, in lieu of or as a bridge to lengthier, definitive surgery is controversial. These procedures are associated with the risk of bile peritonitis; and if the bile is septic, then the patient's prognosis may be significantly worse than before the leakage, so the risks versus benefits of temporary decompression must be carefully weighed.[77,78] In cases in which definitive surgery is not feasible due to extreme operative risk or financial limitations, these techniques may be considered as an alternative to euthanasia. In other cases, this approach may allow time during which the patient can

continue to recover from pancreatitis;[23] and decompression may actually restore pancreatic blood flow, thereby improving tissue pH and acinar cell function and helping to stop the vicious cycle of pancreatitis and EHBDO.[4] Decompression can also buy time for the patient to become a better surgical candidate via systemic stabilization, correction of coagulopathy, improved nutritional plane,[75] partial return of hepatic function,[27] and improved biliary tissue health and gallbladder contractility.[75] Additionally, because sepsis will likely decrease postoperative survival, antibiotic therapy should always be initiated preoperatively.[16] However, it is unlikely to clear an infection if infected bile is not removed mechanically[16] or through improved bile flow, so biliary decompression may facilitate preoperative antibiotic efficacy. Temporary biliary decompression does not improve outcomes in all people with EHBDO, but it has improved outcomes in subpopulations with acute cholecystitis/cholangitis, coagulopathy, and malnutrition.[34,79,80] In addition, it has been shown to improve liver enzymes, hyperbilirubinemia, and clinical signs in cats with experimental EHBDO.[27] Diversion does not address the lack of bile in the intestines, but the bile can be returned to the patient via feeding tube.[75] Therapeutic cholecystocentesis has been described in three dogs with EHBDO due to pancreatitis. Two dogs recovered without surgery, one of which had repeated cholecystocentesis, but the third dog developed bile peritonitis.[81] In patients that can undergo brief anesthesia, laparoscopic (or mini-laparotomy[27]) assisted cholecystostomy tube placement[82] may be considered and provides the advantage of facilitating cholangiography and flushing of the biliary system.[75] However, their successful implementation in cats has been problematic.[82] Biliary stents can also be considered but are reported to require relatively long anesthetic times, and so may not be of much advantage in an unstable patient.[75]

Medical Therapy

Medical therapy is aimed at keeping the patient stable and comfortable while treating possible inflammatory etiologies of EHBDO (e.g., cholangitis, pancreatitis, and biliary sludge). Management of these conditions has been thoroughly reviewed elsewhere,* but the major therapeutic considerations for medical management in the context of EHBDO are highlighted later.

Antibiotics are indicated for all patients, because bacterial infection, whether primary or secondary, is common in EHBDO and its associated conditions, particularly inflammatory liver disease.[1,2,16,33,67,73] In patients with suspected septic shock, broad-spectrum bactericidal antibiotics should be administered as soon as any practical samples have been obtained for culture. In stable patients, antimicrobial choice may wait until the results of bile cytology and Gram stain are available. In general, coverage should be four-quadrant with emphasis on enteric organisms, *Escherichia coli* being the

---

*2, 4-6, 8, 16, 28, 38, 64, 83, 84, 85.

most frequently cultured.[65,67] In a study of 248 hepatobiliary cultures in dogs and cats, amoxicillin/clavulanate provided the best gram-positive coverage (and should effectively treat anaerobes, as well); however, small but not insignificant numbers of isolates are resistant to cephalexin or amoxicillin/clavulanate, so this monotherapy may not be ideal.[33,65] Ciprofloxacin and the aminoglycosides provided the best coverage for *E. coli* and other gram-negative organisms.[65] Due to the risk of nephrotoxicity associated with aminoglycosides, they should be used with extreme caution in this patient population already predisposed to renal complications. Accordingly, rational choices include a fluoroquinolone with either amoxicillin/clavulanate or a combination of ampicillin and metronidazole (7.5 mg/kg twice daily [BID][16,28]).[65] Intravenous (IV) administration of enrofloxacin is off-label in cats and should only be used with caution and informed owner consent due to the risk of retinal toxicity. If clinical response to antibiotics is seen, they should be continued long-term (4 to 8 weeks) to fully clear the infection and minimize the risk of recurrence.[5,28]

Glucocorticoid therapy is often recommended for chronic neutrophilic cholangitis (CNC; mixed inflammatory infiltrates) or LC, as well as associated chronic pancreatitis[38] and IBD.[2,5,28,64] Glucocorticoids may also reduce tissue swelling and therefore cholestasis associated with acute neutrophilic cholangitis (ANC),[5] fluke infestation,[6,7] and neoplasia. Finally, they are an important component of chemotherapy for lymphosarcoma. Ideally, corticosteroid therapy should only be prescribed if indicated by a biopsy diagnosis.

Practically, however, surgical biopsy is not always in a patient's best interest, and corticosteroids may be administered with the goal of "treating the treatable" before pursuing a risky EHBDO surgery. In general, corticosteroids are contraindicated in cases of ANC, ANP, pancreatic abscesses, and confirmed bacterial cholangitis/cholecystitis.[64] However, some authors do advocate the limited use of corticosteroids to ameliorate inflammation and edema associated with ANC that may be narrowing bile ducts.[5,8] Additionally, it can sometimes be difficult to distinguish primary bacterial infection (e.g., ANC) from infection secondary to cholestasis or underlying inflammatory disease (CNC or LC). Although there are no definitive clinical criteria to differentiate these scenarios, cats with ANC tend to be younger,[28,43,53] more commonly febrile, and more acutely ill than cats with CNC or LC.[8,16] They are also more likely to have ultrasonographic pancreatic changes and less likely to have ascites.[28,43]

In the case of EHBDO, if response to antibiotics is incomplete after several days to a week, there is clinical suspicion for underlying chronic inflammatory disease, and bile culture is negative, then anti-inflammatory doses of corticosteroids (e.g., prednisolone 0.5 to 1 mg/kg/day)[5] may be prudent in conjunction with antibiotics. If chronic inflammatory liver disease (CNC, LC) is suspected or confirmed, bacterial infection has been ruled out, and the clinician is certain that surgery will not be pursued, then the dose should be increased to 2 mg/kg/day.[2,5,8,16,28]

Risks of corticosteroid therapy include masking of the underlying disease process, rendering future testing (e.g., biopsy) non-diagnostic; impaired wound and surgical healing; worsening of infection; exacerbation of hepatic lipidosis; insulin antagonism; fluid retention and precipitation of congestive heart failure; and increased risk of thrombotic complications. Accordingly, full owner understanding and informed consent are essential prior to starting empiric corticosteroid therapy.

Other Supportive Care. Intravenous crystalloid fluids are indicated in most cases. Lactated Ringer's solution should theoretically be avoided in cases of significant hepatocellular failure. Colloid therapy should be considered in hypovolemic and/or hypoalbuminemic patients. Hypoglycemia, as well as deficiencies of potassium, phosphorus, and magnesium should also be corrected via IV replacement.[86] Some clinicians also advocate the addition of B-complex vitamins at 1 to 2 mL/L fluids.[87] If hypotension persists despite euvolemia, then pressor therapy should be initiated. Unfortunately, cats with EHBDO may be refractory to pressors.[34,88]

Patients with clinical signs attributable to blood loss or anemia or significantly anemic patients that will be undergoing anesthesia should receive the appropriate blood product.[76] Vitamin K should be administered parenterally (0.5 to 1.5 mg/kg subcutaneously [SC] BID)[5,16] at least 24 hours prior to an invasive procedure to any patient with elevated clotting times or may be given empirically if these tests are not immediately available and is, in fact, advocated by some authors for all patients regardless of clotting time results.[89] In coagulopathic patients with active bleeding or for which an invasive procedure is planned, coagulation factors should be replaced via fresh frozen plasma or fresh whole blood.[76]

Because most conditions associated with EHBDO cause discomfort in other species, and cats are adept at hiding signs of pain, analgesia is advocated for most cases. Pure μ-agonists should theoretically be avoided due to their constrictive effect on the sphincter of Oddi in people[83] and the pancreatic duct in cats.[38] Common analgesics used in cats with hepatobiliary and/or pancreatic disease include buprenorphine and butorphanol. Lidocaine, which may have beneficial intestinal prokinetic effects, and ketamine are sometimes combined with an opioid in a constant rate infusion.[8,38]

Antiemetics should be provided for any vomiting or anorectic cat. Maropitant (1 mg/kg SC every 24 hours; reduce to 0.5 mg/kg SC every 24 hours if severe hepatic dysfunction; the IV route is off-label but frequently used)[28] has been shown to reduce visceral pain in addition to its antiemetic effects.[90] 5-HT$_3$ antagonists, such as ondansetron, are also frequently used although optimal dose and dosing intervals have not been well established in cats.[28,38] Proton pump inhibitor therapy should be administered to any cat with suspected GI bleeding.

Hepatic encephalopathy can be managed with lower protein diet and lactulose (0.5 to 1 mL/kg PO three times daily) with the addition of an oral antibiotic (e.g., amoxicillin, metronidazole, or neomycin) in patients that do not respond to diet and lactulose alone.[28,84] Patients with fulminant HE (uncommon) can be treated with cleansing and lactulose retention enemas.[84] Thiamine and potassium deficiency can present with signs similar to HE and should be ruled out or corrected before limiting a feline patient to a low-protein diet.[87]

Nutritional support is essential in these cases to treat or prevent concurrent hepatic lipidosis and to minimize the deleterious effects of malnutrition on intestinal barrier function,[75] immune function, strength, and overall prognosis.[74] In cats in which oral alimentation is possible, a brief attempt at appetite stimulation can be made, but caloric intake may be inadequate and must therefore be closely monitored. Appetite stimulants most likely only have a place in the stable outpatient. The authors prefer mirtazapine, which may also have an antiemetic effect, at 1.875 mg/cat/day (every other day with renal impairment), although idiosyncratic hepatotoxicity is a rare adverse effect.[91,92] If voluntary intake is insufficient, than assisted feeding via an enteral feeding tube is the next choice. Naso-esophageal and esophagostomy tubes are preferred for assisted feeding due to their ability to be placed in the awake patient (naso-esophageal tube) or with only brief anesthesia (esophagostomy tube) and because feeding into the proximal GI tract is the most physiologic. Parenteral nutrition may be considered in cats with intractable vomiting, severe obtundation or other inability to protect their airway, and with severe malabsorptive/maldigestive intestinal disease.[74] For cats without HE, a diet high in protein, such as a standard recovery diet, is best suited to their metabolic needs.[74] Theoretically, a high-fat recovery diet may be contraindicated due to the effects of EHBDO on fat digestion, and the fat content may need to be minimized if signs of fat intolerance (bloating, abdominal pain, and/or diarrhea) are observed. Highly digestible diets formulated for GI disease may be appropriate. Regardless of nutritional therapy selected, it must be introduced slowly and the patient monitored for refeeding syndrome (hypophosphatemia and other electrolyte derangements).[74]

There are a variety of nutraceuticals and supplements available that may provide hepatic or systemic support.[85] Given the practical problems of administering multiple medications to feline patients, at the authors' institution, the authors tend to use only those that seem to be most beneficial. These include cobalamin,[28,72,87] ursodiol, S-adenosylmethionine (SAMe), milk thistle, and N-acetylcysteine. Ursodiol (ursodeoxycholic acid) has many positive effects and is known to be of benefit with extrahepatic cholestasis in the absence of obstruction. It may be of particular use in cats with cholangitis.[93] Its mechanisms include replacement of more hydrophobic toxic bile acids, stimulation of bile flow, antiapoptotic effects, stabilization of mitochondria, and immunomodulation.[93] It is also cytoprotective to intestinal epithelial cells and cardiomyocytes,[93] so it may theoretically provide protection against endotoxemia and some of its consequences. Biliary obstruction is commonly cited as a contraindication of ursodiol,[23,46,83,64] but this is not based on evidence regarding safety. In fact, in bile duct ligated rats, ursodeoxycholic acid resulted in lower liver enzymes, bilirubin, bile acids, and degree of bile duct

proliferation,[94] as well as decreased hepatocyte apoptosis and oxidative stress.[95] In humans, complete bile duct obstruction due to cholelithiasis is not regarded as a safety contraindication of ursodiol; although surgery is of course the treatment of choice, ursodiol therapy may be considered for patients that refuse surgery.[96] The authors believe that the choleretic effects of ursodiol are unlikely to result in biliary rupture. If a cat ultimately requires biliary surgery, administering ursodiol in the meantime will have improved the bile acid pool, ameliorated secondary liver damage, and perhaps improved intestinal mucosal health and reduced endotoxemia. Additionally, because ursodiol has immunomodulatory properties, it may provide some of the benefits of corticosteroids without the attendant risks.[93] It is also possible that by improving bile flow and reducing inflammation, ursodiol will help to resolve a partial or temporary biliary obstruction due to inflammatory disease or bile sludge, eliminating the need for surgery entirely. Accordingly, the authors believe that ursodiol should be considered as a component of a medical therapeutic trial—with informed owner consent—in cases that do not have a clear indication for surgical intervention. SAMe increases glutathione levels and reduces oxidative stress. It has many of the same benefits as ursodiol, and their effects may be additive.[93] N-acetylcysteine also increases hepatic glutathione levels and is commonly substituted for SAMe during critical illness, because it is administered parenterally and has improved survival in humans with acute liver failure.[16,93] It has also been shown to be cytoprotective in bile duct ligated rats and dogs and may be of particular benefit in cats with severe hepatic lipidosis.[93] Silymarin, the active ingredient in milk thistle, also overlaps mechanistically with the previously mentioned liver protectants, but in particular, it may protect against inflammatory and fibrotic complications associated with the retention of toxins in static bile.[93]

In cats with known or suspected liver fluke infestation, praziquantel is the medical therapy of choice. Dosing regimens described in the literature vary widely, with 20 to 40 mg/kg/day for 5 days seeming reasonable.[8,10,16,71]

Surgical Therapy

The goals of definitive biliary surgery are to confirm a diagnosis, prevent bile leakage and peritonitis, and provide a route for bile flow into the GI tract. Many complications have been associated with the failure to restore bile flow (Box 16-1): pain; gallbladder rupture; duodenal ulceration;[16,26,37] cholelith formation secondary to bile stasis;[33] pancreatitis;[4,16] fat maldigestion and fat-soluble vitamin deficiencies;[16] hypercoagulability or hypocoagulability;[37,62] bacterial overgrowth and translocation, as well as downregulation of the reticuloendothelial system, leading to septicemia, endotoxemia, circulatory shock, acute kidney injury, myocardial damage, decreased wound healing, disseminated intravascular coagulation (DIC), and/or the systemic inflammatory response syndrome (SIRS);[37] and secondary liver damage, including cirrhosis within 6 to 8 weeks of complete obstruction.[16,63]

BOX 16-1 Complications Associated with Failure to Restore Bile Flow

- Pain
- Gallbladder rupture
- Duodenal ulceration[16,26,37]
- Cholelith formation secondary to bile stasis[33]
- Pancreatitis[4,16]
- Fat maldigestion and fat-soluble vitamin deficiencies[16]
- Hypercoagulability or hypocoagulability[37,62]
- Bacterial overgrowth and translocation
- Downregulation of the reticuloendothelial system, leading to the following:
  - Septicemia
  - Endotoxemia
  - Circulatory shock
  - Acute kidney injury
  - Myocardial damage
  - Decreased wound healing
  - Disseminated intravascular coagulation and/or the systemic inflammatory response syndrome[37]
- Secondary liver damage, including cirrhosis within 6 to 8 weeks of complete obstruction[16,63]

BOX 16-2 Surgical Procedures: Definitions and Indications

Access and Catheterization of the Biliary Papilla
- Duodenotomy: Antimesenteric enterotomy over the duodenal papilla
- Sphincterotomy: Incision through the sphincter of Oddi and duodenal papilla

Temporary Biliary Decompression
- Cholecystostomy tube: Tube placement to drain bile from the gallbladder to an external closed collection system; for reversible biliary obstruction when gallbladder and biliary ducts are dilated but otherwise healthy
- Choledochal stent: Tube placed into the CBD and temporarily fixed adjacent to the papilla; for reversible biliary obstruction when the tube is readily placed into the CBD, and gallbladder and duct are dilated but otherwise healthy; or to temporarily decompress the biliary tree if choledochotomy is performed

Removal of Lodged Choleliths in the Common Bile Duct
- Choledochotomy: Incision into the CBD

Removal of Grossly Abnormal Gallbladder or Biliary Calculi when Terminal Biliary Tree is Patent
- Cholecystectomy: Removal of the gallbladder

Biliary Diversion for Irreversible and Permanent Biliary Obstruction or Common Bile Duct Damage
- Cholecystoenterostomy: Gallbladder is anastomosed to the duodenum or jejunum
- Roux-en-Y formation or cholecystojejunoduodenostomy: Interposition of a jejunal segment between the gallbladder and small intestine
- Choledochoduodenostomy: When the gallbladder is not available for bypass, then an anastomosis of a significantly dilated distal CBD to the duodenum is attempted

CBD, Common bile duct.

Available Surgical Procedures

There are limited surgical techniques to restore bile flow to the intestine or relieve the distension and some of the deleterious consequences of EHBDO. Options include temporary procedures, such as choledochal stenting and cholecystostomy tube placement, and permanent procedures, such as cholecystectomy and biliary-enteric diversion. The decision about which procedures to perform is usually straightforward and dictated by intraoperative findings, as described later and in Box 16-2.

The reader is referred to surgical texts[88,97] for the technical aspects of these procedures. The following section describes exploratory findings and intraoperative factors surgeons use to decide the best approach to treat cats with EHBDO.

After a complete abdominal exploration and sampling of any free fluid for cytology and culture, a more detailed visual inspection and palpation of the liver lobes, biliary tree, upper GI tract, and pancreas is undertaken. If there is a diaphragmatic hernia or a proximal GI obstruction that can explain the biliary obstruction, immediate surgical repair is attempted.

When obvious pancreatitis exists causing obstruction of the biliary tract with no other bile duct or gallbladder abnormality, a decision has to be made whether to stent the compressed intrapancreatic portion of the CBD or to place a cholecystostomy tube. It must first be determined, through a duodenotomy, whether a tube can be threaded into the CBD past the obstruction. When the papilla is thickened and a feeding tube will not pass readily, or a cholelith is found lodged at the papilla, a **sphincterotomy** may be considered. A small incision over the intramural CBD is made orad to the papilla. The stone is removed, and an attempt is made to thread a feeding tube through the area. In the case of pancreatitis-related obstruction, if the papilla palpates normally and the duct can be catheterized, the feeding tube can be left in place as a **choledochal stent.** The stent should pass in the feces within several months.[32] The primary indication for stent placement is to temporarily restore bile flow while inflammatory disease is resolving. Stent placement may also be considered as an emergency procedure to help stabilize a patient that is not a good surgical candidate before returning to surgery for a more definitive repair, as a temporary means of decompression after duct repair, or as a palliative measure in the case of neoplasia.[37] In the latter case—and potentially other scenarios, as well—self-expanding or balloon-expanding metallic stents may perform better than feeding tubes, because they expand rather than fill the lumen;[83] however, this technique has been performed in a very limited number of cats

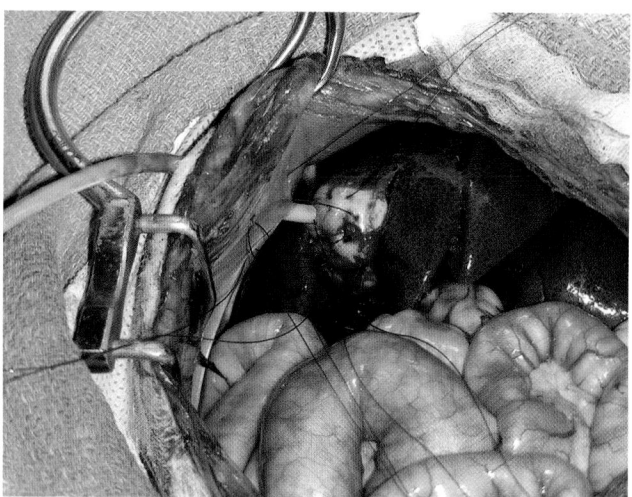

Figure 16-3: Temporary percutaneous biliary drainage via cholecystostomy tube placement.

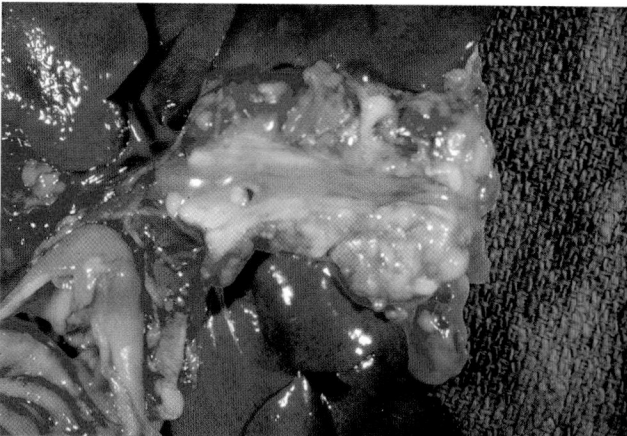

Figure 16-4: Necropsy specimen showing an invasive bile duct carcinoma surrounding the common bile duct (longitudinally sectioned).

at this time (F. Pike, personal communication, August 26, 2014). The advantage of a stent over other temporary decompressive measures that may require shorter anesthesia time is that the bile is not diverted away from the GI tract, thereby preserving the physiology by returning bile to the duodenum.

If the tube will not pass through the obstructed area of the CBD within the substance of the inflamed pancreas, a **cholecystostomy tube** (Figure 16-3) is considered. If the patient does not require definitive repair, the tube should remain in place for at least 3 to 4 weeks to allow for tract formation,[37,75] and in people, drainage is needed for at least 6 weeks to ameliorate some of the hepatic and systemic consequences of biliary obstruction.[98] Maintenance of long-term cholecystostomy tubes is not a reasonable option, because complications due to bactibilia are exceedingly common.[27] Accordingly, this method of diversion should be considered a temporary option only to better stabilize the cat prior to more definitive surgery, or as a means of decompression of the biliary tree with the expectation that the obstructive condition is temporary.

If there is inspissated bile in the CBD causing obstruction and the remaining biliary tree is dilated but healthy, the feeding tube is advanced up the papilla through a **duodenotomy.** Retrograde lavage of the CBD, cystic duct, and gallbladder with sterile saline is performed to flush out inspissated bile. After most of the liquid bile has been aspirated from the tube (and a sample submitted for culture), alternating flushing of the tract and aspirating of the fenestrated tube is conducted. Additionally, the entire tract is irrigated so that it is distended, the tube is removed, and the gallbladder is gently expressed to force any residual sludge or particulate matter from the biliary tree. This is repeated until there is only clear saline seen exiting the papilla, and the biliary tree palpates normally.

If a cholelith is seen or palpated and is causing the obstruction, the viability of the CBD wall must be assessed. If there is evidence of necrosis or leakage at the site of the calculus,

the area is ligated and excised, and a **cholecystoenterostomy** (described later) is performed. Primary anastomosis of the CBD after segmental resection is usually not elected in the cat. Because the duct is small, and the repair is under excessive tension, the procedure carries a high risk of stricture and bile leakage.[99] If the duct is deemed healthy, and the obstructive stone(s) can be milked into the gallbladder, a **cholecystectomy** is performed. It is generally thought that leaving the gallbladder in place (because it is considered the primary region of nidus formation) in cases of cholelithiasis increases the risk of cholelith recurrence in the future.[1,37,67] When a cholelith is immovable even with repeated catheterization and flushing, but the duct is not severely damaged, a **choledochotomy** is performed over the stone. After closing the choledochotomy, the papilla is catheterized, and the biliary tree is flushed and examined for leakage. Although success has been reported with or without stenting following choledochotomy, the authors prefer in this case to leave the tube in place (choledochal stent) as a temporary means of decompression while the incision heals.

If the gallbladder appears grossly abnormal (e.g., presence of a mucocele; if turgid, thickened, or discolored; presence of neoplasia; or if necrotic and/or leaking), the papilla and biliary tree must be confirmed to be patent, and a routine cholecystectomy is performed.

When there is obvious permanent mural or extramural pathology affecting the obstructed bile duct (Figure 16-4) but not the gallbladder or cystic duct, then a biliary-enteric diversion procedure (**cholecystoduodenostomy,** or less ideally, **cholecystojejunostomy**) is necessary. These procedures join the lumen of the gallbladder with the lumen of the small intestine, bypassing the distal CBD. If the patency of the gallbladder or cystic duct is in question, a catheter should be passed normograde through a cholecystostomy site (at an area appropriate for the planned diversion). The preferred biliary-enteric diversion technique in people is a Roux-en-Y (Figure 16-5) or cholecystojejunoduodenostomy (otherwise known as a *jejunal limb interposition*) because of decreased enterobiliary reflux and limited derangement of GI

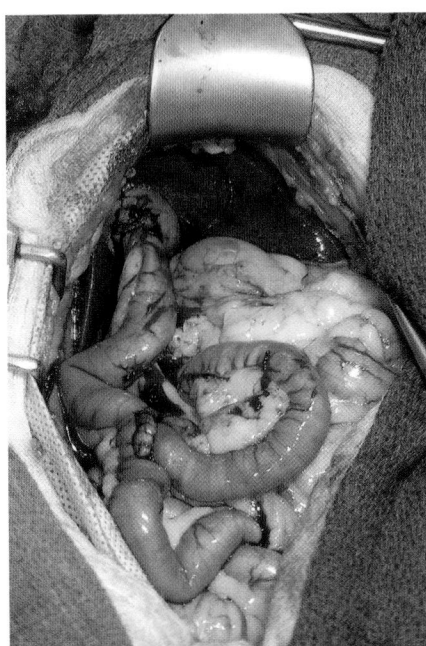

Figure 16-5: Intraoperative image showing cholecystojejunoduodenostomy (Roux-en-Y formation) for treatment of stricture of the terminal common bile duct in a cat.

physiology compared to other procedures. This procedure using a shorter segment of jejunum in cats has not been reported but deserves further evaluation, because biliary reflux and ascending cholangitis are major concerns after biliary-enteric anastomosis in cats.[1]

If neither the distal CBD nor the cystic duct is patent, there are no good options for definitive restoration of bile flow. Direct anastomosis of the CBD to the duodenum (**choledochoduodenostomy**) can be attempted, but this is rarely performed in the cat due to the small CBD lumen. It may be considered when the CBD is significantly dilated, and the intramural bile duct or papilla needs to be bypassed. Any means of biliary-enteric diversion should be considered a salvage procedure to be avoided if possible, due to its high rate of perioperative mortality and long-term complications (Table 16-2).[34]

Although minimally invasive interventions (such as endoscopic retrograde cholangiopancreatography and sphincterotomy or endoscopic stent placement) are commonly performed in people and have been investigated in dogs and four healthy cats, they are technically challenging and not currently clinically available[60]—though further investigation is underway (A. Berent, personal communication). Laparoscopy, however, is commonly performed in cats and is a good alternative for a patient that needs only diagnostic biopsies and culture samples; however, there is some concern about lacerating distended intrahepatic ducts.[16] Some institutions have also placed percutaneous cholecystostomy catheters ("pigtail catheters") under ultrasound guidance or with laparoscopic assistance for temporary gallbladder decompression; but early obstruction, catheter dislodgement, and bile peritonitis are significant risks.[88,82]

Regardless of the biliary surgery being performed, several ancillary procedures should be considered. Because so many EHBDO cases are affected by "triaditis,"[53] and the causal relationships between EHBDO and cholangitis or EHBDO and pancreatitis can be in either direction,[4,103] biopsies of liver, pancreas, and intestines (including ileum)[104] should be obtained and submitted for histopathology. Due to the prevalence of bacteria in the livers and pancreata of cats with inflammatory liver disease[73] and the possibility of opportunistic infection secondary to EHBDO,[16] liver and pancreatic biopsies—as well as bile—should also be submitted for aerobic and anaerobic culture. Any choleliths should be submitted for stone analysis and culture, and the gallbladder or other resected biliary epithelium should be submitted for histopathology and culture. Excisional or incisional biopsies of any mass-like lesions should also be performed. In most cases, placement of a feeding tube should also be considered. Esophagostomy tubes are ideal for cats that are not vomiting or regurgitating, because they generally have high patient and owner acceptance, few complications, and can be used for medication administration. In cats with refractory vomiting or regurgitating patients, a jejunostomy tube will be necessary.

Surgical Timing

In general, it is thought that surgical correction of a complete biliary obstruction should be performed as soon after diagnosis as possible, whereas surgical investigation of a partially obstructed biliary tract should be postponed until the patient is a more ideal surgical candidate.[55] It is commonly assumed that the prognosis associated with biliary surgery is better if surgery is performed before biliary rupture. However, several recent studies have not demonstrated a relationship between aseptic peritonitis secondary to mucocele-associated gallbladder rupture and survival in dogs.[44,45,105,106] However, septic bile peritonitis is in fact associated with worse outcome.[77,78] This has not been assessed directly in cats, and biliary rupture and septic peritonitis are less common in cats than in dogs;[78,107] but regardless, early surgical intervention for complete biliary obstruction seems a reasonable guiding principle. Nevertheless, there are two good reasons to judiciously delay surgery. First, it can be difficult to determine immediately upon presentation whether a patient has a complete EHBDO (versus partial EHBDO or incidental biliary dilation without obstruction, as in some cases of cholangitis; e.g., see Figure 16-6). Because conditions associated with partial EHBDO or incidental biliary dilation may respond to medical therapy alone, a trial of medical therapy should be pursued. The patient's clinical status should be continuously reassessed, and its hemogram and blood chemistries, along with biliary ultrasound, should be rechecked every 24 to 48 hours (or less frequently in the stable outpatient). If the clinical picture is worsening and becoming more convincing for complete EHBDO (e.g., worsening hyperbilirubinemia combined with increased biliary dilation, worsening hemodynamic status[88]), and reasonable means have been attempted at medical therapy, then surgery should be pursued. Others

Table 16-2   **Outcomes of Surgery in Selected Cases of Feline Extrahepatic Biliary Obstruction Associated with Inflammatory Disease, Neoplasia, and Cholelithiasis**

Reason for Biliary Surgery (Number of Cats)	Surgical Procedures Performed (Number of Cats)	Outcomes
Choledocholithiasis (1); pancreatitis (1)[36]	CD plus CC (1); CD plus cholecystostomy (1)	• 100% survival (both euthanized 2 or more years later for other causes)
IBD with obstructive cholelithiasis (3); bile plugs (2); malignant neoplasia (1)[100]	Sphincterotomy (6); plus mass excision, repair of CBD, stricture bougienage in the cat with neoplasia	• Four of six survived longer than 2 months (three of three with cholelithiasis; one of two with bile plugs)
Acute pancreatitis (5); inflammatory gastroduodenal mass (1)[69]	CCD (3); CD plus stent (1); duodenotomy with bile duct flushing (1); mass resection (1)	• Four of six survived longer than 2 weeks and were alive at last follow-up of 4 months to 5 years • Cat requiring mass resection arrested postoperatively • One CCD patient euthanized due to suspected septic peritonitis on day 11
Neoplasia (3); cholangiohepatitis (1)[99]	CCD using endoscopic gastrointestinal anastomosis stapling equipment (4)	• Two of four survived longer than 2 weeks (two euthanized postoperatively due to neoplasia)
Pancreatitis (7)[32]	Choledochal stenting (7); plus CC (2)	• Five of seven survived to discharge (two of seven died postoperatively: one had PTE/pneumonia; one had recurrence of EHBDO) • Two of seven survived longer than 2 years • Short-term complications in survivors: Reobstruction (two cats) • Long-term complications: Ascending cholangitis (stent was retained longer than 6 months in one patient); recurrent vomiting (two cats)
Neoplasia (9): Biliary adenocarcinoma (5), lymphoma (2), squamous cell carcinoma (1), pancreatic adenocarcinoma (1) Inflammatory (13): Chronic hepatitis (10), cholecystitis (8), pancreatitis (7), enteritis (5) >1 organ affected (10) Five had nonneoplastic bile duct mass causing the EHBDO[34]	CCD (13); CCJ (8) Choledochoduodenostomy (1)	• 64% survived to discharge (five of nine neoplasia; nine of 13 inflammatory) • Three of nine neoplasias were grossly metastatic at time of surgery • 27% survived longer than 6 months (all inflammatory) • Common postoperative complications: blood transfusion (15 cats); persistent hypotension in most • All long-term survivors had complications, including recurrent cholecystitis, vomiting, and exocrine pancreatic insufficiency
Cholecystitis with choledocholith (1); choledochitis (1); inflammation of major duodenal papilla (1); traumatic avulsion of CBD (1)[24]	Biliary-enteric diversion (3); CC (1)	• One of three diversion cases survived and was alive at 4 months (cat with inflammatory papilla mass and cholangitis/IBD) • CC survived • The authors also reviewed the literature and reported that of 29 feline biliary diversion cases, 50% were alive at 2 weeks, and 23% were alive at 6 months; the remainder were euthanized in the interim due to recurring bouts of pyrexia, vomiting, and anorexia • Eight of nine nondiversion cases survived postoperatively (follow-up time variable)

Table 16-2	Outcomes of Surgery in Selected Cases of Feline Extrahepatic Biliary Obstruction Associated with Inflammatory Disease, Neoplasia, and Cholelithiasis—cont'd	
Reason for Biliary Surgery (Number of Cats)	**Surgical Procedures Performed (Number of Cats)**	**Outcomes**
Biliary or pancreatic adenocarcinoma (6); inflammatory—at least one of pancreatitis, cholangiohepatitis, cholelithiasis, cholecystitis (15); undiagnosed CBD mass (1)[1]	CCD (10); CCJ (4); choledochal stent (1); CC (2); CD (1); cholecystostomy tube placement (1)	• Zero of six neoplasia cases survived • 60% of inflammatory cases survived at least 1 week • Overall, the immediate (48 hours) postoperative mortality rate was 57%, not including euthanasia • Over 50% of cases required blood transfusion and/or pressor therapy • Cardiopulmonary arrest was common (seven cats) • The single choledochal stent failed (migrated out of CBD, recurrence of EHBDO on postoperative day 3) • Long-term complications included recurrence of cholangitis, EHBDO, and chronic weight loss
Cholelithiasis (9)[33]	CC plus duodenotomy (5); cholecystostomy (1); CCD (2); CCJ (1)	• Seven of nine survived 13 months or longer • Both cases that died perioperatively had hepatic lipidosis • Two of three diversion cases did well for 18 to 27 months and died of other causes • Postoperative anemia requiring blood transfusion was common (four cats)
Biliary carcinoma (1); pancreatic carcinoma (1); bile duct adenoma (1); pancreatic fibrosis (1)[101]	Cholecystostomy and duodenotomy with lavage (1); CC (n = 1); died preoperatively (2)	• None survived
Granulation tissue masses (2); bile duct carcinoma (1); fibrosis due to chronic pancreatitis (1)[31]	CD plus T-tube stent (1); CCD (2); cholecystostomy tube (1)	• One of four survived (granulation tissue polyp treated with stent; the stent was removed after 7 days, and the cat did well for more than 2 years) • Three of four died perioperatively
Ulcerative fibrosing enteritis (1); intestinal adenocarcinoma/previous surgical error (1)[102]	Proximal duodenal resection and CCD (2)	• One of two survived • One euthanized 10 weeks postoperatively due to suspected recurrence of cholangitis and EHBDO • One survived 2 years or longer with frequent episodes of presumptive cholangitis • Both cats developed exocrine pancreatic insufficiency within 1 week

CBD, common bile duct; *CC*, cholecystectomy; *CCD*, cholecystoduodenostomy; *CCJ*, cholecystojejunostomy; *CD*, choledochotomy; *EHBDO*, extrahepatic bile duct obstruction; *IBD*, inflammatory bowel disease; *PTE*, pulmonary thromboembolism.

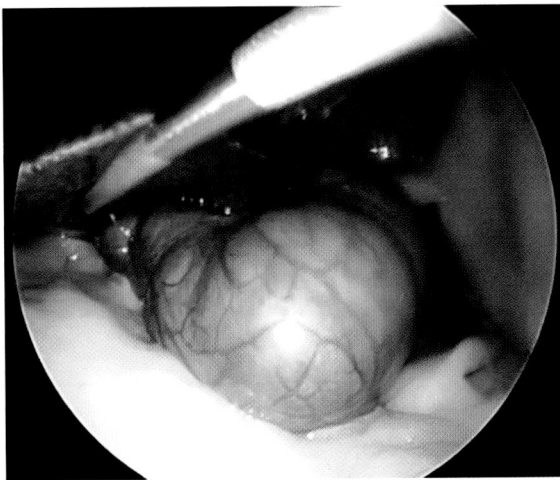

Figure 16-6: Laparoscopic view of a distended gallbladder and cystic duct in a cat with lymphocytic cholangitis.

have recommended surgical intervention (e.g., with pancreatitis) if the obstruction progresses over 1 to 2 weeks,[2,16,88] which seems reasonable as long as the patient remains otherwise stable. Still others advocate an even more conservative approach, as long as the patient's clinical status is improving, because biliary dilation and elevated delta-bilirubin (which has a long half-life because it is protein-bound and increases as a percentage of total bilirubin with increasing duration of hyperbilirubinemia in dogs)[108] may persist for over a month (D. Twedt, personal communication, July 15, 2014). Second, many patients with biliary obstruction are unstable and will be better surgical candidates after a period of medical stabilization. Additionally, passage of choleliths or sludge and spontaneous resolution of the EHBDO are occasionally observed.[6,25,75] However, intentionally waiting for this fortuitous outcome is not advised.

Surgical Complications and Monitoring

As with any abdominal surgery, biliary surgery carries the risks of hemorrhage, dehiscence, seroma, and surgical site infection. Commonly reported adverse events of biliary surgery in cats can be divided into short-term and long-term complications. The reader is referred to other sources for details on surgical techniques to minimize these complications.[37,88,97]

Common short-term complications (see Table 16-2) include anemia, persistent hypotension (especially with prolonged anesthetic time[2,34]), reobstruction (e.g., due to intraoperative error, failure to remove all choleliths, inflammation, residual bile sludge, blood clot, or plugged or dislodged stent or cholecystostomy tube), pancreatitis (e.g., due to surgical manipulation or ductal trauma from stent placement or accidental catheterization), and septic or bile peritonitis (e.g., due to dehiscence of the biliary repair, inadvertent damage to the biliary tree during manipulation or catheterization, or from the duodenotomy and GI biopsy sites). Short-term monitoring should, therefore, include frequent physical examination and measurement of systemic arterial blood pressure, as well as daily CBC and serum biochemistry panel evaluation. The authors expect bilirubin and liver enzymes to decline steadily following a possible brief increase after surgery, although as noted earlier, the delta-bilirubin fraction will take longer to normalize. If anemia or obvious hemorrhage is present, then monitoring of coagulation parameters should be performed and ongoing vitamin K and plasma therapy administered if indicated. A proton pump inhibitor should also be considered, because GI bleeding may be present without overt evidence in the feces. If a cholecystostomy tube or abdominal drain is in place, then daily cytology (and culture, if indicated) of the fluid should be performed. Suspicion of hemoabdomen, bile, septic peritonitis, or repeat obstruction are indications for abdominal ultrasound and diagnostic abdominocentesis. Other than self-limiting hemorrhage, these complications would dictate a return to surgery.

Long-term complications may include reobstruction (e.g., due to stricture of the biliary repair), ascending or descending[24] bacterial cholangitis—particularly common with stents[16] and biliary-enteric diversion (see Table 16-2), exocrine pancreatic insufficiency (uncommonly reported due to accidental ligation of the pancreatic duct),[102] occasional intermittent abdominal pain and diarrhea associated with cholecystectomy,[37] and duodenal ulceration in the case of cholecystojejunostomy[16,88] (proton pump inhibitor therapy is recommended for at least 2 to 4 weeks postoperatively, and possibly indefinitely). Although not a complication of surgery, it is important to note that in cases of cholangitis and/or pancreatitis, with or without IBD, recurrence of clinical illness (and EHBDO) may occur. Similarly, choleliths may form again[2,33] although this risk should be reduced by cholecystectomy and management of any underlying cholangitis.[37] Quarterly physical examinations and minimum database evaluation are therefore recommended in all cases. If clinical signs (e.g., weight loss or steatorrhea) support exocrine pancreatic insufficiency, then serum trypsin-like immunoreactivity should be measured. If a choledochal stent was placed, the feces should be monitored for its passage. If this is not seen within 1 to 2 months, an abdominal radiograph should be performed; if the stent is still present, it should be removed endoscopically to prevent future stent occlusion and ascending cholangitis.[38] Finally, it is important to note that permanent biliary changes may be observed with diagnostic imaging. Previously inflamed and dilated ducts may never return to their normal caliber, and persistent dilation of the CBD has been reported in dogs and humans following cholecystectomy.[45,83,88]

PROGNOSIS

In general, the prognosis for EHBDO is fair-to-guarded in cats. Survival of EHBDO cases with medical management is not well reported in the literature. In general, though, cats with medically treated cholangitis tend to do well in the short term but likely require chronic management and may suffer from disease flares in the future.[2,5,8,53] Cats with ANP have a guarded short-term prognosis but may do well longer term. Cats with chronic pancreatitis may be more difficult to manage and more likely to suffer from irreversible changes (i.e., fibrosis) to their biliary tract.

A survival rate of 40% to 60% with surgery is a conservative estimate, and this approaches 0% with malignant neoplasia.[1,37] However, much of the reported mortality occurs perioperatively, and the prognosis may be better with benign neoplasia and when cats survive the perioperative period.[5] Mortality varies according to the underlying cause of obstruction, as well as the surgical treatment employed, and certain scenarios deserve special mention (see Table 16-2).

Cats with disease that can be surgically corrected without biliary diversion (e.g., cholelithiasis,[23,33] mucocele,[18,19] diaphragmatic hernia,[14] duodenal or biliary foreign body[21,22]) may have an excellent long-term prognosis if they survive the perioperative period.[22,25] Cats tend to tolerate cholecystectomy well long term;[16] however, if they suffer from another EHBDO requiring biliary diversion, it will likely be fatal because most corrective procedures will no longer be possible.[18] Minimal data exists on choledochotomy in cats, but limited evidence suggests that outcomes may be better than previously thought.[36] Choledochal stenting is associated with a better prognosis than biliary-enteric diversion,[83] but stent placement is associated with more complications in cats than dogs,[83,88] and the prognosis with stenting or other temporary biliary diversion procedures remains unclear.

The prognosis for cats that require permanent biliary diversion is guarded—the literature reports approximately only 50% survive to discharge, with only 23% alive at 6 months, and those suffer from intermittent antibiotic-responsive GI upset.[21,34] A subset of patients that may do better following diversion is those with pancreatitis.[69] The prognosis for cats with obstructive and malignant neoplasia requiring diversion is grave, with 100% postoperative mortality reported in the literature. Bile duct adenocarcinoma is the most common hepatobiliary malignancy in cats, and it behaves very aggressively with 67% to 80% metastasis, commonly carcinomatosis, at the time of diagnosis. There is currently no available chemotherapy option for these tumors. However, bile duct adenomas are the most common hepatobiliary tumor in cats, and although they are not as often reported to be the cause of EHBDO, successful surgery could be curative.[29,109] Finally, the prognosis for severe fluke infestation leading to EHBDO must also be regarded as guarded to grave.[7,11,71] However, one cat has been reported to have responded well to choledochojejunostomy.[10] In fact, the prognosis may be worse than some other causes of EHBDO due to the concurrent severe intrahepatic biliary obstruction.[7] Most do not survive surgery.[23,71]

Although published case reports offer some guidance regarding prognosis, they cannot predict how an individual cat will fare with EHBDO treatment. Nevertheless, given the reported outcomes, the decision to pursue surgery in a cat with EHBDO must be weighed very carefully. Consideration of the particular patient's risk factors is imperative. Risk factors for a poor outcome reported in humans include age, malignancy, fever, leukocytosis, hypoalbuminemia, degree of hyperbilirubinemia and ALP elevation, anemia, and acute kidney injury.[37] Poor prognostic indicators reported for cats and dogs are sepsis and septic peritonitis, leukocytosis, renal azotemia, dyspnea, prolonged aPTT or other coagulopathy, and DIC.[37] Refractory hypotension seems to be a predominant risk factor in many studies.[16] Hepatic lipidosis has also been reported to negatively affect outcome if not controlled at the time of surgery.[33] However, in one large case series (22 cats), only the existence of neoplasia significantly affected surgical outcome.[34] Finally, the duration of EHBDO will likely affect long-term prognosis. If the obstruction resolves within a few weeks, secondary liver damage may be reversible, but biliary cirrhosis will set in after 6 weeks of unresolved EHBDO.[16]

SUMMARY

Key points to consider when approaching a case of suspected feline EHBDO are summarized in Box 16-3. EHBDO is uncommon in cats and is usually associated with severe clinical disease. In some cases, prompt surgical intervention is necessary and lifesaving. However, the perioperative mortality rate is high (nearly 100% with malignant neoplasia), and when biliary-enteric diversion is necessary, long-term complications are common. Accordingly, unnecessary surgical procedures should be avoided, with particular emphasis on finding alternatives to biliary-enteric diversion and thoughtful consideration as to whether surgery is prudent in a patient with a known malignant cause of EHBDO. Often, it can be difficult to determine upon initial assessment whether a cat suffers from a permanent, complete cause of EHBDO. If a clear surgical indication is not immediately apparent, then a trial of medical therapy should

> ### BOX 16-3 Key Points to Consider When Approaching a Case of Suspected Feline Extrahepatic Bile Duct Obstruction
>
> - Dilation of the biliary tree seen on ultrasound may not indicate obstruction.
> - Choleliths can be an incidental finding.
> - Biliary surgery is technically challenging, and biliary-enteric diversion has a high rate of perioperative mortality and long-term complications.
> - Cancer leading to EHBDO has a nearly 100% perioperative mortality rate.
> - Simpler surgeries such as cholecystectomy and cholelith removal without biliary-enteric diversion are associated with a good prognosis.
> - Reversible underlying disease (such as pancreatitis) may have a good short-term prognosis even with surgery, but recurrence is possible.
> - Often, the underlying cause of EHBDO may be difficult to determine preoperatively, and lesions observed in surgery should not be presumed to be neoplastic without histopathology.
> - In stable patients without a definitive surgical indication, consider empiric medical therapy for presumptive inflammatory causes of reversible EHBDO (e.g., pancreatitis and cholangitis).
> - In the future, minimally invasive options (e.g., endoscopic retrograde cholangiopancreatography and stent placement) may improve the ability to diagnose and treat cats with EHBDO.
>
> *EHBDO*, Extrahepatic bile duct obstruction.

be considered, with the decision to pursue surgery dependent upon progression of signs consistent with EHBDO. Figure 16-2 is an algorithm for therapeutic decision making in feline EHBDO.

Biliary surgery is technically challenging, and the authors advocate referral to a highly experienced surgeon, as well as minimization of preanesthetic risks and the duration of anesthesia in order to improve the prognosis. Ultimately, the decision to pursue surgery, particularly in ambiguous cases of feline EHBDO, must be made jointly with an owner who has been advised about the possible short-term and long-term outcomes for a given patient and who has carefully weighed the risks and benefits of immediate versus delayed surgical intervention.

ACKNOWLEDGEMENTS

The authors would like to thank Drs. David Twedt, DVM, DACVIM and Angela Marolf, DVM, DACVR for their thoughtful input and review of this chapter.

References

1. Mayhew PD, Holt DE, McLear RC, et al: Pathogenesis and outcome of extrahepatic biliary obstruction in cats. *J Small Anim Pract* 43:247–253, 2002.

2. Rondeau MP: Intrahepatic biliary disorders. In Washabau RJ, Day MJ, editors: *Canine & feline gastroenterology*, St Louis, 2013, Elsevier/Saunders, pp 927–933.

3. Plesman RL, Norris A, Ringwood PB: What is your diagnosis? Pancreatolithiasis. *J Am Vet Med Assoc* 244:647–649, 2014.

4. Washabau RJ: Feline pancreatic disease. In Ettinger SJ, Feldman EC, editors: *Textbook of veterinary internal medicine*, ed 7, St Louis, 2010, Saunders/Elsevier, pp 1704–1709.

5. Harvey AM, Gruffydd-Jones TJ: Feline inflammatory liver disease. In Ettinger SJ, Feldman EC, editors: *Textbook of veterinary internal medicine*, ed 7, St Louis, 2010, Saunders/Elsevier, pp 1643–1648.

6. Aguirre A: Disease of the gallbladder and extrahepatic biliary system. In Ettinger SJ, Feldman EC, editors: *Textbook of veterinary internal medicine*, ed 7, St Louis, 2010, Saunders/Elsevier, pp 1689–1695.

7. Haney DR, Christiansen JS, Toll J: Severe cholestatic liver disease secondary to liver fluke (Platynosomum concinnum) infection in three cats. *J Am Anim Hosp Assoc* 42:234–237, 2006.

8. Hitt ME: Inflammatory liver disease. In August JR, editor: *Consultations in feline internal medicine* (vol 6), St Louis, 2010, Elsevier, pp 213–224.

9. Lewis DT, Malone JB, Taboada J, et al: Cholangiohepatitis and choledochectasia associated with Amphimerus pseudofelineus in a cat. *J Am Anim Hosp Assoc* 27:156–161, 1991.

10. Jenkins CC, Lewis DD, Brock KA, et al: Extrahepatic biliary obstruction associated with Platynosomum concinnum in a cat. *Compend Contin Educ Pract Vet* 10:628–632, 1988.

11. Salomão M, Souza-Dantas LM, Mendes-de-Almeida F, et al: Ultrasonography in hepatobiliary evaluation of domestic cats (Felis catus, L., 1758) infected by Platynosomum Looss, 1907. *Int J App Res Vet Med* 3:271–279, 2005.

12. Satapathy SK, Shifteh A, Kadam J, et al: Acute cholangitis secondary to biliary ascariasis. *Pract Gastroenterol* March:44–46, 2011.

13. Shemesh E, Klein E, Abramowich D, et al: Common bile duct obstruction caused by hydatid daughter cysts—management by endoscopic retrograde sphincterotomy. *Am J Gastroenterol* 81:280–282, 1986.

14. Cornell KK, Jakovljevic S, Waters DJ, et al: Extrahepatic biliary obstruction secondary to diaphragmatic hernia in two cats. *J Am Anim Hosp Assoc* 29:502–507, 1983.

15. Best EJ, Bush DJ, Dye C: Suspected choledochal cyst in a domestic shorthair cat. *J Feline Med Surg* 12:814–817, 2010.

16. Center SA: Diseases of the gallbladder and biliary tree. *Vet Clin North Am Small Anim Pract* 39:543–598, 2009.

17. Grand JG, Doucet M, Albaric O, et al: Cyst of the common bile duct in a cat. *Aust Vet J* 88:268–271, 2010.

18. Bennett SL, Milne M, Slocombe RF, et al: Gallbladder mucocele and concurrent hepatic lipidosis in a cat. *Aust Vet J* 85:397–400, 2007.

19. Woods KS, Brisson BA, Defarges AMN, et al: Congenital duplex gallbladder and biliary mucocele associated with partial hepatic cholestasis and cholelithiasis in a cat. *Can Vet J* 53:269–273, 2012.

20. Gaillot HA, Penninck DG, Webster CRL, et al: Ultrasonographic features of extrahepatic biliary obstruction in 30 cats. *Vet Radiol Ultrasound* 48:439–447, 2007.

21. Della Santa D, Schweighauser A, Forterre F, et al: Imaging diagnosis—extrahepatic biliary tract obstruction secondary to a duodenal foreign body in a cat. *Vet Radiol Ultrasound* 48:448–450, 2007.

22. Brioschi V, Rousset N, Ladlow JF: Imaging diagnosis—extrahepatic biliary tract obstruction secondary to a biliary foreign body in a cat. *Vet Radiol Ultrasound* 55(6):628–631, 2014.

23. Willard MD, Fossum T: Extrahepatic biliary disorders. In Washabau RJ, Day MJ, editors: *Canine & feline gastroenterology*, St Louis, 2013, Elsevier/Saunders, pp 933–936.

24. Bacon NJ, White RAS: Extrahepatic biliary tract surgery in the cat: a case series and review. *J Small Anim Pract* 44:231–235, 2003.

25. Van Geffen C, Savary-Bataille K, Chiers K, et al: Bilirubin cholelithiasis and haemosiderosis in an anemic pyruvate kinase-deficient Somali cat. *J Small Anim Prac* 49:479–482, 2008.

26. Center SA, Baldwin BH, King JM, et al: Hematologic and biochemical abnormalities associated with induced extrahepatic bile duct obstruction in the cat. *Am J Vet Res* 44:1822–1829, 1983.

27. Lawrence D, Bellah JR, Meyer DJ, et al: Temporary bile diversion in cats with experimental extrahepatic bile duct obstruction. *Vet Surg* 21:446–451, 1992.

28. Twedt DC, Armstrong PJ, Simpson KW: Feline cholangitis. In Bonagura JD, Twedt DC, editors: *Current veterinary therapy XV*, St Louis, 2014, Elsevier/Saunders, pp 614–619.

29. Balkman C: Hepatobiliary neoplasia in dogs and cats. *Vet Clin North Am Small Anim Pract* 39:617–625, 2009.

30. Bradley AM, Quimby JM, McCord K, et al: Feline hyperbilirubinemia: a retrospective study of 180 cases. *J Vet Intern Med* 24(3):720, 2010.

31. Martin RA, MacCoy DA, Harvey HJ: Surgical management of extrahepatic biliary tract disease: a report of eleven cases. *J Am Anim Hosp Assoc* 22:301–307, 1986.

32. Mayhew PD, Weisse CW: Treatment of pancreatitis-associated extrahepatic biliary tract obstruction by choledochal stenting in seven cats. *J Small Anim Prac* 49:133–138, 2008.

33. Eich CS, Ludwig LL: The surgical treatment of cholelithiasis in cats: a study of nine cases. *J Am Anim Hosp Assoc* 38:290–296, 2002.

34. Buote NJ, Mitchell SL, Penninck D, et al: Cholecystoenterostomy for treatment of extrahepatic biliary tract obstruction in cats: 22 cases (1994-2003). *J Am Vet Med Assoc* 228:1376–1382, 2006.

35. Webster CRL, Cooper JC: Diagnostic approach to hepatobiliary disease. In Bonagura JD, Twedt DC, editors: *Current veterinary therapy XV*, St Louis, 2014, Elsevier/Saunders, pp 569–575.

36. Baker SG, Mayhew PD, Mehler SJ: Choledochotomy and primary repair of extrahepatic biliary duct rupture in seven dogs and two cats. *J Small Anim Pract* 52:32–37, 2011.

37. Mehler SJ: Complications of extrahepatic biliary surgery in companion animals. *Vet Clin North Am Small Anim Pract* 41:949–967, 2011.

38. Forman MA: Feline exocrine pancreatic disorders. In Bonagura JD, Twedt DC, editors: *Current veterinary therapy XV*, St Louis, 2014, Elsevier Saunders, pp 565–568.

39. Leveille R, Biller DS, Shiroma JT: Sonographic evaluation of the common bile duct in cats. *J Vet Intern Med* 10:296–299, 1996.

40. Nyland TG, Gillett NA: Sonographic evaluation of experimental bile duct ligation in the dog. *Vet Radiol Ultrasound* 23:252–260, 1982.

41. Hittmair KM, Vielgrader HD, Loupal G: Ultrasonographic evaluation of gallbladder wall thickness in cats. *Vet Radiol Ultrasound* 42:149–155, 2001.

42. Harran N, d'Anjou M, Dunn M, et al: Gallbladder sludge on ultrasound is predictive of increased liver enzymes and total bilirubin in cats. *Can Vet J* 52:999–1003, 2011.

43. Marolf AJ, Leach L, Gibbons DS, et al: Ultrasonographic findings of feline cholangitis. *J Am Anim Hosp Assoc* 48:36–42, 2012.

44. Worley DR, Hottinger HA, Lawrence HJ: Surgical management of gallbladder mucoceles in dogs: 22 cases (1999-2003). *J Am Vet Med Assoc* 225:1418–1422, 2004.

45. Pike FS, Berg J, King NW, et al: Gallbladder mucocele in dogs: 30 cases (2000-2002). *J Am Vet Med Assoc* 224:1615–1622, 2004.

46. Berent AC: Acute biliary diseases of the dog and cat. In Silverstein DC, Hopper K, editors: *Small animal critical care medicine*, St Louis, 2009, Saunders/Elsevier, pp 542–546.

47. Gaschen L: Update on hepatobiliary imaging. *Vet Clin North Am Small Anim Pract* 39:439–467, 2009.

48. Rothuizen J: Important clinical syndromes associated with liver disease. *Vet Clin North Am Small Anim Pract* 39:419–437, 2009.

49. Saunders HM, Van Winkle TJ, Drobatz K, et al: Ultrasonographic findings in cats with

clinical, gross pathologic and histologic evidence of acute pancreatic necrosis: 20 cases (1994-2001). *J Am Vet Med Assoc* 221:1724–1730, 2002.

50. Marolf AJ, Kraft SL, Dunphy TR, et al: Magnetic resonance (MR) imaging and MR cholangiopancreatography findings in cats with cholangitis and pancreatitis. *J Feline Med Surg* 15:285–294, 2013.

51. Rademacher N, Ohlerth S, Scharf G, et al: Contrast-enhanced power and color Doppler ultrasonography of the pancreas in healthy and diseased cats. *J Vet Intern Med* 22:1310–1316, 2008.

52. Newell SM, Graham JP, Roberts GD, et al: Quantitative hepatobiliary scintigraphy in normal cats and in cats with experimental cholangiohepatitis. *Vet Radiol Ultrasound* 42:70–76, 2001.

53. Clark JEC, Haddad JL, Brown DC, et al: Feline cholangitis: a necropsy study of 44 cats (1986-2008). *J Feline Med Surg* 13:570–576, 2011.

54. Nyland TG, Koblik PD, Tellyer SE: Ultrasonographic evaluation of biliary cystadenomas in cats. *Vet Radiol Ultrasound* 40:300–306, 1999.

55. Boothe HW, Boothe DM, Komkov A, et al: Use of hepatobiliary scintigraphy in the diagnosis of extra hepatic biliary obstruction in dogs and cats: 25 cases (1982-1989). *J Am Vet Med Assoc* 201:134–141, 1992.

56. Rosenthal SJ, Cox GG, Wetzel LH, et al: Pitfalls and differential diagnosis in biliary sonography. *Radiographics* 10:285–311, 1990.

57. Head LL, Daniel GB: Correlation between hepatobiliary scintigraphy and surgery or postmortem examination findings in dogs and cats with extrahepatic biliary obstruction, partial obstruction, or patency of the biliary system: 18 cases (1995-2004). *J Am Vet Med Assoc* 227:1618–1624, 2005.

58. Forman MA, Marks SL, De Cock HEV: Evaluation of serum feline pancreatic lipase immunoreactivity and helical computed tomography versus conventional testing for the diagnosis of feline pancreatitis. *J Vet Intern Med* 18:807–815, 2004.

59. Gerhardt A, Steiner JM, Williams DA, et al: Comparison of the sensitivity of different diagnostic tests for pancreatitis in cats. *J Vet Intern Med* 15:329–333, 2001.

60. Spillmann T, Willard MD, Ruhnke I, et al: Feasibility of endoscopic retrograde cholangiopancreatography in healthy cats. *Vet Radiol Ultrasound* 55:85–91, 2014.

61. Rothuizen J, Twedt DC: Liver biopsy techniques. *Vet Clin North Am Small Anim Pract* 39:469–480, 2009.

62. Mayhew PD, Savigny MR, Otto CM, et al: Evaluation of coagulation in dogs with partial or complete extrahepatic biliary tract obstruction by means of thromboelastography. *J Am Vet Med Assoc* 242:778–785, 2013.

63. Scherk MA, Center SA: Toxic, metabolic, infectious, and neoplastic liver diseases. In Ettinger SJ, Feldman EC, editors: *Textbook of veterinary internal medicine*, ed 7, St Louis, 2010, Saunders/Elsevier, pp 1672–1689.

64. Rothuizen J: General principles in the treatment of liver disease. In Ettinger SJ, Feldman EC, editors: *Textbook of veterinary internal medicine*, ed 7, St Louis, 2010, Saunders/Elsevier, pp 1629–1637.

65. Wagner KA, Hartmann FA, Trepanier LA: Bacterial culture results from liver, gallbladder, or bile in 248 dogs and cats evaluated for hepatobiliary disease: 1998-2003. *J Vet Intern Med* 21:417–424, 2007.

66. Savary-Bataille KCM, Bunch SE, Spaulding KA, et al: Percutaneous ultrasound-guided cholecystocentesis in healthy cats. *J Vet Intern Med* 17:298–303, 2003.

67. Brain PH, Barrs VR, Martin P, et al: Feline cholecystitis and acute neutrophilic cholangitis: clinical findings, bacterial isolates and response to treatment in six cases. *J Feline Med Surg* 8:91–103, 2006.

68. Rivers BJ, Walter PA, Johnston GR, et al: Acalculous cholecystitis in four canine cases: ultrasonographic findings and use of ultrasonographic-guided, percutaneous cholecystocentesis in diagnosis. *J Am Anim Hosp Assoc* 33:207–214, 1997.

69. Son TT, Thompson L, Serrano S, et al: Surgical intervention in the management of severe acute pancreatitis in cats: 8 cases (2003-2007). *J Vet Emerg Crit Care* 20:426–435, 2010.

70. Chambers G: Abdominal distension, ascites, and peritonitis. In Ettinger SJ, Feldman EC, editors: *Textbook of veterinary internal medicine*, ed 7, St Louis, 2010, Saunders/Elsevier, pp 144–148.

71. Xavier FG, Morato GS, Righi DA, et al: Cystic liver disease related to high Platynosomum fastosum infection in a domestic cat. *J Feline Med Surg* 9:51–55, 2007.

72. Simpson KW, Worhunsky PA: Cobalamin deficiency in cats. In Bonagura JD, Twedt DC, editors: *Current veterinary therapy XV*, St Louis, 2014, Elsevier/Saunders, pp 522–525.

73. Twedt DC, Cullen J, McCord K, et al: Evaluation of fluorescence in situ hybridization for the detection of bacteria in feline inflammatory liver disease. *J Feline Med Surg* 16:109–117, 2014.

74. Chan DL: Critical care nutrition. In August JR, editor: *Consultations in feline internal medicine* (vol 6), St Louis, 2010, Saunders/Elsevier, pp 116–126.

75. Lehner CM, McAnulty JF: Management of extrahepatic biliary obstruction: a role for temporary percutaneous biliary drainage. *Compend Contin Educ Vet* 32(9):E1–E10, 2010.

76. Sullivan L, Hackett TB: Transfusion medicine: best practices. In Bonagura JD, Twedt DC, editors: *Current veterinary therapy XV*, St Louis, 2014, Elsevier/Saunders, pp 309–313.

77. Mehler SJ, Mayhew PD, Drobatz KJ, et al: Variables associated with outcome in dogs undergoing extrahepatic biliary surgery: 60 cases (1988-2002). *Vet Surg* 33:644–649, 2004.

78. Ludwig LL, McLoughlin MA, Graves TK, et al: Surgical treatment of bile peritonitis in 24 dogs and 2 cats: a retrospective study (1987-1994). *Vet Surg* 26:90–98, 1997.

79. Tazawa J, Sanada K, Sakai Y, et al: Gallbladder aspiration for acute cholecystitis in average-surgical-risk patients. *Int J Clin Pract* 59:21–24, 2005.

80. Curro G, Cucinotta E: Percutaneous gall bladder aspiration as an alternative to laparoscopic cholecystectomy in Child-Pugh C cirrhotic patients with acute cholecystitis. *Gut* 55:898–899, 2006.

81. Herman BA, Brawer RS, Murtaugh RJ, et al: Therapeutic percutaneous ultrasound-guided cholecystocentesis in three dogs with extrahepatic biliary obstruction and pancreatitis. *J Am Vet Med Assoc* 227:1782–1786, 2005.

82. Murphy SM, Rodriguez JD, McAnulty JF: Minimally invasive cholecystostomy in the dog: evaluation of placement techniques and use in extrahepatic biliary obstruction. *Vet Surg* 36:675–683, 2007.

83. Richter KP, Pike FS: Extrahepatic biliary tract disease. In Bonagura JD, Twedt DC, editors: *Current veterinary therapy XV*, St Louis, 2014, Elsevier/Saunders, pp 602–605.

84. Hill SL, Armstrong PJ: Feline hepatic lipidosis. In Bonagura JD, Twedt DC, editors: *Current veterinary therapy XV*, St Louis, 2014, Elsevier/Saunders, pp 608–614.

85. Center SA: Acute liver failure. In Bonagura JD, Twedt DC, editors: *Current veterinary therapy XV*, St Louis, 2014, Elsevier/Saunders, pp 580–583.

86. Devey JJ: Crystalloid and colloid fluid therapy. In Ettinger SJ, Feldman EC, editors: *Textbook of veterinary internal medicine*, ed 7, St Louis, 2010, Saunders/Elsevier, pp 487–496.

87. Ruaux CG: Nutritional management of hepatic conditions. In Ettinger SJ, Feldman EC, editors: *Textbook of veterinary internal medicine*, ed 7, St Louis, 2010, Saunders/Elsevier, pp 682–687.

88. Mayhew PD, Weisse C: Liver and biliary system. In Tobias KM, Johnston SA, editors: *Veterinary surgery small animal*, St Louis, 2012, Elsevier/Saunders, pp 1601–1623.

89. Kavanagh C, Shaw S, Webster CRL: Coagulation in hepatobiliary disease. *J Vet Emerg Crit Care* 21:589–604, 2011.

90. Boscan P, Mama K, Monnet E, et al: Effect of maropitant, a neurokinin 1 receptor antagonist, on anesthetic requirements during noxious visceral stimulation of the ovary in dogs. *Am J Vet Res* 72:1576–1579, 2011.

91. Quimby JM, Gustafson DL, Lunn KF: The pharmacokinetics of mirtazapine in cats with chronic kidney disease and in age-matched control cats. *J Vet Intern Med* 25:985–989, 2011.

92. Quimby JM, Lunn KF: Mirtazapine as an appetite stimulant and anti-emetic in cats with chronic kidney disease: a masked

placebo-controlled crossover clinical trial. *Vet J* 197:651–655, 2013.

93. Webster CRL, Cooper J: Therapeutic use of cytoprotective agents in canine and feline hepatobiliary disease. *Vet Clin North Am Small Anim Pract* 39:631–652, 2009.

94. Frezza EE, Gerunda GE, Plebani M, et al: Effect of ursodeoxycholic acid administration on bile duct proliferation and cholestasis in bile duct ligated rat. *Dig Dis Sci* 38:1291–1296, 1993.

95. Serviddio G, Pereda J, Pallardo FV: Ursodeoxycholic acid protects against secondary biliary cirrhosis in rats by preventing mitochondrial oxidative stress. *Hepatology* 39:711–720, 2004.

96. Fromm H: Gallstone dissolution therapy with ursodiol. *Dig Dis Sci* 34:36S–38S, 1989.

97. Martin RA, Lanz OI, Tobias KM: Liver and biliary system. In Slatter D, editor: *Textbook of small animal surgery*, ed 3, Philadelphia, 2003, Saunders, pp 708–726.

98. Pitt HA, Gomes AS, Lois JF, et al: Does preoperative percutaneous biliary drainage reduce operative risk or increase hospital cost? *Ann Surg* 201:445–553, 1985.

99. Morrison S, Prostredny J, Roa D: Retrospective study of 28 cases of cholecystoduodenostomy performed using endoscopic gastrointestinal anastomosis stapling equipment. *J Am Anim Hosp Assoc* 44:10–18, 2008.

100. Furneaux RW: A series of six cases of sphincter of Oddi pathology in the cat (2008-2009). *J Feline Med Surg* 12:794–801, 2010.

101. Fahie MA, Martin RA: Extrahepatic biliary tract obstruction: a retrospective study of 45 cases. *J Am Anim Hosp Assoc* 31:478–482, 1995.

102. Tangner CH, Turrel JM, Hobson HP: Complications associated with proximal duodenal resection and cholecystoduodenostomy in two cats. *Vet Surg* 11:60–64, 1982.

103. Weiss DJ, Gagne JM, Armstrong PJ: Relationship between inflammatory hepatic disease and inflammatory bowel disease, pancreatitis, and nephritis in cats. *J Am Vet Med Assoc* 209:1114–1116, 1996.

104. Scott KD, Zoran DL, Mansell J, et al: Utility of endoscopic biopsies of the duodenum and ileum for diagnosis of inflammatory bowel disease and small cell lymphoma in cats. *J Vet Intern Med* 25:1253–1257, 2011.

105. Crews LJ, Feeney DA, Jessen CR, et al: Clinical, ultrasonographic, and laboratory findings associated with gallbladder disease and rupture in dogs: 45 cases (1997-2007). *J Am Vet Med Assoc* 234:359–366, 2009.

106. Malek S, Sinclair E, Hosgood G, et al: Clinical findings and prognostic factors for dogs undergoing cholecystectomy for gall bladder mucocele. *Vet Surg* 42:418–426, 2013.

107. Volk SW, Holt D: Hepatic and splenic emergencies. In Ettinger SJ, Feldman EC, editors: *Textbook of veterinary internal medicine*, ed 7, St Louis, 2010, Saunders/Elsevier, pp 513–516.

108. Higashijima H, Yamashita H, Makino I, et al: Significance of serum delta bilirubin during obstructive jaundice in dogs. *J Surg Res* 66:119–124, 1996.

109. Liptak JM: Hepatobiliary tumors. In Withrow SJ, Vail DM, Page RL, editors: *Withrow & MacEwen's small animal clinical oncology*, ed 5, St Louis, 2013, Elsevier/Saunders, pp 405–412.

Clinical Remission and Survival in Diabetic Cats: What Has Changed Over the Last Decade

Eric Zini

During the last decade, many new studies have been published in the field of feline diabetology. Some have yielded insights into the disease mechanisms, treatment, or monitoring, and others have given answers to common questions that veterinarians are asked by owners whenever a cat is diagnosed with diabetes. In a clinical setting, questions such as, "How long will my diabetic cat live?" or "Will my diabetic cat need insulin for its entire life?" are very frequent, and knowing the response can help the owner accept the cat's disease and increase willingness to treat. This chapter reviews what is known about the life expectancy and prognostic factors of cats with diabetes. In addition, this chapter reviews what is known about clinical remission of cats with diabetes, and presents an analysis of the factors that can be used to predict remission and how long it will last.

SURVIVAL AND PROGNOSTIC FACTORS

Outline of Past Investigations

Diabetes is one of the most commonly encountered endocrine diseases in cats, with an approximate prevalence of one in 200, based on an insured population in the United Kingdom.[1] Predisposing factors, such as male sex, obesity, indoor confinement, and physical inactivity are well known to contribute to the development of the disease.[1,2] Pathophysiologic features of diabetes and treatment options for affected cats are major topics of research, but few studies have addressed survival and the prognostic factors of the disease.[3-5]

Median survival time after diagnosis seems to vary widely in cats. In a study published in 2008, median life expectancy of 19 diabetic cats was 385 days,[3] whereas in two earlier investigations from the 1990s involving 55 and 104 diabetic cats, respectively, the median survival times were 870 and 780 days.[4,5] The mortality rate was shown to be high soon after diagnosis, with 11% and 12% of cats dying within 3 weeks

from diagnosis or not surviving to the time of discharge from the first hospitalization, respectively.[4,5] Among prognostic factors, age was negatively associated with survival, meaning that older cats had shorter life expectancy,[4] whereas body weight, sex, ketonuria, and glycemic control did not affect outcome.[4,5] Further, the presence of pancreatitis and a higher degree of amyloid deposition in the islets, based on postmortem histologic diagnosis, were not associated with shorter survival.[5]

Current Survival Analysis

In previous reports, comprehensive analysis of medical records was often missing, including data retrieved from signalment, history, hematology, and biochemistry profiles; information pertaining to presence of concurrent diseases or ketoacidosis (i.e., metabolic acidosis and ketonuria); clinical remission of diabetes; and type of insulin administered. All of these factors may affect survival of diabetic cats.

To address survival and outcome predictors in a large population of cats with newly diagnosed diabetes, the author and his colleagues performed a retrospective study at the University of Zurich, Switzerland.[6] In the study, cats were included if they had newly diagnosed diabetes, were treatment naive, and were followed-up at the same institution until death or until the last re-evaluation. Further, cats were excluded if the owners refused a comprehensive diagnostic workup and hospitalization or if referred and previously treated by private practitioners. Thus, of the 275 diabetic cats originally identified, 114 met the inclusion criteria and were used further in the analysis.

The results showed that diabetic cats had a relatively good prognosis. The mortality rate of diabetic cats calculated during the first 10 days from diagnosis was 16.7%; this frequency is relatively high, but it compares favorably to the two previous investigations where observed case fatality rates

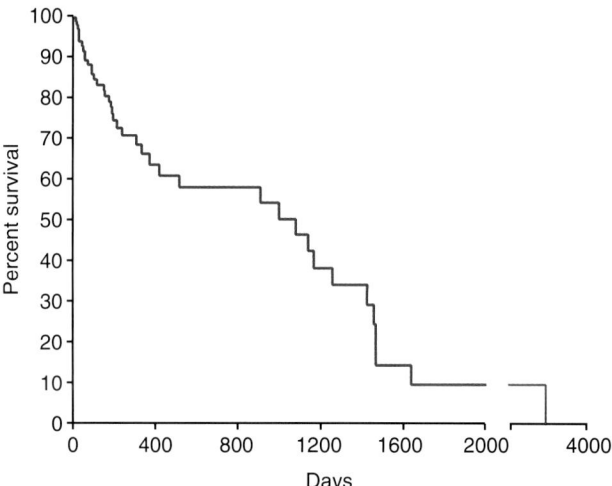

Figure 17-1: Survival of cats with newly diagnosed diabetes discharged from hospitalization.

were 11% and 12% during the first hospitalization period, respectively.[4,5]

Overall median survival in the group of diabetic cats analyzed in Switzerland was 516 days, with 59% living longer than 1 year, and 46% longer than 2 years.[6] Kraus and colleagues[4] had documented a longer median survival time, reaching 870 days. The discrepancy may be because in the latter study, second-opinion cases that had been treated before starting calculation of survival were also included; hence, the estimated survival may have been biased toward longer survival by the exclusion of cats that died soon after diagnosis. Goossens and colleagues[5] calculated median survival time after the first period of hospitalization, yielding 780 days. Cats that died during the first period of hospitalization might have been excluded in this investigation. Of note, to assess whether death before discharge from admission biased the results of the analysis, the author and his colleagues recalculated overall survival excluding cats that died during the first period of hospitalization.[6] Median survival time increased from 516 to 1080 days; 66% of cats lived longer than 1 year, and 57% longer than 2 years (Figure 17-1).

Conclusions: Survival Times of Cats with Diabetes Mellitus

Collectively, the results of the aforementioned studies suggest that survival of diabetic cats is moderately good at admission, but it increases considerably if the cats survive to discharge or if they do not require hospitalization.

Novel Prognostic Factors

With regard to prognostic factors, the author and his colleagues found that higher levels of serum creatinine measured at the time of diagnosis was associated with a significantly shorter life expectancy, with the hazard of dying being about 5% higher for each increase of 10 µg/dL in serum creatinine concentration.[6] This observation may be explained by the fact that higher degrees of azotemia are associated with faster

progression of renal dysfunction in cats, which in turn leads to decreased survival.[7] Of note, 17% of diabetic cats had high serum creatinine concentrations, but it was only mildly elevated in most cases. However, it is possible that polyuria and loss of muscle mass secondary to the diabetic state lead to a decrease in serum creatinine concentration in some cats, which could have masked renal dysfunction.

As it may be predicted, the presence of a concurrent illness at diagnosis tended to decrease life expectancy; cats with concurrent diseases had a mortality rate about 70% higher than those without concurrent diseases.[6] Different reasons may explain this finding, such as the aggravation of insulin resistance induced by the additional disease, the presence of a disorder associated with an unfavorable outcome, and the possible decreased motivation and willingness of owners to treat. No study has been performed to systematically assess whether concurrent diseases affect survival. In the large group of diabetic cats of Goossens and colleagues,[5] the presence of pancreatic disease was not a negative prognostic factor, but this observation was based on necropsy results and not *in vivo* results at diagnosis. Unfortunately, the investigation by the author and his colleagues[6] did not evaluate the effect of specific concurrent diseases on survival. It is possible that some less-relevant disorders had little if any effect on predicting life expectancy of diabetic cats.

In the study, cats that achieved clinical remission of diabetes had a longer median survival time than cats that remained persistently diabetic, suggesting that remission is positively associated with outcome.[6] In particular, considering the 59 diabetic cats that were followed-up until death, the median survival of those with clinical remission was 913 days, whereas the median survival of those that did not achieve clinical remission was only 25 days. In the remaining 55 diabetic cats that were still alive or lost to follow-up, the median survival of those with clinical remission was 244 days, compared to 118 days in those that did not achieve clinical remission.[6] One probable reason for the improved outcome might be that a diabetic cat not needing insulin would be expected to have a better quality of life and less complications (e.g., hepatic lipidosis, urinary tract infection, and/or neuropathy) compared with cats not experiencing remission. It is also likely that owners of diabetic cats, if clinical remission has occurred, are more prone to closely monitor their pets and continue with investigations and treatments if additional disorders develop.

None of the other possible prognostic factors investigated in the study (i.e., sex, breed, body weight, previous administration of corticosteroids or progestagens, hematocrit, leukocyte count, serum glucose, fructosamine, albumin, total proteins, urea, potassium, cholesterol, bilirubin and lipase, type of insulin, and presence of ketoacidosis) were associated with outcome.[6]

Ketoacidosis is a severe complication of diabetes. It developed in 34.2% of the cats at first admission,[6] which is in agreement with an investigation showing a rate of approximately 40%.[8] Practicing veterinarians often consider ketoacidosis to have an unfavorable prognosis as a result of its many

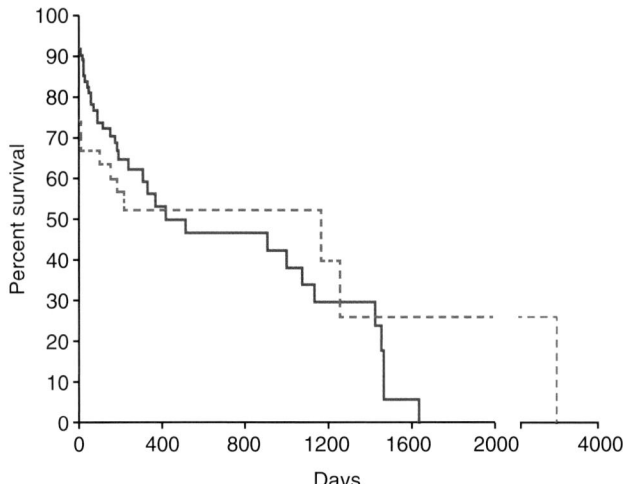

Figure 17-2: Survival of diabetic cats with *(dashed line)* and without ketoacidosis *(solid line)* at admission. Median survival of cats with and without ketoacidosis is similar.

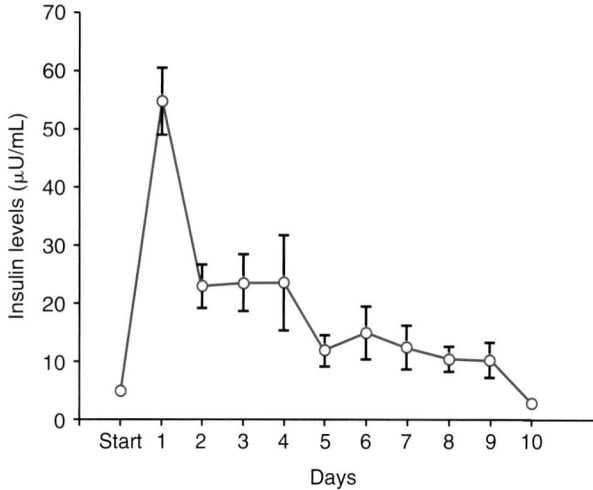

Figure 17-3: Plasma insulin levels in cats infused with glucose for 10 days. Insulin concentrations markedly increased during the first 24 hours and progressively decreased thereafter. Means and standard error are shown.

metabolic derangements and difficult management. However, according to the results, ketoacidosis should not necessarily be considered a predictor for negative outcome.[6] In particular, more than 30% of cats that presented with ketoacidosis survived longer than 3 years[6] (Figure 17-2). Thus, in light of these findings, treatment of diabetic cats with ketoacidosis should always be pursued by clinicians. In support of the favorable outcome of cats with ketoacidosis, reports have demonstrated that clinical remission of diabetes is possible in 50% of cases, irrespective of the complication.[9,10]

Conclusions: Prognosis for Cats with Diabetes Mellitus

In summary, cats with newly diagnosed diabetes have a moderately good prognosis, which becomes very good if they are alive following hospitalization. At diagnosis, increasing age and serum creatinine levels decrease life expectancy, and the presence of concurrent diseases can lead to a poorer outcome.

Because of the extended survival of diabetic cats with remission, clinicians should direct their efforts to achieve this favorable condition. Although ketoacidosis is generally considered a complication leading to shorter survival, based on the most recently available data, it may not represent a negative prognostic factor in cats.

CLINICAL REMISSION AND ITS PREDICTORS

Definition of Clinical Remission

Insulin therapy is the most effective means to achieve glycemic control and to avoid life-threatening complications in diabetic cats.[11] Interestingly, 10% to 67% of affected cats have been reported to maintain normoglycemia without exogenous insulin within weeks to months of beginning therapy.[10,12-15]

The term *diabetic remission,* or *transient diabetes,* is used in cats in which insulin administration can be withdrawn for at

least 4 consecutive weeks with no relapse in clinical signs and maintenance of normal concentrations of glucose and fructosamine.[10] The term *clinical remission* is used because the cat is clinically recovered, based both on owner observations and on routine blood glucose analysis. However, viability of pancreatic beta cells may not have fully recovered from the original damage that caused them to be unable to control glycemia. Indeed, although insulin secretion in diabetic cats shortly after clinical remission was shown to be similar to that of healthy cats, the number of pancreatic islet cells may remain reduced; vacuolar degeneration of islet cells and swollen beta cells may be seen.[12]

Glucotoxicity

The reason why diabetic remission occurs in some cats and not in others is uncertain. It is hypothesized that the diabetic milieu, in particular that associated with uncontrolled hyperglycemia, may contribute to reduce viability of the remaining beta cells in diabetic cats, similar to what has been assumed in humans with type 2 diabetes and in rodent models of the disease.[15] The detrimental effect of sustained high glucose levels on beta cells and insulin secretion is referred to as *glucotoxicity,* and it has been well characterized in cats.

The first study of cats was conducted by the research group of the University of Zurich to verify whether glucotoxicity develops after doing a constant glucose infusion for 10 days, clamping their blood glucose concentrations at the approximate level found in untreated feline diabetes (450 to 540 mg/dL [25 to 30 mmol/L]).[16] This experiment showed that severe beta cell dysfunction is rapidly induced by sustained hyperglycemia in cats. Plasma insulin markedly declined by day 2 of glucose infusion and was below baseline concentrations by day 10 (Figure 17-3); at this time, intravenous (IV) administration of an acute glucose bolus also failed to stimulate insulin secretion. Based on pancreatic histopathology, these hyperglycemic cats had insulin-positive areas reduced by 80% as the result of depletion of insulin stores, and insulin gene transcription was decreased, indicating that chronic overstimulation of beta cells with glucose also led to reduced insulin synthesis.[16] To support this latter observation, pancreatic immunostaining revealed that insulin appeared distributed as a thin rim at the beta cell periphery; because proinsulin is concentrated in the Golgi apparatus of normal beta cells,[17] the lack of perinuclear immunostaining indicated that early steps in insulin synthesis were disturbed.

Altogether, these results confirm that sustained hyperglycemia is toxic in cats by markedly impairing beta cell function, leading to beta cell exhaustion and decreased insulin gene expression.[16] Furthermore, another important result from the same study served to demonstrate that glucotoxicity in the feline species can also cause beta cell loss, as shown by the 50% decrease in beta cell count per pancreatic area, which was not compensated by increased beta cell proliferation in cats infused with glucose. Based on histomorphologic features, hyperglycemic cats had large parts of most islets devoid of nuclei (Figure 17-4).

As for the reason for the reduced number of beta cells in cats made chronically hyperglycemic, it was found that islet transcripts of cytokines or chemokines and the number of islet neutrophils were not increased, excluding a local inflammatory reaction as the cause. However, apoptotic islet cells and beta cells positive for cleaved caspase-3 (i.e., a protein involved in apoptosis) were clearly present in cats infused with glucose (Figure 17-5). Apoptosis may thus be one major mechanism through which hyperglycemia substantially reduces the number of beta cells in cats.[16]

In another experiment, Link and colleagues[18] used two groups of healthy cats that were infused with glucose over 6 weeks, clamping their hyperglycemia either at 300 mg/dL (16.7 mmol/L) or 520 mg/dL (28.9 mmol/L). Results

showed that the suppressive effect of glucose on circulating insulin concentrations was more pronounced at 520 mg/dL (28.9 mmol/L) than at 300 mg/dL (16.7 mmol/L). However, even in cats maintained at a mean glucose concentration of 300 mg/dL (16.7 mmol/L), the circulating insulin response to moderate hyperglycemia was inappropriately low.

Of note, this study also investigated whether recovery of beta cells from glucotoxicity may occur after discontinuation of glucose infusion.[18] After cessation of the glucose infusion, normalization of insulin secretion (based on achievement of normoglycemia) required only a few hours in cats clamped at a glucose concentration of 300 mg/dL (16.7 mmol/L), whereas it took approximately 2 weeks to achieve normoglycemia in cats clamped at 520 mg/dL (28.9 mmol/L). This

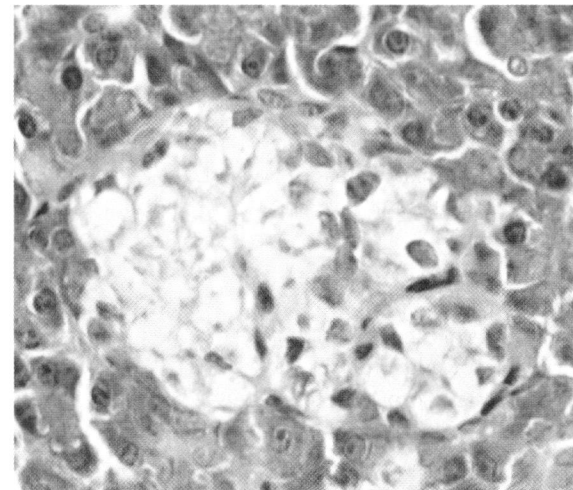

Figure 17-4: Hematoxylin and eosin staining of pancreatic islets in cats infused with glucose for 10 days (magnification ×40). Large areas of the islets appear devoid of nuclei and include several vacuoles.

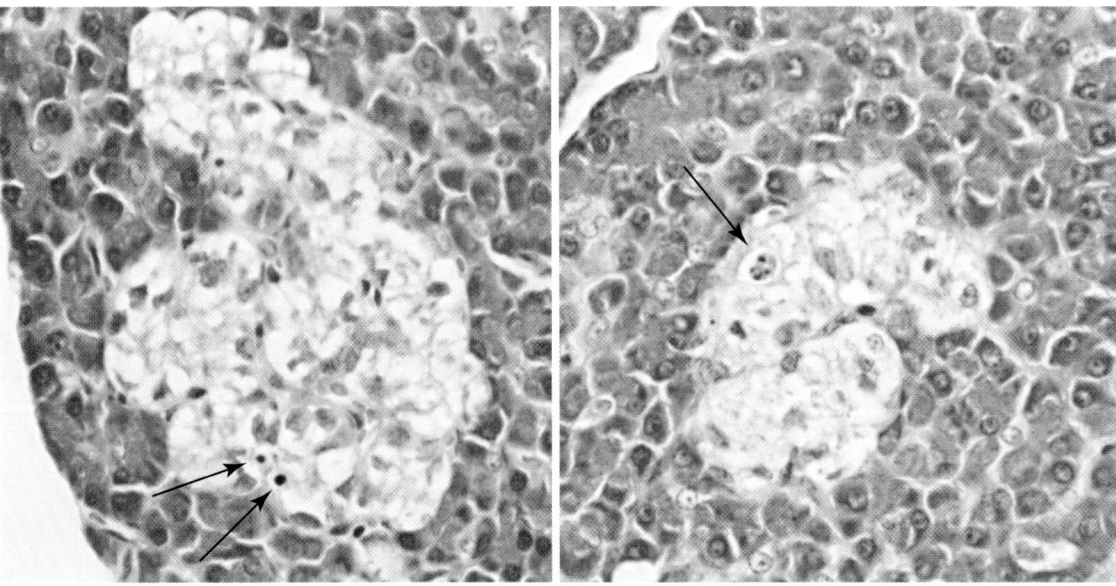

Figure 17-5: Hematoxylin and eosin staining of pancreatic islets in cats infused with glucose for 10 days (magnification ×40). *Arrows* show nuclei with morphologic features of apoptosis.

suggests that more severe elevations in circulating glucose concentration will exert a more profound suppressive effect on beta cells. Histopathology of the pancreas done 3 weeks after cessation of the glucose infusion revealed that beta cells had more insulin immunoreactivity than they did at the end of the period of the 6-week hyperglycemic clamp. However, the histopathology at 3 weeks after the infusion still revealed that beta cells contained less-pronounced insulin immunoreactivity than the healthy control cats, indicating the beta cells were not yet fully recovered from glucotoxicity.[18] Therefore, this study showed that prolonged hyperglycemia results in a dose-dependent suppressive effect on beta cells, with higher glucose concentrations being more detrimental, and that glucotoxicity is at least partially reversible.

In summary, the aforementioned investigations collectively suggest that excess glucose is a major culprit responsible for damage to insulin-secreting beta cells in cats. From a clinical perspective, these results could lead one to hypothesize that prompt and tight control of hyperglycemia in diabetic cats may allow the residual viable beta cells to recover from the glucotoxic damage, possibly anticipating clinical remission of diabetes.

Clinical Remission: When and How Long

Because clinical remission of diabetes may be associated with recovery from glucotoxicity, and prolonged uncontrolled hyperglycemia is expected to progressively cause exhaustion and death of all remaining viable beta cells in cats, it might be assumed that the chances of remission will be higher early in the diabetes disease course.

To verify this hypothesis, a study focused on clinical remission of diabetic cats was performed at the University of Zurich using the same 275 medical records retrieved for the aforementioned survival analysis.[6] For the investigation, cats with newly diagnosed diabetes were included if they were followed-up at least until remission was achieved or until death.[9] Only cats in which insulin was discontinued for at least 4 consecutive weeks while maintaining normal glucose and fructosamine concentrations and showing no clinical signs of diabetes were considered to be in remission.[10]

From the originally identified cases, 90 cats met the inclusion criteria and were used in the analysis. Of these 90 cases, 45 (50%) achieved clinical remission, and 45 (50%) remained permanently diabetic. The calculated median time from discharge to remission was 48 days (range: 8 to 216); 25% of cats achieved remission within 27 days, 75% within 102 days, and only one cat after 6 months[9] (Figure 17-6). These results are in agreement with previous literature showing that the large majority of diabetic cats achieving remission reach it within 6 months from diagnosis,[10,12-15] and they confirm the assumption that chances of remission are high early after diagnosis and largely decrease during the following months, possibly because irreversible damage to the insulin-secreting cells has time to occur.

From the same investigation,[9] the median duration of clinical remission was 114 days (range: 30 to 3370 days) in

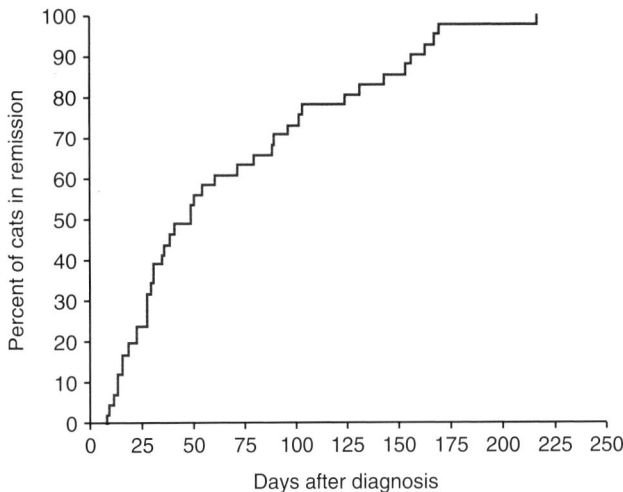

Figure 17-6: Diabetic Cats Achieving Clinical Remission. Cumulative percentage of cats that did not require insulin to maintain normoglycemia over time.

cats that were followed-up until death (*n* = 15), and 151 days (range: 28 to 1180 days) in cats that were still alive (*n* = 30) by the end of the study. Six of the 45 (13%) cats with remission did not require insulin for more than 1000 days; one of them has not received insulin for more than 9 years.

Overall, insulin therapy had to be resumed to control hyperglycemia because of relapse in only 13 (29%) of the 45 cats that had experienced remission, including six of the cats that died and seven of those that were still alive at the study end. None of these 13 cats experienced a further period of clinical remission.[9] These results are also in line with former reports, showing that the duration of diabetic remission varied widely, with some cats not requiring treatment for few months and others for some years.[12,14] Based on another report,[14] insulin therapy had to be restarted in 26% of diabetic cats, which is similar to the study by the author and his colleagues.[9] In both studies, the number of relapses may be underestimated, however, because some of the cats were lost to follow-up.

Based on current knowledge, relapse of diabetes after an initial period of remission may not be an unexpected event in cats. Even during clinical remission, it is well documented that the number of pancreatic islet cells remains reduced and morphologic evidence of beta cell damage is still present.[12] Cats in remission probably have progressed from a clinical to a subclinical diabetic state, but they have not fully recovered from their disease; these cats continue to be susceptible to developing recurrence of clinical diabetes.

Prediction of Clinical Remission with Tests of Beta Cell Function

Several insulin secretagogue tests have been evaluated for measurement of insulin secretion capacity in humans, including the hyperglycemic clamp, the IV and oral glucose tolerance tests, the IV glucagon stimulation test, and the IV arginine stimulation test. In type 1 or 2 diabetic humans, beta cells show progressive deterioration in their responsiveness to various secretagogues (e.g., glucose, glucagon, or amino acids).[19,20] Testing the residual secretory capacity of beta cells with glucose as the secretagogue in an overt diabetic is not appropriate for two reasons. First, the functional reserve of insulin-secreting cells is already being challenged by excess amounts of circulating glucose; and second, hyperglycemia *per se* may lead to glucose-induced desensitization of beta cells, independent from glucotoxicity. Indeed, viable beta cells exposed to hyperglycemia may experience a temporary and reversible state of refractoriness that is expressed at the level of insulin exocytosis either by depleting insulin stores or by making refractory the exocytotic mechanisms responsible for glucose-induced insulin release.[21]

Glucagon is commonly assumed to exert a negative effect on glucose metabolism because it stimulates hepatic glycogenolysis and promotes gluconeogenesis; however, it has been shown to have beneficial effects, as well, by stimulating insulin secretion mediated by receptors distributed on the beta cell surface. Indeed, transgenic mice with a targeted deletion in the glucagon receptor on the beta cells show decreased insulin secretion.[22] From this notion, a study was conducted in diabetic cats to investigate whether a different insulin response to glucagon stimulation could differentiate between diabetic cats achieving clinical remission from those remaining permanently diabetic.[12] Unfortunately, results of that study showed that use of glucagon stimulation cannot discriminate between the diabetic cats that went into remission and the diabetics permanently requiring insulin, indicating that the test is not useful for this purpose.

L-Arginine is known to be the most potent insulin secretagogue of all amino acids and, in cats, increases beta cell secretion by membrane depolarization and a subsequent increase in intracellular calcium.[23] Apart from beta cells, L-arginine also stimulates glucagon from pancreatic alpha cells in cats, and it has been reported to be a valuable tool for yielding information about glucagon secretion in this species.[24] Responsiveness to arginine has been demonstrated to outlast glucose and glucagon stimuli, thus suggesting that it may be used to detect residual beta cell secretory capacity later during the progression of diabetes.[25] Therefore, an investigation of the use of an arginine stimulation test was carried out at the University of Zurich with newly diagnosed diabetic cats.[26] This study showed that the beta cell response to arginine was similar between the cats with newly diagnosed diabetes that latter achieved remission and for the cats that remained permanently diabetic.[26] Interestingly, the arginine-induced secretion of alpha cells was also comparable between groups of diabetic cats. However, the glucagon response tended to be higher in cats that experienced remission (Figure 17-7), and the glucagon-to-insulin ratio was also higher.[26] The reason diabetic cats with remission have an increased secretory reserve of glucagon relative to insulin is unclear, but this might be explained by the fact that pancreatic alpha cells and glucagon seem to be required to maintain beta cell responsiveness to glucose, at least in humans and mice.[22,27] Of note, the study by the author and his colleagues of arginine stimulation testing in cats also showed that glucagon

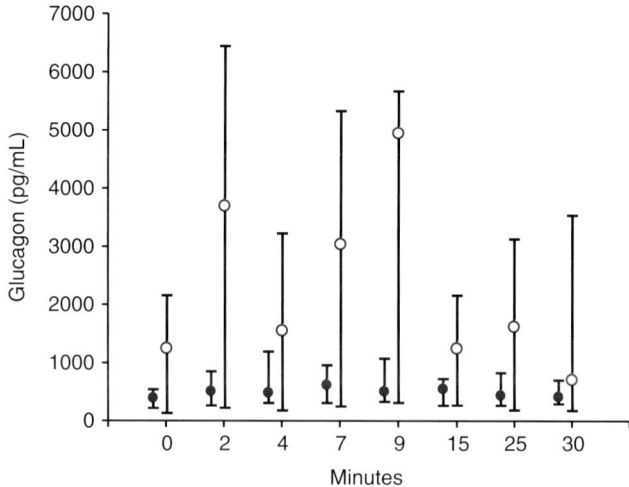

Figure 17-7: Glucagon concentrations at time points up to 30 minutes after arginine injection in diabetic cats that achieved *(white dots)* or did not achieve *(black dots)* clinical remission. Median and interquartile range are shown.

secretion in diabetic cats was similar to healthy cats.[26] However, five of the 17 diabetic cats included had increased glucagon secretion compared to the normal cats, suggesting that diabetes is associated with an absolute increase in the glucagon response to arginine in some diabetic cats. Because four of these five diabetic cats later achieved remission, an increased arginine-induced alpha cell (glucagon) response might be associated with a favorable outcome in diabetic cats.[26] In line with this hypothesis, one of the diabetic cats that achieved remission examined in the previous study of Nelson and colleagues[12] had more alpha cells than the control cats. Further studies are clearly required to verify the role of alpha cells and glucagon secretion in the pathogenesis of diabetes in cats.

In brief, stimulation of insulin-secreting pancreatic cells with either glucagon or arginine failed to predict which diabetic cats have adequate residual beta cell function to eventually achieve clinical remission. However, the higher glucagon-to-insulin ratio observed in diabetic cats that eventually went into clinical remission may indicate that a relative increase of alpha cell function is involved in the mechanisms leading to such remission. Unfortunately, the large overlap in the glucagon-to-insulin ratio between groups prevents the use of this parameter to predict clinical remission in practice.

Prediction of Clinical Remission in Practice

The ability to predict which cats would be likely to experience diabetic remission in practice would be very helpful to increase motivation of owners to treat their diabetic cats. In addition, achieving remission is advantageous because cats benefit from a better quality of life, and the costs of treatment would be decreased. Therefore, a number of investigations have addressed diabetic remission in cats in an effort to identify predictors of this phenomenon at the time of initial diagnosis of the diabetes.

A study published in 2007 reported that baseline serum concentrations of glucose, fructosamine, insulin, glucagon, and insulin growth factor-1 measured at the time of admission were not different in a group of diabetic cats that later achieved remission compared with a group that did not.[13] In another study by Roomp and Rand[14] of diabetic cats treated with a protocol aimed at tight glycemic control with frequent home monitoring of glucose concentrations and change in insulin doses early after diagnosis of diabetes, the following two factors were found to be helpful as predictors of eventual remission: (1) administration of corticosteroids in the 6 months previous to diagnosis and (2) the absence of polyneuropathy at time of diagnosis (e.g., plantigrade stance, walking on the hocks, reduced jumping ability, or an inability to climb stairs). In addition, this study observed that cats that were switched to this tight protocol of glycemic control only after 6 months or longer from the onset of diabetes were less likely to go into clinical remission than those cats treated initially with an intensive insulin regimen (35% versus 84%). This latter finding is in agreement with the studies where remission was unlikely after half a year of treatment.[9] One plausible explanation for the decreased rate of remission in cats with peripheral neuropathies compared to those without neuropathy (30% versus 79%) is that peripheral neuropathy is likely related to a longer duration of severe hyperglycemia. Conversely, cats treated with corticosteroids might have had shorter duration of hyperglycemia, or tapering and discontinuing of the diabetogenic drug might have partially resolved insulin resistance, thus allowing the beta cells to recover.[14] Of note, all cats that received corticosteroids in the study by Roomp and Rand[14] achieved clinical remission after the drugs were discontinued.

In 2010, the author and his colleagues conducted a study at the University of Zurich to explore factors collected at the time of admission that might predict remission in these diabetic cats.[9] The analysis revealed that higher age at admission was associated with an increased chance of diabetic remission (Figure 17-8). Specifically, for each additional year of age at

first diagnosis, remission was 25% more likely.[9] This finding may be unexpected, based on the notion that aging is associated with decreased beta cell function in different mammalian species.[28] However, it has been reported that human patients with type 2 diabetes who are first diagnosed after 65 years of age generally present with a less severe course of disease and show better glycemic control.[29] In contrast, at least in patients with type 1 diabetes, younger age at diagnosis is associated with a faster progression to insulin dependency.[30] Although unlikely, it cannot be excluded that the positive association between older age and eventual clinical remission observed in the cats was not simply due to owners providing better care to the older cats.

In the study, the finding of high serum cholesterol concentration reduced the chance of remission by almost 65% in diabetic cats.[9] Most studies in humans linking hyperlipidemia to the development of type 2 diabetes have focused on the role of serum triglycerides and free fatty acids, but *in vivo* studies with rodents have demonstrated that high cholesterol concentrations can also reversibly impair beta cell function.[31,32] In this transgenic mice model, in addition to impaired insulin secretion, the number and size of pancreatic islets is reduced by more than 50%.[32] Therefore, increased serum cholesterol can exert a direct toxic effect on beta cells.

Therefore, it is possible that hypercholesterolemia also plays a primary role in the progression of diabetes in cats, eventually preventing the recovery of beta cell function or viability. Because the author and his colleagues did not evaluate the concentrations of serum triglycerides or free fatty acids in the study, it is possible that these lipids had a confounding effect on the chance of remission. However, sustained hypertriglyceridemia and increased free fatty acid concentrations did not impair insulin secretion in the study of healthy cats.[16]

In the study, diabetic cats treated with insulin glargine tended to have an increased chance of remission.[9] Because many cats did not survive to discharge and therefore were never treated with a longer-acting insulin, the author and his colleagues could not assess whether the use of insulin glargine independently predicts remission. In another study, Marshall and colleagues[15] have reported that the probability of remission in cats with newly diagnosed diabetes is higher after treatment with insulin glargine than with other insulin types. In particular, by 3 months of treatment, all eight of the cats in the glargine group had achieved remission, while only two of eight cats in the porcine lente insulin group and three of the eight cats in the protamine zinc insulin group had achieved remission. Glargine-treated cats also had better glycemic control based on lower mean blood glucose concentrations by 2 weeks after initiating therapy.[15] Therefore, insulin glargine may increase chance of remission in diabetic cats, possibly by improving metabolic control, although additional studies with larger number of cats are needed to corroborate this finding.

Of note is the finding that cats with ketoacidosis were not any less likely to go into remission than cats without ketoacidosis.[9] This observation also confirms the finding of a

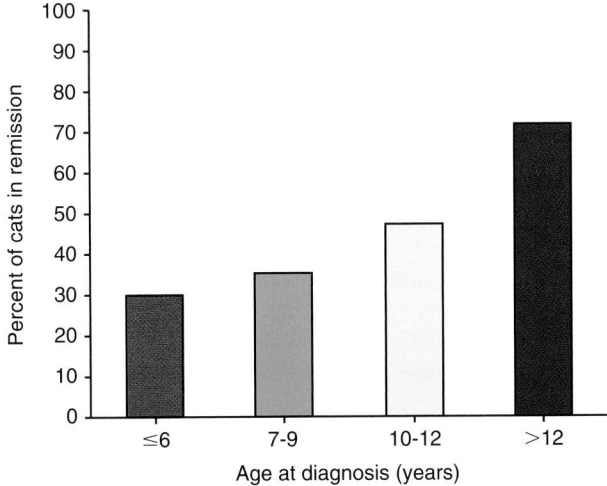

Figure 17-8: Percentage of diabetic cats achieving clinical remission by age at diagnosis.

previous study that documented that cats initially diagnosed with ketoacidosis can achieve remission from diabetes.[10] In that study, seven of 12 cats (58%) with ketoacidosis eventually went into remission. It is worth remarking that, similar to the aforementioned survival investigation,[6] ketoacidosis should not be regarded as an unfavorable complication because the life expectancy and rates of remission are similar to cats that have not had ketoacidosis.

Finally, it has been described that remission can also occur in approximately 50% of diabetic cats with the acromegalic syndrome if treatment of the primary condition is successful. In cats, acromegaly is usually caused by a functional pituitary adenoma that secretes excessive amounts of growth hormone (GH), leading to insulin resistance and beta cell exhaustion. Treatment of the pituitary tumor with external radiation therapy resulted in remission with discontinuation of insulin within 34 weeks of irradiation in five of eight acromegalic cats in one study,[33] and within 24 weeks in six of 14 acromegalic cats in another study.[34] In one diabetic cat with acromegaly that was successfully treated with transsphenoidal hypophysectomy, clinical remission of the diabetes developed 3 weeks after surgery.[35] These reports indicate that clinical remission of diabetes is possible in cats suffering from acromegaly if the cause of the insulin resistance (e.g., GH secreting tumor) can be treated.

Intensive Insulin Protocol and Clinical Remission

In human medicine, a number of trials have evaluated short-term intensive insulin administration in the management of newly diagnosed type 2 diabetic patients.[36-38] Treatment included either multiple daily injections or continuous subcutaneous (SC) insulin infusion for 2 to 3 weeks. In these patients, early intensive insulin therapy was able to improve beta cell function and prolong clinical remission. In addition, remission rates after 1 year were significantly higher in human patients treated with intensive insulin therapy, compared with those treated with oral hypoglycemic agents.[36-38]

In cats, very limited experience exists with intensive insulin therapy. So far, there have been two studies that investigated the effect of frequent adjustment of insulin dose, based on strict home monitoring of blood glucose.[14,15] In both studies, remission rates as high as 64% and 67% were achieved, possibly suggesting a beneficial role of intensive insulin treatments.[14,15]

Because of the well-characterized favorable effect of intensive insulin treatment in type 2 diabetic humans and the promising results achieved in studies in diabetic cats,[14,15] an investigation was carried out at the University of Zurich to assess the feasibility of an intensive protocol of IV insulin therapy in cats with newly diagnosed diabetes and to verify whether the protocol improved the rate of clinical remission compared to standard SC insulin therapy.[39] The experiment was conducted in diabetic cats in the IV group by infusing insulin for 6 consecutive days via a central catheter with rate adjustments performed every 10 to 15 minutes, based on interstitial glucose concentrations measured with a continuous glucose monitoring system. Diabetic cats that were started on SC insulin served as controls and were hospitalized for 6 days. Cats treated with corticosteroids in the 4 months before diagnosis were not included in the analysis to avoid bias on remission.[14] After the 6 days of hospitalization, cats of both groups were discharged on a standard SC insulin protocol and regularly re-evaluated during 6 months to verify the rate of remission and of metabolic control.[39]

The short-term intensive, IV insulin therapy allowed the author and his colleagues to achieve the target glucose concentration of 90 to 180 mg/dL (5 to 10 mmol/L) during most of the cats' hospitalization period, as well as avoiding episodes of hypoglycemia and preventing long periods of marked hyperglycemia. The remission rate in diabetic cats treated with IV insulin was 67%, whereas that of cats started on SC insulin was 50%, meaning a 17% difference between the two groups. However, statistical significance was not reached, presumably due to the relatively low number of cats included in the study.[39]

The rate of remission achieved in cats started on IV insulin was very similar to that obtained in the two reported studies in which frequent adjustments of insulin dose and strict home monitoring of blood glucose was performed.[14,15] However, comparing these two investigations with the study by the author and his colleagues[39] may be difficult because the study designs were very different. Specifically, in the previous investigations, owners were asked to measure glucose concentrations of their diabetic cats at least three times a day at home and to modify the insulin dose regularly, sometimes daily, to maintain blood glucose levels at 50 to 100 mg/dL (2.8 to 5.5 mmol/L).[14,15] To have a cat entered into the previous investigations, owners had to follow a strict web-based protocol and to perform routine examinations by their veterinarians,[14,15] whereas all cats were evaluated at the same institution during 6 consecutive months in the Swiss study.[39] Besides differences in treatment protocols, the criteria for enrolling cats differed among these studies; most importantly, cats treated with glucocorticoids were not excluded in either of the previous investigations.[14,15] It is important to note that by excluding glucocorticoid-treated cats from one of these past investigations,[15] the documented remission rate would have decreased from 64% to 51%, yielding a remission rate similar to the studies of the author and his colleagues performed with standard (rather than intensive) insulin protocols.[9] Therefore, because cases that received glucocorticoids prior to diagnosis were not included in the Swiss study,[39] it might be that the study design of the author and his colleagues more objectively demonstrated an improved rate of remission for intensive protocols aimed at optimally controlling blood glucose concentrations.

In addition to the permissive role on remission, the intensive IV insulin therapy improved metabolic control in diabetic cats.[39] In particular, after exclusion of cats that went into remission, 60% of the cats started with the intensive protocol achieved good metabolic control compared with only 13% of cats started on SC insulin. Furthermore, during the study period, cats started in the intensive treatment group required approximately 40% less insulin than cats started on SC

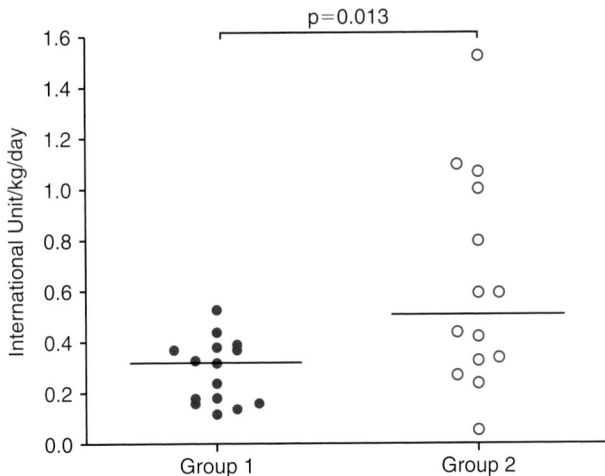

Figure 17-9: Dot Plots of Insulin Dose. Insulin doses administered (per kg per day) during the 6-month study period in cats started on intensive intravenous insulin therapy (group 1) and in cats started on subcutaneous insulin (group 2).

insulin[39] (Figure 17-9). Altogether, these results point to a beneficial effect of prompt and strict glycemic control in diabetic cats early after diagnosis. The reason behind the favorable outcome of treating diabetic cats soon after diagnosis with the intensive IV insulin therapy is not known. However, in human medicine, a consistent finding associated with intensive insulin protocols includes improved beta cell function, as demonstrated by an augmented glucose stimulated first-phase insulin secretion following the intensive protocol.[36-38] The major mechanism by which intensive insulin therapy improves beta cell function is by reversal of glucotoxicity.[36-38] Because the importance of glucotoxicity in the pathogenesis of diabetes in cats has been demostrasted,[9,18] controlling the detrimental effects of hyperglycemia with short-term intensive IV insulin therapy may also improve beta cell viability in cats. This ultimately results in decreased insulin requirements during follow-up and improved rates of remission and of metabolic control in diabetic cats. However, one must remember that the short-term intensive IV insulin therapy, as described earlier, is very demanding, so its use may be limited in clinical practice.

SUMMARY

Clinical remission of diabetes in cats is achievable in approximately 50% of cats within 6 months of initial diagnosis. Glucotoxicity is an important cause of damage to feline insulin-producing cells in experimental conditions, and it probably also exerts detrimental effects on the beta cells of cats with naturally occurring diabetes. If glucotoxicity is not promptly avoided with adequate insulin treatment and strict glycemic control, it may reduce the chance of remission and lead to permanent diabetes. Unfortunately, remission cannot be easily predicted at diagnosis, but factors such as previous administration of corticosteroids, absence of polyneuropathy, higher age, and normal serum cholesterol concentration may be among the most important predictors of this favorable outcome. Diabetic cats with or without ketoacidosis at diagnosis both have a similar chance to achieve remission.

References

1. McCann TM, Simpson KE, Shaw DJ, et al: Feline diabetes mellitus in the UK: the prevalence within an insured cat population and a questionnaire-based putative risk factor analysis. *J Feline Med Surg* 9:289–299, 2007.
2. Slingerland LI, Fazilova VV, Plantinga EA, et al: Indoor confinement and physical inactivity rather than the proportion of dry food are risk factors in the development of feline type 2 diabetes mellitus. *Vet J* 179:247–253, 2009.
3. Little CJ, Gettinby G: Heart failure is common in diabetic cats: findings from a retrospective case-controlled study in first-opinion practice. *J Small Anim Pract* 49:17–25, 2008.
4. Kraus MS, Calvert CA, Jacobs GJ, et al: Feline diabetes mellitus: a retrospective mortality study of 55 cats (1982-1994). *J Am Anim Hosp Assoc* 33:107–111, 1997.
5. Goossens MM, Nelson RW, Feldman EC, et al: Response to insulin treatment and survival in 104 cats with diabetes mellitus (1985-1995). *J Vet Intern Med* 12:1–6, 1998.
6. Callegari C, Mercuriali E, Hafner M, et al: Survival time and prognostic factors in cats with newly diagnosed diabetes mellitus: 114 cases (2000-2009). *J Am Vet Med Assoc* 243:91–95, 2013.

7. Chakrabarti S, Syme HM, Elliott J: Clinico-pathological variables predicting progression of azotemia in cats with chronic kidney disease. *J Vet Intern Med* 26:275–281, 2012.
8. Weingart C, Lotz F, Kohn B: Measurement of β-hydroxybutyrate in cats with nonketotic diabetes mellitus, diabetic ketosis, and diabetic ketoacidosis. *J Vet Diagn Invest* 24:295–300, 2012.
9. Zini E, Hafner M, Osto M, et al: Predictors of clinical remission in cats with diabetes mellitus. *J Vet Intern Med* 24:1314–1321, 2010.
10. Sieber-Ruckstuhl NS, Kley S, Tschuor F, et al: Remission of diabetes mellitus in cats with diabetic ketoacidosis. *J Vet Intern Med* 22: 1326–1332, 2008.
11. Michiels L, Reusch CE, Boari A, et al: Treatment of 46 cats with porcine lente insulin: a prospective, multicentre study. *J Feline Med Surg* 10:439–451, 2008.
12. Nelson RW, Griffey SM, Feldman EC, et al: Transient clinical diabetes mellitus in cats: 10 cases (1989-1991). *J Vet Intern Med* 13:28–35, 1999.
13. Alt N, Kley S, Tschuor F, et al: Evaluation of IGF-1 levels in cats with transient and permanent diabetes mellitus. *Res Vet Sci* 83:331–335, 2007.

14. Roomp K, Rand J: Intensive blood glucose control is safe and effective in diabetic cats using home monitoring and treatment with glargine. *J Feline Med Surg* 11:668–682, 2009.
15. Marshall RD, Rand JS, Morton JM: Treatment of newly diagnosed diabetic cats with glargine insulin improves glycaemic control and results in higher probability of remission than protamine zinc and lente insulins. *J Feline Med Surg* 11:683–691, 2009.
16. Zini E, Osto M, Franchini M, et al: Hyperglycaemia but not hyperlipidaemia causes beta-cell dysfunction and beta-cell loss in the domestic cat. *Diabetologia* 52:336–346, 2009.
17. Orci L, Ravazzola M, Perrelet A: (Pro)insulin associates with Golgi membranes of pancreatic B cells. *Proc Natl Acad Sci U S A* 81:6743–6746, 1984.
18. Link KRJ, Allio I, Rand JS, et al: The effect of experimentally induced chronic hyperglycaemia on serum and pancreatic insulin, pancreatic islet IGF-I and plasma and urinary ketones in the domestic cat (Felis felis). *Gen Comp Endocrinol* 188:269–281, 2013.
19. Druet C, Tubiana-Rufi N, Chevenne D, et al: Characterization of insulin secretion and resistance in type 2 diabetes of adolescents. *J Clin Endocrinol Metab* 91:401–404, 2006.

20. Drucker D, Zinman B: Pathophysiology of beta-cell failure after prolonged remission of insulin-dependent diabetes mellitus (IDDM). *Diabetes Care* 7:83–87, 1984.

21. Robertson RP, Olson LK, Zhang H: Differentiating glucose toxicity from glucose desensitization: a new message from the insulin gene. *Diabetes* 43:1085–1089, 1994.

22. Sørensen H, Winzell MS, Brand CL, et al: Glucagon receptor knockout mice display increased insulin sensitivity and impaired beta-cell function. *Diabetes* 55:3463–3469, 2006.

23. Curry DL, Morris JG, Rogers QR, et al: Dynamics of insulin and glucagon secretion by the isolated perfused cat pancreas. *Comp Biochem Physiol A* 72:333–338, 1982.

24. Furrer D, Kaufmann K, Reusch CE, et al: Amylin reduces plasma glucagon concentrations in cats. *Vet J* 184:236–240, 2010.

25. Brandle M, Lehmann R, Maly FE, et al: Diminished insulin secretory response to glucose but normal insulin and glucagon secretory responses to arginine in a family with maternally inherited diabetes and deafness caused by mitochondrial tRNA (LEU(UUR)) gene mutation. *Diabetes Care* 24:1253–1258, 2001.

26. Tschuor F, Zini E, Schellenberg S, et al: Remission of diabetes mellitus in cats cannot be predicted by the arginine stimulation test. *J Vet Intern Med* 25:83–89, 2011.

27. Huypens P, Ling Z, Pipeleers D, et al: Glucagon receptors on human islet cells contribute to glucose competence of insulin release. *Diabetologia* 43:1012–1019, 2000.

28. Szoke E, Shrayyef MZ, Messing S, et al: Effect of aging on glucose homeostasis: accelerated deterioration of beta-cell function in individuals with impaired glucose tolerance. *Diabetes Care* 31:539–543, 2008.

29. Kolb H, Schneider B, Heinemann L, et al: Type 2 diabetes phenotype and progression is significantly different if diagnosed before versus after 65 years of age. *J Diabetes Sci Technol* 2:82–90, 2008.

30. Achenbach P, Warncke K, Reiter J, et al: Type 1 diabetes risk assessment: improvement by follow-up measurements in young islet autoantibody-positive relatives. *Diabetologia* 49:2969–2976, 2006.

31. Hao M, Head WS, Gunawardana SC, et al: Direct effect of cholesterol on insulin secretion: a novel mechanism for pancreatic beta-cell dysfunction. *Diabetes* 56:2328–2338, 2007.

32. Ishikawa M, Iwasaki Y, Yatoh S, et al: Cholesterol accumulation and diabetes in pancreatic beta-cell-specific SREBP-2 transgenic mice: a new model for lipotoxicity. *J Lipid Res* 49:2524–2534, 2008.

33. Brearley MJ, Polton GA, Littler RM, et al: Coarse fractionated radiation therapy for pituitary tumours in cats: a retrospective study of 12 cases. *Vet Comp Oncol* 4:209–217, 2006.

34. Dunning MD, Lowrie CS, Bexfield JM, et al: Exogenous insulin treatment after hypofractionated radiotherapy in cats with diabetes mellitus and acromegaly. *J Vet Int Med* 23:243–249, 2009.

35. Meij BP, Auriemma E, Grinwis G, et al: Successful treatment of acromegaly in a diabetic cat with transsphenoidal hypophysectomy. *J Feline Med Surg* 12:406–410, 2010.

36. Weng J, Li Y, Xu W, et al: Effect of intensive insulin therapy on β-cell function and glycaemic control in patients with newly diagnosed type 2 diabetes: a multicenter randomised parallel-group trial. *Lancet* 371:1753–1760, 2008.

37. Alvarsson M, Sundkvist G, Lager I, et al: Beneficial effects of insulin versus sulphonylurea on insulin secretion and metabolic control in recently diagnosed type 2 diabetic patients. *Diabetes Care* 26:2231–2237, 2003.

38. Chen HS, Wu TE, Jap TS, et al: Beneficial effects of insulin on glycaemic control and β-cell function in newly diagnosed type 2 diabetes with severe hyperglycaemia after short-term intensive insulin therapy. *Diabetes Care* 31:1927–1932, 2008.

39. Hafner M, Dietiker-Moretti S, Kaufmann K, et al: Intensive intravenous infusion of insulin in diabetic cats. *J Vet Intern Med* 28:1753–1759, 2014.

Management of Idiopathic Hypercalcemia

Joao Felipe de Brito Galvao, Dennis J. Chew, and Valerie J. Parker

Currently, idiopathic hypercalcemia (IHC) is the most common cause of hypercalcemia in cats across the United States, based on diagnoses by endocrinology laboratories; reports of this diagnosis continue to emerge from other parts of the world. IHC has been referred to as the third most common endocrine condition in cats[1] behind diabetes mellitus and hyperthyroidism, though compelling evidence that IHC is an endocrine disorder has not yet been established. Based on the authors' assessment of consultations for cats with hypercalcemia at their respective referral practices, IHC is easily the most common diagnosis, followed in decreasing order by azotemic chronic kidney disease (CKD), neoplasia, and primary hyperparathyroidism. The order for differential diagnosis in cats is considerably different from that in dogs, in which neoplasia accounts for most cases of persistent pathologic hypercalcemia based on either serum total calcium (tCa) or ionized calcium (iCa).[2] Lymphoma is the most common neoplasm accounting for hypercalcemia in the dog, whereas lymphoma and squamous cell carcinoma of the head and neck occur with similar frequency in the cat.[3] The diagnosis of IHC in the dog is very uncommon when adequate medical workup has been performed and analyzed.

DIAGNOSIS OF IDIOPATHIC HYPERCALCEMIA

Discovery of Hypercalcemia

Hypercalcemia is typically discovered fortuitously when a blood sample is taken for other reasons (e.g., wellness examinations, preanesthesia screening, evaluation of urolithiasis, evaluation of minor gastrointestinal signs, minor weight loss). It is traditional to initially evaluate calcium status in cats following measurement of tCa. When serum tCa is increased, iCa is usually then measured to determine if there is also an increase in this fraction of circulating calcium. Most often, cats with increased serum tCa will also have increased iCa. A major exception to this general relationship commonly occurs in cats with azotemic CKD and hypercalcemia. Increased serum tCa in cats with azotemic CKD can be associated with high, normal, or low concentrations of iCa, so it is imperative to measure iCa directly and not try to predict its level, especially in this population.[4] Toxic effects of hypercalcemia only occur from increases in the ionized

fraction of circulating calcium. Many more cases of hypercalcemia are documented in sick cats when iCa is used as the screening analyte rather than when tCa is initially measured.[4]

The magnitude of elevation of serum tCa or iCa cannot be used to establish a diagnosis because there is considerable overlap in the degree of hypercalcemia in cats with IHC and other conditions. Most IHC cats present with mild increases in tCa and iCa concentration (11 to 12 mg/dL; 2.75 to 3.00 mmol/L) and (6 to 6.5 mg/dL; 1.5 to 1.6 mmol/L), respectively, whereas some cats may have tCa and iCa concentrations greater than 15 to 20 mg/dL (3.75 to 5 mmol/L) and 8 to 11 mg/dL (2 to 2.7 mmol/L), respectively.*

Clinical Presentation

Cats with IHC may have persistent elevations in iCa for months without apparent clinical signs, and no relationship has been noted between the magnitude of elevation and occurrence of clinical signs. In a review of 427 cats with IHC diagnosed at an endocrinology referral laboratory, the mean age at presentation was 9.8 years (range 6 months to 20 years), and longhair cats were overrepresented (27% of cases).[5] Both sexes were equally represented. Almost half of the cats had no clinical signs (46%), 18% had mild weight loss, 6% had inflammatory bowel disease, 5% had chronic constipation, 4% presented with vomiting, and 1% were anorectic. Uroliths were reported in 15% of cats with IHC, and calcium oxalate stones were specifically noted in 10% of cases.[5]

Another review of 29 cats with IHC at The Ohio State University Veterinary Medical Center had somewhat different results.* The mean age at presentation was similar to the age previously reported; however, shorthair cats were overrepresented. Both sexes were equally represented. Many cats displayed no clinical signs. Weight loss was the most common clinical sign, followed by decreased appetite, vomiting, increased drinking and urination, constipation, and diarrhea. Other less common clinical signs were mostly associated with urolithiasis (e.g., pollakiuria, stranguria, and hematuria).*

---

*de Brito Galvao JF: *Treatment of idiopathic hypercalcemia in 29 cats (1999-2010)*. Unpublished observations, The Ohio State University, 2013.

Differential Diagnosis, Diagnostic Approach, and Refining the Diagnosis of Idiopathic Hypercalcemia

In some cats, the diagnosis for the cause of hypercalcemia is obvious on analysis of detailed history (e.g., drugs, supplements, and systemic signs) and physical examination (e.g., masses, organomegaly, and small kidneys). There are many potential causes of hypercalcemia in the cat that are beyond detailed discussion in this chapter.[6] Azotemic CKD and neoplasia are the major differential diagnoses to be excluded[3] in order to diagnose IHC. Cats with CKD and hypercalcemia are discussed in more detail in a later section. Assessment of abdominal radiographs is recommended in all cats with chronic hypercalcemia to rule out the presence of nephroliths, ureteroliths, and/or urethroliths that may be associated with the hypercalcemia (Figures 18-1 and 18-2). The possibility of obstructive nephropathy should be further evaluated with ultrasonography when upper urinary tract urolithiasis is detected on radiography. Obstructive nephropathy may contribute a component to an increasing magnitude of azotemia

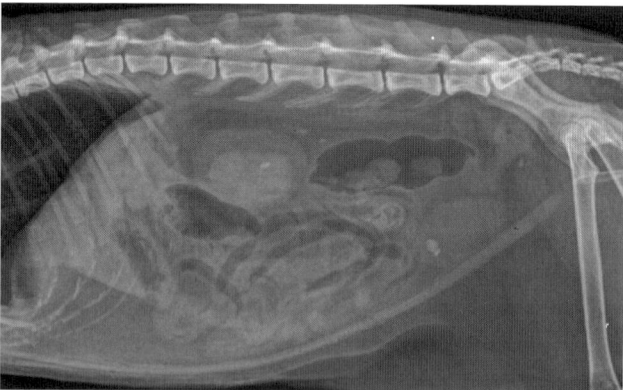

Figure 18-1: Right lateral radiographic view of a 17-year-old female spayed domestic shorthair cat evaluated because of hematuria secondary to a ureterolith. Calcium oxalate uroliths, bilateral nephroliths, and left ureteral obstruction are also present.

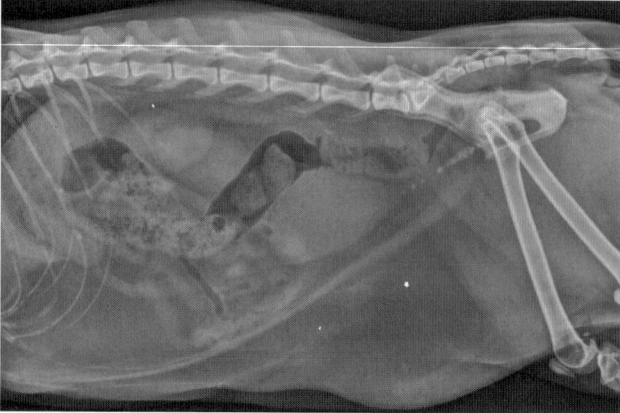

Figure 18-2: Right lateral radiographic view of a 10-year-old female spayed domestic shorthair cat evaluated because of dysuria secondary to urethroliths made of calcium hydrogen phosphate dehydrate (80%) and calcium oxalate monohydrate (20%).

on top of already existing CKD now or in the future. Treatment recommendations and prognosis may change with the presence of stones, so it is important to know of their existence and if they are causing obstruction or not.

The diagnosis of IHC is mostly an exercise in excluding alternative diagnoses after documentation of a circulating iCa concentration above the reference range. Complete blood count, routine serum biochemistry, measurement of parathyroid hormone (PTH), urinalysis, and imaging of the chest and abdomen (radiography and ultrasonography) are considered the minimum database to rule out known causes of hypercalcemia. Because IHC is an example of parathyroid-independent hypercalcemia, the elevation of iCa results in suppression of PTH production. In cats with IHC, PTH values are usually undetectable or within the lower quartile of the reference range.[5,7]

Urine specific gravity (USG) is typically more than 1.030, and it appears that many cats with hypercalcemia can still maximally concentrate their urine if they do not have concurrent CKD. IHC cases seen at The Ohio State University Veterinary Medical Center had an average USG of 1.030 (J.F. de Brito Galvao, unpublished observations, 2013). In a series of cats with various causes of hypercalcemia based on serum tCa, the USG was low mostly in cats with CKD and no other causes of hypercalcemia.[3] In a series of IHC cats, the USG ranged from 1.012 to 1.060.[7]

How extensive a medical workup is needed to establish a likely diagnosis versus the definitive diagnosis of IHC is debatable. An extended database that includes measurement of 25-hydroxyvitamin D could be recommended to exclude the occasional cat that is suffering from overt hypervitaminosis D that would otherwise remain undiagnosed. The authors have not found measurement of parathyroid hormone–related polypeptide (PTHrP) to be particularly useful as it is most often negative. When PTHrP is positive, concerns for underlying cancer as the cause for the hypercalcemia become more pressing. Usually when cancer is the cause of hypercalcemia, the malignancy is obvious, and it is not necessary to measure PTHrP. Additionally, PTHrP is only increased in some malignancies. The concentration of 25-hydroxyvitamin D (calcidiol) is most often within the reference range in cats with IHC, but it should be noted that the reference range is large and has been established in cats consuming diets containing a wide range of vitamin D concentrations. Measurement of $1,25(OH)_2$-vitamin D (calcitriol) is not generally recommended as part of the standard exclusionary diagnostics, because it is most often within the reference range in cats with IHC.[7] Clinical conditions associated with high concentrations of circulating calcitriol in the cat are rare with the exception of granulomatous inflammatory diseases. Calcitriol concentration is within the reference range in most cats with IHC, although this has not been measured in a large number of cats. The magnitude of suppression of circulating calcitriol concentrations that should occur in the presence of ionized hypercalcemia has not been determined in healthy cats. So for both calcidiol and calcitriol, the finding of concentrations within the reference range does not necessarily exclude these vitamin D metabolites as participants in the pathophysiology of the hypercalcemia in IHC.

Circulating calcitonin concentrations have not been measured in cats with IHC to date; however, a new calcitonin assay for use in cats has recently been reported.[8] Interestingly for future consideration of the pathophysiology of IHC, a subgroup of apparently normal experimental cats demonstrated no increase in calcitonin secretion following induction of hypercalcemia. The expression of calcitonin-producing cells in the thyroid gland correlated with the concentration of calcitonin achieved.[8]

Some clients will not be able to afford an exhaustive exclusionary diagnostic evaluation for IHC. In these instances, a likely working diagnosis of IHC is made if the cat has minimal or absent clinical signs in conjunction with low PTH, ionized hypercalcemia, and no findings on physical examination that support the presence of underlying cancer or inflammatory or infiltrative disease. This minimalist approach is safest when treating IHC with diet or alendronate because neither of these treatment modalities will interfere with future potential diagnostics. Most cats with malignancy-associated hypercalcemia have substantial tumor burden, and so they will usually be sick with more obvious clinical signs. Assessment following thoracic radiography and abdominal ultrasonography allows greater confidence that infiltrative neoplastic or granulomatous disease is not accounting for the hypercalcemia. The likely diagnosis of IHC increases the longer the cat lives with its hypercalcemia while demonstrating minimal clinical signs.

TREATMENT

Treatment is currently empiric because the cause of IHC remains unknown. It is not clear whether the hypercalcemia of IHC develops as a consequence of too much intestinal absorption of calcium, too much calcium resorbed from bone, too little renal excretion of calcium, or combinations of these mechanisms.

Should All Cats with Idiopathic Hypercalcemia Receive Treatment?

Minor elevations in serum iCa concentrations are often ignored in clinical practice because many of these cats have mild or no apparent clinical signs. This mild elevation of calcium may continue to increase its magnitude gradually or remain at the initial increased level for long periods of time. The authors and others have observed cats with IHC in which the iCa concentration fluctuates in and out of the reference range; this phenomenon is most likely to be observed in cats in which there are minimal increases in the circulating concentrations of iCa. The possibility for rhythmic change in the concentration of circulating iCa in cats with IHC has not been reported. Excess calcium is toxic to cells, particularly in the central nervous system, gastrointestinal (GI) tract, heart, and kidneys. Mineralization of soft tissues is an important

complication related to the presence of ionized hypercalcemia. The extent of mineralization is in part determined by the concomitant concentration of serum phosphorus. When the calcium (mg/dL) times phosphorus (mg/dL) product is greater than 60, soft tissue mineralization is most severe.[9] The need for therapy in IHC increases when iCa continues to elevate or clinical signs become more obvious (e.g., weight loss, depression, vomiting, constipation, urinary stones, emergence of CKD, and/or development of less-concentrated urine). The consequences of long-standing hypercalcemia can be devastating in those that develop CKD or urolithiasis, and aggressive treatment for hypercalcemia is warranted in these cases. Continued elevation of iCa leads to further development of renal lesions and development of new stones. An algorithm for decision to treat is presented in Figure 18-3. A treatment plan for hypercalcemia is presented in Figure 18-4.

Diet Therapy

A change in diet is usually the first treatment to be given to cats with IHC because normocalcemia is sometimes restored after a change to a different diet. No prospective studies using dietary intervention as treatment of IHC have been reported, so most of the authors' "evidence" for a beneficial effect is anecdotal. Even in cats with an initial salutary response to dietary intervention, the duration of normocalcemia may not be long-lived and hypercalcemia may return. Further dietary modification and/or beginning medical therapy (e.g., with prednisolone or bisphosphonates) should be considered if hypercalcemia recurs.

Dietary factors that have been purported to exert a beneficial effect in lowering circulating calcium in IHC cats include increased concentrations of fiber, sodium, and water and decreased concentrations of calcium, vitamin D, and vitamin A. Non-acidifying diets and those with moderate magnesium concentrations could be beneficial, but there is no reported evidence to support this. Determining which, if any, of these factors are most influential is not currently possible, because there likely are complex interactions within each diet and the individual animal.

Several hypotheses exist regarding the pathophysiology of IHC, which include potential increased sensitivity to vitamin D or increased activity of the nonsaturable pathway for intestinal absorption of calcium.[10] In humans with hypercalciuria and calcium oxalate uroliths, there may be intestinal hyperabsorption of calcium.[11] This not only results in hypercalciuria but also hyperoxaluria, because there is less non-absorbed dietary calcium to combine with intestinal oxalate and, therefore, less of the insoluble calcium oxalate complex.[12,13] Causes of hyperabsorption of calcium from the GI tract are unknown but may be multifactorial, involving both diet and a genetic predisposition.

Fiber

Increased dietary fiber has been reported to successfully lower circulating tCa in five cats with ionized hypercalcemia and calcium oxalate urolithiasis.[10] After diagnosis, four out of five

Chronic Hypercalcemia in the 'Well' Cat:
To Treat or Not to Treat

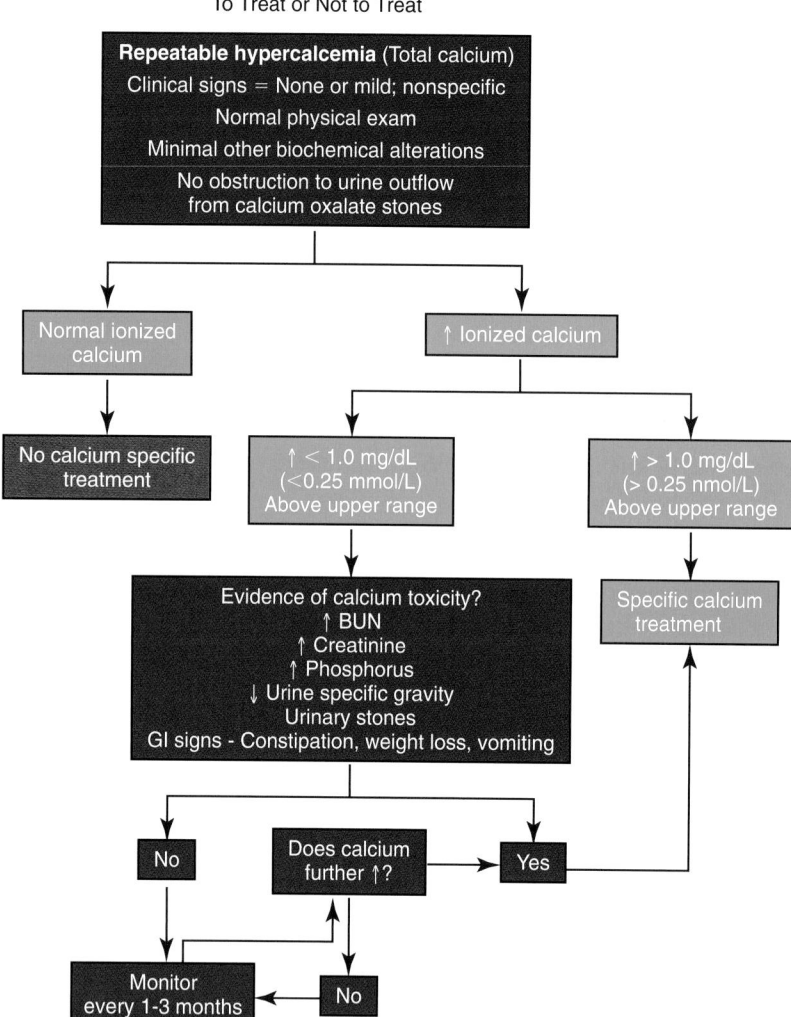

Figure 18-3: Chronic Hypercalcemia in the 'Well' Cat: To Treat or Not to Treat. Algorithm to help decide when idiopathic hypercalcemia (IHC) needs to be treated or if watchful waiting can be considered. *BUN*, Blood urea nitrogen; *GI*, gastrointestinal.

(80%) cats were switched to a veterinary therapeutic diet high in insoluble fiber (Hill's Prescription Diet w/d Feline). One of the cats was fed an over-the-counter feline maintenance diet with added psyllium, a soluble fiber supplement. In the cats with reported follow-up, total hypercalcemia resolved based on measurement of serum tCa; none of the cats had their iCa concentration monitored. However, in another study, there was no beneficial effect of feeding a diet high in insoluble fiber to cats with IHC.[7]

The effects of fiber on intestinal absorption are complex and depend on the type and amount of fiber in the diet and the interactions with other nutrients in the diet. In children receiving prolonged enteral nutrition, those fed a diet supplemented with fiber (mixed fiber sources but predominantly soluble) had significantly lower plasma zinc, calcium, phosphorus, and vitamin D concentrations than those without fiber supplementation.[14] It is theorized that supplemental fiber may lead to increased binding of intestinal calcium, preventing its absorption, and also decreased intestinal transit time through the small intestine, reducing calcium absorp-

tion.[10,15] When cellulose (insoluble fiber) was added to the diet of healthy cats, fecal dry matter and fecal calcium excretion increased, an effect that was greatest with long-fiber cellulose sources.[16] It appears to be common practice for most manufacturers to increase the concentration of calcium in high-fiber diets to offset the potential for decreased absorption. The concept of choosing a "high-fiber" diet can be challenging given that most companies only provide the crude fiber concentration, which is not a good indicator of total dietary fiber.[17] Additional studies investigating the effects of soluble and insoluble fiber on hypercalcemia are warranted.

Renal Diet

Feeding a veterinary therapeutic diet designed for management of CKD may result in normocalcemia in some cats with IHC, but the specific mechanisms as to how this benefit is achieved are not known. Veterinary renal diets are less acidifying than maintenance diets and are lower in calcium and phosphorus. The effect of feeding a non-acidifying diet may

Treatment Considerations for Nonclinical or Minimally
Symptomatic Cats with Ionized Hypercalcemia

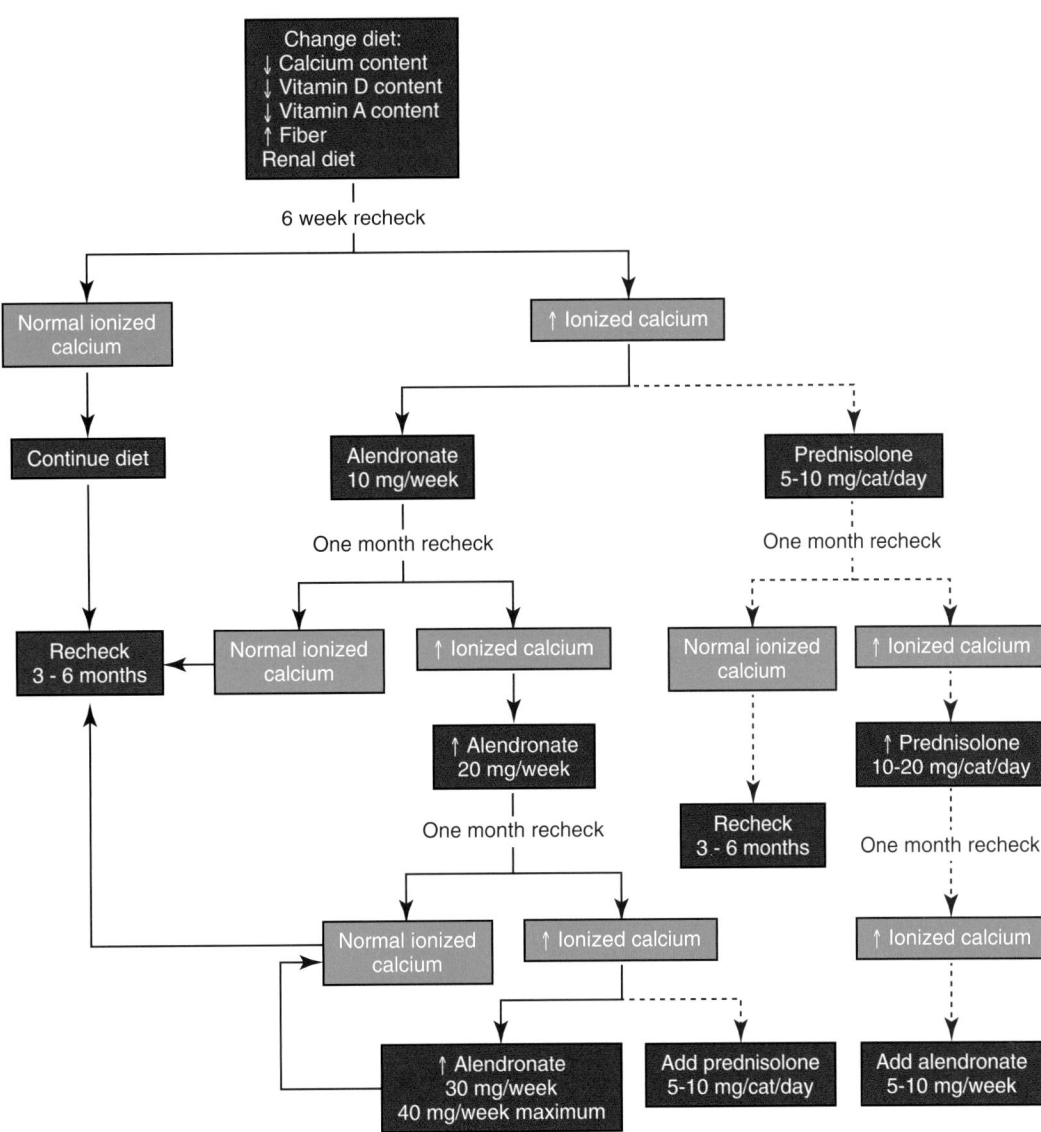

Figure 18-4: Algorithm to help decide treatment path for cats with idiopathic hypercalcemia (IHC) that are minimally ill.

decrease the release of calcium from bone and decrease calcium filtered through the glomerulus.[18] The decreased consumption of dietary calcium could lead to a decrease in the amount of intestinal calcium absorption. However, feeding a reduced-phosphorus diet may enhance renal calcitriol synthesis, thus potentially offsetting the advantage of decreased intestinal calcium absorption. In one study, two out of 15 cats with CKD developed ionized hypercalcemia after being fed a low-phosphorus and low-protein veterinary diet. Ionized calcium normalized after discontinuing dietary phosphorus and protein restriction.[19]

Urolithiasis Diet
Feeding a veterinary therapeutic diet designed to prevent calcium oxalate urolithiasis may restore normocalcemia in some cats with IHC, but most evidence to support their use

is anecdotal. Salutary effects from these diets could be related to reduced calcium content and less urinary acidification (neutral pH urine production) in some diets, but therapeutic formulations of diets for calcium oxalate prevention are quite variable (Table 18-1).

Ionized hypercalcemia resolved after feeding a canned formulation calcium oxalate–prevention diet (Hill's Prescription Diet c/d-oxl Feline; later called Hill's Prescription Diet x/d) in two out of three cats with IHC and calcium oxalate uroliths. The third cat had a reduction in the magnitude of hypercalcemia but did not achieve normocalcemia. Hypercalciuria decreased in these cats that had previously formed a calcium oxalate urinary stone, but none were hypercalcemic based on tCa. Both urinary calcium excretion and concentration significantly decreased with the calcium oxalate prevention diet.[20]

Table 18-1   Dietary Calcium, Vitamin D, and Vitamin A Concentrations in Various Over-the-Counter and Veterinary Therapeutic Diets*

	Calcium (g/1000 kcal)	Vitamin D (International Unit/1000 kcal)	Vitamin A (International Unit/1000 kcal)
Over-the-Counter Diets			
Purina Pro Plan Focus Urinary Tract Health (can)	1.56	579	33,827
Nutro Max Cat Senior Roasted Chicken (dry)	1.68	443	6700
Science Diet Adult Hairball Control (dry)	1.71	147	1510
Royal Canin Persian	1.95	195	6567
Purina ONE Urinary Tract Health (dry)	2.11	493	2972
Wellness CORE Chicken, Turkey & Chicken liver (can)	2.50	500	50,479
Iams Healthy Naturals Weight Control (dry)	2.60	482	37,340
Royal Canin Feline Ultra Light (can)	3.05	180	27,704
Purina Fancy Feast Flaked Tuna Feast (can)	3.25	1305	17,390
Purina Friskies Indoor Chunky Chicken & Turkey Casserole with Garden Greens in Gravy (can)	3.97	555	5171
9Lives Seafood Platter (can)	4.51	372	29,450
Purina Fancy Feast Classic Cod Sole & Shrimp Feast (can)	5.45	781	51,000
EVO Herring & Salmon Formula (dry)	5.61	850	4329
Veterinary Therapeutic Diets			
Iams Veterinary Formula Renal Plus (dry)[†]	1.33	545	6441
Hill's Prescription Diet k/d (can)[‡]	1.45	494	49,990
Royal Canin Veterinary Diet Renal LP Modified-P (dry)	1.50	190	6903
Hill's Prescription Diet g/d (can)	1.52	503	60,260
Hill's Prescription Diet c/d Multicare Oceanfish (can)	1.59	218	25,180
Hill's Prescription Diet k/d (dry)	1.60	494	49,990
Hill's Prescription Diet g/d (dry)	1.63	157	1780
Purina Veterinary Diets NF (dry)	1.64	808	4735
Hill's Prescription Diet d/d venison (can)	1.66	431	78,910
Royal Canin Veterinary Diet Urinary SO (5.8 oz can)	1.70	200	38,947
Iams Veterinary Formula Renal Plus (can)	1.71	203	20,111
Hill's Prescription Diet c/d Multicare Chicken (can)	1.72	277	36,160
Purina Veterinary Diets NF (can)[‡]	1.76	124	17,717
Hill's Prescription Diet c/d Multicare (dry)[‡]	1.80	98	1180
Iams Veterinary Formula Intestinal Plus (can)	1.80	217	6098
Royal Canin Veterinary Diet Calorie Control CC High-fiber (can)	1.80	300	16,226
Hill's Prescription Diet m/d (can)	2.10	399	45,110
Royal Canin Veterinary Diet Urinary SO (dry)	2.20	204	7406
Purina Veterinary Diets DM (can)	2.20	548	61,641
Royal Canin Veterinary Diet Renal LP Modified (6 oz can)	2.20	345	6897

Table 18-1	Dietary Calcium, Vitamin D, and Vitamin A Concentrations in Various Over-the-Counter and Veterinary Therapeutic Diets—cont'd		
	Calcium (g/1000 kcal)	Vitamin D (International Unit/1000 kcal)	Vitamin A (International Unit/1000 kcal)
Hill's Prescription Diet m/d (dry)	2.27	182	2090
Royal Canin Veterinary Diet Diabetic (can)	2.30	258	51,532
Royal Canin Veterinary Diet Diabetic (dry)	2.40	184	5525
Purina Veterinary Diets UR St/Ox (can)	2.42	235	54,982
Hill's Prescription Diet w/d (can)	2.71	582	117,010
Iams Veterinary Formula Glucose & Weight Control Plus	2.88	869	25,989
Purina Veterinary Diets UR St/Ox (dry)	2.89	539	4209
Royal Canin Veterinary Diet Calorie Control (5.8 oz can)	3.00	198	41,226
Iams Veterinary Formula Urinary-O Plus (dry)	3.08	359	9806
Purina Veterinary Diets OM (can)	3.24	363	76,656
Purina Veterinary Diets DM Savory Selects (can)	3.30	203	24,083
Hill's Prescription Diet w/d (dry)	3.32	168	2000
Purina Veterinary Diets OM (dry)	3.40	659	4915
Purina Veterinary Diets DM (dry)	3.50	385	1945
Royal Canin Veterinary Diet Satiety Support (dry)	4.40	239	9231
AAFCO minimum*	1.50	125	1250
AAFCO maximum*	—	2500	187,500

AAFCO, Association of American Feed Control Officials.

*AAFCO minimum and maximum requirements, based on caloric content, for feline adult maintenance are shown for reference. Values contained in these tables are as acquired from the pet food companies in December 2013. It is important to note that the specific nutrient profile for the components of commercial pet foods, as provided here, frequently changes. The abbreviated nutrient profiles in these tables are meant to illustrate a point, not to provide comprehensive lists for long-term reference. Specific nutrient profiles should be acquired at least every 6 to 12 months to keep up with changes that may have occurred.

†This diet meets AAFCO requirements for feline adult maintenance on a dry matter basis.

‡These diets have been substantiated to provide complete and balanced nutrition for feline adult maintenance by AAFCO animal feeding tests.

The addition of sodium chloride is potentially useful in cats with IHC as long as the added salt enhances renal calcium excretion without an increased risk of calcium oxalate uroliths. Increased dietary sodium chloride increased urine volume but did not increase calcium oxalate relative supersaturation in a small number of young healthy cats.[21] However, an increase in urinary excretion of calcium does not always correlate to the development of calcium urolithiasis, because the concentration of calcium in the urine also depends on the degree of water excreted at the same time.[22] The feeding of increased dietary salt is variably effective in creating diuresis that is reflected by decreases in USG and increased water consumption. The USG collected from random urine samples significantly decreased in normal older cats fed a higher salt diet from a baseline of 1.047 to 1.034 by 3 months in one study.[23] USG determined in samples from 24-hour collections more consistently demonstrates decreased USG during high dietary salt intake. Urine specific gravity decreased from 1.051 to 1.045 without an effect on the urinary concentration of calcium in one study of cats fed a higher salt diet.[24] The effects of additional dietary sodium chloride have yet to be reported in cats with IHC. Lastly, the use of canned diets (high moisture) is more beneficial than dry food diets (low moisture) because they have been associated with increased water intake and subsequent lower USG.[25] Lower USG favors prevention of calcium oxalate calculi formation. However, some cats will not readily eat canned diets; therefore the authors have included low-moisture diets in Table 18-1.

Calcium

Some veterinary nutritionists recommend diets to treat IHC based on a decreased amount of calcium evaluated on grams of calcium/1000 kcal energy basis[26] (Table 18-2). Both the Association of American Feed Control Officials (AAFCO)

Table 18-2	AAFCO Minimum and Maximum Nutrient Requirements for Feline Adult Maintenance as Compared to NRC Recommended Allowance and Safe Upper Limit			
Nutrient	**AAFCO Minimum**	**AAFCO Maximum**	**NRC Recommended Allowance**	**NRC Safe Upper Limit**
Calcium (g/1000 kcal)	1.50	None established	0.72	No official guidelines published; 2.6 to 4.6 suggested
Vitamin D (International Unit/1000 kcal)	125	2500	70	7520
Vitamin A (International Unit/1000 kcal)	1250	187,500	833	83,325

National Research Council: Nutrient requirements of dogs and cats. National Academies Press, Washington, DC, 2006.
AAFCO, Association of American Feed Control Officials; *NRC,* National Research Council.

and the National Research Council (NRC) set the minimal and maximal nutrient requirements for cat foods. All diets sold over-the-counter should meet AAFCO requirements; however, veterinary therapeutic diets may be specifically modified in order to provide certain nutrients at concentrations less than AAFCO minimum (e.g., a veterinary renal diet provides a dietary phosphorus concentration less than AAFCO minimum).

The average calcium content of grocery store foods in the United States is often from 2 to 3 g calcium/1000 kcal intake (200 to 300 mg/100 kcal), though some contain up to 6 g calcium/1000 kcal (600 mg/100 kcal) (V. Parker, person communication, 2013). Some of the highest calcium diets are "high-fiber" diets; thus, one must carefully weigh the pros and cons of recommending a high-fiber diet for dietary management of IHC when there is some evidence that reducing dietary calcium may be effective in restoring normocalcemia. Nutrient concentrations of diets can be found either in product guides or by contacting the diet manufacturer. Nutrient profiles are constantly evolving, and this information may change as often as every 6 to 12 months. For adult cats, the NRC's recommended allowance is 0.72 g calcium/1000 kcal, but no safe upper limit (SUL) is provided; the minimal requirement is 0.40 g/1000 kcal.[27] The AAFCO minimum is recommended at 1.5 g calcium/1000 kcal of intake.

In order to rationally choose a diet that is lower in calcium intake, a complete diet history must be obtained; this includes the cat's primary diet, treats, and any supplements. Once this starting dietary calcium concentration has been determined, the veterinarian can determine which diets would provide less calcium, considering potential comorbid conditions. Although a veterinary therapeutic renal diet may be appropriate for a cat with hypercalcemia and CKD, it may not be appropriate to feed a young, otherwise healthy cat a renal diet that contains reduced amounts of phosphorus and protein. A home-prepared diet providing approximately 0.60 g calcium/1000 kcal has been used successfully by one group of nutritionists to restore normocalcemia in some cats with IHC within 1 month of feeding.[26]

It is important to remember that simply prescribing a lower-calcium diet may be too simplistic, because ultimately other factors may influence intestinal calcium absorption. Dietary factors affecting intestinal calcium absorption and bone resorption include concentrations of vitamin D, vitamin A,[28] vitamin K,[29] phytates,[30] fiber,[30] and specific carbohydrates.[31] Individual animal factors (e.g., vitamin D status and its effect on intestinal calcium transport) that affect bioavailability of calcium from the diet are complex and beyond the scope of this chapter.

A More Natural Diet

In a recent review, the feeding of a high-protein and low-carbohydrate food similar to what cats would eat in the wild (i.e., 40% to 60% of calories from protein; 30% to 50% of calories from fat, and less than 15% of calories from carbohydrates) has been recommended to effectively lower serum concentration concentrations in some cats with IHC, especially those with low-magnitude hypercalcemia.[1] The reason why these high-protein, low-carbohydrate diets are sometimes effective is unknown. In any case, these diets are useful in helping to maintain normal lean body (muscle) mass as well as to maintain euglycemia, two factors that become very important if glucocorticoid treatment is needed to control the hypercalcemia in these cats with IHC. High doses of glucocorticoids are catabolic to muscle protein, and their use will predispose treated cats to development of diabetes mellitus.

Vitamin D

IHC is not the result of obvious excess dietary vitamin D intake because serum concentrations of 25-hydroxyvitamin D have been within the reference range in most cats with IHC. However, the minimal requirement for vitamin D in cats is debatable because reference ranges have been established in cats fed vitamin D–supplemented diets. Normal concentrations of 25-hydroxyvitamin D could still potentially be associated with IHC in cats if there are upregulating mutations in the vitamin D receptor. These possibilities have yet to be investigated.

Although the amount of vitamin D supplied in most diets is not listed on the diet label, this information should be obtainable from the pet food manufacturer.[26] Cats may be affected by hypervitaminosis D even when companies claim a certain expected concentration of vitamin D, possibly due to errors in diet formulation.[32] Vitamin D content in commercial diets is the sum of what is provided naturally by animal and plant ingredients, as well as that added by the vitamin premix. It has been recommended to avoid a diet that contains organ meat or oily marine fish as sources that increase vitamin D when formulating a home-prepared diet.[26]

The NRC defines dietary vitamin D_3 (cholecalciferol) adequate intake for adult cats to be 56 International Units (1.4 µg)/1000 kcal, the recommended daily allowance to be 70 International Units (1.75 µg)/1000 kcal, and the SUL to be 7520 International Units (188 µg)/1000 kcal. No minimal requirement for dietary vitamin D is provided by the NRC.[27] AAFCO guidelines require between 125 and 2500 International Units/1000 kcal in order to satisfy a label noted to be complete and balanced[33] (see Table 18-2). In order to meet AAFCO minimum to maximum guidelines, from about two to 45 times the NRC concentration of vitamin D considered "adequate" for maintenance of adult cats could be provided in commercial diets. Feeding a diet formulated to be low in vitamin D content at less than 200 International Units (<5 µg)/1000 kcal has been recommended in a recent review of dietary treatment of cats with IHC.[1]

The vitamin D requirement of adult cats for maintenance has not been studied, so the 56 International Units/1000 kcal considered adequate for growing kittens has been extended to the adult cat population.[27] Determination of toxicity of dietary vitamin D has mostly used the endpoints of hypercalcemia, tissue calcification, and the presence or absence of renal pathology.[27] It has been concluded that cats are more resistant to dietary vitamin D toxicity than other species based on these endpoints because the SUL for cats appears to be nine times higher than that for growing dogs.[27,34] It should be noted that these endpoints for vitamin D toxicity are for advanced changes of overt hypervitaminosis D. Studies are lacking that determine early endpoints marking the development of hypervitaminosis D in cats. Hypercalciuria is a standard early marker of excess vitamin D supplementation in human medicine.[35,36] Hypercalciuria occurs as an early homeostatic mechanism that initially prevents or delays the onset of hypercalcemia. Dietary studies that determine urinary calcium excretion at various levels of dietary intake of vitamin D are sorely needed to further understand the pathophysiology and treatment of IHC.

Vitamin A

Commercial cat foods often contain relatively high vitamin A and vitamin D concentrations that potentially work in concert to affect calcium metabolism in ways that could contribute to the development of IHC in a susceptible population of cats. Most of the focus has been on dietary vitamin D for its potential contribution to the development of IHC, but vitamin A deserves more attention for its possible contribution to the development and maintenance of IHC in cats. The NRC defines adequate intake for vitamin A as 660 International Units (200 µg) retinol/1000 kcal, recommended allowance as 825 International Units (250 µg) retinol/1000 kcal, and the SUL as 82,500 International Units (25,000 µg)/1000 kcal. In order to meet AAFCO guidelines for vitamin A for adult maintenance, the minimum is 1250 International Units/1000 kcal and the maximum is 187,500 International Units/1000 kcal (see Table 18-2). In order to meet AAFCO minimum to maximum guidelines, from about two to 284 times the NRC levels of vitamin A considered adequate for maintenance of adult cats could be provided in commercial diets.

Bisphosphonates

If normocalcemia has not been restored after a dietary feeding trial of 6 to 8 weeks, bisphosphonate treatment should be considered (see Figure 18-4; Box 18-1). Bisphosphonates reduce the activity and number of osteoclasts following binding to hydroxyapatite. Treatment with bisphosphonates may be useful for hypercalcemia in IHC if there is increased

---

BOX 18-1 Summary of Treatment Recommendations

1. Try dietary modification for 6 to 8 weeks if cat is clinically stable.
2. Start with alendronate 10 mg/cat PO once weekly.
   a. Have cat fast for at least 12 hours.
   b. Butter cat's lips.
   c. Give pill and follow with 6 mL of water.
   d. Have cat fast for another 2 hours.
3. Recheck iCa in 3 to 4 weeks.
   a. If normal, recheck in another 4 to 6 weeks.
   b. If low, decrease dosage to 10 mg/cat every other week.
   c. If high, increase dosage to 20 mg/cat/week. Alternatively, can increase to 10 mg/cat and 20 mg/cat on alternate weeks (consider this if iCa is only mildly elevated).
   d. Recheck iCa in 3 to 4 weeks. Consider recommendations listed according to iCa concentration.
4. If iCa remains elevated and if 40 mg/cat of alendronate per week is not enough to control iCa, the authors recommend adding prednisolone. First, the authors recommend rechecking the diagnosis by repeating PTH, PTH-related protein, vitamin D level, abdominal ultrasound (with aspirates of liver and spleen for cytology to rule out mast cell disease and lymphoma), and chest radiographs.
   a. Prednisolone 5 to 10 mg/cat PO every 24 hours.
   b. Recheck iCa in 3 to 4 weeks.
   c. If still elevated, consider increasing prednisolone to 10 to 20 mg PO every 24 hours.

iCa, Ionized calcium; *PO, per os* (by mouth); *PTH,* parathyroid hormone.

osteoclastic bone resorption. Even though not extensively reported, the authors now consider bisphosphonate therapy a safer alternative to glucocorticosteroid use in cats that failed dietary intervention. Alendronate has been shown to lower urinary calcium excretion and reduce calcium oxalate and calcium hydrogen phosphate supersaturation in genetic hypercalciuric rats.[37] Alendronate-induced decrease in urine supersaturation should be beneficial in preventing stone formation in IHC cats. In humans, hypocalcemia, hypophosphatemia, and hypomagnesemia are well-known side effects.[38,39] The package for the alendronate insert includes hypocalcemia and hypophosphatemia as possible adverse effects.

The safety and efficacy of pamidronate given intravenously (IV) to three cats with hypercalcemia have been reported.[40,41] Mild hypocalcemia[41] and severe hypocalcemia and hypophosphatemia[40] were observed in two of the three cats described. Adequate hydration is essential when treating with bisphosphonates because these drugs may cause nephrotoxicity, especially at higher doses given IV. The authors have successfully treated cats with IHC by giving 10 to 40 mg/cat of alendronate orally once weekly.* The longest follow-up on cats undergoing alendronate treatment was over 2 years.* Over 90% of cats had normal iCa at some point during treatment at an average of 15 mg/cat per week of alendronate.* Normocalcemia was restored at some point during treatment in eight out of 12 cats with IHC after a 6-month prospective study on the use of alendronate. Two of the 12 cats developed mild ionized hypocalcemia at 6 months of treatment. These two cats did not have clinical signs of hypocalcemia, and none of the 12 cats showed side effects from the alendronate (dosages ranged from 5 to 20 mg/cat per week) (B. Hardy, unpublished observations, 2008). In another report, a cat diagnosed with IHC was initially treated with pamidronate and subsequently given 5 to 10 mg/cat of alendronate per week to successfully control circulating calcium for 15 months.[40]

Erosive esophagitis is noted as a possibility in women receiving oral bisphosphonates, an effect that has not been reported or observed by the authors. In one study in dogs, the presence of alendronate in the esophagus for 1 hour caused minor mucosal damage, but esophagitis was exacerbated when gastric juice containing alendronate was refluxed into the esophagus.[42] It is thought that alendronate sodium is converted to free acid in the presence of gastric juice. No esophageal lesions and trivial gastric lesions (deemed not clinically significant by the pathologist) were reported from necropsy in cats undergoing relatively high doses (9 mg/kg twice a week in tuna juice) of oral alendronate for 49 weeks.[43] Although the risk for development of esophagitis in cats is low, it is recommended to follow the weekly pill with 6 mL of water given with a dosing syringe and then to dab a small amount of butter on the cat's lips to increase licking and

salivation, which further promote decreased transit time of the pill to the stomach.[44,45]

The oral bioavailability of alendronate administered in water to cats was recently reported to be about 3.0%.[43] This figure reduced approximately tenfold when alendronate was formulated in tuna juice.[43] To maximize intestinal absorption of alendronate, the authors recommend fasting cats overnight for 12 hours prior to the administration of medication, giving the pills in nothing other than tap water, and then feeding the cat 2 hours later. Even better, an 18-hour fast prior and 4-hour fast postpill is recommended to achieve oral bioavailability of 3%. The authors do not recommend any kind of alendronate that has been formulated by compounding pharmacies in flavored solution or suspension due to the severe decreases in intestinal absorption.

As seen with other therapies, hypercalcemia may return after a period of normocalcemia, requiring an increase in dose. Long-term bisphosphonate treatment in humans can lead to osteonecrosis of the jaw in a small number of patients. Osteonecrosis of the jaw is mostly reported in humans given high doses of IV bisphosphonates to treat cancer; it is far less frequently encountered following oral bisphosphonate treatment for postmenopausal osteoporosis. The alveolar bone region of the mandible has a high basal turnover rate for bone and so may be especially prone to necrosis of bone matrix following exposure to bisphosphonates. It is not clear if bisphosphonate exposure creates bone necrosis directly or if this is secondary to reduced bone turnover. Healthy male mongrel dogs treated with 5 mg daily oral alendronate for 23 weeks (average of 1 mg/kg/week) did not have subsequent bone weakness or changes in structural and mechanical properties of bone.[46] Daily oral alendronate at 0.2 mg/kg or 1.0 mg/kg given to skeletally mature female beagles for 3 years resulted in matrix necrosis of the mandible in 25% of the dogs treated with the lower dose and in 33% of the dogs treated with the higher dose. No dogs displayed exposed bone lesions in this study.[47] Intravenous zoledronate given to dogs at 0.06 mg/kg daily for 6 months resulted in more osteonecrosis of the mandible than that encountered with oral alendronate.[48] Osteonecrosis of the jaw was not described in cats with dental lesions treated for 49 weeks with oral alendronate.[43] The authors have not observed Osteonecrosis of the jaw in cats treated with any form of bisphosphonate, including some that have been on oral alendronate for several years.

Glucocorticosteroids

If normocalcemia has not been restored after a dietary feeding trial of 6 to 8 weeks and subsequent treatment with bisphosphonates, glucocorticosteroids should be considered (see Figure 18-4 and Box 18-1). Administration of glucocorticosteroids is thought to decrease serum calcium concentration by decreased intestinal absorption of calcium, decreased renal tubular calcium resorption, and decreased skeletal mobilization of calcium. There is some concern that glucocorticosteroids may increase urinary excretion of calcium, contributing

---

*de Brito Galvao JF: *Treatment of idiopathic hypercalcemia in 29 cats (1999-2010)*. Unpublished observations, The Ohio State University, 2013.

to calcium oxalate urolith formation as occurs in some species. However, little is known regarding the effects of glucocorticosteroids on filtration and tubular resorption of calcium in the cat. Daily prednisolone (oral liquid at average 2.2 mg/kg) treatment did not result in diuresis or an increase in calcium excretion in five healthy female cats.[49] Therefore, according to this study, there must be a different effect on normalization of calcemia after administration of prednisolone in cats. The caveat of this study is that it was performed in cats with normocalcemia for a short period of time (2 weeks). It is possible that results may be different in hypercalcemic cats undergoing prolonged treatment.

Cats usually do not exhibit some of the side effects from glucocorticosteroid treatment seen in dogs, such as severe polyuria and polydipsia and panting. Long-term treatment with prednisolone does contribute to muscle wasting and possible induction of diabetes mellitus in some cats. Oral prednisolone achieves greater maximal concentration in the circulation than oral prednisone in the cat, possibly due to greater GI absorption of prednisolone or less hepatic conversion of prednisone to prednisolone.[50] Prednisolone is given orally at 5 to 10 mg/cat/day for 1 month before re-evaluation (see Figure 18-4 and Box 18-1). If iCa concentration is normal, this dose is continued for several months. If serum iCa concentration is still increased, the dose is increased by 5 mg/cat/day. Some cats may require as much as 15 to 20 mg of prednisolone per day to restore normocalcemia. Approximately 80% of cats with IHC become normocalcemic with 1.5 to 2.0 mg/kg/day prednisolone, but some may require increasing doses to remain normocalcemic over time.[51]

Miscellaneous Treatments

Fluid therapy is a possible treatment option in cats with IHC but has not been evaluated. The administration of subcutaneous fluids on a daily or every-other-day basis potentially could expand the extracellular fluid and promote calciuresis. Diuretics, such as furosemide, have been used effectively to decrease serum iCa during acute rescue protocols for hypercalcemia, usually in combination with IV fluids. Little is known about the effects of chronic furosemide administration regarding calcium status and the development of dehydration. It is a concern that cats receiving chronic diuretics will undergo diuresis but will not increase their water intake, leading to dehydration and electrolyte imbalances.

Calcimimetics are a relatively new class of drug in human medicine that interact with the calcium receptor directly and have been proven effective in lowering iCa, phosphorus, and PTH concentrations in human dialysis patients. The potential future use of calcimimetics in the treatment of IHC is an interesting treatment consideration for future study.

References

1. Peterson ME: Feeding the cat with endocrine disease. American College of Veterinary Internal Medicine Forum, Seattle, 2013, pp 525–528.
2. Messinger JS, Windham WR, Ward CR: Ionized hypercalcemia in dogs: a retrospective study of 109 cases (1998-2003). *J Vet Intern Med* 23(3):514–519, 2009.
3. Savary KC, Price GS, Vaden SL: Hypercalcemia in cats: a retrospective study of 71 cases (1991-1997). *J Vet Intern Med* 14(2):184–189, 2000.
4. Schenck PA, Chew DJ: Prediction of serum ionized calcium concentration by serum total calcium measurement in cats. *Can J Vet Res* 74(3):209–213, 2010.
5. Schenck PA, Chew DJ, Refsal K, et al: Calcium metabolic hormones in feline idiopathic hypercalcemia. *J Vet Intern Med* 18(3):442, 2004. (Abstract).
6. Schenck PA, Chew DJ, Nagode LA, et al: Disorders of calcium: hypercalcemia and hypocalcemia. In DiBartola SP, editor: *Fluid, electrolyte, and acid-base disorders in small animal practice,* ed 4, St Louis, 2011, Saunders/Elsevier, pp 120–194.
7. Midkiff AM, Chew DJ, Randolph JF, et al: Idiopathic hypercalcemia in cats. *J Vet Intern Med* 14(6):619–626, 2000.
8. Pineda C, Aguilera-Tejero E, Raya AI, et al: Assessment of calcitonin response to experimentally induced hypercalcemia in cats. *Am J Vet Res* 74(12):1514–1521, 2013.
9. O'Neill WC: The fallacy of the calcium-phosphorus product. *Kidney Int* 72(7):792–796, 2007.
10. McClain HM, Barsanti JA, Bartges JW: Hypercalcemia and calcium oxalate urolithiasis in cats: a report of five cases. *J Am Anim Hosp Assoc* 35(4):297–301, 1999.
11. Lindsjo M: Oxalate metabolism in renal stone disease with special reference to calcium metabolism and intestinal absorption. *Scand J Urol Nephrol Suppl* 119:1–53, 1989.
12. Ryckelynck JP, Hurault de Ligny B, Beuve-Mery P: [Hypercalcemia induced by dihydroxy-aluminum allantoinate: a further case]. [Article in French] *Nouv Presse Med* 7(22):1953, 1978.
13. Ruml LA, Pearle MS, Pak CY: Medical therapy, calcium oxalate urolithiasis. *Urol Clin North Am* 24(1):117–133, 1997.
14. Gottrand M, Muyshont L, Couttenier F, et al: Micronutrient status of children receiving prolonged enteral nutrition. *Ann Nutr Metab* 63(1–2):152–158, 2013.
15. Parivar F, Low RK, Stoller ML: The influence of diet on urinary stone disease. *J Urol* 155(2):432–440, 1996.
16. Prola L, Dobenecker B, Mussa PP, et al: Influence of cellulose fibre length on faecal quality, mineral excretion and nutrient digestibility in cat. *J Anim Physiol Anim Nutr (Berl)* 94(3):362–367, 2010.
17. de-Oliveira LD, Takakura FS, Kienzle E, et al: Fibre analysis and fibre digestibility in pet foods—a comparison of total dietary fibre, neutral and acid detergent fibre and crude fibre. *J Anim Physiol Anim Nutr (Berl)* 96(5):895–906, 2012.
18. Rosol TJ, Chew DJ, Nagode LA, et al: Pathophysiology of calcium metabolism. *Vet Clin Pathol* 24(2):49–63, 1995.
19. Barber PJ, Rawlings JM, Markwell PJ, et al: Effect of dietary phosphate restriction on renal secondary hyperparathyroidism in the cat. *J Small Anim Pract* 40(2):62–70, 1999.
20. Lulich JP, Osborne CA, Lekcharoensuk C, et al: Effects of diet on urine composition of cats with calcium oxalate urolithiasis. *J Am Anim Hosp Assoc* 40(3):185–191, 2004.
21. Biourge VC, Devois C, Morice G, et al: Increased dietary NaCl significantly increases urine volume but does not increase urinary calcium oxalate relative supersaturation in healthy cats. *J Vet Intern Med* 15(3):301, 2001.
22. Xu H, Laflamme DP, Bartges JW, et al: Effect of dietary sodium on urine characteristics in healthy adult cats. *J Vet Intern Med* 20:738, 2006.
23. Reynolds BS, Chetboul V, Nguyen P, et al: Effects of dietary salt intake on renal function: a 2-year study in healthy aged cats. *J Vet Intern Med* 27(3):507–515, 2013.
24. Hawthorne AJ, Markwell PJ: Dietary sodium promotes increased water intake and urine volume in cats. *J Nutr* 134(8 Suppl):2128S–2129S, 2004.
25. Buckley CM, Hawthorne A, Colyer A, et al: Effect of dietary water intake on urinary

output, specific gravity and relative supersaturation for calcium oxalate and struvite in the cat. *Br J Nutr* 106(Suppl 1):S128–S130, 2011.

26. Fascetti AJ, Delaney SJ: Nutritional management of endocrine disease. In Fascetti AJ, Delaney SJ, editors: *Applied veterinary clinical nutrition*, Chickester, West Sussex, 2012, Wiley-Blackwell, pp 289–300.

27. National Research Council of the National Academies: Nutrient requirements and dietary nutrient concentrations. In *Nutrient requirements of dogs and cats*, Washington, DC, 2006, National Academies Press, pp 354–370.

28. Johansson S, Melhus H: Vitamin A antagonizes calcium response to vitamin D in man. *J Bone Miner Res* 16(10):1899–1905, 2001.

29. Beulens JW, Booth SL, van den Heuvel EG, et al: The role of menaquinones (vitamin K_2) in human health. *Br J Nutr* 110(8):1357–1368, 2013.

30. Camara-Martos F, Amaro-Lopez MA: Influence of dietary factors on calcium bioavailability: a brief review. *Biol Trace Element Res* 89(1):43–52, 2002.

31. Hennequin C, Tardivel S, Medetognon J, et al: A stable animal model of diet-induced calcium oxalate crystalluria. *Urol Res* 26(1):57–63, 1998.

32. Wehner A, Katzenberger J, Groth A, et al: Vitamin D intoxication caused by ingestion of commercial cat food in three kittens. *J Feline Med Surg* 15(8):730–736, 2013.

33. Association of American Feed Control Officials: *Official Publication*, Champaign, Indiana, 2012, AAFCO.

34. Sih TR, Morris JG, Hickman MA: Chronic ingestion of high concentrations of cholecalciferol in cats. *Am J Vet Res* 62(9):1500–1506, 2001.

35. Cranney A, Weiler HA, O'Donnell S, et al: Summary of evidence-based review on vitamin D efficacy and safety in relation to bone health. *Am J Clin Nutr* 88(2):513S–519S, 2008.

36. Parfitt AM, Gallagher JC, Heaney RP, et al: Vitamin D and bone health in the elderly. *Am J Clin Nutr* 36(5 Suppl):1014–1031, 1982.

37. Bushinsky DA, Neumann KJ, Asplin J, et al: Alendronate decreases urine calcium and supersaturation in genetic hypercalciuric rats. *Kidney Int* 55(1):234–243, 1999.

38. Papapetrou PD: Bisphosphonate-associated adverse events. *Hormones* 8(2):96–110, 2009.

39. Tanvetyanon T, Stiff PJ: Management of the adverse effects associated with intravenous bisphosphonates. *Ann Oncol* 17(6):897–907, 2006.

40. Whitney JL, Barrs VR, Wilkinson MR, et al: Use of bisphosphonates to treat severe idiopathic hypercalcaemia in a young Ragdoll cat. *J Feline Med Surg* 13(2):129–134, 2011.

41. Hostutler RA, Chew DJ, Jaeger JQ, et al: Uses and effectiveness of pamidronate disodium for treatment of dogs and cats with hypercalcemia. *J Vet Intern Med* 19(1):29–33, 2005.

42. Peter CP, Handt LK, Smith SM: Esophageal irritation due to alendronate sodium tablets: possible mechanisms. *Dig Dis Sci* 43(9):1998–2002, 1998.

43. Mohn KL, Jacks TM, Schleim KD, et al: Alendronate binds to tooth root surfaces and inhibits progression of feline tooth resorption: a pilot proof-of-concept study. *J Vet Dent* 26(2):74–81, 2009.

44. Griffin B, Beard DM, Klopfenstein KA: Use of butter to facilitate the passage of tablets through the esophagus in cats. *J Vet Intern Med* 17:445, 2003.

45. Westfall DS, Twedt DC, Steyn PF, et al: Evaluation of esophageal transit of tablets and capsules in 30 cats. *J Vet Intern Med* 15(5):467–470, 2001.

46. Fischer KJ, Vikoren TH, Ney S, et al: Mechanical evaluation of bone samples following alendronate therapy in healthy male dogs. *J Biomed Mater Res B Appl Biomater* 76(1):143–148, 2006.

47. Allen MR, Burr DB: Mandible matrix necrosis in beagle dogs after 3 years of daily oral bisphosphonate treatment. *J Oral Maxillofac Surg* 66(5):987–994, 2008.

48. Burr DB, Allen MR: Mandibular necrosis in beagle dogs treated with bisphosphonates. *Orthod Craniofac Res* 12(3):221–228, 2009.

49. Geyer N, Bartges JW, Kirk CA, et al: Influence of prednisolone on urinary calcium oxalate and struvite relative supersaturation in healthy young adult female domestic shorthaired cats. *Vet Ther* 8(4):239–246, 2007.

50. Graham-Mize CA, Rosser EJ, Hauptman J: Absorption, bioavailability and activity of prednisone and prednisolone in cats. *Adv Vet Derm* 5:152–158, 2005.

51. National Research Council: Nutrient Requirements for Adult Dogs: Minimum Requirements and Recommended Allowances. *Nutrient requirements of dogs and cats*, Washington DC, 2006, National Academies Press, p 152.

The Diabetic Cat: Insulin Resistance and Brittle Diabetes

Stijn Niessen

Treating diabetes mellitus in the cat is often a rewarding experience, with relatively high owner acceptance of the need for insulin injections and subsequent fast resolution of the diabetes-associated clinical signs.[1,2] Some diabetic cats can even enter a state of diabetic remission (see Chapter 17).[3] However, in a significant proportion of diabetic cats, treatment success appears challenging to achieve. Broadly speaking, the nature of the problems that make feline diabetics difficult can be divided into four categories (Box 19-1). If clinical signs are present despite effective insulin treatment, clinicians should be alert for the presence of other diseases that share some of the same clinical signs as seen with diabetes mellitus (e.g., polyuria/polydipsia and weight loss with chronic kidney disease (CKD) and hyperthyroidism; polyphagia with gastrointestinal disease, hyperthyroidism, and hypersomatotropism).

This chapter aims to demonstrate the common causes for these problems and to integrate this with a systematic approach to dealing with the difficult diabetic in clinical feline practice.

STRUCTURED STEPWISE APPROACH TO TREATING DIFFICULT DIABETICS

In healthy cats, maintaining euglycemia is established through a complex network of various physiologic systems, with a major role exercised by the pancreatic beta cell and the liver. Within minutes of ingestion of a meal, the beta cell releases preformed active insulin into the circulation and gene transcription is initiated in order to produce newly-formed insulin, which enables the second phase of insulin release. In healthy cats, this process (aided by other body systems and hormones) ensures that only limited blood glucose excursions will occur. When this system fails because of a combination of insulin resistance and beta cell dysfunction, diabetes ensues and insulin injections become necessary. However, these injections of exogenous insulin, often timed to coincide with postprandial hyperglycemia, only partially replace the loss of this previously smoothly and fast operating system. It is therefore understandable that in a proportion of diabetic patients, this relatively limited method of mimicking the

healthy pancreatic function fails, resulting in suboptimal control of hyperglycemia and, thus, associated clinical signs.

Additionally, it is important to realize that diabetes is a dynamic disease, especially in the cat. Beta cell function in some cats might be virtually absent, whereas in other cats it might actually be relatively preserved. Even in one individual cat, beta cell function can be better or worse depending on the time at which it is assessed. One of the reasons for the latter includes the variable influence of glucotoxicity and possibly lipotoxicity.[4] Two weeks of hyperglycemia will cause beta cell dysfunction on its own, which can resolve or improve with effective treatment of the hyperglycemia. It is therefore logical that some cats need different insulin doses at different times in their life, especially initially after diagnosis of their diabetes mellitus and commencement of treatment.

Although less well studied in cats, the severity of insulin resistance also varies significantly, even more so when there is one or more comorbidities.[5,6] The high prevalence of comorbidities among diabetic cats is a clinically accepted fact, as well as documented in the veterinary literature.[2,7,8]

Finally, there are also many variables in the management protocol of feline diabetes. Therefore, it can seem an extremely difficult affair to identify the one factor that could improve the diabetic control in any given patient presented with suboptimal diabetic control. The aforementioned mechanisms can lead to pseudo-insulin resistance, true insulin resistance, variable insulin sensitivity, or brittle diabetes (defined as frequent, extreme swings in blood glucose concentrations, causing hyperglycemia and/or hypoglycemia). Adopting a structured stepwise approach can help in these cats. Such an approach should include a systematic assessment of the main protagonists involved in diabetic management (Box 19-2; Figure 19-1).

Owner and Owner-Related Factors

The number one cause associated with lack of appropriate response to the insulin therapy include factors that are somehow connected with the owner of the diabetic pet.[8] This does not represent true insulin resistance and can more appropriately be called *pseudo-insulin resistance*. A seemingly ever-changing, insulin-dosing requirement, without necessarily reaching a dose qualified as true insulin resistance, could also be the result of these owner factors.

Clinicians should, therefore, try their utmost best to exclude such owner-related management issues prior to undertaking more elaborate and expensive investigations (Box 19-3). In order to achieve this, owners of diabetic pets are encouraged to demonstrate an adequate insulin injection technique and appropriate insulin handling and storage habits. This might seem obvious, but it is the very obvious nature of the issue that leads to its proper assessment often being forgotten or skipped. Clinicians should also not be reluctant to question the owner on these issues, although a

tactful manner of asking the right questions is needed with owners who might take offense if they feel the quality of their management is being doubted. It is not uncommon for owners to initially show fantastic management habits, only to be subsequently forgotten or replaced by suboptimal habits weeks to months later. Continued and repeated assessment is therefore warranted. A good example of an owner-related error is the use of the wrong syringe type for a given insulin type, especially relevant to the use of insulin types that require U-40 syringes. The provision of midday snacks, without an additional injection of insulin to help cope with the induced postsnack hyperglycemia, represents another owner-related factor that might make obtaining good glycemic control difficult to obtain.

Ad libitum feeding can turn out to be an advantage in the management of diabetic cats that tend to graze, because it might be associated with less pronounced blood glucose undulations, especially when used in cats that experience a long-acting effect of the administered insulin type; however, it will not be suited to all diabetic cats. In fact, it could lead to obesity in individual cats that happen to be intrinsic "meal-eaters" or deterioration of glycemic control in cats that experience a short-acting effect to the provided exogenous insulin. It is important to remember that any of the insulin preparations will have an individual glucose-lowering response in a given cat, which often does not match the expected duration of action quoted in drug formularies or other publications. Another example constitutes the lack of variation of injection site, which might induce areas of inflammation, thickening of the skin, and reduced insulin absorption. A range of possible injection sites is shown in Figure 19-2.

It is also of paramount importance that clinicians ensure that all individuals involved in the cat's diabetic care receive

---

BOX 19-1 Broad Categorization of Problems Encountered in Difficult Feline Diabetic Patients

- Clinical signs despite effective insulin treatment
- Lack of glucose response to insulin treatment
- Frequent hypoglycemia
- Periods of good control intermixed with periods of poor control

---

BOX 19-2 A Structured Systematic Approach to the Difficult Diabetic Patient

This approach should include assessment of factors associated with the three main protagonists involved in diabetic management:
- Owner and owner-associated factors
- Veterinarian and veterinarian-associated factors
- Cat and cat-associated factors

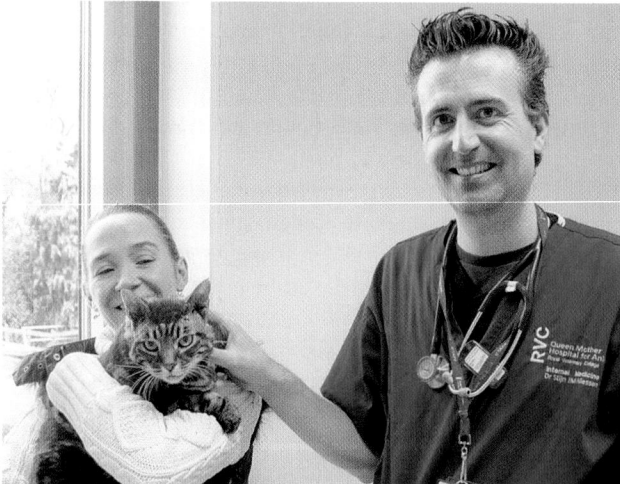

Figure 19-1: The three main protagonists involved in diabetic management. Difficult-to-manage diabetes in a cat can usually be explained by owner, veterinarian, and/or cat-associated factors. The featured uncontrolled diabetic cat, a 10-year-old domestic shorthair, was receiving 8.5 units of lente-type insulin (Caninsulin, MSD Animal Health) twice daily. The cat was subsequently diagnosed with hypersomatotropism.

BOX 19-3 Examples of Owner-Related Reasons for Pseudo-Insulin Resistance or Seemingly Variable Insulin Sensitivity

- Lack of compliance with dietary recommendations
  - Variable timing
  - Variable or incorrect quantity
  - Variable or suboptimal type of food
  - Provision of (unidentified) extras
- Lack of compliance with insulin injection recommendations
  - Variation in timing
  - Lack of injection site variation
  - Insufficient mixing of insulin solution (if required)
  - Use of incorrect syringe type (U-40 vs U-100)
  - Regular inclusion of air bubbles
- Lack of compliance with insulin storage recommendations
  - Refrigeration (if required)
  - Exposure to extreme temperatures
  - Using out of date preparations
  - Use of insulin preparations not recommended for veterinary use, including insulin prepared by compounding pharmacies

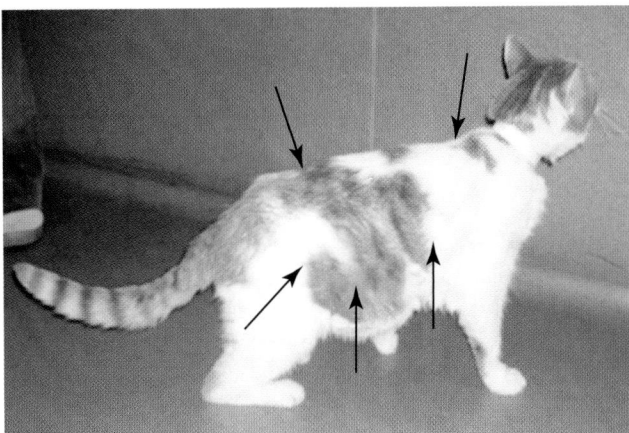

Figure 19-2: Lack of injection site variation can cause variable insulin absorption. Pictured is a diabetic cat suffering from diabetic neuropathy. Possible injection sites are indicated with *black arrows* (scruff of the neck, paralumbar, side of the chest, flank, and hind leg).

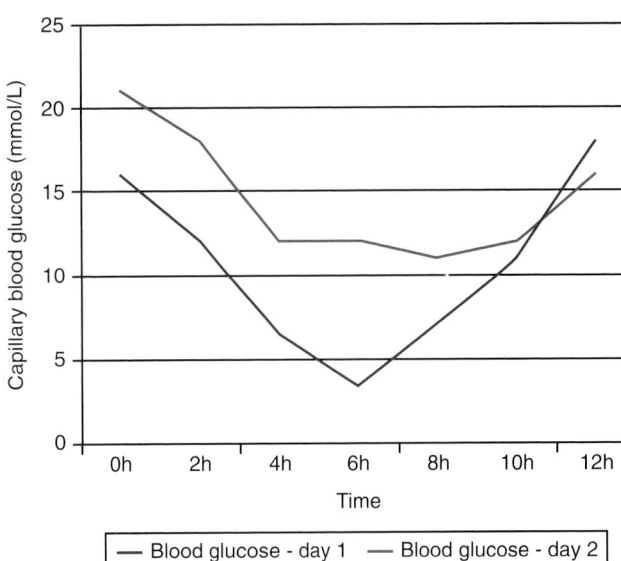

Figure 19-3: Blood glucose curves obtained on 2 consecutive days from the same cat without any change in treatment regimen. The curve on day 2 suggests a dose increase is safe, whereas the curve on day 1 suggests the glucose nadir is too low to recommend an increase in the insulin dose.

and comply with the same veterinary instructions, even if only one member of the family routinely visits the veterinary practice. This includes neighbors or friends who may help care for or are in contact with the cat. A thorough assessment of the quality of life of the diabetic cat and its owner(s) might prove advantageous, because it might reveal those areas that make consistently good management less likely to occur. For instance, if owners are struggling to integrate the diabetic care with their social or work life, it is going to be unlikely that insulin injections are given at regular times. If owners are fearful of injecting the insulin in the first place, perhaps because they are worried about hurting their cat, the overall management can also suffer. A validated structured and individualized quality-of-life tool for insulin-treated diabetic cats to investigate these practical and psychosocial factors has recently become available and can be used by practitioners.[1]

A final specific mention is warranted for the use of insulin preparations that are unreliable or generally not suited for use in cats. A recent study evaluated and compared the characteristics of a commercially-manufactured protamine zinc insulin (PZI) product and PZI products obtained from various compounding pharmacies.[9] A total of 112 vials of PZI (16 vials of commercially-manufactured product and eight vials from each of 12 compounding pharmacies) were tested for appearance, endotoxin concentration, crystal size, supernatant insulin concentration, pH, total insulin and zinc concentrations, and species of insulin origin. Whereas all 16 vials of commercially-manufactured PZI met United States Pharmacopeia specifications, this was not the case for the compounded insulin products. Of the 96 vials of compounded PZI, one contained excess endotoxin, 23 had excessive concentrations of insulin in the supernatant, 45 had pH values that were either too high or too low, 52 did not meet specifications for zinc concentration, and 36 had a total insulin concentration less than 90% of the labeled concentration. Therefore, it is easy to see that the use of these compounded insulin preparations could lead to unexpected, variable, and even dangerous treatment effects.

Veterinarian and Veterinarian-Associated Factors

The number two cause associated with lack of appropriate response to the insulin therapy is in fact clinician-related. Before arriving at a diagnosis of true insulin resistance, it is strongly advised to ensure that we carefully interpret the combination of clinical (i.e., persistent diabetes-related) signs and a range of diagnostic data (e.g., fructosamine, multiple at-home collected urine glucose samples, and multiple hospital and/or home blood glucose curves). A single blood glucose curve indicating consistently high blood glucose concentrations does not prove the presence of insulin resistance, especially not in the cat. In the cat (but also in some dogs), the explanation might be the presence of stress hyperglycemia, although it is also important to realize that blood glucose curves vary significantly from day-to-day without changes in management parameters (Figure 19-3).

Studies comparing the blood glucose curves of two consecutive days demonstrated that different conclusions could be drawn and, therefore, different management interventions planned depending on which of the two consecutive curves was taken as the "true" curve.[10] Evaluation of two home curves conducted on consecutive days led to the same recommendation for adjustment of the insulin dose on only six of 14 occasions, whereas comparison of home and clinic curves done on consecutive days led to the same recommendation on only 14 of 28 occasions. The reproducibility of home curves in diabetic cats with good glycemic control was somewhat better than that of cats with moderate to poor control; four of the six paired home curves in cats with good glycemic control, but only two of the eight paired home curves in cats with poor glycemic control led to the same recommendation. The latter realization might lead us to completely dismiss the use of the blood glucose curve, although this would also mean that we throw away the one single glycemic assessment method that has the potential to demonstrate the duration of insulin action, as well as the daily nadir.

Therefore, it is probably best to not completely abandon the blood glucose curve as a tool but instead adopt a critical attitude in interpreting the glycemic data from a curve. It can, in fact, prove very useful to run a series of curves (instead of one single curve) in a difficult diabetic without necessarily changing a parameter in the management, because it is likely that the overall trend shown by these multiple curves more closely resembles the true glycemic control of the patient.

Other common management-associated issues include insulin underdosing, overdosing, and subsequent hypoglycemia-induced hyperglycemia (Somogyi effect) and short duration of insulin action. Further issues are outlined in Box 19-4. Insulin underdosing is common, and it is important to realize that one should consider true insulin resistance to be present only in diabetic pets that are receiving an insulin dosage in excess of 1.5 to 2 unit/kg per injection on a twice-daily injection protocol. Prior to reaching this point, underdosing remains a possible cause for the inferior clinical control. With the advent of more aggressive insulin protocols aimed (though not yet proven) to foster diabetic remission, hypoglycemia-induced hyperglycemia is likely becoming increasingly common.

Dealing with Hypoglycemia-Induced Hyperglycemia (Somogyi Effect)

Hypoglycemia-induced hyperglycemia can especially be encountered when treating diabetic cats with more aggressive insulin protocols, using relatively high insulin dosages, or through excessively rapid escalation of the insulin dose (more frequently than every 7 days). This phenomenon can also be seen when a diabetic cat temporarily suffers from decreased insulin sensitivity (e.g., after a bout of pancreatitis) and, quite

rightly, the insulin dose is initially progressively increased on documentation of worsening glycemic data. When the cause for the insulin resistance then resolves or improves (and therefore insulin sensitivity improves again), the injected insulin has the potential to produce a rapid drop in blood glucose, with or without actual hypoglycemia. Such rapid falls in blood glucose are thought to be capable of inducing release of catecholamines, glucagon, cortisol, and growth hormone—all insulin-antagonistic hormones, resulting in activation of hyperglycemia-inducing mechanisms. However, the clinician will often merely see the end result of this process (i.e., high blood glucose concentrations) and might wrongly conclude that more (and not less) insulin is needed, further exacerbating the situation and risking fatal hypoglycemia. Three useful strategies for dealing with possible Somogyi effect are shown in Box 19-5. The clinical picture of cats that develop the Somogyi effect is usually that of a mix of periods of good control and periods of suboptimal control, with or without clinical hypoglycemia (although clinical hypoglycemia is difficult to recognize in cats unless severe). Therefore, this is similar to the clinical picture encountered in the presence of any chronic waxing and waning comorbidity causing variable insulin sensitivity (like chronic pancreatitis).

Dealing with Short Duration of Action

Short duration of insulin action is common in the feline diabetic patient. The duration of action of various insulin types have been reported to, on average, fall short of the duration seen in dogs. However, it remains important to realize that the response to insulin, including duration of action, will be unpredictable in an individual cat. On average, the use of neutral protamine Hagedorn (NPH) insulin types is associated with a higher incidence of short duration of action than longer-acting insulin types, such as porcine lente insulin (e.g., Vetsulin/Caninsulin, MSD Animal Health), PZI (e.g., ProZinc, Boehringer Ingelheim Vetmedica, Inc.), and human insulin analogues (e.g., Lantus, Sanofi-Avantis; Levemir, Novo Nordisk). Regardless of the insulin type used, when short duration of action is demonstrated by a blood glucose curve, increasing the insulin dose can help. The latter ceases to be an option, however, when the glucose nadir becomes too low. In such situation, the suggestions shown in Box 19-6 could be considered.

Finally, it is important to realize that the problem of short duration of insulin action can easily go undiagnosed when not using a blood glucose curve. A high fructosamine or high spot blood glucose values, in combination with persistent diabetic signs, could represent underdosing of insulin as well as such short duration of action. This further illustrates the potential crucial role of the blood glucose curve in monitoring the diabetic cat.

Cat and Cat-Associated Factors

The number three cause associated with lack of appropriate response to insulin therapy constitutes concurrent disease in the diabetic pet. Infectious disease is high on this list, with urinary tract infections (UTIs) and dental disease both common problems in the diabetic cat and dog. Inflammatory diseases (e.g., pancreatitis, inflammatory bowel disease [IBD], and gingivostomatitis) are further important considerations, given their prevalence among diabetic cats and their potential to affect insulin sensitivity. Treatment of inflammatory conditions, which often requires the administration of diabetogenic drugs (e.g., glucocorticoids), can pose additional challenges to the clinician—although creative solutions can be explored in many cases and are discussed later.

The connection between inflammation and insulin resistance is the topic of intense research, especially now that obesity is seen as a pro-inflammatory condition.[11] However, the sheer concept of inflammation as a diabetogenic process has been known for over one hundred years, when high doses of salicylates were shown to lower glucose levels in diabetic patients.[12] Endocrinopathies such as hyperthyroidism, hyperadrenocorticism, and iatrogenic hormone administration (including topical preparations) could lead to both overt insulin resistance, as well as reduced insulin sensitivity without actual overt insulin resistance. The diagnosis of hyperthyroidism and especially hyperadrenocorticism can prove challenging in the uncontrolled diabetic cat given the confusion with sick euthyroid syndrome as well as the effects of stress and concurrent disease on pituitary-adrenal axis testing.

An overview of cat and cat-associated factors frequently involved in causing difficult-to-manage diabetes is shown in Box 19-7. The success of any diabetic management protocol depends on correct identification of these comorbidities, as well as successful management. The correct identification starts with a thorough history and physical examination, at times backed up by routine laboratory work, each time

---

BOX 19-6 Possible Strategies to Ameliorate Difficult-to-Control Diabetes Associated with Short Duration of Action of Insulin

1. Increase the insulin dose
   a. Can only be done if nadir allows this
2. Amend the timing of feeding relative to injection of insulin
   a. Injecting insulin prior to feeding ensures presence of active insulin prior to a postprandial increase in blood glucose
   b. Insulin activity is matched better with time of maximal need
   c. Unreliable eaters can be given 25% of food with insulin, 75% later
   d. Exact optimal timing depends on individual cat (expected range of 30 to 90 minutes)
3. Change the insulin type
   a. Options: PZI, porcine zinc, synthetic human insulin analogues (glargine and detemir)
   b. Choice depends on local legislation (cascade system for prescribing medication may dictate choice in many countries), financial implications, and response of individual cat to insulin type
4. Frequency change
   a. BID insulin injections are considered the norm
   b. It is exceptional for SID injection to suffice
   c. TID insulin injections can prove beneficial in some patients
5. Use of a "basal-bolus" system (see also Box 19-8)
   a. BID injection of a longer-acting insulin (PZI, porcine zinc, synthetic human insulins glargine and detemir)
   b. In addition, injection of neutral/soluble/regular insulin (e.g., Actrapid, Novo Nordisk) at meal times
   c. This system is commonly used in human diabetology
6. Changing noninsulin factors
   a. Individual diabetic cats that are true "grazers" (*ad libitum* eaters) can be allowed to graze resulting in less dramatic blood glucose fluctuations
   b. Changing to a low carbohydrate canned food diet
   c. Optimizing insulin sensitivity (appropriate weight loss, ensuring oral health [see Cat and Cat-Associated Factors section])

BID, twice daily; *PZI*, protamine zinc insulin; *SID*, once daily; *TID*, three times daily.

---

looking out for those signs or abnormalities that cannot be explained by mere diabetes alone. For example, weight gain in an uncontrolled diabetic should alert the presence of a different type of diabetes mellitus, such as hypersomatotropism or acromegaly. Furthermore, inappetence is not a sign of uncontrolled diabetes when diabetic ketoacidosis has been excluded and, therefore, warrants a search for inappetence-inducing concurrent diseases (e.g., CKD, pancreatitis, or other gastrointestinal disease). Dealing with inappetence issues is essential because inappetence stands in the way of the successful matching of exogenous insulin dose and

BOX 19-7 Cat-Associated Conditions Frequently Linked with Difficulties in Diabetic Management

1. Infection
   a. Urinary tract infection
   b. Dental infections
2. Inflammation
   a. Pancreatitis
   b. Inflammatory bowel disease
   c. Gingivostomatitis
   d. Obesity
3. Medication
   a. Corticosteroids (including topical medications)
   b. Megestrol acetate
4. Other hormonal disturbances
   a. Hyperthyroidism
5. Misdiagnosis of the type of diabetes mellitus
   a. Hypersomatotropism-induced diabetes mellitus (acromegaly)
   b. Hyperadrenocorticism-induced diabetes mellitus (Cushing's syndrome)
   c. Pancreatic destruction (e.g., neoplasia, abscess, pancreatitis)
6. Other diseases (through known and unknown mechanisms)
   a. Cardiac disease
   b. Chronic kidney disease
   c. Neoplasia
   d. Obesity (also through inflammation)
7. Any disease or condition causing inappetence
   a. Unreliable exogenous insulin requirements result

BOX 19-8 Case Example of Basal-bolus Insulin Dosing

1. Reassess the need for the diabetogenic drug.
   a. Was the comorbidity diagnosis correct? Did the IBD or atopy diagnosis represent food intolerance or hypersensitivity?
   b. Does the comorbidity still need treatment? Is the IBD or immune-mediated hemolytic anemia currently in remission?
   c. Can the disease be treated with other treatment modalities than drugs? Asthma/bronchitis: Could environmental changes or weight reduction help?
2. Replace with a non-diabetogenic drug.
   a. IBD: Could chlorambucil or cyclosporine be used?
   b. Atopy: Could cyclosporine be used?
   c. Asthma/bronchitis: Could metered dose inhalers prove useful?
3. Replace with a less-diabetogenic drug.
   a. Prednisolone could prove less harmful compared to dexamethasone.
   b. Hydrocortisone could prove less harmful than prednisolone.
   c. Topical glucocorticoids could prove less harmful than systemic versions (e.g., eye, ear, and skin preparations).
   d. Oral budesonide might prove useful given the likely more limited systemic exposure to this glucocorticoid (high first-pass effect).
4. Lower the dose of diabetogenic drug.
   a. Use a second immunosuppressive drug along with the glucocorticoid (e.g., azathioprine, mycophenolate mofetil, cyclosporine, or chlorambucil).
   b. Titrate to the lowest clinically acceptable dose.
5. Align the diabetogenic effect with the insulin action.
   a. Give BID short-acting glucocorticoid with BID insulin injections.

postprandial insulin requirements and, thus, hinders any chance of success in the diabetic management.

Dealing with Patients with Pancreatitis

In a study of 29 cats with diabetes mellitus,[7] a likely high prevalence of pancreatitis was demonstrated among diabetic cats. In that study, serum feline pancreatic lipase immunoreactivity (fPLI) concentrations were significantly higher in samples from diabetic cats. A weak association was found between serum fructosamine and fPLI concentrations, indicating the potential for inflammation of the pancreas to interfere with diabetic control. In line with these data, in a study of insulin-treated diabetic cats, 10 of 82 (12.2%) were reported to be suffering from pancreatitis (S. Niessen, unpublished data). The inflammation associated with pancreatitis could indeed result in variable insulin sensitivity and insulin resistance, but the majority of difficulties in cats with pancreatitis is associated with a poor to variable appetite, rendering the choice of an appropriate insulin regimen extremely challenging. The typical clinical image of a diabetic cat with chronic pancreatitis is that of a cat experiencing periods of good control intermixed with periods of suboptimal control, including appetite issues.

Successful management of these cases can therefore prove difficult but is feasible if the clinician follows a number of careful steps. First, the type of pancreatitis needs to be defined as best as possible. Are we dealing with an idiopathic case, or is the cat suffering from a combination of pancreatitis and IBD and/or cholangiohepatitis? Although pancreatitis cannot easily be directly treated, IBD and cholangiohepatitis often can, frequently reducing the frequency and severity of the pancreatitis. If the cat is suffering from a pancreatitis-induced exocrine pancreatic insufficiency (EPI), this should be diagnosed and treated, otherwise glycemic control will remain elusive in light of variable intestinal absorption. The pancreatitis might also be associated with a pancreatic tumor or a cyst, further impacting prognosis but also intervention possibilities. Management should therefore include treating the treatable (e.g., novel protein diet, antibiotics if infectious cholangiohepatitis is demonstrated, and/or draining of a cyst, treatment of EPI including vitamin B_{12}), as well as providing symptomatic treatment. The latter should especially pay attention to pain relief and could include the use of oral buprenorphine or tramadol, because pain inhibits appetite and, therefore, leads to difficult-to-control diabetes. If the cat still suffers from variable appetite, home blood glucose monitoring might prove useful so that adjustments in insulin dosage can be made daily, if needed (also see The Persistently Brittle Diabetic Feline).

Diabetic Cats and Urinary Tract Infections

Several studies have documented a relatively high incidence of UTIs in diabetic cats. One retrospective study reviewed medical records of 141 diabetic cats that had urine obtained for culture by cystocentesis. Urinary tract infection was identified in 18 of 141 diabetic cats (13%),[13] which was similar to another retrospective study in 57 diabetic cats (12%).[14] Interestingly, the latter study reported that many of the cats with a UTI had no clinical signs associated with the lower urinary tract or changes in the laboratory work indicative of

infection. Therefore, it remains prudent to consider running a complete urinalysis, including sediment examination and culture (regardless of sediment findings), in any cat presented with difficult-to-control diabetes. *Escherichia coli* was the most common isolate (67%) in one study,[13] and female cats were at increased risk (prevalence odds ratio 3.7).

Dealing with Patients That Need Diabetogenic Drugs

In some diabetic cats, the use of diabetogenic drugs (e.g., glucocorticoids) can stand in the way of treatment success. Examples include cats needing immunomodulation for treatment of IBD, neoplasia, atopy, or asthma. Simply ignoring the need for treatment of such comorbidities is often not an option, and cessation of the interfering drugs would result in unacceptable quality-of-life consequences. Box 19-9

BOX 19-9   Strategies for Managing a Diabetic Cat Receiving a Diabetogenic Drug

Case Example: "Basal-Bolus" Dosing

Smudge is a 12-year-old, 4.5 kg, male, neutered, domestic shorthair cat diagnosed with diabetes mellitus 2 months earlier. Smudge was started on a low carbohydrate (<7% of metabolizable energy) wet diet (¾ can BID, 12 hours apart) as well as insulin glargine 1 unit BID. Although the clinical signs improved (especially polyuria and polydipsia), the insulin dose was gradually increased on the basis of a combination of some remaining clinical signs and blood glucose curve data obtained by home testing.

The following curve was generated when Smudge was on 3 units of insulin glargine BID. At this stage, Smudge was reported to show polyuria and polydipsia particularly during the few hours immediately after food in both the morning and evening.

Time and Details of Interventions	Blood Glucose (Ear Prick) (mmol/L)
8 AM: ¾ can food + 3 units insulin glargine	9.5 (171.2 mg/dL)
10 AM	19.1 (344.1 mg/dL)
12 PM	16.3 (293.7 mg/dL)
2 PM	11.1 (200.0 mg/dL)
4 PM	8.3 (149.6 mg/dL)
6 PM	5.2 (93.7 mg/dL)
8 PM: ¾ can food + 3 units insulin glargine	9.1 (163.9 mg/dL)

Interpretation

The blood glucose curve was repeated to verify its consistency and gave a similar result. The cat was spending a significant amount of time above the renal threshold for glucose, which would explain the owner's perception of remaining polyuria/polydipsia. This seemed to be especially the case immediately after feeding. Given a nadir of 5.2 mmol/L (93.7 mg/dL), increasing the insulin glargine dose further could have elicited hypoglycemia, and it might not have provided the insulin action seemingly needed immediately after eating. Changing Smudge to a different feeding regimen, such as *ad libitum* eating or grazing

(eating multiple small meals throughout the day) was discussed—although deemed unworkable according to the owner. Changing insulin glargine to porcine lente insulin (Caninsulin/Vetsulin, MSD Animal Health) was attempted, although it resulted in a similar problem.

New Treatment Plan

In order to provide exogenous insulin activity immediately after feeding, Smudge was then started on a "basal-bolus" regimen, receiving initially 0.1 unit/kg of neutral insulin (Actrapid, Novo Nordisk) and 2 units (total dose) of insulin glargine BID at time of his meal.

Outcome

After 1 week, a blood glucose curve (see the following table) suggested an increase in neutral insulin to be beneficial. Smudge was reassessed a week later through a home blood glucose curve and assessment of clinical signs. The postprandial polyuria/polydipsia had resolved, and the blood glucose curve data are shown here. Smudge was, therefore, continued on this regimen.

Time and Details of Interventions	Blood Glucose (Ear Prick) (mmol/L)
8 AM: ¾ can food + 2 units insulin glargine + 1 unit of neutral insulin (Actrapid, Novo Nordisk)	10.1 (181.9 mg/dL)
10 AM	8.3 (149.6 mg/dL)
12 PM	9.5 (171.2 mg/dL)
2 PM	9.1 (163.9 mg/dL)
4 PM	6.7 (120.7 mg/dL)
6 PM	9.3 (167.6 mg/dL)
8 PM: ¾ can food + 2 units insulin glargine + 1 unit of neutral insulin (Actrapid, Novo Nordisk)	10.3 (185.6 mg/dL)

BID, twice daily; *IBD,* inflammatory bowel disease.

highlights some of the strategies that can be used to be successful in treating the comorbidity and the diabetes.

It is also important to realize that some patients show better diabetic control when receiving a diabetogenic drug than without it, which is likely because their untreated comorbidity causes more interference (i.e., through variable insulin sensitivity or inappetence) than the diabetogenic treatment.

Other Types of Diabetes Mellitus

Clinicians should also ensure that the initial diagnosis of type 2 diabetes mellitus in the cat was in fact correct. If not, the subsequent treatment with insulin could often prove difficult. This is especially important when considering the high prevalence of hypersomatotropism or acromegaly in the cat, because such cats could phenotypically look like any other type 2 diabetic cat, especially in the beginning of the disease process.[15,16] The classical acromegalic cat can indeed display broad facial features (Figure 19-4), although this will only become apparent after a period of chronic overexposure to growth hormone (usually produced by a pituitary adenoma) and growth hormone-induced insulin-like growth factor-1 (IGF-1). Additionally, even after such chronic exposure, these gradual changes can be subtle or difficult to recognize by those in daily contact with the cat. Therefore, underdiagnosis of hypersomatotropism-induced diabetes mellitus is common. A screening study conducted in the United Kingdom revealed that 32% of diabetic cats have a serum IGF-1 concentration consistent with presence of hypersomatotropism (or acromegaly).[17] The majority (94%) of these cats with high IGF-1 values were subsequently proven to have a pituitary mass,

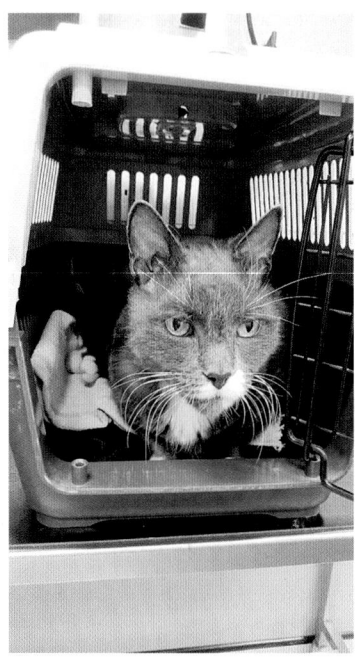

Figure 19-4: A diabetic cat that presented for evaluation of true insulin resistance, subsequently diagnosed with hypersomatotropism. This cat shows the typical broad facial features, although most cats with hypersomatotropism look like any other diabetic cat.

providing further evidence that acromegaly is a common cause of diabetes in cats. A separate study conducted in the United States also highlighted the potential for a high prevalence of hypersomatotropism among diabetic cats.[18] The exact prevalence of the disease among diabetic felines will vary according to the study methods and perhaps also according to geography, although it seems safe to say that it is a common explanation for difficult-to-control diabetes in the cat.

Given this significant prevalence, the author currently advocates screening diabetic cats for hypersomatotropism, just as the author screens for UTIs. The disease should definitely be excluded when the diabetes proves difficult to control in a cat. Weight gain in an uncontrolled diabetic cat, instead of the expected weight loss, is another strong indicator that hypersomatotropism might be present. Determination of serum IGF-1 appears a useful screening tool, although false-negatives can be seen if exogenous insulin has not been started or has been given for less than 6 weeks.[16] Rare false-positives have also been recorded, though an IGF-1 more than 1000 ng/mL was associated with a 94% chance of hypersomatotropism with one particular assay.[8,18]

Fortunately, specific treatment options are increasingly available for hypersomatotropism in the cat, which help turn the difficult diabetic into a well-controlled diabetic or even a non-diabetic. Hypophysectomy is particularly a treatment modality of note here with high diabetic remission rates reported. Pituitary radiotherapy and a new somatostatin analogue called *pasireotide* (Signifor, Novartis) represent the next best treatment modalities, which can also lead to reduced insulin requirements and diabetic remission in some cats.[16]

Spontaneous hyperadrenocorticism-induced diabetes mellitus seems rare among cats, although this condition does represent another situation through which difficult-to-control diabetes can arise. When hyperadrenocorticism does occur, 80% will subsequently develop diabetes mellitus.[16,19-22] Iatrogenic feline hyperadrenocorticism is also rare, certainly less common than it is in dogs. The typical cases of feline hyperadrenocorticism can be identified through their excessive or variable need for insulin and typical physical examination findings, which may include fragile skin (Figures 19-5 and 19-6), muscle wasting, poor wound healing, bruising, and coat changes (see Figure 19-5). A dexamethasone suppression test (using 0.1 mg/kg of dexamethasone intravenously) is generally accepted to be the most useful diagnostic test for this condition, because the adrenocorticotropic hormone stimulation test lacks diagnostic test sensitivity in cats. Nevertheless, given the potential for any concurrent illness to cause false-positive pituitary-adrenal testing (including all causes of uncontrolled diabetes), clinicians should be cautious to avoid overdiagnosing this rare condition. Adrenal and pituitary imaging might improve diagnostic accuracy in suspect cases. Treatment with adrenalectomy (bilateral adrenalectomy for pituitary-dependent diseases, unilateral for adrenal-dependent forms), hypophysectomy, radiotherapy (for pituitary-dependent forms), or trilostane can improve and sometimes, if caught early, cure the diabetes mellitus in a good proportion of cases. Given the rarity of this condition,

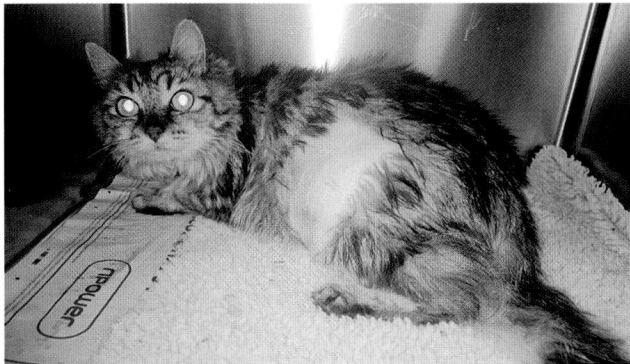

Figure 19-5: A diabetic cat that presented for evaluation of variable insulin sensitivity (brittle diabetes), subsequently diagnosed with pituitary-dependent hyperadrenocorticism. Clues hinting toward this ultimate diagnosis are apparent in the rough hair coat, lack of hair regrowth after clipping for an abdominal ultrasound, and pronounced muscle wastage.

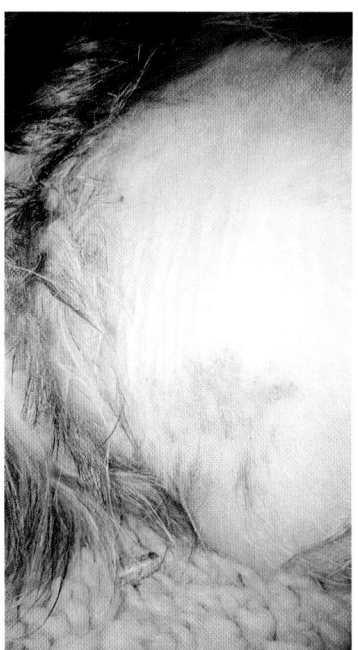

Figure 19-6: The same diabetic cat as in Figure 19-5. Closer inspection of the skin revealed it to be excessively thin.

exact numbers on treatment success are, unfortunately, hard to provide.

The Persistently Brittle Diabetic Cat

In a proportion of diabetic cats, no specific underlying cause can be found for the variable insulin requirements. Additionally, a proportion of diabetic cats will have a documented comorbidity or comorbidities that cannot be cured or have frequent flare-ups. Finally, in an individual cat, beta-cell function can appear to be better or worse, depending on the time at which it is assessed; the same can be true for the cat's insulin sensitivity. Therefore, it is logical that some cats need different insulin doses at different times in their life after diagnosis of their diabetes mellitus. This can lead to the situation where the same insulin dose leads to hypoglycemia one week and underdosing the next.

Brittle diabetes is the term used for this situation in which frequent hypoglycemia and labile glycemic control develop. In human medicine, the term is reserved for those cases in which the instability, whatever its cause, results in disruption of life and often recurrent or prolonged hospitalization.[23] It is most commonly seen in human patients with type 1 diabetes that have little or no preserved beta cell function. A comparable situation can arise in feline diabetic management, resulting in an extremely frustrating situation both for clinician and cat owner. When dose adjustments are needed on a very frequent basis, clients' finances often also become a factor and regular practice visits may not be possible.

If the underlying cause for the brittle diabetes cannot be identified despite the clinician's best efforts, a more empirical approach can be attempted. Home blood glucose monitoring can provide a solution here. Together with the attending clinician, a schedule outlining which insulin dose should be given with which preinjection blood glucose value can be devised and fine-tuned according to the individual cat's response. If home blood glucose monitoring proves not feasible or desirable (because of cat or owner factors), a conservative constant (twice daily) insulin dose could be decided upon, as long as quality of life is continuously monitored. Home morning urine checks for *absence* of glucose can signal overdosing and should still ideally elicit a visit to the veterinarian for blood glucose assessment. It remains inappropriate to *increase* the dose solely on the basis of urine glucose (hypoglycemia-induced hyperglycemia will also cause glucosuria, as will short duration of insulin action). When adopting such a pragmatic approach to the brittle diabetic, quality-of-life tools can prove essential to remain objective about the obtained treatment result.[1] If quality of life cannot be assured, discussions about the validity of continued treatment are indicated.

References

1. Niessen SJ, Powney S, Guitian J, et al: Evaluation of a quality-of-life tool for cats with diabetes mellitus. *J Vet Intern Med* 24:1098–1105, 2010.
2. Callegari C, Mercuriali E, Hafner M, et al: Survival time and prognostic factors in cats with newly diagnosed diabetes mellitus: 114 cases (2000–2009). *J Am Vet Med Assoc* 243:91–95, 2013.
3. Zini E, Hafner M, Osto M, et al: Predictors of clinical remission in cats with diabetes mellitus. *J Vet Intern Med* 24:1314–1321, 2010.
4. Zini E, Osto M, Franchini M, et al: Hyperglycaemia but not hyperlipidaemia causes beta cell dysfunction and beta cell loss in the domestic cat. *Diabetologia* 52:336–346, 2009.
5. Pretty CG, Le Compte AJ, Chase JG, et al: Variability of insulin sensitivity during the first

4 days of critical illness: implications for tight glycemic control. *Ann Intensive Care* 2:17, 2012.

6. Makimattila S, Virkamaki A, Groop PH, et al: Chronic hyperglycemia impairs endothelial function and insulin sensitivity via different mechanisms in insulin-dependent diabetes mellitus. *Circulation* 94:1276–1282, 1996.

7. Forcada Y, German AJ, Noble PJ, et al: Determination of serum fPLI concentrations in cats with diabetes mellitus. *J Feline Med Surg* 10:480–487, 2008.

8. Niessen SJ: Feline acromegaly: an essential differential diagnosis for the difficult diabetic. *J Feline Med Surg* 12:15–23, 2010.

9. Scott-Moncrieff CR, Moore GE, Coe J, et al: Characteristics of commercially manufactured and compounded protamine zinc insulin. *J Am Vet Med Assoc* 240:600–605, 2012.

10. Alt N, Kley S, Haessig M, et al: Day-to-day variability of blood glucose concentration curves generated at home in cats with diabetes mellitus. *J Am Vet Med Assoc* 230:1011–1017, 2007.

11. Shoelson SE, Lee J, Goldfine AB: Inflammation and insulin resistance. *J Clin Invest* 116:1793–1801, 2006.

12. Williamson RT: On the treatment of glycosuria and diabetes mellitus with sodium salicylate. *Br Med J* 1:760–762, 1901.

13. Bailiff NL, Nelson RW, Feldman EC, et al: Frequency and risk factors for urinary tract infection in cats with diabetes mellitus. *J Vet Intern Med* 20:850–855, 2006.

14. Mayer-Roenne B, Goldstein RE, Erb HN: Urinary tract infections in cats with hyperthyroidism, diabetes mellitus and chronic kidney disease. *J Feline Med Surg* 9:124–132, 2007.

15. Lamb CR, Ciasca TC, Mantis P, et al: Computed tomographic signs of acromegaly in 68 diabetic cats with hypersomatotropism. *J Feline Med Surg* 16(2):99–108, 2014.

16. Niessen SJ, Church DB, Forcada Y: Hypersomatotropism, acromegaly, and hyperadrenocorticism and feline diabetes mellitus. *Vet Clin North Am Small Anim Pract* 43:319–350, 2013.

17. Niessen SJ, Petrie G, Gaudiano F, et al: Feline acromegaly: an underdiagnosed endocrinopathy? *J Vet Intern Med* 21:899–905, 2007.

18. Berg RI, Nelson RW, Feldman EC, et al: Serum insulin-like growth factor-I concentration in cats with diabetes mellitus and acromegaly. *J Vet Intern Med* 21:892–898, 2007.

19. Feldman EC, Nelson RW: Hyperadrenocorticism in cats (Cushing's syndrome). In Feldman EC, Nelson RW, editors: *Canine and feline endocrinology and reproduction*, St Louis, 2004, Saunders/Elsevier, pp 358–393.

20. Nelson RW, Feldman EC, Smith MC: Hyperadrenocorticism in cats: seven cases (1978–1987). *J Am Vet Med Assoc* 193:245–250, 1988.

21. Watson PJ, Herrtage ME: Hyperadrenocorticism in six cats. *J Small Anim Pract* 39:175–184, 1998.

22. Peterson M: Feline hyperadrenocorticism. In Mooney CM, Peterson ME, editors: *BSAVA manual of canine and feline endocrinology*, Quedgeley, Gloucester, 2012, BSAVA, pp 190–198.

23. Vantyghem MC, Press M: Management strategies for brittle diabetes. *Ann Endocrinol (Paris)* 67:287–296, 2006.

Continuous Glucose Monitoring in Cats with Diabetes

Amy DeClue and Charles E. Wiedmeyer

Monitoring glycemic control in the cat can be challenging because of the confounding issue of stress-induced hyperglycemia. Several techniques have been developed to circumvent this issue, including the use of central venous catheters, capillary blood sampling, pet owner-performed glucose curves in a home environment, and measurement of long-term markers of glucose homeostasis, such as serum fructosamine. Unfortunately, none of these techniques provides an optimum method for evaluation of glycemic control in cats. Continuous glucose monitoring (CGM) is a new technique for assessing glycemic control, and it could circumvent many issues associated with traditional methods of glycemic evaluation.

CONTINUOUS GLUCOSE MONITORING METHODOLOGY

There are several types of continuous glucose monitoring systems (CGMSs) available commercially (Table 20-1). Only the MiniMed Gold and Guardian Real-Time CGMSs have been critically evaluated in the cat; thus, this chapter focuses on the use of those particular monitors.[1-6] In addition, the i-Pro CGMS, which has effectively replaced the MiniMed Gold CGMS and has the equivalent sensor, methodology, and calibration algorithm, works well for the cat in the authors' experience. The MiniMed Gold CGMS and i-Pro CGMS record interstitial glucose concentrations, but those data are unavailable until the sensor is detached and the information is downloaded onto a computer. In contrast, the Guardian Real-Time CGMS allows for documentation of interstitial glucose concentrations every 5 minutes in real time.

MiniMed Gold, i-Pro, and Guardian Real-Time CGMSs all consist of a flexible electrode sensor, recording or transmitting device, docking station, computer, and appropriate software. The sensor is embedded in an over-the-needle catheter system to allow placement in the subcutaneous space. The MiniMed Gold CGMS recording device is approximately the size of a deck of cards, whereas the i-Pro CGMS recording device is approximately the size of a silver dollar (Figure 20-1). Thus, the major advantage of the i-Pro over the MiniMed Gold is the smaller size of the monitor. The Guardian Real-Time CGMS has a transmitter that attaches to the

sensor that is similar in size to the i-Pro monitor. The transmitter sends a signal to the monitor (again approximately the size of a deck of cards), which provides a real-time display of the interstitial glucose concentration. The monitor must be kept within a tight radius (<1.5 m [<5 ft]) of the transmitter.

The CGMS sensor is an amperometric device designed to measure glucose in the subcutaneous interstitial fluid. The sensor consists of an electroenzymatic three-electrode cell by which a constant potential is maintained between a working electrode and a reference electrode.[7] Glucose concentration is detected by the sensor, based on the generation of hydrogen peroxide from the reaction of glucose and oxygen with the enzyme glucose oxidase[7,8] (Figure 20-2). Oxidation of hydrogen peroxide results in the generation of an electrical signal that is recorded by a recording device.[7]

The sensor is enclosed in the catheter section. It consists of a side window with an electrode covered by a polyurethane membrane. The polyurethane membrane is glucose diffusion-limited to allow for a linear relationship between the glucose concentration and the sensor current. This reaction results in an electrical signal that is converted to a glucose concentration via a mathematical model. The interstitial glucose concentration is recorded in milligrams per deciliter every 10 seconds and is reported as the mean interstitial glucose concentration every 5 minutes.

The relationship between interstitial and plasma glucose concentrations is best described using a two-compartment model. Capillary plasma is separated from the interstitial fluid by the capillary wall barrier. Interstitial fluid glucose concentrations are dependent on the rate of diffusion of glucose across the capillary membrane and then clearance of glucose from the interstitium via insulin-mediated uptake by cells. In most resting situations, glucose uptake by cells has minimal impact on interstitial glucose concentrations; therefore, the predominant determinate of interstitial glucose concentration is diffusion from the capillary plasma. Movement of glucose into the interstitium is not immediate; in cats, there is median delay in equilibration of approximately 11.4 minutes (range 8.8 to 19.7 minutes) after a bolus of dextrose has been administered intravenously (IV).[4] The delay in equilibration is unlikely to be clinically important in most situations unless rapid and dramatic changes in blood glucose are expected.

Table 20-1 Specifications of Available Continuous Glucose Monitoring Systems*

Specifications	MiniMed Gold*	Guardian Real-Time*	i-Pro*	GlucoDay*	FreeStyle Navigator*	Seven Plus
Company	Medtronic	Medtronic	Medtronic	Menarini Diagnostics	Abbott	Dexcom
Availability	FDA approved; no longer manufactured	FDA approved	FDA approved	EU approved; not FDA approved	FDA approved	FDA approved
Evaluated in veterinary patients	Yes	Yes	No	Yes	No	No
Technology	Amperometric electrochemical sensor; glucose oxidase	Amperometric electrochemical sensor; glucose oxidase	Amperometric electrochemical sensor; glucose oxidase	Amperometric microdialysis fiber; glucose oxidase	Amperometric electrochemical sensor; glucose oxidase	Amperometric electrochemical sensor; glucose oxidase
Sensor/transmitter weight	N/A	79 g (2.8 oz)	79 g (2.8 oz)	N/A	13.61 g (0.48 oz)	6.7 g (0.24 oz)
Transmitter/sensor size (L × W × H)	N/A	4.2 × 3.6 × 0.9 cm (1.64 × 1.4 × 0.37 in)	4.2 × 3.6 × 0.9 cm (1.64 × 1.4 × 0.37 in)	N/A	5.2 × 3.1 × 1.1 cm (2.5 × 1.23 × 0.43 in)	3.8 × 2.3 × 1.0 cm (1.5 × 0.9 × 0.4 in)
Monitor weight	113 g (4 oz)	114 g (4 oz)	N/A	245 g (8.6 oz)	100 g (3.5 oz)	100 g (3.5 oz)
Monitor size (L × W × H)	9.1 × 2.3 × 7.1 cm (3.6 × 0.9 × 2.8 in)	8.1 × 2.0 × 5.1 cm (3.2 × 0.8 × 2 in)	N/A	11 × 2.5 × 7.5 cm (4.3 × 1 × 3 in)	8.1 × 2.0 × 5.1 cm (2.5 × 3.2 × 0.9 in)	11.4 × 5.8 × 2.2 cm (4.5 × 2.3 × 0.85 in)
Recording range	40-400 mg/dL (2.2-22.2 mmol/L)	40-400 mg/dL (2.2-22.2 mmol/L)	40-400 mg/dL (2.2-22.2 mmol/L)	20-600 mg/dL (1.1-33.3 mmol/L)	40-400 mg/dL (2.2-22.2 mmol/L)	40-400 mg/dL (2.2-22.2 mmol/L)
Real-time display	No	Yes	No	Yes	Yes	Yes

Retrospective analysis	Yes	Yes	Yes	Yes	Yes	Yes
Wireless transmission	No	Yes	No	Yes	Yes	Yes
Wireless transmission range	N/A	23 m (10 ft)	N/A	N/A	3 m (10 ft)	1.5 m (5 ft)
Sensor needle insertion size	24 gauge	22 gauge (Sof-sensor) 27 gauge (Enlite sensor)	24 gauge	18 gauge	21 gauge	26 gauge
Sensor life	72 h	72 h (Sof-sensor) 144 h (Enlite sensor)	72 h (Sof-sensor) 144 h (Enlite sensor)	48 h	120 h	168 h
Sensor initialization period	1 h	2 h	1 h	1 h	2 h	2 h
Calibration	Two to three times per 24 h	2 h after insertion, within the next 6 h, then every 12 h	1 and 3 h after insertion, then minimum of once every 12 h	Minimum of one time point per 48 h, two if used in real time	10 h after insertion, within the next 2-4 h, then every 12 h	Two calibrations, 2 h after insertion, then every 12 h
Recording frequency	Data collected every 10 sec; mean value reported every 5 min	Data collected every 10 sec; mean value reported every 5 min	Data collected every 10 sec; mean value reported every 5 min	Data collected every 1 sec; mean value reported every 3 min	Data collected every 10 sec; mean value reported every 5 min	Data collected every 10 sec; mean value reported every 5 min

From Surman S, Fleeman L: Continuous glucose monitoring in small animals. *Vet Clin Small Anim* 43:394-395, 2013.
EU, European Union; *FDA,* U.S. Food and Drug Administration: *N/A,* information not available.
*Based on manufacturer's specifications.

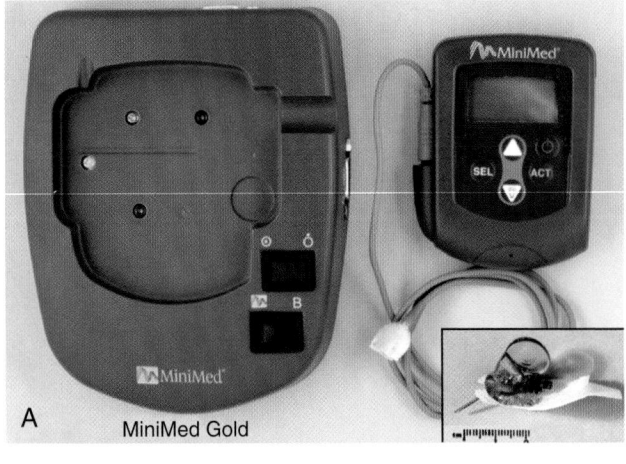

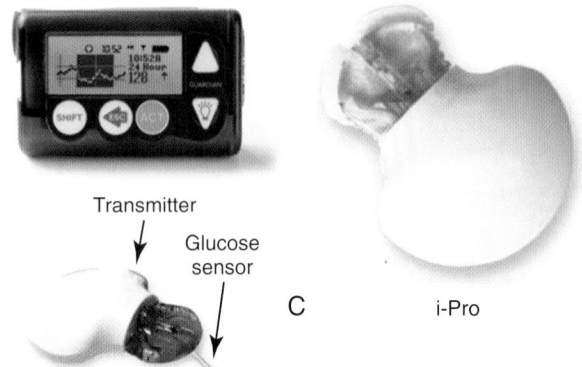

Figure 20-1: Continuous glucose monitoring systems (CGMSs) that have been used in cats. **A,** MiniMed Gold CGMS. **B,** Guardian Real-Time CGMS. **C,** i-Pro CGMS.

Interstitial glucose concentrations have excellent correlation with blood glucose concentrations. Using the MiniMed Gold, interstitial glucose concentrations are highly correlated with blood glucose concentrations in both healthy ($r = 0.974$) and diabetic ($r = 0.932$) cats.[5,8] The range of glucose detection for the CGMS is 40 to 400 mg/dL for the MiniMed Gold, Guardian Real-Time, and i-Pro CGMSs. Interstitial glucose concentrations can be evaluated for up to 72 hours with one sensor. Newer sensor technology has led to development of sensors (Enlite Sensor; Medtronic) that have lifespans of 144 hours in human patients. However, these sensors have not yet been evaluated in cats.

PLACEMENT AND CALIBRATION

The sensor can be placed in any accessible subcutaneous space where there is minimal risk for tissue movement. Typically used placement sites include the area between the shoulder blades on the dorsal aspect of the neck, the lateral chest wall, or the lateral knee fold. In a study of 40 cats, initialization was successful in nine out of 10 neck sensors, 15 out of 20 chest wall sensors, and three out of 10 knee fold sensors.[2] Compared to a reference portable blood glucose meter, sensors placed in the dorsal neck were the least likely to result

in erroneous readings.[2] Thus, the space between the shoulder blades on the dorsal aspect of the neck is the preferred site unless there are factors that would preclude use of that area.

The sensors are disposable, and a new sensor is required for each patient. To place the sensor, the fur should be clipped and the skin cleaned with isopropyl alcohol (see Figure 20-2). Once the skin is dry, the small, flexible sensor is inserted into the subcutaneous tissues using a needle stylet. The stylet is then removed, and the external portion of the sensor is attached to the skin with cyanoacrylate adhesive, tape, suture, or bandaging material. In the authors' experience, cyanoacrylate adhesive works best for sensor attachment because it minimizes displacement. Additionally, a bioclusive covering can be placed over the top of the sensor as added security. Because the insertion needle is small (approximately 24 gauge), sensor insertion is minimally invasive and well tolerated.

Once the sensor is placed and secured to the cat, it is attached to the recording or transmitting device. The recording or transmitting device should also be secured to the cat using cyanoacrylate adhesive, tape, suture, or bandaging material. The i-Pro sensor and Guardian Real-Time transmitter can easily be secured to the cat using cyanoacrylate. The MiniMed Gold monitor can be attached using bandaging material to create a backpack-like wrap. Guardian Real-Time monitor can be attached either to the cat using the backpack method or, for in-hospital use, to the cat's cage door or wall.

After successful sensor placement, one must first wait for an initialization period of 1 to 2 hours and then calibrate the instrument by measuring a blood glucose concentration. The first calibration point should be collected during the first 2 hours after completion of the initialization period. Additional blood glucose measurements for calibration purposes should ideally be performed every 8 hours, with samples collected during periods in which the blood glucose concentration would be expected to be within the glucose detection range of the CGMS (i.e., 40 to 400 mg/dL). In some cases, two calibration points per day may be adequate to maintain appropriate accuracy, although the authors recommend performing three calibrations per day whenever possible.[9]

This calibration data (i.e., blood glucose concentrations) is entered directly into the monitor for the MiniMed Gold and the Guardian Real-Time CGMSs. For these devices, care should be taken to use a rapid and accurate means of glucose evaluation (i.e., handheld glucometer) for calibration points and to enter the calibration data as soon as possible. Delays between blood glucose determination and entry into the CGM should be avoided, because discordance between the measured blood glucose and the interstitial glucose concentrations will result in an error code from the monitor. Owners can be trained to perform at-home blood glucose measurements and to enter this calibration data themselves. Instructional materials should be provided to the client, including a troubleshooting guide (Figure 20-3).

For the i-Pro CGMS, all the calibration points are entered into the computer after the monitoring is completed. Thus,

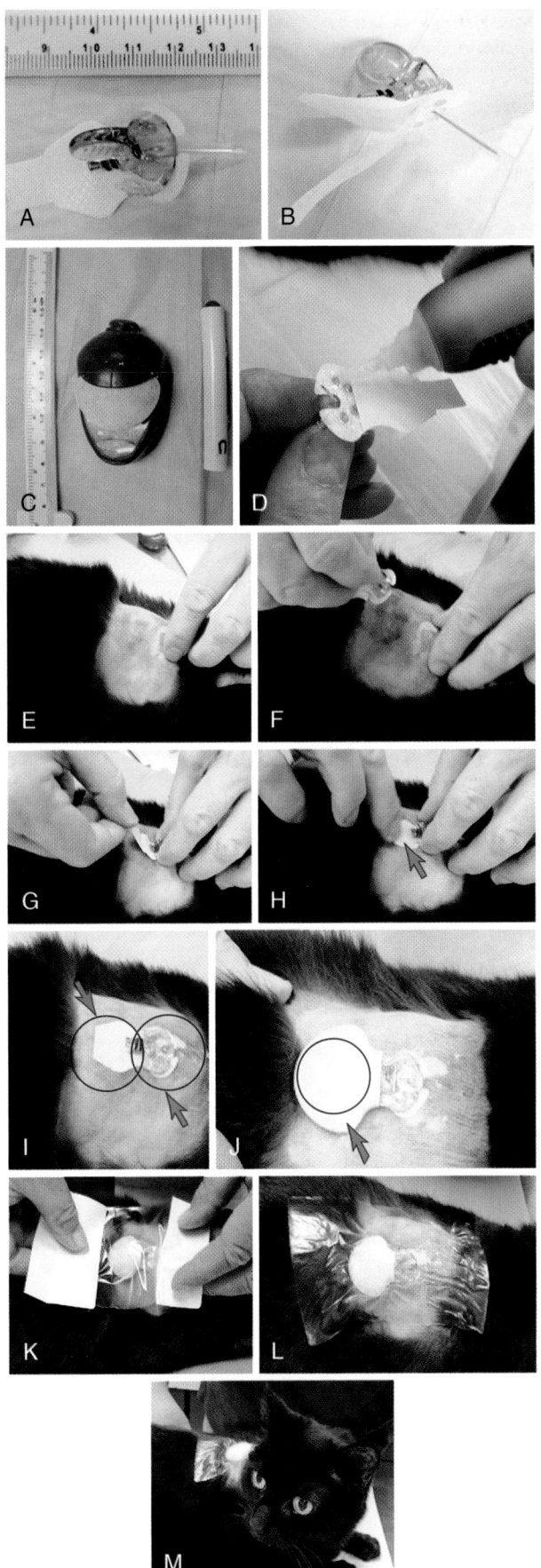

Figure 20-2: Placement of the Continuous Glucose Monitoring System (CGMS) i-Pro Sensor. The disposable sensor (**A** and **B**) and i-Pro monitor (**C**) are small, which facilitate attachment to the cat. The sensors are disposable, and a new sensor is required for each patient. **D,** To place the sensor, the fur should be clipped, and the skin cleaned with isopropyl alcohol. **E,** Once the skin is dry, the small, flexible sensor is inserted into the subcutaneous tissues using a needle stylet. **F,** The stylet is then removed. **G to J,** The sensor and monitor, once attached, are secured with cyanoacrylate adhesive, as indicated by the *red circles* and *blue arrows.* **K** and **L,** Additionally, a bioclusive covering can be placed over the top of the sensor as added security. **M,** The CGMS is well tolerated by cats.

an accurate record of all blood glucose values measured for calibration purposes and time collected should be kept (Figure 20-4). For at-home monitoring, a client information sheet should be provided to the owner so that blood glucose concentrations, food consumption, exercise, and insulin administration can be documented. After the sensor is placed, interstitial glucose concentrations can be monitored for up to 72 continuous hours.

At the end of the monitoring period, the disposable sensor is removed and the recorder is synced with a computer. Software is provided to allow analysis of the measured glucose concentrations. Feeding, exercise, insulin administration, and other notes can be entered into the software as part of the animal's record. The software generates graphs of single- or multiple-day CGM curves that can be inserted into the medical record and shared with the cat's owner. Additional analyses (e.g., mean interstitial glucose concentration, minimum and maximum interstitial glucose concentrations, standard deviation of glucose values, and area under the curve) can also be performed daily or for the entire monitoring period. Advanced features, such as determination of premeal and postmeal average or minimum and maximum glucose concentrations, the area under the curve for time that glucose concentrations are above or below a predetermined high or low limit, and the number of high or low glucose excursions, can also be calculated.

LIMITATIONS

There are some limitations to the use of the CGM. The range of glucose detection of the CGMS is 40 to 400 mg/dL for the models that have been validated for the cat. Concentrations above or below the range of detection are recorded as 400 or 40 mg/dL, respectively. As a result, the CGMS evaluation is not helpful for diabetic patients with persistent, severe hyperglycemia (>400 mg/dL) or severe hypoglycemia (<40 mg/dL). However, from a clinical perspective, persistent hyperglycemia or hypoglycemia should signal a need for a major change in insulin therapy; and thus, CGMS may still have value in such cases.

Recording of glucose concentrations can be interrupted by detachment of the sensor from the skin or from the recorder

MiniMed Gold Continuous Glucose Monitoring Instructions
University of Missouri, College of Veterinary Medicine

Calibration after attachment

1. After attachment, the CGMS needs an hour long initialization period. Following this time, a blood glucose value needs to be entered into the instrument. This is the first calibration point. The process of entering a calibration point in the instrument is as follows:
   a. Obtain a blood glucose value using a handheld glucometer.
   b. The result needs to be entered into the instrument immediately
   c. Press the "SEL" button and the display will show a field called "Meter BG" with dashes (or the last glucose value entered) above this.
   d. Press the "ACT" button and the dashes or numbers will flash.
   e. Enter the blood glucose value by using the up or down button.
   f. Once you have reached the value press the "ACT" button to accept the data.
   g. A field will display "Cal" with "Yes" flashing above.
   h. Press "ACT" a final time and the value will be accepted.
   i. After this, only the time will be showing in the upper left hand corner.
2. **The instrument needs to be calibrated a minimum of THREE times every calendar day the instrument is in place.** More calibration points can be entered in addition to the three at any time.
3. The first blood glucose value entered follow initialization is the first calibration point, two more are necessary before the animal leaves the hospital. The next two can be entered at any time after the first post initialization calibration point. Preferably, the next two are spaced several hours apart. It does not matter if the calibration points are taken before or after insulin/feeding/exercise.
4. On subsequent days, a minimum of **THREE** calibration points need to be entered into the instrument per instructions above. Preferably, first calibration point first thing in the morning, one midday and the last in the evening. Calibration points should be taken at different times of the day and not on a regular schedule.

If the instrument fails

1. If the instrument starts to beep, it means there is a calibration error or has become disconnected. The only thing to do at this point is to take the instrument off and try again.
2. Once the instrument starts to beep, it will not stop or can be shut off without the proper commands. **DO NOT** start pressing buttons or remove the battery to end the beeping.
3. To end the beeping: press "SEL" then "ACT" once than repeat, "SEL" and "ACT". This should make the instrument display the time only. Once this is seen, the instrument can be turned off.
4. To turn off the instrument: press the red power button and the screen will display "confirm" press "ACT" and the instrument will be turned off. All the previous data has been stored at this point and can be downloaded.

To turn off the instrument following the monitoring period

1. To turn off the instrument: press the red power button and the screen will display "confirm" press "ACT" and the instrument will be turned off.
2. DO NOT remove the battery.

To remove the instrument

1. The instrument should be turned off per instructions above.
2. The probe in the skin is held in place by superglue. To remove, just quickly jerk the probe from the skin (like taking tape off your skin).
3. Send the instrument back to the clinic for downloading of data.

Additional notes

1. It is important to note each day when the animal at what time the insulin was given, the dose and when the animal was fed and exercised. This information is important for properly interpreting the results.
2. To obtain the data stored in the instrument, it must be downloaded using the proper software and docking station.

Figure 20-3: MiniMed Gold continuous glucose monitoring instruction sheet for clients.

Continuous Glucose Monitor Information Sheet

University of Missouri, Veterinary Medical Teaching Hospital

Today, we placed a continuous glucose monitor. The procedure involved shaving a small area on your pet's back and inserting the probe under the skin and then securing the monitor to the skin with glue. Your pet will need to wear this monitor for the next 3 days and you will need to perform 3 glucose readings each day with the glucometer. It is important that these readings are no more than 12 hours apart. Please document all of your readings with the designated time. We would also like for you to record food consumption (regular meals and treats), exercise and when you administer insulin.

Please return to the VMTH to have the glucose monitor removed at the end of the three day period. An appointment will be set up for you to have the monitor removed. If the glucose monitor is dislodged at any time, please collect all parts of the monitor and call your pet's doctor. It is very important that you bring all parts of the monitor with you when you return to the hospital.

Glucose readings

Date	Date	Date
Time: Glucose:	Time: Glucose:	Time: Glucose:
Time: Glucose:	Time: Glucose:	Time: Glucose:
Time: Glucose:	Time: Glucose:	Time: Glucose:

Insulin log – Below, please record the time insulin was administered each day.

Time	Time	Time

Food log – Below, please record the type of food, quantity and time the meal or treat was consumed each day

Type of food: Quantity: Time:	Type of food: Quantity: Time:	Type of food: Quantity: Time:
Type of food: Quantity: Time:	Type of food: Quantity: Time:	Type of food: Quantity: Time:

Exercise log – Below, please record when your pet exercises (going for walk, playing fetch etc.).

Time:	Time:	Time:

Figure 20-4: Continuous glucose monitoring data sheet for at-home monitoring.

unit. Occasionally, although no obvious detachment is observed, the sensor fails to read glucose concentrations. Such an event may remain undetected until the monitoring unit is downloaded onto a computer. Sensor placement and maintenance of sensors on lean cats can be more challenging than on obese cats because of failure of the sensor to remain in the interstitial tissue or because of biofouling.[3]

Generally, placement of the sensor is well tolerated, although mild bleeding or bruising of the insertion site is possible. Discomfort or mild dermatitis is possible after sensor removal, particularly if cyanoacrylate adhesive is used to attach the sensor. Typically, the dermatitis is self-limiting and resolves within 24 hours. Application of ointment to the area should be considered if the cat exhibits behavioral signs of irritation.

Other limitations include the fact that CGMS requires 1 to 2 hours of initialization before readings can be acquired, which leads to a delay in glucose evaluation for critically-ill animals. The Guardian Real-Time CGMS has a limited wireless range of 1.5 m (5 ft). Patient factors, such as dehydration or poor subcutaneous perfusion, may alter the accuracy of the CGMS. There is a brief (approximately 11 minutes) lag time between changes in blood glucose concentrations and interstitial glucose concentrations. Finally, the initial cost of the equipment may limit its use to facilities that manage a large number of diabetic patients.

CLINICAL APPLICATIONS

Home Monitoring

The CGMS enables veterinarians to interpret a glucose curve with values provided every 5 minutes, allowing a more accurate description of blood glucose fluctuations. In the authors' practice, almost all diabetic patients are monitored using the CGMS, as opposed to traditional blood glucose curves. The authors feel that it is important to send the cat home with the CGMS to avoid the confounding effects of hospitalization. Because the monitor placement procedure is quick and minimally painful and the majority of the monitoring time is spent in the animal's own home, use of the CGMS helps to circumvent inaccuracies associated with the stress of hospitalization, repeated needlesticks, dietary changes, altered activity patterns, and variations in insulin administration by hospital staff. Therefore, it represents a real-life evaluation of glucose homeostasis. Additionally, CGM reduces technical staff time, because only two to three calibration points are needed per day.

In the authors' practice, CGM is used for initial evaluation of glycemic control after initiation of insulin therapy and for periodic monitoring to confirm optimum insulin treatment. Additionally, the authors use CGM to troubleshoot the cause of poor glycemic control in cats undergoing insulin therapy. Similar to traditional glucose curves, CGM allows for assessment of the effectiveness of insulin, onset of action of insulin, duration of action of insulin, peak blood-glucose concentration, and nadir glucose concentration. The frequency of data

points allows identification of even transient hypoglycemia or hyperglycemia. CGM also gives the added advantage of longer reporting. Previous studies have demonstrated marked day-to-day and day-to-night variation in glucose curves obtained by standard methods, despite similar administration of insulin and feeding schedules.[10] Because the sensor can be left in the patient for up to 3 days, a representation of glucose control that is more accurate as compared with that of a single 12- or 24-hour monitoring period. In complex or challenging cases, repeated sensor placement allows the clinician to evaluate an even longer period to improve detection of transient problems.

When interpreting CGM curves from diabetic cats undergoing insulin therapy, it is important to consider the expected pharmacodynamics of the injected insulin preparation. Some insulin formulations, such as glargine, are designed to have peakless pharmacodynamics unlike more traditional formulations, such as neutral protamine Hagedorn (NPH) (Figure 20-5). Understanding the expected insulin pharmacodynamics helps avoid misinterpretation of insulin effectiveness. However, despite expected differences, interindividual variation in insulin pharmacodynamics is possible and should be considered when interpreting CGM curves.

One of the greatest strengths of evaluating glycemic control using CGMS is the detection of hypoglycemic events, or the Somogyi phenomenon, or both. Traditional methods of evaluating glycemic control, such as intermittent glucose curves or evaluation of serum fructosamine concentrations, often fail to identify transient hypoglycemia or nocturnal hypoglycemia. In one study of 13 hospitalized diabetic cats, CGMS was superior in detecting hypoglycemia, compared with an intermittent ear capillary blood glucose curve performed over 8 to 10 hours.[1] Insulin dose recommendations were different 30% of the time when the CGMS was compared to a traditional glucose curve, with the most common difference being recommendations for a lower insulin dosage with the CGMS.[1]

The use of a monitoring strategy that can identify hypoglycemia is particularly important in the cat. In recent years, many veterinarians have adopted the philosophy of early and aggressive glycemic control for cats with diabetes mellitus, with the goal of inducing diabetic remission. The major risk of this approach is induction of hypoglycemia; previous studies have reported that approximately 10% and 12% of cats undergoing intensive insulin therapy with either glargine or detemir, respectively, develop hypoglycemia.[11,12] Often hypoglycemia is transient or nocturnal in nature, making it challenging to identify using traditional 8- to 12-hour intermittent blood glucose curves. Hypoglycemia can result in irreversible brain damage, neurologic signs, and death. Continuous glucose monitoring could be a method to preemptively identify hypoglycemic events prior to adverse neurologic sequelae.

Additional investigation is needed to determine if CGM is a more effective means to monitor cats undergoing intensive insulin therapy and if outcome (i.e., induction of diabetic remission) is improved when CGM is used as an evaluative strategy. An additional possible strength of CGM is the

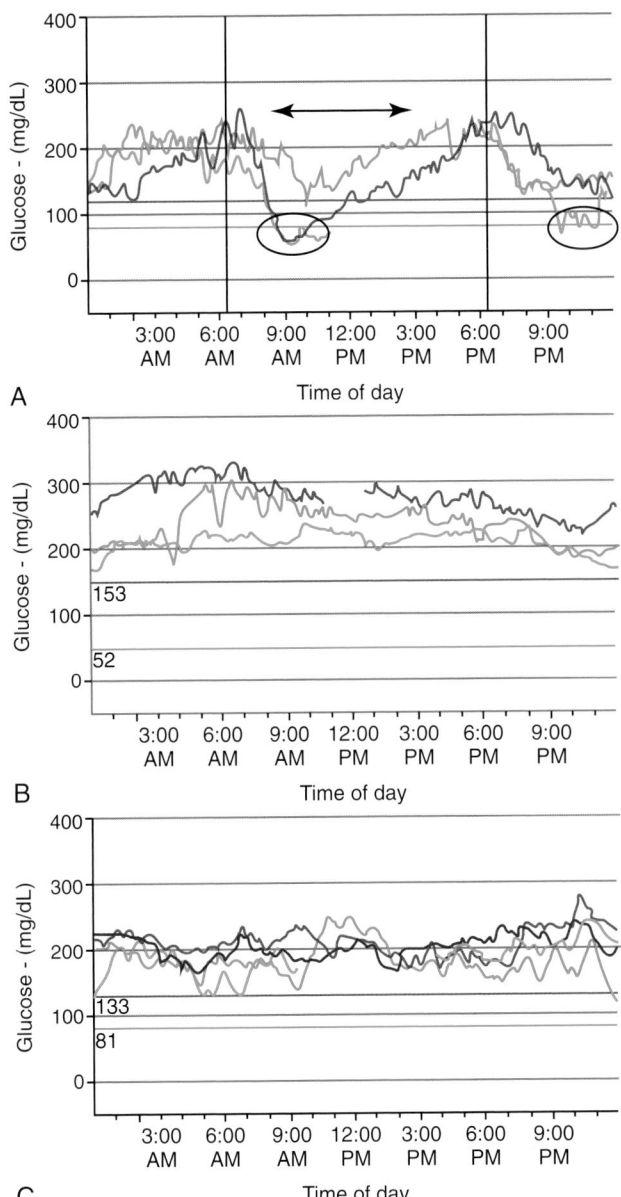

Figure 20-5: Example of Continuous Glucose Monitoring System Tracings. A, The tracings come from a 6-year-old, female spayed, domestic shorthair cat with diabetes mellitus (DM) undergoing treatment with neutral protamine Hagedorn (NPH) insulin (0.7 units/kg every 12 hours, subcutaneously [SC]) and a commercial diet designed for cats with DM. The cat was presented with signs of poor diabetic regulation, including polyuria, polydipsia, polyphagia, and weight loss. Continuous glucose monitoring (CGM) was used to assess glucose homeostasis. The duration of action *(horizontal arrow)* was inadequate, and the cat had two episodes of hypoglycemia *(circles)*. Given the limited duration of action and a need for a dose reduction to avoid hypoglycemia, the cat was transitioned to glargine (1 unit/cat every 12 hours, SC). **B,** Ten days later, the cat's clinical signs did not resolve; therefore, glucose homeostasis was assessed again using a CGM. As expected, glargine administration resulted in peakless pharmacodynamic effect; but in this case, the blood glucose concentrations were inadequately controlled. The dose of insulin was increased. **C,** Ten days later the cat's owners reported improvement in clinical signs. Repeat CGM evaluation indicated good glycemic control.

ability to determine the area under the curve or average glucose concentration over the course of a day or several days. Although there is little information about the use of these parameters in determining optimum insulin therapy, it is possible that these parameters could assist veterinarians in achieving tight glycemic control with the goal of inducing diabetic remission.

In-Hospital Monitoring

The development of the real-time CGMS, which provides a continuous display of the interstitial glucose concentration, has opened new clinical applications for CGM in the hospital setting. The system is wireless, minimizing the impact on patient mobility and necessity for patient interaction. The real-time monitor allows the clinician to detect trends and rapidly identify glucose fluctuations, while avoiding repeated phlebotomies for the patient. In studies of the Guardian Real-Time CGMS in diabetic cats, the diagnostic accuracy of CGMS was 100%, 96.1%, and 91% at normal, high, and low blood glucose concentrations, respectively, when compared to a capillary blood glucose measured via an Alpha-TRAK portable blood glucose meter.[4] The mean delay between capillary blood glucose concentration change and interstitial glucose concentration change after IV infusion of dextrose was 11.4 minutes.[4]

Continuous glucose monitoring can be used for routine in-hospital diabetic monitoring, because it reduces the need for cat handling and technician time. For routine diabetic monitoring in cats undergoing insulin therapy, use the Guardian Real-Time CGMS or retrospective evaluation with either the MiniMed Gold or i-Pro CGMS, because there is only a theoretical advantage to immediately knowing the measured glucose concentration in these patients. Many veterinarians use this in-hospital monitoring approach in situations where cat owners are unable to manage the CGMS at home.

Although CGM reduces the need for cat handling and blood collection, hospital-induced stress hyperglycemia is still possible and should be taken into account when making insulin dose adjustment decisions. For this reason, the authors prefer to perform routine diabetic monitoring in the home setting. However, for clinically ill diabetic cats that require hospitalization and more immediate evaluation of glucose homeostasis, the Guardian Real-Time CGMS provides an effective means to closely monitor interstitial glucose concentrations while minimizing patient stress and the technical demands of frequent blood collections.

One of the most useful applications of CGM in the hospital is for cats with diabetic ketoacidosis (DKA). Managing DKA in the cat can be challenging because frequent blood glucose concentration measurement is needed. Using traditional methods of repeated blood collection for glucose evaluation is associated with multiple problems including stress-induced hyperglycemia, anemia, hypovolemia, pain, tissue trauma, and bruising at the venipuncture site. The use of central venous catheters has helped circumvent stress-induced hyperglycemia, pain, and bruising, but iatrogenic anemia and hypovolemia are still possible complications. The Guardian Real-Time CGMS is an additional option to minimize the stress of repeated phlebotomy. Because blood collection is limited to two to three blood glucose samples per day, the Guardian Real-Time CGMS also eliminates concerns about iatrogenic anemia and hypovolemia related to frequent blood sampling. Blood sampling for glucose calibration points can be timed so that blood collected for electrolyte evaluation is procured concurrently. Fine-tuning of regular insulin administration via either continuous IV infusion or intermittent intramuscular injection can be performed by simply observing the display reading. Furthermore, the real-time system is wireless, so the monitor can be attached to the outside of the cat's cage and the readings can be recorded. This feature is especially appealing for fearful cats, because glucose evaluation does not require any patient interaction. In this capacity, the CGMS may be a more cost effective and less labor-intensive way to closely monitor blood glucose frequently.

The accuracy of CGMS in cats with DKA has been prospectively evaluated in one study of 11 cats. Evaluation of CGMS reading using both the Clarke and Consensus error grids showed that 96.7% and 99% of the CGMS readings were deemed clinically acceptable (Zones A and B errors).[9] However, accuracy was mildly decreased when the cat was dehydrated.[9] Body condition score and severity of ketosis and perfusion did not significantly alter the accuracy of the CGMS.[9] It is important to note that the MiniMed Gold CGMS was evaluated in this study, and not the Guardian Real-Time CGMS; however, it is likely the findings can be extrapolated to the Guardian Real-Time CGMS.[9]

Monitoring During Anesthesia

The CGMS can be used to monitor diabetic cats or cats at risk for either hyperglycemia or hypoglycemia during anesthesia. Glucose homeostatic abnormalities during anesthesia pose a substantial risk, because clinical signs are masked, possibly until hypoglycemia is severe. Because the monitor can be placed and initialized within a couple of hours, placement for emergent surgeries is feasible. Values can be recorded every 5 minutes during anesthesia, along with routine vital parameter assessment to trend changes in interstitial glucose concentrations. This frequent assessment rapidly identifies blood glucose alterations and allows the anesthetist and surgeon to make timely decisions about the use of dextrose or insulin. Additionally, the same CGMS probe can be used postoperatively for 2 to 3 days to monitor for blood glucose fluctuations.

The use of CGMS in the anesthetized cat has not been rigorously evaluated. However, the Guardian Real-Time CGMS has been previously evaluated in anesthetized dogs.[13] In this setting, the Guardian Real-Time CGMS underestimated blood glucose concentrations and inaccurately categorized 24 out of 126 sampling points as hypoglycemic.[13] Although these data are not available for cats, care should be taken when interpreting readings in the hypoglycemic range; in the anesthetized patient, hypoglycemia should be confirmed via traditional blood glucose determinations prior to institution of any therapy. Additionally, reduction in peripheral capillary perfusion related to anesthesia could alter the duration of time needed to see equilibration between blood glucose and interstitial glucose concentrations. Similarly, care should be taken when evaluating response to dextrose infusion under anesthetic conditions.

References

1. Dietiker-Moretti S, Muller C, Sieber-Ruckstuhl N, et al: Comparison of a continuous glucose monitoring system with a portable blood glucose meter to determine insulin dose in cats with diabetes mellitus. *J Vet Intern Med* 25:1084–1088, 2011.
2. Hafner M, Lutz TA, Reusch CE, et al: Evaluation of sensor sites for continuous glucose monitoring in cats with diabetes mellitus. *J Feline Med Surg* 15:117–123, 2013.
3. Hoenig M, Pach N, Thomaseth K, et al: Evaluation of long-term glucose homeostasis in lean and obese cats by use of continuous glucose monitoring. *Am J Vet Res* 73:1100–1106, 2012.
4. Moretti S, Tschuor F, Osto M, et al: Evaluation of a novel real-time continuous glucose-monitoring system for use in cats. *J Vet Intern Med* 24:120–126, 2010.
5. Ristic JM, Herrtage ME, Walti-Lauger SM, et al: Evaluation of a continuous glucose monitoring system in cats with diabetes mellitus. *J Feline Med Surg* 7:153–162, 2005.
6. Wiedmeyer CE, Johnson PJ, Cohn LA, et al: Evaluation of a continuous glucose monitoring system for use in dogs, cats, and horses. *J Am Vet Med Assoc* 223:987–992, 2003.
7. Rebrin K, Steil GM, van Antwerp WP, et al: Subcutaneous glucose predicts plasma glucose independent of insulin: implications for continuous monitoring. *Am J Physiol* 277:E561–E571, 1999.
8. Wiedmeyer CE, DeClue AE: Continuous glucose monitoring in dogs and cats. *J Vet Intern Med* 22:2–8, 2008.
9. Reineke EL, Fletcher DJ, King LG, et al: Accuracy of a continuous glucose monitoring system in dogs and cats with diabetic ketoacidosis. *J Vet Emerg Crit Care* 20:303–312, 2010.
10. Alt N, Kley S, Haessig M, et al: Day-to-day variability of blood glucose concentration curves generated at home in cats with diabetes mellitus. *J Am Vet Med Assoc* 230:1011–1017, 2007.
11. Roomp K, Rand J: Evaluation of detemir in diabetic cats managed with a protocol for intensive blood glucose control. *J Feline Med Surg* 14:566–572, 2012.
12. Roomp K, Rand J: Intensive blood glucose control is safe and effective in diabetic cats using home monitoring and treatment with glargine. *J Feline Med Surg* 11:668–682, 2009.
13. Bilicki KL, Schermerhorn T, Klocke EE, et al: Evaluation of a real-time, continuous monitor of glucose concentration in healthy dogs during anesthesia. *Am J Vet Res* 71:11–16, 2010.

Treatment of Severe, Unresponsive, or Recurrent Hyperthyroidism

Michael R. Broome and Mark E. Peterson

Most cats with hyperthyroidism can be successfully managed by any of the four established treatment options, which include use of antithyroid drugs (i.e., methimazole or carbimazole), nutritional management (i.e., low-iodine diet), surgical thyroidectomy, or radioiodine (^{131}I). Some hyperthyroid cats, however, will fail to respond to therapy or develop recurrence of hyperthyroidism after initial control. This chapter will explore the underlying causes for these treatment failures and will discuss the challenges that accompany the treatment of cats with severe or unresponsive hyperthyroidism.

FACTORS THAT MAY BE INVOLVED IN THE PATHOGENESIS OF FELINE HYPERTHYROIDISM

Hyperthyroidism is currently the most common endocrine disease in the cat. Since the recognition of hyperthyroidism in cats in 1979,[1] this disease has been diagnosed with increasing frequency and evolving global significance.[2-5] Despite more than 30 years of investigation and strong clinical suspicions that environmental and/or dietary factors contribute to its development, the exact cause(s) of feline hyperthyroidism remains unknown.[4-6] A number of potential factors have been implicated in the pathogenesis of the disease, including the feeding of commercial cat foods (e.g., canned food, especially fish flavors), use of cat litter or topical ectoparasite preparations, environmental household chemicals (e.g., polybrominated diphenyl ethers and bisphenol A), dietary goitrogens (e.g., flavonoids), and dietary iodine or selenium deficiency.[4,5]

Hyperthyroidism in cats is most similar to the human disease generally referred to as toxic nodular goiter (i.e., Plummer's disease), which is characterized by one or more thyroid nodules (adenomas) that oversecrete thyroid hormone to produce thyrotoxicosis.[6-10] Historically, chronic dietary iodine deficiency has been implicated as one of the major underlying risk factors for toxic nodular goiter in human patients.[11,12] Interestingly, low-grade iodine deficiency has also been suggested as one of the inciting causes for this condition in hyperthyroid cats.[13-15] In most patients (both human and feline), it is now clear that the added effects of other environmental or nutritional goitrogens also contribute to the disease's pathogenesis.[4,5,9,16,17]

Although dietary iodine deficiency and other goitrogens certainly can play a role in the evolution of toxic nodular goiter, the ultimate cause of this hyperthyroid disease most likely resides within the thyroid gland itself.[6,16-19] The basic lesion appears to be an intrinsic (probably genetic) capacity for autonomous growth and function of some thyroid follicular cells, leading to acquisition of new inheritable qualities by its replicating daughter cells.[20] These changes may be related to somatic mutations which do not produce malignancy *per se*, but that can alter growth and function. For example, constitutively activating mutations of the thyrotropin receptor and G-protein genes are common in both cats and humans with toxic thyroid nodules.[19,21-23] As a consequence of these mutations, chronic activation of the adenylate-cyclase-cyclic adenosine monophosphate (cAMP)-cascade takes place. This results in overexpression of the sodium iodine symporter (i.e., the iodine pump) and enhanced iodine uptake by the thyroid, as well as increased thyroglobulin synthesis, iodine oxidation, and thyroid hormone synthesis and release—all leading to hyperthyroidism.[9,18] Development of autonomous nodules in these cats is a nonreversible, gradual process, leading to the presence of thyroid adenomas and, in some cases, thyroid carcinoma.[5,6,24]

The secondary environmental and/or dietary factors mentioned earlier, however, likely enhance the continued thyroid cell growth and hyperfunction in a susceptible cat, helping to transform the normal thyroid tissue first into hyperplastic nodules and then into the adenomatous nodules (adenomas) associated with hyperthyroidism (Figure 21-1). Given our current lack of understanding of the pathogenesis of hyperthyroidism, it is highly likely that hyperthyroid cats, once diagnosed, would continue to be exposed to the environmental and dietary factors that might contribute to the onset of their disease.[4,5] Whether this continued exposure leads to the formation of new autonomous nodules from previously unaffected thyroid follicular cells or induces further growth and hyperfunction in autonomous nodular tissue that is already present is unknown. However, either of these possibilities could explain the progression of increasing thyroid nodule (goiter) size commonly seen in hyperthyroid cats over time, which ultimately leads to a more severe form of the thyrotoxicosis in these cats.

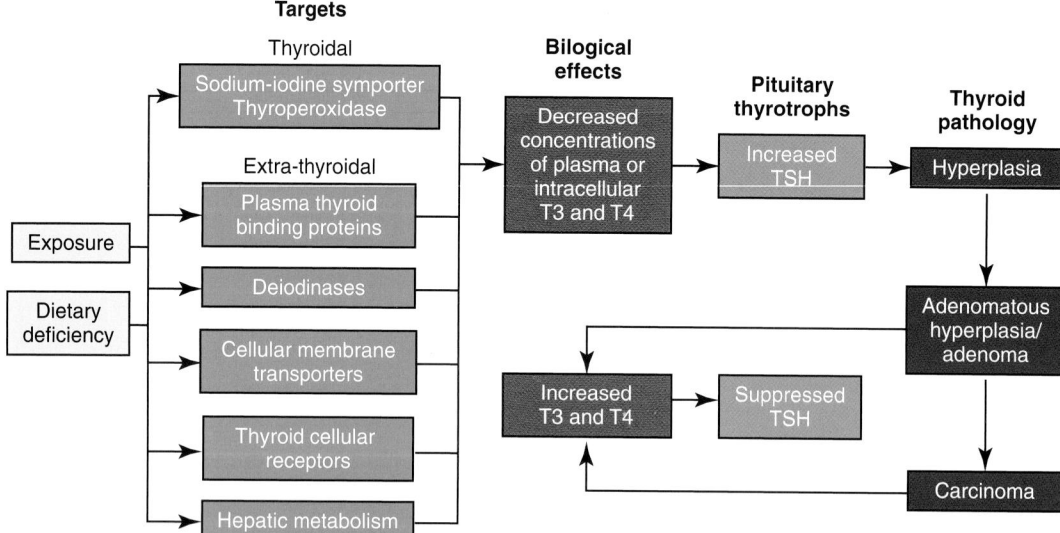

Figure 21-1: Target sites for iodine deficiency and environmental or nutritional disruption of the thyroid, leading to hyperthyroidism. The primary factor involved in development of thyroid autonomy is an inheritable defect in some thyroid follicular cells, leading to acquisition of new inheritable qualities by their replicating daughter cells, as well as somatic mutations of the thyrocytes. In susceptible cats, nutritional (e.g., low iodine) or environmental factors may initially lead to biologic effects of decreased serum thyroid hormone concentrations. This causes a lack of negative feedback (due to low circulating thyroxine [T4] and triiodothyronine [T3]) and leads to increased pituitary thyroid-stimulating hormone (TSH) secretion and thyroid hyperplasia. With time, the thyroid gland can develop gene mutations and become autonomous, resulting in pathological changes of adenomatous hyperplasia or adenoma and the clinical state of hyperthyroidism. With prolonged stimulation, malignant transformation into thyroid carcinoma can occur.

THYROID PATHOLOGY IN CATS WITH HYPERTHYROIDISM

While the exact etiology of hyperthyroidism may still be unclear, the pathologic basis for the disease is somewhat better defined. In the majority of cats that develop hyperthyroidism, the disease is caused by one or more benign autonomously functioning thyroid adenomas, sometimes referred to as adenomatous thyroid hyperplasia.[6,10,25,26] The incidence of thyroid carcinoma causing hyperthyroidism in cats is low, at least at time of diagnosis, typically being reported as less than 2% to 3%[6,27-29] (Figure 21-2).

What most veterinarians do not appreciate is that the pathology, morphology, and function of the hyperthyroid cat's thyroid tumor tissue are not static. Once the adenomatous thyroid gland develops its autonomous state, this leads to continued progression of the cat's goiter size and severity of thyrotoxicosis over time.[24] Again, the exposure to the environmental or nutritional disruptors that helped induce the cat's thyroid disease will likely be ongoing, and this also may contribute to the continued progression of the disease[5] (see Figure 21-1).

Adenomatous Hyperplasia versus Neoplasia: Is There a Difference?

As mentioned previously, the thyroid pathology associated with feline hyperthyroidism is generally benign, most often

reported as either thyroid adenomatous hyperplasia or adenoma.[6,10,25,26] Traditionally, nonneoplastic endocrine hyperplasia results as a response to the excessive secretion of a stimulating or trophic hormone.[30] A common example is the bilateral adrenal hyperplasia associated with pituitary-dependent Cushing's disease, which develops secondary to the chronic, excessive secretion of adrenocorticotropic hormone by the pituitary gland.[31]

Early in the course of nonneoplastic endocrine hyperplasia, the affected gland(s) is typically diffusely enlarged, consistent with a uniform response of its cells to the stimulatory hormone (see Figure 21-1). At this stage of the disease, these hyperplastic changes are largely reversible upon removal of the stimulus or trophic hormone.[30] With prolonged stimulation, however, heterogeneity of the growth pattern may develop, resulting in development of both monoclonal and polyclonal cellular cohorts and ultimately leading to overt nodularity.[7,20] Intrinsic cellular changes associated with genetic mutations may also contribute to the resultant nodular, hyperplasic changes of the endocrine gland.[16,19,21]

A consistent feature of hyperthyroidism in cats (and toxic nodular goiter in humans) is the autonomous growth and function of thyroid tissue during the state of thyrotoxicosis—a period when the thyroid gland's relevant stimulating hormone, namely thyroid-stimulating hormone (TSH), is suppressed rather than increased. Additionally, the formation of adenomatous thyroid nodules, rather than diffuse hyperplasia, is a prominent pathologic feature of hyperthyroidism in cats.[6,10,25,26] Once overt hyperthyroidism has developed,

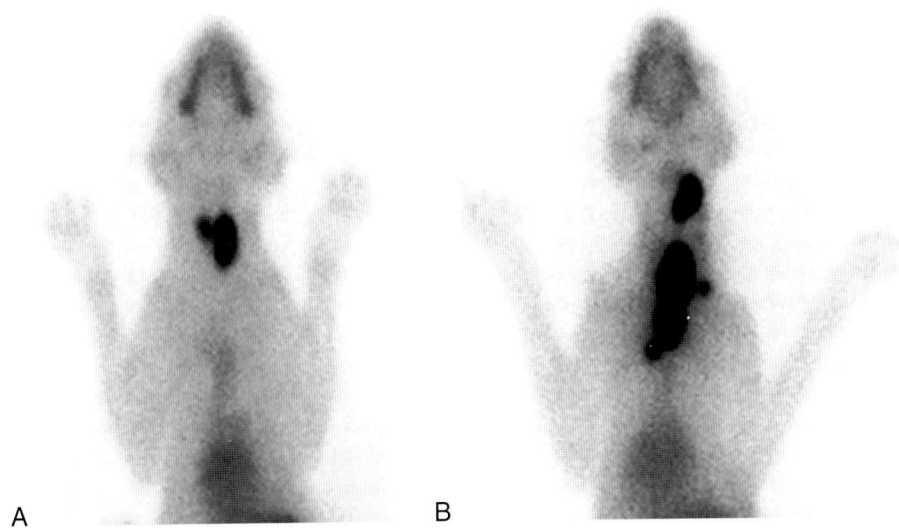

Figure 21-2: Ventral thyroid scintigraphic images of two cats with hyperthyroidism. The scintigraphic images for both cats show an increase in radionuclide uptake in their autonomously functional thyroid tissue (i.e., increased thyroid:salivary uptake ratio), which is diagnostic for hyperthyroidism. **A,** The cat with benign disease has abnormal radionuclide uptake limited to the normal location of both thyroid lobes. **B,** In the cat with thyroid carcinoma, multiple areas of increased radionuclide uptake are noted in areas both cranial and caudal to the normal location of the thyroid lobes, indicative of regional metastases.

extrinsic stimulation from TSH cannot be responsible for the pathologic thyroid abnormalities (e.g., adenomatous hyperplasia or adenoma), as circulating TSH concentrations in these cats are very low to undetectable[32,33] (see Figure 21-1). Again, this suggests that the ultimate mechanisms that cause and perpetuate these pathologic changes must originate within the abnormal thyroid tumor cells themselves.[34] In accord with that, previous studies of adenomatous thyroid tissue transplanted from hyperthyroid cats into nude mice or placed in culture have confirmed that these thyroid nodules continue growing and secreting thyroid hormone outside of the cat—no external stimulation is needed for autonomous growth and hyperfunction of the hyperthyroid cat's thyroid nodule(s).[35,36] Such autonomous growth is a classic feature of neoplasia, whether benign or malignant. Overall, these changes in the hyperthyroid cat's thyroid gland are most consistent with evidence of a transition from early thyroid hyperplasia, which would still be responsive to systemic trophic stimulation, into a true neoplasm (e.g., adenoma), capable of self-perpetuated growth and hyperfunction.[37]

Pathologists have always struggled with the distinction between hyperplasia, hyperplastic nodules, and adenomas of the endocrine tissue of human patients.[38-40] Traditionally, only thyroid adenomas have been considered true tumors, based on the presence of a capsule and a growth pattern that is different from the surrounding, normal parenchyma, but this has turned out to be oversimplistic.[9] Veterinary pathologists have also encountered similar limitations in pathologic diagnosis, with an early review of the histopathologic features of feline thyroid adenomas reporting that "a distinct capsule was seldom present."[41] Other endocrine pathologists have concluded that "cell size and pattern can not be used to distinguish between adenomas and multinodular adenomatous

hyperplasia."[26] These same pathologists reported "no clear gross or microscopic distinction between a nodule interpreted as an adenoma and one or several nodules composing the lesion called multinodular adenomatous hyperplasia."[26]

Modern tools of morphology, such as electron microscopy and immunohistochemistry, have also turned out to be of little assistance in distinguishing hyperplasia of thyroid tissues from true adenomas. Because strict histologic criteria for a thyroid adenoma and its differentiation from an adenomatous nodule are difficult to obtain, the World Health Organization has recommended using a biologic basis for differentiating these thyroid nodules based on clonality.[42] When thyroid nodules of human patients with toxic nodular goiter are classified this way, the majority are true monoclonal neoplasms rather than polyclonal hyperplastic nodules.[16,43,44] However, even this established concept that an endocrine hyperplasia originates from multiple cell precursors and is therefore polyclonal, while an endocrine neoplasia originates from a single cell precursor and is therefore monoclonal, has proven overly simplistic.[43,45,46] The number of cells in normal tissues is normally kept constant by a network of interacting signaling pathways that stimulate proliferation, inhibit excessive growth, and induce apoptosis.[47,48] This balance may be altered by molecular injuries to any of these pathways. Evaluation of all of these findings has led some investigators to conclude that the mechanisms behind the development of nonneoplastic endocrine hyperplasia and true adenomas of endocrine tissues (especially concerning the thyroid gland) are identical and lie within the glandular cells themselves.[30,37]

Overall, it is clear that hyperthyroidism in cats is caused by an autonomous, usually benign, neoplastic process that may take the histopathologic appearance of either adenomatous thyroid hyperplasia or true thyroid adenoma. The use of the term "adenomatous thyroid hyperplasia," however, erroneously implies the dependence on a circulating stimulatory hormone (or other trophic factor) and obscures the fact that the thyroid nodule(s) consistently behaves as true neoplasia. This concept that hyperthyroidism is caused by a neoplastic process is critical to understanding the progressive nature of the disease. With time, the nodular goiter responsible for the hyperthyroid state does change, as reflected both in the expansion of the thyroid nodule size, as well as a worsening of the severity of the hyperthyroid state. In some cats with chronic hyperthyroidism, transformation of benign thyroid nodular changes into thyroid carcinoma may also develop.[24]

Increase in Size of Goiter (Adenoma) over Time

After diagnosis of hyperthyroidism, the thyroid adenomas in these cats will continue to grow autonomously, despite suppression of pituitary TSH secretion resulting in undetectable levels of circulating TSH. In hyperthyroid cats left untreated, the most apparent consequence of this gradual, continued growth of the thyroid adenoma is the progressive increase in circulating T4 and T3 concentrations over time.

In cats chronically managed with methimazole (or carbimazole), this progressive increase in goiter size will continue, because antithyroid drugs act to block thyroid hormone secretion but do not stop or slow tumor growth. Therefore, the gradual increase in the number of adenomatous tumor cells that are overproducing thyroid hormone can also lead to the need for progressive increases in antithyroid drug doses in order to maintain euthyroidism. One recent report confirmed a significant correlation between the duration of medical management of cats with hyperthyroidism and the size of their thyroid tumors, based on thyroid scintigraphy.[24] As the size of the goiter increases, this also leads to a progressive worsening in the severity of the cats' hyperthyroid state and higher serum thyroid hormone concentrations.

Transition of Adenoma to Carcinoma with Time

Specific molecular defects have been associated with the development and progression of thyroid neoplasia in human patients. These models suggest stepwise progression from benign to malignant thyroid tumors, as well as the progression from differentiated to anaplastic malignancies, all secondary to the cumulative effects of multiple genetic events.[49] Less-differentiated thyroid cancers, that is, poorly differentiated carcinoma and anaplastic carcinoma, can develop *de novo*, although many of them also likely arise through the process of stepwise dedifferentiation of papillary and follicular carcinomas.[49]

As in humans, the same stepwise progression from benign to malignant thyroid disease may occur in hyperthyroid cats

as well. Although histopathology is generally considered the gold standard method for the diagnosis of feline thyroid carcinoma, distinguishing between well-differentiated thyroid carcinoma and benign adenoma can be difficult and is not always possible, even by an experienced pathologist.[26,38-40,50,51] Ultimately, differentiated thyroid carcinomas share many histopathologic features in common with benign thyroid tumors. Even after careful histopathologic examination of surgical specimens, it can be difficult to distinguish between the diagnosis of follicular adenoma and carcinoma. In humans, several studies have documented discrepancies between observers in the pathologic diagnosis of thyroid tumors, which have been reported to occur in up to a quarter of cases.[52,53]

One possible reason for such difficulties in interpretation is that malignant transformation of benign adenomatous nodules appears possible in both cats and humans, further complicating the histopathologic diagnosis.[28,51,54] In support of that hypothesis, careful examination of surgical specimens collected from human patients with toxic nodular goiter reveal that 10% to 30% of these patients will be found to harbor a carcinoma.[55-59] Most of these human patients had a long history of nodular thyroid disease and were selected for surgery because of their large goiter size and concern for carcinoma, suggesting progression from benign adenomatous nodules to malignant areas of carcinoma over a long period of time.[60]

In a recent study of feline thyroid carcinoma, histopathologic evaluation of excised thyroid tumor tissue collected from two cats revealed focal areas of both adenoma and carcinoma adjacent to each other, again suggesting that the carcinomas may have arisen from a background of benign neoplasia.[28] The concept of malignant transformation to thyroid carcinoma is further supported by a recent report which found an increase of approximately 4% per year of scintigraphically suspected thyroid carcinomas in cats chronically managed with methimazole.[24]

CORRELATION BETWEEN THE DEGREE OF HYPERTHYROIDISM AND SEVERITY OF CLINICAL SIGNS

In general, the severity of the clinical signs demonstrated by cats with hyperthyroidism is directly proportional to the degree and duration of the hyperthyroid state. Cats with slight increases in serum thyroid hormone concentrations generally show only mild clinical signs, which typically include mild weight loss with occasional bouts of vomiting and/or diarrhea. Cats at this stage of the disease usually have a normal to slightly increased appetite. As the hyperthyroidism worsens, the number and severity of clinical signs attributable to the disease tend to increase. Cats with severe elevations in their serum thyroid hormone values generally show more advanced signs, which commonly include more severe weight loss and overt cardiovascular compromise. Almost all cats presenting with severe clinical features of hyperthyroidism will have severe elevation in serum thyroid hormone values (>20 µg/dL [>257 nmol/L]) and very large, palpable goiters.

Some hyperthyroid cats suffering from a concurrent non-thyroidal illness will present with severe clinical signs, disproportionately worse than expected from the degree of severity of the hyperthyroidism alone. For example, some hyperthyroid cats presenting with extreme weight loss and severe gastrointestinal signs (especially diarrhea) may have only mild elevations in thyroid hormone concentrations; these cats should be carefully screened for the presence of concurrent disease contributing to their clinical signs. Many of these cats have primary gastrointestinal disease, which is difficult to diagnose from the physical examination, laboratory, or radiographic findings. Therefore, the finding of disproportionately severe clinical signs in any cat that has a lower-than-expected serum T4 value should prompt further diagnostics (e.g., abdominal ultrasound and/or endoscopy) to rule out concurrent disease. Even if these hyperthyroid cats are treated and made euthyroid, their clinical signs would not resolve if due to nonthyroidal illness.

In hyperthyroid cats suspected of having concurrent illness, trial therapy with antithyroid drugs can also be used as a diagnostic aid. Use of a methimazole (or carbimazole) trial can be a very useful method to confirm that the clinical signs are in fact caused by hyperthyroidism and are not the result of a concurrent medical disorder. If clinical signs persist despite adequate medical control of the hyperthyroid state with methimazole, then concurrent nonthyroidal disease is very likely.

CAUSES FOR TREATMENT FAILURE

Surgical Thyroidectomy

Surgical thyroidectomy was the first reported therapy for hyperthyroidism in cats and continues to be a useful treatment option.[3,61-63] While a highly effective, curative treatment, persistent or recurrent hyperthyroidism is sometimes observed after surgical thyroidectomy.

Persistent Hyperthyroidism

One of the most common reasons for persistent hyperthyroidism in the immediate postoperative period is the presence of ectopic adenomatous thyroid tissue, which can easily be missed (and therefore not removed) at time of surgery. Ectopic thyroid tissue may be located anywhere along the path of the descent of the thyroid during its embryologic development, although it is most commonly located at the base of the tongue or in the anterior mediastinum.[29,64,65] This ectopic thyroid tissue can develop adenomatous growth and function, just like the two thyroid lobes in the normal cervical location. Indeed, a recent study reported the presence of ectopic adenomatous thyroid disease in approximately 5% of cats diagnosed with hyperthyroidism.[29]

Another reason for persistent hyperthyroidism in the immediate postoperative period is failure to identify and remove all adenoma tissue arising from the two thyroid lobes

located in the midcervical area. Because most hyperthyroid cats have involvement of both thyroid lobes, bilateral thyroidectomy is indicated if long-term cure is the goal. In some hyperthyroid cats, especially those with severe disease, a large thyroid adenoma can migrate caudally (ventrally), falling through the thoracic inlet into the thoracic cavity due to the effects of gravity.[3,29,66,67] In these cats, failure to identify and remove this large thyroid tumor would result in persistent hyperthyroidism. To help avoid this scenario, it is important to identify both thyroid lobes at the time of surgery; if only one lobe can be located, it is possible that the other thyroid lobe is within the anterior mediastinum. These large intrathoracic thyroid tumors can sometimes be pulled back out of the chest through the thoracic inlet in order to be removed. The prevalence of such intrathoracic thyroid masses increases with larger tumor size and longer duration of hyperthyroidism.[24] Such intrathoracic thyroid masses are uncommon in cats with recently diagnosed hyperthyroidism that generally have smaller thyroid nodules.

A third reason for persistent hyperthyroidism in the immediate postoperative period is the presence of thyroid carcinoma.[28,68,69] Many of these malignant thyroid tumors are very large and vascular; thyroid carcinomas may invade adjacent soft tissues and commonly extend through the thoracic inlet into the thoracic cavity. Less commonly, thyroid carcinomas will metastasize to regional lymph nodes or distant sites.

Recurrent Hyperthyroidism

Although disease is bilateral in 70% of cats, some cats have asymmetrical thyroid enlargement, with one thyroid lobe being very large and the other being only minimally enlarged. In these cats, unilateral thyroidectomy generally restores euthyroidism, at least for a few weeks, and it may take many months for the remaining lobe to grow to a size for hyperthyroidism to recur.[3,61,70] However, the client must be warned of the possibility of persistent or recurrent hyperthyroidism whenever unilateral thyroidectomy is contemplated.

The two most common techniques for bilateral thyroidectomy in cats are the intracapsular and extracapsular methods.[3,62,63] The major problem with the intracapsular thyroidectomy technique is that it can be difficult to remove the entire thyroid capsule (and therefore all abnormal thyroid tissue) while concurrently preserving parathyroid function. Small remnants of thyroid tissue that remain attached to the capsule may regenerate and produce recurrent hyperthyroidism. With the extracapsular technique, the incidence of relapse is much less because the entire thyroid capsule is removed at time of surgery.[3,71] When recurrent hyperthyroidism does occur after bilateral thyroidectomy, it generally takes many months to years for the serum T4 to increase or clinical signs of hyperthyroidism to develop.

Preoperative Thyroid Scintigraphy

Use of thyroid scintigraphy to identify the location of all functional thyroid tissue prior to surgery helps avoid persistent hyperthyroidism. Thyroid scintigraphy will differentiate unilateral versus bilateral involvement and can also identify ectopic thyroid disease, large thyroid adenomas or carcinomas that have descended into the chest, and thyroid carcinomas that have metastasized.[29,66]

Antithyroid Drugs (Methimazole or Carbimazole)

Antithyroid drugs are commonly used for treatment of hyperthyroidism in cats. Nowadays, two drugs have been used to manage hyperthyroid cats: methimazole and its prodrug carbimazole (not available in the United States or Canada).[3,72,73] When administered appropriately, antithyroid drugs are actively trapped by the thyroid gland, where they interfere with thyroid peroxidase–mediated iodide oxidation, organification of iodine, and iodotyrosine coupling, thereby lowering serum thyroid hormone concentrations.[2,3,74] On the basis of current evidence and available tablet sizes, starting doses of 2.5 mg (methimazole) once to twice a day or 10 to 15 mg once a day (sustained release formulation of carbimazole) are recommended.[3,72,73] These doses should then be titrated to effect in order to lower serum total T4 concentrations into the middle of the reference interval.

Poor Response to Initial Treatment

Although the majority of hyperthyroid cats respond to these antithyroid drugs with an adequate lowering of circulating T4 concentrations, a few cats appear resistant to initial methimazole treatment. In an early study, 2 of 262 cats treated with methimazole at doses ultimately reaching 20 mg/day failed to respond, even after prolonged treatment.[75] Both of these cats had very large thyroid nodules and extreme T4 elevations, which may explain this apparent resistance to methimazole.

Antithyroid drugs are taken up by the thyroid adenoma(s), where the drugs act on the adenomatous thyrocytes to block thyroid hormone secretion.[3,72,73] If the cat's thyroid tumor volume is too large, it may not be possible to achieve a high enough intrathyroidal drug concentration to adequately inhibit thyroid hormone secretion and restore euthyroidism.[76,77]

Poor Response to Long-Term Treatment

The development of resistance to antithyroid drugs is much more commonly seen in hyperthyroid cats treated on a long-term basis with either methimazole or carbimazole. Because these antithyroid drugs do not slow or stop thyroid tumor growth, thyroid tumors tend to grow progressively larger with time.[24] This increase in the size of the thyroid tumor means that most of these cats will require a progressive increase in the daily antithyroid drug dosage. In support of that, one study found that the final maintenance dosage of methimazole in 80 cats treated with long-term methimazole for up to 1000 days ranged from 5 to 20 mg/day, with a median dose of 10 mg/day.[75] This, of course, is much higher than the dose of 1.25-5 mg/day that will almost always control cats with newly diagnosed hyperthyroidism.[3,72,73]

After 2 to 3 years or longer, many of these cats will develop very large goiters and will become difficult to regulate, even with high daily doses of oral or transdermal methimazole or carbimazole. Eventually, it may be difficult to impossible to raise the antithyroid drug dose to levels high enough to maintain circulating thyroid concentrations to within the reference intervals without inducing toxicity.

Poor Response in Cats with Thyroid Carcinoma

With enough time and as the disease progresses, the thyroid adenoma–adenomatous hyperplasia in some hyperthyroid cats will transform into malignant thyroid carcinoma (Figure 21-1).[24] Again, antithyroid drug therapy cannot stop this malignant transformation.

Many of these cats become increasingly resistant to antithyroid drug treatment, again due, at least in part, to the large amount of carcinomatous thyroid tissue typically found in these cats.[24,27-29] In three reports of cats with hyperthyroidism secondary to histopathologically confirmed thyroid carcinoma, a majority of cats proved to be resistant to the use of antithyroid drugs to control their thyrotoxicosis.[27,28,69]

Radioiodine

Radioiodine therapy is considered by most authorities to be the treatment of choice for most cats with hyperthyroidism.[2,3,78] Since the initial reports describing the first hyperthyroid cats treated with radioiodine (^{131}I) in the early 1980s, many different methods for determining the appropriate dose have been described. These methods can be categorized into either variable or fixed-dose strategies.[78] The variable-dose strategies assume that because cats have varying volumes of adenomatous thyroid tissue, they will be ideally treated by tailoring the dose of radioiodine to their volume of tumor tissue. The fixed-dose strategy, on the other hand, assumes that the majority of hyperthyroid cats can be cured by administration of a standardized, or one-size-fits-all dose of radioactive iodine.[78]

Failure of Standard Radioiodine Treatment

Most hyperthyroid cats treated with radioactive iodine can be cured with administration of a single, relatively low dose (<4 to 5 mCi). Approximately 5% of cats, however, fail to respond completely and remain mildly hyperthyroid after treatment with these standard doses of radioiodine.[78,79] Almost all of these hyperthyroid cats can be cured by a follow-up ^{131}I treatment, although a higher dose of ^{131}I may be needed to achieve euthyroidism. On the other hand, if little or no response to ^{131}I is observed, especially after retreatment with higher ^{131}I doses, thyroid carcinoma must always be considered; in such cases, thyroid scintigraphy and/or thyroid biopsy is strongly recommended.[29,66,78,79]

In both humans and cats, severe hyperthyroidism and large thyroid volume (size) are predictors of ^{131}I treatment failure.[79-82] In support of that, one study reported a higher incidence of failure in cats with larger volumes of tumor tissue, even though these cats received higher ^{131}I doses than the cats with smaller thyroid adenomas.[82]

Relapse After Radioiodine Treatment

Relapse of hyperthyroidism after treatment with ^{131}I is uncommon, with a prevalence of less than 5%. When it does occur, relapse generally develops 3 or more years after treatment.[78,79] In these cats, it is unclear whether such relapse is due to regrowth of the original thyroid tumor tissue or the development of an entirely new thyroid nodule (not related to the original goiter). On the other hand, if relapse develops within a few days to weeks after initial ^{131}I therapy, thyroid carcinoma should be excluded, and thyroid scintigraphy and/or thyroid biopsy are strongly recommended.

Thyroid Carcinoma

Thyroid carcinomas are more resistant to the effect of ^{131}I than benign thyroid disease (i.e., adenomas or adenomatous hyperplasia), and the size of thyroid carcinomas is usually much larger. Therefore, extremely high doses of radioiodine (30 mCi) are almost always needed for destruction of this malignant tissue and cure of the cat's hyperthyroid state.[27,28,69,78]

THERAPY FOR SEVERE, UNRESPONSIVE, OR RECURRENT HYPERTHYROIDISM

Antithyroid Drug Management—No Longer an Option

Despite the fact that radioiodine therapy is widely recognized as the treatment of choice for most cats with hyperthyroidism, various economic and logistical issues, as well as societal phobias, may impede its use in many cases. Therefore, long-term administration of an antithyroid drug is the most common means of treatment used in cats with hyperthyroidism. Successful medical management allows many hyperthyroid cats to live and do relatively well for many years, despite the fact that their thyroid adenomas will continue to grow progressively in size, sometimes developing into very large goiters. Occasionally, these larger thyroid tumors develop areas of cystic degeneration that can lead to further rapid, sometimes massive, growth of the thyroid mass.[83] The additional possibility of malignant transformation of thyroid adenoma to carcinoma is also possible.[24,28] Regardless of the underlying histopathology, medical management may ultimately fail in these cats, either because the high dose of antithyroid drugs needed to control their disease reaches toxic levels or because the cats develop clinical signs (e.g., dysphagia, dyspnea) associated with the large physical size of their goiter. When this happens, definitive (i.e., curative) therapies to remove or destroy the thyroid tumor are indicated.

Surgical Thyroidectomy for Cats with Severe or Unresponsive Disease

When evaluating cats with chronic hyperthyroidism that become resistant to medical management, thyroid scintigra-phy plays a critical role in staging the disease.[29,66,78] While surgery remains a viable option in many of these cats, the presence of adenomatous thyroid tissue within the thoracic cavity, as well as the development of malignant transformation of adenomatous tissue with local tissue invasion or metastasis, often preclude successful surgical intervention. Furthermore, the inability to adequately prepare the cats for surgery by restoring euthyroidism with antithyroid drug therapy increases the risks associated with anesthesia and surgical treatment.[62,63]

Radioiodine Treatment for Cats with Severe or Unresponsive Disease

In the majority of cats that have developed severe or unresponsive hyperthyroidism, radioiodine remains the only viable treatment that will control the disease. However, the standard doses (i.e., 4 to 5 mCi) of ^{131}I used to treat cats with hyperthyroidism typically fail when administered to these cats with very large goiters. The reason for these treatment failures is likely due to the increased number of benign neoplastic cells and a relative radiation resistance of malignant tumors.

Typically large, sometimes ablative doses of [131]I (i.e., 10 to 30 mCi) are needed to resolve these tumors.[78,82] While these ultra-large doses are generally well tolerated, a higher incidence of transient regional clinical signs does occur, including a decreased appetite (presumably secondary to esophageal inflammation) and cervical and/or mediastinal edema. In some cats, use of an appetite stimulant (e.g., mirtazapine) or treatment with anti-inflammatory doses of corticosteroids is indicated.

The majority of cats with severe, unresponsive hyperthyroidism due to development of large goiters or thyroid carcinoma can be cured with use of ultra-large doses of radioiodine and therefore generally have a good prognosis.[28,69,78] The incidence of iatrogenic hypothyroidism is also increased after treatment with these larger, sometimes ablative doses, frequently necessitating the use of chronic thyroid hormone supplementation (see Chapter 23).

SUMMARY

An autonomously functional benign neoplastic process, described as either multinodular adenomatous hyperplasia or thyroid adenoma, usually causes feline hyperthyroidism. The incidence of thyroid carcinoma at the time of initial diagnosis of hyperthyroidism is very low.[6,10,25,26] There is no functional difference between the autonomous thyroid tissues that have the histopathologic appearance of adenomatous hyperplasia and those nodules considered true adenomas. Furthermore, the use of the term *adenomatous thyroid hyperplasia* erroneously implies dependence on a circulating stimulatory hormone (or other systemic factor) and obscures the fact that this condition consistently behaves as a true, autonomous, benign neoplastic growth.[7,20,30]

Treatment with antithyroid drugs will normalize serum T4 values and help resolve clinical signs of hyperthyroidism in most cats, but long-term medical treatment fails to prevent the autonomous growth of their thyroid adenoma responsible for the disease. As a result, chronic medical management often leads to a progressive increase in thyroid tumor size and volume, seen clinically as large, palpable goiters. In addition, some of these long-standing, large thyroid adenomas appear to undergo malignant transformation into thyroid carcinomas.[5,24] In either case, the natural progression of the disease frequently requires gradual increases in the daily doses of antithyroid drugs needed to maintain euthyroidism. Ultimately, the large doses of antithyroid drugs needed in these cats either fail to maintain euthyroidism or reach a level of toxicity, requiring the use of alternative therapies.

Radioiodine and surgery have the potential to either destroy or remove the neoplastic cells responsible for the disease. Because these treatments cure the underlying cause of the hyperthyroidism, they both eliminate the potential for continued thyroid tumor growth and malignant transformation. Once hyperthyroid cats develop a sufficiently large thyroid adenoma or their adenoma transforms into a thyroid carcinoma (or both), the inability to properly prepare the cats with antithyroid drugs increases the risks associated with anesthesia and surgical thyroidectomy. Therefore, radioiodine therapy is frequently the best therapeutic option and is generally quite successful. However, the doses of ^{131}I required to destroy the large to huge thyroid masses in cats with long-standing hyperthyroidism are much larger than the doses typically needed to cure cats that are treated shortly after the initial diagnosis, when the thyroid tumors are much smaller and almost always benign.[78]

Prevention of disease is a primary goal of medicine. Our limited understanding of the underlying etiology of the autonomously functioning, adenomatous thyroid tissue that causes hyperthyroidism does not allow us to prevent the disease at this time. However, we do know that treatment failures and disease recurrence are far more common in cats with long-standing hyperthyroidism that have also developed very large, multicentric or malignant thyroid tumors.[78,79,82]

At this time, we have sufficient evidence to suggest that the progressive growth of small, autonomous thyroid adenomas is responsible for the large, multicentric and possibly malignant thyroid tumors in cats with long-standing hyperthyroidism. The best therapy for severe, unresponsive, or recurrent hyperthyroidism is to prevent a large or malignant goiter from ever developing. Removing or destroying the thyroid tumor early in the course of the disease, at a time when it is still relatively small in size, best accomplishes this goal. While use of antithyroid drugs represents an effective symptomatic treatment for hyperthyroidism, this treatment option allows the underlying adenomatous disease to progress and directly contributes to the development of severe and unresponsive hyperthyroidism in these cats.[80]

References

1. Peterson ME, Johnson JG, Andrews LK: Spontaneous hyperthyroidism in the cat. In *Proceedings. American College of Veterinary Internal Medicine Forum*, 1979, p 108.
2. Baral R, Peterson ME: Thyroid gland disorders. In Little SE, editor: *The cat: clinical medicine and management*, Philadelphia, 2012, Elsevier/Saunders, pp 571–592.
3. Mooney CT, Peterson ME: Feline hyperthyroidism. In Mooney CT, Peterson ME, editors: *Manual of canine and feline endocrinology*, ed 4, Quedgeley, 2012, British Small Animal Veterinary Association, pp 199–203.
4. Peterson ME, Ward CR: Etiopathologic findings of hyperthyroidism in cats. *Vet Clin North Am Small Anim Pract* 37:633–645, 2007.
5. Peterson M: Hyperthyroidism in cats: what's causing this epidemic of thyroid disease and can we prevent it? *J Feline Med Surg* 14:804–818, 2012.
6. Gerber H, Peter H, Ferguson DC, et al: Etiopathology of feline toxic nodular goiter. *Vet Clin North Am Small Anim Pract* 24:541–565, 1994.
7. Studer H, Ramelli F: Simple goiter and its variants: euthyroid and hyperthyroid multinodular goiters. *Endocr Rev* 3:40–61, 1982.
8. Siegel RD, Lee SL: Toxic nodular goiter. Toxic adenoma and toxic multinodular goiter. *Endocrinol Metab Clin North Am* 27:151–168, 1998.
9. Paschke R: Toxic adenoma and toxic multinodular goiter. In Braverman LE, Cooper DS, editors: *Werner & Ingbar's the thyroid: a fundamental and clinical text*, ed 10, Philadelphia, 2013, Lippincott Williams & Wilkins, pp 400–408.
10. Hoenig M, Goldschmidt MH, Ferguson DC, et al: Toxic nodular goitre in the cat. *J Small Anim Pract* 23:1–12, 1982.
11. Laurberg P, Pedersen KM, Vestergaard H, et al: High incidence of multinodular toxic goitre in the elderly population in a low iodine intake area vs. high incidence of Graves' disease in the young in a high iodine intake area: comparative surveys of thyrotoxicosis epidemiology in East-Jutland Denmark and Iceland. *J Intern Med* 229:415–420, 1991.
12. Van de Ven A, Netea-Maier RT, Ross A, et al: Longitudinal trends in thyroid function in relation to iodine intake: ongoing changes of thyroid function despite adequate current iodine status. *Eur J Endocrinol* 170:49–54, 2013.
13. Edinboro CH, Pearce EN, Pino S, et al: Is the iodine content of cat food responsible for "toxic nodular goiter" in older cats? In *Annual 80th Meeting of the American Thyroid Association*, Palm Beach, FL, 2009, p S-27. (Abstract).
14. Edinboro CH, Scott-Moncrieff JC, Glickman LT: Feline hyperthyroidism: potential relationship with iodine supplement requirements of commercial cat foods. *J Feline Med Surg* 12:672–679, 2010.
15. Edinboro CH, Pearce EN, Pino S, et al: Iodine concentration in commercial cat foods from three regions of the USA, 2008-2009. *J Feline Med Surg* 15:717–724, 2013.
16. Krohn K, Paschke R: Clinical review 133: progress in understanding the etiology of thyroid autonomy. *J Clin Endocrinol Metab* 86:3336–3345, 2001.
17. Derwahl M, Studer H: Nodular goiter and goiter nodules: where iodine deficiency falls short of explaining the facts. *Exp Clin Endocrinol Diab* 109:250–260, 2001.
18. Graf H: Multinodular goiter: pathogenesis and management. In Braverman LE, Cooper DS, editors: *Werner & Ingbar's the thyroid: a fundamental and clinical text*, ed 10, Philadelphia, 2013, Lippincott Williams & Wilkins, pp 635–649.
19. Krohn K, Fuhrer D, Bayer Y, et al: Molecular pathogenesis of euthyroid and toxic multinodular goiter. *Endocr Rev* 26:504–524, 2005.
20. Studer H, Peter HJ, Gerber H: Natural heterogeneity of thyroid cells: the basis for understanding thyroid function and nodular goiter growth. *Endocr Rev* 10:125–135, 1989.
21. Krohn K, Paschke R: Somatic mutations in thyroid nodular disease. *Mol Genet Metab* 75:202–208, 2002.
22. Peeters ME, Timmermans-Sprang EP, Mol JA: Feline thyroid adenomas are in part associated with mutations in the G(s alpha) gene and

not with polymorphisms found in the thyro-tropin receptor. *Thyroid* 12:571–575, 2002.

23. Watson SG, Radford AD, Kipar A, et al: Somatic mutations of the thyroid-stimulating hormone receptor gene in feline hyperthyroidism: parallels with human hyperthyroidism. *J Endocrinol* 186:523–537, 2005.

24. Peterson ME, Broome MR: Hyperthyroid cats on long-term medical treatment show a progressive increase in the prevalence of large thyroid tumors, intrathoracic thyroid masses, and suspected thyroid carcinoma. *J Vet Intern Med* 26:1523, 2012.

25. Holzworth J, Theran P, Carpenter JL, et al: Hyperthyroidism in the cat: ten cases. *J Am Vet Med Assoc* 176:345–353, 1980.

26. Carpenter JL, Andrews LK, Holzworth J: Tumors and tumor-like lesions. In Holzworth J, editor: *Diseases of the cat: medicine and surgery*, Philadelphia, 1987, Saunders, pp 406–596.

27. Turrel JM, Feldman EC, Nelson RW, et al: Thyroid carcinoma causing hyperthyroidism in cats: 14 cases (1981-1986). *J Am Vet Med Assoc* 193:359–364, 1988.

28. Hibbert A, Gruffydd-Jones T, Barrett EL, et al: Feline thyroid carcinoma: diagnosis and response to high-dose radioactive iodine treatment. *J Feline Med Surg* 11:116–124, 2009.

29. Peterson ME, Broome MR: Thyroid scintigraphy findings in 2096 cats with hyperthryoidism. *Vet Radiol Ultrasound* 56:84–95, 2015.

30. Studer H: Derwahl M: Mechanisms of non-neoplastic endocrine hyperplasia—a changing concept: a review focused on the thyroid gland. *Endocr Rev* 16:411–426, 1995.

31. Croughs RJ, Rijnberk A, Meyer JC: The pathogenesis of pituitary-dependent Cushing's syndrome. *Neth J Med* 22:80–83, 1979.

32. Peterson ME: More than just T4: diagnostic testing for hyperthyroidism in cats. *J Feline Med Surg* 15:765–777, 2013.

33. Peterson ME: Feline focus: diagnostic testing for feline thyroid disease: hyperthyroidism. *Compend Contin Educ Vet* 35:E3, 2013.

34. Nguyen LQ, Arseven OK, Gerber H, et al: Cloning of the cat TSH receptor and evidence against an autoimmune etiology of feline hyperthyroidism. *Endocrinology* 143:395–402, 2002.

35. Peter HJ, Gerber H, Studer H, et al: Autonomy of growth and of iodine metabolism in hyperthyroid feline goiters transplanted onto nude mice. *J Clin Invest* 80:491–498, 1987.

36. Peter HJ, Gerber H, Studer H, et al: Autonomous growth and function of cultured thyroid follicles from cats with spontaneous hyperthyroidism. *Thyroid* 1:331–338, 1991.

37. Derwahl M, Studer H: Hyperplasia versus adenoma in endocrine tissues: are they different? *Trends Endocrinol Metab* 13:23–28, 2002.

38. DeLellis R, Heitz P, Lloyd R, et al: *WHO Classification of Tumors: Pathology & Genetics of Tumours of Endocrine Organs*, ed 3, Lyon, 2004, International Agency for Research on Cancer (IARC).

39. Chan JKC: Tumors of the thyroid and parathyroid glands. In Fletcher CDM, editor: *Diagnostic histopathology of tumours*, ed 3, Edin-

burgh, 2007, Elsevier/Churchill Livingstone, pp 997–1098.

40. Khan A, Nose V: Pathology of the thyroid gland. In Lloyd RV, editor: *Endocrine pathology: differential diagnosis and molecular advances*, ed 2, New York, 2010, Springer, pp 181–236.

41. Leav I, Schiller AL, Rijnberk A, et al: Adenomas and carcinomas of the canine and feline thyroid. *Am J Pathol* 83:61–122, 1976.

42. Chan JKC, Hirokawa M, Evans H: Follicular adenoma. In DeLellis R, Heitz P, Lloyd R, et al, editors: *WHO classification of tumors: pathology & genetics of tumours of endocrine organs*, ed 3, Lyon, 2004, International Agency for Research on Cancer (IARC), pp 98–103.

43. Namba H, Matsuo K, Fagin JA: Clonal composition of benign and malignant human thyroid tumors. *J Clin Invest* 86:120–125, 1990.

44. Kopp P, Kimura ET, Aeschimann S, et al: Polyclonal and monoclonal thyroid nodules coexist within human multinodular goiters. *J Clin Endocrinol Metab* 79:134–139, 1994.

45. Levy A: Monoclonality of endocrine tumours: What does it mean? *Trends Endocrinol Metab* 12:301–307, 2001.

46. Parsons BL: Many different tumor types have polyclonal tumor origin: evidence and implications. *Mutat Res* 659:232–247, 2008.

47. Kiess W, Gallaher B: Hormonal control of programmed cell death/apoptosis. *Eur J Endocrinol* 138:482–491, 1998.

48. Renehan AG, Bach SP, Potten CS: The relevance of apoptosis for cellular homeostasis and tumorigenesis in the intestine. *Can J Gastroenterol* 15:166–176, 2001.

49. Fagin JA, Nikiforov YE: Molecular genetics of tumors of thyroid follicular cells. In Braverman LE, Cooper DS, editors: *Werner & Ingbar's the thyroid: a fundamental and clinical text*, ed 10, Philadelphia, 2013, Lippincott Williams & Wilkins, pp 681–702.

50. Mete O, Asa SL: Pathological definition and clinical significance of vascular invasion in thyroid carcinomas of follicular epithelial derivation. *Mod Pathol* 24:1545–1552, 2011.

51. Mete O, Asa SL: Pitfalls in the diagnosis of follicular epithelial proliferations of the thyroid. *Adv Anat Pathol* 19:363–373, 2012.

52. Saxen E, Franssila K, Bjarnason O, et al: Observer variation in histologic classification of thyroid cancer. *Acta Pathol Microbiol Immunol Scand [A]* 86A:483–486, 1978.

53. Ron E, Griffel B, Liban E, et al: Histopathologic reproducibility of thyroid disease in an epidemiologic study. *Cancer* 57:1056–1059, 1986.

54. Arora N, Scognamiglio T, Zhu B, et al: Do benign thyroid nodules have malignant potential? An evidence-based review. *World J Surg* 32:1237–1246, 2008.

55. Pelizzo MR, Bernante P, Toniato A, et al: Frequency of thyroid carcinoma in a recent series of 539 consecutive thyroidectomies for multinodular goiter. *Tumori* 83:653–655, 1997.

56. Gandolfi PP, Frisina A, Raffa M, et al: The incidence of thyroid carcinoma in multinodular goiter: retrospective analysis. *Acta Biomed* 75:114–117, 2004.

57. Cerci C, Cerci SS, Eroglu E, et al: Thyroid cancer in toxic and non-toxic multinodular goiter. *J Postgrad Med* 53:157–160, 2007.

58. Luo J, McManus C, Chen H, et al: Are there predictors of malignancy in patients with multinodular goiter? *J Surg Res* 174:207–210, 2012.

59. Smith JJ, Chen X, Schneider DF, et al: Toxic nodular goiter and cancer: a compelling case for thyroidectomy. *Ann Surg Oncol* 20:1336–1340, 2013.

60. Kamran SC, Marqusee E, Kim MI, et al: Thyroid nodule size and prediction of cancer. *J Clin Endocrinol Metab* 98:564–570, 2013.

61. Birchard SJ, Peterson ME, Jacobson A: Surgical treatment of feline hyperthyroidism. Results of 85 cases. *J Am Anim Hosp Assoc* 20:705–709, 1984.

62. Birchard SJ: Thyroidectomy in the cat. *Clin Tech Small Anim Pract* 21:29–33, 2006.

63. Flanders JA: Surgical options for the treatment of hyperthyroidism in the cat. *J Feline Med Surg* 1:127–134, 1999.

64. Noxon JO: An adenoma in ectopic thyroid tissue causing hyperthyroidism in a cat. *J Am Anim Hosp Assoc* 19:369–372, 1983.

65. Patnaik AK, Peterson ME: Hidgon A: Ectopic lingual thyroid tissue in a cat. *J Feline Med Surg* 2:143–146, 2000.

66. Broome MR: Thyroid scintigraphy in hyperthyroidism. *Clin Tech Small Anim Pract* 21:10–16, 2006.

67. Harvey AM, Hibbert A, Barrett EL, et al: Scintigraphic findings in 120 hyperthyroid cats. *J Feline Med Surg* 11:96–106, 2009.

68. Turrel JM, Feldman EC, Hays M, et al: Radioactive iodine therapy in cats with hyperthyroidism. *J Am Vet Med Assoc* 184:554–559, 1984.

69. Guptill L, Scott-Moncrieff CR, Janovitz EB, et al: Response to high-dose radioactive iodine administration in cats with thyroid carcinoma that had previously undergone surgery. *J Am Vet Med Assoc* 207:1055–1058, 1995.

70. Swalec KM: Recurrence of hyperthyroidism after thyroidectomy in cats. *J Am Anim Hosp Assoc* 26:433–437, 1990.

71. Welches CD, Scavelli TD, Matthiesen DT, et al: Occurrence of problems after three techniques of bilateral thyroidectomy in cats. *Vet Surg* 18:392–396, 1989.

72. Trepanier LA: Pharmacologic management of feline hyperthyroidism. *Vet Clin North Am Small Anim Pract* 37:775–788, vii, 2007.

73. Daminet S, Kooistra HS, Fracassi F, et al: Best practice for the pharmacological management of hyperthyroid cats with antithyroid drugs. *J Small Anim Pract* 55:4–13, 2014.

74. Cooper DS: Antithyroid drugs. *N Engl J Med* 352:905–917, 2005.

75. Peterson ME, Kintzer PP, Hurvitz AI: Methimazole treatment of 262 cats with hyperthyroidism. *J Vet Intern Med* 2:150–157, 1988.

76. O'Malley BP, Rosenthal FD, Northover BJ, et al: Higher than conventional doses of carbimazole in the treatment of thyrotoxicosis. *Clin Endocrinol (Oxf)* 29:281–288, 1988.

77. Li H, Okuda J, Akamizu T, et al: A hyperthyroid patient with graves' disease who was strongly resistant to methimazole: Investigation on possible mechanisms of the resistance. *Endocr J* 42:697–704, 1995.

78. Peterson ME, Broome MR: Radioiodine for feline hyperthyroidism. In Bonagura JD, Twedt D, editors: *Kirk's current veterinary therapy XV*, ed 15, Philadelphia, 2013, Elsevier/Saunders.

79. Peterson ME, Becker DV: Radioiodine treatment of 524 cats with hyperthyroidism. *J Am Vet Med Assoc* 207:1422–1428, 1995.

80. Moura-Neto A, Mosci C, Santos AO, et al: Predictive factors of failure in a fixed 15 mci ^{131}I-iodide therapy for graves' disease. *Clin Nucl Med* 37:550–554, 2012.

81. Sharma R, Bhatnagar A, Mondal A, et al: Efficacy of standard ten millicurie dose of radio-iodine in management of autonomously functioning toxic thyroid nodules. *J Assoc Physicians India* 43:167–169, 172, 1995.

82. Forrest LJ, Baty CJ, Metcalf MR, et al: Feline hyperthyroidism: efficacy of treatment using volumetric analysis for radioiodine dose calculation. *Vet Radiol* 37:141–145, 1996.

83. Hofmeister E, Kippenes H, Mealey KL, et al: Functional cystic thyroid adenoma in a cat. *J Am Vet Med Assoc* 219:190–193, 2001.

Diagnostic Testing for Hyperthyroidism in Cats

Carmel T. Mooney

Hyperthyroidism has remained an important and common disorder of older cats since its first description in the early 1970s. Therefore, testing for hyperthyroidism is frequently undertaken in practice. As for most other endocrine diseases, there is no one perfect test capable of confirming the diagnosis in all affected cats and clearly eliminating it in unaffected cases. Each test has its own specific limitations that must be considered when interpreting the results provided.

The clinical syndrome of hyperthyroidism results from excessive circulating concentrations of the active thyroid hormones, thyroxine (T4) and triiodothyronine (T3), produced by an abnormally functioning thyroid gland. The associated clinical signs have been well described.[1,2] To date, confirmation of the diagnosis in highly symptomatic cats has been relatively straightforward. However, presumably because of increased awareness and easier availability of thyroid hormone assays, cats that have few if any clinical signs are now being tested and often as part of a routine annual health examination.[3] Goiter or palpable enlargement of the thyroid gland, once considered a relatively specific indicator of hyperthyroidism, can also be palpated in some euthyroid cats, and it is unknown if all of these cats will eventually succumb to hyperthyroidism or how long this could take.[4] Additionally, hyperthyroidism is a disease of older cats, and concurrent nonthyroidal illness is not unexpected in such a population. Ruling hyperthyroidism in or out is more difficult in early, mild, or subclinical cases and particularly in cats with other illnesses.

Diagnostic test performance can also be affected by the methodology used for the hormone being measured. There has been a move away from the relatively robust radioimmunoassays traditionally used to measure serum thyroid hormone concentrations toward nonisotopic assays that avoid radiation regulations and that can be semiautomated or fully automated or point-of-care in-hospital assays. These may provide quantitative or semiquantitative results and anecdotally, at least, an increased number of false-negative or false-positive results with some of these techniques as compared with radioimmunoassays.

This chapter reviews the diagnostic tests used to confirm a diagnosis of feline hyperthyroidism, particularly highlighting the challenges emerging as less symptomatic cats are tested using newer assay techniques.

THYROID HORMONE CONCENTRATIONS

The diagnostic hallmark of hyperthyroidism is the demonstration of increased circulating concentrations of the thyroid hormones. Measurements of serum concentrations of total and free T4, as well as total T3, have been used frequently in the investigation of hyperthyroidism. The finding of a suppressed serum thyrotropin (thyroid-stimulating hormone [TSH]) concentration can also be used for diagnosis, but this finding is somewhat controversial because no species-specific feline thyroid-stimulating hormone (fTSH) assay has been developed to date. Relevant summary data of the commonly used tests are presented in Figure 22-1, and Tables 22-1 and 22-2.

Total Thyroxine Concentration

Assessment of circulating concentrations of total T4 is considered the most valuable screening test for hyperthyroidism yet offered. It is relatively cheap, has no special sample handling requirements, and is readily available. In older cats with supportive clinical signs, which are highly suspicious for having hyperthyroidism, total T4 has a high sensitivity, and serum concentrations will be increased in over 90% of cases.[1,2,5]

The remaining 10% of hyperthyroid cats have total T4 concentrations that remain within reference limits, usually in the mid- to high-end of the reference interval (e.g., >30 nmol/L [2.3 μg/dL]). As such, hyperthyroidism cannot be ruled out by demonstrating a single normal serum total T4 value, although it is highly unlikely if values are within the lower end of the reference interval.[5] There are several reasons why a serum total T4 value may not be elevated in hyperthyroidism:

- *Subclinical hyperthyroidism:* Hyperthyroidism is an insidiously progressive disease, and it can take many months to years for serum thyroid hormone production to increase in the face of early histopathologic evidence of adenomatous hyperplasia. Such cats have few, if any, clinical signs, and any thyroid nodule present is likely to be small or barely palpable.
- *Mild hyperthyroidism:* Thyroid hormone concentrations fluctuate in all hyperthyroid cats. In cats with markedly

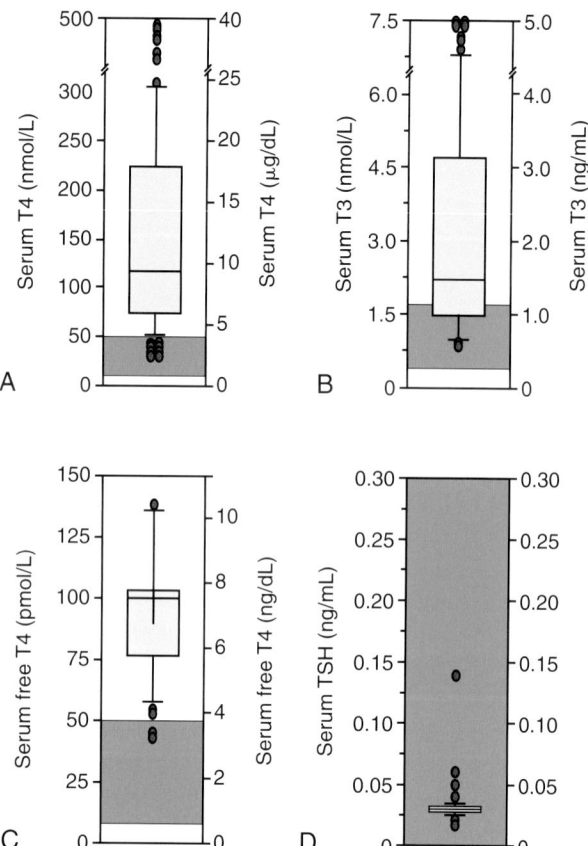

Figure 22-1: Box plots of serum concentrations of total thyroxine (T4), total triiodothyronine (T3), free T4, and thyroid-stimulating hormone (TSH) in 100 cats with untreated hyperthyroidism. These hyperthyroid cats were consecutively diagnosed and ranged in age from 8 to 20 years (median 13 years); almost all were mixed breed (domestic shorthair or domestic longhair), with 45 castrated males and 55 spayed females. **A,** Serum total T4 concentrations, determined by chemiluminescent enzyme immunoassay (CEIA). **B,** Serum total T3 concentrations, determined by CEIA. **C,** Serum free T4 concentrations, determined by equilibrium dialysis. **D,** Serum TSH, determined by canine thyroid-stimulating hormone CEIA. In each graph, the *box* represents the interquartile range (i.e., 25th to 75th percentile range or the middle half of the data). The *horizontal bar* in the box represents the median value. For each box plot, the *T-bars* represent the main body of the data, which in most instances is equal to the range. Outlying data points are represented by *open circles*. The *shaded areas* indicate the reference interval for each hormone. For the TSH assay, the detection limit (not indicated) is 0.03 ng/mL. (Reproduced with permission. From Peterson ME: More than just T4: diagnostic testing for hyperthyroidism in cats. *J Feline Med Surg* 15:765-777, 2013.)

high total T4 concentrations, the degree of fluctuation has little diagnostic significance. However, in mildly affected cats, total T4 concentration may fluctuate in and out of the reference interval.[6,7] Such cats have mild clinical signs and small but usually palpable thyroid nodules. It has been reported that in all cats categorized as having mild disease, approximately 40% will have total T4 concentrations that remain within the reference interval.[5] The majority of hyperthyroid cats (approximately 80%) that have total T4 values that remain within the reference interval have early or mild hyperthyroid disease.

- *Concurrent nonthyroidal illness:* In euthyroid cats, nonthyroidal illness is associated with suppressed total T4 concentrations. In such cats, the degree of suppression is associated with the severity of the illness and can be used as a prognostic marker.[8,9] As with serum T4 fluctuation, the degree of suppression has little diagnostic impact in cats with moderate to severe hyperthyroidism and markedly high total T4 concentrations. However, in cats with milder hyperthyroidism, serum total T4 concentrations may be suppressed into the mid- to high-end of the reference interval.[5,10] Suppression of total T4 values even to the lower end of the reference interval is possible in hyperthyroid cats, but this only occurs in cats with severe, concurrent nonthyroidal illness. While the presence of goiter or other supportive clinical signs may suggest the need for further testing for hyperthyroidism in such cats, the concurrent illness usually dictates the prognosis and primary treatment requirements, at least initially. Concurrent nonthyroidal illness accounts for approximately 20% of the hyperthyroid cats that have total T4 concentrations remaining within the reference interval.[5]
- *Drug therapies:* A large number of drugs are known to suppress circulating total T4 concentrations in dogs, ranging from glucocorticoids and anticonvulsants to certain antibiotics.[11] As with nonthyroidal illness, any suppressive effect of drug therapy is only likely to be of diagnostic significance in mildly hyperthyroid cats. Unfortunately, there are few specific studies assessing the effect of drugs in euthyroid and hyperthyroid cats other than the traditionally used antithyroid agents, carbimazole and methimazole. However, those specific drugs known to suppress thyroid hormone concentrations in dogs (e.g., glucocorticoids, anticonvulsants, potentiated sulphonamides, and certain nonsteroidal anti-inflammatory agents) should always be taken into consideration when evaluating thyroid function in cats.
- *Miscellaneous factors:* The assay methodology used may affect the number of false-negative results obtained. Certainly automated quantitative enzyme immunoassays (EIAs) have been shown to consistently underestimate total T4 concentrations, unlike chemiluminescent methods.[12,13] In hyperthyroid cats with total T4 values above the reference interval but less than 100 nmol/L (7.8 µg/dL), EIA results remain within the reference interval in just over 15% of cases.[12]

The specificity of total T4 for diagnosing hyperthyroidism, while higher than its sensitivity, is not 100%. False-positive results are rare, but they can and do occur. Anecdotally, false-positive T4 results are more common with enzyme-linked immunosorbent assay (ELISA) and EIA methodologies.[12,14] However, many commercial laboratories using chemiluminescent techniques have lowered the upper limit of the reference interval for total T4, partially to account for the lower circulating total T4 values found in some older cats. Although this change in the reference interval will increase the sensitivity of serum T4 to diagnosis hyperthyroidism (e.g., a serum T4 that was in the previous high end of the reference interval

Table 22-1	The Potential Effect of Hyperthyroidism and Nonthyroidal Illness on Thyroid Hormone Concentrations in Both Euthyroid and Hyperthyroid Cats*,†

	HORMONE			
	Total T4	**Total T3**	**Free T4**	**TSH**
Hyperthyroidism				
Subclinical	↔	↔	↔	↓
Mild	↔↑	↔	↑	↓
Mild with significant NTI	↔	↔	↑	↓
Moderate to severe	↑↑	↑↑	↑↑	↓↓
Euthyroidism				
Euthyroidism with no NTI	↔	↔	↔	↔
Euthyroidism with NTI	↔↓↓	↔↓↓	↔↑	↔↓

NTI, Nonthyroidal illness; *T3*, triiodothyronine; *T4*, thyroxine; *TSH*, thyroid-stimulating hormone (thyrotropin); ↓, concentrations decrease; ↔, concentrations remain within reference interval; ↑, concentrations increase.
*These effects are largely known for T3 and T4 and are theoretical for TSH. There is some evidence of the effect of hyperthyroidism and NTI on feline TSH, but this is complicated, as assessment has been using the canine assay.
†The number of arrows indicates severity of changes.

Table 22-2	Summary Characteristics of the Commonly Used Thyroid Hormone Tests for Feline Hyperthyroidism

	Advantages	**Disadvantages**	**Sensitivity**	**Specificity**
Total T4	Widely available Relatively cheap Robust hormone with no special sample handling requirements	Diagnostic performance less than perfect	90% sensitive, but values may remain within reference interval in subclinical and mild hyperthyroidism	Highly specific (approaching 100%); rare high values with particular assay methodologies
Total T3	Widely available Relatively cheap Robust hormone with no special sample handling requirements	Overall, performs poorly as a diagnostic test for hyperthyroidism	Poorly sensitive (≤70%)	Highly specific
Free T4	Not widely available Relatively expensive Special sample handling requirements	Should only be interpreted in association with total T4	≥98% sensitive (dialysis method)	Less specific (≥80%) than total T4
TSH	Canine assay widely available Relatively cheap Robust hormone with no special sample handling requirements Detectable values less likely in hyperthyroidism than euthyroidism	No feline specific assay available Should only be interpreted in association with either total or free T4	>90% sensitive	Poorly specific

T3, Triiodothyronine; *T4*, thyroxine; *TSH*, thyroid-stimulating hormone (thyrotropin).

would now be classified as elevated), it will also make it more likely that euthyroid cats will be misdiagnosed as hyperthyroid.

To interpret the diagnostic test results accurately, all of the aforementioned factors must be considered in light of the history and clinical findings. An apparently healthy cat with no clinical signs and a total T4 concentration that remains within the reference interval is likely to be euthyroid, although the possibility of subclinical hyperthyroidism always remains. Although there are other tests that are considered helpful in diagnosing subclinical hyperthyroidism (see later) in cats, it is questionable whether these should be done. In human patients, subclinical hyperthyroidism can persist for many years and can be detrimental to cardiac and bone health. However, cats with subclinical hyperthyroidism generally show no overt signs apart from the presence of small thyroid nodules. Because we have little evidence that this state has any detrimental effect on other organ systems, treatment for such subclinical hyperthyroidism is not recommended. Indeed, it is unclear if all or only a proportion of cats with subclinical disease will ever develop overt hyperthyroidism. It may be more prudent simply to monitor both the size of any thyroid nodule and circulating total T4 value every 6 months in these cats.

In cats suspected of hyperthyroidism that show mild clinical signs (e.g., weight loss despite good appetite) but maintain serum T4 values within the reference interval, several options exist. Repeating the total T4 value some weeks to months later may be diagnostic, as thyroid hormone concentrations eventually increase into the thyrotoxic range in most cats if the disorder is allowed to progress untreated. If ELISA or EIA methodologies had been used initially, testing via a different method such as radioimmunoassay or chemiluminescence is advisable. Alternatively, other diagnostic tests may be used, although some are more proficient in diagnosing euthyroidism rather than confirming hyperthyroidism (see later). In cats with clinical signs of hyperthyroidism and concurrent moderate to severe nonthyroidal disease, hyperthyroidism is likely if a total T4 concentration is within the upper half of the reference interval. Such cats do not pose a real diagnostic dilemma because sick euthyroid cats would be expected to have total T4 values that are suppressed to low or low-normal values. Alternatively, repeat T4 testing can be carried out upon recovery or after adequate treatment of the nonthyroidal disease. If the diagnosis of hyperthyroidism in a cat on antithyroid medication is questioned, the antithyroid drug should be stopped and T4 testing repeated in several days.

In cats with clinical signs of hyperthyroidism and a total T4 value above the reference interval, hyperthyroidism is confirmed. If there are few or no supportive clinical signs and the diagnosis is based on a high screening total T4 value alone, the diagnosis should be questioned. Again, if ELISAs or EIAs have been used, it may be prudent to verify the total T4 using a different methodology. The upper end of the reference interval should be checked to determine whether it has been substantially lowered, which could increase the rate of false-positive test results. The cat should also be reexamined to assess if any pertinent clinical signs have been missed, and if a thyroid nodule can be palpated. If then deemed appropriate, alternative tests may be selected for further investigation.

Total Triiodothyronine

Measurement of total T3 concentration offers no real advantage over total T4 in the diagnosis of feline hyperthyroidism. Serum total T4 and T3 concentrations are highly correlated in hyperthyroid cats. However, over 30% to 40% of hyperthyroid cats have serum total T3 concentrations that remain

within the reference interval, rendering it a much less sensitive test for diagnosing hyperthyroidism than total T4 determinations.[5,12] The majority of cats with normal total T3 concentrations have serum total T4 concentrations either within the reference interval or only marginally high (e.g., usually <65 nmol/L [<5.0 μg/dL] and always <100 nmol/L [<7.8 μg/dL]). These cats usually have mild disease, and it is likely that total T3 concentrations would increase into the diagnostic thyrotoxic range if the disorder were allowed to progress untreated. It is possible that this phenomenon (high T4 with normal T3) reflects a compensatory decrease in peripheral conversion of T4 to the more active T3 as hyperthyroidism first develops, although in a few cases the suppressive effect of severe concurrent nonthyroidal illness may play a role.

Despite its poor sensitivity, assessment of total T3 concentration, like total T4, is a highly specific test, and high values have only been reported in hyperthyroid cats. However, because total T3 is not commonly measured in cats, it is unclear whether the newer assay methodologies, such as EIA, may give rise to false-positive results.

Free Thyroxine

Estimation of the concentration of free T4 represents the unbound and biologically active portion of total T4. In human thyrotoxicosis, assessment of free T4 is considered a more sensitive diagnostic test for hyperthyroidism because it provides a more accurate reflection of thyroid status and is less affected by the myriad nonthyroidal factors that can suppress total T4. Concentrations of free T4 are disproportionately increased compared with total T4, which may be related in part to relative saturation of binding proteins or subnormal concentration of the major thyroid hormone binding proteins. Additionally, serum free T4 concentration remains elevated in hyperthyroid patients with nonthyroidal illnesses when total T4 concentration is suppressed into the reference interval.

Accurate measurement of free T4 concentrations remains mired in controversy in human medicine. There are many different methodologies employed, which can be broadly divided into direct and indirect methods. Direct methods employ equilibrium dialysis or filtration to separate free from bound T4, followed by quantification of the separated hormone by an ultrasensitive immunoassay. The most commonly used indirect method is a one-step method that can be fully automated; this method uses a hormone analogue that supposedly does not react with binding proteins but will compete with free T4 for unoccupied binding sites. However, because these analog methods tend to retain protein-binding capability, they can, at best, only estimate free hormone concentrations and probably offer minimal if any advantage over measurement of total T4 alone. The direct methods are considered as reference methods but are not immune to the possibility of erroneous results.

Measurement of free T4 concentration for diagnosing feline hyperthyroidism has been evaluated in many studies. As it is in humans, free T4 appears to be a more sensitive diagnostic test compared with total T4 measurement. This test is most useful in hyperthyroid cats that maintain serum total T4 concentrations within the reference interval as a result of mild thyroid disease or the suppressive effect of concurrent nonthyroidal illness.[5] Overall, the sensitivity of free T4 (by equilibrium dialysis) for hyperthyroidism exceeds 98%, compared with a test sensitivity of approximately 90% for total T4.[5] Determination of free T4 is most useful in mildly affected cats, where serum concentrations are high in over 95% of cases; by comparison, the corresponding total T4 is elevated in just over 60% of these cases.[5] In cats with markedly high total T4 concentrations, free T4 will also be elevated, but its measurement provides no more additional information and is therefore unnecessary.

The increased diagnostic sensitivity of free T4 measurement, however, is complicated by a loss of specificity because up to 30% of sick euthyroid cats will also have high concentrations.[5,8,15] It is unclear if such high free T4 values are truly reflective of circulating concentrations. Certainly, in humans, a transient increase in free T4 concentration is an uncommon but possible consequence of nonthyroidal illness.[16] However, falsely high values are possible with prolonged storage (50% increase over 5 days at 37° C [98.6° F]) and in lipemic samples.[17]

Given the poor specificity of free T4 for diagnosing feline hyperthyroidism, results should be interpreted with caution, especially in cats with normal T4 values. It is not recommended as a sole diagnostic criterion for confirmation of the disease. Free T4 concentrations should only be measured in cats with suspicious clinical signs and then always interpreted with a corresponding total T4 concentration. Hyperthyroidism is likely if the total T4 concentration is within the upper half of the reference interval and a free T4 concentration is high. This combination reflects either mild thyroid disease or hyperthyroidism with concurrent nonthyroidal illness. By comparison, nonthyroidal illness alone is usually only associated with high free T4 concentrations when total T4 concentrations are suppressed to the lower half or below the reference interval. Cats with few if any clinical signs and total and free T4 concentrations that remain within the reference intervals are likely euthyroid; however, the possibility of subclinical thyroid disease remains.

Despite widespread recommendation of indirect automated analog methods for free T4 measurement by commercial laboratories, there is limited published data available. Overall, it appears that their diagnostic performance is similar to that of total T4 concentrations (i.e., lower sensitivity and higher specificity than free T4 by equilibrium dialysis). This might reflect that such assays measure a proportion of total T4, but that this measured amount is not necessarily the true free concentration. As such, there is no real advantage in using these assays over those that measure the total T4 concentration.

Feline Thyroid-Stimulating Hormone

In humans, measurement of circulating TSH concentration is firmly established as a first-line diagnostic test of thyroid function. Commercially available assays have a functional sensitivity up to 30 times lower than the lower limit of the reference interval; therefore, these human assays are capable of accurately measuring both extremely mild and severe suppression of the TSH concentration. Moreover, there is a log-linear negative feedback relationship between TSH and free T4, such that marked changes in TSH concentration can be induced by relatively small changes in free T4.

A feline-specific TSH assay has not yet been developed. The greater homology of feline with canine rather than human TSH[18] has meant that most studies in cats have focused on using the assay designed for dogs.

One of the first studies measured TSH concentrations (using the canine thyroid-stimulating hormone [cTSH] assay) in healthy cats, cats with mild chronic kidney disease, and cats suffering from both hyperthyroidism and chronic kidney disease.[19] All of the hyperthyroid cats had circulating TSH concentrations lower than the limit of detection of the assay (0.03 ng/mL), thereby suggesting a diagnostic test of excellent sensitivity. Other studies have investigated the possibility of using TSH as a marker of subclinical disease when serum T4 concentrations have not yet increased. In support of this approach, one study reported that euthyroid cats having TSH concentrations deemed as undetectable (below the limit of detection of the cTSH assay) were more likely to have histopathologic evidence of thyroid nodular hyperplasia than euthyroid cats with detectable TSH concentrations.[20] Similarly, another study found that cats with undetectable TSH concentrations were significantly more likely to develop hyperthyroidism within 14 months than those with detectable concentrations.[21]

On the other hand, the specificity of TSH for diagnosing hyperthyroidism is less than optimal, with approximately 10% of euthyroid sick cats and 15% of healthy cats having suppressed concentrations similar to those seen in hyperthyroidism.[19] In sick cats, such a situation is not unexpected because suppression of TSH is a well-known component of the nonthyroidal illness syndrome in humans.[16] Additionally, most cats with initially undetectable TSH concentrations do not go on to develop hyperthyroidism.[21]

However, cats with detectable TSH concentrations rarely develop hyperthyroidism, at least in the short term.[21] Even though this might suggest that measurement of TSH is more valuable in eliminating a diagnosis of hyperthyroidism when detectable concentrations are found, individual hyperthyroid cats can occasionally have detectable TSH concentrations.[12] In cats being treated with antithyroid drugs in which there is a question about the original diagnosis, measurement of TSH as a diagnostic tool is not recommended. Even after the antithyroid drugs are stopped, it is not known how long it may take for TSH concentrations to become suppressed as the serum T4 concentrations increase.

Overall, the use of the cTSH assay to diagnose hyperthyroidism in cats is controversial. Thyroid-stimulating hormone is species-specific, and even though there may be good homology between cTSH and fTSH, there is only an approximate 36% cross reactivity to recombinant fTSH in the canine assay.[22] Additionally, the cTSH assay is already known to be incapable of distinguishing normal from low values in dogs, so it cannot be expected to reveal subtle suppression of TSH in cats. Overreliance on TSH should therefore be avoided until a functionally sensitive, species-specific fTSH assay is developed. If a canine assay is considered at all, results should be interpreted in light of clinical findings. In cats without clinical signs (apart from palpation of small thyroid nodules) that maintain serum TSH concentrations within the reference interval, hyperthyroidism is unlikely at least for the foreseeable short-term future.

Dynamic Thyroid Function Tests

If mild hyperthyroidism is suspected clinically but the total T4 concentration is within the reference interval, a diagnosis of hyperthyroidism or euthyroidism may be achieved by the simultaneous measurement of free T4 or TSH concentrations or by repeat testing of total T4 at some future date. As such, further diagnostic tests are rarely required. However, a number of dynamic tests have previously been suggested to be useful in such cats. Occasionally, these tests may still play a role in diagnosis, especially if repeated serum total T4 concentrations remain equivocal and serum free T4 or TSH measurement is unavailable or unhelpful. Commonly used protocols for dynamic thyroid function tests in cats are found in Table 22-3.

Thyroid-Stimulating Hormone Stimulation Test
There is a limited total T4 response to exogenous TSH in hyperthyroid cats, a finding that may be useful in diagnosis. Whereas early studies used bovine TSH,[1,23] it is no longer commercially available as a pharmaceutical preparation and has largely been replaced by recombinant human TSH (rhTSH), which is significantly more expensive.[24-27]

There are two potential explanations for this lack of T4 response to TSH stimulation; either these hyperthyroid cats are secreting T4 independently of TSH control or they are producing T4 at a maximal rate, with minimal reserve

capacity. The former is the least likely, given the response of feline hyperthyroid cells *in vitro* to rhTSH and the increased radioactive iodine uptake induced by rhTSH in hyperthyroid cats.[25,28] Thus hyperthyroid cats with equivocal basal total T4 concentrations exhibit a response indistinguishable from that in healthy cats, suggesting that this test is of more limited value diagnostically in mild cases.[23] Given the expense of rhTSH and its poor performance in mildly affected cats, the test has significant limitations in the evaluation of hyperthyroidism.

Thyrotropin-Releasing Hormone Stimulation Test
As with TSH stimulation, there is also a limited total T4 response to thyrotropin-releasing hormone (TRH) stimulation in hyperthyroid cats. In the first published study, it was reported that the percentage increase in total T4 after TRH administration was considerably less in hyperthyroid cats compared with healthy cats and those with other diseases.[29] However, a later study reported that the TRH stimulation test failed to differentiate severely sick hyperthyroid and euthyroid cats.[30] A further problem with this test is that adverse reactions to TRH administration appear to be relatively common in cats. These include vomiting, excessive salivation, tachypnea, and defecation. These reactions are transient, developing within a few minutes of TRH administration, and they are usually resolved by the end of the 4-hour test. Given its problem differentiating hyperthyroidism from euthyroidism in sick cats, coupled with the adverse effects, the TRH stimulation test is rarely recommended now.

Triiodothyronine Suppression Test
Theoretically, exogenous T3 suppresses thyroidal T4 production through negative feedback of the hypothalamic-pituitary-thyroid axis. In hyperthyroidism, because excess circulating thyroid hormone concentrations have already suppressed TSH production and secretion, additional T3 has minimal effect on T4 production. Therefore, serum total T4 concentration remains significantly higher after T3

Table 22-3	Commonly Used Protocols for Dynamic Thyroid Function Tests in Cats*		
	T3 Suppression	**TSH Stimulation**	**TRH Stimulation**
Drug	Liothyronine	TSH	TRH
Dose	20 µg every 8 h for 7 doses	25 µg/cat	0.1 mg/kg
Route	Oral	Intravenous	Intravenous
Sampling times	0 and 2 to 4 h after last dose	0 and 6 h	0 and 4 h
Assay	Total T4†	Total T4	Total T4
Reference interval	<20 nmol/L (<1.5 µg/dL) with >50% suppression	>100% increase	>60% increase

T3, Triiodothyronine; *T4*, thyroxine; *TRH*, thyrotropin-releasing hormone; *TSH*, thyroid-stimulating hormone (thyrotropin).
*Values quoted for interpretation are guidelines only. Individual laboratories should furnish their own reference interval and criteria for diagnosing hyperthyroidism.
†Concurrent assessment of total T3 is recommended to ensure adequate owner compliance in administration and sufficient gastrointestinal absorption of liothyronine.

(liothyronine) administration in hyperthyroid, compared with euthyroid (both healthy and sick) cats, and the percentage decrease is consequently significantly lower.[31,32]

Although the T3 suppression test is capable of diagnosing hyperthyroidism, it has been suggested to be more useful in confirming euthyroidism and therefore in ruling out hyperthyroidism. Unlike the TRH response test, it is not associated with any adverse reactions. However, it is a relatively prolonged test that is dependent on good owner compliance in reliably administering liothyronine tablets, a reasonable temperament of the cat in accepting and swallowing the tablets, and adequate gastrointestinal absorption. Because of these factors, it is usually recommended that T3 concentrations be measured simultaneously with T4. This obviously increases the expense of the test, but it ensures greater confidence in interpreting the results. Overall, despite its limitations, it is the preferred dynamic test over either the TSH or TRH stimulation tests for investigating hyperthyroidism in cats.

THYROIDAL RADIOISOTOPE UPTAKE

Uptake of radioactive iodine isotopes (^{131}I or ^{123}I) and technetium-99m as pertechnetate (^{99m}TcO$_4^-$) is increased in hyperthyroid cats.[33-37] Both radioactive iodine isotopes and pertechnetate are trapped and concentrated within the thyroid gland, although unlike ^{131}I and ^{123}I, pertechnetate is not organically bound to thyroglobulin nor stored within the thyroid gland. The relatively long half-life, higher gamma energy and beta emission of ^{131}I, and the higher expense of ^{123}I make their routine use in feline thyroid scintigraphy uncommon. Because of its availability, lower cost, superior image quality, and reduced radiation risks, pertechnetate is preferred.

There are many ways in which uptake of radioisotopes can be assessed. A quantitative percentage uptake can be calculated, provided that the administered dose and background activity is measured.[34] Values are significantly higher in hyperthyroid compared with healthy cats, and they correlate well with circulating thyroid hormone concentrations.[36] Similar, if not more diagnostically efficient results are obtained if the thyroid to salivary (T:S) ratio is calculated, either subjectively by observation or by drawing regions of interest and comparing both areas. It is generally accepted that the T:S ratio in healthy cats is less than 1,[36] although the upper limit for the reference interval in older, euthyroid cats has been reported to be as high as 1.5.[37] Although routinely used intravenously, pertechnetate may be administered subcutaneously.[37,38]

It is clear that quantitative thyroid imaging is not required for the diagnosis of hyperthyroidism in the majority of cats. However, it is considered the most sensitive diagnostic test that is less influenced by nonthyroidal factors, as compared with other tests of thyroid function. Thus it has successfully been used to diagnose hyperthyroidism in those cats with thyroid hormone concentrations that remain within the reference interval and has confirmed euthyroidism in sick cats with falsely high serum free T4 concentrations.[39,40] On the other hand, thyroid scintigraphy is not without its drawbacks. It is expensive and it requires access to sophisticated nuclear medicine equipment and may require sedation of the cats under investigation. Additionally, like most other diagnostic tests, it is not completely sensitive or specific. False-positive results have been reported in a few cats that had no histopathologic evidence of thyroid disease,[41] and recent administration of methimazole may increase measured uptake values, at least in euthyroid cats.[42,43]

Despite some diagnostic shortcomings, scintigraphic imaging remains a useful procedure to determine unilateral or bilateral involvement, the position of enlarged thyroid lobes, the site of hyperfunctioning accessory or ectopic thyroid tissue, or the presence of distant metastases from a functioning thyroid carcinoma in hyperthyroid cats.[44] It may also provide some useful predictive information for therapeutic radioactive iodine dose calculations and expected response to such treatment.[45,46]

OTHER DIAGNOSTIC TESTS

Ultrasonography has been used to document the dimensions and volume of the thyroid glands in euthyroid and hyperthyroid cats.[47,48] There is good agreement between ultrasonography and scintigraphy in defining normal and abnormal thyroid lobes.[47] Additionally, thyroid volume determined by scintigraphy is comparable to that obtained by ultrasonography, which may be useful in predicting the success of radioactive iodine therapy.[48-50] Computed tomography has also been used to determine the dimensions and volume of thyroid tissue in clinically healthy cats.[51] However, although capable of correctly identifying the more active thyroid lobe, it is considered less reliable than scintigraphy is in differentiating unilateral from bilateral involvement in hyperthyroid cats.[52] It must be stressed that these imaging modalities do not provide reliable information on hyperfunctioning of the thyroid gland *per se*. They are most useful in anatomically depicting abnormal thyroid tissue when a diagnosis of hyperthyroidism has already been confirmed.

SUMMARY

Hyperthyroidism remains a common endocrine disorder of cats. Although relatively easy to diagnose in cats presenting with classical overt hyperthyroidism, the increased frequency of routine testing of cats with few if any clinical signs of the disease, which are just as likely to be euthyroid as mildly hyperthyroid, has had significant implications for the diagnostic performance of many of the traditional tests used. Further advances in accurately predicting subclinical thyroid disease is only likely with the development of a species-specific fTSH assay, which is not available at this time.

References

1. Peterson ME, Kintzer PP, Cavanagh PG, et al: Feline hyperthyroidism: pretreatment clinical and laboratory evaluation of 131 cases. *J Am Vet Med Assoc* 183:103–110, 1983.
2. Thoday KL, Mooney CT: Historical, clinical and laboratory features of 126 hyperthyroid cats. *Vet Rec* 131:257–264, 1992.
3. Broussard JD, Peterson ME, Fox PR: Changes in clinical and laboratory findings in cats with hyperthyroidism from 1983 to 1993. *J Am Vet Med Assoc* 206:302–305, 1995.
4. Norsworthy GD, Adams VJ, McElhaney MR, et al: Relationship between semi-quantitative thyroid palpation and total thyroxine concentration in cats with and without hyperthyroidism. *J Feline Med Surg* 4:139–143, 2002.
5. Peterson ME, Melian C, Nichols R: Measurement of serum concentrations of free thyroxine, total thyroxine, and total triiodothyronine in cats with hyperthyroidism and cats with nonthyroidal disease. *J Am Vet Med Assoc* 218:529–536, 2001.
6. Peterson ME, Graves TK, Cavanagh I: Serum thyroid hormone concentrations fluctuate in cats with hyperthyroidism. *J Vet Int Med* 1:142–146, 1987.
7. Broome MR, Feldman EC, Turrel JM: Serial determination of thyroxine concentrations in hyperthyroid cats. *J Am Vet Med Assoc* 192:49–51, 1988.
8. Mooney CT, Little CJ, Macrae AW: Effect of illness not associated with the thyroid gland on serum total and free thyroxine concentrations in cats. *J Am Vet Med Assoc* 208:2004–2008, 1996.
9. Peterson ME, Gamble DA: Effect of nonthyroidal illness on serum thyroxine concentrations in cats: 494 cases. *J Am Vet Med Assoc* 197:1203–1208, 1988.
10. McLoughlin MA, DiBartola SP, Birchard SJ, et al: Influence of systemic nonthyroidal illness on serum concentration of thyroxine in hyperthyroid cats. *J Am Anim Hosp Assoc* 29:1227–1234, 1993.
11. Daminet S, Ferguson DC: Influence of drugs on thyroid function in dogs. *J Vet Intern Med* 17:463–472, 2003.
12. Peterson ME: More than just T4: diagnostic testing for hyperthyroidism in cats. *J Feline Med Surg* 15:765–777, 2013.
13. Higgs P, Costa M, Freke A, et al: Measurement of thyroxine and cortisol in canine and feline blood samples using two immunoassay analysers. *J Small Anim Pract* 55:153–159, 2014.
14. Lurye JC, Behrend EN, Kemppainen JC: Evaluation of an in-house enzyme-linked immunosorbent assay for quantitative measurement of serum total thyroxine concentration in dogs and cats. *J Am Vet Med Assoc* 221:243–249, 2002.
15. Wakeling J, Moore K, Elliott J, et al: Diagnosis of hyperthyroidism in cats with mild chronic kidney disease. *J Small Anim Pract* 49:287–294, 2008.
16. Warner MH, Beckett GJ: Mechanisms behind the non-thyroidal illness syndrome: an update. *J Endocrinol* 205:1–13, 2010.
17. Refsal KR, Nachreiner RF: Hormone assays and collection of samples. In Mooney CT, Peterson ME, editors: *BSAVA manual of canine and feline endocrinology*, ed 4, Gloucester, 2012, British Small Animal Veterinary Association, pp 1–7.
18. Rayalam S, Eizenstat LD, Hoenig M, et al: Cloning and sequencing of feline thyrotropin (fTSH): heterodimeric and yoked constructs. *Domest Anim Endocrinol* 30:203–217, 2006.
19. Wakeling J, Moore K, Elliott J, et al: Diagnosis of hyperthyroidism in cats with mild kidney disease. *J Small Anim Pract* 49:287–294, 2008.
20. Wakeling J, Smith K, Scase T: Subclinical hyperthyroidism in cats: a spontaneous model of subclinical toxic nodular goiter in humans. *Thyroid* 17:1202–1340, 2007.
21. Wakeling J, Elliott J, Syme H: Evaluation of predictors for the diagnosis of hyperthyroidism in cats. *J Vet Int Med* 25:1057–1065, 2011.
22. Rayalam S, Eizenstat LD, Davis RR, et al: Expression and purification of feline thyrotropin (fTSH): immunological detection and bioactivity of heterodimeric and yoked glycoproteins. *Domest Anim Endocrinol* 30:185–202, 2006.
23. Mooney CT, Thoday KL, Doxey DL: Serum thyroxine and triiodothyronine responses of hyperthyroid cats to thyrotropin. *Am J Vet Res* 57:987–991, 1996.
24. Stegeman JR, Graham PA, Hauptman JG: Use of recombinant human thyroid-stimulating hormone for thyrotropin-stimulation testing of euthyroid cats. *Am J Vet Res* 64:149–152, 2003.
25. van Hoek I, Daminet S, Vandermeulen E, et al: Recombinant human thyrotropin administration enhances thyroid uptake of radioactive iodine in hyperthyroid cats. *J Vet Intern Med* 22:1340–1344, 2008.
26. van Hoek IM, Peremans K, Vandermeulen E, et al: Effect of recombinant human thyroid stimulating hormone on serum thyroxine and thyroid scintigraphy in euthyroid cats. *J Feline Med Surg* 11:309–314, 2009.
27. van Hoek IM, Vandermeulen E, Peremans K, et al: Thyroid stimulation with recombinant human thyrotropin in healthy cats, cats with non-thyroidal illness and in cats with low serum thyroxin and azotaemia after treatment of hyperthyroidism. *J Feline Med Surg* 12:117–121, 2010.
28. Ward CR, Windham WR, Dise D: Evaluation of activation of G proteins in response to thyroid stimulating hormone in thyroid gland cells from euthyroid and hyperthyroid cats. *Am J Vet Res* 71:643–648, 2010.
29. Peterson ME, Broussard JD, Gamble DA: Use of the thyrotropin releasing hormone stimulation test to diagnose mild hyperthyroidism in cats. *J Vet Intern Med* 8:279–286, 1994.
30. Tomsa K, Glaus TM, Kacl GM, et al: Thyrotropin-releasing hormone stimulation test to assess thyroid function in severely sick cats. *J Vet Intern Med* 15:89–93, 2001.
31. Peterson ME, Graves TK, Gamble DA: Triiodothyronine (T3) suppression test: an aid in the diagnosis of mild hyperthyroidism in cats. *J Vet Intern Med* 4:233–238, 1990.
32. Refsal KR, Nachreiner RF, Stein BE, et al: Use of the triiodothyronine suppression test for diagnosis of hyperthyroidism in ill cats that have serum concentration of iodothyronines within normal range. *J Am Vet Men Assoc* 199:1594–1601, 1991.
33. Mooney CT, Thoday KL, Nicoll JJ, et al: Qualitative and quantitative thyroid imaging in feline hyperthyroidism using technetium-99m as pertechnetate. *Vet Radiol Ultrasound* 33:313–320, 1992.
34. Nap AM, Pollak YW, van den Brom WE, et al: Quantitative aspects of thyroid scintigraphy with pertechnetate (99mTcO4−) in cats. *J Vet Intern Med* 8:302–303, 1994.
35. Sjollema BE, Pollak YW, van den Brom WE, et al: Thyroidal radioiodine uptake in hyperthyroid cats. *Vet Q* 11:165–170, 1989.
36. Daniel GB, Sharp DS, Nieckarz JA, et al: Quantitative thyroid scintigraphy as a predictor of serum thyroxin concentration in normal and hyperthyroid cats. *Vet Radiol Ultrasound* 243:374–382, 2002.
37. Peterson ME, Broome MR: Thyroid scintigraphy findings in 2,096 cats with hyperthyroidism. *Vet Radiol Ultrasound* 56:84–95, 2015.
38. Page RB, Scrivani PV, Dykes NL, et al: Accuracy of increased thyroid activity during pertechnetate scintigraphy by subcutaneous injection for diagnosing hyperthyroidism in cats. *Vet Radiol Ultrasound* 47:206–211, 2005.
39. Smith TA, Bruyette DS, Hoskinson JJ, et al: Total thyroxine, free thyroxine, pertechnetate scan, and T3 suppression test results in cats with occult hyperthyroidism. *J Vet Intern Med* 10:185, 1996.
40. Marsolais ME, Mott J, Berry CR: Diagnosis of feline hyperthyroidism using thyroid scintigraphy. *J Vet Intern Med* 17:393, 2003.
41. Tomsa K, Hardeggar R, Glaus T, et al: 99mTc-pertechnetate scintigraphy in hyperthyroid cats with normal serum thyroxine concentrations. *J Vet Intern Med* 15:299, 2001.
42. Nieckarz JA, Daniel GB: The effect of methimazole on thyroid uptake of pertechnetate and radioiodine in normal cats. *Vet Radiol Ultrasound* 42:448–457, 2001.
43. Fischetti AJ, Drost WT, DiBartola SP, et al: Effects of methimazole on thyroid gland uptake of 99mTC-pertechnetate in 19 hyperthyroid cats. *Vet Radiol Ultrasound* 46:267–272, 2005.
44. Harvey AM, Hibbert A, Barrett EL, et al: Scintigraphic findings in 120 hyperthyroid cats. *J Feline Med Surg* 11:96–106, 2009.
45. Forrest LJ, Batt CJ, Metcalfe MR, et al: Feline hyperthyroidism: efficacy of treatment using volumetric analysis for radioiodine dose

calculation. *Vet Radiol Ultrasound* 37:141–145, 1996.

46. Wallack S, Metcalf M, Skidmore A, et al: Calculation and usage of the thyroid to background ratio on pertechnetate thyroid scan. *Vet Radiol Ultrasound* 51:554–560, 2010.

47. Wisner ER, Theon AP, Nyland TG, et al: Ultrasonographic examination of the thyroid gland of hyperthyroid cats: comparison to $^{99m}TcO_4^-$ scintigraphy. *Vet Radiol Ultrasound* 35:53–58, 1994.

48. Volckaert V, Vandermeulen E, Saunders JH, et al: Scintigraphic thyroid volume calculation

in hyperthyroid cats. *J Feline Med Surg* 14:889–894, 2012.

49. Barberet V, Baeumlin Y, Taeymans O, et al: Pre-and posttreatment ultrasonography of the thyroid gland in hyperthyroid cats. *Vet Radiol Ultrasound* 51:324–330, 2010.

50. Peterson ME, Broome MR: Radioiodine for feline hyperthyroidism. In Bonagura JD, Twedt DC, editors: *Kirk's current veterinary therapy XV*, Philadelphia, 2014, Elsevier/ Saunders, pp e112–e122.

51. Drost WT, Mattoon JS, Weisbrode SE: Use of helical computed tomography for measure-

ment of thyroid glands in clinically normal cats. *Am J Vet Res* 67:467–471, 2006.

52. Lautenschlaeger IE, Hartmenn A, Sicken J, et al: Comparison between computed tomography and ^{99m}Tc-pertechnetetae scintigraphy characteristics of the thyroid gland in cats with hyperthyroidism. *Vet Radiol Ultrasound* 54:666–673, 2013.

Diagnosis and Management of Iatrogenic Hypothyroidism

Mark E. Peterson

In cats, as in other species, hypothyroidism is the clinical syndrome that results from the chronic deficient secretion of the two thyroid hormones: thyroxine (T4) and triiodothyronine (T3).[1-4] Unlike the situation in dogs, in which primary hypothyroidism is common, naturally occurring hypothyroidism is extremely rare in the adult cat, with only two documented cases reported.[5,6] Most commonly, feline hypothyroidism is an iatrogenic complication associated with overtreatment of hyperthyroidism. Spontaneous hypothyroidism, when it does develop in cats, is seen most commonly as a congenital form in dwarf kittens.[1-4]

CLINICAL FEATURES OF FELINE HYPOTHYROIDISM

Although many of the clinical features that develop in hypothyroid cats are similar to those seen in dogs with the disorder, there are some major differences that can make diagnosis more difficult in the cat.[1-4] First, hypothyroid cats may develop a poor appetite, a sign not reported in dogs with hypothyroidism. Second, hypothyroid cats rarely develop severe hair loss or total alopecia, which are relatively common signs in dogs. The major clinical signs of hypothyroidism in adult cats are not specific but can include lethargy, dullness, decreased appetite, and weight gain[1-4] (Table 23-1). Nonspecific cutaneous changes (e.g., nonpruritic seborrhea sicca, dull hair coat, excessive shedding or matting of hair) and obesity can develop, whereas hypothermia and bradycardia are less common[1-4] (Figure 23-1).

Iatrogenic hypothyroidism is a recognized complication of treatment of hyperthyroidism in cats and can develop during therapy with antithyroid drugs,[7-9] after thyroidectomy,[7,9,10] or following radioiodine (^{131}I) treatment.[7,11-14] Although early reports suggested that clinical signs associated with severe iatrogenic hypothyroidism in cats were uncommon and that most cats did not require treatment, it is now realized that milder degrees of iatrogenic hypothyroidism are relatively common and that these cats may benefit from thyroid replacement therapy (especially if concurrent chronic kidney disease [CKD] is present). Many of these cats with mild or subclinical iatrogenic hypothyroidism fail to develop any overt clinical features that are noticeable to either the owner or veterinarian (see Table 23-1). With enough time

(i.e., months to years), most cats with iatrogenic hypothyroidism will develop some clinical signs of the disease; however, in many of these cats, signs develop so gradually that they are not always noticed by the owners.

HYPOTHYROIDISM AND THE KIDNEY

A major potential benefit of treating iatrogenic hypothyroidism in cats is that doing so may help maintain renal function. It is well known that untreated feline hyperthyroidism leads to a reversible increase in glomerular filtration rate (GFR) and that successful treatment of hyperthyroidism results in a decrease in GFR, which can lead to the development of azotemia if underlying CKD is present.[2,15] To make matters worse, when iatrogenic hypothyroidism develops in these cats with underlying CKD, GFR may fall even further, which leads to an additional decline in renal function.[2,15-17]

A report concluded that cats that developed iatrogenic hypothyroidism after treatment with antithyroid drugs or surgical thyroidectomy were at higher risk for development of azotemia and also had reduced survival times.[9] Even if severe clinical signs associated with hypothyroidism are not present in these cats, treatment of hypothyroidism might help increase GFR, improve kidney function, and improve survival.[9,18] Therefore, it may be important to avoid or at least minimize iatrogenic hypothyroidism when treating hyperthyroid cats because many of these cats will have some degree of pre-existing CKD at the time of diagnosis with hyperthyroidism.[9,15,17]

DIAGNOSING CATS WITH HYPOTHYROIDISM

Correctly diagnosing feline hypothyroidism can be challenging regardless of its etiology. Again, this syndrome rarely develops spontaneously.[1-6] Because hypothyroidism in the adult cat is almost always iatrogenic, diagnosing this disorder starts with a history of the cat being treated for hyperthyroidism. Thereafter the presumptive diagnosis of overt hypothyroidism is based on a combination of clinical features (e.g., lethargy, weight gain despite normal or decreased appetite), physical examination findings (e.g., poor hair coat, obesity),

Table 23-1	Clinical Features of Congenital, Iatrogenic, and Spontaneous Adult-Onset Hypothyroidism in Cats		
	Iatrogenic	**Congenital**	**Adult Onset**
Lethargy	+	+++	++
Dermatologic signs	+	+	++
Weight gain or obesity	++	+	+
Poor appetite	+	+	++
Constipation	+	+++	+
Goiter	− or +	− or +++	−
Disproportionate dwarfism	−	+	−
Delayed closure of growth plates	−	+	−
No obvious clinical signs	+	−	−

+, Present; −, absent.
The number of plus signs indicates severity of change.

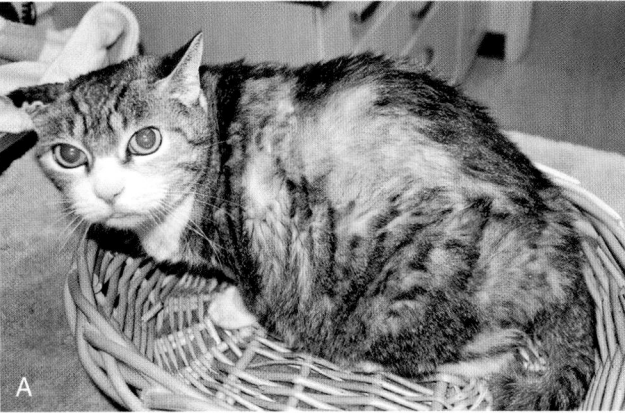
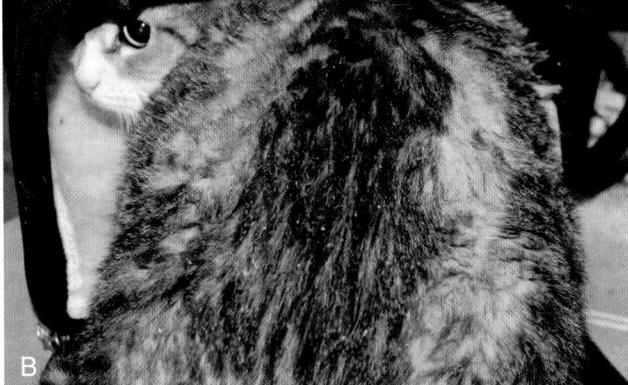

Figure 23-1: A 14-year-old female, neutered, domestic shorthair cat with iatrogenic hypothyroidism that developed 15 months after treatment with radioiodine (^{131}I). Notice the diffuse scaling, unkempt hair coat, and bilateral hair thinning on the lateral flanks.

routine laboratory tests (e.g., mild, nonregenerative anemia), and low to low-normal circulating thyroid hormone concentrations[1-4] (see Table 23-1).

A range of thyroid function tests is available to aid in diagnosis of feline hypothyroidism. Currently, the diagnosis of hypothyroidism relies largely on assessment of basal thyroid hormone analyses (i.e., serum T4, T3, and free T4), as well as serum thyroid-stimulating hormone (TSH) determinations. The greatest problem in interpretation of all of these laboratory tests is the number of factors other than intrinsic thyroid function that can affect hormone concentrations, including assay technique, nonthyroidal illness, and certain drugs (e.g., sulfonamides).[1,19-21] In clinical practice, we have to deal with four major factors that can make the diagnosis of iatrogenic hypothyroidism difficult to confirm in cats.

1. First, concurrent diseases, which are common in older cats, can result in a "euthyroid sick syndrome" characterized by falsely low serum thyroid hormone concentrations.[19-21] Serum TSH concentrations may also be high in some of these cats,[7] as in the situation in dogs,[22] which may lead to an incorrect diagnosis of hypothyroidism.
2. Second, one should expect a cat to gain weight and decrease its activity level after successful treatment of hyperthyroidism. Therefore, the clinical signs associated with iatrogenic hypothyroidism can overlap with those expected from a return to a euthyroid state.[2-4,9]
3. Third, the classical routine laboratory abnormalities associated with hypothyroidism (e.g., anemia, hypercholesterolemia) are inconsistent and may not develop, especially in adult cats with mild or subclinical hypothyroidism.[1-4]
4. Finally, many cats develop a marked transient decrease in total T4 within the first month of therapy with ^{131}I or

thyroidectomy.[23] This transient hypothyroid state is followed by a return to euthyroidism over the next 3 to 6 months as the remaining normal thyroid tissue recovers and starts to function once again.

Specific Thyroid Function Tests Used in Cats

Serum Thyroxine Concentration

By definition, cats with hypothyroidism have deficient thyroid hormone secretion. Therefore, finding a low serum T4 concentration is key in establishing a preliminary diagnosis of overt feline hypothyroidism. Like dogs,[24] however, it is possible for a cat with mild hypothyroidism to maintain a normal serum T4 concentration in the lower third of the reference range (e.g., 0.8 to 1.5 µg/dL [10 to 20 nmol/L]).[25-27] In human patients, the combination of normal serum thyroid hormone concentrations in combination with high TSH values is referred to as subclinical hypothyroidism.[28] In our series of cats with iatrogenic hypothyroidism,[25] half of the cats had a low serum T4 concentration (overt hypothyroidism) and half maintained a low-normal T4 value (subclinical hypothyroidism).

Although extremely important in establishing a diagnosis, a subnormal (or borderline low) T4 concentration alone is never definitive for hypothyroidism for two reasons—laboratory error and nonthyroidal illness. Serum T4 results must always be interpreted in light of the cat's history, clinical signs, and other laboratory findings. If a low serum T4 value is found in a cat that lacks clinical signs of hypothyroidism, especially if there is no history of treatment for hyperthyroidism or obvious nonthyroidal illness, one should never hesitate to repeat the serum T4 test using a different technique, if possible. Radioimmunoassay (RIA) and chemiluminescent enzyme immunoassay (Immulite, Siemens) may be the preferred assay techniques in such cases. In addition, the determination of a complete thyroid panel, especially measuring serum TSH concentration, will be very helpful in this situation[25-27] (see later).

Secondly, the serum T4 concentration will commonly be falsely low in cats with nonthyroidal illness, such as diabetes mellitus, hepatic disease, renal disease, and systemic neoplasia.[19-21] In general, the severity of the illness correlates inversely with the serum T4 concentration (i.e., sicker cats have lower serum T4 concentrations). Because multiple diseases and other factors can falsely lower the serum T4 concentration in cats, the veterinarian must always first rule out nonthyroidal disease before considering a diagnosis of hypothyroidism.

Once assay error and nonthyroidal illness have been excluded, cats with suspected hypothyroidism and a low to low-normal T4 concentration still require additional testing before one can establish a definitive diagnosis. Further thyroid function tests, such as determination of serum free T4, T3, and canine TSH (cTSH), are recommended. In some cats in which difficulties are encountered in confirming (or excluding) a diagnosis of hypothyroidism using these thyroid function tests, thyroid scintigraphy (imaging) or TSH stimulation testing may be indicated to confirm the disease.[25,27]

Serum Triiodothyronine Concentration

In most cats with hypothyroidism, serum total T3 concentrations are low to subnormal, correlating fairly well with the low T4 values.[25,27] This is in contrast to the situation in dogs with hypothyroidism, in which serum T3 generally remains within the reference range limits.[24]

The feline thyroid gland lacks the deiodinase enzyme (i.e., type 1 iodothyronine deiodinase) needed to convert T4 to T3.[29] Therefore, cats may not secrete very much T3 directly from the thyroid gland, and circulating T3 may be primarily derived from peripheral deiodination of T4 in the liver and kidney. As thyroid function abates, it appears that cats cannot compensate—as dogs and humans initially do—by increasing the thyroidal secretion of T3 such that circulating concentrations fall. Like total T4, however, T3 concentrations can also be suppressed in euthyroid cats suffering from a variety of nonthyroidal illnesses.[2,21]

Serum Free Thyroxine Concentration

Free T4 is the nonprotein-bound fraction of circulating T4 that can enter cells, producing the biologic effect of thyroid hormone and regulating the pituitary feedback mechanism. Free T4 accounts for less than 1% of circulating T4. Because only the free T4 component is biologically active, measuring

free T4 is generally considered a more sensitive test for diagnosing hypothyroidism. In addition, nonthyroidal illness influences free T4 less than it influences the total T4.[2,20,21] Therefore, free T4 should be theoretically better at distinguishing a euthyroid cat with nonthyroidal disease from a hypothyroid cat.

Although measuring free T4 concentration may be a more sensitive stand-alone test than total T4 concentration for diagnosis of hyperthyroidism, free T4 is less helpful for confirming feline hypothyroidism. First, like total T4, it is possible for a cat with hypothyroidism to maintain a normal serum free T4 concentration, especially a value in the lower half of the reference range. Second, moderate to severe nonthyroidal illness can also falsely lower the free T4 concentration, although to a lesser degree than seen with total T4.[20,21] Finally, at least when measured by dialysis, up to 20% of cats with nonthyroidal disease develop a falsely high free T4 concentration, further confusing the interpretation.[20,21,30] However, such a high free T4 result, even if falsely high, would completely exclude a diagnosis of hypothyroidism.

As a thyroid function test, free T4 does not appear to be very helpful in diagnosing feline hypothyroidism. In our series of cats with iatrogenic hypothyroidism,[27] only 20% of the cats had a low serum free T4 concentration (when measured by dialysis), whereas 60% had a low-normal value and 20% maintained a mid-normal free T4 value. Many hypothyroid cats that develop a low serum total T4 value will maintain a normal free T4 concentration, a combination that might be expected in cats with nonthyroidal illness rather than in cats with iatrogenic hypothyroidism.

Obviously, finding a low free T4 value combined with a low total T4 and a high TSH concentration is consistent with overt hypothyroidism (see Serum Thyroid Hormone Panels [Thyroxine, Free Thyroxine, Triiodothyronine, Thyroid-Stimulating Hormone]). However, like serum T4, the finding of a low free T4 value alone is not diagnostic for hypothyroidism because it could also be low in cats with nonthyroidal disease. Finally, because many hypothyroid cats will maintain free T4 concentrations within reference range limits, the finding of a normal value can never rule out hypothyroidism.

Serum Thyroid-Stimulating Hormone Concentration

In human patients, measurement of serum TSH concentration is commonly used as a front-line test of thyroid function.[31] The pituitary gland constantly monitors the circulating levels of T4 and T3, and if it senses the slightest decrease in serum thyroid hormone concentrations, it increases the secretion of TSH. Therefore, the finding of a high serum TSH value in a human patient is considered diagnostic for hypothyroidism, even if serum T4 concentrations remain normal.[28,31]

A specific assay for feline TSH is not yet available, but the commercially available cTSH assay cross-reacts with feline TSH enough to enable its use as a diagnostic test for hypothyroid cats. In one of the reported adult cats with spontaneous hypothyroidism, the serum TSH concentration was high when measured with the cTSH assay.[6] Similarly, cats with suspected iatrogenic hypothyroidism will also develop high serum TSH concentration as measured by the cTSH assay.[7,9,25-27] Based on these results, the cTSH assay has been touted as a good diagnostic test for feline hypothyroidism.[29,32] However, one must remember that the measurement of TSH concentrations is a relatively new test for cats, and no one has published results of a large case series documenting the true predictive value of serum cTSH as a diagnostic test for feline hypothyroidism.

In a cat suspected of hypothyroidism, the finding of a high serum TSH value in combination with low serum concentrations of total and free T4 can be considered diagnostic for hypothyroidism. This assay, however, is far from perfect. Like the situation in dogs with nonthyroidal illness in which high TSH values are found in about 10% of cases,[22] some cats with mild nonthyroidal illness—in particular obese cats and cats with poorly controlled diabetes—will show high (false-positive) cTSH concentrations, even when these cats have mid-normal to high-normal T4 and free T4 concentrations. Similar findings have been reported in euthyroid, obese human patients.[33]

Finally, the high serum TSH concentrations in some cats with suspected iatrogenic hypothyroidism fail to decrease after adequate levothyroxine (L-T4) or liothyronine (L-T3) replacement (see later). Physiologically, the rise in T4 and T3 should provide negative feedback to the pituitary gland to decrease TSH secretion.[31] The failure of TSH to fall despite high circulating T4 and T3 makes one question the accuracy of the cTSH assay in these cats.

Thyroid-stimulating hormone is a heterogeneous molecule and different isoforms of TSH may circulate in the blood.[34] The current TSH assay would likely detect these different isoforms, including those with little to no biologic activity.[34-37] Therefore, it is possible that the finding of a high measured serum TSH concentration in some cats with hypothyroidism (especially the TSH values that fail to decrease after adequate thyroid hormone replacement therapy) may actually represent secretion of high amounts of TSH isoforms with reduced biologic activity.

Obviously, a better TSH assay for feline hyperthyroidism is needed—particularly a feline-specific TSH assay that hopefully will better resolve these issue. However, until better TSH assays for cats are available, caution is advised in over-interpreting values in cats.

Serum Thyroid Hormone Panels (Thyroxine, Free Thyroxine, Triiodothyronine, Thyroid-Stimulating Hormone)

Differentiating hypothyroid from euthyroid cats can be challenging and may require evaluation of more than a single thyroid function test. The use of thyroid panels, which include serum total T4, free T4, total T3, and cTSH, are now commonly offered by many commercial laboratories. Evaluation of panels that measure multiple thyroid hormones can be very helpful in improving diagnostic sensitivity for hypothyroidism.

However, although complete thyroid panels are helpful in diagnosis, discordant results are very common. For example,

as noted earlier, it is not uncommon to see high cTSH concentrations with completely normal T4 and free T4 values in cats that have been treated for hyperthyroidism.[25-27] In one study, high serum TSH values developed in over one third of hyperthyroid cats treated with methimazole.[26] However, 17% of these cats had a high TSH value despite low-normal T4 and completely normal free T4 concentrations. We have seen similar findings in cats treated with ^{131}I, in which a subgroup of cats with low-normal T4 values (<20 nmol/L [<1.6 µg/dL]) will develop high cTSH levels, suggestive of mild or partial hypothyroidism.[27] These cats remain totally asymptomatic and show no clinical signs suggestive of hypothyroidism (although some may develop mild azotemia).

The clinical significance of these high serum TSH values is unclear and raises a number of questions:
1. Are these cats with low-normal T4/free T4 values but high TSH concentrations really hypothyroid?
2. Is this a form of "biochemical" subclinical hypothyroidism, as reported in humans?[28,37]
3. Should the methimazole dosage (or the ^{131}I dose) be reduced to prevent (and correct) the rise in serum TSH?
4. Should these cats be started on thyroid hormone supplementation despite their normal circulating thyroid hormone values? Or are these serum TSH values falsely high, simply representing a TSH laboratory artifact?

At this time, the answers to these questions remain unknown. Further studies and research are needed to answer them.

Thyroid-Stimulating Hormone Response Test

The TSH stimulation test provides important information for diagnosing hypothyroidism because it directly tests the thyroid's secretory reserve. In normal cats, administering exogenous TSH produces a consistent rise in serum T4 concentration. In contrast, hypothyroid cats show little, if any, rise in the low basal serum T4 concentrations after TSH stimulation.[1-4,38] In the past, bovine TSH was the preferred preparation for TSH stimulation testing in cats. However, bovine TSH is no longer available.

A recombinant human thyroid-stimulating hormone (rhTSH) preparation has been validated for TSH stimulation testing in cats.[39,40] The testing protocol involves collecting samples for serum total T4 concentration before and 6 hours after intravenous administration of 25 to 200 µg of rhTSH. Administrating rhTSH to clinically normal cats generally increases the basal T4 concentration by at least twofold. Further studies are needed to validate the use of this test for diagnosing feline hypothyroidism, but one would expect these cats to experience little to no rise in serum T4. The major disadvantage of this test is that rhTSH is extremely expensive, making it cost prohibitive for most owners.

Thyroid Scintigraphy

Thyroid scintigraphy is a nuclear medicine procedure that produces a visual display of functional thyroid tissue based on the selective uptake of various radionuclides by thyroid tissue.[41,42] Thyroid scintigraphy is considered the best imaging technique for cats (and dogs) with suspected hypothyroidism because it can distinguish animals with hypothyroidism from those with a falsely low serum T4 concentration.[43,44]

In cats with hypothyroidism secondary to treatment with thyroidectomy or ^{131}I, thyroid imaging typically reveals decreased or even absent radionuclide uptake (i.e., the thyroid volume may be less than normal or no thyroid tissue may be visible on the scan).[6,27] In human patients treated for hyperthyroidism, about one third of normal residual thyroid tissue is needed to maintain euthyroidism. Therefore, it may not be that surprising that many cats treated with bilateral thyroidectomy or ^{131}I might not have enough normal residual thyroid tissue left to maintain euthyroidism once the thyroid tumor tissue has been removed or destroyed.

In contrast, cats with a falsely low serum thyroid hormone concentration secondary to illness or drug therapy will have a normal thyroid image. Thyroid scintigraphy is of no benefit in diagnosis of hypothyroidism, however, in cats overtreated with methimazole.[8]

Unfortunately, apart from expense and the difficulties in dealing with radioisotopes, few veterinarians have access to the equipment needed to obtain thyroid images or perform thyroid uptake determinations.

Diagnostic Protocol for Cats with Suspected Iatrogenic Hypothyroidism

After treatment of cats with ^{131}I, surgical thyroidectomy, or methimazole, the author recommends monitoring with a complete physical examination as well as routine laboratory testing (e.g., complete blood count, serum chemistry panel, complete urinalysis) and total T4 determinations. No matter what treatment is chosen, the ideal post-treatment serum T4

concentration is a value in the mid-normal range (i.e., if the T4 reference range is listed as 10 to 50 nmol/L [0.8 to 4.0 µg/dL], the goal is to maintain the T4 values between 20 to 40 nmol/L [1.5 to 3.0 µg/dL]). Research indicates that both mild hyperthyroidism and hypothyroidism are deleterious to kidney function and may worsen already present CKD.[9,45,46]

If a low to low-normal serum total T4 (<20 nmol/L [<1.5 µg/dL]) is found during treatment with antithyroid drug therapy, the daily dosage should be reduced and the cat rechecked in a month. If a low to low-normal serum total T4 develops after therapy with surgery or ^{131}I, however, a complete thyroid panel is recommended. As in dogs and human patients with hypothyroidism, the finding of a high serum TSH concentration, together with low serum thyroid hormone values (i.e., total T4, free T4, and T3), is consistent with "overt" primary hypothyroidism. Cats with nonthyroidal illness (e.g., CKD) commonly have low serum total and free T4 concentrations, but these sick cats generally maintain normal values for serum TSH, which helps exclude iatrogenic hypothyroidism.

If, after treatment, the serum T4 remains normal but falls into the low-normal range, a complete thyroid profile is needed to rule out mild or subclinical hypothyroidism. This is especially important to do in cats that develop posttreatment azotemia or show marked worsening of existing CKD. Even if the serum thyroid values remain in the low-normal range, the finding of a high serum TSH concentration is consistent with a diagnosis of subclinical hypothyroidism and thyroid hormone replacement should be considered (Table 23-2).

In most cats, the author recommends waiting at least 3 months after ^{131}I or thyroidectomy before embarking on a workup for permanent iatrogenic hypothyroidism, especially

Table 23-2	When to Institute Thyroid Hormone Replacement in Cats with Suspected Hypothyroidism, Based on Serum Thyroxine and Thyroid-Stimulating Hormone Concentrations and Degree of Azotemia			
Serum Thyroxine	**Serum Thyroid-Stimulating Hormone**	**Worsening Azotemia**	**Diagnosis**	**Thyroid Hormone Supplementation**
Low	High	No	Overt hypothyroidism	Yes
Low	High	Yes	Overt hypothyroidism	Yes
Low	Normal	No	Nonthyroid illness Early hypothyroidism?	No
Low	Normal	Yes	Nonthyroid illness Early hypothyroidism?	Yes?
Low-normal	High	No	Subclinical hypothyroidism	No
Low-normal	High	Yes	Subclinical hypothyroidism	Yes
Low-normal	Normal	No	Subclinical hypothyroidism	No
Low-normal	Normal	Yes	Subclinical hypothyroidism	Yes?
High-normal	High	No	Subclinical hypothyroidism?	No
High-normal	High	Yes	Subclinical hypothyroidism?	No

if the cat is not presenting with the clinical features of hypothyroidism. However, the veterinarian should diagnose or exclude hypothyroidism as soon as possible in cats with renal disease inasmuch as hypothyroidism, treatment for hyperthyroidism, and CKD all lower the GFR. The combined effect of these three factors can lead to severe azotemia or even total renal failure. In hypothyroid cats with concurrent CKD, instituting T4 replacement therapy and increasing serum thyroid hormone concentrations back into the reference range may help raise the GFR to an acceptable level and reduce azotemia.[47,48]

TREATING CATS WITH NATURAL OR IATROGENIC HYPOTHYROIDISM

If hypothyroidism is diagnosed in a cat treated with methimazole, the daily dosage should be lowered. In contrast, if overt hypothyroidism developed after treatment with ^{131}I or surgical thyroidectomy, it is likely that the hypothyroid state is permanent and treatment with thyroid hormone supplementation should be considered. Likewise, if spontaneous hypothyroidism develops, treatment with thyroid hormone must be instituted.

Deciding Which Cats Should Be Treated or Just Monitored

If overt hypothyroidism is present (low serum concentrations of total T4, free T4, and T3, together with high levels of TSH), treatment should be instituted (see Table 23-2). In contrast, if subclinical hypothyroidism is present (i.e., normal serum concentrations of total T4, free T4, and T3, together with high TSH), then one should base the decision about whether to supplement or "wait and see" based on presence and degree of azotemia (see Table 23-2).

Choice of Thyroid Hormone Preparation

All cats with permanent, overt hypothyroidism require chronic thyroid hormone replacement therapy. A variety of thyroid hormone preparations are available, including synthetic sodium L-T4, synthetic sodium L-T3, or natural thyroid hormone preparations (desiccated thyroid).[49,50]

Synthetic Levothyroxine
Supplementation with L-T4 is the treatment of choice for most species (i.e., humans, dogs, cats) because T4 is the principal secretory product of the thyroid gland and is the physiologic "prohormone" for T3, the most potent or biologically active thyroid hormone.[49,51] Therefore, normalizing circulating concentrations of T4 and T3 in cats with hypothyroidism can be best achieved by administration of L-T4, which ends up replacing T3 as well as T4. However, some cats that do not respond adequately to replacement with L-T4 alone will benefit with the addition of L-T3; this is especially true if serum T3 concentrations remain low on

L-T4 supplementation (see Dose Adjustments and Therapeutic Failure).

Many L-T4 products (both brand name and generic) are available, although none are currently marketed for cats. Most of these are made available as tablets, but an oral solution (Leventa, Merck Animal Health; 100 µg/mL) is licensed for use in dogs. This liquid formulation is preferred over L-T4 tablets by many owners because the small volume formulation of the L-T4 solution may be easier to administer or hide in the cat's food.

Synthetic Liothyronine
Administration of L-T3 tablets (e.g., Cytomel, Tertroxin, generic L-T3) as the sole treatment for hypothyroidism circumvents the normal physiologic process of T4 deiodination to T3. Consequently, although circulating total and free T3 concentrations may be within the reference range limits after L-T3 administration, total and free T4 concentrations remain subnormal. Administration of purely T3-containing products may result in adequate tissue concentrations in organs such as the liver and kidneys, tissues which derive their T3 from the circulation.[51,52] However, the brain and pituitary gland, tissues that depend on circulating T4, may be deficient in T3 if circulating concentration of free T4 is subnormal. Conversely, it has been suggested that administration of sufficient T3 to provide adequate brain and pituitary concentrations may result in excessive concentrations in other organs.

In human patients that fail to adequately respond to replacement with L-T4 alone, combination L-T4 and L-T3 therapy is sometimes required.[53,54] Similarly, some cats that have persistently low serum T3 concentrations (and high TSH values) on adequate doses of L-T4 will benefit from addition of L-T3 to the L-T4 supplementation (see Dose Adjustments and Therapeutic Failure). One major disadvantage of prescribing L-T3 products, however, is the high cost of this drug.

Desiccated Thyroid Preparations
Desiccated thyroid or thyroid extract refers to porcine thyroid glands, dried and powdered for therapeutic use.[50] This product is sometimes referred to as *natural* thyroid hormone, pork thyroid, or by the name of a commercial brand, such as Armour Thyroid, Nature-Throid, WP Thyroid, or Erfa.

All brands of desiccated thyroid tablets contain a mixture of T4 and T3 in the proportion usually present in pig thyroids (a 4:1 ratio of T4:T3); each grain (about 60 to 65 mg) of desiccated thyroid contains 38 µg of T4 and 9 µg of T3. In normal cats, the ratio of circulating T4 to T3 is much higher (approximately 15:1), with much more T4 secreted than T3. Because the amount of T3 in desiccated thyroid products is high, postpill serum T4 and free T4 concentrations generally remain low, whereas serum T3 frequently rises to high-normal or even high values. Again, these postpill thyroid results are similar to those expected after supplementation with L-T3 alone.

In problem hypothyroid cats that maintain persistently low serum T3 concentrations and high serum TSH values on L-T4 therapy, however, the addition of desiccated thyroid to L-T4 therapy provides an inexpensive means to provide supplemental T3 to these cats (see Dose Adjustments and Therapeutic Failure).

Choice of Dosing Regimen

Pharmacokinetic studies of oral L-T4 in young, clinically normal cats indicate that L-T4 is rapidly cleared from the circulation with an average half-life of only 5.5 hours (range: 3.0 to 10.7 hours).[55] In that study, the time to reach peak L-T4 concentrations occurred shortly after administration (i.e., 1.5 to 3.0 hours) and reached peak plasma concentrations of 57 nmol/L (4.4 µg/dL). Based on those results, an oral L-T4 dosage of 100 µg/cat given once daily was recommended. A liquid L-T4 preparation (Leventa, Merck Animal Health) was administered to the normal cats of that study.[55] To the author's knowledge, no feline studies evaluating L-T4 tablets have been reported; however, it is well known that the bioequivalence can vary among different human thyroid products,[56,57] so it is also likely that the absorption kinetics of various thyroid preparations could also differ in cats.

In contrast to young, clinically normal cats, our clinical studies of cats with iatrogenic hypothyroidism treated with the same oral liquid formulation of L-T4 (i.e., Leventa) demonstrate that it may difficult to achieve high enough post-treatment serum T4 values in many of these senior or geriatric cats, even after administration of Leventa doses higher than the 100 µg/day.[49] Although the reason for this is not clear, it is well known that many factors can interfere with L-T4 absorption, including gastrointestinal disease, oral medications (e.g., calcium carbonate, aluminum hydroxide), and food, including high-fiber diets.[58-62] In addition, the inclusion of the various inert ingredients in the formulation of an individual L-T4 product may also hamper absorption of L-T4. Finally, senior and geriatric cats may have a reduced ability to absorb nutrients from the gastrointestinal tract,[63] which could also play a role in this apparent L-T4 malabsorption.

Because of this poor apparent absorption of L-T4 in many of our senior or geriatric cats, coupled with the short plasma half-life of T4 in cats, the author recommends that one initiate supplementation with twice daily administration of 75 µg of L-T4 (either as solution or tablet), given on an empty stomach, if possible (see later).[48] If the owner cannot administer the L-T4 twice a day, once daily administration (100 to 150 µg orally) can be attempted, but this regimen will not result in adequate thyroid replacement in all older cats with iatrogenic hypothyroidism.

Timing of Feeding and Thyroid Replacement Dosing

Simultaneous administration of L-T4 with food can markedly delay and inhibit the absorption of the drug in both humans[58,59,61] and dogs,[64] and this likely also occurs in cats.

In one study of dogs, giving the L-T4 with food decreased its absorption by about 45%.[64] The standard of care for human patients requiring L-T4 is to administer the drug on an empty stomach, generally an hour before meals.[65]

Food, as well as some commonly used medications (e.g., phosphate binders),[62] also appear to impair L-T4 absorption in cats.[48] All balanced commercial cat foods have added minerals (e.g., calcium), which may bind to L-T4 to form an insoluble or nonabsorbable complex reducing its absorption.[60] There is a marked individual variation in the absorption of L-T4 among senior cats; in some cats, the L-T4 will be well absorbed even when given at the time of feeding, but most cats will have higher post-treatment serum T4 concentrations when the L-T4 is given on an empty stomach. Therefore, to ensure optimal absorption and consistent serum thyroid hormone concentrations, L-T4 is best given by mouth at least 1 hour before or 3 hours after feeding (and administration of other medications).[48]

Depending on lifestyle, not all cat owners can easily follow these recommendations concerning the timing between the L-T4 dose and feeding. However, even if the L-T4 dose must be given with food, it is always important to standardize the time in which the L-T4 dose is given in relation to feeding. Once a protocol is established, it should be used for each dosing period, especially on the day of thyroid hormone monitoring (see later).

If the L-T4 must be given in food because of difficulties in directly administering the L-T4 into the cat's mouth, the owners can place the liquid solution or crushed tablet into a small amount of a favorite food (e.g., chicken or beef baby food works well for many cats) and then feed the main meal 1 hour later. Again, it is important for owners to be consistent in the amount of favorite food fed as well as the timing between the L-T4 dose and main meal to avoid marked variations in L-T4 absorption from day to day.

Clinical and Laboratory Monitoring

Clinical Signs

If clinical signs of overt hypothyroidism are present, metabolic signs, such as mental dullness and lethargy, are the first to improve, generally within a few days of starting thyroid hormone replacement therapy. Weight loss and increased activity may also be noted within a few weeks, whereas an improvement in the hair coat (e.g., shedding, dandruff, matted coat) should occur within 3 to 4 months of starting replacement therapy.

Routine Clinical Pathology Testing

Improvements in the routine clinicopathologic abnormalities associated with hypothyroidism following thyroid hormone replacement therapy can be expected to occur broadly in parallel with the clinical response. Circulating cholesterol and triglyceride values, if high, should decrease within just 2 to 4 weeks of starting therapy. If anemia is present, red blood cell values also start to improve quickly but may take 3 months to normalize.

The most important serum chemistry values to follow are the serum urea nitrogen and creatinine. Many untreated older cats with iatrogenic hypothyroidism will develop mild to moderate azotemia (International Renal Interest Society stage 2 to 3 CKD).[25,38,46] Of these, most will show improvement in their azotemia as the hypothyroidism resolves and euthyroidism is restored.[38,47,48] Even if the level of azotemia does not improve, adequate L-T4 replacement should slow progression of the CKD and stabilize the azotemia.

Thyroid Hormone Testing

Because most hypothyroid cats will display few, if any, overt clinical signs, we need to monitor serum thyroid hormone and TSH concentration to adequately judge the efficacy of thyroid hormone replacement therapy in these cats. Such laboratory monitoring is especially important given the wide variation in absorption of L-T4 (and therefore the final daily dose) among individual cats.

Therapeutic monitoring should be performed 4 weeks after starting L-T4 therapy or after making any subsequent dosage adjustment. Once the dose has been shown to be adequate, monitoring every 3 to 6 months thereafter is generally adequate.

Timing for Serum Thyroid Monitoring. Hypothyroid cats receiving L-T4 supplementation should demonstrate an increase in circulating total T4 and T3 values, which peak only a few hours after treatment and then progressively decline until the next dose.[55] In order to identify "peak" serum thyroid concentrations, it is therefore essential that posttreatment samples be collected approximately 4 hours after administration of the morning L-T4 dose.

If this monitoring time is not convenient because of the owner's life schedule, measurement of "trough" thyroid hormone concentrations (i.e., 10 to 12 hours after L-T4 dose; just prior to next dose) can also be used to evaluate adequacy of treatment.

No matter what monitoring protocol is chosen, owners should never modify the dosing schedule on the day before or the morning of thyroid testing in order to fit the correct timing for the blood draw at the veterinary office.

Ideal Post-treatment Serum Thyroid Concentrations. Laboratory monitoring is aimed at showing a rise of serum thyroid hormone values into the normal range together with lowering of the cTSH values into the reference range. Use of a complete thyroid panel (total T4, T3, free T4, and cTSH) for monitoring is ideal for a complete picture of thyroid function, but use of total T4 and TSH measurements are most important.[48]

During L-T4 treatment, the optimal peak circulating total T4 concentrations are between 30 to 45 nmol/L (2.5 to 3.5 µg/dL), whereas our goal for serum TSH is to have values fall to normal. Peak total T4 values <30 nmol/L (<2.5 µg/dL) are usually associated with low serum T3 and very high serum TSH concentrations, indicating that an increase in dosage is needed or that L-T4 administration be changed to empty-stomach dosing. Marked increases in peak total T4

values to ≥50 nmol/L (≥4.0 µg/dL) are generally unnecessary; in these cats, the L-T4 dose should be lowered, especially if the serum concentrations of T3, free T4, or both are also high.

If trough testing is used, the serum total T4 and T3 concentrations will be much lower than expected peak values but should remain within the lower end of the reference range limits. Ideally, serum TSH values should remain within reference range limits when tested at trough time.

Dosage Adjustments and Therapeutic Failure

In hypothyroid cats that fail to achieve the desired circulating thyroid hormone concentrations after L-T4 treatment, the L-T4 dosage should be increased. Such dosage adjustments will be needed in many cats, especially those on once-daily therapy or those in which the L-T4 is administered with food. However, there appears to be a wide variation in daily L-T4 dosage requirements among individual hypothyroid cats, with some showing lower than expected peak serum T4 and T3 levels with very high TSH concentrations, despite the administration of adequate doses of L-T4 on an empty stomach.[48] In most of these cats, the reason for this apparent malabsorption of L-T4 is unknown.

After any dosage adjustment or change in dosing protocol (i.e., timing between L-T4 and feeding), the cat should be scheduled for a recheck and thyroid monitoring in 4 weeks. This process should be repeated until the serum thyroid hormone and TSH concentrations are found to be acceptable.

In cats that do not respond adequately to L-T4 supplementation, the addition of L-T3 (5 to 10 µg/cat orally, twice daily) to the L-T4 supplementation may be helpful. This is especially true in cats that have persistently low serum T3 concentrations with high TSH values despite adequate posttreatment T4 levels (i.e., in the high-normal range). This can be achieved by adding in either L-T3 or a desiccated thyroid preparation to the current L-T4 regimen. The author generally uses desiccated thyroid because it is less expensive than L-T3 products but still provides an adequate dose of T3. For example, twice-daily administration of 1 grain of desiccated thyroid provides 9 µg of T3 as well as 38 µg of T4 at each dose. When this dose of desiccated thyroid is combined with the L-T4 supplement, the twice-daily dosage of L-T4 should be reduced accordingly (i.e., from 75 to 100 µg down to 30 to 50 µg).

Finally, the high serum TSH concentrations in some cats with suspected iatrogenic hypothyroidism fail to decrease after adequate L-T4 replacement with L-T3 or even combination L-T4/L-T3 therapy. In these cats, serum TSH concentrations remain very high despite a rise in postpill T4 and T3 concentrations to the upper half of the reference range. Physiologically, the rise in T4 and T3 should feed back to the pituitary gland to decrease TSH secretion.[30] The failure of TSH to fall despite high circulating T4 and T3 makes one question the accuracy of the cTSH assay in these cats.

References

1. Daminet S: Feline hypothyroidism. In Mooney CT, Peterson ME, editors: *BSAVA manual of canine and feline endocrinology*, ed 4, Quedgeley, Gloucester, 2012, British Small Animal Veterinary Association, pp 111–115.

2. Baral RM, Peterson ME: Thyroid gland disorders. In Little SE, editor: *The cat: clinical medicine and management*, St Louis, 2012, Elsevier/Saunders, pp 571–592.

3. Peterson ME: Feline hypothyroidism. In Kirk RW, Bonagura JD, editors: *Current veterinary therapy X*, Philadelphia, 1989, WB Saunders Co, pp 1000–1001.

4. Peterson ME, Randolph JF, Mooney CT: Endocrine diseases. In Sherding RG, editor: *The cat: diseases and clinical management*, ed 2, New York, 1994, Churchill Livingstone, p 1403.

5. Rand JS, Levine J, Best SJ, et al: Spontaneous adult-onset hypothyroidism in a cat. *J Vet Intern Med* 7:272–276, 1993.

6. Blois SL, Abrams-Ogg AC, Mitchell C, et al: Use of thyroid scintigraphy and pituitary immunohistochemistry in the diagnosis of spontaneous hypothyroidism in a mature cat. *J Feline Med Surg* 12:156–160, 2010.

7. Graham P: Measurement of feline thyrotropin using a commercial canine-specific immunoradiometric assay. *J Vet Intern Med* 14:342, 2000.

8. Fischetti AJ, Drost WT, DiBartola SP, et al: Effects of methimazole on thyroid gland uptake of ^{99m}TC-pertechnetate in 19 hyperthyroid cats. *Vet Radiol Ultrasound* 46:267–272, 2005.

9. Williams TL, Elliott J, Syme HM: Association of iatrogenic hypothyroidism with azotemia and reduced survival time in cats treated for hyperthyroidism. *J Vet Intern Med* 24:1086–1092, 2010.

10. Welches CD, Scavelli TD, Matthieson DT, et al: Occurrence of problems after three techniques of bilateral thyroidectomy in cats. *Vet Surg* 18:392–396, 1989.

11. Meric SM, Rubin SI: Serum thyroxine concentrations following fixed-dose radioactive iodine treatment in hyperthyroid cats: 62 cases (1986-1989). *J Am Vet Med Assoc* 197:621–623, 1990.

12. Jones BR, Cayzer J, Dillon EA, et al: Radioiodine treatment of hyperthyroid cats. *N Z Vet J* 39:71–74, 1991.

13. Peterson ME, Becker DV: Radioiodine treatment of 524 cats with hyperthyroidism. *J Am Vet Med Assoc* 207:1422–1430, 1995.

14. Nykamp SG, Dykes NL, Zarfoss MK, et al: Association of the risk of development of hypothyroidism after iodine 131 treatment with the pretreatment pattern of sodium pertechnetate Tc-99m uptake in the thyroid gland in cats with hyperthyroidism: 165 cases (1990-2002). *J Am Vet Med Assoc* 226:1671–1675, 2005.

15. Langston CE, Reine NJ: Hyperthyroidism and the kidney. *Clin Tech Small Anim Pract* 21:17–21, 2006.

16. Panciera DL, Lefebvre HP: Effect of experimental hypothyroidism on glomerular filtration rate and plasma creatinine concentrations in dogs. *J Vet Intern Med* 23:1045–1050, 2009.

17. Boag AK, Neiger R, Slater L, et al: Changes in the glomerular filtration rate of 27 cats with hyperthyroidism after treatment with radioactive iodine. *Vet Rec* 161:711–715, 2007.

18. Gommeren K, van Hoek I, Lefebvre HP, et al: Effect of thyroxine supplementation on glomerular filtration rate in hypothyroid dogs. *J Vet Intern Med* 23:844–849, 2009.

19. Peterson ME, Gamble DA: Effect of nonthyroidal illness on serum thyroxine concentrations in cats: 494 cases (1988). *J Am Vet Med Assoc* 197:1203–1208, 1990.

20. Mooney CT, Little CJ, Macrae AW: Effect of illness not associated with the thyroid gland on serum total and free thyroxine concentrations in cats. *J Am Vet Med Assoc* 208:2004–2008, 1996.

21. Peterson ME, Melian C, Nichols R: Measurement of serum concentrations of free thyroxine, total thyroxine, and total triiodothyronine in cats with hyperthyroidism and cats with nonthyroidal disease. *J Am Vet Med Assoc* 218:529–536, 2001.

22. Kantrowitz LB, Peterson ME, Melian C, et al: Serum total thyroxine, total triiodothyronine, free thyroxine, and thyrotropin concentrations in dogs with nonthyroidal disease. *J Am Vet Med Assoc* 219:765–769, 2001.

23. Peterson ME, Broome MR: Radioiodine for feline hyperthyroidism. In Bonagura JD, Twedt DC, editors: *Kirk's current veterinary therapy XV*, Philadelphia, 2014, Elsevier/Saunders, pp e112–e122.

24. Peterson ME, Melián C, Nichols R: Measurement of serum total thyroxine, triiodothyronine, free thyroxine, and thyrotropin concentrations for diagnosis of hypothyroidism in dogs. *J Am Vet Med Assoc* 211:1396–1402, 1997.

25. Peterson ME: Feline focus: Diagnostic testing for feline thyroid disease: hypothyroidism. *Compend Contin Educ Vet* 35:E4, 2013.

26. Chciuk K, Behrend EN, Martin L, et al: Evaluation of thyroid-stimulating hormone, total thyroxine and free thyroxine concentrations in 65 hyperthyroid cats receiving methimazole therapy. *J Vet Intern Med* 27:691–692, 2013.

27. Peterson ME, Guterl JN: Overt or subclinical iatrogenic hypothyroidism in cats: clinical, laboratory, and thyroid scintigraphic findings in 35 cases. In *Proceedings of the 24th Congress of the ECVIM-CA (European College of Veterinary Internal Medicine—Companion Animal)*, Mainz, Germany, September 5, 2014.

28. Biondi B, Cooper DS: The clinical significance of subclinical thyroid dysfunction. *Endocr Rev* 29:76–131, 2008.

29. Foster DJ, Thoday KL, Beckett GJ: Thyroid hormone deiodination in the domestic cat. *J Mol Endocrinol* 24:119–126, 2000.

30. Wakeling J, Moore K, Elliott J, et al: Diagnosis of hyperthyroidism in cats with mild chronic kidney disease. *J Small Anim Pract* 49:287–294, 2008.

31. Ross DS: Serum thyroid-stimulating hormone measurement for assessment of thyroid function and disease. *Endocrinol Metab Clin North Am* 30:245–264, 2001.

32. Wakeling J: Use of thyroid stimulating hormone (TSH) in cats. *Can Vet J* 51:33–34, 2010.

33. Michalaki MA, Vagenakis AG, Leonardou AS, et al: Thyroid function in humans with morbid obesity. *Thyroid* 16:73–78, 2006.

34. Magner JA: Thyroid-stimulating hormone: biosynthesis, cell biology, and bioactivity. *Endocr Rev* 11:354–385, 1990.

35. Pickles AJ, Peers N, Robertson WR, et al: Different isoforms of human pituitary thyroid-stimulating hormone have different relative biological activities. *J Mol Endocrinol* 9:251–256, 1992.

36. Beck-Peccoz P, Persani L: Variable biological activity of thyroid-stimulating hormone. *Eur J Endocrinol* 131:331–340, 1994.

37. Khandelwal D, Tandon N: Overt and subclinical hypothyroidism: who to treat and how. *Drugs* 72:17–33, 2012.

38. van Hoek IM, Vandermeulen E, Peremans K, et al: Thyroid stimulation with recombinant human thyrotropin in healthy cats, cats with non-thyroidal illness and in cats with low serum thyroxin and azotaemia after treatment of hyperthyroidism. *J Feline Med Surg* 12:117–121, 2010.

39. Stegeman JR, Graham PA, Hauptman JG: Use of recombinant human thyroid-stimulating hormone for thyrotropin-stimulation testing of euthyroid cats. *Am J Vet Res* 64:149–152, 2003.

40. van Hoek IM, Peremans K, Vandermeulen E, et al: Effect of recombinant human thyroid stimulating hormone on serum thyroxin and thyroid scintigraphy in euthyroid cats. *J Feline Med Surg* 11:309–314, 2009.

41. Daniel GB, Sharp DS, Nieckarz JA, et al: Quantitative thyroid scintigraphy as a predictor of serum thyroxin concentration in normal and hyperthyroid cats. *Vet Radiol Ultrasound* 43:374–382, 2002.

42. Peterson ME, Broome MR: Thyroid scintigraphy findings in 2096 cats with hyperthyroidism. *Vet Radiol Ultrasound* 56(1):84–95, 2015.

43. Diaz Espineira MM, Mol JA, Peeters ME, et al: Assessment of thyroid function in dogs with low plasma thyroxine concentration. *J Vet Intern Med* 21:25–32, 2007.

44. Shiel RE, Pinilla M, McAllister H, et al: Assessment of the value of quantitative thyroid scintigraphy for determination of thyroid function in dogs. *J Small Anim Pract* 53:278–285, 2012.

45. Williams TL, Peak KJ, Brodbelt D, et al: Survival and the development of azotemia after treatment of hyperthyroid cats. *J Vet Intern Med* 24:863–869, 2010.

46. Williams TL, Elliott J, Syme HM: Iatrogenic hypothyroidism (IH) contributes to the

development of azotemia in hyperthyroid cats. *J Vet Intern Med* 24:684, 2010.

47. Williams TL, Elliott J, Syme H: Restoration of euthyroidism in medically treated hyperthyroid cats with iatrogenic hypothyroidism (IH) improves renal function. *J Vet Intern Med* 2753–2754, 2012.

48. Peterson ME, Guterl JN: Iatrogenic feline hypothyroidism: challenges and complexities of thyroid hormone replacement in cats. In *Proceedings of the 24th Congress of the ECVIM-CA (European College of Veterinary Internal Medicine—Companion Animal)*, Mainz, Germany, September 5, 2014.

49. Fadeyev VV, Melnichenko GA, Morgunova TB: Options of replacement therapy in hypothyroidism. In Springer D, editor: *Hypothyroidism—influences and treatments*, Rijecka, 2010, InTech, pp 181–202.

50. Hoang TD, Olsen CH, Mai VQ, et al: Desiccated thyroid extract compared with levothyroxine in the treatment of hypothyroidism: a randomized, double-blind, crossover study. *J Clin Endocrinol Metab* 98:1982–1990, 2013.

51. Marsili A, Zavacki AM, Harney JW, et al: Physiological role and regulation of iodothyronine deiodinases: a 2011 update. *J Endocrinol Invest* 34:395–407, 2011.

52. Silva JE, Dick TE, Larsen PR: The contribution of local tissue thyroxine monodeiodin-ation to the nuclear 3,5,3′-triiodothyronine in pituitary, liver, and kidney of euthyroid rats. *Endocrinology* 103:1196–1207, 1978.

53. Biondi B, Wartofsky L: Combination treatment with T4 and T3: toward personalized replacement therapy in hypothyroidism? *J Clin Endocrinol Metab* 97:2256–2271, 2012.

54. Wartofsky L: Combination L-T3 and L-T4 therapy for hypothyroidism. *Curr Opin Endocrinol Diabetes Obes* 20:460–466, 2013.

55. Le Traon G, Burgaud S, Horspool L: Pharmacokinetics of L-thyroxine after oral administration to healthy cats. In *Proceedings of the 19th ECVIM-CA Congress (European College of Veterinary Internal Medicine—Companion Animals)*, 2009, p 209.

56. Eisenberg M, Distefano JJ: TSH-based protocol, tablet instability, and absorption effects on L-T4 bioequivalence. *Thyroid* 19:103–110, 2009.

57. Hennessey JV: Generic vs name brand L-thyroxine products: interchangeable or still not? *J Clin Endocrinol Metab* 98:511–514, 2013.

58. Singh N, Hershman JM: Interference with the absorption of levothyroxine. *Curr Opin Endocrinol Diabetes Obes* 10:347–352, 2003.

59. Liwanpo L, Hershman JM: Conditions and drugs interfering with thyroxine absorption.

Best Pract Res Clin Endocrinol Metab 23:781–792, 2009.

60. Zamfirescu I, Carlson HE: Absorption of levothyroxine when coadministered with various calcium formulations. *Thyroid* 21:483–486, 2011.

61. Lamson MJ, Pamplin CL, Rolleri RL, et al: Quantitation of a substantial reduction in levothyroxine (T4) absorption by food. *Thyroid* 14:876, 2004.

62. Diskin CJ, Stokes TJ, Dansby LM, et al: Effect of phosphate binders upon TSH and L-thyroxine dose in patients on thyroid replacement. *Int Urol Nephrol* 39:599–602, 2007.

63. Teshima E, Brunetto MA, Vasconcellos RS, et al: Nutrient digestibility, but not mineral absorption, is age-dependent in cats. *J Anim Physiol Anim Nutr (Berl)* 94:e251–e258, 2010.

64. Le Traon G, Burgaud S, Horspool LJ: Pharmacokinetics of total thyroxine in dogs after administration of an oral solution of levothyroxine sodium. *J Vet Pharmacol Ther* 31:95–101, 2008.

65. Bach-Huynh TG, Nayak B, Loh J, et al: Timing of levothyroxine administration affects serum thyrotropin concentration. *J Clin Endocrinol Metab* 94:3905–3912, 2009.

Treatment of Hyperthyroidism and Concurrent Renal Disease

Michael R. Broome

Between 14% and 49% of cats with hyperthyroidism have pre-existing chronic kidney disease (CKD).[1-9] Therapy to resolve thyrotoxicosis in these cats may potentially unmask the presence of previously occult CKD or result in the worsening of pre-existing azotemia. Initial reports focused on blunting the development or progression of azotemia in these cats by limiting control of their thyrotoxicosis.[10] Subsequent investigations demonstrated that the resolution of thyrotoxicosis in hyperthyroid cats results in the normalization of markers of renal injury that had been elevated while these cats were thyrotoxic, suggesting that thyrotoxicosis itself may actually contribute to the progression of kidney disease.[11-14]

Iatrogenic hypothyroidism may accompany medical therapy with antithyroid drugs[11,15-18] or definitive therapy with surgery[11,15] or radioiodine.[19-23] Hypothyroidism has been associated with low cardiac output leading to a decrease in renal blood flow and subsequently reduced glomerular filtration rate (GFR). Furthermore, iatrogenic hypothyroidism contributes to worsening of azotemia and shortened life expectancy in cats with pre-existing CKD.[11]

This chapter will explore the treatment of cats with hyperthyroidism and concurrent CKD with an emphasis on preventing further renal injury by resolving thyrotoxicosis while avoiding iatrogenic hypothyroidism.

IDENTIFYING HYPERTHYROID CATS WITH CONCURRENT CHRONIC KIDNEY DISEASE

Thyrotoxicosis can effectively mask the presence of concurrent CKD by increasing GFR, leading to potential normalization of laboratory measurements of renal function. Concurrent CKD should prompt adjustments in the management of hyperthyroid cats undergoing treatment. The first step in altering patient management is to recognize which hyperthyroid cats have CKD. There is, however, no single test that will accurately predict which hyperthyroid cats will become azotemic following a return to persistent euthyroidism. An early report suggested that GFR as estimated by renal scintigraphy was predictive in determining which cats with hyperthyroidism will become azotemic following radioiodine therapy.[1] Subsequent reports have been mixed, with some finding value in pretreatment GFR measurement[24,25] and other reports failing to confirm the value.[5,8,12]

In response to the inability to accurately predict which hyperthyroid cats will become azotemic following a return to euthyroidism, the use of a trial course of medical therapy, usually referred to as the *methimazole trial*, has been advocated (see Chapter 25).[10,26] However, hyperthyroid cats that develop azotemia following a return to euthyroidism have a similar survival to hyperthyroid cats that do not develop post-treatment azotemia,[11,27] and are unlikely to progress more than one International Renal Interest Society (IRIS) stage.[28] A recent consensus opinion of a panel of veterinary experts no longer recommends the routine use of a therapeutic trial in non-azotemic hyperthyroid cats to assess the effect of treatment on renal function.[29]

INITIATION OF SYMPTOMATIC THERAPY FOR CHRONIC KIDNEY DISEASE CONCURRENT WITH ANTITHYROID THERAPY

Nevertheless, cats with pretreatment laboratory evaluations that identify the presence of, or suggest the potential for, concurrent CKD will benefit from the initiation of standard supportive therapies based on IRIS staging. Some reports have shown limited value attempting to predict which hyperthyroid cats will become azotemic following a return to euthyroidism using more routinely available laboratory parameters, including serum creatinine, urine specific gravity, and thyroxine (T4) levels.[12,24,25] One report that evaluated pretreatment creatinine levels using a logistic regression model identified a pretreatment creatinine concentration of more than 1.4 mg/dL (123.8 μmol/L) as predictive of the development of post-treatment azotemia with 77% sensitivity and 76% specificity.[25]

Iatrogenic Hypothyroidism

While spontaneous hypothyroidism in the adult cat is uncommon,[30] iatrogenic hypothyroidism is a recognized complication that has been reported relatively commonly following treatment with antithyroid drugs,[11,15-18] surgical thyroidectomy,[11,15] and treatment with radioiodine.[19-23] Many clinical signs of hypothyroidism in the cat are similar to those in the dog, including lethargy, obesity, and cold intolerance.[31-34] The bilaterally symmetric alopecia and the normochromic, normocytic, nonregenerative anemia and hypercholesterolemia, classic in the hypothyroid dog, may be absent in the hypothyroid cat.[35] The severity of the clinical signs observed in the hypothyroid cat may also be less than typically observed in the hypothyroid dog. Indeed a low total T4 concentration secondary to treatment for hyperthyroidism is not always associated with any clinical signs of hypothyroidism, which can make the diagnosis of iatrogenic hypothyroidism challenging.[36,37] Furthermore, because spontaneous hypothyroidism in adult cats is rare, it may reduce the clinician's index of suspicion for this differential diagnosis.[35,38,39]

The diagnosis of iatrogenic hypothyroidism may be complicated by the presence of concurrent CKD. The effects of nonthyroidal illness on circulating levels of thyroid hormones may be to suppress levels of total T4 and free T4 (fT4) in euthyroid patients, resulting in subnormal thyroid hormone values. As a result, the finding of a low total T4 and/or fT4 level in a cat with azotemia must be interpreted in light of the possibility that this finding is due entirely to the effect of the concurrent CKD. Hence the tentative diagnosis of iatrogenic hypothyroidism in a cat with a low total T4 and concurrent azotemia requires confirmation. While no assay for feline thyroid-stimulating hormone is currently available, the canine thyroid-stimulating hormone (cTSH) assay has shown value in diagnosing iatrogenic hypothyroidism.[15,18,40,41] The finding of a decreased total T4 in conjunction with an elevated cTSH level following treatment of a hyperthyroid cat is generally considered diagnostic of iatrogenic hypothyroidism.[18,42,43] For more on diagnosis of iatrogenic hypothyroidism, see Chapter 23.

Iatrogenic Hypothyroidism Worsens Chronic Kidney Disease

Initial reports failed to identify the negative impact of iatrogenic hypothyroidism following therapy for hyperthyroidism. Indeed, until recently, the importance of iatrogenic hypothyroidism was largely unrecognized. Recent reports however, have alerted us to the relative frequency and clinical importance of this condition in cats with pre-existing CKD.[11,34,41,44] Hypothyroidism has been associated with significant decreases in renal function in every species evaluated, including the rat, cat, dog, and human.[11,42,45-57] Systemic responses to hypothyroidism include reduced cardiac output, decreased renal blood flow, and ultimately a reduced GFR. Direct renal responses to hypothyroidism include glomerular lesions such as thickening of the basement membrane and increased mesangial matrix.[58,59] The increased transcapillary leaking of plasma proteins that occurs in hypothyroidism can lead to proteinuria and the subsequent renal injury.[50]

In cats with otherwise normal renal function, the effect of hypothyroidism is frequently subtle (i.e., normal or only slightly increased blood urea nitrogen and serum creatinine levels) and may go unrecognized. However, in patients with concurrent renal dysfunction, the additional decrease in GFR that accompanies the development of hypothyroidism can

result in a significant worsening of azotemia and shortened survival time.[11] Furthermore, the restoration of euthyroidism has been shown to improve renal function in spontaneously hypothyroid dogs and people, as well as in medically treated hyperthyroid cats with iatrogenic hypothyroidism.[48,56,60,61]

Transient Iatrogenic Hypothyroidism Following Radioiodine Therapy

In the majority of cats with hyperthyroidism, the disease is caused by one or more benign, autonomously functioning thyroid adenomas, sometimes referred to as adenomatous thyroid hyperplasia. Only a small percentage of hyperthyroidism is caused by autonomously functional, differentiated thyroid carcinoma. Regardless of the exact histopathologic characterization of the thyroid tissue responsible for thyrotoxicosis, the one consistent clinical characteristic is autonomous function and growth. This autonomous thyroid hormone production causes a persistent and progressive thyrotoxicosis. Chronically elevated levels of circulating thyroid hormones lead to feedback suppression of the hypothalamus and the pituitary gland, resulting in chronically low thyroid-stimulating hormone (TSH) levels. Ultimately, chronically decreased TSH levels lead to atrophy of the normal thyroid tissue, which is dependent on TSH for its function and growth. Subclinical elevations in circulating thyroid hormone levels occurring at the earliest stages of hyperthyroidism will lead to feedback suppression of TSH release from the anterior pituitary long before clinical signs of thyrotoxicosis develop. As a result, cats with hyperthyroidism are typically diagnosed following months of suppression of normal thyroid tissue by persistently low TSH levels. This atrophy of normal thyroid tissue can lead to a period of transient hypothyroidism following curative radioiodine therapy.[22,41,62-65] The declining levels of circulating thyroid hormones that follow radioiodine therapy lead to an increase in TSH release from the anterior pituitary. The reactivation and/or regeneration of the previously atrophied thyroid tissue that occurs in response to the increased TSH levels are not instantaneous; an interval of transient iatrogenic hypothyroidism is possible following radioiodine therapy. Ultimately, the elevated TSH levels that occur in response to declining levels of circulating thyroid hormones following radioiodine therapy lead to reactivation and/or regeneration of the previously atrophied thyroid tissue, returning the majority of these cats to persistent euthyroidism.

The duration of this transient iatrogenic hypothyroidism ranges from days to months. When the duration of transient hypothyroidism is less than the interval used to recheck the patient following treatment, it may go undetected. The majority of hyperthyroid cats with normal kidney function tolerate an interval of iatrogenic hypothyroidism without negative consequences. Hyperthyroid cats with concurrent CKD will likely become azotemic during this interval, motivating the initiation of thyroid hormone supplementation to limit the progression of CKD that occurs in response to iatrogenic hypothyroidism.[44] The persistence of low GFR levels in hypothyroid dogs following the re-establishment of euthyroidism by oral thyroid hormone supplements suggests the possibility of an irreversible renal injury that accompanied the hypothyroidism in these dogs.[56] In hyperthyroid cats with more advanced CKD resulting in the presence of azotemia while they are thyrotoxic, the transient hypothyroidism that follows radioiodine therapy may similarly contribute to irreversible renal function decline and shortened survival.[11] In support of this premise, a recent study found that avoiding iatrogenic hypothyroidism following radioiodine therapy in hyperthyroid cats with concurrent azotemia by the administration of oral thyroid hormone supplements blunted the progression of azotemia.[66]

There is mounting evidence that iatrogenic hypothyroidism contributes to the progression of CKD, as well as shortened survival. The previous approach that focused on resolving thyrotoxicosis without consideration of the effects of iatrogenic hypothyroidism can no longer be supported. Current recommendations for the management of hyperthyroid cats must include a realization of the negative effects of both thyrotoxicosis and hypothyroidism on the kidney.

Hyperthyroid Cats with Concurrent Azotemia

Cats with documented azotemia while thyrotoxic will often have an interval with worsening of azotemia following a return to persistent euthyroidism. The decline in GFR that accompanies a resolution of thyrotoxicosis is potentially more clinically significant in hyperthyroid cats with pre-existing azotemia at the time of diagnosis. In a previous study of 300 hyperthyroid cats treated with medical therapy or medical therapy in combination with thyroidectomy, 32 cats with pretreatment azotemia (creatinine >2 mg/dL [176.8 μmol/L]) were identified, and these cats had significantly shorter survival times (median 178 days, range 0 to 1505 days) than cats that were not azotemic at the time of treatment (median 612 days, range 0 to 2541 days).[67] It is not surprising that hyperthyroid cats with more advanced CKD at the time of diagnosis would have shortened survival times relative to hyperthyroid cats with lesser degrees of CKD. Chronic kidney disease is, after all, a leading cause of death in geriatric cats.[68] However, the progression of CKD is widely variable among cats, with many cats demonstrating stable levels of azotemia for extended periods.[69] Experimentally, cats appear to have relatively stable renal function for at least 12 months following the induction of reduced renal function by partial (five-sixths) renal ablation.[70] Furthermore, cats with naturally occurring CKD will die from illness other than their kidney disease approximately 50% of the time.[71]

Cats with concurrent azotemia at the time of diagnosis of hyperthyroidism can demonstrate extended survival times. A recent report evaluated 181 hyperthyroid cats with concurrent CKD (IRIS stage 2 to 3) that were treated with radioiodine therapy.[72] All of the cats in this report were treated with individualized doses of iodine-131 that were calculated with the goal of resolving adenomatous disease while minimizing iatrogenic hypothyroidism. Furthermore, 131 cats in this report were supplemented with oral levothyroxine sodium (0.1 mg, by mouth [PO], every 24 hours) at discharge following radioiodine therapy. This supplementation was designed to avoid the transient iatrogenic hypothyroidism that might follow successful radioiodine therapy. The remaining 50 cats served as controls and received no thyroxine supplementation. All of the cats in this study, both the levothyroxine sodium–supplemented and control groups, were discharged on subcutaneous fluids administered at home, every other day for the immediate post-therapy (20 days) interval. Despite the pretreatment azotemia demonstrated by these cats (median creatinine = 2.5 mg/dL [221 μmol/L], range = 2.0 to 4.7 mg/dL [176.8 to 415.5 μmol/L]), the median survival times for both the supplemented (1094 days) and control (643 days) cats in this study parallel median survival times from previous reports of nonazotemic hyperthyroid cats following radioiodine therapy.[6,22,73]

There are several possible explanations for the extended survival noted in these azotemic hyperthyroid cats treated with radioiodine. All cats in this report were managed with subcutaneous fluids during hospitalization for radioiodine therapy (3 to 6 days) and the subsequent 20 days following discharge. Subcutaneous fluids were administered with the goal of improving hydration and supporting renal function during the period of thyroid hormone decline and subsequent GFR reduction. Hyperthyroid cats may undergo a period of reduced food and water consumption following radioiodine therapy. This reduction in food and water intake is generally attributed to the psychological responses to the experience of hospitalization for radioiodine therapy and readjustment following return home. Subcutaneous fluid therapy could therefore avoid episodes of suboptimal hydration that could otherwise contribute to worsening kidney function and shortened survival.

An additional explanation for the disparity in survival times of the hyperthyroid cats with pretreatment azotemia between these two studies could be the effectiveness of the therapy to control thyrotoxicosis. Many of the medically treated cats were inadequately treated. Only 123 of 300 cats (41%) were documented to have good control of their disease (T4 <3.1 μg/dL [40 nmol/L]) in the 2 to 6 month period following treatment.[67] Of the 181 cats treated with radioiodine, 152 (84%) were documented to have total T4 levels less than 3.1 μg/dL (40 nmol/L) at the three-month post–radioiodine therapy interval.[72] Persistent, uncontrolled thyrotoxicosis may have contributed to a reduced survival in the medically managed cats with pretreatment azotemia.

Finally, in light of the reduced survival that accompanies the development of iatrogenic hypothyroidism in cats without pre-existing azotemia,[11] the development of iatrogenic hypothyroidism in cats with pre-existing azotemia may contribute to an even more significantly reduced survival. Management of hyperthyroid cats with concurrent azotemia with the goal of avoiding iatrogenic hypothyroidism can result in survival times that parallel that of nonazotemic hyperthyroid cats.[72]

Current Recommendations

The current literature supports several key concepts that are important for optimizing survival when treating hyperthyroid cats with concurrent CKD. The first key concept is the importance of resolving the thyrotoxicosis. Thyrotoxicosis has been shown to cause progressive and potentially terminal cardiovascular changes in hyperthyroid cats since shortly following documentation of the disease in the cat.[74-80] More recently, reports suggest the contribution that thyrotoxicosis makes to the progression of CKD in hyperthyroid cats.[12,14] The previous recommendation to allow hyperthyroid cats with concurrent renal disease to remain mildly thyrotoxic in an effort to improve numerical creatinine levels has been abandoned.[29]

While initial reports suggested that the large majority of cats on medical therapy for hyperthyroidism achieved adequate control,[36] subsequent reports and clinical experience demonstrate that medical therapy frequently leads to inadequate control of thyrotoxicosis. In a recent study of 1428 cats treated with methimazole or carbimazole, total T4 levels remained above the reference range in 52.9% and 49.0%, respectively, of the samples analyzed.[17] Curative therapies including both thyroidectomy and radioiodine therapy are more consistently effective in resolving the thyrotoxicosis associated with hyperthyroidism. Radioiodine therapy results in a permanent resolution of thyrotoxicosis in approximately 95% of the hyperthyroid cats treated.[41] The permanent resolution of thyrotoxicosis that occurs following radioiodine therapy was associated with survival times approximately twice as long[72] as those measured in hyperthyroid cats treated with methimazole.[67]

The second key concept is the importance of preventing iatrogenic hypothyroidism. While unrecognized until recently, the avoidance of iatrogenic hypothyroidism is of major importance in maximizing survival following therapy for hyperthyroidism in cats. Hypothyroidism has been shown to reduce renal function in every species evaluated. And iatrogenic hypothyroidism has been shown to worsen azotemia and shorten survival following treatment of cats with hyperthyroidism.[11,34,44] Iatrogenic hypothyroidism has been documented during medical therapy using methimazole or carbimazole, as well as following the definitive therapies of thyroidectomy and radioiodine. Regardless of the treatment modality utilized, efforts to avoid inducing iatrogenic hypothyroidism are critical to avoid further renal injury in these cats.

When treating hyperthyroid cats with radioiodine, the use of individualized dosages that are determined with the goal of resolving adenomatous disease while avoiding iatrogenic hypothyroidism is recommended.[41] Furthermore, the transient use of levothyroxine sodium supplementation initiated upon discharge has been shown to blunt the progression of azotemia in hyperthyroid cats with concurrent pretreatment azotemia.[72]

When treating hyperthyroid cats with thyroidectomy, the transient use of levothyroxine sodium supplementation is recommended even following unilateral thyroid lobectomies. This supplementation will help to avoid the transient period of hypothyroidism that occurs prior to the reactivation and regeneration of the remaining normal, but previously suppressed, thyroid tissue. The use of permanent levothyroxine sodium supplementation is similarly indicated following bilateral thyroid lobectomies.

Medical management of the hyperthyroid cat with concurrent renal disease may be the most problematic form of therapy. Ideally, the dose of antithyroid medication needs to be adjusted to achieve persistent control of the patient's thyrotoxicosis while avoiding the negative effects of iatrogenic hypothyroidism. In addition to consistently overcoming the variable tolerance of hyperthyroid cats for the process of being medicated with either oral or transdermal forms of antithyroid drugs, there are numerous other limitations to achieving this goal. These limitations include the progressive nature of hyperthyroidism, requiring regular increases in drug dosage,[41] increasing incidence of gastrointestinal side effects associated with increasing antithyroid drug dosage,[81] and the limited absorption of transdermal forms of antithyroid drugs.[82] The difficulty in achieving persistent euthyroidism in hyperthyroid cats managed medically may explain the reduced survival times in cats managed with methimazole when compared to cats managed with radioiodine.[3,67,72]

The task of ensuring persistent euthyroidism using levothyroxine sodium supplementation in cats with iatrogenic hypothyroidism following either radioiodine therapy or thyroidectomy is, by comparison, relatively straightforward. The nature of the condition is relatively static. Once euthyroidism is achieved on oral thyroid hormone supplements there is rarely a need for ongoing dose adjustments. Thyroxine is a hormone naturally produced by the patient's thyroid gland. As such, there are no idiosyncratic reactions or other side effects associated with the administration of appropriate doses of the synthetic supplement. Levothyroxine sodium is both odorless and tasteless[83] and therefore easily concealed in small volumes of highly palatable foods or treats. Finally, levothyroxine sodium is available in both tablet and liquid forms.

The third key concept is the importance of the use of the standard supportive therapies traditionally utilized in cats with CKD. The reduction in GFR that accompanies a resolution of thyrotoxicosis should be anticipated and standard supportive therapies for pre-existing renal disease should be initiated to ensure tolerance for the incremental change in renal function that accompanies the return to euthyroidism. Most cats with concurrent CKD and hyperthyroidism will benefit from the administration of subcutaneous fluids following the initiation of antithyroid therapy. Many cats will benefit from the initiation of other standard therapies, including possible dietary phosphorus restriction, phosphate binders, histamine (H_2) blockers, potassium supplementation, antihypertensive therapy when indicated, treatment of proteinuria when indicated, and supplemental B vitamin administration. For more on treatment of CKD, see Chapter 47.

In conclusion, hyperthyroid cats with concurrent azotemia can be successfully treated, leading to relatively long-term survival by resolving their thyrotoxicosis while avoiding the consequences of iatrogenic hypothyroidism and simultaneously initiating the standard supportive therapies utilized in cats with CKD.

References

1. Adams WH, Daniel GB, Legendre AM, et al: Changes in renal function in cats following treatment of hyperthyroidism using [131]I. *Vet Radiol Ultrasound* 38:231–238, 1997.
2. Broussard JD, Peterson ME, Fox PR: Changes in clinical and laboratory findings in cats with hyperthyroidism from 1983 to 1993. *J Am Vet Med Assoc* 206:302–305, 1995.
3. Milner RJ, Channell CD, Levy JK, et al: Survival times for cats with hyperthyroidism treated with iodine 131, methimazole, or both: 167 cases (1996-2003). *J Am Vet Med Assoc* 228:559–563, 2006.
4. Bucknell DG: Feline hyperthyroidism: spectrum of clinical presentations and response to carbimazole therapy. *Aust Vet J* 78:462–465, 2000.
5. Boag AK, Neiger R, Slater L, et al: Changes in the glomerular filtration rate of 27 cats with hyperthyroidism after treatment with radioactive iodine. *Vet Rec* 161:711–715, 2007.
6. Slater MR, Geller S, Rogers K: Long-term health and predictors of survival for hyperthyroid cats treated with iodine 131. *J Vet Intern Med* 15:47–51, 2001.
7. Graves TK, Olivier NB, Nachreiner RF, et al: Changes in renal function associated with treatment of hyperthyroidism in cats. *Am J Vet Res* 55:1745–1749, 1994.
8. Riensche MR, Graves TK, Schaeffer DJ: An investigation of predictors of renal insufficiency following treatment of hyperthyroidism in cats. *J Feline Med Surg* 10:160–166, 2008.
9. Becker TJ, Graves TK, Kruger JM, et al: Effects of methimazole on renal function in cats with hyperthyroidism. *J Am Anim Hosp Assoc* 36:215–223, 2000.
10. Feldman EC, Nelson RW: Feline hyperthyroidism (thyrotoxicosis). In Feldman EC, Nelson RW, editors: *Canine and feline endocrinology and reproduction*, ed 3, Philadelphia, 2004, Saunders, pp 152–218.
11. Williams TL, Elliott J, Syme HM: Association of iatrogenic hypothyroidism with azotemia and reduced survival time in cats treated for hyperthyroidism. *J Vet Intern Med* 24:1086–1092, 2010.
12. van Hoek I, Lefebvre HP, Peremans K, et al: Short- and long-term follow-up of glomerular and tubular renal markers of kidney function in hyperthyroid cats after treatment with radioiodine. *Domest Anim Endocrinol* 36:45–56, 2009.
13. van Hoek I, Lefebvre HP, Kooistra HS, et al: Plasma clearance of exogenous creatinine, exoiohexol, and endo-iohexol in hyperthyroid cats before and after treatment with radioiodine. *J Vet Intern Med* 22:879–885, 2008.
14. Lapointe C, Belanger M, Dunn M, et al: N-acetyl-beta-D-glucosaminidase index as an early biomarker for chronic kidney disease in cats with hyperthyroidism. *J Vet Intern Med* 22:1103–1110, 2008.
15. Graham PA, Refsal KR, Nachreiner RF, et al: The measurement of feline thyrotropin (TSH) using a commercial canine immunoradiometric assay. *J Vet Intern Med* 14:342, 2000. (Abstract).
16. Fischetti AJ, Drost WT, DiBartola SP, et al: Effects of methimazole on thyroid gland uptake of [99m]TC-pertechnetate in 19 hyperthyroid cats. *Vet Radiol Ultrasound* 46:267–272, 2005.
17. Gallagher B, Mooney C, Graham P: Efficacy of two oral antithyroid medications used once daily: a laboratory survey. In *British Small Animal Veterinary Association (BSAVA) Congress, Scientific Proceedings*, Birmingham, 2011, p 457.
18. Chciuk K, Behrend EN, Martin L, et al: Evaluation of thyroid-stimulating hormone, total thyroxine and free thyroxine concentrations in 65 hyperthyroid cats receiving methimazole therapy. *J Vet Intern Med* 27:691–692, 2013.
19. Jones BR, Cayzer J, Dillon EA, et al: Radioiodine treatment of hyperthyroid cats. *N Z Vet J* 39:71–74, 1991.
20. Meric SM, Rubin SI: Serum thyroxine concentrations following fixed-dose radioactive iodine treatment in hyperthyroid cats: 62 cases (1986-1989). *J Am Vet Med Assoc* 197:621–623, 1990.
21. Nykamp SG, Dykes NL, Zarfoss MK, et al: Association of the risk of development of hypothyroidism after iodine 131 treatment with the pretreatment pattern of sodium pertechnetate Tc99m uptake in the thyroid gland in cats with hyperthyroidism: 165 cases (1990-2002). *J Am Vet Med Assoc* 226:1671–1675, 2005.
22. Peterson ME, Becker DV: Radioiodine treatment of 524 cats with hyperthyroidism. *J Am Vet Med Assoc* 207:1422–1428, 1995.
23. Boshoven EW, Conway TS: Surprising bloodwork results following treatment of 90 hyperthyroid cats with radioactive iodine-131 (^{131}I). In *Proceedings, American College of Veterinary Radiology Annual Scientific Conference*, Las Vegas, 2012, p 96.
24. Morrison J, Jergens A, Deitz K, et al: Investigation of prognostic factors for the development of renal disease following I-131 therapy in feline hyperthyroidism. *J Vet Intern Med* 24:745, 2010. (Abstract).
25. Morrison J, Jergens A, Deitz K, et al: Comparison of models for predicting renal disease following I-131 therapy for feline hyperthyroidism. *J Vet Intern Med* 24:744–745, 2010. (Abstract).
26. Mooney CT, Peterson ME: Feline hyperthyroidism. In Mooney CT, Peterson ME, editors: *Manual of canine and feline endocrinology*, ed 4, Quedgeley, 2012, British Small Animal Veterinary Association, pp 199–203.
27. Wakeling J, Rob C, Elliott J, et al: Survival of hyperthyroid cats is not affected by posttreatment azotaemia. *J Vet Intern Med* 20:1523, 2006.
28. Harley LS, Peterson ME, Langston CE, et al: IRIS stages of chronic kidney disease before and after treatment with radioiodine in cats with hyperthyroidism. *J Vet Intern Med* 25:678–679, 2011.
29. Daminet S, Kooistra HS, Fracassi F, et al: Best practice for the pharmacological management of hyperthyroid cats with antithyroid drugs. *J Small Anim Pract* 55:4–13, 2014.
30. Greco DS: Diagnosis of congenital and adult-onset hypothyroidism in cats. *Clin Tech Small Anim Pract* 21:40–44, 2006.
31. Peterson ME: Feline hypothyroidism. In Kirk RW, Bonagura JD, editors: *Current veterinary therapy X*, Philadelphia, 1989, Saunders, pp 1000–1001.
32. Peterson ME, Randolph JF, Mooney CT: Endocrine diseases. In Sherding RG, editor: *The cat: diagnosis and clinical management*, ed 2, New York, 1994, Churchill Livingstone, pp 1404–1506.
33. Daminet S: Feline hypothyroidism. In Mooney CT, Peterson ME, editors: *BSAVA manual of canine and feline endocrinology*, Quedgeley, 2011, British Small Animal Veterinary Association, pp 111–115.
34. Baral R, Peterson ME: Thyroid gland disorders. In Little SE, editor: *The cat: clinical medicine and management*, Philadelphia, 2012, Elsevier/Saunders, pp 571–592.
35. Rand JS, Levine J, Best SJ, et al: Spontaneous adult-onset hypothyroidism in a cat. *J Vet Intern Med* 7:272–276, 1993.
36. Peterson ME, Kintzer PP, Hurvitz AI: Methimazole treatment of 262 cats with hyperthyroidism. *J Vet Intern Med* 2:150–157, 1988.
37. Mooney CT, Thoday KL, Doxey DL: Carbimazole therapy of feline hyperthyroidism. *J Small Animal Pract* 33:228–235, 1992.
38. Gillen PL: Coping with an uncommon condition: hypothyroidism in a cat. *Vet Med* 80:46–53, 1986.
39. Blois SL, Abrams-Ogg AC, Mitchell C, et al: Use of thyroid scintigraphy and pituitary immunohistochemistry in the diagnosis of spontaneous hypothyroidism in a mature cat. *J Feline Med Surg* 12:156–160, 2010.
40. van Hoek IM, Vandermeulen E, Peremans K, et al: Thyroid stimulation with recombinant human thyrotropin in healthy cats, cats with nonthyroidal illness and in cats with low serum thyroxin and azotaemia after treatment of hyperthyroidism. *J Feline Med Surg* 12:117–121, 2010.

41. Peterson M, Broome MR: Radioiodine for feline hyperthyroidism. In Bonagura JD, Twedt D, editors: *Kirk's current veterinary therapy XV*, St Louis, 2014, Elsevier/Saunders, pp e112–e122.
42. Wakeling J: Use of thyroid stimulating hormone (TSH) in cats. *Can Vet J* 51:33–34, 2010.
43. Peterson ME: Feline focus: Diagnostic testing for feline thyroid disease: hypothyroidism. *Compend Contin Educ Vet* 35:E4, 2013.
44. Williams TL: Is hyperthyroidism damaging to the feline kidney? PhD thesis, Royal Veterinary College, University of London, 2013.
45. Ford RV, Owens JC, Curd GW, Jr, et al: Kidney function in various thyroid states. *J Clin Endocrinol Metab* 21:548–553, 1961.
46. Katz AI, Lindheimer MD: Renal sodium- and potassium-activated adenosine triphosphatase and sodium reabsorption in the hypothyroid rat. *J Clin Invest* 52:796–804, 1973.
47. Capasso G, Lin JT, De Santo NG, et al: Short term effect of low doses of tri-iodothyronine on proximal tubular membrane Na-K-ATPase and potassium permeability in thyroidectomized rats. *Pflugers Arch* 403:90–96, 1985.
48. Montenegro J, Gonzalez O, Saracho R, et al: Changes in renal function in primary hypothyroidism. *Am J Kidney Dis* 27:195–198, 1996.
49. Moses AM, Scheinman SJ: The kidneys and electrolyte metabolism in hypothyroidism. In Braverman LE, Utiger RD, editors: *Werner and Ingbar's the thyroid, a fundamental and clinical text*, ed 7, Philadelphia, 1996, Lippincott-Raven, pp 812–815.
50. Villabona C, Sahun M, Roca M, et al: Blood volumes and renal function in overt and subclinical primary hypothyroidism. *Am J Med Sci* 318:277–280, 1999.
51. den Hollander JG, Wulkan RW, Mantel MJ, et al: Correlation between severity of thyroid dysfunction and renal function. *Clin Endocrinol (Oxf)* 62:423–427, 2005.
52. Kaptein E: The kidneys and electrolyte metabolism in hypothyroidism. In Braverman LE, Utiger RD, editors: *Werner & Ingbar's the thyroid, a fundamental and clinical text*, ed 9, Philadelphia, 2005, Lippincott Williams & Wilkins, pp 789–795.
53. Elgadi A, Verbovszki P, Marcus C, et al: Long-term effects of primary hypothyroidism on renal function in children. *J Pediatr* 152:860–864, 2008.
54. Iglesias P, Diez JJ: Thyroid dysfunction and kidney disease. *Eur J Endocrinol* 160:503–515, 2009.
55. Panciera DL, Lefebvre HP: Effect of experimental hypothyroidism on glomerular filtration rate and plasma creatinine concentration in dogs. *J Vet Intern Med* 23:1045, 2009.
56. Gommeren K, van Hoek I, Lefebvre HP, et al: Effect of thyroxine supplementation on glomerular filtration rate in hypothyroid dogs. *J Vet Intern Med* 23:844–849, 2009.
57. Mariani LH, Berns JS: The renal manifestations of thyroid disease. *J Am Soc Nephrol* 23:22–26, 2012.
58. Lafayette RA, Costa ME, King AJ: Increased serum creatinine in the absence of renal failure in profound hypothyroidism. *Am J Med* 96:298–299, 1994.
59. Katz AI, Emmanouel DS, Lindheimer MD: Thyroid hormone and the kidney. *Nephron* 15:223–249, 1975.
60. Williams TL, Elliott J, Syme H: Restoration of euthyroidism in medically treated hyperthyroid cats with iatrogenic hypothyroidism (IH) improves renal function. *J Vet Intern Med* 26:753–754, 2012. (Abstract).
61. Basu G, Mohapatra A: Interactions between thyroid disorders and kidney disease. *Indian J Endocrinol Metab* 16:204–213, 2012.
62. MacFarlane IA, Shalet SM, Beardwell CG, et al: Transient hypothyroidism after iodine-131 treatment for thyrotoxicosis. *Br Med J* 2:421, 1979.
63. Sawers JS, Toft AD, Irvine WJ, et al: Transient hypothyroidism after iodine-131 treatment of thyrotoxicosis. *J Clin Endocrinol Metab* 50:226–229, 1980.
64. Connell JM, Hilditch TE, McCruden DC, et al: Transient hypothyroidism following radioiodine therapy for thyrotoxicosis. *Br J Radiol* 56:309–313, 1983.
65. Theon AP, Van Vechten MK, Feldman E: Prospective randomized comparison of intravenous versus subcutaneous administration of radioiodine for treatment of hyperthyroidism in cats. *Am J Vet Res* 55:1734–1738, 1994.
66. Broome MR, Peterson ME: Use of L-thyroxine supplementation after radioiodine therapy helps blunt the worsening of azotemia in hyperthyroid cats with pre-existing kidney disease. *J Vet Intern Med* 27:686, 2013.
67. Williams T, Peak K, Brodbelt D, et al: Survival and the development of azotemia after treatment of hyperthyroid cats. *J Vet Intern Med* 24:863–869, 2010.
68. Lulich JP, Osborne CA, O'Brien TD, et al: Feline renal failure: questions, answers, questions. *Compen Contin Educ Pract Vet* 14:127–152, 1992.
69. Elliott J, Barber PJ: Feline chronic renal failure: clinical findings in 80 cases diagnosed between 1992 and 1995. *J Small Anim Pract* 39:78–85, 1998.
70. Adams LG, Polzin DJ, Osborne CA, et al: Influence of dietary protein/calorie intake on renal morphology and function in cats with 5/6 nephrectomy. *Lab Invest* 70:347–357, 1994.
71. Elliott J, Rawlings JM, Markwell PJ, et al: Survival of cats with naturally occurring chronic renal failure: effect of dietary management. *J Small Anim Pract* 41:235–242, 2000.
72. Broome MR, Peterson ME: Use of L-thyroxine supplementation after radioiodine therapy in hyperthyroid cats with pre-existing kidney disease reduces the incidence of iatrogenic hypothyroidism and reduces the progression of azotemia, Unpublished data, 2014.
73. Vagney M, Desquilbet L, Reyes-Gomez E, et al: Survival times for cats with hyperthyroidism treated with a fixed low-dose of iodine 131. *J Vet Intern Med* 28:742–743, 2014.
74. Liu SK, Peterson ME, Fox PR: Hypertrophic cardiomyopathy and hyperthyroidism in the cat. *J Am Vet Med Assoc* 185:52–57, 1984.
75. Jacobs G, Hutson C, Dougherty J, et al: Congestive heart failure associated with hyperthyroidism in cats. *J Am Vet Med Assoc* 188:52–56, 1986.
76. Moise NS, Dietze AE: Echocardiographic, electrocardiographic, and radiographic detection of cardiomegaly in hyperthyroid cats. *Am J Vet Res* 47:1487–1494, 1986.
77. Bond BR, Fox PR, Peterson ME, et al: Echocardiographic findings in 103 cats with hyperthyroidism. *J Am Vet Med Assoc* 192:1546–1549, 1988.
78. Fox PR, Peterson ME, Broussard JD: Electrocardiographic and radiographic changes in cats with hyperthyroidism: comparison of populations evaluated during 1992-1993 vs. 1979-1982. *J Am Anim Hosp Assoc* 35:27–31, 1999.
79. Weichselbaum RC, Feeney DA, Jessen CR: Relationship between selected echocardiographic variables before and after radioiodine treatment in 91 hyperthyroid cats. *Vet Radiol Ultrasound* 46:506–513, 2005.
80. Altay UM, Skerritt GC, Hilbe M, et al: Feline cerebrovascular disease: clinical and histopathologic findings in 16 cats. *J Am Anim Hosp Assoc* 47:89–97, 2011.
81. Trepanier LA: Pharmacologic management of feline hyperthyroidism. *Vet Clin North Am Small Anim Pract* 37:775–788, vii, 2007.
82. Sartor LL, Trepanier LA, Kroll MM, et al: Efficacy and safety of transdermal methimazole in the treatment of cats with hyperthyroidism. *J Vet Intern Med* 18:651–655, 2004.
83. Plumb DC: Levothyroxine sodium. In *Plumb's veterinary drug handbook*, ed 6, Stockholm, 2008, PharmaVet, pp 534–536.

Are Methimazole Trials Really Necessary?

Harriet M. Syme

Hyperthyroidism and chronic kidney disease (CKD) are both very common problems of the old cat and may occur concurrently in the same individual.[1,2] Hyperthyroidism increases glomerular filtration rate (GFR) and so, in some cats, the presence of CKD is masked and only revealed once the cat is rendered euthyroid and azotemia is documented. This has led to the recommendation that trial treatment with methimazole (or carbimazole) should be routinely performed before definitive therapy with radioactive iodine or thyroidectomy. A few important implications result from this recommendation. First, if azotemia develops following medical treatment, then it would be best to subsequently leave the hyperthyroidism untreated (or at least undertreat it) to maximize renal function. Second, if the patient develops azotemia, the client should then be counseled against having definitive therapy for their cat's hyperthyroidism because of a poor long-term prognosis. However, evidence suggests that both of these conjectures are misguided, as will be outlined later.

To understand the arguments for and against doing methimazole trials before definitive treatment for hyperthyroidism, it is helpful to first review the effect of thyroid hormones on renal function and the changes that can be anticipated following treatment of hyperthyroidism.

EFFECT OF THYROID HORMONES ON RENAL FUNCTION

Both hyper- and hypothyroidism cause changes in renal function, and these are usually opposite in nature. For example, hyperthyroidism increases GFR, and hypothyroidism decreases it. These changes have been demonstrated in rodents, dogs, cats, and humans.[3-5] The changes that occur in association with thyroid disease in humans and dogs have received relatively little attention because, in general, these patients have adequate renal reserve and so the development of azotemia is relatively uncommon in spite of the changing GFR.[3,6] By contrast, in elderly cats where the prevalence of clinical and subclinical CKD is very high,[7] alterations in renal function that occur coincident with changes in thyroid status are a source of great clinical concern to veterinarians.

Thyroid hormones alter renal blood flow (RBF) and GFR via many different mechanisms. Cardiac output is increased in hyperthyroidism because of positive chronotropic and ionotropic effects on the heart. This occurs in part because of the direct effects of thyroid hormones, and in part in response to a marked reduction in systemic vascular resistance.[8,9] The increase in cardiac output tends to increase RBF, an effect that is augmented by increased cortical production of the vasodilator nitric oxide and reduced production of the vasoconstrictor endothelin.[10,11] Glomerular hemodynamics are also influenced by the activation of the renin-angiotensin-aldosterone system that occurs with hyperthyroidism.[12] This results in relative efferent arteriolar vasoconstriction and consequently an increase in filtration fraction; this means that GFR is increased over and above what would be predicted from alterations in RBF. In addition, thyroid hormones directly stimulate sodium and chloride reabsorption from the proximal nephron,[13] which decreases delivery of chloride to the macula densa and stimulates tubuloglomerular feedback mechanisms, which also serve to increase GFR.

Hyperthyroidism causes proteinuria. Increased glomerular pressure is one potential cause of this. There is some evidence to suggest, however, that the proteinuria that occurs in hyperthyroidism is not entirely glomerular in origin since it may also result from changes in the tubular handling of filtered protein.[14,15]

In the hyperthyroid state, renal tubules hypertrophy and several different carrier-mediated transport processes are activated. In addition to the insertion of chloride channels described earlier, thyroid hormones also modulate the expression of the sodium hydrogen exchanger and sodium-phosphate transporters in the proximal nephron.[16] These changes result in impaired urinary acidification mechanisms in hypothyroidism and a tendency for hyperphosphatemia in hyperthyroidism. Hyperphosphatemia, in turn, may lead to hyperparathyroidism in hyperthyroid cats.[17,18]

CHANGES IN GLOMERULAR FILTRATION RATE, CREATININE, AND UREA WITH TREATMENT OF HYPERTHYROIDISM IN CATS

Several studies have shown that GFR declines markedly following treatment of hyperthyroidism in cats. This is associated with the resolution of the hyperthyroid state, rather than adverse effects of any particular treatment modality. It has been demonstrated in cats treated with radioiodine,[19,20] by surgery,[21] or with medical therapy.[22] The changes in GFR are marked, ranging from a 44% to 51% decrease from pretreatment values.[19-22] The GFR stabilizes by 30 days following treatment, with no further significant change noted for up to 6 months.[19,20]

In routine clinical practice, measurement of GFR is uncommon, and the plasma or serum concentration of creatinine is used instead to provide a measure of renal function. Creatinine concentration is a hybrid parameter that is not only a function of GFR but also of the distribution of creatinine within the body, and also its endogenous rate of production. The rate of production of creatinine in hyperthyroid cats has not been measured. However, it is notable that although in general GFR has stabilized by 1 month after treatment of hyperthyroidism, creatinine concentration continues to increase for longer than this.[19,23] This may be due to increases in muscle mass that result from the cats becoming euthyroid or may be due to other, as yet uncharacterized influences of thyroid hormones on the rate at which creatinine is generated in the body. In dogs with experimentally induced hypothyroidism, creatinine production rate is decreased, meaning that the creatinine concentration underestimates the reduction in GFR that occurs.[4] This effect may also be relevant to cats that develop iatrogenic hypothyroidism following treatment for hyperthyroidism.

The proportion of cats that develop azotemia (i.e., creatinine concentration above the laboratory reference interval) following treatment for hyperthyroidism is dependent on the degree to which the hyperthyroidism is controlled. In a study of 268 initially nonazotemic cats, 28 of 106 (26.4%) cats considered well controlled (total thyroxine <40 nmol/L [3.1 μg/dL] for 6 months) developed azotemia, compared with only three of 39 (7.7%) cats with poor control of hyperthyroidism.[15] Of the cats for which control of hyperthyroidism fluctuated or could not be assessed because of a lack of follow-up, 10 of 123 (8.1%) developed azotemia.

Urea concentrations in cats with hyperthyroidism are often mildly increased, in spite of the increased GFR that occurs with this condition. This increase is thought to relate to increases in dietary protein intake and protein catabolism. This means that urea/creatinine ratios tend to be high initially in hyperthyroid cats and normalize with treatment.

ARGUMENTS FOR PERFORMING METHIMAZOLE TRIALS

Prediction of Cats That Will Develop Azotemia Is Not Possible without Treatment

The proportion of cats that become azotemic following treatment of hyperthyroidism has been quite variable in different studies, ranging from 17% to 49%.[19,21,22,24-28] One reason for this disparity may be that azotemia is more likely to occur if iatrogenic hypothyroidism develops following treatment for hyperthyroidism,[27] and the incidence of this may have differed among the published studies. It will also depend, to some extent, on how long after treatment the assessment of renal

function was made, because it will take some time for azotemia to develop. As discussed earlier, creatinine concentrations may not peak until as long as 3 months after treatment.[19,23]

Treatment trials with methimazole would not be necessary if it were possible to predict reliably which cats will develop azotemia with treatment of hyperthyroidism; cats unlikely to develop azotemia could have permanent treatment immediately. Unfortunately, currently no single test currently exists that will reliably predict renal function after treatment for hyperthyroidism. Measurement of GFR was reported in one early study to predict the cats that will develop azotemia following treatment for hyperthyroidism.[25] However, this relationship has not been borne out in other studies in which GFR has been measured. Although pretreatment GFR values generally have been lower in cats that subsequently develop azotemia than in those that do not, there has been significant overlap between the groups.[19,23] This might be anticipated because the decline in GFR is presumably going to depend, to some extent, on the severity of hyperthyroidism before treatment.

Pretreatment creatinine concentrations perform in a similar manner to measurement of GFR in predicting development of azotemia. In the largest study reported to date, the pretreatment creatinine concentration (median [25th, 75th] percentiles) was significantly greater ($P < 0.001$) in those cats that developed azotemia with treatment (1.31 [1.18, 1.69], $n = 34$) than in those that did not (1.07 [0.90, 1.28], $n = 183$).[15] In spite of this observation, baseline creatinine was not considered to be a reliable indicator for the development of azotemia following treatment in individual patients because there was considerable overlap between the groups. Urea performed in a similar manner.

It has sometimes been suggested that cats with good renal concentrating ability (urine specific gravity >1.035) are less likely to develop azotemia following treatment. However, the studies that have objectively evaluated this claim have not found that urine specific gravity is a useful predictor of the post-treatment development of azotemia.[15,26]

Proteinuria is common in hyperthyroid cats, and it declines with treatment. However, the magnitude of proteinuria does not predict the subsequent development of azotemia.[15] It is correlated with overall survival time; however, this association is relatively weak in hyperthyroidism by comparison with studies of cats with CKD and/or hypertension.[29,30]

ARGUMENTS AGAINST PERFORMING METHIMAZOLE TRIALS

Undertreatment of Hyperthyroidism Is Common with Medical Treatment

If trial treatment is to be successful in predicting the cats that will develop azotemia when treated with permanent therapies (radioiodine or surgical thyroidectomy), then it must reduce the thyroid hormone concentration to a comparable extent, and for long enough to allow azotemia to develop. This is difficult to do in practice because with medical treatment (e.g., drug therapy or iodine-restricted diet) of hyperthyroidism, undertreatment is relatively common. In addition, reversible treatments for hyperthyroidism are likely to result in more day-to-day variation in thyroid hormone concentrations.

In one of the earliest studies of methimazole treatment, failure to control the thyroid hormone concentration was only reported in two out of 262 cats treated, although doses as high as 20 mg/day (divided) were given.[31] However, subsequent clinical experience would suggest that failure to control hyperthyroidism with drugs is relatively common, perhaps because lower initial doses tend to be given and owners become disheartened when serial increases in dose have to be made. Even in the original study, almost one third of the cats treated for more than 100 days had a total thyroxine value above the reference range on one to four occasions,[31] demonstrating that while treatment with drugs could be effective, consistency of therapeutic effect was difficult to maintain.

In one large study of samples submitted to a laboratory following once-daily administration of methimazole ($n = 543$) or carbimazole ($n = 883$), total thyroxine values were above the therapeutic target (10 to 50 nmol/L [0.78 to 3.89 µg/dL]) in 52.9% and 49.0%, and below the therapeutic target in 17.3% and 10.5% of samples, respectively.[32] This might reflect a conservative approach by practitioners with an incremental increase in dosage at the start of treatment, submission bias owing to samples being taken from cats that were showing persistent signs of hyperthyroidism, and results might have been better if patients on twice-daily therapy had been included in the study. Even so, the results suggest that many cats treated medically for hyperthyroidism are not well controlled. This is especially true, as the therapeutic target in that study was quite wide; optimal control of hyperthyroidism would usually be considered a total thyroxine concentration within the lower half of the laboratory reference range.

Side effects are reported in 18% of cats treated with methimazole.[31] Most often this consists of simple gastrointestinal (GI) upset, which resolves with a dose reduction. More serious adverse drug reactions such as blood dyscrasias and facial excoriations necessitate drug withdrawal. Similar side effects have been reported for carbimazole,[33] which is expected because it is a pro-drug, converted to methimazole *in vivo*. Development of side effects with medical treatment is therefore a relatively common reason for cats to be referred for radioactive iodine therapy. This, together with the difficulty of consistently controlling hyperthyroidism with medical treatment for a period of several weeks to months, means that a relatively high proportion of cats receiving permanent treatment for hyperthyroidism have never received an effective methimazole trial. Although this has not been studied in any objective manner, anecdotally, there have been very few reported complications from this lack of "trial treatment".

Transdermal drug application has been associated with a lower rate of GI side effects than the orally administered drug.[34] Even so, the efficacy of treatment with transdermal formulations has been lower than with tablet treatments in some,[34] but not all,[35] studies. Transdermal administration of methimazole is not appropriate in cats that have previously developed a serious adverse drug reaction to methimazole or carbimazole because these drug reactions are considered idiosyncratic and are not classically dose related. Transdermal treatment will therefore allow for successful methimazole trials in some, but by no means all, cats.

It is also now possible to treat hyperthyroidism in cats by the exclusive feeding of an iodine-restricted diet (Hill's Prescription Diet y/d). There are only limited reports of the efficacy of this treatment, with many studies having only been published as abstracts. However, in one study of 225 cats treated by feeding this diet, 25% of the cats were still hyperthyroid after 8 weeks of treatment.[36] It is hard to be certain because of the manner in which the results are reported, but it appears that the majority of cats had total thyroxine concentrations that were within the upper half of the laboratory reference range. Creatinine concentrations were actually reduced 4 weeks after introduction of the diet in that study. The authors speculate that this could be because of the low heat-processed meat content of the diet.[36] Alternatively, it could be due to poor control of the hyperthyroidism; approximately half of the cats in the study had been receiving antithyroid drugs before the diet being introduced, so it is possible that the thyroid hormone concentration increased in some of the cats after introduction of the diet. These results suggest that dietary management of hyperthyroidism is unlikely to suppress thyroid levels to the same extent as permanent therapies and is therefore less likely to "unmask" underlying CKD than are other forms of treatment.

If Iatrogenic Hypothyroidism Occurs Following Definitive Treatment, Then Azotemia May Still Develop

Iatrogenic hypothyroidism can occur following radioactive iodine therapy, bilateral thyroidectomy, or treatment with antithyroid medication. It is also theoretically possible for hypothyroidism to occur in cats fed an iodine-restricted diet, but it appears to be much less common.[36] It used to be thought that iatrogenic hypothyroidism was of very little clinical consequence. However, it has since been shown that cats with iatrogenic hypothyroidism are more likely to be azotemic than those that remain euthyroid following treatment.[27] In another study, restoration of euthyroidism in cats with iatrogenic hypothyroidism resulted in a significant reduction in plasma creatinine concentration, with azotemia resolving in half of the cats.[37]

These observations emphasize the point that unless the degree of control of hyperthyroidism is equivalent with different treatments the effect on renal function will not be comparable. Thus, it is quite possible for a cat that has been pretreated with methimazole to have a significant increase in creatinine concentration following the administration of radioactive iodine because of the development of iatrogenic hypothyroidism. It has been reported that approximately 30% of cats treated with radioactive iodine develop hypothyroidism.[38] In humans treated with radioactive iodine, the development of hypothyroidism continues to occur for many years following treatment.[39]

Undertreatment of Hyperthyroidism May Be Damaging to the Kidney

Why do so many cats treated for hyperthyroidism develop azotemia? Hyperthyroidism and CKD are both very common feline problems, and both increase in prevalence with advancing age, which may explain the association between these two conditions. Alternatively, it is possible that the frequency with which CKD is diagnosed following treatment is because hyperthyroidism is actually damaging to the feline kidney.

One mechanism by which hyperthyroidism could cause injury is through the process of hyperfiltration. In patients with CKD, the remaining functional nephrons hyperfiltrate; this means that although the global GFR for the patient is decreased, each of the remaining nephrons individually has an increased filtration rate. This process is largely due to an increase in filtration pressure across the glomerular barrier.[40] This increase in glomerular pressure has been associated with proteinuria and with accelerated nephron loss, resulting in progressive renal injury. Hyperthyroidism has the potential to exacerbate these processes. Ameliorating this glomerular hypertension is the rationale for treating patients with CKD with angiotensin-converting enzyme inhibitors. Although the effectiveness of such therapies in management of (predominantly tubulointerstitial) CKD in cats is questionable,[41] it does not seem logical to deliberately undertreat hyperthyroidism with the aim of causing renal hyperfiltration. Such an approach will inevitably decrease the patient's creatinine value; however, it does nothing to improve nephron health.

Other possible mechanisms by which hyperthyroidism could cause renal injury include activation of the renin-angiotensin-aldosterone system, development of hyperparathyroidism, and increases in renal oxidative stress. These mechanisms have been implicated in progression of CKD, either in cats with naturally occurring disease and/or in experimental models of renal injury. It has been shown that plasma renin activity and aldosterone concentrations are increased in cats with hyperthyroidism.[42] Hyperthyroid cats also have increased plasma phosphate and parathyroid hormone concentrations, although this is not associated with the development of azotemia following treatment.[17,18] Urinary concentrations of 8-isoprostanes, eicosanoids generated by lipid peroxidation, are increased in cats with hyperthyroidism and decrease with treatment, suggesting that hyperthyroidism causes reversible oxidative stress.[43]

Even If Azotemia Develops, Effective Treatment for Hyperthyroidism Is Still Advised

In most cats that develop newly diagnosed azotemia following treatment for hyperthyroidism, the degree is mild (usually International Renal Interest Society [IRIS] stage 2) and associated with few, if any, clinical signs other than mild polyuria

or polydipsia. Owners of cats that have developed azotemia still usually report that the clinical condition of their cat is improved overall following treatment, and notice weight gain and reversal of other clinical signs of hyperthyroidism.

The survival time of cats that develop azotemia following treatment of hyperthyroidism is not significantly different from that of those that do not.[27] This finding may be surprising to practitioners who will tend to assume that the development of azotemia is associated with a worse prognosis. However, CKD is relatively slowly progressive in cats, and only about half of all cats diagnosed with mild CKD will ultimately succumb to the disease, with many dying from other causes.[44] Additionally, the cut point between azotemic and nonazotemic is somewhat arbitrary, and it is likely that many old cats, even among those that are classified nonazotemic, have a degree of renal compromise. Therefore, the distinction between these two groups (azotemic and nonazotemic) may not be as great as initially thought.

In contrast to the situation in cats that are euthyroid following effective treatment of hyperthyroidism, the development of azotemia in cats with iatrogenic hypothyroidism appears to have a negative effect on patient welfare. In one study, survival of hypothyroid, azotemic cats was significantly worse (median 456 [25th, 75th percentiles; 362, 841] days) than that of the hypothyroid, nonazotemic (905 [625, 1701] days) cats.[27] Thus, the current treatment recommendation is to maintain total thyroxine concentrations within the lower half of the laboratory reference range, but not below it, to ensure that hyperthyroidism is being effectively treated.

Progression of Chronic Kidney Disease Is Inherently Unpredictable

Many cats with CKD have nonprogressive or slowly progressive disease, and the magnitude of azotemia remains very stable for months or even years. When cats are diagnosed with azotemic CKD, approximately half will die from unrelated causes.[44] In a study of cats with naturally occurring CKD, only a minority of the cats with IRIS stage 2 disease progressed to IRIS stage 4 before death.[45] Similarly, studies of cats with surgical reduction of renal mass have shown that renal function remains stable for protracted periods.[46]

Although risk factors for progressive renal disease have been identified on a population basis (e.g., proteinuria, phosphate concentration, and packed cell volume),[30,45] it remains very difficult to predict longevity in any individual patient. Cats with CKD often seem to demonstrate a "stepwise" progression of their azotemia, with their renal function remaining stable for a long period and then seemingly showing an abrupt increase. Given the inherent unpredictability of when this deterioration in renal function occurs, this means that occasionally a cat is treated with radioactive iodine and shows an abrupt clinical decline. This is possible whether the patient has previously completed a methimazole trial. In fact, in some ways, if an abrupt decline does occur this can be worse for the owner if the patient has been through a methimazole trial because they thought they were protected from this eventuality.

SPECIAL CIRCUMSTANCES IN WHICH METHIMAZOLE TREATMENT IS STRONGLY ADVISED BEFORE DEFINITIVE TREATMENT

Treatment Trials before Surgery

Radioiodine is considered to be the treatment of choice for hyperthyroidism based on its high efficacy and lack of complications, although initial cost and length of hospital stay may be a deterrent for some owners.[47] Surgical thyroidectomy is also an effective and permanent treatment option, particularly in cats where thyroid scintigraphy has been performed first to exclude the possibility of ectopic hyperplastic thyroid tissue.[48]

In cats treated by surgical thyroidectomy, prior medical treatment not only allows for the assessment of renal function in the euthyroid state but also has the added benefit of potentially reducing the risks associated with general anesthesia. In this situation, medical treatment is not so much a trial therapy as a consideration for preoperative stabilization of the patient's clinical condition. Even so, recommendations for prior medical treatment of hyperthyroidism vary. Some authors recommend initial medical treatment routinely,[49,50] whereas others recommend this approach only for cats with cardiac hypertrophy, arrhythmias, or tachycardia,[48,51] or cats that are severely clinically affected.[52] In the author's practice, medical treatment of hyperthyroidism is usually advised before surgery unless the cat has a history of adverse reactions to antithyroid medications, or the cat shows no clinical signs.

Treatment of Cats with Pre-existing Azotemia

In cats that are azotemic before treatment for hyperthyroidism, it is generally recommended that they be treated medically initially (and with a gradually escalating dose), so that if their condition deteriorates the antithyroid medications can be discontinued and the cat will return to a hyperthyroid state. If the biochemical deterioration is mild following treatment, and the well-being of the cat is improved, then permanent treatment for hyperthyroidism (thyroidectomy or radioiodine therapy) can be considered. However, in general, the survival of cats that have azotemic CKD before treatment of hyperthyroidism is poor; in one study performed in first-opinion practices (and so likely to have included an unselected population of cats), the median survival time for azotemic cats was only 178 days (range 0 to 1505 days).[15]

It is worth remembering that the relationship between GFR and creatinine is not linear; once renal function is poor, small changes in GFR will result in large changes in creatinine concentration. Thus, when treating hyperthyroidism, a comparable decrement in GFR in a cat that is initially nonazotemic will result in a much smaller change in creatinine concentration than in a cat that is already azotemic at baseline.

In cats with elevated creatinine concentrations before treatment for hyperthyroidism, starting with a low dose of medication initially is prudent; the dose can then gradually be escalated if this is necessary and well tolerated.

SUMMARY

In summary, in the opinion of the author, treatment trials with reversible therapies (i.e., methimazole, carbimazole, or diet) need not be routinely recommended for all hyperthyroid cats. This was also the consensus opinion of a panel of European key opinion leaders,[53] because medical treatment may not be immediately successful, necessitating an adjustment in dose or a change in modality because of side effects or poor owner and patient compliance. Even if euthyroidism is achieved, this state needs to be maintained for a reasonable length of time (more than one month) to determine if azotemia will develop. The requirement for multiple visits to the veterinary clinic and the cost associated with repeated blood tests during this period are likely to lead to owner frustration and may make subsequent permanent treatment unaffordable for some. Added to which, when permanent treatment (radioiodine or surgical thyroidectomy) is performed, azotemia may still develop because the thyroid hormone concentration may not be identical to that achieved with medical management. In any case, survival of cats that develop azotemia following treatment for hyperthyroidism is no different from that of those that remain nonazotemic, provided that the cats are not hypothyroid; clinically, many of these patients do very well. Even though there is no direct evidence that hyperthyroidism is actually damaging to the feline kidney, maintaining cats in a mildly hyperthyroid state to improve numerically their creatinine values is no longer recommended.

Treatment trials with methimazole or other reversible therapies should be reserved for cats that are azotemic when hyperthyroidism is diagnosed and before any treatment is instigated. Consideration should also be given to providing thyroid hormone replacement in cats with iatrogenic hypothyroidism following radioiodine therapy or bilateral thyroidectomy (see Chapter 23).

References

1. Wakeling J, Elliott J, Syme HM: Evaluation of predictors for the diagnosis of hyperthyroidism in cats. *J Vet Intern Med* 25:1057–1065, 2011.
2. Jepson RE, Brodbelt D, Vallance C, et al: Evaluation of predictors of the development of azotemia in cats. *J Vet Intern Med* 23:806–813, 2009.
3. den Hollander JG, Wulkan RW, Mantel MJ, et al: Correlation between severity of thyroid dysfunction and renal function. *Clin Endocrinol* 62:423–427, 2005.
4. Panciera DL, Lefebvre HP: Effect of experimental hypothyroidism on glomerular filtration rate and plasma creatinine concentration in dogs. *J Vet Intern Med* 23:1045–1050, 2009.
5. Adams WH, Daniel GB, Legendre AM: Investigation of the effects of hyperthyroidism

on renal function in the cat. *Can J Vet Res* 61:53–56, 1997.

6. Gommeren K, van Hoek I, Lefebvre HP, et al: Effect of thyroxine supplementation on glomerular filtration rate in hypothyroid dogs. *J Vet Intern Med* 23:844–849, 2009.

7. Lulich JP, O'Brien TD, Osborne CA, et al: Feline renal failure: questions, answers, questions. *Compend Cont Educ Pract Vet* 14:127–152, 1992.

8. Klein I, Ojamaa K: Thyroid hormone and the cardiovascular system. *N Engl J Med* 344:501–509, 2001.

9. Kahaly GJ, Wagner S, Nieswandt J, et al: Stress echocardiography in hyperthyroidism. *J Clin Endocrinol Metab* 84:2308–2313, 1999.

10. Quesada A, Sainz J, Wangensteen R, et al: Nitric oxide synthase activity in hyperthyroid and hypothyroid rats. *Eur J Endocrinol* 147:117–122, 2002.

11. Singh G, Sharma AC, Thompson EB, et al: Renal endothelin mechanism in altered thyroid states. *Life Sci* 54:1901–1908, 1994.

12. Montiel M, Jimenez E, Navaez JA, et al: Aldosterone and plasma renin activity in hyperthyroid rats: effects of propranolol and propylthiouracil. *J Endocrinol Invest* 7:559–562, 1984.

13. Santos Ornellas D, Grozovsky R, Goldenberg R, et al: Thyroid hormone modulates ClC-2 chloride channel gene expression in rat renal proximal tubules. *J Endocrinol* 178:503–511, 2003.

14. Vargas F, Moreno JM, Rodriguez-Gomez I, et al: Vascular and renal function in experimental thyroid disorders. *Eur J Endocrinol* 154:197–212, 2006.

15. Williams TL, Peak KJ, Brodbelt D, et al: Survival and the development of azotemia after treatment of hyperthyroid cats. *J Vet Intern Med* 24:863–869, 2010.

16. Yusufi ANK, Murayama N, Keller MJ, et al: Modulatory effect of thyroid hormones on uptake of phosphate and other solutes across luminal brush border membrane of kidney cortex. *Endocrinology* 116:2438–2449, 1985.

17. Barber PJ, Elliott J: Study of calcium homeostasis in feline hyperthyroidism. *J Small Anim Pract* 37:575–582, 1996.

18. Williams TL, Elliott J, Syme HM: Calcium and phosphate homeostasis in hyperthyroid cats—associations with development of azotaemia and survival time. *J Small Anim Pract* 53:561–571, 2012.

19. Boag AK, Neiger R, Slater L, et al: Changes in the glomerular filtration rate of 27 cats with hyperthyroidism after treatment with radioactive iodine. *Vet Rec* 161:711–715, 2007.

20. van Hoek I, Lefebvre HP, Kooistra HS, et al: Plasma clearance of exogenous creatinine, exoiohexol, and endo-iohexol in hyperthyroid cats before and after treatment with radioiodine. *J Vet Intern Med* 22:879–885, 2008.

21. Graves TK, Olivier NB, Nachreiner RF, et al: Changes in renal function associated with treatment of hyperthyroidism in cats. *Am J Vet Res* 55:1745–1749, 1994.

22. Becker TJ, Graves TK, Kruger JM, et al: Effects of methimazole on renal function in cats with hyperthyroidism. *J Am Anim Hosp Assoc* 36:215–223, 2000.

23. van Hoek I, Lefebvre HP, Peremans K, et al: Short- and long-term follow-up of glomerular and tubular renal markers of kidney function in hyperthyroid cats after treatment with radioiodine. *Domest Anim Endocrinol* 36:45–56, 2009.

24. Slater MR, Geller S, Rogers K: Long-term health and predictors of survival for hyperthyroid cats treated with iodine 131. *J Vet Intern Med* 15:47–51, 2001.

25. Adams WH, Daniel GB, Legendre AM, et al: Changes in renal function in cats following treatment of hyperthyroidism using I-131. *Vet Radiol Ultrasound* 38:231–238, 1997.

26. Riensche MR, Graves TK, Schaeffer DJ: An investigation of predictors of renal insufficiency following treatment of hyperthyroidism in cats. *J Feline Med Surg* 10:160–166, 2008.

27. Williams TL, Elliott J, Syme HM: Association of iatrogenic hypothyroidism with azotemia and reduced survival time in cats treated for hyperthyroidism. *J Vet Intern Med* 24:1086–1092, 2010.

28. Milner RJ, Channell CD, Levy JK, et al: Survival times for cats with hyperthyroidism treated with iodine 131, methimazole, or both: 167 cases (1996-2003). *J Am Vet Med Assoc* 228:559–563, 2006.

29. Syme HM, Markwell PJ, Pfeiffer D, et al: Survival of cats with naturally occurring chronic renal failure is related to severity of proteinuria. *J Vet Intern Med* 20:528–535, 2006.

30. Jepson RE, Elliott J, Brodbelt D, et al: Effect of control of systolic blood pressure on survival in cats with systemic hypertension. *J Vet Intern Med* 21:402–409, 2007.

31. Peterson ME, Kintzer PP, Hurvitz AI: Methimazole treatment of 262 cats with hyperthyroidism. *J Vet Intern Med* 2:150–157, 1988.

32. Gallagher B, Mooney C, Graham P: Efficacy of two oral anti-thyroid medications used once-daily: a laboratory survey. *British Small Animal Veterinary Association (BSAVA) Congress, Scientific Proceedings*. 457, 2011.

33. Frénais R, Rosenberg D, Burgaud S, et al: Clinical efficacy and safety of a once-daily formulation of carbimazole in cats with hyperthyroidism. *J Small Anim Pract* 50:510–515, 2009.

34. Sartor LL, Trepanier LA, Kroll MM, et al: Efficacy and safety of transdermal methimazole in the treatment of cats with hyperthyroidism. *J Vet Intern Med* 18:651–655, 2004.

35. Hill KE, Gieseg MA, Kingsbury D, et al: The efficacy and safety of a novel lipophilic formulation of methimazole for the once daily transdermal treatment of cats with hyperthyroidism. *J Vet Intern Med* 25:1357–1365, 2011.

36. van der Kooij M, Becvárová I, Meyer HP, et al: Effects of an iodine-restricted food on client-owned cats with hyperthyroidism. *J Feline Med Surg* 16(6):491–498, 2014.

37. Williams TL, Elliott J, Syme HM: Effect on renal function of restoration of euthyroidism in hyperthyroid cats with iatrogenic hypothyroidism. *J Vet Intern Med* 28(4):1251–1255, 2014.

38. Nykamp SG, Dykes NL, Zarfoss MK, et al: Association of the risk of development of hypothyroidism after iodine 131 treatment with the pre-treatment pattern of sodium pertechnetate Tc 99m uptake in the thyroid gland in cats with hyperthyroidism: 165 cases (1990-2002). *J Am Vet Med Assoc* 226:1671–1675, 2005.

39. Metso S, Jaatinen P, Huhtala H, et al: Long-term follow-up study of radioiodine treatment of hyperthyroidism. *Clin Endocrinol* 61:641–648, 2004.

40. Brown SA, Brown CA: Single-nephron adaptations to partial renal ablation in cats. *Am J Physiol* 269:R1002–R1008, 1995.

41. King JN, Gunn-Moore DA, Tasker S, et al: Tolerability and efficacy of benazepril in cats with chronic kidney disease. *J Vet Intern Med* 20:1054–1064, 2006.

42. Williams TL, Elliott J, Syme HM: Renin-angiotensin-aldosterone system activity in hyperthyroid cats with and without concurrent hypertension. *J Vet Intern Med* 27:522–529, 2013.

43. Branter E, Drescher N, Padilla M, et al: Antioxidant status in hyperthyroid cats before and after radioiodine treatment. *J Vet Intern Med* 26:582–588, 2012.

44. Elliott J, Rawlings JM, Markwell PJ, et al: Survival of cats with naturally occurring chronic renal failure: effect of dietary management. *J Small Anim Pract* 41:235–242, 2000.

45. Chakrabarti S, Syme HM, Elliott J: Clinicopathological variables predicting progression of azotemia in cats with chronic kidney disease. *J Vet Intern Med* 26:275–281, 2012.

46. Adams LG, Polzin DJ, Osborne CA, et al: Influence of dietary protein/calorie intake on renal morphology and function in cats with 5/6 nephrectomy. *Lab Invest* 70:347–357, 1994.

47. Trepanier LA: Pharmacologic management of feline hyperthyroidism. *Vet Clin North Am Small Anim Pract* 37:775–788, 2007.

48. Naan EC, Kirpensteijn J, Kooistra HS, et al: Results of thyroidectomy in 101 cats with hyperthyroidism. *Vet Surg* 35:287–293, 2006.

49. Radlinsky MG: Thyroid surgery in dogs and cats. *Vet Clin North Am Small Anim Pract* 37:789–798, 2007.

50. Flanders JA: Surgical options for the treatment of hyperthyroidism in the cat. *J Feline Med Surg* 1:127–134, 1999.

51. Padgett S: Feline thyroid surgery. *Vet Clin North Am Small Anim Pract* 32:851–859, 2002.

52. Birchard SJ: Thyroidectomy in the cat. *Clin Tech Small Anim Pract* 21:29–33, 2006.

53. Daminet S, Kooistra HS, Fracassi F, et al: Best practice for the pharmacological management of hyperthyroid cats with antithyroid drugs. *J Small Anim Pract* 55:4–13, 2014.

Christine L. Cain, DVM

Cutaneous Manifestations of Internal Disease

Darcie Kunder and J.D. Foster

In addition to its roles in barrier function, thermoregulation, immunoregulation, and sensory perception the skin is also an indicator of general health. When hormonal shifts or medications influence systemic health or internal organs, the skin can serve as a signal that the patient's well-being is affected. This is particularly helpful with feline patients that may hide signs until they reach a critical point. Many cutaneous signs are clinically distinctive and can lead to diagnosis with thorough dermatologic examination. Recognizing these signals in the skin can lead to appropriate treatment that may make long-term management or cure possible. The skin, being easy to evaluate, sample, and monitor, often provides a noninvasive way of assessing internal health. For a list of differential diagnoses based on clinical appearance of a skin lesion, see Table 26-1.

CUTANEOUS PARANEOPLASTIC SYNDROMES

Paraneoplastic syndromes (PNS) are non-neoplastic, cancer-related disorders that cause alterations in body function or structure and occur at sites distant from the primary neoplasm or its metastasis.[1,2] The signs of PNS are related to the remote effects of neoplasia rather than from any direct effects of tumor growth or invasion. Causes are variable but are thought to be from the production of small molecules (e.g., cytokines, hormones, peptides) by the tumor cells or by other body cells in response to the biologic action of the tumor.[1,2] Paraneoplastic syndromes can often be the first sign of any internal disturbance or malignancy; recognizing these signs can result in early cancer detection and appropriate therapy. However, PNS can also carry their own morbidity and may cause more problems and concerns than the underlying disease.

Greater than 50% of human patients will experience symptoms of PNS during the course of a malignancy.[2] The incidence is less well known for veterinary patients. This may be related to the fact that clinical signs may precede, coexist with, or follow a diagnosis of neoplasia, making a direct correlation between onset of lesions and underlying disease difficult.

Two PNS are recognized only in feline patients and will be discussed here.

Feline Paraneoplastic Alopecia

Feline paraneoplastic alopecia is a syndrome of middle-aged to older cats with a median age of 13 years and has been reported with pancreatic carcinoma (12 cases), biliary carcinoma (two cases), and a single case of hepatocellular carcinoma.[2-6] There does not appear to be any breed or sex predilection.[7] Skin lesions occur with the presence of the tumor, but neoplasia does not involve the skin and typically no endocrine changes are present.

Cats present with a several weeks' to months' history of acute-onset, rapidly progressive alopecia. Most cats have concurrent signs of gastrointestinal illness, including weight loss, decreased appetite, listlessness, and variable degrees of vomiting and diarrhea. Hair loss typically begins on the ventrum (neck and/or abdomen) and progresses to involve the head, limbs, especially the medial aspect of the extremities, and eventually the face (Figure 26-1). Hair from the dorsum is generally spared but can be dry, brittle, thinning, or unkempt. Hair from adjacent skin is easily epilated and the alopecic skin is glistening, not fragile. Depending on the amount of self-grooming, there can be erythema, scale, and crust on the alopecic skin. Some cats have been reported to excessively overgroom, and it is suspected that the glistening appearance of the skin is a result of exfoliation of stratum corneum secondary to this overgrooming.[2,3,7] Footpad involvement is common with crusting, fissuring, and brown-black keratosebaceous buildup interdigitally and within the nail beds. Pain and reluctance to walk is reported when footpad lesions are present. The brown-black waxy material is secondary to *Malassezia* spp. dermatitis (see Chapter 33). Mauldin and colleagues[4] found generalized *Malassezia* spp. in 7 of 15 feline

Table 26-1	Differential Diagnoses Based on Dermatologic Examination or Presenting Complaint of Cutaneous Symptom
Cutaneous Symptom	**Differential Diagnoses**
Unkempt coat	Endocrine disease (hyperthyroidism, diabetes mellitus); infectious (dermatophytosis, bacterial, fungal, protozoal, viral); allergic (adverse food reaction, atopic dermatitis, flea allergy dermatitis); neoplasia
Erythroderma and erythema	Paraneoplastic syndromes (paraneoplastic alopecia, thymoma-associated exfoliative dermatitis); cutaneous drug reaction; allergic (adverse food reaction, atopic dermatitis, flea allergy dermatitis); neoplasia
Alopecia	Endocrine disease (hypercortisolism, diabetes mellitus, hyperthyroidism); infectious (dermatophytosis, bacterial, fungal, viral); neoplasia/paraneoplastic syndromes
Excessive scaling	Infectious (dermatophytosis, bacterial, fungal); paraneoplastic (thymoma-associated exfoliative dermatitis); seborrheic disorders
Pruritus	Infectious (bacterial, fungal, viral, parasitic); allergic
Ulcers	Cutaneous drug reaction; autoimmune
Thin skin	Endocrine (exogenous or endogenous hypercortisolism); adverse drug reaction (topical glucocorticoids)

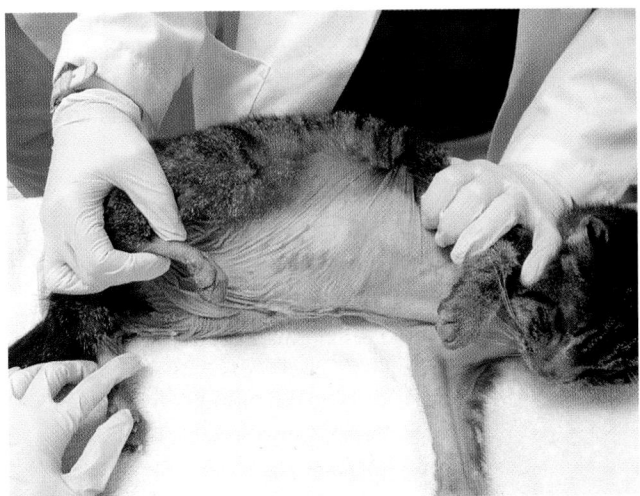

Figure 26-1: Well-demarcated alopecia with erythema and mild superficial scale on the ventrum of a 9-year-old female cat with paraneoplastic alopecia.

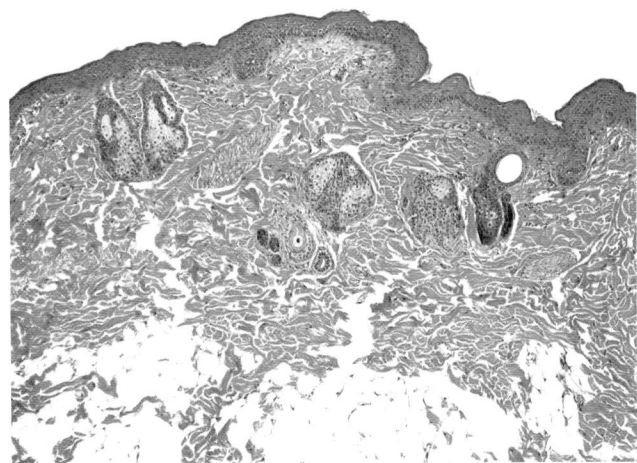

Figure 26-2: Cutaneous histopathology of feline paraneoplastic alopecia. The epidermis is moderately hyperplastic with acanthosis, hair follicles are faded, but sebaceous glands are unaffected. There is a large arrector pili muscle in the center of the sample with minimal dermal inflammation. (Hematoxylin and eosin, 10×)

biopsy specimens that were consistent with paraneoplastic alopecia.[2,4,7] It is important to keep paraneoplastic alopecia in mind when generalized *Malassezia* spp. are found on histopathologic specimens from cats. Although paraneoplastic alopecia is nonpruritic, secondary *Malassezia* dermatitis may dramatically increase itch and discomfort in these patients.

Although this syndrome is visually distinctive, differential diagnoses include feline hypercortisolism (endogenous or iatrogenic), hyperthyroidism, dermatophytosis, self-induced alopecia, telogen defluxion, or alopecia areata.[2,8] Hematologic and biochemical results do not aid in diagnosis; skin biopsy is the preferred diagnostic test and has characteristic changes that can confirm diagnosis. A region of maximal alopecia with the typical shiny appearance of the skin should be sampled. Histopathology shows alopecia with diffuse telogenization of hair follicles with a "miniaturized," atrophied appearance.[8] Sebaceous glands and epitrichial sweat glands are typically unaffected. Moderate acanthosis is observed, and the stratum corneum can be absent or can exhibit parakeratotic or orthokeratotic hyperkeratosis. Dermal inflammation is largely absent, unless secondary erosion or crusts are present[8] (Figure 26-2).

To rule out other differential diagnoses, dexamethasone suppression test, thyroid hormone measurement, Wood's lamp evaluation, fungal culture, superficial and deep skin scrapings, and trichograms can be helpful. When paraneoplastic alopecia is suspected, abdominal radiography and/or ultrasound, thoracic radiography, computed tomography, or exploratory laparotomy can aid in finding the underlying visceral neoplasia.[2,7]

Prognosis is grave for these patients. The majority of reported cases were found to have exocrine pancreatic carcinoma.[2-4,7] Often there are intraperitoneal metastases, commonly to the liver, or metastasis to lungs and/or regional lymph nodes by the time of initial evaluation or diagnosis.[1]

Greater than 80% of reported cases were euthanized or died within 8 weeks of the onset of clinical signs.[2] There is one report of resolution of cutaneous signs following partial pancreatectomy in a feline patient. Pancreatic and skin biopsies confirmed exocrine pancreatic carcinoma with concurrent paraneoplastic alopecia. Within 4 weeks of surgery, the patient was regrowing hair and had lost the shiny appearance to the skin; within 10 weeks, there was significant hair regrowth over all previously alopecic areas. Unfortunately, 18 weeks postsurgery, the cat represented for a 2-week history of ventral alopecia and weight loss. Adenocarcinoma of the remaining pancreas, liver, spleen, and peritoneum were found on necropsy examination, and histopathology confirmed their similarity to the original neoplasia.[5] This case does demonstrate that cutaneous signs can resolve when the underlying neoplasia is treated or resected. Early surgical intervention may prove curative if neoplasia can be completely excised.

Feline Thymoma-Associated Exfoliative Dermatitis

Paraneoplastic exfoliative dermatitis is reported in cats associated with presence of a thymoma. In humans with paraneoplastic exfoliative dermatitis, leukemia and lymphoma are the most common underlying neoplasms; exfoliative dermatitis

has not been reported with thymomas in humans.[1] Thymomas in humans are shown to generate new autoantigen-responsive CD4+ T cells. In graft-versus-host disease and erythema multiforme (EM), autoreactive T cells attack keratinocytes; the same process is suspected for thymoma-associated exfoliative dermatitis. This is supported by similar histopathologic findings in these diseases as well as the discovery of CD3+ T lymphocytes within the epidermis of feline patients with thymoma-associated exfoliative dermatitis, leading to the hypothesis that the pathogenesis of exfoliative dermatitis may involve a T cell–mediated process.[7,9] Myasthenia gravis and megaesophagus are also related to presence of thymoma in veterinary patients, and these syndromes may also be T cell–driven.[2,7]

Generally, middle-aged to older cats are affected, but thymoma-associated exfoliative dermatitis has been reported in one cat as young as 4 years old.[7] Breed or sex predilections have not been reported. Skin lesions in cats are typically recognized prior to discovery of a mediastinal mass or any signs associated with the cancer. Regions of erythema and exfoliation develop, typically on the head, pinnae, and neck, before becoming generalized (Figure 26-3A). At presentation, marked scaling with or without crusting and thickening of the skin is typically found. The scale can be large, and sheets of exfoliated stratum corneum can be more than 1 cm

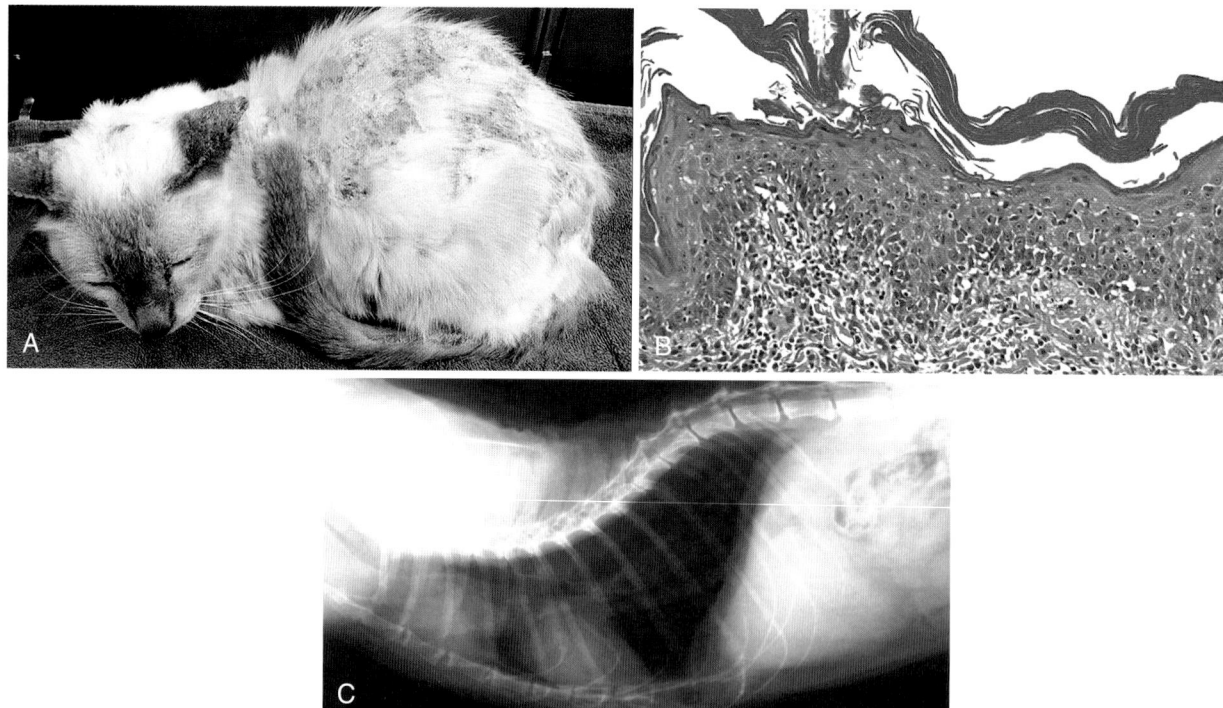

Figure 26-3: A, Generalized erythema, alopecia, superficial crusts, and thick scale in a domestic shorthair cat with thymoma-associated exfoliative dermatitis. **B,** Cutaneous histopathology of feline thymoma-associated exfoliative dermatitis. This biopsy was taken from the cat seen in **A.** Compact orthokeratotic hyperkeratosis with acanthosis and a hydropic interface dermatitis is present that obscures the normal dermal-epidermal junction. There is a mild superficial dermal inflammatory infiltrate consisting primarily of lymphocytes. (Hematoxylin and eosin, 40×) **C,** Lateral thoracic radiograph from the same cat as in **A** showing a cranial mediastinal soft tissue opacity consistent with thymoma.

in diameter.[9] Alopecia develops in erythematous areas as the disease progresses and will sometimes be the presenting complaint. Although initially nonpruritic, *Malassezia* dermatitis can cause waxy keratosebaceous debris that is then associated with overgrooming and intense itch.[2,7] Periocular, perioral, and interdigital spaces, and the external ear canal are often found to have brown-black waxy debris associated with *Malassezia* spp. infections.[7] Secondary pyoderma is another common clinical finding. When present, systemic signs include coughing, dyspnea, anorexia, weight loss, and lethargy.[9] Differential diagnoses for erythema and exfoliation of this nature include drug reaction, EM, epitheliotropic T-cell lymphoma, pemphigus foliaceus, primary bacterial, fungal, or dermatophyte infection, demodicosis, allergic skin disease, or endocrine disorder, such as hypercortisolism. Skin biopsy along with chest radiographs followed by fine-needle aspirates of a mediastinal mass allow for definitive diagnosis. To obtain the best skin biopsy, areas of erythema and exfoliative material should be targeted.[2,9]

Histopathology reveals a hydropic interface dermatitis with basal cell and keratinocyte apoptosis that extends into the hair follicle at the level of the infundibulum or isthmus.[2,9] Lymphocytes and macrophages are found most often in an otherwise cell-poor interface pattern. Sebaceous glands are often absent with either orthokeratotic or parakeratotic epidermal hyperkeratosis (resulting in the scale seen clinically)[2] (see Figure 26-3B). *Malassezia* spp. may be present. These changes are similar to what would be seen histologically for graft-versus-host disease and EM; however, both of those diseases typically have more apoptosis present in the samples.[7] In addition to skin biopsy, routine tests that may help rule out other differential diagnoses include superficial and deep skin scrapings, trichograms, Wood's lamp evaluation, and fungal culture. If thymoma-associated lesions are suspected, thoracic imaging should be the next step (see Figure 26-3C). If found, fine-needle aspirate or core biopsies can confirm a diagnosis of thymoma. These can often be safely obtained with ultrasound guidance.[1,2] There are reports of feline patients with clinical skin lesions that were histologically identical to thymoma-associated exfoliative dermatitis, but thymoma or other neoplastic disease was not present with postmortem examination. This supports the hypothesis that this disease is a T cell–driven reaction pattern and may not always be specific for thymoma.[9]

The treatment of choice is surgical removal of the thymoma, and there are numerous reports of exfoliative dermatitis resolving after successful thoracic surgery to remove a thymoma.[2,7,9,10] As for paraneoplastic alopecia, recognizing exfoliative dermatitis as an indicator of thymoma can result in prompt and successful management of both systemic and cutaneous lesions and result in better overall prognosis for the patient. In a review of thymomas that were surgically excised in dogs and cats, Zitz and colleagues[10] found that 74% of cats had a 3-year survival rate after surgery. Radiation could also be considered as primary or adjunctive treatment. Metastasis is not common.[2,10]

CUTANEOUS MANIFESTATIONS OF HORMONAL CHANGES

Feline Hypercortisolism

Hypercortisolism or hyperadrenocorticism is rare in the cat and can be both naturally occurring and iatrogenic.[11,12] Approximately 80% of reported cases of primary hypercortisolism are caused by an adrenocorticotropic hormone (ACTH)–secreting pituitary tumor, and approximately 20% are caused by functional adrenal tumors. If a pituitary tumor is present, the majority are adenomas; when an adrenal tumor is present, 50% are benign adenomas and 50% are malignant adenocarcinomas.[13] The scarcity of reported cases of iatrogenic hypercortisolism in cats is explained by the relative insensitivity of cats to the deleterious side effects of glucocorticoids (see Chapter 30).[14]

Hypercortisolism is a disease of middle-aged to older cats, although iatrogenic hypercortisolism can occur in cats of any age. Ten years is the mean age of endogenous hypercortisolism presentation; cats with adrenal tumors tend to be slightly older compared with those with pituitary-dependent tumors.[12] There may be a female predilection, but it does occur in both males and females and neutered and intact cats. The majority of cases are in domestic shorthair or domestic longhair cats, but many other breeds have been affected by naturally occurring hypercortisolism.[14]

The most common presenting complaint of owners is difficult to control diabetes mellitus with polyuria, polydipsia, and polyphagia. However, an unkempt coat, easy bruising, poor grooming habits, thinning hair coat, spontaneous alopecia, or failure to regrow hair after clipping are also frequently found.[13,14] Hair loss was an owner complaint in 60% of cases of feline hypercortisolism. Based on physical examination findings, alopecia was found in 60%, skin fragility in 50%, pyoderma in 40%, and seborrhea in 20% of feline patients with hypercortisolism.[12,14]

Alopecia of feline hypercortisolism is most often a failure to regrow hair after clipping. Abnormal and excessive grooming is also reported, but it may be difficult to know if overgrooming is occurring. If cats are grooming normally but this behavior is now resulting in broken, easily shed hairs, it may appear as if a cat is causing the hair loss when the hair loss is actually due to atrophy of the hair follicles from excess cortisol.[14]

Thin skin, increased susceptibility to infection, and poor wound healing are caused by suppression of the keratinocyte and dermal fibroblast proliferation and suppression of fibroblast-derived proteins. Glucocorticoid-induced suppression of collagen synthesis as well as suppression of early inflammatory mediators is suspected to be responsible for the poor wound healing.[12,15] Chronic skin infections occur secondary to impaired immune defenses against pathogens. Glucocorticoids generally stifle the immune response by decreasing macrophage cytokine expression, increasing expression of inflammatory cytokines, impairing dendritic cell function and maturation, decreasing T cell and B cell function, and decreasing antibody formation.[12]

There are some dermatologic abnormalities associated with feline hypercortisolism that are considered serious and potentially life threatening. In certain cases, dermal atrophy and thinning of the skin is so severe that even normal handling, grooming, or restraint can result in skin tearing and large wounds. Affected skin can appear paper thin and may even seem translucent prior to trauma. Sepsis can be a confounding sequela if the wound is large enough, and this complication as well as patient discomfort and poor quality of life can lead to euthanasia.[12,14] Data are limited, but skin fragility may be more likely in cats with adrenal tumors as compared with those with pituitary-dependent disease.[11]

Medial curling of the ear tips has been reported in cats with iatrogenic but not endogenous hypercortisolism (see Chapter 30). Weakened cartilage from chronic excess cortisol is thought to be the cause. Because it has not been recognized with endogenous hypercortisolism, it is either under recognized or could be of diagnostic significance between the iatrogenic and endogenous forms of the disease.[11,14]

For a feline patient that presents for alopecia and thin fragile skin, endogenous or iatrogenic hypercortisolism should be suspected and appropriate screening tests performed. If alopecia is the primary concern, differential diagnoses include self-induced alopecia (see Chapter 32), paraneoplastic alopecia, other endocrinopathy (diabetes mellitus or hyperthyroidism), or telogen defluxion. Fragile skin is more characteristic of hypercortisolism, but differential diagnoses also include inherited collagen defects (Ehlers-Danlos syndrome) or other causes of acquired skin fragility[8,11] (see later).

Serum chemistry, complete blood count, and urinalysis findings may be nonspecific in feline patients. Often there is evidence of diabetes mellitus with persistent glucosuria and hyperglycemia. Isosthenuria is not a common finding; most cats are able to maintain a urine specific gravity above 1.035 even after long-term, high-dose glucocorticoid administration. Liver enzymes can be abnormal but reflections of steroid hepatopathy on a serum chemistry screen are inconsistent.[12]

Skin biopsy may aid in diagnosis; samples should be taken from areas of significant alopecia. If skin fragility is severe, skin biopsy should be avoided because it may lead to secondary infections and complications from abnormal wound healing. Histopathology shows atrophy of the epidermis and epithelium of the hair follicle infundibulum, although some cats will only show hair follicles in early telogen with no atrophic changes. Consistently there is decreased dermal collagen with widely separated thinner than normal collagen bundles that lack organization. Excessive tricholemmal keratinization that results in a brightly eosinophilic core of an atrophic hair follicle can be characteristic of feline hypercortisolism.[8,11]

Although both ACTH stimulation test and low-dose dexamethasone suppression test (LDDST) are used for diagnosis of hypercortisolism in cats, the ACTH stimulation test is not as sensitive, with reports ranging from 30% to 50% diagnostic sensitivity. Because of this variability, the ACTH stimulation test is not recommended for diagnosis of hypercortisolism in feline patients.[12] The urine cortisol-to-creatinine ratio (UCCR) is the easier test to perform because it requires urine collection that can be done at home. Measurement of 24-hour urine cortisol secretion is the standard test for diagnosis of hypercortisolism is humans because it evaluates the cortisol secreted by the adrenal glands over time instead of in a minute-to-minute fashion as can be seen in plasma concentrations. This may be of particular interest in feline patients that are stressed or nervous in a hospital setting. The UCCR is highly sensitive, but specificity data are lacking, making it more efficient as a screening test rather than a diagnostic test. A negative UCCR can be used to rule out hypercortisolism, but a positive result will need to be further investigated.[12,14] An elevated UCCR has been documented in hyperthyroid, sick, and stressed cats. A LDDST can be used to confirm the presence of excess endogenous cortisol. It is recommended to use 0.1 mg/kg dexamethasone intravenously and collect serum samples prior to injection as well as at 4 and 8 hours postinjection. Normal cats will have a cortisol level suppressed to less than 1 µg/dL. The LDDST is not helpful at differentiating between pituitary- and adrenal-dependent disease in the cat, but test results do not appear to be different when testing normal, diabetic, or non-diabetic systemically ill patients.[11] The LDDST and the UCCR can be combined for outpatients by giving dexamethasone at a dose of 0.1 mg/kg by mouth (PO) every 8 to 12 hours for 2 to 3 days with urine samples being collected at home both before and after administration of the oral medication.[12]

Prognosis for cats with hypercortisolism is variable, and no studies have compared outcome and survival among treatments. A retrospective study demonstrated successful management with trilostane (Vetoryl, Dechra), resulting in median survival time of 20 months.[16] Mitotane (Lysodren, Bristol-Myers Squibb Oncology) has been shown to be inconsistent in suppressing adrenocortical function or clinical signs of hypercortisolism. Variable results are reported for surgical intervention when either one adrenal gland or both are removed. Surgery is certainly contraindicated in a patient with fragile skin; laparoscopic procedures for adrenalectomy could be considered as an alternative to laparotomy and could be preferable for patients with thin skin or poor wound healing. Radiation therapy can also be considered, especially for large pituitary tumors or for those cats with neurologic signs secondary to a pituitary tumor.[12]

Feline Acquired Skin Fragility

Acquired skin fragility is a rare condition with multiple underlying causes. The skin of cats with this condition is remarkably thin and very fragile; the skin may tear even with gentle handling, restraint, or normal grooming. Trauma results in irregular tears where large sheets of skin can be shed (Figure 26-4). The skin may have a paper thin, almost translucent quality and secondary alopecia can occur.[17] For

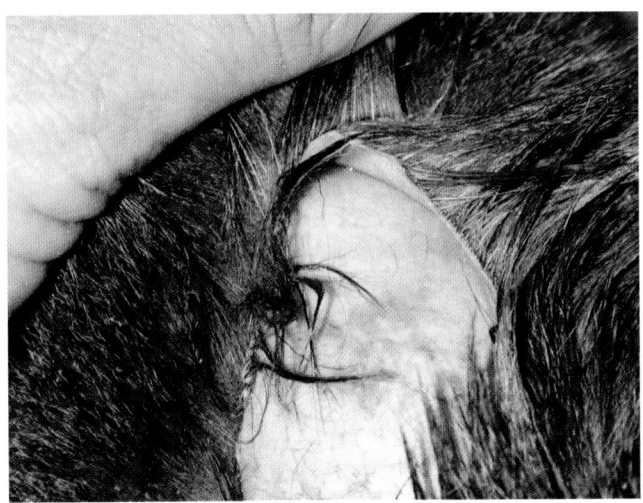

Figure 26-4: Torn skin with a resultant large cutaneous defect in a domestic shorthair cat with skin fragility syndrome. The skin is very thin along the dorsal edge of the tear.

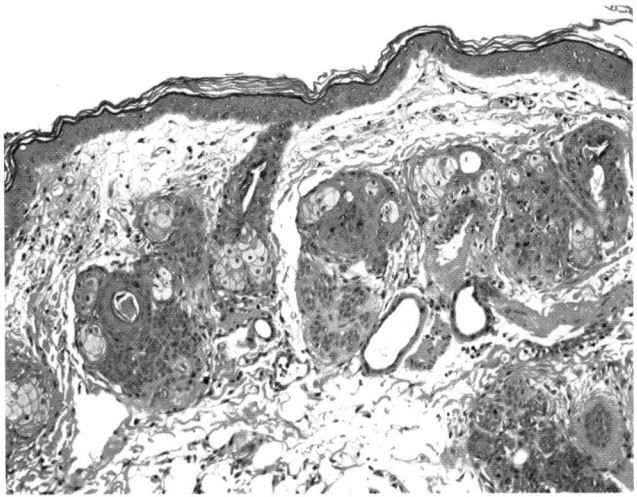

Figure 26-5: Cutaneous histopathology of feline skin fragility syndrome. Adnexal units are prominent in a relatively thin, edematous noninflammatory dermis. (Hematoxylin and eosin, 20×)

unknown reasons, tears are more common on the dorsum. Repair of wounds can be difficult because surrounding skin is also atrophic and attempts to suture can result in larger areas of trauma.[18] It is most often recognized in middle-aged or older cats with no breed or sex predilection. The exact pathogenesis is unknown, but it is most commonly seen in cats with either iatrogenic or endogenous hypercortisolism, diabetes mellitus, or use of progestational compounds.[17] It has also been reported in cats with feline infectious peritonitis, disseminated histoplasmosis, multicentric follicular lymphoma, cholangiocarcinoma, nephrosis, feline dysautonomia, and liver disease such as cholangiohepatitis and hepatic lipidosis.[19-23] There is one case report of a cat developing dermal atrophy after receiving daily oral phenytoin for a period of 3 weeks. The dermal signs resolved when phenytoin was discontinued and reappeared when the drug was restarted.[24] There are a small number of cases where no underlying cause was found and the skin fragility was deemed idiopathic.[18]

Underlying causes include endogenous or iatrogenic hypercortisolism, diabetes mellitus, paraneoplastic alopecia, drug reaction, or liver disease and patients with skin fragility should be screened for these disorders. Cutaneous asthenia (Ehlers-Danlos syndrome) can present with similar signs, but it typically becomes evident in patients at a very young age and exhibits marked skin hyperextensibility that is not present in skin fragility syndrome.[18] Serum chemistries, complete blood count, and urinalysis may be unremarkable or nondiagnostic but can indicate if diabetes mellitus or liver disease is contributing to the cutaneous signs. A complete medication history should be taken, and LDDST may be indicated.

Obtaining a skin biopsy can be very difficult in these patients. The sample should be taken from intact rather than pieces of previously torn or lacerated skin. The samples often fold and twist, making histopathologic review difficult. All attempts should be made to include underlying adipose tissue

and to keep the skin layers together. Microscopically, the epidermis appears very thin with severely atrophic underlying dermis. Adipose tissue is not always present, but when seen, provides a stark contrast to the extremely thin dermis. Dermal atrophy is more striking than adnexal atrophy, but some samples show small, thin, and short hair follicles. Arrector pili muscles often appear enormous when compared with atrophied adnexal units. Inflammation is scant unless older, scarred lesions are sampled[18] (Figure 26-5).

Prognosis is grave regardless of underlying cause. If the inciting cause can be found and treated, there is a better chance of lesion improvement or resolution. There are some data that support the use of oral retinoids for healing when glucocorticoids are the cause of the wound or the reason for poor wound healing. They work by restoring the levels of growth factors (transforming growth factor-β and insulin-like growth factor-1) that reinvigorate the production of collagen.[25]

Hyperthyroidism

Hyperthyroidism is the most common endocrinopathy seen in middle-aged to older cats.[26] The underlying cause is typically functional adenomatous hyperplasia or adenoma of both glands; thyroid carcinoma is possible but very rare.[11] Secretion of thyroxine and triiodothyronine by the abnormal glands provides negative feedback to the pituitary gland that then suppresses the release of thyroid-stimulating hormone; any normal thyroid gland atrophies in response to this suppression.[27] The underlying cause of hyperthyroidism is not known, though many hypotheses exist, including nutritional, environmental, genetic, autoimmune, or altered hormone responses.[26-28] Thyroid hormones are responsible for temperature regulation; carbohydrate, protein, and lipid metabolism; as well as increasing sympathetic drive via interactions with the nervous system. Because of this broad range of functions, many different organ signs can be affected by an increase in thyroid hormone synthesis.[28] An overall increase in metabolic rate is a reason for many of the clinical signs of the disease.

The majority of affected cats are 8 years of age or older; less than 5% of documented cases affect patients younger than 8 years old, although cases in cats younger than 4 years have been reported.[26] There are no breed or sex predilections, but Siamese and Himalayan cats may have a decreased risk of developing hyperthyroidism.[26,29]

Clinical signs tend to be slowly progressive and include weight loss, polyphagia, polydipsia, polyuria, restlessness, hyperactivity, vomiting, diarrhea, change in respiratory rate or effort, and tachycardia. Cutaneous changes are recognized in approximately 36% of feline patients with hyperthyroidism and include unkempt or matted hair coat, excessive shedding or grooming, thin hair coat or hair loss, abnormal appearance of nails or increased nail growth and turnover, seborrhea, and thin skin.[11,26] In chronic cases, flank alopecia and thin skin can sometimes mimic hypercortisolism.[11] Thyrotoxicosis in humans can result in skin changes secondary to increased protein synthesis and vasodilation, with an increased production of heat. In feline patients, body temperature may rise and the skin may feel damp or moist. Vasodilation from a dynamic circulatory state is thought to occur and can account for the aggressive grooming and tearing out of hair that can sometimes be observed in feline patients. Overgrooming may help remove hair to release heat as well as distribute saliva over the surface of the skin that acts as a cooling behavior.[26] Because of the broad range of cutaneous signs for cats with hyperthyroidism, when a patient presents with an unkempt, matted, or overgroomed coat, differential diagnoses include hypercortisolism, diabetes mellitus, infections (bacterial pyoderma, *Malassezia* dermatitis), parasites, allergic skin disease, and neoplasia. Diagnosis and treatment of hyperthyroidism are reviewed in the section on Endocrine and Metabolic Diseases. Return to a euthyroid state should result in resolution of the cutaneous signs of the disease.

Diabetes Mellitus

Diabetes mellitus may be caused by either circulating autoantibodies to the insulin producing beta cells of the pancreas (type 1) or by insulin resistance related to abnormal beta cells (type 2). In human diabetic patients, a number of dermatologic conditions are associated with undiagnosed, untreated, or unregulated disease or as secondary complication from immune compromise. Approximately one third of human diabetic patients will have cutaneous manifestations, including hemodynamic changes, vasculopathies, acanthosis nigricans, necrobiosis lipoidica, scleroderma, diabetic neuropathy, infections (bacterial and fungal) of the skin and nails, wound development, poor wound healing, cellulitis, xerosis, seborrhea, and alopecia.[11,30,31] In dogs and cats, secondary infections are the most common cutaneous manifestation of diabetes mellitus, reported in up to one third of cases.[11] Human diabetic patients are more likely to have cutaneous colonization by methicillin-resistant *Staphylococcus* spp.[30] This can make treatment more difficult and present concerns for

systemic spread. Cats with diabetes were not shown to have a higher incidence of *Malassezia* spp. colonization from skin and mucosal sites.[32] However, diabetic patients are predisposed to dermatophyte infections.[11]

Physical examination of feline patients suspected to have diabetes may reveal dry, lusterless, unkempt, or matted hair coats.[33] This is thought to be secondary to decreased grooming from lethargy or neuropathy (Figure 26-6). Cats may also develop seborrhea, thin skin, and multiple areas of alopecia that are explained by protein catabolism. Protein catabolism also accounts for poor wound healing and lipid metabolism that contribute to seborrheic skin disease.[11,34] The propensity of diabetics to develop secondary infections is related to altered neutrophil recruitment and phagocytosis, abnormal T cell–mediated immunity, and increase in the release of certain cytokines (interleukin-8).[11,35] These abnormalities can be corrected with a state of normoglycemia but because diabetic patients tend to have higher than normal serum glucose concentrations, even mild hyperglycemia causes alterations in

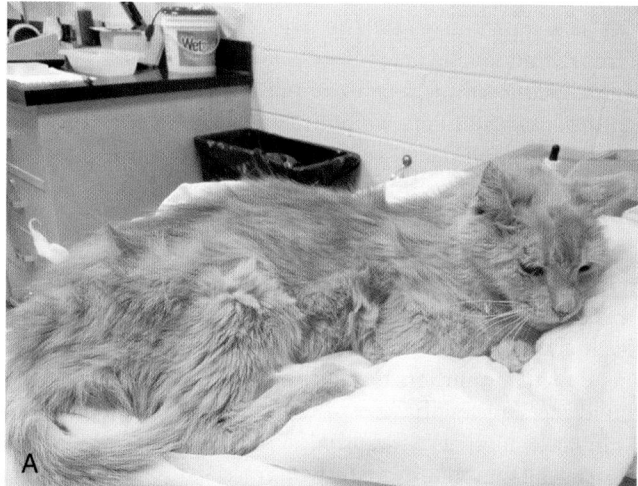

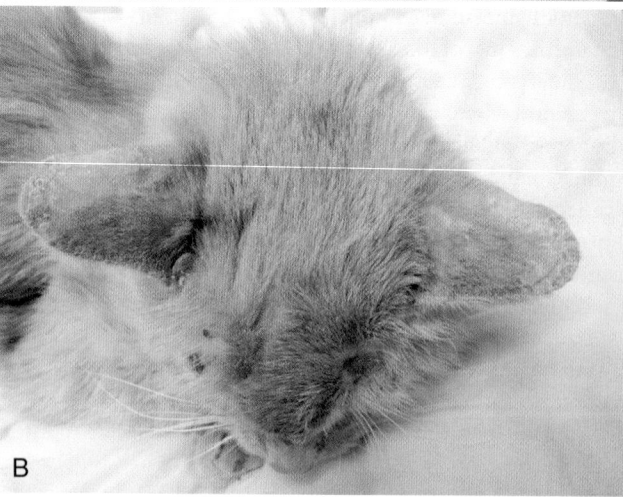

Figure 26-6: A, Unkempt coat with focal areas of alopecia, erosion, and erythema on the pinnae and face secondary to dermatophytosis in a domestic shorthair cat with diabetes mellitus. **B,** Closer view of the alopecia, erythema, and superficial scale on the dorsal head and pinnae of the same patient.

wound healing and persistent cutaneous abnormalities.[11,34] In addition to a predisposition to bacterial and fungal infections, diabetic patients may develop focal or generalized *Demodex* infections.[18]

Cutaneous signs for diabetes mellitus can be generalized and nonspecific. For a newly diagnosed diabetic patient, bacterial, fungal, and parasitic infections should be ruled out. Once appropriate therapy is initiated, hair coat and skin changes should improve. However, any new skin lesions in diabetic patients should be screened for evidence of infections.

CUTANEOUS XANTHOMAS

Xanthomas are benign, typically multifocal, granulomatous deposits in the skin.[11,36] They contain lipoprotein-derived components and are associated with a derangement of lipid metabolism. Abnormal plasma levels of cholesterol, lipoproteins, and triglycerides are found in patients that develop xanthomas. Most often the underlying cause is natural or drug-induced diabetes mellitus. However, they have also been associated with diets high in fats or triglycerides, hyperlipoproteinemia, and hyperchylomicronemia, as well as one report of idiopathic xanthoma formation in a cat.[11,37-39] Lipoproteins are assemblies of both proteins and lipids; they transport fat both inside and out of cells, allowing for movement of cholesterol and triglycerides in the blood. An elevation in the blood is called hyperlipoproteinemia. With increased blood levels, deposition of lipoproteins into other body tissues produces xanthomas. The pathogenesis of the association of hyperlipoproteinemia with xanthoma is not clear; it is possible that trauma contributes to xanthoma formation.[36,40]

Cats with xanthomatosis are presumed to have a defect in lipid metabolism. These cats cannot tolerate high-fat meals and have high levels of triglycerides, cholesterol, or low-density lipoproteins, even when fasted. A derangement of lipid metabolism plays a role in development and complications of diabetes mellitus from a lack of insulin, causing accelerated lipid catabolism. Although xanthoma formation is related to diabetes mellitus, cats with familial lipoprotein deficiencies do not tend to develop xanthomas. Other metabolic factors are likely to be affecting these patients.[36,41] In one report, a cat with a history of hyperlipoproteinemia and long-term use of glucocorticoids developed xanthomas.[36,38]

On clinical evaluation, xanthomas appear as multifocal, yellow to white papules, plaques, or nodules that may have erythematous borders and surrounding skin. They are often found on the head, especially in the periauricular area or on the pinnae, and can extend to the periocular region, but they can also develop on the paw pads and over bony prominences. Bruising of lesions is common due to friability of affected skin and ulceration can occur. Lesions often have bilateral symmetry.[36,37] Some cats develop peripheral neuropathy, presumably from lipid deposits. There do not appear to be any breed, age, or sex predilections.

Differential diagnoses include allergic skin disease, dermatophytosis, and infectious, noninfectious, or neoplastic granulomas.[11,36] Serum chemistry, urinalysis, and complete blood count tests should be performed looking for evidence of diabetes mellitus as well as evaluating fasted cholesterol and triglyceride levels. Fasting 24-hour lipid profile and lipoprotein electrophoresis can be performed for levels and/or activity of lipoproteins in serum.[36] Histopathology is required for a definitive diagnosis of xanthoma. Nonulcerated nodules or plaques should be sampled. Paw pads should be avoided, if possible, due to generally poor healing and discomfort for the patient. Skin biopsy samples have a generally normal to mildly acanthotic epidermis. An abundance of foamy, lipid-laden macrophages are found between collagen fibers; they may also be found in sheets that destroy normal collagen architecture (Figure 26-7). Multinucleated giant cells, eosinophils, and rarely neutrophils, lymphocytes, and plasma cells can also be observed. Often eosinophils are plentiful. Lipid deposits are present as large "lakes" of extracellular,

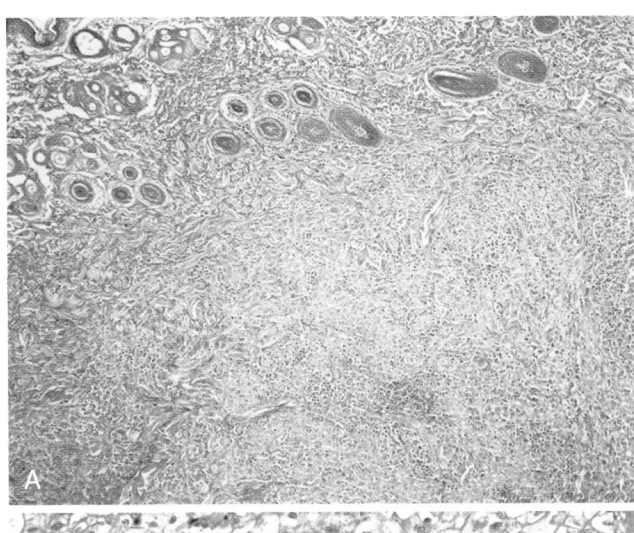
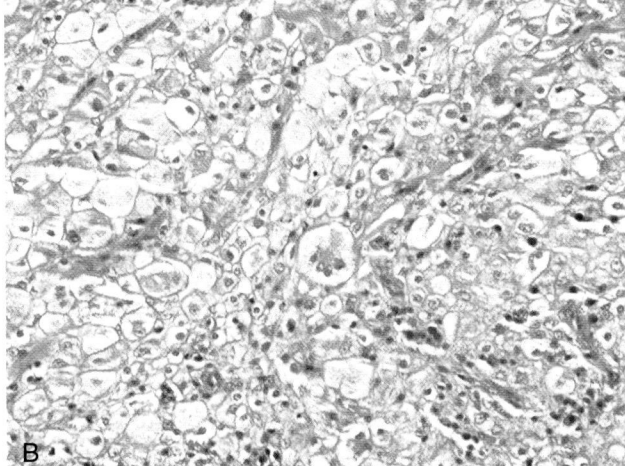

Figure 26-7: A, Cutaneous histopathology of feline xanthoma. In the mid to deep dermis there is dense inflammatory infiltrate obscuring normal collagen architecture. (Hematoxylin and eosin [H&E], 10×) **B,** Close up of **A** showing lipid-laden macrophages and few multinucleated giant cells. (H&E, 40×)

pale-staining deposits but are not observed in all lesions.[36] Oil red O staining can confirm lipid deposition within macrophages so that extracellular deposits are not a requirement for definitive diagnosis.[36] Low-fat diets with fiber or fish oil supplementation and correction of any underlying abnormalities of lipid metabolism are recommended for these patients. Treatment is lifelong, but control of associated diabetes mellitus or hyperlipoproteinemia can lead to resolution of cutaneous xanthomas. Surgical removal is an option but usually leads to recurrence if no other measures are taken. In one feline patient, a low-fat diet resolved lesions; each time a commercial diet was reintroduced, there was a relapse of the cutaneous xanthomas.[11,42]

SUPERFICIAL NECROLYTIC DERMATITIS

Superficial necrolytic dermatitis (SND) is also commonly called metabolic epidermal necrosis, necrolytic migratory erythema, or hepatocutaneous syndrome, and is a necrotizing skin disorder associated with underlying metabolic disease, often involving the liver. It is rare in the cat, uncommon in the dog, and frequently identified in humans.[43] In dogs, it is most often associated with hepatic dysfunction, pancreatic glucagonoma, phenobarbital administration, mycotoxins, or diabetes mellitus.[43,44] In humans with glucagonoma syndrome secondary to a glucagon-secreting islet cell tumor, 70% of patients will develops SND as a complicating syndrome.[2] Humans can also develop SND secondary to pancreatitis, zinc or fatty acid deficiency, and inflammatory bowel disease. In dogs with metabolic hepatic abnormalities, the skin lesions are thought to be related to cutaneous nutritional deprivation, though the exact pathogenesis is unknown. Keratinocytes degenerate, possibly from cellular starvation that leads to edema.[11] Serum amino acid measurements in these patients reveal profound hypoaminoacidemia of many amino acids. Increase in glucagon from a pancreatic endocrine tumor has been investigated, but only a few cases of SND have been associated with high levels of glucagon. In cats, SND has been seen with pancreatic carcinoma, thymic amyloidosis, hepatopathy, intestinal lymphoma, and hepatic carcinoid.[43,44] At least one case of pancreatic carcinoma was thought to be of endocrine origin; immunohistochemical staining of glucagon was not diagnostic and plasma glucagon levels were not measured.[45] In one case of hepatopathy, serum amino acid levels were low, suggesting that the underlying pathogenesis may be related to some forms of this disease in dogs and humans.[43,44]

Classic SND lesions in dogs consist of thick, adherent, often fissured crusts on the paw pads, around mucocutaneous junctions, areas of high trauma such as the lateral aspect of the elbows, and on the ventral abdomen. The muzzle, pinnae, vulva, and scrotum are also commonly involved. Erosions, ulcers, alopecia, and exudate are secondary sequelae. Secondary infections with bacterial and *Malassezia* spp. are very common, and pruritus and pain can be variable but are often present.[44] Scaling and alopecia of the trunk and limbs with

pruritus were the only cutaneous lesions found in two feline cases of SND.[4,44,45] Initial lesions started out on the proximal front limbs, dorsum, and the axillae but spread to the ventrum, lateral thorax, and groin. In one case associated with hepatopathy, alopecia of the ventrum, flanks, and inguinal region with underlying erythema and mild crusting was initially observed.[46] Another patient with hepatic disease presented with alopecia of the neck which spread to the flanks with pigmented crusts of the feet and tail. *Malassezia* infections have been diagnosed in multiple cases of cats with SND.[4,44] Lesion distribution in cats may be related to grooming habits.[46]

Differential diagnoses include thymoma-associated exfoliative dermatitis, paraneoplastic alopecia, feline leukemia virus– or feline immunodeficiency virus–associated dermatitis, skin fragility syndrome, EM, and cutaneous lymphoma.[11,44] All cats reported in the literature presented with systemic as well as cutaneous signs, which included weight loss, appetite changes, gastrointestinal upset, lethargy, or dyspnea. One cat presented with alopecia, erythema, mild crusting, and pruritus but had a recent episode of vomiting, diarrhea, and inappetence.[46]

Obtaining a skin biopsy paired with abdominal ultrasonographic findings should lead to diagnosis. Biopsy should be performed on erythematous plaques with mild to moderate crust. The crusts should be left in place and no scrubbing or disinfection of the superficial skin surface should be performed prior to sampling. If paws and paw pads are involved, biopsy should be performed at the margin of the paw pad; this prevents lameness and trauma to the site but still allows for sampling of a site that may aid in diagnosis.[44] When SND is suspected in feline patients, multiple biopsy samples should be collected; case reports of cats with SND have shown a large amount of variation in the histopathologic appearance and sometimes only one section may show uniform characteristics of SND that leads to definitive diagnosis.[46] Histopathologically, the most distinctive feature of SND is the "red, white, and blue layering": parakeratosis and serocellular crusting comprises the top, "red" layer, pallor of keratinocytes creates the middle or "white" layer, and a hyperplastic basal and suprabasal layer creates a deeply basophilic layer that causes the "blue" stripe.[44] It is not uncommon to find bacteria, dermatophyte spores, or yeast organisms embedded in the thick parakeratotic plaques. A mixed inflammatory pattern may be seen in the superficial dermis, mainly around vessels, with variable amounts of dermal edema.[44]

In dogs with SND, the ultrasonographic appearance of the liver has been described as "Swiss cheese-like" or "honeycomb" with areas of hyperechoic parenchyma surrounding hypoechoic areas with an overall reticular appearance to the liver.[46-48] A similar reticular pattern of the liver was reported in one feline case report of SND, whereas other feline cases were associated with pancreatic carcinoma.[44,46] Histopathologically, the liver of both dogs and cats with SND secondary to hepatic disease is identical with metabolic vacuolar hepatopathy observed.[44] If ultrasound evaluation does not reveal the expected findings, plasma glucagon measurements can be considered; however, a normal reference range has not been established in healthy cats.[48]

The prognosis is guarded to poor. There is not enough published data to comment specifically on survival time in cats, but it appears to be similar to canine patients that died or were euthanized anywhere from 1.6 to 5 months following diagnosis.[11,46] One cat with SND secondary to hepatic neuroendocrine carcinoma was euthanized 11 months after diagnosis with no treatment.[43] Because a proposed pathogenesis for SND involves elevated glucagon concentration that leads to amino acid deficiency, supplementation with amino acids may be helpful. These can be administered intravenously or orally; often a combination is recommended. Some dogs do well with a treatment regimen developed at the University of California that recommends high-quality protein, zinc supplementation, and fatty acid supplementation.[11]

IMMUNE-MEDIATED SKIN DISEASE ASSOCIATED WITH INTERNAL DISEASE

Erythema Multiforme

Erythema multiforme is a disease of cutaneous inflammation from immunologic dysregulation characterized by epidermal apoptosis.[49,50] It is rare in the cat and can be secondary to a drug reaction, infection, or neoplasia; drug reactions and herpesvirus infection are most commonly implicated in the cat.[50] Erythema multiforme is thought to be a host-specific T cell–mediated hypersensitivity reaction where cellular response is directed at keratinocyte-associated antigens.[9] In the case of herpesvirus infection, viral particles are found in epidermal keratinocytes; herpes-specific CD4+ type-1 helper T cell are attracted by virus particles, and the result is an upregulation of interferon-gamma. In the case of drug-induced EM, a tumor necrosis factor-alpha response by lymphocytes leads to keratinocyte apoptosis.[50] Either way, lymphocytes bind to these altered keratinocytes, triggering cell death. Alteration of the keratinocyte might be a primary factor in disease pathogenesis, although the exact mechanism remains unknown. The three most common drug classes associated with EM in dogs and cats are all antibiotics: trimethoprim-potentiated sulfonamides, cephalosporins, and penicillins.[9] Other medications (e.g., aurothioglucose, griseofulvin, and propylthiouracil), combinations of drugs, and vaccines (e.g., rabies) have also been suspected causes in the cat.[51,52] Currently, EM is subclassified into EM minor and EM major according to the percentage of body surface affected and severity of clinical presentation. Erythema multiforme minor, the milder form, has an acute onset of target lesions (the typical lesion seen in humans that is uncommon in dogs and cats) involving extremities with less systemic signs and only mild mucocutaneous involvement.[50] Erythema multiforme minor tends to be self-limiting. Erythema multiforme major is more severe with more mucocutaneous involvement and generalized systemic illness. Erythema multiforme overlaps clinically with Stevens-Johnson syndrome (SJS) and toxic epidermal necrolysis (TEN). In veterinary

medicine, the diagnosis of EM, SJS, or TEN is typically made on histopathologic findings, whereas in human medicine there are stricter clinical criteria to separate the diseases.

Skin lesions of EM in cats are described as symmetrical in onset with overwhelmingly vesicular, bullous, and/or ulcerative lesions. The trunk and mucocutaneous junctions are commonly involved, but generalized lesions are possible.[9,50] Erythematous macules, papules, or urticaria may also be seen, and in a report of six cats with EM, lesions were also seen on the pinnae, in the external ear canals, the head, and on the paws[50,51] (Figure 26-8). Systemic signs, such as fever, lethargy, and anorexia may be described, and it is reported that the more severe the clinical presentation, the more likely the eruption is due to a drug reaction.[37] A generalized exfoliative dermatitis with associated alopecia as a manifestation of EM in cats has also been reported. No breed or sex predilections are documented.

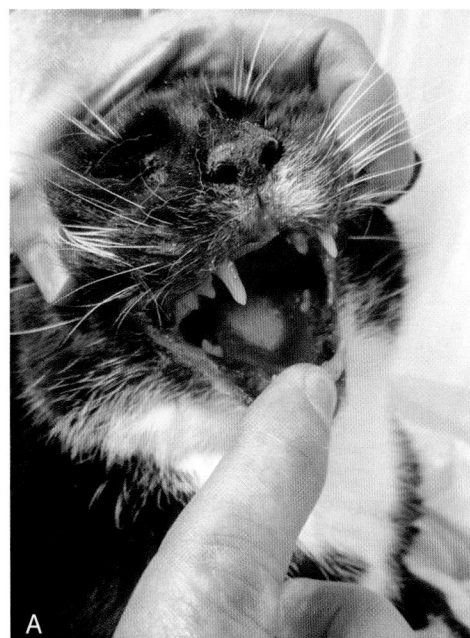

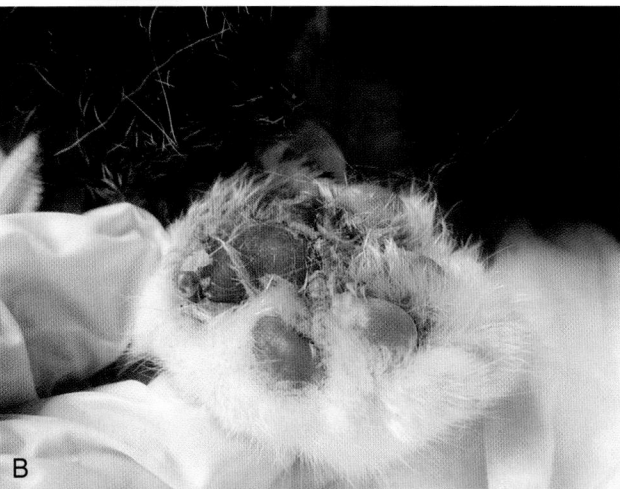

Figure 26-8: A, Severe ulceration on the tongue and mucocutaneous junctions in a domestic shorthair cat with erythema multiforme following antibiotic administration. **B,** Ulcer involving almost the entire carpal paw pad of the same patient.

Differential diagnoses are numerous given the variable clinical presentation of EM. Bacterial pyoderma, dermatophytosis, or demodicosis may be considered for milder cases; autoimmune disease (e.g., pemphigus foliaceus, pemphigus vulgaris, and epidermolysis bullosa), burns, feline idiopathic ulcerative dermatosis, eosinophilic granuloma complex, SND, thymoma-associated exfoliative dermatitis, and cutaneous neoplasia may be considered for more severe lesions.[9,50] Biopsy is the diagnostic test of choice. An intact epidermis or mucosa is essential for the demonstration of keratinocyte apoptosis, so ulcers should be avoided for sampling. Biopsies should be obtained from erythematous areas with or without crusting.[9,37] The most characteristic histopathology shows keratinocyte apoptosis with lymphocyte satellitosis, but often an interface dermatitis is also present with lymphocytes and macrophages obscuring the dermal-epidermal junction. Apoptosis is seen at all levels of the epidermis, which helps to differentiate it from thymoma-associated exfoliative dermatitis.[9] A thorough history, including all medications and vaccines given and any recent travel, paired with these histopathologic changes can lead to diagnosis. Polymerase chain reaction for the presence of herpesvirus in the skin may be indicated and can give additional treatment options to target the underlying trigger.[50] No characteristic abnormalities are found on routine laboratory testing.

Signs may spontaneously resolve after a variable length of time, typically weeks. Drug-induced EM may markedly improve within 1 to 2 weeks after discontinuing the causative medication.[51] If lesions are aggressive, especially vesiculobullous and ulcerative lesions, hospitalization and supportive care may be indicated. Immunosuppressive agents, such as glucocorticoids or modified cyclosporine, may be needed and intravenous immunoglobulin can be considered in serious, life-threatening cases.[50,52]

PANNICULITIS ASSOCIATED WITH PANCREATITIS

Panniculitis is an inflammatory condition of the subcutaneous fat. It is not uncommon in cats and has a number of underlying causes, including bacterial, fungal, or protozoal infections (from penetrating trauma or foreign bodies, cat fights, or environmental wound contamination), vasculitis, drug or vaccine reactions, nutritional deficiencies, and trauma.[17] The panniculus is primarily made up of lipocytes, which are particularly susceptible to trauma and secondary inflammation and ischemia. Any damage to the blood supply or to the cells themselves can lead to lipid release by lipocytes, which can be broken down into fatty acids that have profound inflammatory effects in the surrounding tissue. Sterile nodular panniculitis does not have an underlying infectious cause but may still be related to other systemic illness. Pancreatitis and pancreatic tumors in the cat have been reported to cause sterile panniculitis. Any cat presenting for clinical signs consistent with panniculitis should be evaluated for underlying pancreatic disease as well as performing diagnostics for other possible causes.[17,53]

In humans with pancreatitis, panniculitis is caused by the release of active pancreatic enzymes (phospholipase, trypsin, amylase). One theory is that these activated pancreatic enzymes cause vessel wall damage, leading to increased vascular permeability that can negatively affect the fat cells leading to inflammation and possible necrosis.[53]

Panniculitis secondary to pancreatitis is rare in the cat with no breed, sex, or age predilections.[53] Clinically, panniculitis presents as subcutaneous nodules that may be focal or generalized, firm or soft, well circumscribed or ill-defined. Some nodules may rupture and extend to the skin surface, leading to draining tracts and/or ulcers; there may be erythema of the overlying epidermis. When nodules rupture or are aspirated, a purulent, hemorrhagic, or oily material may be extracted. Most lesions are found on the trunk, and some can be quite painful. Cats with pancreatitis-associated panniculitis are often systemically ill with nonspecific signs, such as lethargy and inappetence, as well as signs consistent with pancreatitis, such as abdominal pain and distention, clinical dehydration, vomiting or diarrhea, and fever.[17,53]

Because systemic and cutaneous signs are concurrent, blood work (complete blood count, chemistry profile, urinalysis), measurement of feline pancreatic lipase immunoreactivity, and abdominal ultrasonography are indicated. Direct impressions of draining tracts or aspirates from nodules may show suppurative or pyogranulomatous inflammation. Although a sterile process, secondary infection from surface bacteria, typically staphylococci, may be seen.

Panniculitis can only be diagnosed by skin biopsy. When planning for skin biopsies, multiple samples should be collected and samples should be deep enough to evaluate the panniculus; any lesion that is ulcerated or necrotic should be avoided. On histopathology, the panniculus will have severe, nodular to diffuse suppurative or pyogranulomatous inflammation. Lipocytes may be necrotic and necrotic fat may become saponified; saponification leads to amorphic basophilic material within or around lipocytes. To make a definitive diagnosis of sterile panniculitis, the histopathologic changes must be paired with negative tissue cultures (aerobic, anaerobic, fungal, and mycobacterial cultures recommended); special stains for infectious organisms performed by a pathologist can also aid in the diagnosis of a sterile process.[17,53]

Not much is known regarding the timing of resolution of panniculitis associated with pancreatitis; there is only one report in a dog, where panniculitis resolved with successful treatment of the underlying pancreatitis.[54] Systemic glucocorticoids are commonly prescribed for treatment of sterile nodular panniculitis not associated with pancreatitis. Systemic steroid therapy is not indicated for pancreatitis without panniculitis, and it should be avoided in patients with concurrent illness, such as diabetes mellitus. Intralesional glucocorticoids could be considered in patients where systemic glucocorticoids may be contraindicated. The focus of treatment should be on the underlying pancreatitis. The treatment of pancreatitis is reviewed elsewhere (see Chapter 15) and is based upon maintaining proper hydration and perfusion, analgesics, and nutritional support.

References

1. Bergman PJ: Paraneoplastic syndromes. In Withrow SJ, Vail DM, Page RL, editors: *Small animal clinical oncology*, ed 5, St Louis, 2013, Elsevier, pp 83–97.

2. Turek MM: Cutaneous paraneoplastic syndromes in dogs and cats: a review of the literature. *Vet Dermatol* 14(6):279–296, 2003.

3. Pascal-Tenorio A, Olivry T, Gross TL, et al: Paraneoplastic alopecia associated with internal malignancies in the cat. *Vet Dermatol* 8(1):47–52, 1997.

4. Mauldin EA, Morris DO, Goldschmidt MH: Retrospective study: the presence of *Malassezia* in feline skin biopsies. A clinicopathological study. *Vet Dermatol* 13(1):7–13, 2002.

5. Tasker S, Griffon DJ, Nuttall TJ, et al: Resolution of paraneoplastic alopecia following surgical removal of a pancreatic carcinoma in a cat. *J Small Anim Pract* 40(1):16–19, 1999.

6. Marconato L, Albanese F, Viacava P, et al: Paraneoplastic alopecia associated with hepatocellular carcinoma in a cat. *Vet Dermatol* 18(4):267–271, 2007.

7. Frank LA: Miscellaneous alopecias. In Miller WH, Griffin CE, Campbell KL, editors: *Muller and Kirk's small animal dermatology*, ed 7, St Louis, 2013, Elsevier, pp 554–572.

8. Atrophic diseases of the adnexa. In Gross TL, Ihrke PJ, Walder EJ, et al, editors: *Skin diseases of the dog and cat clinical and histopathologic diagnosis*, ed 2, Ames, IA, 2005, Blackwell, pp 480–517.

9. Interface diseases of the dermal-epidermal junction. In Gross TL, Ihrke PJ, Walder EJ, et al, editors: *Skin diseases of the dog and cat clinical and histopathologic diagnosis*, ed 2, Ames, IA, 2005, Blackwell, pp 49–74.

10. Zitz JC, Birchard SJ, Couto GC, et al: Results of excision of thymoma in cats and dogs: 20 cases (1984-2005). *J Am Vet Med Assoc* 232(8):1186–1192, 2008.

11. Endocrine and metabolic diseases. In Miller WH, Griffin CE, Campbell KL, editors: *Muller and Kirk's small animal dermatology*, ed 7, St Louis, 2013, Elsevier, pp 501–553.

12. Graves TK: Hypercortisolism in cats (feline Cushing's syndrome). In Ettinger SJ, Feldman EC, editors: *Textbook of veterinary internal medicine*, vol 2, ed 7, St Louis, 2010, Elsevier/Saunders, pp 1840–1847.

13. Gunn-Moore D, Simpson K: Hyperadrenocorticism in cats. In Rand J, editor: *Clinical endocrinology of companion animals*, ed 1, Ames, IA, 2013, Wiley-Blackwell, pp 71–79.

14. Feldman EC, Nelson RW: Hyperadrenocorticism in cats (Cushing's syndrome). In Feldman EC, Nelson RW, editors: *Canine and feline endocrinology and reproduction*, ed 3, St Louis, 2004, Saunders/Elsevier, pp 358–393.

15. Lowe AD, Campbell KL, Graves T: Glucocorticoids in the cat. *Vet Dermatol* 19(6):340–347, 2008.

16. Mellett Keith AM, Bruyette D, Stanley S: Trilostane therapy for treatment of spontaneous hyperadrenocorticism in cats: 15 cases (2004-2012). *J Vet Intern Med* 27:1471–1477, 2013.

17. Miscellaneous skin diseases. In Miller WH, Griffin CE, Campbell KL, editors: *Muller and Kirk's small animal dermatology*, ed 7, St Louis, 2013, Elsevier, pp 695–723.

18. Degenerative, dysplastic and depositional diseases of dermal connective tissue. In Gross TL, Ihrke PJ, Walder EJ, et al, editors: *Skin diseases of the dog and cat clinical and histopathologic diagnosis*, ed 2, Ames, IA, 2005, Blackwell, pp 373–403.

19. Crosaz O, Vilaplana-Grosso F, Alleaume C, et al: Skin fragility syndrome in a cat with multicentric follicular lymphoma. *J Feline Med Surg* 15(10):953–958, 2013.

20. Tamulevicus AM, Harkin K, Janardhan K, et al: Disseminated histoplasmosis accompanied by cutaneous fragility in a cat. *J Am Anim Hosp Assoc* 47(3):e36–e41, 2011.

21. Daniel AGT, Lucas SRR, Júnior AR, et al: Skin fragility syndrome in a cat with cholangiohepatitis and hepatic lipidosis. *J Feline Med Surg* 12(2):151–155, 2010.

22. Trotman TK, Mauldin E, Hoffmann V, et al: Skin fragility syndrome in a cat with feline infectious peritonitis and hepatic lipidosis. *Vet Dermatol* 18(5):365–369, 2007.

23. Fernandez CJ, Scott DW, Erb HN: Staining abnormalities of dermal collagen in eosinophil- or neutrophil-rich inflammatory dermatoses of horses and cats as demonstrated with Masson's trichrome stain. *Vet Dermatol* 11(1):43–48, 2000.

24. Barthold SW, Kaplan BJ, Schwartz A: Reversible dermal atrophy in a cat treated with phenytoin. *Vet Pathol* 17(4):469–476, 1980.

25. Wicke C, Halliday B, Allen D, et al: Effects of steroids and retinoids on wound healing. *Arch Surg* 135(11):1265–1270, 2000.

26. Feline hyperthyroidism (thyrotoxicosis). In Feldman EC, Nelson RW, editors: *Canine and feline endocrinology and reproduction*, ed 3, St Louis, 2004, Saunders/Elsevier, pp 152–218.

27. Gunn-Moore D: Feline endocrinopathies. *Vet Clin North Am Small Anim Pract* 35(1):171–210, 2005.

28. Mooney CT: Hyperthyroidism. In Ettinger SJ, Feldman EC, editors: *Textbook of veterinary internal medicine*, vol 2, ed 7, St Louis, 2010, Elsevier/Saunders, pp 1761–1796.

29. Broussard JD, Peterson ME, Fox PR: Changes in clinical and laboratory findings in cats with hyperthyroidism from 1983 to 1993. *J Am Vet Med Assoc* 206(3):302–305, 1995.

30. Levy L, Zeichner JA: Dermatologic manifestation of diabetes. *J Diabetes* 4(1):68–76, 2012.

31. Goyal A, Raina S, Kaushal SS, et al: Pattern of cutaneous manifestations in diabetes mellitus. *Indian J Dermatol* 55(1):39–41, 2010.

32. Perrins N, Gaudiano F, Bond R: Carriage of *Malassezia* spp. yeasts in cats with diabetes mellitus, hyperthyroidism and neoplasia. *Med Mycol* 45(6):541–546, 2007.

33. Feline diabetes mellitus. In Feldman EC, Nelson RW, editors: *Canine and feline endocrinology and reproduction*, ed 3, St Louis, 2004, Saunders/Elsevier, pp 539–579.

34. Reusch CE: Feline diabetes mellitus. In Ettinger SJ, Feldman EC, editors: *Textbook of veterinary internal medicine*, vol 2, ed 7, St Louis, 2010, Elsevier/Saunders, pp 1796–1816.

35. Lan C-CE, Wu C-S, Huang S-M, et al: High-glucose environment enhanced oxidative stress and increased interleukin-8 secretion from keratinocytes: new insights into impaired diabetic wound healing. *Diabetes* 62(7):2530–2538, 2013.

36. Noninfectious nodular and diffuse granulomatous and pyogranulomatous diseases of the dermis. In Gross TL, Ihrke PJ, Walder EJ, et al, editors: *Skin diseases of the dog and cat clinical and histopathologic diagnosis*, ed 2, Ames, IA, 2005, Blackwell, pp 320–341.

37. Outerbridge CA: Cutaneous manifestations of internal diseases. *Vet Clin North Am Small Anim Pract* 43(1):135–152, 2013.

38. Wisselink MA, Koeman JP, Wensing T, et al: Hyperlipoproteinaemia associated with atherosclerosis and cutaneous xanthomatosis in a cat. *Vet Q* 16(4):199–202, 1994.

39. Chanut F, Colle MA, Deschamps JY, et al: Systemic xanthomatosis associated with hyperchylomicronaemia in a cat. *J Vet Med A Physiol Pathol Clin Med* 52(6):272–274, 2005.

40. Johnstone AC, Jones BR, Thompson JC, et al: The pathology of an inherited hyperlipoproteinaemia of cats. *J Comp Pathol* 102(2):125–137, 1990.

41. Jones BR: Inherited hyperchylomicronaemia in the cat. *J Small Anim Pract* 34:493–499, 1993.

42. Grieshaber TL, McKeever PJ, Conroy JD: Spontaneous cutaneous (eruptive) xanthomatosis in two cats. *J Am Anim Hosp Assoc* 27(5):509–512, 1991.

43. Asakawa MG, Cullen JM, Linder KE: Necrolytic migratory erythema associated with a glucagon-producing primary hepatic neuroendocrine carcinoma in a cat. *Vet Dermatol* 24(4):466–469, e109–e110, 2013.

44. Necrotizing diseases of the epidermis. In Gross TL, Ihrke PJ, Walder EJ, et al, editors: *Skin diseases of the dog and cat clinical and histopathologic diagnosis*, ed 2, Ames, IA, 2005, Blackwell, pp 75–104.

45. Patel A, Whitbread TJ, McNeil PE: A case of metabolic epidermal necrosis in a cat. *Vet Dermatol* 7(4):221–225, 2008.

46. Kimmel SE, Christiansen W, Byrne KP: Clinicopathological, ultrasonographic, and histopathological findings of superficial necrolytic dermatitis with hepatopathy in a cat. *J Am Anim Hosp Assoc* 39(1):23–27, 2003.

47. Jacobson LS, Kirberger RM, Nesbit JW: Hepatic ultrasonography and pathological findings in dogs with hepatocutaneous syndrome: new concepts. *J Vet Intern Med* 9(6):399–404, 1995.

48. Outerbridge CA, Marks SL, Rogers QR: Plasma amino acid concentrations in 36 dogs with histologically confirmed superficial

necrolytic dermatitis. *Vet Dermatol* 13(4):177–186, 2002.

49. Merchant SR: The skin as a sensor of internal medicine disorders. In Ettinger SJ, Feldman EC, editors: *Textbook of veterinary internal medicine*, vol 1, ed 7, St Louis, 2010, Saunders/Elsevier, pp 64–66.

50. Halliwell REW: Autoimmune and immune-mediated dermatoses. In Miller WH, Griffin CE, Campbell KL, editors: *Muller and Kirk's small animal dermatology*, ed 7, St Louis, 2013, Elsevier, pp 432–500.

51. Scott DW, Miller WH: Erythema multiforme in dogs and cats: literature review and case material from the Cornell University College of Veterinary Medicine (1988-96). *Vet Dermatol* 10:297–309, 1999.

52. Byrne KP, Giger U: Use of human immunoglobulin for treatment of severe erythema multiforme in a cat. *J Am Vet Med Assoc* 220(2): 197–201, 2002.

53. Diseases of the panniculus. In Gross TL, Ihrke PJ, Walder EJ, et al, editors: *Skin diseases of the dog and cat clinical and histopathologic diagnosis*, ed 2, Ames, IA, 2005, Blackwell, pp 538–558.

54. O'Kell AL, Inteeworn N, Diaz SF, et al: Canine sterile nodular panniculitis: a retrospective study of 14 cases. *J Vet Intern Med* 24(2):278–284, 2010.

Diagnostically Challenging Dermatoses of Cats

Christine L. Cain and Elizabeth A. Mauldin

This chapter outlines the clinical features, diagnosis, and treatment of several unusual feline dermatoses. Some of these diseases have been described in the veterinary literature for decades, whereas others are more recently recognized, but all may present a diagnostic challenge due to their rare occurrence or poorly elucidated etiologies. Most of these dermatoses are definitively diagnosed based on characteristic clinical and histopathologic features, as well as ruling out other more common differential diagnoses. When performing histopathology of the skin, care should be taken in biopsy site selection to maximize diagnostic yield, and biopsy samples should be sent to a pathologist skilled in dermatopathologic interpretation.

PLASMA CELL PODODERMATITIS

Clinical Features

Plasma cell pododermatitis is a localized dermatosis of cats characterized by soft swelling of the paw pads, most commonly the metacarpal or metatarsal pads.[1-7] Affected paw pads may have an inflated "pillow-like" appearance with erythema, prominent striae, and/or fine scaling[2,5,6] (Figure 27-1A). The paw pad changes may be accompanied by lameness or may be asymptomatic.[6,7] With chronicity, ulceration and hemorrhage of the paw pads can occur, which may exacerbate lameness[3,7,8] (see Figure 27-1B).

Most reports of plasma cell pododermatitis cite no definitive age, sex, or breed predilections[1,3]; one retrospective study of 26 cats found neutered males to be overrepresented in the patient population.[6] Most reported cases have been in domestic shorthair cats.[5,6] In addition to the footpad changes and possible lameness, some affected cats will present with other clinical signs, including poor body condition[4,6,8] and hypersalivation (presumably related to concurrent stomatitis).[6] Concurrent plasmacytic stomatitis,[1,6] renal and hepatic amyloidosis,[3] or immune-mediated glomerulonephritis[9] have been infrequently reported. Plasmacytic nasal dermatitis presenting as diffuse swelling of the bridge of the nose has been described in cats with plasma cell pododermatitis.[10,11] A similar plasmacytic nasal dermatitis has also been reported in

two cats without accompanying pododermatitis.[12,13] In one cat, onset of nasal swelling was associated with clinical signs of upper respiratory infection.[12]

Although recognized as a clinical entity since the 1980s,[1,4,9] the etiology of feline plasma cell pododermatitis is still unknown. Infectious agents, including bacteria, fungi, and protozoa, have been investigated as a cause of plasma cell pododermatitis.[1,14] In a study of 14 skin biopsies collected from the paw pads of cats with plasma cell pododermatitis, Bettenay and colleagues failed to identify infectious agents (including *Bartonella* spp., *Ehrlichia* spp., *Anaplasma phagocytophilum*, *Chlamydophila felis*, *Mycoplasma* spp., *Toxoplasma gondii*, and feline herpesvirus) in tissue samples by immunohistochemistry and polymerase chain reaction (PCR).[14] The absence of demonstrable infectious agents from the skin of cats with plasma cell pododermatitis does not rule out the possibility that the disease has an inciting infectious cause. It has been suggested that the inflammatory response may persist beyond elimination of the triggering infectious agent from the tissue.[12,14] A possible link between feline immunodeficiency virus (FIV) and plasma cell pododermatitis has also been suggested. Several studies of plasma cell pododermatitis have included FIV-positive cats in the patient population.[2,3,5,6,15] Simon and colleagues reported histopathologic features of plasma cell pododermatitis from the paw pads of four of six cats with natural FIV infection. Additionally, clusters of FIV-infected cells were detected by immunohistochemistry within the inflammatory infiltrate of the paw pad of one cat with plasma cell pododermatitis.[15] Infiltration of the lungs, liver, and kidneys by plasma cells was also demonstrated in one FIV-positive cat with plasma cell pododermatitis by Guaguere and colleagues.[6] Plasma cell pododermatitis may also be diagnosed in cats tested negative for FIV infection.[5,6] Some authors have suggested that plasma cell pododermatitis is a cutaneous reaction pattern in cats with multiple possible causes; FIV infection may be one contributing factor.[6]

At this time, plasma cell pododermatitis appears to have an immune-mediated pathogenesis.[7,8,14] This is supported not only by the lack of consistent evidence of infectious agents from the skin of affected cats but also by the favorable

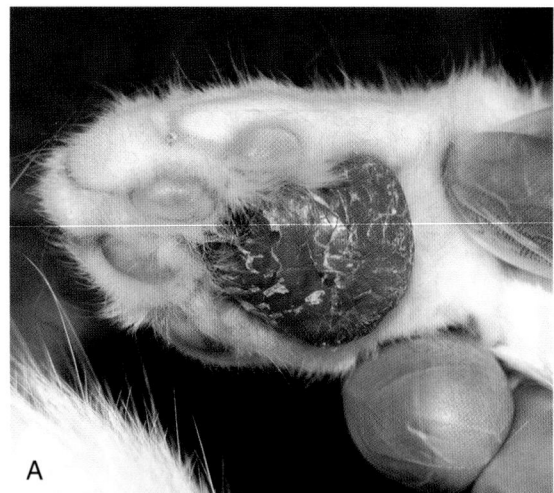

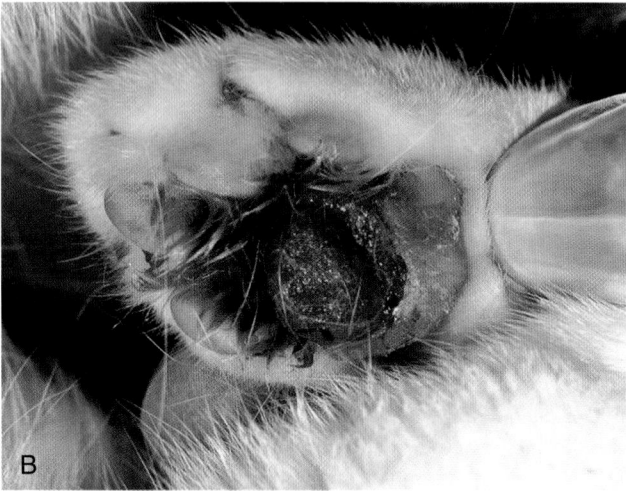

Figure 27-1: A, Swelling of the metacarpal paw pad (note the inflated "pillow-like" appearance) with prominent striae and fine scale in a cat with plasma cell pododermatitis. **B,** Ulcerated metacarpal paw pad with granulation tissue protrusion in the same cat with chronic plasma cell pododermatitis.

response to treatment with immunomodulatory medications.[1,2,3,5,8,10,16] An allergic etiology has also been suggested due to seasonal recurrence in some patients.[4,7,12]

Diagnosis

A tentative diagnosis of feline plasma cell pododermatitis may be made based on typical clinical appearance. Plasma cell pododermatitis is clinically distinct; the primary differential diagnosis is eosinophilic granuloma of the paw pad. Frequently, eosinophilic granulomas of the paw pads will present with erythema, erosions, and crusts of the surrounding interdigital skin as well as the paw pad.[17] By contrast, plasma cell pododermatitis is typically restricted to the paw pad itself. See Chapter 32 for further discussion of eosinophilic granuloma complex.

Clinical pathologic findings may be supportive of a diagnosis of feline plasma cell pododermatitis. Complete blood count may reveal anemia (associated with chronic inflammatory disease or blood loss through hemorrhage of ulcerated

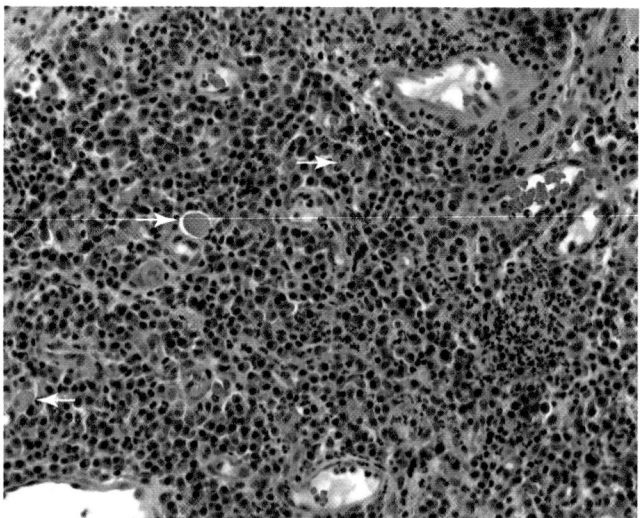

Figure 27-2: Photomicrograph: Plasma Cell Pododermatitis. The dermis of the paw pad is infiltrated by large numbers plasma cells and fewer neutrophils and lymphocytes. Many plasma cells contain cytoplasmic Russell bodies *(arrows)*. (Hematoxylin and eosin, 20×)

paw pads),[8] thrombocytopenia, and leukocytosis.[5] Serum chemistry analysis frequently reveals hypergammaglobulinemia,[5,7,8,16] which has been further characterized as a polyclonal gammopathy.[8] Hypergammaglobulinemia may be a persistent finding even in cats undergoing treatment.[5] Testing for FIV is recommended during workup of cats with suspected plasma cell pododermatitis.

Cytologic evaluation of fine-needle aspirates from affected paw pads may show plasma cells, but histopathology is required for definitive diagnosis. Histopathologic features include diffuse infiltration of the dermis and subcutis by plasma cells, with variable numbers of lymphocytes, neutrophils, and eosinophils[6,17] (Figure 27-2). Mott cells (plasma cells containing Russell bodies) are common.[17] Mitotic figures and binucleated plasma cells may be noted.[3] Ulcers, granulation tissue, and dermal fibrosis may be present in chronic lesions.[17] Every attempt should be made to avoid sampling ulcerated skin to obtain the most diagnostic samples. Leukocytoclastic vasculitis has also been described in skin biopsies from affected cats.[1,3]

Treatment

Immunomodulatory therapy is the current mainstay of treatment for feline plasma cell pododermatitis. Doxycycline has been reported to be effective as a monotherapy in two studies.[2,5] In one uncontrolled trial, doxycycline was administered to 17 cats at a dose of 25 mg/cat orally every 24 hours. After 3 to 4 weeks of therapy, complete remission was noted in 4 of 17 cats, with two additional cats achieving complete clinical remission after 6 to 8 weeks of treatment.[2] In another uncontrolled trial of 10 cats, doxycycline was administered at a dose of 10 mg/kg orally every 24 hours for 40 days. After 30 days, one cat had achieved complete clinical remission, with four additional cats achieving complete remission after 60 days.[5] Clinical benefits of doxycycline therapy are presumably due to its immunomodulatory effects, though improvement due to antimicrobial activity against an unidentified infectious agent cannot be completely ruled out.[2,14] Because of the potential for esophagitis and esophageal stricture with doxycycline administration in tablet or capsule form, a liquid formulation should be used or care should be taken to follow tablets or capsules with food and/or water.[18] Other reportedly effective therapies are glucocorticoids (e.g., prednisolone at a starting dose of 2 to 4 mg/kg/day orally),[3,8,10] injectable gold salts,[1,16] or surgical excision of affected paw pads.[6,7,19] Modified cyclosporine at the approved feline starting dose of 7 mg/kg orally every 24 hours is also a promising therapy for management of plasma cell pododermatitis.[20] Modified cyclosporine has been shown to be effective for treatment of plasmacytic stomatitis in cats.[21] Immunosuppressive therapy (such as with systemic glucocorticoids or modified cyclosporine) should be undertaken with caution in FIV-positive cats. Spontaneous regression of paw pad changes has also been reported.[1,3]

URTICARIA PIGMENTOSA-LIKE DERMATITIS

Clinical Features

Urticaria pigmentosa-like dermatitis (also called papular eosinophilic and mastocytic dermatitis) is a dermatosis of Sphynx and Devon Rex cats.[22-24] There is controversy regarding whether urticaria pigmentosa-like dermatitis is a distinct clinical entity and whether an identical disorder affects both Sphynx and Devon Rex cats. In humans, urticaria pigmentosa is the most common form of cutaneous mastocytosis diagnosed in children. Mastocytoses in humans are the result of clonal expansion of mast cells and subsequent infiltration of the skin and/or systemic sites. Development of mastocytosis in humans has been linked to mutations in *c-kit*, the gene encoding for the mast cell surface receptor kit. Despite its name, urticaria pigmentosa is not generally associated with urticaria in humans; lesions are most commonly maculopapular and are frequently pruritic.[25] Similar maculopapular lesions, crusts, and variable hyperpigmentation have been described in three related Sphynx cats[22] and several Devon Rex cats.[23,24] Due to the similar clinical presentation, as well as histopathologic findings, homology with urticaria pigmentosa in humans has been suggested.[22]

Similar to urticaria pigmentosa in humans, which primarily affects children, the three affected Sphynx cats described by Vitale and colleagues were young (between 5 and 7 months of age at the time of lesion onset). A genetic basis was proposed because the cats had a common sire.[22] A familial relationship in Devon Rex cats with a similar clinical presentation has not been demonstrated.[23,24] Dermatophytosis was diagnosed in three reported cases of urticaria pigmentosa-like dermatitis in Devon Rex cats.[24] Urticaria pigmentosa-like dermatitis, more appropriately referred to as "papular eosinophilic and mastocytic dermatitis" in this breed, may be a

reaction pattern with multiple potential causes (including dermatophytosis) in Devon Rex cats and not a true correlate of human urticaria pigmentosa.[23,24] Dermatophytosis has not been reported as a cause of cutaneous mastocytosis in Sphynx cats, but urticaria pigmentosa-like dermatitis may represent a cutaneous reaction pattern to multiple underlying causes in this breed as well. It is unknown whether the conditions described in Sphynx cats and Devon Rex cats represent the same disease,[22] although the genetic relatedness of the two breeds (the Sphynx breed is derived from the Devon Rex breed) suggests that this is the case.[25]

Diagnosis

Differential diagnoses for papular eosinophilic and mastocytic dermatitis (urticaria pigmentosa-like dermatitis) in cats include allergic dermatitis, dermatophytosis, ectoparasitic infestation (cheyletiellosis, *Demodex cati* or *Demodex gatoi* infestation), pemphigus foliaceus, pyoderma, or multifocal cutaneous mast cell tumors.[22,23] Impression smears and/or acetate tape preparations should be collected from the skin surface to investigate for bacteria, *Malassezia* spp. yeasts, or acantholytic keratinocytes. Superficial and deep skin scrapings should be performed to investigate for superficial mites and *D. cati*. Wood's lamp examination may be performed as a screening test for dermatophytosis; fungal culture should be performed on all cats with suspected papular eosinophilic and mastocytic dermatitis to rule out dermatophytosis.[24]

A CBC may reveal peripheral eosinophilia and/or basophilia in affected cats.[22] Histopathology, in conjunction with the clinical presentation, provides the definitive diagnosis. It should be kept in mind that in more eosinophil-rich lesions, histopathology may not be able to distinguish between papular eosinophilic and mastocytic dermatitis of the Sphynx or Devon Rex and other eosinophilic diseases of cats (e.g., flea allergy dermatitis, food allergy, or atopic dermatitis).[23] Biopsies should be sent to a pathologist who is skilled in dermatopathology interpretation. Histopathology shows a perivascular to interstitial infiltrate consisting of well-differentiated mast cells[17] (Figure 27-3); variable numbers of eosinophils may also been seen.[23,24] Luminal folliculitis and fungal hyphae within or spores surrounding hair shafts may be seen with dermatophytosis.[17,24]

Treatment

In children with urticaria pigmentosa, treatment is mainly symptomatic because the disease typically spontaneously regresses with puberty.[26] Commonly employed symptomatic therapies for children include topical glucocorticoids and mast cell stabilizers, such as cromolyn sodium or oral antihistamines.[26] In cats with papular eosinophilic and mastocytic dermatitis, an attempt should be made to identify and control underlying causes. If identified by fungal culture or histopathology, dermatophytosis should be treated with topical and systemic antifungal therapy.[24] Complete lesion remission with antifungal therapy has been described in

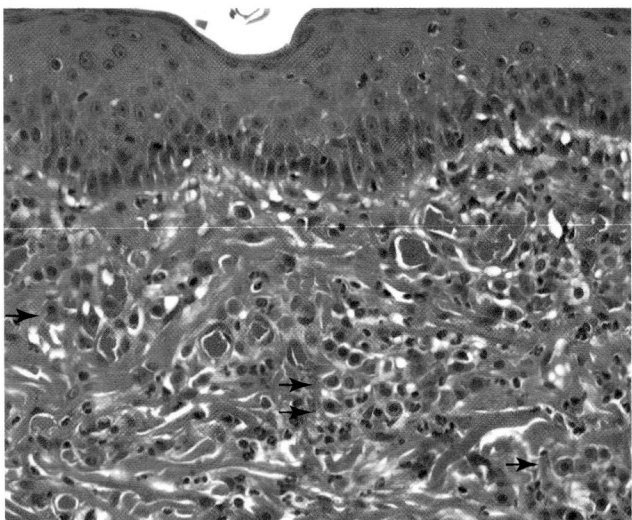

Figure 27-3: Photomicrograph: Urticaria Pigmentosa-Like Dermatitis. The dermis contains an inflammatory infiltrate rich in mast cells *(arrows)* with fewer eosinophils. (Hematoxylin and eosin, 20×)

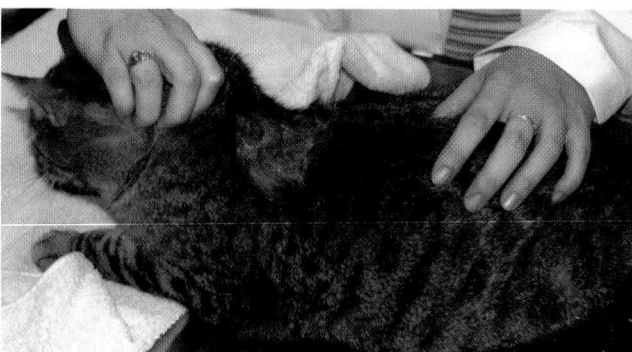

Figure 27-4: Well-demarcated ulcer with adherent crust in the interscapular region of a cat with idiopathic ulcerative dermatosis.

Devon Rex cats with dermatophytosis. Antihistamine therapy (oral cetirizine) and essential fatty acid supplementation was used in conjunction with antifungal therapy for management of papular eosinophilic and mastocytic dermatitis in one Devon Rex cat with dermatophytosis described by Colombo and colleagues. In this case, all medications were discontinued following two negative fungal cultures, and no relapse occurred over the next 2 years.[24] Strict ectoparasite control and workup for allergic dermatoses (such as an elimination diet trial to investigate food hypersensitivity) are also recommended. Glucocorticoids (e.g., prednisolone at a starting dose of 1 to 2 mg/kg/day orally) have also been reported to be effective for inducing lesion remission,[22,23] as have antihistamines,[22-24] oral essential fatty acid supplementation,[23,24] and cyclosporine at a starting dose of 7.5 mg/kg orally every 24 hours.[27] Treatment with immunosuppressive medications, such as systemic glucocorticoids or modified cyclosporine, should not be undertaken until dermatophytosis has been ruled out via negative fungal culture, particularly in Devon Rex cats.

IDIOPATHIC ULCERATIVE DERMATOSIS

Clinical Features

Cats with idiopathic ulcerative dermatosis present with single or, less commonly, multiple cutaneous ulcers over the dorsal neck, shoulders, or interscapular region[28,29] (Figure 27-4). Ulcers are usually covered by adherent crusts[28,29] and are typically 0.5 to 1 cm in diameter.[27] Lesions may enlarge over time, with some ulcers progressing to 5 to 7 cm in diameter.[28] Pruritus and lymphadenopathy may be accompanying clinical features.[29] Age and breed predilections have not been reported[28,29]; in one report of eight cases, 75% of affected cats were male.[28]

The etiology of idiopathic ulcerative dermatosis is not known. Given the typical location of lesions, an underlying reaction to trauma, contact irritants, vaccines, or subcutaneous injections has been suggested.[28,29] Due to the large number of sensory nerves on the dorsal neck of cats, idiopathic ulcerative dermatosis may also represent a cutaneous reaction pattern to a number of pruritic or painful stimuli resulting in self-trauma of this region.[17] A focal vasculopathy, possibly due to immune complex deposition, has been suggested due to the presence of thrombi within dermal blood vessels on histopathologic examination of skin biopsies from some affected cats.[29] An underlying neuropathy associated with feline herpesvirus infection has also been suggested.[30]

Diagnosis

The clinical finding of a well-demarcated ulcer on the dorsal neck or interscapular region, usually with an overlying adherent crust, is distinctive for idiopathic ulcerative dermatosis. Differential diagnoses for focal cutaneous ulcers in this region include thermal or chemical burn.[17] Underlying causes of pruritus or pain leading to self-trauma and development of ulcers include dermatophytosis, parasitic infestations (*Cheyletiella* spp., *D. gatoi* or *D. cati*, *Notoedres cati*, *Otodectes* dermatitis, fleas), allergic dermatitis, foreign bodies, wounds, contact dermatitis, neoplasia, or injection-site reactions.[20,29] Impression smears should be performed from the surface of lesions and under crusts to assess for secondary bacterial infection. Bacterial culture and susceptibility should be performed from infected lesions of cats with a history of empiric antimicrobial treatment failure. Superficial and deep skin scrapings should be performed from the edge of ulcers to assess for surface mites and *D. cati*. Fungal culture should be considered to rule out dermatophytosis.

Complete blood counts and serum chemistry analyses may reveal leukocytosis and hyperglobulinemia in affected cats.[29] Histopathology is supportive of a clinical diagnosis of idiopathic ulcerative dermatosis. As for other ulcerative diseases, an attempt should be made to sample the junction of ulcerated and nonulcerated skin in order to evaluate intact epidermis.[17] Typical histopathologic features include an ulcer covered by a serocellular crust containing necrotic granulocytes. Bacteria may also be found on the surface of the ulcer and embedded within serocellular crusts. A perivascular to interstitial inflammatory cell infiltrate consisting mainly of neutrophils may be found within the superficial dermis below the ulcer. In more chronic lesions, a linear band of superficial dermal fibrosis may be found.[17,28,29] Although initially reported as a distinctive feature, this linear subepidermal fibrosis is not consistently noted in newer lesions.[17,28] In one report of three cases, superficial dermal vascular congestion and intraluminal thrombi were also seen.[29]

Treatment

In the authors' opinion, the healing phase presents the greatest challenge to treatment. As the wound begins to contract, cats may become more intensely pruritic, creating a vicious cycle of wound contracture and expansion. Some lesions can expand to occupy a large portion of the dorsal thorax. As with papular eosinophilic and mastocytic dermatitis in cats, idiopathic ulcerative dermatosis may represent a cutaneous reaction to various conditions. As such, an attempt should be made to identify and treat underlying causes. Particularly in pruritic cats, strict ectoparasite control and workup for allergic dermatoses (such as an elimination diet trial to investigate food hypersensitivity) should be considered. Reportedly effective therapies include complete surgical resection of lesions,[28] systemic glucocorticoids (including subcutaneous injections of methylprednisolone acetate or oral prednisolone [at a starting dose of 2.2 mg/kg/day]),[28,29] and application of protective bandages.[30] Treatment with glucocorticoids, however, should not be considered a substitute for identification and control of an underlying cause. Secondary infections of ulcers should also be addressed with systemic antibiotics and/or topical antibacterial or antiseptic therapy. Silver sulfadiazine cream may be an effective sole or adjunctive therapy for secondary bacterial infection.[20] Antiviral therapy targeting a possible herpesvirus-associated peripheral neuropathy has been suggested as a potential treatment, but efficacy has not been documented.[30]

PROLIFERATIVE AND NECROTIZING OTITIS EXTERNA

Clinical Features

Proliferative and necrotizing otitis externa is characterized by adherent, verrucous, proliferative plaques on the concave pinnae and extending to the vertical ear canals[31-33] (Figure 27-5A). Involvement of the ear canals alone without pinnal involvement has also been reported.[34] Proliferative plaques are often covered by brown to black crusts and are friable on manipulation with underlying erosions and ulcers.[31-34] Secondary suppurative otitis externa and bacterial or yeast infection are common.[31,32,34] Although frequently reported in kittens less than 6 months of age,[17,33] the condition has been diagnosed in adult cats as well.[31,34] The reason for the increased incidence in kittens is unknown at this time, though an

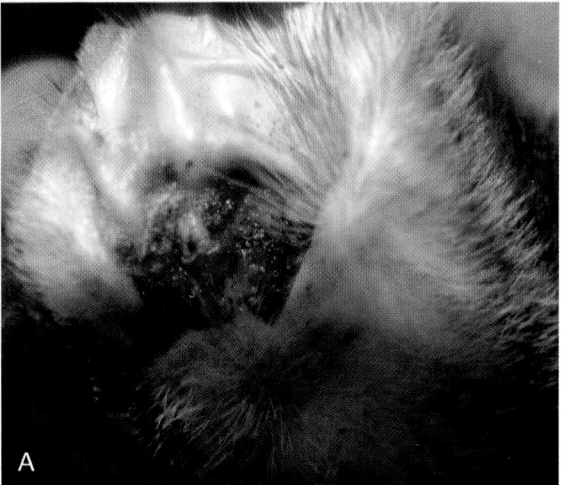
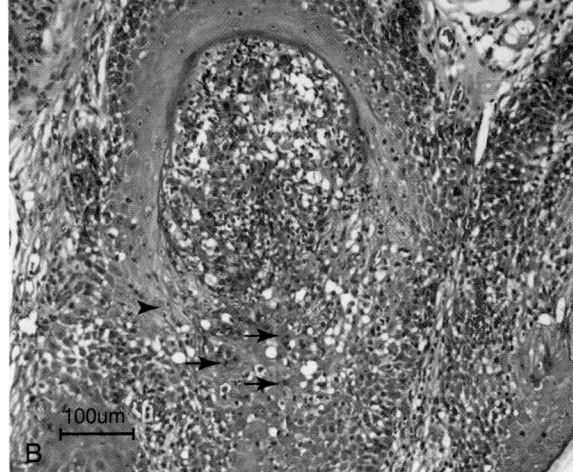

Figure 27-5: **A,** Proliferative, adherent plaque with overlying crust on the concave pinna of a cat with proliferative and necrotizing otitis externa. **B,** Photomicrograph: proliferative and necrotizing otitis externa. The follicular external root sheath is markedly hyperplastic and contains apoptotic keratinocytes *(arrows)*. The hair follicle lumen is filled with cell debris, neutrophils, and nucleated corneocytes. A few keratinocytes in the spinous layer have enlarged nuclei and swollen cytoplasm *(arrowhead)*. (Hematoxylin and eosin, 10×)

aberrant viral infection or cutaneous drug eruption has been proposed.[31] No sex or breed predilection has been reported. Affected cats are otherwise healthy.[31]

The pathogenesis of proliferative and necrotizing otitis externa is not known. An immune-mediated basis is suspected due to the favorable response to topical tacrolimus, an immunomodulatory medication[31-34] and the typical histopathologic feature of numerous individual pyknotic keratinocytes with hypereosinophilic cytoplasm within hair follicle outer root sheaths.[31-33] These hypereosinophilic, shrunken keratinocytes have been demonstrated to be the products of T cell–mediated apoptosis through immunohistochemistry for CD3+ and active caspase-3. Lymphocytes infiltrating the epidermis were shown to be predominantly positive for CD3+ (a T cell surface protein), and cytoplasmic and nuclear staining of pyknotic keratinocytes for active caspase-3 (an enzyme involved in apoptosis induction) was also shown.[33]

Multifocal individual keratinocyte apoptosis is also a feature of erythema multiforme (EM), a T cell–mediated disorder in which the cytotoxic response is directed at keratinocytes; triggering factors include drugs and infectious agents.[17,35] Some cats with proliferative and necrotizing otitis externa have a history of drug administration or vaccination prior to diagnosis. Although a focal cutaneous drug eruption is possible, other cats do not have a history of medication administration or vaccination prior to lesion onset.[31] An unusual presentation of viral infection has also been investigated in cats with proliferative and necrotizing otitis externa; immunohistochemical stains for feline herpesvirus, feline calicivirus, and papillomavirus on tissue samples from lesional skin have been negative.[31] As is speculated for feline plasma cell pododermatitis, this does not rule out that the disease has an inciting infectious cause, with the immune-mediated response persisting beyond elimination of the triggering infectious agent from the tissue.[31] In one affected cat, food hypersensitivity was demonstrated as the cause of aural pruritus following resolution of proliferative aural plaques. It is unknown whether food hypersensitivity was related to this cat's proliferative and necrotizing otitis because the plaques did not recur with dietary rechallenge.[31]

Diagnosis

When there is involvement of the concave pinna, proliferative and necrotizing otitis externa is visually distinctive. Differential diagnoses for a vegetative plaque on the concave pinna of a cat include dermatophytosis, neoplasia (e.g., ceruminous gland adenoma and adenocarcinoma or squamous cell carcinoma), or a viral plaque. Diagnosis of proliferative and necrotizing otitis may be more challenging if there is involvement of the ear canals in the absence of pinnal involvement.[34] In this case, differential diagnoses for feline otitis externa include *Otodectes cynotis* infestation, an obstructive inflammatory polyp, ear canal neoplasia, allergic otitis externa, irritant or allergic contact otitis externa secondary to topical products, and secondary bacterial or yeast infection. Ear swabs should be obtained from all affected cats to evaluate for ear mites and for cytologic assessment of bacteria, yeast, and inflammatory cells.

Histopathology is required for definitive diagnosis of proliferative and necrotizing otitis externa. Typical histopathologic features include follicular outer root sheath hyperplasia with multifocal individually pyknotic and hypereosinophilic (apoptotic) keratinocytes, dilated hair follicle infundibula with parakeratotic hyperkeratosis, and luminal folliculitis[17,31-33] (see Figure 27-5B). Lymphocytes located adjacent to shrunken, hypereosinophilic keratinocytes (satellitosis), a typical feature of EM, may also be seen.[33]

Treatment

The most successful treatment for feline proliferative and necrotizing otitis externa appears to be topical tacrolimus ointment applied every 12 to 24 hours to affected areas.[31-34]

Although 0.1% tacrolimus ointment has been used successfully in most reported cases, 0.03% tacrolimus ointment applied twice daily was successful for treatment of one kitten.[33] Tacrolimus 0.1% ointment was diluted in mineral oil to facilitate treatment of the ear canals in one cat with ear canal but not pinnal involvement.[34] Tacrolimus is a calcineurin inhibitor (similar to cyclosporine but with superior penetration through the stratum corneum when applied topically) with immunomodulatory activity through inhibition of T cell activation.[36] Additionally, tacrolimus may inhibit T cell–mediated keratinocyte apoptosis.[37] In one case reported by Mauldin and colleagues, oral prednisolone was used in combination with 0.1% tacrolimus ointment to control aural pruritus.[31] In pruritic patients, particularly those refractory to therapy or in which aural pruritus extends beyond resolution of proliferative plaques, a diet trial to investigate underlying food hypersensitivity should be considered.[31] Topical treatment of secondary yeast or bacterial otitis externa should also be undertaken based on cytologic findings.[31,34] Bacterial culture and susceptibility should be performed as a basis for therapy from the ear canals in cases of refractory otitis externa and from the middle ear cavity in cases of concurrent otitis media. Spontaneous resolution of lesions within 12 to 24 months has been reported in kittens[17]; spontaneous resolution does not appear to occur in all cases with juvenile onset and has not been documented in adult onset cases of proliferative and necrotizing otitis externa.[31]

IDIOPATHIC FACIAL DERMATITIS

Clinical Features

Idiopathic facial dermatitis occurs in young adult Persian and Himalayan cats.[30,38-40] The cats develop an accumulation of dark brown to black keratosebaceous debris on the face, particularly around the eyes, mouth, and chin[38-40] (Figure 27-6). Dark waxy debris may cause matting of the hair on the face;

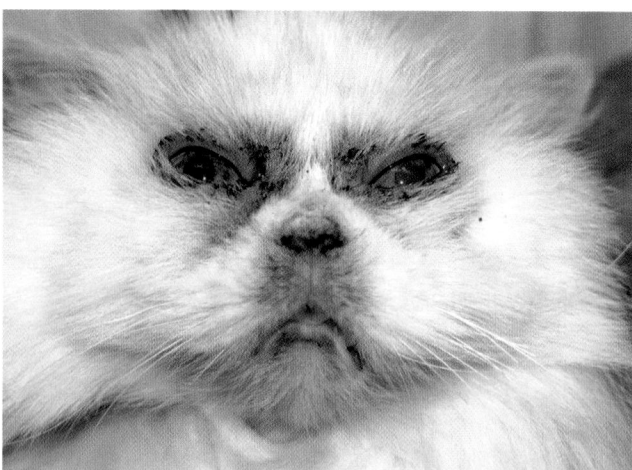

Figure 27-6: Symmetrical accumulation of dark brown to black keratosebaceous material around the eyes, lips, and chin of a Persian cat with idiopathic facial dermatitis.

erosions, ulcers, and crusts may also be seen in affected areas.[38,39] Concurrent ceruminous otitis externa is also common.[38-40] Pruritus is generally not a feature early in the disease course, but chronically affected cats may be pruritic.[38,39] With long-standing lesions, pruritus may be severe and lead to facial excoriations.[38] Secondary bacterial or *Malassezia* spp. infections are common and may contribute to pruritus development.[38,39]

The etiology of idiopathic facial dermatitis is not known. A genetic basis has been suggested given the association with the Persian and Himalayan breeds.[30,38] Workup for underlying allergic dermatitis, including strict ectoparasite control, elimination diet trials, and intradermal testing, have not been rewarding in reported cases.[38,39]

Diagnosis

Clinical features of idiopathic facial dermatitis, particularly symmetrical accumulation of dark waxy debris in the facial folds, and perioral and periocular regions, are striking. In cats presenting with evidence of facial pruritus (excoriations, erosions, or ulcers), differential diagnoses include *N. cati* or *O. cynotis* infestation, dermatophytosis, and allergic dermatitis (flea allergy dermatitis, food allergy, or atopic dermatitis). Impression smears and/or acetate tape preparations should be performed from lesional areas to assess for secondary bacterial or yeast infections. Ear swabs should be collected from cats with ceruminous otitis for cytologic evaluation and to screen for ear mites (*O. cynotis* or *D. cati*). Wood's lamp examination and fungal culture should be performed to rule out dermatophytosis as a cause of facial dermatitis.

A CBC may reveal peripheral eosinophilia in affected cats.[38] Histopathology is supportive of a diagnosis of idiopathic facial dermatitis but must be interpreted together with clinical presentation. The facial dermatosis lesion consists of an interface-type reaction (i.e., hydropic degeneration of basal keratinocytes), epidermal hyperplasia and spongiosis (often marked), neutrophil and eosinophil exocytosis, and microabscess formation.[38] The epidermis may have scattered individually shrunken and hypereosinophilic (dyskeratotic) keratinocytes. Surface crust or scale may be seen, often containing bacteria or *Malassezia* spp. yeasts. Within the dermis, perivascular to interstitial infiltrates of neutrophils, eosinophils, lymphocytes, plasma cells, and mast cells may be prominent. Sebaceous glands are often hyperplastic.[17,38,39]

Treatment

Secondary bacterial or yeast infections should be identified and treated with systemic antimicrobial therapy; treatment of secondary infections may partially alleviate clinical signs and decrease pruritus.[38,39] Antibiotic treatment should be based on bacterial culture and susceptibility in cats with an extensive antimicrobial history or a history of empiric antimicrobial treatment failure. Topical antimicrobial or antiseptic therapy may be a helpful adjunct for clearance or prevention of secondary infections if cats are amenable.[38,39] In pruritic cats, idiopathic facial dermatitis is often a diagnosis of exclusion. Although it may be strongly suspected based on the breed and clinical signs, workup for other causes of facial pruritus (strict ectoparasite control, elimination diet trials, and possible intradermal or serologic allergy testing) should be considered prior to making a final diagnosis of idiopathic facial dermatitis. Systemic corticosteroids, including oral prednisolone (1 to 3 mg/kg/day) or methylprednisolone acetate injections, have not been helpful for inducing disease remission in affected cats.[38] Topical tacrolimus 0.1% ointment applied every 12 hours to affected areas helped decrease lesion severity in one Persian cat; this cat was also bathed every 3 days with a 4% chlorhexidine shampoo for maintenance prevention of secondary infections.[39] Oral modified cyclosporine at a starting dose of 6 to 7 mg/kg/day was also reported to be effective for disease control in three Persian cats.[40] The good clinical response to cyclosporine and tacrolimus, calcineurin inhibitors with immunomodulatory activity by decreasing T cell activation, supports an immune-mediated pathogenesis of idiopathic facial dermatitis.[36,41] An underlying hypersensitivity disorder cannot be ruled out.

DEGENERATIVE MUCINOTIC MURAL FOLLICULITIS

Clinical Features

Degenerative mucinotic mural folliculitis is an idiopathic alopecic disorder documented in seven adult cats.[42] The "mural" in the disease name refers to specific targeting of inflammatory cells within the wall or outer root sheath of the hair follicle, rather than the more typical "luminal" inflammation of bacterial folliculitis. All documented cases have occurred in mixed breed rather than purebred cats (i.e., domestic longhair or shorthair cats).[42] Affected cats have progressive hair loss, often starting over the head and neck, and advancing to generalized alopecia in some cats (Figure 27-7A). Scales or crusts may also be noted in alopecic regions. Pruritus is a variable feature and can be severe and refractory.[42] The cats may develop systemic signs: lethargy, fever, weight loss, and polyarthropathy. The most striking clinical feature in all affected cats is swelling of the facial skin and narrowing of the palpebral fissures.[42] The cause of this skin thickening is currently unknown; although mucin accumulation is a typical feature of the disease, this may not be the cause of facial swelling because it is found within follicular outer root sheaths and only mild amounts may be present.[42]

The etiology of degenerative mucinotic mural folliculitis is unknown. Signs of illness (i.e., lethargy and weight loss) in some affected cats are suggestive of an underlying systemic disease.[42] As is the case for plasma cell pododermatitis, there may be a link between FIV infection and development of degenerative mucinotic mural folliculitis. In the case series reported by Gross and colleagues, three of seven cats were documented to be FIV positive.[42] All of the cats were

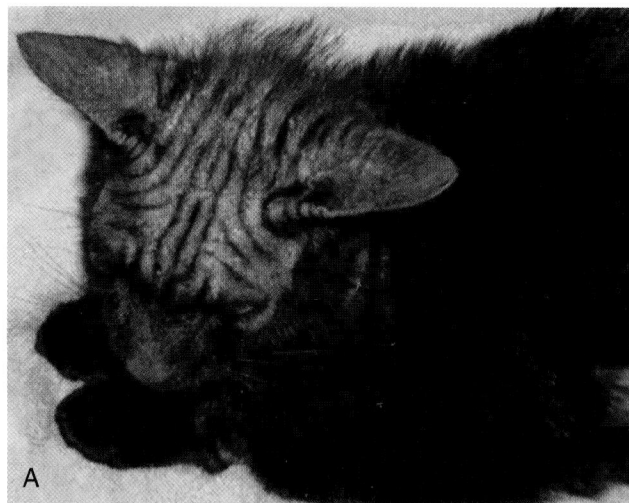

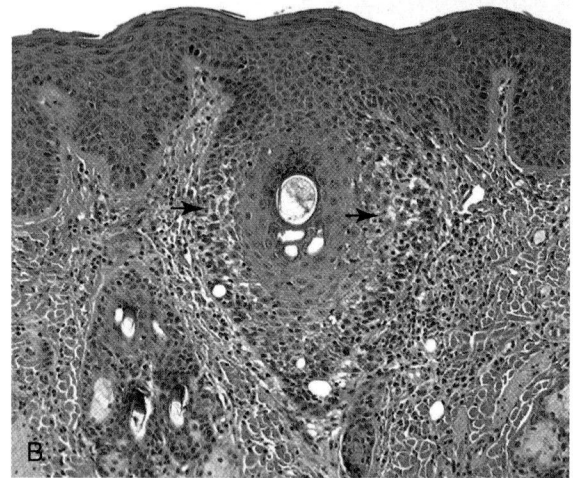

Figure 27-7: **A,** Alopecia, scale, and swelling of the skin with exaggerated folds on the head of a cat with degenerative mucinotic mural folliculitis. **B,** Photomicrograph: degenerative mucinotic mural folliculitis. Marked hyperplasia and edema/mucin *(arrows)* in hair follicle outer root sheath with lymphocyte exocytosis and loss of crisp outer root sheath/dermal distinction. (Hematoxylin and eosin, 10×)

mented in any of the cases reported by Gross and colleagues, suggesting that alopecia mucinosa may represent a distinct clinical entity or a unique variant of degenerative mucinotic mural folliculitis.[42]

Diagnosis

Differential diagnoses for alopecia secondary to degenerative mucinotic mural folliculitis in cats include dermatophytosis, demodicosis, other causes of mural folliculitis (pseudopelade, sebaceous adenitis), alopecia mucinosa, epitheliotropic cutaneous lymphoma, or paraneoplastic alopecia.[17,42] Impression smears and acetate tape preparations should be performed from areas of scale or crust to investigate for secondary bacterial or yeast infections. Deep skin scrapings should be performed to assess for *D. cati*. Wood's lamp examination and fungal culture should be performed to rule out dermatophytosis.

In cats presenting with concurrent lethargy, weight loss, or inappetence, CBC and serum chemistry analysis, as well as urinalysis, may be helpful to screen for signs of systemic illness. Consistent abnormalities have not been documented in previously reported cases of degenerative mucinotic mural folliculitis.[42] FIV testing should be pursued in all cats with suspected or confirmed mucinotic mural folliculitis.

In cats with alopecia of the head and neck, swelling of the facial skin, and narrowing of the palpebral fissures, degenerative mucinotic mural folliculitis may be strongly suspected.[17] Histopathology is necessary to confirm the diagnosis. Skin biopsy samples should be collected from the most severe areas of hair loss and skin thickening to maximize results.[17] Typical histopathologic features include infiltration of hair follicle outer root sheaths (by lymphocytes, plasma cells, macrophages, and neutrophils), follicular mucin accumulation characterized by accumulation of pale basophilic material within clear spaces between keratinocytes, and occasional neutrophilic luminal folliculitis[42] (see Figure 27-7B). Mural folliculitis may progress to complete follicular degeneration and replacement by pyogranulomas containing multinucleated giant cells.[17,42]

Treatment

No effective treatment has been identified for feline degenerative mucinotic mural folliculitis. One cat in the case series reported by Gross and colleagues had partial hair regrowth with monthly administration of a reposital injectable glucocorticoid.[42] This cat was euthanized after 5 months due to development of oral ulcers and inappetence.[42] In another report, one cat was managed for 3 years with triamcinolone and cyclosporine with resultant partial hair regrowth prior to being lost to follow-up.[20] The authors are aware of several other cases anecdotally responsive to oral cyclosporine. Use of immunosuppressive medications, such as glucocorticoids and cyclosporine, should be undertaken with caution in cats with FIV infection due to the potential for additive immunosuppression.

eventually euthanized due to worsening alopecia and lethargy (six of seven cats) or due to severe and unresponsive pruritus (one of seven cats). A full postmortem examination was performed on one cat that was FIV positive. Necropsy findings included bronchopneumonia, hepatitis, pancreatitis, and lymph node atrophy. It is unknown whether any of these findings are specific for degenerative mucinotic mural folliculitis or nonspecific findings in a 10-year-old cat with immunosuppression due to FIV infection.[42]

Although an immune-mediated basis for mucinotic mural folliculitis has been suggested, response to immunosuppressive therapy is poor.[42] Alopecia mucinosa, a disease with similar histopathologic and clinical features, was reported in two cats.[9] In both of these cats there was progression within months from follicular mucinosis to epitheliotropic cutaneous lymphoma.[9] Malignant transformation was not docu-

CUTANEOUS LYMPHOCYTOSIS (INDOLENT CUTANEOUS LYMPHOMA)

Clinical Features

Cutaneous lymphocytosis in cats is characterized by skin lesions associated with dermal lymphocyte proliferation that should be regarded as a form of indolent lymphoma.[43] The disease is seen in older cats, with a mean age of 12 years. No breed predilection has been identified. In one report of 23 cats, female cats were overrepresented.[43] Affected cats typically present with solitary or multifocal areas of alopecia, erythema, and scaling (Figure 27-8), erythematous plaques, or single or multiple cutaneous nodules. Skin lesions are frequently located on the thorax but may also be found on any region of haired skin or the nasal planum. Pruritus is a common clinical feature. Although lesions are typically slowly progressive, an acute onset may be noted.[43]

Cutaneous lymphocytosis in cats is considered to be a form of indolent cutaneous lymphoma that may disseminate late in the disease course.[43] It was initially suggested to be a possible correlate of cutaneous lymphoid hyperplasia (CLH) in humans.[43] In humans, CLH is a benign lymphoproliferative disorder that may arise in response to triggering antigens, including drugs, vaccines, tick-borne disease, insect bites or stings, or tattoos.[44] Cutaneous lymphoid hyperplasia is generally associated with dermal proliferation of polyclonal populations of B cells and admixed T cells.[44] By contrast, in cats with cutaneous lymphocytosis, lymphoid infiltrates consist mainly of CD3+ T cells and smaller numbers of admixed B cells.[43] Furthermore, PCR for the feline T cell receptor gamma has demonstrated clonality of T cells in lesions from 14 of 20 cats with cutaneous lymphocytosis, confirming a neoplastic population of lymphocytes.[45] Cutaneous lymphocytosis in cats may possibly arise in response to one or more antigenic triggers, although none have been identified at this time.[43,45]

Lymphoma can also be found in the viscera of some cats with cutaneous lymphocytosis.[43] In cats with visceral lymphoma, clinical signs of systemic disease, such as lethargy,

inappetence, and weight loss, may be noted, often a year or more after initial diagnosis.[43] Lymphoid infiltrates consist mainly of CD3+ T cells, although B cells predominated in one cat reported by Gilbert and colleagues.[43] Monoclonal populations of T cells have been further demonstrated within the internal organs and skin of three of five cats using PCR for the feline T cell receptor γ.[45] The clinical course of cutaneous lymphocytosis is long, with most cats reported to survive 1 to 2 years following diagnosis.[43]

Diagnosis

Due to the variable clinical presentation of cutaneous lymphocytosis in cats, there are multiple possible differential diagnoses for skin lesions. In cats presenting with focal or multifocal areas of erythema, alopecia, and scale, differentials include dermatophytosis, demodicosis, cheyletiellosis, secondary superficial pyoderma or *Malassezia* dermatitis, epitheliotropic cutaneous lymphoma, or allergic dermatitis (flea allergy dermatitis, food allergy, atopic dermatitis). In cats presenting with erythematous plaques or nodules (with or without surface ulcers or crusts), differentials include eosinophilic plaques or granulomas, viral plaques, or neoplastic diseases (mast cell tumors, squamous cell carcinoma or bowenoid carcinoma *in situ*, nonepitheliotropic or epitheliotropic cutaneous lymphoma). Recommended initial diagnostic tests include impression smears or acetate tape preparations to assess for secondary bacterial or yeast infection, deep and superficial skin scrapings to assess for surface mites or *D. cati*, and Wood's lamp examination and fungal culture to rule out dermatophytosis.

Complete blood counts and serum chemistry panels are generally not helpful in diagnosis of cutaneous lymphocytosis. Routine bloodwork and urinalysis should be considered in cats with lethargy, inappetence, or weight loss to screen for signs of systemic disease. A CBC may reveal leukocytosis and lymphocytosis in affected cats.[43] Infection with feline leukemia virus (FeLV) or FIV has not been documented in cats with cutaneous lymphocytosis.[43]

Histopathology is required for diagnosis of cutaneous lymphocytosis. Typical histopathologic features include a diffuse to nodular infiltrate of small lymphocytes within the superficial to deep dermis (Figure 27-9A). Small numbers of lymphocytes may infiltrate the epidermis and hair follicle epithelia, but epitheliotropism is not a common feature. Mitotic figures are usually rare to absent (see Figure 27-9B). Immunohistochemistry reveals a predominantly CD3+ T cell population with small aggregates of CD79a+ B cells.[17,43] The major distinguishing features of cutaneous lymphocytosis from "typical" nonepitheliotropic cutaneous T cell lymphoma are the uniform population of small lymphocytes, the relative lack of mitoses, and the less-pronounced cellular pleomorphism in the former as compared with the latter.[17,43]

In cats diagnosed with cutaneous lymphocytosis, particularly those with clinical signs suggestive of systemic disease, workup for internal organ involvement should be considered.[43] This workup may include imaging (radiography,

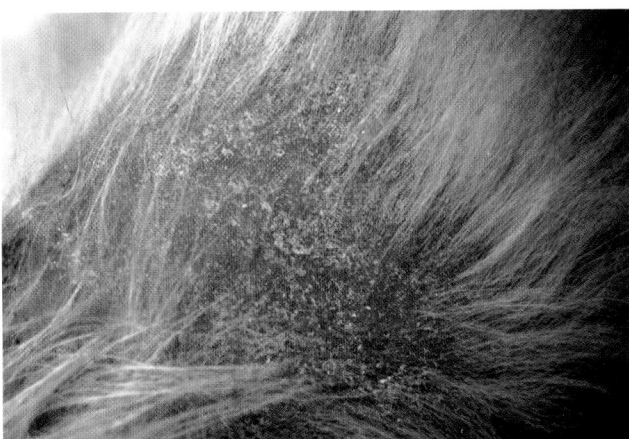

Figure 27-8: Focal area of alopecia, erythema, and scale on the flank of a cat with cutaneous lymphocytosis.

ultrasound) of the thoracic and abdominal cavities as well as fine-needle aspirate or biopsy of internal organs with ultrasonographic abnormalities for cytologic or histopathologic evaluation.

Treatment

No uniformly effective treatment of cutaneous lymphocytosis has been described. Skin lesions have been reported to wax and wane or to spontaneously regress in some affected cats.[43] Recurrence of lesions after several weeks has been reported following spontaneous resolution. Surgical resection of solitary skin lesions has also been described, though lesions may recur after surgery in the same or distant sites.[43] Most reported cases have been treated with topical or systemic glucocorticoids (administered orally or by repositol injection); response to glucocorticoid therapy is variable with some cats showing a complete response and others no response.[43] Some cats with cutaneous lymphocytosis have also been treated with glucocorticoids in combination with

an alkylating agent. Lomustine (CCNU) and chlorambucil were administered in combination with glucocorticoids in five cats reported by Gilbert and colleagues; three of these cats showed complete lesion resolution, one showed partial lesion resolution, and one cat had no response to treatment.[43]

FELINE PROGRESSIVE HISTIOCYTOSIS

Clinical Features

Feline progressive histiocytosis (FPH), regarded as an indolent form of malignant histiocytic neoplasia, is characterized by focal or more commonly multifocal cutaneous papules and nodules (Figure 27-10). Lesions are most frequently located on the head and extremities, though any portion of the haired skin, nasal planum, lips, or pinnae may be involved.[46] Early in the disease course, lesions are usually alopecic but nonpainful and nonpruritic. Ulceration and secondary bacterial infection, with resultant pain or pruritus, may occur as lesions progress.[46] No breed or age predilections have been identified. In one report of 30 cases, female cats were overrepresented.[46]

Feline progressive histiocytosis was initially described as multiple cutaneous histiocytomas in a case report of a 15-year-old domestic longhair cat by Day and colleagues. In contrast to the typical behavior of cutaneous histiocytomas in dogs, this cat's cutaneous nodules did not spontaneously regress and continued to progress despite medical therapy and surgical excision.[47] The histiocytic origin of the round cell infiltrate in affected cats has been demonstrated by immunohistochemistry. The cells stain positively for the integrin subunit CD18 but negatively for T cell (CD3+) and B cell (CD79a) markers, confirming a population of histiocytes.[46-48] Furthermore the histiocytes show positive staining for major histocompatibility complex II as well as CD1a and CD1c (proteins involved in antigen presentation), which further categorizes the cells into a dendritic cell

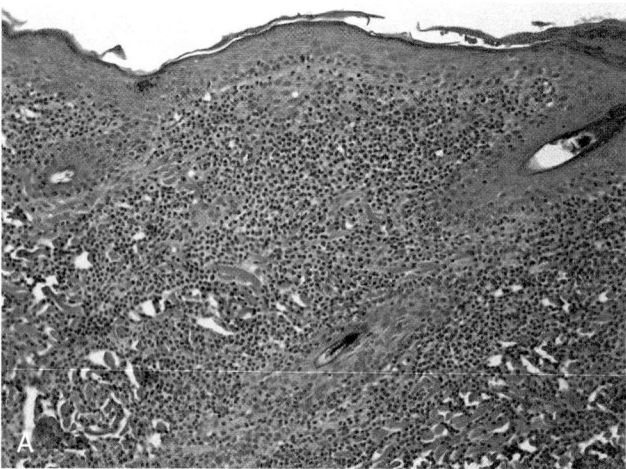
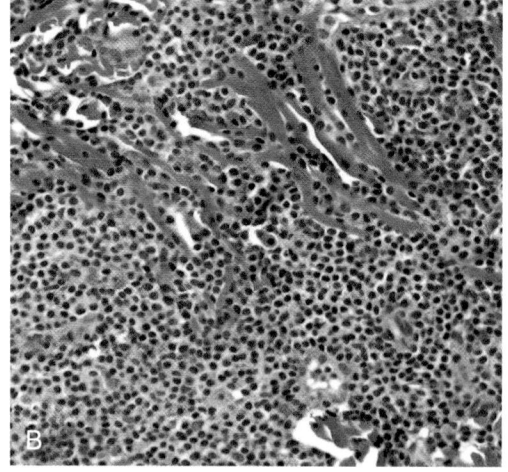

Figure 27-9: Photomicrograph: Cutaneous Lymphocytosis. A, The dermis is infiltrated by sheets of small lymphocytes with few mast cells and plasma cells. (Hematoxylin and eosin [H&E], 4×) **B,** The lymphocytes have small heterochromatic nuclei and mitoses are not evident. (H&E, 20×)

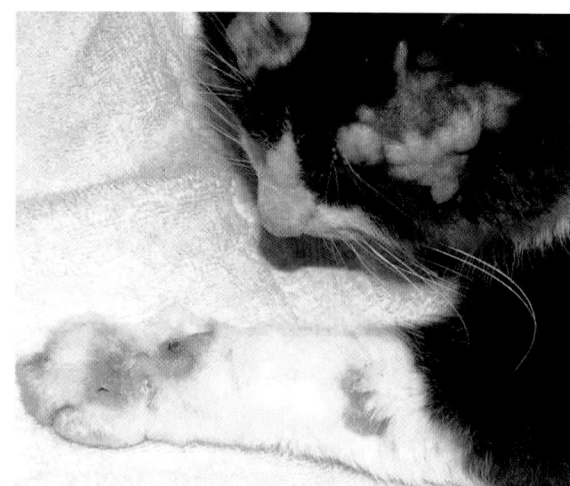

Figure 27-10: Coalescing alopecic and eroded nodules on the head and forelimb of a cat with feline progressive histiocytosis.

lineage.[46] Most biopsy samples from affected cats have stained negatively for E-cadherin, an adhesion protein expressed by Langerhans cells.[46] By contrast, canine histiocytomas express E-cadherin, consistent with Langerhans cell origin.[17,46,47] It is unclear if the dendritic cells in FPH arise from epidermal Langerhans cells with downregulated expression of E-cadherin or from dermal dendritic cells.[46]

Feline progressive histiocytosis may have a protracted clinical course. In the 30 cases reported by Affolter and Moore, the average survival time was over 1 year, with some cats surviving up to 3 years following diagnosis.[46] With time, systemic involvement may occur. Cats with internal disease may present with weight loss, lethargy, inappetence, dyspnea, or lymph node enlargement. On necropsy, effacement of internal organs, including the lungs, lymph nodes, liver, spleen, and pancreas, by masses of round cells may be found.[46] Like cutaneous lymphocytosis, FPH is best classified as an indolent cutaneous neoplasm with the potential for systemic dissemination late in the disease course.[46,48] Due to its more aggressive clinical behavior, as well as the unidentified dendritic cell origin of the neoplastic histiocytes, FPH is now considered to be a distinct entity from multiple cutaneous histiocytomas.

Diagnosis

Because most affected cats present with intradermal nodules, other neoplastic diseases, such as epitheliotropic or nonepitheliotropic cutaneous lymphoma, cutaneous lymphocytosis, cutaneous mast cell tumors, basal cell tumors, melanomas, or plasma cell tumors, are the primary differential diagnoses for FPH.[48]

Cytologic evaluation of fine-needle aspirates from cutaneous nodules may reveal histiocytes, but histopathology is required for definitive diagnosis. Typical histopathologic features include a nodular to diffuse dermal cellular infiltrate (Figure 27-11A) composed of round cells with ovoid to round or reniform ("bean-shaped") nuclei and a moderate amount of lightly eosinophilic cytoplasm, morphologically consistent with histiocytes[17,46,48] (see Figure 27-11B). Infiltration of the epidermis (epitheliotropism) by histiocytes may be observed.[17,46,48] Mild cellular pleomorphism and a low number of mitotic figures may be seen early in the disease course.[46] Sampling of later skin lesions or infiltrated internal organs may reveal a higher number of mitotic figures or bizarre mitoses, marked anisocytosis and anisokaryosis, or multinucleated giant cells. Later or disseminated lesions of FPH cannot be distinguished histopathologically from histiocytic sarcoma.[46,48]

In cats diagnosed with FPH, particularly those with clinical signs suggestive of systemic disease, a workup for internal organ involvement should be considered. This workup may include imaging (radiography, ultrasound) of the thoracic and abdominal cavities as well as fine-needle aspirate or biopsy of internal organs with ultrasonographic abnormalities or enlarged lymph nodes for cytologic or histopathologic evaluation.

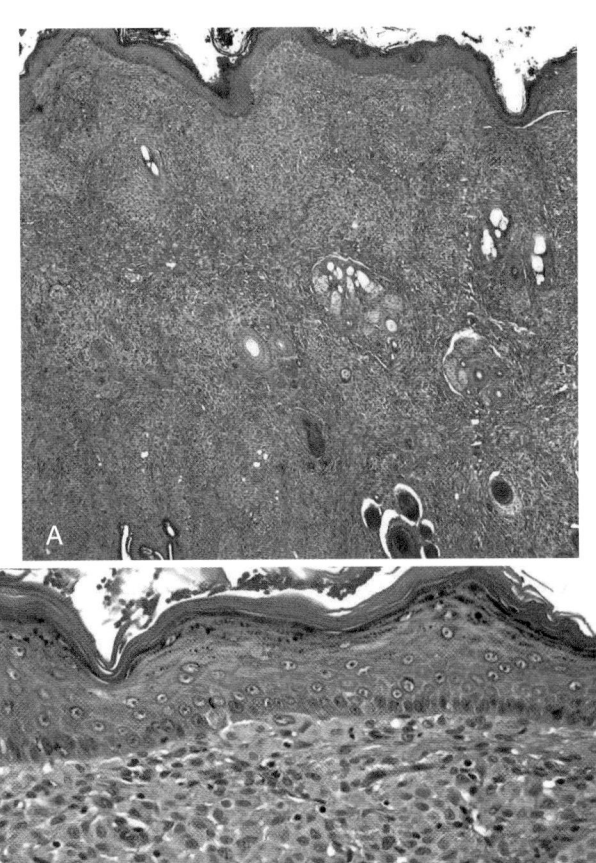

Figure 27-11: Photomicrograph: Feline Progressive Histiocytosis. A, The entire dermis is infiltrated by sheets of histiocytoid round cells. (Hematoxylin and eosin [H&E], 4×) **B,** The infiltrate abuts the epidermis. The cells have large ovoid to reniform nuclei and abundant lightly staining eosinophilic cytoplasm. (H&E, 20×)

Treatment

No effective treatment for FPH has been identified. Surgical resection of solitary lesions is generally not successful due to lesion recurrence locally or distant from the original site.[46,47] Immunomodulatory or immunosuppressive medications, including chemotherapeutics, glucocorticoids, cyclosporine, and leflunomide, have not been reported to be helpful to prevent progression of skin lesions or dissemination of disease.[46] Antibiotic therapy and analgesics may be temporarily helpful for managing secondary bacterial infection of the skin or discomfort associated with ulcerated lesions, respectively. Euthanasia is often elected in cats with progressive skin lesions or systemic signs, such as lethargy, inappetence, weight loss, or anemia, associated with internal disease spread.[46]

References

1. Scott DW: Feline dermatology 1979–82: introspective retrospections. *J Am Anim Hosp Assoc* 20:537–564, 1984.

2. Bettenay SV, Mueller RS, Dow K, et al: Prospective study of the treatment of feline plasmacytic pododermatitis with doxycycline. *Vet Record* 152:564–566, 2003.

3. Pereira PD, Faustino AMR: Feline plasma cell pododermatitis: a study of 8 cases. *Vet Dermatol* 14:333–337, 2003.

4. Drolet R, Bernard J: Plasma cell pododermatitis in a cat. *Can Vet J* 25:448–449, 1984.

5. Scarampella F, Ordeix L: Doxycycline therapy in 10 cases of feline plasma cell pododermatitis: clinical, haematological, and serological evaluations. *Vet Dermatol* 15(Suppl 1):27, 2004. (Abstract).

6. Guaguere E, Prelaud P, Degorce-Rubiales F, et al: Feline plasma cell pododermatitis: a retrospective study of 26 cases. *Vet Dermatol* 15(Suppl 1):27, 2004. (Abstract).

7. Guaguere E, Hubert B, Delabre C: Feline pododermatoses. *Vet Dermatol* 3:1–12, 1992.

8. Taylor JE, Schmeitzel LP: Plasma cell pododermatitis with chronic footpad hemorrhage in two cats. *J Am Vet Med Assoc* 197:375–377, 1990.

9. Scott DW: Feline dermatology 1983-85: 'The secret sits.' *J Am Anim Hosp Assoc* 23:255–274, 1987.

10. De Man M: What is your diagnosis? *J Feline Med Surg* 5:245–247, 2003.

11. Declercq J, De Man M: Swelling of the nose in three cats with plasmacytic pododermatitis. *Vlaams Diergeneeskundig Tijdschrift* 71:277–281, 2002.

12. Declercq J, De Bosschere H: Nasal swelling due to plasma cell infiltrate in a cat without plasma cell pododermatitis. *Vet Dermatol* 21:412–414, 2010.

13. Bensignor E, Merven F: Nasal plasma cell dermatitis in cats [letter to the editor]. *Vet Dermatol* 22:286, 2011.

14. Bettenay SV, Lappin MR, Mueller RS: An immunohistochemical and polymerase chain reaction evaluation of feline plasmacytic pododermatitis. *Vet Pathol* 44:80–83, 2007.

15. Simon M, Horvath C, Pauley D, et al: Plasma cell pododermatitis in feline immunodeficiency virus-infected cats. *Vet Pathol* 30:477, 1993.

16. Medleau L, Kaswan RL, Lorenz MD, et al: Ulcerative pododermatitis in a cat: immunofluorescent findings and response to chrysotherapy. *J Am Anim Hosp Assoc* 18:449–451, 1982.

17. Gross TL, Ihrke PJ, Walder EJ, et al: *Skin diseases of the dog and cat*, ed 2, Ames, IA, 2005, Blackwell Science.

18. German AJ, Cannon MJ, Dye C, et al: Oesophageal strictures in cats associated with doxycycline therapy. *J Feline Med Surg* 7:33–41, 2005.

19. Yamamura Y: A surgically treated case of feline plasma cell pododermatitis. *J Japanese Vet Med Assoc* 51:669–671, 1998.

20. Miller WH, Griffin CE, Campbell KL: *Muller & Kirk's small animal dermatology*, ed 7, St Louis, 2013, Elsevier, p 570, 718–719.

21. Vercelli A, Raviri G, Cornegliani L: The use of cyclosporine to treat feline dermatoses: a retrospective analysis of 23 cases. *Vet Dermatol* 17:201–206, 2006.

22. Vitale CB, Ihrke PJ, Olivry T, et al: Feline urticarial pigmentosa in three related Sphinx cats. *Vet Dermatol* 7:227–233, 1996.

23. Noli C, Colombo S, Abramos F, et al: Papular eosinophilic/mastocytic dermatitis (feline urticarial pigmentosa) in Devon Rex cats: a distinct disease entity or a histopathological reaction pattern? *Vet Dermatol* 15:253–259, 2004.

24. Colombo S, Scarampella F, Ordeix L, et al: Dermatophytosis and papular eosinophilic/mastocytic dermatitis (urticaria pigmentosa-like dermatitis) in three Devon Rex cats. *J Feline Med Surg* 14:498–502, 2012.

25. Lipinski MJ, Froenicke L, Baysac KC, et al: The ascent of cat breeds: genetic evaluations of breeds and worldwide random-bred populations. *Genomics* 91:12–21, 2008.

26. Fried AJ, Akin C: Primary mast cell disorders in children. *Curr Allergy Asthma Rep* 13:693–701, 2013.

27. Guagere E, Fontaine J: Efficacy of cyclosporine in the treatment of feline urticarial pigmentosa: two cases. *Vet Dermatol* 15(Suppl 1):63, 2004.

28. Scott DW: An unusual ulcerative dermatitis associated with linear subepidermal fibrosis in eight cats. *Feline Pract* 18:8–11, 1990.

29. Spaterna A, Mechelli L, Rueca F, et al: Feline idiopathic ulcerative dermatosis: three cases. *Vet Res Commun* 27(Suppl 1):795–798, 2003.

30. Power HT: Newly recognized feline skin diseases. In *14th Proceedings. AAVD & ACVD Annual Members Meeting*, 1998, pp 27–32.

31. Mauldin EA, Ness TA, Goldschmidt MH: Proliferative and necrotizing otitis externa in four cats. *Vet Dermatol* 18:370–377, 2007.

32. Stevens BJ, Linder KE: Pathology in practice. *J Am Vet Med Assoc* 241:567–569, 2012.

33. Videmont E, Pin D: Proliferative and necrotising otitis in a kitten: first demonstration of T-cell-mediated apoptosis. *J Small Anim Pract* 51:599–603, 2010.

34. Borio S, Massari F, Abramo F, et al: Proliferative and necrotising otitis externa in a cat without pinnal involvement: video-otoscopic features. *J Feline Med Surg* 15:353–356, 2013.

35. Halliwell REW: Autoimmune and immune-mediated dermatoses. In Miller WH, Griffen CE, Campbell KL, editors: *Muller & Kirk's small animal dermatology*, ed 7, St Louis, 2013, Elsevier, p 473.

36. Carr WW: Topical calcineurin inhibitors for atopic dermatitis: review and treatment recommendations. *Pediatr Drugs* 15:303–310, 2013.

37. Trautmann A, Akdis M, Schmid-Grendelmeier P, et al: Targeting keratinocyte apoptosis in the treatment of atopic dermatitis and allergic contact dermatitis. *J Allergy Clin Immunol* 108:839–846, 2001.

38. Bond R, Curtis CF, Ferguson EA, et al: An idiopathic facial dermatitis of Persian cats. *Vet Dermatol* 11:35–41, 2000.

39. Chung TH, Ryu MH, Kim DY, et al: Topical tacrolimus (FK506) for the treatment of feline idiopathic facial dermatitis. *Aust Vet J* 87:417–420, 2009.

40. Fontaine J, Heimann M: Idiopathic facial dermatitis of the Persian cat: three cases controlled with cyclosporine. *Vet Dermatol* 15(Suppl 1):64, 2004.

41. Palmeiro BS: Cyclosporine in veterinary dermatology. *Vet Clin Small Anim* 43:153–171, 2013.

42. Gross TL, Olivry T, Vitale CB, et al: Degenerative mucinotic mural folliculitis in cats. *Vet Dermatol* 12:279–283, 2001.

43. Gilbert S, Affolter VK, Gross TL, et al: Clinical, morphological and immunohistochemical characterization of cutaneous lymphocytosis in 23 cats. *Vet Dermatol* 15:3–12, 2004.

44. Nihal M, Mikkola D, Horvath N, et al: Cutaneous lymphoid hyperplasia: a lymphoproliferative continuum with lymphomatous potential. *Hum Pathol* 34:617–622, 2003.

45. Gilbert S, Affolter VK, Schmidt P, et al: Clonality studies of feline cutaneous lymphocytosis. *Vet Dermatol* 15(Suppl 1):24, 2004.

46. Affolter VK, Moore PF: Feline progressive histiocytosis. *Vet Pathol* 43:646–655, 2006.

47. Day MJ, Lopatkin I, Lucke VM, et al: Multiple cutaneous histiocytomas in a cat. *Vet Dermatol* 11:305–310, 2000.

48. Gelberg HB: Diagnostic exercise: multiple skin nodules in a cat. *Vet Pathol* 50:569–571, 2013.

Feline Food Allergy

Jill L. Abraham

Food allergy or food hypersensitivity is an immune-mediated type of adverse food reaction that is a common differential diagnosis in cats with nonseasonal pruritus, various cutaneous lesions, and/or gastrointestinal (GI) symptoms. The most commonly reported food allergens in cats are beef, dairy products, and fish. While the exact incidence is unknown, food allergy may account for 1% to 6% of all feline dermatoses and 11% of cases of miliary dermatitis. Although there are no pathognomonic clinical signs for food allergy in cats, pruritus is the most commonly reported clinical sign and may be nonresponsive to systemic glucocorticoid therapy. Up to 30% of cats with food allergy may have a concurrent hypersensitivity disorder. Confirming or refuting the presence of food allergy in cats is challenging, as the only accurate means of diagnosis is to institute a strict elimination dietary trial followed by a provocative dietary challenge. Despite these difficulties, cats with food allergy often have a very good long-term prognosis through avoidance of the causative food allergen(s).

PATHOGENESIS

"Adverse food reaction" is a broad term that signifies a link between the ingestion of an otherwise harmless dietary component and a clinically abnormal response. This term encompasses both immunologic and nonimmunologic reactions. Food allergy (food hypersensitivity) describes an immune-mediated process. Food intolerance describes nonimmune-mediated reactions and includes food idiosyncrasy, food toxicity and food poisoning, anaphylactic food reaction, and pharmacologic and metabolic food reactions (Figure 28-1).

Food idiosyncrasy is an abnormal response to a food component or additive that involves nonimmune mechanisms but resembles food allergy. A food idiosyncrasy is responsible for most reactions to food additives and can occur on the first exposure to a substance. Food intoxication and food poisoning are caused by the presence of infection or toxins in foods, such as *Salmonella* species or botulism. An anaphylactoid food reaction is not immune-mediated but resembles true anaphylaxis. Ingesting large amounts of histamine (i.e., from spoiled tuna) can cause an anaphylactoid reaction. A metabolic food reaction involves a reaction of the host's metabolism after ingestion of a particular food; lactose intolerance is one example.[1,2]

A key role of the GI tract is to differentiate between nutrients, which have to be tolerated, and potentially harmful substances such as bacteria, viruses, and parasites, which have to be expelled. There are four mechanisms that are essential for both the tolerance and exclusion of antigens: the mucosal barrier, elimination of antigens, regulation of the immune response, and tolerance of antigens reaching the mucosa. Disruption of these defense mechanisms predisposes patients to developing food allergy. Various immunologic and nonimmunologic factors contribute to the integrity of the mucosal barrier, including the morphology and functionality of the enterocytes, the presence of immunoglobulin A (IgA), the presence of inflammation, the quality and composition of the food, and effective digestion.[2,3]

Even when defense mechanisms are intact and fully functional, the mucosal barrier is not entirely impervious to macromolecules. Food proteins can cross an intact intestinal mucosa in small but significant amounts, which can result in the formation of immune complexes. Antigens that pass through the lamina propria are removed by the mononuclear-macrophage phagocyte (reticuloendothelial) system of the liver and mesenteric lymph nodes. In some situations oral tolerance to the absorbed protein is maintained, but in other situations hypersensitivity develops.[2,3]

The body is exposed to huge quantities of food antigens and must remain unresponsive to these antigens. Oral tolerance is the state of both local and systemic immune unresponsiveness that is induced by exposure to antigens such as food proteins.[4] Oral tolerance develops at a young age and involves T cell suppressor activity, anergy, and cell deletion. The basis of this phenomenon is the suppressor function of the gut-associated lymphoid tissue (GALT). Four distinct lymphoid compartments compose GALT:

- Peyer's patches, which contain specialized antigen-presenting epithelial cells called M cells, and aggregates of lymphoid follicles throughout the intestinal mucosa
- Lymphocytes and plasma cells scattered throughout the lamina propria
- Intraepithelial lymphocytes interlaced between enterocytes
- Mesenteric lymph nodes

In the GI tract of patients with food allergy, an antigen-specific immune reaction occurs and leads to the formation of immunoglobulin (Ig) M (IgM), IgG, or IgE.[2,3]

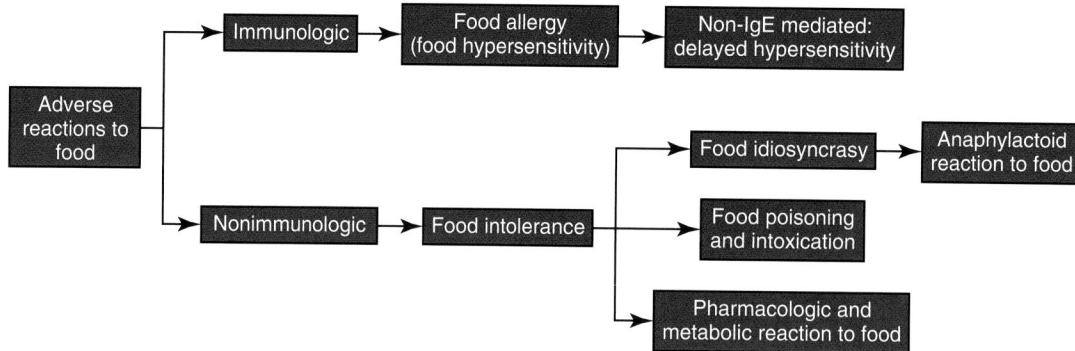

Figure 28-1: Categories of Adverse Reactions to Food. (Adapted from Verlinden A, Hesta M, Millet S, et al: Food allergy in dogs and cats: a review. *Crit Rev Food Sci Nutr* 46:259-273, 2006; and Roudebush P, Guilford WG, Jackson HA: Adverse reactions to food. In Hand MS, Thatcher CD, Remillard RL, et al., editors: *Small animal clinical nutrition*, ed 5, Topeka, KS, 2010, Mark Morris Institute, pp 609-627.)

Studies detailing the etiopathogenesis of food hypersensitivity in cats are lacking, so information is often extrapolated from either human or canine data. The specific immunologic mechanisms behind food allergy have not been fully elucidated, but type I, III, and IV hypersensitivity reactions are thought to be involved.[2,3]

FOOD ALLERGENS

The major food allergens identified in people are almost always water-soluble glycoproteins that range in molecular weight from 10 to 70 kDa. They are typically stable when treated with heat, acid, and proteases.[5,6] In cats, the most commonly reported food allergens are beef, dairy products, and fish. These proteins account for nearly 90% of the cases documented in 10 different studies.[7] Chicken, lamb, pork, rabbit, egg, corn, wheat, and clam juice have also been implicated as food allergens in cats.[2,7-9] There are reports of multiple food sensitivities in cats with cutaneous signs,[10] and one report of a cat previously diagnosed with a fish hypersensitivity that developed a lamb hypersensitivity after being fed an exclusive lamb diet for 2 years.[9] In a study of cats with chronic GI symptoms, 50% of cats with food allergy were allergic to more than one ingredient.[11] Nonprotein allergens may include fungi, preservatives, and colorings,[12] but there are only two confirmed feline cases of sensitivity to food additives.[8,11]

CLINICAL FEATURES

Incidence

While several studies report the incidence of food allergies as 1% to 6% of all dermatoses in cats,[10,13,14] the exact incidence is unknown. Food allergy may account for 11% of cases of miliary dermatitis.[10] In one prospective study, 17% of cats with chronic pruritus, chronic vomiting, chronic diarrhea, or concomitant pruritus and vomiting and/or diarrhea were diagnosed with food allergy.[8] There are various explanations why the exact incidence is difficult to establish. Food allergy can be a difficult diagnosis to confirm, as dietary elimination trials are the only reliable method of diagnosis, and up to 30% of cats with food allergies may have concurrent flea bite hypersensitivity and/or atopy.[15,16] There may be geographic differences among study populations and variations in criteria among studies, and there have been a variety of eliminations diets used in different studies.

Clinical Signs

There is no confirmed breed or sex predilection for food allergy in cats,[15] but a higher risk for Siamese and Siamese crosses has been noted.[13,16] The age of onset ranges from 3 months to 11 years, with a mean of 4 to 5 years reported.[10,15,17,18] There is no established connection between the onset of clinical signs and a recent change in diet,[13,15] and in many cases the food to which the cat was proven allergic had been fed for over 2 years.[9,15] This has led to the thought that a long period of sensitization is involved, but in one study, 38.5% of cases developed clinical symptoms before 2 years of age.[17] Furthermore, cases have been noted to occur in cats less than 1 year of age.[12,13,18] The clinical signs of food allergies are typically nonseasonal. They consist primarily of dermatologic and/or GI symptoms, but food allergies have been reported to affect other organ systems.[2,11]

Dermatologic Signs

The most commonly encountered clinical sign is pruritus, which was reported as present in 100% of cats with food allergy in more than one study.[13,15,16] Pruritus may be localized or generalized, but in one study 42% of cats with food allergy had pruritus localized primarily to the head, neck, or ear region,[15] and in another study 100% of cats with confirmed food allergy had pruritus of the head and neck.[19] Although the degree of pruritus can vary from cat to cat, some cats will experience intense pruritus that leads to severe self-trauma. In an individual cat, the degree of pruritus may be fairly constant from day to day,[20] and treatment with systemic glucocorticoids may or may not reduce pruritus

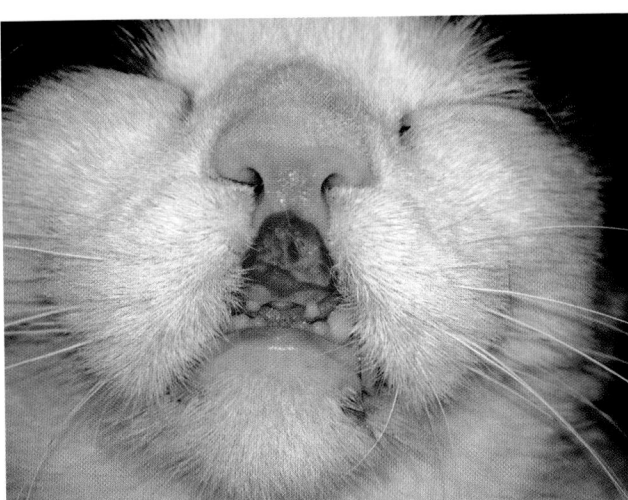

Figure 28-2: Feline indolent ulcer with secondary bacterial infection in an 8-year-old cat with cutaneous adverse food reactions confirmed to codfish, chicken, and duck.

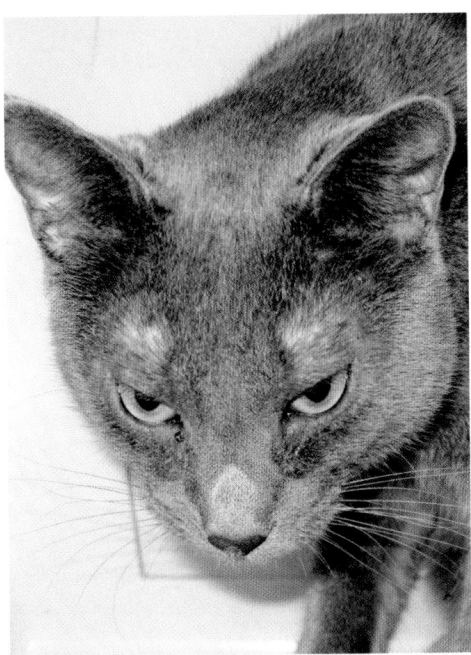

Figure 28-3: Moderate to severe erythema on the face, head, and the concave surfaces of the pinnae in a 4-year-old cat with cutaneous adverse food reaction.

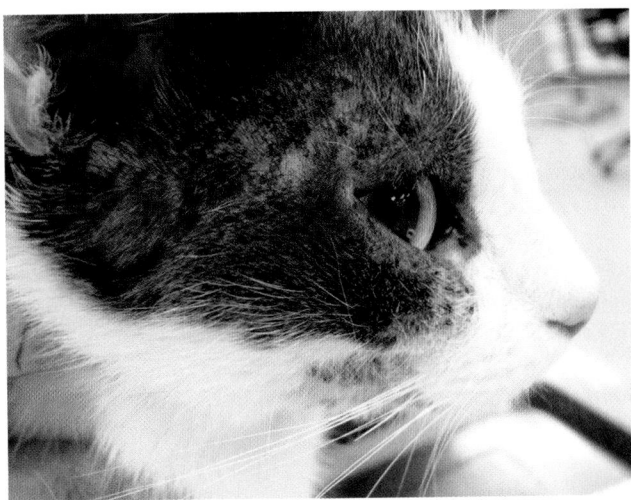

Figure 28-4: Partial alopecia, mild erythema, excoriations, and crusts on the face and head of a 1½-year-old cat with cutaneous adverse food reaction and concomitant atopy.

associated with food allergy. In three separate studies, 10 out of 10, four out of 14, and four out of 11 cats with confirmed food allergy had either no response or only a partial response to systemic glucocorticoid therapy.[13,16,21]

Primary lesions such as erythema, maculae, and papules may be seen. Cats may present with one or more of the following reactions patterns: miliary dermatitis, self-induced or symmetric alopecia, facial or neck dermatitis, eosinophilic plaques, granulomas, or indolent ulcers; or exfoliative dermatitis.[9,12-15,22,23] Figure 28-2 is an example of a cat with an indolent ulcer caused by food allergies. In a case series published in 2006 investigating possible medical causes of presumed "psychogenic alopecia" in 21 cats, 57% were confirmed to have an adverse food reaction.[24] Although there are no specific clinical signs that are pathognomonic for an individual hypersensitivity disorder of nonflea origin,[14,23,25] a multicenter study of cats with various hypersensitivity disorders found that cats with food allergies were presented more often with lesions affecting the head, face, and neck than cats with other types of hypersensitivity disorders.[25] Figure 28-3 represents a cat with erythema on the head, face, and pinnae secondary to food allergy, and Figure 28-4 demonstrates a cat with erythema and other cutaneous lesions of the head and face secondary to both food allergy and atopy. Otitis externa and/or aural pruritus may occur in conjunction with more generalized pruritus and cutaneous lesions or may be the sole clinical sign(s) seen.

Other dermatologic signs, such as chin acne, vasculitis, angioedema, urticaria, and plasma cell pododermatitis, have been associated rarely to uncommonly with food allergies in cats.[12,20]

Gastrointestinal Signs

Gastrointestinal signs may occur concurrently with dermatologic signs in 10% to 23% of cats with food allergies.[8,13] Signs may include weight loss, vomiting, diarrhea, abdominal pain, flatulence, and inflammatory bowel disease, including lymphocytic-plasmacytic colitis.[11,13,15,22] Large bowel diarrhea may be observed more commonly than small bowel diarrhea.[11] While not pathognomonic, the simultaneous occurrence of dermatologic and GI signs appears to be the clinical feature most suggestive of food allergy in cats.[11]

Other Clinical Signs

Rarely rhinitis, conjunctivitis, bronchoconstriction, seizures, lower urinary tract disease, glomerulonephritis, lethargy, and behavior changes have been associated with food allergies in cats.[2,11] Lymphadenopathy has been reported in approximately 30% of cats with food allergies.[2,10] There are no specific hematologic or serum biochemical markers or changes specific to food allergies, but a peripheral eosinophilia can be seen in 20% to 50% of cases.[2,11,26]

Histopathology Findings

Skin biopsies are not diagnostic for food allergies in cats but can be helpful in ruling out other diseases with similar clinical presentations. Histopathology findings often vary with the specific clinical lesions that are sampled. One common reaction pattern is superficial perivascular inflammation with primarily eosinophils and/or mast cells, although lymphocytes and histiocytes may also be seen. Rarely, cases involving large numbers of mast cells infiltrating the superficial and middle dermis have been confused with mast cell neoplasia.[10,27] In one study, an infiltrative lymphocytic mural folliculitis was identified in the majority of skin biopsies from cats with food allergies.[28] The presence and number of neutrophils may depend on the degree of self-trauma or on the presence of pyoderma. Biopsies from lesions of the eosinophilic granuloma complex often show histopathological changes typical for those lesions (see Chapter 32). Eosinophilic folliculitis and furunculosis, and extension of perivascular inflammation into the deep dermis and upper layers of the panniculus—particularly in lesions confined to the head and neck—are also patterns suggestive of food allergy in cats.[10,27] However, there are documented cases of self-induced alopecia caused by food allergy that did not show any histopathologic abnormalities.[24]

DIFFERENTIAL DIAGNOSES

Given the variety of symptoms that may be seen in cats with food allergy, there are numerous potential differential diagnoses (Table 28-1). A detailed history and careful evaluation of the specific dermatologic findings aid in organizing which differentials are more likely in an individual cat.

DIAGNOSIS

Diagnosing food allergies in cats can prove quite challenging. Unfortunately there are no specific clinical or laboratory tests currently available that are able to accurately confirm or refute the presence of a food allergy. Serum testing for food allergen-specific IgE is commercially available, but multiple studies demonstrate low specificity or sensitivity.[11,29-32] Intradermal allergen testing, salivary allergen-specific antibody testing, and gastroscopy testing have been shown to be inaccurate as well.[11,33] While patch testing for food allergens has been performed in dogs (with a negative predictive value of 99.3% and a positive predictive value of 63.0%),[34] to the author's knowledge there are no published studies of patch testing for food allergies in cats.

A diagnosis of food allergy is made based on the history, dermatologic examination findings, and response to an

Table 28-1	**Examples of More Commonly Encountered Differential Diagnoses for Food Allergy**
Category	**Differential Diagnoses**
Ectoparasites	Fleas *Cheyletiella* spp. Demodicosis *Notoedres* *Otodectes* Reaction to tick bites
Immune-mediated diseases	Atopy Flea bite hypersensitivity Mosquito bite hypersensitivity Contact hypersensitivity Pemphigus foliaceus Erythema multiforme Cutaneous adverse drug reaction
Infections	Staphylococcal pyoderma *Malassezia* dermatitis Dermatophytosis Herpesvirus Calicivirus Poxvirus Cryptococcus
Neoplasia	Mast cell neoplasia Squamous cell carcinoma Cutaneous lymphoma Basal cell tumor
Other	Trauma or bite wound Foreign body Behavioral/"psychogenic" Idiopathic facial dermatitis of Persian cats

elimination dietary trial and provocative dietary challenge. The "gold standard" diagnostic approach is to feed a strict novel protein or hydrolyzed diet until significant improvement or resolution of clinical signs is noted, and then reintroduce previously fed foods and monitor for worsening or recurrence of clinical signs. The success of this test relies greatly on diet selection, the duration of the diet trial, and owner and patient compliance. As there is nothing inherently hypoallergenic about any particular protein,[2] it is necessary to obtain a thorough dietary history in order to select the best elimination diet for an individual cat. The diet history should include the main diet fed as well as any treats or table food, flavored medications, and possible access to foods given to other pets in the household.

Elimination Diet Options

There are three categories of elimination diets: commercial novel protein diets, home-cooked novel protein diets, and hydrolyzed diets.

Commercial Novel Protein Diets

There are several "novel" protein sources that can be considered for use in an elimination diet. Examples include venison, duck, lamb, rabbit, goat, lobster, kangaroo, pork, and ostrich, and potentially fish for cats that have not previously eaten fish.[2,12,35] Meat from species that have close taxonomic relationships to the triggering food may have a greater risk of cross-reactivity, so the selection of a novel protein must be based on the diet history. For example, the presence of common allergens in avian meat sources such as chicken, turkey, dove, and quail has been demonstrated.[36] Even though this has not been studied specifically in cats, it is advisable to avoid using duck in an elimination diet in cats previously exposed to chicken.[35] In cats, green peas are a common carbohydrate source used in an elimination diet, but potatoes, pumpkin, lentils, and bananas may be used.[37]

At the time of writing, several commercial prescription novel protein diets were available for cats: Hill's Prescription Diet offers d/d Feline Skin Support Duck & Green Pea Formula and d/d Venison & Green Pea Formula, and Royal Canin Veterinary Diet offers Hypo Selected Protein PD (pea and duck), PV (pea and venison), and PR (pea and rabbit). Rayne Clinical Nutrition produces limited whole-ingredient diets that undergo less processing than other commercial diets, and it avoids the use of cans in its packaging of soft foods. The methods by which foods are processed, preserved, and packaged may play a role in the etiopathogenesis of food allergy in a small percentage of cats. In one study of 22 cats with confirmed food allergy, four were found to be sensitive to canned foods, and one cat was found to be sensitive to a mixed panel of food additives.[8] Novel protein diets offered by Rayne Clinical Nutrition include kangaroo, rabbit, pork, and cod, mixed with either squash, potato, or chickpea (depending on the protein).

In recent years, numerous over-the-counter (OTC) "limited"-ingredient and novel protein diets have become available. Although OTC diets are less expensive and more readily accessible to cat owners than prescription diets, they are not recommended for use as a test diet. In a study published in 2011, three out of four OTC venison dry dog foods that did not list beef or soy on their ingredient labels tested positive for beef, soy, or both via enzyme-linked immunosorbent assay (ELISA) testing. All four diets were found to contain common pet food proteins, and all were considered unsuitable for use in a diagnostic elimination food trial.[38] Even though only dog foods were tested, there are similar concerns of protein contamination in OTC limited-ingredient cat foods.

Home-Cooked Novel Protein Diets

The gold standard elimination diet is a home-cooked novel protein diet. One main advantage over a commercial diet is that the veterinarian and owner have complete control over the ingredients. Also, these diets can be more specifically tailored to each patient. Home-cooked diets do not contain additives or preservatives found in commercial diets, and they will be much less likely to be contaminated with other proteins. Some cats may not show improvement or may exhibit worsening of their clinical signs on commercial diets and will only improve on a home-cooked diet. In one study, 20 cats with pruritus and skin lesions demonstrated complete resolution of clinical signs when fed home-cooked diets consisting of goat, lamb, or turkey and had recurrence of clinical signs when challenged with their original dietary components. When challenged with a commercial diet, eight of these cats relapsed on a lamb-and-rice diet and 13 cats relapsed on a chicken-and-rice diet. But since only three cats showed recurrence of signs on both diets, it was concluded that while neither commercial diet was as effective as the home-cooked diets at controlling pruritus and skin lesions, commercial diets can successfully be used for long-term management.[12]

One major concern with home-cooked diets is proper nutritional balance. In a survey of veterinarians in North America in 1992, 92% of the home-cooked diets recommended for an initial elimination diet for cats were considered nutritionally inadequate for adult maintenance. The diets tended to be higher in protein and lower in calcium, thiamin, and iron than what is recommended. Levels of taurine and phosphorus were deemed insufficient, and sodium and potassium levels varied widely among the diets.[39] Therefore, it is advisable to have a nutritionally balanced recipe formulated by a board-certified veterinary nutritionist, particularly if the diet will be fed for more than 3 weeks or if the cat is not fully grown or has concurrent medical conditions. Although in-person access to veterinary nutritionists is limited, balanced recipes in veterinary textbooks[40,41] and Internet-based nutrition consultation services are currently available (Box 28-1).

Other concerns with home-cooked diets include palatability and the potential for GI upset. Cats may more readily accept a diet consisting of a protein source only, without a carbohydrate. Introducing a new diet slowly may increase acceptance of the diet and decrease the chance for GI problems.

Client compliance is a principle obstacle to the completion of a home-cooked elimination diet. The time, effort, and expense involved in preparing and feeding a home-cooked diet are main reasons why owners elect to feed a commercial diet. Other reasons for choosing a commercial diet are patient factors, including intolerance or refusal of a home-cooked diet. Investigators in France obtained follow up on 45 cats 1 year after a homemade elimination diet was prescribed and found that only 42.2% of the cats were receiving the prescribed diet exclusively. The top reasons cited by clients for not feeding the prescribed diet were cost and refusal by the cat to eat the diet.[42] However, another investigator revealed that when clients were asked to prepare home-cooked diets for their dogs, the number of cases lost to follow-up decreased from 52% to 27% after establishing better client education practices.[43] Thus detailed client education and frequent client communication prior to and during the diet trial period may significantly increase owner compliance.

Some cat owners express interest in feeding raw meat diets. A raw meat diet offers no advantage over a home-cooked diet in terms of diagnosing or managing food allergies.[44] Additionally, there are significant public health concerns, as contamination of raw meat with bacteria such as *Salmonella, Clostridium, Campylobacter,* and *Escherichia coli* is common.[44,45] Although owners can take precautions to reduce the risks, and there are commercial raw diets that utilize high-pressure pasteurization to try to eliminate bacterial contamination, many dermatologists and nutritionists do not recommend the use of raw meat diets in cats. A raw meat diet is not advisable for cats receiving cyclosporine, because of the risk of *Toxoplasma gondii* exposure.

Hydrolyzed Diets

Hydrolyzed protein diets have been available for cats for over 10 years now, but studies investigating the use of hydrolyzed diets in cats with allergic dermatitis are lacking. The primary goal of hydrolysis of proteins is to disrupt the protein structure by breaking peptide bonds in amino acid chains to generate smaller peptide fragments. This process reduces the molecular weight of the original protein, reduces the antigenicity and allergenicity of the protein, and may increase digestibility.[2,46] The molecules created by hydrolysis should be too small to cross-link two IgE antibodies bound to the surface of mast cells. Failure to cross-link IgE antibodies prevents mast cell degranulation, thereby preventing an IgE-mediated (type I) hypersensitivity.[47] However, hydrolyzed proteins will not have any effect on non-IgE–mediated forms of food allergy.

The minimum molecular weight required to reduce or potentially eliminate antigenicity and allergenicity is not known and may vary among protein sources. Most major food allergens in humans range from 10 to 60 kDa, but peptides as small as 4.5 kDa may still retain allergenicity.[2,46] In one study in dogs, proteins that were identified as major food allergens all weighed over 25 kDa,[48] but similar studies in cats are lacking. Creating a hydrolysate that does not contain any peptides greater than 1 kDa would provide the best chance of eliminating any residual allergens. It is possible that peptides even up to 3 kDa may be tolerated in the majority of patients sensitized to the parent protein. But molecular weight is not the only determinant of allergenicity.

Complete nutritionally balanced hydrolyzed diets also contain carbohydrate and lipid ingredients, either of which may contain small quantities of intact protein allergens. Corn (maize) zein proteins are the major food allergens in humans allergic to maize and can be found in cornstarch.[49] Refined vegetable oils used in hydrolyzed diets may also contain lipophilic protein allergens.[50]

The palatability, digestibility, and osmolarity of a protein can be altered significantly with hydrolysis. As peptides are broken down smaller and smaller, bitterness may increase. Both digestibility and osmolarity increase as well. A high-osmolarity solution in the intestines can attract large amounts of water and result in diarrhea.[2,46] Palatability and GI upset are problems that can be seen with the use of hydrolyzed diets in cats.

Currently there are three types of hydrolyzed diets available for cats: Hill's Prescription Diet z/d Low Sensitivity and z/d ULTRA, Royal Canin Hypoallergenic HP, and Purina Veterinary Diets HA Hypoallergenic Feline Formula (Box 28-2). Hill's Prescription Diet z/d ULTRA is a canned formula, while the others are available as dry kibble only.

Several studies support the use of hydrolyzed diets in dogs and demonstrate significant improvement or complete resolution of clinical signs.[29,51,52] But it is possible to see reactions or lack of improvement of clinical signs with hydrolyzed diets. In a review of studies investigating hydrolyzed diets in dogs, it was found that up to 50% of dogs with food allergies enrolled in three of the studies demonstrated worsening of clinical signs after ingesting partial hydrolysates that originated from foods to which they were hypersensitive.[53] Similar studies evaluating the efficacy of hydrolyzed diets in cats with cutaneous signs are lacking, but anecdotal evidence suggests that successful diagnosis of food allergy in cats with pruritus or skin lesions can be attained utilizing a hydrolyzed diet. However, to achieve the best success with a hydrolyzed protein diet, it is essential to obtain a full dietary history and avoid feeding a hydrolyzed diet that contains parent proteins and/or carbohydrates that the cat has been fed previously.

Other Dietary Trial Considerations

There are some key factors that may be overlooked by many pet owners that are essential for the completion of a proper elimination diet trial. All treats and table food must be eliminated from the diet. Exposure to food from other pets and from family members (e.g., toddlers) must be restricted. Gelatin used in medication capsules may contain beef, pork, or fish proteins; therefore, medication in capsules, as well as flavored medications, should be avoided. For cats receiving oral medications, the use of flavored Feline Greenies Pill Pockets and the use of other foods to hide medications must be avoided as well. Cats that are allowed outside should be restricted to indoors to prevent hunting or scavenging.

Duration of the Diet Trial

Advice on the recommended duration of an elimination diet trial varies in the literature. While many cats with food allergies will show improvement within 3 to 4 weeks of starting an elimination diet, others may not improve for 10 to 13 weeks.[2,13-16,18,21] Improvement in GI symptoms may be seen within 2 weeks,[2,35] but the reason why GI signs may resolve faster than cutaneous signs is not known. For cats with relapsing clinical signs, the duration of the elimination diet must extend beyond the time during which the cat is typically symptom free.[2] Extending the diet trial period is required to determine if resolution of the clinical signs was due to the elimination diet or to the relapsing nature of the condition. Most veterinary dermatologists recommend feeding an elimination diet for at least 12 to 16 weeks, to reduce the chance of misdiagnosing cats that may take longer to respond.

Interpreting the Response to the Dietary Trial

A complete lack of response to a properly conducted elimination diet trial likely indicates that food allergy is not the correct diagnosis. Once food allergy has been ruled out, further investigation for the cause of the pruritus and/or skin lesions is required. If only partial improvement is achieved with an elimination diet and recrudescence of clinical signs occurs with dietary challenge, this may indicate that the cat has both a food allergy and a concurrent hypersensitivity disorder such as atopy. If food allergy is highly suspected but no improvement is seen, lack of owner and/or patient compliance may be the cause. An alternative explanation is that the diet may have contained a protein to which the cat is allergic or which cross-reacts with the protein to which the cat is allergic.

In cases where food allergies are highly suspected but the cat fails to improve with an initial elimination diet, a second elimination diet trial may be warranted. If a second trial is needed, many dermatologists elect to use a completely different type of diet. For example, if a novel protein diet was utilized first, then a hydrolyzed diet may be selected for the second trial, or if a commercial diet was fed, then a home-cooked diet may be recommended next. Figure 28-5 gives a protocol for the diagnosis and management of food allergy utilizing an elimination dietary trial followed by provocative dietary challenge.

Provocative Dietary Challenge

Although ideally one would anticipate 100% resolution of pruritus and other clinical signs in a food-allergic cat treated with an appropriate elimination diet, if pruritus and lesions are reduced at least 50%, many dermatologists consider this to be a positive response.[15,30] But to definitively confirm the diagnosis of a food allergy, the cat must be challenged with the food ingredients it was eating prior to the elimination diet and exhibit relapse or worsening of clinical signs. One study noted that recurrence of pruritus and skin lesions may occur anywhere from 1 to 18 days after a provocative dietary challenge.[12] Other researchers found that while most cats recrudesced within 3 to 5 days, other cats did not show recurrence of symptoms for up to 10 days after the dietary challenge.[11] Based on this information, provocation testing should last at least 10 to 14 days.

Up to 26% of cats that have complete resolution of either cutaneous or GI symptoms on an elimination diet will not relapse when their previous diet is reintroduced.[8,11,12] This may be from failure to challenge with the protein to which the cat is allergic, spontaneous remission or a change in immune response, the reestablishment of a more normal intestinal permeability, the misdiagnosis of food allergy (e.g., food intolerance, ectoparasites, or other hypersensitivity disorder), coincidence, or other therapies that may have been used just prior to or during the beginning of the elimination diet trial.[2,8,11,12,37]

Provocative Testing with Individual Food Components
Once the diagnosis of food allergy has been established, provocative testing with individual food ingredients can be performed. Identification of the offending food components will allow for both avoidance of the proteins to which the cat is allergic and for selection of a maintenance diet for long-term management of the patient.

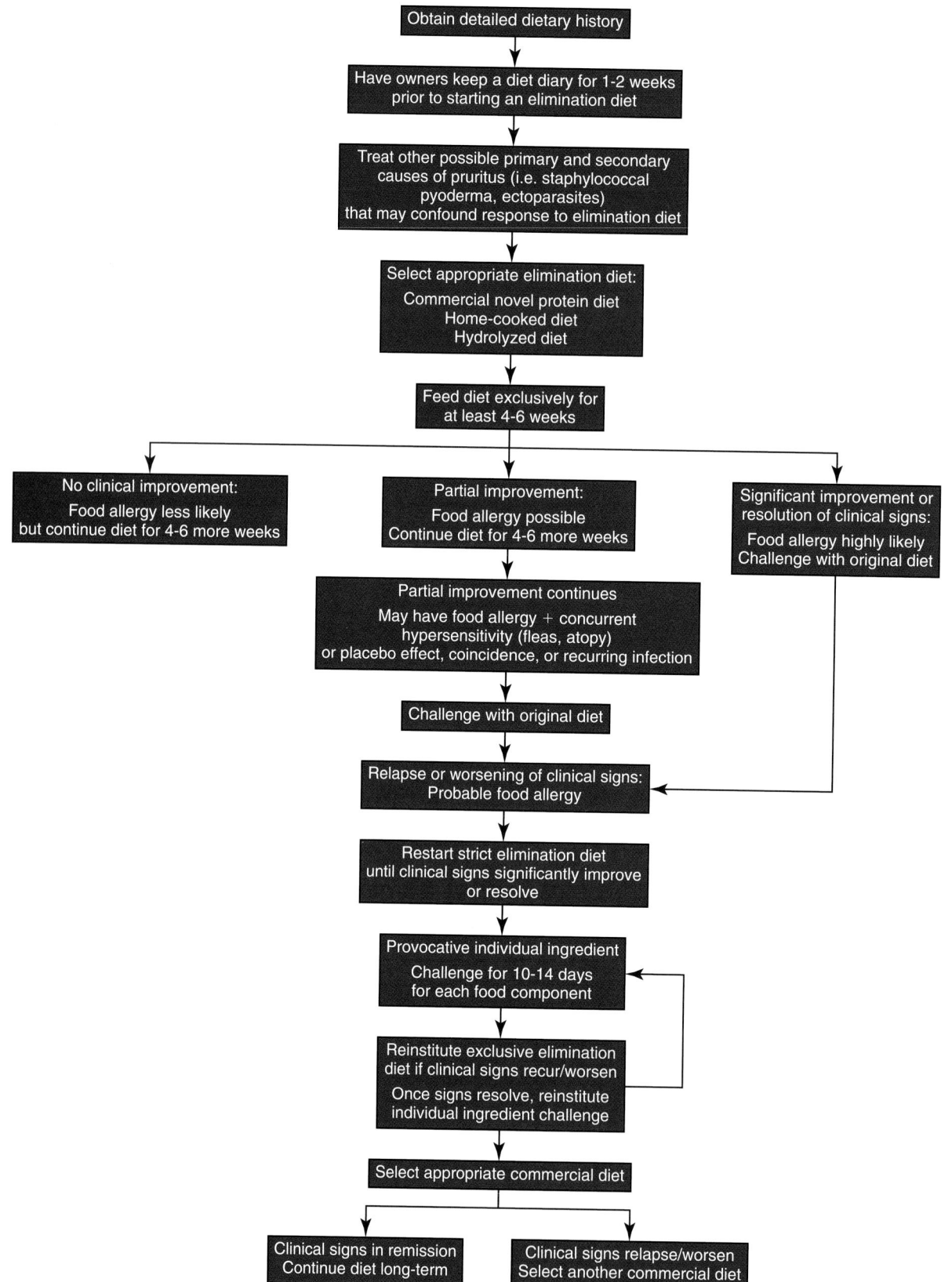

Figure 28-5: Protocol for the diagnosis and management of food allergy utilizing an elimination dietary trial followed by provocative dietary challenge. (Adapted from Roudebush P, Guilford WG, Jackson HA: Adverse reactions to food. In Hand MS, Thatcher CD, Remillard RL, et al., editors: *Small animal clinical nutrition,* ed 5, Topeka, KS, 2010, Mark Morris Institute, pp 609-627.)

Other Diagnostic Tests

As different types of allergic dermatoses cannot be distinguished based on clinical findings alone,[23,25] and as infectious and parasitic dermatoses can be confused with or complicate lesions associated with allergic dermatoses, it is important to perform basic dermatologic diagnostic tests prior to embarking on an elimination diet trial. Flea combings, skin scrapings, skin cytology, and fungal culture form a dermatologic minimum database for cats.[23] Otic mite preparations and otic cytology are indicated if ear disease is present. Cats should be treated for fleas and ectoparasites prior to starting an elimination diet trial. But since flea combings and skin scrapings may lead to false negative results, excluding fleas and other ectoparasites may require a therapeutic trial. It is also essential to treat any existing secondary bacteria or *Malassezia* skin infections. While secondary infections occur less commonly in cats than dogs, they can contribute to pruritus, complicate skin lesions, and prevent resolution of symptoms. If a cat presents with severe pruritus or severely inflamed skin lesions, treatment with short-acting glucocorticoids or other anti-inflammatory medications such as antihistamines or cyclosporine may be warranted. But the elimination diet trial period should extend at least 2 weeks after medications have been discontinued in order to evaluate the cat's response to the elimination diet alone.[35]

PROGNOSIS AND LONG-TERM MANAGEMENT

The prognosis for cats with food allergy alone is very good, as long as the cat avoids the offending allergen(s). Many cases can eventually be managed with an OTC commercial diet, but some cats may need to be fed a prescription commercial diet or home-cooked diet long term. Attempts should be made to find an acceptable commercial diet, as this will lead to improved owner compliance and minimize the risk of nutritional imbalances long term. Also, a significant proportion of cats may tolerate their original diet after successful resolution of clinical signs during an elimination dietary trial. Although seemingly rare in cats, it is possible to develop an allergy to another or a new food component over time, so if a relapse in clinical signs occurs, re-evaluation is needed. If other causes of pruritus, such as ectoparasites, skin infections, and other hypersensitivities have been ruled out, then a new elimination dietary trial may be needed.

References

1. Anderson JA: The establishment of common language concerning adverse reactions to foods and food additives. *J Allergy Clin Immunol* 78:140–144, 1986.
2. Verlinden A, Hesta M, Millet S, et al: Food allergy in dogs and cats: a review. *Crit Rev Food Sci Nutr* 46:259–273, 2006.
3. Roudebush P, Guilford WG, Jackson HA: Adverse reactions to food. In Hand MS, Thatcher CD, Remillard RL, et al, editors: *Small animal clinical nutrition*, ed 5, Topeka, KS, 2010, Mark Morris Institute, pp 609–627.
4. Pabst O, Mowat AW: Oral tolerance to food protein. *Mucosal Immunol* 5:232–239, 2012.
5. Taylor SL, Lemanske RF, Bush KR, et al: Food allergens: structure and immunologic properties. *Ann Allerg* 59:93–99, 1987.
6. Taylor SL, Lehrer SB: Principles and characteristics of food allergens. *Crit Rev Food Sci Nutr* 36(S):91–118, 1996.
7. Roudebush P: Ingredients and foods associated with adverse reactions in dogs and cats. *Vet Dermatol* 24:293–294, 2013.
8. Guilford WB, Markwell PJ, Jones BR: Prevalence and causes of food sensitivity in cats with chronic pruritus, vomiting or diarrhea. *J Nutr* 128(12 Suppl):2790S–2791S, 1998.
9. Reedy LM: Food hypersensitivity to lamb in a cat. *J Am Vet Med Assoc* 1(204):1039–1040, 1994.
10. Miller WH, Griffin CE, Campbell KL, editors: *Muller & Kirk's small animal dermatology*, ed 7, St Louis, 2013, Elsevier, pp 404–405.
11. Guilford WG, Jones BR, Markwell PJ, et al: Food sensitivity in cats with chronic idiopathic gastrointestinal problems. *J Vet Intern Med* 15:7–13, 2001.
12. Leistra M, Willemse T: Double-blind evaluation of two commercial hypoallergenic diets in cats with adverse food reactions. *J Feline Med Surg* 4:185–188, 2002.
13. Carlotti DN, Remy I, Prost C: Food allergy in dogs and cats: a review and report of 43 cases. *Vet Dermatol* 1:55–62, 1990.
14. Wills J, Harvey R: Diagnosis and management of food allergy and intolerance in dogs and cats. *Aust Vet J* 71:322–326, 1994.
15. White SD, Sequoia D: Food hypersensitivity in cats: 14 cases (1982-1987). *J Am Vet Med Assoc* 194:692–695, 1989.
16. Rosser EJ: Food allergy in the cat: a prospective study of 13 cats. In Ihrke PJ, Mason I, Shite SD, editors: *Advances in veterinary dermatology*, vol 2, Oxford, England, 1993, Pergamon, pp 33–39.
17. Guaguère E: Intolérance alimentaire à manifestations cutanées: à propos de 17 cas chez le chat. *Prat Méd Chir Anim Comp* 28:451–460, 1993.
18. Rosser EJ: Food allergy in dogs and cats: a review. *Vet Allerg Clin Immunol* 6:21–35, 1998.
19. Marin A, Crosaz O, Hubert B, et al: Retrospective study of homemade elimination diets prescribed during 1 year in a university consultation: (2) clinical signs of 28 canine and feline cases. *Vet Dermatol* 23(Suppl 1):2–104, 2012.
20. Bryan J, Frank L: Food allergy in the cat: a diagnosis of elimination. *J Feline Med Surg* 12:861–866, 2010.
21. Guaguere E: Food intolerance in cats with cutaneous manifestations: a review of 17 cases. *Vet Allergy Clin Immunol* 4:90–98, 1996.
22. Medleau L, Latimer KS, Duncan JR: Food hypersensitivity in a cat. *J Am Vet Med Assoc* 189:692–693, 1986.
23. Favrot C: Feline non-flea induced hypersensitivity dermatitis: clinical features, diagnosis, and treatment. *J Feline Med Surg* 15:778–784, 2013.
24. Waisglass SE, Landsberg GM, Yager JA, et al: Underlying medical conditions in cats with presumptive psychogenic alopecia. *J Am Vet Med Assoc* 228:1705–1709, 2006.
25. Hobi S, Linek M, Marignac G, et al: Clinical characteristics and causes of pruritus in cats: a multicentre study on feline hypersensitivity-associated dermatoses. *Vet Dermatol* 22:406–413, 2011.
26. Hirt R, Iben C: Possible food allergy in a colony of cats. *J Nutr* 128:2792S–2794S, 1998.
27. Gross TL, Ihrke PJ, Walder EJ, editors: *Skin diseases of the dog and cat: clinical and histopathologic diagnosis*, ed 2, Ames, IA, 2005, Blackwell Science, pp 207–208.
28. Rosenberg AS, Scott DW, Erb HN, et al: Infiltrative lymphocytic mural folliculitis: a histopathological reaction pattern in skin-biopsy specimens from cats with allergic skin disease. *J Feline Med Surg* 12:80–85, 2010.
29. Jackson HA, Jackson MW, Coblentz L, et al: Evaluation of the clinical and allergen specific serum immunoglobulin E responses to oral challenge with cornstarch, corn, soy and a soy hydrolysate diet in dogs with spontaneous food allergy. *Vet Dermatol* 14:181–187, 2003.
30. Jeffers JG, Shanley KJ, Meyer EK: Diagnostic testing of dogs for food hypersensitivity. *J Am Vet Med Assoc* 198:245–250, 1991.

31. Mueller RS: Tsohalis J: Evaluation of serum allergen-specific IgE for the diagnosis of food adverse reactions in the dog. *Vet Dermatol* 9:167–171, 1998.

32. Foster AP, Knowles TG, Hotston Moore A, et al: Serum IgE and IgG responses to food antigens in normal and atopic dogs, and dogs with gastrointestinal disease. *Vet Immunol Immunopathol* 92:113–124, 2003.

33. Kunkle G, Horner S: Validity of skin testing for diagnosis of food allergy in dogs. *J Am Vet Med Assoc* 200:677–680, 1992.

34. Bethlehem S, Bexley J, Mueller RS: Patch testing and allergen-specific serum IgE and IgG antibodies in the diagnosis of canine adverse food reactions. *Vet Immunol Immunopathol* 145:582–589, 2012.

35. Gaschen F, Merchant S: Adverse food reactions in dogs and cats. *Vet Clin North Am Small Anim Pract* 41:361–379, 2011.

36. Kelso JM, Cockrell GE, Helm RM, et al: Common allergens in avian meats. *J Allergy Clin Immunol* 104:202–204, 1999.

37. Guaguere E, Prelaud P: Food hypersensitivity in the cat. *Eur J Comp Anim Pract* 19:234–241, 2009.

38. Raditic DM, Remillard RL, Tater KC: ELISA testing for common food antigens in four dry dog foods used in dietary elimination trials. *J Anim Physiol Anim Nutr* 95:90–97, 2011.

39. Roudebush P, Cowell CS: Results of a hypoallergenic diet survey of veterinarians in North America with a nutritional evaluation of homemade diet prescriptions. *Vet Dermatol* 3:23–28, 1992.

40. Roudebush P: Nutritional management of the allergic patient. In August JR, editor: *Consultations in feline internal medicine*, ed 2, Philadelphia, 1994, Saunders, pp 201–208.

41. Remillard RL, Paragon BM, Crane SW, et al: Making pet foods at home. In Hand MS, Thatcher CD, Remillard RL, et al, editors: *Small animal clinical nutrition*, ed 4, Topeka, KS, 2000, Mark Morris Institute, p 163.

42. Marin A, Crosaz O, Hubert B, et al: Retrospective study of homemade elimination diets prescribed during one year in a university consultation: one observance of 155 canine and feline cases. *Vet Dermatol* 23(Suppl 1):2–104, 2012.

43. Chesney CJ: Food sensitivity in the dog: a quantitative study. *J Small Anim Pract* 43:203–207, 2002.

44. Jackson HL: Hypoallergenic diets: principles in therapy. In Bonagura JD, Twedt DC, editors: *Kirk's current veterinary therapy XIV*, ed 14, St Louis, 2009, Saunders/Elsevier, pp 395–397.

45. Weese JS, Rousseau J, Arroyo L: Bacteriological evaluation of commercial canine and feline raw diets. *Can Vet J* 46(6):513–516, 2005.

46. Cave NJ: Hydrolyzed protein diets for dogs and cats. *Vet Clin North Am Small Anim Pract* 36:1251–1268, 2006.

47. Cordle CT: Control of food allergies using protein hydrolysates. *Food Technol* 48:72–76, 1994.

48. Martin A, Sierra MP, Gonzalez JL, et al: Identification of allergens responsible for canine cutaneous adverse food reactions to lamb, beef, and cow's milk. *Vet Dermatol* 15:349–356, 2004.

49. Frisner H, Rosendal A, Barkholt V: Identification of immunogenic maize proteins in a casein hydrolysate formula. *Pediatr Allergy Immunol* 11:106–110, 2000.

50. Zitouni N, Errahali Y, Metche M, et al: Influence of refining steps on trace allergenic protein content in sunflower oil. *J Allergy Clin Immunol* 106:962–967, 2000.

51. Loeffler A, Lloyd DH, Bond R, et al: Dietary trials with a commercial chicken hydrolysate diet in 63 pruritic dogs. *Vet Rec* 154:519–522, 2004.

52. Biourge VC, Fontaine J, Vroom MW: Diagnosis of adverse reactions to food in dogs: efficacy of a soy-isolate hydrolysate-based diet. *J Nutr* 134(8 Suppl):2062S–2064S, 2004.

53. Olivry T, Bizikova P: A systematic review of the evidence of reduced allergenicity and clinical benefit of food hydrolysates in dogs with cutaneous adverse food reactions. *Vet Dermatol* 21:32–41, 2010.

Cyclosporine in Feline Dermatology

Katherine Irwin

Cyclosporine is a fat-soluble, cyclic polypeptide metabolite of the fungus *Beauveria nivea* (formerly *Tolypocladium inflatum*). It is also referred to as cyclosporine A, cyclosporin, cyclosporin A, and ciclosporin. Cyclosporine has potent immune-modulating properties and was initially employed in human medicine to prevent organ rejection in transplant patients. Soon after, it was adopted for use as part of immunosuppressive protocols for feline renal transplant patients.[1] Cyclosporine also became increasingly used for dermatologic conditions in people, such as atopic dermatitis and psoriasis, and in the late 1980s, reports of its use for skin disease in animals began to be published.[2-4] The efficacy of cyclosporine in managing a number of allergic and immune-mediated dermatologic diseases in dogs and cats has been investigated.[2] The strongest data has been with regard to its efficacy in managing atopic dermatitis in dogs and manifestations of allergic dermatitis in cats. Its usefulness in treatment of these conditions is now widely accepted, and veterinary-specific formulations of cyclosporine labeled for use in managing allergic dermatitis, Atopica for Dogs and Atopica for Cats (Elanco, Greensboro, NC), are now available.

Cyclosporine was initially released in the early 1980s as a vegetable oil-based formulation. Absorption of this formulation (Sandimmune, Novartis Pharmaceuticals) was highly influenced by bile excretion, gastrointestinal (GI) motility, and the presence of food in the GI tract, leading to poor oral bioavailability and significant intraindividual and interindividual pharmacokinetic variability and response.[5] In the 1990s, the product was reformulated to a modified version that immediately forms a microemulsion in an aqueous environment. This modification improved the speed and consistency of absorption, reduced the impact of feeding, reduced intrapatient and interpatient variation in serum concentrations, and provided more consistent correlation between serum trough concentrations and total drug exposure.[5,6] The modified and unmodified versions of cyclosporine are not considered bioequivalent and are not directly interchangeable. Atopica for Cats is a modified version of cyclosporine and is available as a 100 mg/mL concentration oral solution.

MECHANISM OF ACTION

Cyclosporine is a calcineurin inhibitor with far-reaching immunosuppressive effects.[7,8] It enters the target cell (most notably T lymphocytes) and binds to cyclophilin, a cytosolic protein. This cyclosporine-cyclophilin complex is then able to bind to calcineurin, a cytosolic, calcium-dependent enzyme that, via dephosphorylation, activates the nuclear factor of activated T cells (NFAT).[6-8] When activated, NFAT can then enter the cell's nucleus to initiate transcription of a variety of cytokine genes involved in the activation, function, and proliferation of a number of cells involved in the immune response. Blocking the ability of calcineurin to dephosphorylate NFAT means these cytokines are not produced, thus preventing progression of the immune response.

Cyclosporine is most recognized as suppressing the production of interleukin (IL)-2 and its receptor, to which much of its immunosuppressive and antiallergic activity is attributed.[3,7] This cytokine is produced by a number of cells including type-1 helper T cells. It is a significant contributor to the activation and proliferation of T cells and their differentiation into CD4+ and CD8+ cells. Activation of T cells then in turn upregulates production of additional cytokines and induces the activation and proliferation of a number of other immune-effector cells such as B lymphocytes, macrophages, eosinophils, mast cells, and even keratinocytes.[3] Suppression of IL-2 occurs in a dose-dependent manner, and at *in vitro* concentrations of 450 ng/mL and above, its production is significantly reduced in cat peripheral blood mononuclear cells (PBMC).[8]

In cats, cyclosporine has also been documented (both *in vitro* and *in vivo*) to suppress the transcription and production of additional cytokines including IL-4, interferon-gamma (IFN-γ), tumor necrosis factor-alpha (TNF-α), granulocyte-marcophage colony-stimulating factor (GM-CSF), and IL-10.[8,9] This suppression also appears to occur in a dose-dependent manner, although the degree of suppression of IL-10 is less than that seen with the other cytokines.[9] As will be discussed later, effects of these cytokines may further explain cyclosporine's ability to impact a number of immune-mediated and allergic skin diseases in cats.

Although not specifically documented in cats, additional mechanisms by which cyclosporine influences the immune response have been confirmed and characterized in other species. It stands to reason these same processes likely occur in cats as well. In addition to blocking the activation of NFAT, cyclosporine has also been shown to affect the activities of activator protein-1 and nuclear factor κB (NF-κB), two additional transcription factors that may influence immunologic and inflammatory cascades.[7] In humans, it has also been shown to increase transforming growth factor-beta which can stimulate cells to increase production of extracellular matrix and decrease extracellular matrix degrading proteases.[7] Cyclosporine has also been documented to inhibit keratinocyte proliferation and secretion of inflammatory mediators and chemotactic factors, reduce lipopolysaccharide-induced prostaglandin E2 synthesis, inhibit production of keratinocyte chemoattractant and chemokine ligand 2 chemokines, and reduce production of the proinflammatory mediator IFN-γ-inducible protein 10.[10] Finally, cyclosporine can also block calcium-dependent signal transduction in mast cells, which prevents mediator release; inhibits eosinophil function, recruitment, and survival; and reduces the numbers of Langerhans cells in the skin and inhibits their antigen-presenting functions.[3,5,11]

PHARMACOKINETICS

Following oral administration in cats, cyclosporine is rapidly absorbed, with peak blood concentrations reported to occur from as early as 1 hour up to 3 to 4 hours.[6,12] Administering it with food does not appear to significantly change oral bioavailability as compared with administration in a fasted state.[13] Following absorption, it is extensively distributed to all tissues, including glandular tissues, fat, and skin.[6,12] Mean terminal half-life has been reported to be 8.2 hours, with a range of 6.8 to greater than 40 hours noted in some cats.[6,12,13] Oral bioavailability has been reported to be approximately 25% to 35%, which is about the same or slightly less than that seen in dogs where bioavailability of around 35% has been reported.[6,11,12] Studies assessing the disposition of cyclosporine in cats following multiple oral dosing observed marked variation in all pharmacokinetic parameters assessed both between and within individual cats.[6,12,13] One of these studies concluded that the degree of variation present makes therapeutic drug monitoring challenging.[6] In one study where patients received microemulsion cyclosporine at 3 mg/kg orally every 12 hours, the maximum serum concentrations (C_{max}) ranged between 320 and 716 ng/mL.[6] In an older study using the unmodified version of cyclosporine at an oral dose of 10 mg/kg every 12 hours, the trough (C12) serum concentrations ranged from 134 to 902 ng/mL, with a mean of 576 ng/mL.[12]

Cyclosporine is absorbed in the small intestine by passive diffusion; absorption is impacted both via metabolism by intestinal cytochrome P450 (CYP450) oxidases and first-pass elimination via intestinal P-glycoprotein efflux pumps.[5,11,14-16] Clearance is primarily through the liver where it is extensively metabolized by hepatic CYP450 3A enzymes into a number of metabolites.[5,12,14] It is then excreted in the bile. In cats, after 28 days of oral dosing, serum levels were undetectable within a week following discontinuation of the medication.[12]

Due to the difficulty that can be encountered when giving cats oral medications, the effectiveness of administering cyclosporine transdermally has been explored.[5,17] Because of its lipophilic nature and high molecular weight, absorption

through keratinized skin is poor. It gets trapped in the stratum corneum, preventing penetration to the deeper skin layers. A pilot study comparing blood cyclosporine concentrations following both oral dosing and transdermal application (at a dose of 5.1 to 7.4 mg/kg in pluronic lecithin organogel) revealed very poor absorption after the transdermal application, with a resulting mean serum concentration of only 58 ng/mL. Only one of six cats in this study had a 2-hour serum concentration that could be considered therapeutic (878 ng/mL).[17] The study's conclusion was that transdermal application could not be recommended because of inconsistent and poor absorption.

DRUG INTERACTIONS

The absorption, metabolism, and excretion of cyclosporine in cats can vary greatly, not only as a function of the formulation used and individual variability, but also with concomitant use of other medications. Because of its extensive metabolism by CYP450 enzymes and intestinal transport via P-glycoprotein, any other medications that also participate in these processes can potentially affect the bioavailability of cyclosporine. Those drugs that inhibit CYP450 or compete for P-glycoprotein transport can increase cyclosporine serum levels. Those that upregulate CYP450 activity can reduce serum levels of the drug. In human medicine, there are numerous drugs and other compounds that have been implicated or confirmed to affect cyclosporine absorption and metabolism, including a variety of antibiotics, azole antifungals, calcium channel blockers, grapefruit juice, and steroids.[5,14] Drug interactions that have been substantiated in cats include ketoconazole, itraconazole, and clarithromycin.[14-16]

Drug interaction studies have been primarily performed with regard to renal transplant patients as a means to find ways to increase serum blood concentrations of cyclosporine so that maintenance dosing can be reduced from twice daily to once daily. The azole antifungal ketoconazole is an inhibitor of both CYP450 and intestinal P-glycoprotein. One study assessing ketoconazole's influence on cyclosporine pharmacokinetics found that 10 mg/kg ketoconazole orally once daily approximately doubled serum blood cyclosporine concentrations at 12 and 24 hours compared with cyclosporine dosed alone, and also reduced the rate of systemic clearance, increasing the half-life from 12.1 to 19.7 hours.[14] In this study, the authors were able to successfully manage renal transplant cats on once-daily cyclosporine via the addition of ketoconazole. In addition, the total dose of cyclosporine needed to maintain goal serum levels was reduced by 50% to 85%. Although hepatotoxicity is of concern in cats receiving ketoconazole, liver values were monitored in patients in the study and the authors noted the medication was well tolerated.[14,15,18]

Itraconazole is another azole antifungal that also inhibits CYP450 enzymes and P-glycoprotein transport pumps. A study assessing the impact of 10 mg/kg once daily oral itraconazole on cyclosporine pharmacokinetics in cats also found that it significantly increased the oral bioavailability of cyclosporine, again about two times higher than with cyclosporine alone.[15] A third study assessed the impact of oral clarithromycin on cyclosporine pharmacokinetics in cats.[16] Clarithromycin is a macrolide antibiotic that is also known to inhibit CYP450 and P-glycoprotein. At 10 mg/kg orally once daily, the addition of clarithromycin also significantly increased the oral bioavailability of cyclosporine, reduced a renal transplant cat's cyclosporine dose by approximately 65%, and allowed dosing to be reduced to once daily. At the time the study was published, the patient had been successfully maintained on the protocol for 10 months with the clarithromycin well tolerated.

As most cyclosporine dosing regimens for dermatologic disease already utilize once daily dosing, the value of incorporating the aforementioned drug regimens for skin disease in cats appears limited. However, awareness of these interactions is important as they are drugs that can be used with some frequency in cats, and dosing adjustments of cyclosporine may need to be considered if used concurrently. In addition, although specific data for cats are lacking, oral administration of fluconazole has also been documented to increase cyclosporine blood levels in beagles and thus may very well impact cyclosporine metabolism in cats as well.[19]

APPLICATIONS IN FELINE DERMATOLOGY

Given the global immunologic impact cyclosporine exhibits on both cellular and humoral immune processes in cats (reduction in IL-2, IL-4, IFN-γ, TNF-α, GM-CSF, and IL-10), it stands to reason that it can be effective in modulating disease processes for a number of inflammatory, allergic, and immune-mediated conditions. By suppressing IL-2 production, T cells are not stimulated to differentiate into CD4+ and CD8+ cells, which are found in lesional skin of allergic cats.[6,20] Activated IL-4–producing T cells, which promote B cell differentiation and secretion of immunoglobulins (Ig), have also been recognized in the skin of these patients.[8] By reducing IL-4 production, secretion of allergen specific IgE may be reduced in cats with allergic skin disease. Additional modulation of the activities of keratinocytes, Langerhans cells, mast cells, and eosinophils can also contribute to reduction of allergic reactions in the skin. Furthermore, although their roles in cats have not been fully defined, IFN-γ and TNF-α are recognized in both humans and dogs as contributing to the development of chronic skin lesions and playing a role in the pathogenesis of chronic inflammatory and autoimmune diseases.[21] If this is also the case in cats, reduction in these cytokines may be the basis for cyclosporine-induced improvement in skin conditions not associated with allergy. In summary, given the combination and extent of cytokine suppression and immune-cell modulation exhibited by cyclosporine, there has been much interest in utilizing it for a number of dermatologic diseases in cats.

By far, the most in-depth research and strongest data to support efficacy involve the use of cyclosporine to control nonseasonal pruritus and lesions (eosinophilic granuloma complex [Figure 29-1]), head and neck excoriations (Figure 29-2), self-induced alopecia (Figure 29-3), and miliary dermatitis (Figure 29-2) associated with feline allergic skin disease not due to food or flea allergy.[20,22-26] This is also referred to by some as feline atopic dermatitis, although others will argue much is still to be learned about this disease in cats and whether their syndromes of allergic dermatitis truly correlate with what is known about atopic dermatitis in dogs and humans.[18] (See Chapter 32 for further discussions on manifestations of allergic dermatitis in cats.)

An early abstract reported the efficacy of cyclosporine in managing 12 cats with eosinophilic granuloma complex (consisting of indolent ulcers, eosinophilic plaques, and eosinophilic granulomas).[26] Patients were dosed at 25 mg/cat (4.9 to 12.5 mg/kg/day) for 60 days. Significant improvement was seen in the cats with eosinophilic plaques and granulomas, with only partial regression seen in the three cats

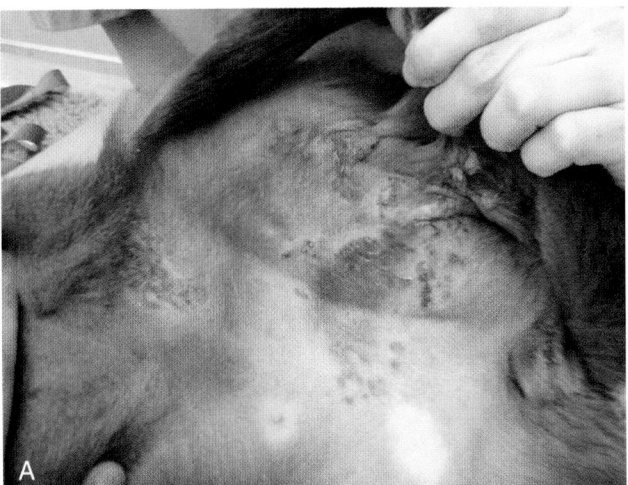
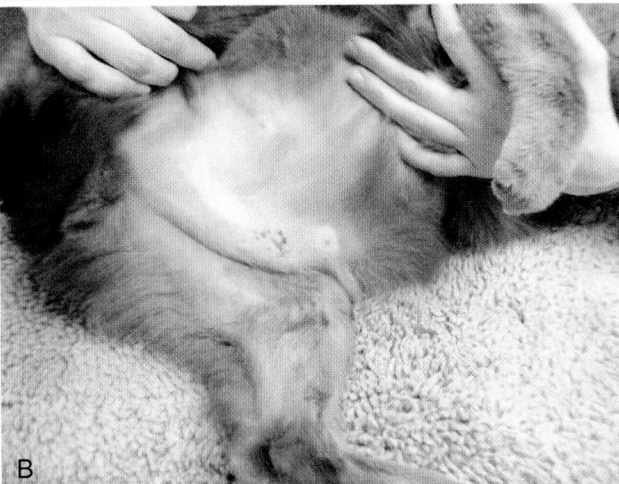

Figure 29-1: A, Eosinophilic granulomas on the belly and medial left rear leg of a cat with allergic dermatitis. *Head is to the left.* **B,** Same cat 4 weeks after starting cyclosporine. This cat was also treated with an oral antibiotic for concurrent infection. *Head is now to the right.*

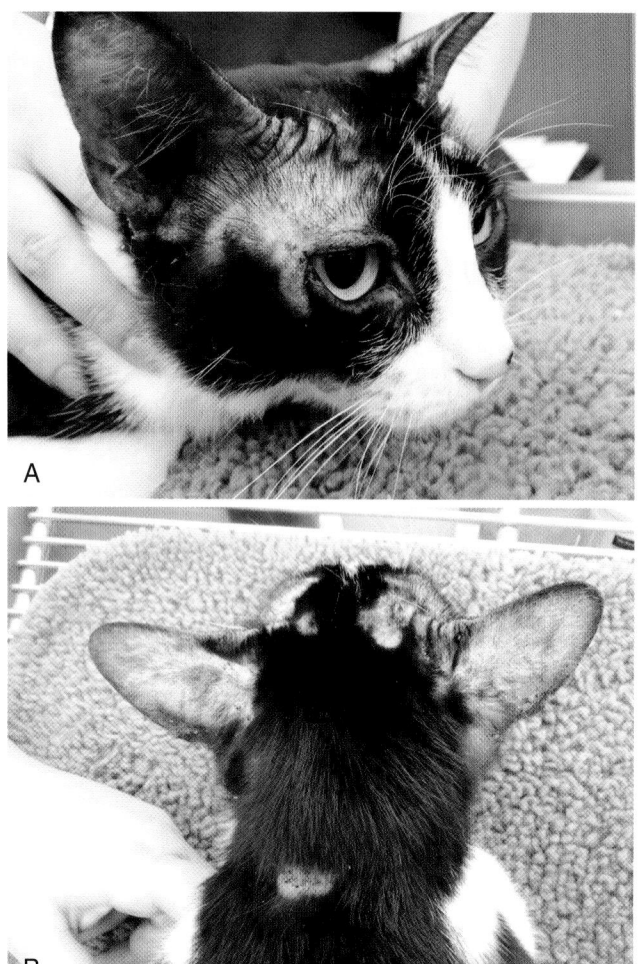

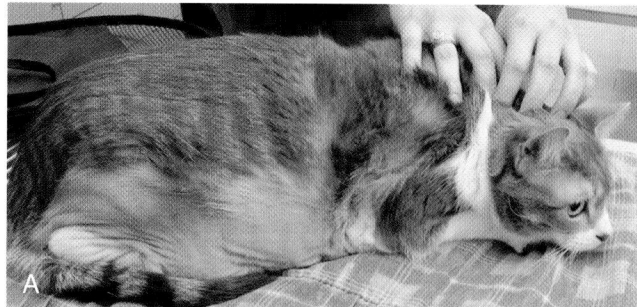

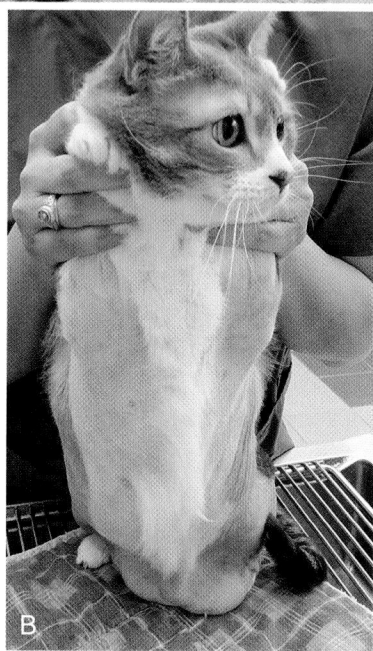

Figure 29-2: A, Cat with allergic dermatitis exhibiting miliary dermatitis and excoriations secondary to head and neck pruritus. **B,** Same cat as shown in **A.**

Figure 29-3: A, Bilaterally symmetric self-induced alopecia on the ventrum and flanks of a cat with allergies. **B,** Same cat as shown in **A.**

with indolent ulcer. Recent or concurrent antimicrobial therapy was not allowed during the study. It is unknown if the patients with indolent ulcer would have exhibited better response if potential secondary bacterial infection had also been addressed, as it is now recognized that infection can contribute significantly to these lesions.[18]

A retrospective study described the responses of 23 cats with dermatologic disease to cyclosporine.[24] These cats had lesions and/or clinical signs consisting of eosinophilic granuloma complex (eosinophilic granuloma, eosinophilic plaque, indolent ulcer, and linear granulomas), idiopathic pruritus, and/or stomatitis. Doses of cyclosporine used ranged from 5.8 to 13.3 mg/kg/day and patients were monitored for a minimum of 3 months. All cats with lesions of eosinophilic granuloma complex or pruritus ($n = 16$) exhibited significant improvement and could be maintained on alternate day therapy (every other day or twice weekly). Of eight cats with stomatitis, four went into complete remission. The remaining four were noted to exhibit fair to good improvement, and overall response by the cat owners was noted as acceptable due to improved quality of life. Only one cat presented with an indolent ulcer, and although response was slower than in

the other patients, it did resolve with cyclosporine therapy. In this study, all cats had been treated with oral antibiotics for 4 weeks before starting the cyclosporine to eliminate secondary bacterial infections. This may account for the better response seen with the indolent ulcer. Cats in this study were treated with either a microemulsion-based capsule or the oil-based liquid. All cats with stomatitis were treated with the oil-based formulation while cats with the other lesions were treated with both. The same response was seen in cats with similar lesions whether the liquid or the microemulsion capsule was used, but the mean dose needed for response was lower with the capsules than with the liquid (8.6 mg/kg versus 11.8 mg/kg).

A prospective pilot study with 10 cats dosed with 3.6 to 8.3 mg/kg/day cyclosporine for 1 month provided additional early support for utilizing cyclosporine for feline allergic skin disease, again manifested by pruritus, self-induced alopecia, miliary dermatitis, and/or lesions of eosinophilic granuloma complex.[23] In this study, 50% of patients were assessed as responding well by 30 days of treatment. Compared with the previously noted studies, this study was of much shorter duration, and it is possible greater improvement would have been seen with longer courses of therapy.

As a means to compare its efficacy with other accepted therapies for feline allergic skin disease, cyclosporine was compared with oral prednisolone in a double-blind randomized study of cats with presumed atopic dermatitis.[20] For 4 weeks, 18 cats were treated with 5 mg/kg/day cyclosporine while 11 were treated with 1 mg/kg/day oral prednisolone. Approximately 70% of the cats treated with cyclosporine showed more than 25% improvement (range 30% to 100%, mean 62.3%). There was no significant difference among groups in degree of response or number of cats that improved, and it was concluded cyclosporine is an effective alternative to prednisolone in these patients.

The largest study to date focused on establishing a safe and effective dose of modified cyclosporine to control the symptoms of feline allergic dermatitis.[22] In this multicenter, double-blind, placebo-controlled study, 100 client-owned cats were treated for 6 weeks with microemulsion cyclosporine at 2.5 or 7 mg/kg/day or with a placebo. During the course of the study, 28 cats were withdrawn, significantly more of those from the placebo and 2.5 mg/kg/day groups than from the 7 mg/kg/day dose group. Most withdrawals were due to a lack of efficacy. Only one cat was withdrawn because of an adverse event (anorexia). Those cats treated with 7 mg/kg/day cyclosporine exhibited significantly greater improvement in total lesion scores, extent of lesions, and pruritus as compared with those receiving 2.5 mg/kg/day or placebo. Inadequate or complete lack of response was reported in 24% of cats in the 7 mg/kg/day group. Overall, little improvement was appreciated in the cats receiving 2.5 mg/kg/day. In this study, the cyclosporine could be administered directly by mouth or mixed in food. The degree of efficacy was similar regardless of the route of administration.

In a follow-up to the aforementioned study, cyclosporine dose-tapering was assessed in 88 cats.[25] The cats were given 7 mg/kg/day cyclosporine for 4 weeks. Depending on response, frequency was then reduced to every other day for 4 weeks and then if possible to twice weekly for 4 weeks. By the study's end, 65 cats remained and clinical signs were controlled with twice weekly dosing in 57%, in 15% with every-other-day dosing, and in 22% with daily dosing.

In summary, the aforementioned studies support cyclosporine as an effective therapy to control the clinical signs and lesions of feline allergic skin disease. The labeled starting dose for the licensed product (Atopica for Cats, Elanco) is 7 mg/kg/day, and it can be administered with food or just after feeding. Daily dosing is continued for a minimum of 4 to 6 weeks, or until clinical remission, at which point gradual tapering of the dosing frequency to every other day and then twice weekly can be attempted. The author also finds that for those cats in which frequency can be reduced, if relapse occurs on twice-weekly dosing, some will respond favorably to three-times-per-week dosing versus returning to an every-other-day or daily dosing regimen.

Although there has been great interest in and anecdotal reports of utilizing cyclosporine to manage other immune-mediated and inflammatory skin conditions in cats, there is still limited published information. An abstract reported on utilizing oral cyclosporine to manage urticaria pigmentosa-like dermatitis in two cats, a Sphynx and a Devon Rex.[27] (See Chapter 27 for further discussions on clinical signs and treatment of this condition.) Both cats in that study exhibited marked pruritus along with skin lesions. They were treated with 7.5 mg/kg cyclosporine once daily and within 4 weeks there was approximately 75% reduction in lesions and pruritus.

An early study investigated the use of cyclosporine to manage six patients (three dogs, three cats) with immune-mediated skin disease and three patients with epitheliotropic lymphoma.[4] In this study, there were two cats with immune-mediated disease (one with pemphigus foliaceus [PF] and one with pemphigus erythematosus [PE]), and one cat with epitheliotropic lymphoma. All patients began treatment with unmodified cyclosporine at 15 mg/kg/day. None of the dogs or the cat with lymphoma responded well to the therapy. The cat with PE exhibited complete response within 2 weeks. The cat with PF showed initial partial improvement but then relapsed despite increases in the cyclosporine dose.

A later retrospective study compared the use of microemulsion cyclosporine with chlorambucil to manage PF in cats whose illness could not be controlled with glucocorticoids alone.[28] There were no significant differences in time to disease remission or overall disease response between the two therapies. Of the nine cats that received cyclosporine, eight were maintained on it for disease control; of these, six cats were eventually weaned off systemic glucocorticoids and maintained on the cyclosporine alone. Doses of cyclosporine used ranged from 4.4 to 7.4 mg/kg; frequency ranged from daily to twice weekly. Five of the eight cats remained controlled on some form of alternate-day dosing of the cyclosporine.

In another report, an Oriental Shorthair cat diagnosed with sebaceous adenitis was successfully managed with cyclosporine.[29] Initial dose was 5 mg/kg/day with complete remission noted at 3 months. The frequency was slowly tapered until the cat relapsed when the cyclosporine was administered every 72 hours. Treatment was then maintained at every-other-day dosing. In this same report, another cat was managed with cyclosporine for nonpruritic alopecia of 6 months' duration.[29] Biopsy results were supportive of an immune-mediated follicular disease but were not consistent with any previously described conditions. Cyclosporine was started at 5 mg/kg/day with almost complete hair regrowth noted within 2 months. It was continued on an alternate-day basis for 4 months, at which time it was discontinued with the cat remaining in remission. Another report on using cyclosporine to manage an immune-mediated folliculitide regarded a cat with disease resembling pseudopelade in people.[30] The cat was treated with 5 mg/kg cyclosporine twice daily. Improvement was noted at 1 month, at which time the dose was reduced by approximately half. The cat became difficult to medicate and relapsed, and the medication was discontinued within several months.

An abstract also reported on the use of cyclosporine to manage three Persian cats with idiopathic facial dermatitis.[31]

(See Chapter 27 for further discussions on clinical signs and treatment of this condition.) Treatment was initiated with 6 to 7 mg/kg/day microemulsion cyclosporine with control noted by 4 to 6 weeks. Two cats were followed up for 6 months. The lesions were noted to be more resistant to cyclosporine therapy during that time and the cats experienced secondary bacterial and *Malassezia* yeast infections. An additional cat in one of the previously presented allergic dermatitis studies was also reported to have this condition.[23] This cat's facial disease did not improve with cyclosporine therapy.

SIDE EFFECTS/ADVERSE EVENTS

The safety of using cyclosporine in cats has been assessed in a number of studies.* Fortunately, it appears to be well tolerated in the majority of treated cats. By far the most common side effects are GI in nature (e.g., vomiting, diarrhea, anorexia). In many patients these side effects are reported as mild and/ or self-limiting and do not require discontinuation of the drug.[20,22-24] In the largest studies assessing cyclosporine safety and tolerability in cats (the Atopica for Cats clinical trials and a retrospective analysis of adverse events in cats treated with cyclosporine for allergic dermatitis), GI events were seen in up to 35.1% of patients.[13,22,25,32,33] The greatest incidence of these adverse events was reported during the initial weeks of treatment and/or with daily dosing.[25] In many cases, adverse events resolved with continued therapy and/or reduction in frequency of administration.

In the Atopica for Cats clinical studies, mild temporary weight loss, particularly when on initial daily 7 mg/kg dosing, was reported in 20.5% of cats receiving cyclosporine.[13,33] Two of the 205 cats in those studies developed hepatic lipidosis due to excessive weight loss.[13] In the study assessing adverse events in allergic cats receiving cyclosporine, 14% (7 of 50 cats) exhibited weight loss.[32] Most lost between 4% and 14% of starting body weight, although one cat with concurrent diabetes mellitus lost half its body weight over 2 years of treatment. To avoid complications from excessive weight loss, monitoring of body weight is advised for cats receiving cyclosporine.[13]

Additional adverse reactions noted with greater than 2% frequency in cyclosporine-treated cats included lethargy and malaise, hypersalivation, behavioral disorders (hiding, hyperactivity, aggression), ocular discharge and conjunctivitis, sneezing and rhinitis, gingival hyperplasia (Figure 29-4), and polydipsia.[13,22,25,33] One cat of 50 receiving cyclosporine for allergic dermatitis developed a urinary tract infection (UTI) during therapy that was considered potentially related to drug administration.[32] Currently, there are limited data on the incidence of UTIs in cats receiving cyclosporine, although a recent study reported 15% of dogs receiving cyclosporine for 5 months or more had positive bacterial urine cultures.[34] In

*References 5, 12, 20, 22-25, 32, 33.

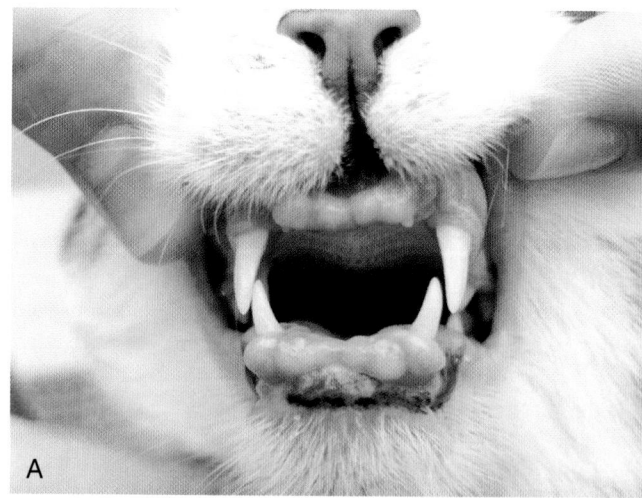

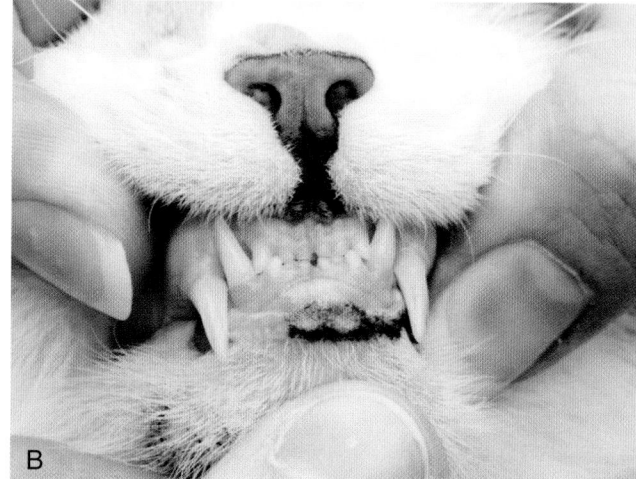

Figure 29-4: A, Gingival hyperplasia and/or overgrowth in a cat being treated with cyclosporine for allergic skin disease. **B,** Same cat as shown in **A.** Resolution of the gingival overgrowth following discontinuation of the cyclosporine.

the largest studies, therapy was discontinued in 14 of 205 cats and five of 50 cats due to unacceptable severity of cyclosporine-related adverse events.[13,32,33]

With the global immunomodulatory effects exhibited by cyclosporine, there is concern about impact on the immunosurveillance required to minimize risk of infection and development of neoplasia. Infection rates have been assessed extensively in large case series of renal transplant cats receiving cyclosporine; infections, both fatal and nonfatal, are frequent in this group of cats.[35-37] Incidence of infections was also monitored in the Atopica for Cats clinical studies. In these studies, one cat was diagnosed with the effusive form of feline infectious peritonitis and died 2 weeks after the normal study exit date.[13,33] Another cat was diagnosed with clinical toxoplasmosis but recovered with treatment and discontinuation of the cyclosporine.[33] Other infections noted in these studies included UTI, bacterial dermatitis, and otitis externa (of which the last two could also be a direct manifestation of the patient's dermatologic disease). All were reported in less than 2% of the study patients. In addition, clinical signs of rhinitis and conjunctivitis exhibited by some cats in these studies may support recrudescence of viral-associated upper respiratory tract infections. There is evidence that cyclosporine can lead to clinical signs of activated feline herpesvirus type 1 infection, although disease in affected cats most commonly appears to be mild and self-limiting.[38]

There have been additional reports in the literature of fulminant, fatal, systemic infections (e.g., toxoplasmosis, mycobacteriosis, and actinobacillosis) in cats receiving cyclosporine for skin disease or following renal transplantation.* Many of these have been for a single patient or a small number of cases, although even in larger series, disseminated toxoplasmosis and mycobacterial infections were uncommon. In one report of 169 transplant patients, there were five patients diagnosed with mycobacterial infections (two of which were disseminated) and two patients diagnosed with toxoplasmosis.[35] Another large series of 60 cases identified systemic mycobacteriosis in only one cat.[37]

There has been particular focus upon toxoplasmosis risk in cats treated with cyclosporine as cats are definitive hosts for this parasite *(Toxoplasma gondii)* and exposure is high in the United States with seroprevalence rates of approximately 30% to 32%.[39,43] In most cats, infection remains latent, but if active systemic infection develops (either via recrudescence of a latent infection or due to a new primary infection in a naïve cat), it can be very difficult to treat and can be life threatening. Common clinical signs that can indicate systemic or disseminated toxoplasmosis are fever, respiratory abnormalities (e.g., tachypnea, increased respiratory effort, increased lung sounds on auscultation, pleural effusion, abnormal thoracic radiographs) and evidence of liver dysfunction (e.g., elevated liver enzymes, hyperbilirubinemia, jaundice). Currently, the greatest risk appears to be in naïve cats that become exposed to *T. gondii* while being treated with cyclosporine.[13] In particular, the risk appears to be greatest in seronegative cats with serum cyclosporine levels greater than 1000 ng/mL.[44] In two studies, cats previously exposed to *T. gondii* did not exhibit recurrence of oocyst shedding nor signs of disseminated clinical disease when treated with cyclosporine.[33,43] It is not yet fully clear if there is absolutely no risk for cats that are seropositive and treated with cyclosporine, and risk may be a function of serum cyclosporine concentrations in individual cats.[44] Thus monitoring serum concentrations and ensuring that they are below 1000 ng/mL may be prudent in *T. gondii*–seropositive cats treated with cyclosporine. Furthermore, all cats treated with cyclosporine should be prevented from becoming exposed to *T. gondii.* They should be kept strictly indoors, prevented from hunting (including rodents and other hosts that may enter the home), fed only cooked or processed foods, and be quarantined for a period of time from any other cats newly introduced into the home.

The risk of developing neoplasia secondary to therapy has been another concern relative to cyclosporine use in cats. Certainly in cyclosporine-treated renal transplant patients there appears to be a greater risk of developing neoplasia post-transplantation.[45] However, there are a number of other factors unique to this population of cats (e.g., metabolic and systemic abnormalities directly related to the renal disease, chronic antigenic stimulation from the allograft, and generalized immune suppression) that may also be contributing to higher cancer risk. Studies of human transplant patients have shown increased incidence of cancer regardless of whether or not cyclosporine was used as a part of the immunosuppressive protocol.[45,46] At this time it is difficult to say if there is a definitive increased cancer risk in cats treated with cyclosporine for dermatologic disease. Currently, it is advisable not to use cyclosporine in cats with a history of malignant disorders, and it should be noted that it may exacerbate subclinical neoplastic conditions.[13] As more cats are managed with cyclosporine for skin disease (allergic and immune mediated), it would be useful to compare the incidence of malignant neoplasia in treated cats with the general feline population.

MONITORING

In the large-scale clinical trials assessing efficacy of cyclosporine in allergic cats, tolerability and safety were also closely monitored. Mean alkaline phosphatase, amylase, cholesterol, creatinine, glucose, and urea nitrogen were higher in cyclosporine-treated cats than in those treated with placebo.[33] Mean eosinophil count, magnesium, and chloride were lower.[33] However, all means remained within normal ranges. Other studies have also failed to identify any significant abnormalities in serum biochemistries or blood cell counts in cats treated with cyclosporine.[20,23,24] Various monitoring protocols have been advised by different authors for patients treated with cyclosporine.[2,11] Currently, before starting the medication, the author advises a thorough physical examination, ensuring that the cat is negative for feline leukemia virus (FeLV) and feline immunodeficiency virus (FIV), and indoor only, and evaluating baseline serum chemistries and complete blood count (CBC) with or without urinalysis with initial reassessment at 6 weeks. For cats maintained and stable on cyclosporine, reassessments (physical examinations with CBC, serum chemistries, urinalysis and/or urine cultures) are performed at 6 to 12 month intervals. The author reassesses cats that remain on daily dosing at the shorter end of the interval; reassessments for those on alternate-day dosing may not need to be as frequent.

The manufacturer of the licensed product (Elanco) advises that cats should be tested and found negative for FeLV and FIV before starting therapy and should not be treated with this medication if seropositive.[13] However, in one case series, two FIV-positive cats treated with cyclosporine did not express signs of active viral disease, and there

---

*References 28, 35-37, 39, 40-42.

are other anecdotal reports of using it successfully in retroviral-infected cats.[24] The use of cyclosporine in these cats warrants further investigation. However, until such information is available, the risk-benefit ratio of using the medication in FIV- or FeLV-positive cats should be carefully weighed and owners clearly informed that this is off-label use of the medication and may exacerbate viral disease.

When used for skin disease, monitoring cyclosporine serum concentrations is not routinely advocated. In the Atopica for Cats studies, oral bioavailability was highly variable both within and among cats and there was no correlation between serum concentrations and clinical response.[13] Instances where monitoring of serum concentrations may be advised would be to ensure that serum concentrations remain below 1000 ng/mL in cats seropositive for *T. gondii* or in naïve cats with potential risk of exposure to *T. gondii*.

SUMMARY

In summary, cyclosporine is an immune-modulating agent that is effective in managing manifestations of allergic skin disease in a significant portion of treated cats. There is also some support for its effectiveness in controlling other inflammatory and/or immune-mediated skin conditions, although additional research is needed to better characterize its efficacy for these conditions. In most cats, cyclosporine is well tolerated, although close to one third may exhibit some degree of GI upset, albeit of limited severity. Monitoring body weight is advised during treatment to prevent excessive weight loss and resulting complications. Monitoring for infections is also prudent and controlling exposure risk is important in treated cats.

References

1. Bernsteen L, Gregory CR, Kyles AE, et al: Renal transplantation in cats. *Clin Tech Small Anim Pract* 15:40–45, 2000.
2. Robson DC, Burton GG: Cyclosporin: applications in small animal dermatology. *Vet Dermatol* 14:1–9, 2003.
3. Marsella R: Calcineurin inhibitors: a novel approach to canine atopic dermatitis. *J Am Anim Hosp Assoc* 41:92–97, 2005.
4. Rosenkrantz WS, Griffin CE, Barr RJ: Clinical evaluation of cyclosporin in animal models of cutaneous immune-mediated disease and epitheliotropic lymphoma. *J Am Anim Hosp Assoc* 25:377–384, 1989.
5. Robson D: Review of the pharmacokinetics, interactions and adverse reactions of cyclosporin in people, dogs and cats. *Vet Rec* 152:739–748, 2003.
6. Mehl ML, Kyles AE, Craigmill AL, et al: Disposition of cyclosporine after intravenous and multi-dose oral administration in cats. *J Vet Pharmacol Therap* 26:349–354, 2003.
7. Matsuda S, Koyasu S: Mechanims of action of cyclosporine. *Immunopharmacology* 47:119–125, 2000.
8. Kuga K, Nishifuji K, Iwasaki T: Cyclosporin A inhibits transcription of cytokine genes and decreases the frequencies of IL-2 producing cells in feline mononuclear cells. *J Vet Med Sci* 70:1011–1016, 2008.
9. Aronson LR, Stumhofer JS, Drobatz KJ, et al: Effect of cyclosporine, dexamethasone, and human CTLA4-Ig on production of cytokines in lymphocytes of clinically normal cats and cats undergoing renal transplantation. *Am J Vet Res* 72:541–549, 2011.
10. Baumer W, Kietzmann M: Effects of cyclosporin A and cilomilast on activated canine, murine, and human keratinocytes. *Vet Dermatol* 18:107–114, 2007.
11. Kovalik M, Thoday KL, van den Broek AHM: The use of ciclosporin A in veterinary dermatology. *Vet J* 193:317–325, 2012.
12. Latimer KS, Rakich PM, Purswell BJ, et al: Effects of cyclosporin A administration in cats. *Vet Immunol Immunopathol* 11:161–173, 1986.
13. Atopica for cats [product insert]. Greensboro, NC, 2011, Elanco.
14. McAnulty JF, Lensmeyer GL: The effects of ketoconazole on the pharmacokinetics of cyclosporine A in cats. *Vet Surg* 28:448–455, 1999.
15. Katayama M, Katayama R, Kamishina H: Effects of multiple oral dosing of itraconazole on the pharmacokinetics of cyclosporine in cats. *J Feline Med Surg* 12:512–514, 2010.
16. Katayama M, Nishijima N, Okamura Y, et al: Interaction of clarithromycin with cyclosporine in cats: pharmacokinetic study and case report. *J Feline Med Surg* 14:257–261, 2012.
17. Miller R, Schick A, Booth D, et al: Absorption of transdermal cyclosporine versus orally administered cyclosporine in six healthy cats. In *Proceedings, 26th North American Veterinary Dermatology Forum*, 2011, p 198.
18. Miller WH, Griffin CE, Campbell KL, editors: *Muller and Kirk's small animal dermatology*, ed 7, St Louis, 2013, Elsevier.
19. Katayama M, Igarashi H, Tani K, et al: Effect of multiple oral dosing on fluconazole on the pharmacokinetics of cyclosporine in healthy beagles. *J Vet Med Sci* 70:85–88, 2008.
20. Wisselink MA, Willemse T: The efficacy of cyclosporin A in cats with presumed atopic dermatitis: a double blind, randomized prednisolone-controlled study. *Vet J* 180:55–59, 2009.
21. Kobayashi T, Momoi Y, Iwasaki T: Cyclosporin A inhibits the mRNA expressions of IL-2, IL-4 and IFN-gamma, but not TNF-alpha, in canine mononuclear cells. *J Vet Med Sci* 69:887–892, 2007.
22. King S, Favrot C, Messinger L, et al: A randomized double-blinded placebo-controlled study to evaluate an effective ciclosporin dose for the treatment of feline hypersensitivity dermatitis. *Vet Dermatol* 23:440–e84, 2012.
23. Noli C, Scarampella F: Prospective open pilot study on the use of ciclosporin for feline allergic skin disease. *J Small Anim Pract* 47:434–438, 2006.
24. Vercelli A, Raviri G, Cornegliani L: The use of oral cyclosporin to treat feline dermatoses: a retrospective analysis of 23 cases. *Vet Dermatol* 17:201–206, 2006.
25. Steffan J, Roberts E, Cannon A, et al: Dose tapering of ciclosporin in cats with nonflea-induced hypersensitivity dermatitis. *Vet Dermatol* 24:315–e70, 2013.
26. Guaguere E, Prelaud P: Efficacy of cyclosporin in the treatment of 12 cases of eosinophilic granuloma complex. *Vet Dermatol* 11(Suppl 1):31, 2000.
27. Guaguere E, Fontaine J: Efficacy of cyclosporin in the treatment of feline urticaria pigmentosa: two cases. *Vet Dermatol* 15(Suppl 1):63, 2004.
28. Irwin KE, Beale KM, Fadok VA: Use of modified ciclosporin in the management of feline pemphigus foliaceus: a retrospective analysis. *Vet Dermatol* 23:403–e76, 2012.
29. Noli C, Toma S: Three cases of immune-mediated adnexal skin disease treated with cyclosporin. *Vet Dermatol* 17:85–92, 2006.
30. Olivry T, Power HT, Woo JC, et al: Anti-isthmus autoimmunity in a novel feline acquired alopecia resemping pseudopelade of humans. *Vet Dermatol* 11:261–270, 2000.
31. Fontaine J, Heimann M: Idiopathic facial dermatitis of the Persian cat: three cases controlled with cyclosporine. *Vet Dermatol* 15(Suppl 1):64, 2004.
32. Heinrich NA, McKeever PJ, Eisenschenk MC: Adverse events in 50 cats with allergic dermatitis receiving ciclosporin. *Vet Dermatol* 22:511–520, 2011.
33. U.S. Food and Drug Administration: Freedom of information summary—original new animal

drug application: NADA 141-329—Atopica for cats (cyclosporine oral solution, USP) modified cats (PDF online): www.fda.gov/downloads/AnimalVeterinary/Products/ApprovedAnimalDrugProducts/FOIADrugSummaries/UCM287922.pdf. Accessed May 6, 2015.

34. Peterson A, Torres S, Rendahl A, et al: Frequency of urinary tract infection in dogs with inflammatory skin disorders treated with ciclosporin alone or in combination with glucocorticoid therapy: a retrospective study. *Vet Dermatol* 23:201–e43, 2012.

35. Kadar E, Sykes JE, Kass PH, et al: Evaluation of the prevalence of infections in cats after renal transplantation: 169 cases (1987-2003). *J Am Vet Med Assoc* 227:948–953, 2005.

36. Mathews KG, Gregory CR: Renal transplants in cats: 66 cases (1987-1996). *J Am Vet Med Assoc* 211:1432–1436, 1997.

37. Schmiedt CW, Holzman G, Schwarz T, et al: Survival, complications, and analysis of risk factors after renal transplantation in cats. *Vet Surg* 37:683–695, 2008.

38. Lappin MR, Roycroft L: Effect of cyclosporine and methylprednisolone acetate on cats with chronic feline herpesvirus 1 infection. *J Vet Intern Med* 3:709, 2011.

39. Barrs VR, Martin P, Beatty JA: Antemortem diagnosis and treatment of toxoplasmosis in two cats on cyclosporin therapy. *Aust Vet J* 84:30–35, 2006.

40. Last RD, Suzuki Y, Manning T, et al: A case of fatal systemic toxoplasmosis in a cat being treated with cyclosporin A for feline atopy. *Vet Dermatol* 15:194–198, 2004.

41. Bernsteen L, Gregory CR, Aronson LR, et al: Acute toxoplasmosis following renal transplantation in three cats and a dog. *J Am Vet Med Assoc* 215:1123–1126, 1999.

42. Griffin A, Newton AL, Aronson LR, et al: Disseminated Mycobacterium avium complex infection following renal transplantation in a cat. *J Am Vet Med Assoc* 222:1097–1101, 2003.

43. Lappin MR, Scorza V: Toxoplasma gondii oocyst shedding in normal cats and cats treated with cyclosporine. *J Vet Intern Med* 3:709, 2011.

44. Lappin MR: Infectious disease complications of cyclosporine use in cats. In *Proceedings, 26th North American Veterinary Dermatology Forum*, 2011, pp 14–17.

45. Schmiedt CW, Grimes JA, Holzman G, et al: Incidence and risk factors for development of malignant neoplasia after feline renal transplantation and cyclosporin-based immunosuppression. *Vet Comp Oncol* 7:45–53, 2009.

46. Wooldridge JD, Gregory CR, Mathews KG, et al: The prevalence of malignant neoplasia in feline renal-transplant recipients. *Vet Surg* 31:94–97, 2002.

Glucocorticoids in Feline Dermatology

Andrew Lowe

Glucocorticoids (GCs) are effective anti-inflammatory agents but have additional, unwanted effects on most other systems in the body. Despite advances in anti-inflammatory therapy, GCs remain one of the most commonly prescribed drug classes in feline medicine and in one study were employed in 16.68% of feline consultations in the United Kingdom.[1] Glucocorticoids are more likely to be used for dermatologic conditions than other clinical problems.[1] Cats are considered less susceptible to GC-induced side effects than other species, though potentially serious side effects do still occur. While there are a wide variety of synthetic GCs available for use, feline-specific pharmacologic and clinical studies of these drugs are scarce. Many currently recommended GC-dosing regimens for cats are therefore extrapolated from studies in other species and modified through clinical experience, though newer studies on this long-standing form of therapy are becoming available. Knowledge of how these drugs work, as well as the cat's unique dosing requirements and response to GCs, is essential for optimal case management.

MECHANISM OF ACTION

Glucocorticoids can exert their effects through a variety of mechanisms, including genomic and nongenomic interactions.[2] Genomic interactions involve binding of a GC to an intracellular glucocorticoid receptor (GR), located primarily in the cytoplasm (Figure 30-1). Once bound, the GR disassociates from a series of chaperone proteins including heat shock protein 90 (Hsp90), Hsp70, Hsp40, co-chaperone p23, and immunophilins FKBP52 and Cyp40.[2,3] This disassociation was thought to expose nuclear localization domains on the GR. Binding of these localization domains by proteins known as importins was believed to prompt the migration of the ligand-bound GR into the nucleus. However, it has been suggested that the binding of importins with GRs can be independent of GC binding, drawing this theory into question.[4] An alternative theory is that the protein 14-3-3 serves as a cytoplasmic tether for the GR in the absence of GC, and release from 14-3-3 may also be an important factor in GR migration.[2,3] Once present within the nucleus, the GR binds as a homodimer to specific regions of DNA known as glucocorticoid response elements (GREs) and may then either upregulate or downregulate transcription.[2,3] Many upregulated proteins, such as lipocortin-1, IκB, interleukin (IL)-10, and the glucocorticoid-induced leucine zipper, have potent anti-inflammatory actions while others, such as tyrosine amino transferase and phosphoenolpyruvate carboxykinase, are responsible for gluconeogenic effects.[2,3,5]

Squelching, tethering, and interaction with negative glucocorticoid response elements (nGREs) are all possible methods by which GCs can downregulate gene transcription.[2,3] Squelching involves the competitive inhibition by a GR of transcriptional activators for necessary co-activating molecules. Tethering involves the GR interfering with DNA-bound transcriptional activators with no direct GR-DNA interaction, but rather a protein-protein interaction between the GR and another transcriptional activator. Squelching and tethering are possible mechanisms by which GCs interfere with nuclear factor kappa B and activator protein-1, two transcriptional activators with products that include a host of inflammatory products.[2,3] Negative GREs are regions of DNA at which GR binding causes direct repression of gene transcription. Negative GREs regulate the expression of many proteins including corticotropin-releasing hormone and proopiomelanocortin.[2,3,5,6]

Genomic effects take some time to occur and are dependent on many factors such as the transportation time of the GC in the blood, the activation of the cytosolic GR, translocation of the GC/GR complex to the nucleus, binding of the complex to a GRE, and finally the transcription and translation of the protein itself.[7] However, some GC-induced events occur rapidly, within minutes, and cannot be explained by such mechanisms. These rapid changes may be mediated by nongenomic means.[7,8] Possible mechanisms by which GCs may mediate these nongenomic effects include specific interaction with the cytosolic GRs, direct GC interactions with cellular membranes, and specific interactions with membrane-bound GRs.[2,7,8] The chaperone proteins released from the cytosolic GR on GC binding may possess signaling properties of their own. Src, for example, is a protein released from the GR upon GC binding that leads to activation of lipocortin-1, which in turn possesses anti-inflammatory properties.[2,8] Glucocorticoids have also been shown to inhibit mitogen-stimulated respiration of cells such as thymocytes, and it has been proposed that this effect is due in part to GCs incorporating into the plasma membrane, altering its physicochemical properties and leading to inhibition of membrane-associated ion channels.[2,8] Such GC-induced alterations in transmembrane currents could have myriad effects.[8] Finally, a membrane-bound variant of the GR, arising from the gene which encodes for the cytosolic GR, has been detected.[7]

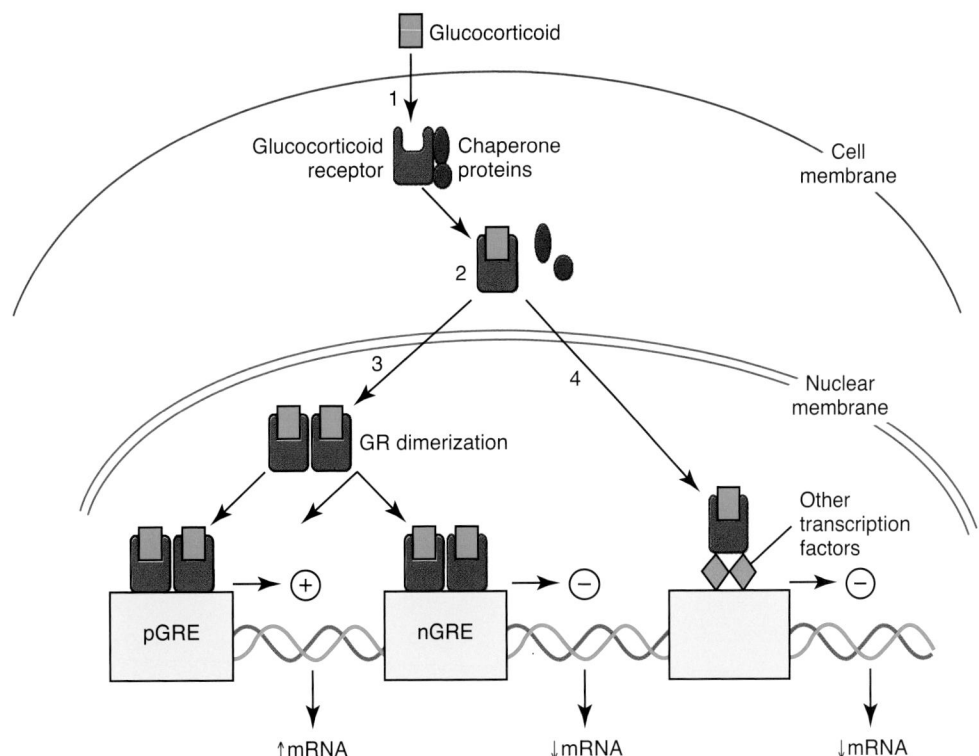

Figure 30-1: Mechanism of Action of Glucocorticoids. *1*, Glucocorticoids (GCs) enter the cell and bind to glucocorticoid receptors (GRs) in the cytoplasm. *2*, GR-associated chaperone proteins are released and the GC/GR complex moves through the nuclear membrane into the nucleus. *3*, The GC/GR complexes dimerize and bind to positive or negative glucocorticoid response elements (positive glucocorticoid response elements [GREs] and negative GREs) on genes in the DNA leading to increased or decreased messenger ribonucleic acid (mRNA) production respectively. *4*, GC/GR complexes may also interfere with the action of other transcription factors bound to DNA. (Reprinted with permission. From Lowe AD, Campbell KL, Graves T: Glucocorticoids in the cat. *Vet Dermatol* 19:340-347, 2008.)

Though the full role of the membrane-bound GR is unknown, it has been shown to be active and to cause rapid phosphorylation or dephosphorylation of at least 51 different kinase substrates after activation, which could alter signal transduction and influence gene expression.[7]

DOSING

In feline dermatology, GCs are most commonly used for anti-inflammatory purposes when treating diseases such as feline hypersensitivity dermatitis, or immunosuppressive purposes when treating diseases such as pemphigus foliaceus (PF). Divisions into anti-inflammatory and immunosuppressive ranges are somewhat arbitrary however, and it is probably more important that GCs be administered to desired effect given the lack of published evidence. There are a large number of synthetic GCs available for this purpose, but information is scarce as to which is best for the feline patient. The relative potencies of some of the more common GCs used in veterinary medicine are given in Table 30-1. These potency values are derived primarily from human studies. Although similar relative potencies likely exist in cats, there are few studies to

Table 30-1	Relative Glucocorticoid Potencies and Duration of Action of Selected Glucocorticoids

	Glucocorticoid Potency Relative to Hydrocortisone	Duration of Action (hours)
Short Acting		
Hydrocortisone	1	>12
Cortisone	0.8	>12
Intermediate Acting		
Prednisolone	4	12-36
Methylprednisolone	5	12-36
Triamcinolone	5-40	12-36
Long Acting		
Dexamethasone	30	>48
Betamethasone	25-40	>48
Paramethasone	10	>48

From Lowe AD, Campbell KL, Graves T: Glucocorticoids in the cat. *Vet Dermatol* 19:340-347, 2008.

validate this assumption. There is a particular discrepancy in the veterinary literature on the relative potency of triamcinolone. While it is typically cited as being five times more potent than hydrocortisone, some dermatologists claim that triamcinolone may be up to 40 times more potent than hydrocortisone.[9] In general these synthetic GCs have been developed to maximize beneficial anti-inflammatory activity and minimize unwanted side effects such as the sodium and water retention associated with mineralocorticoid activity.

One of the most commonly prescribed GCs in veterinary medicine is prednisone or prednisolone, though this is more because of familiarity rather than proven increased efficacy of this particular GC.[1] Prednisone is an inactive prodrug that must undergo hepatic conversion to the biologically active drug prednisolone. In dogs this process occurs efficiently, and these two drugs are considered bioequivalent. However, in cats the absorption or metabolism of prednisone is inefficient and approximately four to five times greater plasma concentrations of prednisolone are obtained when oral prednisolone is administered than when cats are given oral prednisone.[10,11] In cats, therefore, there is a clear preference for oral prednisolone over oral prednisone. Either prednisone or prednisolone can be used in dogs, but only prednisolone should be used for cats. Veterinarians may choose to stock only prednisolone, which is appropriate for both species, to avoid confusion. There are conflicting opinions as to whether prednisolone should be administered once or twice daily, although supportive studies are lacking. In the absence of any indication to the contrary, once-daily dosing is reasonable in a species as notoriously difficult to medicate as the cat.

Comparative studies are lacking, but it has been noted anecdotally that cats seem to require higher doses of GCs than dogs to achieve equivalent effects. This clinical experience is supported by work which showed that in two tissues evaluated, liver and skin, cats have approximately half the density of GRs as dogs.[12] Additionally, the GRs that were present had a lower binding affinity for GCs.[12] This mirrors the common clinical practice of recommending that cats receive approximately twice the dose of GCs necessary for a dog to achieve equivalent effects.[13-16]

One early study of four cats suggested a circadian rhythm of cortisol secretion with peak concentrations occurring in the evening, indicating that evening dosing was most appropriate for cats.[17] Subsequent larger studies have documented episodic secretion however, with no circadian rhythm of feline cortisol secretion; therefore, time of day is probably not a key consideration with GC dosing in cats.[18-20]

Center and colleagues[11] have shown that body condition is also an important consideration when dosing a feline patient, at least for prednisolone, which may not distribute well to adipose tissue. Obese cats, when dosed based on their actual body weight, achieved plasma prednisolone concentrations that were approximately twice as high as those of cats with an ideal body condition given a similar dose.[11] This correlated with the dosage based on the experimentally determined lean body mass of the obese patients, which was approximately twice that of the cats with an ideal body

---

BOX 30-1   Key Features of Glucocorticoid Dosing in Cats

- Use prednisolone instead of prednisone
- Cats require twice the glucocorticoid dose that dogs do
- Dosage based on lean body weight
- Time of day is unimportant for dosing

---

condition.[11] As obese cats may already be at risk for diabetes mellitus, further exacerbating this risk by not adjusting the dosage for lean body mass should be avoided. Key features of GC dosing in cats are summarized in Box 30-1.

Glucocorticoids are normally classified as short, intermediate, or long acting by the expected durations of their biologic activities, which may exceed the plasma half-lives of the drugs. In people, the potency and duration of a GC's anti-inflammatory effects roughly parallel the potency and duration of its suppression of the hypothalamic-pituitary-adrenal (HPA) axis.[21,22] Such information is summarized in Table 30-1. Again, similar studies are lacking for cats. Table 30-2 summarizes published studies of pharmacokinetics and duration of HPA suppression of GCs in cats.[23-26] None of these studies examined biologic half-lives. Pending further studies, it is assumed—and supported by clinical experience—that biologic half-lives in cats are similar to those in people.

Formulation also affects the duration of action of a GC. Although oral GC preparations usually contain the free steroid alcohol form of the drug and have the duration of action of the base GC, parenteral formulations come in variety of forms that affect drug solubility.[16] Sodium phosphate and sodium succinate are commonly bound to parenterally administered GCs. These compounds are highly water soluble, giving the drug a rapid onset of action. The duration of action is similar to that of the base GC. Acetate and diacetate are poorly water soluble, while pivalate, dipropionate, hexacetate, and acetonide are the least soluble. Glucocorticoids bound to poorly soluble compounds are slowly released from tissue and absorbed over periods of days to months, resulting in long-lasting, low concentrations. One of the most commonly used, poorly soluble GCs is methylprednisolone acetate. Methylprednisolone is an intermediate-acting GC with a duration of action of approximately 12 to 36 hours, but when given as methylprednisolone acetate the duration of action ranges from 3 to 6 weeks.[27] In general, rapidly acting oral or parenteral formulations are preferred over repositol GCs because there is less prolonged suppression of the HPA axis, a greatly enhanced ability to monitor and adjust the dosage, and possibly less pronounced side effects.[16] The use of repositol GCs should be reserved for those cats in which oral dosing is not possible because of patient or owner noncompliance. When treating any chronic condition over the long term with GCs, it is thought that the goal should be to achieve alternate-day dosing using an intermediate-acting GC to allow the HPA axis to recover on the "off" days. While the importance of alternate-day dosing has not been proven

Table 30-2	Available Pharmacokinetic Parameters of Various Glucocorticoids in Cats*			
	Time to Peak Plasma Concentration after Oral Administration (T_{max})	**Elimination Half-Life ($T_{1/2}$)**	**Bioavailability after Oral Administration**	**Duration of Hypothalamic-Pituitary-Adrenal Suppression**
Prednisone	1.44 h[10]	2.46 h[10]	21%[†]	N/A
Prednisolone	0.77 h[10]	0.66 h[10]	100%[10]	N/A
Methylprednisolone	0.5 h[22]	Multiphasic: From 0 to 30 min $T_{1/2} = 0.25$ h From 60 to 120 min $T_{1/2} = 1.7$ h[23]	82%[22]	4 mg/kg/day for 7 days: <7 days after the drug withdrawal[24]
Methylprednisolone acetate	0.75 h[22]	N/A	93%[22]	N/A
Dexamethasone	0.25 h[25]	1.41 h[25‡]	N/A	0.01 mg/kg: 6-12 h[26] 0.1 mg/kg: 32 h[18]

N/A, Information not available.
*Superscript numbers in table are citation numbers that correlate with the References section at the end of this chapter.
†Relative bioavailability of the active metabolite, prednisolone, after administration of prednisone.
‡Information not calculated by authors and graphically estimated from manuscript.

to be significant, such a strategy is not possible using repository forms of GCs.

Despite a lack of validation, reported GC dosage ranges do provide a useful starting point when choosing an initial GC dosage for cats, depending on the condition to be treated. In general, recommended anti-inflammatory dosages of prednisolone in cats range from 0.55 to 2.2 mg/kg every 24 hours, divided once or twice daily.[13-16] Anti-inflammatory dosages for other GCs can be extrapolated using the information in Table 30-1. In feline dermatology, the most common indication for anti-inflammatory GC use is likely hypersensitivity dermatitis. Wisselink and Willemse[28] found that only 45% of such cats experienced a reduction in pruritus at a dosage of 1 mg/kg daily by mouth (PO) of prednisolone, suggesting the upper end of this dosage range, or alternate GCs, may be most appropriate to induce remission of pruritus. Ganz and colleagues[29] compared methylprednisolone with triamcinolone for the induction and maintenance of pruritus treatment in allergic cats. Mean dosages of 1.41 mg/kg/day PO of methylprednisolone and 0.18 mg/kg/day PO of triamcinolone were found to be effective at inducing remission in 90.6% of cats. Mean dosages of 0.54 mg/kg every other day PO and 0.08 mg/kg every other day PO of methylprednisolone and triamcinolone respectively were effective in maintaining remission. These dosages are consistent with triamcinolone having a potency approximately seven times greater than methylprednisolone for treating pruritus in allergic cats, supporting the earlier reported opinion that triamcinolone is significantly more potent than often cited.[29] Allergen-specific immunotherapy (ASIT) is also frequently prescribed for the treatment of hypersensitivity dermatitis in cats. To generate such a prescription, allergy testing is necessary, though GCs may interfere with such testing. Cats given prednisolone (10 mg/cat/day PO for 1

month) were found to have decreased intradermal skin test reactivity for 2 weeks, though there was no effect on serum IgE reactivity.[30] GCs may also diminish the efficacy of concurrently administered ASIT, as suggested by studies in cats with experimentally induced asthma.[31]

Immunosuppressive dosages of prednisolone recommended for the cat range from 2.2 to 8.8 mg/kg/day.[15,32] At these higher dosages, some authors believe that division of the daily dose is indicated to decrease gastrointestinal (GI) irritation.[27] In feline dermatology, immunosuppressive GC dosages are indicated for the treatment of cutaneous autoimmune diseases, the most common of which is proposed to be PF.[33] There are few comparative studies to establish a superior GC type or dosage for treating such diseases, though the current recommendation is 4 to 5 mg/kg/day PO of prednisolone to induce remission of feline PF.[34,35] It has been previously estimated that only 35% to 50% of patients with PF are controlled with GCs alone.[36,37] Concurrent use of additional steroid-sparing drugs is therefore commonly prescribed. In a retrospective study of 15 cats, when combined with either cyclosporine or chlorambucil, prednisolone dosages of between 1.6 and 8.0 mg/kg/day PO or dexamethasone dosages between 0.10 and 0.38 mg/kg/day PO were found to be sufficient to induce remission of PF.[33] In contrast to the low success rate of GCs suggested by other studies, Simpson and Burton[35] found that prednisolone monotherapy, at a mean dosage of 2 mg/kg/day PO, was effective at inducing remission in 97% of cats with PF by 8 weeks. Most (67%) of these cats could be maintained on prednisolone monotherapy at a median dosage of 1.2 mg/kg/week.[35] Finally, a retrospective study of 57 cats with PF indicated that triamcinolone (dosage range 0.6 to 2.0 mg/kg/day PO) resulted in a higher remission rate than prednisone (dosage range 4 to 5 mg/kg/day PO), with remission rates of

100% and 62%, respectively.[38] The low bioavailability of prednisone may have contributed to the lower remission rate in this study.

SIDE EFFECTS

Carbohydrate Metabolism

Glucocorticoids interfere with a variety of pathways that result in insulin resistance and can potentially lead to overt diabetes mellitus.[39] Glucocorticoids antagonize the effects of insulin on the liver and increase hepatic glucose production, in large part by upregulating a rate-limiting enzyme in the gluconeogenesis pathway (phosphoenolpyruvate carboxykinase).[39] Glycogen synthesis is also stimulated through inhibition of glycogen phosphorylase and activation of glycogen synthase.[5] In peripheral tissues (primarily skeletal muscle), the insulin-dependent transportation of the glucose transporter type 4 to the cell membrane is inhibited by GCs, resulting in a decreased cellular uptake of glucose.[39] As well as inhibiting the action of insulin, GCs also directly inhibit insulin release from the pancreas.[2] Through these mechanisms as well as others, GCs may induce or worsen a diabetic state.

There is a strong association between high endogenous GC levels and diabetes mellitus in cats. In fact, approximately 80% of cats with naturally occurring hyperadrenocorticism suffer from diabetes mellitus.[40] Exogenous GCs have also been associated with diabetes mellitus in cats, and some authors believe GCs are more potent hyperglycemic agents in cats than in other species.[16,41] Studies directly comparing cats with other species would be required to validate this belief. However, some support for this theory exists in the literature comparing separate studies that showed no changes in blood glucose concentrations or glucose tolerance measurements after 28 days of treatment with prednisone at a dosage of 1.1 mg/kg/day in dogs, whereas cats treated with similar dosages of prednisolone (2 mg/kg/day) developed hyperglycemia and impaired glucose tolerance after only 8 days.[42,43] Glucose tolerance is defined as the ability of an animal to dispose of an oral or intravenous glucose load. Measurement of insulin sensitivity, defined as the ability of insulin to dispose of glucose, is a common method to assess changes in carbohydrate metabolism associated with diabetes mellitus. Diabetic cats have been shown to have decreased insulin sensitivity values compared with healthy cats.[44] In a recent study, cats administered immunosuppressive doses of prednisolone and dexamethasone showed significant decreases in insulin sensitivity values.[45] In addition, a greater decrease in insulin sensitivity was seen with dexamethasone, suggesting that at the dosages tested, this GC may possess greater diabetogenic effects in the cat than prednisolone.[45] The hyperglycemia and glucosuria induced by GCs should resolve in normal cats with drug withdrawal; however, in cases of pre-existing subclinical diabetes mellitus, or potentially with sufficient duration of therapy, glucocorticoid treatment may be enough to push a patient into a permanent diabetic state.

Skin

Glucocorticoids exhibit atrophic effects on the skin that may lead to epidermal and dermal thinning, follicular atrophy, easy bruising, and poor wound healing.[5] These effects are due to the suppression of both keratinocyte and dermal fibroblast proliferation, as well as suppression of various fibroblast-derived proteins.[5] Perhaps the most important of the suppressed proteins is collagen, but other components of the extracellular matrix such as tenascin-C, hyaluronic acid, sulfated glycosaminoglycans, and elastin are also downregulated by GCs.[5] Suppression of collagen synthesis and the necessary early inflammatory phase is likely responsible for the deleterious effect of GCs on wound healing.[5] A decrease in epidermal lipids and an increase in transepidermal water loss have also been documented with GC use, which contribute to the dry, scaly skin that can accompany use.[5] Similar clinical signs of cutaneous atrophy, alopecia, and easy bruising have been observed in cats secondary to both endogenous and exogenous GC excess.[46] In a non–peer-reviewed series of 62 cats with naturally occurring hyperadrenocorticism, 61% of cats were reported to have thin skin, 23% had hair loss, and 14% displayed bruising.[40]

Published reports of iatrogenic hyperadrenocorticism are rare for the cat. The cutaneous signs observed in 18 cats reported in the literature[47-52] are summarized in Table 30-3. The reason for GC administration in many of these cases was a pruritic skin disorder, and it is therefore unclear in some cases whether the cutaneous signs noted were due to the

Table 30-3	**Reported Cutaneous Signs in 18 Cats with Iatrogenic Hyperadrenocorticism**
Cutaneous Sign	**Number and Percentage of Affected Cats**
Hair loss	15 (83%)
Thin or inelastic skin	8 (44%)
Skin tears	4 (22%)
Hyperpigmentation	4 (22%)
Medially curled pinna	3 (17%)
Bruising	2 (11%)
Poor hair coat	2 (11%)

Data from Lowe AD, Campbell KL, Graves T: Glucocorticoids in the cat. *Vet Dermatol* 19:340-347, 2008; Scott DW, Manning TO, Reimers RJ: Iatrogenic Cushing's syndrome in the cat. *Feline Pract* 12:30-36, 1982; Lowe AD: Glucocorticoid use in cats, *Vet Med* 105:56-62, 2010; Ferasin L: Iatrogenic hyperadrenocorticism in a cat following a short therapeutic course of methylprednisolone acetate. *J Feline Med Surg* 3:87-93, 2001; Schaer M, Ginn PE: Iatrogenic Cushing's syndrome and steroid hepatopathy in a cat. *J Am Anim Hosp Assoc* 35:48-51, 1999; Lien Y, Huang H, Chang P: Iatrogenic hyperadrenocorticism in 12 cats. *J Am Anim Hosp Assoc* 42:414-423, 2006; Greene CE, Gratzek A, Carmichael KP: Iatrogenic hyperadrenocorticism in a cat. *Feline Pract* 23:7-12, 1995; and Smith SA, Freeman LC, Bagladi-Swanson M: Hypercalcemia due to iatrogenic secondary hypoadrenocorticism and diabetes mellitus in a cat. *J Am Anim Hosp Assoc* 38:41-44, 2002.

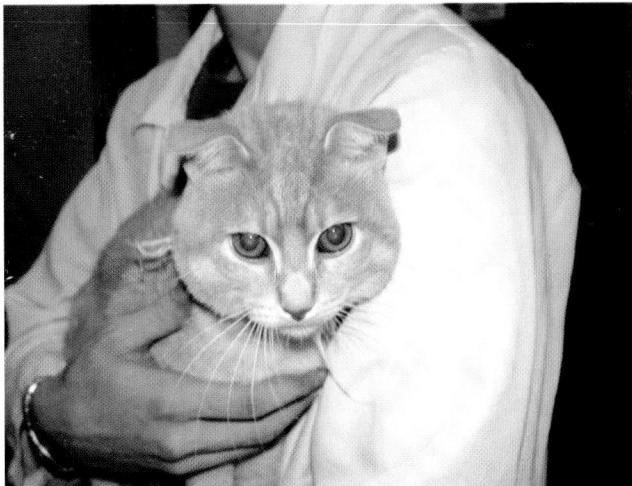

Figure 30-2: Curling of the pinnae in a cat administered immunosuppressive doses of dexamethasone for 2 months.

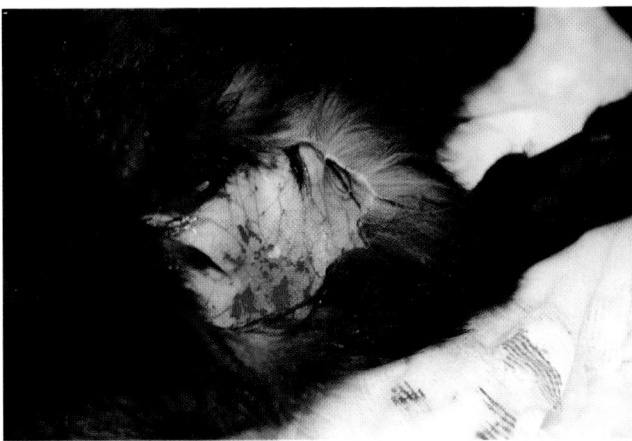

Figure 30-3: Glucocorticoid-induced cutaneous atrophy and fragility in a cat leading to a large tear in the skin with exposure of the underlying fascia.

disease being treated, or the GCs themselves. Two unique side effects of GCs in cats are fragile, easily torn skin and curling of the pinna[46] (Figures 30-2 and 30-3). The skin can become so fragile that even routine handling and restraint may lead to tearing and sloughing of large areas of skin, resulting in large wounds that are difficult to repair. Curling of the pinna is rare and may occur more commonly with iatrogenic disease.[46]

Liver

Cats do not possess the GC-induced isoenzyme of alkaline phosphatase (ALP), which is present in dogs.[53] The half-life of feline ALP is also only half that of dogs.[53] Consequently, GC-induced elevations in ALP concentrations, common in dogs, are rare in cats. Mild to moderate, and rarely marked, elevations of hepatic enzymes are however occasionally seen in cats secondary to GC use.[41,48,49,54,55] Additionally, palpable enlargement of the liver is not a common feature of GC use in cats as it is in dogs. Glucocorticoid-induced hepatomegaly

in dogs has been shown to be due to a vacuolar hepatopathy from glycogen deposition. These changes have been termed a steroid hepatopathy, which has been said to be unique to dogs.[16] Such steroid hepatopathy may be either asymptomatic, or the hepatic swelling and vacuolization can lead to cholestasis. Several studies have examined liver biopsies of cats either with natural hyperadrenocorticism or after GC treatment. Each has consistently shown excessive glycogen deposition in a typical vacuolar pattern, characteristic of a steroid hepatopathy.[40,41,49,54,55] Steroid hepatopathy does therefore seem to occur in cats, but may be less frequent or more difficult to induce or detect. Invasive tests such as liver biopsies may be necessary to document feline steroid hepatopathy as even abdominal ultrasound may fail to identify typical hepatic changes in some affected cats.[55]

Cardiovascular

Glucocorticoids have been associated with hypertension in both dogs and people.[5,14] The mechanisms are unclear but could include increased vascular sensitivity to the vasoconstrictive effects of catecholamines, sodium and water retention by the kidney due to mineralocorticoid activity, and decreased amounts of vasodilatory substances such as nitric oxide.[5,14] In cats, GCs have been associated with congestive heart failure (CHF) in a number of cases, even in the absence of known cardiac disease.[56,57] The most common GC associated with this side effect was methylprednisolone acetate, and signs were seen as quickly as 1 day following administration.[57] Congestive heart failure in affected cats was associated with hypertrophic changes; however, provided cats survived the initial crisis, the hypertrophic changes resolved over time upon withdrawal of GCs.[56,57] Cats surviving the initial crisis had prolonged survival times relative to cats with CHF due to other forms of disease, leading the authors to propose that cats may develop a unique form of GC-associated CHF.[57] A study investigating the mechanism of CHF in cats administered methylprednisolone acetate suggested that plasma volume expansion due to the hyperosmotic effect of hyperglycemia was the most likely cause.[58] In that study, despite the increase in plasma volume, systemic hypertension was not observed, nor was there an increase in total body water or a decrease in potassium concentration to suggest that a significant mineralocorticoid effect was involved.[58] A small but significant increase in interventricular septal thickness was also noted, although its clinical significance was unclear.[58]

Behavior

Though not as frequently considered as other side effects, GCs can also have significant effects on behavior. In both people and animal models, prolonged GC exposure leads to signs associated with depression.[59] Approximately one third of dogs treated with GCs have also been shown to develop some form of behavioral abnormality ranging from nervousness to aggression.[60] Though there are no feline-specific studies on the behavioral effects of GCs, it is reasonable to suspect, and anecdotally supported, that this species may also experience behavioral changes with GC use that would be important to communicate to owners.

Polyuria and Polydipsia

Dogs treated with GCs usually develop a rapid onset of polyuria and polydipsia (PU/PD) accompanied by a decrease in the urine specific gravity. Similar changes have not been documented in cats and in multiple studies GCs caused no significant changes in feline urine specific gravity.[17,40,41,55] Polyuria and polydipsia can occur in GC-treated cats, however longer treatment courses and higher GC dosages seem to be necessary to generate these signs than with dogs.[41,55] Consequently, interference with the release or action of antidiuretic hormone does not appear to be a major factor in the onset of GC-induced PU/PD in cats as it is for dogs.

Glucocorticoid-induced glucosuria has been documented in cats, and osmotic diuresis may be involved in the PU/PD seen in some cases.[40,41,45,61] In other cases however, PU/PD has been seen in the absence of concurrent glucosuria, suggesting additional mechanisms may be involved for some cats.[40,45]

SUMMARY

Species differences are important to keep in mind when designing effective GC treatment plans for cats. Key differences in the absorption, metabolism, potency, and expected side effects of GCs between cats and other species affect everything from the choice of GC, the GC dose, and necessary monitoring regimens. Knowledge of these differences is necessary for proper case management.

References

1. O'Neil D, Hendricks A, Summers J, et al: Primary care veterinary usage of systemic glucocorticoids in cats and dogs in three UK practices. *J Small Anim Pract* 53:217–222, 2013.
2. Lowe AD, Campbell KL, Graves T: Glucocorticoids in the cat. *Vet Dermatol* 19:340–347, 2008.
3. Tuckerman JP, Kleiman A, McPherson KG, et al: Molecular mechanisms of glucocorticoids in the control of inflammation and lymphocyte apoptosis. *Crit Rev Clin Lab Sci* 42: 71–104, 2005.
4. Freedman ND, Yamamoto KR: Importin 7 and importin α/importin β are nuclear import receptors for the glucocorticoid receptor. *Mol Biol Cell* 15:2276–2286, 2004.
5. Schacke H, Docke W, Asadullah K: Mechanisms involved in side effects of glucocorticoids. *Pharmacol Ther* 96:23–43, 2002.
6. Saklatvala J: Glucocorticoids: do we know how they work? *Arthritis Res* 4:146–150, 2002.
7. Strehl C, Buttgereit F: Optimized glucocorticoid therapy: teaching old drugs new tricks. *Mol Cell Endocrinol* 380:32–40, 2013.
8. Buttgereit F, Scheffold A: Rapid glucocorticoid effects on immune cells. *Steroids* 67:529–534, 2002.
9. Scott DW: Rational use of glucocorticoids in dermatology. In Kirk RW, Bonagura JD, editors: *Current veterinary therapy XII: small animal practice*, ed 12, Philadelphia, 1995, Saunders, pp 573–580.
10. Graham-Mize CA, Rosser EJ, Hauptman J: Absorption, bioavailability and activity of prednisone and prednisolone in cats. In Hiller A, Foster AP, Kwochka KW, editors: *Advances in veterinary dermatology*, ed 5, Oxford, 2005, Blackwell, pp 152–158.
11. Center SA, Randolph JF, Warner KL, et al: Influence of body condition on plasma prednisolone and prednisone concentrations in clinically healthy cats after single oral dose administration. *Res Vet Sci* 95:225–230, 2013.
12. Broek AHM, Stafford WL: Epidermal and hepatic glucocorticoid receptors in cats and dogs. *Res Vet Sci* 52:312–315, 1992.
13. Bondy PJ, Cohn LA: Choosing an appropriate glucocorticoid treatment plan. *Vet Med* 97:841–849, 2002.
14. Behrend EN, Kemppainen RJ: Glucocorticoid therapy: pharmacology, indications and complications. *Vet Clin North Am Small Anim Pract* 27:187–213, 1997.
15. Rhodes KH: Feline immunomodulators. In Kirk RW, Bonagura JD, editors: *Current veterinary therapy XII: small animal practice*, ed 12, Philadelphia, 1995, Saunders, pp 581–584.
16. Feldman EC, Nelson RW: Glucocorticoid therapy. In Feldman ED, Nelson RW, editors: *Canine and feline endocrinology and reproduction*, ed 3, St Louis, 2004, Saunders, pp 464–483.
17. Scott DW, Kirk RW, Bentinck-Smith J: Some effects of short-term methylprednisolone therapy in normal cats. *Cornell Vet* 69:104–115, 1979.
18. Johnston SK, Mather EC: Feline plasma cortisol (hydrocortisone) measured by radioimmunoassay. *Am J Vet Res* 40:190–192, 1979.
19. Kemppainen RJ, Peterson ME: Domestic cats show episodic variation in plasma concentrations of adrenocorticotropin, alpha-melanocyte-stimulating hormone (alpha-MSH), cortisol and thyroxine with circadian variation in plasma alpha-MSH concentrations. *J Endocrinol* 137:602–609, 1996.
20. Leyva H, Addiego L, Stabenfeldt G: The effect of different photoperiods on plasma concentration of melatonin, prolactin, and cortisol in the domestic cat. *Endocrinol* 11:1729–1736, 1984.
21. Melby JC: Clinical pharmacology of systemic corticosteroids. *Annu Rev Pharmacol Toxicol* 17:511–527, 1977.
22. Garg DC, Ng P, Weidler DJ, et al: Preliminary in vitro and in vivo investigations on methyl-prednisolone and its acetate. *Res Commun Chem Pathol Pharmacol* 22:37–48, 1978.
23. Braughler JM, Hall ED: Pharmacokinetics of methylprednisolone in cat plasma and spinal cord following a single intravenous dose of sodium succinate ester. *Drug Metab Dispos* 10:551–552, 1982.
24. Crager CS, Billon AR, Kemppainen RJ, et al: Adrenocorticotropic hormone and cortisol concentrations after corticotrophin-releasing hormone stimulation testing in cats administered methylprednisolone. *Am J Vet Res* 55: 704–709, 1994.
25. Willis-Goulet HS, Schmidt BA, Nicklin CF, et al: Comparison of serum dexamethasone concentrations in cats after oral or transdermal administration using Pluronic Lecithin Organogel (PLO): a pilot study. *Vet Dermatol* 14:83–89, 2003.
26. Peterson ME, Graves TK: Effects of low dosages of intravenous dexamethasone on serum cortisol concentrations in the normal cat. *Res Vet Sci* 44:38–40, 1988.
27. Cohn LA: Glucocorticoid therapy. In Ettinger SJ, Feldman EC, editors: *Textbook of veterinary internal medicine*, ed 6, St Louis, 2005, Saunders, pp 503–508.
28. Wisselink MA, Willemse T: The efficacy of cyclosporine A in cats with presumed atopic dermatitis: a double blind, randomised prednisolone-controlled study. *Vet J* 180:55–59, 2009.
29. Ganz EC, Griffin CE, Keys DA, et al: Evaluation of methylprednisolone and triamcinolone for the induction and maintenance treatment of pruritus in allergic cats: a double-blinded, randomized, prospective study. *Vet Dermatol* 23:387–e72, 2012.
30. Chang C, Lee-Fowler TM, DeClue AE, et al: The impact of oral versus inhaled glucocorticoids on allergen specific IgE testing in experimentally asthmatic cats. *Vet Immunol Immunopathol* 144:437–441, 2011.

31. Chang C, Cohn LA, DeClue AE, et al: Oral glucocorticoids diminish the efficacy of allergen-specific immunotherapy in experimental feline asthma. *Vet J* 197:268–272, 2013.

32. Cohn LA: Glucocorticosteroids as immunosuppressive agents. *Semin Vet Med Surg (Small Anim)* 12:150–156, 1997.

33. Irwin KE, Beale KM, Fadok VA: Use of modified ciclosporin in the management of feline pemphigus foliaceus: a retrospective analysis. *Vet Dermatol* 23:403–e76, 2012.

34. Halliwell REW: Autoimmune and immune-mediated dermatoses. In Miller WH, Jr, Griffin CE, Campbell KL, editors: *Mueller and Kirk's small animal dermatology*, ed 7, St Louis, 2013, Elsevier, pp 432–500.

35. Simpson DL, Burton GG: Use of prednisolone as monotherapy in the treatment of feline pemphigus foliaceus: a retrospective study of 37 cats. *Vet Dermatol* 24:298–e144, 2013.

36. Manning TO, Scott DW, Smith CA: Pemphigus diseases in the feline: seven case reports and discussion. *Vet Dermatol* 18:433–443, 1982.

37. Rosenkrantz WS: Pemphigus: current therapy. *Vet Dermatol* 15:90–98, 2004.

38. Preziosi DE, Goldschmidt MH, Greek JS, et al: Feline pemphigus foliaceus: a retrospective analysis of 57 cases. *Vet Dermatol* 14:313–321, 2003.

39. Andrews RC, Walker BR: Glucocorticoids and insulin resistance: old hormones, new targets. *Clin Sci* 96:513–523, 1999.

40. Feldman EC, Nelson RW: Hyperadrenocorticism in cats (Cushing's syndrome). In Feldman EE, Nelson RW, editors: *Canine and feline endocrinology and reproduction*, ed 3, St Louis, 2004, Saunders, pp 643–652.

41. Scott DW, Manning TO, Reimers RJ: Iatrogenic Cushing's syndrome in the cat. *Feline Pract* 12:30–36, 1982.

42. Middleton DJ, Watson AD: Glucose intolerance in cats given short-term therapies of prednisolone and megestrol acetate. *Am J Vet Res* 46:263–265, 1985.

43. Moore GE, Hoenig M: Effects of orally administered prednisone on glucose tolerance and insulin secretion in clinically normal dogs. *Am J Vet Res* 54:126–129, 1993.

44. Feldhahn JR, Rand JS, Martin G: Insulin sensitivity in normal and diabetic cats. *J Feline Med Surg* 1:107–115, 1999.

45. Lowe AL, Graves TK, Campbell KL, et al: A pilot study comparing the diabetogenic effects of dexamethasone and prednisolone in cats. *J Am Anim Hosp Assoc* 45:215–224, 2009.

46. Helton-Rhodes K: Cutaneous manifestations of hyperadrenocorticism. In August JR, editor: *Consultations in feline internal medicine*, ed 3, Philadelphia, 1997, Saunders, pp 191–198.

47. Lowe AD: Glucocorticoid use in cats. *Vet Med* 105:56–62, 2010.

48. Ferasin L: Iatrogenic hyperadrenocorticism in a cat following a short therapeutic course of methylprednisolone acetate. *J Feline Med Surg* 3:87–93, 2001.

49. Schaer M, Ginn PE: Iatrogenic Cushing's syndrome and steroid hepatopathy in a cat. *J Am Anim Hosp Assoc* 35:48–51, 1999.

50. Lien Y, Huang H, Chang P: Iatrogenic hyperadrenocorticism in 12 cats. *J Am Anim Hosp Assoc* 42:414–423, 2006.

51. Greene CE, Gratzek A, Carmichael KP: Iatrogenic hyperadrenocorticism in a cat. *Feline Pract* 23:7–12, 1995.

52. Smith SA, Freeman LC, Bagladi-Swanson M: Hypercalcemia due to iatrogenic secondary hypoadrenocorticism and diabetes mellitus in a cat. *J Am Anim Hosp Assoc* 38:41–44, 2002.

53. Hoffman WE, Renegar WE, Dorner JL: Alkaline phosphatase and alkaline phosphatase isoenzymes in the cat. *Vet Clin Pathol* 6:21–27, 1977.

54. Fulton R, Thrall MA, Weiser MG, el al: Characterization of hepatic pathology, serum chemistry and immunologic effects of prednisolone acetate administration in the cat. In Proceedings of the 29th Annual Meeting of American College of Veterinary Pathologists, 1988, p 18.

55. Lowe AD, Campbell KL, Barger A, et al: Clinical, clinicopathological and histological effects observed in 14 cats treated with glucocorticoids. *Vet Rec* 162:777–783, 2008.

56. Smith SA, Tobias AH, Fine DM, et al: Corticosteroid-associated congestive heart failure in 29 cats. *J Vet Intern Med* 16:371, 2002.

57. Smith SA, Tobias AH, Fine DM, et al: Corticosteroid-associated congestive heart failure in 12 cats. *Int J Appl Res Vet Med* 2:159–170, 2004.

58. Ployngam T, Tobias AH, Smith AS, et al: Hemodynamic effects of methylprednisolone acetate administration in cats. *Am J Vet Res* 67:583–587, 2006.

59. Sterner EY, Kalynchuk LE: Behavioral and neurobiological consequences of prolonged glucocorticoid exposure in rats: relevance to depression. *Prog Neuropsychopharmacol Biol Psychiatry* 34:777–790, 2010.

60. Notari L, Mills D: Possible behavioral effects of exogenous corticosteroids on dog behavior: a preliminary investigation. *J Vet Behav* 6:321–327, 2011.

61. Middleton DJ, Watson AD, Howe CJ, et al: Suppression of cortisol responses to exogenous adrenocorticotrophic hormone, and the occurrence of side effects attributable to glucocorticoid excess, in cats during therapy with megestrol acetate and prednisolone. *Can Vet J* 51:60–65, 1987.

Dermatophytosis: Decontamination Recommendations

Karen A. Moriello

Dermatophytosis is the most common infectious and contagious skin disease of cats, especially kittens. All cats are susceptible, but the most at-risk cats are those at the age extremes, cats with systemic illnesses that encounter another infected cat (e.g., the new kitten or cat), cats that suffer poor husbandry, and cats with chronic skin diseases that predispose them to self-trauma (e.g., chronically pruritic cats). It is not within the scope of this chapter to discuss details of diagnosis and treatment, and thus the reader is referred to references for further details.[1,2] However, successful treatment involves concurrent use of systemic and topical therapy, reasonable confinement to easily cleaned areas, and decontamination of the environment. Much has been written about decontamination of the environment; however, little is based upon actual controlled studies and/or field studies. Early controlled studies that led to many of the author's previous recommendations for decontamination were conducted before the importance of hard cleaning was known.[3] The two major goals of this chapter are to summarize known facts about environmental contamination and to present evidence-based information for best-practices recommendations (Box 31-1).

ENVIRONMENTAL CONTAMINATION

The Source of Environmental Contamination

A very common statement from clients when informed about the real possibility that environmental contamination is likely to occur is, *"You mean it's in my house!"* This comment is reasonable, given that most lay people are familiar only with mildew and media coverage of black mold (*Stachybotrys chartarum*), mold and sick building syndrome, or mold contamination after flooding. It is important to make it explicitly clear to owners that *Microsporum canis* requires keratin to grow and multiply, and the home environment does not support its growth. The only source is from the infected cat. Naturally infective spores are called arthroconidia. These are asexual spores formed by segmentation of existing hyphae. Their formation is a survival response to the depletion of nutrients or other environmental stressors.[4,5]

Disease Pathogenesis and Its Effect on Environmental Contamination

Studies on the pathogenesis of *M. canis* infection highlight important information relative to environmental contamination. Briefly, active infection requires exposure of susceptible skin to an unknown critical mass of viable arthrospores. To establish an infection, the spores must first adhere to the stratum corneum. After successful adherence, infection progresses with penetration of corneocytes via fungalysins (proteases), followed by the emergence of germ tubes and spreading hyphae. In the case of *M. canis*, adhesion is time dependent, starting 2 hours after exposure and increasing up to 6 hours after exposure.[6,7] Studies using feline reconstructed epidermis exposed to *M. canis* spores have shown that inoculation sites are culture positive, and the sites have fungal hyphae in the stratum corneum within 5 days after inoculation.[7] The clinically important points from these studies are as follows:

1. The incubation period from exposure to early infection in sites capable of shedding infective material is days not weeks.
2. The time from first active infection to clinically obvious lesions is 2 to 3 weeks.
3. Environmental contamination starts to occur long before clinical signs are noted.

Why Decontaminate the Environment?

The most commonly cited reason for environmental decontamination is to prevent infection of people and susceptible animals via naturally infective material in the environment.[1,2] In people, a major mode of transmission of tinea pedis (*Trichophyton* spp.) is through contact with contaminated objects (e.g., socks) or by walking barefoot in public areas such as showers or pools.[8] However, well-documented cases of human infection with *M. canis* from casual contact with a contaminated environment are rare in the literature. One well-documented case involved a 5-year-old boy who contracted *M. canis* from the interior of a used car.[9] There was no known contact with an infected animal, and investigation

BOX 31-1 Key Decontamination Recommendations

- Primarily, decontamination is necessary because a contaminated environment will result in false-positive fungal culture results, which make it difficult, if not impossible, to determine mycologic cure.
- Contaminated laundry items can be decontaminated via washing. It is generally not necessary to discard exposed pet blankets and towels.
- Exposed items that cannot be routinely laundered can be decontaminated via dry cleaning.
- Although vacuuming cannot decontaminate carpets, it is strongly recommended because it will remove hairs that may protect spores from carpet cleaning procedures.
- Water bowls, food dishes, and litter boxes can be easily decontaminated by aggressive cleaning and washing with detergent and hot water, followed by a thorough rinsing.
- Hair clippers are best decontaminated by hard cleaning, followed by autoclaving.

later found that child had contracted the infection from contact with contaminated textiles in the car. The car's previous owner had a dog with generalized *M. canis* dermatophytosis. There is little doubt that exposure to contaminated environments will result in cats being fungal-culture positive for *M. canis* via mechanical carriage of spores on the hair coat. Given that most cases of dermatophytosis are usually traced to some contact with another infected animal, it is hard to provide clients with factual estimates of the risk of another cat in the home developing true disease from contact with naturally infective material.

A study on cohabitant infection development as part of a treatment study had some interesting findings regarding the risk of infection from the environment. In the experimental study evaluating the protective effect of pretreatment with lufenuron, 24 specific pathogen-free juvenile cats housed in groups of eight cats per room were exposed to a single infected cat.[10] The infected cat had been experimentally infected with a strongly fluorescent strain of *M. canis* and was allowed to self-cure until the clinical lesions had resolved and only Wood's lamp-positive hairs remained in the preauricular area. Environmental and individual cat cultures were monitored weekly, along with examination for the development of lesions using a Wood's lamp. All environments and cats became readily fungal-culture positive shortly after introduction of the infected cat. However, infection-site development was slow, with lesions developing in a clear pattern. The cats that were most social became infected first, and the shy cats were infected last. The first place that lesions developed was on cat-to-cat contact sites (i.e., the face and ears). If casual exposure to spores in the environment were a high risk factor for contracting disease, it is reasonable to postulate that infection should have developed in all of the 24 cats in a similar period, but it did not. In other studies with group-housed cats, heavily contaminated environments never resulted in

reinfection.[11-15] Contaminated fomites are a known source of inoculation of infective spores and subsequent lesion development; however, the fomites invariably are items that not only deposit spores but also induce microtrauma to the skin (i.e., clippers, brushes, and gloved hands restraining cats). It is conceivable that a susceptible cat, especially a kitten or immunocompromised cat, could contract *M. canis* dermatophytosis solely from exposure to a contaminated environment, but this author believes it to be an uncommon source of infection. Excluding traumatic induction of lesions, one plausible scenario is a cat with an actively pruritic skin being exposed to a contaminated environment.

If *M. canis* infection in people almost always involves contact with an infected animal or an infected person and the environment is not a significant source of infection for cats, then why the emphasis on environmental decontamination?[16] The primary reason decontamination is necessary is that a contaminated environment will result in false-positive fungal culture results, which make it difficult, if not impossible, to determine mycologic cure. False-positive cultures may result in unnecessary confinement, which can be highly stressful for cats and/or interfere with the socialization of newly acquired cats or kittens. Moreover, unnecessary confinement can cause prolonged topical treatment of cats, as well as prolonged administration of systemic antifungal drugs. False-positive fungal culture results also increase the total cost of treatment of the infected cat. As will be detailed later in this chapter, research has shown that spores are more readily removed than what is currently believed. Environmental cleaning focusing on removal of spores to prevent false-positive fungal cultures is equally adequate to protect susceptible people or animals from infection.

Spores in the Environment: Are They Merely Viable or Truly Infective?

One of the earliest English-language publications documenting the long-term viability of *M. canis* spores was in 1960.[17] In the report, hairs from three different kittens with strongly fluorescing Wood's lamp-positive *M. canis* infected hairs were fungal cultured once weekly until there were six consecutive negative fungal cultures. The first negative cultures were noted at 6 to 9 months, and the last positive fungal culture was reported at 10 to 14 months. The remaining hairs were unable to infect susceptible kittens in an experimental infection attempt. These findings were very similar to those of another study, where 25 specimens were periodically fungal cultured. The first negative fungal culture was found at 14 months, and the last fungal positive culture was found at 18 months.[18] Very recently, this author found a cache of Wood's lamp-positive hairs in the laboratory that had been stored at room temperature in plastic vials. The oldest hairs were 21 years old. For pure academic interest, every possible attempt was made to determine if there were any viable spores present; after several months of effort, a single *M. canis* colony was isolated. A lay person reading this would conclude that *M. canis* spores live for over two decades in the environment.

This author's experience with thousands of hair and tooth-brush specimens from cats over the last 25 years is that some isolates will remain culture positive for up to 24 months, but clearly not all.[19] What is more commonly observed in the author's laboratory is for isolates to lose viability and become culture negative within months of collection. For example, in one study the carpet culture technique was used to collect infective hairs and spores from Wood's lamp-positive culture positive cats.[20] Specimens were logged and cultured within days of collection, using a cotton-tip applicator to confirm culture status; all specimens had too many to count (TMTC) colonies per plate. However, within 5 months of collection, 30% (45 of 150) of samples were culture-negative, including cultures made by direct inoculation of the carpet surface onto the surface of a fungal culture plate. In addition, another 10% of specimens had less than 10 colonies per carpet square.

In the author's experience with stored specimens, over time, the number of viable colonies that can be isolated from a sample markedly decreases. Often within months, the number of days from inoculation to positive culture becomes longer than 21 days, and laboratory manipulation (hydration and growth on enriched medium) is commonly needed to reach culture-positive status. Even then, the number of colony-forming units (CFUs) per plate is often less than 10. In addition, these colonies often have abnormal gross colony characteristics and microscopic features, and they are poorly sporulating. Finally, the hair shaft is protective (as in the 21-year-old viable arthrospore), but even arthrospores within hair shafts are very vulnerable to environmental conditions. For example, as the laboratory humidity increases, spore viability decreases. Specimens from containers that are repeatedly opened and closed are less viable than those that are sampled less frequently.[19] If spores are removed from hair shafts, as is done in one testing model,[21] spores remain viable for 1 week to 3 months if stored at 4°C, but, at room temperature, they rarely survive for more than 1 week.[19]

It is indisputable that arthrospores, particularly those protected within hairs and debris, may remain viable for years. Any client searching the literature will find this fact; however, several important things need to be impressed upon clients. First, all of the studies citing "culture-positive status" are reporting viability of spores on fungal culture medium; it is unknown how infective these spores are under natural conditions. Second, all of these studies stored spores under laboratory conditions, not in homes with temperature and humidity fluctuations. Third, these studies have used infected hairs, and the hair shafts protect spores. Simple mechanical removal of shed hairs removes the bulk of infective material and decreases risk. Fourth, spores not in hair shafts are vulnerable to mechanical cleaning and disinfectants. Finally, there is great variability in how long spores remain viable.

What Are "Reasonable Confinement" and An "Easily Cleaned Room"?

Owners are much more cooperative with respect to confinement when it is properly explained. Confinement will help shorten treatment time because it will make cleaning easier and minimize the spread of infective material that could lead to false-positive fungal culture results. The goal of treatment is to shorten the course of the infection and return the cat to its normal family life. "Reasonable confinement" means selecting how widely the cat can roam in the home, relative to its age and other conditions. Reasonable confinement does not preclude interaction with the cat. For example, kittens should not be left alone in a home unsupervised. It is important to remember that this disease occurs in kittens at the same time that socialization is needed. Older cats may not move around much to begin with, and thus strict confinement may be less of a problem. In addition, older cats may have other diseases that require intense monitoring. Some older cats will not eat or will not be easy to medicate if not in close contact with the owner. The human-animal bond cannot be ignored. Simple instructions on how to interact with the cat while it is undergoing treatment are needed. Owners should wear old clothes when they play with the cat and wash their clothes immediately afterward. Owners should avoid rubbing the body of the cat or kitten. Gloves are a reasonable recommendation, especially during the early stages of treatment. If children are in the home, the author prefers lime sulfur as a topical therapy for the infected cat. It is rapidly sporicidal and, after several treatments, it accumulates on the hair coat and provides a short-term barrier from spore contact.

Rooms can be converted to "easily cleaned rooms" with some minimal changes. Keep closet doors and furniture drawers closed. Long drapes can be temporarily removed or tied so that they are above the cat's reach. Remove any area rugs to minimize the need to clean these later. Plastic drop cloths placed over furniture are not recommended because of the risk of asphyxiation should the cat be wrapped up or tangled in it; moreover plastic drop cloths are unnecessary and excessive. If an owner has a cherished piece of upholstered furniture, simply remove it or cover it with a bed sheet to prevent it from collecting cat hair. All other furniture items need only be dusted. Washable cat beds should be placed in highly desirable places (e.g., in front of windows). Until the infection is resolved, replace all soft toys with washable plastic toys (e.g., balls). When explaining the meaning of confinement and an easily cleaned room, simply reframe the situation and ask the client, "what would you do if the cat had diarrhea that requires several weeks to resolve?" because this scenario would require similar preparations.

ENVIRONMENTAL SAMPLING

When to Obtain Environmental Samples

A common question from clients is, "When do we sample the environment?" In this author's opinion, the only time it is cost effective to sample the environment for contamination is when it is pertinent to the treatment plan. Based upon environmental culturing of homes where infected cats are living, environmental contamination is an expected finding.[22,23] Contamination was most severe in homes where there were kittens; *M. canis* dermatophytosis is more common in kittens, and often more severe than in adults.[22] There is no reason to sample the environment to document that contamination is present at the time of diagnosis. The cat merely needs to be confined to areas that are easily cleaned, and any exposed areas (especially where there is visible cat hair) simply need to be cleaned (see later). If a client has a strong reason to know that a specific exposed area is decontaminated (e.g., a child's bedroom), then environmental sampling is indicated.

Environmental sampling is most often recommended when false-positive fungal cultures are suspected because cats have been appropriately treated and the client has been compliant with reasonable confinement and cleaning. The problem of false-positive fungal cultures is most common when cultures are not performed in house and results are being reported as "positive" or "negative." In-house fungal cultures allow one to determine the number of CFUs per plate. If the cat is clinically cured, there are no glowing shafts on Wood's lamp examination, but the fungal culture is positive and there are 1 to 9 CFUs per plate, environmental contamination is most probable. Clinically normal cats with an active site of infection, appropriately fungal cultured, have more than 10 CFUs per plate (usually TMTC), even if the active infection site is limited to one whisker.

In the author's experience, cats that are culture-positive because of fomite carriage readily become culture-negative within 48 to 72 hours after being removed from the environment. Merely wiping the cat's coat with a damp towel is not always effective in removing spores. The best way to remove spores mechanically is to let the cat groom itself in a clean environment. In the home, the cat is housed in an unexposed room for 72 hours and then fungal cultured. Over the next 72 hours while the cat is living in a different room, the owner decontaminates the exposed rooms with two or three hard cleanings. The efficacy of decontamination is determined by two environmental fungal cultures: one obtained from the floor and the other obtained from surfaces above the floor that the cat can reach. If the cat is culture-negative, environmental contamination was the problem. If not, then the cat is infected, and a change to the treatment plan is needed. If the owner is appropriately compliant with cleaning, the environmental cultures should be negative. If environmental cultures are not negative, cleaning protocols need to be reviewed with the client and the "hot spot" of contamination should be identified.

Environmental Cultures of Nonporous Surfaces

Institutional and industry environmental sampling is done with a specialized culture plate called a *contact plate*. It is pressed against the surface of the target area. This is not a practical method for home environmental sampling. Using contact plates as the control, cotton-tip swabs, sterile gauze squares, toothbrushes, and disposable dust cloths (Swiffer, Proctor & Gamble) were compared. If surfaces were heavily contaminated, there was no difference between contact plates and any of these other sampling methods. When surfaces were less contaminated, sampling with Swiffer cloths correlated best with contact plates for hard surfaces and textiles.[20] Only one side of the Swiffer sheet is used, and an "X" is placed on that side. Target sites are dusted or swept until visibly soiled. Even if the client has just cleaned, surfaces almost invariably have some debris present. The sample is placed in a self-closing plastic bag. At the laboratory, the entire surface of the Swiffer with the X is pressed against a fungal culture plate. Samples should be stored until results are final in case the plate is readily swarmed with contaminant so that plates can be recultured. Fungal culture plates must be examined daily because they are often swarmed with other contaminants. If the environment is heavily contaminated, plates may show growth of just *M. canis*, often with highly suspect colonies within 7 days. Gross colonies compatible with *M. canis* morphology typically are seen in the second week of contamination. With the two-sample technique, the goal is to determine the efficacy of decontamination. Excluding carpeting (see later), repeated hard cleaning would readily decontaminate environments. If environmental contamination is found, it is important to remind the client that this represents what was present on the day of sampling. If cleaning has continued, a common finding is that repeat cultures of the target site are negative.

DECONTAMINATION OF NONPOROUS SURFACES

Hard Cleaning

The term *hard cleaning* refers to the mechanical removal of all gross debris via vacuuming, sweeping, or dusting of surfaces, as well as the mechanical washing of the surface with a detergent in water and thorough rinsing of the detergent from the surface. It is important to rinse surfaces thoroughly to remove detergent residue because some detergents inactivate disinfectants. Disinfectants are used to kill any spores not removed by hard cleaning.

M. canis spores are protected in hairs and debris, and they readily bond to dust particles; thus removal of this material is critical to cleaning. Surfaces must be hard cleaned until they are visibly clean. Hard cleaning alone can decontaminate *M. canis* contaminated surfaces, objects, or rooms. At one shelter, dermatophytosis was introduced into a group-housed room of cats. After the cats were removed, environmental cultures were obtained, before and after cleaning. Culture results revealed widespread contamination and that hard cleaning alone decontaminated the room.[24]

Special Surfaces: Wood Floors

The hard cleaning of wood floors is always a concern for clients. It is important to remind clients that fungal spores do not grow in the environment and therefore will not grow in wood. To the author's knowledge, there are no safe disinfectants for use on wood floors, especially because a contact time of 10 minutes is needed. The author has worked with many clients who have had environmental contamination of wood floors. The wood floors in homes were successfully decontaminated by daily removal of hair and dust using commercial dusting items (Swiffers and "sticky Swiffers"—see later). Floors were damp mopped using commercial wood oil soap for wood floors (Murphy Oil Soap, Colgate Palmolive).

Helpful Tools for Hard Cleaning

A number of cleaning implements can make hard cleaning less onerous. General dusting is best done using electrostatically charged dust cloths to remove cat hair and spore-laden dust from surfaces and items above the floor. Large amounts of gross debris are best removed with a vacuum cleaner. The ideal vacuum cleaner has a bag that will collect and trap debris, which is easily discarded, and does not vent excessive amounts of air. This is a common problem with canister wet-dry vacuums. If the vacuum cleaner has a bin, this could potentially contain a large amount of infective material, so gloves should be worn and care taken to discard contents directly into a paper bag (or similar) that is immediately placed in the trash for pick up. Brooms are problematic because cat hair becomes trapped in the bristles and is difficult to remove, so they need to be decontaminated after use. Alternatively, floors can be cleaned with Swiffers. Another excellent cleaning tool is a tacky dust cloth (e.g., 3M Easy Trap Duster, 3M, Minneapolis, Minnesota). The cleaning sheets are slightly "sticky," and thus they remove more floor debris than cloth or disposable floor cleaning sheets. The sheets are perforated so smaller sections can be quickly used to remove hair and debris from upholstery if vacuuming is not easily possible. Lint rollers are expensive to use on upholstery, but duct tape is an excellent inexpensive alternative. Floors can be washed with disposable floor cleaning pads (e.g., Swiffer Mopping Cloths, Proctor & Gamble). Another very helpful tool, especially in veterinary clinics, is a flat mop with reusable pads (e.g., 3M Easy Scrub Flat Mop, 3M). These come with an easily changed cleaner-on-demand dispenser. One pad and one detergent cleaner can be used for the hard clean, and a second pad can be used with the disinfectant. These are particularly helpful because they are very effective cleaning tools that prevent the use of a mop and buckets and excessive wetting of surfaces and decrease cleaning time. Over time, the cost of a reusable flat-mop system is less expensive than using commercial disposable wet mops. All of these cleaning tools are readily available on major Internet shopping sites or at cleaning supply stores.

Disinfectants

What to Look for on the Label

A common misconception among clients is that disinfectants are a first-line step in decontamination. To the contrary, disinfectants are used after hard cleaning to kill any spores not removed by mechanical cleaning. There is a much wider range of effective disinfectants so that enilconazole and various dilutions of household sodium hypochlorite (1:10, 1:32, and 1:100) are no longer the only options.[1] *Trichophyton mentagrophytes* is the most common test pathogen for labeling of antifungal activity although it was widely assumed that antifungal efficacy against the naturally infective form did not correlate. This was because early studies tested disinfectants in the presence of organic debris. Studies by the author found good correlation between disinfectant testing using the conidial form of *Trichophyton* and *M. canis* and *Trichophyton* isolated infective spores without organic debris.[20,25] From a practical perspective, this means that disinfectants with a label claim against *T. mentagrophytes* are an option if coupled with hard cleaning. It is important to read these labels because some products have multiple uses (e.g., cleaning versus disinfection) and require different concentrations and/or contact times.

"One-Step" Cleaners

The term *one-step*, often found on many disinfectants, is very confusing. Many clients will assume this means, "it is all I have to do." One-step cleaners are those that can clean a lightly soiled surface and sanitize it in one wipe. Test studies require documentation that shows 99% efficacy within 5 minutes against selective bacteria (e.g., *Staphylococcus*), but not against fungal spores.[26] Careful reading of products labeled as "one-step" cleaners will reveal a statement that if the surface is contaminated by organic material, the material should be removed via hard cleaning prior to the use of the cleaner. In addition, product labels may state that the disinfectant does not need to be rinsed from the surface. One-step cleaners can be used by clients for cleaning on days between hard cleanings.

Effective Antifungal Disinfectants

There are many effective antifungal disinfectants; however, several are worth special mention because of their widespread use in homes or in veterinary clinics. These compounds were also found to be consistently antifungal (no growth or less than 10 colonies per plate) when used at 1:10, 1:5, or 1:1 spore-to-disinfectant dilutions.[20]

Sodium Hypochlorite. The antifungal efficacy of household sodium hypochlorite has been well established, and either 1:10 or 1:32 dilutions are commonly used as a treatment control in disinfectant studies. Sodium hypochlorite at 1:10 and 1:32 is consistently antifungal, even after short contact times.[20] The only time household sodium hypochlorite has failed in the author's laboratory was when the stock solution was opened and out of date or the dilution was not freshly prepared. If household sodium hypochlorite is the disinfectant of choice, the stock bottles should be used within the "use-by date," and dilutions should be prepared once a week. Reasons not to use sodium hypochlorite include, but are not limited to: lack of detergency, potential to react with other chemicals to create toxic gases, unpleasant odor, damage to hard surfaces, discoloration of fibers and colored surfaces, damage to floor finishes, and rapid loss of efficacy once diluted.

Enilconazole. The antifungal efficacy of enilconazole is well established, and it is commonly used as a treatment control for disinfectant studies. It is available as concentrated spray or as a fogger. It is widely available in many countries, and in the United States is available as Clinafarm spray or fogger (Eli Lilly and Company). A major obstacle to more widespread use in the United States is that it is not available in reasonably priced small quantities. A 10-minute contact time is recommended even though enilconazole was antifungal at shorter contact times.

Accelerated Hydrogen Peroxide. This is one of the newer broad-spectrum disinfectants to gain widespread use in hospitals, veterinary clinics, and homes. Over-the-counter 3% stabilized hydrogen peroxide is antifungal, but it rapidly loses its stability.[25] Accelerated hydrogen peroxide (AHP) is a proprietary compound that is increasingly available worldwide. What makes this product different from over-the-counter hydrogen peroxide is that it contains surfactants (wetting agents) and chelating agents that help to reduce metal content and/or hardness of water. Water hardness may affect the efficacy of some disinfectants if high. This product has been tested using isolated infective spore suspensions of both *Trichophyton* and *M. canis*, and it is an effective disinfectant.[25,27] It is available as a concentrate or an over-the-counter ready-to-use form under several trade names. A 10-minute contact time is recommended even though AHP was antifungal at shorter contact times.[20] Of important note is that the Materials Safety Data Sheet (MSDS) states that it should not be mixed with a concentrated sodium hypochlorite product. When recommending this product to clients, it is important to make this clear. If a veterinary clinic were making the decision to use AHP as a disinfectant, it would be advisable to give serious consideration as to whether household sodium hypochlorite should be kept in the clinic.

Potassium Peroxymonosulfate. This is the main component of Trifectant (Vetoquinol) and has broad-spectrum antibacterial and antiviral properties. Early studies on the antifungal efficacy of potassium peroxymonosulfate did not reveal good efficacy; however, in those studies, the contact time was less than 5 minutes, and the spore-to-disinfectant challenge was robust.[21] In subsequent studies, this product was found to be antifungal against both *M. canis* and *Trichophyton* spp. when applied liberally and with a minimum contact time of 10 minutes.[27] Additional studies found a 2% solution to be more effective than a 1% solution.[20]

Over-the-Counter Products. One study investigated the efficacy of ready-to-use over-the-counter products as alternatives to sodium hypochlorite.[27] The criteria for selection were easy access by the consumer, preferably ready-to-use formulation, and label claim as antifungal against *T. mentagrophytes*. Active ingredients included sodium hypochlorite, quaternary ammonium, lactic acid, AHP, and an ethoxylated alcohol mixture. Products were tested with one and five sprays; all products were effective with a more liberal application and 10-minute contact time.

Frequency of Cleaning of "Easily Cleaned Rooms"

Again, the major concern of contamination in the home is false-positive fungal culture results. Even though infection in one or two cats can show large numbers of spores on environmental cultures,[22] contamination in the environment can easily be managed.[23] With the exception of completely noncompliant owners, the author has not encountered a home situation where decontamination was not possible.[28] In several instances, contamination was never documented even though infected cats were present in the home. In one field study, environmental culturing (*n* = 20) once weekly for 8 weeks in a treatment ward housing 16 to 30 cats showed zero to two sites of contamination 6 of 8 weeks and four sites of contamination 2 of 8 weeks (Figure 31-1). The ward was thoroughly cleaned and disinfected only twice weekly, with routine cleaning on other days.

For the pet owner with one or two infected cats receiving topical and systemic antifungal therapy that are reasonably confined, twice weekly hard cleaning followed by disinfectant is sufficient. Twice weekly decontamination is recommended early in the course of treatment, with once weekly decontamination being adequate as the cat(s) are curing. Between hard cleanings, it is important to remove hair and debris mechanically. One-step cleaners (e.g., AHP ready-to-use sprays or AHP wipes) can be used on days between cleanings. More aggressive cleaning can be done if indicated (e.g., because of false-positive fungal cultures).

Although not the focus of this chapter, it is appropriate to emphasize the importance of topical therapy. This will kill spores on the hair coat and greatly decrease spore shedding. Prior to the application of topical therapy, the hair coat should be combed to remove fragile hairs.

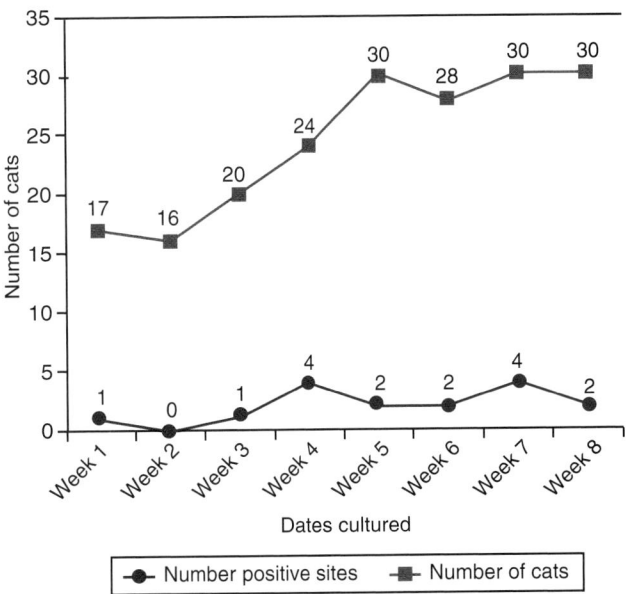

Figure 31-1: **Number of Cats and Number of Positive Sites over the 8-Week Sampling Period.**

DECONTAMINATION OF TEXTILES

Information in the veterinary literature on decontamination of textiles exposed to *M. canis* contamination is lacking. What is in the published literature describes findings associated with *Trichophyton* spp. because this is the most common cause of tinea pedis in people. Care must be taken when extrapolating this information to *M. canis* because it is a different pathogen, and spore contact with socks worn all day and/or contaminated shoes has no direct counterpart in cats.

The decontamination recommendations mentioned later are based upon experimental and field studies.[20,29] Almost all studies involving laundry items were conducted with a 15-year-old domestic top-loading washer and front-loading dryer to best simulate what might be in an *average* home. One field study was conducted using contaminated laundry washed in a 2-year-old front-loading washer and dryer. Pilot studies were conducted using both hot and cold water, with and without added bleach, to determine the most economical way to clean laundry items. Experimental contamination was done using isolated infected hair suspensions containing no less than 500,000 spores per mL and using sterile towels contaminated with infected hairs collected from toothbrushes. Laundry items simulating natural contamination used either actual soiled laundry from the cages of cats under treatment for dermatophytosis in a shelter or sterilized terry cloth wash cloths intentionally rubbed over untreated infected cats to simulate a "high challenge." As many "mistake protocols" were tested as could be conceived and included both the following single and combination events: the detergent was not added, the cycle length was short, the laundry tub was overfilled, the water level was low, and the laundry tub was not disinfected postcleaning. Suspensions of common laundry detergents were tested for antifungal efficacy, as were samples of wash water containing half cup of household bleach in a "regular" laundry load. Studies involving dry cleaning as a decontamination method were done using both experimentally contaminated items and naturally exposed items temporarily donated to the author; dry cleaning was done with informed verbal consent of the merchant. Hard surfaces (i.e., inside laundry tubs) were cultured using the Swiffer technique. Textiles were cultured using enough 90-mm diameter fungal cultures so that the entire surface of the item could be cultured by direct inoculation.

Please note while reading the following that studies showed that contaminated laundry items could be decontaminated via washing. It is generally not necessary to discard exposed pet blankets and towels.

Mixing of Contaminated and Uncontaminated Laundry Prewashing

Experimental studies looking at risk situations before washing used combinations of wet or dry contaminated laundry and wet or dry uncontaminated laundry.[29] Testing revealed contamination in all possible combination scenarios when tumbled in a dryer for 30 seconds in a large biohazard bag. The highest risk scenarios involved wet laundry items, especially wet contaminated laundry mixed with wet uncontaminated laundry (100% contamination of all towels).

Recommendation

Known or potentially contaminated laundry should be kept separate from all other laundry items. At-risk items should be stored in a plastic bag until washed and not allowed contact with other household laundry. From a practical perspective, this means changing bedding or towels in contact with the pet at the end of the day and just before it is feasible to wash these items. Wet contaminated laundry represents the highest risk situation, so it should be handled carefully.

Water Temperature

In the literature regarding humans, the recommended temperature for decontamination of *T. rubrum* from contaminated textiles is 60°C (140°F) versus 40°C (105°F) because this was consistently more effective.[30,31] Pilot studies conducted in a home setting revealed that to reach this temperature, the hot water heater needed to be set at "very hot." Although the temperature of the water entering the washtub was more than 60°C (140°F), this temperature was never maintained throughout the wash cycle no matter how low the water setting or short the wash cycle. In a home setting, this water temperature could result in accidental thermal injuries to family members if the hot water heater was not reset into a safe zone. In addition, to do several loads of laundry or repeat a washing of contaminated material, adequate time would need to be allowed for the hot water to heat. In multiple animal facilities, it is impractical to use this temperature. Finally, this is not energy efficient.

Using experimentally contaminated textiles likely to come into contact with pets (e.g., linen, terry cloth, and denim), twenty 90-mm swatches of each were washed in hot water (greater than or equal to 60°C [140°F], while the tub was filling) or cold water on a 14-minute cycle and cultured immediately after washing. This was repeated three separate times. All postwashing samples were culture-negative, regardless of water temperature.

Recommendation

M. canis contaminated laundry can be washed in either hot or cold water.

Bleach and Commercial Laundry Detergents

Commercial laundry detergent was not found to be sporicidal using an isolated fungal spore suspension test. Aliquots of tub water containing 4 or 8 ounces of bleach at this dilution were also not sporicidal. When the earlier experiment was repeated with 4 or 8 ounces of household bleach added to the water, there was no significant difference in the findings.

Recommendation

There is no preferred laundry detergent, and the use of household bleach as a laundry additive is optional.

Transfer of Contaminated Spores to Unexposed Laundry During the Wash Cycle

Experimentally contaminated and uncontaminated textiles were washed together to look for transfer of infective material during the wash cycle. Samples were cultured immediately after washing. Transfer of infective spores from either direct contact during agitation or in the wash water was not detected.

Recommendation

Transfer of infective material to nonexposed laundry is rare, but possible. This can be avoided by washing contaminated and unexposed laundry items separately.

Contamination of the Laundry Tub and Dryer after Washing

Experimental studies using textiles contaminated with spore suspensions showed no contamination of either the laundry tub immediately after washing or the inside of the dryer or lint trap. Contamination of the inside of the laundry tub or lint trap was found in the top-loading washer when heavily contaminated towels were washed. These towels had large amounts of visible hairs, many Wood's lamp positive, caught in the fibers before washing. When the surfaces of Swiffers used to sample the laundry tub were examined, intact hairs were commonly found. Contamination of the inside of the dryer was rare. Contamination of the lint trap (less than 10 CFUs per sample) occurred when laundry items contained large amounts of infective material; however, the air vented to the outside was more often heavily contaminated (e.g., more than 20 CFUs per plate).

The laundry tub of the top-loading washing machine was easily decontaminated after mechanical removal of hair via wiping with a towel and application of a disinfectant for 10 minutes. The lint trap was decontaminated by washing it in an all-purpose household detergent.

In a shelter with a dedicated building for the treatment of infected cats that used front-loading washers and dryers, contamination of the laundry tub, dryer, or lint trap was never found. This suggests that the newer high-capacity laundry machines are more efficient at removal of spores and contaminated hairs.

In a small field study, the insides of top-loading laundry tubs at three different public laundry sites were cultured. Pertinent to this study, small numbers of CFUs per plate of *T. rubum* were isolated several times, and samples were often culture-positive for a wide range of yeast and gram-positive and gram-negative bacteria.

Recommendation

For all laundry situations, assume that there is possible contamination of the inside of the laundry tub after washing. Mechanically clean and remove all hairs from the inside of the tub, spray the surface with a disinfectant, and keep wetted for 10 minutes. After disinfection, the tub can be rinsed by running a water-only wash cycle. Clean and wash the dryer lint traps after washing pet laundry. Be sure that dryer vents are not clogged and that there is adequate venting of air. The inside of the dryer is not likely contaminated, but, like all nonporous surfaces, it be cleaned mechanically. Suitable disinfectants include any over-the-counter bathroom disinfectants.

Efficacy of Routine Laundering to Decontaminate Laundry

Field studies washing towels from either the cages of cats being treated or towels rubbed over infected kittens consistently showed that the mechanical agitation of routine laundering was an effective method of decontamination of towels. In the most robust challenge, 50 face cloths were intentionally contaminated and washed in cold water on a long cycle, followed by drying on the highest dryer temperature.[20] Fourteen of fifty face cloths had 1 or 2 CFUs per plate, per side. When repeated, face cloths were completely decontaminated after two washings.

Even when the laundry tub did not reveal visible hairs when environmental cultures were obtained, the lint trap from the same load of laundry often had large numbers of hairs in it. Removal of hair is important in all decontamination procedures. In experimental studies and field studies, denim was the fabric most likely to be heavily contaminated with hairs, and in one experiment, it was the textile with the most number of positive cultures after washing. Denim is also one fabric that is most likely to be air dried by a client. Two washings were required to decontaminate exposed denim jeans.[29]

In laundry error studies, the conditions that resulted in residual contamination were predictable: short laundry cycles and overfilled laundry tubs. Even so, the contamination was never large (i.e., more than 10 CFUs per plate, per item).

Summary Recommendations

Although laundry detergent is not sporicidal, detergents have wetting factors that aid in removal of dirt from surfaces, and therefore their use is recommended. The use of bleach is optional. Laundry can be washed in hot or cold water. Agitation is the most important part of decontamination; therefore, wash laundry on the longest possible machine cycle, taking extra care not to overfill the machine. In most situations, one washing followed by drying is sufficient especially if a high capacity washing machine is used. Two washings immediately following each other are recommended if textiles are heavily contaminated with hair or organic material (e.g., food, feces, urine, or blood). Two washings for exposed denim items are recommended. After washing, the inside of the laundry tub and lint trap should be cleaned and disinfected. Follow this with a rinsing of the tub with a short cycle water wash. The inside of the dryer should be mechanically wiped clean with a detergent and soap. (Residual disinfectants may stain or discolor clothing if not thoroughly removed from inside the dryer.)

Dry Cleaning

Silk ties intentionally contaminated by rubbing them with infected cat hair and temporarily donated client-owned dry-clean-only items were successfully decontaminated by dry cleaning. All pet hair was visibly removed before having the item cleaned.

Recommendation

Exposed items that cannot be routinely laundered can be decontaminated via dry cleaning. It is important to remove hair from the fabric mechanically with a lint roller. Although the human health risk is low and dry cleaner personnel routinely handle clothing with gloves, place the items in a plastic bag and inform the merchant that the samples have been soiled by animals.

DECONTAMINATION OF CARPETS

Decontamination recommendations for carpets are based upon laboratory and field studies.[20] For these studies, sterile carpet squares were contaminated by vigorously brushing the coat of Wood's lamp–positive *M. canis*-infected cats. For the studies involving area carpets, Wood's lamp–positive *M. canis*-infected hairs were deliberately placed on the surface and rubbed into the carpet fibers using a sterile toothbrush, or carpets were contaminated by rubbing confirmed contaminated carpet squares or contaminated toothbrushes without hairs in the bristles on the surface to simulate areas where hairs had been removed but spores remained.

Pilot studies were conducted to determine both the best method of culturing contaminated carpets and whether or not repeat sampling had a significant effect on the culture results. Contact plates, toothbrush cultures, and Swiffer sampling were compared, and all were found to be equivalent in detecting heavy contamination. As few as 10 light Swiffer swipes detected heavy contamination; however, 20 hard Swiffer swipes consistently detected any degree of contamination. Gauze squares were also tested, but often spores were trapped in the fibers and not consistently inoculated onto the surface of a fungal culture plate. Two infected carpet squares were repeat cultured 25 times, either by repeated direct impression onto fungal culture plates or repeated culturing with a new toothbrush. Neither repeated-impression culturing nor toothbrush culturing decreased the number of CFUs per plate; the first and last fungal culture plate had TMTC CFUs per plate.

Carpets and Spore Viability

Research studies on carpet decontamination revealed some interesting findings. On carpets, spores may not be as viable as originally believed. As mentioned previously, 30% of samples previously having TMTC CFUs per plate at the time of receipt were culture-negative within less than 5 months, and another 10% had less than 10 CFUs per plate. Another interesting finding was that thorough wetting of carpets appeared to have a negative effect on the viability of spores. During review of the data, it was noted that carpet samples that had low numbers of CFUs per plate showed one of three patterns when cultured 24 hours after wetting. There was no growth, contaminant growth, or a sudden increase in the number of *M. canis* colonies at 24 hours (i.e., a "bloom"). The day 7 post-treatment samples were always culture-negative for *M. canis*. One can hypothesize that wetting rehydrates dormant spores and triggers sporulation, and, because of the lack of suitable nutrients (i.e., keratin), the spores die. The one thing worth noting is that these samples were free of visible cat hair. In addition, if naturally infected carpets (i.e., carpets infected after kittens have been playing on them) are cultured, different sites on the carpet will reveal vastly different culture results. At best, carpet sampling reveals what is found at that site of sampling; cultures can underestimate or overestimate the amount of contamination, depending upon sampling.

Vacuuming

Vacuuming carpets is commonly recommended as a means to decrease contamination.[2] The efficacy of vacuuming as a method to decrease contamination of carpets was tested on carpet samples ($n = 20$) that had been rubbed over infected kittens. There was no difference in the number of CFUs per plate cultured from any of the samples, even after a cumulative vacuuming time of 60 seconds. Cat hairs (often Wood's lamp–positive hairs) were present in the bin, and it was culture positive.

Recommendation

In light of the findings described earlier, under "Carpets and Spore Viability," although vacuuming cannot decontaminate carpets, it is strongly recommended because it will remove hairs that may protect spores from carpet cleaning procedures.

Commercial Steam Cleaning and Carpet Shampooers

A very common question is whether steam cleaning or carpet shampooing will decontaminate carpets. Steam cleaning or hot water extraction uses a combination of pressure, agitation, and hot water to remove debris. Depending upon the equipment, the water can be heated at the source (i.e., truck) to over 100°C (212°F); however, as it travels through the equipment, much of the heat is lost. With carpet shampooers, cleaning is achieved via mechanical brushing of carpets combined with vacuuming of soiled water. Both cleaning methods were tested using large area rugs, each of which had been contaminated in 10 sites with infected cat hair. In one site on each carpet, a larger quantity of infected cat hair was used so that it was easily visible from a distance. Carpets were cleaned within 24 hours of contamination. In both situations, contamination sites had TMTC CFUs per plate before cleaning, but culture samples after cleaning were different. The 20 contamination sites from the carpets cleaned with the carpet shampooer had TMTC CFUs per plate, per site. In contrast, only 2 of 20 contamination sites cleaned by steam cleaning had marked contamination (21 and 40 CFUs per plate). The remaining sites were either culture negative or had less than 10 CFUs per plate. One week later, all sites were not culture negative, but there was a continued increase in the number of culture-negative sites along with decreasing CFUs. In a final experiment, all four carpets were thoroughly soaked with water until it seeped through the backing and then cultured at 7 days after water treatment. Water treatment did decontaminate the carpets, but it took nearly 5 days for the carpets to dry, which is far from ideal in homes.

Chemical Decontamination of Carpets

Area rugs were contaminated as described earlier, but, in this study, the carpet surface was thoroughly wetted with water, and one of the following disinfectant chemicals was applied to the surface: AHP (AccelTB, Virox Technologies), enilconazole, potassium peroxymonosulfate (Trifectant, Vetoquinol), a quaternary ammonium disinfectant, 3.2% lactic acid (Lysol, Reckitt Benckiser), ethoxylated alcohol mixture (Simple Green, Sunshine Makers), a miconazole dog shampoo, a climbazole dog shampoo, and a ketoconazole dog shampoo. After the area was thoroughly wet with the disinfectant, each carpet was scrubbed with a deck brush and was then allowed a contact time of 15 minutes. After this, a carpet shampooer filled only with water was used to remove the chemical disinfectant and any debris. This took a significant amount of time because many of the products were sudsy. After the carpets were thoroughly dry, they were repeatedly cultured. Samples taken before treatment revealed TMTC CFUs per plate on all carpets. All of the commercial disinfectants decontaminated the carpets, and all three antifungal shampoos were effective. It is important to note that the carpets were not vacuumed before cleaning.

General Recommendations

Given that carpets are more difficult to decontaminate than other household items, the best way to decontaminate carpets is to prevent contamination from happening in the first place (i.e., keep carpets and infected cats separated). Vacuuming will not decontaminate carpets, but the mechanical removal

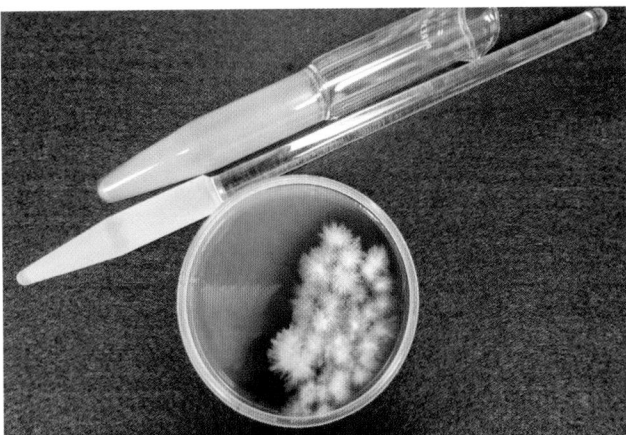

Figure 31-2: This figure shows the contaminated laboratory glassware decontaminated with a detergent and hot water, before and after culture (no growth).

of hair is important in minimizing contamination. It is very likely that over time, spores will spontaneously die in carpets. If carpet decontamination is necessary, it is important to keep small children away from wet carpeting. Infection occurs via microtrauma and inoculation of spores onto the skin. The bloom seen after wetting may represent a risk to children playing on carpets. Although proprietary carpet cleaners are not sporicidal, repeated carpet cleaning with water and detergent is one option. Another option is to vacuum, apply a chemical disinfectant, and then clean the carpets. Clients with concerns about using chemicals on carpets may want to consider using a commercial antifungal dog shampoo instead of a disinfectant. If a client is concerned about the safety of a disinfectant, refer them to the product label, and the MSDS can be consulted.

DECONTAMINATION OF BOWLS

Water bowls, food dishes, and litter boxes can be easily decontaminated by aggressive cleaning and washing with detergent and hot water, followed by a thorough rinsing. This protocol consistently completely decontaminates glassware used to prepare fungal spore suspensions (Figure 31-2).[19]

DECONTAMINATION OF HAIR CLIPPERS

Hair clippers are best decontaminated by hard cleaning, followed by autoclaving. If this is not possible, contaminated clippers can be decontaminated if gross debris is meticulously removed from all of the surfaces and then sprayed with an appropriate disinfecting product (e.g., Clippercide, King Research). The surfaces should be wetted for 10 minutes, and then the procedure repeated. It is important to remember to clean the plastic base and electric cord, as well.

SUMMARY

The best summary statement for decontamination is "if you can wash it, you can decontaminate it." The most important part of decontamination is the mechanical removal of debris and the washing of the surface with a surface-safe detergent until visibly clean (i.e., hard clean). This step removes the vast majority of infective material on hard surfaces. Disinfectants are only needed to kill spores remaining after the "hard clean." Many alternatives to household bleach are safer for people, cats, and home surfaces. One example is AHP. Cat owners can use any product registered as efficacious against *T. mentagrophytes*. Laundry can be effectively decontaminated with two washings, using either hot or cold water, if the laundry tub is not overfilled and the longest wash cycle is used. The primary goal of decontamination is the mechanical removal of spores to prevent false-positive fungal culture results, which make it difficult, if not impossible, to determine mycologic cure.

ACKNOWLEDGMENTS

Studies described in this chapter were funded by the Winn Feline Foundation, Merck Merial Scholarship Program, Companion Animal Fund (University of Wisconsin-Madison), an unrestricted gift from Maddie's Fund, and private donations. The author would like to thank the following people for providing the field specimens needed to complete these studies: Laura Mullen and the volunteers of the SPORE program at the San Francisco SPCA; Beth Rodger; Dr. Sandra Newbury and Dr. Rebecca Stunteveck from the Felines In Treatment Center (Fit Center) at the Dane County Humane Society, Madison, Wisconsin, and Hanna Hondzo for her laboratory assistance. Finally, the author is grateful to all of the cat owners and shelters that participated in field studies for this chapter.

References

1. Moriello K, DeBoer DJ: Dermatophytosis. In Greene CE, editor: *Infectious diseases of the dog and cat*, ed 4, St Louis, 2012, Elsevier/Saunders, pp 599–601.

2. Frymus T, Gruffydd-Jones T, Pennisi MG, et al: Dermatophytosis in cats ABCD guidelines on prevention and management. *J Feline Med Surg* 15:598–604, 2013.

3. Moriello KA, DeBoer DJ: Environmental decontamination of *Microsporum canis*: in vitro studies using isolated infected cat hair. In Kwochka KW, Willemse T, Von Tscharner C, editors: *Advances in veterinary dermatology*, Oxford, 1998, Butterworth-Heinemann, pp 309–318.

4. Aljabre SH, Richardson MD, Scott EM, et al: Dormancy of *Trichophyton* mentagrophytes arthroconidia. *J Med Vet Mycol* 30:409–412, 1992.

5. Barrera CR: Formation and germination of fungal arthroconidia. *Crit Rev Microbiol* 12:271–292, 1986.

6. Baldo A, Tabart J, Vermout S, et al: Secreted subtilisins of *Microsporum canis* are involved in adherence of arthroconidia to feline corneocytes. *J Med Microbiol* 57:1152–1156, 2008.

7. Tabart J, Baldo A, Vermout S, et al: Reconstructed interfollicular feline epidermis as a model for *Microsporum canis* dermatophytosis. *J Med Microbiol* 56:971–975, 2007.

8. Hsu AR, Hsu JW: Topical review: skin infections in the foot and ankle patient. *Foot Ankle Int* 33:612–619, 2012.

9. Thomas P, Korting H, Strassl W, et al: *Microsporum canis* infection in a 5-year-old boy: transmission from the interior of a second-hand car. *Mycoses* 37:141–142, 1994.

10. DeBoer DJ, Moriello KA, Blum JL, et al: Effects of lufenuron treatment in cats on the establishment and course of *Microsporum canis* infection following exposure to infected cats. *J Am Vet Med Assoc* 222:1216–1220, 2003.

11. DeBoer DJ, Moriello KA, Blum JL, et al: Safety and immunologic effects after inoculation of inactivated and combined live-inactivated dermatophytosis vaccines in cats. *Am J Vet Res* 63:1532–1537, 2002.

12. DeBoer DJ, Moriello KA: Investigations of a killed dermatophyte cell-wall vaccine against infection with *Microsporum canis* in cats. *Res Vet Sci* 59:110–113, 1995.

13. Moriello KA, DeBoer DJ: Efficacy of griseofulvin and itraconazole in the treatment of experimentally induced dermatophytosis in cats. *J Am Vet Med Assoc* 207:439–444, 1995.

14. Moriello KA, Deboer DJ, Schenker R, et al: Efficacy of pre-treatment with lufenuron for the prevention of *Microsporum canis* infection in a feline direct topical challenge model. *Vet Dermatol* 15:357–362, 2004.

15. DeBoer DJ, Moriello KA: Inability of two topical treatments to influence the course of experimentally induced dermatophytosis in cats. *J Am Vet Med Assoc* 207:52–57, 1995.

16. Snider R, Landers S, Levy ML: The ringworm riddle: an outbreak of *Microsporum canis* in the nursery. *Pediatr Infect Dis J* 12:145–148, 1993.

17. Keep JM: The viability of *Microsporum canis* on isolated cat hair. *Aust Vet J* 36:277–278, 1960.

18. Sparkes AH, Werrett G, Stokes CR, et al: *Microsporum canis*: Inapparent carriage by cats and the viability of arthrospores. *J Small Anim Pract* 35:397–401, 1994.

19. Moriello KA: Unpublished laboratory observations. University of Wisconsin-Madison.

20. Moriello KA: Unpublished decontamination studies. University of Wisconsin-Madison, 2013.

21. Moriello KA, Deboer DJ, Volk LM, et al: Development of an *in vitro*, isolated, infected spore testing model for disinfectant testing of *Microsporum canis* isolates. *Vet Dermatol* 15:175–180, 2004.

22. Mancianti F, Nardoni S, Corazza M, et al: Environmental detection of *Microsporum canis* arthrospores in the households of infected cats and dogs. *J Feline Med Surg* 5:323–328, 2003.

23. Heinrich K, Newbury S, Verbrugge M, et al: Detection of environmental contamination with *Microsporum canis* arthrospores in exposed homes and efficacy of the triple cleaning decontamination technique. *Vet Dermatol* 16:204–205, 2005.

24. Moriello KA, Newbury SN: Unpublished data. 2005.

25. Moriello KA, Hondzo H: Efficacy of disinfectants containing accelerated hydrogen peroxide against conidial arthrospores and isolated infective spores of *Microsporum canis* and *Trichophyton* spp. *Vet Dermatol* 25:191–194, 2014. doi: 10.1111/vde.12122.

26. United States Environmental Protection Agency Sanitizer Test For Inanimate Surfaces 2012: <http://www.epa.gov/>, (Accessed April 1, 2014.)

27. Moriello KA, Kunder D, Hondzo H: Efficacy of eight commercial disinfectants against *Microsporum canis* and *Trichophyton* spp. infective spores on an experimentally contaminated textile surface. *Vet Dermatol* 24:621–e152, 2013.

28. Moriello K: Unpublished field study data. University of Wisconsin-Madison, 2003-2013.

29. Moriello K: Decontamination of laundry exposed to *Microsporum canis* hairs and spores. *J Feline Med Surg* 2015. [ahead of print].

30. Hammer TR, Mucha H, Hoefer D: Infection risk by dermatophytes during storage and after domestic laundry and their temperature-dependent inactivation. *Mycopathologia* 171:43–49, 2011.

31. Amichai B, Grunwald MH, Davidovici B, et al: The effect of domestic laundry processes on fungal contamination of socks. *Int J Dermatol* 52:1392–1394, 2013.

Recognition of and Approach to Feline Cutaneous Reaction Patterns

Adam P. Patterson and Alison Diesel

With regard to the manifestations of feline skin disease, the phrase "cats are not small dogs" cannot be overemphasized. Feline patients present a unique clinical challenge in terms of dermatologic abnormalities. Their clinical lesions are often visibly more severe, more striking, and more marked with regard to improvement seen with successful therapy when compared to their canine counterparts. Likewise, the recognition of pruritus, by the owner and veterinarian alike, can be frustratingly difficult compared with the dog because of the normal grooming tendencies of cats. After retrieving and uncovering pertinent historical clues, diagnosis of skin disease in the cat first begins by surveying the cutaneous landscape from a bird's eye vantage in hopes of observing one or more clinically recognizable reactive patterns. Cutaneous reaction patterns are common arrangements of lesions in cats that reflect the skin's response to various inflammatory stimuli, which may or may not manifest with concurrent pruritus. The reaction patterns themselves are just that: patterns, not definitive diagnoses. Indeed, cutaneous reaction patterns are often indicative of feline allergic skin disease (Table 32-1), but other differentials, namely infectious and parasitic etiologies, must be considered and systematically excluded (Table 32-2) before a making diagnosis of allergy.

CLINICAL PRESENTATION OF CUTANEOUS REACTION PATTERNS

Self-Induced Alopecia

Also termed "feline symmetrical alopecia" and "fur mowing," cats with self-induced alopecia (SIA) will overgroom and barber to the point of partial to near complete alopecia of the affected body region (Figure 32-1). On close inspection, hairs typically appear broken (barbered) where the cat has chewed them off. The skin in the alopecic areas may or may not be erythematous or excoriated. Excessive hairball production may also be reported as cats will ingest a large amount of hair as they overgroom; in fact, the owners may initially present them for the clinical complaint of vomiting. This reaction pattern has historically been overdiagnosed as feline psychogenic alopecia. However, when cats fitting the pattern of SIA were evaluated more closely in one study, the majority were noted to have various medical conditions that responded favorably to antipruritic agents, as opposed to behavior

modifying medications. Cutaneous adverse reaction to food, atopic dermatitis, and other undefined hypersensitivity reactions were reported most commonly in the group of cats evaluated in the study.[1]

Based on the location of the SIA, other nondermatologic conditions should be considered. For example, SIA centered on the ventral abdomen may be indicative of bladder discomfort, abdominal pain, or even spinal or back pain. Therefore, a complete, thorough physical examination is indicated for these patients.

Miliary Dermatitis

Named for lesions resembling millet seeds (small grains), miliary dermatitis (MD) will often best be palpated as opposed to visualized. The lesions are small, pinpoint, erythematous, crusted papules present on any haired body region, normally on pericervical skin or along the dorsal topline (Figure 32-2). Lesions are usually more identifiable with tactile examination (analogous to reading Braille) as opposed to visible observation because of the dense undercoat of the cat and the frequent paucity of associated alopecia. These lesions will feel like small grits or grains on the skin, giving the palpable impression of petting coarse sandpaper. However, the sparsely haired region of preauricular skin can be a good location to visualize the crusted papules of MD. This reaction pattern is more commonly seen in cats with flea allergy dermatitis than other allergic conditions,[2] but as with the cat presenting with SIA, other etiologies should be considered. Mastocytosis (urticaria pigmentosa-like dermatitis; see Chapter 27 for further discussion) and Bowenoid *in situ* carcinoma are differential diagnoses to consider, particularly if miliary lesions do not respond to appropriate antibiotic therapy and/or antipruritic interventions.

Cervicofacial Dermatitis

Cats presenting with cervicofacial dermatitis (CFD) have lesions that are restricted to the cranial portion of the patient. Caudal to the neck, the skin will generally appear normal; however, the face, ears, and neck may be marked with excoriation, erythema, crusts, and alopecia (Figure 32-3). Frequently, these lesions are partially symmetrically distributed in the affected body regions. Because this cutaneous reaction pattern

Table 32-1 Cutaneous Reaction Patterns Associated with Allergic Skin Disease in Cats*

Allergic Skin Disease	Fleabite ($n = 146$)	Food Related ($n = 61$)	Environmental ($n = 100$)
Miliary dermatitis (%)	35	20	18
Eosinophilic granuloma complex (%)	14	25	26
Cervicofacial dermatitis (%)	38	64	56
Self-induced alopecia (%)	39	43	57
At least one of previous four presentations (%)	91	94	95
Multiple patterns (%)	28	46	46

*Results of a multicenter prospective study[2] involving 502 pruritic cats of which 381 were diagnosed with hypersensitivity dermatitis. Regardless of the offending allergen (flea, food, or environmental), at least one type of reaction pattern was observed in 90% of study cats. Several cats presented with more than one cutaneous reaction pattern.

Table 32-2 Probable Differential Diagnoses for Feline Cutaneous Reaction Patterns

	Self-Induced Alopecia	Miliary Dermatitis	Cervicofacial Dermatitis	Eosinophilic Granuloma Complex
Infectious	Pyoderma *Malassezia* dermatitis Dermatophytosis	Pyoderma Dermatophytosis Papillomavirus Feline cowpox virus	Pyoderma *Malassezia* dermatitis Dermatophytosis feline herpesvirus type 1 (FHV-1)	Deep pyoderma Mycobacteriosis Deep mycosis Feline cowpox virus FHV-1 Calicivirus
Parasitic	Fleas Pediculosis Trombiculiasis Cheyletiellosis Demodicosis *(D. gatoi)*	Fleas Pediculosis Trombiculosis Cheyletiellosis Otodectosis Notoedric mange Demodicosis	Fleas Pediculosis Trombiculosis Cheyletiellosis Otodectosis Notoedric mange Sarcoptic mange Demodicosis	Fleas *Cutereba*
Allergy	Fleabite Mosquito bite Food related Environmental	Fleabite Mosquito bite Food related Environmental	Fleabite Mosquito bite Food related Environmental	Fleabite Mosquito bite Food related Environmental
Autoimmune/immune-mediated		Pemphigus foliaceus Erythema multiforme Drug reaction	Pemphigus foliaceus Erythema multiforme Vasculitis Drug reaction	Erythema multiforme Vasculitis Drug reaction
Metabolic	Hyperthyroidism Hyperadrenocorticism Diabetes mellitus	Fatty acid deficiency Biotin deficiency		Xanthoma
Neoplastic	Paraneoplastic	Bowenoid *in situ* Squamous cell carcinoma Hair follicle tumor	Bowenoid *in situ* Squamous cell carcinoma Mast cell tumor	Squamous cell carcinoma Mast cell tumor Cutaneous lymphoma Mammary adenocarcinoma Hair follicle tumor
Other	Psychogenic Interstitial cystitis Anal sacculitis Orthopedic pain Hyperesthesia syndrome	Mastocytosis or urticaria pigmentosa Hypereosinophilic syndrome	Burn Mastocytosis or urticaria pigmentosa Hypereosinophilic syndrome Methimazole side effect	Burn Trauma Foreign body Mastocytosis or urticaria pigmentosa Hypereosinophilic syndrome Idiopathy

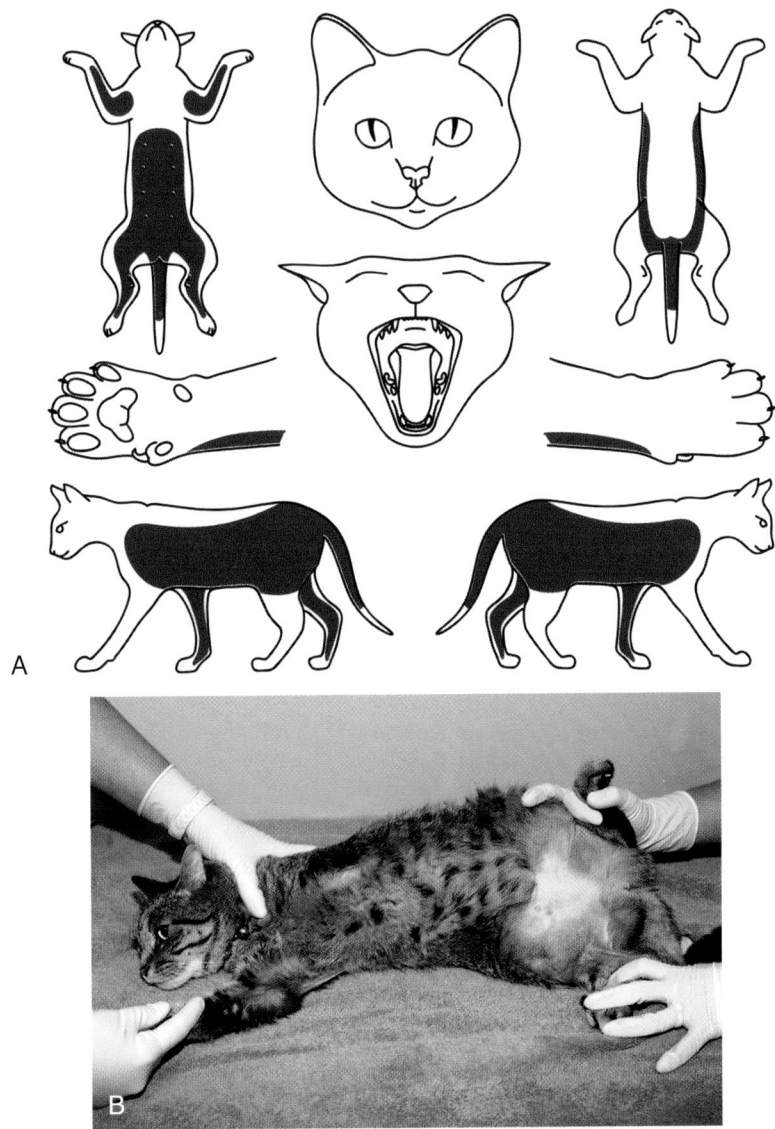

Figure 32-1: Self-Induced Alopecia. A, Cutaneous distribution pattern of self-induced alopecia (SIA). Partial to complete alopecia, which is most often symmetrically distributed, is depicted in *red.* Note that alopecic areas are where the cat can reach to overgroom. **B,** Clinical example of SIA in a cat diagnosed with environmental allergy. Alopecia is present along inguinal skin with extension down the medial thighs. Partial alopecia is also seen on the medial antebrachium of the right forelimb. The left forelimb was amputated because of a prior traumatic injury.

is most often accompanied by pruritus, CFD is also referred to as head, neck, and pinnal pruritus. In some cases, pruritus can be so severe and relentless that self-mutilation can result in disfigurement of the patient. Many cats with cutaneous adverse reaction to food or food-related allergy will display this pattern of disease[2]; however, other allergic and nonallergic diseases should be considered before initiating a strict hypoallergenic diet trial.

Eosinophilic Granuloma Complex

A constellation of clinical entities, which includes indolent (rodent) ulcer (IU), eosinophilic plaques (EPs), and eosinophilic granulomas (EGs), falls under the subheading of eosinophilic granuloma complex (EGC), also termed feline

eosinophilic dermatitis. Indolent ulcer is a focal crateriform ulceration of the upper lips that is often present in the absence of any clinical signs, including pruritus (Figure 32-4); this lesion may be an incidental finding on physical examination. Lesions may be unilateral or bilateral on the upper lips opposite the canine teeth; extension up the philtrum to the nasal planum is not uncommon. Eosinophilic plaque lesions on the other hand are typically *severely* pruritic and will commonly be seen with concurrent SIA. These elevated erythematous lesions have a glistening and often moist and eroded surface (Figure 32-5). Eosinophilic plaques tend to affect the ventral abdomen with an asymmetric or symmetric distribution; occasionally, multiple lesions will coalesce to form a large EP. Peripheral blood eosinophilia may be a concurrent finding in cats with EP lesions. Eosinophilic granuloma lesions will

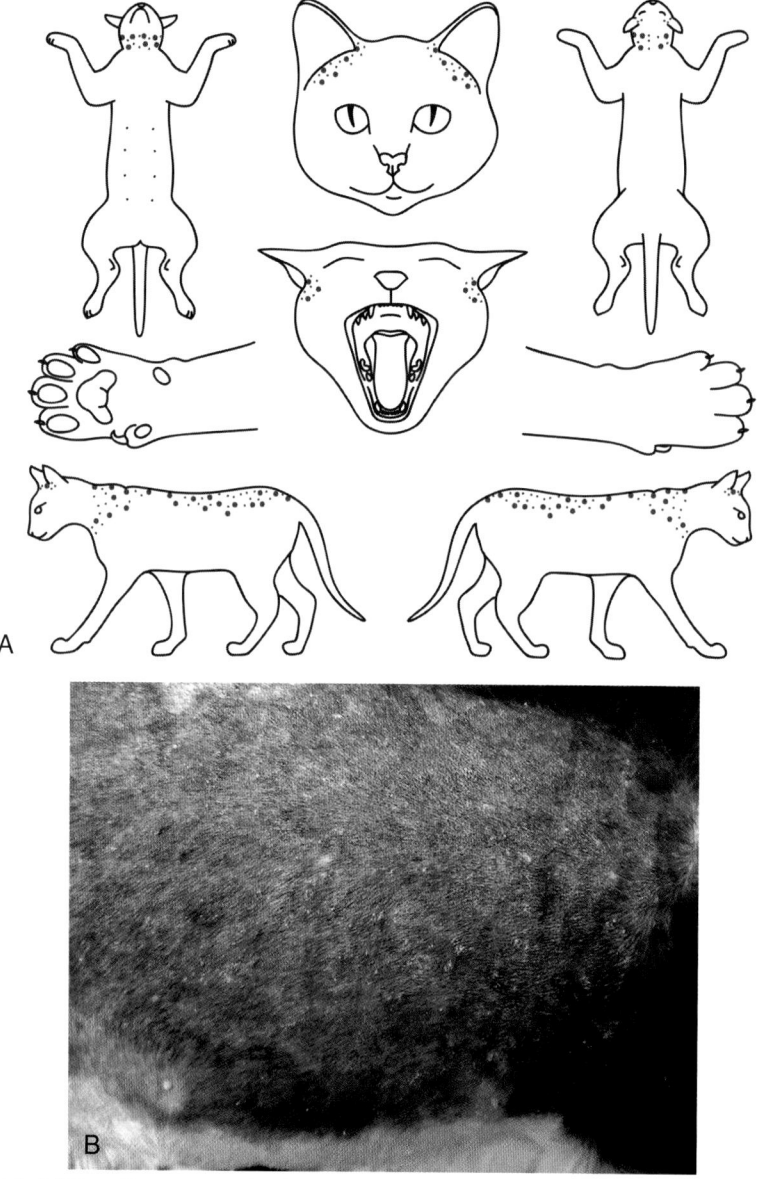

Figure 32-2: **Miliary Dermatitis. A,** Cutaneous distribution pattern of miliary dermatitis (MD). Asymmetrically to symmetrically distributed crusted papular lesions tend to predominate on peri-cervical skin, but lesions can also be elsewhere. Affected areas are depicted in *red.* **B,** Clinical example of MD present along the left lateral flank of a cat. The coat has been clipped in order to show the diseased skin. Note the lesion of this reaction pattern is a crusted papule, which can be pruritic.

often present on the chin, caudal thigh, or be associated with a paw pad. Eosinophilic granulomas are well-demarcated, fairly firm, dermal nodules that when raised will have an erythematous to yellowish surface hue and a gritty texture (Figure 32-6). Alopecia and pruritus may or may not be associated with these lesions. Eosinophilic granulomas can also be found in the oral cavity; affected cats may initially present with clinical signs of dysphagia, drooling, decreased appetite, or even dyspnea depending on the size and location of the lesion present. It is generally accepted by many veterinary dermatologists that these eosinophilic lesions, especially IU and EP, are manifestations of feline bacterial pyoderma (as opposed to the papules, pustules, epidermal collarettes,

and crusting seen with staphylococcal pyoderma in the dog). These lesions will often improve, or even resolve, solely with antibiotic therapy.[3]

DIAGNOSIS

It cannot be overstated that the aforementioned cutaneous reaction patterns are not definitive diagnoses, but rather clinically observable lesions that are arranged in a predictive way on the skin. Indeed, the aim of diagnosis is therefore to determine, "What is the underlying reason for the pattern?"—not to name the pattern of disease. This begins with a

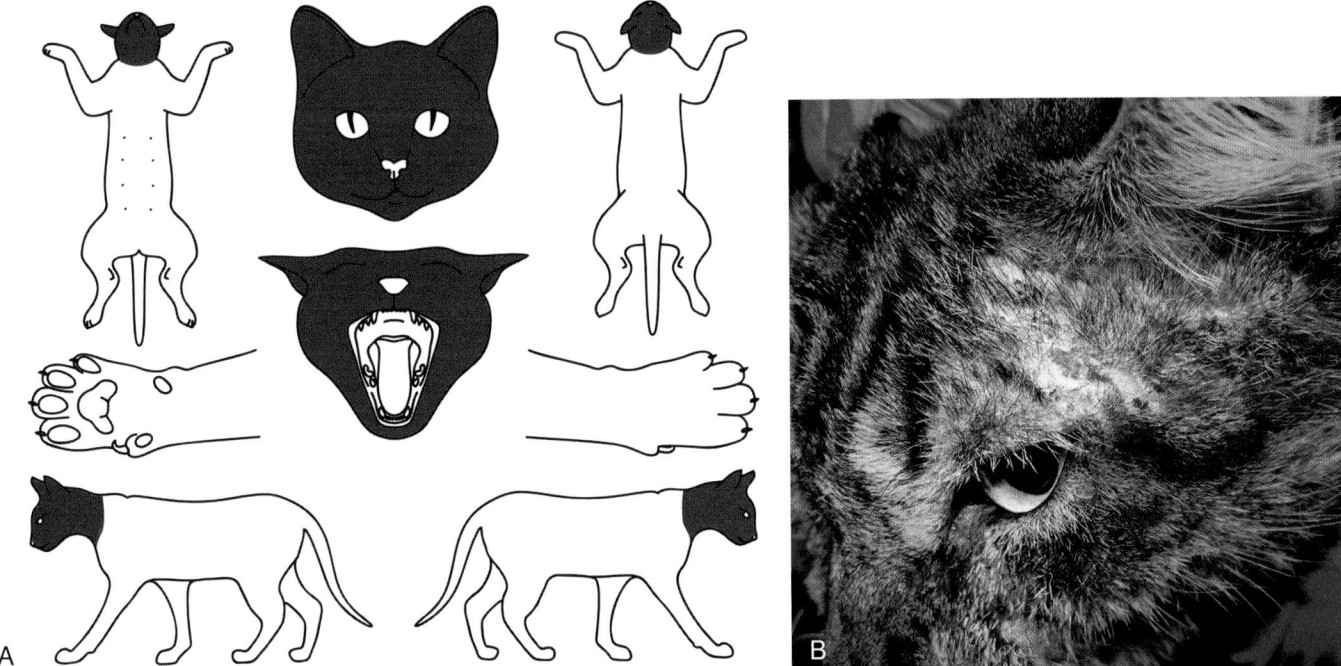

Figure 32-3: Cervicofacial Dermatitis. A, Cutaneous distribution pattern of cervicofacial dermatitis (CFD). Lesions are reflective of pruritus (e.g., excoriations) and are distributed anywhere along the haired skin of the face, pinnae, and neck as depicted in *red*. **B,** Clinical example of CFD in a cat diagnosed with food-related and environmental allergy. Preaural, periocular, and perinasal skin is excoriated and partially alopecic.

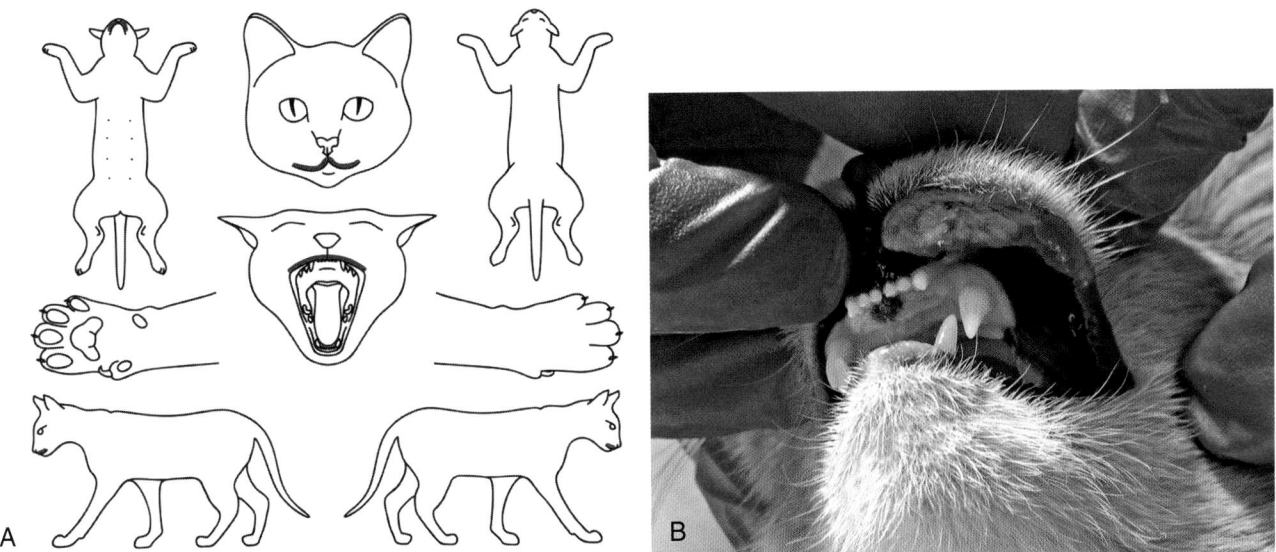

Figure 32-4: Indolent Ulcer. A, Cutaneous distribution pattern of indolent (rodent) ulcer (IU). A focal crateriform ulcerative lesion with surrounding edema occurs along the mucocutaneous junction of the upper lip, often opposite the canine teeth. Unilateral or bilateral (depicted in *red*) ulcers may be present. **B,** Clinical example of a unilateral IU on the left upper lip of a cat diagnosed with flea allergy dermatitis. Rarely is this lesion pruritic or painful.

thorough and complete dermatologic history, with particular attention paid to the following:

- Age at disease onset (e.g., young, middle-aged, geriatric)
- Duration of skin disease (e.g., first occurrence, chronic, seasonal)

- Patient lifestyle (e.g., indoor, outdoor, travel history)
- Changes in behavior (e.g., in relation to a new dwelling place, a different litter box, addition or loss of an individual in the household)
- Presence of pruritus (Box 32-1)

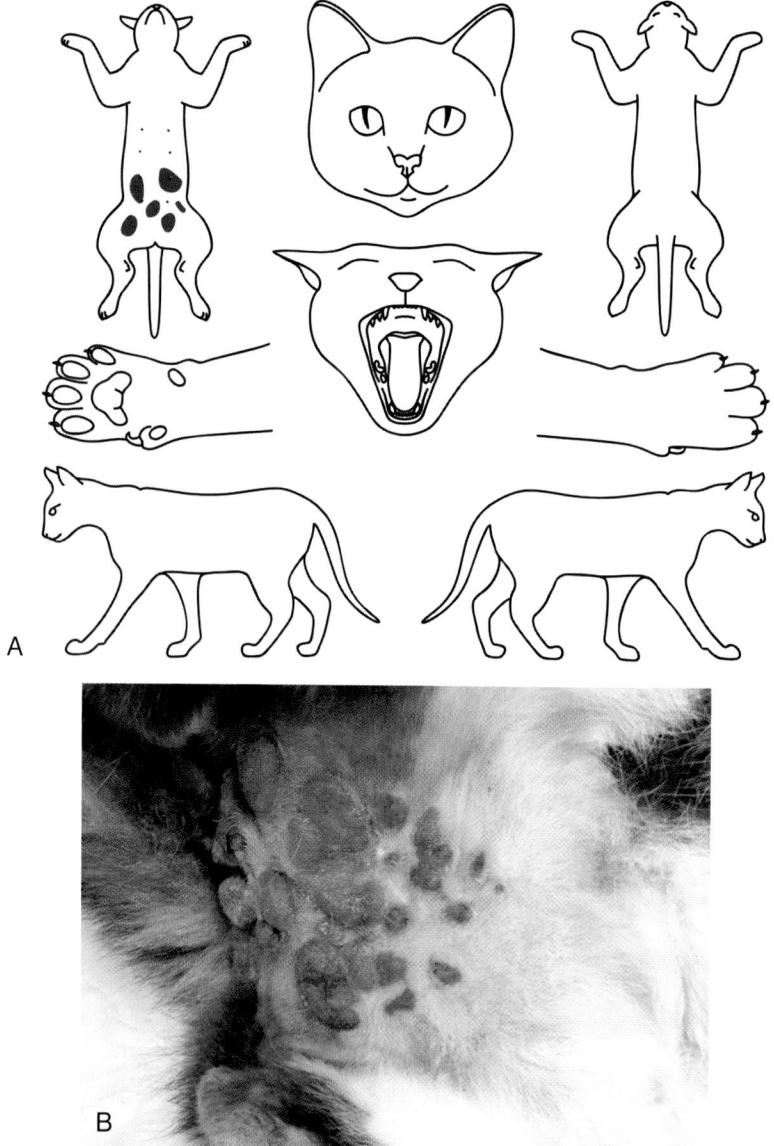

Figure 32-5: Eosinophilic Plaque. A, Cutaneous distribution pattern of eosinophilic plaque (EP). Focal or grouped erythematous plaques are asymmetrically to symmetrically distributed along ventral abdominal skin as depicted in *red*. **B,** Clinical example of EPs in a cat diagnosed with flea allergy dermatitis. Grouped and coalescing, eroded and erythematous, elevated lesions (plaques) are on the ventral abdominal and inguinal skin. These lesions are extremely pruritic. This strictly indoor cat had flea allergy dermatitis.

- Dietary history
- Signs of systemic disease (e.g., lethargy, changes in body weight, inappetence or polyphagia, sneezing, oculonasal discharge, vomiting, diarrhea, polyuria or polydipsia)
- Other individuals in the same environment that are similarly affected
- Response to previous treatments
- Consistent and correct use of adulticidal flea prevention (when applicable depending on the geographical location)

A complete physical examination is performed to determine if the presenting condition is limited to the skin. When examining the cutaneous landscape, the pattern of the patient's disease is marked by the type of lesions, the distribu-

tion of lesions (asymmetrically or symmetrically distributed), and the type of epithelia affected (e.g., haired skin, nonhaired skin, lightly pigmented skin, mucocutaneous junctions).

Although commonly recognized as manifestations of feline allergic skin disease,[2,4,5] other differential diagnoses for cutaneous reaction patterns, specifically those which are clinically similar to allergy, must be considered and systematically excluded (see Table 32-2). Clearly, cutaneous infections (bacterial and fungal) and ectoparasitism, both of which mimic allergic skin disease, must be ruled out with the use of skin surface and/or otic cytology, dermatophyte culture, flea combings, and skin scrapings (Figure 32-7). Trial antimicrobial therapy can be beneficial when IUs and/or EPs are present, as these patterns of disease may be reflections of

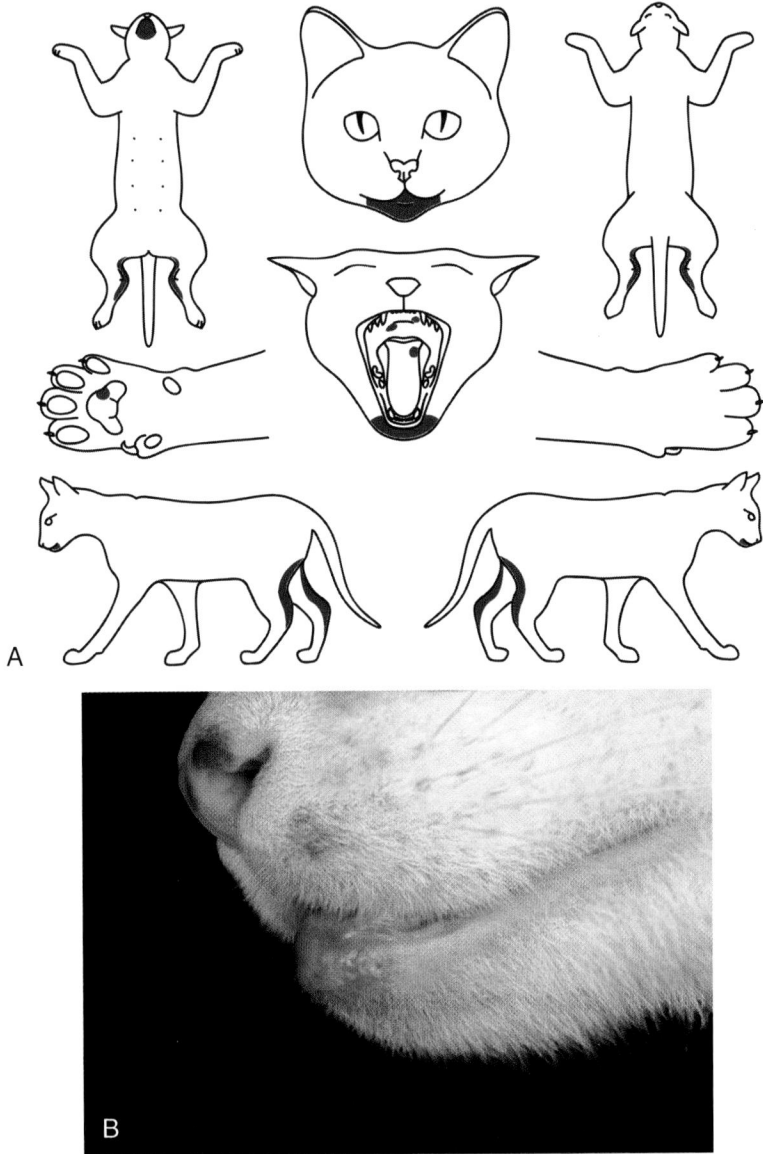

Figure 32-6: Eosinophilic Granuloma. A, Cutaneous distribution pattern of eosinophilic granuloma (EG). Granulomas, usually focal, raised, well-demarcated nodules, are yellow to erythematous and often gritty in texture and are typically present in the oral cavity (hard palate or tongue), on the chin, along the caudal thigh (linear granuloma), or associated with a paw pad. **B,** Clinical example of an EG on the chin of a cat ("pouty" cat). EGs are not usually pruritic or painful. (Image courtesy of Dr. John August.)

BOX 32-1 Helpful Clues for Distinguishing Overgrooming from Normal Grooming

- Cats tend not to scratch, but rather show pruritic behaviors by licking and rubbing affected areas, as well as by the pulling of hair
- There is a recent history of vomiting hair balls or excessive hair in the cat's stool when a cat is overgrooming
- Other household animals, particularly cats, show more overt signs of pruritus when the cat in question is overgrooming
- Barbered hair can be appreciated in the pruritic cat by rubbing a hand against the direction of fur growth

- Self-induced excoriations are not seen with normal grooming
- The presence of a cutaneous reaction pattern, especially self-induced alopecia, cervicofacial dermatitis, and/or eosinophilic plaque, often provides circumstantial evidence for pruritus
- Microscopic examination of the hair (trichogram) can help determine if the distal hair shaft is fractured, which is associated with overgrooming

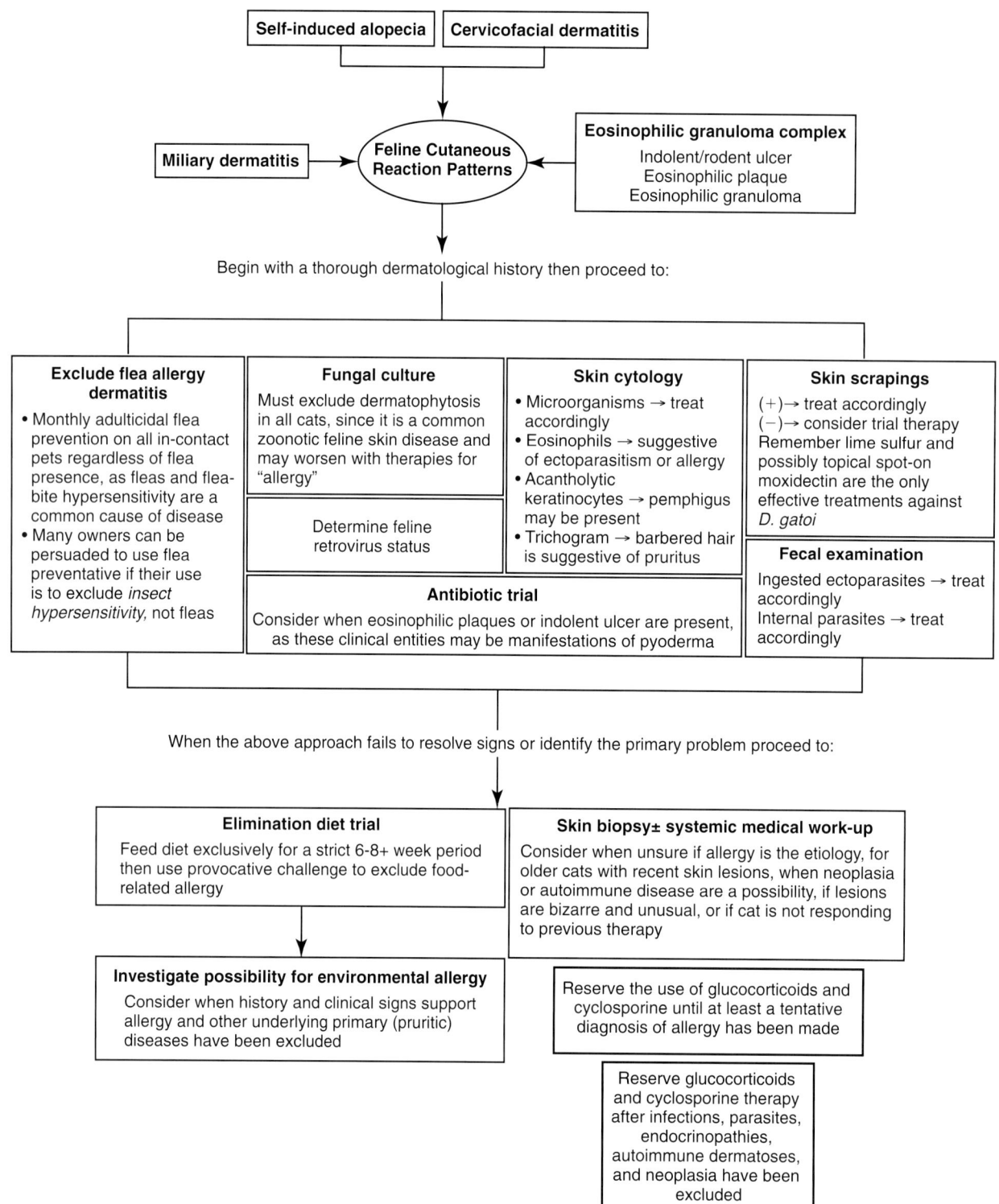

Figure 32-7: Diagnostic Algorithm for Feline Cutaneous Reaction Patterns.

staphylococcal pyoderma in the cat.[3] Similarly, trial therapy with parasiticidal treatment directed against superficial, and often pruritic, parasites (e.g., *Ctenocephalides felis*, *Otodectes*, *Notoedres*, *Sarcoptes*, *Cheyletiella*, *Demodex gatoi*) may be needed when the history is suggestive of ectoparasitism but the parasite of interest cannot be found. Importantly, in most cases, all household animals will require the same or similar parasiticidal therapy for the entire duration of the trial in an

attempt to exclude the possibility of ectoparasitism. If signs remain despite the exclusion of infections and parasites, then a tentative diagnosis of allergic skin disease can be made, diagnostics to identify the allergenic trigger can be performed (e.g., elimination diet trial and provocative challenge to exclude food-related allergy, intradermal testing to select candidate allergens for immunotherapy), and symptomatic therapy tailored to the individual can be prescribed (e.g., glucocorticoids, cyclosporine). Readers are referred to Chapters 29 and 30 for further discussion of the use of cyclosporine and glucocorticoids, respectively, for treatment of feline dermatologic disease.

Skin biopsy is performed to confirm that a lesion is likely associated with allergy, when the diagnosis of allergic skin disease is in question, or if lesions are extending onto non-haired epithelia (e.g., oral cavity, nasal planum, paw pads). By and large, skin biopsy helps to exclude the possibility of deep-seated infection or neoplasia masquerading as an EP or EG, or a viral-related dermatitis, autoimmune skin disease (e.g., pemphigus foliaceus) or neoplasia posing as MD, CFD, or IU. Potential histopathologic findings of each cutaneous reaction pattern are described later, but results of individual skin biopsies must be interpreted in light of the patient's history and clinical presentation.

Histopathologic Findings of Self-Induced Alopecia

With psychogenic alopecia, there are no specific histopathologic abnormalities.[6] Rarely, broken or twisted hair shafts, as a result of barbering or hair pulling, are found within amorphous tricholemmal keratin. These findings with histologic evidence of dermal inflammation, especially a superficial eosinophilic to lymphohistiocytic perivascular infiltrate, suggest a condition associated with pruritus, such as allergy. The presence of neutrophilic or eosinophilic follicular pustules or lymphocytic interface dermatitis at the level of the follicular isthmus is typical histopathologic pattern of dermatophytosis; fungal hyphae may be present. Paraneoplastic alopecia (see Chapter 26 for further discussion), a differential diagnosis for this pattern of disease, is characterized by an absent stratum corneum, moderate to severe acanthosis, follicular telogenization, minimal dermal inflammation, and possibly the presence of superficial *Malassezia* spp. yeast.[7]

Histopathologic Findings of Miliary Dermatitis

Histopathologic separation between MD and the clinical entities of EGC can be difficult, as the former is regarded as a milder and more superficial histopathologic variant of the latter. Because both clinical reaction patterns are often manifestations of feline allergic skin disease, histopathologic separation is not critical. Basically, discrete serocellular crusts are atop foci of mild to moderate acanthosis and accompanying spongiosis within the epidermis and superficial follicles.[6] Eosinophilic exocytosis and a superficial dermal infiltrate composed of eosinophils, neutrophils, mast cells, histiocytes, and lymphocytes further complete the histopathologic picture. Differential diagnoses outside the realm of allergy will usually have disease-specific findings (e.g., neutrophilic pustular dermatitis with acantholytic keratinocytes as seen with pemphigus foliaceus, or an abundance of monomorphic cells typically seen with neoplasia) that a dermatopathologist will recognize.

Histopathologic Findings of Cervicofacial Dermatitis

There are no specific histopathologic findings associated with this gross clinical pattern of disease. Often the histopathol-

ogy is reflective of allergy with the findings of varying degrees of acanthosis, spongiosis, eosinophilic exocytosis, and dermal inflammation, particularly in resolving or ulcerative lesions.[6] An important clinical and histopathologic differential diagnosis to consider with these findings is feline herpesvirus type 1 ulcerative dermatitis, a dermatosis that commonly affects, but is not limited to, the face.[8] Eosinophilic necrotizing folliculitis with severe exudation is typical of this viral dermatitis. When present, intranuclear inclusion bodies are best identified in intact epithelium adjacent to areas of necrosis. Immunostaining, possibly with accompanying polymerase chain reaction testing, may be required when viral inclusion bodies are absent.[9]

Histopathologic Findings of Eosinophilic Dermatoses

Eosinophilic granuloma complex encompasses a group of clinically distinct lesions (IU, EP, EG) that are indistinguishable histopathologically.[6,10] The unifying histopathologic characteristic of these eosinophilic dermatoses is the presence of varying numbers of collagen flame figures—eosinophilic debris surrounding dermal collagen bundles as a consequence of degranulating eosinophils. Granulomatous inflammation may be centered on flame figures, whereas an erosive to ulcerative dermatitis is superficial to them. In addition, a hyperplastic epidermis with a diffuse eosinophilic infiltrate spanning the entire dermis, and possibly deeper, is observed. All of these findings are suggestive of allergic skin disease in the cat.

A minimum extracutaneous diagnostic database is performed at the discretion of the clinician and is based on the signalment, history, physical exam, and/or a lack of response to seemingly appropriate treatment, but often will include retrovirus testing, complete blood count, serum biochemical analysis, and urinalysis. Other diagnostics, such as screening tests for endocrine disorders or radiographic/ultrasonographic imaging to exclude neoplasia, are considered on a case-by-case basis.

SUMMARY

When approaching the feline patient with dermatologic disease, pattern recognition can be a clinician's best friend. Identification of the lesions present, where they are located, and how they are arranged can help the practitioner prioritize a list of differential diagnoses to consider. Complete and accurate history and physical examination will further narrow the list of selected diseases to investigate. Box 32-2 provides a summary of the approach to feline cutaneous reaction patterns, highlighting the importance of ruling out other possibilities before leaping to a diagnosis of allergy. Accurate interpretation of the history, clinical findings, and select diagnostic tests allows for the best chance to correctly identify the underlying disease process, thereby thwarting unnecessary, and potentially harmful, therapy in favor of more directed, and likely successful, therapeutic recommendations.

BOX 32-2 Important Points to Consider When Evaluating Feline Cutaneous Reaction Patterns

- Self-induced symmetrical alopecia, miliary dermatitis, cervicofacial pruritus, and eosinophilic granuloma complex (indolent ulcer, eosinophilic plaque, and eosinophilic granuloma) are clinically recognized reactive patterns of feline skin
- Cutaneous reaction patterns are not definitive diagnoses, but rather the skin's response to a variety of antigenic stimuli
- The reaction patterns of feline skin rarely affect the paws
- Many differential diagnoses can present as, or mimic, a cutaneous reaction pattern
- Pruritus may be subtle to severe depending on the underlying primary disease
- Identifying and managing the underlying primary disease, when possible, will result in the best chance for clinical improvement

- When confronted with a cutaneous reaction pattern, infection and ectoparasitism must first be excluded—although there are different geographical differences, most cases should receive monthly adulticidal flea prevention
- Once cutaneous infections and ectoparasitism have been excluded, allergy (insect, food-related, or environmental allergy) is most likely the underlying cause of disease
- Skin biopsy and a medical workup are indicated when disease onset occurs later in life, systemic signs are present, therapy (symptomatic or targeted) for allergy is ineffective, or the clinical presentation is bizarre and unusual in appearance
- A relapsing and remitting course of disease is not uncommon, most notably with allergy, and the disease manifested as a cutaneous reaction pattern may become refractory to therapy over time

References

1. Waisglass SE, Landsberg GM, Yager JA, et al: Underlying medical conditions in cats with presumptive psychogenic alopecia. *J Am Vet Med Assoc* 228:1705–1709, 2006.
2. Hobi S, Linek M, Marignac G, et al: Clinical characteristics and causes of pruritus in cats: a multicenter study on feline hypersensitivity-associated dermatoses. *Vet Dermatol* 22:406–413, 2011.
3. Wildermuth BE, Griffin CE, Rosenkrantz WS: Response of feline eosinophilic plaques and lip ulcers to amoxicillin trihydrate-clavulanate potassium therapy: a randomized, double-blinded placebo-controlled prospective study. *Vet Dermatol* 23:110–118, 2011.
4. King S, Favrot C, Messinger L, et al: A randomized double-blinded placebo-controlled study to evaluate an effective ciclosporin dose for the treatment of feline hypersensitivity dermatitis. *Vet Dermatol* 23:440–447, 2012.
5. Vercelli A, Raviri G, Cornegliani L: The use of oral cyclosporine to treat feline dermatoses: a retrospective analysis of 23 cases. *Vet Dermatol* 17:201–206, 2006.
6. Gross TL, Ihrke PJ, Walder EJ, et al: *Skin diseases of the dog and cat, clinical and histopathologic diagnosis*, ed 2, Oxford, 2005, Blackwell Science.
7. Mauldin EA, Morris DO, Goldschmidt MH: Retrospective study: the presence of *Malassezia* in feline skin biopsies. A clinicopathological study. *Vet Dermatol* 13:7–13, 2002.
8. Sánchez MD, Goldschmidt MH, Mauldin EA: Herpesvirus dermatitis in two cats without facial lesions. *Vet Dermatol* 23:171–173, 2012.
9. Persico P, Roccabianca P, Corona A, et al: Detection of feline herpes virus 1 via polymerase chain reaction and immunohistochemistry in cats with ulcerative facial dermatitis, eosinophilic granuloma complex reaction patterns and mosquito bite hypersensitivity. *Vet Dermatol* 22:521–527, 2011.
10. Fondati A, Fondevila D, Ferrer L: Histopathological study of feline eosinophilic dermatoses. *Vet Dermatol* 12:333–338, 2001.

Malassezia spp. in Feline Dermatology

Darren Berger

EPIDEMIOLOGY AND PATHOGENESIS

Malassezia spp. are nonmycelial, lipid-dependent (requiring lipids as a source of carbon) yeasts that reproduce asexually through monopolar or sympodial budding and reside within the family Cryptococcaceae.[1-3] *Malassezia* spp. are considered a normal part of the commensal microbiota of both human and animal skin.[3,4] The commensal nature of the yeast is further substantiated as it is primarily isolated from the mucosa and skin of animals and seldom recovered from the environment.[1] The organism is confined to the outer layer of the epidermis (stratum corneum) and follicular openings, where it is present in the yeast form with only three species known to form rudimentary filaments.[2] *Malassezia* spp. have a characteristic elliptical to globose appearance that measures 2 to 4 μm by 3 to 7 μm in size, with slight variations observed in size and shape among the different species (Figure 33-1).[1,3] They also have a distinct thick, multilamellar cell wall (2 to 4 layers depending on the lipid composition of the growth environment) with corrugations on the inner cell surface, which is characteristic of fungi from their particular phylum.[1,3]

Although *Malassezia* spp. are a commensal part of the skin's normal microenvironment, they have been associated with disease in both humans and animals. *Malassezia* spp. (i.e., *Pityrosporum*) were first described in 1846, associated with scale taken from human patients with pityriasis versicolor, and originally classified as a new species of dermatophyte.[3] The original description of *Malassezia* from animals transpired in 1925 and was associated with scales from an Indian rhinoceros with exfoliative dermatitis.[4] The first description in companion small animals did not take place until 1955, when it was seen associated with canine otitis.[5] True recognition of *Malassezia* spp. as pathogens in companion animals is relatively recent, with an explosion of information on the subject being witnessed since Dufait's initial report in 1983.[6] Today, in human medicine, *Malassezia* spp. are known to be associated with conditions such as pityriasis versicolor, *Malassezia* folliculitis, and seborrheic dermatitis and dandruff.[7,8] In veterinary medicine, the yeast is primarily associated with *Malassezia* dermatitis and otitis externa.[9]

Since their first description, the genus *Malassezia* has undergone major taxonomic revisions, specifically in the last decade with the development and utilization of molecular genetic techniques. At present, the genus *Malassezia* encompasses 14 species, including *caprae, cuniculi, dermatis, equina,* *furfur, globosa, japonica, nana, obtusa, pachydermatis, restricta, slooffiae, sympodialis,* and *yamatoensis.*[10,11] *M. pachydermatis* is unique among this genus in being lipophilic but not lipid dependent. It is the only species within the genus that readily grows *in vitro* on Sabouraud dextrose agar, aiding in the easy identification of this organism.[1] Molecular techniques utilizing large subunit ribosomal ribonucleic acid sequencing have also demonstrated that *M. pachydermatis* is composed of seven sequevars (types Ia through Ig), the importance of which is likely related to host-specific adaptations.[1,2]

Healthy cats are most commonly colonized with *M. pachydermatis,* but an ever-growing body of research suggests that colonization with lipid-dependent species is more prevalent than previously thought. Lipid-dependent species recovered from the skin and ears of healthy cats include *M. furfur, M. globosa, M. nana, M. obtusa, M. restricta, M. slooffiae,* and *M. sympodialis.*[12-22] *Malassezia* spp. have also been shown in limited studies to compose the normal microbiota of the auditory canal of captive wild felids, with *M. sympodialis* recovered exclusively from larger cats (specifically lions, *Panthera leo*) and *M. pachydermatis* from smaller species.[23] *M. globosa* has also been recovered from a healthy cheetah (*Acinonyx jubatus*).[12]

Factors that favor proliferation of *Malassezia* spp. and the transition from commensal to pathogen are still not completely understood. However, *Malassezia* overgrowth likely results from alterations in the skin's normal microenvironment or host defenses involved in the natural restriction of microbial colonization.[1] Comparatively little is still known about the predisposing factors involved in feline *Malassezia* dermatitis and otitis, but it is likely that factors similar to those described in the dog are shared to a certain degree by the cat. Primary disorders associated with *Malassezia* dermatitis and otitis in the dog include allergic hypersensitivities, keratinization disorders, endocrinopathies, metabolic diseases, and neoplasia.[11,24,25] *Malassezia* dermatitis also appears to be more common in warm, humid climates or when the skin environment favors these conditions, such as within skin folds.[3] Although antibiotic use has been proposed as a cause of exacerbation of candidiasis in humans, similar findings have not been the case with *Malassezia* overgrowth in veterinary medicine.[2] *Malassezia* spp. are believed to have a symbiotic relationship with *Staphylococcus* spp., whereby the organisms produce mutually beneficial growth factors and alterations to the skin microenvironment. Because of this, it is common to see concurrent pyoderma and *Malassezia*

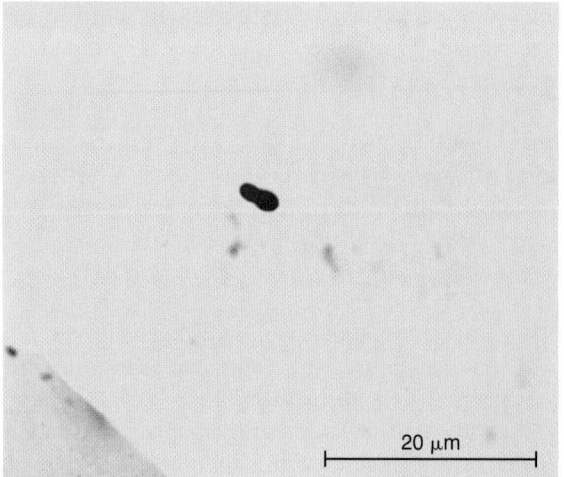

Figure 33-1: Direct impression cytology stained with a modified Wright's stain and observed under oil immersion (magnification ×1000), demonstrating characteristic morphology and size of *Malassezia pachydermatis.*

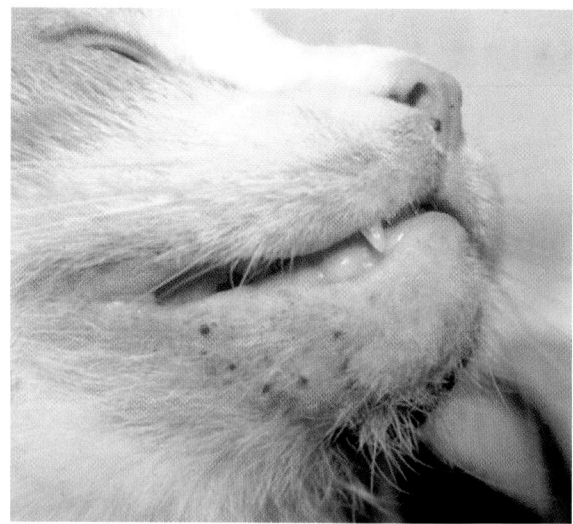

Figure 33-2: A Clinical Case of Feline Acne with a Secondary *Malassezia* Infection. (Photo courtesy of James Noxon, Iowa State University, Ames, Iowa.)

overgrowth in the same patient.[24] This finding is further supported by observations from a recent *in vivo* study, where in the control group, mean *Malassezia* yeast counts on the skin were found to be decreased following therapy with cephalexin for concurrent pyoderma.[26]

Although secondary *Malassezia* infections in cats are being recognized more frequently by veterinary dermatologists, they are still encountered considerably less frequently than in dogs. This may stem from the relatively low carriage rate in clinically normal and healthy cats or it may be the result of differences in primary disease pathogenesis and syndromes observed in the two species. Traditionally, *Malassezia* dermatitis or overgrowth in cats has been considered a cutaneous manifestation of a more serious systemic illness. Conditions classically associated with secondary *Malassezia* infections have been paraneoplastic syndromes (thymoma or pancreatic and bile duct carcinomas), hyperadrenocorticism, diabetes mellitus, hyperthyroidism, hepatocutaneous syndrome (superficial necrolytic dermatitis, metabolic epidermal necrosis, or necrolytic migratory erythema), systemic toxoplasmosis, and other neoplastic conditions (e.g., multicentric lymphoma).[27-30] Chapter 26 discusses further several of these conditions. Even though anecdotal and case reports have described associations between these syndromes and *Malassezia* overgrowth, a recent report failed to demonstrate increased carriage of *Malassezia* spp. in cats with several of these conditions.[31]

In other studies, both aural and cutaneous colonization with *Malassezia* spp. were significantly increased in cats with natural retroviral infections (feline immunodeficiency virus [FIV] and feline leukemia virus [FeLV]) compared with their healthy counterparts. Even more specifically, cats that were FIV-infected and colonized with *Malassezia* spp. had significantly lower CD4+/CD8+ lymphocyte ratios than FIV-infected cats without secondary *Malassezia* colonization.[32,33] The significance of these findings is questionable, as none of

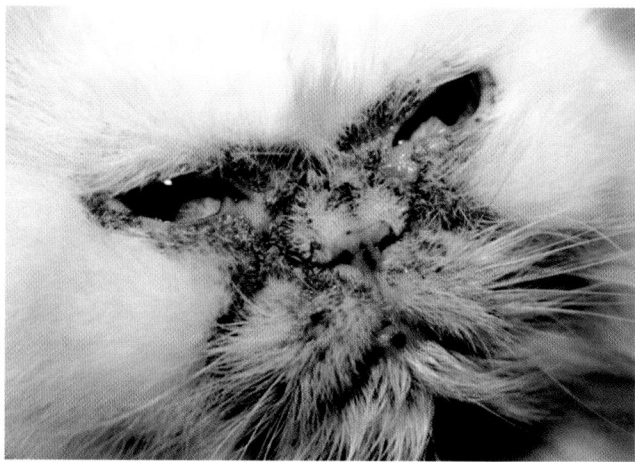

Figure 33-3: A Himalayan Cat with Idiopathic Facial Dermatitis Complicated by *Malassezia* Overgrowth. (Photo courtesy of James Noxon, Iowa State University, Ames, Iowa.)

the culture-positive animals demonstrated cutaneous lesions. However, based on the current information that FeLV and FIV positive cats are more likely to be colonized, these animals should be considered to have a higher risk for developing *Malassezia* dermatitis. Other conditions where the importance of *Malassezia* overgrowth and colonization is being recognized more frequently include hypersensitivity dermatitides (e.g., atopic-like disease, cutaneous adverse food reaction, and parasitic hypersensitivities), refractory chin acne, and idiopathic facial dermatitis (Figures 33-2 and 33-3).[34-36] Ceruminous otitis externa appears to be the most common clinical presentation of *Malassezia*-associated disease in the cat and is normally associated with an underlying allergic disease. As is the case in dogs, *Malassezia* can be commonly recovered from the auditory canals of cats with and without otitis, with significantly higher colonization rates observed in cases of otitis externa.[12-16,37] The occurrence rate of secondary

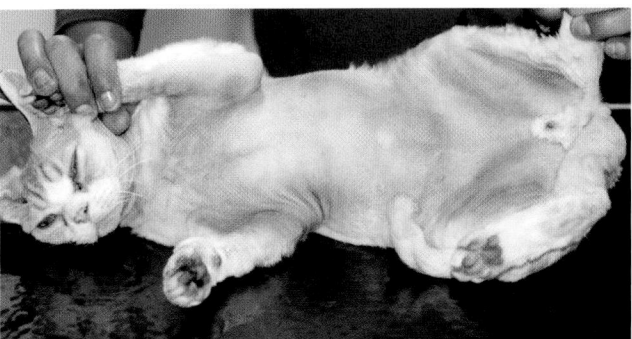

Figure 33-4: A 2-Year-Old Devon Rex Cat with Mild Seborrheic Dermatitis and Secondary *Malassezia* Overgrowth.

Malassezia otitis externa in the cat does not appear to be dependent on the underlying primary cause.[13] Regardless of ear disease state, *M. pachydermatis* is the predominant species recovered and identified. Co-isolation of lipid- and nonlipid-dependent *Malassezia* spp. from cases of feline otitis has also been demonstrated. The clinical relevance of this phenomenon is unknown at this time.[12-16] Unlike in dogs, lipid-dependent species are recovered more commonly in cats, specifically in cases of feline otitis, where they may play a more prominent role in disease pathogenesis.[12,13,15,16,37]

Regarding canine *Malassezia* dermatitis, certain breeds such as the Basset Hound, Cocker Spaniel, West Highland White Terrier, and Poodle are recognized as having higher colonization rates that are not always associated with a concurrent underlying disease compared to other breeds of dogs.[9] Recent studies evaluating various breeds of cats have also demonstrated similar findings. Studies have revealed that both healthy and seborrheic Devon Rex cats (DRC) and Sphynx cats have higher colonization rates than that of healthy domestic shorthair cats (DSH) (Figure 33-4).[38-41] In these studies, lipid- and nonlipid-dependent species were recovered with *M. pachydermatis* being significantly more common independent of seborrheic status.[39,40] A similar study looking at the rate of colonization in Cornish Rex cats found the rate was not different from that of DSH.[42] Given these findings, current studies would suggest that the Rex mutation alone does not favor susceptibility to colonization with *Malassezia* and that additional factors or genetic components may account for the overgrowth seen with DRC and Sphynx cats. Unlike similar studies with Basset Hounds, an elevated rate of aural carriage was not seen with the DRC and Sphynx cats in comparison with DSH cats.[39-41]

The mechanism(s) by which *Malassezia* spp. propagate disease is not fully understood at this time. Because the agent does not invade deeper than the stratum corneum, dermatitis is thought to arise from inflammatory or allergic reactions to yeast products and antigens.[24] The current body of research does not support an individual mechanism but rather an intricate interplay between the host's immune system and *Malassezia*'s virulence factors. Adhesion of the yeast appears to be mediated through trypsin-sensitive proteins and glycoproteins on the organism's cell wall and carbohydrate residues on corneocytes.[1,3] This is likely true for the cat, as well,

although differences in the exact species of *Malassezia* involved and adhesion studies suggest that slight alterations in the exact molecules may exist in the feline species.[43] *Malassezia* spp. also have been shown to produce various enzymes including zymogen, phospholipases, lipases, acid and alkaline phosphatase, azelaic acid, lipoxygenase, protease, and urease. Each of these various enzymes in some way contributes to the activation of the innate immune system, inflammation, pruritus, or alters the skin microenvironment to create a favorable niche for the organism.[3,24,44] The adaptive immune response has also been implicated in disease pathogenesis. In both humans and dogs, hypersensitivity reactions (head and neck syndrome, *Malassezia* hypersensitivity) in atopic patients are believed to exist that exacerbate disease.[3,7-9] This has been demonstrated through numerous studies evaluating immunoglobulin levels and immediate hypersensitivity reactions in patients with and without atopy, along with the simultaneous occurrence of *Malassezia* dermatitis.[45-49] Although not demonstrated at this time in cats, it is conceivable to think that such mechanisms may exist, specifically in cats with hypersensitivity dermatitides or in breeds such as the Sphynx and DRC, where seborrheic conditions have been described.

CLINICAL PRESENTATION

As previously stated, *Malassezia* dermatitis and otitis in the cat appear to occur much less frequently than in the dog and tend to have a more variable clinical presentation. The primary lesion traditionally associated with *Malassezia* dermatitis is erythema, with secondary lesions such as excoriations, scale, greasy exudate, traumatic alopecia, hyperpigmentation, and lichenification.[9,11,24] The latter two lesions are not encountered as frequently in cats as in dogs.[34] Another consistent feature of *Malassezia* dermatitis is pruritus, which also appears more variable in cats, ranging from very mild to severe. Lesion distribution may be localized or generalized and typically affects the face, ventral neck, axillary region, abdomen, claw folds, and interdigital skin (Figure 33-5).[11,34,39] Those lesions that are reported to occur most commonly in the cat are erythema, paronychia with reddish-brown discoloration of the proximal claw, excessive buildup of keratosebaceous debris at the claw fold, matting and staining of the hair coat with red-brown exudate, tightly adherent scale with follicular casts or lightly adherent scale, and exfoliative lesions (Figures 33-6 and 33-7).[11,24,34,38,39]

Malassezia otitis, the more common clinical presentation of *Malassezia*-associated skin disease in the cat, is primarily associated with an increase in ceruminous debris, canal erythema, and swelling or stenosis (Figure 33-8).[11,24] The ceruminous exudate in cases of feline *Malassezia* otitis has been observed to vary in consistency and color, ranging from opaque, moist, and adherent to reddish-brown or black, dry, and granular. These observations underscore the importance that veterinarians should avoid relying on the physical character of the exudate and odor when making a diagnosis and selecting therapy. Pruritus with periauricular excoriations and

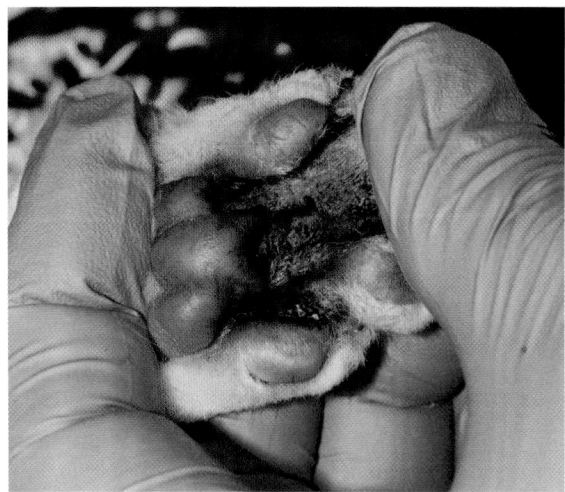

Figure 33-5: Interdigital Erythema, Increased Keratosebaceous Debris, and Reddish-Brown Discoloration Associated with *Malassezia* Pododermatitis in a Cat.

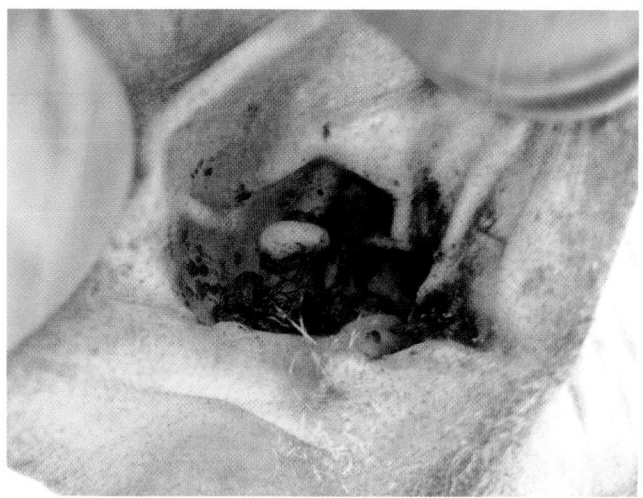

Figure 33-8: Excessive Brown to Black Ceruminous Exudate Associated with *Malassezia* Otitis in a Cat.

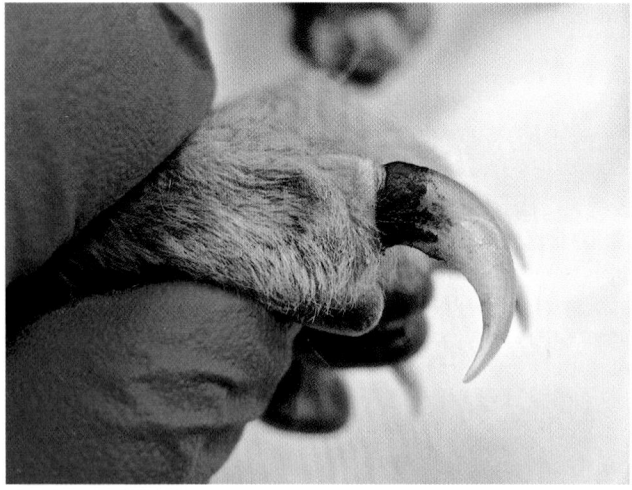

Figure 33-6: Excessive Dark-Brown Waxy Exudate Along the Proximal Claw from a Cat with Paronychia Associated with a Secondary *Malassezia* Infection.

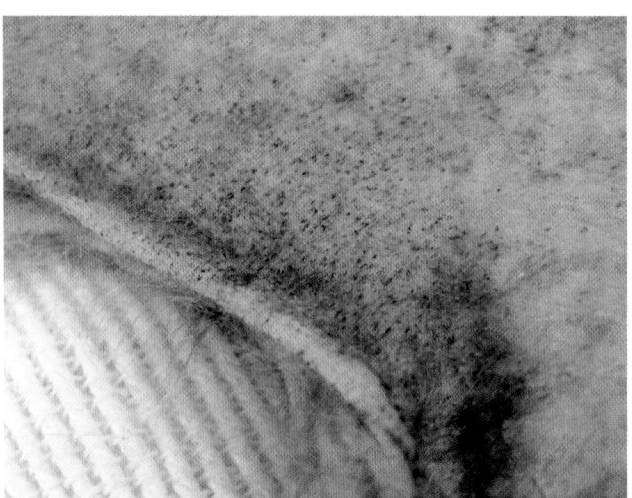

Figure 33-7: Erythema, Tightly Adherent Brown Scale, and Discoloration of the Skin in the Inguinal Region from a Cornish Rex Cat with Secondary *Malassezia* Overgrowth.

secondary pinnal alopecia also seem to be a consistent clinical feature of *Malassezia* otitis in the cat with variable degrees of headshaking reported by owners.

DIAGNOSIS

The diagnosis of *Malassezia* dermatitis and otitis is based on consistent clinical signs, demonstration of *Malassezia* organisms from lesional skin, and response to specific antifungal therapy.[9,24,25] *Malassezia* organisms can be demonstrated from feline skin via culture, histopathologic, or cytological techniques. The former two techniques are seldom- if at all-used in the clinical setting. Although *M. pachydermatis* grows well on Sabouraud dextrose agar, the lipid-dependent species recovered more frequently from cats fail to grow on this media. Given this, if culture is elected in a feline patient, a lipid-supplemented media such a modified Dixon agar should be used, which supports growth of lipid-dependent species. Regardless, *Malassezia* spp. are normal cutaneous habitants, so recovery alone via culture is of little diagnostic value. However, culture techniques do offer an advantage of providing potential quantitative information, which can be useful in clinical trials evaluating the efficacy of various treatment modalities.[11] With regard to biopsy and histopathology, *Malassezia* reside on or in the stratum corneum and rarely penetrate past this epidermal layer. During routine processing of samples, this layer is commonly disrupted, leading to a loss of the organism and a high rate of false-negative results. This scenario leads to a very low sensitivity for this diagnostic method and a lack of practical application in comparison to cytology.[29]

The most useful method for detection of *Malassezia* in a clinical setting is cytological examination, and numerous collection techniques have been used. The various techniques all have advantages and disadvantages. Studies investigating dogs with and without *Malassezia* dermatitis have

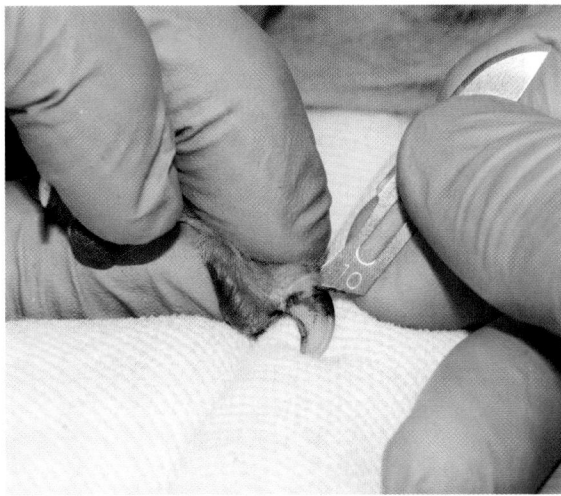

Figure 33-9: A photo demonstrating the use of the back end of a scalpel blade to acquire a dry scrape sample of waxy exudate from the proximal claw for evaluation of the presence of *Malassezia* organisms.

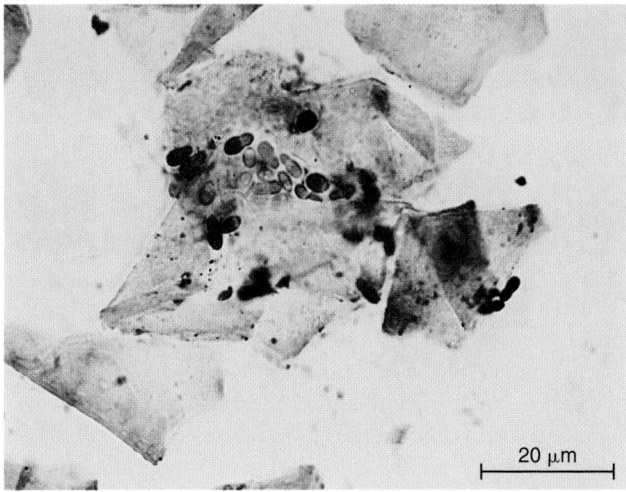

20 μm

Figure 33-10: Tape-strip sample stained with a modified Wright's stain observed under oil immersion (magnification ×1000) demonstrating the morphology, variable stain uptake, and clustering around keratinocytes that are typical of *Malassezia* yeasts.

demonstrated that all the techniques yield similar results. Clinical experience and trials have also shown that the nature of the clinical lesion and its anatomical location should be the determining criteria for selection of the collection method.[3,24,25] Some of the methods used include direct impression cytology with a nonadhesive glass slide (moist or seborrheic lesions), dry skin scraping (claws), cotton-tipped swabs (intertriginous regions or ears), adhesive slides (Delasco, Council Bluffs, Iowa), and tape-stripping using clear acetate tape (3M Corp., St. Paul, Minneapolis) (Figure 33-9). In the author's clinical practice, the latter two techniques are most commonly used for acquisition of clinical samples for evaluation of *Malassezia* dermatitis, with a preference for the tape-strip method, as it is effective regardless of lesion location and exudate character. To acquire a tape-strip sample, the overlying hair may either be parted or clipped, and a strip of clear adhesive tape is firmly applied to the skin, removed, and repeated several times. Following staining, the tape is placed on a glass slide and observed under oil immersion.[50]

For collection and examination of exudate for otic cytology from feline ears, use of a cotton-tipped swab is preferred. To acquire an appropriate sample, a cotton-tipped swab is inserted into the ear canal in order to obtain a sample from the distal horizontal canal or the junctional region where the horizontal and vertical canals meet. Once obtained, the swab is gently rolled across a glass slide, attempting to distribute the material evenly in a uniform thin layer. Samples may be heat fixed, however, a single study looking into the effects of heat-fixing samples from cases of canine *Malassezia* otitis demonstrated that there was no obvious effect on the visual appearance of samples after staining or in *Malassezia* counts between the fixed and unfixed slides.[51] Clinicians should remember to acquire separate specimens from each ear even if the patient presents with a unilateral problem, as this allows comparison between the sides and potential early detection of a problem in the less obviously affected side.

Samples are stained with a modified Wright's stain such as JorVet Dip Quick Stain (Jorgensen Laboratories, Loveland, Colorado) and examined microscopically under oil immersion (magnification ×1000) for the presence of yeast organisms of appropriate size and shape, and the demonstration of monopolar budding. The organism has been described as having a "peanut," "snowman," or "footprint" appearance and is commonly found in clusters or adhered to keratinocytes (Figure 33-10). Because *Malassezia* is a normal cutaneous inhabitant, it can be recovered from the skin and ear canals of clinically normal animals. Various criteria have been proposed to constitute what should be considered pathogenic overgrowth of the organism. Published criteria include the following:[3,24,25,52]

- The finding of 10 or more yeast organisms per 0.5 square inches of a glass slide
- Ten organisms in 15 random consecutive oil immersion fields
- An average of four organisms per oil immersion field
- An average of one or more organisms per oil immersion field
- Greater than two organisms per magnification ×40 field
- Equal to or greater than five organisms per magnification ×40 field in otic samples

Given the varying nature of these criteria, prior studies demonstrating population size differences at various anatomical sites, breed-specific differences, and the existence of hypersensitivity reactions in which low numbers of organisms may be causing disease, considerable overlap is present with these criteria.[9,11] As a result, the author takes a very practical approach to interpreting cytological results from patients. If *Malassezia* yeasts are recovered from lesional skin and ear canals in patients with consistent clinical signs or if inflammatory cells are observed concurrently, the author considers the agent to be contributing to the condition and treats accordingly, regardless of the number of organisms seen.

TREATMENT

There is a significant void in the literature on specific therapies for both *Malassezia* dermatitis and otitis in the cat, with most therapeutic recommendations being extrapolated from trials in dogs or anecdotal experiences. Regardless, the hallmark of therapy is identification and treatment of the underlying factors that initially led to overgrowth. Failure to identify and address properly the primary condition is the most common cause for recurrent or persistent disease. Specific treatment of *Malassezia* infections is centered around topical, systemic, or combination therapy. The route of treatment and specific product(s) chosen are commonly based on severity, extent and lesion location, and owner and animal compliance.

Topical therapy is routinely effective and can be delivered via a variety of formulations such as shampoos, creams, ointments, lotions, sprays, medicated wipes, or mousse applications. Active ingredients commonly incorporated into these products include miconazole, clotrimazole, ketoconazole, acetic acid, boric acid, thiabendazole, nystatin, climbazole, and chlorhexidine. Cats present several unique hurdles to the application of many of these products. The most problematic is their fastidious grooming behavior, which does not allow adequate contact time for many leave-on products or the vehicle and inactive ingredients present a potential toxicity issue (e.g., propylene glycol), along with their objection to being bathed. When practical and amenable to both the owner and cat, the author prefers to use a shampoo containing 2% miconazole nitrate and 2% chlorhexidine gluconate (Malaseb, Bayer HealthCare). This decision is based on information in the only systematic review on interventions for *Malassezia* dermatitis in dogs. A shampoo containing these two active ingredients is the only treatment modality that qualified as having good evidence for its use.[53] A comparative study looking at a 3% chlorhexidine digluconate shampoo versus 2% miconazole nitrate-2% chlorhexidine gluconate showed promising results in the treatment of canine *Malassezia* dermatitis, suggesting that shampoos containing 3% chlorhexidine may also be a sound choice for topical treatment.[54] Anecdotally, shampoos containing various concentrations of ketoconazole have also been effective. Bathing with medicated shampoos is most effective when used two to three times per week and when adequate contact time is allowed before rinsing (8 to 10 minutes). With cats that are not amenable to bathing, other topical delivery systems may provide clinical benefit. Those used most commonly by the author have been spray-on products (one to two times daily until clinical resolution), medicated wipes (once to twice daily application), and a topical massage-in mousse product containing 3% chlorhexidine and 0.5% climbazole (Douxo Chlorhexidine + Climbazole Mousse, Sogeval Laboratories).

Specific studies investigating systemic treatment of *Malassezia* dermatitis in cats have been limited to oral itraconazole (Sporanox, Janssen Pharmaceuticals). In both studies,

oral itraconazole at 5 to 10 mg/kg every 24 hours by mouth (PO) appears to be effective at reducing mycologic counts and improving associated clinical lesions.[55,56] This would be in agreement with the systematic review in dogs that also found fair evidence for the use of oral itraconazole in canine *Malassezia* dermatitis. At this time, itraconazole is the drug of choice in cats, based on the results of these limited studies, the drug's pharmacokinetics, and overall tolerability. However, cost of the trade name product has likely limited its widespread use. Anecdotal evidence suggests that fluconazole at 5 mg/kg every 24 hours PO may also be a reasonable option as it provides a better safety margin. The use of terbinafine in veterinary medicine is growing, and it has been investigated in pilot studies for the treatment of canine *Malassezia* dermatitis.[26,57] However, because of an overall lack of studies showing appropriate dosing, efficacy, and potential adverse events in cats, this medication currently should be used only in refractory cases or in those in which adverse events to azole derivatives have been documented. Although there are reports of ketoconazole used for the treatment of *Malassezia* overgrowth in cats, use of this medication is commonly discouraged because of concerns of gastrointestinal upset and hepatotoxicity, and griseofulvin is ineffective in the treatment of *Malassezia* infections.[24,34] Finally, newer triazole derivatives such as voriconazole and posaconazole have become available. The use of these agents for the treatment of *Malassezia* infections is limited, and potential hepatotoxic and neurotoxic adverse reactions have been reported.[58] The author would also contend that as these drugs are commonly used to treat resistant and invasive fungal infections in people, their use should be avoided for the treatment of *Malassezia* infections in veterinary medicine. Treatment length for most cases of *Malassezia* dermatitis consists of approximately 30 days, but a more accurate time frame should be 1 week beyond clinical and cytological resolution.

With specific attention to the treatment of *Malassezia* otitis, similar principles to those for *Malassezia* dermatitis must be considered to prevent recurrence or persistence of infection. Appropriate treatment of *Malassezia* otitis is dependent upon choosing an effective ear cleaner and topical medication. Cleaning is important for the removal of exudate to prevent inactivation of medications and to facilitate effective penetration of the chosen medication throughout the length of the ear canal. Numerous commercial ear cleaner preparations are available, and investigations have shown that several have significant anti-*Malassezia* effects.[59,60] Products more commonly used include Epi-Otic Advance (Virbac, Ft. Worth, Texas), MalAcetic ULTRA otic cleanser (Dechra, Overland Park, Kansas), and T8 Keto (Bayer HealthCare, Shawnee Mission, Kansas). Ear canals should be flushed one to two times per week to avoid excessive fluid being instilled into the ear, possibly leading to maceration of the epidermal lining and worsening normal epidermal barrier function. Following therapeutic resolution, transition to routine cleaning is commonly employed as maintenance therapy or until the inciting cause is resolved. Specific topical antifungal therapy is also commonly needed, and numerous commercial otic preparations exist, including those containing clotrimazole, miconazole, thiabendazole, or nystatin. Preparations utilizing clotrimazole or miconazole are normally preferred over the latter agents because of a lower minimum inhibitory concentration against *Malassezia* demonstrated in limited *in vitro* studies.[61,62] Medicated drops should be instilled into the ear canals once or twice daily, using an appropriate volume of medication (approximately 0.5 mL). Follow-up at 2 to 4 weeks is recommended to re-evaluate if changes or additional therapy are needed.

ZOONOTIC CONSIDERATIONS

M. pachydermatis has been associated with problems in a neonatal intensive care unit where it was cultured from the blood, urine, and cerebral spinal fluid of low–birth-weight patients. The route by which *M. pachydermatis* was introduced into this unit is not certain, but it is suspected to have occurred via transient carriage on a health care worker following casual contact with a pet dog.[63] A study by Morris et al.[64] demonstrated that *M. pachydermatis* could be detected from 93% of the dog owners' hands, regardless of their pets' skin disease status.[64] This finding underscores the importance of good standard hand hygiene by health care professionals, which was credited with the abatement of problems in the previously mentioned intensive care unit. Despite this information, there are no current reports indicating that immunocompromised or human immunodeficiency virus-positive individuals are at an increased risk of infection with *M. pachydermatis*.[11] The same cannot be said for lipid-dependent

species of *Malassezia*. Individuals that are immunocompromised secondary to acquired immunodeficiency syndrome, immunomodulatory therapy, or other debilitating diseases have been shown to have an elevated rate of lipid-dependent *Malassezia*-associated diseases.[65] Given that cats are more likely to be colonized by lipid-dependent *Malassezia* species, extra consideration may need to be given in situations where a cat's owner is immunocompromised, to remind them about standard hygiene practices following interactions with their pet.

SUMMARY

Feline otitis and dermatitis secondary to both lipid and non-lipid dependent *Malassezia* spp. overgrowth are being recognized more frequently in veterinary medicine. Primary conditions resulting in secondary *Malassezia* infections appear to include hypersensitivity dermatitides, refractory chin acne, idiopathic facial dermatitis, retroviral infections, and neoplastic conditions. In addition, Devon Rex and Sphynx cats have been shown to have higher colonization rates with *Malassezia* spp., likely predisposing these two breeds to a higher rate of secondary infections with the organism. Clinical diagnosis of *Malassezia* otitis and dermatitis in the cat is based on cytological recovery of the organism from skin and ear canals with compatible lesions. Therapy at this time is primarily extrapolated from therapeutic interventions in dogs and anecdotal experiences, with specific interventions in the cat limited to small pilot studies utilizing systemically administered itraconazole.

References

1. Guillot J, Bond R: *Malassezia pachydermatis*: a review. *Med Mycol* 37:295–306, 1999.
2. Matousek JL, Campbell KL: *Malassezia* Dermatitis. *Compend Contin Educ Vet* 24:224–232, 2002.
3. Chen T, Hill PB: The biology of *Malassezia* organisms and their ability to induce immune responses and skin disease. *Vet Dermatol* 16:4–26, 2005.
4. Weidman FD: Exfoliative dermatitis in the Indian rhinoceros (*Rhinoceros unicornis*), with description of a new species: *Pityrosporum pachydermatis*. In *Report of the laboratory museum comparative pathology Zoological Society*, Philadelphia, 1925, Comparative Pathology Zoological Society, pp 36–43.
5. Gustafson B: Otitis externa in the dog. A bacteriological and experimental study. Thesis. Stockholm, 1955, Royal Veterinary College of Sweden.
6. Dufait R: *Pityrosporum canis* as the cause of canine chronic dermatitis. *Vet Med Small Anim Clin* 78:1055–1057, 1983.
7. Hay RJ: *Malassezia*, dandruff and seborrhoeic dermatitis: an overview. *Br J Dermatol* 165:2–8, 2011.
8. Gupta AK, Batra R, Bluhm R, et al: Skin diseases associated with *Malassezia* species. *J Am Acad Dermatol* 51:785–798, 2004.
9. Bond R: Superficial veterinary mycoses. *Clin Dermatol* 28:226–236, 2010.
10. Castellá G, DeBellis F, Bond R, et al: Molecular characterization of *Malassezia nana* isolates from cats. *Vet Microbiol* 148:363–367, 2011.
11. Bond R: *Malassezia* dermatitis. In Greene CE, editor: *Infectious diseases of the dog and cat*, ed 4, St Louis, 2012, Elsevier/Saunders, pp 602–606.
12. Crespo MJ, Abarca ML, Cabañes FJ: Occurrence of *Malassezia* spp. in the external ear canals of dogs and cats with and without otitis externa. *Med Mycol* 40:115–121, 2002.
13. Nardoni S, Mancianti F, Rum A, et al: Isolation of *Malassezia* species from healthy cats and cats with otitis. *J Feline Med Surg* 7:141–145, 2005.
14. Cafarchia C, Gallo S, Capelli G, et al: Occurrence and population size of *Malassezia* spp. in the external ear canal of dogs and cats both healthy and with otitis. *Mycopathologia* 160:143–149, 2005.
15. Dizotti CE, Coutinho S: Isolation of *Malassezia pachydermatis* and *M. sympodialis* from the external ear canal of cats with and without otitis externa. *Acta Vet Hung* 55:471–477, 2007.
16. Shokri H, Khosravi A, Rad M, et al: Occurrence of *Malassezia* species in Persian and domestic short hair cats with and without otitis externa. *J Vet Med Sci* 72:293–296, 2010.
17. Bond R, Anthony RM, Dodd M, et al: Isolation of *Malassezia sympodialis* from feline skin. *J Med Vet Mycol* 34:145–147, 1996.
18. Bond R, Howell SA, Haywood PJ, et al: Isolation of *Malassezia sympodialis* and *Malassezia globosa* from healthy pet cats. *Vet Rec* 141:200–201, 1997.
19. Raabe P, Mayser P, Weib R: Demonstration of *Malassezia furfur* and *M. sympodialis* together with *M. pachydermatis* in veterinary specimens. *Mycoses* 41:493–500, 1998.
20. Crespo MJ, Abarca ML, Cabañes FJ: Isolation of *Malassezia furfur* from a cat. *J Clin Microbiol* 37:1573–1574, 1999.
21. Hirai A, Kano R, Makimura K, et al: A unique isolate of *Malassezia* from a cat. *J Vet Med Sci* 64:957–959, 2002.

22. Cabañes FJ, Hernandez JJ, Castellá G: Molecular analysis of *Malassezia sympodialis*—related strains from domestic animals. *J Clin Microbiol* 43:277–283, 2005.

23. Coutinho S, Fedullo J, Corrêa S: Isolation of *Malassezia* spp. from cerumen of wild felids. *Med Mycol* 44:383–387, 2006.

24. Miller WH, Griffin CE, Campbell K: *Malassezia* dermatitis. In *Muller & Kirk's small animal dermatology*, ed 7, St Louis, 2013, Elsevier, pp 243–249.

25. Morris DO: *Malassezia* dermatitis and otitis. *Vet Clin North Am Small Anim Pract* 29:1303–1310, 1999.

26. Rosales MS, Marsella R, Kunkle G, et al: Comparison of the clinical efficacy of oral terbinafine and ketoconazole combined with cephalexin in the treatment of *Malassezia* dermatitis in dogs—a pilot study. *Vet Dermatol* 16:171–176, 2005.

27. Foster-Van Hute MA, Curtis CF, White RN: Resolution of exfoliative dermatitis and *Malassezia pachydermatis* overgrowth in a cat after surgical thymoma resection. *J Small Anim Pract* 38:451–454, 1997.

28. Godfrey DR: A case of feline paraneoplastic alopecia with secondary *Malassezia*-associated dermatitis. *J Small Anim Pract* 39:394–396, 1998.

29. Mauldin EA, Morris DO, Goldschmidt MH: Retrospective study: the presence of *Malassezia* in feline skin biopsies. A clinicopathological study. *Vet Dermatol* 13:7–14, 2002.

30. Turek MM: Cutaneous paraneoplastic syndrome in dogs and cats: a review of the literature. *Vet Dermatol* 14:279–296, 2003.

31. Perrins N, Gaudiano F, Bond R: Carriage of *Malassezia* spp. yeasts in cats with diabetes mellitus, hyperthyroidism and neoplasia. *Med Mycol* 45:541–546, 2007.

32. Sierra P, Guillot J, Jacob H, et al: Fungal flora on cutaneous and mucosal surfaces of cats infected with feline immunodeficiency virus or feline leukemia virus. *Am J Vet Res* 61:158–161, 2000.

33. Reche A, Daniel A, Strauss T, et al: Cutaneous mycoflora and CD4:CD8 ratio of cats infected with feline immunodeficiency virus. *J Feline Med Surg* 12:355–358, 2010.

34. Ordeix L, Galeotti F, Scarampella F, et al: *Malassezia* spp. overgrowth in allergic cats. *Vet Dermatol* 18:316–323, 2007.

35. Jazic E, Coyner KS, Loeffler DG, et al: An evaluation of the clinical, cytological, infectious and histopathological features of feline acne. *Vet Dermatol* 17:134–140, 2006.

36. Bond R, Curtis CF, Ferguson EA, et al: An idiopathic facial dermatitis of Persian cats. *Vet Dermatol* 11:35–41, 2000.

37. Crespo MJ, Abarca ML, Cabañes FJ: Otitis externa associated with *Malassezia sympodialis* in two cats. *J Clin Microbiol* 38:1263–1266, 2000.

38. Colombo S, Nardoni S, Cornegliani L, et al: Prevalence of *Malassezia* spp. yeasts in feline nail folds: a cytological and mycological study. *Vet Dermatol* 18:278–283, 2007.

39. Åhman S, Perrins N, Bond R: Carriage of *Malassezia* spp. yeasts in healthy and seborrhoeic Devon Rex cats. *Med Mycol* 45:449–455, 2007.

40. Åhman S, Bergström K: Cutaneous carriage of *Malassezia* species in healthy and seborrhoeic Sphynx cats and a comparison to carriage in Devon Rex cats. *J Feline Med Surg* 11:970–976, 2009.

41. Volk A, Belyavin C, Varjonen K, et al: *Malassezia pachydermatis* and *M. nana* predominate amongst the cutaneous mycobiota of Sphynx cats. *J Feline Med Surg* 12:917–922, 2010.

42. Bond R, Stevens K, Perrins N, et al: Carriage of *Malassezia* spp. yeasts in Cornish Rex, Devon Rex and Domestic short-haired cats: a cross-sectional survey. *Vet Dermatol* 19:299–304, 2008.

43. Bond R, Wren L, Lloyd D: Adherence of *Malassezia pachydermatis* and *Malassezia sympodialis* to canine, feline and human corneocytes in vitro. *Vet Rec* 147:454–455, 2000.

44. Cafarchia C, Otranto D: The pathogenesis of *Malassezia* yeasts. *Parassitologia* 50:65–67, 2008.

45. Morris D, Olivier B, Rosser E: Type-1 hypersensitivity reactions to *Malassezia pachydermatis* extracts in atopic dogs. *Am J Vet Res* 59:836–841, 1998.

46. Nuttal T, Halliwell R: Serum antibodies to *Malassezia* yeasts in canine atopic dermatitis. *Vet Dermatol* 12:327–332, 2001.

47. Bond R, Curtis C, Hendricks A, et al: Intradermal test reactivity to *Malassezia pachydermatis* in atopic dogs. *Vet Rec* 150:448–449, 2002.

48. Morris D, DeBoer D: Evaluation of serum obtained from atopic dogs with dermatitis attributable to *Malassezia pachydermatis* for passive transfer of immediate hypersensitivity to that organism. *Am J Vet Res* 64:262–266, 2003.

49. Bond R, Patterson-Kane J, Lloyd D: Intradermal test reactivity to *Malassezia pachydermatis* in healthy basset hounds and bassets with *Malassezia* dermatitis. *Vet Rec* 151:105–109, 2002.

50. Bensignor E, Jankowski F, Seewald W, et al: Comparison of two sampling techniques to assess quantity and distribution of *Malassezia* yeasts on the skin of Basset Hounds. *Vet Dermatol* 13:237–241, 2002.

51. Griffin J, Scott D, Erb H: *Malassezia* otitis externa in the dog: the effect of heat-fixing otic exudate for cytological analysis. *J Vet Med A Physiol Pathol Clin Med* 54:424–427, 2007.

52. Angus J: Otic cytology in health and disease. *Vet Clin North Am Small Anim Pract* 34:411–424, 2004.

53. Negre A, Bensignor E, Guillot J: Evidence-based veterinary dermatology: a systematic review of interventions for *Malassezia* dermatitis in dogs. *Vet Dermatol* 20:1–12, 2009.

54. Maynard L, Rème C, Viaud S: Comparison of two shampoos for the treatment of canine *Malassezia* dermatitis: a randomized controlled trial. *J Small Anim Pract* 52:566–572, 2011.

55. Åhman S, Perrins N, Bond R: Treatment of *Malassezia pachydermatis*-associated seborrhoeic dermatitis in Devon Rex cats with itraconazole—a pilot study. *Vet Dermatol* 18:171–174, 2007.

56. Bensignor E: Treatment of *Malassezia* overgrowth with itraconazole in 15 cats. *Vet Rec* 167:1011–1012, 2010.

57. Berger D, Lewis T, Schick A, et al: Comparison of once-daily versus twice-weekly terbinafine administration for the treatment of canine *Malassezia* dermatitis—a pilot study. *Vet Dermatol* 23:418–425, 2012.

58. Quimby J, Hoffman S, Duke J, et al: Adverse neurological events associated with voriconazole use in 3 cats. *J Vet Intern Med* 24:647–649, 2010.

59. Swinney A, Fazakerley J, McEwan N, et al: Comparative *in vitro* antimicrobial efficacy of commercial ear cleaners. *Vet Dermatol* 19:373–379, 2008.

60. Mason C, Steen S, Paterson S, et al: Study to assess *in vitro* antimicrobial activity of nine ear cleaners against 50 *Malassezia pachydermatis* isolates. *Vet Dermatol* 24:362–366, 2013.

61. Kiss G, Radvanyi S, Szigeti G: New combination for the therapy of canine otitis externa microbiology of otitis externa. *J Small Anim Pract* 38:51–56, 1997.

62. Peano A, Beccati M, Chiavassa E, et al: Evaluation of the antifungal susceptibility of *Malassezia pachydermatis* to clotrimazole, miconazole and thiabendazole using a modified CLSI M27-A3 microdilution method. *Vet Dermatol* 23:131–135, e29, 2012.

63. Chang HJ, Miller HL, Watkins N, et al: An epidemic of *Malassezia pachydermatis* in an intensive care nursery associated with colonization of health care workers' pet dogs. *N Engl J Med* 338:706–711, 1998.

64. Morris D, O'Shea K, Shofer F, et al: *Malassezia pachydermatis* carriage in dog owners. *Emerg Infect Dis* 11:83–88, 2005.

65. Tragiannidis A, Bisping G, Koehler G, et al: Minireview: *Malassezia* infections in immunocompromised patients. *Mycoses* 53:187–195, 2010.

Cardiac Blood Tests

Mark A. Oyama

The assessment of feline cardiac function relies traditionally on electrocardiography, radiography, and echocardiography. These diagnostic modalities are relatively time consuming, expensive, and in the case of echocardiography may be of limited availability. Blood-based cardiac testing is a growing field offering important advantages over traditional diagnostic tests, including lower financial cost and wider availability. The clinical utility of blood-based testing relies on the specificity and sensitivity of the assay to detect underlying heart disease and provide information regarding disease severity, response to treatment, and prognosis.

Sensitivity refers to the ability of a test to detect affected individuals, whereas specificity refers to the ability to detect individuals not affected by the condition in question. Clinical tests are often considered as a yes or no (i.e., binary) result. The parameter being tested is either above or below a critical cutoff value. This represents a conflicting balance between sensitivity and specificity. That is, gains in sensitivity typically are offset by losses of specificity and vice versa. Sensitivity and specificity are properties that describe the assay. The performance of the test in a clinical setting is represented by an assay's positive and negative predictive values (respectively, PPVs and NPVs). These values represent the proportion of individuals that are truly positive when the test result is positive (PPV) or truly negative when the test result is negative (NPV). Unlike sensitivity and specificity, PPVs and NPVs are affected by the underlying prevalence of disease. In general, the PPV of an assay increases as prevalence of disease increases, and it decreases as the prevalence of disease decreases. In an opposite fashion, NPV increases as disease prevalence decreases, and it decreases as disease prevalence increases. The relationship between PPV, NPV, and disease prevalence is illustrated in Figure 34-1. Thus interpretation of a diagnostic test involves not only the test result but also the pretest risk that the individual has the disease in question.

Cardiac blood testing is widely accepted in human medicine, and blood-based detection of cardiac "biomarkers" represents the diagnostic standard for detection of acute myocardial infarction and congestive heart failure (CHF).[1,2]

A biomarker is defined as a substance elaborated by a specific tissue, detected in circulation, and released in proportion to a particular disease process that provides information regarding presence and severity of disease and is relatively stable and easy to detect by routine clinical laboratory methods. Detection of biomarkers for disease of organs other than the heart is both familiar and routine. For example, bilirubin is a commonly used biomarker to detect hepatic disease. In cats B-type natriuretic peptide (BNP), atrial natriuretic peptide (ANP), and cardiac troponin have demonstrated the greatest potential as cardiac biomarkers.

NATRIURETIC PEPTIDES

Atrial natriuretic peptide and BNP, released from the myocardium primarily in response to elevated wall stress, elicit vasodilation, diuresis, and natriuresis. In this respect the biologic activity of ANP and BNP counters that of the renin-angiotensin-aldosterone system, which also is activated in cats with heart disease and heart failure. Production of ANP occurs primarily within the atrial myocardium, whereas in cats with heart disease both the atrial and ventricular myocardia secrete BNP.[3-5] Both hormones are produced initially as prohormones and upon secretion subsequently are cleaved by serum proteases to form the active hormones (C-terminal ANP and C-terminal BNP), as well as an inactive N-terminal portion (NT-proANP and NT-proBNP). Detection of circulating N-terminal fragments is facilitated by their longer half-life and greater stability as compared with the C-terminal molecules. Thus the current commercially available feline ANP and BNP tests detect the N-terminal molecules specifically.

In human beings, ANP and BNP assays are used to (1) detect asymptomatic disease in high-risk populations, (2) assess severity of disease, (3) confirm or exclude a diagnosis of heart failure in emergent patients, (4) provide prognosis, and (5) guide treatment through use of sequential measurements.[2,6,7]

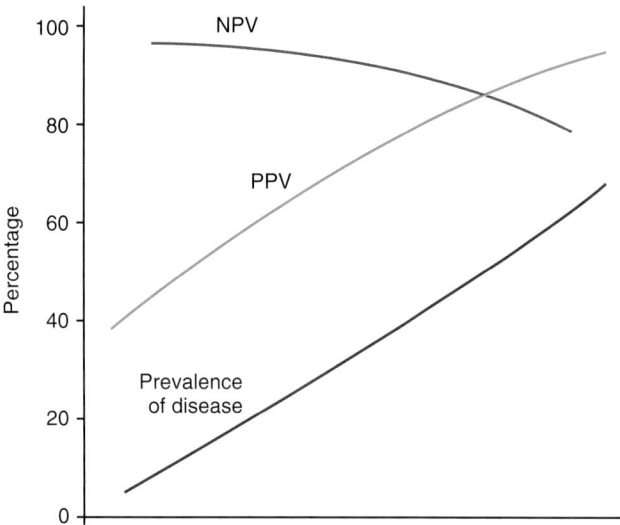

Figure 34-1: Hypothetical Performance of an Assay over a Range of Disease Prevalence Values. The positive predictive value (PPV), or the proportion of individuals who test positive that are truly positive, increases as disease prevalence increases. The negative predictive value (NPV), or the proportion of individuals who test negative that are truly negative tends to increase as disease prevalence decreases. Thus interpretation of the assay depends not only on the test result (positive or negative) but also on the prevalence of disease in the population to which the individual being tested belongs.

DETECTION OF UNDERLYING HEART DISEASE

Circulating concentrations of C-ANP and C-BNP are elevated in cats with heart disease,[8] and plasma C-ANP concentrations correlate strongly with left atrial pressure in cats.[9] NT-proANP and NT-proBNP are similarly elevated in affected cats.[10] Median (95% confidence interval [CI]) concentrations of NT-proANP in healthy control cats, cats with heart disease without heart failure, and cats with heart disease and heart failure were 682 (530 to 834) pmol/L, 1176 (810 to 1543) pmol/L, and 1865 (1499 to 2231) pmol/L, respectively.[10] Using a cutoff value of 960 pmol/L, NT-proANP assay possessed a sensitivity of 84% and specificity of 82% in distinguishing healthy controls from cats with heart disease or heart failure. Overall, NT-proANP assay classified 83% of the 78 cats correctly in the study. In the same study,[10] the median (95% CI) concentrations of NT-proBNP in healthy control cats, cats with heart disease without heart failure, and cats with heart disease and heart failure were 34 (11 to 56) pmol/L, 184 (111 to 257) pmol/L, and 525 (437 to 612) pmol/L, respectively. Using a cutoff value of 49 pmol/L, NT-proBNP assay possessed 100% sensitivity and 89% specificity, and 96% of all cats were classified correctly. Thus every cat with heart disease or heart failure ($n = 50$) was detected by NT-proBNP assay. The detection of heart disease in cats using NT-proBNP assay is further supported by a study of 80 healthy control cats and 86 cats with asymptomatic heart disease.[11] In this population, an NT-proBNP cutoff value of 40 pmol/L yielded 90% sensitivity and 85% specificity for detecting cats with asymptomatic heart disease. These results indicate that detection of asymptomatic or occult cardiomy-

opathy is possible using natriuretic peptide assay, and in particular the NT-proBNP assay. In 2013, use of a point-of-care feline NT-proBNP assay (SNAP Feline proBNP, IDEXX Laboratories, Westbrook, Maine) was described.[12] The device uses enzyme-linked immunosorbent assay to produce two blue spots on the test surface, and the relative optical density (i.e., darkness) of the colored spots indicates whether the patient sample contains elevated or normal NT-proBNP concentrations based on a cutoff value of 200 pmol/L. The use of this point-of-care device to rapidly evaluate NT-proBNP concentration in cats suspected to have heart disease merits further study.

Cats with preclinical cardiomyopathy are a particularly important subpopulation, because by definition they demonstrate no clinical signs referable to their underlying disease. Cats with preclinical disease frequently escape detection until overt sequelae (i.e., pulmonary edema, pleural effusion, systemic thromboembolism) develop, at which time prognosis is often very poor.

In general, screening tests to rule in disease benefit from high sensitivity and, when applied to a high-risk population with a relatively high prevalence of disease, yield high PPV.[13] Screening tests to rule out disease benefit from high specificity and high NPV.

ASSESSMENT OF DISEASE SEVERITY

In cats with cardiomyopathy, circulating NT-proANP and NT-proBNP concentrations correlate with traditional indices of disease severity, such as vertebral heart size seen on thoracic radiographs, left ventricular wall thickness, and left atrial size.[10,14] These results agree with findings in humans with hypertrophic cardiomyopathy (HCM).[15,16] It should be noted, however, that the precise clinical utility of circulating BNP concentrations for quantification of disease severity in any *individual* patient is still a subject of great debate.[17,18] Importantly, NT-proBNP may not detect very early and mild disease (i.e., a false-negative result). More studies in this specific population are needed. The importance of detecting very early disease can be viewed in different ways. On the one hand, a false-negative result would allow mild disease in a cat to remain undetected, and this may negatively impact breeding decisions made for animals young enough to be in breeding programs. In this regard, identification and screening for specific causative genetic mutations remain the gold standard (see Chapter 74). On the other hand, proponents of cardiac blood testing argue that the impact of a false-negative result on any individual animal outside of breeding considerations is relatively low, because very mild disease is not typically associated with clinical signs, nor are there proven medical interventions that alter the course of disease at this early stage. Thus no practical intervention other than rechecking disease at a later date is typically performed in cats with very mild disease. Based on previous studies indicating a high degree of sensitivity and specificity in cats with moderate to severe disease,[10,11,14] one could reasonably expect that serial

Table 34-1	Values of NT-proBNP Concentration from Three Different Clinical Studies Associated with Cause of Respiratory Signs in Cats*				
Population Tested	**NT-proBNP Cutoff Value**	**Sensitivity (%)**	**Specificity (%)**	**Positive Predictive Value (%)**	**Negative Predictive Value (%)**
Cats with respiratory signs in which either CHF or primary respiratory disease is possible	220[10]	94	88	NR	NR
	265[13]	90	88	92	85
	277[18]	95	85	NR	NR

NR, not reported.

*Values above the assay cutoff indicate that congestive heart failure is more likely and values below the cutoff indicate that primary respiratory disease is more likely. NT-proBNP results should be interpreted in conjunction with other appropriate diagnostic tests such as the physical exam and radiography. Echocardiography remains the gold standard for diagnosis of feline heart disease. NT-proBNP assay might be particularly helpful in deciding whether pursuit of echocardiography is likely to reveal underlying heart disease or to help formulate a preliminary treatment plan in the absence of readily available echocardiography.

NT-proBNP assay in these cats could be used to detect progressive disease.

DETECTING HEART FAILURE IN THE CAT WITH RESPIRATORY SIGNS

In cats with respiratory signs, BNP assay helps to differentiate causes of dyspnea. In three different clinical studies, NT-proBNP values differentiated cardiac (i.e., CHF) from noncardiac (i.e., asthma, pneumonia, neoplasia, etc.) etiologies in cats that presented with respiratory signs[19] (Table 34-1). When NT-proBNP assay was added to a diagnostic workup that included chest radiographs and electrocardiogram (ECG), the ability of practitioners to correctly diagnose cause of respiratory signs in cats significantly improved from 69.2% to 87.0%.[20] Cats with elevated NT-proBNP concentrations likely suffer from CHF, whereas those with lower values are more likely to have primary respiratory disease. The value of such testing is especially pertinent to patients who are not stable enough for routine diagnostic tests (e.g., thoracic radiography, echocardiography, transtracheal wash). In a small study, measurement of NT-proBNP concentration in pleural fluid helped differentiate between cats with cardiac and noncardiac causes of pleural effusion.[21] This and other applications such as the potential use of a rapid point-of-care NT-proBNP assay for use in the emergent patient are areas of interest and require further study.

PROGNOSTIC VALUE AND GUIDE TO TREATMENT

Few data regarding the use of cardiac biomarkers as guides to therapy or prognostic indicators are available for cats. One report indicated that NT-proBNP was associated with 1-month survival of cats with CHF.[22] In humans, however, BNP measurement has proven to be useful in risk stratification and as a predictor of survival. In one study[23] of 48,629 hospitalizations in people with heart failure, BNP possessed a strong linear relationship to in-hospital mortality. Patients

with the highest BNP concentrations were 2.2 times more likely to die than those with the lowest values. Importantly, this study included a large number ($n = 18,164$) of people with heart failure but preserved systolic function, which is similar to the most common forms of feline cardiomyopathy (i.e., hypertrophic and restrictive cardiomyopathy). In a study of human patients with HCM, Magga and colleagues[24] reported that BNP concentration correlated with the degree of pathological myocardial remodeling, and this may help to explain the correlation between elevated BNP and decreased survival.

In cats, prediction of either survival or risk of morbid events such as CHF or thromboembolism is particularly difficult. It is generally believed, however, that both the severity of left ventricular hypertrophy and the degree of atrial enlargement are predictive of outcome in cats with heart disease.[25] Therefore, biomarkers that are released in response to atrial and ventricular stretch, such as NT-proBNP, may have prognostic value. Treatment of feline heart disease generally is guided by clinical signs and echocardiographic findings. In human patients with HCM, progressively elevated BNP concentration is associated with clinical deterioration,[26] and BNP-directed treatment may improve outcome. In one study[27], therapy designed specifically to decrease BNP concentration to less than 100 ng/L resulted in a 50% reduction of death from heart failure or rehospitalization versus control.

CARDIAC TROPONINS

Contraction of the cardiac muscle is initiated by release of intracellular calcium ions and the subsequent cross-bridging of actin and myosin filaments. The cardiac troponin complex, which acts in conjunction with the actin filament, is a critical regulator of this process. The troponin complex is formed by three distinct units, cardiac troponins I (cTnI), T (cTnT), and C. During the initiation of contraction, cardiac troponin-C binds intracellular calcium and relieves the inhibitory effect of cTnI on the actin and myosin, thus allowing cross-bridging to begin. Subsequent disassociation of calcium from troponin-C effectively ends contraction and allows the muscle to relax.

In cases of cardiac injury, the troponin subunits detach from the actin filament, leak into the interstitial space, and gain entry into the general circulation. The cTnI and cTnT isoforms present in cardiac muscle are distinct from those in skeletal muscle, and detection of either cardiac isoform in plasma or serum is a highly specific and sensitive indicator of cardiac injury. Although the exact kinetics of troponin release from feline myocardium are relatively unknown, the characteristics of cardiac troponin release appear similar in most mammalian species.[28,29] In humans, the release kinetics of cardiac troponin are biphasic, with rapid leakage of small amounts of cytosolic troponin followed by greater and more sustained release of bound troponin, allowing detection of rising troponin levels within 4 hours of injury and peaking between 12 and 48 hours. Elevated concentrations can persist after acute myocardial infarction for as long as 2 weeks.[30]

Because of the high degree of homology between human and veterinary species,[31] detection of feline cardiac troponin can be accomplished using immunoassays designed for detection of human troponin.[32] The majority of studies performed in cats use assays that test specifically for cTnI. Although results among different commercial immunoassay machines are not likely to be directly comparable, the concentration of circulating cTnI in healthy cats should be uniformly low. Most healthy cats possess cTnI concentrations below any particular assay's detection limit (typically <0.03 to 0.05 ng/mL).[33] The particular sample type that is used (i.e., plasma, serum, or whole blood) depends on each manufacturer's assay. It is important to note that elevated cardiac troponin is indicative of myocardial cell damage, but is not specific for any particular etiology. Thus a variety of causes have been associated with increased cTnI in cats, including cardiomyopathy,[34,35] blunt myocardial trauma,[36] hyperthyroidism,[37] and renal disease.[38]

In human beings, troponin testing is used primarily for the diagnosis of acute myocardial infarction secondary to atherosclerotic disease. In cats, this particular cause of myocardial infarction is rare; however, small infarctions secondary to coronary artery and myocardial hypertrophy are a prominent feature of feline cardiomyopathy.[39,40] Acute infarction in cats would result in a biphasic release of troponin similar to that seen in human beings. This release pattern is in contrast to cases of chronic cardiac disease in which chronic low-level myocardial injury produces mild but persistently elevated troponin concentrations.[41] In human patients with chronic heart disease, elevated troponin is associated with increased mortality and hospitalization.[42,43] In cats with moderate to severe HCM, cTnI is elevated and is correlated to ventricular wall thickness, as well as the presence or absence of CHF.[34,35] Therefore, higher elevations of cTnI are thought to signify greater myocardial injury, and it is tempting to speculate whether cTnI values correlate with survival. In human patients, persistently elevated troponin levels predict worse

outcomes, whereas treatment producing a decrease in troponin is associated with a corresponding decrease in mortality.[44-46] These data suggest that cTnI has prognostic value and potentially could be used to guide treatment.

Due to its specificity for cardiac muscle, cTnI assay can assist in the differentiation of cardiac and noncardiac causes of dyspnea in cats.[34,47] In patients with respiratory distress, the median plasma cTnI concentration in cats with CHF was 10-fold greater than in cats with primary respiratory disease such as asthma. Plasma cTnI concentration greater than 1.43 ng/mL was 100% specific (but only 58% sensitive) for identifying cats with CHF.[47] Thus detecting a very elevated cTnI will reliably signal heart failure; however, because of the relatively low sensitivity, use of this cutoff point will generate many false-negatives. The use of cardiac blood tests in combination, such as performing both NT-proBNP and cTnI assays, may help to improve sensitivity and specificity, but specific clinical studies are lacking.

In cats, cTnI is elevated in cases of blunt myocardial trauma,[36] hyperthyroidism,[37] and renal disease.[38] In the case of trauma or hyperthyroidism, the underlying myocardial cell injury producing these elevations is thought to be limited. Thus cTnI levels presumably would return to normal once the primary condition is remedied. In a study of hyperthyroid cats,[37] elevated cTnI values tended to return to normal after successful radioactive iodine treatment. Cardiac troponin is cleared from circulation by the reticuloendothelial system and by renal excretion. In a small study involving cats with azotemia, cTnI was elevated in 8 of 14 cats (57%),[38] and these findings are consistent with human cases of chronic kidney disease where troponin is elevated in approximately 50% of cases.

LIMITATIONS OF CARDIAC BLOOD TESTING

Many unknowns exist regarding the clinical application of natriuretic peptide and cardiac troponin testing in cats. To date, studies investigating the diagnostic potential of these assays have been promising, but many important limitations remain. As with any diagnostic assay, the results of cardiac blood tests should be interpreted in conjunction with the patient signalment, history, physical examination findings, and other diagnostic test results. In this regard cardiac blood tests should augment, not replace, conventional diagnostic tests such as ECG, radiography, and echocardiography. In many instances, blood-based testing may help to increase confidence in pursuing further diagnostic tests; however, the information obtained by natriuretic peptide or troponin assay is not a substitute for further evaluation. Proper sample collection, handling, and shipping are particularly important for feline NT-proBNP assay, and strict adherence to the manufacturer's instructions is required to obtain accurate results.

For both NT-proBNP and cardiac troponin, little is known about the assay's ability to guide therapy and improve outcome. Ideally, improved cardiac function could be detected by serial cardiac blood tests, much in the same way that improved renal function is detected by serial declines in serum creatinine values. In human beings, BNP-guided therapy leads to improved outcome in patients with heart failure,[27] but these types of studies in veterinary species are lacking. In cases of renal or thyroid[48] disease, both NT-proBNP and cardiac troponin may be falsely elevated, and results must be interpreted cautiously. This limitation is particularly germane to an older population of cats in whom concurrent renal and cardiac disease is common.

In summary, feline cardiac blood tests represent a rapidly developing field from which several indications appear reasonable. Preclinical (occult) cardiomyopathy can be detected in cats with an acceptable level of positive and negative predictive value if populations with increased likelihood for disease are tested. Initial blood testing in cats with suspected disease may help to determine which patients should undergo further diagnostic tests such as ECG, radiography, or echo-cardiography. Blood testing can help to determine the etiology of respiratory signs in cats, and use of blood testing may permit more specific and timely treatment. In cats with heart disease, the natriuretic peptides and cardiac troponin are correlated with severity of underlying morphological and functional changes. Further studies are needed to determine if this relationship can predict risk of death or morbid events and if cardiac blood tests can be used to help tailor individualized treatments aimed at minimizing the severity of, or preventing, these outcomes.

ACKNOWLEDGMENT

The author consults for and has received funding for clinical studies involving feline NT-proBNP from IDEXX Laboratories, Inc., Westbrook, Maine, USA.

References

1. Wu AH, Apple FS, Gibler WB, et al: National Academy of Clinical Biochemistry Standards of Laboratory Practice: recommendations for the use of cardiac markers in coronary artery diseases. *Clin Chem* 45:1104, 1999.
2. Arnold JM, Howlett JG, Dorian P, et al: Canadian Cardiovascular Society Consensus Conference recommendations on heart failure update 2007: prevention, management during intercurrent illness or acute decompensation, and use of biomarkers. *Can J Cardiol* 23:21, 2007.
3. Mifune H, Suzuki S, Noda Y, et al: Fine structure of atrial natriuretic peptide (ANP)-granules in the atrial cardiocytes in the hamster, guinea pig, rabbit, cat and dog. *Jikken Dobutsu* 41:321, 1992.
4. Biondo AW, Liu ZL, Wiedmeyer CE, et al: Genomic sequence and cardiac expression of atrial natriuretic peptide in cats. *Am J Vet Res* 63:236, 2002.
5. Biondo AW, Ehrhart EJ, Sisson DD, et al: Immunohistochemistry of atrial and brain natriuretic peptides in control cats and cats with hypertrophic cardiomyopathy. *Vet Pathol* 40:501, 2003.
6. Heart Failure Society of America: HFSA 2006 comprehensive heart failure practice guideline. *J Card Fail* 12:e1, 2006.
7. Tang WH, Francis GS, Morrow DA, et al: National Academy of Clinical Biochemistry Laboratory Medicine practice guidelines: clinical utilization of cardiac biomarker testing in heart failure. *Circulation* 116:e99, 2007.
8. Sisson DD, Oyama MA, Solter PF: Plasma levels of ANP, BNP, epinephrine, norepinephrine, serum aldosterone, and plasma renin activity in healthy cats and cats with myocardial disease. *J Vet Intern Med* 17:438, 2003 (Abstract).
9. Hori Y, Yamano S, Iwanaga K, et al: Evaluation of plasma C-terminal atrial natriuretic peptide in healthy cats and cats with heart disease. *J Vet Intern Med* 22:135, 2008.
10. Connolly DJ, Magalhaes RJ, Syme HM, et al: Circulating natriuretic peptides in cats with heart disease. *J Vet Intern Med* 22:96, 2008.
11. Fox PR, Rush JE, Reynolds CA, et al: Multi-center evaluation of plasma N-terminal pro-brain natriuretic peptide (NT-pro BNP) as a biochemical screening test for asymptomatic (occult) cardiomyopathy in cats. *J Vet Intern Med* 25:1010, 2011.
12. Machen MC, Gordon SG, Rush JE, et al: Multi-centered investigation of a point-of-care NT-proBNP ELISA assay to detect moderate to severe occult (pre-clinical) feline heart disease in cats referred for cardiac evaluation. *J Vet Cardiol* 16:245–255, 2014.
13. Nakamura M, Tanaka F, Sato K, et al: B-type natriuretic peptide testing for structural heart disease screening: a general population-based study. *J Card Fail* 11:705, 2005.
14. Fox PR, Oyama MA, Reynolds CA, et al: Utility of plasma N-terminal pro-brain natriuretic peptide (NT-pro BNP) to distinguish between congestive heart failure and non-cardiac causes of acute dyspnea in cats. *J Vet Cardiol* 11(Suppl 1):S51, 2009.
15. Kaski JP, Tome-Esteban MT, Mead-Regan SJ, et al: B-type natriuretic peptide predicts disease severity in children with hypertrophic cardiomyopathy. *Heart* 94:1478, 2008.
16. Panou FK, Kotseroglou VK, Lakoumentas JA, et al: Significance of brain natriuretic peptide in the evaluation of symptoms and the degree of left ventricular diastolic dysfunction in patients with hypertrophic cardiomyopathy. *Hellenic J Cardiol* 47:344, 2006.
17. Binder J, Ommen SR, Chen HH, et al: Usefulness of brain natriuretic peptide levels in the clinical evaluation of patients with hypertrophic cardiomyopathy. *Am J Cardiol* 100:712, 2007.
18. Arteaga E, Araujo AQ, Buck P, et al: Plasma amino-terminal pro-B-type natriuretic peptide quantification in hypertrophic cardiomyopathy. *Am Heart J* 150:1228, 2005.
19. Wess G, Daisenberger P, Hirschberger J: The utility of NT-proBNP to differentiate cardiac and respiratory causes of dyspnea in cats. *J Vet Intern Med* 22:707, 2008 (Abstract).
20. Singletary GE, Rush JE, Fox PR, et al: Effect of NT-pro-BNP assay on accuracy and confidence of general practitioners in diagnosing heart failure or respiratory disease in cats with respiratory signs. *J Vet Intern Med* 26:542, 2012.
21. Hassdenteufel E, Henrich E, Hildebrant N, et al: Assessment of circulating N-terminal pro B-type natriuretic peptide concentration to differentiate between cardiac from noncardiac causes of pleural effusion in cats. *J Vet Emerg Crit Care* 23:416, 2013.
22. Fox PR, Ettinger SJ, Lamb KE, et al: Evaluation of NT-pro-brain natriuretic peptide as a prognostic indicator of short-term outcome in cats with heart failure. *J Vet Intern Med* 27:637, 2013 (Abstract).
23. Fonarow GC, Peacock WF, Phillips CO, et al: Admission B-type natriuretic peptide levels and in-hospital mortality in acute decompensated heart failure. *J Am Coll Cardiol* 49:1943, 2007.
24. Magga J, Sipola P, Vuolteenaho O, et al: Significance of plasma levels of N-terminal Pro-B-type natriuretic peptide on left ventricular remodeling in non-obstructive hypertrophic cardiomyopathy attributable to the Asp175Asn mutation in the alpha-tropomyosin gene. *Am J Cardiol* 101:1185, 2008.
25. Fox PR, Liu SK, Maron BJ: Echocardiographic assessment of spontaneously occurring feline hypertrophic cardiomyopathy. An animal model of human disease. *Circulation* 92:2645, 1995.

26. Pieroni M, Bellocci F, Sanna T, et al: Increased brain natriuretic peptide secretion is a marker of disease progression in non-obstructive hypertrophic cardiomyopathy. *J Card Fail* 13:380, 2007.

27. Jourdain P, Jondeau G, Funck F, et al: Plasma brain natriuretic peptide-guided therapy to improve outcome in heart failure: the STARS-BNP Multicenter Study. *J Am Coll Cardiol* 49:1733, 2007.

28. Cummins B, Cummins P: Cardiac specific troponin-I release in canine experimental myocardial infarction: development of a sensitive enzyme-linked immunoassay. *J Mol Cell Cardiol* 19:999, 1987.

29. O'Brien PJ, Smith DE, Knechtel TJ, et al: Cardiac troponin I is a sensitive, specific biomarker of cardiac injury in laboratory animals. *Lab Anim* 40:153, 2006.

30. Mair J, Thome-Kromer B, Wagner I, et al: Concentration time courses of troponin and myosin subunits after acute myocardial infarction. *Coron Artery Dis* 5:865, 1994.

31. Rishniw M, Barr SC, Simpson KW, et al: Cloning and sequencing of the canine and feline cardiac troponin I genes. *Am J Vet Res* 65:53, 2004.

32. Langhorn R, Willesen JL, Tarnow I, et al: Evaluation of high-sensitivity assay for measurement of canine and feline serum cardiac troponin I. *Vet Clin Pathol* 42:490–498, 2013.

33. Adin DB, Milner RJ, Berger KD, et al: Cardiac troponin I concentrations in normal dogs and cats using a bedside analyzer. *J Vet Cardiol* 7:27, 2005.

34. Connolly DJ, Cannata J, Boswood A, et al: Cardiac troponin I in cats with hypertrophic cardiomyopathy. *J Feline Med Surg* 5:209, 2003.

35. Herndon WE, Kittleson MD, Sanderson K, et al: Cardiac troponin I in feline hypertrophic cardiomyopathy. *J Vet Intern Med* 16:558, 2002.

36. Kirbach B, Schober KE, Oechtering G: Diagnosis of myocardial cell injuries in cats with blunt thoracic trauma using circulating biochemical markers. *Tieraerztl Prax* 28:30, 2000.

37. Connolly DJ, Guitian J, Boswood A, et al: Serum troponin I levels in hyperthyroid cats before and after treatment with radioactive iodine. *J Feline Med Surg* 7:289, 2005.

38. Porciello F, Rishniw M, Herndon WE, et al: Cardiac troponin I is elevated in dogs and cats with azotaemic renal failure and in dogs with non-cardiac systemic disease. *Aust Vet J* 86:390, 2008.

39. Kittleson MD, Meurs KM, Munro MJ, et al: Familial hypertrophic cardiomyopathy in Maine coon cats: an animal model of human disease. *Circulation* 99:3172, 1999.

40. Cesta MF, Baty CJ, Keene BW, et al: Pathology of end-stage remodeling in a family of cats with hypertrophic cardiomyopathy. *Vet Pathol* 42:458, 2005.

41. Healey JS, Davies RF, Smith SJ, et al: Prognostic use of cardiac troponin T and troponin I in patients with heart failure. *Can J Cardiol* 19:383, 2003.

42. Metra M, Nodari S, Parrinello G, et al: The role of plasma biomarkers in acute heart failure. Serial changes and independent prognostic value of NT-proBNP and cardiac troponin-T. *Eur J Heart Fail* 9:776, 2007.

43. Horwich TB, Patel J, MacLellan WR, et al: Cardiac troponin I is associated with impaired hemodynamics, progressive left ventricular dysfunction, and increased mortality rates in advanced heart failure. *Circulation* 108:833, 2003.

44. Mueller C: Risk stratification in acute decompensated heart failure: the role of cardiac troponin. *Nat Clin Pract Cardiovasc Med* 5:680, 2008.

45. Peacock WF, De Marco T, Fonarow GC, et al: Cardiac troponin and outcome in acute heart failure. *N Engl J Med* 358:2117, 2008.

46. La Vecchia L, Mezzena G, Zanolla L, et al: Cardiac troponin I as a diagnostic and prognostic marker in severe heart failure. *J Heart Lung Transplant* 19:644, 2000.

47. Herndon WE, Rishniw M, Schrope D, et al: Assessment of plasma cardiac troponin I concentration as a means to differentiate cardiac and non-cardiac causes of dyspnea in cats. *J Am Vet Med Assoc* 233:1261, 2008.

48. Menault P, Connolly DJ, Volk A, et al: Circulating natriuretic peptide concentrations in hyperthyroid cats. *J Small Anim Pract* 53:673, 2012.

Treatment and Prevention of Feline Arterial Thromboembolism

Daniel F. Hogan

INTRODUCTION

Feline arterial thromboembolism (ATE) is a devastating clinical condition most commonly associated with underlying cardiac disease (Figure 35-1).[1-9] Studies have identified a relatively small (2.5% to 6%) but consistent number of cats with ATE associated with neoplasia in the absence of cardiac disease.[3,6,9,10] Possible underlying mechanisms could include paraneoplastic thrombocytosis, platelet hyperreactivity, and tumor embolism.[10-13]

These clinical events appear to be exclusively due to ATE, which is distinctly different from arterial thrombosis (AT). Arterial thromboembolism is the result of obstruction of a normal artery by a fragment of a larger thrombus located distant from the site of arterial obstruction (i.e., dilated left atrium), whereas AT results in arterial obstruction because of the formation of a thrombus at the site of arterial obstruction because of some form of endothelial injury (i.e., fractured atherosclerotic plaque). The human corollaries would be cardiogenic ATE secondary to a condition such as atrial fibrillation versus coronary arterial thrombosis associated with longstanding atherosclerosis leading to acute myocardial infarction.

Formation of the thrombi distant from the site of arterial obstruction is most often described through a cumulative thrombotic risk paradigm called Virchow's triad or triangle. Virchow's triad states that there are three major contributors for thrombosis risk: blood stasis, endothelial injury, and hypercoagulability. Each of these contributors adds to the overall cumulative thrombosis risk but may do so in an unequal manner. Clinical examples of blood stasis include a dilated left atrium from underlying cardiac disease, and extramural vascular compression from a tumor. Endothelial injury is most commonly associated with left atrial dilation resulting in exposure of subendothelial collagen or fibrosis, where platelet adhesion, aggregation, and activation of the coagulation cascade is initiated. Hypercoagulability is a more difficult contributor to assess objectively. Suggested hypercoagulable conditions in cats include platelet hyperreactivity, increase in factor VIII, and reduced antithrombin and protein C.[14-16]

In ATE, the primary thrombus can become dislodged entirely or fragments of the thrombus can travel down the arterial tree to a point where their size is larger than the arterial lumen, causing infarction of the vascular bed distal from the obstruction. Cerebral, renal, splanchnic, brachial, and terminal aortic infarction have all been reported, with terminal aortic infarction accounting for more than 90% of ATE events in cats.[9] A major contributing factor for infarction appears to be the release of vasoactive substances from activated platelets, reducing potential collateral flow around the site of arterial obstruction. Experimental models have revealed that simple ligation of the distal feline aorta does not result uniformly in the classical clinical signs of terminal aortic infarction.[17-19] With aortic ligation, blood flow is maintained through an extensive collateral circulation in the vertebral system and epaxial muscles. However, in the presence of a thrombus, this collateral circulation is absent, and clinical signs are present. Platelet release products, such as serotonin, appear to be the agents primarily responsible for the loss of the collateral circulation. Experimental models have shown that the presence of serotonin was associated with loss of the collateral circulation, and pretreatment with cyproheptadine (a serotonin antagonist) or clopidogrel (an antiplatelet agent) resulted in improved collateral circulation and reduced clinical signs.[20,21] Platelet release products appear to play a similar role in humans suffering from thrombotic stroke, cardiogenic thromboembolic stroke, and pulmonary thromboembolism.[22-27]

As mentioned previously, ATE is most commonly associated with underlying cardiac disease, and according to a previous survey from the veterinary medical database, ATE occurs in 0.1% of all cats that present for medical care at North American veterinary teaching hospitals.[28] From that same survey, approximately 6% of cats with underlying cardiac disease presented with ATE. In addition, two retrospective studies reported an ATE frequency of 12% to 17% in cats with hypertrophic cardiomyopathy.[4,7] Arterial thromboembolism occurs most commonly in males, but this parallels the frequency of males with underlying myocardial disease and most likely accounts for this sex bias. Breeds that appear to have an increased risk include Ragdoll, Birman, Tonkinese, Abyssinian, and Maine Coon.[9,28]

CLINICAL SIGNS

Clinical signs attributable to ATE are dependent upon the infarcted arterial bed. Renal infarction can result in acute

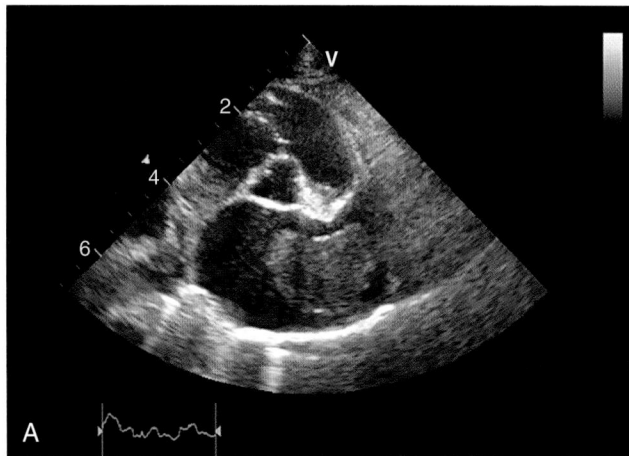

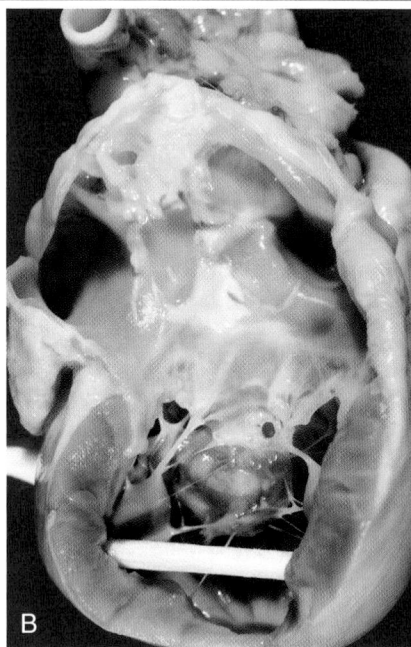

Figure 35-1: **A,** Two-dimensional echocardiographic image demonstrating a large mural thrombus within the left atrium and auricle of a cat with unclassified cardiomyopathy. **B,** Large antemortem thrombus can be seen entangled in moderator bands within the left ventricle of a cat with restrictive cardiomyopathy. Note the large area of fibrosis along the endothelium of the left atrium. (Left lateral aspect, lateral wall of left atrium removed.)

kidney injury and renal pain, whereas mesenteric infarction can manifest with abdominal pain and vomiting. Profound central neurological deficits, seizures, or sudden death can be associated with cerebral infarctions (Figure 35-2).[29]

Terminal aortic infarction (i.e., saddle thrombus) induces ischemic neuromyopathy of the pelvic limbs, which results in paresis or paralysis with absence of segmental reflexes (i.e., lower motor neuron), firm and very painful pelvic limb musculature, and cold limbs with cyanotic nail beds and either reduced strength or complete absence of the femoral arterial pulse (Figure 35-3). These changes can be bilateral and symmetrical, bilateral and asymmetrical, or unilateral depending upon the degree of obstruction and collateral circulation (Figure 35-4). Clinical signs develop acutely and can worsen over the first 12 to 24 hours but typically remain stagnant or

improve over the next several days to 3 weeks. However, improvement can be dramatically quick (i.e., 2 to 4 hours) in some cats. Approximately 50% of cats will regain some to all motor function of the pelvic limbs within 4 to 6 weeks because of establishment of the collateral circulation, recanalization of the aorta, or intrinsic dissolution of the embolus.[30] For these reasons, owners should be encouraged to at least consider therapy for these cats and not immediate euthanasia. More chronic complications with terminal aortic infarction might include self-mutilation, limb necrosis requiring amputation, and limb contracture.[9] The clinical signs associated with brachial infarction are very similar to terminal aortic infarction, although they are asymmetric, with the right forelimb more commonly affected.[30]

Tachypnea or dyspnea can also be seen with ATE, typically associated with pain or with congestive heart failure (CHF) in many cats. Congestive heart failure is reported in 44% to 66% of cats at presentation, although this is less common in the author's experience, and radiographs are required to discriminate CHF from tachypnea or dyspnea caused by ATE.[3,9,31] Inappropriate treatment of tachypnea with diuretics should be avoided, as this may result in volume contraction and negatively affect perfusion of the tissue at risk.

MANAGEMENT

Arterial thromboembolism results in dramatic and disturbing clinical signs. However, treatment for at least 48 to 72 hours should be suggested strongly to the owner. This recommendation is based upon the author's experience where within a 72-hour time window some cats will remain stable or improve, whereas others may worsen. Even though this may seem intuitive, the majority of cats are euthanized before treatment is attempted. Euthanasia can be performed later in those cats that worsen, but, if performed immediately, cats are not given the chance to remain stable or improve. The key points in the management of acute ATE are (1) reduction in continued thrombus formation associated with the embolus, (2) improvement in arterial blood flow (either aortic or collateral), (3) pain management, (4) treatment of concurrent CHF, if present, and (5) supportive care.

Reduction in Thrombus Formation

The focus here is not necessarily to reduce the size of the primary thrombus, but instead to reduce continued thrombus formation on the surface of the embolus within the arterial lumen. The emboli will typically activate the coagulation cascade, further increasing the size of the embolus, as well as inducing the release of vasoactive substances.

Unfractionated Heparin

Unfractionated heparin (UH) is an anticoagulant and inhibits the activated forms of factors X (FXa) and II (IIa or thrombin). Ideally, a coagulation panel including platelet count, prothrombin time (PT), and activated partial

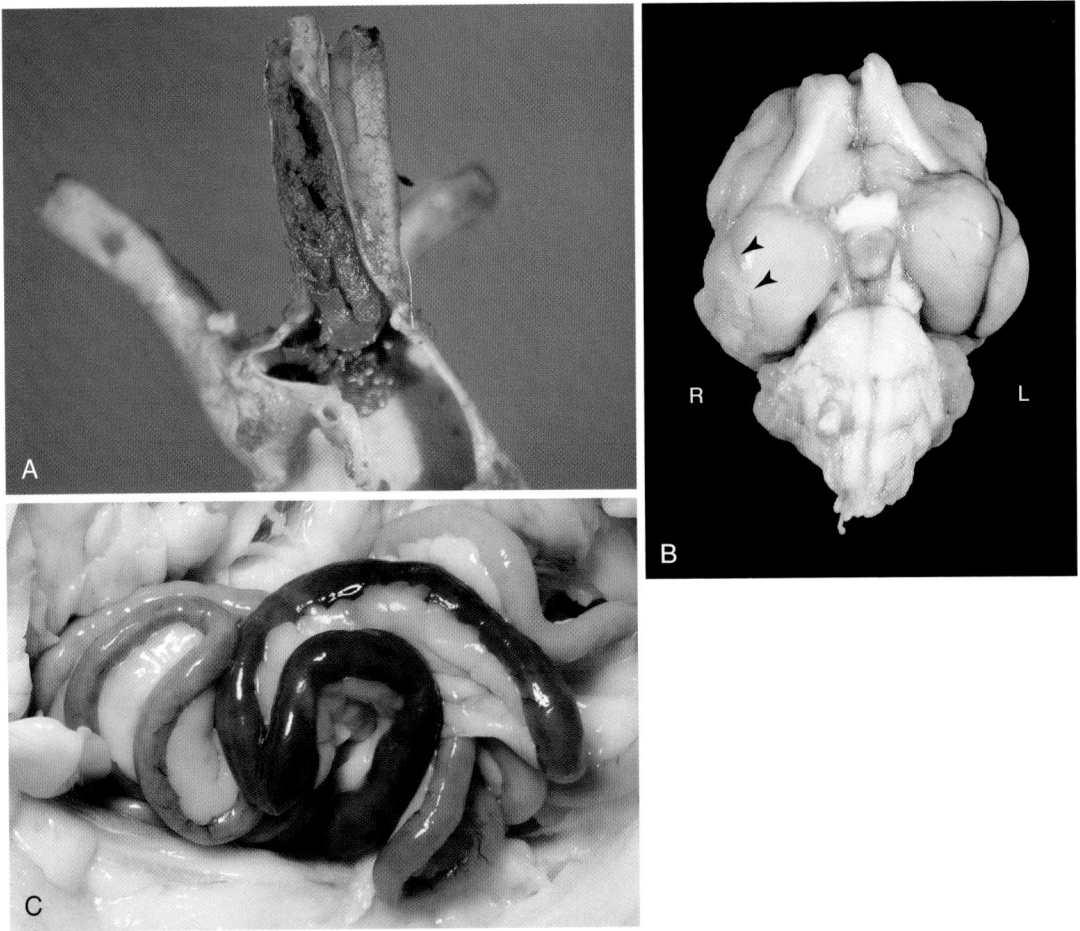

Figure 35-2: **A,** Large occlusive embolus within the right common carotid artery. **B,** Brain (ventral aspect) of the cat in **A**. Reduced vascularity along the right side of the brain (*arrowheads*) because of the embolism of the right common carotid artery. **C,** Necropsy image from a cat with hypertrophic cardiomyopathy that died from an ATE. Note the devitalized segment of jejunum secondary to a splanchnic infarction.

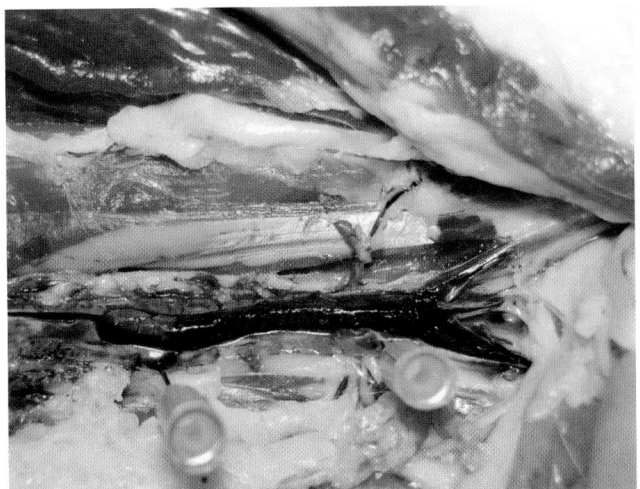

Figure 35-3: Large occlusive embolus can be seen at the aortic trifurcation.

thromboplastin time (aPTT) should be submitted before administering UH to monitor therapy. Response to UH in cats with thromboembolic disease is variable, but a prudent beginning dosing regimen is 250 to 375 International Unit (IU)/kg intravenously (IV) initially, followed by 150 to 250 IU/kg subcutaneously (SC) every 6 to 8 hours.[32] Plasma UH levels may not correlate well with the aPTT, but a goal of 1.5 to 2.0 times the baseline aPTT value has been suggested.

Low Molecular Weight Heparins

The low molecular weight heparins (LMWH) are smaller than UH but maintain a critical peptide sequence that inhibits FXa, and to a lesser degree factor IIa. These drugs have no effect on the aPTT or PT, given the reduced inhibition of IIa. Dalteparin (Fragmin) and enoxaparin (Lovenox) have been used in cats at 100 to 200 IU/kg SC every 24 to 12 hours and 1.0 to 1.5 mg/kg SC every 24 to 12 hours, respectively.[33,34] The cost for these agents is considerably more expensive than UH, and, in the author's opinion, they do not provide any benefit over UH for the short duration of acute management.

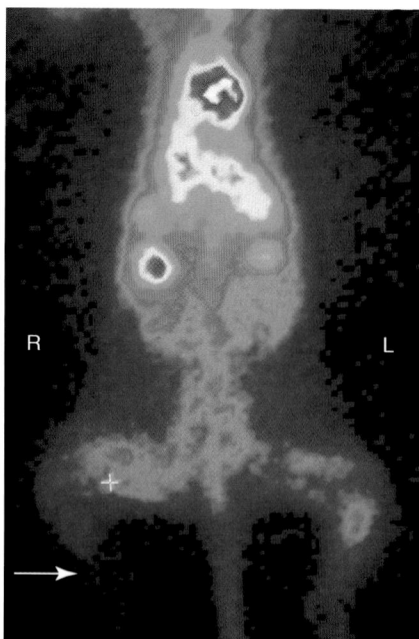

Figure 35-4: Nuclear perfusion study using free (unbound) technetium-99m demonstrating lack of perfusion distal to the midtibial region (*arrow*) in the right hind limb of a cat approximately 48 hours after a terminal aortic infarction.

Improvement in Arterial Blood Flow

Thrombolytic Therapy

Establishing arterial flow to the infarcted organ is the ideal therapeutic goal. This can be accomplished by removal of the embolus, through either embolectomy or dissolution by using thrombolytic drugs. The use of rheolytic embolectomy equipment in cats with ATE has been evaluated in one study.[35] The embolus was successfully removed in five of six cats with three surviving to discharge, but such an approach is unlikely to be applicable widely in veterinary medicine. Thrombolytic drugs such as streptokinase,[6,36] urokinase,[37] and tissue plasminogen activator (tPA)[38-40] have been used in cats to dissolve emboli and re-establish aortic flow. Ideally, thrombolytics should be administered as soon as possible, but thrombolysis has been noted as late as 18 hours after initial clinical signs. Severe adverse effects might be associated with thrombolytic therapy; therefore, the use of these drugs should be done with some consideration. The sudden resumption of arterial flow to infarcted tissue can result in life-threatening hyperkalemia and metabolic acidosis (reperfusion injury), which may require immediate and aggressive therapy. Reperfusion injury occurs in 40% to 70% of cats receiving thrombolytic therapy, with survival rates ranging from 0% to 43%.[6,36,38,39] Given that approximately 50% of cats will regain some motor function over 4 to 6 weeks following an ATE event with conservative treatment,[30] the benefit-to-risk ratio for thrombolytic therapy must be determined for each individual cat. Although cats with more complete infarction have a greater risk for reperfusion injury,[6,38] they are more likely to have a poor outcome and therefore possibly have a higher benefit-to-risk ratio for thrombolytic therapy than that of

less severely affected cats. Thrombolytics should be strongly considered in cases of cerebral, splanchnic, or bilateral renal infarction, as the re-establishment of arterial flow is critical for survival.

Streptokinase. Streptokinase combines with plasminogen to form an activator complex that converts plasminogen to the proteolytic enzyme plasmin. Plasmin degrades fibrin, fibrinogen, plasminogen, coagulation factors, and streptokinase. The streptokinase-plasminogen complex converts circulating and fibrin-bound plasminogen and is therefore considered a nonspecific activator of plasmin. Streptokinase is typically administered IV at 90,000 IU over 1 hour, followed by an IV infusion of 45,000 IU/hour IV for up to 8 hours. Currently, streptokinase is not commercially available.

In one retrospective study of 46 cats, approximately 50% of cats had a return of femoral pulses within 24 hours, with return of motor function in 30%.[6] Spontaneous bleeding from oral, rectal, or catheter sites was seen in 24% of cats. Transfusions were required in 27% of the bleeding cats, and only 18% of these cats survived. Hyperkalemia and reperfusion injury developed in approximately 40% of cats, and the overall survival rate was 33%.

Urokinase. Urokinase is similar in activity to streptokinase but is considered more fibrin specific. Urokinase is typically administered as a loading dose of 4400 IU/kg IV given over 10 minutes, followed by another 4400 IU/kg per hour IV for 12 hours.[37] Urokinase is not currently commercially available.

There is one retrospective study reporting the use of urokinase in 12 cats with ATE where return of pulses was seen in three of 10 cats and return of motor function in five of nine cats.[37] There were no bleeding complications, but hyperkalemia developed in three of 12 cats. Total survival with urokinase therapy was five of 12 (42%), with euthanasia as the cause of death for all cats.

Tissue Plasminogen Activator. Plasminogen and tPA each have a high affinity for fibrin, which results in their binding to thrombi and emboli in close proximity. This confers a relatively thrombus/embolus-specific conversion of plasminogen to plasmin. The recommended dosing protocol for human recombinant tPA (Activase, Genentech, San Francisco, California) is 0.25 to 1 mg/kg per hour IV for a total dose of 1 to 10 mg/kg.[38] Activase is supplied in 50 mg and 100 mg bottles, with an estimated cost of $1500 USD (U.S. dollars) and $3000 USD, respectively. The average cat will not require more than 50 mg, and smaller amounts of tPA can be purchased (Cathflo Activase, Genentech, San Francisco, California) for approximately $100 USD per 2 mg.

There have been two clinical trials of tPA in cats with ATE.[39,40] In the original study,[40] return of pulses was noted within 36 hours and return of motor function within 48 hours. Minor bleeding was noted in 50% of cats, with 33% of cats experiencing fever and reperfusion injury. The acute survival rate was 50%, with deaths attributable to reperfusion injury and cardiogenic shock. The second and more recent study involving 11 cats[39] reported a return of arterial pulses at 4 hours in 50% of surviving cats, which increased to 62% at 24 hours. Complications occurred in 100% of cats and included azotemia, neurological signs, arrhythmias, hyperkalemia, acidosis, and sudden death. The study ended early because of the high rate of complications, and the overall survival was 64% at 24 hours and 27% at discharge.

Collateral Flow Improvement

As mentioned previously, loss of terminal aortic flow alone does not result in reduced perfusion of the pelvic limbs or clinical signs of terminal aortic infarction because of the presence of a collateral circulatory network. However, with ATE, platelet release products result in vasoconstriction of this collateral circulation and reduced perfusion. Maintaining this collateral circulation may help maintain perfusion to the pelvic limbs even in the presence of an aortic embolus. Vasodilatory drugs, such as acepromazine, should not be used, as they are not effective and may actually worsen the clinical picture by causing hypotension. Cyproheptadine improved collateral circulation in an experimental model of feline ATE,[20] but it has not been clinically evaluated. Antiplatelet drugs may have a beneficial effect on the collateral circulation through platelet inhibition and reduction in platelet release of vasoactive substances, and they should be administered as soon as possible.

Aspirin. Aspirin has been shown to reduce the amount of released thromboxane A_2 from activated cat platelets and improve collateral flow in an experimental cat model of terminal aortic infarction.[41,42] However, the dose of aspirin used was quite high and could induce toxicity. Given that antiplatelet effects can be seen at 20 to 50 µg/mL, and this can be accomplished with a dose of 10.5 mg/kg in the cat,[43] it would seem prudent to administer no more than the standard dose of 25 mg/kg orally (PO) every 72 hours.

Clopidogrel. Clopidogrel (Plavix) has been shown to reduce serotonin release from activated platelets in cats and exert a vasomodulating effect in rats, rabbits, dogs, and cats.[21,44,45] This vasomodulating effect in cats was demonstrated through improved pelvic limb perfusion and reduced clinical signs of terminal aortic infarction in an experimental model using a 75 mg/cat dose.[21] This dose represents an approximately 16 mg/kg dose in an average-sized cat and a fourfold increase over the currently recommended daily dose in cats.[46] Although not evaluated in cats, a fourfold increase in the daily clopidogrel dose in humans results in maximal platelet inhibition within 90 minutes of administration.[47-49] Similarly, a dose of 10 mg/kg resulted in maximal platelet inhibition within 90 minutes in dogs.[50] Therefore, the author recommends administering 75 mg/cat of clopidogrel PO upon presentation for ATE.

Pain Management

Arterial thromboembolism often results in severe pain, and the need for effective control of this pain cannot be overstated. Although some cats may demonstrate clear and dramatic signs such as vocalization and self-mutilation, others may be more stoic, exhibiting only anorexia, elevated heart rate, or mild anxiety, so one should assume that all cats are experiencing clinically relevant pain. Narcotics are very effective analgesics and are the most commonly used agents. Butorphanol tartrate (0.2 to 0.4 mg/kg SC, intramuscularly (IM) or IV every 1 to 4 hours), hydromorphone (0.08 to 0.3 mg/kg SC, IM, or IV every 2 to 6 hours), buprenorphine HCl (0.005 to 0.01 mg/kg SC, IM, or IV every 6 to 12 hours), and oxymorphone HCl (0.05 to 0.1 mg/kg SC, IM, or IV every 1 to 3 hours) have been widely used in cats and appear to provide good analgesia with little adverse effects.[51] In severe or refractory cases, fentanyl citrate (4 to 10 µg/kg IV bolus, followed by 4 to 10 µg/kg per hour infusion) can be used.[51]

Treatment of Concurrent Congestive Heart Failure

Decompensated CHF can occur with ATE, complicating the clinical situation.[3,6,9,31] Acute management utilizing diuretics, oxygen, and possibly nitroglycerin is important and will frequently result in resolution of the congestive state. The reader is directed to Chapter 41 for review of treatment options for CHF.

Supportive Care

A low rectal temperature is commonly associated with ATE, but this is typically related to reduced perfusion of the pelvic limbs and not true hypothermia. Heating pads should not be used, as thermal injury may occur, but blankets or increased air temperature may be considered. Fluid therapy may be helpful in assisting in the removal of metabolic toxins, such as potassium and organic acids, but overaggressive rates may induce or worsen CHF. Therefore, it is recommended to use parenteral fluid therapy cautiously when deemed beneficial and in cats without active CHF. Physical therapy to maintain flexibility of joints and encourage collateral flow is recommended but may not be possible in the early painful period.

SURVIVAL

The average reported survival rates for initial ATE events are remarkably similar, whether conservative (37%)[3,9,31] or thrombolytic (38%)[6,37,39,40] therapy is used. Cats with single pelvic limb infarction do dramatically better (68% to 93%) compared with cats with bilateral pelvic limb infarction (15% to 36%), regardless of therapy used.[3,6,9,31] Nonsurvival rates range from 61% to 67%, with natural death rates (28% to 40%) similar to euthanasia rates (25% to 35%).[3,6,9,31] Nonsurvival has been significantly associated with hypothermia,[6,9] reduced heart rate,[9] and absence of motor function.[9] The author believes that survival rates can quickly improve through a reduction in immediate euthanasia and new-found hope of reduced ATE recurrence rate with newer antithrombotics (see Prevention of Arterial Thromboembolism).

PREVENTION OF ARTERIAL THROMBOEMBOLISM

Primary prevention of ATE is defined as preventing the first event in a cat at risk for ATE. However, there has been no such study performed in veterinary medicine to date, so no firm therapeutic recommendations can be made with any scientific support. Considering the cumulative thrombotic risk described by Virchow's triad, and clinical judgment of experienced cardiologists, blood stasis induced by a dilated left atrium could confer greater risk for ATE. In fact, a large retrospective study of cats with hypertrophic cardiomyopathy demonstrated that cats that experienced ATE had a significantly larger left atrial size than asymptomatic cats or cats with CHF.[7] These findings combined with clinical experience have led to the recommendation that primary prevention be considered in cats with echocardiographic evidence of moderate to marked left atrial enlargement. Echocardiographic measurements of end-systolic left atrial diameter greater than 1.7 cm or left atrium-to-aortic ratios greater than 2.0[52] are examples of recommendations that have been proposed. Primary prevention is also indicated in cats with spontaneous contrast or "smoke" in the left atrium on echocardiography.[52] Secondary prevention of ATE is defined as preventing a subsequent ATE event in a cat that has a history of ATE. Secondary prevention is recommended in all cats given the high prevalence of ATE recurrence and poor survival rates. There are a number of retrospective studies evaluating secondary prevention of ATE, as well as one prospective study. The recurrence rate for ATE in a small number of cats not receiving antithrombotic therapy was 40%, with a 1-year recurrence rate of 25%,[31] whereas reported recurrence rates for cats receiving an antithrombotic range from 17% to 75%,[3,6,9,31,38,53] with a 1-year recurrence rate of 25% to 61%.[6,31,53]

Antithrombotic Drugs

Because the underlying cardiac disease can only rarely be reversed, antithrombotic agents have become a mainstay for both primary and secondary prevention of ATE. The two major categories of antithrombotics are antiplatelet agents and anticoagulants.

Antiplatelet Agents

These agents inhibit some aspect of platelet function and impair the formation of the initial platelet-rich thrombus at the injured endothelial site. Some of these agents also exhibit some vasomodulating effects by interfering with vasoactive substances such as serotonin. These drugs have been used extensively in humans for primary and secondary prevention of AT, and for primary prevention of ATE in specific circumstances.

Aspirin. Aspirin irreversibly acetylates platelet cyclooxygenase preventing the formation of thromboxane A_2, which has potent proaggregating and vasoconstrictive properties. Aspirin is considered a modest and indirect antiplatelet agent. The prophylactic effect of aspirin on AT in humans is well established,[54] whereas the prophylactic effect on ATE is less clear. For primary prevention in low-risk patients, aspirin has been shown to provide some benefit in some studies.[55,56] With respect to secondary prevention of ATE in humans, aspirin is inferior to the standard treatment of warfarin.[57,58]

The pharmacological, analgesic, and antiplatelet effects of aspirin have been well studied in the cat. Aspirin has been shown to inhibit platelet aggregation in response to arachidonic acid,[59,60] but the author has not been able to demonstrate this effect using whole blood aggregometry (D.F. Hogan, unpublished data). The standard dose of aspirin is 25 mg/kg PO every 72 to 48 hours or one low-dose adult aspirin (81 mg) in the average-sized cat. Adverse effects are typically gastrointestinal (GI), such as anorexia and vomiting, and have been reported in up to 22% of treated cats.[9] The use of a low-dose aspirin protocol (5 mg/cat PO every 48 hours) has been associated with reduced adverse GI effects but shows no treatment benefit over the standard 25 mg/kg dosing protocol.[9] Aspirin has been used for primary and secondary prevention of ATE in cats for more than 30 years, with recurrence rates ranging from 17% to 75%,[3,9,31,38] with median survival times from 117 to 192 days.[9,31,53] A prospective study demonstrated that aspirin was inferior to clopidogrel for secondary prevention of ATE in cats.[53] The cost of aspirin therapy is extremely low, and even though platelet aggregation can be used to monitor drug effect, it is rarely performed.

Clopidogrel. Clopidogrel (Plavix) causes irreversible antagonism of the adenosine diphosphate $(ADP)_{2Y12}$ receptor along the platelet membrane. The ADP-induced conformational change of the glycoprotein IIb/IIIa receptor complex is also inhibited, which reduces binding of fibrinogen and von Willebrand factor.[61,62] Clopidogrel is a potent and direct antiplatelet agent exhibiting antiplatelet effects that are more potent than those of aspirin. Clopidogrel is a prodrug that must undergo hepatic biotransformation to an active metabolite.[63-65] Clopidogrel has been shown to be more effective than aspirin in humans with AT, by decreasing rates of stroke, myocardial infarction, or vascular death.[66-68] Clopidogrel has been shown to be superior to aspirin alone for primary prevention of ATE in humans with atrial fibrillation, but the combination of aspirin and clopidogrel were inferior to warfarin.[69,70]

In a short-term pharmacodynamic study in normal cats, clopidogrel was shown to induce a 95% inhibition in platelet aggregation in response to ADP, 92% inhibition in serotonin release, and a 3.9-fold prolongation in oral mucosal bleeding time when dosed at 18.75 mg, 37.5 mg, or 75 mg PO per cat every 24 hours.[46] The maximal antiplatelet effect was seen by day 3 of drug administration and was lost by 7 days after drug discontinuation. Given the equipotent effect of the studied doses, the current recommended dosing protocol for clopidogrel is 18.75 mg/cat (1/4 of a 75 mg tablet) PO every 24 hours. There were no adverse effects noted during the pharmacodynamic study. Clopidogrel was shown to be superior to aspirin for the secondary prevention of ATE in cats, with a reduced recurrence rate of 39% versus 61% at 1 year, and a significantly prolonged survival time of 443 days versus 192 days.[53] One cat receiving clopidogrel developed icterus and elevated liver enzymes during the study, which has also rarely been reported in humans.

Anticoagulants

Anticoagulant drugs inhibit the coagulation cascade by interfering with the formation of one or more active coagulation factors. These drugs are used in the acute management of stroke and myocardial function, as well as being the preferred choice for secondary prevention of ATE in humans.

Warfarin. Warfarin inhibits the formation of the vitamin K-dependent coagulation factors II, VII, IX, and X, as well as the anticoagulant proteins C and S. Warfarin has been considered the drug of choice for ATE prevention in humans with atrial fibrillation.[55-58,71-75] Bleeding is the most common complication in humans, with clinical trials reporting a 1.3% to 2.5% occurrence rate for major bleeding and 16% to 21% for minor bleeding.[55-58,71,72,74,75] Warfarin has numerous interactions with other medications that may increase or decrease the anticoagulation effect. Warfarin therapy is adjusted to obtain a desired degree of anticoagulation as measured by the PT or International Normalized Ratio (INR). Medium anticoagulation intensity (INR of 2 to 3) is recommended for the prevention of ATE in humans. A standard protocol for monitoring INR in humans is daily for the first 5 days, then 3 times weekly for up to 2 weeks. Once the steady-state warfarin dose is determined, the INR is measured every 4 to 6 weeks.

Pharmacokinetic studies of warfarin in cats demonstrate a wide interindividual and intraindividual variable anticoagulant response.[76] The suggested starting dose for warfarin is 0.06 mg/kg to 0.09 mg/kg PO every 24 hours.[76,77] Warfarin is not evenly distributed throughout the tablet, so the tablet should be crushed and compounded by a pharmacist to enable dosing in cats. Although unsubstantiated, a goal of PT prolongation of 1.3 to 1.6 from baseline or an INR of 2 to 3 has been considered as adequate anticoagulation in the cat. The recommended protocol for monitoring the INR or PT in the cat is daily for 5 to 7 days, then at least twice weekly for 2 to 3 weeks, once weekly for 2 months, and then at least once every 6 to 8 weeks. Bleeding is seen in 13% to 20% of cats, with fatal hemorrhage reported in up to 13% of cats.[3,6,34,52] The published ATE recurrence rates for cats receiving warfarin range from 42% to 53%, with estimated mean survival times from 210 to 471 days.[3,6,52] Even though warfarin has been the drug of choice for ATE prevention in humans for decades, the issues with variability in clinical response, requirement for frequent monitoring, and bleeding complications have usually limited it to a secondary consideration in cats.

Low Molecular Weight Heparins. As mentioned previously, the LMWH inhibit FXa and, to a much lesser degree, IIa. Because of the reduced inhibition of IIa, common hemostatic assays such as PT, aPTT, INR, and thromboelastography are not altered and are ineffective for drug monitoring. Therapeutic monitoring can be done by measuring anti-Xa

activity, but this is not commonly recommended in humans because of the poor correlation between anti-Xa activity and the development of bleeding or thrombosis. There is no standard monitoring protocol in cats and, similar to humans, there was poor correlation between measured anti-Xa activity and thrombus inhibition in an experimental cat model.[78] Therefore, the author does not recommend anti-Xa activity to monitor LMWH treatment. The LMWH are noninferior to UH and better than warfarin or placebo in the prevention of deep venous thrombosis and pulmonary embolism in humans.[79-83] In humans, bleeding is the most common complication with the LMWH, with a reported incidence of 5% to 27% for minor bleeding and 0% to 6.5% for major bleeding.[79-81,84-87]

The current recommended protocols for dalteparin and enoxaparin in cats are 100 to 200 IU/kg SC every 24 to 12 hours and 1.0 to 1.5 mg/kg SC every 24 to 12 hours, respectively. Although there are no efficacy studies evaluating the LMWH with ATE in cats, an experimental feline venous thrombosis model demonstrated that there was a 100% thrombus inhibition at 4 hours and 91% inhibition at 12 hours after administering 1 mg/kg enoxaparin SC every 12 hours. In the author's practice, the LMWH are administered once daily for ATE prevention. The LMWH appear to have very few adverse effects, as bleeding is only rarely reported.[34,88] There is one retrospective study that demonstrated no significant difference between dalteparin and warfarin with respect to ATE recurrence (43% versus 24%, respectively) or median survival time (255 days versus 69 days, respectively).[34] The main limitations for the LMWH are their high cost and need for subcutaneous injection.

Future Direction of Antithrombotics

A number of new antithrombotics have been developed for the human market. The advantages of these new drugs are excellent efficacy with no monitoring requirement and minimal bleeding risk.

Dabigatran (Pradaxa) is a direct thrombin inhibitor and the first drug shown to be noninferior to warfarin for the prevention of ATE associated with atrial fibrillation.[89] A larger class of drugs that have been coming to market are the Xa inhibitors. These drugs inhibit FXa, either directly or through antithrombin, and have been shown to be noninferior to warfarin.[90,91] These drugs have not been critically evaluated in cats to date. Fondaparinux (Arixtra), a synthetic Xa inhibitor that works through antithrombin, has been evaluated in a small number of cats, where anti-Xa activity approximated that achieved in humans when administered at 0.06 mg/kg SC every 12 hours.[92] However, this dosing protocol is more expensive than the LMWH protocol and therefore has no appreciable benefit. Rivaroxaban (Xarelto) is an orally administered direct Xa inhibitor that has been shown to inhibit coagulation in cat blood *in vitro*.[93] The Xa inhibitors are likely to have a major effect on the prevention of ATE in cats in the next few years. If a drug can be identified that is orally available, requires no monitoring, has minimal adverse effects, and is efficacious and cost-effective, this would be a major advance in the field of ATE prevention in cats.

Current Antithrombotic Recommendations

The following recommendations reflect author bias based on mechanistic drug effects, comparative data from humans, and currently available data in cats.

Primary Prevention

Clopidogrel. Clopidogrel (Plavix) has more potent antiplatelet effects than aspirin, and in the only prospective clinical trial of ATE prevention in cats, it was superior to aspirin in both recurrence rate and median survival time.

Secondary Prevention

Low Molecular Weight Heparins. Through their anticoagulant action, these drugs theoretically have a better mechanism of action for the stagnant blood flow associated with a dilated left atrium. They have exhibited good efficacy in humans for the prevention of deep venous thrombosis and pulmonary embolism. They appear to be safe in cats and in one retrospective study, had similar ATE recurrence rate compared with warfarin. They are expensive and require SC injections, so owners must be prepared, but the injections are no different than treating a diabetic cat.

Clopidogrel. Antiplatelet agents are considered inferior to anticoagulants in secondary prevention of ATE in humans.

However, if the owner is unwilling to give injections or cost is a concern, then clopidogrel is a viable alternative to the LMWH.

Low Molecular Weight Heparin, Clopidogrel Combination Therapy. This protocol would have combined antiplatelet and anticoagulant properties and theoretically have an enhanced antithrombotic profile. The risk for bleeding would be theoretically increased, although the author has not seen bleeding in approximately 20 to 30 cats treated with this protocol.

SUMMARY

In summary, ATE secondary to underlying cardiac disease is a clinically devastating condition in cats with an extremely high mortality rate, which is heavily influenced by the perceived inability to prevent future recurrences. Given that clopidogrel has been shown to be superior to aspirin for the prevention of recurrent ATE, there should be new hope for these cats, and immediate euthanasia rates should be reduced. The development of newer anticoagulant drugs that can be given orally and do not require clinical monitoring holds great promise and is likely to have a dramatic effect on the management of ATE in the near future.

References

1. Harpster NK: Feline myocardial diseases. In Kirk RW, editor: *Current veterinary therapy IX*, Philadelphia, 1986, Saunders, pp 380–398.
2. Bonagura JD, Fox PR: Restrictive cardiomyopathy. In Bonagura JD, editor: *Kirk's current veterinary therapy XII*, Philadelphia, 1995, Saunders, pp 863–867.
3. Laste NJ, Harpster NK: A retrospective study of 100 cases of feline distal aortic thromboembolism: 1977–1993. *J Am Anim Hosp Assoc* 31:492, 1995.
4. Atkins CE, Gallo AM, Kurzman ID, et al: Risk factors, clinical signs, and survival in cats with a clinical diagnosis of idiopathic hypertrophic cardiomyopathy: 74 cases (1985–1989). *J Am Vet Med Assoc* 201:613, 1992.
5. Baty CJ, Malarkey DE, Atkins CE, et al: Natural history of hypertrophic cardiomyopathy and aortic thromboembolism in a family of domestic shorthair cats. *J Vet Intern Med* 15:595, 2001.
6. Moore KE, Morris N, Dhupa N, et al: Retrospective study of streptokinase administration in 46 cats with arterial thromboembolism. *J Vet Emerg Crit Care* 10:245, 2000.
7. Rush JE, Freeman LM, Fenollosa NK, et al: Population and survival characteristics of cats with hypertrophic cardiomyopathy: 260 cases (1990–1999). *J Am Vet Med Assoc* 220:202, 2002.
8. Peterson EN, Moise NS, Brown CA, et al: Heterogeneity of hypertrophy in feline hypertrophic heart disease. *J Vet Intern Med* 7:183, 1993.
9. Smith SA, Tobias AH, Jacob KA, et al: Arterial thromboembolism in cats: acute crisis in 127 cases (1992–2001) and long-term management with low-dose aspirin in 24 cases. *J Vet Intern Med* 17:73, 2003.
10. Hogan DF, Dhaliwal RS, Sisson DD, et al: Paraneoplastic thrombocytosis-induced systemic thromboembolism in a cat. *J Am Anim Hosp Assoc* 35:483, 1999.
11. John WJ, Foon KA, Patchell RA: Paraneoplastic syndromes. In DeVita VT, Hellman S, Rosenberg SA, editors: *Cancer: principles and practice of oncology*, ed 5, Philadelphia, 1997, Lippincott-Raven.
12. Bick RL, Strauss JF, Frenkel EP: Thrombosis and hemorrhage in oncology patients. *Hematol Oncol Clin North Am* 10:875, 1996.
13. McNiel EA, Ogilvie GK, Fettman MJ, et al: Platelet hyperfunction in dogs with malignancies. *J Vet Intern Med* 11:178, 1997.
14. Helenski CA, Ross JN: Platelet aggregation in feline cardiomyopathy. *J Vet Intern Med* 1:24, 1987.
15. Stokol T, Brooks M, Rush JE, et al: Hypercoagulability in cats with cardiomyopathy. *J Vet Intern Med* 23:546, 2009.
16. Hogan DF: Markers of thrombotic risk in cats. In *Proceedings of the American College of Veterinary Internal Medicine Forum*, Seattle, Washington, 2007.
17. Schaub RG, Meyers KM, Sande RD, et al: Inhibition of feline collateral vessel development following experimental thrombotic occlusion. *Circ Res* 39:736, 1976.
18. Butler HC: An investigation into the relationship of an aortic emboli to posterior paralysis in the cat. *J Small Anim Pract* 12:141, 1971.
19. Imhoff RK: Production of aortic occlusion resembling acute aortic embolism syndrome in cats. *Nature* 192:979, 1961.
20. Olmstead ML, Butler HC: Five-hydroxytryptamine antagonists and feline aortic embolism. *J Small Anim Pract* 18:247, 1977.
21. Hogan DF, Widmer WR, Ward MP: Clopidogrel (Plavix) and collateral vessel development in experimental feline aortic thrombosis. *J Vet Intern Med* 20:731, 2006.
22. Bisschops RH, Klijn CJ, Kappelle LJ, et al: Collateral flow and ischemic brain lesions in patients with unilateral carotid artery occlusion. *Neurology* 60:1435, 2003.
23. Kim JJ, Fischbein NJ, Lu Y, et al: Regional angiographic grading system for collateral flow: correlation with cerebral infarction in patients with middle cerebral artery occlusion. *Stroke* 35:1340, 2004.
24. Tohgi H, Takahashi S, Chiba K, et al: Cerebellar infarction. Clinical and neuroimaging analysis in 293 patients. The Tohoku Cerebellar Infarction Study Group. *Stroke* 24:1697, 1993.

25. Haimovici H: Cardiogenic embolism of the upper extremity. *J Cardiovasc Surg (Torino)* 23:209, 1982.

26. Endys J, Hayat N, Cherian G: Comparison of bronchopulmonary collaterals and collateral blood flow in patients with chronic thromboembolic and primary pulmonary hypertension. *Heart* 78:171, 1997.

27. Todd MH, Forrest JB, Cragg DB: The effects of aspirin and methysergide on responses to clot-induced pulmonary embolism. *Am Heart J* 105:769, 1983.

28. Veterinary Medical Data Base (VMDB). 1980–2003. <www.vmdb.org>. (Accessed August 2, 2014.)

29. Green HW, Hogan DF: Suspected iatrogenic paradoxical embolism in a cat. *J Am Anim Hosp Assoc* 41:193, 2005.

30. Fox PR: Feline cardiomyopathies. In Fox PR, Sisson DD, Moise NS, editors: *Textbook of canine and feline cardiology: principles and clinical practice*, ed 2, Philadelphia, 1999, Saunders.

31. Schoeman JP: Feline distal aortic thromboembolism: a review of 44 cases (1990–1998). *J Feline Med Surg* 1:221, 1999.

32. Smith SA, Lewis DC, Kellerman DL: Adjustment of intermittent subcutaneous heparin therapy based on chromogenic heparin assay in 9 cats with thromboembolism. *J Vet Intern Med* 12:200, 1998 [Abstract].

33. Goodman JS, Rozanski EA, Brown D, et al: The effects of low-molecular weight heparin on hematologic and coagulation parameters in normal cats. *J Vet Intern Med* 13:268, 1999 [Abstract].

34. DeFrancesco TC, Moore RR, Atkins CE, et al: Comparison of dalteparin and warfarin in the long-term management of feline arterial thromboembolism. *J Vet Intern Med* 17:448, 2003 [Abstract].

35. Reimer SB, Kittleson MD, Kyles AE: Use of rheolytic thrombectomy in the treatment of feline distal aortic thromboembolism. *J Vet Intern Med* 20:290, 2006.

36. Ramsey CC, Riepe RD, Macintire DK, et al: Streptokinase: a practical clot-buster? In *Proceedings of the 5th International Veterinary Emergency and Critical Care Symposium*, 225, 1996.

37. Whelan MF, O'Toole TE, Chan DL, et al: Retrospective evaluation of urokinase use in cats with arterial thromboembolism (four cases: 2003–2004). *J Vet Emerg Crit Care* 15:S8, 2005.

38. Pion PD, Kittleson MD: Therapy for feline aortic thromboembolism. In Kirk RW, editor: *Current veterinary therapy X*, Philadelphia, 1989, Saunders.

39. Welch KM, Rozanski EA, Freeman LM, et al: Prospective evaluation of tissue plasminogen activator in 11 cats with arterial thromboembolism. *J Feline Med Surg* 12:122, 2010.

40. Pion PD, Kittleson MD, Peterson S, et al: Thrombolysis of aortic thromboemboli in cats using tissue plasminogen activator: clinical data. In *Proceedings of the American College of Veterinary Internal Medicine Forum*, San Diego, California, 1987 [Abstract].

41. Schaub RG, Gates KA, Roberts RE: Effect of aspirin on collateral blood flow after experimental thrombosis of the feline aorta. *Am J Vet Res* 43:1647, 1982.

42. De Clerk F, Loots W, Somers Y, et al: 5-Hyroxytryptamine and arachidonic acid metabolites modulate extensive platelet activation induced by collagen in cats in vivo. *Br J Pharmacol* 99:631, 1990.

43. Davis LE: Clinical pharmacology of salicylates. *J Am Vet Med Assoc* 176:65, 1980.

44. Yang LH, Fareed J: Vasomodulatory action of clopidogrel and ticlopidine. *Thromb Res* 86:479, 1997.

45. Yang LH, Hoppensteadt D, Fareed J: Modulation of vasoconstriction by clopidogrel and ticlopidine. *Thromb Res* 92:83, 1998.

46. Hogan DF, Andrews DA, Green HW, et al: Antiplatelet effects and pharmacodynamics of clopidogrel in cats. *J Am Vet Med Assoc* 225:406, 2004.

47. Cadroy Y, Bossavy JP, Thalamas C, et al: Early potent antithrombotic effect with combined aspirin and a loading dose of clopidogrel on experimental arterial thrombogenesis in humans. *Circulation* 101:2823, 2000.

48. Muller I, Seyfarth M, Rudiger S, et al: Effect of a high loading dose of clopidogrel on platelet function in patients undergoing coronary stent placement. *Heart* 85:92, 2001.

49. Matsagas M, Jagroop IA, Geroulakos G, et al: The effect of a loading dose (300 mg) of clopidogrel on platelet function in patients with peripheral arterial disease. *Clin Appl Thromb Hemost* 9:115, 2003.

50. Goodwin JC, Hogan DF, Green HW: The pharmacodynamics of clopidogrel in the dog. *J Vet Intern Med* 21:609, 2007.

51. Plumb DC: *Veterinary drug handbook*, ed 7, Ames, IA, 2011, Wiley-Blackwell.

52. Harpster NK, Baty CJ: Warfarin therapy of the cat at risk of thromboembolism. In Bonagura JD, editor: *Current veterinary therapy XII*, Philadelphia, 1995, Saunders.

53. Hogan DF: Analysis of the feline arterial thromboembolism: clopidogrel vs. aspirin trial (FAT CAT). In *Proceedings of the American College of Veterinary Internal Medicine Forum*, Seattle, Washington, 2013.

54. Antiplatelet Trialists' Collaboration: Collaborative overview of randomized trials of antiplatelet therapy-I: prevention of death, myocardial infarction, and stroke by prolonged antiplatelet therapy in various categories of patients. *Br Med J* 308:81, 1994.

55. Warfarin versus aspirin for prevention of thromboembolism in atrial fibrillation: stroke prevention in atrial fibrillation II study. *Lancet* 343:687, 1994.

56. Hellemons BS, Langenberg M, Lodder J, et al: Primary prevention of arterial thromboembolism in non-rheumatic atrial fibrillation in primary care: randomised controlled trial comparing two intensities of coumarin with aspirin. *Br Med J* 319:958, 1999.

57. Secondary prevention in non-rheumatic atrial fibrillation after transient ischaemic attack or minor stroke. EAFT (European Atrial Fibrillation Trial) Study Group. *Lancet* 342:1255, 1993.

58. Adjusted-dose warfarin versus low-intensity, fixed-dose warfarin plus aspirin for high-risk patients with atrial fibrillation: stroke prevention in atrial fibrillation III randomised clinical trial. *Lancet* 348:633, 1996.

59. Greene CE: Effects of aspirin and propranolol on feline platelet aggregation. *Am J Vet Res* 46:1820, 1985.

60. Behrend EN, Grauer GF, Greco DS, et al: Comparison of the effects of diltiazem and aspirin on platelet aggregation in cats. *J Am Anim Hosp Assoc* 32:11, 1996.

61. Di Minno G, Cerbone AM, Mattioli PL, et al: Functionally thrombasthenic state in normal platelets following the administration of ticlopidine. *J Clin Invest* 75:328, 1985.

62. Fareed J, Messmore HL: Clopidogrel. *Semin Thromb Hemost* 25:1, 1999.

63. Picard-Fraire C: Ticlopidine hydrochloride: relationship between dose, kinetics, plasma concentration and effect on platelet function. *Thromb Res Suppl* 4:119, 1983.

64. Savi P, Herbert JM, Pflieger AM, et al: Importance of hepatic metabolism in the antiaggregating activity of the thienopyridine clopidogrel. *Biochem Pharmacol* 44:527, 1992.

65. Savi P, Pereillo JM, Uzabiaga MF, et al: Identification and biological activity of the active metabolite of clopidogrel. *Thromb Haemost* 84:891, 2000.

66. Gent M, Blakely JA, Easton JD, et al: The Canadian American ticlopidine study (CATS) in thromboembolic stroke. *Lancet* 1:1215, 1989.

67. Hass WK, Easton JD, Adams HP, Jr, et al: A randomized trial comparing ticlopidine hydrochloride with aspirin for the prevention of stroke in high-risk patients. Ticlopidine Aspirin Stroke Study Group. *N Engl J Med* 321:501, 1989.

68. CAPRIE Steering Committee: A randomised, blinded, trial of clopidogrel versus aspirin in patients at risk of ischaemic events (CAPRIE). *Lancet* 348:1329, 1996.

69. The ACTIVE Investigators: The effect of clopidogrel added to aspirin in patients with atrial fibrillation. *N Engl J Med* 360:2066, 2009.

70. ACTIVE Writing Group of the ACTIVE Investigators: Clopidogrel plus aspirin versus oral anticoagulation for atrial fibrillation in the Atrial Fibrillation Clopidogrel Trial with Irbesartan for Prevention of Vascular Events (ACTIVE W): a randomized controlled trial. *Lancet* 367:1903, 2006.

71. Petersen P, Boysen G, Godtfredsen J, et al: Placebo-controlled, randomised trial of warfarin and aspirin for prevention of thromboembolic complications in chronic atrial fibrillation. The Copenhagen AFASAK Study. *Lancet* I:175, 1989.

72. Stroke Prevention in Atrial Fibrillation Study. Final results. *Circulation* 84:527, 1991.

73. The Boston Area Anticoagulation Trial for Atrial Fibrillation Investigators: The effect of low dose warfarin on the risk of stroke in

patients with nonrheumatic atrial fibrillation. *N Engl J Med* 323:1505, 1990.

74. Connolly SJ, Laupacis A, Gent M, et al: Canadian atrial fibrillation anticoagulation (CAFA) study. *J Am Coll Cardiol* 18:349, 1991.

75. Ezekowitz MD, Bridgers SL, James KE, et al: Warfarin in the prevention of stroke associated with non-rheumatic atrial fibrillation. *N Engl J Med* 327:1406, 1992.

76. Smith SA, Kraft SL, Lewis DC, et al: Plasma pharmacokinetics of warfarin enantiomers in cats. *J Vet Pharmacol Therap* 23:329, 2000.

77. Smith SA, Kraft SL, Lewis DC, et al: Pharmacodynamics of warfarin in cats. *J Vet Pharmacol Therap* 23:339, 2000.

78. Van De Wiele CM, Hogan DF, Green HW, et al: Antithrombotic effect of enoxaparin in clinically healthy cats; a venous stasis model. *J Vet Intern Med* 24:185, 2010.

79. Low-molecular-weight heparin in the treatment of patients with venous thromboembolism. The Columbus Investigators. *N Engl J Med* 337:657, 1997.

80. Agnelli G, Piovella F, Buoncristiani P, et al: Enoxaparin plus compression stockings compared with compression stockings alone in the prevention of venous thromboembolism after elective neurosurgery. *N Engl J Med* 339:80, 1998.

81. Samama MM, Cohen AT, Darmon JY, et al: A comparison of enoxaparin with placebo for the prevention of venous thromboembolism in acutely ill medical patients. Prophylaxis in Medical Patients with Enoxaparin Study Group. *N Engl J Med* 341:793, 1999.

82. Hull RD, Pineo GF, Francis C, et al: Low-molecular-weight heparin prophylaxis using dalteparin in close proximity to surgery vs warfarin in hip arthroplasty patients: a double-blind, randomized comparison. The North American Fragmin Trial Investigators. *Arch Intern Med* 160:2199, 2000.

83. Hull RD, Pineo GF, Francis C, et al: Low-molecular-weight heparin prophylaxis using dalteparin extended out-of-hospital vs in-hospital warfarin/out-of-hospital placebo in hip arthroplasty patients: a double-blind, randomized comparison. North American Fragmin Trial Investigators. *Arch Intern Med* 160:2208, 2000.

84. Klein W, Buchwald A, Hillis SE, et al: Comparison of low-molecular-weight heparin with unfractionated heparin acutely and with placebo for 6 weeks in the management of unstable coronary artery disease. Fragmin in unstable coronary artery disease study (FRIC). *Circulation* 96:61, 1997.

85. Cohen M, Demers C, Gurfinkel EP, et al: A comparison of low-molecular-weight heparin with unfractionated heparin for unstable coronary artery disease. Efficacy and Safety of Subcutaneous Enoxaparin in Non-Q-Wave Coronary Events Study Group. *N Engl J Med* 337:447, 1997.

86. Long-term low-molecular-mass heparin in unstable coronary-artery disease: FRISC II prospective randomised multicentre study. Fragmin and fast revascularisation during instability in coronary artery disease. Investigators. *Lancet* 354:701, 1999.

87. Kontny F, Dale J, Abildgaard U, et al: Randomized trial of low molecular weight heparin (dalteparin) in prevention of left ventricular thrombus formation and arterial embolism after acute anterior myocardial infarction: the Fragmin in Acute Myocardial Infarction (FRAMI) Study. *J Am Coll Cardiol* 30:962, 1997.

88. Smith CE, Rozanski EA, Freeman LE, et al: Use of low molecular weight heparin in cats: 57 cases (1999–2003). *J Am Vet Med Assoc* 225:1237, 2004.

89. Connolly SJ, Ezekowitz MD, Yusuf S, et al: Dabigatran versus warfarin in patients with atrial fibrillation. *N Engl J Med* 361:1139, 2009.

90. Patel MR, Mahaffey KW, Garg J, et al: Rivaroxaban versus warfarin in nonvalvular atrial fibrillation. *N Engl J Med* 365:883, 2011.

91. Granger CB, Alexander JH, McMurray JJ, et al: Apixaban versus warfarin in patients with atrial fibrillation. *N Engl J Med* 365:981, 2011.

92. Fiakpui NN, Hogan DF, Whittem T, et al: Dose determination of fondaparinux in healthy cats. *Am J Vet Res* 73:556, 2012.

93. Brainard BM, Cathcart CJ, Dixon AC, et al: *In vitro* effects of rivaroxaban on feline coagulation indices. In *Proceedings of the American College of Veterinary Internal Medicine Forum*, Denver, Colorado, 2011.

Feline Lungworm Infection

Viktor Szatmári

Lungworm infection in cats is found worldwide. It is caused by various species. The infection is probably more common in cats with exposure to intermediate hosts, and it may be particularly common in free-roaming cats that depend on hunting. Common clinical signs include coughing, tachypnea, and respiratory distress. Thoracic radiographs commonly document a diffuse or patchy bronchointerstitial to bronchoalveolar pattern. Diagnosis is most frequently confirmed by identification of larvae in a Baermann fecal flotation. Treatment with selected anthelmintics is typically effective.

ETIOLOGY

Aelurostrongylus abstrusus is considered the main feline lungworm. Adult worms reside in the alveoli, alveolar ducts, and terminal bronchioles.[1-4] Males are 5 to 6 mm long and 70 μm wide, whereas females are 9 to 10 mm by 100 μm wide.[1-4] *A. abstrusus* has been reported from Asia, Australia, Europe, and North and South America.[1-7] It belongs to the phylum Nematoda (roundworms), order Strongylida, superfamily Metastrongyloidea, and family Angiostrongylidae.[8,9]

Troglostrongylus brevior and *Troglostrongylus subcrenatus* have so far only been reported from Asia and Europe.[1,8] Morphological similarities between the first stage larvae (L1) of *A. abstrusus* and *Troglostrongylus* spp., as well as inconsistencies in descriptions, suggest that these worms have been misdiagnosed for a long time.[9] The adults of *T. brevior* reside in the bronchi and bronchioles. The males are 5 to 7 mm long and 294 to 365 μm wide, whereas the females are 6 to 16 mm long by 335 to 430 μm wide.[1,8] The adults of *T. subcrenatus* reside in the trachea and bronchi. The males are 9 to 10 mm long and 285 to 305 μm wide, whereas the females measure 20 to 24 mm long by 486 to 542 μm wide.[8] *Troglostrongylus* spp. also belong to the superfamily Metastrongyloidea, but to the family of Crenosomatidae.[8,9]

Eucoleus aerophilus (synonym *Capillaria aerophila*) adult worms reside in the trachea and bronchi. The males are 10 to 25 mm long, and the females are 16 to 41 mm long.[10,11] It has been documented in Asia, Australia, Europe, and North and South America and it belongs to the phylum Nematoda (roundworms), order Enoplida, superfamily Trichinelloidea, and family Trichuridae or Capillariidae.[10-14] *E. aerophilus* can infect cats, dogs, foxes, and humans.[14]

Oslerus rostratus (synonym *Anafilaroides rostratus*) has been reported from Asia, Europe, and North America.[1,15,16]. The adult males are 2.1 to 3 cm long and 240 to 290 μm wide, whereas the females are 3.5 to 5 cm long and 690 μm wide.[1,15] They belongs to the superfamily Metastrongyloidea, and the family Filaroidae.[8]

Paragonimus kellicotti, the American lung fluke, can parasitize, among others, the feline, canine, and human lung.[17] *Paragonimus* species are hermaphroditic, and they belong to the phylum Platyhelminthes (flatworms), class Trematoda (flukes), and family Paragonimidae.[17] Their length is 7.5 to 12 mm, and their width is 4 to 6 mm.[17] *P. kellicotti* can only be found in a restricted area of North America.[18] *P. westermani* has, however, been described in Asia and Africa.[19]

Toxocara cati, *Toxocara canis*, *Strongyloides felis*, and *Strongyloides stercoralis* are intestinal nematodes that may also damage the pulmonary arteries and parenchyma during their migration.[20-22]

LIFE CYCLE AND PATHOGENESIS

Aelurostrongylus abstrusus

The females lay their eggs in the alveolar ducts.[2] After the eggs hatch, L1 larvae move toward the trachea, where they are then coughed up and subsequently swallowed. After a gastrointestinal (GI) passage, they end up in the feces, and in the environment. Terrestrial snails and slugs are obligatory intermediate hosts.[23] There are no specific species required for the development of the infectious third-stage larvae (L3). The L1 larvae penetrate the integument of the muscular foot of the snails or slugs.[24] The larvae coil up in the muscular layer and a tubercle will develop.[24] The development of L3 from L1 in the intermediate hosts takes from 9 to 11 days at 22° to 30°C (71.6° to 86°F), but stops below 8°C (46.4°F).[1,2] The L1 larvae die if they are swallowed by mollusks.[24] After a cat ingests a snail or slug with L3 larvae, these larvae are released in the cat's upper GI tract, where they perforate the intestinal wall.[4] Ingestion of L3 larvae induces vomiting usually within 5 minutes, regardless of whether isolated L3 or L3-containing intermediate hosts are taken up, and it occurs even in anesthetized cats when the L3 are administered via a stomach tube.[2] However, vomiting does not prevent infection.[4] After perforating the esophageal, gastric, or duodenal wall, the L3 larvae travel via blood vessels or lymphatic vessels into the smallest pulmonary artery branches, which they perforate to get into the alveoli. The L3 larvae can reach the lungs within 1 day after ingestion.[4] By the seventeenth day after infection, adults are present, and, by the twenty-eighth day, they lie in pairs and start laying eggs.[2,4] From day 28 to 37, L1 larvae appear in the feces. The largest number can be found 60 to 120 days after infection.[1,2,7] Fecal shedding of L1 larvae spontaneously disappears between 6 and 9 months after infection, but, in some cats, L1 larvae excretion can persist for 15 months.[7] Adult worms may live for years.[25]

Frogs, toads, lizards, snakes, sparrows, chickens, ducklings, mice, and rats are documented transport and paratenic hosts.[2,4,6] These nonobligatory intermediate hosts have many strategic advantages for the parasite: (1) paratenic hosts can keep the L3 larvae alive during the cold months when slugs and snails are inactive, (2) cats prefer eating these animals to snails and slugs, (3) ingesting L3 larvae-containing mice does not always induce vomiting, and (4) L3 larvae may live in snails up to 2 years, but probably longer in the paratenic hosts.[2,15]

Necropsy of infected cats reveals pale nodules of 1 to 2 mm in all lung lobes, most of them containing worms.[2] The bronchiolar mucosa is invaded by eosinophils, lymphocytes, and plasma cells (bronchiolitis); in addition, the terminal bronchioles and alveolar ducts show smooth muscle hypertrophy.[3,26,27] The pulmonic arteries and arterioles show smooth muscle hypertrophy, which can cause complete obliteration of the lumen.[3,28] The muscular layer is invaded by eosinophils, and the endothelial cells show proliferation and vacuolization. In addition, subendothelial and perivascular fibrosis may be seen.[3,28] Prolonged vasoconstriction together with the aforementioned arterial changes can cause pulmonary hypertension.[3,28,29]

Troglostrongylus spp. and Oslerus rostratus

The life cycles of *Troglostrongylus* spp. and *Oslerus rostratus* are comparable to that of *A. abstrusus*.[8,9,30] However, the life cycle of *T. brevior* differs from that of *A. abstrusus* at several points. Direct transmission has been documented from queen to offspring via milk; adult worms develop in the kittens in 25 days, and L1 larvae appear in the feces from day 40.[31] *T. brevior* has the shortest development time among the metastrongyloids in mollusks: L3 larvae can be found from the eighth day at 22° to 27°C (71.6° to 80.6°F), and from the fortieth day at 4° to 8°C (39.2° to 46.4°F).[1] The L3 larvae continue to develop at low temperatures when *A. abstrusus* does not, even when they are maintained for 7 months.[1,8] Snails can retain the infection throughout their winter hibernation.[32] Mice are documented paratenic hosts of *T. brevior* and *O. rostratus*.[1,15]

Eucoleus aerophilus (Synonym Capillaria aerophila)

E. aerophilus has a direct life cycle. Earthworms are believed to act as transport and paratenic hosts.[14,30] The adults live under the cat's bronchial and tracheal epithelium, deeply embedded in the mucosa.[10,11,30] Eggs are coughed up and swallowed by the cat, and, after passage through the GI tract, they are excreted into the feces.[30] The eggs become infective in 30 to 45 days in the environment.[14] Infection occurs after ingestion of embryonated eggs containing the infective L1 larvae.[14,30] The eggs hatch in the cat's GI tract, and, after penetration of the wall, the larvae migrate via the bloodstream or lymphatics to the lungs.[30] The worms become sexually mature 3 to 6 weeks after infection.[14]

Paragonimus kellicotti

For *P. kellicotti*, the usual definitive host is believed to be the mink, but cats, dogs, and humans may also become infected.[17,18] Eggs are shed in the feces of the final host. At temperatures below 7°C (44.6°F) no development takes place, but at 27°C (80.6°F) miracidia (ciliated larvae) develop within 2 to 3 weeks.[17] If the eggs are frozen for more than 30 minutes, no further development takes place.[17] The miracidia (100 by 50 μm) leave the eggs and infect the first intermediate host, a small (1 to 5 mm long) amphibious snail (*Pomatiopsis lapidaria*), by penetration.[17] The miracidia multiply in the snail and produce cercaria (tailed larvae) within 78 to 93 days.[17] Cercariae leave the snail and infect the second intermediate host, a crayfish (*Orcocentes* spp.), by penetration.[17,33] The cercaria reach the heart of the crayfish, where they develop into metacercaria within 46 days.[17,33] The definitive host becomes infected after ingesting an infected crayfish or another definitive host containing flukes that have not yet entered the lungs.[17] The metacercariae (600 by 200 μm) are excysted in the stomach or duodenum, and they penetrate the host's intestinal wall within 24 hours after oral infection.[17,18] Most immature flukes (about 1 mm long) move from the peritoneal into the pleural space 10 to 14 days after infection by penetrating the diaphragm.[18,33,34] Between days 10 and 23, the flukes arrive in the lungs by penetration of the visceral pleura. In the lungs they produce cystic cavities, where they can be found in pairs 21 days postinfection.[18,34] Most flukes are found in the caudal and right lung lobes, most likely because of the proximity of these lobes to the descending duodenum, the site of penetration.[18] The pulmonary lesions are 10 to 15 mm in size by 29 to 34 days after infection, and they contain immature flukes (2 to 4 mm long) surrounded by eosinophilic exudate.[34] By day 39 after infection, the pulmonary cysts contact the bronchial tree, and the adult flukes start producing eggs.[34] The eggs are coughed up and swallowed. Eggs appear in the feces from the thirty-sixth day after metacercaria ingestion.[18,33] A fluke produces 1000 to 2000 eggs/day and can live at least 6 years.[18]

Strongyloides felis

The parasitic adults of *S. felis* (only females) live in the cat's small intestine. They lay eggs, which hatch and become L1 larvae.[22] The L1 larvae are shed into the environment with feces, where they become free-living males and females.[22]

These produce larvae, which infect cats by skin penetration. The larvae are carried via the bloodstream to the pulmonary capillaries, which they perforate; from the alveoli, they migrate up the trachea and are coughed up and swallowed.[22] The migrating larvae may cause interstitial pneumonia, granulomas and vasculitis.

Toxocara cati and Toxocara canis

Oral administration of infective eggs (containing L3 larvae) of *T. cati* may cause severe pulmonary changes in kittens and in some adult cats.[20] These larvae are about 400 μm long and are present in the highest number in the lungs 6 to 21 days after infection.[20] Despite the changes in bronchoalveolar lavage (BAL) fluid (60% eosinophils), on thoracic radiographs (diffuse peribronchial pattern and mildly enlarged pulmonary arteries), and on computed tomography (CT) scans (patchy interstitial pattern), cats remain clinically healthy.[20] Because the pulmonary damage is not accompanied or always followed by the presence of adult worms in the intestines, identifying the etiology of pulmonary changes in a clinical case is impossible.[20] Histopathology reveals occlusion of the pulmonary arteries caused by markedly thickened walls 6 weeks after infection.[35] The pulmonary arteries show intimal and smooth muscle hyperplasia.[20] Patent infection in adult cats probably results after ingestion of an infected rodent paratenic host, in which the prerequisite pulmonary migration had already taken place.[36] The larvae then mature without migrating to the lungs.

Oral administration of 5000 infective eggs (containing L3 larvae) of *T. canis* to cats causes similar pathological and histopathologic pulmonary changes as that of *T. cati* (i.e., eosinophilic granulomas and medial hypertrophy of the pulmonary arteries).[21] Cats though merely function as paratenic hosts for *T. canis*. In addition to eosinophilic endarteritis, bronchiolitis, peribronchiolitis, and focal pleural fibrosis may also be found.[21]

CLINICAL SIGNS

Cats experimentally infected with low worm burdens of *A. abstrusus* (less than 1600 L3 larvae) show no clinical signs; however, high worm burdens (more than 1600 L3 larvae) can lead to chronic cough, dyspnea, and emaciation starting 5 weeks after infection.[37] Silent infections may contribute to unexpected anesthetic-associated deaths, although the mechanism is unclear.[38] Severe infection can lead to a cardiac murmur caused by tricuspid valve regurgitation as a result of severe pulmonary hypertension, and rarely even to ascites (M. Dirven, personal communication, November 25, 2013).[29]

T. brevior infection may cause fatal respiratory distress in kittens.[8,31] *E. aerophilus* infection can cause chronic cough, but may also be asymptomatic.[12] There are very few clinical reports about *T. brevior* and *E. aerophilus* in cats. *O. rostratus* seems to cause no obvious clinical signs.[1,16]

P. kellicotti infection may be clinically silent but may also cause chronic cough from the twenty-ninth day after infection.[33] In some cats dyspnea develops, as early as 39 days after infection, because of a spontaneous pneumothorax after rupture of a pulmonary cavitary lesion.[33,34]

No clinical signs are present during the pulmonary migration of larvae of *T. cati* and *T. canis*.[20,21] The damage to the pulmonary arteries may lead to pulmonary hypertension later, when the etiology cannot be revealed.[20] The clinical significance of *S. felis* infection is unclear.[22]

DIAGNOSTIC EVALUATION

Radiography

Performing thoracic radiographs is usually the first diagnostic step in any cat with chronic cough or dyspnea. The radiographic signs of *A. abstrusus* infection are nonspecific, and they depend on the length of infection, as well as the worm burden.[26,39] The first changes starting from 5 to 6 weeks after infection vary from bronchial thickening with a focal alveolar pattern (poorly defined nodules) to a generalized alveolar pattern.[39] Multifocal bronchial and unstructured interstitial patterns can be seen in mild cases.[26] In severe cases, multiple nodules throughout the lungs are present with areas of alveolar pattern (Figure 36-1).[26,39] From as early as 11 to 17 weeks and as late as 20 to 40 weeks, partial resolution of the alveolar pattern occurs, and thickened bronchial walls and increased interstitial opacity remains.[39] The interstitial density is the result of interalveolar smooth muscle hypertrophy, cellular infiltration, and collagen deposition, as well as medial hypertrophy and hyperplasia of the small arteries and arterioles.[39] The right caudal lobar artery may be enlarged from the sixth to beyond the fortieth week after infection.[39] The changes on radiographs and CT scans are similar.[26] Pulmonary changes resulting from *Troglostrongylus* spp. and *E. aerophilus* infections may be similar to those of *A. abstrusus*. None of the

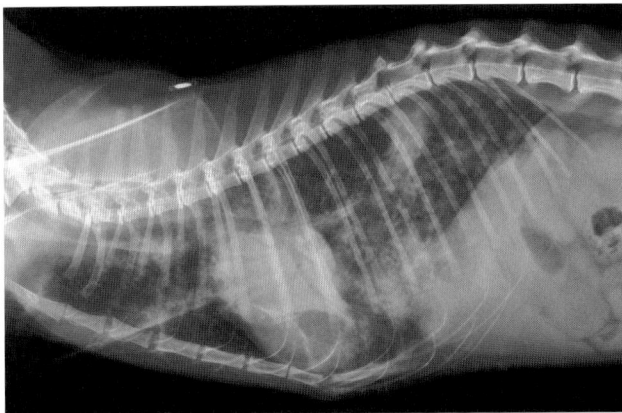

Figure 36-1: Lateral thoracic radiograph of a 2-year-old cat with severe respiratory distress resulting from *A. abstrusus* infection. Multiple poorly emarginated nodular densities, and patchy alveolar infiltrates (with negative bronchogram) can be seen, the latter in the caudoventral and caudodorsal pulmonary regions, and overlying the cardiac shadow. (Courtesy Division of Diagnostic Imaging. Utrecht University.)

radiographic changes are specific for lungworm infection, which necessitates further diagnostics.

P. kellicotti causes solid pulmonary nodules with small (2 to 4 cm) air cavities.[33] The earliest lesions appear 2 to 3 weeks after infection.[33] The cavities are divided by thin septae into several chambers.[33] By the sixty-fifth day after infection, cystic nodular pulmonary densities develop, the appearance of which does not change thereafter.[33] Spontaneous pneumothorax may also develop.[33]

Bronchoalveolar Lavage

Microscopic examination of BAL fluid is less sensitive than the Baermann technique for detection of L1 larvae of *A. abstrusus*. Moreover, it requires general anesthesia in an animal with a high procedure-related morbidity and mortality risk because of respiratory compromise.[38,40] Although eggs or (rarely) adult worms of *E. aerophilus* can be found in the BAL fluid with microscopic examination, fecal examination is preferred and should always be performed first.[12]

Fecal Examination

Fecal examination is a very good method to diagnose lungworm infections. Disadvantages are the need for a well-trained microscopist, the inability to diagnose infection during the prepatent period, the intermittent shedding of larvae or eggs, and contamination of the sample with free-living nematodes (leading to false-positive results).[25] Heavy infections may be diagnosed by direct fecal smear, but if no L1 larvae or eggs are found, the following methods to examine feces should be used.

Baermann Technique

The Baermann technique is the cheapest, most sensitive (after polymerase chain reaction [PCR]), noninvasive, and widely available method for diagnosing *A. abstrusus* and *Troglostrongylus* spp. infections. It utilizes the positive hydrotaxis of L1 larvae.[4,25] A glass with a pointed bottom is first filled with tap water, and then about 5 g of feces is wrapped in gauze and partially immersed in the water (Figure 36-2). After 18 to 24 hours at room temperature, a few milliliters of fluid are drawn from the very bottom of the glass using a long pipette. This sample is placed in a Petri dish and examined under a microscope at 40× magnification. Characteristics of L1 larvae of feline lungworm species are given in Table 36-1 (Figures 36-3 and 36-4). To increase the sensitivity, fecal samples from 3 consecutive days should be examined, as larval counts are highly variable among different fecal samples of an individual cat, and also among cats.[23,41] Finding larvae of *Oslerus* spp. with the Baermann technique is unlikely because these larvae do not tend to migrate out of the feces.[23]

Free-living or plant-parasitic nematodes or their larvae may also be found using the Baermann technique if the fecal sample was collected from the ground. Contamination should be suspected if larvae are found that are out of the size range of parasitic L1 larvae (i.e., 150 to 415 μm long) or when adult

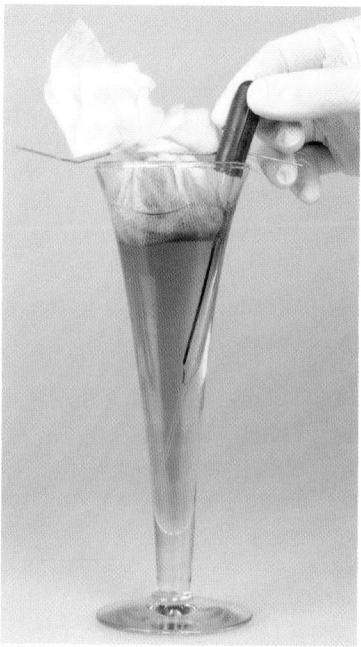

Figure 36-2: The Baermann technique is the best way to find first stage larvae in the feces of *A. abstrusus* and *Troglostrongylus* spp. It can easily be performed in any veterinary practice by using a champagne glass, a straightened paper clip, and a piece of gauze. Do not let the edges of the gauze stick outside the glass as they can induce a heave-effect. After 18 to 24 hours of partial immersion of the feces (wrapped in the gauze) in the glass filled with tap water, a sample of a few milliliters is taken with a long pipette from the bottom of the glass, which subsequently is examined in a Petri dish with a light or stereo microscope.

stages (i.e., males with spicules or females with an egg-containing uterus) are identified.[23] Nonparasitic L1 larvae have a rhabditiform esophagus (i.e., with a narrow central region and a terminal bulb).[23]

Survival of L1 larvae of *A. abstrusus* in feces was documented to be 36 days when temperature varied from –6° C to 22° C (21.2 to 71.6° F) and when freezing and thawing occurred many times.[42] At 0° C (32° F), L1 larvae survived in feces for 33 days.[42] In water, L1 larvae survived at 4° C (39.2° F); at room temperature for 226 and 72 days, respectively; and in feces at both temperatures for 48 days.[42] The L1 of *T. brevior* survive at 26° C (78.8° F) in water and feces up to 7 days, whereas at 4° C (39.2° F) in feces for 49 days.[32]

Flotation Techniques

About 5 g of feces is dispersed in 20 mL of zinc sulfate solution (specific gravity 1.350) and centrifuged at 600 g for 5 minutes. The top layer of the supernatant (around 100 μL) is placed on a slide and examined at 20× magnification with light microscopy.[14] This is the best method to find eggs of *E. aerophilus*. The eggs are 60 to 83 μm long by 25 to 40 μm wide; they have a lemon-like morphology, with asymmetrical bipolar plug position on their ends, and the outer shell is densely striated with a network of anastomosing ridges (Figure 36-5).[10,14,30] Flotation with zinc sulfate solution (specific gravity 1.200) is preferred to the Baermann technique

Table 36-1	Characteristics of L1 Larvae of Parasitic Nematodes That May Be Encountered in Feline Fecal Samples	
Species	**Size**	**Comments**
A. abstrusus[1,2,8,9,30]	Length: 360-415 µm (mean 399.1 ± 11.3 µm) width:18-19 µm	L1 larvae are very motile; thorough examination may require immobilization with heat or chemical agents. The oral opening is terminal; the tail is ventrally curved or coiled with dorsal and ventral incisures, a ventral kink, and an evident knob-like appendage (Figures 36-3 and 36-4A)
T. brevior[1,8,9,31]	Length: 300-357 µm (mean 338.8 ± 15.6 µm) width: 16-19 µm	The oral opening is dorsal; the tail is ventrally coiled with dorsal and ventral incisures, no ventral kink, and a less pronounced knob-like appendage (Figure 36-4B)
T. subcrenatus[8]	Mean length: 280.7 µm (±17.9 µm) Mean width: 15.5 µm (±1.7 µm)	
O. rostratus[1,16,30]	Length: 300-320 µm Width: 17-18 µm	The tail has a kinked end, as well as a constriction anterior to the end
S. felis[22,23]	Length: 217-238 µm	
S. stercoralis[22,23]	Length: 290-360 µm	The tail is straight and pointed

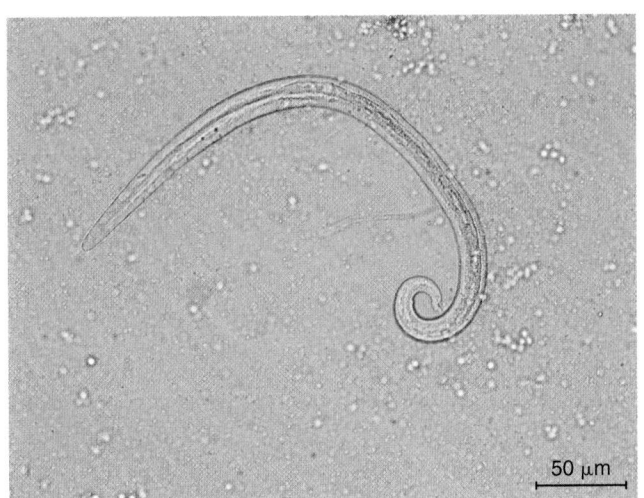

Figure 36-3: Light microscopic image of a first stage larva of *A. abstrusus*. Note the ventrally coiled tail, the terminal oral opening, and the nonrhabditiform esophagus (i.e., uniform in length without a bulb). (Courtesy of Dr. Rolf Nijsse, Veterinary Microbiology Diagnostic Centre, Faculty of Veterinary Medicine, Utrecht University, the Netherlands.)

when looking for L1 larvae of *Oslerus* spp.[23] However, flotation is less optimal for finding L1 larvae of *A. abstrusus* and *Troglostrongylus* spp. because the larvae get dehydrated and damaged in hypertonic solutions, making identification difficult.[6,25] Hypertonic solutions can also damage the eggs of *P. kellicotti*; therefore sedimentation is the preferred diagnostic method for this parasite.[33]

With the traditional flotation method, not all of the floating parasitic elements adhere to the underside of the cover slip. The FLOTAC apparatus is a cylindrical device with two 5-mL flotation chambers, and it overcomes the shortcoming of the traditional method by cutting the top portion of the flotation suspension transversally.[43] The FLOTAC technique was found to be more sensitive and less time consuming than the Baermann technique in detecting L1 larvae of *A. abstrusus*.[44] The mini-FLOTAC apparatus offers an even quicker, less labor-intensive, and simpler flotation technique without the need of centrifugation, but its sensitivity is yet to be determined.

Sedimentation Technique

A sedimentation technique is used to find eggs of *P. kellicotti*. Feces are first emulsified in water and passed through one layer of gauze.[18,33] Then 1 mL of fecal emulsion is mixed with 5 mL of water. After sedimentation for at least 6 minutes, the supernatant is decanted and discarded. After adding two drops of 1:1000 aqueous methylene blue, 0.1 mL of sample is examined under light microscopy using 100× magnification. The eggs have a gold-brown color and a single operculum (Figure 36-6). Their size varies depending on the host: 75 to 118 µm long by 46 to 62 µm wide.[17,33]

Molecular Techniques and Serology

Diagnosing *A. abstrusus* infection with a PCR assay from pharyngeal swab and fecal samples has been shown to be 100% specific, and it is more sensitive (96.6%) than the Baermann technique (90%), but it was not yet commercially available as of January 2015.[45] A duplex-PCR could detect simultaneous infection with *A. abstrusus* and *T. brevior* in feces.[46] *E. aerophilus* infection can be detected with a semi-nested PCR assay from feces with 100% specificity and 97% to 100% sensitivity.[13]

Only two studies have investigated serological techniques in diagnosis of *A. abstrusus* infection. Because of the persistence of antibodies for a long period, present and past infec-

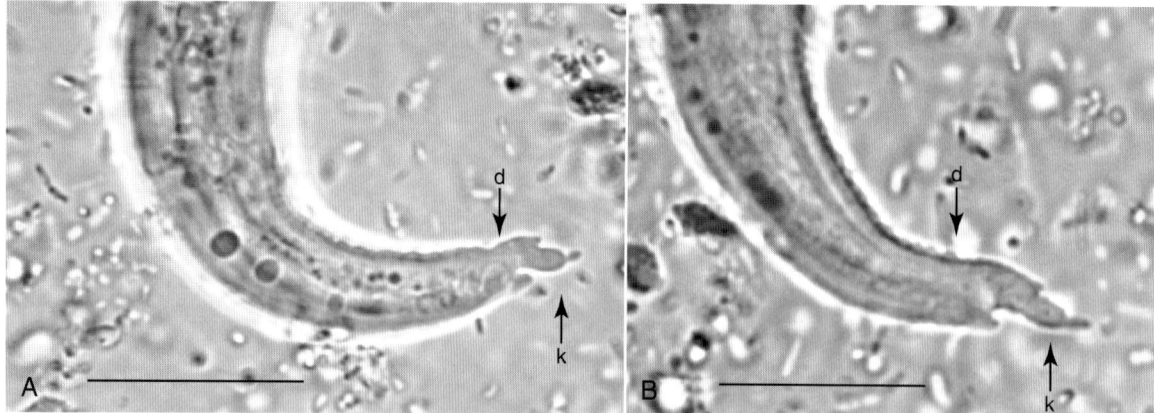

Figure 36-4: Light microscopic images show the difference between the tail morphology of the first stage larvae of *A. abstrusus* (**A**) and *T. brevior* (**B**).[8] The bar is 20 μm long. The larva of *A. abstrusus* has a dorsal kink (*d*) and a knob-like terminal end (*k*) and the larva of *T. brevior* does not. (From Jefferies R, Vrhovec MG, Catalan DR: *Aelurostrongylus abstrusus* and *Troglostrongylus* sp. (Nematoda: Metastrongyloidea) infections in cats inhabiting Ibiza, Spain. *Vet Parasitol* 173:344-348, 2010.)

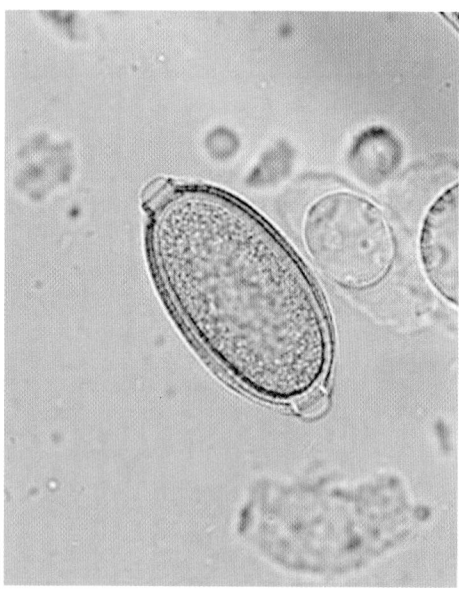

Figure 36-5: **Light Microscopic Image of** *E. aerophilus* **(Synonym** *C. aerophila*) **Egg.** (From Ettinger SJ, Feldman EC, editors: *Textbook of veterinary internal medicine*, vol. 1, St Louis, 2010, Elsevier Saunders.)

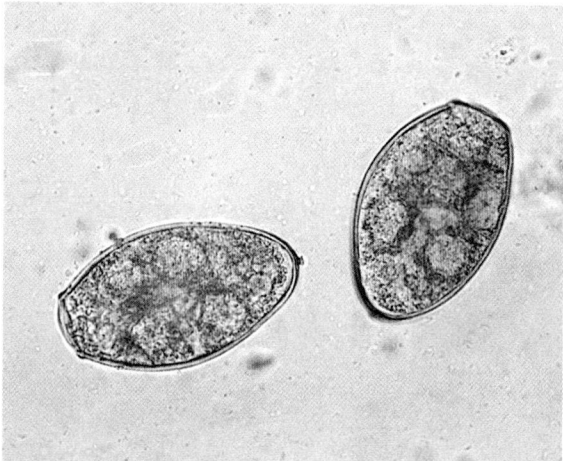

Figure 36-6: **Light Microscopic Image of** *Paragonimus kellicotti* **Eggs Found with Sedimentation Technique.** (From Hendrix CM, Sirois M: *Laboratory procedures for veterinary technicians*, ed 5, St Louis, 2007, Elsevier Mosby.)

tions cannot be readily differentiated.[25,47] Currently, no commercial assay is available.

TREATMENT AND PROGNOSIS

Aelurostrongylus abstrusus and *Troglostrongylus* spp.

Fenbendazole (20 mg/kg every 24 hours, orally [PO], for 5 days), a benzimidazole anthelminthic, was shown to be effective in eradicating *A. abstrusus* in eight kittens.[48] The therapy was started 8 weeks after an infection with 450 L3 larvae. At 2 and 4 weeks after treatment, no L1 larvae were found in the feces, and necropsy failed to reveal adult worms.[48] Another study tested fenbendazole (50 mg/kg every 24 hours, PO, for 3 days) in 15 experimentally infected cats.[41] No L1 larvae

were found on the fourteenth day after treatment; however, between days 14 and 25, five cats began shedding L1 larvae.[41] Longer (e.g., 14 days) administration of fenbendazole (50 mg/kg every 24 hours, PO) eradicated the worms with success.[5] Fenbendazole given to seven clinically healthy kittens in a fivefold overdose (250 mg/kg every 24 hours, PO) for 9 consecutive days caused no clinical, subclinical (determined by serum biochemical and blood hematologic analysis), gross, or histopathologic changes.[49]

Moxidectin is an endectocide macrolytic lactone.[50] A randomized, blinded, controlled multicenter field trial showed no L1 larvae in the feces 28 days after a single dose of 1% moxidectin spot-on solution in 12 cats, whereas out of 12 other cats that received fenbendazole (50 mg/kg every 24 hours, PO, for 3 days), only 11 became negative in the same period.[51] No adverse effects have been reported in any cat.

Emodepside 2.1% and/or praziquantel 8.6% spot-on was tested on 24 naturally infected cats in a randomized, blinded, controlled, multicenter field trial.[52] Twelve cats were treated with a single dose of spot-on, and 12 cats were treated with fenbendazole (50 mg/kg every 24 hours, PO, for 3 days). Four weeks after therapy, the number of larvae reduced by 99% in both groups.[52]

Selamectin 45 mg spot-on given twice with a 23-day interval was tested on 10 naturally infected cats.[53] Ten days after the first dose, nine cats were negative, and 15 days after the second dose, one cat was still positive. All 10 cats became negative 37 days after the second treatment.

The Baermann technique should always be performed on fecal samples from 3 consecutive days after completing any anthelmintic therapy to check whether the infection has successfully been cleared. Within a month after eradication of the infection, the clinical signs usually disappear. The radiographic changes are partly reversible, and the echocardiographic changes are fully reversible.[29]

Eucoleus aerophilus

A randomized, controlled, multicenter field trial investigated the effect of moxidectin spot-on on 36 naturally infected

cats.[50] One week after a single dose, the number of eggs per gram of feces reduced in the 16 treated cats from 152.9 (±128.1) to 2.9 (±12.1).[50]

Paragonimus kellicotti

Praziquantel given to five experimentally infected kittens (23 mg/kg every 8 hours, PO, for 3 days) days resulted in the disappearance of eggs from the feces by the eleventh day after therapy, and the radiographic pulmonary lesions were resolved.[19] Surgical lung-lobe resection might be necessary to treat cats with pneumothorax to remove the ruptured parasitic cyst(s).

ACKNOWLEDGMENTS

The author is grateful to Dr. Rolf Nijsse for his valuable comments on this manuscript, to the Division of Diagnostic Imaging, Utrecht University for Figure 36-1, and to Mr. Joop Fama for photography.

References

1. Gerichter CB: Studies on the nematodes parasitic in the lungs of *Felidae* in Palestine. *Parasitology* 39:251–262, 1949.
2. Mackerras J: Observations on the life history of the cat lungworm, *Aelurostrongylus abstrusus. Aust J Zool* 5:188–195, 1957.
3. Hamilton JM: *Aelurostrongylus abstrusus* infestation of the cat. *Vet Rec* 75:417–422, 1963.
4. Hobmaier M, Hobmaier A: Mammalian phase of the lungworm *Aelurostrongylus abstrusus* in the cat. *J Am Vet Med Assoc* 87:191–198, 1935.
5. Grandi G, Calvi LE, Venco L, et al: *Aelurostrongylus abstrusus* (cat lungworm) infection in five cats from Italy. *Vet Parasitol* 134:177–182, 2005.
6. Scott DW: Current knowledge of aelurostrongylosis in the cat—literature review and case reports. *Cornell Vet* 63:483–500, 1973.
7. Ribeiro VM, Lima WS: Larval production of cats infected and re-infected with *Aelurostrongylus abstusus* (Nematoda: Protostrongylidae). *Revue Méd Vét* 152:815–820, 2001.
8. Brianti E, Gaglio G, Giannetto S, et al: *Troglostrongylus brevior* and *Troglostrongylus subcrenatus* (Strongylida: Crenosomatidae) as agents of broncho-pulmonary infestation in domestic cats. *Parasit Vectors* 5:178–189, 2012.
9. Otranto D, Brianti E, Dantas-Torres F: *Troglostrongylus brevior* and a nonexistent "dilemma". *Trends Parasitol* 29:517–518, 2013.
10. Holmes PR, Kelly JD: *Capilaria aerophila* in the domestic cat in Australia. *Aust Vet J* 49:472–473, 1973.
11. Lalošević V, Lalošević D, Capo I, et al: High infection rate of zoonotic Eucoleus aerophila infection in foxes from Serbia. *Parasite* 20:1–3, 2013.

12. Barrs VR, Martin P, Nicoll RG, et al: Pulmonary cryptococcosis and *Capillaria aerophila* infection in an FIV-positive cat. *Aust Vet J* 78:154–158, 2000.
13. Di Cesare A, Castagna G, Otranto D, et al: Molecular detection of *Capillaria aerophila*, an agent of canine and feline pulmonary capillariosis. *J Clin Microbiol* 50:1958–1963, 2012.
14. Traversa D, Di Cesare A, Lia RP, et al: New insights into morphological and biological features of *Capillaria aerophila* (Trichocephalida, Trichuridae). *Parasitol Res* 109:S97–S104, 2011.
15. Seneviratna P: Studies on *Anafilaroides rostratus* Gerichter, 1949 in cats—II. The life cycle. *J Helminthol* 33:109–122, 1959.
16. Juste RA, Garcia AL, Mencia L: Mixed infestation of a domestic cat by *Aelurostrongylus abstrusus* and *Oslerus rostratus. Angew Parasitol* 33:56–60, 1992.
17. Ameel DJ: Paragonimus, its life history and distribution in North America and its taxonomy (Trematoda: Troglotrematidae). *Am J Hyg* 19:279–317, 1934.
18. Stromberg PC, Dubey JP: The life cycle of *Paragonimus kellicotti* in cats. *J Parasitol* 64:998–1002, 1978.
19. Bowman DD, Frongillo MK, Johnson RC, et al: Evaluation of praziquantel for treatment of experimentally induced paragonimiasis in dogs and cats. *Am J Vet Res* 52:68–71, 1991.
20. Dillon AR, Tillson DM, Hathcock J, et al: Lung histopathology, radiography, high-resolution computed tomography, and bronchio-alveolar lavage cytology are altered

by *Toxocara cati* infection in cats and is independent of development of adult intestinal parasites. *Vet Parasitol* 193:413–426, 2013.
21. Parsons JC, Bowman DD, Grieve RB: Pathological and haematological responses of cats experimentally infected with *Toxocara canis* larvae. *Internat J Parasitol* 19:479–488, 1989.
22. Speare R, Tinsley DJ: *Strongyloides felis*: an "old" worm rediscovered in Australian cats. *Aust Vet Practit* 16:10–18, 1986.
23. Traversa D, Di Cesare A, Conboy G: Canine and feline cardiopulmonary parasitic nematodes in Europe: emerging and underestimated. *Parasit Vectors* 3:1–22, 2010.
24. Hobmaier A, Hobmaier M: The route of infestation and the site of localization of lungworms in mollusks. *Science* 80:229, 1934.
25. Traversa D, Guglielmini C: Feline aelurostrongylosis and canine angiostrongylosis: A challenging diagnosis for two emerging verminous pneumonia infections. *Vet Parasitol* 157:163–174, 2008.
26. Dennler M, Bass DA, Gutierrez-Crespo B, et al: Thoracic computed tomography, angiographic computed tomography, and pathology findings in six cats experimentally infected with *Aelurostrongylus abstrusus. Vet Radiol Ultrasound* 54:459–469, 2013.
27. Stockdale PHG: The pathogenesis of the lesions elicited by *Aelurostrongylus abstrusus* during its prepatent period. *Path Vet* 7:102–115, 1970.
28. Naylor JR, Hamilton JM, Weatherley AJ: Changes in the ultrastructure of feline pulmonary arteries following infection with the lungworm *Aelurostrongylus abstrusus. Br Vet J* 140:181–190, 1984.

29. Dirven M, Szatmári V, van den Ingh T, et al: Reversible pulmonary hypertension associated with lungworm infection in a young cat. *J Vet Cardiol* 14:465–474, 2012.
30. Traversa D, Di Cesare A: Feline lungworms: what a dilemma. *Trends Parasitol* 29:423–430, 2013.
31. Brianti E, Gaglio G, Napoli E, et al: Evidence for direct transmission of the cat lungworm *Troglostrongylus brevior* (Strongylida: Crenosomatidae). *Parasitology* 140:821–824, 2013.
32. Ramos RAN, Gianelli A, Dantas-Torres F, et al: Survival of first-stage larvae of the cat lungworm *Troglostrongylus brevior* (Strongylida: Crenosomatidae) under different conditions. *Exp Parasitol* 135:570–572, 2013.
33. Dubey JP, Stromberg PC, Toussant MJ, et al: Induced paragonimiasis in cats: clinical signs and diagnosis. *J Am Vet Med Assoc* 173:734–742, 1978.
34. Hoover EA, Dubey JP: Pathogenesis of experimental pulmonary paragonimiasis in cats. *Am J Vet Res* 39:1827–1832, 1978.
35. Weatherley AJ, Hamilton JM: Possible role of histamine in the genesis of pulmonary arterial disease in cats infected with *Toxocara cati*. *Vet Rec* 114:347–349, 1984.
36. Sprent JFA: The life history and development of *Toxocara cati* (Schrank 1788) in the domestic cat. *Parasitology* 46:54–78, 1956.
37. Hamilton JM: The number of *Aelurostrongylus abstrusus* larvae required to produce pulmonary disease in the cat. *J Com Path* 77:343–346, 1967.
38. Gerdin JA, Slater MR, Makolinski KV, et al: Post-mortem findings in 54 cases of anesthetic associated death in cats from two spay-neuter programs in New York state. *J Feline Med Surg* 13:959–966, 2011.
39. Losonsky JM, Thrall DE, Prestwood AK: Radiographic evaluation of pulmonary abnormalities after *Aelurostrongylus abstrusus* inoculation in cats. *Am J Vet Res* 44:478–482, 1983.
40. Lacorcia L, Gasser RB, Anderson G, et al: Comparison of bronchoalveolar lavage fluid examination and other diagnostic techniques with the Baermann technique for detection of naturally occurring *Aelurostrongylus abstrusus* infection in cats. *J Am Vet Med Assoc* 235:43–49, 2009.
41. Roberson EL, Burke TM: Evaluation of granulated fenbendazole (22.2%) against induced and naturally occurring helminths infections in cats. *Am J Vet Res* 41:1499–1502, 1980.
42. Hamilton JM, McCaw AW: An investigation into the longevity of first stage larvae of *Aelurostrongylus abstrusus*. *J Helminthol* 41:313–320, 1967.
43. Cringoli G: FLOTAC, a novel apparatus for a multivalent faecal egg count technique. *Parassitologia* 48:381–384, 2006.
44. Gaglio G, Cringoli G, Rinaldi L, et al: Use of the FLOTAC technique for the diagnosis of *Aelurostrongylus abstrusus* in the cat. *Parasitol Res* 103:1055–1057, 2008.
45. Traversa D, Iorio R, Otranto D: Diagnostic and clinical implications of a nested PCR specific for ribosomal DNA of the feline lungworm *Aelurostrongylus abstrusus* (Nematoda, Strongylida). *J Clin Microbiol* 46:1811–1817, 2008.
46. Annoscia G, Latrofa MS, Campbell BE, et al: Simultaneous detection of the feline lungworms Troglostrongylus brevior and Aelurostrongylus abstrusus by a newly developed duplex-PCR. *Vet Parasitol* 199:172–178, 2014.
47. Briggs KR, Yaros JP, Liotta JL, et al: Detecting *Aelurostrongylus abstrusus*-specific IgG antibody using an immunofluorescence assay. *J Feline Med Surg* 15:1114–1118, 2013.
48. Hamilton JM, Weatherley A, Chapman AJ: Treatment of lungworm disease in the cat with fenbendazol. *Vet Rec* 114:40–41, 1984.
49. Schwartz RD, Donoghue AR, Baggs RB, et al: Evaluation of the safety of fenbendazol in cats. *Am J Vet Res* 61:330–332, 2000.
50. Traversa D, Di Cesare A, Di Giulio E, et al: Efficacy and safety of imidacloprid 10%/moxidectin 1% spot-on formulation in the treatment of feline infection by *Capillaria aerophila*. *Parasitol Res* 111:1793–1798, 2012.
51. Traversa D, Di Cesare A, Di Milillo P, et al: Efficacy and safety of imidacloprid 10%/moxidectin 1% spot-on formulation in the treatment of feline aelurostrongylosis. *Parasitol Res* 105:S55–S62, 2009.
52. Traversa D, Milillo P, Di Cesare A, et al: Efficacy and safety of emodepside 2.1%/praziquantel 8.6% spot-on formulation in the treatment of feline aelurostrongylosis. *Parasitol Res* 105:S83–S89, 2009.
53. Iannino F, Iannetti L, Paganico D, et al: Evaluation of the efficacy of selamectin spot on in cats infested with *Aelurostrongylus abstrusus* (Strongylida, Filaroididae) in Central Italy cat shelter. *Vet Parasitol* 197:258–262, 2013.

Feline Laryngeal Disease

Samantha Taylor and Andrea Harvey

Feline laryngeal diseases are generally uncommon. However, they are an important group of disorders because clinical signs may arise acutely, and affected cats frequently present with life-threatening dyspnea, despite having potentially treatable underlying etiologies.[1] This results in tracheostomy sometimes being required urgently, prior to further diagnostics being possible.[1,2] The sedentary behavior of cats may contribute to their usually presenting later on in the course of disease than dogs do. In addition, earlier clinical signs, such as exercise intolerance, that are often observed in dogs are not frequently observed in cats. Prompt recognition, diagnosis, and treatment are therefore vital to the success in managing feline laryngeal disease. Once there was a lack of published data on feline laryngeal disease, with most publications consisting of small numbers of cats with specific laryngeal disorders. Now, three large series of cases from different parts of the world have been published, giving rise to a wealth of further information on the importance of different etiologies of feline laryngeal disease, their diagnosis, treatments, and outcomes.[3,4,5]

ETIOLOGY OF LARYNGEAL DISEASE

In studies from the United Kingdom[3] and Australia[5], the most frequent causes of laryngeal disease were reported to be laryngeal paralysis (LP) and neoplasia. Inflammatory laryngeal disease was the third most common etiology in these reports, whereas it was the most frequently identified cause of laryngeal disease in a French study, accounting for more than 50% of cases.[4]

The most common laryngeal neoplasm in cats is lymphoma, followed by squamous cell carcinoma (SCC), with occasional other neoplasms encountered, including adenocarcinoma, other carcinomas, and round cell tumors or sarcomas. Feline immunodeficiency virus (FIV) appears to be relatively prevalent in cats with laryngeal neoplasia, with 5 out of 22 cases (23%) of laryngeal lymphoma over three studies,[3,5,6] and 3 out of 11 cases (27%) of laryngeal SCC over two studies,[3,6] occurring in FIV-positive cats. In many of the other studies reporting laryngeal neoplasia, retroviral status was not evaluated in all cats, and so it is possible that the prevalence of FIV infection in cases of laryngeal neoplasia is even higher than this.

Laryngeal paralysis is most commonly bilateral. Even though unilateral LP has also been described with some frequency, it may be less commonly recognized because cats are less likely to become significantly symptomatic. Underlying etiologies for LP were described in about one third of reported cases, with iatrogenic trauma to the recurrent laryngeal nerve after thyroidectomy being the most common cause, comprising around 10% of all cases of LP. Other reported etiologies include neuropathy, tick paralysis, brainstem lesions, neoplasia, idiopathic, or congenital causes.

Tick paralysis is an important etiology in parts of the world where paralysis ticks are encountered. In the Australian case series,[5] it only accounted for 4 out of 29 (14%) cases of LP; however, this is likely to be significantly underestimated because laryngeal examination was an inclusion criterion for this study, and the majority of cats with tick paralysis would not undergo laryngeal examination unless they were requiring intubation. It is likely that tick paralysis is in fact the most common cause of LP in cats in this region.

Inflammatory laryngeal disease is an especially interesting group of diseases because it is common in cats, and to date, no consistent or definite underlying etiology has been identified. The nature of inflammation in described cases has been extremely diverse, from mixed inflammation, to lymphoplasmacytic, neutrophilic, or granulomatous inflammation,[1-4,6,7] suggesting that multiple different etiologies likely exist. In some studies, laryngeal "swelling" was not classified as inflammatory if cytology or histopathology was unavailable, so this group of laryngeal diseases is likely to be underestimated in published studies. Searches for infectious etiologies have generally been unrewarding; no organisms were identified with special stains in cases of granulomatous inflammation.[7] Foreign body penetration or other trauma has been postulated as a cause, but, interestingly, in cases of granulomatous inflammation, a narrow zone of tissue that was less inflamed was present immediately beneath the epithelium, suggesting that inflammation was originating deep in the tissue, making trauma a less likely cause.[7] Upper respiratory tract (URT) viruses are a feasible etiologic agent in some cases, and several reported cases have had concurrent clinical signs of URT infection and/or calicivirus infection identified.[1-5,8] No reported cases have had herpesvirus identified, but it could also be a possible inciting cause. Primary or secondary bacterial infection may also occur.[1,3,7] Some cases of inflammatory laryngeal disease have developed following a procedure requiring intubation, and this could be an inciting cause[1]; however, this is not a consistent finding. One case with regional collagen lysis had a history of eosinophilic granulomas, and, although not previously reported on the larynx, the etiology may be similar.[1] Other reported causes of laryngeal disease include laryngeal spasm, cyst, hypoplasia, tear, and swelling.

SIGNALMENT

There have been no sex or breed predispositions reported for most etiologies of feline laryngeal disease. However, Burmese cats accounted for 50% of the cases of inflammatory laryngeal disease in one study,[5] and 16% in another report.[3] Acute laryngeal swelling was also reported in two young Burmese siblings, and, on repeat laryngeal evaluation once the swelling had subsided, it was suspected that they had laryngeal hypoplasia.[3] The authors have also encountered other Burmese cats with laryngeal swelling or edema of unknown etiology. It is possible that the breed is predisposed to inflammatory laryngeal disease.

The age range of presentation of cats with laryngeal disease is wide. The median age of cats with laryngeal neoplasia is older than cats with inflammatory laryngeal disease and LP; however, older cats can be equally afflicted with inflammatory disease or LP. Neoplasia is much less likely in cats less than 7 years of age. The reported age range for cats with LP is 1 to 19 years, with a median of 10 years, whereas cats with laryngeal neoplasia ranged from 7 to 18 years (median 13 years), and cats with inflammatory laryngeal disease ranged from 9 months to 18 years (median 7 years).[3,5]

CLINICAL FINDINGS

The most common presenting signs of any laryngeal disease in cats include inspiratory stridor, dyspnea, and dysphonia, with dysphagia, gagging, and coughing reported less frequently.[1,3-7] In unusual cases, a palpable mass in the laryngeal region may be identified, suggestive of neoplasia of that region (e.g., thyroid carcinoma). No association between clinical signs and disease category has been reported.[3-5]

A history of dysphonia and inspiratory stridor localizes pathology to the laryngeal region and should prompt investigation of that area, but these signs are not present in all cases. Only between one third and one half of reported cases of laryngeal disease were dysphonic in the three largest case series reported.[3-5]

The vast majority of cases of upper airway disease will show primarily inspiratory signs, but a fixed obstruction in the laryngeal area may result in both inspiratory and expiratory signs. Nonspecific clinical signs, such as weight loss, are also reported frequently.[5] Some cats may cough and wheeze, and may initially be suspected of lower airway disease. Cases with neuromuscular pathology may show signs of generalized weakness. In geographic locations where paralysis ticks occur, the presence of an attached tick in a cat presenting with compatible clinical signs such as weakness, ataxia, and pupillary dilation indicates tick paralysis,[9] but an attached tick is not always present, and this disorder should be at the top of the differential diagnosis list in any cat with signs of laryngeal dysfunction in such geographical regions.

It is common for cats to present in acute respiratory distress because preceding signs, such as exercise intolerance, as reported in dogs with laryngeal disease, are rarely noted, and the small diameter of the glottis in cats predisposes to the development of severe dyspnea. An acute presentation is more common in cats with inflammatory laryngeal disease because cats with LP and neoplasia may have a more subacute or chronic history of clinical signs.[1,3,5]

DIAGNOSTICS

Clinical signs often localize disease to the larynx but in most cases, do not allow the identification of a specific disease etiology, with the exception of tick paralysis,[5,9] and other causes of more generalized neuromuscular disease. Therefore, making a definitive diagnosis can be challenging. Cats in acute respiratory distress make poor candidates for restraint for diagnostic procedures, and clinician reticence to anesthetize such cases is understandable. However, making a diagnosis is important to allow specific treatment, and it is possible at times when less invasive techniques are in use. The clinician should be prepared to proceed to more involved diagnostics if required. Direct visualization of the larynx is the most useful diagnostic evaluation in these cases, and these cats are usually more stable under anesthesia when an endotracheal tube can be placed. Further diagnostics as required can then be performed, with severity of laryngeal disease used to help determine whether tracheotomy or tracheostomy is required before recovery from anesthesia. A number of small endotracheal tubes and smaller diameter tubes such as red rubber urinary catheters or polypropylene catheters should be ready before anesthesia in preparation for potential difficulty with intubation, and equipment should be readily available for an emergency tracheotomy if required. Generally, hematology, biochemistry, and urinalysis do not have a high diagnostic yield in feline laryngeal disease but may identify concurrent disease or involvement of other organ systems in the laryngeal pathology (e.g., lymphoma). Other tests such as *Cryptococcus* antigen testing or retroviral serology, for example, may be indicated in certain cases. Feline immunodeficiency virus serology is particularly useful in cases of laryngeal lymphoma or SCC, given that a significant proportion of these cases to date appear to be FIV positive. In some cases, inflammatory laryngeal disease may be the result of respiratory viral infections (herpesvirus or calicivirus), and therefore testing for viral infection may be appropriate, although the carrier state must be taken into account, and detection of the virus does not always imply a causal relationship.

Noninvasive diagnostic techniques such as radiography or echolaryngography allow identification of a lesion in the region of the larynx in the majority of cases but importantly do not provide a definitive diagnosis. More invasive procedures such as biopsy are needed for this, and, in the majority of cases, a biopsy may be performed safely and without resulting in clinical deterioration.[3,5]

Diagnostic Imaging

Diagnostic imaging can be useful in cases of upper airway disease, to allow localization of pathology, evaluation of the patient for disease away from the larynx (e.g., aspiration pneumonia in cases of LP), and as a screening modality before more invasive diagnostics.

Radiography is commonly used in the investigation of laryngeal disease, but more advanced imaging techniques are being investigated (e.g., computed tomography [CT]) as they become more widely available.

Radiography

Radiography can be useful in the investigation of laryngeal disease, but it has some significant limitations. Superimposition of other soft tissue structures in the region of the larynx on lateral cervical projections can mask lesions, and cats with laryngeal masses may have normal cervical radiographs.[3,6,10] Tumors of the larynx may present as generalized thickening in the laryngeal region rather than a discrete mass, creating only subtle radiographic changes. Similarly, cats with inflammatory laryngeal disease may show radiographic signs of soft tissue swelling in the larynx that may be indistinguishable from neoplastic lesions but again may be radiographically unremarkable, necessitating further investigation (e.g., laryngoscopy) in all cases.[1,3,7] Identification of a mass in the laryngeal region (Figure 37-1) may be useful in cases where clinical signs are less localizing. In rare cases of a laryngeal or pharyngeal foreign body, radiography may identify radiopaque objects (needles in particular).

All cases undergoing radiography would benefit from thoracic imaging in addition to cervical views. These views may demonstrate thoracic pathology associated with the laryngeal disease; for example, aspiration pneumonia in cases of LP,

metastasis, or a primary lesion affecting the recurrent laryngeal or vagus nerve causing LP. A ventrodorsal and two lateral thoracic projections should be evaluated for metastases.

Echolaryngography

Echolaryngography is a noninvasive technique requiring minimum restraint that with adequate user experience can consistently identify laryngeal masses and cysts.[3,11] Laryngeal paralysis and vocal fold thickening can also be documented, but diagnosis requires more skill, and laryngoscopic confirmation. In dogs with LP, echolaryngography has not been shown to be superior to direct laryngoscopy *per os* (PO),[12] and the same is likely true for cats.

However, in selected cases, particularly where a laryngeal mass is suspected, echolaryngography affords the clinician a noninvasive diagnostic test and an opportunity to plan further investigation, such as sampling for histopathology, as is required for a definitive diagnosis. As with radiography, the similarity between the appearance of neoplastic and inflammatory laryngeal lesions means further diagnostics (e.g., histopathology) should always be undertaken, and neoplasia should not be assumed when a mass is identified.

Computed Tomography

Computed tomography is not commonly used to image the feline upper airway but can identify mass lesions (Figure 37-2) or underlying etiologies for LP, and be used in non-anesthetized cats as shown in one study.[13] Computed tomography was also used to identify an invasive thyroid mass in one study,[5] but it failed to identify LP in two other cats.

In the former study,[13] cats with upper airway masses, laryngotracheitis, and LP were identified using CT, with diagnoses confirmed with further investigation. It is noted by the authors that although CT could be helpful for

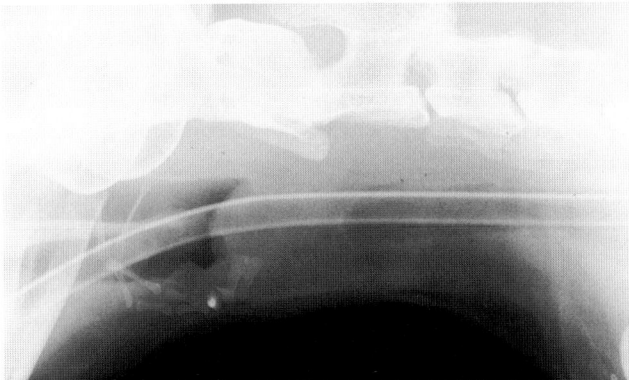

Figure 37-1: Lateral pharyngeal radiograph showing a soft tissue mass in the region of the larynx. Subsequent histopathology confirmed squamous cell carcinoma. (From Taylor SS, Harvey AM, Barr FJ, et al: Laryngeal disease in cats: a retrospective study of 35 cases. *J Feline Med Surg* 11:954-962, 2009.)

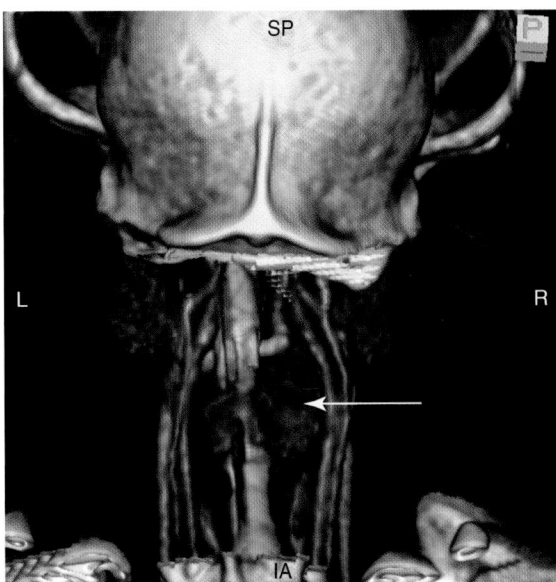

Figure 37-2: Reconstructed CT image (with spinal column removed from image) of the laryngeal region of a cat with a laryngeal chondroma (*arrow*). (Image courtesy of Andrew Holloway.)

preliminary investigation, a definitive diagnosis still requires techniques that are more invasive, such as biopsy, as not all mass lesions are neoplastic. In nonanesthetized dogs with LP, CT has been described as an effective diagnostic test,[14] and the same maybe true for cats. However, the mixed results mentioned previously indicate the need for further investigation of this imaging modality in cats with upper airway disease. Concurrent thoracic CT may be useful for identification of thoracic pathology, and it has been evaluated in conscious cats.[15] As mentioned previously, however, anesthesia to secure an airway is usually safer in these cats than is attempting diagnostics with the cat conscious.

Laryngoscopy

Laryngoscopy can be performed PO, using minimal equipment (a laryngoscope), and it is usually the most high-yield and cost-effective diagnostic evaluation, allowing visualization of the larynx and observation of laryngeal motility. For example, discrete masses may be observed (Figure 37-3), or diffuse thickening of the vocal folds (which notably can indicate inflammation and neoplasia).[10] Observable disease may be unilateral or bilateral, and, again, this does not distinguish between an inflammatory or neoplastic lesion.[5] Alternatively, an endoscope can be used to observe the larynx, but this technique is not usually required, given the view of the larynx afforded by direct visualization. As mentioned earlier, laryngoscopy is required in most cases, along with further diagnostic testing, because of the limitations of diagnostic imaging. Laryngoscopy allows the operator to biopsy abnormal areas of laryngeal and/or surrounding soft tissue.

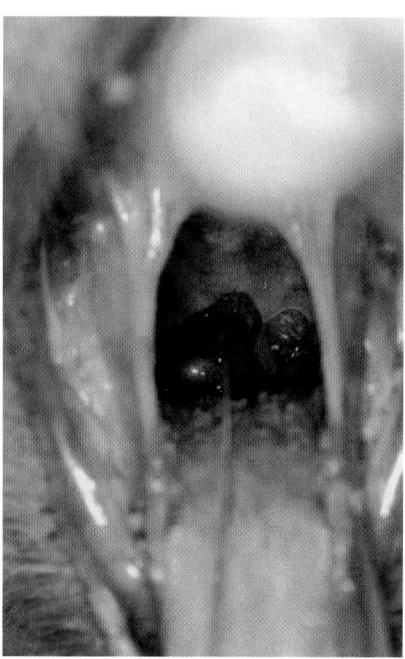

Figure 37-3: A laryngeal mass observed with a laryngoscope (note guide wire in place to aid intubation). Subsequent histopathology diagnosed laryngeal squamous cell carcinoma.

Biopsy

Cytology or histopathology are required to make a definitive diagnosis because of the similarities in the appearance of inflammatory and neoplastic lesions and the vastly different reported outcomes.[1,3,5-7] Previous studies have demonstrated discordant results between cytology and histopathology,[3,6] and therefore tissue biopsy is preferred. Fine-needle aspiration (FNA) may be diagnostic in cases with exfoliative neoplasia, but it can be misleading, particularly when inflammatory lesions are suspected. Percutaneous FNA with prior echolaryngographic or CT planning may be possible. It allows for avoidance of anesthesia but it is technically demanding.

Tissue samples obtained PO are adequate for diagnosis in the majority of reported cases,[1,3,5-7] and they are not technically challenging to obtain. Simple equipment can be used, such as endoscopy cup biopsy forceps. Understandable concern is often raised regarding the consequences to the patient of laryngeal biopsy; however, the two largest studies of laryngeal disease in cats reported no clinical deterioration after biopsy.[3,5] In contrast, in a small case series by Costello,[1] it was noted that emergency tracheostomy was required after biopsy in the majority of cases. Equipment should certainly be available for urgent tracheostomy should it become necessary, and cats should be monitored closely in recovery for any deterioration in respiratory pattern. Administration of a short-acting corticosteroid prior to obtaining a biopsy may reduce morbidity after surgery, but further study is required.

Procedures that are more invasive, such as ventral laryngotomy, are rarely required, and they may be associated with risks to the cat that are more significant.

Diagnosis of Laryngeal Paralysis

Definitive diagnosis of LP requires laryngoscopy and observation of laryngeal motility directly with laryngoscopy, using echolaryngography (see earlier), or using video-endoscopy. Echolaryngography and CT have not been shown to be superior to direct laryngoscopy in dogs,[12] but they have not been directly compared in cats. They do allow assessment without sedation or anesthesia, negating the effect of drugs on laryngeal motility. For a diagnosis of LP, the larynx should be observed PO under a light plane of anesthesia. A lack of arytenoid abduction on inspiration or paradoxical laryngeal motion confirms the diagnosis. Diagnosis can be affected by choice of anesthetic agent, and the effect of various agents on laryngeal motility in cats has not been well documented. A light plane of anesthesia should be maintained during laryngeal observation, and importantly spontaneous ventilation should be maintained. In dogs the use of doxapram has been advocated to increase respiratory rate during laryngoscopy,[16] but doxapram use has not been evaluated in feline LP.

In dogs, there is evidence that acquired LP is part of a generalized peripheral neuropathy,[17] and as such, all cats with suspected and confirmed LP without any other identifiable underlying etiology should ideally undergo a full neurological evaluation and further testing as indicated. This could include acetylcholine receptor antibody assay for myasthenia gravis, and electromyography and nerve conduction velocity for peripheral neuropathy.

TREATMENT OF LARYNGEAL DISEASE

Cats presenting in acute respiratory distress because of upper airway obstruction or partial obstruction will require emergency treatment (Box 37-1). Once the specific etiology has been determined, targeted treatment can be selected according to the individual case.

Laryngeal Paralysis

In some cases, the underlying cause of LP may be managed with curative results. Treatment of tick paralysis requires a variable intensity of treatment depending on severity of clinical signs, varying from administration of tick antiserum, application of fipronil spray, and rest with or without light sedation, to intubation, and even ventilation in severely affected cases. Complications of LP must be aggressively managed (e.g., bronchopneumonia and aspiration pneumonia).

Where the primary cause cannot be directly treated, further options include conservative or surgical treatment. Conservative treatment is indicated for less severely affected cats (usually those with unilateral LP), and it includes weight management and restricted excitement and exercise. This

---

BOX 37-1 Management of Acute Respiratory Distress Caused by Laryngeal Disease

- Initial patient triage should be performed promptly and efficiently to avoid further stressing an already compromised cat.
- Oxygen supplementation should be provided, again in a way to avoid stress (e.g., oxygen tent rather than mask).
- Light sedation, for example with butorphanol +/– acepromazine, can help to reduce severity of dyspnea during initial stabilization.
- Clinical signs may localize disease to the upper airway but are unlikely to be specific to one diagnosis; further investigations will inevitably be required.
- Cats with severe upper airway obstruction should be anesthetized to secure a patent airway, after which further diagnostics may proceed.
- Equipment to aid intubation (e.g., guide wire or urinary catheter to be used to facilitate intubation) or to perform an emergency tracheostomy should be easily accessible.
- Emergency tracheostomy should be reserved for patients that cannot be intubated.
- Less severely affected patients may be treated medically (e.g., with oxygen supplementation and corticosteroids) and undergo diagnostic imaging conscious or under sedation before further investigations.

---

approach can be effective. It is associated with prolonged survival times,[3,18] and is perhaps more applicable to cats than dogs, given cats' lifestyle (e.g., generally less active) and differences in type of exercise (e.g., cats are rarely taken for walks).

Successful surgical management of LP in cats has been described,[3,5,18-20] and it may be indicated for those with severe respiratory compromise, which often includes bilateral cases. Unilateral arytenoid lateralization is the technique of choice in most cases, and surgical success rates are variable. Complications during and after surgery are common. Complications arose in 50% of cases after surgery in one study,[20] a figure similar to that reported previously.[19] Complications that occur during and after surgery include aspiration pneumonia (most commonly), persistent laryngeal obstruction, and laryngeal swelling necessitating tracheotomy in some cases, and less commonly, Horner syndrome and recurrence of signs of upper respiratory obstruction.[3,18-21] Given the potential for complications, it is advised that the decision for surgery is taken based on the severity of the clinical signs, and bilateral arytenoid lateralization is avoided because of the increased risk of aspiration pneumonia.[19] Other surgical procedures such as partial laryngectomy and ventriculocordectomy have also been reported,[18,21] but generally they have been replaced with unilateral arytenoid lateralization.

Laryngeal Neoplasia

The management of laryngeal neoplasia greatly depends on the type of tumor diagnosed. Management of squamous cell and other types of carcinoma is usually palliative and may include permanent tracheotomy.[2] Aggressive surgical interventions, usually with airflow bypass (such as complete laryngectomy and tracheostomy) are rarely indicated in veterinary medicine, although small lesions may be amenable to surgical management.

Laryngeal lymphoma may respond to chemotherapy with protocols including cyclophosphamide, vincristine, and prednisolone, and long-term survival has been reported (see Prognosis). Radio-responsive tumors such as laryngeal lymphoma might be managed with radiotherapy, but limited reports of response are available.[6]

Laryngeal Inflammation

The underlying cause of laryngeal inflammation is usually not identified, and cases are generally managed symptomatically.

Granulomatous laryngitis in three cats was managed with a combination of medical (corticosteroids and antibiotics) and surgical (excision of laryngeal tissue) treatment in one study, with encouraging results.[7] The majority of cats diagnosed with laryngeal inflammation in other studies have been treated with combinations of corticosteroids and antibiotics with favorable responses, if the cat survived the period of acute upper airway obstruction, for which some cases required tracheostomy.[1,3,5] Even though corticosteroids are generally contraindicated in cases of upper respiratory viral

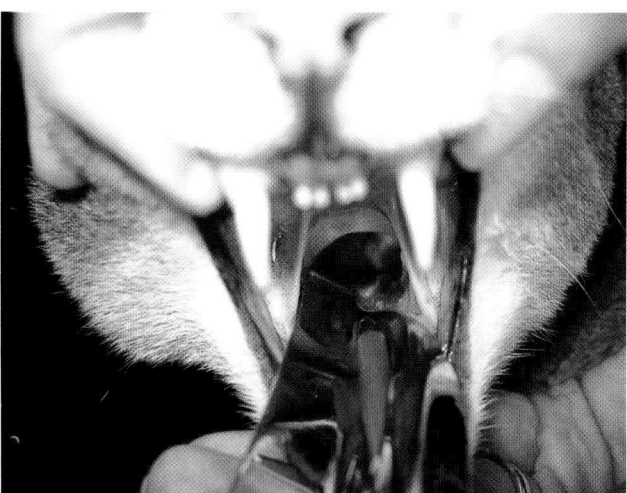

Figure 37-4: A cat with a laryngeal mass diagnosed as laryngeal lymphoma prior to treatment. (Photo courtesy of Dan Holden. In Taylor SS, Harvey AM, Barr FJ, et al: Laryngeal disease in cats: a retrospective study of 35 cases. *J Feline Med Surg* 11:954-962, 2009.)

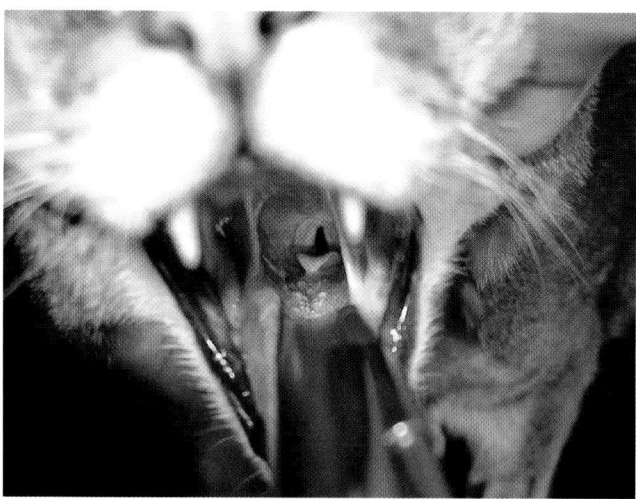

Figure 37-5: The cat in Figure 37-4 with laryngeal lymphoma, 7 days after starting treatment with cyclophosphamide, vincristine, and prednisolone. Laryngoscopy revealed a normal larynx, and the cat went on to survive for 1440 days. (Photo courtesy of Dan Holden. In Taylor SS, Harvey AM, Barr FJ, et al: Laryngeal disease in cats: a retrospective study of 35 cases. *J Feline Med Surg* 11:954-962, 2009.)

infection (e.g., herpesvirus), their use is justified in cases of URT obstruction caused by laryngeal inflammation, because they seem to greatly reduce potentially life-threatening laryngeal inflammation and edema.[8] Consideration should be given to the use of short-acting corticosteroids when viral infection is suspected or diagnosed.

If herpesvirus infection is the suspected cause of the pathology, then management with antiviral drugs such as famciclovir may be indicated,[22] but further evaluation of the benefit of this treatment in inflammatory laryngeal disease is required.

PROGNOSIS

Depending on the underlying cause of the laryngeal disease, long-term survival is possible. Long survival times have been reported for LP treated either conservatively (120 to 2520

days; median 811 days)[3] or surgically (approximately 150 days).[3,19,20]

Survival times reported for inflammatory laryngeal disease can also be prolonged.[1,3,5] In general, the prognosis for cats with LP and inflammatory laryngeal disease depends on the severity of clinical signs at presentation and decisions to treat aggressively (possibly with tracheostomy) at that stage. If affected cats survive the acute period of treatment or surgery and avoid complications after surgery in the case of LP, then long-term survival is possible.

The prognosis for cats with laryngeal tumors depends on the type of neoplasia and choice of treatment. Survival of cats with laryngeal carcinoma managed with tracheostomy is generally short (2 to 281 days),[2] with progression of disease or tracheostomy complications resulting in death or euthanasia. Management of laryngeal lymphoma with chemotherapy may result in longer survival times (up to 1440 days[3]; Figures 37-4 and 37-5), and a median survival time of 112 days.[23]

References

1. Costello MF, Keith D, Hendrick M, et al: Acute upper airway obstruction due to inflammatory laryngeal disease in 5 cats. *J Vet Emerg Crit Care* 11:205–211, 2001.
2. Guenther-Yenke CL, Rozanski EA: Tracheostomy in cats: 23 cases (1998-2006). *J Feline Med Surg* 9:451–457, 2007.
3. Taylor SS, Harvey AM, Barr FJ, et al: Laryngeal disease in cats: a retrospective study of 35 cases. *J Feline Med Surg* 11:954–962, 2009.
4. Bertolani C, Bota I, Hernandez L: Feline laryngeal disease: 40 cases (2000-2001). In *Proceeding of 21st Congress of the European College of Veterinary Internal Medicine*, 2011, p 248. (Abstract).

5. Lam AL, Beatty JA, Moore L, et al: Laryngeal disease in 69 cats: a retrospective multicentre study. *Aust Vet Pract* 42:321–326, 2012.
6. Jakubiak MJ, Siedlecki CT, Zenger E, et al: Laryngeal, laryngotracheal, and tracheal masses in cats: 27 cases (1998-2003). *J Am Anim Hosp Assoc* 41:310–316, 2005.
7. Tasker S, Foster DJ, Corcoran BM, et al: Obstructive laryngeal disease in three cats. *J Feline Med Surg* 1:53–59, 1999.
8. Malik R, Pearson M, Davis P, et al: Airway obstruction due to laryngeal oedema in a cat. *Aust Vet Pract* 21:64–66, 1991.
9. Schull D, Litster A, Atwell R: Tick toxicity in cats caused by *Ixodes* species in Australia: a

review of published literature. *J Feline Med Surg* 9:487–493, 2007.
10. Carlisle CH, Biery DN, Thrall DE: Tracheal and laryngeal tumors in the dog and cat: literature review and 13 additional patients. *Vet Radiol Ultrasound* 5:229–235, 1991.
11. Rudorf H, Barr F: Echolaryngography in cats. *Vet Radiol Ultrasound* 43:353–357, 2002.
12. Radlinsky MG, Williams J, Frank PM, et al: Comparison of three clinical techniques for the diagnosis of laryngeal paralysis in dogs. *Vet Surg* 38:434–438, 2009.
13. Stadler K, O'Brien R: Computed tomography of nonanesthetized cats with upper airway

obstruction. *Vet Radiol Ultrasound* 54:231–236, 2013.

14. Stadler K, Hartman S, Matheson J, et al: Computed tomographic imaging of dogs with primary laryngeal or tracheal airway obstruction. *Vet Radiol Ultrasound* 52:377–384, 2011.

15. Oliveira CR, Mitchell MA, O'Brien RT: Thoracic computed tomography in feline patients without use of chemical restraint. *Vet Radiol Ultrasound* 52:368–376, 2011.

16. Jackson AM, Tobias K, Long C, et al: Effects of various anesthetic agents on laryngeal motion during laryngoscopy in normal dogs. *Vet Surg* 33:102–106, 2004.

17. Jeffery ND, Talbot CE, Smith PM, et al: Acquired idiopathic laryngeal paralysis as a prominent feature of generalised neuromuscular disease in 39 dogs. *Vet Rec* 158:17–21, 2006.

18. Schachter S, Norris CR: Laryngeal paralysis in cats: 16 cases (1990-1999). *J Am Vet Med Assoc* 216:1100–1103, 2000.

19. Hardie RJ, Gunby J, Bjorling DE: Arytenoid lateralization for treatment of laryngeal paralysis in 10 cats. *Vet Surg* 38:445–451, 2009.

20. Thunberg B, Lantz GC: Evaluation of unilateral arytenoid lateralization for the treatment of laryngeal paralysis in 14 cats. *J Am Anim Hosp Assoc* 46:418–424, 2010.

21. White RAS, Littlewood JD, Herritage ME, et al: Outcome of surgery for laryngeal paralysis in four cats. *Vet Rec* 118:103–104, 1986.

22. Malik R, Lessels NS, Webb S, et al: Treatment of feline herpesvirus-1 associated disease in cats with famciclovir and related drugs. *J Feline Med Surg* 11:40–48, 2009.

23. Taylor SS, Goodfellow MR, Browne WJ, et al: Feline extranodal lymphoma: response to chemotherapy and survival in 110 cats. *J Small Anim Pract* 50:584–592, 2009.

Feline Hypertension

Brian A. Scansen

DEFINITION OF HYPERTENSION

By definition, systemic arterial hypertension (henceforth referred to as hypertension) is an elevation from normal systemic arterial blood pressure (ABP). Therefore, making a diagnosis of hypertension requires knowledge of what the normal ABP is in this species. In a study of six apparently normal awake cats with an implanted telemetric device, blood pressures at rest were reported as a systolic pressure of 126 ± 4 mm Hg, a mean pressure of 106 ± 5 mm Hg, and a diastolic pressure of 91 ± 6 mm Hg.[1] Although from a small sample, these values are comparable to normal ABP in other species and serve as a useful approximation of the normal ABP in cats. However, given the small size of feline arteries and the invasiveness of direct arterial pressure measurements, nearly all estimates of feline ABP in clinical patients are made with noninvasive devices—either Doppler or oscillometric, the details of which are outlined below.

Oscillometric devices have been evaluated for ABP measurement in apparently healthy cats with mean values reported from 115 to 139 mm Hg for systolic pressure, 96 to 99 mm Hg for mean pressure, and 74 to 77 mm Hg for diastolic pressure.[2,3] Using Doppler ultrasound devices in a clinical setting, systolic ABP measured in healthy awake cats has been reported to be from 118 to 162 mm Hg.[4-6] In nearly all of these studies, standard deviations of the measured ABP are wide, suggesting high variability in ABP measurement with current noninvasive devices. Poor agreement is also found when noninvasive ABP measurements are compared with direct ABP measurements, particularly in awake cats.[7,8] In one study[8] comparing simultaneous measurements of direct ABP to noninvasive oscillometric and Doppler ABP measurements in awake cats, the Doppler method had the best agreement with invasive measurements ($R^2 = 0.82$), while the oscillometric method was relatively poorly correlated in this population of awake cats ($R^2 = 0.26$). In anesthetized cats, both devices performed better. This variability and lack of accuracy must be kept in mind when interpreting measurements of ABP in cats.

As ABP is nearly always measured in a clinic or hospital setting, elevations in ABP are common and related to stress or excitement, an effect that was been termed *white coat hypertension*. The stress of the examination leads to peripheral vasoconstriction, increased cardiac output, and an elevated value of ABP, which may not be reflective of the animal's ABP at home or the true risk of complications from hypertension. Both the variability in ABP measurement and the effect of stress can be seen in a recent study evaluating ABP in 30 cats measured both at home and at the hospital, where the mean difference between ABP measured at home versus the hospital was a 6 mm Hg increase, though the individual differences ranged from a decrease of 26 mm Hg to an increase of 31 mm Hg.[9] The reality of white coat hypertension complicates ABP measurement in cats and requires the veterinarian to interpret a cat's ABP within the context of the animal's age, the environment in which the ABP is taken, the cat's level of perceived anxiety, and the likelihood that any measured elevation in ABP is real. This is discussed further in the section describing the diagnosis of feline hypertension.

In studies of dogs,[10] humans,[11] and cats[3,12,13] a relationship between ABP and age is often reported, with a gradual increase in the expected ABP with advancing age. Although the effect of age on ABP is not confirmed in all studies of cats, it is likely that the reference interval for blood pressure in cats varies to a small degree with the age of the animal. Definitive reference intervals based upon age are not available for the cat at this time. The effect of sex is also poorly defined, though one study found increased systolic ABP in male cats compared with females.[6]

The prevalence of hypertension in the feline population is not defined. However, a recent prospective study of 100 middle-age and geriatric cats found 8 of 100 cats with an ABP greater than 160 mm Hg.[13] Epidemiologic studies of the feline population at large evaluating the prevalence of hypertension have not been performed.

ETIOLOGY OF HYPERTENSION

The etiology of systemic hypertension is complex and multifactorial. In general, the ABP measured in an animal reflects an interplay between cardiac output and systemic vascular resistance (ABP = cardiac output × systemic vascular resistance). A myriad of local and global neurohormonal systems exist in the body to maintain normal arterial pressure by varying cardiac output (via modulation of the heart rate and contractility) and systemic vascular resistance (via modulation of arteriolar constriction and dilation). When a disease state alters the balance of these neurohormonal systems, pathological increases in ABP may develop.

Causes of Systemic Hypertension

Hypertension in the cat appears to develop primarily in the setting of concurrent systemic disease. Conditions that have been associated with hypertension in the cat include renal disease,[2,5,12,14,15] hyperthyroidism,[5,14] hyperaldosteronism,[16] hyperadrenocorticism,[17] pheochromocytoma,[18] chronic anemia,[19] and high salt intake.[20] Of these conditions, renal disease appears to be the most common underlying disorder resulting in hypertension in cats, with at least 60% of hypertensive cats presenting with azotemia or inappropriate urine concentration.[21] The prevalence of hypertension among hyperthyroid cats is variable in the literature, ranging from roughly 10% to 20% of hyperthyroid cats[22-24] with approximately an additional 20% of cats developing hypertension after therapy for their hyperthyroidism.[24] Diabetes mellitus has been suspected as a cause in some cases of feline hypertension,[25] with other studies suggesting hypertension is not a common finding in the diabetic cat.[26] Diabetes mellitus in cats also appears to be associated with a tenfold greater risk of cardiac death compared to the normal population, though the exact pathogenesis involved in this finding is not clear.[27]

As noted above, white coat hypertension complicates the diagnosis of hypertension, and effort must be expended to confirm the diagnosis before treatment is initiated, particularly if there is no evidence of target organ injury nor an underlying condition that is known to be associated with hypertension. Interestingly, a proportion of cats diagnosed with hypertension, including those with retinal lesions or other evidence of target organ injury, do not have a clear underlying cause for the elevated ABP.[14,25] The finding of hypertension without a causative systemic condition is common in humans and termed essential or primary hypertension. Dietary salt intake has been proposed as a contributing mechanism in the development of essential hypertension in humans[28] and, as noted above, has been reported to cause hypertension in a cat receiving a high dietary salt intake.[29] However, a short-term study[30] of increased salt intake in cats did not find a relationship between salt intake and ABP, and the relationship between dietary salt intake and development of hypertension in cats remains unresolved. Early, nonazotemic renal disease has been proposed as an explanation for these cases of hypertension without overt concurrent disease, but definitive studies proving this theory are not available. For the feline practitioner, it is important to keep in mind that a small percentage of cats with hypertension will not have a readily identifiable cause.

TARGET ORGAN INJURY

Target organ injury is defined as clinical signs or diagnostic findings of disease that may be related to pathological elevations in ABP. Those organs at greatest risk for hypertensive damage are the eyes, brain, kidney, and heart, and the presence of lesions compatible with hypertensive damage in one or more of these organs strongly supports a diagnosis of hypertension (Figures 38-1 to 38-3). The eyes, brain, and kidneys are organs with extensive vascular networks, whereas the heart is the organ that must work against an elevation in ABP and is therefore affected by hypertension.

In the eye (see Figure 38-1), hypertensive changes manifest in three ways: hypertensive retinopathy, hypertensive choroidopathy, and hypertensive optic neuropathy.[31] Hypertensive retinopathy refers to changes in the retinal arterioles (e.g., tortuosity, beading), as well as the development of retinal hemorrhage or periarteriolar edema (see Figure 38-1C), while hypertensive choroidopathy reflects changes associated with the choroidal vascular bed including changes to the retinal pigment epithelium, fluid leakage into the retina from the choroid, and development of serous retinal detachment (see Figures 38-1C and 38-1D).[31] Hypertensive optic neuropathy refers to changes in the optic nerve head including papilledema in early disease, progressing to ischemia and eventual atrophy of the optic disk in chronic cases.[31] In addition to these changes, hemorrhage into the anterior chamber or vitreous is also possible.[22,25,31] Hypertensive ocular disease appears to be among the most common manifestations of hypertension, occurring in roughly half of all hypertensive cats,[15,21,22,32] and studies suggest that retinal changes in hypertension can develop at a systolic ABP of 168 mm Hg and above.[12]

Neurological signs associated with hypertension appear less frequently than ocular changes, but were reported in 15% of cases in one study[32] and in 20% of cases in another.[25] Neurological manifestations of hypertension occur as a result of disruption of the blood-brain barrier and development of cerebral edema, which may progress to elevated intracranial pressure and even cerebellar herniation.[33,34] Neurological signs may include disorientation, vestibular signs, ataxia, seizures, tremor, or paraparesis.[25] Although the presence of neurological signs in a cat with documented hypertension strongly supports a diagnosis of hypertensive encephalopathy, there are few reports correlating clinical signs to imaging[35] or postmortem[33] findings.

Renal side effects of hypertension can be challenging to distinguish from the renal dysfunction that typically underlies the development of hypertension (see Figure 38-2). However, it is clear that hypertension can overwhelm the kidney's autoregulatory mechanism, resulting in the transmission of high ABP to the renal glomerulus, which leads to glomerular capillary stretch, endothelial damage, proteinuria, and progressive glomerulosclerosis that accelerate the underlying nephropathy.[36] In one experimental study, the severity of proteinuria was directly proportional to elevations in ABP.[37]

Cardiac side effects of hypertension reflect the increased afterload that the left ventricle must pump against (see Figure 38-3). As a result of the increased left ventricular wall stress from the elevated systemic vascular resistance, concentric left ventricular hypertrophy develops and auscultatory abnormalities of a gallop sound, heart murmur, or arrhythmia may manifest (see Figures 38-3A and 38-3B). In rare cases, hypertensive cats may present with an aortic dissection, in which

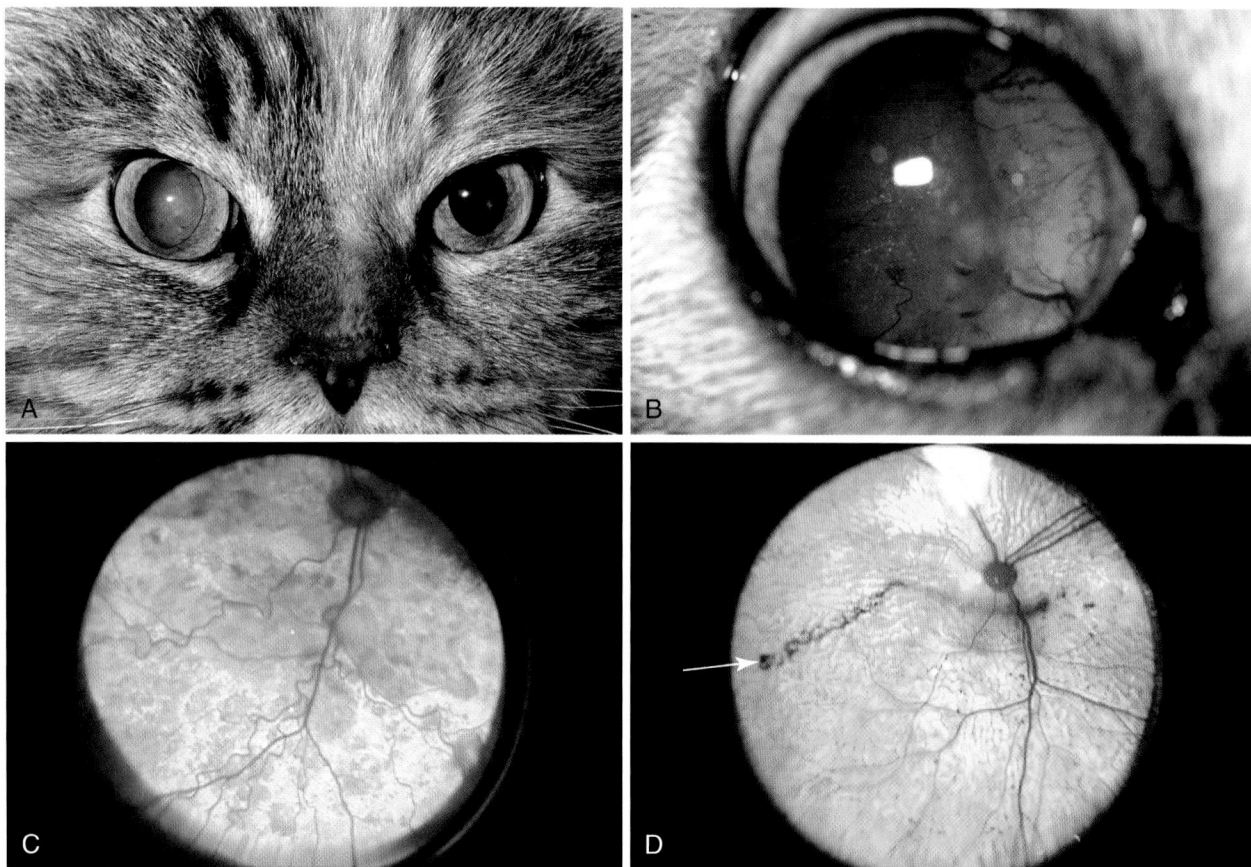

Figure 38-1: Target Organ Injury to the Eye in Feline Hypertension. A, An extraocular photograph of a cat with right leukocoria secondary to severe bullous retinal detachment. **B,** A close-up of the same cat's right eye in which tortuous retinal vessels are apparent without the aid of ophthalmoscopy as the detached retina is displaced to the posterior aspect of the lens. **C,** An image captured during indirect ophthalmoscopy of a feline fundus from a hypertensive cat showing arteriolar tortuosity, diffuse intraretinal edema, and several focal areas of subretinal edema and bullous detachment. **D,** An image captured during indirect ophthalmoscopy of a feline fundus from a hypertensive cat following antihypertensive therapy showing a wrinkled appearance of the fundus as the previously-detached retina reattaches. The linear area of pigmentation (*arrow*) reflects either an area of prior hemorrhage or pigmentation of the retinal pigment epithelium. (Images courtesy of DA Wilkie, DVM, MS, Dipl. ACVO, The Ohio State University College of Veterinary Medicine; used with permission.)

an intimal tear extends within the wall of the aorta and dissects the tunica media, resulting in a true lumen of blood flow surrounded by a false lumen of the dissection (see Figures 38-3C and 38-3D). While cardiac abnormalities on physical examination have been reported in 62% of hypertensive cats,[32] both functional and pathological murmurs are common in geriatric cats and are neither sensitive nor specific to a diagnosis of systemic hypertension. Hypertensive cats have been documented to have left ventricular hypertrophy and reduced left ventricular internal dimensions when compared with normotensive cats,[32,38] with variable resolution of this hypertrophy following therapy.[38] Experimentally, myocardial fibrosis and local activation of angiotensin II have also been documented in the left ventricle of cats with pressure overload.[39] Although evidence of cardiac target organ injury can be documented in hypertensive cats, life-threatening complications related to hypertensive heart disease appear uncommon. Cases of congestive heart failure, malignant arrhythmias,

or aortic dissection have been reported in the literature in association with feline hypertension, but are infrequent in the author's experience.[40]

The earlier descriptions of target organ injury are seen in clinical cases of feline hypertension; however, predicting the development of such lesions in an individual animal is challenging. This is likely related to interindividual variation in target organ susceptibility, lability and temporal variability of ABP measurement, and other as yet unrecognized factors. The American College of Veterinary Internal Medicine convened an expert panel to form a consensus statement on hypertension in dogs and cats in 2007, and this panel formalized an approach to prediction of target organ injury based upon documented ABP.[41] In this approach, the categorization of risk for target organ injury is related to measured ABP (Table 38-1). Although these values are largely based on clinical experience and have not been derived from large-scale epidemiological studies, they provide useful guidelines

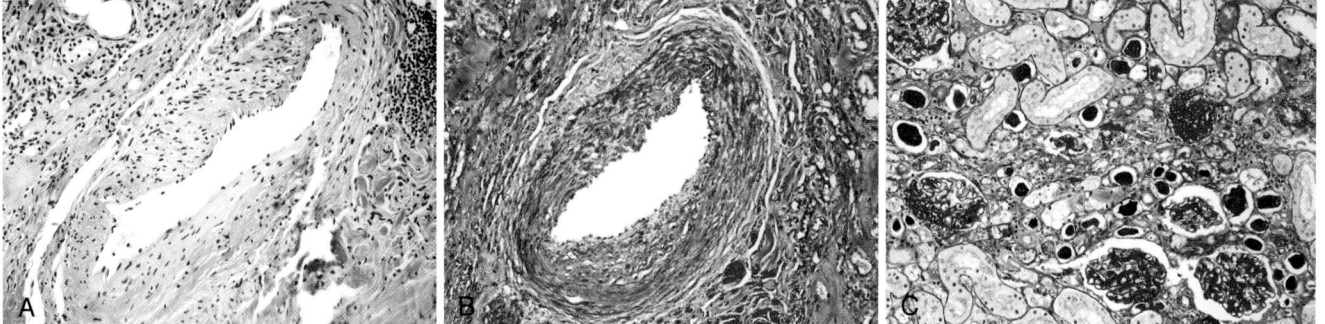

Figure 38-2: Target Organ Injury to the Kidney in Feline Hypertension. A and **B,** Photomicrographs of a renal arcuate artery from a 14-year-old spayed female domestic shorthaired cat with hypertension (systolic ABP of 220 mm Hg at time of diagnosis) that had been treated with amlodipine for 1.5 years before euthanasia. During this time the systolic blood pressure varied between 155 and 185 mm Hg. The duplication of the internal elastic lamina is difficult to appreciate in routine hematoxylin and eosin stained sections **(A),** but the trichrome stain **(B)** reveals fragmentation and duplication of the internal elastic lamina deep to a proliferation of endothelial cells and fibroblasts—changes consistent with hypertension-induced arteriosclerosis. **C,** A photomicrograph of the renal cortex from a 6-year-old castrated male domestic shorthaired cat that was diagnosed with hypertension (systolic ABP of 185 mm Hg) but not treated during the 8 months before euthanasia. The periodic acid Schiff stained section highlights the segmental and global sclerosis of multiple glomeruli, as well as numerous cross sections of atrophied tubules that contain protein casts. These changes are presumed secondary to transmission of high arterial pressure to the renal arterioles and glomerular capillaries. In addition, there is mild diffuse interstitial fibrosis. (Images courtesy of SM McLeland, DVM, Colorado State University College of Veterinary Medicine & Biomedical Sciences; used with permission.)

to the feline practitioner when assessing the risk of injury in cats with hypertension.

DIAGNOSIS OF FELINE HYPERTENSION

The evaluation of the cat with suspected hypertension should begin with a thorough history and a general physical examination. Importantly, most cats with hypertension are geriatric at the time of diagnosis, having a median age of 13 to 15 years,[21,25,32] though the diagnosis has been reported in cats as young as 7 years.[25,35] Given these results, the diagnosis of hypertension in a young or middle-aged cat should be considered cautiously and the result verified before therapy. The history should evaluate for evidence of target organ injury such as sudden-onset blindness, seizure activity or neurological deficits, syncope, etc. Additional aspects of the history can be pertinent and direct diagnostic investigation by providing clues to the presence of other systemic disease that may result in hypertension. These historical findings may include polyuria or polydypsia in the cat with diabetes mellitus or renal dysfunction, symptoms of a hypermetabolic state (e.g., muscle wasting, polyphagia, nocturnal vocalization) in the hyperthyroid cat, or signs of muscle weakness in the cat with hyperaldosteronism.

Physical examination of the cat with suspected hypertension should focus on documentation of vital parameters, careful auscultation of all heart and lung fields, evaluation of the jugular veins for distension and/or pulsation, palpation of the femoral pulse, inspection of the mucous membranes and capillary refill time, palpation of the ventral neck for a

palpable goiter, careful abdominal palpation for changes in kidney shape and size, and an ophthalmic examination including the fundus. The jugular veins are useful as a sign of volume overload, which causes visible jugular venous distension. The fundic examination is useful as the retina is often the earliest, and most easily visualized, target organ of hypertension. In a study in New Zealand, 16% of cats more than 8 years of age had hypertensive ocular lesions; from this, the authors conclude that hypertensive ocular disease occurs frequently enough to recommend routine fundic evaluation in all geriatric cats.[42] Auscultation may reveal a heart murmur, gallop sound, or abnormality in cardiac rhythm. Older cats (>10 years of age) may occasionally have a gallop sound related to an aging and stiff ventricle without overt cardiovascular disease or documented hypertension. However, a gallop sound in any cat should prompt further diagnostic testing for underlying heart disease or hypertension.

Measurement of ABP in the cat may be done by direct arterial monitoring, typically by placement of a 22- or 24-gauge catheter into the dorsal pedal artery. However, the small size of feline arteries makes placement of an arterial line challenging even in the anesthetized cat and is impractical in the awake cat. As such, noninvasive techniques are employed for measurement of ABP in the clinic setting. The author prefers Doppler interrogation using a Parks Model 811-B ultrasonic flow detector with the cat lightly restrained in lateral recumbency (Figure 38-4). Some authors advocate measurement of ABP in cats in a sitting position or sternal recumbency; when doing so, it is important to maintain the limb in which the ABP is measured at the level of the right atrium to avoid erroneous changes in ABP related to

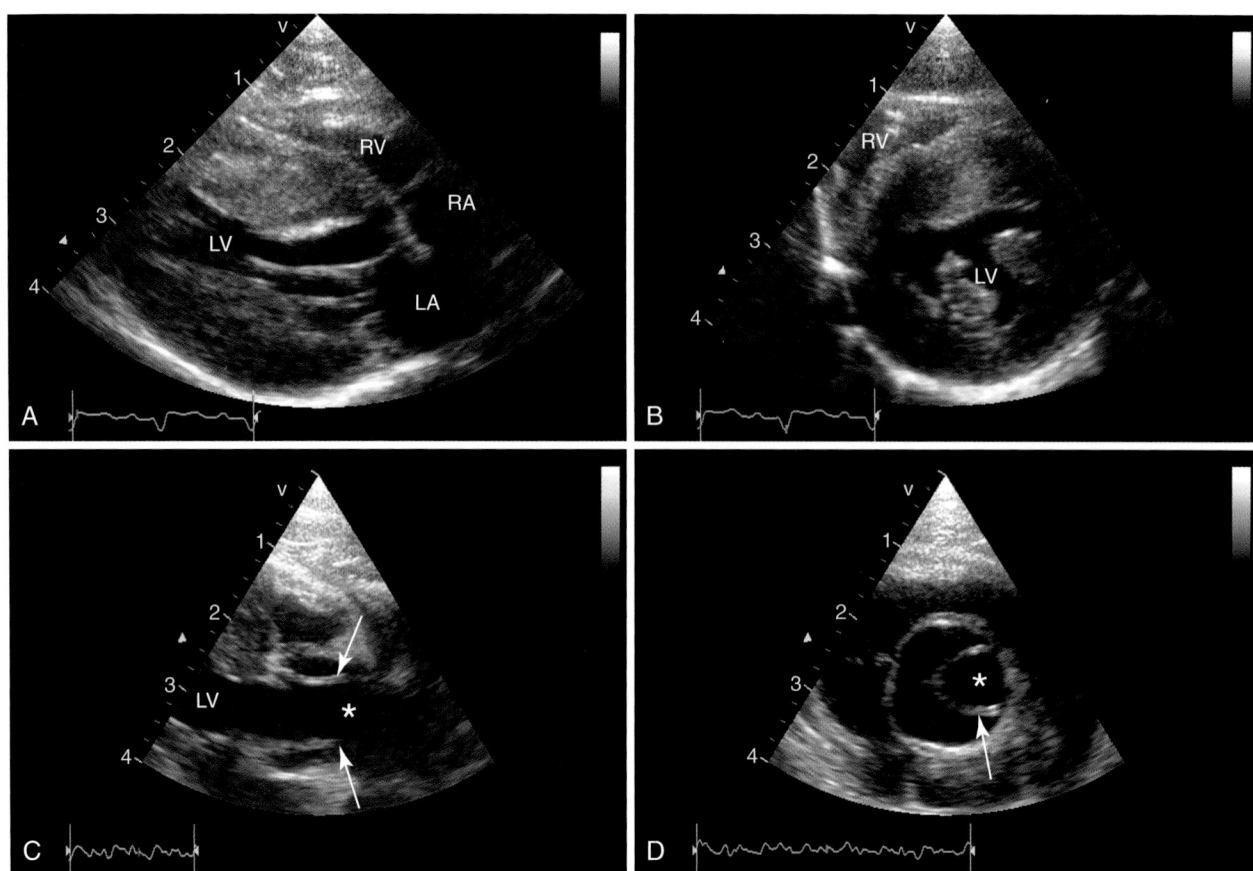

Figure 38-3: Target Organ Injury to the Heart in Feline Hypertension. A and **B,** A 17-year-old cat presented for dullness with a systolic ABP of 210 mm Hg and a prominent gallop sound; renal disease was detected on blood testing and presumed to be the underlying cause for the hypertension. In both the long-axis **(A)** and short-axis **(B)** images, moderate to severe left ventricular hypertrophy is observed secondary to the increased systemic vascular resistance. **C** and **D,** A 15-year-old cat presented for acute collapse and vocalization. A systolic ABP of 215 mm Hg was measured on examination and echocardiography revealed an aortic dissection. In the long-axis **(C)** view of the aorta, separation of the aortic wall is seen as two distinct lines (*arrows*). The short-axis image **(D)** of the ascending aorta shows the true aortic lumen (*) separated from the false aortic lumen by the dissection (*arrow*), which begins as an intimal tear and extends within the tunica media. *LA,* left atrium; *LV,* left ventricle; *RA,* right atrium; *RV,* right ventricle.

Table 38-1	**Risk Stratification for Target Organ Injury Based on BP (mm Hg) in Cats**		
Risk Category	**Systolic BP**	**Diastolic BP**	**Risk of Injury**
I	<150	<95	Minimal
II	150-159	95-99	Mild
III	160-179	100-119	Moderate
IV	>179	>119	Severe

Adapted from Brown S, Atkins C, Bagley R, et al: Guidelines for the identification, evaluation, and management of systemic hypertension in dogs and cats. *J Vet Intern Med* 21(3):542-588, 2007.

hydrostatic pressure.[43] Most cats can be comfortably restrained in lateral recumbency, and this position is preferred by the author. Doppler techniques have been shown to be more accurate than standard oscillometric measurements when compared with direct ABP measurement; for this reason, the author prefers Doppler measurement of ABP in conscious cats.[7,8] Recent data using high definition oscillometry reported good correlation to invasive measurements with reasonable limits of agreement, suggesting this device may also be useful in awake cats.[44] With respect to the limb chosen, the author prefers the forelimb for the Doppler measurement of ABP in cats both for ease of measurement and because prior studies in the cat found a stronger correlation between Doppler and directly measured ABP from the forelimb as compared with the hind limb.[8] If oscillometric methods are chosen, a recent study found better tolerance of oscillometric ABP measurement from the tail as compared with the forelimb of conscious cats.[45] The optimal site for measurement of ABP in cats likely varies by the experience of the operator, the tolerance of the patient, and the characteristics of the measurement device. Whichever method and site are chosen, it is important to note both in the medical record and to use the same methodology for future measurements in the same cat when monitoring an animal over time. In general, each practice should select a method of ABP measurement, a

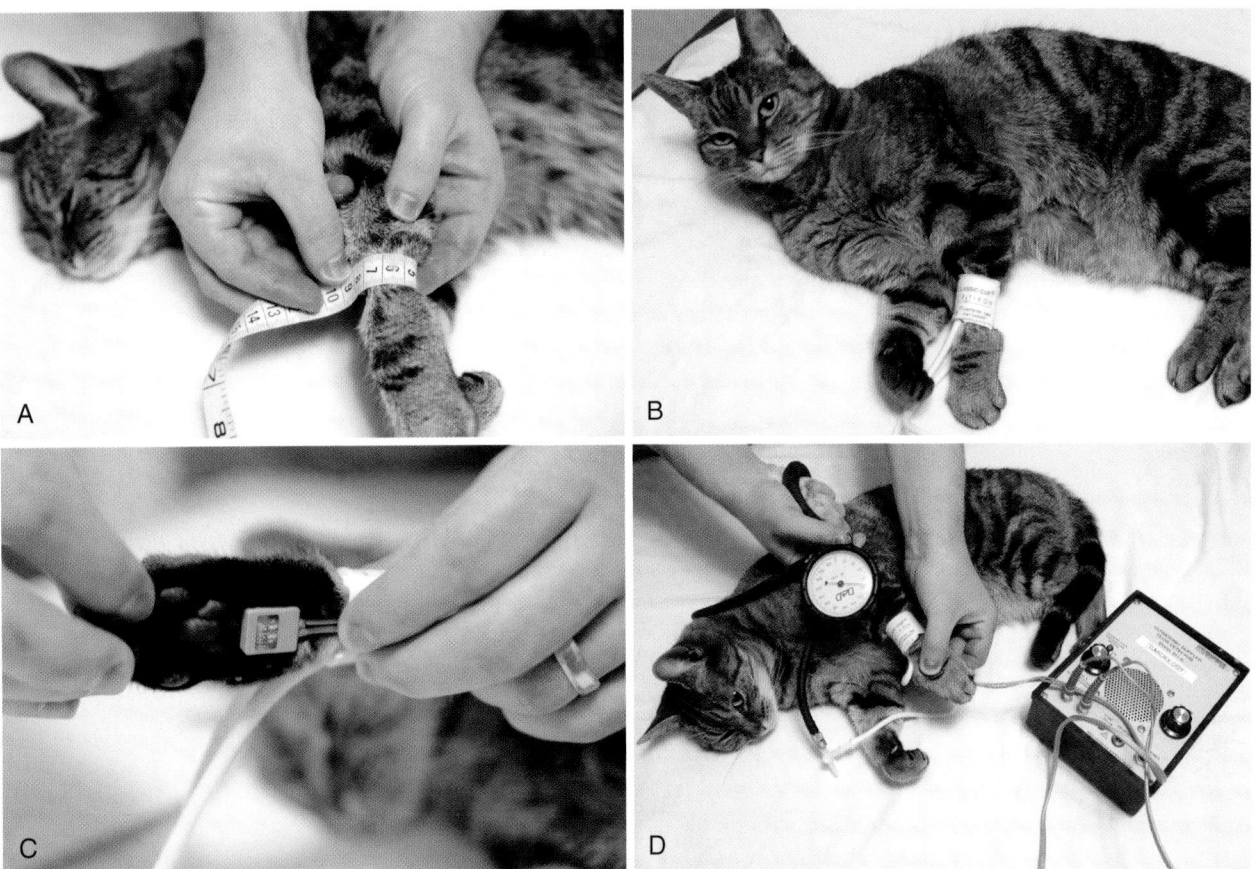

Figure 38-4: Measurement of ABP in the cat by the Doppler ultrasound technique. The cat should be positioned in a comfortable position that allows the limb to be held at the level of the right atrium; lateral recumbency is preferred. The circumference of the limb is measured at the mid-antebrachium **(A)**. A cuff width equal to 30% to 40% of the limb circumference is chosen and tightly wrapped around the limb **(B).** The sphygmomanometer is connected to the cuff and the Doppler crystal is placed over the median palmar artery, just proximal to the metacarpal pad **(C)**. Improved contact with the skin is achieved by shaving the fur, wetting the fur with alcohol, and by applying ultrasound gel. The cuff is inflated to a pressure at which the Doppler signal can no longer be heard and then slowly released, with the systolic arterial pressure reflected by the pressure at which the sound first returns **(D)**. The first measurement is discarded and a minimum of three consecutive measurements are recorded once minimal variance in the measurement is observed.

preferred location, and a preferred position, and then try to adhere to that method as much as possible for consistency in measurement and interpretation of ABP.

An appropriately-sized Velcro cuff (typically #1 or #2 in cats, determined by the cuff width equal to approximately 30% to 40% of the limb circumference) is then placed around the antebrachium of the nonrecumbent forelimb.[46] The pulse is found by an audible Doppler signal on the ventral aspect of the distal forelimb, typically just proximal to the metacarpal pad. Improvement in picking up the audible pulse signal is achieved by clipping the fur, wetting the measurement site with alcohol, and using gel to maximize coupling between the skin and the Doppler crystal. Additionally, headphones attached to the Doppler unit are useful to block out extraneous noise to the operator and to minimize the effect of movement artifact and loud Doppler signals on the cat. The cuff is lightly inflated with a sphygmomanometer until the pulse is lost, and then pressure in the cuff is gradually released until the pulse is again audible, which indicates the cat's systolic

ABP. This measurement should be repeated approximately five times until consistent values are achieved (varying by <10%); often, the first measurement is rejected as the cat is not yet used to having the cuff inflated and the ABP may be falsely elevated. If repeat measurements continue to drop as the cat becomes accustomed to the procedure, the measurement is repeated until consistent values are obtained.

Oscillometric devices are, in the author's opinion, most useful in very compliant or sedated patients. Such devices are more sensitive to patient movement and can provide false readings in the cat that cannot lie perfectly still. The benefit of the oscillometric devices, as described earlier, is that they provide diastolic and mean blood pressure readings in addition to the systolic measurement; however, isolated diastolic hypertension has not been described in the cat and the systolic pressure is therefore likely sufficient to screen all cats for hypertension. It is preferable to have one or two dedicated technicians perform all ABP measurements in a given practice, with a recent study showing much greater variability in

ABP measurements performed by less-experienced operators.[47] The variability that is inherent in the technique can likely be reduced by practice and consistency between measurements and a dedicated technician who performs all ABP measurements.

Given the variability in reported values for normal ABP in cats and the likelihood of a white coat effect elevating APB, most experts recommend a cautious approach to the diagnosis of hypertension in cats.[41] This means that the diagnosis of hypertension should be confirmed either by repeated measurement of a consistently elevated value and/or by the presence of target organ injury. Care should be taken to confirm that the measured ABP is reproducible, and efforts should be made to minimize the cat's stress during measurement. This is optimally performed at the start of an appointment, in the room with the client, once the cat is acclimated to the surroundings, and with a technician who is proficient in the technique. Admittedly, this will not eliminate white coat hypertension for all cats, but expending the effort to minimize stress and handling is critical to an accurate measurement of ABP. Last, many hypertensive cats have an underlying condition that has causally been associated with hypertension, and documentation of a concurrent disease known to be associated with hypertension (see Etiology of Hypertension) is also strongly supportive of the diagnosis.

Once hypertension is diagnosed, screening tests for diseases that have been associated with hypertension, as well as tests to evaluate for target organ injury are advised. In general, this should include renal parameters, urinalysis, thyroid hormone panel, and an ophthalmologic (including fundic) examination. If target organ injury is documented and an ABP > 160 mm Hg is measured, then antihypertensive therapy is indicated. Similarly, if a disease known to be associated with hypertension is documented and ABP > 160mm Hg is consistently measured, therapy for hypertension is also warranted. If there is no evidence of underlying disease to explain the hypertension and no evidence of target organ injury, the author recommends a repeat ABP measurement to confirm the diagnosis before starting therapy. The cat is reevaluated in 7 to 10 days and the ABP measurement is performed at the very start of the visit, with the client present to minimize stress as outlined above. If the ABP remains elevated in the absence of target organ injury or clear evidence of an underlying condition, a discussion about antihypertensive therapy is begun. In general, the author advises treatment if the systolic ABP is >180 mm Hg and will often reevaluate the ABP in another 2 to 3 weeks to confirm consistent elevation if it is between 160 and 180 mm Hg.

There is recent interest in the use of cardiac biomarkers in small animal practice. B-type natriuretic peptide (BNP) is a hormone that has natriuretic (salt-wasting) and vasodilating properties. It is released by the myocardium in response to stretch, hypertrophy, and hypoxia. Although the cardiac changes that occur in hypertension may suggest an elevation in N-terminal pro-brain natriuretic petide (NT-proBNP) is possible in the hypertensive cat, at this time the role of NT-proBNP in the evaluation of cats with hypertension is not defined as no studies have comprehensively addressed this clinical question.

TREATMENT STRATEGIES FOR FELINE HYPERTENSION

As noted above, hypertension is often documented in cats with renal disease or hyperthyroidism. Primary therapy for those disease states is required, concurrent with antihypertensive therapy. Antihypertensive treatment is directed at reducing systemic vascular resistance; the currently preferred medication in the cat is amlodipine besylate, which is a calcium channel blocker with vascular selectivity. Several studies have documented the efficacy of oral amlodipine in decreasing ABP in hypertensive cats.[14,38,48,49] The optimal ABP for a cat on amlodipine is poorly defined, but reduction to levels that minimize the risk of target organ injury (e.g., 130 to 160 mm Hg systolic ABP) is recommended. Amlodipine is typically given at 0.625 mg/cat every 12 to 24 hours (roughly 0.1 mg/kg/day). Higher doses are occasionally required for cats with resistant hypertension (rarely exceeding 0.3 mg/kg/day). Transdermal amlodipine administration has been described in the cats with fair efficacy, although it appears to be not as effective as oral administration, and therefore oral administration is recommended.[50]

In other species, angiotensin-converting enzyme (ACE) inhibition is considered a first-line therapy for hypertension. However, ACE inhibitors, by themselves, have only weak antihypertensive properties in cats and should not be used as sole therapy for systemic hypertension.[51,52] As many cats develop systemic hypertension secondary to renal disease, ACE inhibition is frequently prescribed to most cats with hypertension as a secondary agent for its renal-protective properties. Benazepril is considered by many clinicians to be the preferred angiotension-converting enzyme inhibtor (ACE-I) for cats with renal dysfunction. The standard dose for benazepril is 0.5 mg/kg orally (PO) every 12 hours; however, the author often starts at a lower dose (0.1 to 0.2 mg/kg every 12 hours) in cats with renal dysfunction and escalates to the full dose in 10 to 14 days if renal function remains stable as assessed by serum urea nitrogen and creatinine concentrations.

Beta-adrenergic blocking agents have also been studied as sole agents in feline hypertension. In one study of hyperthyroid cats with hypertension, atenolol at 1 to 2 mg/kg PO every 12 hours was unable to reduce ABP to <160 mm Hg in 70% of cats and, as a result, usually cannot be recommended as sole therapy for the hyperthyroid cat with hypertension.[53]

Most cats with hypertension can be controlled with up titration of amlodipine as a sole agent or by the addition of an ACE-I or a beta-blocker. In human and canine hypertension, and rarely in cats, therapy with multiple agents is necessary to achieve a target blood pressure <160 mm Hg. The author has also found prazosin, an alpha-blocking agent, to be effective in reducing ABP in cats typically given at a dose of 0.25 to 0.5 mg/cat PO every 8 to 12 hours. Experimental data also support the efficacy of prazosin as an ABP-lowering agent in cats.[54] Owners of cats that are consuming high-sodium diets should be counseled about the possible beneficial effect of switching to a diet moderated in sodium, although firm recommendations relative to ideal dietary sodium content for hypertension are lacking.

It cannot be overly emphasized that the initiation of therapy should be reserved for cats with evidence of target organ injury or those cats for which the risk of injury is likely (see Table 38-1). In general, this means that treatment should be initiated for hypertensive cats with hypertensive retinopathy or choroidopathy, left ventricular hypertrophy, and/or signs of neurological dysfunction. Treatment for the cat with no evidence of organ dysfunction secondary to hypertension is more problematic. Once initiated, antihypertensive therapy will almost certainly require lifelong medication, so the diagnosis should be confirmed before initiating treatment as discussed earlier. For the cat with an acute hypertensive crisis (e.g., blood pressure >200 mm Hg with evidence of target organ injury), additional strategies are required as discussed in Chapter 87.

PROGNOSIS FOR FELINE HYPERTENSION

Few studies have documented an improved prognosis for cats treated with antihypertensive medications. However, this lack of evidence may reflect a lack of adequately powered studies to prove such benefit. Additionally, there may be improvements in quality of life during antihypertensive therapy that are less easily quantified, but important for the cat and client. With respect to target organ injury, it is uncommon for cats with hypertensive retinopathy or choroidopathy to regain vision if blindness is documented at the presenting visit; however, return of some vision occurs in some cats. Partial to complete retinal reattachment and gradual resolution of retinal hemorrhage and edema have been observed.[22] In cats with neurological signs, antihypertensive medications and

supportive therapy often result in gradual improvement. In a case study of two cats with findings of hypertensive encephalopathy on magnetic resonance imaging, neurological improvement was observed within 24 to 48 hours of initiation of antihypertensive medication.[35] In cats with hypertensive heart disease, no correlation was apparent between the severity of left ventricular hypertrophy and survival,[32] although a reduction in the degree of left ventricular hypertrophy has been reported with amlodipine therapy.[38] In a prospective study of feline hypertension, therapy with amlodipine and reduction in ABP did not show a significant effect on survival.[21] However, in the same study, therapy with amlodipine did significantly reduce the degree of proteinuria in these cats, and proteinuria itself was found to be a significant predictor of survival in hypertensive cats.[21]

SUMMARY

The consequences of systemic hypertension in the cat can be devastating (e.g., retinal detachment, hyphema, neurological sequelae, cardiac hypertrophy, aortic dissection, progressive renal dysfunction). The most common cause of systemic hypertension in cats is renal disease; hyperthyroidism is also variably associated with this condition. Rare causes include aldosterone-secreting tumors and essential (e.g., idiopathic) hypertension. All cats with elevated serum thyroid hormone concentrations or renal disease, regardless of severity, should have their ABP evaluated. Additionally, any cat over the age of 7 years with a heart murmur or gallop rhythm should have its ABP measured to rule out hypertensive heart disease. Fundic examinations should be considered in all cats more than 8 years of age to screen for hypertensive ocular lesions. Treatment is initiated in the setting of target organ injury or consistently elevated ABP measurements taken over several time points and in a minimally stressful environment. Prognosis for ABP control over time is good, though survival benefits from antihypertensive therapy in cats have not been proven.

References

1. Belew AM, Barlett T, Brown SA: Evaluation of the white-coat effect in cats. *J Vet Intern Med* 13(2):134–142, 1999.
2. Mishina M, Watanabe T, Fujii K, et al: Noninvasive blood pressure measurements in cats: clinical significance of hypertension associated with chronic renal failure. *J Vet Med Sci* 60(7):805–808, 1998.
3. Bodey AR, Sansom J: Epidemiological study of blood pressure in domestic cats. *J Small Anim Pract* 39(12):567–573, 1998.
4. Sparkes AH, Caney SM, King MC, et al: Inter- and intraindividual variation in Doppler ultrasonic indirect blood pressure measure-

ments in healthy cats. *J Vet Intern Med* 13(4):314–318, 1999.
5. Kobayashi DL, Peterson ME, Graves TK, et al: Hypertension in cats with chronic renal failure or hyperthyroidism. *J Vet Intern Med* 4(2):58–62, 1990.
6. Lin CH, Yan CJ, Lien YH, et al: Systolic blood pressure of clinically normal and conscious cats determined by an indirect Doppler method in a clinical setting. *J Vet Med Sci* 68(8):827–832, 2006.
7. Binns SH, Sisson DD, Buoscio DA, et al: Doppler ultrasonographic, oscillometric sphygmomanometric, and photoplethysmographic

techniques for noninvasive blood pressure measurement in anesthetized cats. *J Vet Intern Med* 9(6):405–414, 1995.
8. Haberman CE, Morgan JD, Kang CW, et al: Evaluation of Doppler ultrasonic and oscillometric methods of indirect blood pressure measurement in cats. *Intern J Appl Res Vet Med* 2(4):279–289, 2004.
9. Quimby JM, Smith ML, Lunn KF: Evaluation of the effects of hospital visit stress on physiologic parameters in the cat. *J Feline Med Surg* 13(10):733–737, 2011.
10. Bodey AR, Michell AR: Epidemiological study of blood pressure in domestic

dogs. *J Small Anim Pract* 37(3):116–125, 1996.

11. Franklin SS, Gustin Wt, Wong ND, et al: Hemodynamic patterns of age-related changes in blood pressure. The Framingham Heart Study. *Circulation* 96(1):308–315, 1997.

12. Sansom J, Rogers K, Wood JL: Blood pressure assessment in healthy cats and cats with hypertensive retinopathy. *Am J Vet Res* 65(2):245–252, 2004.

13. Paepe D, Verjans G, Duchateau L, et al: Routine health screening: findings in apparently healthy middle-aged and old cats. *J Feline Med Surg* 15(1):8–19, 2013.

14. Elliott J, Barber PJ, Syme HM, et al: Feline hypertension: clinical findings and response to antihypertensive treatment in 30 cases. *J Small Anim Pract* 42(3):122–129, 2001.

15. Syme HM, Barber PJ, Markwell PJ, et al: Prevalence of systolic hypertension in cats with chronic renal failure at initial evaluation. *J Am Vet Med Assoc* 220(12):1799–1804, 2002.

16. Ash RA, Harvey AM, Tasker S: Primary hyperaldosteronism in the cat: a series of 13 cases. *J Feline Med Surg* 7(3):173–182, 2005.

17. Brown AL, Beatty JA, Lindsay SA, et al: Severe systemic hypertension in a cat with pituitary-dependent hyperadrenocorticism. *J Small Anim Pract* 53(2):132–135, 2012.

18. Wimpole JA, Adagra CF, Billson MF, et al: Plasma free metanephrines in healthy cats, cats with non-adrenal disease and a cat with suspected phaeochromocytoma. *J Feline Med Surg* 12(6):435–440, 2010.

19. Morgan RV: Systemic hypertension in four cats: ocular and medical findings. *J Am Anim Hosp Assoc* 22:615–621, 1985.

20. Turner JL, Brogdon JD, Lees GE, et al: Idiopathic hypertension in a cat with secondary hypertensive retinopathy associated with a high-salt diet. *J Am Anim Hosp Assoc* 26:647–651, 1990.

21. Jepson RE, Elliott J, Brodbelt D, et al: Effect of control of systolic blood pressure on survival in cats with systemic hypertension. *J Vet Intern Med* 21(3):402–409, 2007.

22. Stiles J, Polzin DJ, Bistner SI: The prevalence of retinopathy in cats with systemic hypertension and chronic renal failure or hyperthyroidism. *J Am Anim Hosp Assoc* 30(6):564–572, 1994.

23. Williams TL, Peak KJ, Brodbelt D, et al: Survival and the development of azotemia after treatment of hyperthyroid cats. *J Vet Intern Med* 24(4):863–869, 2010.

24. Williams TL, Elliott J, Syme HM: Renin-angiotensin-aldosterone system activity in hyperthyroid cats with and without concurrent hypertension. *J Vet Intern Med* 27(3):522–529, 2013.

25. Maggio F, DeFrancesco TC, Atkins CE, et al: Ocular lesions associated with systemic hypertension in cats: 69 cases (1985-1998). *J Am Vet Med Assoc* 217(5):695–702, 2000.

26. Sennello KA, Schulman RL, Prosek R, et al: Systolic blood pressure in cats with diabetes mellitus. *J Am Vet Med Assoc* 223(2):198–201, 2003.

27. Little CJL, Gettinby G: Heart failure is common in diabetic cats: findings from a retrospective case-controlled study in first-opinion practice. *J Small Anim Pract* 49(1):17–25, 2007.

28. Aaron KJ, Sanders PW: Role of dietary salt and potassium intake in cardiovascular health and disease: a review of the evidence. *Mayo Clin Proc* 88(9):987–995, 2013.

29. Turner JL, Brogdon JD, Lees GE, et al: Idiopathic hypertension in a cat with secondary hypertensive retinopathy associated with a high-salt diet. *J Am Anim Hosp Assoc* 26(6):647–651, 1990.

30. Luckschander N, Iben C, Hosgood G, et al: Dietary NaCl does not affect blood pressure in healthy cats. *J Vet Intern Med* 18(4):463–467, 2004.

31. Crispin SM, Mould JR: Systemic hypertensive disease and the feline fundus. *Vet Ophthalmol* 4(2):131–140, 2001.

32. Chetboul V, Lefebvre HP, Pinhas C, et al: Spontaneous feline hypertension: clinical and echocardiographic abnormalities, and survival rate. *J Vet Intern Med* 17(1):89–95, 2003.

33. Brown CA, Munday JS, Mathur S, et al: Hypertensive encephalopathy in cats with reduced renal function. *Vet Pathol* 42(5):642–649, 2005.

34. Kent M: The cat with neurological manifestations of systemic disease. Key conditions impacting on the CNS. *J Feline Med Surg* 11(5):395–407, 2009.

35. O'Neill J, Kent M, Glass EN, et al: Clinicopathologic and MRI characteristics of presumptive hypertensive encephalopathy in two cats and two dogs. *J Am Anim Hosp Assoc* 49(6):412–420, 2013.

36. Ljutic D, Kes P: The role of arterial hypertension in the progression of non-diabetic glomerular diseases. *Nephrol Dial Transplant* 18(Suppl 5):v28–v30, 2003.

37. Mathur S, Syme H, Brown CA, et al: Effects of the calcium channel antagonist amlodipine in cats with surgically induced hypertensive renal insufficiency. *Am J Vet Res* 63(6):833–839, 2002.

38. Snyder PS, Sadek D, Jones GL: Effect of amlodipine on echocardiographic variables in cats with systemic hypertension. *J Vet Intern Med* 15(1):52–56, 2001.

39. Uechi M, Tanaka Y, Aramaki Y, et al: Evaluation of the renin-angiotensin system in cardiac tissues of cats with pressure-overload cardiac hypertrophy. *Am J Vet Res* 69(3):343–348, 2008.

40. Wey AC, Atkins CE: Aortic dissection and congestive heart failure associated with systemic hypertension in a cat. *J Vet Intern Med* 14(2):208–213, 2000.

41. Brown S, Atkins C, Bagley R, et al: Guidelines for the identification, evaluation, and management of systemic hypertension in dogs and cats. *J Vet Intern Med* 21(3):542–558, 2007.

42. Carter JM, Irving AC, Bridges JP, et al: The prevalence of ocular lesions associated with hypertension in a population of geriatric cats in Auckland, New Zealand. *N Z Vet J* 62(1):21–29, 2014.

43. Pickering TG, Hall JE, Appel LJ, et al: Recommendations for blood pressure measurement in humans and experimental animals. Part 1: Blood pressure measurement in humans: a statement for professionals from the Subcommittee of Professional and Public Education of the American Heart Association Council on High Blood Pressure Research. *Circulation* 111(5):697–716, 2005.

44. Martel E, Egner B, Brown SA, et al: Comparison of high-definition oscillometry—a non-invasive technology for arterial blood pressure measurement—with a direct invasive method using radio-telemetry in awake healthy cats. *J Feline Med Surg* 15(12):1104–1113, 2013.

45. Cannon MJ, Brett J: Comparison of how well conscious cats tolerate blood pressure measurement from the radial and coccygeal arteries. *J Feline Med Surg* 14(12):906–909, 2012.

46. Henik R, Dolson M, Wenholz L: How to obtain a blood pressure measurement. *Clin Tech Small Anim Pract* 20(3):144–150, 2005.

47. Gouni V, Tissier R, Misbach C, et al: Influence of the observer's level of experience on systolic and diastolic arterial blood pressure measurements using Doppler ultrasonography in healthy, conscious cats. *J Feline Med Surg* April 29, 2014. [Epub ahead of print].

48. Henik RA, Snyder PS, Volk LM: Treatment of systemic hypertension in cats with amlodipine besylate. *J Am Anim Hosp Assoc* 33(3):226–234, 1997.

49. Snyder PS: Amlodipine: a randomized, blinded clinical trial in 9 cats with systemic hypertension. *J Vet Intern Med* 12(3):157–162, 1998.

50. Helms SR: Treatment of feline hypertension with transdermal amlodipine: a pilot study. *J Am Anim Hosp Assoc* 43(3):149–156, 2007.

51. Brown SA, Brown CA, Jacobs G, et al: Effects of the angiotensin converting enzyme inhibitor benazepril in cats with induced renal insufficiency. *Am J Vet Res* 62(3):375–383, 2001.

52. Steele JL, Henik RA, Stepien RL: Effects of angiotensin-converting enzyme inhibition on plasma aldosterone concentration, plasma renin activity, and blood pressure in spontaneously hypertensive cats with chronic renal disease. *Vet Ther* 3(2):157–166, 2002.

53. Henik RA, Stepien RL, Wenholz LJ, et al: Efficacy of atenolol as a single antihypertensive agent in hyperthyroid cats. *J Feline Med Surg* 10(6):577–582, 2008.

54. Kellar KJ, Quest JA, Spera AC, et al: Comparative effects of urapidil, prazosin, and clonidine on ligand binding to central nervous system receptors, arterial pressure, and heart rate in experimental animals. *Am J Med* 77(4a):87–95, 1984.

Nutritional Management of Heart Disease

Lisa M. Freeman

Traditionally, nutritional modifications have been considered only in cats with congestive heart failure (CHF), and few (if any) nutritional recommendations have been made for cats in earlier stages of heart disease. However, if one waits to address nutrition until this later stage of disease, the benefits of optimizing nutrition during the longer, and more common, earlier stages are lost. Nutrition may play a role in the development of heart disease, so careful attention to nutrition even before heart disease develops is important. Modulation of certain nutrients (either reducing or increasing amounts) may be beneficial in asymptomatic disease. In addition, optimizing body composition, preventing deficient or excessive intake of various nutrients, and avoiding nutritionally unbalanced diets may help to slow progression of disease and improve quality of life. Therefore, nutrition should be considered as an integral part of the overall care for *all* stages of heart disease, from cats with a predisposition for heart disease, to cats with asymptomatic heart disease, to cats with CHF.

IMPORTANT ISSUES FOR ALL CATS WITH HEART DISEASE

No matter what the stage of disease, there are some general but critical features of optimal nutritional therapy for cats with heart disease:
- Perform a complete nutritional assessment on every cat at every visit
- Make individualized nutritional recommendations
- Address all components of the diet
- Monitor the cat carefully
- Ensure clear client communication

Perform a Complete Nutritional Assessment on Every Cat at Every Visit

A nutritional assessment helps determine whether the current diet is optimized or what specific modifications might be beneficial for a cat with heart disease. A nutritional assessment includes an assessment of the cat and its current diet. Nutritional assessment consists of a screening evaluation and, if any "red flags" are identified, an extended evaluation.[1] Standardized diet history forms make gathering complete information more efficient and ensure that the required information is collected for every patient. The screening evaluation can be achieved by having the owner complete a short diet history form[2] and by performing a physical examination. This screening evaluation can quickly identify nutritional issues in the cat with heart disease that require further evaluation,[1] such as:
- Diet
  - Unconventional diets (e.g., home-prepared, vegetarian, or raw): Unless formulated by a board-certified veterinary nutritionist, home-prepared diets are nearly always nutritionally unbalanced (including home-prepared cooked, vegetarian, and raw diets). Commercial vegetarian and raw diets also commonly have nutritional imbalances. In addition, raw-meat diets carry numerous nutritional, health, safety, and public health risks.[3]
  - Unfamiliar commercial diets: Quality control varies widely among pet food companies. Even if you recognize the manufacturer and are confident in its quality, further investigation may be required to determine whether the levels of sodium and other nutrients in that diet are optimal for the individual cat (e.g., based on stage of disease, clinical signs, laboratory values, and body composition).
  - Cat foods designed for "intermittent or supplemental use": All over-the-counter pet foods should be nutritionally complete and balanced. If the nutritional adequacy statement on the label reads "for intermittent or supplemental use," it is not complete and balanced, which may be acceptable if it is a veterinary therapeutic diet and is being used for a specific purpose (e.g., in a case of severe kidney disease) but should be avoided in over-the-counter cat foods.
  - Dietary supplements: Cats with heart disease are more likely to be receiving dietary supplements than cats in the general population.[4] Some dietary supplements may be useful for cats with heart disease (see later), but it is always important to ask if owners are administering any supplements so that further investigation can be conducted on dose, quality control, side effects, or potential interactions with medications.
  - Snacks, treats, and table food: If the snacks, treats, and table food comprise more than 10% of total calorie intake, it is likely that the nutritional balance of the overall diet is adversely affected.

- Medication administration: Asking owners about how they administer medications can reveal suboptimal approaches (e.g., high-sodium foods like cheese or lunch meats being used to hide medications).
- Physical examination
  - Alterations in body composition are common and important issues in cats with heart disease or heart failure and can negatively affect the outcome and quality of life.
  - Weight loss: Use a consistent scale at each visit to identify subtle changes in body weight.
  - Body condition score (BCS) less than 4 or more than 5 (on a 9-point scale)[5]: Use a consistent method to determine BCS to assess current status and changes over time (either a 9-point scale or a 5-point scale). The BCS evaluates body fat, with a goal for most cats of 4 to 5 on a 9-point scale. However, in cats with CHF, a BCS of 5 to 6 may be more desirable.
  - Muscle loss: The muscle condition score (MCS)[6] differs from the BCS in that the MCS evaluates muscle mass (Figure 39-1). Cats can be very obese and yet have severe muscle loss, and conversely, cats can be thin but have normal muscle mass. Evaluation of muscle mass includes visual examination and palpation over the temporal bones, scapulae, lumbar vertebrae, and pelvic bones. Assessing MCS is important because cats with CHF lose primarily muscle—compared to a healthy animal that would lose fat. Early identification of muscle loss at the "mild muscle wasting" stage is valuable for successful intervention.
- Other
  - Presence of other medical conditions that also require dietary modifications (e.g., feline lower urinary tract disease, gastrointestinal disease, and/or chronic kidney disease [CKD]).

If any of these issues are identified on the screening evaluation, an extended evaluation to gather necessary additional information is recommended so that an optimal individualized nutritional plan can be developed.[1]

Make Individualized Nutritional Recommendations

Always make a specific recommendation for diet. This may be only to say that the diet the cat is currently eating is a good choice and that the owner is feeding an appropriate amount to keep the cat in ideal body condition. It is important to reinforce good nutritional choices that owners are making, because there are so many myths about cat nutrition.[7,8]

In addition to the importance of making a recommendation, it also is important to design it specifically for an individual cat. Just as one would not recommend an angiotensin-converting enzyme inhibitor (ACE-I) or furosemide for every cat with heart disease, the same nutritional recommendations are not ideal for all cats. Therefore, it is important to individualize recommendations based not only on the stage of disease (see later) but also on the cat's nutritional assessment, physical examination, laboratory results,

and individual food preferences. For example, some cats with heart disease will be obese and some will have lost body weight and muscle mass, which will affect the nutritional profile of the optimal diet(s). Cats with heart disease can be hyperkalemic, normokalemic, or hypokalemic, which also influences the choice of diet. Therefore, the same diet will not meet the requirements of all cats with heart disease. Concurrent diseases also alter diet choice and were shown in one study to be present in 56% of cats with heart disease.[4] The optimal diet is very different for a cat with concurrent heart disease and CKD compared to a cat with heart disease and struvite urolithiasis or inflammatory bowel disease. In complicated cases, consider referring the cat to a board-certified veterinary nutritionist, which can be found by consulting the American College of Veterinary Nutrition[9] (http://www.acvn.org) or the European College of Veterinary and Comparative Nutrition (http://www.esvcn.eu/college).

Address All Components of the Diet

Be sure to address all components of the diet, not only the cat food, but also the treats, table food, and foods used for medication administration. In some cases, cats may be eating an ideal cat food but are getting large amounts of sodium from treats or table food. One study showed that over 30% of cats with heart disease received treats.[4] Therefore, a diet must be selected that has the desired nutritional properties and palatability, but it also is important to devise an overall dietary plan that includes appropriate treats, if desired by the owner.[10] Many cat owners (34%) use food to administer medications, and the most commonly used foods are high in sodium (e.g., cheese, hot dogs, or lunch meats).[4] Including all sources of dietary sodium intake in the overall diet plan is important to achieve success with nutritional modifications.

Fewer cats (13%) than dogs (31%) with cardiac disease receive dietary supplements,[4] but addressing this issue with the owner is important because surfing the Internet for alternative treatments for cardiac disease is common. It is important to be aware that dietary supplements do not require proof of safety, efficacy, or quality control before being marketed. Therefore, careful selection of type, dose, and brand is important to avoid toxicities or complete lack of efficacy.

Because the use of dietary supplements is common in this patient population and the risks of side effects or interactions is even more common, it is important to *specifically ask* owners if they are giving them to their cats. Owners often do not consider dietary supplements to be either a part of the diet or a medication, and so they may not offer the information unless specifically asked. Because there is little governmental regulation over dietary supplements, cat owners should consider selecting dietary supplements for their cats (and themselves) that have the United States Pharmacopeial Convention Dietary Supplement Verification Program logo if the supplement can provide an appropriate form and dose for a cat. This program tests supplements for ingredients, concentrations, dissolvability, and contaminants. Another resource is Consumerlab.com (http://www.consumerlab.com;

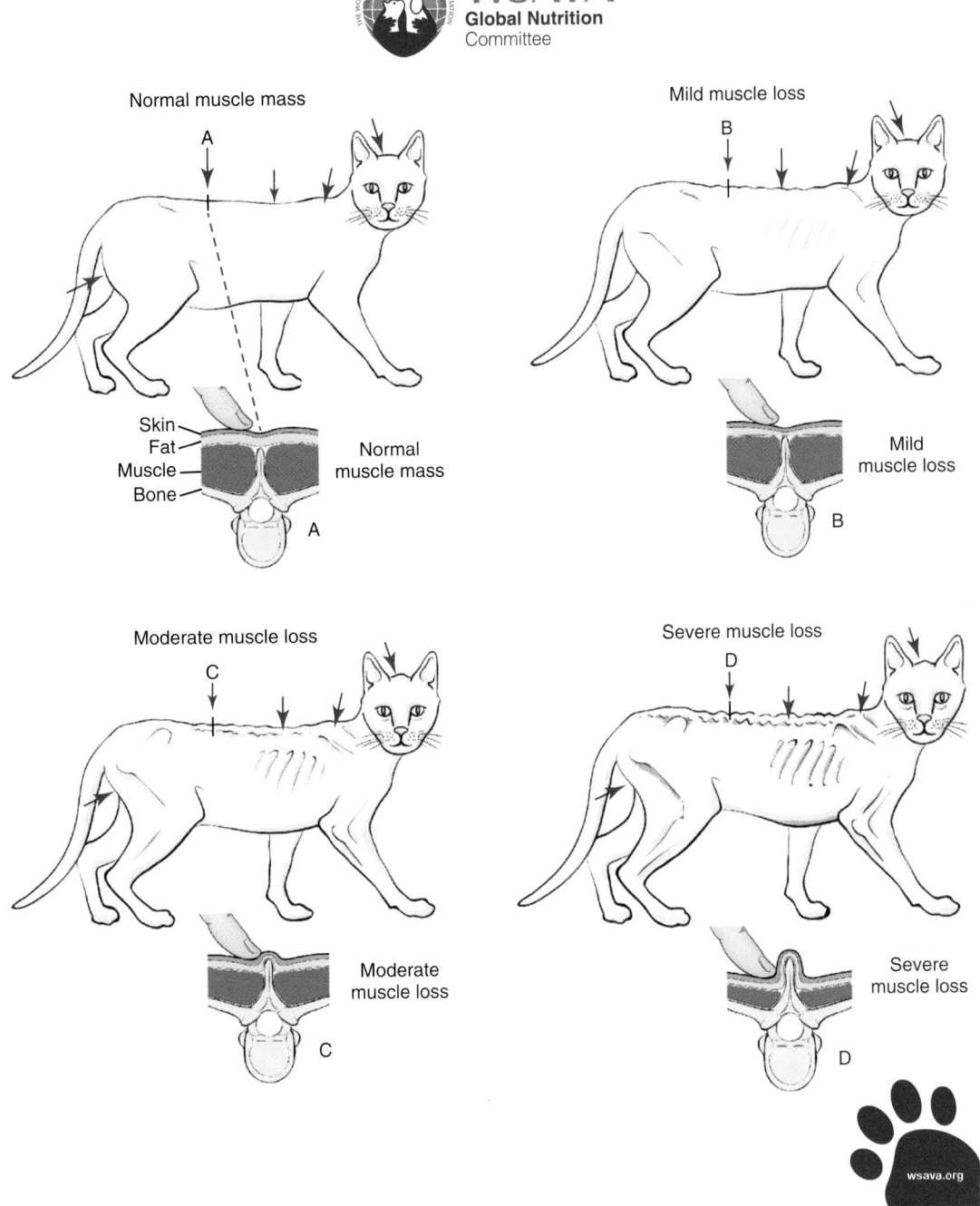

Figure 39-1: Muscle condition score (MCS) is assessed by visualization and palpation of the spine, scapulae, skull, and wings of the ilia. MCS is graded as normal **(A)**, mild loss **(B)**, moderate loss **(C)**, or severe loss **(D)**. Note that cats can have significant muscle loss even when overweight or obese. (Global Nutrition Committee Toolkit provided courtesy of the World Small Animal Veterinary Association.)

accessed May 11, 2015), which performs independent testing of health and nutrition products.

Monitor the Cat Carefully

Reductions in food intake may indicate the need for dietary modifications but also may be an early sign of decompensation of the cardiac disease or the need for medication adjustment. Body weight, BCS, and MCS should be monitored carefully at every visit and addressed if not optimal. Also, it is important to reassess the diet to ensure that it remains optimal for the cat's stage of disease, laboratory values, and clinical signs. Owners often change the diet (e.g., the cat food, treats, and/or table food), add supplements, or use different methods for administering medications. Therefore, just because the diet was appropriate at a previous visit does not mean that it is still optimal.

Ensure Clear Client Communication

Good client communication is important for achieving desired outcomes, particularly in cats with cardiac disease. Discussion of diet, treats, table food, dietary supplements, and effective medication administration is beneficial for both the owner's and the cat's quality of life. Try to engage the client in decision making and defining expectations so that recommendations can address the cat's preferences, as well as the client's time, lifestyle, and financial limitations.

Owners appear much more likely to change dietary factors (e.g., diet, treats, and/or supplements) than they would a medication. Therefore, it is relatively common to have various aspects of the diet change from one visit to the next. This is why it is important to perform a screening nutritional evaluation and to make specific recommendations at every visit (even if just to say that what the owner is doing is ideal). Demonstrating and teaching the client to effectively administer medications and to evaluate the body weight, BCS, and MCS is beneficial for engaging the client in their cat's care.

Communication Tips

A few tips for communicating with the cat's owner are:
- For cats with CHF, warn the owner about the potential for variable or cyclical appetite and have multiple appropriate dietary options available for the owner to provide.
- Specifically discuss (and demonstrate, if necessary) appropriate methods for medication administration.
- Provide owners with skills for searching the Internet about nutrition topics[7] and useful websites[10] to help them avoid the many common myths about pet food.

NUTRITIONAL GOALS BASED ON THE STAGE OF DISEASE

Depending on the stage of disease, there are some specific goals that should be considered. However, the goals for all cats with cardiac disease are:

- Maintain optimal body condition
- Avoid nutritional deficiencies
- Avoid nutritional excesses
- Avoid drug-nutrient interactions
- Consider administration of certain nutrients in levels above those required for nutritional needs (i.e., nutritional pharmacology)

Feeding the Cat at Risk for Heart Disease

Because heart disease is so common in cats, finding ways to reduce the risk is important. Although it is not possible to identify cats at risk (other than predisposed breeds, such as the Maine Coon or Ragdoll), the changes that may help reduce the phenotype of cardiac disease are easily achieved and are good general recommendations for feeding cats in general.

One of the challenges in heart disease is the wide phenotypic variation among cats with cardiomyopathies—some cats have asymptomatic hypertrophic cardiomyopathy (HCM), which never progresses, whereas others have rapid progression of disease with early death. This phenotypic variation also occurs in people with HCM. Genetic mutations have been identified in half of people with HCM, but the phenotypic expression of the disease is highly variable—even in people within the same family with the same genetic mutation. The cause for this phenotypic disparity is unknown, but environmental modifiers, especially gene-nutrient interactions, may play a major role. Nutrient deficiencies and excesses during the *in utero* and early postnatal period influence the cardiovascular system through alterations in the growth hormone/insulin-like growth factor-1 (IGF-1) system and glucose metabolism. These gene-nutrient interactions suggest that the phenotype of genetically based heart disease may be modifiable depending upon early nutrition or other environmental factors.

Our group has shown that cats with HCM are significantly larger (i.e., body weight, head length and width, and humeral and vertebral length) than healthy controls.[11,12] In addition, cats with HCM had higher IGF-1 concentrations compared to healthy controls.[12] Obesity also was significantly associated with HCM in a case-control study of Maine Coon cats[12] but not in a study of cats of other breeds.[11] Also, in the study of Maine Coon cats,[12] body weight at 6 and 12 months was significantly higher in cats with HCM compared to controls, suggesting that the larger size was already developing at an early age. These data suggest a relationship between early nutrition, body size, and HCM.

A great deal of additional information is needed in this area. For example, it is unclear whether the *in utero* growth period or postnatal nutrition and growth have the greatest influence. Until this information is further clarified, general recommendations can be made for young cats. Although these recommendations may not prevent heart disease, they are good recommendations for all cats and may also help to reduce the risk for other medical conditions (e.g., obesity, diabetes mellitus, and osteoarthritis).

Recommendations for the *In Utero* and Growth Periods in Cats

Queens

- Feed queens a cat food made by a well-known, reputable manufacturer throughout gestation and lactation.[8] Food during this period should be nutritionally complete and balanced for growth or all life stages (if formulated to meet Association of American Feed Control Officials [AAFCO] Cat Food Nutrient Profiles) or for gestation and lactation (if tested by feeding trials, which is ideal).
- Keep the queen trim throughout gestation (5 on a 9-point BCS scale).[5]

Kittens

- Feed a food made by a well-known, reputable manufacturer throughout growth (until 1 year of age).[8] Food during this period should be nutritionally complete and balanced for growth or all life stages (if formulated to meet AAFCO Cat Food Nutrient Profiles) or for growth (if tested by feeding trials, which is ideal).
- Keep kittens trim from weaning through adulthood (and beyond; 4 to 5 on a 9-point BCS scale).[5]
- Encourage clients to meal feed (feeding a measured amount of food two to three times a day), rather than feeding *ad libitum*. Few cats can eat *ad libitum* and remain trim.
- Reduce the kitten's calorie intake at time of neutering, because energy requirements decrease 15% to 20% at this time.
- Perform a nutritional assessment at each visit (i.e., complete diet history, BCS, MCS, and body weight). Make specific nutritional recommendations, even if this is just to say the owner is feeding the right food in the right amount. If the diet is not optimal (e.g., too many treats, unconventional diet, more than 5 on a 9-point BCS scale), make specific recommendations for a more appropriate food and/or an adjusted amount of food.
- If the kitten is becoming overweight during the growth phase, do not change to an "adult" cat food before the cat is 1 year of age. Instead, switch to a lower calorie density food (kitten foods can range from 281 kcal/cup to more than 600 kcal/cup).
- Consider referring challenging cases to a board-certified veterinary nutritionist.[9]

Cat with Asymptomatic Disease

In the 1960s and 1970s, very low sodium diets were recommended to be fed when a heart murmur was first detected. Later, the prevailing belief was that severe sodium restriction may not be ideal at this stage because of early activation of the renin-angiotensin-aldosterone system, and this led to the idea that no nutritional modifications can or should be made for animals with asymptomatic heart disease. However, more recent research indicates that dietary modification in early heart disease might be beneficial, and the nutritional management of cats with asymptomatic heart disease should not be ignored. For example, a study (Freeman et al., unpublished data) showed that cats with asymptomatic HCM randomized to one of three diets for 6 months had significantly different responses in biochemical and echocardiographic variables. The diets varied in carbohydrate content, calorie density, and ingredients. Whether nutritional modifications can slow progression in cats with asymptomatic heart disease is not yet known, but these findings are promising.

Severe sodium restriction is not recommended in early (asymptomatic) heart disease. In early heart disease, the goal should be to avoid excessive sodium intake and to educate the owner about treats and table foods high in sodium. The author counsels owners of cats with asymptomatic heart disease to avoid diets high in sodium (>100 mg sodium/100 kcal of diet) and to avoid high-sodium treats and table food. However, this is an opportune time to begin talking to the owner about the animal's overall dietary patterns (i.e., the cat food, treats, table food, and how medications are administered), because it is generally much easier to institute dietary modifications (e.g., a degree of sodium restriction) when the cat is asymptomatic. Also, owners sometimes do a great deal of Internet "research" when their cat is first diagnosed with heart disease and may make significant dietary changes or begin administering dietary supplements at this time. Most owners do not know what foods are high or low in sodium. This information is not available on cat food or treat labels; and even when it is listed on human foods, it is difficult for owners to determine how much sodium is too much for a cat. Therefore, it is important to provide specific and clear information on appropriate cat foods, treats, table foods, and methods to administer medications.

In addition to mild sodium restriction, another main goal is to achieve or maintain optimal body condition. Goals for body condition in animals with CHF may be different (see later), but in asymptomatic heart disease, veterinarians should assess the animal's body weight, BCS, and MCS at every visit as part of a nutritional screening. A BCS of 4 to 5 on a 9-point scale should be the goal. If the cat is above an optimal body condition (i.e., more than 5 on a 9-point scale), a gradual and comprehensive weight loss program should be instituted with careful monitoring.

Adequate protein intake is recommended for cats with heart disease, unless severe concurrent kidney disease is present. The AAFCO minimum for protein for adult cats is 6.5 g protein/100 kcal of diet.[13] Over-the-counter cat foods are often well over this amount, with some of the newer trend of "high protein, low carbohydrate foods" having protein contents well over 13.0 g protein/100 kcal of diet. In the healthy cat, there is no documented benefit to very high-protein, low-carbohydrate diets, and little is known about the effects of long-term feeding of these diets. However, ensuring adequate protein intake should be a goal in cats with heart disease.

Although dilated cardiomyopathy (DCM) is now uncommonly seen in cats, taurine deficiency and DCM can still occur, particularly in cats fed vegetarian diets, nutritionally unbalanced home-made diets, commercial foods that are designed to be for "intermittent or supplemental use," or foods made by small companies that do not have stringent quality-control practices. One study showed that commercial vegetarian cat foods were deficient in taurine, even though the label stated that the food is nutritionally complete and balanced.[14] Collecting a complete diet history can identify cats eating diets that could predispose them to taurine deficiency (as well as a variety of other deficiencies).

At this time, there are no dietary supplements that have been shown to have a benefit for cats with asymptomatic heart disease. However, the supplement that may have the most potential is omega-3 fatty acids. In addition to being a source of calories and essential fatty acids, fat also can have significant effects on immune function, inflammatory mediator production, and hemodynamics.[15] The omega-3 fatty acids, eicosapentaenoic acid (EPA) and docosahexaenoic acid (DHA), are normally are found in very low concentrations in cell membranes compared to the omega-6 fatty acids, but they can be increased by a food or supplement enriched in omega-3 fatty acids. The benefit of having a higher concentration of omega-3 fatty acids in the membranes is that breakdown products of the omega-3 fatty acids (eicosanoids) are less potent inflammatory mediators than eicosanoids derived from n-6 fatty acids. This decreases the production of cytokines and other inflammatory mediators. Fish oil also reduces the production of the inflammatory cytokines, tumor necrosis factor (TNF) and interleukin-1 (IL-1). The antiinflammatory, antiarrhythmic, and antithrombotic effects of omega-3 fatty acids have many potential benefits in cats with cardiac disease. Omega-3 fatty acid supplementation can reduce muscle loss and improve appetite via its antiinflammatory effects, and studies have shown benefits in dogs from omega-3 fatty acid supplementation.[16-18]

Although studies have been conducted in cats with omega-3 fatty acids to assess effects on coagulation,[19,20] little work has been done to determine whether omega-3 fatty acid supplementation would have similar benefits in cats as in humans and dogs. Although dogs with CHF have been shown to have a relative deficiency of omega-3 fatty acids (which can be corrected by supplementation),[16] a recent study showed that cats with heart disease actually have significantly *higher* serum omega-3 fatty acid concentrations, particularly DHA.[21] Future studies will help to build a better understanding of the role of supplementation of omega-3 fatty acids and other nutrients for nutritional modification in cats with early stage heart disease.

Cat with Congestive Heart Failure

Body Composition
When CHF develops, additional nutritional concerns arise for the cat with heart disease. Maintaining optimal body condition is of primary importance in the animal with CHF. Although obesity still can be present at this stage, animals with CHF commonly begin to demonstrate weight loss. This weight loss, or cardiac cachexia, is unlike that seen in a healthy animal where primarily fat is lost. In an animal with CHF, the primary tissue lost is lean body mass. The term *cachexia* does not necessarily equate with an emaciated, end-

stage patient; there is a spectrum of severity with cachexia. In the early stages, it can be very subtle and may even occur in obese cats (i.e., a cat may have excess fat stores but still lose lean body mass). Loss of lean body mass usually is first noted in the epaxial, gluteal, scapular, or temporal muscles. Cardiac cachexia can occur with any underlying cause of CHF (e.g., HCM, DCM, restrictive cardiomyopathy, congenital heart disease) but typically does not occur until CHF has developed. Marked muscle loss in cats is most commonly observed when recurrent pleural effusion has developed. The loss of lean body mass in cardiac cachexia is a multifactorial process caused by anorexia, increased energy requirements, and an increased production of inflammatory cytokines, such as TNF and IL-1. These cytokines cause anorexia, increase energy requirements, and increase the catabolism of lean body mass. In addition, TNF and IL-1 also cause cardiac myocyte hypertrophy and fibrosis and have negative inotropic effects. Cardiac cachexia is a common finding in cats with CHF and has deleterious effects on strength, immune function, and survival; thus, it is important to recognize cachexia at an early stage for better opportunities to manage it effectively.[22]

The nutritional management of cats with cardiac cachexia consists primarily of providing adequate calories and protein and modulating cytokine production. One of the most important issues for managing anorexia (complete loss of appetite) or hyporexia (partial loss of appetite or changes in food preference) is to optimize medical therapy. An early sign of worsening CHF or the need for medication adjustment is a reduction in food intake in a cat that has previously been eating well. Medication side effects such as azotemia secondary to ACE-Is or overzealous diuretic use also can cause anorexia or hyporexia, so the current drug doses and regimen should be reconsidered. Recurrent CHF is another cause for a reduction in food intake, thus thoracic radiographs should be considered. Providing a more palatable diet can help to improve appetite (e.g., switching from a dry food to a canned food, changing to a different brand, or having a balanced cooked home-made diet formulated by a veterinary nutritionist). It also may be useful to use flavor enhancers to increase food intake (e.g., home-cooked meats or fish, not lunch meats or canned tuna fish). Modulation of cytokine production also can be beneficial for managing cardiac cachexia. Supplementation of fish oil, which is high in omega-3 fatty acids, can decrease inflammatory cytokine production and improve cachexia.

As CHF progresses, cardiac cachexia becomes more common; thus it is critical to maintain adequate calorie and protein intake. This can be a challenge because appetite in severe CHF is often cyclical, and owners should be warned that appetite can be highly variable. In addition to optimization of medical therapy, offering multiple choices of appropriate cat foods can be very useful. Palatability enhancers also can be very helpful for cats with severe CHF (e.g., cooked unsalted meat or fish, not lunch meats). Encouraging the owner to try offering foods at different temperatures may increase food intake in some animals (e.g., warmed versus room temperature). Omega-3 fatty acid supplementation also can be beneficial in some animals in which appetite is reduced. Other tips that may increase food intake include providing smaller, more frequent meals, feeding the recommended diet(s) from the owner's plate, or putting the recommended diet(s) into a treat jar. The author generally tries to recommend multiple diets so that the owner can determine which is most palatable to the cat.

In contrast to the healthy cat, obesity may actually be associated with a protective effect once CHF is present—this is known as the *obesity paradox*.[23] Although there are a number of hypothesized reasons for the obesity paradox, the benefit of obesity in CHF is likely due more to a *lack* of cachexia, rather than to the obesity *per se,* given the adverse effects associated with cachexia. However, even in cats with CHF, a BCS over 7 was still associated with shorter survival times.[23] Therefore, the author recommends maintaining a BCS of 5 to 6 on a 9-point scale for cats with CHF.

Protein

Protein restriction is actually detrimental to the cat with CHF because it can contribute to lean body mass loss and malnutrition. Animals with CHF should not be protein restricted unless they have concurrent severe kidney disease. Although protein-restricted renal diets are sometimes recommended for cats with heart disease because these diets often (but not always) are moderately sodium restricted, this is *not* a recommended practice. Unless concurrent advanced kidney disease dictates otherwise, diets fed to cats with cardiac disease should meet feline minimums (6.5 g protein/100 kcal of diet); this is particularly important for cats with CHF and muscle loss.

Although taurine deficiency-induced DCM is uncommon, it should still be suspected whenever the diagnosis of DCM is made. A complete diet history should be obtained because cats that are eating a vegetarian, unbalanced homemade, or other unconventional diet are at higher risk for taurine deficiency. Plasma and whole blood taurine should be analyzed in cats with DCM, and treatment with taurine (125 to 250 mg orally [PO] every 12 hours) should begin concurrent with medical therapy. If the cat is eating an unconventional diet, the owner also should be counseled to switch to a well-known, nutritionally balanced, meat-based commercial cat food.

Fat

The anti-inflammatory, antiarrhythmic, and antithrombotic effects of omega-3 fatty acids may be beneficial in animals with heart disease, although the metabolic differences in cats compared to dogs make it more difficult to know whether supplementation in an individual cat will be beneficial. Despite the lack of evidence in cats, many owners wish to supplement with omega-3 fatty acids, and supplementation may be particularly useful in cats with reduced appetite or muscle loss. The optimal dose of omega-3 fatty acids has not been determined; however, the author currently recommends a daily dosage of fish oil to provide 40 mg/kg EPA and 25 mg/kg DHA for cats with CHF. Most cat foods do not achieve this dose, so supplementation is often necessary. Fish oil supplements vary in their concentration of EPA and DHA, so the author recommends a 1-gram capsule that contains 180 mg EPA and 120 mg DHA. At this concentration, fish oil can be administered at a dose of one capsule per 10 lbs (4.5 kg) of body weight. The capsule can be administered whole (although it is very large) or the oil can be expressed from the capsule and given as a treat or in the food. It should be noted that if the owner cannot administer the capsule intact, the cat will be exposed to the very strong flavor of the fish oil. Although some cats appear to enjoy the taste, others do not. In cats that dislike the flavor, administration of omega-3 fatty acids should be discontinued due to adverse effects on food intake. Fish oil supplements should contain vitamin E as an antioxidant, but other nutrients should not be included to avoid toxicities. Cod liver oil and flax oil should not be used to provide omega-3 fatty acids. Cod liver oil is high in vitamins A and D, which can cause toxicity at this dose, whereas cats are unable to convert the omega-3 fatty acids in flax oil to EPA and DHA.

Sodium

In the 1960s, when few medications were available for treating animals with CHF, dietary sodium restriction was one of the few methods of reducing fluid accumulation. However, with the current availability of newer and more effective medications, the role of severe sodium restriction is no longer clear, although a degree of sodium moderation is appropriate. The author currently recommends moderate sodium restriction (i.e., less than 80 mg sodium/100 kcal of diet) for cats with CHF; although as CHF worsens, additional sodium restriction may be useful if it is difficult to control with medications alone.

Most owners are unaware of the sodium content of cat and human foods and need very specific instructions regarding appropriate cat foods, acceptable low-salt treats, and methods for administering medications. Owners also should be counseled on specific foods to avoid, such as baby food, cheeses, including "squirtable" cheeses, lunch meats and cold cuts (e.g., ham, corned beef, salami, sausages, bacon, and hot dogs), and most cat foods and treats.

There are currently no veterinary therapeutic diets marketed specifically for cats with heart disease. Diets designed for cats with kidney disease sometimes are recommended for cats with heart disease, but the author recommends against this practice because of the protein restriction (to varying degrees) inherent in these diets. Be careful not to recommend senior diets uncategorically for cats with heart disease. If a diet designed for senior cats is to be used, it is very important to look at the characteristics of the individual product. Because there is no legal definition for senior diets, the levels of calories, protein, sodium, and other nutrients can vary dramatically among products from different companies. The sodium content of senior cat foods can range from 64 to 346 mg sodium/100 kcal of diet;[24] the AAFCO minimum for cats is 50 mg sodium/100 kcal of diet.

Potassium and Magnesium

Potassium and magnesium are nutrients of concern in cats with heart disease because depletion of these electrolytes can cause cardiac arrhythmias, decreased myocardial contractility, and muscle weakness and can potentiate the adverse effects of cardiac medications. Cats with CHF can have low, normal, or high serum potassium concentrations, depending upon severity of disease and medications being administered. Medications that can contribute to hyperkalemia include ACE-Is and spironolactone, whereas other medications can lead to hypokalemia (e.g., loop diuretics). In addition, feline diets have a wide range of potassium content, so using one appropriate for the individual patient is important (e.g., avoiding high-potassium diets would be recommended for cats with hyperkalemia). Consequently, serum potassium should be monitored, especially as more medications arc administered to a cat with CHF. Recommended dietary potassium modifications will depend upon medications being administered and serum potassium concentrations. Serum magnesium concentrations also should be measured, but clinicians should be aware that serum magnesium concentrations are a relatively poor indicator of total body magnesium stores. Nonetheless, serial evaluations in an individual patient may be useful, especially in patients with arrhythmias or in those taking high doses of diuretics. Diets high in magnesium or an oral magnesium supplement should be used in cats with hypomagnesemia. These drug-nutrient interactions are important to consider in cats with CHF, particularly as more medications are being administered.

B Vitamins

If high doses of diuretics are being administered, B vitamin supplementation may be indicated, particularly if anorexia or hyporexia are present.

Clinical Pearls for Cats with Heart Disease

1. Making changes: Make all dietary changes gradually over a period of 3 to 7 days. However, major dietary changes should not be made while the cat is acutely ill or hospitalized. Usually it is better to wait several days until the cat's condition has improved and then initiate the change to reduce the risk for food aversions. It also is important to instruct the owner to notify the veterinarian if the cat does not eat adequate amounts of the new food so that other options can be devised. Some cats transition to new foods best by mixing the old food and the new food in varying proportions over the course of 3 to 7 days (gradually reducing the amount of the old food and gradually increasing the amount of the new food, until the cat has completely transitioned to the new food). However, for other cats, a preferable way to transition is to offer the two foods (i.e., the old food and the new food) side-by-side for several days to ensure the cat is eating the new food well before removing the old food.

2. Treats: It is important to make specific recommendations to owners regarding cat treats that are appropriate (and those that should not be fed) if owners wish to provide treats. Foods to be avoided include most commercial cat treats (unless specifically determined to be low in sodium), baby food, lunch meats and cold cuts, canned fish, and most cheeses. Acceptable treats (in limited quantities) include cat treats that are determined to be low in sodium (less than 5 mg sodium/treat). Note that even low-sodium treats and foods can provide large doses of sodium if fed in large quantities.

3. Medication administration: It also is important to provide the owner with appropriate methods for administering medications because cats are difficult to pill and many common foods used to administer medications are high in sodium. Owners can be taught to administer the pill without using foods (either by hand or using a device designed for this purpose, such as a pet piller or pet pill gun). Alternatively, foods such as low-sodium canned cat food or home-cooked meat (cooked without salt, not lunch meats) can be used. Many owners find that reserving a tasty, low-sodium canned food only for administering medications can make life easier. Pill administration treats also can be used, but be sure to check the individual brand for content of sodium and other nutrients of concern for an individual patient. This becomes particularly important if many of these treats per day are used for medication administration. Finally, a compounded liquid medication can be considered, although the pharmacokinetics of medications may be significantly altered by compounding.

4. Tips for increasing palatability: Cats with CHF often have variable appetites (i.e., they may eat a food well for a week but then stop eating that food and will only eat if a different food is offered). Although reductions in appetite in a cat that was previously eating well can indicate the need for reassessment and medication adjustment, sometimes providing a different food will increase appetite again. Communicating with the owner about these issues before they occur can help to reduce anxiety, and it is important to provide the owner with specific strategies to address the problem (and determine when to bring the cat in for reassessment). Home-made, low-sodium broth (e.g., chicken, beef, or fish) can enhance palatability. Most store-bought broths are high in sodium, even if they are labeled as "low sodium." Small amounts of cooked chicken, beef, or fish can be added to the food. Omega-3 fatty acids will often improve appetite in cats with CHF; however, effects will take several weeks. If CHF is well controlled and if drug doses are felt to be appropriate (e.g., no hypotension, bradycardia, or hypothermia), then appetite stimulants can be considered (e.g., mirtazapine). Cats with CHF often prefer warmed foods, but encourage the owner to experiment to determine which food temperature works best for their cat. Sometimes feeding the cat from a dinner plate (rather than the pet bowl) and in a place in the home that is different from their usual site can improve appetite.

References

1. WSAVA Nutritional Assessment Guidelines Task Force Members, Freeman L, Becvarova I, et al: WSAVA nutritional assessment guidelines. *J Small Anim Pract* 52(7):385–396, 2011.

2. World Small Animal Veterinary Association (WSAVA) Global Nutrition Committee: *Short diet history form.* (PDF online): <http://www.wsava.org/sites/default/files/Diet%20History%20Form.pdf>. Accessed May 11, 2015.

3. Freeman LM, Chandler ML, Hamper MA, et al: Current knowledge about the risks and benefits of raw meat based diets. *J Am Vet Med Assoc* 243:1549–1558, 2013.

4. Torin DS, Freeman LM, Rush JE: Dietary patterns of cats with cardiac disease. *J Am Vet Med Assoc* 230:862–867, 2007.

5. BCS chart for cats: *World Small Animal Veterinary Association Global Nutrition Committee Nutrition Toolkit.* <http://www.wsava.org/nutrition-toolkit>. Accessed August 6, 2014.

6. World Small Animal Veterinary Association (WSAVA) Global Nutrition Committee: *Muscle condition score chart.* (PDF online): <http://www.wsava.org/sites/default/files/Muscle%20condition%20score%20chart-Cats.pdf>. Accessed May 11, 2015.

7. World Small Animal Veterinary Association (WSAVA) Global Nutrition Committee: *The savvy cat owner's guide: nutrition on the internet.* (PDF online): <http://www.wsava.org/sites/default/files/nutrition%20on%20the%20internet%20cats.pdf>. Accessed May 11, 2015.

8. World Small Animal Veterinary Association (WSAVA) Global Nutrition Committee: *Selecting the best food for your pet.* (PDF online): <http://www.wsava.org/sites/default/files/Recommendations%20on%20Selecting%20Pet%20Foods.pdf>. Accessed May 11, 2015.

9. American College of Veterinary Nutrition. <http://www.acvn.org>. Accessed August 6, 2014.

10. Cummings Veterinary Medical Center at Tufts University: *HeartSmart: information on pets with heart disease.* <http://vet.tufts.edu/heartsmart>. Accessed May 11, 2015.

11. Yang VK, Freeman LM, Rush JE: Morphometric measurements and insulin-like growth factor in normal cats and cats with hypertrophic cardiomyopathy. *Am J Vet Res* 69:1061–1066, 2008.

12. Freeman LM, Rush JE, Meurs KM, et al: Body size and metabolic differences in Maine Coon cats with and without hypertrophic cardiomyopathy. *J Feline Med Surg* 15:74–80, 2013.

13. Association of American Feed Control Officials: *2013 official publication*, West Lafayette, IN, 2012, Association of American Feed Control Officials, Inc.

14. Gray CM, Sellon RK, Freeman LM: Nutritional adequacy of two vegan diets for cats. *J Am Vet Med Assoc* 225:1670–1675, 2004.

15. Freeman LM: Beneficial effects of omega-3 fatty acids in cardiovascular disease. *J Small Anim Pract* 51:462–470, 2010.

16. Freeman LM, Rush JE, Kehayias JJ, et al: Nutritional alterations and the effect of fish oil supplementation in dogs with heart failure. *J Vet Intern Med* 12:440–448, 1998.

17. Slupe JL, Freeman LM, Rush JE: The relationship between body weight, body condition, and survival in dogs with heart failure. *J Vet Intern Med* 22:561–565, 2008.

18. Smith CE, Freeman LM, Rush JE, et al: Omega-3 fatty acids in Boxer dogs with arrhythmogenic right ventricular cardiomyopathy. *J Vet Intern Med* 21:265–273, 2007.

19. Bright JM, Sullivan PS, Melton SL, et al: The effects of n-3 fatty acid supplementation on bleeding time, plasma fatty acid composition, and in vitro platelet aggregation in cats. *J Vet Intern Med* 8:247–252, 1994.

20. Saker KE, Eddy AL, Thatcher CD, et al: Manipulation of dietary (n-6) and (n-3) fatty acids alters platelet function in cats. *J Nutr* 128:2645S–2647S, 1998.

21. Hall DJ, Freeman LM, Rush JE, et al: Comparison of serum fatty acid concentrations in cats with cardiomyopathy and healthy controls. *J Feline Med Surg* 16:631–636, 2013.

22. Freeman LM: Cachexia and sarcopenia: Emerging syndromes of importance in dogs and cats. *J Vet Intern Med* 26:3–17, 2012.

23. Finn E, Freeman LM, Rush JE, et al: The relationship between body weight, body condition, and survival in cats with heart failure. *J Vet Intern Med* 24:1369–1374, 2010.

24. Hutchinson D, Freeman LM: Optimal nutrition for older cats. *Compend Contin Educ Vet* 33(5):e1–e3, 2011.

Genetics of Feline Heart Disease

Kathryn M. Meurs

Feline heart disease may develop as the result of a variety of different etiologies, including nutritional, infectious, endocrine, and inherited—among others.[1] This chapter focuses on what is known about inherited heart disease in cats.

CONGENITAL HEART DISEASE

Congenital heart disease in the cat is fairly uncommon; and although some breed predispositions have been suggested as described later, an inherited etiology has not been proven for any defect.

Mitral Valve Dysplasia

Mitral valve dysplasia is the most common congenital defect in the cat.[2] It is characterized by an abnormally formed mitral valve that typically results in secondary mitral valve insufficiency, and left atrial and ventricular enlargement.[3] Although the etiology of mitral valve dysplasia is unknown, one study found it to be frequently diagnosed in the Sphynx breed, which may suggest a possible heritable etiology.[4] Six of the 16 Sphynx cats with this defect also had an atrial or ventricular septal defect.

Endomyocardial Fibrosis

Endomyocardial fibrosis is an uncommon congenital heart disease characterized by left atrial and ventricular dilation with severe endocardial thickening. It has been shown to be inherited in the Siamese and Burmese breeds as well as in a colony of domestic shorthair cats.[5,6] The mode of inheritance is not known.

CARDIOMYOPATHY

Cardiomyopathies are the most common forms of heart disease in the cat.[1] There are several different forms of cardiomyopathy, including hypertrophic, restrictive, unclassified, dilated, and arrhythmogenic.[1] In human beings, hypertrophic, dilated, restrictive, and arrhythmogenic have all been found to be of inherited etiology.[7] However, at this time, only the hypertrophic form of cardiomyopathy has been determined to be inherited in the cat.[4,8-15] Dilated cardiomyopathy has previously been shown to be frequently associated with

a nutritional (i.e., taurine deficiency) etiology, although there is some evidence that there may be genetic influences as well.[16,17]

Hypertrophic Cardiomyopathy

Hypertrophic cardiomyopathy (HCM) is the most common form of cardiomyopathy in the cat.[1] It is an adult onset myocardial disease known to be inherited in the Maine Coon, Ragdoll, British Shorthair, and Sphynx breeds.[4,8-12] Several reports also exist for familial HCM in mixed breed cats.[13-15] Causative genetic mutations have now been identified in both the Ragdoll and the Maine Coon.[8,9] A number of small families of cats with several affected members have been observed in a few additional breeds, including the Norwegian Forest Cat, American Shorthair, Siberian, Bengal, and Scottish Fold. This suggests that HCM is an inherited disease in these breeds as well, although conclusive genetic studies have not yet been performed. A useful and frequently updated website for veterinarians and cat breeders interested in future developments in familial feline HCM, as well as other feline inherited diseases, is maintained by International Cat Care (http://www.icatcare.org/advice/cat-breeds/inherited-disorders-cats).

Maine Coon Hypertrophic Cardiomyopathy

A familial form of HCM in the Maine Coon cat was reported by Dr. Mark Kittleson at the University of California Davis in 1999.[11] Breeding studies demonstrated that it was an autosomal dominant trait as defined by the following criteria: males and females were fairly equally affected, every affected individual had at least one affected parent, and the trait was observed in every generation.

In the Maine Coon, a genetic mutation (A31P) has been identified in the myosin binding protein C (MYBPC3) gene.[8] Myosin binding protein C is a cardiac sarcomeric protein involved in cardiac contraction. Mutations in this gene are also frequently implicated in human familial HCM as well.[7] In the Maine Coon cat, the mutation is a single base pair change from a guanine to a cytosine (Figure 40-1) in the 31st codon of the gene. The mutation changes the highly conserved amino acid that is produced from alanine to proline. Additionally, the alteration of the amino acid is predicted to change the structure of myosin binding protein C in this region and alters the ability of the cardiac protein to interact with other contractile proteins.[8] Affected animals

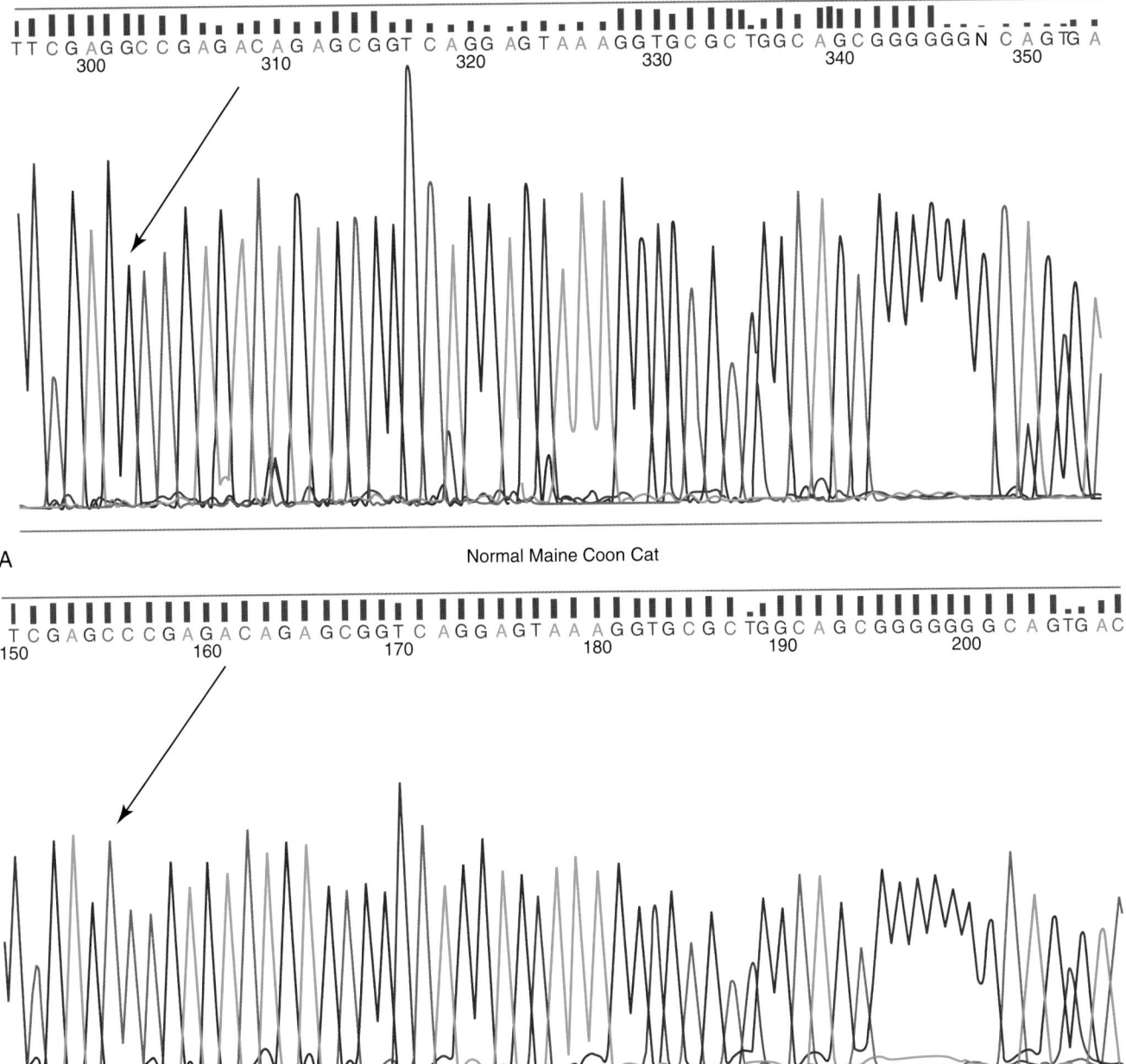

Figure 40-1: In the Maine Coon cat, the known causative mutation is a single base pair change in the myosin binding protein C gene, from a guanine (**A**) to a cytosine (**B**), in the 31st codon of the gene. The mutation changes the highly conserved amino acid that is produced from alanine to proline.

may carry the genetic mutation on one copy of the gene (heterozygous) or both copies (homozygous) of the gene. Heterozygous cats have a 50% chance of passing on the genetic mutation to their offspring. This does not mean that 50% of a litter of kittens will have the mutation but rather that each kitten has a 50% chance of having the mutation. The individual litter may actually have from zero to 100% of kittens born with the mutation. Homozygous cats pass on the mutation to 100% of their kittens.

Although a second causative mutation for HCM was reported to be identified in the Maine Coon cat, this variant (A74T) was later found to be a normal variant in the cat population and not causative for the disease. There is no value to testing for the A74T variant.[18]

A very important, but poorly understood, aspect of the inheritance of HCM in the cat is that the disease appears to be inherited with incomplete penetrance.[8,19,20] This means that cats that have the mutation will have different levels of disease severity depending on the "penetrance" of the trait in that individual cat. Even within the same litter, two litter-mates may have the same mutation, but one may show a more severe form of the disease than the other. Some cats with the mutation may never actually show a clinical form of the disease at all. Homozygous Maine Coon cats have a higher penetrance of the trait and are much more likely to develop the disease.[19] In fact, the odds ratio for homozygous cats has been estimated to be 26.4 (i.e., cats that are homozygous for the mutation are 26 times more likely to develop the disease than cats without the mutation).[20] Additionally, they may develop a more severe form of HCM and may show clinical signs before 4 years of age.[8] Cats that are heterozygous for the mutation are more likely to develop the disease (odds ratio of 1.8) than cats without the mutation but are much less likely than homozygous cats.[20] Heterozygous cats may develop the disease at a later age and have milder signs. As mentioned earlier, a small percentage of cats, even homozygous cats, with the mutation may not ever show clinical signs of the disease due to incomplete penetrance. Genetic and environmental modifiers that affect the expression and penetrance of the disease are likely but have yet to be determined.

The prevalence of the mutation in the Maine Coon population has been estimated to be between 30% to 40%, with the majority of cats with the mutation being positive heterozygotes.[19,21,22] Due to the high frequency of the mutation in the breed, careful recommendations should be made to breeders to gradually decrease the prevalence of the mutation in the breed. Attempts to rapidly decrease the prevalence of the mutation within a family line could have negative effects on the breed by altering the gene pool. Suggestions for making recommendations to owners of cats with the mutation are described later in the Breeding Recommendations section.

Although the Maine Coon mutation appears frequently in the Maine Coon population, it is quite breed specific. It is very uncommonly observed in other breeds and is unlikely to be associated with HCM in other cat breeds—unless they are closely related to the Maine Coon breed. Very rarely mutations have been found in a small number of Siberian, Ragdoll, and British Longhair cats.[19,21]

Ragdoll Hypertrophic Cardiomyopathy

A substitution mutation has also been identified in the myosin binding protein C gene in the Ragdoll cat.[9] Although identified in the same gene, the Ragdoll mutation is at a very different location than the Maine Coon mutation. The Ragdoll cat has a substitution mutation from a cytosine to a thymine (Figure 40-2) at the 820th codon of the gene, whereas the Maine Coon mutation is at the 31st codon. Given this very different location, it is extremely unlikely that the Maine Coon and Ragdoll mutations were inherited from a common ancestor; but rather, they are more likely to be two novel mutations that developed independently.

Although the mode of inheritance of this mutation in the Ragdoll has not been identified through breeding studies, it is most likely an autosomal dominant trait as well.

As in the Maine Coon, Ragdoll cats that are homozygous for the mutation appear to be much more severely affected than cats that are heterozygous for the mutation.[23] Homozygous cats are more likely to succumb to cardiac disease than heterozygous cats or cats without the mutation.

The Ragdoll mutation also appears to be very breed specific to the Ragdoll.[20]

Hypertrophic Cardiomyopathy in Other Breeds of Cats

The Sphynx cat has been recognized as a breed with a familial form of HCM in both Europe and North America.[4,10] In the Sphynx, both males and females were frequently affected with an average age of onset of 4 years (range of 1 to 10 years).[4] Although extensive breeding studies were not performed, an autosomal dominant pattern of inheritance was suggested.[4,10]

The British Shorthair has also been reported to have a familial form of HCM with an average age of onset of 2.7 years. The mode of inheritance is not known, although almost half of the affected cats had at least one affected parent, which is consistent with an autosomal dominant trait.[12]

Neither the Sphynx nor British Shorthair has either the Maine Coon or the Ragdoll mutation.[24]

There appear to be examples of familial HCM in additional breeds of cats, including the Norwegian Forest Cat, American Shorthair, Siberian, Bengal, and Scottish Fold among others, although extensive breeding studies have not been done. There is no evidence that any of these breeds share the same mutations as the Maine Coon or Ragdoll, and screening these breeds for the mutations is not likely to be useful. There may be some benefit to performing DNA screening of affected cats from breeds that have a known familial relationship to the Maine Coon or Ragdoll breed.

Additional Causes of Hypertrophic Cardiomyopathy in the Maine Coon and Ragdoll

Unfortunately, not all Maine Coon cats or Ragdolls with HCM have one of the identified mutations. The cause of the disease in these individual cases is unknown as of yet. In human beings, there are over 400 genetic mutations that lead to the development of HCM; therefore, it is likely that cats may have many genetic causes (and nongenetic causes) as well.[7]

Mutation Screening

Genetic testing is now available to test both Maine Coons and Ragdolls for their respective mutations by submitting a DNA sample to a reputable genetic screening laboratory. Good quality DNA samples can be obtained either from a blood sample submitted in an ethylenediaminetetraacetic acid (EDTA) tube or by brushing the gums of the cat with a special buccal swab, although many laboratories will even accept samples submitted on a cotton swab. Buccal swabbing is particularly helpful for testing young kittens in which it may be difficult to obtain a blood sample. Additionally, an owner can perform the buccal swabbing at home without stressing a difficult adult cat and mail the swabs directly to the screening laboratory.

Once the sample is provided to the laboratory, it can be analyzed in a number of ways. The gold standard for testing is to perform polymerase chain reaction (PCR)-based sequencing for actual visualization of the DNA sequence.

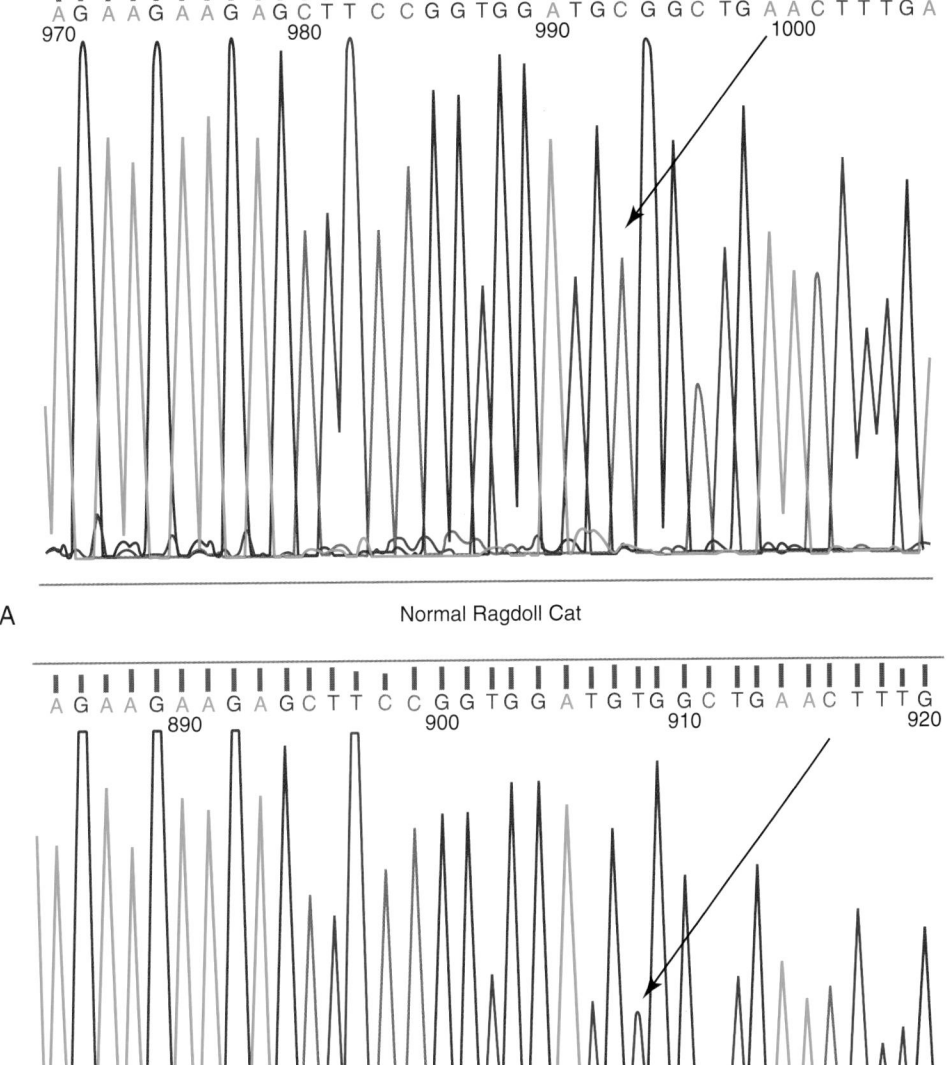

A   Normal Ragdoll Cat

B   Homozygous Positive Ragdoll Cat

Figure 40-2: In the Ragdoll cat, the known causative mutation is in the same gene as the Maine Coon mutation (myosin binding protein C) but at a different location. The Ragdoll cat has a substitution mutation from a cytosine (**A**) to a thymine (**B**) at the 820th codon of the gene.

The test results should indicate if the cat is negative, positive heterozygous, or positive homozygous for the mutation. Cats that test negative do not have the mutation. This does not mean that they cannot ever develop HCM; it simply means that they will not develop the form of the disease caused by that specific genetic mutation. Although the mutations described have been shown to be the cause of HCM in many Maine Coon and Ragdoll cats, there are some cats that are echocardiographically positive for HCM that do not have either of these known mutations and likely have the disease due to other causes of familial or other origin.

Breeding Recommendations

Due to the apparent fairly high prevalence of the known mutations for HCM in both breeds (over 30%), it would be unwise to recommend that all cats with the mutations be removed from breeding programs. A reduction of 30% of the breeding animals from a closed, purebred gene pool could dramatically alter the genetic makeup of these breeds. Additionally, it should be emphasized that not all cats that have the mutation, particularly if they are heterozygous, will develop a clinical form of the disease because of the variable penetrance of the disease. Therefore, guidelines for counseling owners about the results of their genetic testing could be as follows:

Negative. A negative test result indicates that the individual cat does not carry the known genetic mutation that can lead to HCM. Because there are likely other possible causes for HCM, it does not mean that this cat can never develop the disease. It only means that they cannot develop the disease from the mutation tested.

Positive Heterozygous. Positive heterozygous cats have one copy of the normal gene and one copy of the mutated gene. These cats can develop the disease, but many do not. If they do, it is generally at an older age. Therefore, in some cases where the cat has other exceptional traits, it may be reasonable to consider keeping the cat in a breeding program. In those situations, the cat should be evaluated annually with an echocardiogram by a cardiologist to evaluate for any evidence of cardiomyopathy. Breeding only should be considered if the cat appears to be clear of disease and then only to a negative cat. The offspring of this mating of a positive heterozygous and a negative should be screened for the mutation, and if possible, a mutation-negative kitten with the desirable traits of the parents should be selected to replace the mutation-positive parent in the breeding colony. Over a few generations, this will decrease the prevalence of the disease mutation in the population, hopefully without greatly altering the genetic makeup of the breed too significantly.

However, if there is evidence of cardiomyopathy on the annual evaluation, the cat should be removed from the breeding program for the health of the cat as well as to keep the mutation out of the bloodline.

There is certainly the substantial risk with this approach that additional positive heterozygous cats will be born and go on to develop the disease. However in both breeds, the positive heterozygous cats have lower penetrant disease, so they are much less likely to develop the disease. Additionally, this approach will allow the gene pool of the breed to be somewhat preserved.

It should be remembered that this is an adult onset disease, and some cats will be selected for breeding based on a clear echocardiogram evaluation one year only to be diagnosed with the disease the next year. Therefore, this approach should only be used for exceptional cats, and they should be clinically evaluated for the disease every year. If they develop the clinical disease, they should no longer be kept in the breeding program.

Positive Homozygous. The author's current recommendations for both breeds are not to use cats that are homozygous for the mutation for breeding purposes, because they will certainly pass on the mutation to all of their offspring, and they have the highest risk of developing the disease.

References

1. MacDonald K: Myocardial disease. In Ettinger SJ, Feldman EC, editors: *Textbook of veterinary internal medicine,* ed 7, St Louis, 2010, Elsevier, pp 1328–1342.
2. MacDonald K: Congenital heart disease in puppies and kittens. *Vet Clin North Am Small Anim Pract* 36:503–531, 2006.
3. Oyama MA, Sisson DD, Thomas WP, et al: Myocardial disease. In Ettinger SJ, Feldman EC, editors: *Textbook of veterinary internal medicine,* ed 7, St Louis, 2010, Elsevier, pp 1250–1299.
4. Chetboul V, Petit A, Gouni V, et al: Prospective echocardiographic and tissue Doppler screening of a large Sphynx cat population: reference ranges, heart disease prevalence and genetic aspects. *J Vet Cardiol* 14:497–509, 2012.
5. Zook BC, Paasch LH: Endocardial fibroelastosis in Burmese cats. *Am J Pathol* 106:435–438, 1982.
6. Fox PR: Feline cardiomyopathies. In Fox PR, Sisson DD, Moise NS, editors: *Textbook of canine and feline cardiology,* ed 2, Philadelphia, 1999, Saunders, pp 621–678.
7. Cahill TJ, Ashrafian H, Watkins H: Genetic cardiomyopathies causing heart failure. *Circ Res* 113:660–675, 2013.
8. Meurs KM, Sanchez X, David RM, et al: Identification of a missense mutation in the cardiac myosin binding protein C gene in a family of Maine Coon cats with hypertrophic cardiomyopathy. *Hum Mol Genet* 14:3587–3593, 2005.
9. Meurs KM, Norgard MM, Ederer MM, et al: A substitution mutation in the myosin binding protein C gene in Ragdoll cats. *Genomics* 90:261–264, 2007.
10. Silverman SJ, Meurs KM, Stern JA: Hypertrophic cardiomyopathy in the Sphynx cat: a retrospective evaluation of phenotype and etiology. *J Feline Med Surg* 14:246–249, 2012.
11. Kittleson MD, Meurs KM, Munro MJ, et al: Familial hypertrophic cardiomyopathy in Maine Coon cats: an animal model of human disease. *Circulation* 24:3172–3180, 1999.
12. Granstro S, Nyberg MT, Godiksen M, et al: Prevalence of hypertrophic cardiomyopathy in a cohort of British Shorthair cats in Denmark. *J Vet Intern Med* 25:866–871, 2011.
13. Nakagawa K, Takemura N, Machida N, et al: Hypertrophic cardiomyopathy in a mixed breed cat family. *J Vet Med Sci* 64:619–621, 2002.
14. Kraus MS, Calvert CA, Jacobs GJ: Hypertrophic cardiomyopathy in a litter of five mixed-breed cats. *J Am Anim Hosp Assoc* 35:293–296, 1999.
15. Baty CJ, Malarkey DE, Atkins CE, et al: Natural history of hypertrophic cardiomyopathy and aortic thromboembolism in a family of domestic shorthair cats. *J Vet Intern Med* 15:595–599, 2001.
16. Pion PD, Kittleson MD, Thomas WP, et al: Clinical findings in cats with dilated cardiomyopathy and relationship of findings to taurine deficiency. *J Am Vet Med Assoc* 15:267–285, 1992.
17. Lawler DF, Templeton AJ, Monti KL: Evidence for genetic involvement in feline dilated cardiomyopathy. *J Vet Intern Med* 7:383–387, 1993.
18. Longeri M, Ferrari P, Knafelz P, et al: Myosin-binding protein C DNA variants in domestic cats (A31P, A74T, R820W) and their association with hypertrophic cardiomyopathy. *J Vet Intern Med* 27:275–285, 2013.
19. Mary J, Chetboul V, Sampedrano CC, et al: Prevalence of the MYBPC3-A31P mutation in a large European feline population and association with hypertrophic cardiomyopathy in the Maine Coon breed. *J Vet Cardiol* 12:155–161, 2010.
20. Longeri M, Ferrari P, Knafelz P, et al: Myosin-Binding Protein C DNA variants in domestic cats (A31P, A74T, R820W) and their association with hypertrophic cardiomyopathy. *J Vet Intern Med* 27:275–285, 2013.
21. Fries R, Heaney AM, Meurs KM: Prevalence of the myosin binding protein C in Maine Coon cats. *J Vet Intern Med* 22:893–896, 2008.
22. Casamian-Sorrosal D, Chong SK, Fonfara S, et al: Prevalence and demographics of the MYBPC3-mutations in ragdolls and Maine coons in the British Isles. *J Small Anim Pract* 55(5):269–273, 2014.
23. Borgeat KA, Casamian D, Helps CR, et al: Outcome of 174 ragdoll cats tested for the myosin binding protein C3 mutation. *J Vet Intern Med* 27:683, 2013.
24. Meurs KM, Norgard MM, Kuan M, et al: Analysis of eight sarcomeric candidate genes for feline hypertrophic cardiomyopathy mutations in cats with hypertrophic cardiomyopathy. *J Vet Intern Med* 23:840–843, 2009.

Update on the Management of Feline Cardiomyopathy

Sonya G. Gordon

Cardiomyopathies represent primary diseases of the myocardium that are characterized by a variety of phenotypes that may or may not be progressive and, thus, may or may not lead to the development of clinical signs. Other comorbid conditions, such as systemic hypertension and hyperthyroidism, can mimic feline cardiomyopathy and/or contribute to progression if left unmanaged in cats with cardiomyopathy and, thus, should always be ruled out in cats with known or suspected cardiomyopathy. Initial clinical signs of cardiomyopathy can be acute and life threatening. Clinical signs associated with feline cardiomyopathies include those associated with congestive heart failure (CHF), syncope, or arterial thromboembolism (ATE). Treatment and prevention of ATE is covered in Chapter 35. This chapter deals predominantly with the treatment and potential prevention of signs of CHF (e.g., dyspnea, tachypnea, weakness, and collapse) with emphasis on areas where new data has been published.

HEART DISEASE/FAILURE CLASSIFICATION

The American College of Veterinary Internal Medicine (ACVIM) consensus statement guidelines for the diagnosis and treatment of canine chronic valvular heart disease put forth a staging scheme for heart disease and failure in 2009.[1] Since that time, others have broadened the use of this grading scheme to include the staging of canine dilated cardiomyopathy[2] and feline cardiomyopathies.[3] The ACVIM grading scheme in general, when adapted for cats, recognizes that some apparently healthy cats either have or are at increased risk of developing cardiomyopathy and that some of these cats are at risk for CHF or ATE and can be identified based on knowledge of signalment (e.g., age, sex, and breed) and physical examination findings (e.g., presence of a murmur, gallop heart sound, and/or arrhythmia). The use of this information to identify "at-risk" cats facilitates development of recommendations to owners regarding the most financially savvy approaches to screening for cardiomyopathy in apparently healthy cats. This group of cats is considered Stage A. It is important to recognize that not all cats with heart murmurs or other auscultatory abnormalities have cardiomyopathy and, thus, further testing is required to establish a diagnosis of cardiomyopathy. Many cardiac murmurs are benign (e.g., due to dynamic right ventricular outflow tract obstruction) or innocent (i.e., no identifiable etiology based on echocardiogram). Cats in Stage A have no signs of heart disease or failure and are not currently known to have cardiomyopathy, but they simply have some sort of "clue" identified from the signalment and/or physical examination that causes them to be at increased risk of cardiovascular disease. Genetic predispositions are recognized in some cat breeds, and the role of genetics in feline heart disease is covered in Chapter 40.

Stage B includes all cats that are known to have a cardiomyopathy (typically based on an echocardiogram) but have no current or previous signs or symptoms of heart disease or failure. This group can be stratified into Stage B1 and Stage B2 based on the presence and magnitude of structural and/or functional changes to the heart. Cats are categorized as Stage B1 if cardiac remodeling is mild and Stage B2 if the cardiovascular changes are moderate to severe. Although these categories are somewhat subjective, most observers would use the presence and magnitude of left atrial enlargement, the magnitude of left ventricular hypertrophy, the degree of systolic dysfunction, and the presence or severity of left ventricular outflow tract obstruction (LVOTO) to aid in classification of B1 versus B2.

Stage C includes all cats that currently have or historically had clinical signs as a consequence of their heart disease. Clinical signs of CHF include dyspnea, tachypnea, orthopnea, and infrequently cough. A diagnosis of CHF should be established from the history and physical examination, combined with thoracic radiography, echocardiography, and perhaps biomarker testing (blood levels of N-terminal pro-brain natriuretic peptide [NT-proBNP] and/or cardiac troponin-I). Affected cats have pulmonary edema, pleural effusion, pericardial effusion, or less commonly ascites found in combination with cardiac disease sufficient enough to be the cause for congestion. It is important to recognize that Stage C cats remain Stage C even if treatment completely resolves the clinical signs of CHF.

Cats classified as Stage D were formerly Stage C, but the heart disease has progressed; and despite appropriate therapy (e.g., furosemide, an angiotensin-converting enzyme inhibitor [ACE-I], and/or pimobendan), they continue to experience clinical signs of congestion. This is the refractory stage of heart failure, and less commonly used drugs are often added at this stage to control signs of CHF. A summary of this adapted heart failure classification scheme can be seen in Figure 41-1. The advantages of utilizing a classification scheme of this nature are that it provides a useful framework to discuss heart disease with colleagues and clients, and it provides an easy way to develop and communicate stage specific recommendations. An overview of stage specific recommendations can be seen in Figure 41-2 and Table 41-1. Drugs commonly used in cats with cardiomyopathy are given in Table 41-2.

CLASSIFICATION-BASED DIAGNOSTIC, TREATMENT, AND FOLLOW-UP STRATEGIES

Using the aforementioned outlined classification scheme for cats with cardiomyopathy, specific diagnostic, treatment, and monitoring recommendations can be offered. To some degree, these recommendations follow from the practice patterns of the author, but many veterinary cardiologists follow a similar plan in their clinical practice. Emphasis is placed on topics for which clinically relevant new information has been recently published.[4-10] Some of the recommendations are based on echocardiographic findings or laboratory results. For specific details regarding the echocardiographic diagnosis of feline cardiomyopathy and the utility of NT-proBNP, see Chapters 46 and 34, respectively.

Diagnosis, Therapy, and Monitoring of Stage A Patients—Cats at Risk for Having or Developing Cardiomyopathy

Several recent reports have documented that 10% to 15% of presumed healthy cats have evidence of cardiovascular disease. Not all of these cats will develop CHF, but the pool of cats that might develop cardiovascular disease is quite large. Cats with a murmur, gallop, or other cardiac arrhythmia; those who have a close relative with cardiomyopathy; and those with a genetic predisposition for cardiomyopathy are clearly candidates for additional cardiovascular disease screening. There are a variety of diagnostic tests available to evaluate or screen cats suspected to have an asymptomatic form of cardiomyopathy. Cardiac ultrasound (echocardiography) is considered the gold standard. Other screening strategies, in particular the use of cardiac biomarkers such as NT-proBNP,

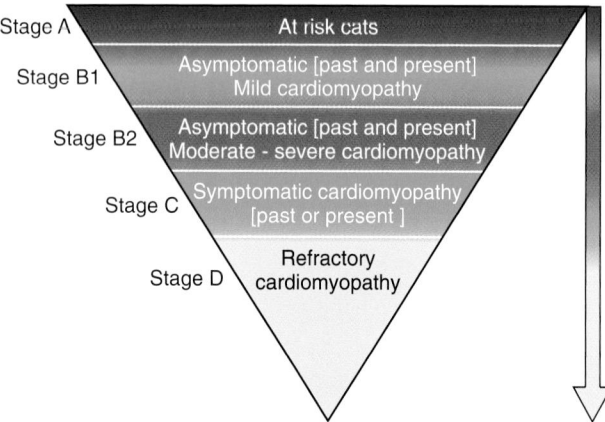

Figure 41-1: Feline cardiomyopathy classification scheme. (Modification of American College of Veterinary Internal Medicine Congestive Heart Failure Classification Scheme: Atkins C, Binaural J, Hettinger S, et al: Guidelines for the diagnosis and treatment of canine chronic alular heart disease. *J Vet Intern Med* 23(6):1142-1150, 2009; Gordon SG, Estrada AH: *The ABCDs of small animal cardiology: a practical manual,* Guelph, 2013, LifeLearn.)

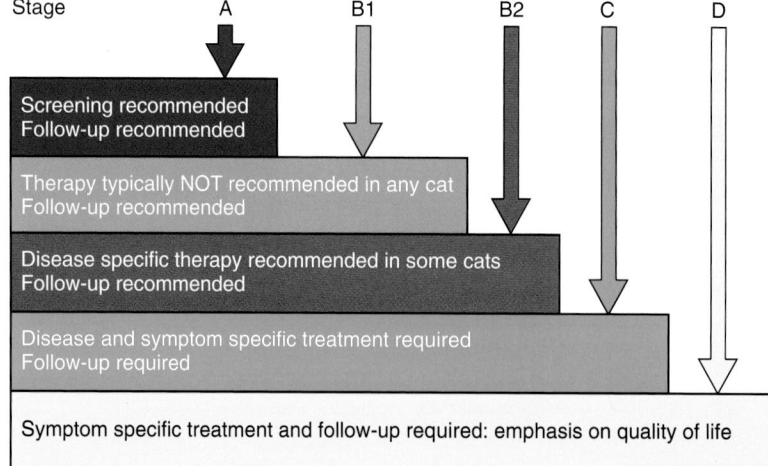

Figure 41-2: Cardiomyopathy classification-based diagnostic, treatment, and follow-up strategies. (Modification of American College of Veterinary Internal Medicine Congestive Heart Failure Classification Scheme: Atkins C, Binaural J, Hettinger S, et al: Guidelines for the diagnosis and treatment of canine chronic alular heart disease. *J Vet Intern Med* 23(6):1142-1150, 2009; Gordon SG, Estrada AH: *The ABCDs of small animal cardiology: a practical manual,* Guelph, 2013, LifeLearn.)

Table 41-1 Summary of Stage-Based Recommendations on Diagnosis, Treatment, and Follow-Up

Stage	Diagnostics	Treatment	Follow-Up
A	Definitive diagnostics*: Echocardiogram§ Screening: NT-proBNP (see Chapter 34)	None	Re-evaluation: Typically every 1 year
B1	Definitive diagnostics*‡: Echocardiogram§	Typically none	Re-evaluation: Every 6 to 12 months
B2	Definitive diagnostics*‡†: Echocardiogram§ Thoracic radiographs	None Antithrombotic if significant left atrial enlargement No evidence of LVOTO on echocardiogram; consider an ACE-I Evidence of LVOTO on echocardiogram; consider atenolol ± ACE-I	Client education: Signs of CHF and ATE HRR Re-evaluation: Every 4 to 8 months Sooner if clinical signs develop or HRR >30 breaths/min
C	Definitive diagnostics*‡†: Thoracic radiographs Echocardiogram§ Response to CHF treatment	No evidence of LVOTO on echocardiogram; Pleurocentesis as needed, furosemide, ACEI, antithrombotic, pimobendan† Evidence of LVOTO on echocardiogram; Pleurocentesis as needed, furosemide, ACEI, antithrombotic†	Client education: Signs of CHF and ATE HRR Re-evaluation: Every 3 to 4 months Sooner if major change in medication or clinical status Sooner if new clinical signs develop or HRR >30 breaths/min
D	As required to work up clinical signs that are contributing to a poor quality of life	As per Stage C with appropriate dosage adjustments ± add pimobendan Addition of other medications on a case-by-case basis as needed Discontinuation of medications may be indicated in some cases	As needed; similar to Stage C

ACE-I, Angiotensin-converting enzyme inhibitor; *ATE,* arterial thromboembolism; *CHF,* congestive heart failure; *HRR,* home resting/sleeping respiration rate; *LVOTO,* left ventricular outflow tract obstruction; *NT-proBNP,* N-terminal pro-brain natriuretic peptide.
*Other conditions (e.g., systemic hypertension and hyperthyroidism) can mimic feline cardiomyopathy and/or contribute to progression if left unmanaged as comorbidities in cats with cardiomyopathy and should always be ruled out in cats with known or suspected cardiomyopathy.
†Listed in order of priority.
‡Ancillary tests may be indicated in individual cases (e.g., thoracic radiographs/orthogonal views, electrocardiogram, routine blood work, and/or urinalysis).
§Echocardiogram ideally with Doppler.

may provide additional information when cardiac ultrasound is not available or is declined by the owner. Thoracic radiographs and electrocardiography (ECG) are poor screening tests for cardiomyopathy due to their low sensitivity and should not be used in lieu of more definitive tests. Measurement of arterial blood pressure or thyroid hormone testing may be indicated in older cats when heart disease becomes a differential diagnosis. There is no therapy recommended for cats in Stage A. Periodic evaluation, via echocardiography or natriuretic peptide testing, may be indicated in cats with a known predisposition to cardiomyopathy, even if the current echocardiographic examination is normal.

Stage B1 Patients—Asymptomatic Cats with Minimal Remodeling Secondary to Cardiomyopathy

By definition, Stage B1 cats have no overt clinical signs of CHF, and identification is typically the result of screening Stage A cats.

Diagnosis of Stage B1 Patients

Definitive diagnosis of Stage B1 cardiomyopathy requires an echocardiogram (ideally with Doppler studies). Although the definition of minimal remodeling secondary to cardio-

Table 41-2	Drugs Typically Used in the Treatment of Feline Cardiomyopathy	
Drug	**Dose**	**Comments**
Atenolol	PO: 1.0-2.5 mg/kg every 12 h, or 6.25-12.5 mg/cat every 12 h	Target heart rate is approximately 160 bpm in hospital Do not initiate in face of active CHF Up-titration to target dose is required Dose may need to be reduced or discontinued in cats that develop CHF Down-titration is recommended; abrupt discontinuation should be avoided Adverse effects: Possible bradycardia, hypotension, and new or recurrent CHF
Benazepril	PO: 0.25-0.5 mg/kg every 12 h, or 0.5 mg/kg every 24 h	Start at the lower end of the dosage range and increase to maximal dose with monitoring of renal function and serum potassium and blood pressure Adverse effects: Possible azotemia, acute renal failure, and hyperkalemia

Diltiazem	Regular formulation:
	    PO: 7.5 mg/cat every 8 h
	Sustained release:
	    PO: 30-60 mg/cat every 12 to 24 h
		The sustained release formulations cannot be made into a suspension
		Adverse effects: Possible hyporexia and vomiting with the sustained release formulations; possible hypotension and bradycardia with all formulations

Enalapril	PO: 0.25-0.5 mg/kg every 12 h, or 0.5 mg/kg every 24 h	Start at the lower end of the dosage range and increase to maximal dose with monitoring of renal function and serum potassium and blood pressure Adverse effects: Possible azotemia, acute renal failure, and hyperkalemia
Furosemide	Parenteral: 0.5-2.0 mg/kg every 1 to 8 h IV/IM/SC CRI: 0.25-0.6 mg/kg/h PO: 1-2 mg/kg every 12 to 24 h to a maximum total daily dose of 4-6 mg/kg	For parenteral dosing, interval depends on response to therapy Initial boluses are typically every 2 hours, thereafter every 6 to 8 hours Compounded suspensions from tablets are typically better tolerated than commercial alcohol-based elixirs Adverse effects: Possible azotemia, renal failure, hypotension, hypochloremia, hypokalemia, and hyponatremia
Pimobendan	PO: 0.625-1.25 mg/cat every 12 h	Do not reformulate into a suspension Relatively contraindicated in cats with LVOTO Adverse effects: None consistently reported; tachycardia and hypotension possible in cats with LVOTO
Spironolactone	PO: 1-2 mg/kg every 12 to 24 h	Weak diuretic effect May have antifibrotic effects that are cardioprotective May help limit severity of hypokalemia Adverse effects: Possible facial excoriations

CHF, Congestive heart failure; *CRI,* continuous rate infusion; *IM,* intramuscularly; *IV,* intravenously; *LVOTO,* left ventricular outflow tract obstruction; *PO, per os* (by mouth); *SC,* subcutaneously.

myopathy is subjective, these cats are typically characterized by normal to minimal increases in left atrial size, mild increases in interventricular septal and/or left ventricular free wall thickness, minimal evidence of LVOTO, and perhaps mild impairment of diastolic function. In some cases, echocardiography may not be able to discriminate between normal and mild cardiomyopathy, especially in cats over 9 years old where age-related echocardiographic changes can be difficult to differentiate from a mild form of cardiomyopathy. In general, establishing a diagnosis of Stage B1 cardiomyopathy represents a clinical challenge and significant echocardiographic skill is required. Other tests may be indicated to assess organ systems that may be affected by

treatment for heart disease (e.g., routine blood tests and/or urinalysis) or contribute to the progression of heart disease/failure (e.g., thyroid function testing and/or blood pressure measurement).

Treatment of Stage B1 Patients
For cats with Stage B1 cardiomyopathy, therapy is almost never recommended, unless an underlying cause (e.g., hyperthyroidism, systemic hypertension, and/or taurine deficiency) is identified. Certain cats with mild cardiomyopathy can have rapid progression, even if many cats have rather slow progression of heart disease. Thus, scheduled surveillance to assess for worsening heart disease is recommended.

Monitoring of Stage B1 Patients

Typically, re-evaluation for Stage B1 includes an echocardiogram once every 6 to 12 months. Six-month or shorter intervals are typically recommended in young (less than 5 years old) purebred cats with a recognized predisposition to cardiomyopathy.

Stage B2 Patients—Asymptomatic Cats with Moderate to Severe Remodeling Secondary to Cardiomyopathy

By definition, Stage B2 cats are free of overt signs of CHF, and identification is typically either the result of screening Stage A cats or as a consequence of re-evaluation of Stage B1 cats.

Diagnosis of Stage B2 Patients

Definitive diagnosis of Stage B2 cardiomyopathy requires an echocardiogram (ideally with Doppler studies). Although the definition of moderate to severe remodeling secondary to cardiomyopathy is subjective, these cats are typically characterized by some combination of left atrial enlargement, regional or diffuse thickening (hypertrophy) of the left ventricular walls and papillary muscles, evidence of myocardial fibrosis, altered left ventricular contractile function, evidence of LVOTO, or impaired diastolic function. The number and type of these abnormalities may depend upon the form of cardiomyopathy and the degree of progression of the disease. Establishing a definitive diagnosis may ultimately affect therapeutic recommendations, although for many cardiologists the degree of left atrial enlargement, the severity of left ventricular hypertrophy, or the magnitude of LVOTO are the factors most likely to affect treatment recommendations. Other tests may be indicated to assess organ systems that may be affected by treatment for heart disease (e.g., routine blood tests and/or urinalysis) or contribute to the progression of heart disease/failure (e.g., thyroid function testing and/or blood pressure measurement).

Treatment of Stage B2 Patients

Given that the first sign(s) of heart disease in cats can be life threatening, there is often a strong urge to initiate treatment when heart disease is discovered. Unfortunately, with the possible exception of dilated cardiomyopathy secondary to taurine deficiency, there is no published evidence demonstrating that initiation of any medication in asymptomatic cats with cardiomyopathy can prolong symptom-free life and/or survival. The decision to treat should be considered in light of the owner's ability and willingness to chronically medicate the cat and the cat's tolerance of the medication(s).

Although ACE-Is (e.g., enalapril and benazepril) have not been demonstrated to reduce left ventricular hypertrophy or prolong survival in cats with CHF secondary to a variety of cardiomyopathies, they have been demonstrated to be relatively safe and well tolerated. Because the renin angiotensin system is likely activated as a cat gets closer to CHF, many veterinary cardiologists advocate initiation of ACE-Is in

Stage B2 cats with moderate to marked left atrial enlargement, regardless of the form of cardiomyopathy. Empirical antithrombotic therapy is likewise often initiated in Stage B2 cats with moderate to marked left atrial enlargement, in those with spontaneous contrast (smoke) in the left atrium, or in those with reduced left atrial function because these findings have been demonstrated to be associated with increased risk of ATE (see Chapter 35).

The most common cardiomyopathy diagnosed in the cat is hypertrophic cardiomyopathy (HCM). Cats with HCM can be subdivided into those without LVOTO and those with LVOTO; the latter is sometimes referred to as *hypertrophic obstructive cardiomyopathy (HOCM)*. Left ventricular outflow tract obstruction can be a consequence of systolic anterior motion (SAM) of the mitral valve and/or hypertrophy at the top of the interventricular septum that is causing an obstruction to the ejection of blood out of the left ventricle. Left ventricular outflow tract obstruction can occur with other forms of cardiomyopathy and with disease of the mitral valve, but it is most commonly seen in cats with HCM. Historically, beta-blockers have often been used to treat cats with Stage B2 HCM, especially in those cats with LVOTO or in cats with tachycardia or ventricular arrhythmias. The premise for this treatment strategy is based in part on extrapolation from human patients with HCM and clinical signs during excitement or exercise. In cats, atenolol, a beta-1 specific beta-blocker, has been demonstrated to blunt the severity of LVOTO and reduce the associated mitral regurgitation, limit myocardial oxygen consumption, and limit progressive hypertrophy in selected cases. However, there have been concerns raised that beta blockade could result in decompensation to CHF and potentially increase the risk of ATE as a consequence of impaired left atrial systolic function. Publication of a prospective, observational, open-label, non-randomized, clinical cohort study has provided some much-needed evidence regarding the effect of long-term atenolol treatment in cats with preclinical (Stage B) HCM with or without obstruction (HOCM).[6] Although there were some cited limitations to this study, there was no significant difference in all-cause mortality and cardiac mortality between cats with HCM that were treated with atenolol versus those cats that were untreated. The percentage of cats that died and the time to death for cats that died during the study in the atenolol treated group was 45% and 1133 ± 503 days (mean ± standard deviation); and in the untreated group, it was 38% and 1043 ± 659 days. Age and left atrial size were the only predictors of 5-year outcome. In this study, atenolol was well tolerated with no recognized adverse effects. The results of this study suggest that the use of atenolol is likely to be well tolerated, although atenolol use was not associated with any obvious prolongation in survival in cats with preclinical (Stage B) HCM. Additional studies are warranted in this area.

Calcium channel blockers, such as diltiazem, have also been used to treat Stage B2 HCM not characterized by LVOTO. Calcium channel blockers as a class can improve relaxation directly, and diltiazem has been reported in one study to reduce the severity of ventricular hypertrophy in cats with HCM. However, the nonsustained release formulation requires dosing every 8 hours, and the sustained release formulation frequently causes clinically significant gastrointestinal (GI) complications, including hyporexia and vomiting, and still requires dosing every 12 hours. For these reasons, diltiazem is often not the agent of choice for the treatment of HCM in the cat.

The potential role of nutritional management of Stage B2 cats is covered in Chapter 39.

Monitoring of Stage B2 Patients

Given the potential for progression of Stage B2 patients to Stage C, client education and scheduled follow-up remain the cornerstone of management regardless of whether treatment is initiated or not.

Client education should include information regarding potential clinical signs with emphasis on those signs that could be associated with ATE or CHF, such as lameness, weakness, paralysis, pain, abnormal behavior, syncope, weight loss, labored breathing, rapid breathing, and cough (rare). Measurement of home resting (or ideally sleeping) breathing rate by the owner is widely used in the dog as a sensitive tool to identify the onset or recurrence of CHF.[4] Although it has not been proven to be similarly useful in the cat, there is reason to believe that it may be, and reference ranges for normal adult cats have been reported (≤30 breaths per minute).[5] Cats with sleeping home respiration rates repeatedly greater than 30 breaths/min are abnormal and likely warrant re-evaluation by their veterinarian.[5] There are a variety of free smartphone applications that have been developed to facilitate owner measurement of resting/sleeping respiration rate. Home resting/sleeping respiration rates should be performed regularly (daily or weekly) in a Stage B2 cat. Typically, more frequent evaluations are recommended in cats which are judged to have a high risk developing of CHF in the near future (e.g., the next 3 to 6 months).

Periotic re-evaluations to track the progression of disease and potentially detect early signs of decompensation should be recommended. Typically, appointments of this type are scheduled every 4 to 8 months with shorter intervals elected in the most advanced cases. In addition to a thorough history and physical examination, a variety of other diagnostics tests may be valuable including thoracic radiographs, echocardiogram, blood pressure, NT-proBNP measurement, routine blood tests, and ECG.

Stage C Patients—Cats with Past or Present Signs of Heart Failure Attributable to Cardiomyopathy

By definition, Stage C cats currently have or previously experienced signs of CHF attributable to heart disease.

Diagnosis of Stage C Patients

Definitive diagnosis of Stage C cardiomyopathy is made in a cat with appropriate clinical signs (e.g., respiratory distress, dyspnea or orthopnea, increased home breathing rate, weakness, or collapse) in combination with supportive thoracic radiographic evidence of CHF, or other conclusive evidence of CHF (e.g., jugular distention with modified transudate pleural effusion and echocardiographic evidence of advanced heart disease). In severely compromised cats, when optimum diagnostic tests are declined or when routine test results are ambiguous, response to emergency CHF therapy may be used to establish a diagnosis. A rapid, brief cage-side ultrasound examination in a dyspneic cat may help determine whether there is sufficient fluid for thoracocentesis, or whether left atrial enlargement is present. Other diagnostic tests may be done to help establish the diagnosis (e.g., complete echocardiogram and/or NT-proBNP measurement), stage the severity of the heart disease (e.g., echocardiogram, blood pressure measurement, and/or ECG), and assess organ systems that may be affected by treatment for CHF (e.g., routine blood tests and/or urinalysis) or contribute to the progression of heart disease/failure (e.g., thyroid function testing and/or blood pressure measurement).

Treatment of Stage C Patients

Congestive heart failure is associated with significant morbidity and is life threatening; thus, treatment is always recommended. Like many feline diseases, there are few evidence-based publications reporting the best methods to manage CHF in cats, so much of the therapeutic approach is empirical and based on clinical experience. One cornerstone of CHF treatment in cats with moderate to large volume pleural effusion is pleurocentesis to relieve the signs of respiratory distress associated with pleural effusion.

Furosemide is the diuretic most frequently used for management of CHF. Furosemide is usually given parenterally (intravenous, intramuscular, or subcutaneous) for acute CHF and orally for chronic management of heart failure. The dose and frequency is adjusted as needed until a sufficient dose has been given to resolve signs of congestion (e.g., pulmonary edema and/or pleural effusion). For acute decompensated CHF, furosemide can be administered at 0.5 to 2 mg/kg parenterally and repeated every 2 hours as needed until dyspnea is starting to improve. The dose often needs to be adjusted downward once respiratory rate and effort are improving. In cats with developing or worsening azotemia, increased packed cell volume, or elevated total solids, the furosemide dose may need to be withheld for 1 to 2 days to avoid excessive hemoconcentration. Similarly, the chronic oral dose often requires a degree of experimentation because the furosemide dose in cats can range from 1 mg/kg every 48 hours up to 2 to 4 mg/kg every 12 hours; the maximum total chronic daily dose of furosemide should not exceed 4 to 6 mg/kg. Chronic CHF in cats is often also treated with an ACE-I (e.g., enalapril, benazepril or lisinopril), in part to blunt the anticipated up-regulation of the renin-angiotensin-aldosterone system. In addition, given that most cats with CHF have atrial enlargement and thus are at an increased risk of developing ATE, initiation of an antithrombotic medication is usually recommended once CHF has been diagnosed. For most veterinarians, this combination of medications (furosemide, ACE-I, and antithrombotics) is considered standard CHF therapy in the cat and is employed regardless of the form of cardiomyopathy.

If the results of an echocardiogram are available, and they confirm the presence of ventricular systolic dysfunction with no LVOTO, then (based on recent publications) pimobendan may be added to standard CHF therapy. The drug is usually well tolerated, and observational reports indicate the potential empirical benefit in cats with obvious echocardiographic ventricular systolic dysfunction.[8,9] The chronic median oral dose reported is approximately 0.25 mg/kg every 12 hours and a range of 0.18 to 0.35 mg/kg.[7-10] A feline pharmacokinetic study reported that following a single oral dose of pimobendan (mean ± standard deviation; 0.28 mg/kg ± 0.04) it was rapidly absorbed with an absorption half-life of 0.2 ± 0.08 hours (mean ± standard deviation) and an elimination half-life of 1.3 ± 0.2 hours. Maximum plasma concentration was high and predicted by the model to occur at 0.9 hours after drug administration.[10] Whether to add pimobendan to the therapeutic plan for cats whose echocardiogram does not identify systolic dysfunction and whether to use the drug in cats with documented LVOTO (e.g., HOCM) are more problematic to determine. Theoretically, a drug with positive inotropic action and vasodilator properties could worsen the physiology associated with LVOTO, possibly creating hypotension, worsening obstruction, or increasing mitral regurgitation. One retrospective study of pimobendan use in cats, along with a variety of background therapies, included cats with various forms of cardiomyopathy, some without obvious echocardiographic evidence of ventricular systolic dysfunction.[7] Only five out of 170 cats experienced potential side effects (i.e., unusual agitation [$n = 2$], anorexia [$n = 1$], vomiting [$n = 1$], or constipation [$n = 1$]). In only one cat was the side effect considered severe enough (unusual agitation) to discontinue the pimobendan, and agitation resolved when the drug was discontinued.[7] The absence of a control group in all three of the retrospective pimobendan studies precludes any definitive comments on whether pimobendan favorably influences survival time.[7-9] However, pimobendan does appear to be well tolerated in cats with CHF due to most forms of cardiomyopathy that are not associated with LVOTO regardless of the presence or absence of ventricular systolic dysfunction. However, safety in cats with LVOTO (e.g., HOCM) cannot be assumed based on available data because too few treated cats with LVOTO have been reported. In one of the retrospective studies, one cat with LVOTO secondary to SAM of the mitral valve experienced tachycardia and hypotension 2 hours after the initial oral dose of pimobendan, which resolved after the drug was discontinued.[8] Thus, pending additional data, use of pimobendan for treatment of CHF characterized by LVOTO should be carried out with caution and likely used predominantly as rescue treatment (e.g., Stage D patients). Likewise, in cats with no echocardiographic diagnosis, LVOTO cannot be ruled out; thus, pimobendan should be reserved for Stage D in this case as well. If used, vital signs and blood pressure should be measured 1 to 2 hours after administration of the first dose.

Some cats with CHF may have previously been treated with atenolol for LVOTO, and some cats with CHF have LVOTO at the time of diagnosis of CHF. If atenolol was previously started in Stage B2, it can be continued in Stage C, although the dose might need to be reduced by 50% if CHF is severe. If control of CHF becomes difficult, some cats may no longer have LVOTO by the time CHF develops, which is likely due to ventricular dilation. Discontinuing atenolol with a subsequent echocardiogram to see if LVOTO has resolved following discontinuation of the drug is one approach to these patients. Atenolol should not be discontinued abruptly, if possible. Most veterinary cardiologists would recommend that atenolol should not be initiated in the face of active CHF. If atenolol is a desired as an adjunctive therapy in a cat with Stage C cardiomyopathy, it should ideally be initiated once the cat is free of clinical signs of CHF (e.g., no evidence of active pulmonary edema, pleural effusion, or pericardial effusion). Likewise, if cats with CHF have been previously treated with diltiazem, it can be continued as long as significant ventricular hypertrophy remains and the drug is well tolerated by the cat. Initiation of diltiazem as adjunctive therapy in a cat with Stage C HCM should only be done once the cat is stable on more standard therapies.

All therapeutic options should be considered in light of the owner's ability and willingness to chronically medicate the cat and the cat's tolerance of the medication(s). Furosemide and ACE-Is can be compounded into a variety of formulations (but not transdermal). There is no data to support the oral bioavailability or stability of compounded pimobendan. The potential role of nutritional management is covered in Chapter 39.

Monitoring of Stage C Patients
Given the potential for recurrence of CHF and disease progression, client education and scheduled follow-up is critical for successful of management of CHF. Stage C cats should have breathing rates assessed daily at home. Development of new clinical signs, or an elevated breathing rate at home (greater than 30 breaths/min), represents an indication for re-evaluation. Periodic re-evaluations, every 3 to 4 months, should be recommended even if the cat remains free of clinical signs and apparently stable to the owner. These appointments provide an opportunity to track disease progression and detect early signs of decompensation or complications of CHF treatment as well as the opportunity to assess owner compliance issues. Infrequently, individual cats may experience stress during appointments or travel, leading to decompensation of CHF. In these cats, limiting the frequency of appointments may be appropriate. In general, if significant changes are made in medications, or following clinical decompensation, a re-evaluation should be made in 7 to 14 days to check for clinical improvement or changes in kidney values or electrolytes. Depending upon the individual case, re-evaluation testing (e.g., thoracic radiographs,

echocardiogram, blood pressure measurement, routine blood tests, and ECG) may be periodically indicated.

Stage D Patients—Cats with Recurrent Clinical Signs of Cardiomyopathy Despite Standard Treatment

Stage D is defined as CHF that has progressed from Stage C and is now refractory to standard CHF therapies and requires additional medication or management. Diagnostic strategies are similar to those discussed previously in Stage C. Specific diagnostic recommendations are based on the prevailing clinical signs that are adversely affecting some aspect of quality of life, but often include thoracic radiographs, echocardiography, and laboratory testing. Management strategies may involve discontinuing medications that might be associated with side effects, escalation of doses of the currently employed medications, use of medications that are less commonly used in cats, trying to find novel ways to deliver medications for owners having difficulty with compliance, and treating anorexia and cachexia (see Chapter 39). If pimobendan has not yet been initiated, this is likely the stage to try the drug. For cats already on pimobendan, a trial of a higher dose can be attempted. In cats with recurrent signs of congestion, higher doses of furosemide can be used (up to 2 to 3 mg/kg every 8 to 12 hours), or replacing one or more daily oral doses of furosemide by subcutaneous injection can be attempted. Spironolactone can be added, although this drug may not be tolerated by all cats (i.e., dermatologic or GI side effects). Hypokalemia contributing to lethargy and weakness can be addressed by the addition of spironolactone and/or potassium supplementation. Sildenafil may be tried in selected cases, especially cats with documented pulmonary hypertension. There is no standard therapy recommended for this stage but rather an opportunity to tailor management strategies to limit clinical signs in each individual cat and discuss possible outcomes with the owner. Consultation with a veterinary cardiologist always has value, but in Stage D it may be of particular benefit.

References

1. Atkins C, Binaural J, Hettinger S, et al: Guidelines for the diagnosis and treatment of canine chronic alular heart disease. *J Vet Intern Med* 23(6):1142–1150, 2009.
2. Bonagura J, Gordon SG, Luethy M, et al: The ABCDs of canine cardiology, *The Cardiac Education Group* (website): <http://www.cardiaceducationgroup.org/recommendations/abcd-chart>, (Accessed May 12, 2015).
3. Gordon SG, Estrada AH: *The ABCDs of small animal cardiology: a practical manual*, Guelph, 2013, LifeLearn.
4. Schober KE, Hart TM, Stern JA, et al: Effects of treatment on respiratory rate, serum natriuretic peptide concentration, and Doppler echocardiographic indices of left ventricular filling pressure in dogs with CHF secondary to degenerative mitral valve disease and dilated cardiomyopathy. *J Am Vet Med Assoc* 239(4):468–479, 2011.
5. Ljungvall I, Rishniw M, Porciello J, et al: Sleeping and resting respiratory rates in healthy adult cats and cats with subclinical heart disease. *J Feline Med Surg* 16(4):281–290, 2014.
6. Schober KE, Zientek J, Li X, et al: Effect of treatment with atenolol on 5-year survival in cats with preclinical (asymptomatic) hypertrophic cardiomyopathy. *J Vet Cardiol* 15(2):93–104, 2013.
7. Macgregor JM, Rush JE, Laste NJ, et al: Use of pimobendan in 170 cats (2006-2010). *J Vet Cardiol* 13(4):251–260, 2011.
8. Gordon SG, Saunders AB, Roland RM, et al: Effect of oral administration of pimobendan in cats with CHF. *J Am Vet Med Assoc* 241(1):89–94, 2012.
9. Hambrook LE, Bennett PF: Effect of pimobendan on the clinical outcome and survival of cats with non-taurine responsive dilated cardiomyopathy. *J Feline Med Surg* 14(4):233–239, 2012.
10. Hanzlicek AS, Gehring R, Kukanich B, et al: Pharmacokinetics of oral pimobendan in healthy cats. *J Vet Cardiol* 14(4):489–496, 2012.

Radiographic and Computed Tomography Imaging of the Feline Thorax

Robert T. O'Brien

Thoracic imaging plays an important part in the clinical evaluation of a cat with suspected cardiopulmonary disease. The decision when, and with what modality, to perform imaging is changing as new technologies allow more sophisticated imaging earlier in the course of patient care. Although radiography will remain the most common modality for some time to come, computed tomography (CT) provides opportunities to improve upon conventional imaging. As described here, CT allows imaging of the upper airway and lungs without an indwelling intravenous catheter anytime in the clinical course.[1,2] Survey CT may also be useful for the evaluation of left atrial size.[3,4] With intravenous access, CT angiography provides better characterization of many diseases with a vascular basis.

This chapter reviews the common radiographic basis of intrathoracic imaging. The advantages and disadvantages of conventional imaging are discussed in comparison with additional modalities. The utility of CT and ultrasound are discussed in the relevant anatomic location. The discussion of echocardiography is beyond the scope of this chapter, but comparative radiographic and CT appearance of heart and heart failure is discussed. More details on echocardiographic imaging may be found in Chapter 46.

IMAGING MODALITIES

Radiography has been the mainstay of thoracic imaging. Most clinicians are able to use the data derived from a radiograph in a positive and productive manner. Radiography is especially valuable for pulmonary disease. However, there are many limitations to the utility of radiography in the clinical setting, especially in emergency situations. The frequent need for orthogonal views requires handling that may pose stress to a feline patient in respiratory distress. The time to take two or more radiographic views is greater than may be necessary for other modalities, such as focused echocardiography or CT. Many diseases lead to border effacement with surrounding structures, including pleural free fluid, alveolar lung disease, and large mass lesions. This limits our ability to view adjacent structures, including the heart and mediastinal organs, via

thoracic radiograph. Fat in the mediastinum may cause border effacement with the heart affecting our ability to accurately judge heart size[5] (Figure 42-1).

Thoracic ultrasound often overcomes many, if not all, of the limitations previously listed for radiography. Ultrasound is used successfully as a part of the extended emergency physical examination in the dyspneic cat. A focused ultrasound examination for pleural free fluid or enlarged left atrium seems warranted early in the work up, assuming that the patient can tolerate the increased handling and that the clinician has sufficient skills to perform focused ultrasonographic imaging efficiently. In many emergency settings, clinicians have variable skill sets with ultrasound. The most basic ultrasound skill is the detection of large volumes of free pleural fluid, which may be drained for both diagnostic and therapeutic purposes. With improved skills, a very limited echocardiogram to evaluate the size of the left atrium is possible. A more extended scan would provide additional characterization of pleural free fluid, alveolar lung disease, and mass lesions. And when these coexisting conditions are present, ultrasound can use these lesions as a window to provide clinically useful images of the mediastinal space and heart. Echocardiography is the gold standard for imaging the heart. Additionally, ultrasound often provides the best means to not merely provide the image of lesions but also to guide needle biopsy or drainage of the lesion. Given the synergy and complementary nature of these two modalities and greater comfort with these two techniques, one might not immediately see the advantage of CT imaging.

In routine nonemergent patients, no other modalities provide the sum of information provided by the combination of radiography and ultrasound. However, these modalities both suffer from many limitations in the emergency clinical situation. First, they both require substantial patient restraint, which is often deemed ill-advised in the distressed feline patient. They both require substantial time, even though limited studies or partial scans can yield valuable data. Both have their technical expertise requirements for image acquisition and image interpretation. Even with the advent of teleradiology and tele-echocardiology, many of these limitations hinge on the skills of the "-ographer" obtaining the image

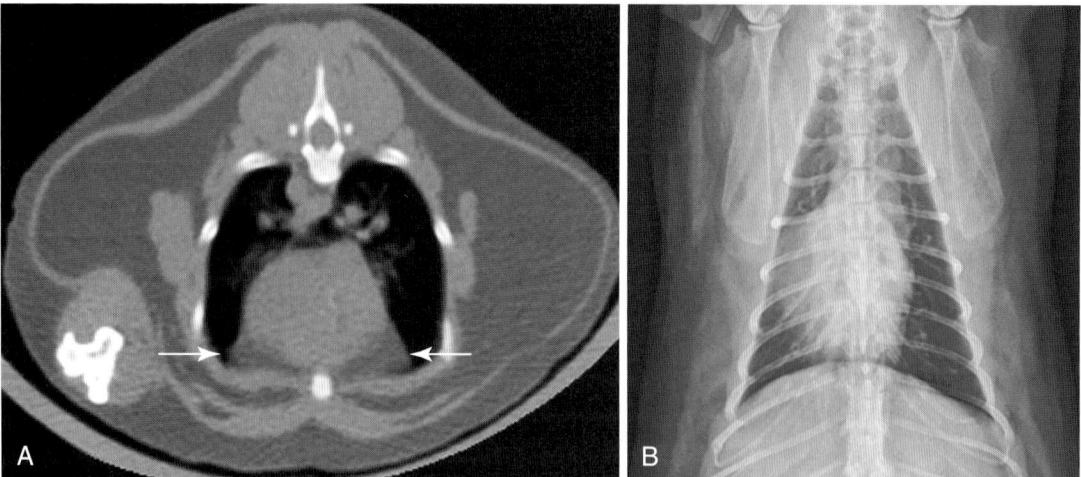

Figure 42-1: Transverse plane computed tomography **(A)** and ventrodorsal (VD) radiograph of obese cat **(B).** Note mediastinal fat *(arrows)* that would artificially augment a vertebral heart scale measurement on a VD radiograph.

set—not the "-ologist" providing the interpretation. The question asked in our clinical environment was as follows: Is there an imaging modality that (1) provides excellent quality lung imaging and can assist with the differentiation of primary heart or secondary lung disease versus other forms of intrathoracic disease causing respiratory distress and (2) provides very fast imaging—with minimal to no patient handling and restraint—and is, therefore, useful in the first few minutes or hours of the clinical evaluation of any feline patient, regardless of the level of respiratory distress?

Computed tomography may provide many of those features, especially in an emergency situation. Depending on the system available, CT can image an entire cat within a few seconds.[1,2] Multislice CT scan systems provide fast images at very high resolution and form the basis of an image set that also allows imaging in additional planar views (e.g., sagittal, dorsal) and three-dimensional image sets that mimic virtual endoscopy (e.g., laryngoscopy, bronchoscopy).[6] Additionally, a recent study has demonstrated potential for evaluating the left atrium : aorta (LA : Ao) ratio of cats using survey CT[3,4] (Figure 42-2).

Augmenting the multislice CT with a motion-limiting device that minimizes handling is necessary for imaging cats in respiratory distress. Based on multiple research and clinical projects, this author has observed that most cats in respiratory distress are more tolerant of being in a limited space than most normal cats. Many institutions have created novel restraint-limiting devices, some of which provide an oxygen enriched environment and visualization of the patient throughout the CT imaging.[2] The imaging features of CT will be contrasted and compared to conventional imaging for each anatomic location in the subsequent subsections. It may be that practices with access to high-speed multislice CT equipment, a suitable restraint device, and a highly experienced technologist may find that the ability to image an alert cat with limited restraint compares favorably with routine radiography and ultrasound from a diagnostic perspective.

THE HEART

Using either subjective or objective criteria, radiography is both insensitive and nonspecific for cardiomegaly in cats. Many cats have substantial disease on echocardiography, but the heart appears to be of normal size on radiographs. Similarly, if fat within the mediastinum is not accounted for, the size of the cardiac silhouette will appear large in obese cats without heart enlargement.[6] If the viewer accounts for body condition, radiographs can be used more accurately. Subjective assessment of cardiac enlargement is challenging; however, a "lordotic" (concave shape) caudal heart border on a lateral projection is commonly associated with left atrial enlargement. The vertebral heart scale (VHS) system has been used with varying success in cats. The normal cat has an upper limit of 8.0 vertebra (combined length and width) on the lateral projection and 3.9 vertebra based on the heart width on the ventrodorsal (VD) view.[7] A recent manuscript reinforced the principle that measuring the heart on a lateral projection poses limitations.[8] In this study, 22% of cats with an enlarged heart had a VHS of less than 8.1 and a highly-specific diagnosis of cardiomegaly was reached only using a VHS greater than 9.3. In this author's opinion, using the VHS system on the VD projection is more clinically useful. A VHS greater than 4.0 is highly specific for cardiomegaly, assuming that mediastinal fat can be accounted for.[9]

If radiographs are often equivocal for cardiac enlargement, can we do better without echocardiography? Preliminary information indicates that CT may be better than radiography. In cats, there is a persistent fat density surrounding the aorta at the level of the aortic valve, allowing differentiation between the left atrium and aorta[4] (see Figure 42-2). Even without correcting for obliquity and nontraditional echocardiography plane imaging, good correlation was seen between echocardiography and CT for LA : Ao ratio.[3] Survey CT also provided excellent definition of the lungs and pleural and

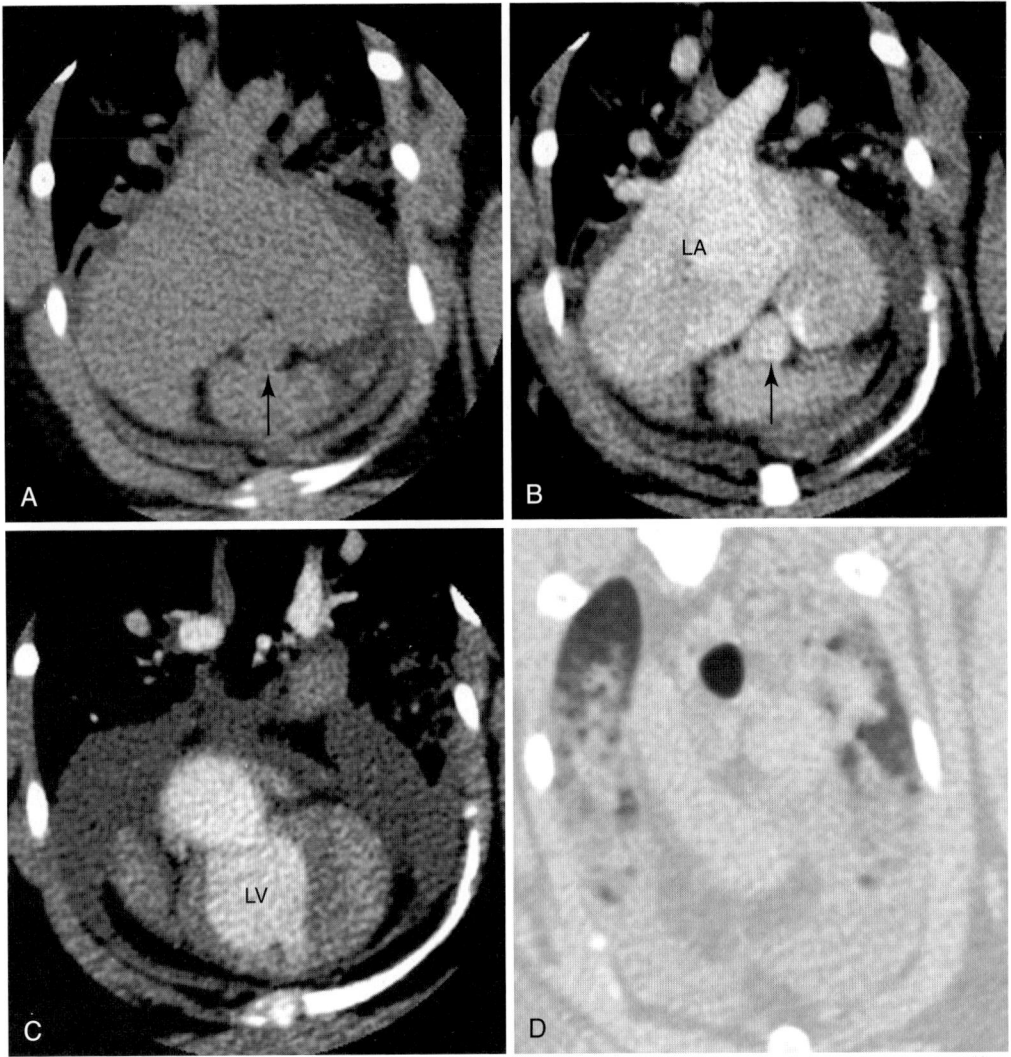

Figure 42-2: Computed tomography (CT) images of a cat with restrictive cardiomyopathy. Note well delineated aorta *(black arrow)* on survey CT image **(A)**. On postcontrast CT images, note enlarged left atrium *(LA)* compared to size of aorta *(black arrow)* **(B)** and normal thickness left ventricular *(LV)* free wall **(C)**. Note concurrent severe pulmonary edema on lung windowed image **(D)**.

mediastinal spaces, adding to the information derived from this quite quick study (approximately 10 seconds). Adding a contrast CT angiographic phase to the study provided information of left ventricular wall thicknesses. This study was performed with a multislice CT scanner (16 slices) and using a unique motion-limiting device (VetMouseTrap).

LUNGS

Radiography is the mainstay of lung disease characterization. The most common and traditional method of lung interpretation is the "pattern approach." The patterns used to characterize disease on radiographs include alveolar, bronchial, structured interstitial, and unstructured interstitial. Following the assignation of a pattern is the characterization of a distribution, which may be valuable in redefining disease categorization.

The alveolar pattern may be, at the same time, the most commonly missed pattern and the most prevalent clinically significant pattern in cats. That means the diseases causing this pattern are often not listed as differentials, thereby limiting the value of radiography. Any disease that fills alveoli will cause border effacement with adjacent structures, such as the bronchial wall (causing air bronchograms), pulmonary vessels, heart, and diaphragm. Air bronchograms are not necessary components of an alveolar pattern, but they are helpful when present. The differentials for an alveolar pattern are recalled using the acronym "HELP" (i.e., hemorrhage, edema, lymphoma [or other pulmonary neoplasia], pneumonia).

Of particular note is the prevalence of multifocal patchy alveolar patterns in cats (Figure 42-3). This pattern and distribution is quite common and can be caused by cardiogenic pulmonary edema, atypical infectious pneumonia, or primary pulmonary neoplasia. The three are indistinguishable unless concurrent lesions, such as cardiomegaly, are present.[10]

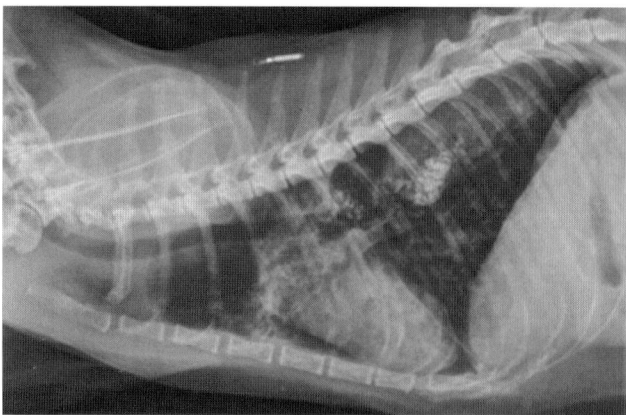

Figure 42-3: Lateral radiograph of cat with bronchogenic carcinoma. Note patchy alveolar pattern in multiple lobes with evidence of mineralization.

Mineralization within the lesions is not seen with cardiogenic edema and would limit the differential to more chronic infiltration lesions. The confidence of characterizing a cat having congestive heart failure, based on the size of the left atrium and concurrent compatible lung lesions, is substantially higher with CT or focused echocardiography than with radiography alone (see Figure 42-2).

As cats age, there is a certain prevalence and variable severity of dystrophic mineralization of bronchial walls, and thus assessment of a bronchial pattern can become tricky. In other words, "how much mineralization is too much?" The author uses clinical features to sway image interpretation as much as the images themselves. More severe clinical signs (e.g., cough), more severe respiratory effort, and the lack of any other lesions on thoracic and lateral neck images suggest a diagnosis of lower airway disease. The classic radiographic findings with lower airway disease are often listed as either hyperinflation (in the acute severe manifestation) or moderate-to-severe diffuse bronchial pattern. However, the author also adds a "normal" radiographic appearance to the list of possibilities for a cat afflicted with lower airway disease. Additional features of lower airway disease include lung lobe collapse (Figure 42-4) and bronchiectasis. Lung lobe collapse, if severe and chronic, takes on the appearance of a pleural fissure line and there is often no mediastinal shift. Bronchiectasis and concurrent bronchial plug formation are important factors affecting prognosis.

Structured interstitial lesions are basically masses. Ranging in size from a millet seed (i.e., miliary pattern) to a very large mass, differentials for structured interstitial lesions can be listed using the acronym "CHANG" (i.e., cyst, hematoma, abscess, neoplasia, granuloma). In cats, the most prevalent differentials seem to be granuloma and neoplasia.

The last pattern has traditionally been the most commonly applied pattern, albeit it may be the least prevalent in cats. Similar to the bronchial pattern, a certain amount of pulmonary fibrosis is a normal aging change. So, many clinicians assign an assessment of "mild bronchointerstitial" pattern

rather than accepting the pattern as a normal age-related event. Again, the challenge is correctly assessing "how much is too much?" The unstructured interstitial pattern, as a standalone pattern, is quite unusual in cats. Lymphoma is reported to have this pattern, as does mild edema. However, understanding that all edema begins adjacent to the capillaries in the interstitial space, the author believes that cats with clinically-relevant pulmonary edema also have an alveolar component. The author and colleagues have recently encountered a few cats with forms of pulmonary fibrosis without an underlying known cause. These cats have a very intense, diffuse reticular interstitial pattern (Figure 42-5).

Ultrasound is uncommonly used as an initial test to assess the lung for parenchymal disease. Ultrasound is especially helpful when there is pleural fluid to assess the thoracic cavity for concurrent pulmonary abnormalities. The differentiation of various forms of infiltrative lung disease is very difficult using ultrasound. There is very little in the literature that makes us confident that ultrasound description alone provides a prioritized differential diagnosis. However, ultrasound is the gold standard for guiding fluid drainages and minimally-invasive needle biopsy sampling of mass lesions.

Does CT provide any advantages over conventional imaging for pulmonary diseases? In one study, CT was superior to radiographs for the characterization of lung lesions and for the characterization of concurrent lung lesions in cats with pleural free fluid.[1] In this study, the value of CT was aided by combining survey and postcontrast imaging. Computed tomography has improved sensitivity for detecting pulmonary lesions, although the clinical significance of very small lesions or very mild disease could be debated. In this same report of cats with respiratory-related signs, CT was superior for characterizing pulmonary disease, including the detection of regional emphysema (regional lung density less than −900 HU) in cats with lower airway disease. Again, the clinical significance of these lesions was not known. Computed tomography seems the best modality for detection and characterization of thickened bronchial wall, bronchial plugs, and lobe collapse (see Figure 42-4). Probably the most important aspect of this clinical study was the positive clinical attributes of CT. Computed tomography imaging was performed earlier and with less perceived stress to cats in respiratory distress compared to radiography. In a motion-limiting device, cats were imaged without any perceived morbidity. Although many image sets had nontraditional original image planes (oblique transverse), CT provided more detailed imaging and more accurate information compared to radiography. As a tool for imaging cats in respiratory distress, clinicians at the author's institution often prefer CT over radiography. The only disadvantage of CT imaging, depending on the hospital fee schedule, is cost to the client.

PLEURAL SPACE

Radiography is quite sensitive for detection of moderate and severe pleural free fluid. However, small volumes may be

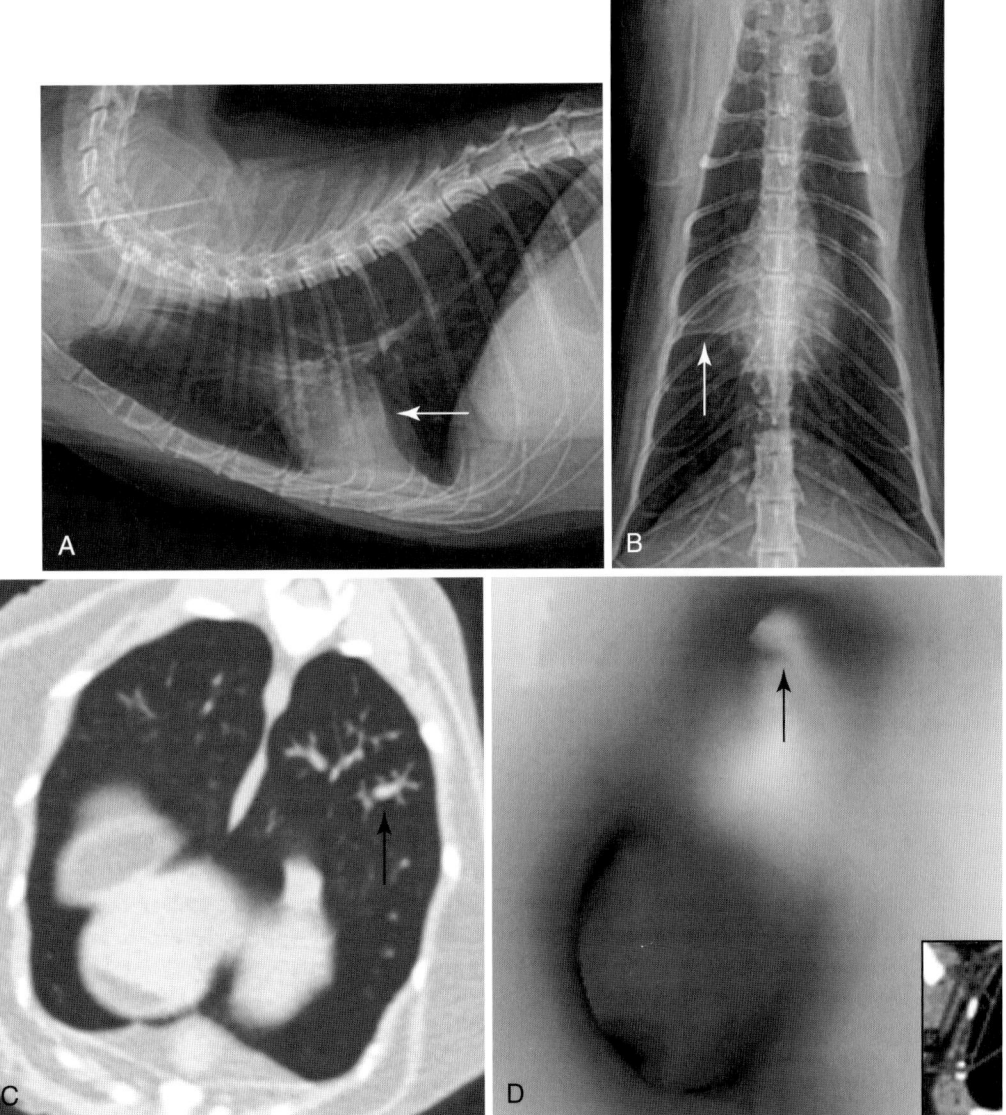

Figure 42-4: Radiographs **(A** and **B)** and computed tomography (CT) **(C** and **D)** images of cat with asthma. Note collapse of the right middle lung lobe *(white arrows)* on the radiographs **(A** and **B)** and three-dimensional internal volume rendered *(black arrow)* **(D).** Note thickened bronchi with plugged lumen *(black arrow)* on transverse plane CT image **(C).**

occult or confused with other diseases. The radiographic features of pleural fluid include (1) pleural fissure lines (fluid between two layers of visceral pleura), (2) retraction of the lung from the body wall (fluid between visceral and parietal pleura), (3) widening of the mediastinum (fluid between visceral and mediastinal pleura), and (4) border effacement. Unfortunately, these features are shared by many other diseases. Fissure lines are seen as a normal age-related change (pleural fibrosis) and are often mistakenly identified with severe lung lobe atelectasis (especially the right middle lobe). Lung lobes are retracted from the chest wall in very obese cats by adipose tissue. Widening of the mediastinum has many causes, including mediastinal masses. Finally, border effacement is seen with all causes of the alveolar pattern and

some large mass lesions. Although quite rare, pleural mass lesions are usually occult with radiography.

Radiography can often provide additional clinical information beyond the mere diagnosis of pleural free fluid. Rounding of lung lobes may be pathologic. Many normal lung lobes have rounded margins (e.g., the cranial aspect of the cranial lobes and ventral margins of most lobes). However, the caudodorsal margins of the caudal lobe should be very angular, and the angle should be even sharper when the lung retracts with pleural free fluid. Therefore, rounding of the caudodorsal lung margins is a sign of fibrosing pleuritis (i.e., restrictive pleuritis) (Figure 42-6). The most common differential diagnoses include chylothorax and pyothorax, although any chronic fluid may predispose to fibrin deposition. Aggressive testing, including fluid cytology and evaluation of concurrent heart and mediastinal lesions, should be undertaken to reach the underlying diagnosis.

Ultrasound is superior for detecting, characterizing, and providing the means of acquiring pleural free fluid. Although the echogenicity of the fluid does not always correlate with cellularity, very echogenic fluid with linear echogenic lesions is associated with chronic inflammatory fluids. Ultrasound often provides valuable information on underlying causes of pleural free fluid, including primary lung, mediastinal, body wall, and cardiac lesions.

One of the big advantages of CT imaging is the ability to characterize separate but concurrent lesions. Computed tomography is vastly superior to radiography for "seeing through the fluid." For this benefit to be realized, the addition of contrast is often necessary. Without contrast enhancement, a collapsed and infiltrated lung may have the same attenuation as pleural fluid. With contrast enhancement, the lung will have higher attenuation, providing differentiation between the lung and surrounding fluid (Figure 42-7). Similarly, many foreign bodies have higher attenuation values than surrounding soft tissues, allowing identification of the cause of pyothorax (Figure 42-8).

MEDIASTINAL MASSES

The radiographic diagnosis of a mediastinal mass depends on the size and location of the mass. Masses in the ventral mediastinum (e.g., sternal lymph nodes or cysts) are detected at smaller sizes than similar-sized masses more dorsally located, especially on lateral projections. The sternal lymph node is typically located dorsal to the junction of the second and third sternebrae and bears particular mention due to an unobvious drainage origin. The sternal lymph node drains the cranial abdomen, pleural space, diaphragm, body wall, and pericardium. Lesions in the midcranial mediastinum may be occult until they reach a moderate size and cause widening, and convex shape, of the left and right borders on VD and dorsoventral projections and ventral deviation of the mediastinal border on lateral projections. Ultrasound is a very useful tool to confirm a mediastinal lesion and guide interventional procedures. As previously noted, CT is superior to radiography for characterizing the size of the normal structures and lesions in the mediastinum (Figure 42-9). Computed tomography angiography is often very valuable for characterizing the vascular characteristics of mass or primary vascular lesions.

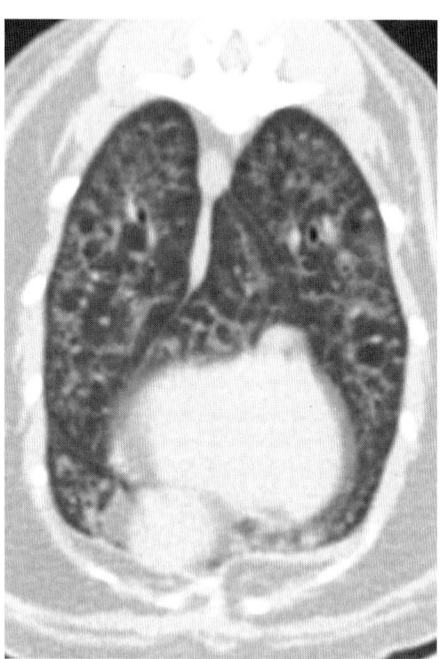

Figure 42-5: Computed tomography transverse plane image of cat with idiopathic fibrosis. Note severe, diffuse, reticular interstitial lung pattern.

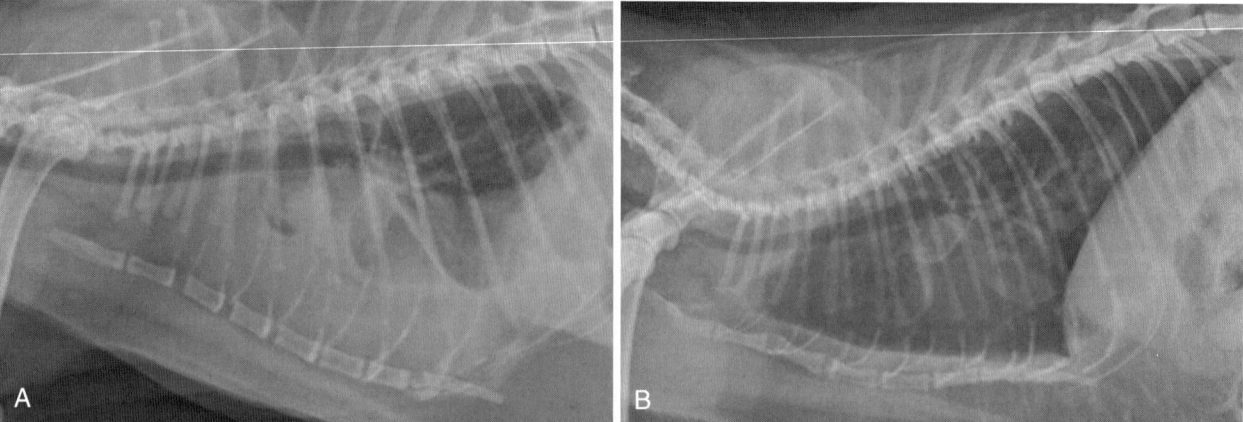

Figure 42-6: Prethoracocentesis **(A)** and post-thoracocentesis **(B)** lateral projection radiographic images of cat with fibrosing pleuritis secondary to chronic chylothorax. Note lack of lung expansion on post-thoracocentesis image **(B)** and iatrogenic pneumothorax.

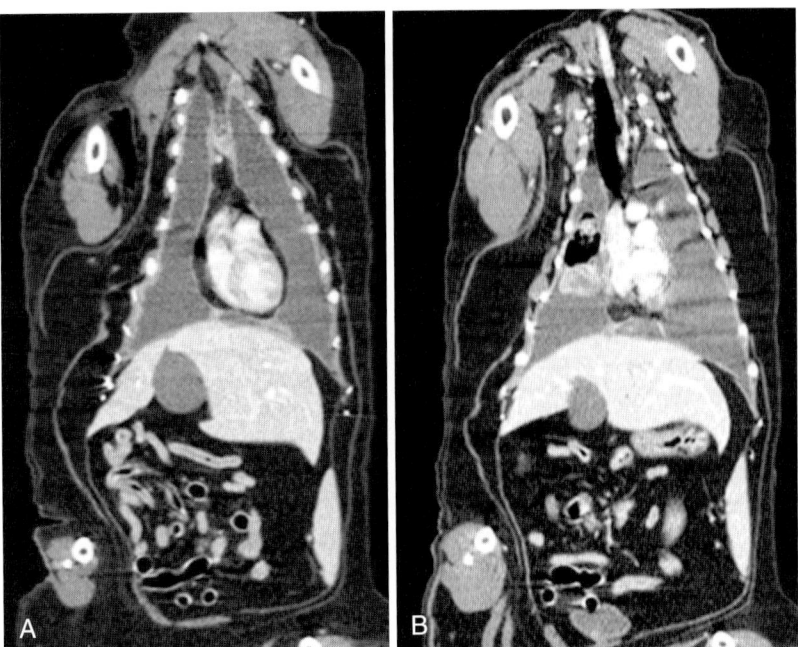

Figure 42-7: A and **B,** Dorsal plane computed tomography multiplanar reconstruction images of a cat with bronchogenic carcinoma and pleural free fluid. Note contrast-enhanced mass in right lung.

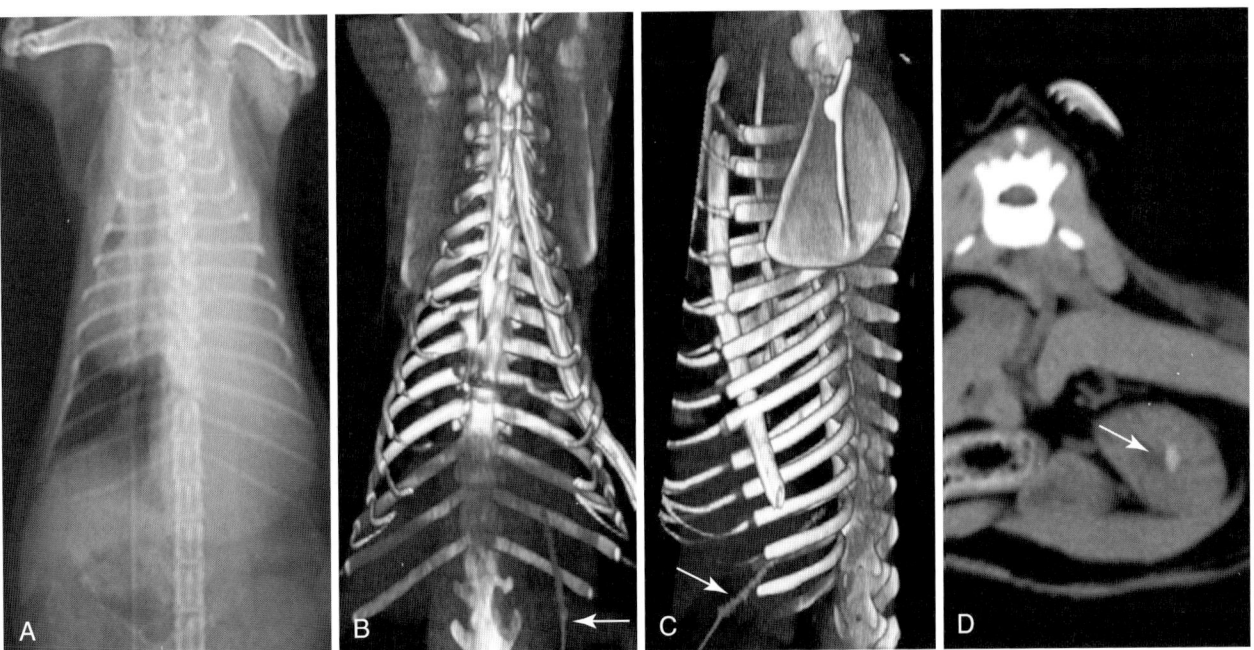

Figure 42-8: Ventrodorsal radiograph **(A)** prethoracocentesis and post–chest tube placement computed tomography images **(B through D)** of a cat with pyothorax due to penetrating wood (stick) foreign body. Note linear foreign object in three-dimensional reconstruction images (**B** and **C,** *white arrows*) originating from gastric lumen (**D,** *white arrow*).

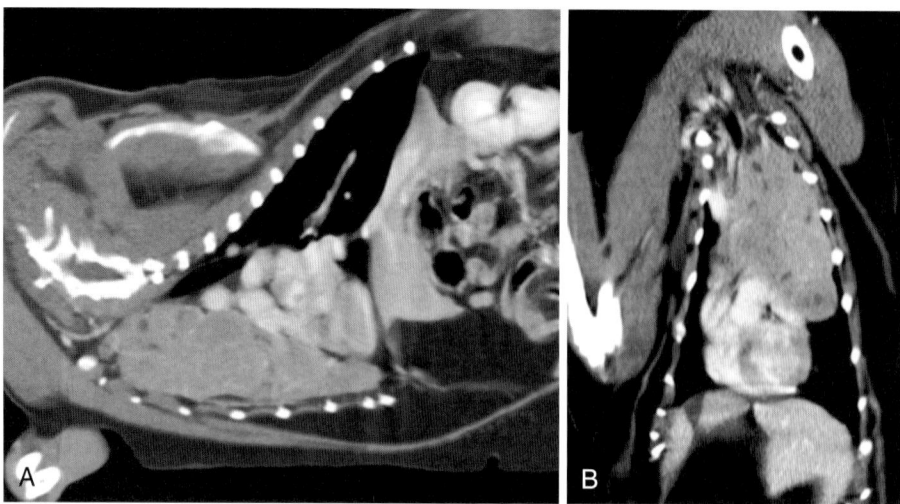

Figure 42-9: A and **B,** Computed tomography reconstructed images of a large mediastinal mass (thymoma) in a cat.

References

1. Oliveira CR, Mitchell MA, O'Brien RT: Thoracic computed tomography in feline patients without use of chemical restraint. *Vet Radiol Ultrasound* 52(4):368–376, 2011.
2. Oliveira CR, Ranallo FN, Pijanowski GJ, et al: The VetMousetrap: a device for computed tomographic imaging of the thorax of awake cats. *Vet Radiol Ultrasound* 52(1):41–52, 2011.
3. O'Brien RT, O'Brien MA, Rapoport G: *Comparison of microdose computed tomographic cardiac angiography and echocardiography in cats with cardiomyopathy,* Portugal, 2013, Cascais.
4. Rodriguez KT, O'Brien MA, Hartman SK, et al: Microdose computed tomographic cardiac angiography in normal cats. *J Vet Cardiol* 16:19–25, 2014.
5. Litster AL, Buchanan JW: Radiographic and echocardiographic measurement of the heart in obese cats. *Vet Radiol Ultrasound* 41(4):320–325, 2000.
6. Stadler K, O'Brien RT: Computed tomography of nonanesthetized cats with upper airway obstruction. *Vet Radiol Ultrasound* 54(3):231–236, 2013.
7. Litster AL, Buchanan JW: Vertebral scale system to measure heart size in radiographs of cats. *J Am Vet Med Assoc* 216(2):210–214, 2000.
8. Sleeper MM, Roland R, Drobatz KJ: Use of the vertebral heart scale for differentiation of cardiac and noncardiac causes of respiratory distress in cats: 67 cases (2002-2003). *J Am Vet Med Assoc* 242(3):366–371, 2013.
9. Litster AL, Buchanan JW: Radiographic and echocardiographic measurement of the heart in obese cats. *Vet Radiol Ultrasound* 41(4):320–325, 2000.
10. O'Brien RT: *Thoracic radiology for the small animal practitioner,* Jackson, WY, 2001, Teton NewMedia.

Feline Heartworm Disease

SeungWoo Jung and Ray Dillon

EPIDEMIOLOGY AND LIFE CYCLE

Dirofilaria immitis (*D. immitis*) infection has been reported worldwide in cats wherever canine heartworms have been observed. Cats are at greatest risk in endemic areas where repeated bites by infected mosquitoes occur. Indoor and outdoor cats are at similar risk for infection. There is no difference in prevalence between male and female cats, although in experimental infections, male cats have a tendency toward a higher worm burden than females when infected with an equal number of larvae.[1] When mosquitoes carrying microfilariae feed on a cat, the infective third-stage larvae (L3) enter the cat through the bite wound. The L3 moult to the infected fourth and fifth stages (L4 and L5, respectively) and migrate to the pulmonary arteries as immature adults, approximately 70 to 90 days after infection.[2] The frequency of fully mature adult feline heartworm infection correlates with that of dogs in the same geographic area, but at a lower incidence.[3] Serological studies of randomly selected cats using a commercial feline heartworm antibody test found an antibody prevalence of 4.2% to 15.9%.[2,4] Reasons for the lower prevalence of adult heartworms in the cat include an innate resistance and poor host susceptibility to *D. immitis*.[5] The belief that adult heartworms in cats have a shortened life span was based on limited experimental studies. However, by evaluating infected cats using antigen testing and echocardiography, Venco and colleagues demonstrated that client-owned cats infected with mature adult heartworms required approximately 4 years or longer to clear the infections.[6]

Once infected, the cat's natural resistance results in a shortened period of patent microfilaremia. Experimentally, the percentage of infective L3 developing into adult worms is lower in cats than it is in dogs.[7] The clinical adult worm burden typically is less in the cat (usually one to nine worms) than it is in the dog. The average time for infective larvae to develop into circulating microfilariae in experimental feline infections is about 8 months.[7] Thus, microfilaremia is uncommon (<20%), inconsistent, and transient in cats (1 to 2 months), and very low numbers are usually produced.[7] The comparable development period in the dog is 5 to 6.5 months. The immature adult heartworm is only 1 to 2 cm in length when it arrives in the pulmonary arteries 70 to 90 days after infection.[5] There is higher mortality of the L5 that arrive in the distal pulmonary arteries in the cat compared with those in the dog. High mortality of immature adult heartworms is

associated with an intense pulmonary bronchial and parenchymal response, which has been termed heartworm-associated respiratory disease (HARD; Figure 43-1).[7] Residual pulmonary pathology related to HARD persists even after immature heartworms die. Thus many heartworm infections in cats may be misdiagnosed as feline asthma.

When positive heartworm infections are defined by the presence of fully mature adult heartworms, the prevalence in cats is less common than it is in canine heartworm infections. However, if assessed by respiratory diseases secondary to immature adult worms, then the incidence of heartworm disease in the cat and the dog is typically identical for any given area.[1-4]

PATHOPHYSIOLOGY AND CLINICAL FEATURES

Heartworm disease in cats is characterized by pulmonary eosinophilic bronchial and interstitial reaction associated with immature adults (3 to 6 months after infection), chronic lung changes associated with mature adult heartworms (6 months to 4 years after infection), and acute respiratory distress associated with the death of worms of any age. The initial arrival of immature adults in the small pulmonary vessels of the lungs is associated with an intense eosinophilic pulmonary reaction and chronic bronchial damage, resulting in clinical signs at 3 to 4 months after infection.[8] These initial responses are documented not only in cats that develop fully mature adult heartworms 6 months after infection but also in those that never develop mature adult heartworm infections.[9] Lesions associated with HARD are initiated by immature larvae as early as 70 to 90 days after infection.[7] The lesions in HARD are characterized by peribronchial fibrosis, interstitial actin-positive myofibroblasts, and fibrosis of alveolar struts (see Figure 43-1).[10] Muscular hypertrophy, villous endarteritis, and adventitial cellular infiltrates are common histopathological findings in all pulmonary arteries, although the caudal pulmonary arteries are most often identified radiographically.[11] However, pulmonary hypertension rarely occurs, and right-sided congestive heart failure is infrequent, indicating that severe cor pulmonale is uncommon. A bronchial ring reactivity study reported the increased wall-to-lumen ratios in bronchioles and peripheral arterioles in heartworm-infected cats, and decreased response of the bronchioles to contraction or relaxation.[12] The respiratory disease in these cats was more attributable to infiltrative interstitial lung

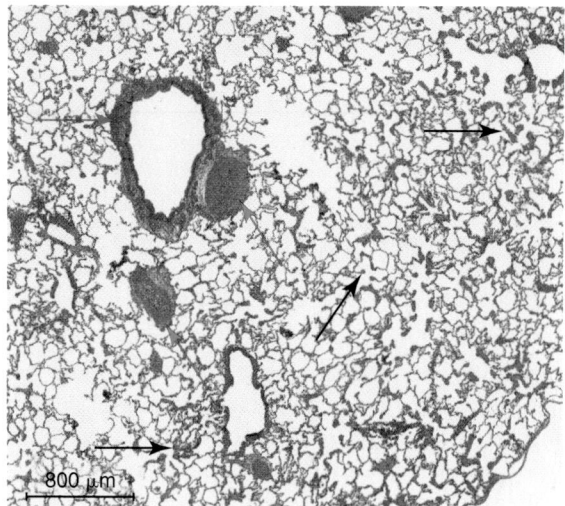

Figure 43-1: Pulmonary histopathology consistent with heartworm-associated respiratory disease in a cat with occult infection; notice the severe peribronchial interstitial lesions (*blue arrow*), pulmonary arterial hypertrophy (*green arrows*), and interstitial fibrosis (*black arrows*). Hematoxylin and eosin stain.

disease and reduced clearance of mucus and inflammatory debris, rather than substantially increased bronchiolar wall reactivity as proposed in asthma models.[12] A subsequent study demonstrated that heartworm homogenate alone in heartworm-negative cats blunted normal bronchial ring contraction and relaxation, which suggests a direct innate response of the lung to heartworm by-products.[11]

Wolbachia are gram-negative bacteria that reside within the body of *D. immitis* and belong to the order Rickettsiales.[13] In both experimental and natural heartworm infections in cats, circulating antibodies against a major surface protein of *Wolbachia* appear within 2 months of exposure to infective larvae.[14] *Wolbachia* have been postulated to produce an acute inflammatory response at bronchial, vascular, and parenchymal levels.[15] The release of bacteria following worm death has shown to cause upregulation of proinflammatory cytokines, neutrophil recruitment, and an increase in specific immunoglobulins, although the role of this intracellular bacteria alone in the pathogenesis of feline heartworm infection is unclear.[16,17] Heartworm-positive dogs treated with doxycycline for *Wolbachia* and melarsomine for *D. immitis* had less pulmonary pathology than dogs treated with melarsomine alone.[18]

Clinical features of heartworm disease are nonspecific but often include intermittent coughing or vomiting, and these signs are most commonly associated with immature heartworms arriving in the lungs or death of adult heartworms. The initial arrival of L5 in the distal pulmonary arteries induces diffuse pulmonary infiltrates and often eosinophilic pneumonitis.[19] Clinical signs associated with this acute phase subside as the worms mature, but histopathological lesions are apparent even in those cats that clear the infection. Cats developing adult heartworm infections have a downregulation of the pulmonary intravascular macrophages that suppress the inflammatory reaction in the lung.[8] Most cats with

mature adult heartworm infections will be asymptomatic during most of the infection. Adult heartworm death, however, may induce acute, potentially fatal disease. In a linear study of client-owned cats with adult heartworms, approximately 75% of cats eliminated adult heartworm infections without any life-threatening disease over a 48-month observation.[6] However, approximately 20% of the cats died in response to adult heartworms in the study. The death of as little as one adult worm can cause acute circulatory collapse, clinically significant respiratory distress, and death of the infected cat.

Anorexia and lethargy may be the only presenting signs. In chronic infections, vomiting or respiratory signs predominate. In a regional study of client-owned cats presented to veterinary practices for coughing or intermittent vomiting, 40% were antibody positive for feline heartworm infection.[20] When vomiting occurs, it tends to be sporadic and unrelated to eating. Release of inflammatory mediators and stimulation of the chemoreceptor trigger zone have been postulated as the cause of vomiting.[2]

DIAGNOSTIC TESTS

Because of low worm burdens, a definitive diagnosis of feline heartworm infection is often challenging. A heart murmur or a gallop sound may be heard over the sternum.[21] Exercise intolerance and right-sided congestive heart failure are rare, although pleural effusion and even chylothorax have been documented. The peripheral eosinophilia is transient, and it depends on the stage of infective larvae, occurring most commonly 4 to 7 months after infection, and it does not correlate with an eosinophilic bronchoalveolar lavage (BAL) cytology.[22] The absence of eosinophilia does not exclude a diagnosis of feline heartworms, but the presence of eosinophilia and basophilia together is highly suggestive. Clinical diagnosis of early disease is difficult at this stage in the cat because the radiographic lesion is a diffuse bronchial to interstitial pattern.[21] Serum biochemistries and urinalysis are usually normal.[22] Hyperglobulinemia occurs in some cats but not consistently or predictably.

Because microfilaremia is characterized by short duration and low numbers, most cats with heartworms are not microfilaremic when evaluated.[1,7] A positive blood test for microfilariae is unlikely but diagnostic when present. Diagnostic accuracy is increased when large quantities of blood are evaluated by concentration tests such as modified Knott's tests or filter techniques. Even with repetitive testing, the majority of cats with heartworm disease are amicrofilaremic (occult infection).

Given the high incidence of occult infection in the cat, serological tests can be valuable. Because antibody is produced by the cat in response to the early migration of the L3 or L4, positive titers are detected about 2 to 3 months after infection, even if the L4 die and never become L5.[23] Most cats will be antibody positive for 3 to 6 months after infection. If all immature adults induce HARD and die, the antibody titer will gradually become negative over the next 3 to 8 months.[19] Most cats with fully mature adult heartworms will be antibody positive for the duration of the infection. Generally, cats will be antibody negative 6 to 9 months after all adult worms are eliminated.

A positive antibody result indicates that a cat has been infected with L3, the L3 has moulted into L4, and the parasite has lived at least 2 to 3 months.[23] Adult heartworms may or may not have developed from this infection. When the use of macrolides as a preventive medication has been initiated 30 days after infection, larvae can live long enough to initiate positive antibody response and yet be killed by the macrolide with no immature adults developing in the pulmonary arteries. This produces an antibody-positive response in cats on preventative medications after the mosquito season, although the cat does not have adult heartworms. Treatment with preventative medication at least 1 month before infection will kill the infective larvae before detectable antibody has developed, and cats on year-round prevention should be antibody negative even if bitten by a mosquito with infective larvae.[11] However, for a variety of reasons, occasionally a cat with fully mature adult heartworms will be antibody negative on all diagnostic platforms. Infected cats can also produce antibodies against the surface protein of *Wolbachia*.[14,16] However, serological testing for *Wolbachia* has no clinical diagnostic advantage over heartworm antibody testing because both become positive during L4 to L5 subcutaneous migration.

The use of enzyme-linked immunosorbent assay for antigen detection to confirm infections has been helpful. Because antigen tests are specific for glycoproteins mainly associated with the reproductive tract of fully mature adult female worms, false-negative results are common. The antigen test is usually positive if there are three or more mature female worms. False-negative test results may be found in sexually immature infections (less than 7 months old), low worm burden, or male-only infections. Thus, cats presented with HARD from immature adults will be antigen negative, and 3 to 6 months after immature adult worm death, they also will be antibody negative.[8,19] Cats with active adult heartworm disease often test negative for antigen because adult heartworm infection classically involves low numbers of worms. Thus a positive antigen test can be considered diagnostic, but a negative test does not rule out heartworms.

Eosinophilic cytology (greater than 16% of nucleated cells) on BAL fluid is associated with the precardiac migrating stages of heartworms, arrival of immature adults in pulmonary arteries, adult heartworm infections, and the death of adult heartworms. The most intense eosinophilic response is typically 3 to 6 months after infection and is intermittent in chronic infections. Peripheral eosinophilia does not correlate with eosinophilic BAL cytology. Further, eosinophilic cytology on BAL was demonstrated in cats that were experimentally infected, despite being on preventative medication.[24]

Radiology is a useful adjunctive test in cats with high index of suspicion of heartworm infection. Pulmonary parenchymal changes are nonspecific and can change rapidly in infected

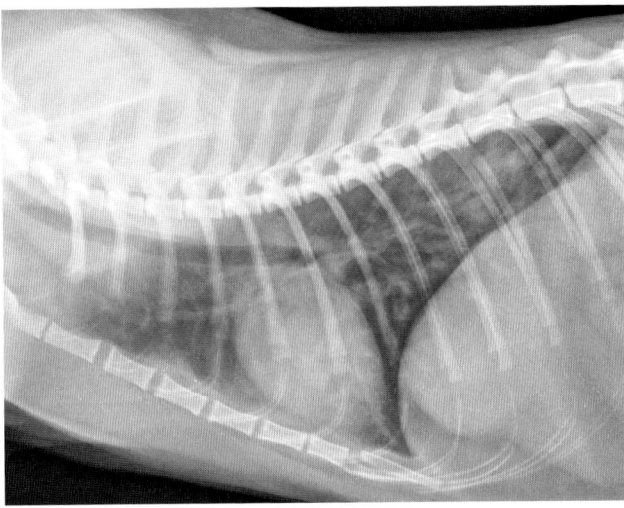

Figure 43-2: Right lateral radiograph taken 110 days after L3 infection in a cat that did not receive preventative medication; notice the enlarged pulmonary arteries and increased interstitial density.

cats. These changes include interstitial infiltrates, peribronchial disease, and enlarged pulmonary arteries associated with perivascular densities (Figure 43-2).[25] The most consistent radiographic sign is enlarged pulmonary arteries, although this finding is not specific for feline heartworm disease. This finding is most prominent in the caudal lung lobes on the ventrodorsal view. Blunted or tortuous pulmonary arteries are occasionally noted but not as commonly as in the dog. Heartworm-associated respiratory disease associated with immature adults that do not develop into adult infections have the identical radiographic lesions seen in cats with fully mature adult heartworms. Further, the histopathological changes in the lung parenchyma, bronchiole, and pulmonary artery are indistinguishable.

The enlargement of the caudal pulmonary artery may disappear even in the presence of adult heartworms over a period of several months as the initial inflammatory disease abates. Nonselective angiography may demonstrate enlarged pulmonary arteries and pulmonary occlusion. Cardiac changes such as right-side heart enlargement on radiographs are rare. In the cat with respiratory signs, heartworm disease must be differentiated from *Aelurostrongylus abstrusus* infection, *Paragonimus kellicotti* infection, *Toxocara cati* infection, bronchitis, asthma, pleural effusion, pulmonary edema, and other systemic disorders.[26,27] In particular, lungworm and roundworm infections can mimic clinical manifestations and radiographic changes seen in heartworm disease (e.g., pulmonary parenchymal infiltrates, bronchial pattern, and enlarged pulmonary arteries).[27]

When adult heartworms are present in the right ventricle or main pulmonary artery, they are readily detectable by echocardiography. Parallel hyperechoic lines, representing an image from the heartworm cuticle, may be observed in the proximal pulmonary arteries, the right ventricle, or rarely the right atrium (Figure 43-3).[23,25] Heartworms in the most distal pulmonary arteries often cannot be visualized. Attempts to distinguish between viable worms and dead worms have been

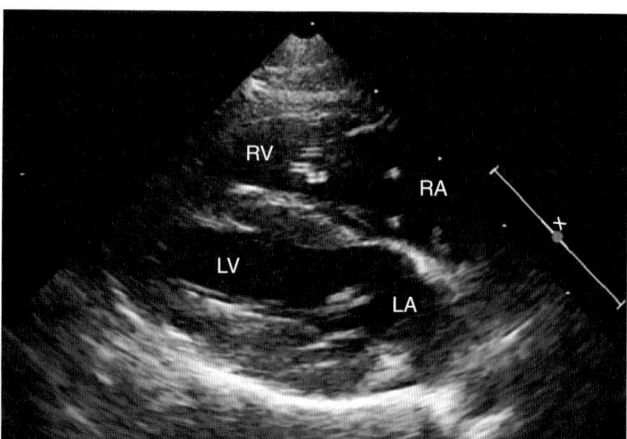

Figure 43-3: Right parasternal echocardiogram visualizing adult heartworms demonstrated as double-lined echodensities in the right side of the heart. *LA*, Left atrium; *LV*, left ventricle; *RA*, right atrium; *RV*, right ventricle.

unsuccessful. Detection of a right axis deviation or right ventricular hypertrophy is rarely present on a standard six-lead surface electrocardiography. Ectopic ventricular beats and other arrhythmias rarely occur.

PREVENTION

The best prevention strategy is to start cats on a monthly preventive product as young as possible and to continue administration for life. Prescribing preventatives year-round or at least recommending prevention methods before the predicted season of transmission will avoid heartworm infection and also should result in negative antibody test results even when the cat is bitten by a mosquito with infective larvae. The reservoir for infection would be mosquitoes actively feeding on infected wildlife or unprotected dogs. Infection from *D. immitis* can be prevented with a macrocyclic lactone formulated for monthly administration (e.g., ivermectin, milbemycin, selamectin, or moxidectin).[28] All prophylactic drugs can be administered in cats without prior testing for heartworm infection. This is because a definitive negative diagnosis is not straightforward, microfilariae are infrequent in cats, and the drugs can be safely administered in cats with adult heartworms. Most preventative agents also have a broad spectrum of activity against a variety of endoparasites and ectoparasites.

In cats, heartworm-preventative drugs should be considered to both prevent a patent infection and prevent HARD. When cats were infected with L3 heartworms experimentally and treated with monthly selamectin 28 days after infection, selamectin treatment prevented the development of adult heartworms, but these cats still seroconverted to an antibody-positive status.[29] One study demonstrated that cats pretreated with selamectin 32 and 2 days before the L3 infection did not develop HARD, and this treatment prevented seroconversion to a positive heartworm antibody titer. The clinical

implication of the study is that successful elimination of heartworm larvae with heartworm preventatives initiated at least 1 month before the risk of infection may prevent seroconversion to heartworm antibody and HARD.[24,30]

CLINICAL MANAGEMENT

The decision to treat feline heartworm infection is often complicated by the unpredictable nature of the disease and the risks of treatment.[22] The drug-induced death of adult heartworms frequently results in acute respiratory distress in cats.[1] Melarsomine dihydrochloride should not be administered to cats because no safe protocol has been determined. Symptomatic alleviation of coughing or vomiting with corticosteroids is generally successful, but it will not prevent the acute clinical signs associated with adult heartworm death. Conservative management of adult worms allows worms to die spontaneously over months to years, with the residual risk of acute crisis. The majority of cats will tolerate the eventual elimination of adult worms. Although the natural death of the adult worms can be associated with severe respiratory signs, most cats will recover without severe complications. In cases of intermittent clinical signs, owners should be educated about the nature of acute signs related to heartworm death. Prednisolone (1 to 2 mg/kg orally, daily for 10 days) can be used successfully in some infected cats to treat coughing and vomiting; however, radiographic lesions usually progress, and acute respiratory distress and death are not prevented. The onset of acute respiratory signs is a true emergency requiring immediate care, including oxygen therapy, cage rest, small volumes of intravenous fluids, and injectable corticosteroids. This therapy may improve clinical and radiographic signs within 24 hours in most cats with life-threatening dyspnea and collapse. However, peracute deaths are not uncommon in the absence of any previous clinical signs.

Because *Wolbachia* is considered a potential complication of pulmonary inflammation in the course of filarial disease, elimination with antibiotic therapy may be beneficial.[31] Combined ivermectin and doxycycline treatment has shown microfilaricidal and adulticidal effects against *D. immitis* in experimentally infected dogs.[32] Doxycycline treatment in combination with monthly preventative medications may, as in the dog, shorten the expected life span of adult heartworms in cats. If this method is attempted, the owner should be advised of the risk that doxycycline capsules or tablets could cause esophageal strictures unless administered with a bolus of food or water.

Invasive procedures to remove adult worms should be reserved for cats in which heartworms have been visualized by echocardiography, because complications such as vascular trauma, hemorrhage, and worm breakage resulting in acute anaphylactic reaction and intraoperative death are possible. Removal of heartworms by jugular venotomy has been used successfully with an endoscopic basket, a Swan-Ganz catheter, or an Ishihara forcep.[33] Silk suture loops on the end of a 5-French red rubber urinary catheter have been successfully used to wrap up worms for extraction, and it is a safe method where fluoroscopic access is not possible. Removal of the heartworms by right ventricular incision, pulmonary arteriotomy, or right atriotomy using total venous inflow occlusion has also been successful.[34,35]

SUMMARY

Heartworm disease remains a significant problem in cats because of complications such as HARD, respiratory distress, and sudden death. Diagnostic confirmation usually requires a combination of tests, and treatment is often limited to alleviation of clinical signs. The emerging role of *Wolbachia* in the pathogenesis of heartworm disease offers the potential for a novel therapy that may reduce the complication rate, as

well as the adverse effects associated with treatment. The misconception that heartworm disease is less common in the cat than it is in the dog has led to the under-recognition of respiratory diseases caused by the immature heartworms. In addition, the respiratory disease associated with HARD and heartworms is often overlooked or mistakenly attributed to lungworm infection, migrating roundworm infection, or asthma. Adult heartworms have a shorter longevity in the cat than in the dog, and spontaneous recovery is always possible. However, elimination of heartworm larvae with preventative medications before they reach the lungs can prevent the clinical and pathological changes associated with both HARD and adult heartworm infections. Therefore, the best approach to feline heartworm disease is preventative medications administered either before the transmission season or year-round.

References

1. Litster AL, Atwell RB: Feline heartworm disease: a clinical review. *J Feline Med Surg* 10:137–144, 2008.
2. Dillon AR: Feline dirofilariasis. *Vet Clin North Am Small Anim Pract* 14:1185–1199, 1984.
3. Levy JK, Snyder PS, Taveres LM, et al: Prevalence and risk factors for heartworm infection in cats from northern Florida. *J Am Anim Hosp Assoc* 39:533–537, 2003.
4. Lorentzen L, Caola AE: Incidence of positive heartworm antibody and antigen tests at IDEXX Laboratories: trends and potential impact on feline heartworm awareness and prevention. *Vet Parasitol* 158:183–190, 2008.
5. Donahoe JM: Experimental infection of cats with *Dirofilaria immitis*. *J Parasitol* 61:599–605, 1975.
6. Venco L, Genchi C, Genchi M, et al: Clinical evolution and radiographic findings of feline heartworm infection in asymptomatic cats. *Vet Parasitol* 158:232–237, 2008.
7. Dillon AR, Brawner WR, Grieve RB, et al: The chronic effects of experimental *Dirofilaria immitis* infection in cats. *Semin Vet Med Surg* 2:72–77, 1987.
8. Dillon AR, Warner AE, Brawner W, et al: Activity of pulmonary intravascular macrophages in cats and dogs with and without adult *Dirofilaria immitis*. *Vet Parasitol* 158:171–176, 2008.
9. Maia FC, McCall JW, Jr VA, et al: Structural and ultrastructural changes in the lungs of cats *Felis catus* (Linnaeus, 1758) experimentally infected with *D. immitis* (Leidy, 1856). *Vet Parasitol* 176:304–312, 2011.
10. Holmes RA, Clark JN, Casey HW, et al: Histopathologic and radiographic studies of the development of heartworm pulmonary vascular disease in experimentally infected cats. In *Proceedings of the Heartworm Symposium '92*, Batavia, 1992, American Heartworm Society, pp 81–89.
11. Dillon AR, Tillson DM, Wooldridge AA, et al: Effects of intravenous and subcutaneous heartworm homogenate from doxycycline-treated and untreated donor dogs on bronchial reactivity and lung in cats. *Vet Parasitol* 206:14–23, 2014.
12. Wooldridge AA, Dillon AR, Tillson DM, et al: Isometric responses of isolated intrapulmonary bronchioles from cats with and without adult heartworm infection. *Am J Vet Res* 73:439–446, 2012.
13. Sironi M, Bandi C, Sacchi L, et al: Molecular evidence for a close relative of the arthropod endosymbiont Wolbachia in a filarial worm. *Mol Biochem Parasitol* 74:223–227, 1995.
14. Morchon R, Ferreira AC, Martin-Pacho JR, et al: Specific IgG antibody response against antigens of *Dirofilaria immitis* and its Wolbachia endosymbiont bacterium in cats with natural and experimental infections. *Vet Parasitol* 125:313–321, 2004.
15. Garcia-Guasch L, Caro-Vadillo A, Manubens-Grau J, et al: Is Wolbachia participating in the bronchial reactivity of cats with heartworm associated respiratory disease? *Vet Parasitol* 196:130–135, 2013.
16. Taylor MJ, Cross HF, Ford L, et al: Wolbachia bacteria in filarial immunity and disease. *Parasite Immunol* 23:401–409, 2001.
17. Kramer L, Grandi G, Leoni M, et al: Wolbachia and its influence on the pathology and immunology of *Dirofilaria immitis* infection. *Vet Parasitol* 158:191–195, 2008.
18. Kramer L, Grandi G, Passeri B, et al: Evaluation of lung pathology in *Dirofilaria immitis*-experimentally infected dogs treated with doxycycline or a combination of doxycycline and ivermectin before administration of melarsomine dihydrochloride. *Vet Parasitol* 176:357–360, 2011.
19. Dillon AR, Brawner AR, Robertson-Plouch CK, et al: Feline heartworm disease: correlations of clinical signs, serology, and other diagnostics—results of a multicenter study. *Vet Ther* 1:176–182, 2000.
20. Browne LE, Carter TD, Levy JK, et al: Pulmonary arterial disease in cats seropositive for *Dirofilaria immitis* but lacking adult heartworms in the heart and lungs. *Am J Vet Res* 66:1544–1549, 2005.
21. Atkins CE, DeFrancesco TC, Coats JR, et al: Heartworm infection in cats: 50 cases (1985–1997). *J Am Vet Med Assoc* 217:355–358, 2000.
22. Donahoe JM, Kneller SK, Lewis RE: Hematologic and radiographic changes in cats after inoculation with infective larvae of *Dirofilaria immitis*. *J Am Vet Med Assoc* 168:413–417, 1976.
23. Murray MJ: Canine and feline dirofilariasis. *Compendium* 30:442–443, 2008.
24. Dillon AR, Tillson DM, Wooldridge AA, et al: Effect of pre-cardiac and adult stages of *Dirofilaria immitis* in pulmonary disease of cats: CBC, bronchial lavage cytology, serology, radiographs, CT images, bronchial reactivity, and histopathology. *Vet Parasitol* 206:24–37, 2014.
25. Calvert CA, Mandell CP: Diagnosis and management of feline heartworm disease. *J Am Vet Med Assoc* 180:550–552, 1982.
26. Naylor JR, Hamilton JM, Weatherley AJ: Changes in the ultrastructure of feline pulmonary arteries following infection with the lungworm *Aelurostrongylus abstrusus*. *Br Vet J* 140:181–190, 1984.
27. Dillon AR, Tillson DM, Hathcock J, et al: Lung histopathology, radiography, high-resolution computed tomography, and bronchio-alveolar lavage cytology are altered by *Toxocara cati* infection in cats and is independent of development of adult intestinal parasites. *Vet Parasitol* 15;193(4):413–426, 2013.
28. Bowman DD, Atkins CE: Heartworm biology, treatment, and control. *Vet Clin North Am Small Anim Pract* 39:1127–1158, 2009.
29. Dillon AR, Blagburn B, Tillson DM, et al: Immature heartworm infection produces pulmonary parenchymal, airway, and vascular disease in cats. *J Vet Intern Med* 21:608–609, 2007.
30. Little SE, Raymond MR, Thomas JE, et al: Heat treatment prior to testing allows

detection of antigen of *Dirofilaria immitis* in feline serum. *Parasit Vectors* 13(7):1, 2014.

31. Rossi MI, Paiva J, Bendas A, et al: Effects of doxycycline on the endosymbiont Wolbachia in *Dirofilaria immitis* (Leidy, 1856)—naturally infected dogs. *Vet Parasitol* 174:119–123, 2010.

32. Bazzocchi C, Mortarino M, Grandi G, et al: Combined ivermectin and doxycycline treat-ment has microfilaricidal and adulticidal activity against *Dirofilaria immitis* in experimentally infected dogs. *Int J Parasitol* 38:1401–1410, 2008.

33. Borgarelli M, Venco L, Piga PM, et al: Surgical removal of heartworms from the right atrium of a cat. *J Am Vet Med Assoc* 211:68–69, 1997.

34. Iizuka T, Hoshi K, Ishida Y, et al: Right atriotomy using total venous inflow occlusion for removal of heartworms in a cat. *J Vet Med Sci* 71:489–491, 2009.

35. Small MT, Atkins CE, Gordon SG, et al: Use of a nitinol gooseneck snare catheter for removal of adult *Dirofilaria immitis* in two cats. *J Am Vet Med Assoc* 233:1441–1445, 2008.

Approach to Feline Cardiorespiratory Disease in Shelter Medicine

Martha Smith-Blackmore

ANIMAL SHELTERING

Animal sheltering is the activity of providing care to society's "unwanted" animals. The diversity of facilities influences how cats may be sheltered. Cat sheltering may happen in a bricks and mortar building, such as a municipal impound facility ("pound") or a private, nonprofit animal welfare organization. Loose knit, grassroots efforts are increasingly playing a role in saving the lives of cats, and this activity may happen in private foster homes or other unconventional "shelter" settings. Shelter medicine is considered the practice of veterinary medicine in this wide variety of animal shelter settings. In the practice of shelter medicine, a unique and recently growing veterinary specialty, the focus must be simultaneously on the health of the population and the health and care of the individual animal.

Shelter veterinarians and program managers must work together closely to appropriately distribute the available resources for care of sheltered animals within the constraints of each particular setting. Some suggest that shelter medicine is analogous to herd management but this is not entirely the case. The major difference from herd health science is that in an animal shelter, cats come from diverse backgrounds on a rolling admission basis. There is not the benefit of an "all in, all out" management process.

Not all animal shelters can afford to have a veterinarian on staff. In some communities, veterinary guidance is completely unavailable to the animal shelter. But, often, a veterinarian in the community works as an advisor to the facility or will make regular visits to the animal shelter. In these settings, standing protocols are often established to guide shelter staff in decision making.

The population of cats presented to animal shelters for care is as diverse as the variety of shelters engaged in caring for them. Health conditions (e.g., pregnancy, retroviral infections, or parasitism) may challenge their immune systems and make them more vulnerable to infectious disease.

CARDIOPULMONARY RECOMMENDATIONS FOR FELINES IN SHELTER FACILITIES

Because of the variety of settings and cat populations, it is difficult to make sweeping specific recommendations for feline shelter health policies to support optimal cardiorespiratory cat health. Ideally, each animal shelter should work closely with a shelter veterinarian or veterinarian with specific shelter training to develop the best approach for the health of the individual cats in that particular setting, as well as the policies for the population.[1]

Basic necessary allocations of resources include the vaccination of animals on intake, surgical sterilization, parasite treatment, and microchip implantation. Some facilities routinely perform retroviral and heartworm testing, whereas others will do so only on symptomatic animals. Other facilities use evidence of disease as a sorting and selection mechanism to identify individuals for quarantine or euthanasia. Because of this, some shelters completely avoid diagnostic testing and make decisions based on clinical appearance and adoptability. If disease incidence is low, testing every incoming cat for a particular infectious or cardiopulmonary disease may sideline resources that could be redirected for greater positive impact for the population. The necessary allocation of basic resources for all admitted animals reduces available resources for diagnostics and treatment of individual animals showing signs of cardiac and respiratory diseases.[2]

SHELTERING TO MITIGATE FELINE INFECTIOUS UPPER RESPIRATORY TRACT DISEASE

The number one respiratory challenge for sheltered cats is infectious upper respiratory tract disease. Feline herpesvirus (FHV) and feline calicivirus (FCV), the agents that most frequently cause upper respiratory infection (URI) in cats, are ubiquitous and highly infectious.[3] The virus is often already present within the cat, and viral expression and release occurs because of the distress of the major life change.[4] Whether the cat is a stray picked up from the streets or a pet surrendered from a home setting, the move into a shelter is a radical and stressful shift regardless of how accommodating the setting may be.

Vaccination on intake with a modified live vaccine, along with stress reduction, the avoidance of crowding, keeping the length of stay (LOS) within the facility to the shortest time possible, and appropriate cleaning and disinfection methods are the means by which animal shelters can most effectively prevent the expression and transmission of infectious respiratory disease within the facility.[5]

Vaccination on Intake

Rapid onset of protection against FHV and FCV is critical for cats coming into an animal shelter. Administration of a modified live vaccine should be done for all cats at the time of intake or even before, if possible.[6] Vaccines help to mitigate signs of respiratory disease but do not entirely prevent them. The decision to use an intranasal versus a parenteral vaccine is one that should be made with consideration of shelter resources. Panleukopenia vaccination by the intranasal route is never appropriate in a shelter setting,[7] so a shelter may or may not desire to split the respiratory components out for intranasal administration.

Because intranasal vaccines activate local immunity, maternal antibody interference is not an issue; therefore, intranasal FHV and FCV vaccination may be helpful for the young kitten population.[8] In animal shelters, vaccinations are indicated at an earlier age and should be administered at shorter intervals, compared with schedules for pet cats.[6] Transient, mild signs of URI may develop following administration of vaccine by the intranasal route. Vaccines will be administered by animal shelter staff, not necessarily veterinary technicians, so training should cover the basics of vaccine handling, mixing, administration, and storage. Vaccination should begin as early as 4 to 6 weeks of age and be repeated every 2 to 3 weeks until 16 weeks of age.[6] When possible, kittens younger than 8 weeks of age should be kept in foster care, away from the unavoidable disease exposure in the shelter environment.

Vaccinate in the Face of Disease Symptoms

All shelter kittens and cats should be vaccinated on intake regardless of physical condition. If the cat's immune system is so weakened that a modified live vaccine will induce disease, exposure to the wide variety of infectious pathogens present in most shelters will cause serious illness and may even kill the cat. In general, if a cat cannot be safely vaccinated, it should not be admitted and cared for in the animal shelter. Cats that are injured or ill at the time of initial vaccination should be revaccinated when healthy, at least 2 weeks later.[6]

Non-Core Vaccines

Routine vaccination of shelter-housed cats against other respiratory agents, such as *Bordetella bronchiseptica* and *Chlamydophila felis*, has proven to be of limited benefit.[6] The association between a positive culture or polymerase chain reaction test result for these agents and disease in shelter cats is inconsistent. These vaccines should only be considered if the pathogens have been demonstrated as a current problem by clinical signs in the population and confirmed with laboratory diagnostics. It may be appropriate to introduce the vaccine for a limited period of time to break a cycle of disease transmission within the cat shelter. *B. bronchiseptica* vaccination should be used where there is potential direct or indirect

contact between cats and dogs on the same site—most appropriately when the dogs have a recent or current history of infectious respiratory disease. Further information on immunization strategies for shelter cats is found in Chapter 70.

Stress Reduction

Negative stress or distress (hereinafter referred to simply as "stress") has come to be appreciated as the major contributor to the occurrence of respiratory disease in shelter cats.[9] One study demonstrated that cats with high stress scores during the first week in shelter housing were 5.6 times as likely to develop URI as were cats with low stress scores. Poorly designed cat housing is one of the greatest shortcomings observed in animal shelters (Figure 44-1); the resulting stress has a substantially negative impact on physical and mental health. Unfortunately, signs of stress in cats are subtle and can be hard to appreciate without careful observation by well-trained observers. Because stress can be difficult to assess in the individual cat, the best approach is to assume if a cat is in an animal shelter, it is stressed, and measures should be taken to help the cat accommodate to that stress.

Existing housing can be modified to improve feline welfare (e.g., cutting portholes between cages) to increase available space and create multicompartment housing units. A second stress reduction benefit to double-sided cages is that it reduces disruption of the cat's environment during cage cleaning. The ability to hide significantly decreases cat stress;[10] simple offerings such as paper bags or shoeboxes will help cats adjust

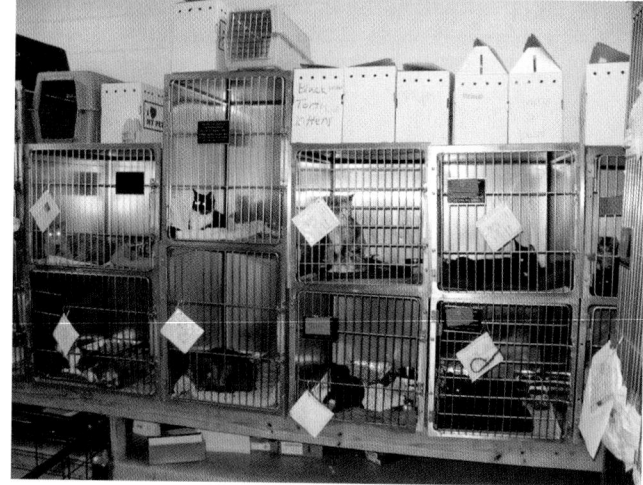

Figure 44-1: Stressful feline shelter housing has insufficient space to allow separation among food, elimination, and resting areas. Cats require space large enough to accommodate places to hide (e.g., paper bag or box large enough to provide concealment), to have a litter box large enough to comfortably accommodate their entire body, and should have high points to perch upon. Cats should be able to turn freely and to easily stand, sit, stretch, move their head—all without touching the top of the enclosure—and to lie in a comfortable position with limbs and tail extended. A lack of separation between primary enclosures increases stress and the risk of infectious disease spread. (Courtesy of Dr. Brenda Griffin.)

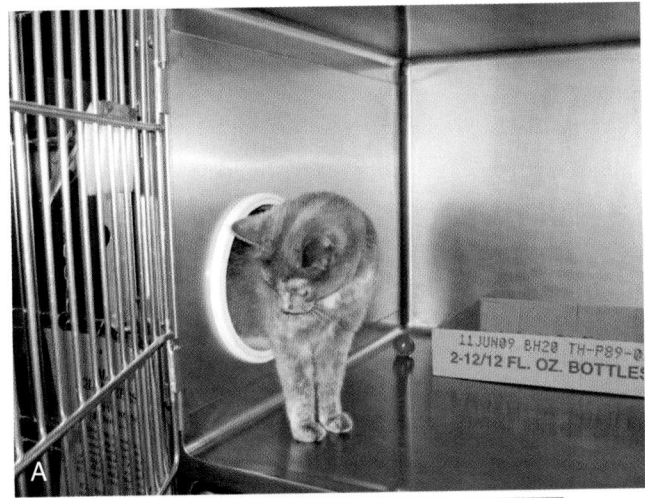

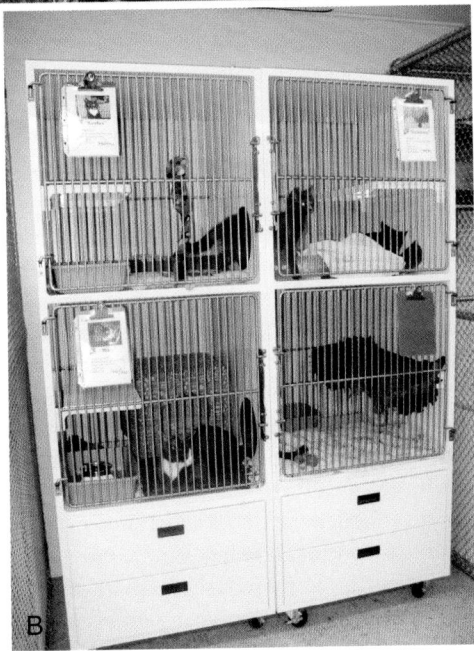

Figure 44-2: A, Insufficiently sized stainless steel or fiberglass caging can be modified to allow cats to have double-sided compartments, thereby significantly increasing available living space and decreasing stress. **B,** Commercially-available cat condo units are increasingly available with features that decrease cat kennel stress. They are elevated with room for storage and cleaning supplies below and are of sufficient size to allow the cat to have some choice and therefore a sense of control over the environment. (**A** and **B,** Courtesy of Dr. Brenda Griffin.)

to the shelter environment. Elevated perches also help to give choice and a sense of control over the environment (Figure 44-2).

The use of a synthetic feline facial pheromone diffuser in cat housing rooms, or the use of a synthetic feline facial pheromone spray on a cloth, placed in the cats' primary enclosure may also help to reduce stress.[11] Other stressful features of animal shelters are elevated noise levels including forced air ventilation, use of power hoses, metal kennel gates, metal food bowls, and nonporous building materials. Cats are particularly adversely affected by the sound of barking dogs.[9]

Air Handling

Separate air exchange for feline housing areas is a lesser priority in the reduction of viral transmission because cats do not readily aerosolize their respiratory pathogens over great distances.[12,13] In order to prevent droplet transmission of respiratory viruses when cages face each other, they should be spaced at least 4 feet apart. Adequate ventilation to provide good air quality, however, is essential. The understanding should be that good ventilation reduces loose fur and dander, which act as fomites, and it provides healthy air to breathe. The reduction of aerosolized cell wall components from bacteria in dust, and chemical irritants (e.g., ammonia and bleach) reduces associated respiratory inflammation, which predisposes cats to infection. However, even optimal ventilation will not overcome the harmful effects of inadequate housing.

Length of Stay

The longer a cat stays in an animal shelter, the more likely it is to fall ill with infectious respiratory disease.[14] The longer the average LOS in an animal shelter for a population of cats, the greater the incidence of respiratory disease. It is imperative that the LOS be managed to the shortest time feasible in order to maintain the healthiest population of cats possible. When analyzing an outbreak of infectious respiratory tract disease in shelter cats, the LOS should be examined; if increased over the average ordinary LOS for that facility, the reason for this change should be addressed. Bottlenecks in the population flow typically include waiting for examination, moving up to adoption, or moving out to spay or neuter; every effort should be made to remove restrictions to flow. Longer stays also mean more crowded shelters; the more crowded a shelter, the less space and care are available for each cat.

Appropriate Cleaning and Disinfection Methods

Appropriate cleaning and disinfection techniques in cat shelters reduce the amount of infectious materials in the shelter and must take into account the need for as few stressors as possible in the cat's day. As a general rule, a cat's primary enclosure can be "spot-cleaned" during the entirety of the cat's stay (Figure 44-3). This is the process of removing visible debris and replacement of soiled litter and bedding, without the introduction of chemical cleaning or disinfecting agents. This minimizes stress and allows the cat to remain in its own familiar environmental scent. The cleaning process should be done quietly and efficiently, with a concerted effort not to raise dust when changing litter pans or bedding. Paper towels and squeeze or squirt bottles (that produce a stream of cleaner rather than a spray are preferred) can be used to clean spots of food, mucus, or feces. Sponges or rags and buckets should never be used in cage cleaning, because these will transmit infectious organisms from one enclosure to the next[15] (Figure 44-4).

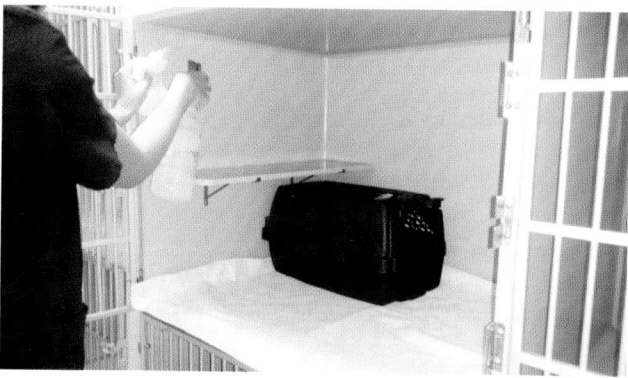

Figure 44-3: Spot cleaning should be used to tidy a primary enclosure while the same cat is resident within that cage. The cat should be able to hide from the cleaning activity in a box within the cage. Care should be taken to minimize aerosolization of chemicals for respiratory safety of staff and cats. Also, because cats may be distressed by the noise of a spray bottle, care should be taken to apply cleaning agents quietly or, alternatively, a squeeze bottle producing a stream may be used. (Courtesy of Dr. Brian DiGangi.)

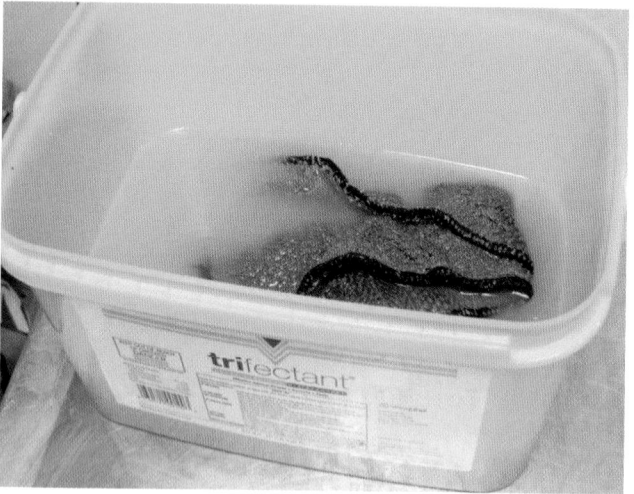

Figure 44-4: Rag and bucket cleaning methods create a toxic "soup" of potentially infectious pathogens. If the same rag and fluid is used from cage to cage, there is a risk of spreading disease instead of the intended effect of disease reduction. (Courtesy of Dr. Brian DiGangi.)

Each cage should be thoroughly cleaned and disinfected after its occupant moves out. Attention should be paid to scrubbing all biological materials from the cage walls, floor, ceiling, and especially the cage door with many crevices to hold debris, which is often overlooked. Disinfectants should be chosen based on the infectious disease elements present in the shelter. Quaternary ammonium agents are broad spectrum and do a good job of general disinfection. Surfaces must remain wet with the appropriate disinfectant for the period of time specified by the manufacturer, usually 10 minutes. During a period of FCV outbreak, the disinfectant should be changed to one that can kill this nonenveloped agent.[16] Bleach is most effective but is also a respiratory irritant and corrosive agent. An alternative disinfectant that is gaining ground in animal shelters is accelerated hydrogen peroxide, because it has many of the disinfection benefits of bleach without the corrosive and irritant drawbacks.[17] Many shelters

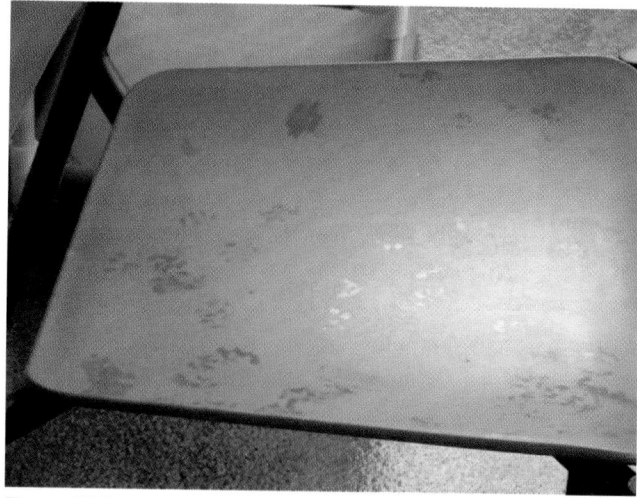

Figure 44-5: If cats walk on damp surfaces, they will track the moisture around. If the source of moisture is disinfectant, the cat will be exposed to the toxin while grooming. If cats are allowed to exercise on the floor after cleaning is completed, the floor should be dry and, depending on disease incidence in that shelter, potentially cleaned between cats. (Courtesy of Dr. Brian DiGangi.)

routinely rotate among types of disinfectant in order to ensure the broadest spectrum of disinfection.

It is important to remember to disinfect food bowls, brushes, litter boxes, carriers, toys, smocks, and hands between cats. Again, items limited to the cat's primary enclosure do not need to be disinfected every day, but when there is an increase in incidence of respiratory disease in a cat shelter, shared items are an area to examine as a possible source of spread. Common areas and objects frequently touched by people (e.g., telephones and doorknobs) should be disinfected in times of disease outbreak. Long-handled squeegees should be used to collect litter, loose hairs, and debris from floors because this eliminates the dust raising that is inherent in dry sweeping.[18]

Cats must not be allowed to contact surfaces wet with disinfectant (Figure 44-5). Oral exposure to quaternary ammonium compounds can cause ulceration that mimics FCV ulcers.[19] This should be suspected when cats that have oral ulcers are reluctant to eat but have no fever, nasal, or ocular discharge. Phenols are never an appropriate disinfection choice for use in cat shelters because they are hepatotoxic.[20]

What Does Not Work

Disinfecting without cleaning first is ineffective; all surfaces to be disinfected should look perfectly clean before applying disinfectant. Disinfectants do not work in the presence of biological materials. Some steam cleaning equipment does not ensure that surfaces attain high enough temperatures, and in most uses, surfaces are not exposed long enough to achieve true disinfection. Steam cleaning can be effective if the right equipment is used appropriately, but this equipment and staff training is rare in animal shelters. Ultraviolet lights may inactivate airborne bacteria and viruses, but they do not clean the air of particulate or vapor irritants. Additionally, because the source of infectious respiratory disease for shelter cats tends to be autogenously or fomite transmitted, the purchase of ultraviolet lights is usually not the best expenditure of resources.[21]

MANAGING INFECTIOUS UPPER RESPIRATORY INFECTION

Polymerase chain reaction surveys of URI in shelter cats attribute the vast majority of cases to FHV and/or FCV.[22] Cats can harbor FHV for their entire life and experience a recrudescence in times of stress. Similarly, cats may be healthy transmitters of FCV for prolonged periods of time so a "Trojan horse" nidus of infection is often present within a population at any given time. Cats with predominantly ocular signs, particularly with corneal ulcers, are much more likely to have FHV infection.[23] Conversely, cats with oral ulceration (e.g., glossitis, pharyngitis, faucitis, or stomatitis) are most likely have FCV infection.[24] Other important players include *Bordetella*, *Chlamydophila*, and *Mycoplasma* species. Differentiation among the causes of URI may have more importance in shaping the cleaning and disinfection protocol than in the caregiving response.

Despite our best efforts to lessen the inciting causes of infectious upper respiratory tract disease among shelter cats, it will always remain a challenge of cat sheltering. Cats with respiratory difficulty or a painful mouth or throat have to choose between eating, drinking, grooming, and breathing. For this reason, many cats with viral or other respiratory disease will have an unkempt appearance and may be both anorectic and dehydrated. Staff should be trained in the observation of a cat's eating, drinking, litter box, and grooming habits as a part of assessing the animal's well-being; attending to the sick cat's individual care needs must be a priority.

Nursing Care

Regardless of the etiology of URI in cats, supportive care is the most essential part of nursing cats through their illness. Eyes should be kept clean of discharges and lubricated with a hydrogel-based eye lubricant (e.g., GenTeal, Alcon) four times per day.[25] This water-soluble solution does not cause ocular irritation that can be seen in cats when using petrolatum-based eye ointments. Oxytetracycline (e.g., Terramycin) and other petrolatum-based ophthalmic ointments can cause contact conjunctivitis in cats; ongoing treatment may be perpetuating chemosis after the infectious component has resolved and may even cause anaphylaxis.[26]

Nares should be kept clean of discharges. Cats unable to smell their food are often unwilling to eat.[27] They will act hungry, approach the food when offered, but after attempting to sniff the food, they will not eat. Some cats will eat when encouraged, after a grooming session, or when the food is heated to enhance the smell. Simply crushing some dry food

between the fingers in the food dish will stimulate some cats to start eating. Cats that are not eating will benefit from the administration of subcutaneous fluids; well-hydrated cats will produce a moister mucous discharge and maintain more effective mucociliary apparatus function.[28] Oral ulcers are very painful; analgesic medications and oral sucralfate slurry can help a cat to resume eating.[29]

Antibiotics

Antibiotics are often considered the least important factor in dealing with URI in shelter cats. The additional stress induced by the handling necessary for administration of medication may do more harm than good. Antibiotics should only be introduced in cats after evidence of secondary bacterial infection is apparent with purulent discharges. Doxycycline is the most frequently used antibiotic in shelter cats with secondary bacterial URI. This antibiotic tends to be effective against *Bordetella*, *Chlamydophila*, and *Mycoplasma* species, commonly cultured from upper respiratory tracts of shelter cats.[30] It has the added operational and financial benefits of once daily administration and historically relatively low cost. A compounded liquid formulation is recommended in order to avoid the risk of esophageal stricture associated with tablet and capsule formulations.[31]

Kitten Concerns

Queens will often readily accept kittens from other litters; however, mixing litters of kittens is risky in the shelter setting.[32] Kittens may be harboring one disease causative agent and coping well. When litters are mixed, super-infections may be introduced, leading to severe respiratory disease, sometimes expressing as a fulminant or even lethal pneumonia. Whenever possible, kittens should be moved to foster homes out of the institutional animal shelter setting in order to reduce exposure to infectious disease agents.[33]

Housing Zones

In order to reduce the risk and impact of infectious disease outbreaks, the cat shelter should be divided into at least three individual sections or zones (e.g., quarantine area for incoming cats, isolation facilities for sick or potentially infectious cats, and accommodation for apparently healthy cats).[34] Adult cats which have been vaccinated and observed in the shelter for 2 weeks, are free of clinical signs of respiratory tract disease, and are socially appropriate can be introduced into group or colony housing.[35]

The Intake Exam

Because the animal shelter is not a setting in which advanced diagnostics can commonly be performed, a careful clinical examination is essential to rule out or diagnose and localize cardiorespiratory disease in the shelter cat. Radiographs, echocardiography, electrocardiogram, and blood pressure monitoring are all considered advanced diagnostics in the animal shelter setting. If there is no veterinarian on staff or if intake numbers exceed the capacity of the veterinary staff, lay intake personnel should be trained on the detection of disease. Cats showing clinical signs should be referred for veterinary examination. Clinical signs that point to cardiorespiratory disease in cats include nasal discharge, an unkempt or ungroomed appearance, cough, respiratory noise, tachypnea, dyspnea, and exercise intolerance. If they cannot be appropriately treated, cats with tachypnea, dyspnea, or exercise intolerance should be euthanized rather than allowing them to suffer without treatment. Some consulting veterinarians maintain treatment protocols for staff to implement when signs of infectious upper respiratory tract disease are noted. Any cat that fails to respond to preliminary treatment should be referred for evaluation by a veterinarian.

CARDIAC DISORDERS

Cardiac murmurs indicate turbulence within the heart or great vessels.[36] A packed cell volume and total solids test should be considered as part of the diagnostic workup when a murmur is detected in an asymptomatic kitten. The anemia that accompanies many diseases of young felines can be associated with a murmur due to a decrease in blood viscosity.[37] Although congenital heart disease must always be suspected when a murmur is detected in a kitten, some kittens have innocent murmurs that resolve by 6 months of age. These "innocent" physiologic murmurs are due to disparities in the size of the great vessels receiving the blood volume ejected by the growing heart. Physiologic murmurs tend to be soft (usually grade I to III/VI), early to mid-systolic high frequency murmurs.[38] The point of maximum intensity is generally at the left heart base or the sternum, and they tend not to radiate extensively. Cardiac murmurs that are particularly loud (greater than III/VI), associated with a palpable thrill, murmurs that contain a diastolic component, and those associated with an arrhythmia, cardiac gallop, abnormal membrane color or arterial pulses, and those resulting in cardiac enlargement on radiographs are most likely to result from congenital heart disease.[39] Murmurs, gallop rhythms, and cardiac arrhythmias detected in mature cats are more likely to result from acquired heart diseases, such as cardiomyopathy, hyperthyroidism, systemic hypertension, or feline heartworm disease.[40] Anemia should also be ruled out as a contributor to cardiac murmur in an adult cat. The reported incidence of heart murmurs in apparently healthy cats can be as high as 21% to 50%.[41]

Diagnosis of cardiac disease can be challenging in a shelter medicine setting due to the limited finances available and the high cost of some cardiac diagnostics (e.g., echocardiography). Thoracic radiographs can be useful to screen for cardiac enlargement or changes in the lungs of cats with significant cardiac disease. Unfortunately, the concentric nature of the hypertrophy in cats with hypertrophic cardiomyopathy limits the utility of thoracic radiographs, because this most common form of feline heart disease often does not result in appreciable radiographic cardiomegaly until there is notable left atrial enlargement.[42]

A recently developed test, N-terminal pro-brain natriuretic peptide (NT-proBNP), may provide some utility in identification of cats with innocent murmurs or mild cardiac disease compared to cats with more impressive cardiac disease.[43] A commercially-available test is available for this cardiac biomarker, and NT-proBNP concentrations above 100 to 200 pmol/L are often associated with significant heart disease. In addition, a relatively inexpensive, patient-side test kit for NT-proBNP has been developed (SNAP Feline proBNP Test, IDEXX Laboratories, Westbrook, ME). This may prove to be an economical approach to evaluation of cats with heart murmurs. The test helps to differentiate which cats are likely to have moderate to severe heart disease from those lacking significant clinical changes to the heart. A shelter veterinarian could use this test in adult cats with heart murmurs to determine which cats are at low risk for having pathologic changes to their hearts and which ones might benefit from additional cardiac diagnostics. If cats with murmurs are made available for adoption without further diagnostics, the potential owners can be made aware of the possibility of significant heart disease before adoption.

CARDIOPULMONARY PARASITES

Lungworms and migrating larval forms of gastrointestinal (GI) parasites may account for a substantial proportion of respiratory disease in cats.[44] Larvae of various GI ascarids migrating through the lungs induce pulmonary inflammation and include *Toxocara cati* (feline roundworm) and *Ancylostoma tubiforme* (feline hookworm). These worms have been found to be present in shelter cat populations at approximately 30% in national survey studies.[45] Feline lungworm infection is covered in Chapter 36.

Heartworm disease is another concern in shelter settings, especially as it relates to the adoptability of affected cats. *Dirofilaria immitis* has been demonstrated to cause heartworm-associated respiratory disease (HARD) in cats.[46] Heartworm infection takes place when a mosquito carrying infective, microscopic-size heartworm larvae bites a cat. Clinical signs develop when the immature adult worms enter the pulmonary arteries, which may result in acute inflammation of the vessels or the lung parenchyma. Because cats are not definitive hosts for *D. immitis*, heartworms may not reach maturity, and pulmonary inflammation and fibrosis may develop even if the infection is never patent.[47] Cats with HARD express coughing, asthma-like signs, dyspnea, and lethargy. When degeneration of dead adult worms begins, it may cause inflammation of the lungs and pulmonary thromboembolism.

Approaches to heartworm testing in the shelter medicine situation vary greatly, depending upon the prevalence of heartworm in that region of the world and based on the financial resources available for screening at the shelter.[48]

Current antigen tests will not detect male worms but are capable of detecting a single mature female heartworm in cats.[49] Because the average worm burden in a cat is only one to two worms, approximately 30% of infections will be only male worms and thus undetected by antigen testing.[50] Antibody testing will detect male and female worms, as well as fourth stage larvae and juvenile worms.[51] Unfortunately, surveys of necropsy-confirmed, heartworm infected cats have shown that test sensitivity is only in the 50% to 80% range.[52] A negative antibody test does not rule out heartworm infection, but it does lower the index of suspicion. A positive antigen test indicates the presence of at least one adult female worm. A positive antibody test indicates that the cat was infected at some point, most likely in the previous 18 months,[50] and the cat may or may not currently harbor live heartworms. Necropsy surveys of shelter cats have placed the prevalence of adult heartworm infections at 5% to 15% of the rate in unprotected dogs in a given area.[53]

Because testing of cats for heartworm disease for the purposes of diagnostic screening is ambiguous, the best use of resources in the shelter setting is to put all cats on preventive medication. The American Heartworm Society recommends heartworm prevention for all cats, even indoor only cats, year round. Heartworm prevention in cats, with one of the many proven preventive drug choices, is recommended for cats living in heartworm endemic regions of the country. Shelters in heartworm endemic areas should start preventive medications in kittens at 8 weeks of age and administer preventive medication to all cats.[49] Feline heartworm disease is covered further in Chapter 43.

SUMMARY

Given the variety of cat sheltering situations, veterinary guidance should be customized to the particular setting, population, and resources available. Some general principles to support optimal feline cardiorespiratory health include vaccination on intake with modified live vaccines, an emphasis on reducing stress, the administration of broad spectrum anthelmintics, and the careful evaluation of each cat as an individual patient within the context of the population to be managed. Whatever the level of evaluation of the adoptable cat (by a veterinarian or by shelter staff), transparent communication of the findings (and who made them) is essential along with the possible implications and outcomes. This open dialogue creates trust with potential adopters and helps to make optimal and more lasting adoptions. The importance of establishing a relationship with a private practice veterinarian should be emphasized to the new owner at the time of adoption.

References

1. Newbury SP, Blinn MK, Bushby PA, et al: Guidelines for standards of care in animal shelters, *The Association of Shelter Veterinarians* (PDF online): <http://www.sheltervet.org/assets/docs/shelter-standards-oct2011-wforward.pdf>. Accessed May 14, 2015.
2. Hurley KF, Pesavento P: Disease Recognition and Diagnostic Testing. In Miller L, Zawistowski S, editors: *Shelter medicine for veterinarians and staff*, ed 2, Ames, IA, 2012, Wiley-Blackwell, p 329.
3. Scarlett JM: Feline upper respiratory disease. In Miller L, Hurley KF, editors: *Infectious disease management in animal shelters*, Ames, IA, 2009, Wiley-Blackwell, p 125.
4. Binns SH, Dawson S, Speakman AJ, et al: A study of feline upper respiratory tract disease with reference to prevalence and risk factors for infection with feline calicivirus and feline herpesvirus. *J Feline Med Surg* 2:123–133, 2000.
5. Miller L: A blend of science and art: what every shelter should know about shelter medicine. *Animal Sheltering* Jan/Feb:49–51, 2007.
6. Scherk MA, Ford RB, Gaskell RM, et al: 2013 American Association of Feline Practitioners Feline Vaccination Advisory Panel Report. *J Feline Med Surg* 15(9):785–808, 2013.
7. Schultz RD: A commentary on parvovirus vaccination. *J Feline Med Surg* 11:163–164, 2009.
8. Edinboro CH, Janowitz LK, Guptill-Yoran L, et al: A clinical trial of intranasal and subcutaneous vaccines to prevent upper respiratory infection in cats at an animal shelter. *Feline Pract* 27(6):7–13, 1999.
9. McCobb EC, Patronek GJ, Marder AM, et al: Assessment of stress levels among cats in four animal shelters. *J Am Vet Med Assoc* 226(4):548–555, 2005.
10. Griffin B: Wellness. In Miller L, Hurley KF, editors: *Infectious disease management in animal shelters*, Ames, IA, 2009, Blackwell, pp 17–38.
11. Beck A: Use of pheromones to reduce stress in sheltered cats. *J Feline Med Surg* 15:829–830, 2013.
12. Gaskell RM, Povey RC: Transmission of feline viral rhinotracheitis. *Vet Rec* 111:359–362, 1982.
13. Wardley RC, Povey RC: Aerosol transmission of feline caliciviruses: an assessment of its epidemiological importance. *Br Vet J* 133:504–508, 1977.
14. Dinnage JD, Scarlett JM, Richards JR: Descriptive epidemiology of feline upper respiratory tract disease in an animal shelter. *J Feline Med Surg* 11(10):816–825, 2009.
15. Smith M: *Operational guide: sanitation and disease control in the shelter environment*, Denver, CO, 2010, American Humane Association. (PDF online): <http://www.americanhumane.org/assets/pdfs/animals/operational-guides/op-guide-diseasecontrol.pdf>. Accessed May 13, 2015.
16. Schorr-Evans EM, Poland A, Johnson WE, et al: An epizootic of highly virulent feline calicivirus disease in a hospital setting in New England. *J Feline Med Surg* 5(4):217–226, 2003.
17. Omidbakhsh N, Sattar SA: Broad-spectrum microbicidal activity, toxicologic assessment, and materials compatibility of a new generation of accelerated hydrogen peroxide-based environmental surface disinfectant. *Am J Infect Control* 34:251–257, 2006.
18. Sansone EB, Losikoff AM, Pendleton RA: Sources and dissemination of contamination in material handling operations. *Am Ind Hyg Assoc J* 38(9):433–442, 1977.
19. Hurley KF: When is a virulent calicivirus really a virulent calicivirus? *Animal Sheltering* Nov:53–56, 2007.
20. Aronson AL: Chemical poisonings in small animal practice. *Vet Clin North Am* 2(2):379–395, 1972.
21. Petersen CA, Dvorak G, Spickler AR: *Maddie's infection control manual for animal shelters*, Des Moines, IA, 2008, Center for Food Security and Public Health, Iowa State University, College of Veterinary Medicine.
22. Burns RE, Wagner DC, Leutenegger CM, et al: Histologic and molecular correlation in shelter cats with acute upper respiratory infection. *J Clin Microbiol* 49(7):2454–2460, 2011.
23. Gaskell R, Dawson S, Radford AD, et al: Feline herpesvirus. *Vet Res* 38(2):337–354, 2007.
24. Coyne KP, Dawson S, Radford AD, et al: Long-term analysis of feline calicivirus

prevalence and viral shedding patterns in naturally infected colonies of domestic cats. *Vet Microbiol* 118(1–2):12–25, 2006.

25. Glaze MB: Feline conjunctival and corneal disease. In *Proceedings of the Northeast Veterinary Conference*, 2004.

26. Hume-Smith KM, Groth AD, Rishniw M, et al: Anaphylactic events observed within 4 h of ocular application of an antibiotic-containing ophthalmic preparation: 61 cats (1993-2010). *J Feline Med Surg* 13(10):744–751, 2011.

27. Tanaka A, Wagner D, Kass P, et al: Associations among weight loss, stress, and upper respiratory tract infection in shelter cats. *J Am Vet Med Assoc* 240(5):570–576, 2012.

28. Gaskell RM, Dawson S, Radford A: Feline respiratory disease. In Greene CE, editor: *Infectious diseases of the dog and cat*, ed 4, St Louis, 2012, Elsevier/Saunders, p 155.

29. Plumb DC: Sucralfate. In *Plumb's veterinary drug handbook*, ed 7, Ames, IA, 2011, Wiley.

30. Bannasch MJ, Foley JE: Epidemiologic evaluation of multiple respiratory pathogens in cats in animal shelters. *J Feline Med Surg* 7(2):109–119, 2005.

31. German AJ, Cannon MJ, Dye C, et al: Oesophageal strictures in cats associated with doxycycline therapy. *J Feline Med Surg* 7(1):33–41, 2005.

32. Smith-Blackmore M, Newbury S: Foster care. In Miller L, Hurley KF, editors: *Infectious disease management in animal shelters*, Ames, IA, 2009, Wiley-Blackwell, p 498.

33. Levy JK: Breeding and rescue catteries—managing infectious disease in kittens. In *Proceedings of the International Society of Feline Medicine*, 2013.

34. Möstl K, Egberink H, Addie D, et al: Prevention of infectious diseases in cat shelters: ABCD guidelines. *J Feline Med Surg* 15(7):546–554, 2013.

35. Griffin BG: Feline care in the animal shelter. In Miller L, Hurley KF, editors: *Infectious disease management in animal shelters*, Ames, IA, 2009, Wiley-Blackwell, p 174.

36. Kittleson MD: The approach to the feline patient with a cardiac auscultatory abnormality. In *Small animal cardiovascular medicine textbook*, St Louis, 1998, Mosby.

37. Rentko VT, Cotter SM: Feline anemia: the classifications, causes, and diagnostic procedures. *Vet Med* 85(6):584, 1990.

38. Johnson L: *Clinical canine and feline respiratory medicine*, Ames, IA, 2010, Wiley-Blackwell.

39. Durham EH: A review of congenital heart disease. In *Proceedings of the Western Veterinary Conference*, 2013.

40. Côté E, Manning AM, Emerson D, et al: Assessment of the prevalence of heart murmurs in overtly healthy cats. *J Am Vet Med Assoc* 225:384–388, 2004.

41. Drourr LT, Gordon SG, Roland RM: Prevalence of heart murmurs and occult heart disease in apparently healthy adult cats. In *ACVIM Forum Proceedings*, 2010, p 159.

42. Paige CF, Abbott JA, Elvinger F, et al: Prevalence of cardiomyopathy in apparently healthy cats. *J Am Anim Hosp Assoc* 234(11):1398–1403, 2009.

43. Fox PR, Rush JE, Reynolds CA, et al: Multicenter evaluation of plasma N-terminal pro-brain natriuretic peptide (NT-pro BNP) as a biochemical screening test for asymptomatic (occult) cardiomyopathy in cats. *J Vet Intern Med* 25(5):1010–1016, 2011.

44. Bowman DD: Pulmonary disease from canine- and feline-associated intestinal helminths. In *ACVIM Forum Proceedings*, 2012.

45. Hill S, Lappin MR, Cheney J, et al: Prevalence of enteric zoonotic agents in cats. *J Am Vet Med Assoc* 216:687–692, 2000.

46. Blagburn BL, Dillon RA: Feline heartworm disease: solving the puzzle. *Vet Med* 102(3 Suppl):7–14, 2007.

47. Dingman P, Levy JK, Kramer LH, et al: Association of Wolbachia with heartworm disease in cats and dogs. *Vet Parisitol* 170(1–2):50–60, 2010.

48. Dunn KF, Levy JK, Colby KN, et al: Diagnostic, treatment, and prevention protocols for feline heartworm infection in animal sheltering agencies. *Vet Parasitol* 176(4):342–349, 2011.

49. Atkins C, Carithers D, Clyde E, et al: Current feline guidelines for the diagnosis, prevention, and management of heartworm (*Dirofilaria immitis*) infection in cats, American Heartworm Society (PDF online): <https://www.heartwormsociety.org/images/pdf/2014-AHS-Feline-Guidelines.pdf>. Accessed May 14, 2015.

50. Nelson CT: Heartworm disease. In Miller L, Hurley KF, editors: *Infectious disease management in animal shelters*, Ames, IA, 2009, Wiley-Blackwell, pp 341–347.

51. Berdoulay P, Levy JK, Snyder PS, et al: Comparison of serological tests for the detection of natural heartworm infection in cats. *J Am Anim Hosp Assoc* 40(5):376–384, 2001.

52. Nelson CT, Young TS: Incidence of *Dirofilaria immitis* in shelter cats from southeast Texas. In Seward RL, editor: *Recent advances in heartworm disease: symposium '98*, Batavia, IL, 1998, American Heartworm Society.

53. Levy JK, Snyder PS, Taveres LM, et al: Prevalence and risk factors for heartworm infection in cats from northern Florida. *J Am Anim Hosp Assoc* 39(6):533–537, 2003.

Feline Lower Airway Disease

Elizabeth Rozanski

Respiratory disease is common in cats and may be classified based upon either localization (e.g., upper, lower, parenchymal, or pleural space) or by etiology (e.g., nasal tumor, congestive heart failure, chylothorax, etc.). Typically, the first step is to localize the lesion, and then further classify the specific cause. Treatment for a specific cause is preferable to simple supportive care, and it typically results in a better outcome. Feline lower airway disease (or "asthma") is a common cause of respiratory distress and/or coughing in cats.[1-3] The actual number of affected cats is unknown, but is estimated to be 1% to 5% of the feline population. However, coughing, which is more common than overt respiratory distress, is commonly misidentified as "hairballs" so the actual prevalence of airway disease is unknown and may be much higher. It is common for owners of a cat with lower airway disease to identify similar signs in subsequent feline additions to the family, so the author's perception is that a higher number of cats are affected than generally estimated. Importantly, lower airway disease is *rarely* identified as a new problem in geriatric cats; a suspicion of lower airway disease in old cats should be confirmed, and diseases that are more nefarious excluded.

CLINICAL SIGNS

Clinical signs of lower airway disease most commonly include coughing, but may include periodic respiratory distress.[1-3] Occasional coughing, perhaps once per week, may not warrant extensive evaluation, but more frequent cough, or any distress should prompt further testing. The independent nature of cats may preclude a complete understanding of the frequency of the clinical signs. Audible wheezes may be present, or may be identified on auscultation. Lower airway disease results in thickening of the lower airways and subsequent difficulty on exhalation. This may be hard to appreciate in cats given their relatively rapid respiratory rate, but cats with a clear prolongation of expiration or an expiratory push should be suspected of having lower airway disease.

DIFFERENTIAL DIAGNOSES

Cats with cough most often have lower airway disease. Cough in cats may be distinguished from hairballs by lack of vomit-

ing of hair (e.g., no hairballs ever found despite apparent frequent attempts to "cough them up") and lack of response to hairball medications. In addition, most cats with cough will have an increased tracheal sensitivity on palpation, and have a briefly productive cough after gentle pressure is placed on the trachea. Cardiac disease is an uncommon cause of cough in cats, although it is common for airway disease and cardiomyopathy to coexist. Other differential diagnoses for cough include lungworm (see Chapter 36) or heartworm infection, bacterial infection (e.g., *Bordetella bronchiseptica*), lung or tracheal tumors, and rarely, pleural effusion.

Acute respiratory distress may also be a presenting sign in cats with lower airway disease and should be excluded from other causes of respiratory distress including upper airway disease, parenchymal disease, and pleural space disease. Common upper airway diseases include laryngeal masses or paralysis and nasal disease.[4] Upper airway obstruction should result in a prolonged inspiratory phase, although this may be mistaken for an expiratory effort, and an audible "wheeze" is often heard, which may further inadvertently support lower airway disease.

Parenchymal diseases primarily include congestive heart failure, but also trauma, atypical infections (e.g., toxoplasmosis), and neoplasia. Pleural space diseases include congestive heart failure, neoplasia, chylothorax, pyothorax, feline infectious peritonitis, and pneumothorax or chest wall instability (such as bite wounds).

PHYSIOLOGY

Normal lung function is dependent upon adequate lung mechanics and gas exchange. *Lung mechanics* are defined as the mechanical properties of the pulmonary system and are comprised of ratios of airflow rate, airway pressures, and lung volumes. Compliance represents the distensibility of the lungs, and primarily reflects the lung parenchyma; low compliance is associated with clinical entities such as pulmonary contusions and edema. Lung compliance is not typically affected by lower airway disease. Lung resistance primarily represents ease of airflow; most of the airway resistance (due to branching airway generations) is in the larger airways. Lower airway disease should increase airway resistance. Lower airway disease results in narrowed airway lumen and subsequent increase in airway resistance due to bronchoconstriction (typically reversible), increased airway mucus, and/or airway smooth muscle hypertrophy.

Gas exchange may be impaired by flow limitation and would be expected to result in hypoxemia; however, arterial blood gases are rarely measured in cats with respiratory distress. Pulse oximetry and end-tidal carbon dioxide analysis may be substituted for blood gas analysis, but may also be inaccurate or difficult to obtain in the distressed cat.

CHRONIC BRONCHITIS VERSUS "ASTHMA"

Feline airway disease is often considered a spectrum, with some cats having a syndrome more consistent with true asthma, with reversible bronchoconstriction in response to inhaled allergens, and other cats having a clinical syndrome more similar to chronic bronchitis with cough, excessive mucus, and bronchial thickening.[5] Cats with more asthma-like disease, with true bronchoconstriction, are more likely to develop respiratory distress, and more likely to respond to bronchodilators. Asthma is considered to have more eosinophilic bronchoalveolar lavage fluid (BALF), whereas chronic bronchitis will be associated with BALF containing nondegenerative neutrophils. However, clinically, it may be challenging to distinguish the two syndromes. One study involving the use of biomarkers was unable to distinguish asthma and chronic bronchitis based upon BALF biomarkers.[5]

CAUSES

The underlying cause surrounding the development of lower airway disease remains undetermined in most cats. The typical changes of feline asthma are reversible flow limitation, excessive mucus production, and airway remodeling. Local type I hypersensitivity reactions within the airways are thought to induce these changes. Subsequent re-exposure to the airborne antigen results in local airway responses including histamine and leukotriene release from mast cells, and degranulation of eosinophils. Eosinophils in asthmatic cats are considered especially crucial in the development of true asthma, but similar to most biological systems, eosinophils may also suppress some local inflammatory responses.[3] Siamese cats have been described as over-represented with lower airway disease, but it is unclear if this is a real increase or if Siamese cats may be more likely to be presented for ongoing veterinary care.[3] Viral respiratory infections are a common cause of asthma in genetically susceptible infants and children. Although viral respiratory infections are common in kittens, the role that respiratory infections may have in the development of later lower airway disease in cats is unclear. Lower airway disease is suspected to represent allergy to some inhaled allergen in most cases, but how or why a specific cat becomes sensitized remains unclear. Some cats appear to worsen seasonally, whereas others appear to have year-round clinical signs. Certain cats appear to react to more dusty kitty litters or the presence of indoor pollution,

including environmental tobacco smoke or potpourri scent. Some cats with lower airway disease also appear to have chronic rhinitis, although this syndrome has not been formally evaluated as it has been in people.[6] Allergy testing is rarely performed in cats with suspected asthma, but one pilot study in cats showed a high rate of positive responses to skin testing.[7] Serum immunoglobulin E (IgE) assays have variable reliability in cats, and care should be taken in interpreting the results.[8]

Experimentally, cats may be sensitized to various antigens, such as Bermuda grass or *Ascaris suum*, and a clinical syndrome similar to lower airway disease may be stimulated with re-exposure.[9] While experimental models are useful to elucidate some mechanistic aspects of airway disease, validation of any results in naturally occurring cases in a home environment may be more useful clinically.

Secondary spontaneous pneumothorax has been reported in cats with lower airway disease. Medical therapy is typically adequate, but care should be taken to carefully monitor and aggressively treat underlying inflammatory disease.[10]

DIAGNOSTIC IMAGING

Thoracic radiographs are a mainstay of diagnosis, with affected cats demonstrating a bronchial or bronchointerstitial pattern (Figure 45-1). Radiograph interpretation may also demonstrate hyperinflation due to air-trapping and occasionally collapse of the right middle lung lobe due to mucus plugging. Importantly, cats with severe airway disease are occasionally thought to have metastatic disease. Thoracic metastatic disease, as is seen in dogs, is less common in cats. Computed tomography (CT) may also be used to document lower airway disease, but has to date not been used commonly for this approach in cats because of the cost, availability, and potential requirement for anesthesia (Figure 45-2). A restraint chamber (VetMouse Trap) has been introduced for awake CT scanning and is covered in Chapter 42.

Lung function, and specifically airway resistance, will be affected by lower airway disease. Airway resistance is increased

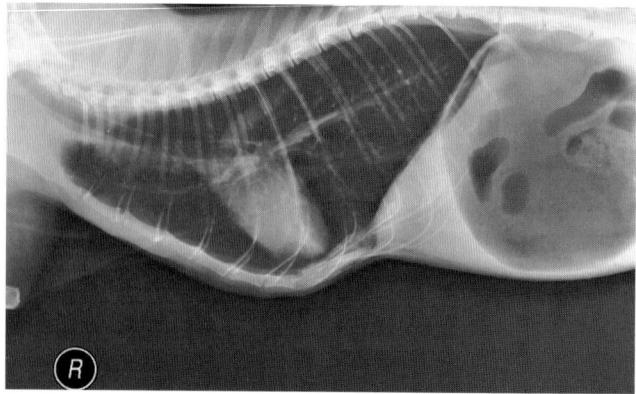

Figure 45-1: A Lateral Thoracic Radiograph from a Cat with Severe Lower Airway Disease. Note in specific the marked hyperinflation and bronchial pattern.

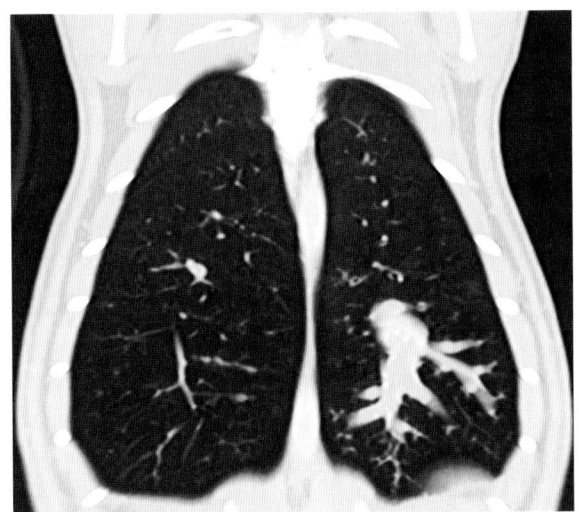

Figure 45-2: A Reconstructed Computed Tomography Scan from a Cat with Severe Bronchial Disease, with Bronchiectasis.

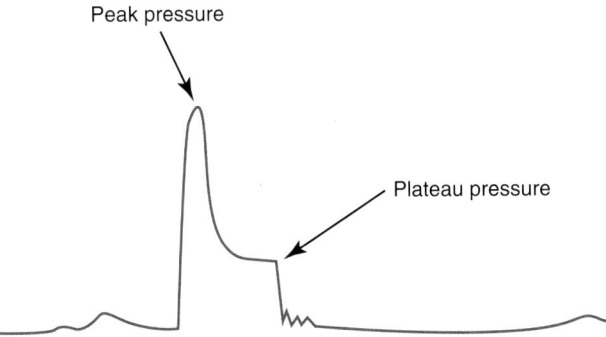

Figure 45-3: Severe Bronchoconstriction (Increased Resistance) as Demonstrated by a Large Peak-to-Plateau Pressure Difference, Measured Using a Commercial Critical Care Ventilator (Puritan Bennett 840).

due to narrowing of the airways from smooth muscle hypertrophy and excessive mucus. Bronchoconstriction, when present, will also increase airway resistance. Historically, lung function has been difficult to measure in the clinical setting, but with the emergence of the critical care ventilators it has become easier to measure lung function using built-in algorithms (Figure 45-3).

OTHER DIAGNOSTIC TESTS

Routine laboratory testing is commonly unremarkable in cats with lower airway disease, but it should be performed to exclude systemic diseases. In addition, because cats may be treated with glucocorticoids, it is prudent to evaluate for hyperglycemia and potential for insulin resistance. Heartworm antibody and antigen testing is indicated in endemic areas, even in indoor cats. Baermann fecal sedimentation may also be performed to evaluate for lungworms. Older cats may

be evaluated for hyperthyroidism, which may worsen control of a previously well-controlled patient.

Tracheal cytology (and perhaps culture) may be performed to evaluate cats for airway eosinophilia, and lack of other causes of respiratory distress (e.g., infection, neoplasia, etc.). Biomarkers in BALF have been evaluated in cats with asthma and chronic bronchitis, but initial results have been disappointing in their ability to distinguish asthma from chronic bronchitis.[5] Bronchoscopy may be useful to more completely evaluate the airways and to collect samples. Airway cytology is collected by performing a tracheal wash or bronchoalveolar lavage under brief anesthesia. Briefly, a cat should be preoxygenated. Propofol is commonly used, but any anesthetic protocol is acceptable. The cat should be intubated using a sterile endotracheal tube, and airway cytology collected by infusing sterile saline. Volume of saline to infuse ranges from 3 to 20 mL total. Airway cytology should usually not be collected from cats showing marked respiratory distress, as the procedure may temporarily worsen lung function and in rare cases may be associated with severe complications.

TREATMENT

Acute therapy includes supplemental oxygen therapy, glucocorticoids, and bronchodilators. Cats with airway disease should improve within 4 to 6 hours of starting therapy. Some cats do not easily convert prednisone to prednisolone, so prednisolone is preferred in cats with lower airway disease. In an emergency setting, treatment usually includes 2 to 4 mg/cat of dexamethasone intravenously (IV) or 5 to 10 mg/cat of prednisolone orally, as well as supplemental oxygen, ideally via an oxygen cage if available. As respiratory distress is typically associated with bronchoconstriction, therapy with either inhaled albuterol (1 to 2 puffs every 6 hours) or parenteral terbutaline (0.01 mg/kg subcutaneously [SC]) is often beneficial.

Occasionally, it may be challenging to determine if respiratory distress is airway or cardiac (e.g., pulmonary edema) in origin; if in doubt, a single dose of furosemide (2 to 4 mg/kg IV) may be given. Rapid assessment by echocardiography is ideal; however, use of the cardiac biomarker N-terminal pro-brain natriuretic peptide may be helpful to establish or exclude a diagnosis of heart failure, particularly now that this is available as point-of-care test. In cats where bacterial infection cannot be excluded, antibiotics may be administered, although pulmonary infection is uncommon in cats.

Chronic therapy includes removing any identifiable trigger, and glucocorticoids, either orally or by inhalation. Because of the lack of voluntary patient cooperation, aerosol therapy requires the use of a face mask and spacer (e.g., Aerokat, Trudell Medical, London, and Ontario). The feline nasopharynx is much smaller and more complex than in humans, which results in aerosolized medications being deposited in the nasal passage, where subsequently it may be swallowed. A study by Schulman and colleagues with aerosolized radiopharmaceuticals showed there was deposition of the radiopharmaceutical in the lung, although in most of the cats, the radiopharmaceuticals were also visualized in the stomach.[11]

Inhaled glucocorticoids affected the hypothalamic pituitary axis in a study by Cohn and colleagues, although there were limited effects on the immune system.[12] The diabetogenic effect of inhaled corticosteroids has not been evaluated to date in cats, although they do increase the risk of diabetes in people.

Many proprietary products are available as inhaled glucocorticoids, although most studies have used fluticasone. As an unknown amount of drug reaches the airways, the appropriate starting dose is unknown. One study in cats supported a starting fluticasone dose of 44 μg/cat twice daily, whereas other investigators suggest 110 μg/cat twice daily up to a maximum of 440 μg twice daily.[1,13,14] There are also combination products such as fluticasone and the long-acting beta-2 agonist salmeterol (Advair); a study by Leemans showed improved efficacy in an experimental model of feline asthma with this combination.[13] Most commonly, oral glucocorticoid therapy is continued for about 10 to 14 days, with a tapering overlap as inhalant therapy is started.

The advantages of inhaled medications may include less systemic effects and limitation of potential complications. Potential disadvantages include requirements for daily therapy, training the cat to accept therapy, and the current high cost of fluticasone. If a cat does not respond well to oral glucocorticoid therapy, it is very unlikely to see a response to inhaled glucocorticoid therapy.

Inhaled glucocorticoids should be discussed with owners of all affected cats, and strong consideration given for use in cats with diabetes or cardiomyopathy. Clients should learn of the options for inhaled medications from their primary care veterinarian, who can effectively counsel them on their specific pet. Other therapeutic options, such as stem cell therapy, or desensitization may become available in the coming years as the understanding of feline lower airway disease expands. Key therapeutic points for feline lower airway disease are summarized in Box 45-1.

For cats that do not have a good response to glucocorticoids, it is prudent to reassess compliance, as well as to consider alterative diagnoses. Cyclosporine has been described as a potential therapy, at 10 mg/kg orally every 12 hours, with improvement in airway hyperresponsiveness and evidence of amelioration of cytological inflammation.[3] Cyclosporine is a potent immunosuppressive agent. Drug levels should be monitored, and adjusted as needed.

WHAT DOES NOT WORK

A variety of drugs has been evaluated in experimental asthma models in cats, but have not been shown to be beneficial. These include cyproheptadine, cetirizine, and zafirlukast.[3] In abstract form, data were presented showing that maropitant (Cerenia, Zoetis) was also ineffective in research cats.[15]

BOX 45-1 Key Therapeutic Points for Feline Lower Airway Disease

1. Limit exposure to airway irritants in the environment.
2. Oral steroids: prednisolone 5 mg/cat every 12 hours for 10 days, then taper to 2.5 to 5 mg/cat once a day. It is likely that cats will need lifelong therapy, and the goal is NOT to wean the patient from the medication, but rather to control airway inflammation.
3. Inhaled steroids: fluticasone 110 to 220 μg every 12 hours, using feline mask and spacer (e.g., Aerokat) may be substituted for oral glucocorticoids. In this case, fluticasone and oral prednisolone may be given together for about 14 days, after which the oral prednisolone is tapered and discontinued.
4. Doxycycline or azithromycin is prescribed if bacterial infection is suspected (uncommon).
5. Bronchodilation may be provided in the acute setting with either injectable terbutaline (0.01 mg/kg, subcutaneously) or inhaled albuterol.
6. If respiratory distress is present, treat with dexamethasone 1 to 4 mg/cat, a beta-2 agonist such as albuterol, and supplemental oxygen until the crisis resolves, and then initiate or continue steroid maintenance therapy.

FUTURE DIRECTIONS IN THERAPY

Therapeutic options for cats with difficult-to-control asthma are being developed and evaluated. Although in most cases a specific allergen is not identified, in cases with severe disease, a specific hunt for allergens may be warranted, including skin testing or serum IgE evaluation. In research cats, allergen-specific rush immunotherapy has been evaluated with good results.[16] Briefly, the cat is rapidly desensitized to the specific allergen by exposure to rapidly increasing allergen concentrations. Allergen-specific rush immunotherapy has not been evaluated in pet cats to date, but it might be an exciting opportunity in cases where a particular antigen can be identified. Almost 20 years ago, a study evaluated the effect of hyposensitization on cats with allergy based upon radioallergosorbent testing and identified that many cats (86.1%) improved with immunotherapy.[17] For severely affected cats, this might be a potential therapeutic option.

Fish oil, specifically omega 3 polyunsaturated fatty acids, has been shown to reduce airway hyperresponsiveness in an experimental model of feline asthma, and it may have a role as an adjuvant therapy.[18] A recent article described therapeutic benefit in research cats receiving masitinib, a tyrosine kinase inhibitor, but this has not been evaluated in clinical patients.[19] Masitinib is associated with side effects in cats, so its safety profile should be carefully considered before use.

Stem cell therapy represents an exciting avenue in veterinary therapeutics. Limited studies in experimentally asthmatic cats have shown only minor benefits in controlling airway remodeling.[20] However, further studies are ongoing, and ultimately stem cells may be useful. Stem cells act primarily to modulate inflammation, so it is likely they will be more useful for long-term disease control than as a short-term crisis medication.

In evaluating a cat with new onset of hard to control asthma, it is prudent to re-evaluate the cat; occasionally, cats with long-standing airway disease develop another syndrome such as a laryngeal mass or heart failure.

SUMMARY

Feline lower airway disease represents a heterogeneous mixture of lower airway diseases; some cats have a more compelling "asthma" phenotype with acute bronchoconstriction, and some have a more "chronic bronchitis" picture with cough and excessive airway mucus. Diagnostic efforts should be directed at excluding other potential causes of cough or respiratory distress. Effort should be made to limit the exposure to controllable aeroallergens in the home and toward

prevention of the development of respiratory infection. Therapy revolves around the use of anti-inflammatory steroids, with oral or inhaled forms both being acceptable. Key facts about lower airway disease in cats are summarized in Box 45-2.

> **BOX 45-2 Key Facts about Lower Airway Disease in Cats**
>
> 1. Feline lower airway disease is uncommon in kittens and rare as a new-onset diagnosis in geriatric cats.
> 2. Longterm therapy with steroids is the most effective treatment if the underlying trigger cannot be removed.
> 3. Inhaled fluticasone is an appealing and effective form of therapy, but it does not work immediately. Therefore, concurrent therapy with oral prednisolone is required for at least 14 days when inhaled medication is initiated. Further studies evaluating its clinical efficacy are warranted.
> 4. Bronchodilators should be given concurrent with clinical signs, not daily.
> 5. Cough is the most common clinical sign.

References

1. Padrid P: Use of inhaled medications to treat respiratory diseases in dogs and cats. *J Am Anim Hosp Assoc* 42(2):165–169, 2006.
2. Corcoran BM, Foster DJ, Fuentes VL: Feline asthma syndrome: a retrospective study of the clinical presentation in 29 cats. *J Small Anim Pract* 36(11):481–488, 1995.
3. Venema CM, Patterson CC: Feline asthma what's new and where might clinical practice be heading? *J Feline Med Surg* 12(9):681–692, 2010.
4. Reed N, Gunn-Moore D: Nasopharyngeal disease in cats: 2. Specific conditions and their management. *J Feline Med Surg* 14(5):317–326, 2012.
5. Nafe LA, DeClue AE, Lee-Fowler TM, et al: Evaluation of biomarkers in bronchoalveolar lavage fluid for discrimination between asthma and chronic bronchitis in cats. *Am J Vet Res* 71(5):583–591, 2010.
6. Navarro A, Valero A, Juliá B, et al: Coexistence of asthma and allergic rhinitis in adult patients attending allergy clinics: ONEAIR study. *J Investig Allergol Clin Immunol* 18(4):233–238, 2008.
7. Moriello KA, Stepien RL, Henik RA, et al: Pilot study: prevalence of positive aeroallergen reactions in 10 cats with small-airway disease without concurrent skin disease. *Vet Dermatol* 18(2):94–100, 2007.
8. Delgado C, Lee-Fowler TM, DeClue AE, et al: Feline-specific serum total IgE quantita-

tion in normal, asthmatic and parasitized cats. *J Feline Med Surg* 12(12):991–994, 2010.
9. Norris Reinero CR, Decile KC, et al: An experimental model of allergic asthma in cats sensitized to house dust mite or Bermuda grass allergen. *Int Arch Allergy Immunol* 135(2):117–131, 2004.
10. Mooney E, Rozanski EA, King R, et al: Spontaneous pneumothorax in 35 cats (2001-2010). *J Feline Med Surg* 14(6):384–391, 2012.
11. Schulman RL, Crochik SS, Kneller SK, et al: Investigation of pulmonary deposition of a nebulized radiopharmaceutical agent in awake cats. *Am J Vet Res* 65(6):806–809, 2004.
12. Cohn LA, DeClue AE, Reinero CR: Endocrine and immunologic effects of inhaled fluticasone propionate in healthy dogs. *J Vet Intern Med* 22(1):37–43, 2008.
13. Leemans J, Kirschvink N, Clercx C, et al: Effect of short-term oral and inhaled corticosteroids on airway inflammation and responsiveness in a feline acute asthma model. *Vet J* 192(1):41–48, 2012.
14. Cohn LA, DeClue AE, Cohen RL, et al: Effects of fluticasone propionate dosage in an experimental model of feline asthma. *J Feline Med Surg* 12(2):91–96, 2010.
15. Grobman M, Dodam JR, Outi H, et al: Acute and chronic neurokinin-1 antagonism fail to dampen airflow limitation or airway eosinophilia in asthmatic cats. In *Proceedings from the 32nd Annual Veterinary Comparative*

Respiratory Society Meeting, Kennett Square, Pennsylvania, Oct 2014.
16. Reinero CR, Byerly JR, Berghaus RD, et al: Rush immunotherapy as an experimental model of feline allergic asthma. *Vet Immunol Immunopathol* 110:141–153, 2006.
17. Halliwell RE: Efficacy of hyposensitization in feline allergic diseases based upon results of in vitro testing for allergen-specific immunoglobulin E. *J Am Anim Hosp Assoc* 33(3):282–288, 1997.
18. Leemans J, Cambier C, Chander T, et al: Prophylactic effects of omega-3 polyunsaturated fatty acids and luteolin on airway hyperresponsiveness and inflammation in cats with experimentally-induced asthma. *Vet J* 184(1):111–114, 2010.
19. Lee-Fowler TM, Guntur V, Dodam J, et al: The tyrosine kinase inhibitor Mastinib blunts airway inflammation and improves associated lung mechanics in a feline model of chronic allergic asthma. *Int Arch Allergy Immunol* 158:369–374, 2012.
20. Trzil J, Masseau I, Webb TL, et al: Long term evaluation of mesenchymal stem cell therapy in a feline model of chronic allergic asthma. *Clin Exp Allergy* 2014. Epub ahead of print [November 30, 2014].

Ultrasound Imaging for Diagnosis and Staging of Feline Cardiomyopathy

Virginia Luis Fuentes

Cardiomyopathy is very common in cats. Recent studies suggest around 15% of apparently healthy cats are affected.[1,2] Fortunately, many cats remain clinically normal, but some cats develop signs of congestive heart failure (CHF) or aortic thromboembolism, and in other cats sudden death may be the first sign.[3,4] The term *cardiomyopathy* is used to refer to conditions primarily affecting the myocardium and includes idiopathic myocardial diseases as well as those of known etiology (e.g., a genetic or nutritional cause).[5,6] The myocardium can also be affected by a number of systemic diseases, such as hyperthyroidism,[7,8] hypertension,[9] and hypersomatotropism.[10] Recognition of these causes of myocardial disease is extremely important, because treatment of the underlying disease is necessary for optimum management.

Echocardiography is the most important method for classifying cardiomyopathy phenotypes, using a combination of morphologic and functional measurements, such as ventricular wall thickness, chamber diameters, left ventricular (LV) systolic function, and diastolic filling patterns. Hypertrophic cardiomyopathy (HCM) is the most common cardiomyopathy and is characterized by increased LV wall thickness (≥6 mm) at end-diastole. Restrictive cardiomyopathy (RCM) is less common and is associated with normal LV wall thickness and systolic function, but with enlargement of both atria and a restrictive diastolic filling pattern. Dilated cardiomyopathy (DCM) is uncommon with the principle characteristic of global LV systolic dysfunction. Arrhythmogenic right ventricular cardiomyopathy (ARVC) results in dilation of the right atrium and right ventricle and is often associated with arrhythmias. There is a degree of overlap among phenotypic categories, so that classification among clinicians is not always consistent. As the genetic basis for human cardiomyopathies becomes better understood, there is increasing recognition that phenotypic expression can be highly varied even among individuals with the same mutation. A more logical priority for feline clinicians is to identify cats with a phenotype that carries a high risk of cardiac mortality, rather than focusing on the "correct" classification of cardiomyopathy type.

PROGNOSTIC FACTORS

Echocardiography is an extremely valuable tool for gauging prognosis in cats with cardiomyopathy. The association between left atrial (LA) enlargement and a poor prognosis has long been recognized in cats with cardiomyopathy.[4,11] Left atrial dysfunction (i.e., reduced LA contractile function) is also a useful marker for risk of cardiac death, although this has been less widely reported.[12,13] Other echocardiographic prognostic markers include LV systolic dysfunction, extreme LV hypertrophy (>9 mm), presence of spontaneous echocontrast or a thrombus, regional LV wall hypokinesis, and a restrictive diastolic filling pattern.[12] Presence of dynamic left ventricular outflow tract obstruction (DLVOTO) has not been linked to a worse prognosis in cats, in contrast with human HCM patients.[11,14]

Although ultrasonography is one of the most powerful tools available to identify "high-risk" cats, echocardiography in cats provides many challenges. Cats are not always cooperative, the feline heart presents a small echocardiographic target, and their diseases are difficult to characterize. Some aspects of feline echocardiography are inevitably limited to those with extensive training and experience (i.e., veterinary cardiologists), but there are other very useful echocardiographic skills that can be acquired by anyone prepared to devote the necessary time and practice.

ECHOCARDIOGRAPHIC TECHNIQUE IN CATS

Equipment
Echocardiography machines used for imaging the feline heart should be capable of high frame rates in order to deal with the fast heart rates of cats. This is mainly a limiting factor for older, more basic machines when measuring LV wall thickness using two-dimensional (2D) echocardiography and is not a problem for most new echocardiography machines. High frequency ultrasound transducers (between 5 to 10 MHz) are needed for adequate resolution, and phased

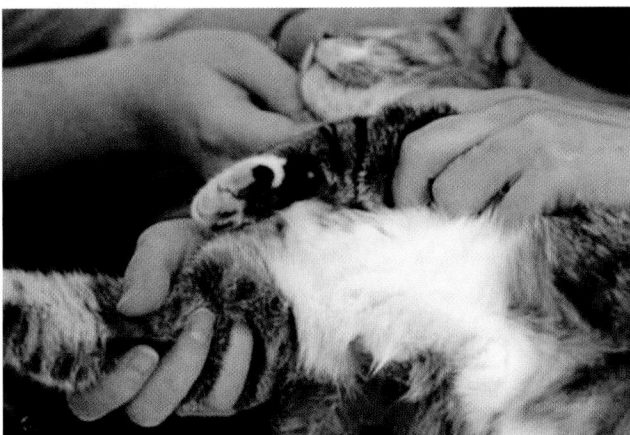

Figure 46-1: Preferred method for restraining a cooperative cat in lateral recumbency using a table cut-out, with the probe placed on the right chest wall from underneath. Note the right forelimb is "pushed" forward from above the elbow. For cats with respiratory distress or less cooperative cats, it may be necessary to scan the cat in a standing or sitting position.

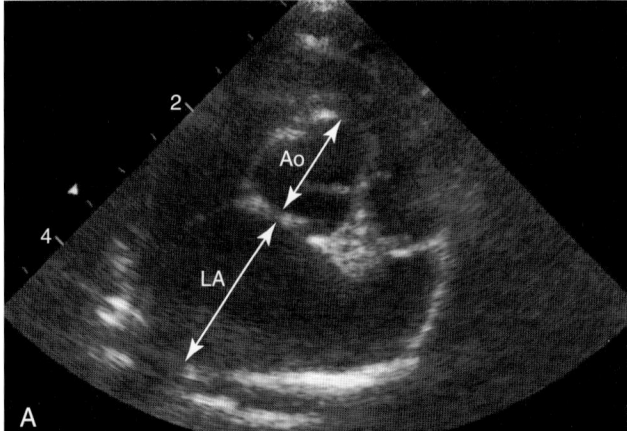

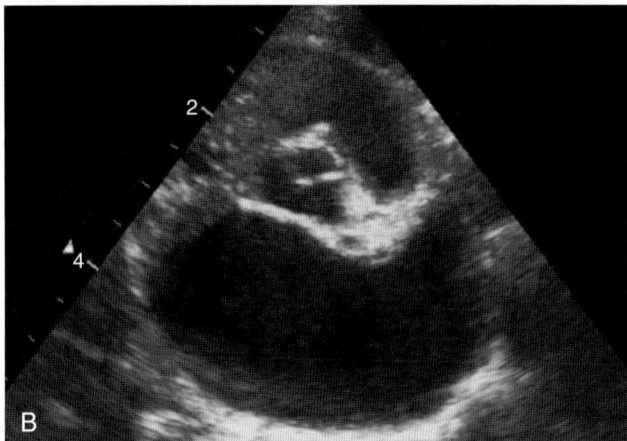

Figure 46-2: Right parasternal short axis views at the aortic (Ao)/left atrial (LA) level in two cats with cardiomyopathy. **A,** Shows a cat with a normal *LA:Ao* ratio. **B,** Shows a cat with the LA dilated.

array sector transducers with a square footprint are ideal, because curvilinear probes may result in rib-shadowing in short axis views.

Patient Preparation/Restraint

Clipping the hair coat is not necessary in all cats if copious quantities of alcohol and ultrasound gel are used. With sympathetic restraint, most cats can be scanned without sedation. Many clinicians prefer to position the cat in lateral recumbency using a table with a cut-out section to allow access to the dependent chest wall. Most cats tolerate lateral recumbency better if the lowermost forelimb is pushed forward proximal to the elbow rather than pulled forward (see Figure 46-1). For less cooperative cats, it may be preferable to allow the cat to select the position, because patient immobility is of prime importance. Ideally, electrocardiography (ECG) cables are attached during the scan, but not if this compromises patient cooperation. If an arrhythmia is auscultated, an ECG can always be recorded separately. Sedation is sometimes required, but a combination should be used that does not affect cardiac chamber dimensions or systolic function.[15] Sometimes butorphanol (0.25 mg/kg intramuscularly) is sufficient to improve patient tolerance.

Echocardiographic Exam Protocol
Two-Dimensional and M-Mode
The most essential prognostic information can be obtained from right parasternal views using 2D echocardiography. The most valuable views are those that include the LA, such as the right parasternal long axis views and a right parasternal short axis view at the level of the aortic valve (Figure 46-2). M-mode can be useful for assessing LV systolic function (Figure 46-3) and is also useful for assessment of LA function (Figure 46-4). It is less useful for assessing LV wall thickness,

because it is difficult to position the M-mode cursor without including papillary muscles, and false tendons often mimic endocardial borders, confounding accurate measurement of LV walls.

Doppler Echocardiography
Additional expertise is required for Doppler echocardiography, and the incremental prognostic value for feline cardiomyopathies may not warrant the additional necessary training. Color Doppler echocardiography can help to localize the source of murmurs, which are often associated with dynamic left or right ventricular outflow tract obstruction, but in cats with a functional murmur, the origin sometimes remains unclear. Spectral Doppler can be used to record blood flow velocity for estimation of pressure gradients across the LV outflow tract with DLVOTO. A higher pressure gradient is predicted to result in increased myocardial work and increased risk of ischemia, but the clinical implications of DLVOTO in cats are not clear. Treatment with atenolol did not affect 5-year survival rates in one study of cats with HCM.[16] In human HCM patients with dynamic obstruction, only symptomatic individuals are treated.[14] It is unknown whether cats with DLVOTO experience chest pain associated with

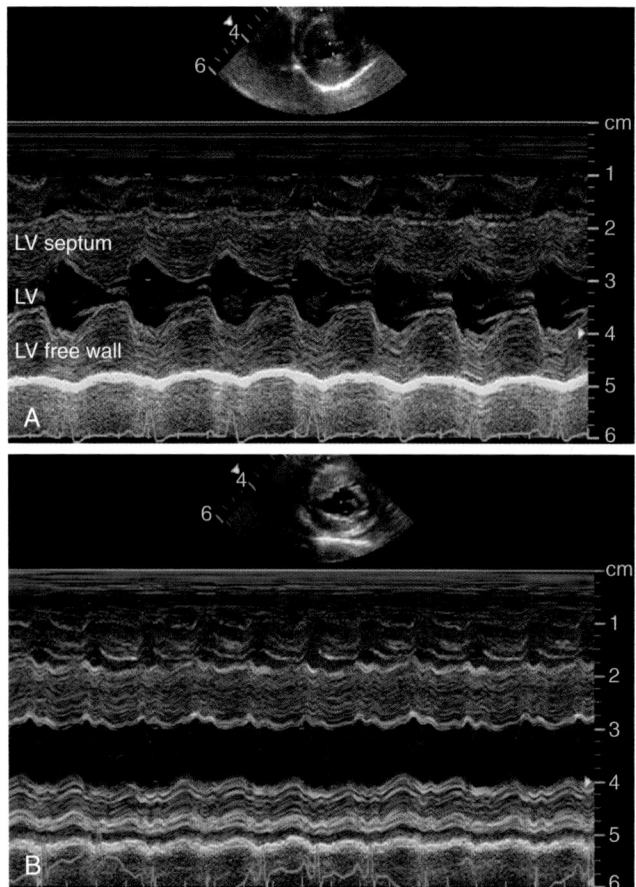

Figure 46-3: **A** and **B,** M-mode images of the left ventricle of two cats with hypertrophic cardiomyopathy. **B,** This cat has reduced left ventricular (LV) systolic function, which is associated with a worse prognosis.

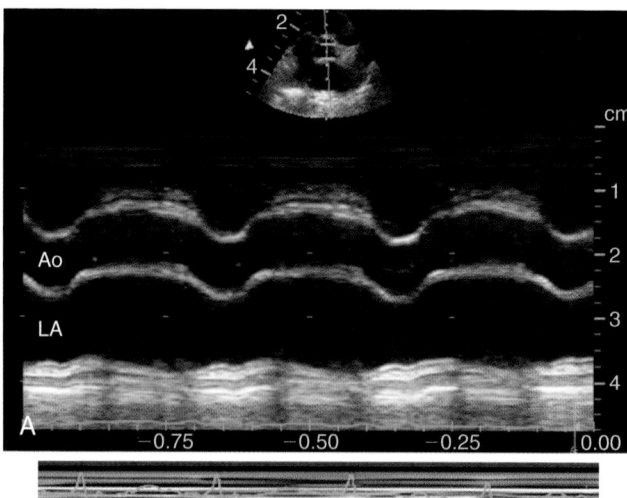

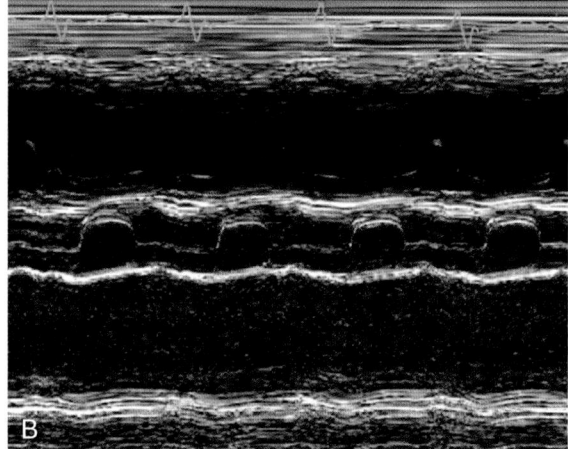

Figure 46-4: M-mode images of the left atrium (LA) and aorta (Ao) in two cats with hypertrophic cardiomyopathy. **A,** This cat has normal *LA* size and function. **B,** This cat has LA dilation and contractile dysfunction.

myocardial ischemia, and it is possible some signs in cats go unnoticed.

An even greater level of echocardiographic skill is required to investigate diastolic filling patterns. Doppler echocardiography can help to identify cats with suspicion of high LV filling pressures by demonstrating a restrictive filling pattern (where the majority of LV filling occurs early in diastole). More advanced echocardiographic imaging techniques (e.g., Doppler tissue imaging and strain imaging) have been reported in cats with cardiomyopathy, but their prognostic value has not been proven.[17-20]

ROLE OF ECHOCARDIOGRAPHY VERSUS OTHER DIAGNOSTIC TESTS

The value of echocardiography with respect to other tests depends on the technical and interpretive skills of the echocardiographer. In experienced hands, echocardiography is generally the most valuable tool for assessing cats with cardiomyopathy in almost all settings. For the novice echocardiographer, it may be sufficient to limit the echocardiography focus to LA size and the presence of pleural effusion. Whatever the operator's level of skill and experience, it is important to interpret echocardiographic findings in the context of other diagnostic tests (including physical examination findings). Arguably, among the most important adjunct tests are those for systemic diseases affecting the myocardium (e.g., anemia, hyperthyroidism, and hypertension) that require a definitive diagnosis for appropriate treatment, because management is aimed more at the underlying systemic disease than the heart.

Echocardiography can be used to help differentiate between cardiac and noncardiac causes of respiratory distress and, with increasing levels of echocardiographic skill, between normal healthy cats and cats with occult cardiomyopathy. The choice of other diagnostic tests, an echocardiographic examination "in-house," or referral to a cardiologist depends on the level of echocardiographic expertise available, as well as the specific clinical question and owner's finances.

The Cat with Respiratory Distress: Determining Congestive Heart Failure or Respiratory Disease

Decisions on management of cats with respiratory distress are frequently based on a brief physical examination with judicious use of imaging. Echocardiography offers a number of advantages in the assessment of dyspneic cats and requires minimal patient manipulation compared with conventional radiography. In cases with convincing physical exam evidence of CHF, such as presence of a gallop sound with pulmonary crackles and tachypnea, diuretic treatment may be started immediately.

Ultrasound can be used to identify pleural fluid and may even be used to help increase suspicion of pulmonary edema when B-lines ("comet-tail artifacts") are present. The diagnostic priority for cats with suspected CHF is not necessarily to obtain a cardiac diagnosis or to determine whether cardiac disease is present—but to *determine whether cardiac disease is present of sufficient severity to result in signs of CHF*. The majority of cats with pulmonary edema or pleural effusion due to cardiomyopathy have LA enlargement, so evaluation of LA size is of paramount importance. A right parasternal short axis view allows a comparison of the LA and aortic (Ao) diameter; the LA : Ao ratio should not exceed 1:6 in diastole (see Figure 46-2). An enlarged LA in this view or in a right parasternal long axis view (Figure 46-5) provides supporting evidence for CHF as the cause of respiratory distress, whether

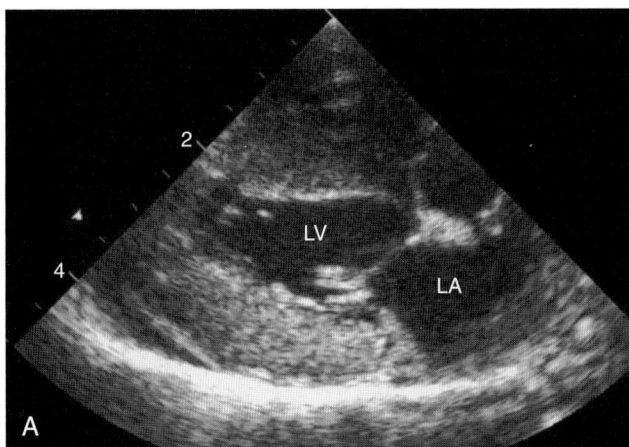

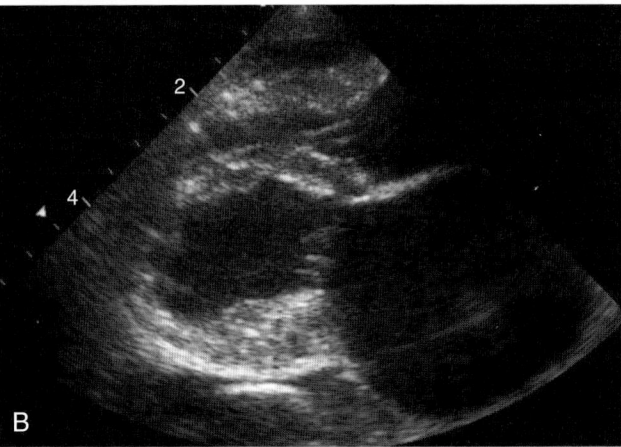

Figure 46-5: Right parasternal long axis view in two cats with cardiomyopathy. **A,** This cat has substantial left ventricle *(LV)* hypertrophy but normal left atrium *(LA)* size and shape. Such cats appear to have a relatively low risk of congestive heart failure (CHF) or aortic thromboembolism but may still be at risk of sudden death. **B,** This cat has less severe LV hypertrophy but severe LA enlargement. The risk of CHF or aortic thromboembolism is likely to be high.

or not there are ventricular changes characteristic of one of the main cardiomyopathy phenotypes.

An alternative to echocardiography or radiography (providing a blood sample can be safely obtained) is a patient-side test for N-terminal pro-brain natriuretic peptide (NT-proBNP), which identifies cats at low risk of CHF if plasma concentrations are less than 100 pmol/L (e.g., negative patient-side test). A cat with respiratory distress and NT-proBNP concentrations below this value should be investigated further for respiratory disease.

For more on the approach to the cat with respiratory distress. see Chapter 76.

The Asymptomatic Cat with a Heart Murmur

Determining Functional Murmur or Structural Heart Disease

Functional (or innocent) systolic murmurs are very common in cats, and in young adult cats functional murmurs may be more common than pathologic murmurs. Anemia should be excluded, and blood pressure and serum thyroxine concentrations should always be measured in older cats with a murmur. In the absence of other suggestive signs of heart disease (e.g., a gallop sound or arrhythmia), further testing is necessary to differentiate normal cats from those with various forms of cardiomyopathy. Biomarkers can be considered as an initial screening tool for cardiac disease; elevated NT-proBNP or cardiac troponin-I concentrations increase suspicion, but echocardiography is the gold standard test. *Identifying mild myocardial disease can be challenging and requires substantial echocardiography skills.* Mild focal LV hypertrophy is easily missed. Many cats with HCM and a murmur will have DLVOTO associated with systolic anterior motion of the mitral valve, which is best seen by viewing a right parasternal long axis loop in slow motion but is easily missed.

Fortunately, in most situations, a cat with mild LV hypertrophy and normal LA size is not managed very differently from a normal cat. Such cats appear to be at low risk for CHF or aortic thromboembolism and will often (though not always) cope with general anesthesia or intravenous fluid therapy without developing CHF. Dynamic left ventricular outflow tract obstruction appears to be well tolerated by many cats, and a subgroup that benefits from treatment to reduce outflow tract pressure gradients has not yet been identified. Overall, the prognosis remains fair for cats with HCM and normal LA size, but a risk of sudden death remains. We currently know of no therapy that decreases this risk.

The main group where it is important to differentiate normal cats from cats with a "mild" form of cardiomyopathy is pedigreed breeding cats. Veterinary cardiologists should carry out HCM screening of these cats.

Structural Heart Disease: Determining High Risk or Low Risk of Congestive Heart Failure/Aortic Thromboembolism

Although a murmur can be present in cats with advanced cardiomyopathies, some severely affected cats are completely normal on physical exam and so remain unidentified until presenting with CHF or aortic thromboembolism, which is worrisome. A gallop sound or audible arrhythmia may in fact be a better indication of a "high-risk" cat than a heart murmur.[12] Echocardiographic factors independently associated with a high risk of CHF or aortic thromboembolism include LA enlargement, reduced LA contractile function, LV systolic dysfunction, and extreme LV hypertrophy.[12] Additional echocardiographic findings in "high-risk" cats include presence of spontaneous echo-contrast (or thrombus) and regional LV wall hypokinesis, which is often associated with LV replacement fibrosis (presumably from ischemic damage). Although there are no medications known to decrease the risk of CHF in "high-risk" cats, it may be worth considering antithrombotic treatment in an attempt to reduce the risk of aortic thromboembolism (see Chapter 35).

SUMMARY

Echocardiography remains the gold standard test for evaluating cardiomyopathy in cats, even though it is highly dependent on user training and experience. Although specialized echocardiography skills are often needed for identifying subtle myocardial disease, such cats generally have a good prognosis; in nonbreeding animals, it is more important to rule out anemia, hypertension, and hyperthyroidism. More common and important clinical problems are to identify CHF in cats with respiratory distress and to identify cats with occult cardiomyopathy that are at high risk of future cardiac complications. These cats can often be identified using 2D echocardiography, with assessment of LA size playing a crucial role.

References

1. Paige CF, Abbott JA, Elvinger F, et al: Prevalence of cardiomyopathy in apparently healthy cats. *J Am Vet Med Assoc* 234:1398–1403, 2009.
2. Wagner T, Fuentes VL, Payne JR, et al: Comparison of auscultatory and echocardiographic findings in healthy adult cats. *J Vet Cardiol* 12:171–182, 2010.
3. Atkins CE, Gallo AM, Kurzman ID, et al: Risk factors, clinical signs, and survival in cats with a clinical diagnosis of idiopathic hypertrophic cardiomyopathy: 74 cases (1985-1989). *J Am Vet Med Assoc* 201:613–618, 1992.
4. Rush JE, Freeman LM, Fenollosa NK, et al: Population and survival characteristics of cats with hypertrophic cardiomyopathy: 260 cases (1990-1999). *J Am Vet Med Assoc* 220:202–207, 2002.
5. Maron BJ, Towbin JA, Thiene G, et al: Contemporary definitions and classification of the cardiomyopathies: an American Heart Association Scientific Statement from the Council on Clinical Cardiology, Heart Failure and Transplantation Committee; Quality of Care and Outcomes Research and Functional Genomics and Translational Biology Interdisciplinary Working Groups; and Council on Epidemiology and Prevention. *Circulation* 113:1807–1816, 2006.
6. Elliott P, Andersson B, Arbustini E, et al: Classification of the cardiomyopathies: a position statement from the european society of cardiology working group on myocardial and pericardial diseases. *Eur H J* 29:270–276, 2008.
7. Weichselbaum RC, Feeney DA, Jessen CR: Relationship between selected echocardiographic variables before and after radioiodine treatment in 91 hyperthyroid cats. *Vet Radiol Ultrasound* 46:506–513, 2005.
8. Menaut P, Connolly DJ, Volk A, et al: Circulating natriuretic peptide concentrations in hyperthyroid cats. *J Small Anim Pract* 53:673–678, 2012.
9. Sampedrano CC, Chetboul V, Gouni V, et al: Systolic and diastolic myocardial dysfunction in cats with hypertrophic cardiomyopathy or systemic hypertension. *J Vet Intern Med* 20(5):1106–1115, 2006.
10. Peterson ME, Taylor RS, Greco DS, et al: Acromegaly in 14 cats. *J Vet Intern Med* 4:192–201, 1990.
11. Payne J, Luis Fuentes V, Boswood A, et al: Population characteristics and survival in 127 referred cats with hypertrophic cardiomyopathy (1997 to 2005). *J Small Anim Pract* 51:540–547, 2010.
12. Payne JR, Borgeat K, Connolly DJ, et al: Prognostic indicators in cats with hypertrophic cardiomyopathy. *J Vet Intern Med* 27:1427–1436, 2013.
13. Linney CJ, Dukes-McEwan J, Stephenson HM, et al: Left atrial size, atrial function and left ventricular diastolic function in cats with hypertrophic cardiomyopathy. *J Small Anim Pract* 55:198–206, 2014.
14. Maron BJ, Maron MS, Wigle ED, et al: The 50-year history, controversy, and clinical implications of left ventricular outflow tract obstruction in hypertrophic cardiomyopathy from idiopathic hypertrophic subaortic stenosis to hypertrophic cardiomyopathy. *J Am Coll Card* 54:191–200, 2009.
15. Ward JL, Schober K, Luis-Fuentes V, et al: Effects of sedation on echocardiographic variables of left atrial and left ventricular function in healthy cats. *J Fel Med Surg* 14:678–685, 2012.
16. Schober KE, Zientek J, Li X, et al: Effect of treatment with atenolol on 5-year survival in cats with preclinical (asymptomatic) hypertrophic cardiomyopathy. *J Vet Cardiol* 15:93–104, 2013.
17. Koffas H, Dukes-McEwan J, Moran CM: Myocardial velocities measured by pulsed Doppler Tissue Imaging (DTI) in normal cats and cats with hypertrophic cardiomyopathy. *J Vet Intern Med* 16:627, 2002.
18. MacDonald KA, Kittleson MD, Kass PH, et al: Tissue Doppler imaging in Maine Coon cats with a mutation of myosin binding protein C with or without hypertrophy. *J Vet Intern Med* 21:232–237, 2007.
19. Carlos Sampedrano C, Chetboul V, Mary J, et al: Prospective echocardiographic and tissue Doppler imaging screening of a population of Maine Coon cats tested for the A31P mutation in the myosin-binding protein C gene: a specific analysis of the heterozygous status. *J Vet Intern Med* 23:91–99, 2009.
20. Wess G, Sarkar R, Hartmann K: Assessment of left ventricular systolic function by strain imaging echocardiography in various stages of feline hypertrophic cardiomyopathy. *J Vet Intern Med* 24:1375–1383, 2010.

Chronic Kidney Disease: An Update

Scott A. Brown

STAGING OF CHRONIC KIDNEY DISEASE

The International Renal Interest Society (IRIS) has proposed that the terms *chronic renal failure* and *chronic renal insufficiency* be replaced by *chronic kidney disease (CKD)* and that a staging system be used to facilitate the management of feline patients with CKD.[1] This classification scheme is based on a three-step process:

1. Establish a diagnosis of a chronic (greater than 3 months) disease affecting the kidney.
2. Determine the stage of the disease in a euvolemic cat.
3. Substage the patient based on assessment of proteinuria and blood pressure.

The term *CKD* refers to any disease process in which there is a loss of functional renal tissue due to a prolonged (generally greater than 2 months in duration), usually progressive process. Chronic kidney disease generally produces dramatic changes in renal structure as well, although the correlation between structural and functional changes in this organ is imprecise. This is partly because of the tremendous renal functional reserve; cats can survive for long periods of time (months to years) with only a small fraction of initial renal tissue, perhaps as little as 10%. Thus, CKD often smolders for many months or years before it becomes clinically apparent.

Most feline CKDs are not reversible and, once acquired, CKD rarely resolves. Although congenital disease causes a transient increase in incidence of CKD in cats less than 3 years of age, the prevalence of CKD increases with advancing age from 5 to 6 years upward. In geriatric populations at referral institutions, CKD affects up to 35% of cats.[2,3] Chronic kidney disease is common in clinical practice,[4] and the most common metabolic disease of cats, with a reasonable estimate of the prevalence of CKD in the general feline population being 1% to 3%.

ESTABLISHING A DIAGNOSIS OF CHRONIC KIDNEY DISEASE

The first step in the IRIS staging scheme is to establish a diagnosis of CKD. Any disease that affects the kidney of a cat is likely to alter both renal structure and function. It is the adequacy of renal functions, however, that dictates the impact of this disease on the patient. Although the kidney has many biological functions of importance to a cat, the most basic and central renal function is filtration and the glomerular filtration rate (GFR) serves as the "gold standard" for assessment of kidney function in cats. It is generally fair to assume that the level of most renal functions parallels changes in GFR in a clinical patient.

There are a variety of clinical signs and risk factors that may cause a clinician to suspect that a cat has CKD, such as polyuria, polydipsia, weight loss, inappetence, inactivity, unkempt hair coat, vomiting, dental disease, and halitosis. Interestingly, these clinical findings may also herald the subsequent development of CKD.[5] The presence of a reduced GFR is a highly reliable test, although it must be remembered that reductions of GFR can be caused by renal, prerenal, and postrenal factors and that renal function may be lost due to acute kidney injury (AKI, formerly known as *acute renal failure*) or CKD. In the research laboratory, GFR is assessed as urinary clearance of marker substances, such as inulin or creatinine. In clinical patients, urinary clearance tests are generally not practical, and the measurement of the disappearance from plasma of a renally-cleared marker substance such as creatinine, inulin, iohexol, or diethylenetriamine penta-acetic acid, following intravenous administration, can provide an approximation of GFR as well.[6-11]

In addition to blood creatinine and blood urea nitrogen (BUN), there are blood biomarkers for estimation of GFR that hold promise. In particular, cystatin C[12] and symmetric

Findings that Establish the Presence of a Renal Disease
Renal azotemia
Renal structural changes
Renal infection

Findings Suggestive of the Presence of a Renal Disease
Serial increases of serum creatinine (≥0.3 mg/dL [23 μmol/L])
   concentration within the reference range
Otherwise unexplained low urine specific gravity (USG)
   (<1.035)
Persistent renal proteinuria

*Distinguishing acute kidney injury (formerly known as *acute renal failure*) from chronic kidney disease (CKD) is generally based on disease duration, with CKD being any renal disease present for 3 months or longer.

dimethylarginine[13] may prove useful in cats with CKD, particularly those that are losing lean body mass, which is a common change in the latter stages of CKD and one that lowers creatinine without a change in GFR.

The IRIS recommendations recognize that in most clinical patients, GFR is assessed by the measurement of creatinine. The BUN is of less utility because it is affected by several nonrenal factors, including protein intake, liver function, and urine flow rate, making creatinine a better index of GFR. Classically, CKD in cats was diagnosed as the presence of renal azotemia (elevated creatinine) accompanied by low urine specific gravity (USG; <1.035) (Box 47-1). The broad nature of reference ranges for creatinine has led to the oversimplified assertion that three-quarters of nephrons must be destroyed before creatinine (and BUN) rises out of the reference range. This "75%" figure is indicative of how much decline in GFR would have to occur in an average cat for it to fall outside of the broad reference range, but this number does not apply to serial measurements in an individual. There is a strong correlation between creatinine (or BUN) and GFR; and in a given cat, any structural damage that reduces GFR will almost always be reflected as an increase in creatinine, initially within the reference range. Increases in creatinine in a patient that are not of prerenal or postrenal origin and that exceed 0.3 mg/dL (23 μmol/L) are suggestive of a declining GFR and the presence of a renal disease, even when the creatinine remains within the reference range.

In early feline CKD, when azotemia and clinical signs are absent, the diagnosis of CKD is sometimes made serendipitously as a result of imaging studies, laparotomy, or urinalyses conducted for other purposes. Structural changes appreciated by palpation, radiography, ultrasonography, or histopathology are generally taken as diagnostic of CKD. The urinalysis may provide clues to the presence of a renal disease. A urinary tract infection localized to the kidney is one example. A potentially useful early indicator of the presence of CKD is a USG less than 1.035 despite dehydration. Cats with early CKD often have a USG less than 1.020. However, cats with early CKD, and some with CKD of any severity, may retain the ability to concentrate urine to a specific gravity greater than or equal to 1.035. Whereas measuring USG is a simple and readily-available test, interpretation of a finding of a low USG can be complicated by the presence of conditions that lead to retention of solute in tubular fluid (e.g., diuretic administration and diabetes mellitus), central diabetes insipidus, and nephrogenic diabetes insipidus (e.g., hyperadrenocorticism, hypercalcemia, and diseases causing septicemia). Recently, tests for identification of proteinuria in cats that are both sensitive and specific have been developed.[14] These include the urine protein-creatinine (UPC) ratio and feline-specific albuminuria tests. The ability to identify persistent renal proteinuria with these tests offers promise for identifying early CKD.[14] The presence of persistent renal proteinuria in a cat is suggestive of the presence of renal disease.

IRIS grading and treatment of AKI and IRIS staging and management of CKD differ; this chapter addresses the latter. Distinguishing AKI from CKD is based on disease duration, with CKD generally being defined as any renal disease that is present for 3 months or longer. Although AKI may progress to CKD, it is generally identified soon (less than 2 weeks) after the insult. History, physical examination, hemogram, and renal imaging studies are also useful in distinguishing AKI from CKD. Some findings that are suggestive of CKD, such as the presence of renal osteodystrophy, may assist in establishing a diagnosis but are generally not useful for identifying the presence of an otherwise masked case of CKD.

INITIAL EVALUATION OF ANIMALS WITH CHRONIC KIDNEY DISEASE

For all animals with CKD, a thorough history and physical examination should be accompanied by complete clinical pathology testing that includes a biochemical panel, hematology, urinalysis with sediment examination, and aerobic bacterial urine culture. Unless these tests reveal evidence of urinary tract inflammation, hemorrhage, or infection, specific tests to quantify the magnitude of proteinuria (typically the UPC) should also be performed. Survey radiography and/or abdominal ultrasonography and blood pressure measurements should be performed. This initial battery of tests allows the veterinarian to stage and substage the disease, which leads to the proper therapeutic and diagnostic considerations.

ESTABLISHING THE CHRONIC KIDNEY DISEASE STAGE OF THE PATIENT'S DISEASE

Chronic kidney disease in cats often progresses along a continuum from an initial nonazotemic stage (IRIS CKD Stage 1) to end-stage uremia (IRIS CKD Stage 4). In many cats with CKD, the rate of progression is remarkably slow. As veterinarians, we are obligated to address the specific problems and patient needs that characterize the animal's disease, and this varies from stage to stage. Staging of an animal with

Table 47-1	International Renal Interest Society Staging of Feline Chronic Kidney Disease			
Creatinine*	**Stage 1: Nonazotemic Chronic Kidney Disease**	**Stage 2: Mild Renal Azotemic**	**Stage 3: Moderate Renal Azotemia**	**Stage 4: Severe Renal Azotemia**
(µmol/L)	<140	140 to 250	251 to 440	>440
(mg/dL)	<1.6	1.6 to 2.8	2.9 to 5.0	>5.0

*Blood creatinine measured in a euvolemic patient with stable renal function.

Table 47-2	Blood Pressure: Substaging of Feline Chronic Kidney Disease			
	RISK OF FUTURE TARGET ORGAN DAMAGE			
	Minimal Risk	**Low Risk**	**Moderate Risk**	**High Risk**
Blood Pressure (mm Hg)				
Systolic	<150	150-159	160-179	≥180
Diastolic	<95	95-99	100-119	≥120
IRIS Substage	Normotension	Borderline Hypertension	Hypertension	Severe Hypertension

IRIS, International Renal Interest Society.

an established diagnosis of CKD is based on measurement of creatinine in a well-hydrated patient with stable renal function using a four-stage classification system (Table 47-1).[1] As outlined later, staging enables an individualized prognosis and an approach to diagnostic and therapeutic procedures that is tailored to disease severity.

PROGNOSIS

International Renal Interest Society CKD staging enables a veterinarian to offer stage-specific prognostic information. Median survival in a study of 208 cats with CKD varied dramatically among IRIS CKD Stage 2 (median survival of 1151 days), Stage 3 (679 days), and Stage 4 (35 days) patients.[15] As in other species, the renal lesion that correlates best with progression of CKD is interstitial fibrosis;[16] hyperphosphatemia, anemia, and proteinuria are positively correlated with the extent of renal interstitial fibrosis in cats. In general, negative prognostic factors in cats with CKD include the presence of persistent renal proteinuria (elevated UPC), systemic hypertension, and increased severity of hyperphosphatemia and anemia.[16-19] In cats with CKD, fibroblast growth factor 23 (FGF-23) is positively correlated with parathyroid hormone and blood phosphate levels and inversely related to hematocrit. Elevated levels of FGF-23 predict the development of azotemia in geriatric cats,[20-22] and thus FGF-23 appears to be another negative prognostic factor in cats with CKD. A role for oxidative stress as a cause of progression, as noted in dogs,[23] remains uncertain in cats.[24] Some of these negative prognostic factors—notably proteinuria,

hypertension, hyperphosphatemia, elevated FGF-23, and anemia—may be both predictors and causes of progression in feline CKD.

SUBSTAGING CHRONIC KIDNEY DISEASE ON BASIS OF BLOOD PRESSURE

Cats with CKD frequently exhibit elevations of systemic arterial blood pressure.[25,26] The American College of Veterinary Internal Medicine consensus statement defined systemic hypertension as any elevation of blood pressure that leads to target organ damage (TOD) and defined blood pressure ranges associated with minimal, low, moderate, and severe risk of TOD (Table 47-2).[25] The target organs of concern in cats with the associated TOD are the kidneys (progression of CKD, proteinuria), eyes (blindness, intraocular hemorrhage, retinal detachment, retinal vessel tortuosity), brain (seizures, depression), and cardiovascular system (congestive heart failure, vessel rupture). Left ventricular hypertrophy (LVH) is commonly observed in hypertensive cats, although there is controversy as to whether this constitutes true TOD or is simply an adaptive change. Nonetheless, the presence of LVH in a cat with CKD should be taken as presumptive evidence of clinically significant hypertension unless proven otherwise. Systemic hypertension is linked to glomerulosclerosis in cats with CKD[16] and is a negative prognostic factor. The IRIS recommends that blood pressure be measured, using a device and method individualized for each clinical practice, in every cat with CKD and that target organs be carefully evaluated for the presence of TOD. Although some devices provide both systolic and diastolic blood pressure, staging is most often done on the basis of systolic blood pressure measurements because recent evidence suggests that systolic hypertension may be the most important determinant of TOD in other species.[27] For more on hypertension in cats, see Chapter 38.

SUBSTAGING CHRONIC KIDNEY DISEASE ON BASIS OF PROTEINURIA

Recent findings have suggested that renal protein leak is not only a marker of severity of renal disease but also of prognostic value and potentially a cause of renal injury.[14,19] We now recognize that proteinuria (UPC >0.4) is associated with increased risk of developing end-stage CKD in cats[28,29] and that there is an increased risk of mortality in aged cats when proteinuria is present (UPC >0.2). Proteinuria is associated with the presence of intraglomerular hypertension[30] even when the primary renal lesion does not involve the glomerulus, which seems to be the usual case in cats. Further, studies in a variety of species have shown that therapies that reduce the magnitude of proteinuria are often renoprotective.

Proper substaging based on proteinuria mandates following a multistep approach.[14] A positive finding of proteinuria in a urinalysis with routine dipstick evaluation is often the first step, and because of frequent false positives, most clinical pathology laboratories follow up a positive dipstick test with an acid precipitation test (e.g., sulfosalicylic acid test). The clinician should carefully evaluate the urine sediment and other patient data to determine if prerenal (e.g., hemolysis) or postrenal (e.g., inflammation, hemorrhage, or infection) causes may be causing proteinuria. If a renal proteinuria is still suspected, then a more specific test (UPC or species-specific albuminuria test) should be conducted. When monitoring a feline patient with renal proteinuria, it is important to determine if the proteinuria is transient or persistent (at least two tests at 2-week intervals). If persistent renal proteinuria is present in a patient with CKD, further management is generally based on the UPC (Table 47-3). Although not useful for urine cultures, fresh, carefully-collected, properly-stored urine can be used to monitor changes in UPC in a patient. Substantial within-individual variation in UPC occurs. There is utility in pooling multiple urine samples, collected over 2 to 3 days and stored in the refrigerator, to limit the influence of this variation on patient management. Nonetheless, a change of at least 50% in the UPC must be observed before one can conclude that the magnitude of proteinuria has changed in a patient (e.g., as evidence of a positive response to therapy).

RENAL EVALUATION AND SPECIFIC THERAPY

Every CKD is caused by a primary renal disease. In cats with early CKD (IRIS CKD Stages 1 and 2), identification of the primary renal disease is an important focus (Figure 47-1). Examples of renal evaluation that may be appropriate at these early stages include renal imaging (survey and/or contrast radiographic studies, ultrasonography), urinalysis with specific tests for proteinuria and urine culture, and renal biopsy. Known causes of CKD that may be diagnosed through this approach include diseases of the macrovascular compartment (e.g., systemic hypertension, coagulopathies, chronic hypoperfusion), microvascular compartment (e.g., systemic and glomerular hypertension, glomerulonephritis, developmental disorders, congenital collagen defects, amyloidosis), interstitial compartment (e.g., pyelonephritis, neoplasia, neoplastic, obstructive uropathy, allergic and immune-mediated nephritis), and tubular compartment (e.g., tubular reabsorptive defects, chronic low grade nephrotoxicity, obstructive uropathy). These conditions may be acquired or heritable. A variety of breeds are afflicted with heritable CKD that may have pathognomonic clinical and histopathologic findings, including the Abyssinian (medullary amyloidosis)[31,32] and Persian (polycystic kidney disease) cats.[33,34]

Specific therapy is defined as a treatment that is directed at elimination of the primary renal disease. The goal of specific therapy is to reduce injury caused by the primary renal disease in order to prevent progression of the CKD to the latter stages. Examples of specific therapy (Table 47-4) include antibiotic therapy in cases of CKD caused by pyelonephritis, antihypertensives for cats with hypertensive nephropathy, dietary calcium restriction for animals with hypercalcemic nephropathy, immunosuppressive medications for immune complex glomerulonephritis, and surgery for obstructive uropathy. Nonetheless, remarkably little is known about the prevalence of primary renal diseases in cats and, as a result, biopsy and specific therapy are rarely employed in this species.

Interstitial fibrosis and alterations in renal shape and size occur in most animals with IRIS CKD Stages 3 or 4, regardless of inciting primary renal disease.[35,36] The severity of interstitial fibrosis is positively correlated to the magnitude

Table 47-3	Proteinuria: Substaging of Feline Chronic Kidney Disease*		
	INTERNATIONAL RENAL INTEREST SOCIETY SUBSTAGE		
	Nonproteinuric	**Borderline Proteinuric**	**Proteinuric**
Urine protein-to-creatinine ratio	<0.2	0.2-0.4	>0.4

*If urine protein is not measured, the patient is categorized with the substage of risk not determined (P-RND).

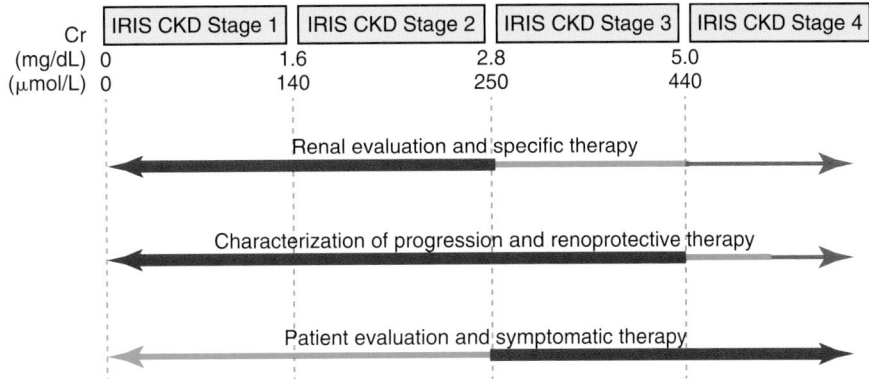

Figure 47-1: Diagnostic and therapeutic emphases in different stages of feline chronic kidney disease *(CKD)*. Once a diagnosis of CKD is established, the International Renal Interest Society *(IRIS)* recommends staging (see Table 47-1) the disease on the basis of a measurement of blood creatinine *(Cr)* concentration in a cat that is hydrated with stable renal function and then substaging on the basis of blood pressure (see Table 47-2) and proteinuria (see Table 47-3). There are three sets of linked diagnostic and therapeutic considerations, with the importance of each set being reflected by the thickness of the corresponding arrow in this diagram. See the text for further details.

of decline of GFR and negatively correlated with the prognosis. Factors associated with enhanced interstitial fibrosis in cats include hyperphosphatemia, proteinuria, and anemia.[16] Chronic interstitial nephritis, also known as *chronic tubulointerstitial fibrosis,* describes the morphologic appearance of kidneys with IRIS Stages 3 or 4 CKD of any cause and renal evaluation (e.g., biopsy) is unlikely to yield clues as to the identity of the primary disease. Consequently, for cats in Stages 3 and 4, renal evaluation and specific therapy are a lower priority.

EVALUATION OF PROGRESSION AND RENOPROTECTIVE THERAPY

A critical consideration in the treatment of cats with CKD is the progressive nature of the disease.[37] Because the only effective therapy for end-stage uremia (i.e., intensive fluid therapy, renal transplantation, and/or dialysis) is often prohibitively expensive, a goal of therapy should be to prevent progression of CKD through the IRIS stages to end-stage uremia. There are several reasons that renal function progressively deteriorates in an animal with CKD. As outlined earlier, in Stage 1 and early Stage 2, the goal of specific therapy is to minimize damage that occurs from the primary renal disease. However, there are two additional types of processes that contribute to progressive destruction of renal tissue in the middle stages of CKD (Stages 2 to 3): (1) abnormalities caused by a disruption of renal homeostatic mechanisms (e.g., complications of kidney dysfunction such as systemic hypertension and hyperphosphatemia) and (2) maladaptive changes in remaining renal tissue (e.g., glomerular hypertension and associated proteinuria).[30] These two types of processes are common to CKD of any cause and lead to a vicious cycle of self-perpetuating renal injury referred to as *inherent progression.* Therapeutic intervention can modify renal adaptations and limit the extent of some complications

of kidney dysfunction, theoretically limiting progressive renal injury by interrupting this vicious cycle.

Although the rate of progressive decline of renal function varies, studies to date suggest that inherent progression occurs in all animals with IRIS Stages 2 to 3, albeit very slowly in many cats. Characterization of the rate of progression of CKD through serial determinations of creatinine is a high priority at this time (see Figure 47-1). Measures that may slow inherent progression are referred to as *renoprotective therapies* (see Table 47-4), and these include dietary phosphate restriction,[38,39] antihypertensive agents in animals with high blood pressure,[40-42] antiproteinuric therapy,[43,44] and dietary therapy.[45] Although some recommend the incorporation of modifications, such as a phosphate binder and fish oil supplementation, to a maintenance feline diet in IRIS CKD Stage 2, this approach is untested and current evidence[45] suggests that a renal diet is appropriate for this stage. In any case, dietary changes instituted in IRIS CKD Stages 2 to 4 generally include reduced phosphate intake,[38] fish oil supplementation,[46] and (based on studies in dogs[23]) dietary antioxidants. There is evidence[47] that calcitriol administration slows progression in dogs with IRIS CKD Stages 3 to 4, and this approach is often recommended in cats in these stages as well. When given, calcitriol is initiated in cats that are normocalcemic with serum phosphate less than 6.0 mg/dL (1.9 mmol/L) at an ultralow dosage (2.5 ng/kg orally, [PO] given once daily separately from meals).

Control of hyperphosphatemia is widely accepted to be renoprotective in cats with CKD.[48] Adjustments of therapy are based on measurement of serum phosphate concentration and therapeutic targets vary by IRIS stage (Table 47-5), with evidence suggesting that the therapeutic goal is the lowest achievable blood phosphate concentration. Although cats with IRIS CKD Stage 1 generally do not require therapeutic intervention, and where needed, the addition of an intestinal phosphate binder to a feline maintenance diet or the use of a specially formulated ("renal") diet is usually effective. In

Table 47-4 **Diagnostic and Therapeutic Focus of Staged Management of Feline Chronic Kidney Disease**

Process	Primary Focus in IRIS Stage(s)	Diagnostic Assessment	Therapeutic Considerations
Primary renal disease	IRIS CKD Stages 1 to 2	**Renal Evaluation** Renal palpation Radiography Ultrasonography Urinalysis with sediment exam ± quantification of urine protein Renal biopsy	**Specific Therapies (Examples)** Antibiotics for pyelonephritis Antihypertensive for hypertensive nephropathy Immunosuppressive medications for immune complex glomerulonephritis
Progressive loss of kidney function	IRIS CKD Stages 2 to 3	**Evaluation of Progression** Serial measurements of Cr	**Renoprotective Therapies** Dietary phosphate restriction, intestinal phosphate binders Antihypertensive therapy (see later) Antiproteinuric therapy (see later) Dietary n-3 PUFA supplementation Calcitriol Dietary antioxidants
Uremia	IRIS CKD Stages 3 to 4	**Patient Evaluation** History Physical examination Body condition scoring Hematology Biochemical panel Urinalysis Urine culture	**Symptomatic Therapies** "Renal diet" formulated for feline renal disease Manage acid-base and electrolyte disorders Antiemetics; appetite stimulant Darbepoietin Fluid therapy Calcitriol Treat postrenal factors, such as uroliths, where identified Feeding tube placement Renal replacement therapy
Elevated blood pressure	IRIS CKD Stages 1 to 4	Serial measurements of blood pressure	**Antihypertensive Therapies** Calcium channel blocker (e.g., amlodipine 0.25-0.50 mg/kg once daily orally [PO]) ACE-I (e.g., enalapril or benazepril 0.5 mg/kg once or twice daily PO) ARB (e.g., telmisartan 1-3 mg/kg once daily PO)
Proteinuria	IRIS CKD Stages 1 to 4	Urinalysis with sediment exam Urine culture Urine protein-to-creatinine ratio Albumin-specific tests	**Antiproteinuric Therapies** ACE-I or angiotensin receptor blocker (dosage as earlier) Dietary protein restriction ("renal diet") Dietary n-3 PUFA supplementation (renal diet ± 0.25 g/kg n-3 PUFA containing fish oil)

ACE-I, Angiotensin-converting enzyme inhibitor; *ARB,* angiotensin receptor blocker; *CKD,* chronic kidney disease; *Cr,* creatinine; *IRIS,* International Renal Interest Society, *PUFA,* polyunsaturated fatty acid.

IRIS CKD Stages 2 to 4, a special renal diet is indicated. If dietary restriction of phosphate is unsuccessful in maintaining the target level of serum phosphate within 2 to 3 months, phosphate-binding gels containing lanthanum, aluminum, or calcium salts should be administered with meals (e.g., initial dosage for calcium and aluminum salts is 30 mg/kg with dosage increased as needed to achieve desired effect, up to 180 mg/kg). Calcium-containing phosphate binding agents should be used with caution in cats receiving calcitriol. By late Stage 2 and in Stages 3 and 4, the addition of an intestinal phosphate binding agent is generally required to reach the target serum phosphate concentration.

Approximately 20% of cats with CKD exhibit elevations of blood pressure, which may be observed in any IRIS stage. This is not effectively controlled by feeding a low-salt diet. In cats with a blood pressure in the moderate or high risk category and those with a low risk exhibiting ocular or central nervous system (CNS) TOD, antihypertensive therapy is appropriate (see Table 47-2). Unless emergency therapy is required (e.g., acute blindness due to retinal detachment), it is important to document elevated blood pressure on at least two occasions, because this therapy is often lifelong. Because of the importance of maintaining renal perfusion in animals with CKD, the usual antihypertensive

Table 47-5	Therapeutic Targets for Management of Hyperphosphatemia in Cats with Chronic Kidney Disease	
IRIS CKD Stage	**Target Serum Phosphate**	**Management Options**
1	2.5-4.5 mg/dL (0.81-1.45 mmol/L)	Normal diet ± intestinal phosphate binder or dietary phosphate restriction
2	2.5-5.0 mg/dL (0.81-1.61 mmol/L)	Dietary phosphate restriction ("renal diet") and/or intestinal phosphate binder
3	2.5-4.5 mg/dL (0.81-1.45 mmol/L)	Dietary phosphate restriction plus intestinal phosphate binder
4	2.5-6.0 mg/dL (0.81-1.94 mmol/L)	Dietary phosphate restriction plus intestinal phosphate binder

CKD, Chronic kidney disease; *IRIS*, International Renal Interest Society.

medications are vasodilatory agents. The most commonly employed agents are calcium channel blockers (CCBs), specifically amlodipine besylate (0.25 to 0.50 mg/kg PO once daily). Others include angiotensin-converting enzyme inhibitors (ACE-Is) such as enalapril or benazepril (0.5 to 1.0 mg/kg PO every 12 to 24 hours), and angiotensin receptor blockers (ARBs) such as telmisartan (1 to 3 mg/kg PO once daily). Although it is generally agreed that the most appropriate initial agent is amlodipine, some recommend the coadministration of an inhibitor of the renin-angiotensin-aldosterone system (ACE-I or ARB), because CCBs activate the renin-angiotensin-aldosterone system. Although these may be coadministered at the recommended dosages, it is important to include a CCB as part of the initial therapy in cats (particularly in Substage AP3).[49] An ACE-I or ARB certainly should be added if the highest recommended dosage of amlodipine (0.5 mg/kg PO once daily) is ineffective or if proteinuria (UPC >0.4) persists. See Chapter 38 for more on diagnosis and management of feline hypertension. The institution of antihypertensive therapy and any dosage adjustments should be followed in 5 to 10 days with a re-evaluation of creatinine, blood pressure, and UPC. Although it is reasonable to conclude that the best markers of efficacy of antihypertensive therapy are a reduction in blood pressure (preferably of at least one risk category; see Table 47-2) and a reduction in the UPC (preferably to <0.4), the UPC is the single best indicator of therapeutic success (or failure).

Proteinuria confers a poorer prognosis when the UPC ratio exceeds 0.4 in cats with CKD. If proteinuria of this magnitude is persistent and renal in origin in a cat with CKD, the clinician should consider antiproteinuric therapy (e.g., ACE-I or ARB, low protein renal diet, and/or omega-2 n-3 polyunsaturated fatty acid [PUFA] supplementation). In this situation, antiproteinuric therapy is considered renoprotective and is, thus, of high priority in Stages 2 and 3. Specially-formulated renal diets are already supplemented with n-3 PUFA. If the aforementioned measures do not reduce the magnitude of proteinuria to the target UPC of 0.4, the diet may be further supplemented with of 0.25 g/kg of n-3 PUFA containing fish oil. Serial determinations of the level of

proteinuria by a complete urinalysis with measurement of the UPC should be used to evaluate the success of this approach. The therapeutic goal is a UPC less than 0.4.

In dogs[50,51] and to a lesser extent cats[45,46] there is a rationale for the inclusion of dietary n-3 PUFA in IRIS Stages 2 and 3, regardless of the level of blood pressure or UPC. This may be accomplished with the use of renal diets and/or additional n-3 PUFA (as earlier). Although renoprotective therapy is a high priority in IRIS Stages 2 and 3, it becomes increasingly less important in late Stage 4 as the focus of therapy becomes management of the complications of uremia (see the next section).

The use of agents with potential nephrotoxicity, such as aminoglycoside antibiotics, generally should be avoided in CKD. Interestingly, laboratory studies indicate that nonsteroidal anti-inflammatory drugs (NSAIDs) do not reduce GFR in normal cats[52] or those with reduced renal function.[53] Furthermore, results of recent clinical investigations support the contention that these agents can be used safely in affected cats[54] and, further, that low-dosage NSAIDs (e.g., meloxicam at 0.015 to 0.033 mg/kg PO once daily) may actually slow the rate of progression of feline CKD.[55] Until evaluated in a prospective, blinded, placebo-controlled clinical trial, the use of NSAIDs as renoprotective therapy seems unwarranted. However, these agents may be less nephrotoxic in cats with CKD than previously thought.

PATIENT EVALUATION AND SYMPTOMATIC THERAPY

Patient evaluations, which include efforts to identify developing complications (e.g., systemic hypertension, disorders of potassium homeostasis, metabolic acidosis, proteinuria, anemia, and bacterial urinary tract infections), should be aggressively and prospectively pursued during all routine visits regardless of IRIS stage.

As CKD progresses into IRIS Stage 4, clinical consequences of the reduction of GFR become apparent and thorough patient evaluations followed by appropriate symptomatic therapy (see Table 47-4) become increasingly important (see Figure 47-1). Initially, uremia causes occasional vomiting and lethargy. As CKD progresses within Stage 4 (generally over many months or years in cats), anorexia, weight loss, dehydration, oral ulceration, vomiting, and diarrhea may become more frequent and severe. Loose teeth, deformable maxilla and mandible, or pathologic fractures may be seen with renal secondary osteodystrophy, but these are not common in cats. Physical examination and imaging studies of animals in IRIS Stages 3 and 4 usually reveal small, irregular kidneys, although normal to large kidneys can be observed in cats with tumors, hydronephrosis, or glomerulonephritis. Mucous membranes are pale in late IRIS Stages 3 and 4 due to the presence of a nonregenerative, normocytic, normochromic anemia.

Symptomatic therapy is a high priority at this time. As dietary restriction of protein may relieve some of the signs of uremia, a high-quality protein (e.g., egg protein) should be fed at a level of 2.8 to 3.8 g/kg/day. Commercial diets formulated for cats with CKD generally meet this recommendation. Cats with Stage 4 CKD often exhibit acid-base and electrolyte disorders; these should be aggressively treated. Although commercial renal diets are supplemented with potassium and alkali, hypokalemia and acidemia are common observations in cats with IRIS Stage 4 CKD. Potassium citrate or sodium bicarbonate, given PO to effect, may be indicated if the animal is acidemic (plasma bicarbonate less than 18 mEq/L [18 mmol/L]). Potassium supplementation (1 to 3 mEq/kg/day) may be required to maintain eukalemia, particularly in polyuric cats or cats with inappetence. The therapeutic goals are the reference ranges for potassium and bicarbonate, with no known benefit of additional supplementation of potassium or alkali once this goal is achieved.

Gastric hyperacidity and the adverse effects of uremic toxins on the gastric mucosa lead to mucosal erosions and ulcerations, which contribute to inappetence and vomiting. The administration of a proton pump inhibitor (e.g., omeprazole 1 mg/kg PO once daily) or a histamine-2 receptor agonist, such as famotidine (0.5 mg/kg PO every 6 to 12 hours) or ranitidine (2 mg/kg PO every 8 to 12 hours), may decrease gastric acidity and thus enhance appetite and reduce the frequency of vomiting. Other antiemetics such as prokinetic agents (e.g., metoclopramide at 0.2 mg/kg PO every 8 to 12 hours), phenothiazine derivatives (e.g., meclizine), and/or maropitant (1 mg/kg PO once daily) may prove useful in the management of uremic cats. Anabolic steroids, such as oxymetholone or nandrolone, have been administered to stimulate red blood cell (RBC) production in animals that are anemic, but this approach is not effective. Human recombinant erythropoietin (e.g., darbepoetin alfa, 1 to 2 mcg/kg subcutaneously (SC) weekly initially, dosed every 2 to 3 weeks to effect after hematocrit reaches the target range of 25% to 35% with supplemental iron administration and weekly hematocrit determinations)[56,57] is often effective in stimulating RBC production (sustained response observed in 56% of treated cats in one study).[58] An increase in systolic blood pressure of approximately 30 mm Hg may be observed in cats that respond to recombinant erythropoietin adminis-

tration.[58] Darbepoetin has a longer half-life than erythropoietin and appears to be less likely to induce antibody formation. Administration is recommended for animals showing apparent clinical signs of anemia (e.g., weakness, lack of sociability, and lethargy not attributable to other factors), which generally occurs at a hematocrit less than or equal to 20%.

In latter Stage 3 and Stage 4, canned foods are generally preferred to reduce the extent of dehydration. Furthermore, fluid therapy with polyionic solutions or 5% dextrose, given intravenously (IV) or SC in the hospital or SC by owners at home (10 to 50 mL/kg every 1 to 3 days), may prove beneficial in cats with intermittent signs of uremia. Renal secondary hyperparathyroidism may contribute to uremia in cats, and calcitriol may be a useful adjunct to dietary phosphate restriction and intestinal phosphate binders to manage this condition. The use of pharmacologic agents for appetite stimulation is appropriate in late Stage 4. In particular, mirtazapine (initial dosage of 2 mg/cat PO every 2 days) can be effective as both an appetite stimulant and an antiemetic.[59,60] Cyproheptadine (0.5 to 1 mg/cat PO once daily) has also been advocated as an appetite stimulant in Stage 4 CKD, although its efficacy has not been established. Veterinarians should be prepared to provide counseling to owners on approaches to enhance food intake, including the use of multiple renal diet preparations, warming of food, flavor enhancers, and the pluses and minuses of home-made diets. Cats with CKD may develop ureteroliths, and obstructive uropathy should be considered in any cat with CKD that develops a sudden, unexpected increase in creatinine. Placement of feeding tubes, such as nasogastric or percutaneous endoscopic gastrostomy tubes, can be an effective approach to the management of cats with chronic inappetence in late Stage 4. Renal replacement therapy (e.g., renal transplantation and/or dialytic therapy) should be discussed with owners in early Stage 4 with implementation considered in late Stage 4.

Patient evaluation and symptomatic therapy are lower priorities in the earlier stages (1 and 2). However, as noted earlier, systemic hypertension, proteinuria, and urinary tract infections are three patient problems that may be encountered in any IRIS stage.

FOLLOW-UP PATIENT EVALUATIONS

Scheduled evaluations of cats with CKD should include a thorough history and physical examination, complete biochemical panel, hematology, urinalysis, assessment of UPC and blood pressure, and annual aerobic bacterial urine culture. It should be noted that systemic hypertension, proteinuria, and urinary tract infections may be observed in any IRIS stage. In IRIS Stages 1 and 2, annual evaluations may suffice. Evaluations should be done on a semiannual basis in Stage 3, regardless of the health of the animal. Uremic animals in late Stage 3 and animals in Stage 4 should be evaluated at 1- to 3-month intervals. Cats with unstable renal function, ocular or CNS TOD, or undergoing adjustments to therapy should be seen more frequently.

SUMMARY

The proper management of a cat with CKD requires a clear understanding of the diagnostic and therapeutic priorities in the stage of disease at the time the patient is being managed (see Figure 47-1). Early in the disease process (IRIS CKD Stage 1), a careful evaluation of the kidneys to identify the primary disease process and specific therapy to eliminate this disease is appropriate. In the middle stages (2 and 3), inherent progression and renoprotective therapy are paramount. In the final stage of CKD, IRIS Stage 4, more frequent and thorough evaluations of the patient with institution of appropriate symptomatic therapy become the primary considerations of the veterinarian.

References

1. Elliott J, Watson A: Chronic kidney disease: staging and management. In Bonagura J, Twedt D, editors: *Current veterinary therapy XIV*, St Louis, 2009, Saunders/Elsevier, pp 883–892.
2. Polzin DJ, Osborne CA: Update: conservative medical management of chronic renal failure. In Kirk RW, editor: *Current veterinary therapy IX*, Philadelphia, 1986, Saunders, pp 1167–1173.
3. Krawiec D, Gelberg H: Chronic renal disease in cats. In Kirk RW, editor: *Current veterinary therapy X*, Philadelphia, 1989, Saunders, pp 1170–1173.
4. Lund E, Armstrong P, Kirk C, et al: Health status and population characteristics of dogs and cats examined at private veterinary practices in the United States. *J Am Vet Med Assoc* 214:1336–1342, 1999.
5. Greene JP, Lefebvre SL, Wang M, et al: Risk factors associated with the development of chronic kidney disease in cats evaluated at primary care veterinary hospitals. *J Am Vet Med Assoc* 244:320–327, 2014.
6. Labato MA, Ross LA: Plasma disappearance of creatinine as a renal function test in the dog. *Res Vet Sci* 50:253–258, 1991.
7. Finch NC, Heiene R, Elliott J, et al: A single sample method for estimating glomerular filtration rate in cats. *J Vet Intern Med* 27:782–790, 2013.
8. Brown SA, Finco DR, Boudinot D, et al: Evaluation of a single injection method, using iohexol, for estimating glomerular filtration rate in cats and dogs. *Am J Vet Res* 57:105–110, 1996.
9. Moe L, Heiene R: Estimation of glomerular filtration rate in dogs with 99m-Tc-DTPA and iohexol. *Res Vet Sci* 52:138, 1995.
10. Heiene R, Moe L: Pharmacokinetic aspects of measurement of glomerular filtration rate in the dog: a review. *J Vet Intern Med* 12:401–414, 1998.
11. Finch NC, Syme HM, Elliott J, et al: Glomerular filtration rate estimation by use of a correction formula for slope-intercept plasma iohexol clearance in cats. *Am J Vet Res* 72:1652–1659, 2011.
12. Almy FS, Christopher MM, King DP, et al: Evaluation of cystatin C as an endogenous marker of glomerular filtration rate in dogs. *J Vet Intern Med* 16:45–51, 2002.
13. Jepson RE, Syme HM, Vallance C, et al: Plasma asymmetric dimethylarginine, symmetric dimethylarginine, l-arginine, and nitrite/nitrate concentrations in cats with chronic kidney disease and hypertension. *J Vet Intern Med* 22:317–324, 2008.
14. Lees GE, Brown SA, Elliott J, et al: Assessment and management of proteinuria in dogs and cats: 2004 ACVIM Forum Consensus Statement (small animal). *J Vet Intern Med* 19:377–385, 2005.
15. Boyd LM, Langston C, Thompson K, et al: Survival in cats with naturally occurring chronic kidney disease (2000-2002). *J Vet Intern Med* 22:1111–1117, 2008.
16. Chakrabarti S, Syme HM, Brown CA, et al: Histomorphometry of feline chronic kidney disease and correlation with markers of renal dysfunction. *Vet Pathol* 50:147–155, 2013.
17. Chakrabarti S, Syme HM, Elliott J: Clinicopathological variables predicting progression of azotemia in cats with chronic kidney disease. *J Vet Intern Med* 26:275–281, 2012.
18. King JN, Tasker S, Gunn-Moore DA, et al: Prognostic factors in cats with chronic kidney disease. *J Vet Intern Med* 21:906–916, 2007.
19. Syme HM, Markwell PJ, Pfeiffer D, et al: Survival of cats with naturally occurring chronic renal failure is related to severity of proteinuria. *J Vet Intern Med* 20:528–535, 2006.
20. Finch NC, Geddes RF, Syme HM, et al: Fibroblast growth factor 23 (FGF-23) concentrations in cats with early nonazotemic chronic kidney disease (CKD) and in healthy geriatric cats. *J Vet Intern Med* 27:227–233, 2013.
21. Geddes RF, Elliott J, Syme HM: The effect of feeding a renal diet on plasma fibroblast growth factor 23 concentrations in cats with stable azotemic chronic kidney disease. *J Vet Intern Med* 27:1354–1361, 2013.
22. Geddes RF, Finch NC, Elliott J, et al: Fibroblast growth factor 23 in feline chronic kidney disease. *J Vet Intern Med* 27:234–241, 2013.
23. Brown SA: Oxidative stress and chronic kidney disease. *Vet Clin North Am Small Anim Pract* 38:157–166, 2008.
24. Krofic Zel M, Tozon N, Nemec Svete A: Plasma and erythrocyte glutathione peroxidase activity, serum selenium concentration, and plasma total antioxidant capacity in cats with IRIS stages I-IV chronic kidney disease. *J Vet Intern Med* 28:130–136, 2014.
25. Brown S, Atkins C, Bagley R, et al: Guidelines for the identification, evaluation, and management of systemic hypertension in dogs and cats. *J Vet Intern Med* 21:542–558, 2007.
26. Syme HM, Barber PJ, Markwell PJ, et al: Prevalence of systolic hypertension in cats with chronic renal failure at initial evaluation. *J Am Vet Med Assoc* 220:1799–1804, 2002.
27. Mentari E, Rahman M: Blood pressure and progression of chronic kidney disease: importance of systolic, diastolic, or diurnal variation. *Curr Hypertens Rep* 6:400–404, 2004.
28. Syme HM, Elliott J: Urinary protein excretion in cats with renal failure and/or hypertension. *J Vet Int Med* 17:405A, 2003.
29. Syme HM, Elliott J: Relation of survival time and urinary protein excretion in cats with renal failure and/or hypertension. *J Vet Int Med* 17:405A, 2003.
30. Brown SA: Renal pathophysiology: lessons learned from the canine remnant kidney model. *J Vet Emerg Crit Care (San Antonio)* 23:115–121, 2013.
31. Boyce J, DiBartola SP, Chew DJ, et al: Familial renal amyloidosis in Abyssinian cats. *Vet Pathol* 21:33–38, 1984.
32. DiBartola SP, Reiter JA, Cornacoff JB, et al: Serum amyloid A protein concentration measured by radial immunodiffusion in Abyssinian and non-Abyssinian cats. *Am J Vet Res* 50:1414–1417, 1989.
33. Pedersen KM, Pedersen HD, Haggstrom J, et al: Increased mean arterial pressure and aldosterone-to-renin ratio in Persian cats with polycystic kidney disease. *J Vet Intern Med* 17:21–27, 2003.
34. Bonazzi M, Volta A, Gnudi G, et al: Prevalence of the polycystic kidney disease and renal and urinary bladder ultrasonographic abnormalities in Persian and Exotic Shorthair cats in Italy. *J Feline Med Surg* 9:387–391, 2007.
35. Perico N, Codreanu I, Schieppati A, et al: The future of renoprotection. *Kidney Int Suppl* S95–S101, 2005.
36. Schnaper HW: Renal fibrosis. *Methods Mol Med* 117:45–68, 2005.
37. Finco DR, Brown SA, Brown CA, et al: Progression of chronic renal disease in the dog. *J Vet Intern Med* 13:516–528, 1999.
38. Ross LA, Finco DR, Crowell WA: Effect of dietary phosphorus restriction on the kidneys of cats with reduced renal mass. *Am J Vet Res* 43:1023–1026, 1982.
39. Brown SA, Finco DR, Crowell WA, et al: Beneficial effect of moderate phosphate restriction in partially nephrectomized dogs on a low protein diet. *Kidney Int* 31:380, 1987.

40. Jacob F, Polzin DJ, Osborne CA, et al: Association between initial systolic blood pressure and risk of developing a uremic crisis or of dying in dogs with chronic renal failure. *J Am Vet Med Assoc* 222:322–329, 2003.

41. Mathur S, Brown CA, Dietrich UM, et al: Evaluation of a technique of inducing hypertensive renal insufficiency in cats. *Am J Vet Res* 65:1006–1013, 2004.

42. Mathur S, Syme H, Brown CA, et al: Effects of the calcium channel antagonist amlodipine in cats with surgically induced hypertensive renal insufficiency. *Am J Vet Res* 63:833–839, 2002.

43. Grauer G, Greco D, Gretzy D, et al: Effects of enalapril treatment versus placebo as a treatment for canine idiopathic glomerulonephritis. *J Vet Intern Med* 14:526–533, 2000.

44. Gunn-Moore D: Influence of proteinuria on survival time in cats with chronic renal insufficiency. *J Vet Int Med* 17:405A, 2003.

45. Ross SJ, Osborne CA, Kirk CA, et al: Clinical evaluation of dietary modification for treatment of spontaneous chronic kidney disease in cats. *J Am Vet Med Assoc* 229:949–957, 2006.

46. Plantinga EA, Everts H, Kastelein AM, et al: Retrospective study of the survival of cats with acquired chronic renal insufficiency offered different commercial diets. *Vet Rec* 157:185–187, 2005.

47. Polzin D, Ross S, Osborne C: Calcitriol. In Bonagura J, Twedt D, editors: *Current veterinary therapy XIV*, St Louis, 2009, Saunders/Elsevier, pp 892–895.

48. Elliott J, Rawlings JM, Markwell PJ, et al: Survival of cats with naturally occurring chronic renal failure: effect of dietary management. *J Small Anim Pract* 41:235–242, 2000.

49. Elliott J, Barber PJ, Syme HM, et al: Feline hypertension: clinical findings and response to antihypertensive treatment in 30 cases. *J Small Anim Pract* 42:122–129, 2001.

50. Brown SA, Brown CA, Crowell WA, et al: Beneficial effects of chronic administration of dietary omega-3 polyunsaturated fatty acids in dogs with renal insufficiency. *J Lab Cin Med* 131:447–455, 1998.

51. Brown SA, Brown CA, Crowell WA, et al: Effects of dietary polyunsaturated fatty acid supplementation in early renal insufficiency in dogs. *J Lab Clin Med* 135:275–286, 2000.

52. Goodman LA, Brown SA, Torres BT, et al: Effects of meloxicam on plasma iohexol clearance as a marker of glomerular filtration rate in conscious healthy cats. *Am J Vet Res* 70:826–830, 2009.

53. Surdyk KK, Brown CA, Brown SA: Evaluation of glomerular filtration rate in cats with reduced renal mass and administered meloxicam and acetylsalicylic acid. *Am J Vet Res* 74:648–651, 2013.

54. Gowan RA, Baral RM, Lingard AE, et al: A retrospective analysis of the effects of meloxicam on the longevity of aged cats with and without overt chronic kidney disease. *J Feline Med Surg* 14:876–881, 2012.

55. Gowan RA, Lingard AE, Johnston L, et al: Retrospective case-control study of the effects of long-term dosing with meloxicam on renal function in aged cats with degenerative joint disease. *J Feline Med Surg* 13:752–761, 2011.

56. Cowgill LD: Clinical experience and the use of recombinant human erythropoietin in uremic dogs and cats. In *Proceedings of 9th ACVIM Forum*, 1991, pp 147–149.

57. Cowgill LD, James KM, Levy JK, et al: Use of recombinant human erythropoietin for management of anemia in dogs and cats with renal failure. *J Am Vet Med Assoc* 212:521–528, 1998.

58. Chalhoub S, Langston CE, Farrelly J: The use of darbepoetin to stimulate erythropoiesis in anemia of chronic kidney disease in cats: 25 cases. *J Vet Intern Med* 26:363–369, 2012.

59. Quimby JM, Lunn KF: Mirtazapine as an appetite stimulant and anti-emetic in cats with chronic kidney disease: a masked placebo-controlled crossover clinical trial. *Vet J* 197:651–655, 2013.

60. Quimby JM, Gustafson DL, Lunn KF: The pharmacokinetics of mirtazapine in cats with chronic kidney disease and in age-matched control cats. *J Vet Intern Med* 25:985–989, 2011.

Phosphate and the Kidney

Rosanne E. Jepson

PHOSPHORUS HOMEOSTASIS

Phosphorus is found in the body in either an organic (e.g., phospholipids or phosphoesters) or inorganic form (e.g., orthophosphoric and pyrophosphoric acid) and is an important component of many cellular structures and functions. Approximately 85% of total body phosphorus is present in an organic form as hydroxyapatite in bone ($Ca_{10}[PO_4]_6OH_2$) with a further 14% located intracellularly. Only 1% of organic phosphate is active extracellularly and within serum. Organic phosphate comprises approximately two-thirds of total serum phosphate with the remainder being inorganic phosphate (e.g., H_3PO_4, $H_2PO_4^-$, HPO_4^{2-}). Eighty-five percent of inorganic phosphate circulates unbound in an ionized form, 10% is bound to protein, and 5% is complexed with either calcium or magnesium.[1,2] Laboratory analyzers typically quantify total inorganic phosphorus with normal plasma phosphorus concentrations ranging from 2.5 to 6.0 mg/dL (0.81 to 1.94 mmol/L), depending on the age of the patient and the specific instrument.[2-4]

Phosphorus homeostasis is incompletely understood but is coupled to the reciprocal regulation of calcium and is dependent on parathyroid hormone (PTH) and calcitriol (1,25-dihydroxycholecalciferol, which is abbreviated 1,25[OH]$_2$D).[2,5] More recent evidence suggests independent regulation of phosphorus by compounds referred to as *phosphatonins*, such as fibroblast growth factor 23 (FGF-23). In health, net total body phosphorus is controlled by three major body organ systems: intestine, bone, and kidney. Active intestinal absorption of inorganic phosphate occurs predominantly within the duodenum via the sodium-phosphate type IIb co-transporter (NaPi-IIb) under direct control of calcitriol.[6] Parathyroid hormone also indirectly increases intestinal phosphorus absorption by stimulating 1α-hydroxylase activity and increasing calcitriol production.[6] Calcium and phosphorus can be quickly mobilized from bone to the extracellular fluid compartment with calcitriol and PTH acting synergistically to stimulate osteoclastic activity, bone resorption, and hence release of calcium and phosphorus from skeletal stores.[2]

The kidneys are the primary regulators of neutral phosphate balance and are able to perform this role by modulating tubular phosphate reabsorption and excretion. Free and complexed inorganic phosphate ions are filtered by glomeruli with up to 80% to 95% reabsorbed within the proximal tubule and a questionable, smaller component reabsorbed within the distal tubule.[2] The resorptive capacity of the proximal tubules reflects serum phosphorus concentrations. During periods of hypophosphatemia, nearly 100% of phosphate ions are reabsorbed from tubular filtrate, whereas with normophosphatemia or hyperphosphatemia, phosphate ion reabsorption is proportional to serum phosphate concentrations and is ultimately dependent on glomerular filtration rate (GFR).[2,7] Phosphate transport across the apical proximal tubular cell membrane occurs against the electrochemical gradient via the type II sodium-phosphate co-transporters (NaPi-IIa and NaPi-IIc) located on the brush border. Approximately 80% of phosphate reabsorption occurs via the NaPi-IIa, with the remaining 20% via the NaPi-IIc.[2] This active process of phosphate uptake is a rate-limiting step, with phosphate subsequently transported to the bloodstream by a phosphate carrier utilizing the electrochemical gradient.[2]

Expression of the NaPi-IIa in the proximal tubule is under control of intestinal phosphate, PTH, and phosphaturic factors (e.g., FGF-23). An increase in intestinal inorganic phosphate results in a rapid increase in renal fractional excretion of phosphorus.[6,8] This effect is independent of plasma phosphate concentrations, PTH, and phosphaturic factors (e.g., FGF-23) and is believed to be the result of a putative "enteric phosphatonin."[6,8] Parathyroid hormone increases endocytosis of the NaPi-IIa into lysosomes for degradation and therefore increases urinary phosphate excretion. Finally, phosphatonins (e.g., FGF-23) play an important role in renal phosphate regulation. Fibroblast growth factor 23 decreases expression of the NaPi-IIa within the proximal tubule, resulting in phosphaturia.[9-11] Fibroblast growth factor 23 also decreases 1α-hydroxylase activity, decreasing calcitriol production, which has a net effect of decreasing intestinal absorption of phosphorus and release of phosphorus from bone.[12,13]

Fibroblast Growth Factor 23

Fibroblast growth factor 23 is produced by osteoblasts and osteocytes. The physiological effects of FGF-23 occur through interaction with receptor complexes (FGFR1, FGFR3c, and FGFR4) with subsequent intracellular signaling dependent on co-expression of a transmembrane β-glucuronidase, α-klotho (αK1). FGF-23 binds more avidly to its receptors in the presence of αK1, and the limited tissue expression of αK1 within the parathyroid, kidney, and pituitary contributes

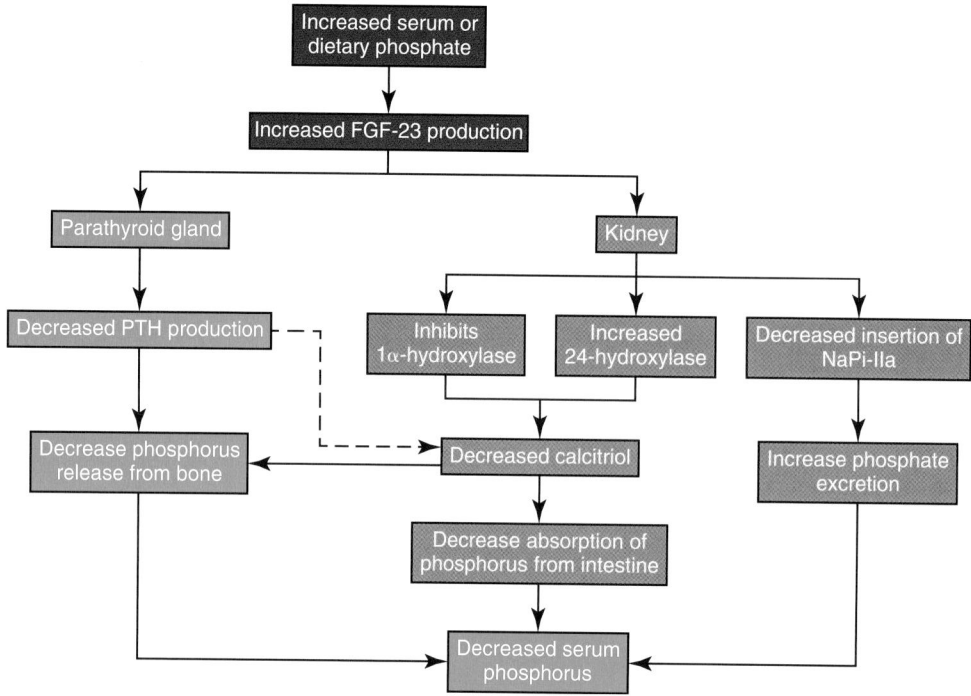

Figure 48-1: The role of fibroblast growth factor 23 *(FGF-23)* in phosphorus regulation in health. *NaPi-IIa,* Sodium-phosphate type IIa co-transporter a; *PTH,* parathyroid hormone.

to the tissue specificity of the actions of FGF-23.[10,14] The main physiological functions of FGF-23 are downregulation of transcription and translation of the NaPi-IIa promoting phosphaturia and decreasing production of calcitriol.[11] This latter action occurs through inhibition of 1α-hydroxylase required for conversion of calcidiol (25-hydroxycholecalciferol) to calcitriol and stimulation of 24-hydroxylase activity required for inactivating calcidiol to 24,25(OH)$_2$-cholecalciferol. Fibroblast growth factor 23 also has an inhibitory effect on PTH production (Figure 48-1).[10,14] The factors regulating FGF-23 production are incompletely understood; however, studies support that increased dietary phosphate intake stimulates FGF-23 production and that a negative feedback loop exists between FGF-23 and calcitriol.[13,15,16] Fibroblast growth factor 23 is a low molecular weight molecule (32 kilodaltons), freely filtered by the kidney with the potential for accumulation in patients with reduced renal function.[17]

HYPERPHOSPHATEMIA AND RENAL SECONDARY HYPERPARATHYROIDISM

Pathophysiology

With loss of functional mass, renal capacity to excrete phosphorus is impaired. Increasing plasma phosphate concentrations result in a relative reduction in ionized calcium, which stimulates PTH production by the law of mass action. Increasing inorganic phosphorus concentrations may also directly stimulate PTH production. Whilst sufficient functional renal reserve remains, the net effect of increasing PTH concentrations is renal excretion of phosphate. With progres-

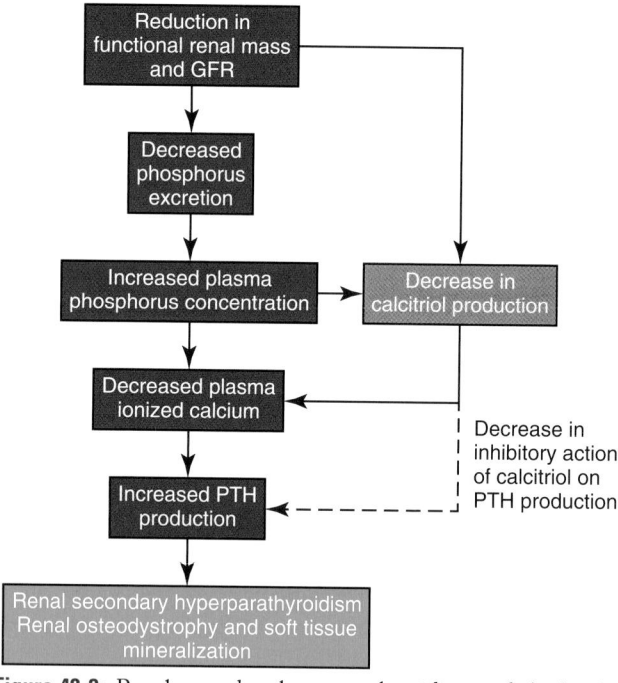

Figure 48-2: Renal secondary hyperparathyroidism and the "trade-off" hypothesis. *GFR,* Glomerular filtration rate; *PTH,* parathyroid hormone.

sive tubular loss and reduction in total GFR, renal phosphorus excretion is impaired, leading to whole body phosphorus retention. The "trade-off" for maintenance of phosphate excretion by the remaining nephrons is a chronic increase in PTH (Figure 48-2) and development of renal secondary hyperparathyroidism (RHPTH).

Ionized calcium and calcitriol have a negative influence on gene transcription of PTH. Reduced availability of calcitriol is an important factor in the uncontrolled production of PTH. Loss of functional renal mass decreases the availability of 1α-hydroxylase for production of calcitriol, and increasing phosphorus concentrations have a direct inhibitory effect on 1α-hydroxylase activity. Decreased availability of calcitriol limits calcium release from bone and absorption from the gastrointestinal (GI) tract, providing a further stimulus for PTH production. In chronic kidney disease (CKD), increased PTH production sustains calcitriol synthesis by upregulating 1α-hydroxylase such that calcitriol concentrations are initially maintained in the face of chronically increased PTH.

Fibroblast growth factor 23 plays a role in the early reduction of calcitriol production in CKD due to inhibitory action of FGF-23 on 1α-hydroxylase.[18] An updated "trade-off" hypothesis that incorporates FGF-23 in phosphorus regulation is proposed. In the early stages of CKD, increased FGF-23 has a phosphaturic effect. Increasing FGF-23 inhibits 1α-hydroxylase activity, decreasing calcitriol production and limiting intestinal absorption and release of phosphorus from bone. Increased FGF-23 has a direct inhibitory action on production of PTH. In the early stages of CKD, increase in FGF-23 concentration acts to maintain normophosphatemia and limits development of RHPTH (Figure 48-3).[19-21]

In the later stages of CKD, FGF-23 continues to increase due to reduced renal excretion with declining GFR and as a consequence of increasing phosphorus concentrations, which stimulate FGF-23 production. End-organ resistance to FGF-23, secondary to decreased expression of FGFR and αK1, develops such that the inhibitory action of FGF-23 on PTH is lost. In this later stage of disease, increasing phosphorus concentrations, calcitriol deficiency, and loss of the inhibitory action of FGF-23 promote PTH synthesis, ultimately leading to the development of overt RHPTH (Figure 48-4).[14,19,21]

Prevalence in Feline Chronic Kidney Disease

Hyperphosphatemia is a commonly recognized biochemical abnormality in cats with CKD.[22,23] Early histopathologic studies demonstrated evidence of parathyroid gland hyperplasia in cats with advanced CKD and a correlation between duration of clinical disease, parathyroid gland weight, and the severity of any bone changes as a consequence of renal osteodystrophy.[24] A study by Elliott and colleagues evaluated the evidence for RHPTH in 80 cats with CKD.[25] Cats were divided into three groups based on whether they were deemed to have compensated (no clinical or historical features but CKD confirmed on biochemical and urine assessment with mean plasma creatinine of 2.6 mg/dL [229 μmol/L]), uremic (compatible historical, physical examination, and biochemical and urine assessment creatinine of 3.6 mg/dL [316 μmol/L]), or end-stage CKD (showing clinical signs of end-stage disease and surviving less than 21 days after diagnosis with mean creatinine of 10.3 mg/dL [909 μmol/L]). Hyperphosphatemia

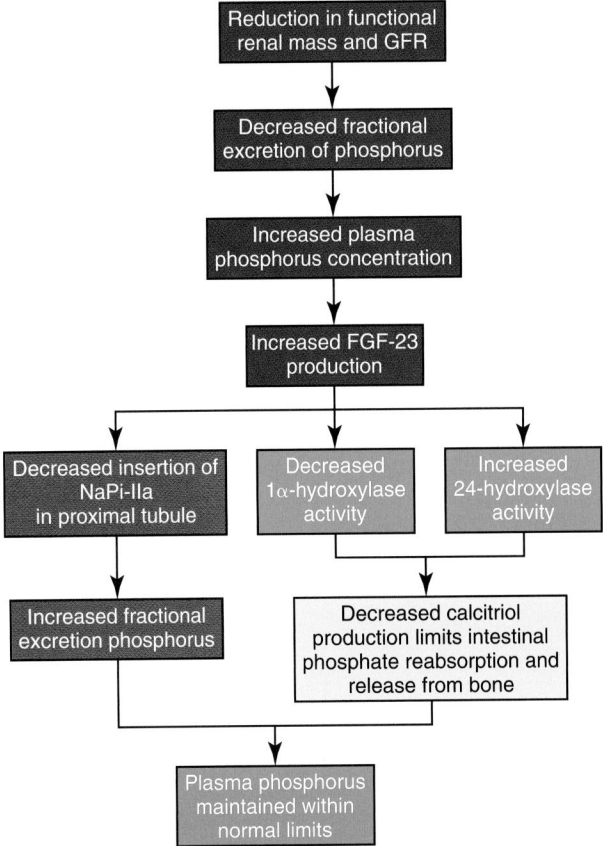

Figure 48-3: An updated "trade-off" hypothesis incorporating fibroblast growth factor 23 *(FGF-23)* in early chronic kidney disease (CKD). *GFR,* Glomerular filtration rate; *NaPi-IIa,* sodium-phosphate type IIa co-transporter.

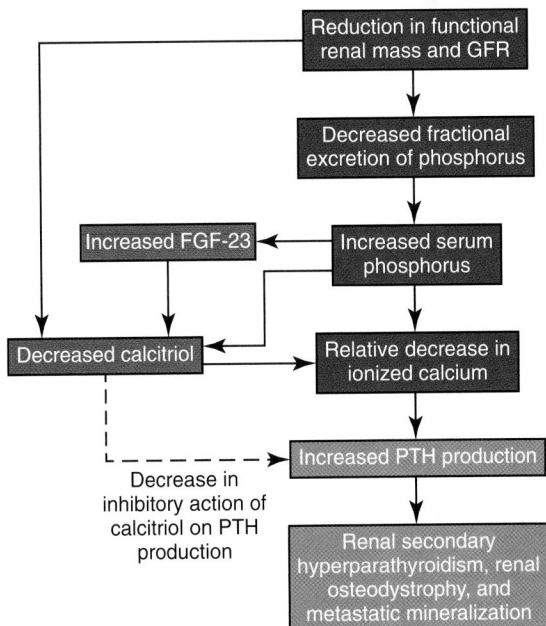

Figure 48-4: An updated "trade-off" hypothesis incorporating fibroblast growth factor 23 *(FGF-23)* in late stage chronic kidney disease. *GFR,* Glomerular filtration rate; *PTH,* parathyroid hormone.

was identified in 20% of compensated, 49% of uremic, and 100% of the end-stage cats. The prevalence of hyperparathyroidism overall in cats diagnosed with CKD was 84%, with 47% of the compensated, 87% of the uremic, and 100% of the end-stage cats demonstrating increased PTH concentrations. Blood ionized calcium concentrations were variable, being below the laboratory reference interval in 14% of cats with uremic CKD and 56% of cats with end-stage CKD. However, 9% of uremic cats and 6% of end-stage cats demonstrated ionized hypercalcemia. Calcitriol concentrations were significantly decreased in the uremic (17 ± 3 pg/mL) and end-stage groups (6 ± 2 pg/mL) compared to healthy age-matched control cats (28 ± 3 pg/mL) and were below the laboratory reference interval (9-57 pg/mL) in 35% (11 out of 31) of cats including 8 out of 10 cats with end-stage disease. Renal secondary hyperparathyroidism was documented in nine cats (13% of RHPTH cases) with normal concentrations of total and ionized calcium, calcitriol ($n = 3$) and plasma phosphate.[25] Based on this study, the prevalence of hyperphosphatemia and RHPTH increase with declining renal function and the prevalence of RHPTH is higher than hyperphosphatemia for any given stage of CKD. Furthermore, a recent study has demonstrated that PTH concentrations are significantly higher in nonazotemic cats, which are known to develop azotemia within a 12-month period (median: 82.8 pg/mL, range: 14.11-3269.24 pg/mL), than in cats remaining non-azotemic over the same time period (median: 44.37 pg/mL, range: 7.62-265.22 pg/mL). Hyperparathyroidism was identified in 19.4% of nonazotemic cats that went on to develop azotemia within 12 months.[26] This study further supports that alteration in phosphate homeostasis and hyperparathyroidism occurs early in the course of CKD, often before the onset of overt azotemia, and precedes the development of hyperphosphatemia.[26]

A commercially-available human enzyme-linked immunosorbent assay for quantification of FGF-23 has been validated for use with feline plasma.[27] Fibroblast growth factor 23 concentrations have been shown to be significantly higher in nonazotemic cats that develop azotemia within a 12-month period than those remaining nonazotemic over the same period. After a diagnosis of CKD, FGF-23 concentrations continue to increase with declining renal function.[27,28] Furthermore, FGF-23 concentrations have been shown to be significantly higher in cats within International Renal Interest Society (IRIS) Stages 2 and 3 CKD when their plasma phosphate concentrations exceed the IRIS target for phosphate, compared to normophosphatemic cats within the same IRIS stage.[27] These data together indicate that, similar to the situation in humans, alteration in FGF-23 occurs early in the course of CKD and that not only GFR, but also phosphorus concentrations, are likely to be determinants of FGF-23 in cats.[29,30] On the basis of studies performed to date, it seems likely that PTH and FGF-23 are important in the regulation of phosphate in cats with CKD and integral to the development of RHPTH. However, the full temporal relationship among PTH, FGF-23, phosphate, calcium, and calcitriol in cats requires further study.

Clinical Consequences, Associations, and Outcome

The presence of hyperphosphatemia *per se* may not be directly associated with apparent clinical signs, and yet the clinical consequences of this abnormality as a marker of RHPTH can be significant. Clinical manifestations occurring as a consequence of hyperphosphatemia can include soft tissue metastatic mineralization and, although rarely reported, in the late stages of CKD, renal osteodystrophy (Figure 48-5).[22] Enlargement of parathyroid glands may also be identified in cats with CKD and can occasionally, if marked, be mistaken for the presence of a thyroid goiter. Postmortem examination of 74 cats with CKD identified bone demineralization in 9.8% and soft tissue mineralization in 9.3% of cats.[22] The process of metastatic mineralization is particularly evident in proton-secreting organs, such as the kidney and stomach, but has also been reported to affect the tunica media of thoracic and abdominal aorta, liver, and pulmonary vessels.[22] Soft tissue mineralization occurs with greater frequency when the

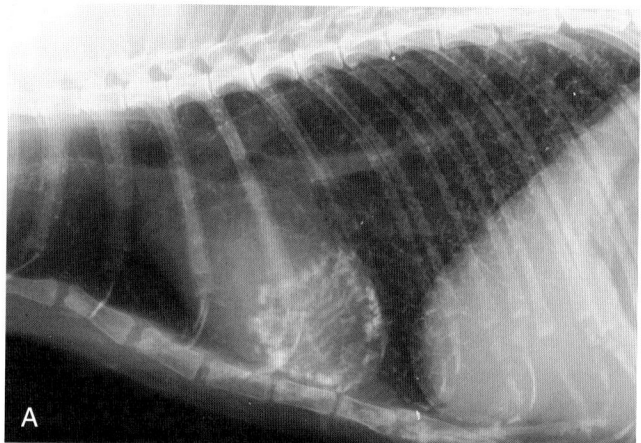
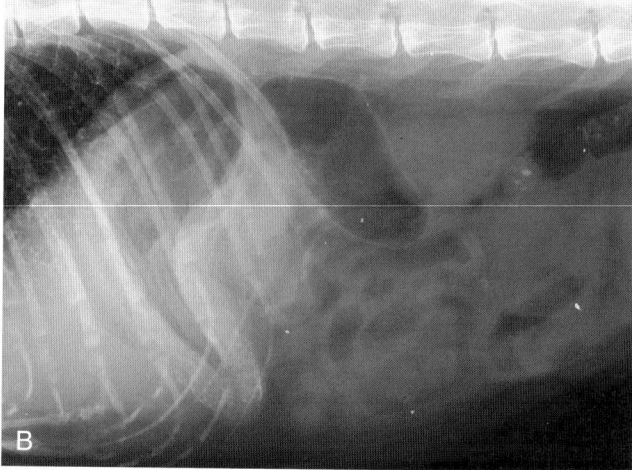

Figure 48-5: Lateral thoracic **(A)** and abdominal **(B)** radiographs of a 12-year-old, neutered, male, domestic shorthair cat with chronic kidney disease. There is metastatic calcification of the myocardium, aorta, abdominal arteries, and gastric mucosa. (Reproduced with permission from Lamb CR: *Self-assessment picture tests in veterinary medicine: diagnostic imaging of the dog and cat*, London, 1994, Mosby-Year Book Europe.)

calcium phosphorus product exceeds 70 mg²/dL² in conjunction with elevated PTH concentrations, although total calcium may be within the reference interval. Nephrocalcinosis has been proposed to contribute to the progression of kidney disease because deposition of calcium products within the interstitium may initiate an inflammatory response exacerbating tubulointerstitial nephritis, fibrosis, and tubular atrophy. A recent study evaluating renal histopathology in 80 cats with variable renal function identified tubular mineralization in approximately 50% of cats in IRIS Stages 2 and 3 CKD and 58% in IRIS Stage 4 CKD.[31] Metastatic mineralization of the paws has also been reported, appearing often as intact or ulcerating nodules in the interdigital space or on footpads, causing discomfort and lameness.[32,33] A single case report has documented resolution of metastatic paw calcification with appropriate management of RHPTH, 179 days after diagnosis.[33]

Survival of cats with naturally occurring CKD has been associated with serum phosphorus concentrations.[34,35] Phosphorus concentrations have also been identified as a risk factor for progressive CKD in cats, defined as an increase in plasma creatinine greater than 25%, such that an increase in plasma phosphorus of 1 mg/dL (0.32 mmol/L) was associated with a 41% increase in risk of disease progression.[36] In addition, dietary phosphate restriction and control of RHPTH have been demonstrated to improve survival of cats with CKD.[37,38]

In human medicine, PTH is considered a uremic toxin that contributes to a number of other clinical manifestations and pathophysiological mechanisms affecting the progression of CKD, including osmotic fragility of red blood cells, inhibition of mitochondrial respiration with adverse effects on myocardial function, impaired motor nerve velocity, and glucose tolerance.[39] Increased PTH may affect the immune system with direct effects on lymphocyte and polymorphonuclear cell function.[39] These additional actions of PTH in cats with CKD have not been explored.

Targets and Management

The IRIS targets for phosphate control in cats with CKD have been widely accepted (Table 48-1).[40] These guidelines were initially proposed by a group of veterinary nephrologists based on the evidence and guidelines advocated in human medicine (Kidney Disease Outcome Quality Initiative) in conjunction with information available from studies in veterinary medicine.[37,38,41,42] The IRIS phosphate targets reflect not only achieving a plasma phosphorus concentration within laboratory reference interval but, for early stages of CKD, achieving phosphorus concentrations within the mid to lower half of the reference interval. The rationale for this more stringent target reflects that not all cats will be hyperphosphatemic at diagnosis of azotemic CKD, and yet a proportion of these normophosphatemic cats will have evidence of RHPTH.[26] Whilst the IRIS targets are based on control of phosphate concentrations, elevated PTH and FGF-23 may be secondary markers of alteration in phosphate homeostasis in the early stages of CKD. However, it remains unknown whether normalization of PTH or potentially FGF-23 would be clinically superior to the use of phosphate as a therapeutic target.

Dietary Phosphate Restriction

When urinary fractional excretion of phosphorus is impaired due to declining renal function, restriction of intestinal phosphate absorption can be used to regulate serum phosphate concentrations. The use of a phosphate-restricted renal diet is considered the current standard of care for cats with both normophosphatemic and hyperphosphatemic IRIS Stages 2 to 4 CKD. Commercially-available renal diets achieve phosphate restriction through limiting dietary protein. In addition, renal diets are often supplemented in potassium, polyunsaturated fatty acids, B vitamins, antioxidants, and soluble fiber; may be sodium restricted; and are usually designed to have a neutral effect on acid-base balance.[40] In the early stages of CKD, dietary phosphate restriction alone may be sufficient to control hyperphosphatemia and RHPTH. However, in the later stages, additional use of intestinal phosphate binders may be required. There is currently no published evidence supporting the use of a phosphate-restricted diet in cats with nonazotemic, nonproteinuric IRIS Stage 1 CKD.

An early experimental nephrectomy study provided evidence that feeding a phosphate-restricted diet significantly reduced phosphate concentrations.[41] Cats receiving the phosphate-restricted diet maintained plasma phosphorus concentrations between 4.0 to 5.0 mg/dL (1.3 to 1.6 mmol/L) and demonstrated a renoprotective effect in terms of reduced renal fibrosis, mineralization, and mononuclear cell infiltrates compared to cats eating a maintenance diet.[41] Similarly, a study examining naturally occurring feline CKD demonstrated that feeding a phosphate-restricted renal diet resulted in a significant decline in plasma phosphate and PTH concentrations over the 5-month study period but without any significant impact on calcitriol concentrations.[43] In contrast, those cats that continued to be fed a commercial adult maintenance diet demonstrated persistence of hyperphosphatemia and significant increase in PTH concentrations.[43]

The use of a phosphate-restricted diet has been demonstrated to improve survival in cats with CKD.[37,38,44] In a

Table 48-1	International Renal Interest Society Staging of Creatinine and Targets for Phosphate Control in Cats				
	CREATININE CONCENTRATION			PHOSPHORUS TARGET	
IRIS Stage	mg/dL	μmol/L		mg/dL	mmol/L
2	1.6-2.7	140-249		<4.5	<1.45
3	2.8-4.9	250-440		<5.0	<1.6
4	>4.9	>440		<6.0	<1.9

IRIS, International Renal Interest Society.

nonblinded, nonrandomized study, cats ($n = 29$) that were fed a phosphate-restricted diet had significantly longer survival times (median: 633 days) compared to cats ($n = 21$) that refused to eat the renal diet and were therefore maintained on adult maintenance diets (median: 264 days) despite being matched at entry to the study for age, body weight, packed cell volume, plasma creatinine, phosphate, and PTH concentrations.[37] A further study followed cats in IRIS Stages 2 and 3 CKD randomized in a blinded manner to receive either a phosphate-restricted renal diet or adult maintenance diet.[38] A significantly greater proportion of cats fed the maintenance diet had uremic episodes (26%, 6 out of 23) or died (22%, 5 out of 23) during the 24 months of follow-up compared to cats eating the renal diet (uremic episodes 0%, 0 out of 22; died 0%, 0 out of 22 cats).[38]

Recently published data report that a restricted renal diet also regulates FGF-23 production in cats with CKD.[45] Hyperphosphatemic cats fed a phosphate-restricted diet demonstrated significant reduction in plasma phosphorus, PTH, and FGF-23 concentrations, whilst normophosphatemic cats with CKD demonstrated a significant decline in FGF-23 concentrations without significant change in phosphate or PTH.[45] Further work is required to determine whether modulation of FGF-23 confers any clinical or survival advantage and whether in the future FGF-23 may be a useful target for the regulation of RHPTH.[45]

Phosphorus concentrations should be monitored in cats started on a phosphate-restricted renal diet. Due to the presence of whole body phosphate retention, the overall effect of introducing a phosphate-restricted diet may not be evident until the patient has been consuming the diet for several weeks.[43] Plasma phosphate concentrations should be assessed

3 to 4 weeks after introduction of a phosphate-restricted diet. If dietary phosphate restriction has not enabled the IRIS phosphate target to be met, then intestinal phosphate binders should be introduced and used in conjunction with the phosphate-restricted diet. Serial monitoring of plasma phosphorus concentrations should be performed on approximately a monthly basis until targets are reached and thereafter every 2 to 4 months to ensure continued phosphate control.

Intestinal Phosphate Binders

In the later stages of CKD, intestinal phosphate binders in addition to a phosphate-restricted renal diet may be required to meet the IRIS targets (see Table 48-1). The cations present within intestinal phosphate binders complex with dietary phosphate forming an insoluble compound, reducing intestinal phosphate absorption and thereby increasing fecal phosphate excretion. Intestinal phosphate binders work optimally when administered with food and should ideally be given in divided doses at every meal. There are few published studies available evaluating the role, safety, and efficacy of intestinal phosphate binders in feline CKD, although it is widely accepted that their use is beneficial. Intestinal phosphate binders that have commonly been used in feline clinical practice include aluminum hydroxide/acetate, calcium carbonate (± chitosan), lanthanum carbonate octahydrate, and sevelamer hydrochloride/carbonate (Table 48-2). Rarely, use of more than one intestinal phosphate binder may be required in order to avoid toxicity related to individual agents.

Aluminum Salts. Aluminum salts (aluminum hydroxide or aluminum carbonate) are both effective and inexpensive (see Table 48-2). Sucralfate, which contains a complex of aluminum hydroxide and sulfated sucrose, has anecdotally

Table 48-2 Commonly Used Intestinal Phosphate Binders in Feline Chronic Kidney Disease

Drug*	Dosage	Comment
Aluminum hydroxide	30-90 mg/kg/day PO in divided doses	Can cause constipation Aluminum toxicity with high doses
Chitosan and calcium carbonate	1 g/5 kg every 12 hours PO	Can cause constipation Monitor for hypercalcemia
Calcium carbonate	30-90 mg/kg/day PO in divided doses	Can cause constipation Monitor for hypercalcemia Efficacy influenced by pH
Calcium acetate	60-90 mg/kg/day PO in divided doses	Can cause constipation Efficacy less influenced by pH Monitor for hypercalcemia
Lanthanum carbonate octahydrate	400-800 mg/cat/day PO in divided doses	Also contains kaolin and vitamin E Gastrointestinal side effects above recommended doses
Lanthanum carbonate	12.5-25 mg/kg/day PO in divided doses	Gastrointestinal side effects above recommended doses
Sevelamer hydrochloride	90-160 mg/kg/day PO in divided doses	Pills are hygroscopic Can cause constipation

PO, per os (orally).
*All phosphate binders must be administered in divided dosages with each meal.

been used, although no studies have evaluated this product as a phosphate binder. The use of aluminum salts in human medicine has been limited by concern regarding aluminum toxicity, with clinical signs including osteomalacia, adynamic bone disease, microcytic anemia, and neurological signs as a consequence of associated encephalopathy.[42,46,47] Side effects of aluminum hydroxide administration have not been systematically investigated in veterinary patients, but the clinical consensus is that they are rarely appreciated, although constipation is occasionally identified. A single case series has documented aluminum toxicity in two dogs presenting with clinical signs of tetraparesis, reduced menace response, absent patellar and withdrawal reflexes, and evidence of microcytosis on complete blood count.[48] Serum aluminum concentrations were markedly increased in both patients, and the doses reported in this case series were in excess of the published dose ranges for patients with CKD.

Calcium Salts. Calcium-based phosphate binders (e.g., calcium carbonate and calcium acetate) have been used in the cat (see Table 48-2). The affinity of calcium carbonate for phosphate is pH dependent, being most effective within an acid environment. Consideration should therefore be given to timing of administration, particularly when patients are receiving concurrent antacid therapy.[49] Calcium acetate is reported to be more effective than calcium carbonate and to have a superior action across a wider range of pH conditions.[50] Antacid therapy may therefore be of less concern with this agent. However, care should be taken when administering calcium-based intestinal phosphate binders because elevated calcium intake may contribute to the development of hypercalcemia.[51] Such an effect has been reported in human medicine contributing to an elevated calcium-phosphate product and, as a consequence, soft tissue and vascular calcification.[51-53] Calcium-based phosphate binders should ideally be avoided in patients with either idiopathic or renal-related hypercalcemia and in those patients with prior evidence of calcium oxalate nephrolithiasis/ureterolithiasis. Patients receiving calcium-based phosphate binders should be carefully monitored for the development of hypercalcemia, or alternative phosphate binding agents should be used. Ipakitine/Epakitin (Vétoquinol) containing the combination of calcium carbonate (10%), chitosan (8% shell and crab shell extract), and lactulose (82%) is licensed as a food additive in both Europe and the United States. Given the presence of calcium carbonate within this product, care must be similarly taken regarding monitoring of calcium concentrations.

Lanthanum Compounds. Lanthanum carbonate has been used as a phosphate binder in human medicine particularly for patients with end-stage renal disease and to date has a high safety profile for this use.[46,54] Lanthanum carbonate binds phosphate over a very broad pH range (pH of 1 to 7), giving it a long period of activity within the GI tract. Absorption of lanthanum across the intestinal tract is extremely low, with any lanthanum that is absorbed subsequently undergoing hepatic and biliary rather than renal excretion.[55,56] In Europe, lanthanum carbohydrate octahydrate (Renalzin,

Bayer; see Table 48-2) is licensed as a food additive with the product being administered as a paste formulation. Renalzin also contains kaolin and vitamin E with the speculated benefits of binding uremic toxins and antioxidant activity, respectively, although studies documenting the benefits of these additional actions have not been published. When lanthanum carbonate octahydrate was administered to healthy cats receiving a maintenance diet, a dose-dependent increase in fecal and decrease in urinary phosphate excretion occurs, although no change in serum phosphate concentration was reported in these healthy cats.[57,58] Lanthanum dioxycarbonate when administered to young healthy growing cats did not cause changes in bone morphology, although vomiting was reported at higher doses.[59]

Sevelamer Compounds. Sevelamer hydrochloride and carbonate are organic polymers that bind phosphate. They are not systemically absorbed from the intestinal tract and are excreted entirely by the fecal route. Information on the use of sevelamer-based compounds in cats is limited.[58] Side effects reported in human patients with CKD include constipation and, at high doses, the possibility of impaired absorption of folic acid and fat soluble vitamins. Sevelamer hydrochloride may contribute to metabolic acidosis which led to the development of sevelamer carbonate to limit this effect.[60] An additional reported benefit of sevelamer compounds in human medicine is their capacity to bind and sequester bile acids, modifying the lipid profile.[61] However, none of these potential effects of sevelamer compounds have been investigated in cats.

With introduction of any intestinal phosphate binder, monitoring of serum phosphorus concentration and, in the case of calcium-containing phosphate binders, calcium concentrations is important. This can initially be performed every 3 to 4 weeks with dose titration to desired IRIS phosphate target and subsequently every 2 to 4 months dependent on severity and rate of progression of CKD. Phosphate binders may have a variable effect on the absorption of other medications from the intestinal tract. Therefore, medications should preferably be given either 1 hour prior to or more than 3 hours after administration of an intestinal phosphate binder.

The high concentration of phosphorus within commercially-available feline maintenance diets means that control of phosphorus with use of intestinal phosphate binders alone when feeding a maintenance diet is challenging.[58] In addition, the use of intestinal phosphate binders in conjunction with maintenance diet does not provide the additional nutritional advantages that are widely incorporated into commercially-available renal diets. A single study has evaluated the use of Ipakitine/Epakitin in combination with a maintenance diet in cats (n = 10) that had undergone experimental 11/12th nephrectomy.[62] In a crossover design study lasting 112 days, cats received either maintenance diet alone or in combination with the phosphate binder. Cats had stable kidney function as assessed by serum urea, creatinine, renal plasma flow, and GFR over the duration of the study and were classified with IRIS Stages 1 and 2 CKD. During the period of Ipakitine/Epakitin administration, a significant decrease in serum phosphorus and PTH concentrations was demonstrated compared to receiving the maintenance diet alone, although the IRIS phosphate targets were not met.[62] Parathyroid hormone concentrations also remained significantly increased compared to prenephrectomy levels.[62] Following a 3-month washout period, six cats were then studied for a further year, receiving Ipakitine/Epakitin for 9 months with biochemical and GFR monitoring performed. Cats maintained stable IRIS Stage 1 and 2 CKD, and phosphate concentrations were significantly reduced during the 9 months of Ipakitine/Epakitin administration, reaching IRIS phosphate targets at the 6- and 9-month time points.[62] To date, studies have not evaluated the efficacy of phosphate binders in combination with adult maintenance or senior diets to enable phosphate control in later stages of CKD when it can be envisaged that efficacy may be limited.

Calcitriol Therapy

Calcitriol therapy is proposed as an adjunctive therapy for patients with RHPTH where the combination of dietary phosphate restriction and intestinal phosphate binders fail to control PTH production or maintain calcitriol concentrations. Decreased calcitriol concentrations in CKD occur as a consequence of reduced functional renal mass and the inhibitory action of both increasing phosphate and FGF-23 concentrations on 1α-hydroxylase activity, which is required for the synthesis of calcitriol.[20] Calcitriol has an inhibitory action on the gene transcription and production of PTH, and persistent reduction in calcitriol concentration can therefore contribute to sustained, autonomous secretion of PTH, a situation sometimes referred to as *tertiary hyperparathyroidism*.[40] Exogenous calcitriol can be administered to combat the effects of a relative or absolute decrease in calcitriol concentration. Although the effects of calcitriol therapy are perceived to relate to regulation of PTH, recent studies in human patients suggest that beneficial effects may be more diverse and include suppression of renin production and left ventricular hypertrophy, preservation of the slit-diaphragm morphology limiting albuminuria, decreasing transforming growth factor-β and hence renal fibrosis, and contributing to maintenance of the immune system.[63]

In human medicine, calcitriol therapy is widely used in the management of renal osteodystrophy and meta-analyses confirm that use of calcitriol or vitamin D analogues significantly decreases PTH concentrations in both dialysis and predialysis CKD patients.[64,65] In human patients with CKD, low calcitriol concentrations have been significantly associated with all-cause mortality and progression of CKD.[66,67] A number of studies have demonstrated the significant benefit of calcitriol therapy in terms of slowing progression to end-stage renal disease and improving survival.[68,69]

Based on a survey of veterinarians, a number of clinical benefits are reported to occur in dogs and cats with calcitriol therapy, including increased activity and improved appetite and social interaction.[70] Furthermore, in a randomized controlled clinical trial performed at the University of Minnesota, calcitriol therapy was shown to increase survival of dogs

with IRIS Stages 3 and 4 CKD.[71] To date, published data on the use of calcitriol therapy in cats is very limited. An unpublished 1 year randomized, controlled clinical trial performed at the University of Minnesota did not demonstrate a survival advantage for cats with IRIS Stage 2, 3, or 4 CKD.[71] However, short duration of follow up, in what is often a slowly progressive disease and where survival can be protracted, may have limited the ability of this study to demonstrate a significant impact of calcitriol therapy in cats. A single published study has evaluated daily (2 ng/kg/day orally [PO]) and intermittent (8.75 ng/kg every 84 hours [twice weekly] PO) calcitriol therapy in normal healthy cats ($n = 10$) and those with CKD ($n = 10$).[72] Cats received these doses of calcitriol for a period of 14 days with a 7-day wash out period in between them. Although PTH concentrations were significantly higher in cats with CKD compared to the control cats, there was no significant change in PTH concentration with either daily or intermittent calcitriol therapy in either group.[72] A recommendation for the use of calcitriol therapy in cats, therefore, cannot be made based on currently available evidence, and further study is warranted to explore this avenue of therapy.

Nevertheless, information is available regarding the use of calcitriol in cats, and anecdotally clinical improvements in terms of demeanor and quality of life are reported.[20,71,73] A major limitation is the availability of calcitriol formulations appropriate for dosing in small patients. Overdosage must be avoided in order to prevent calcitriol-induced hypercalcemia and its secondary consequences, in particular renal and vascular metastatic mineralization. Calcitriol is available as a capsule preparation or alternatively as a pediatric oral solution (Rocaltrol, Roche; 250 ng or 500 ng capsules, 1 mcg/mL solution). In the United States and Canada, reputable pharmacies may be used for appropriate compounding of calcitriol in order to allow accurate dosing for small animals. Availability of reliable quantification of PTH may also be a limitation.

Close monitoring is required because hyperphosphatemia, hypercalcemia, and an elevated calcium x phosphorus product are contraindications for the administration of calcitriol. Therefore, patients must be carefully stabilized and adequate control of hyperphosphatemia, according to the IRIS targets (<6 mg/dL [<1.94 mmol/L]), achieved through dietary phosphate restriction and intestinal phosphate binders before administration of calcitriol. Calcitriol doses reported in cats range from 2.5 to 5 ng/kg/day with the recommendation to start at the lowest end of the dose range, monitor response to therapy, and titrate upward as required. Careful monitoring of phosphorus, ionized calcium, and PTH concentrations, and renal function is required (e.g., 2, 5, and 8 weeks after introduction of calcitriol therapy and after each dose adjustment).[20,40,73] Cautious dose adjustments of calcitriol should be made with increments of approximately 1 ng/kg/day if an inadequate response is seen. Calcitriol dose should not exceed 5 ng/kg/day with the ultimate goal being to normalize PTH concentrations without inducing hypercalcemia.[20,40,73] Life-long therapy with calcitriol is required if the speculated reductions in renal disease progression and survival advantage are to be achieved.

In order to limit absorption of calcium and phosphorus and decrease the risk of calcitriol associated hypercalcemia, calcitriol should be administered separate from meals (e.g., last thing at night) and should not be administered with calcium-based intestinal phosphate binders. Calcitriol therapy should be discontinued if hypercalcemia is documented. If reintroduction is considered, a reduced dose or intermittent dosing schedule may help to limit the development of calcitriol-related hypercalcemia. In human medicine, the use of calcitriol analogues has been advocated to decrease the risk of calcitriol-associated hypercalcemia. Use of these analogues has not been evaluated in veterinary medicine.[20]

References

1. DiBartola SP, Willard MD: Disorders of phosphorus: hypophosphatemia and hyperphosphatemia. In DiBartola SP, editor: *Fluid, electrolyte and acid base disorders in small animal practice*, ed 3, St Louis, 2006, Saunders/Elsevier, pp 195–209.
2. Schropp DM, Kovacic J: Phosphorus and phosphate metabolism in veterinary patients. *J Vet Emerg Crit Care* 17(2):127–134, 2007.
3. Pineda C, Aguilera-Tejero E, Guerrero F, et al: Mineral metabolism in growing cats: changes in the values of blood parameters with age. *J Feline Med Surg* 15(10):866–871, 2013.
4. Bates JA: Phosphorus: a quick reference. *Vet Clin North Am Small Anim Pract* 38(3):471–475, 2008.
5. Guyton AC, Hall JE: Parathyroid hormone, calcitonin, calcium, phosphate metabolism, vitamin D, bone and teeth. In Hall JE, editor: *Guyton and Hall textbook of medical physiology*, ed 12, Philadelphia, 2011, Saunders/Elsevier, pp 955–973.
6. Marks J, Debnam ES, Unwin RJ: The role of the gastrointestinal tract in phosphate homeostasis in health and chronic kidney disease. *Curr Opin Nephrol Hypertens* 22(4):481–487, 2013.
7. Guyton AC, Hall JE: Renal regulation of potassium, calcium, phosphate, magnesium; integration of renal mechanisms for control of blood volume and extracellular fluid volume. In Hall JE, editor: *Guyton and Hall textbook of medical physiology*, ed 12, Philadelphia, 2011, Saunders/Elsevier, pp 367–369.
8. Berndt T, Thomas LF, Craig TA, et al: Evidence for a signaling axis by which intestinal phosphate rapidly modulates renal phosphate reabsorption. *Proc Natl Acad Sci U S A* 104(26):11085–11090, 2007.
9. Shimada T, Urakawa I, Yamazaki Y, et al: FGF-23 transgenic mice demonstrate hypophosphatemic rickets with reduced expression of sodium phosphate cotransporter type IIa. *Biochem Biophys Res Comm* 314(2):409–414, 2004.
10. Bhattacharyya N, Chong WH, Gafni RI, et al: Fibroblast growth factor 23: state of the field and future directions. *Trends Endocrinol Metab* 23(12):610–618, 2012.
11. Baum M, Schiavi S, Dwarakanath V, et al: Effect of fibroblast growth factor-23 on phosphate transport in proximal tubules. *Kidney Int* 68(3):1148–1153, 2005.
12. Shimada T, Hasegawa H, Yamazaki Y, et al: FGF-23 is a potent regulator of vitamin D metabolism and phosphate homeostasis. *J Bone Miner Res* 19(3):429–435, 2004.

13. Antoniucci DM, Yamashita T, Portale AA: Dietary phosphorus regulates serum fibroblast growth factor-23 concentrations in healthy men. *J Clin Endocrinol Metab* 91(8):3144–3149, 2006.
14. Wolf M: Update on fibroblast growth factor 23 in chronic kidney disease. *Kidney Int* 82(7):737–747, 2012.
15. Ferrari SL, Bonjour J-P, Rizzoli R: Fibroblast growth factor-23 relationship to dietary phosphate and renal phosphate handling in healthy young men. *J Clin Endocrinol Metab* 90(3):1519–1524, 2005.
16. Collins MT, Lindsay JR, Jain A, et al: Fibroblast growth factor-23 is regulated by 1α,25-dihydroxyvitamin D. *J Bone Miner Res* 20(11):1944–1950, 2005.
17. Isakova T, Xie H, Yang W, et al: Fibroblast growth factor 23 and risks of mortality and end-stage renal disease in patients with chronic kidney disease. *JAMA* 305(23):2432–2439, 2011.
18. Gutierrez O, Isakova T, Rhee E, et al: Fibroblast growth factor-23 mitigates hyperphosphatemia but accentuates calcitriol deficiency in chronic kidney disease. *J Am Soc Nephrol* 16(7):2205–2215, 2005.
19. Geddes RF, Finch NC, Syme HM, et al: The role of phosphorus in the pathophysiology of chronic kidney disease. *J Vet Emerg Crit Care* 23(2):122–133, 2013.
20. De Brito Galvao JF, Nagode LA, Schenck PA, et al: Calcitriol, calcidiol, parathyroid hormone, and fibroblast growth factor-23 interactions in chronic kidney disease. *J Vet Emerg Crit Care* 23(2):134–162, 2013.
21. Quarles LD: Role of FGF23 in vitamin D and phosphate metabolism: implications in chronic kidney disease. *Exp Cell Res* 318(9):1040–1048, 2012.
22. Dibartola SP, Rutgers HC, Zack PM, et al: Clinicopathologic findings associated with chronic renal disease in cats: 74 cases (1973-1984). *J Am Vet Med Assoc* 190(9):1196–1202, 1987.
23. Lulich JP, Osborne CA, O'Brien TD, et al: Feline renal failure: questions, answers, questions. *Compend Cont Educ Pract Vet* 14(2):127–152, 1992.
24. Lucke VM: Renal disease in the domestic cat. *J Pathol Bacteriol* 95(1):67–91, 1968.
25. Elliott J, Barber PJ: Feline chronic renal failure: calcium homeostasis in 80 cases diagnosed between 1992 and 1995. *J Small Anim Pract* 39(3):108–116, 1998.
26. Finch NC, Syme HM, Elliott J: Parathyroid hormone concentration in geriatric cats with

various degrees of renal function. *J Am Vet Med Assoc* 241(10):1326–1335, 2012.
27. Geddes RF, Finch NC, Elliott J, et al: Fibroblast growth factor 23 in feline chronic kidney disease. *J Vet Intern Med* 27(2):234–241, 2013.
28. Finch NC, Geddes RF, Syme HM, et al: Fibroblast growth factor 23 (FGF-23) concentrations in cats with early nonazotemic chronic kidney disease (CKD) and in healthy geriatric cats. *J Vet Intern Med* 27(2):227–233, 2013.
29. Levin A, Bakris GL, Molitch M, et al: Prevalence of abnormal serum vitamin D, PTH, calcium, and phosphorus in patients with chronic kidney disease: results of the study to evaluate early kidney disease. *Kidney Int* 71(1):31–38, 2007.
30. Isakova T, Wahl P, Vargas GS, et al: Fibroblast growth factor 23 is elevated before parathyroid hormone and phosphate in chronic kidney disease. *Kidney Int* 79(12):1370–1378, 2011.
31. Chakrabarti S, Syme HM, Brown CA, et al: Histomorphometry of feline chronic kidney disease and correlation with markers of renal dysfunction. *Vet Pathol* 50(1):147–155, 2012.
32. Bertazzolo W, Toscani L, Calcaterra S, et al: Clinicopathological findings in five cats with paw calcification. *J Feline Med Surg* 5(1):11–17, 2003.
33. Jackson HA, Barber PJ: Resolution of metastatic calcification in the paws of a cat with successful dietary management of renal hyperparathyroidism. *J Small Anim Pract* 39:495–497, 1998.
34. King JN, Tasker S, Gunn-Moore DA, et al: Prognostic factors in cats with chronic kidney disease. *J Vet Intern Med* 21(5):906–916, 2007.
35. Boyd LM, Langston C, Thompson K, et al: Survival in cats with naturally occurring chronic kidney disease (2000-2002). *J Vet Intern Med* 22(5):1111–1117, 2008.
36. Chakrabarti S, Syme HM, Elliott J: Clinicopathological variables predicting progression of azotemia in cats with chronic kidney disease. *J Vet Intern Med* 26(2):275–281, 2012.
37. Elliott J, Rawlings JM, Markwell PJ, et al: Survival of cats with naturally occurring chronic renal failure: effect of dietary management. *J Small Anim Pract* 41(6):235–242, 2000.
38. Ross SJ, Osborne CA, Kirk CA, et al: Clinical evaluation of dietary modification for the treatment of spontaneous chronic kidney disease in cats. *J Am Vet Med Assoc* 229(6):949–957, 2006.
39. Rodriguez M, Lorenzo V: Progress in uremic toxin research: parathyroid hormone, a uremic toxin. *Semin Dial* 22(4):363–368, 2009.

40. Polzin DJ: Chronic kidney disease. In Ettinger SJ, Feldman EC, editors: *Textbook of veterinary internal medicine*, vol 2, ed 7, St Louis, 2010, Saunders/Elsevier, pp 1990–2021.

41. Ross LA, Finco DR, Crowell WA: Effects of dietary phosphorus restriction on the kidneys of cats with reduced renal mass. *Am J Vet Res* 43(6):1023–1026, 1982.

42. Eknoyan G, Levin A, Levin NW: Bone metabolism and disease in chronic kidney disease. *Am J Kidney Dis* 42(Suppl 3):1–201, 2003.

43. Barber PJ, Rawlings JM, Markwell PJ, et al: Effect of dietary phosphate restriction on renal secondary hyperparathyroidism in the cat. *J Small Anim Pract* 40:62–70, 1999.

44. Plantinga EA, Everts H, Kastelein J, et al: Retrospective study of the survival of cats with acquired chronic renal insufficiency offered different commercial diets. *Vet Rec* 157:185–187, 2005.

45. Geddes RF, Elliott J, Syme HM: The effect of feeding a renal diet on plasma fibroblast growth factor 23 concentrations in cats with stable azotemic chronic kidney disease. *J Vet Intern Med* 27:1354–1361, 2013.

46. Hutchison AJ: Oral phosphate binders. *Kidney Int* 75(9):906–914, 2009.

47. Cannata Andía JB, FernándezMartín JL: The clinical impact of aluminium overload in renal failure. *Nephrol Dial Transplant* 17(Suppl 2):9–12, 2002.

48. Segev G, Bandt C, Francey T, et al: Aluminum toxicity following administration of aluminum-based phosphate binders in 2 dogs with renal failure. *J Vet Intern Med* 22(6):1432–1435, 2008.

49. Cervelli MJ, Shaman A, Meade A, et al: Effect of gastric acid suppression with pantoprazole on the efficacy of calcium carbonate as a phosphate binder in haemodialysis patients. *Nephrol* 17(5):458–465, 2012.

50. Schaefer K, Scheer J, Asmus G, et al: The treatment of uraemic hyperphosphatemia with calcium acetate and calcium carbonate: a comparative study. *Nephrol Dial Transplant* 6(3):170–175, 1991.

51. Braun J, Asmus HG, Hozer H, et al: Long-term comparison of a calcium-free phosphate binder and calcium carbonate-phosphorus metabolism and cardiovascular calcification. *Clin Nephrol* 62(2):104–115, 2004.

52. Goodman WG, London G, Amann K, et al: Vascular calcification in chronic kidney disease. *Am J Kid Dis* 43(3):572–579, 2004.

53. Navaneethan SD, Palmer SC, Craig JC, et al: Benefits and harms of phosphate binders in CKD: a systematic review of randomized controlled trials. *Am J Kid Dis* 54(4):619–637, 2009.

54. Persy VP, Behets GJ, Bervoets AR, et al: Lanthanum: a safe phosphate binder. *Semin Dial* 19(3):195–199, 2006.

55. Albaaj F, Hutchison AJ: Lanthanum carbonate (Fosrenol®): a novel agent for the treatment of hyperphosphataemia in renal failure and dialysis patients. *Int J Clin Pract* 59(9):1091–1096, 2005.

56. Damment SJP: Pharmacology of the phosphate binder, lanthanum carbonate. *Ren Fail* 33(2):217–224, 2011.

57. Schmidt B, Dribusch U, Delport P, et al: Tolerability and efficacy of the intestinal phosphate binder Lantharenol in cats. *BMC Vet Res* 8(1):14, 2012.

58. Kidder AC, Chew D: Treatment options for hyperphosphatemia in feline CKD: what's out there? *J Feline Med Surg* 11(11):913–924, 2009.

59. Nunamaker EA, Sherman JG: Oral administration of lanthanum dioxycarbonate does not alter bone morphology of normal cats. *J Vet Pharmacol Ther* 35(2):193–197, 2012.

60. Pai AB, Shepler BM: Comparison of sevelamer hydrochloride and sevelamer carbonate: risk of metabolic acidosis and clinical implications. *Pharmacotherapy* 29(5):554–561, 2009.

61. Braunlin W, Zhorov E, Guo A, et al: Bile acid binding to sevelamer HCl. *Kidney Int* 62(2):611–619, 2002.

62. Brown SA, Rickertsen M, Sheldon S: Effects of an intestinal phosphorus binder on serum phosphorus and parathyroid hormone concentration in cats with reduced renal function. *Intern J Appl Res Vet Med* 6(3):155–160, 2008.

63. Melamed ML, Thadhani RI: Vitamin D therapy in chronic kidney disease and end stage renal disease. *Clin J Am Soc Nephrol* 7(2):358–365, 2012.

64. Palmer SC, McGregor DO, Craig JC, et al: Vitamin D compounds for people with chronic kidney disease requiring dialysis. *Cochrane Database Syst Rev* (4):CD005633, 2009.

65. Palmer SC, McGregor DO, Craig JC, et al: Vitamin D compounds for people with chronic kidney disease not requiring dialysis. *Cochrane Database Syst Rev* (4):CD00008175, 2009.

66. Ravani P, Malberti F, Tripepi G, et al: Vitamin D levels and patient outcome in chronic kidney disease. *Kidney Int* 75(1):88–95, 2008.

67. Drechsler C, Verduijn M, Pilz S, et al: Vitamin D status and clinical outcomes in incident dialysis patients: results from the NECOSAD study. *Nephrol Dial Transplant* 26(3):1024–1032, 2011.

68. Kovesdy CP, Ahmadzadeh S, Anderson JE, et al: Association of activated vitamin D treatment and mortality in chronic kidney disease. *Arch Intern Med* 168(4):397–403, 2008.

69. Shoben AB, Rudser KD, de Boer IH, et al: Association of oral calcitriol with improved survival in nondialyzed CKD. *J Am Soc Nephrol* 19(8):1613–1619, 2008.

70. Nagode LA, Chew DJ, Podell M: Benefits of calcitriol therapy and serum phosphorus control in dogs and cats with chronic renal failure. Both are essential to prevent or suppress toxic hyperparathyroidism. *Vet Clin North Am Small Anim Pract* 26(6):1293–1330, 1996.

71. Polzin DJ: Chronic kidney disease in small animals. *Vet Clin North Am Small Anim Pract* 41(1):15–30, 2011.

72. Hostutler RA, DiBartola SP, Chew DJ, et al: Comparison of the effects of daily and intermittent-dose calcitriol on serum parathyroid hormone and ionized calcium concentrations in normal cats and cats with chronic renal failure. *J Vet Intern Med* 20(6):1307–1313, 2006.

73. Korman RM, White JD: Feline CKD: current therapies—what is achievable? *J Feline Med Surg* 15(1 Suppl):29–44, 2013.

Chronic Kidney Disease: Stem Cell Therapy

Jessica M. Quimby

REGENERATIVE MEDICINE

Regenerative medicine refers to the process of using living tissues to repair or replace organs that are functionally damaged. Stem cell therapy in particular is an innovative new field of scientific investigation and clinical application that holds promise for a variety of diseases in veterinary medicine as well as human medicine. Recent years have brought increased interest in the potential for adult stem cells to help in the treatment of many diseases through both their regenerative properties as well as their apparent ability to alter the environment in injured and diseased tissues. In particular, adult stem cells called *mesenchymal stem cells (MSCs)* can migrate to affected areas and may be able to support the growth of other stem cells as well as moderate the response of the immune system. This type of therapy may therefore be useful in acute kidney injury (AKI) and chronic kidney disease (CKD).

A *stem cell* is a generic term referring to any unspecialized cell that is capable of long-term self-renewal through cell division but that can be induced to differentiate into a specialized, functional cell. Stem cells are generally divided into two groups, embryonic stem cells and adult stem cells. Adult stem cells can be obtained from many differentiated tissues, including but not limited to bone marrow, bone, fat, and muscle. Obtaining adult stem cells does not raise ethical concerns, and stem cells are most commonly obtained from bone marrow or adipose sources. For most studies, the adult stem cell in question is actually a MSC or mesenchymal stromal cell. Mesenchymal stem cells are multipotent but not pluripotent, which means they can differentiate into some, or "multiple," but not all tissue types.[1]

MESENCHYMAL STEM CELL SOURCES

Mesenchymal stem cells can be isolated from virtually every tissue in the body. In cats, sources of MSCs that have been explored for expansion and clinical utility include bone marrow, adipose tissue, and fetal membrane tissues discarded from pregnant ovariohysterectomy.[2-5] The tissue source with the highest MSC proliferation potential appears to vary from species to species,[6,7] and a recent study in cats compared the proliferative capacities of MSCs from different sources.[4] In addition to a relatively easier collection procedure, adipose-derived MSCs (aMSCs) were found to be superior in proliferative potential to bone marrow-derived MSCs (bmMSCs) and are considered by most to be the preferred source for cats.[4] Although the majority of studies of MSC therapy in AKI and CKD rodent models utilize bmMSCs, more recent studies indicate similar efficacy with aMSCs.[8,9] Characterization and immunologic properties also appear to be similar between the sources,[10] with recent literature even suggesting an added advantage of using aMSCs for immunomodulatory indications.[11]

Two different types of MSC products are currently being investigated as a novel therapy for CKD in cats; aMSCs expanded in culture and stromal vascular fraction (SVF) or nonexpanded aMSCs. Stromal vascular fraction is the initial product of adipose tissue processing and is the type of cellular product produced from point-of-care processors and several private companies. Although isolation and expansion in culture allow the expanded aMSC product to have a purer population of MSCs, the SVF product contains multiple cell types. These are thought to include MSCs as well as a mixture of B and T lymphocytes, endothelial cells, fibroblasts, macrophages, pericytes, and preadipocytes.[12] Currently, not enough information is known about SVF to determine if a cellular product with a mixed cellular type is a therapeutic advantage or disadvantage. Culture-expanded MSCs (both bmMSCs and aMSCs) are the type predominantly used in the rodent model literature; however, more recent rodent studies have started to explore the therapeutic potential of the SVF cellular product with promising results.[13,14]

Stem cells that are harvested from the patient with the intention of administering them back to the same patient are termed *autologous MSCs*. Stem cells that are harvested from healthy donors for administration to a clinical patient are termed *allogeneic MSCs*. The relative efficacy of autologous versus allogeneic cells is an area of controversy. Although allogeneic MSCs are immune-privileged and are not expected to incite an immune response, according to some authors they may not be as effective as autologous cells.[15] It is argued that autologous MSCs may survive longer in the body in comparison to allogeneic cells, which could reduce efficacy of the latter. Decreased efficacy of allogeneic MSCs in comparison to autologous MSCs has been observed in one AKI rodent study.[15] However, allogeneic MSCs have been widely used in experimental stem cell transfer investigations, including clinical trials in humans, with positive results.[15,16] The advantages of using allogeneic MSCs include sparing the patient from undergoing the harvest procedure as well as the use of MSCs from young healthy donor animals. Recent studies in humans and rodents support the view that MSCs obtained from young healthy individuals have greater proliferation potential and have greater therapeutic potential than those collected from elderly diseased individuals.[17-20]

MESENCHYMAL STEM CELL CHARACTERIZATION

Mesenchymal stem cells are plastic adherent and assume a fibroblast-like morphology during culture (Figure 49-1). They proliferate easily in culture and can be cryopreserved without loss of phenotype or differentiation potential[21] but

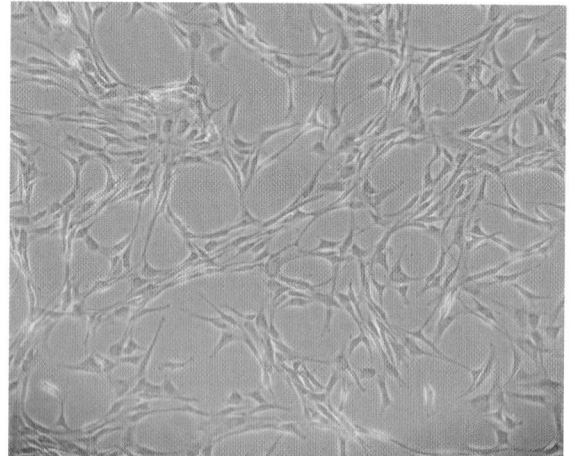

Figure 49-1: Phenotype of feline adipose-derived mesenchymal stem cells. Stem cells are plastic adherent and assume a fibroblast-like morphology during culture (magnification ×10).

whether cryopreservation affects their immunomodulatory capabilities has not been fully investigated. Cell surface marker characterization via flow cytometry differentiates them from hematopoietic cells, but no truly unique MSC molecule has been identified.[22] For the most part, feline MSCs have been reported to be CD44 positive, CD90 positive, CD105 positive, CD45 negative, and HLA-DR negative. These markers are similar in both bmMSCs and aMSCs.[2,4,22-24] In part, the lack of definitive markers probably reflects the diverse lineage of MSCs and the fact that each MSC population reflects to some degree the characteristics of tissues from which they were derived. Most importantly, stem cells from both adipose and bone marrow sources possess the ability to differentiate into cell types of multiple lineages, including adipocytes, chondrocytes, and osteocytes demonstrating their multipotent potential (Figure 49-2).[1,22]

MESENCHYMAL STEM CELL IMMUNOLOGIC PROPERTIES

Mesenchymal stem cells clearly modulate immune responses, as demonstrated by both *in vitro* and *in vivo* studies.[25,26] For example, MSCs are poor antigen-presenting cells and do not express major histocompatibility complex (MHC) class II or costimulatory molecules and only low levels of MHC class I molecules.[1] Thus, MSCs are very nonimmunogenic and can be transferred to fully allogeneic recipients and still mediate their immunologic effects.[27] Among their other immunological properties, MSCs inhibit lymphocyte proliferation and cytokine production, suppress dendritic cell function and alter dendritic cell cytokine production, and decrease interferon gamma production by natural killer cells.[1] *In vitro* studies have demonstrated that MSCs can produce growth factors, cytokines, and anti-inflammatory mediators, all of which could help maintain or improve renal function and suppress intrarenal inflammation.[16,28,29] The ability of MSCs to suppress inflammation appears to be mediated both by

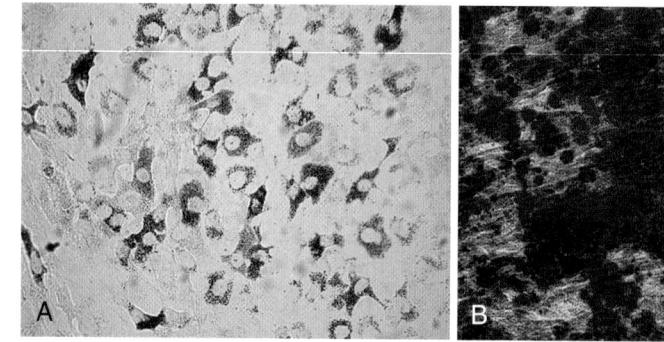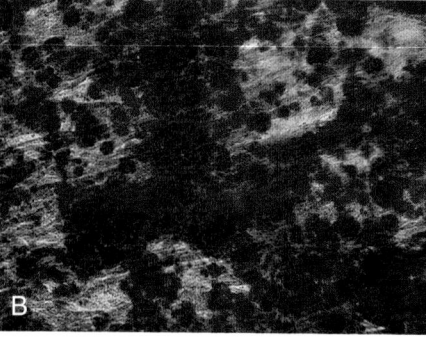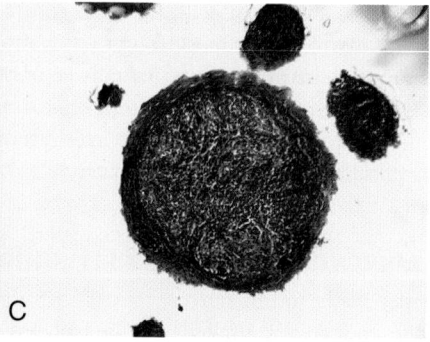

Figure 49-2: Trilineage differentiation of feline adipose-derived mesenchymal stem cells (aMSCs). **A,** aMSCs formed intracellular lipid vacuoles when incubated in adipocytic differentiation media for 21 days (Magnification ×20). **B,** aMSCs stained positive for calcium with alizarin red following differentiation into osteocytic phenotype after 21 days of incubation in differentiation media (Magnification ×20). **C,** Cryosection of pellets of cartilage matrix (stained with toluidine blue) formed by aMSCs when exposed to chondrocytic differentiation media for 21 days (Magnification ×10).

secreted factors and by direct contact with inflammatory cells.[16,29] These properties of MSCs could potentially be harnessed therapeutically.

MESENCHYMAL STEM CELL THERAPY FOR CHRONIC KIDNEY DISEASE: RODENT MODELS

The question is frequently asked why it might be thought that MSC therapy would be beneficial for CKD in cats. The potential of MSC therapy has been illustrated by literally dozens of studies assessing MSC therapy in rodent models of renal disease, although most studies have focused on models of short-term protection from AKI.[14,28,30-32] The majority of these studies provide evidence that systemic administration of bmMSCs or aMSCs (both culture-expanded and SVF products) can help preserve renal function in the face of acute insults (e.g., ischemic injury, toxic insult, and obstruction) and can also help reduce tubular injury and fibrosis.[14,28,30-32] Several studies have also demonstrated incorporation of small numbers of MSCs into the renal parenchyma.[31,33,34] It has been proposed that some of these MSCs may actually differentiate into functional renal tubular epithelial cells, although this theory remains controversial. Other investigators propose that paracrine effects from the injected MSCs are more important than the effects of direct cellular incorporation into the kidney.[28,35] Thus, the available data indicate that systemically-administered MSCs can help improve or stabilize renal function in AKI by a variety of mechanisms.

Fewer studies have investigated the effects of MSC therapy in CKD rodent models.[23,24,36-41] Rodent models of CKD are most commonly created by performing a $5/6$ nephrectomy, and a limitation of these models is that frequently MSC therapy is administered a relatively short time after nephrectomy (days to weeks). In the majority of CKD rodent model studies that have been performed, administration of both bmMSCs and aMSCs has demonstrated significant renoprotective effects, including reduction of intrarenal inflammatory infiltrate, decreased fibrosis, and glomerulosclerosis.[23,24,36,40,41] Parameters of renal function and clinical health, including weight, serum creatinine, blood urea nitrogen, proteinuria, blood pressure, and hematocrit have also been demonstrated to improve as a result of MSC therapy.[23,24,36,40,41] Several routes of administration—intraparenchymal, subcapsular, intravenous (IV)—have been explored and all seem to be effective. Multiple repeated injections of MSCs appear to be even more effective than single injections.[23,36]

Small numbers of administered MSCs have been shown to home to renal parenchyma in several studies,[23,24,36,39] but as for AKI, mechanism of action is thought to be paracrine in nature.[23] MSC effects appear to come both from anti-inflammatory capabilities as well as protection of vascular integrity as mediated by vascular endothelial growth factor (VEGF).[23,36,37,39,41] Pro-fibrotic molecules and cytokines and pro-inflammatory cytokines, specifically transforming growth factor beta, monocyte chemotactic protein 1, and interleukin

(IL)-6, are found to be decreased in MSC-treated rodents, particularly when multiple injections are administered.[23,36] Anti-inflammatory cytokines (e.g., IL-10 and vasculoprotective factor VEGF) have been shown to increase as a result of MSC therapy.[36,37,39,41] Although this body of literature demonstrates the immense potential of MSC therapy for CKD, results of rodent models should be evaluated with care because administration of MSCs immediately after surgical nephrectomy is likely not representative of long standing naturally occurring disease.

MESENCHYMAL STEM CELL THERAPY FOR CHRONIC KIDNEY DISEASE: FELINE CLINICAL TRIALS

At present, there is little published work regarding MSC therapy for CKD in cats and dogs. A series of pilot studies for cats with CKD has been conducted at the Center for Immune and Regenerative Medicine at Colorado State University,[3,42] and a clinical trial is also currently underway at the Animal Medical Center in New York.[43] The progress of these studies is summarized here to provide an overview of the current state of knowledge with regard to feline clinical trials.

Studies at Colorado State University have focused on assessing the safety and efficacy of intrarenal administration of autologous culture-expanded MSCs in CKD cats, as well as the safety and efficacy of IV administration of allogeneic cryopreserved culture-expanded aMSCs in CKD cats. In the first pilot study, the feasibility of autologous intrarenal MSC therapy was investigated.[42] Six cats (two healthy and four with CKD) received a single unilateral intrarenal injection of autologous bmMSCs or aMSCs via ultrasound guidance. Minimum database and glomerular filtration rate (GFR) via nuclear scintigraphy were determined preinjection, at 7 days and at 30 days postinjection. Intrarenal injection did not induce immediate or longer-term adverse effects. Two International Renal Interest Society (IRIS) Stage 3 CKD cats that received aMSCs experienced modest improvement in GFR and a mild decrease in serum creatinine concentration. It was concluded that MSCs could be transferred safely by ultrasound-guided intrarenal injection in cats, but that alternative sources and routes of MSC therapy should be investigated because the number of sedations and interventions required to implement this approach would likely preclude widespread clinical application. Additional information obtained during this pilot study was the relative difficulty of expanding MSCs in culture from elderly diseased patients.

In a second series of pilot studies, the feasibility of allogeneic IV culture-expanded MSC therapy was investigated.[3] The goal of these studies was to assess the feasibility of an "off the shelf" cellular product. Stable CKD cats with no concurrent illness were enrolled in these studies and received an IV infusion of allogeneic aMSCs collected and cryopreserved from healthy young specific pathogen-free cats every 2 weeks (Figure 49-3). Cats in pilot study 1 received 2×10^6 cryopreserved aMSCs per infusion, cats in pilot study 2

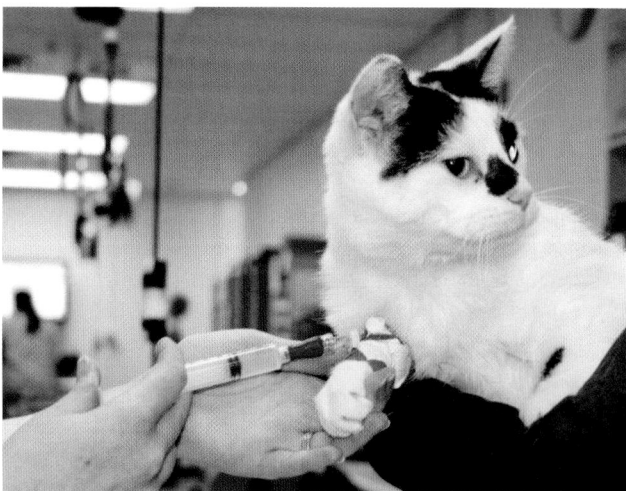

Figure 49-3: Cat with stable chronic kidney disease receiving an intravenous infusion of allogeneic adipose-derived mesenchymal stem cells.

received 4×10^6 cryopreserved aMSCs per infusion, and cats in pilot study 3 received 4×10^6 aMSCs cultured from cryopreserved adipose tissue. Serum biochemistries, complete blood count, urinalysis, urine protein, GFR, and urinary cytokine concentrations were monitored during the treatment period. Cats in pilot study 1 had few adverse effects from the aMSC infusions, and there was a statistically significant decrease in serum creatinine concentrations during the study period; however, the degree of decrease seemed unlikely to be clinically relevant.

Adverse effects of cryopreserved aMSC infusion in pilot study 2 cats included vomiting (two out of five cats) during infusion and increased respiratory rate and effort (four out of five cats). Cats in pilot study 3 that received aMSCs cultured from cryopreserved adipose did not experience any adverse side effects. Serum creatinine concentrations, urinary cytokines, and GFRs did not change significantly in pilot study 2 or 3 cats, although individual cats experienced potentially significant changes, including some cats that had adverse effects. Based on the results of the three pilot studies, it appeared that use of higher doses of aMSCs taken directly from cryopreservation was the source of the treatment-related adverse effects in pilot study 2 because similar doses of aMSCs cultured from cryopreserved adipose tissue did not result in any adverse effects. The most likely explanation for this reaction is an instant blood-mediated inflammatory reaction (IBMIR), which results in clumping of the cells as they contact the blood and potential subsequent micro pulmonary thromboembolism.[44] The IBMIR phenomenon has been described previously with cryopreserved cells in humans and increases in severity with dose and passage number.[44] It can result in lysis of the administered MSCs and subsequent poor efficacy. Although all cells given in pilot study 2 were of the same passage 3 as those used in the other two pilot studies, the reaction was only seen in the pilot group where cells were taken directly from cryopreservation and used at the higher dose. In pilot study 3, no complications during or after administration of aMSCs cultured from cryopreserved fat were appreciated. Thus, it was concluded that the administration

of a higher dose of aMSCs taken directly from cryopreservation, despite careful washing, was the source of the toxic reactions observed, and this form of administration is not recommended. To further explore the potential of MSC therapy for feline CKD, a placebo-controlled clinical trial is currently underway that focuses on assessing the efficacy of allogeneic MSCs expanded from cryopreserved adipose and administered repeatedly at a cell/kg dosage. No adverse effects have been seen in cats who have participated in this trial. Long-term follow-up of cats participating in all clinical trials is still underway and will provide additional information about the effects of MSC therapy on disease progression.

Studies at the Animal Medical Center in New York have focused on assessing the safety and efficacy of autologous intra-arterial nonexpanded MSC therapy for cats with CKD.[43] In these studies, cats were treated with autologous SVF injected into the renal artery via the use of minimally-invasive image-guided interventional radiologic techniques. This delivery method is particularly advantageous because it bypasses the initial uptake of the stem cells by other organs and delivers a larger number of cells directly to the diseased renal tissue. When MSCs are given IV (usually via the cephalic vein), the cells must first pass through the pulmonary capillary bed and the entire dose administered likely does not reach the kidney. In addition, MSCs have the ability to home to any injured or inflamed tissue, and because elderly patients are likely to have multiple comorbidities, cells may be directed to nonrenal tissues.

The safety and efficacy of the intra-arterial delivery system is currently being assessed in a two phase pilot study. In phase 1, six cats with stable IRIS Stage 3 CKD received unilateral intra-arterial injections of MSCs and were followed for 3 months. No adverse effects on renal blood flow or creatinine were noted as a result of intra-arterial injection. The median procedure time for intra-arterial injection was 37.5 minutes (range: 25 to 75 minutes). The median hospitalization time was $1\frac{1}{2}$ days (range: $\frac{1}{4}$ to 3 days). Two cats had evidence of partial renal artery embolism at the time of MSC administration with no clinical consequence. A mild improvement in serum creatinine was observed, but the degree of decrease is unlikely to be of clinical significance. Other parameters, including GFR estimated by iohexol clearance and proteinuria, were unchanged after 3 months. Long-term follow-up of phase 1 cats, currently $2\frac{1}{2}$ years post-treatment, demonstrates stable disease with no indication of progression. In phase 2, cats will be enrolled in a placebo-controlled randomized trial in which the effects of MSCs administered via the renal artery are compared to the effects of MSCs administered IV, as well as a placebo group. These cats will be followed for a period of 3 years. This trial is currently underway and, thus, data on efficacy is still forthcoming. In addition to the two clinical trials, data has been collected on a group of cats with CKD and ureteral obstruction that received IV nonexpanded MSC therapy at the time their ureteral obstruction was surgically addressed. Few adverse effects were seen as a result of MSC injection, with the only complications being two cats that vomited after administration with no clinical consequences. Serum creatinine was seen to improve after relief of ureteral obstruction and MSC injection, as would be expected. Comparison to cats that only received ureteral surgery and long-term follow-up are necessary to fully assess efficacy.

SUMMARY

The fields of stem cell therapy and regenerative medicine are expanding rapidly. Veterinary medicine is poised to take a leading role in these fields, because there are a number of chronic inflammatory diseases in companion animals that would be amenable to stem cell therapy. Among the challenges facing these emerging fields are standardization of treatment protocols and adherence to strict principles of evidence-based medicine in reporting study results and conclusions. Nonetheless, it is likely that stem cell therapy will make significant progress in changing treatment paradigms for a number of important feline diseases in the relatively near future.

References

1. Reinders ME, Fibbe WE, Rabelink TJ: Multipotent mesenchymal stromal cell therapy in renal disease and kidney transplantation. *Nephrol Dial Transplant* 25:17–24, 2010.
2. Martin DR, Cox NR, Hathcock TL, et al: Isolation and characterization of multipotential mesenchymal stem cells from feline bone marrow. *Exp Hematol* 30:879–886, 2002.
3. Quimby JM, Webb TL, Habenicht LM, et al: Safety and efficacy of intravenous infusion of allogeneic cryopreserved mesenchymal stem cells for treatment of chronic kidney disease in cats: results of three sequential pilot studies. *Stem Cell Res Ther* 4:48, 2013.
4. Webb TL, Quimby JM, Dow SW: *In vitro* comparison of feline bone marrow–derived and adipose tissue–derived mesenchymal stem cells. *J Feline Med Surg* 14:165–168, 2012.
5. Iacono E, Cunto M, Zambelli D, et al: Could fetal fluid and membranes be an alternative source for mesenchymal stem cells (MSCs) in the feline species? A preliminary study. *Vet Res Commun* 36:107–118, 2012.
6. Kisiel AH, McDuffee LA, Masaoud E, et al: Isolation, characterization, and *in vitro* proliferation of canine mesenchymal stem cells derived from bone marrow, adipose tissue, muscle, and periosteum. *Am J Vet Res* 73:1305–1317, 2012.
7. Ribitsch I, Burk J, Delling U, et al: Basic science and clinical application of stem cells in veterinary medicine. *Adv Biochem Eng Biotechnol* 123:219–263, 2010.
8. Kim JH, Park DJ, Yun JC, et al: Human adipose tissue–derived mesenchymal stem cells protect kidneys from cisplatin nephrotoxicity in rats. *Am J Physiol Renal Physiol* 302:F1141–F1150, 2012.
9. Furuichi K, Shintani H, Sakai Y, et al: Effects of adipose-derived mesenchymal cells on ischemia-reperfusion injury in kidney. *Clin Exp Nephrol* 16:679–689, 2012.
10. Strioga M, Viswanathan S, Darinskas A, et al: Same or not the same? Comparison of adipose tissue–derived versus bone marrow–derived mesenchymal stem and stromal cells. *Stem Cells Dev* 21:2724–2752, 2012.
11. Ivanova-Todorova E, Bochev I, Mourdjeva M, et al: Adipose tissue–derived mesenchymal stem cells are more potent suppressors of dendritic cells differentiation compared to bone marrow–derived mesenchymal stem cells. *Immunol Lett* 126:37–42, 2009.

12. Gimble JM, Bunnell BA, Guilak F: Human adipose-derived cells: an update on the transition to clinical translation. *Regen Med* 7:225–235, 2012.
13. Riordan NH, Ichim TE, Min WP, et al: Non-expanded adipose stromal vascular fraction cell therapy for multiple sclerosis. *J Transl Med* 7:29, 2009.
14. Yasuda K, Ozaki T, Saka Y, et al: Autologous cell therapy for cisplatin-induced acute kidney injury by using non-expanded adipose tissue–derived cells. *Cytotherapy* 14:1089–1100, 2012.
15. Togel F, Zhang P, Hu Z, et al: VEGF is a mediator of the renoprotective effects of multipotent marrow stromal cells in acute kidney injury. *J Cell Mol Med* 13:2109–2114, 2009.
16. McTaggart SJ, Atkinson K: Mesenchymal stem cells: immunobiology and therapeutic potential in kidney disease. *Nephrology (Carlton)* 12:44–52, 2007.
17. Scruggs BA, Semon JA, Zhang X, et al: Age of the donor reduces the ability of human adipose-derived stem cells to alleviate symptoms in the experimental autoimmune encephalomyelitis mouse model. *Stem Cells Transl Med* 2:797–807, 2013.
18. Lei L, Liao W, Sheng P, et al: Biological character of human adipose-derived adult stem cells and influence of donor age on cell replication in culture. *Sci China C Life Sci* 50:320–328, 2007.
19. Kretlow JD, Jin YQ, Liu W, et al: Donor age and cell passage affects differentiation potential of murine bone marrow–derived stem cells. *BMC Cell Biol* 9:60, 2008.
20. Wang J, Liao L, Wang S, et al: Cell therapy with autologous mesenchymal stem cells-how the disease process impacts clinical considerations. *Cytotherapy* 15:893–904, 2013.
21. Martinello T, Bronzini I, Maccatrozzo L, et al: Canine adipose-derived-mesenchymal stem cells do not lose stem features after a long-term cryopreservation. *Res Vet Sci* 91:18–24, 2011.
22. Schaffler A, Buchler C: Concise review: adipose tissue–derived stromal cells—basic and clinical implications for novel cell-based therapies. *Stem Cells* 25:818–827, 2007.
23. Semedo P, Correa-Costa M, Antonio Cenedeze M, et al: Mesenchymal stem cells attenuate renal fibrosis through immune modulation and remodeling properties in a rat remnant kidney model. *Stem Cells* 27:3063–3073, 2009.

24. Cavaglieri RC, Martini D, Sogayar MC, et al: Mesenchymal stem cells delivered at the subcapsule of the kidney ameliorate renal disease in the rat remnant kidney model. *Transplant Proc* 41:947–951, 2009.
25. English K, Barry FP, Mahon BP: Murine mesenchymal stem cells suppress dendritic cell migration, maturation and antigen presentation. *Immunol Lett* 115:50–58, 2008.
26. McIntosh KR, Frazier T, Rowan BG, et al: Evolution and future prospects of adipose-derived immunomodulatory cell therapeutics. *Expert Rev Clin Immunol* 9:175–184, 2013.
27. Togel F, Cohen A, Zhang P, et al: Autologous and allogeneic marrow stromal cells are safe and effective for the treatment of acute kidney injury. *Stem Cells Dev* 18:475–485, 2009.
28. Togel F, Weiss K, Yang Y, et al: Vasculotropic, paracrine actions of infused mesenchymal stem cells are important to the recovery from acute kidney injury. *Am J Physiol Renal Physiol* 292:F1626–F1635, 2007.
29. Barry FP, Murphy JM, English K, et al: Immunogenicity of adult mesenchymal stem cells: lessons from the fetal allograft. *Stem Cells Dev* 14:252–265, 2005.
30. Semedo P, Wang PM, Andreucci TH, et al: Mesenchymal stem cells ameliorate tissue damages triggered by renal ischemia and reperfusion injury. *Transplant Proc* 39:421–423, 2007.
31. Morigi M, Imberti B, Zoja C, et al: Mesenchymal stem cells are renotropic, helping to repair the kidney and improve function in acute renal failure. *J Am Soc Nephrol* 15:1794–1804, 2004.
32. Little MH, Rae FK: Review article: Potential cellular therapies for renal disease: can we translate results from animal studies to the human condition? *Nephrology (Carlton)* 14:544–553, 2009.
33. Kim SS, Park HJ, Han J, et al: Improvement of kidney failure with fetal kidney precursor cell transplantation. *Transplantation* 83:1249–1258, 2007.
34. Kitamura S, Yamasaki Y, Kinomura M, et al: Establishment and characterization of renal progenitor like cells from S3 segment of nephron in rat adult kidney. *FASEB J* 19:1789–1797, 2005.
35. Togel F, Yang Y, Zhang P, et al: Bioluminescence imaging to monitor the *in vivo* distribution of administered mesenchymal stem

cells in acute kidney injury. *Am J Physiol Renal Physiol* 295:F315–F321, 2008.

36. Lee SR, Lee SH, Moon JY, et al: Repeated administration of bone marrow–derived mesenchymal stem cells improved the protective effects on a remnant kidney model. *Ren Fail* 32:840–848, 2010.

37. Villanueva S, Ewertz E, Carrion F, et al: Mesenchymal stem cell injection ameliorates chronic renal failure in a rat model. *Clin Sci (Lond)* 121:489–499, 2011.

38. Kirpatovskii VI, Kazachenko AV, Plotnikov EY, et al: Functional aftereffects of intraparenchymatous injection of human fetal stem and progenitor cells to rats with chronic and acute renal failure. *Bull Exp Biol Med* 141:500–506, 2006.

39. Choi S, Park M, Kim J, et al: The role of mesenchymal stem cells in the functional improvement of chronic renal failure. *Stem Cells Dev* 18:521–529, 2009.

40. Ninichuk V, Gross O, Segerer S, et al: Multipotent mesenchymal stem cells reduce interstitial fibrosis but do not delay progression of chronic kidney disease in collagen4A3-deficient mice. *Kidney Int* 70:121–129, 2006.

41. Villanueva S, Carreno JE, Salazar L, et al: Human mesenchymal stem cells derived from adipose tissue reduce functional and tissue damage in a rat model of chronic renal failure. *Clin Sci (Lond)* 125:199–210, 2013.

42. Quimby JM, Webb TL, Gibbons DS, et al: Evaluation of intrarenal mesenchymal stem cell injection for treatment of chronic kidney disease in cats: a pilot study. *J Feline Med Surg* 13:418–426, 2011.

43. Berent A: Selective renal intra-arterial and non-selective intravenous delivery of autologous mesenchymal-derived stem cells in canine and feline patients with acute and chronic kidney disease. *ACVIM Forum*. Seattle, WA. 2013.

44. Moll G, Rasmusson-Duprez I, von Bahr L, et al: Are therapeutic human mesenchymal stromal cells compatible with human blood? *Stem Cells* 30:1565–1574, 2012.

Acute Kidney Injury

Cathy Langston and Adam Eatroff

ETIOLOGY AND PATHOPHYSIOLOGY

Acute kidney injury (AKI) has traditionally been classified into hemodynamic (prerenal), renal parenchymal (intrinsic), and postrenal etiologies. Although conceptually these categories provide a framework for understanding the pathophysiology of various renal insults, the clinical relevance of this taxonomy is questionable, because AKI is often the culmination of systemic, extra-renal disease, and renal-specific insults. Recent work has questioned whether azotemia secondary to volume depletion truly results in kidney injury *per se* or whether it represents an appropriate, physiologic renal response (i.e., marked reduction in glomerular filtration) to the need for extracellular fluid conservation.[1] Furthermore, the diagnosis of hemodynamic (prerenal) azotemia is often made in retrospect, limiting its clinical utility. Nonetheless, in people, hemodynamic azotemia (referred to as *transient azotemia*) is associated with a higher odds ratio for mortality, similar to persistent azotemia.[2] Although postrenal etiologies of AKI are typically recognized as structural or functional alterations in the urinary tract that prevent urine outflow, the pathophysiologic processes that result in uremia may be unrelated to renal excretory function (e.g., lower urinary tract rupture) or may be comprised of multiple components of this classification scheme. For example, in the case of a ureteral obstruction, azotemia may be the result not only of blockade of urine outflow from the renal pelvis, but also the maladaptive renal response to such obstruction, consisting of intense arteriolar vasoconstriction and influx of inflammatory cells.[3] The inflammatory response to ureteral obstruction may in itself produce significant, intrinsic renal parenchymal injury sufficiently severe to affect renal excretory function.

Classically, the clinical course of AKI proceeds through four phases: the initiation phase, the extension phase, the maintenance phase, and the recovery phase. These phases are defined by experimental models of AKI and may not be representative of the multifactorial nature of the disease. In clinical cases of AKI, the pathophysiologic process resulting in renal dysfunction is often multifactorial, with overlapping ischemic, inflammatory, toxic, and septic components in many cases; partitioning of AKI into these phases has little clinical utility.

There are a myriad of possible etiologies of feline AKI (Box 50-1). The most frequently encountered, diagnosed, or discussed etiologies in feline medicine are discussed in the following sections.

Ureteral Obstruction

Obstruction of the upper urinary tract has become a common cause of feline AKI in the last 20 years. The inner diameter of the feline ureter is approximately 0.4 mm (0.016 inches), making this structure highly prone to obstruction due to stricture, intraluminal concretion, mural inflammation or edema, muscular spasm, or extramural compression.[4,5] Although calcium oxalate nephroliths and ureteroliths are most frequently implicated as obstructive lesions,[6] the emergence of blood stones,[7] inflammation and fibrosis with smooth muscle hypertrophy of the ureteral wall (strictures),[8] and circumcaval ureters[9] have made advanced imaging techniques paramount for accurate presurgical identification of the cause of ureteral obstruction. This information can inform whether referral to select institutions for specific interventions (e.g., subcutaneous [SC] ureteral bypass) is indicated. The pathophysiology of AKI secondary to ureteral obstruction is complex, and most of the available information has been obtained from species other than the cat.[3,10] Pathophysiologic processes shared among various species include vasoconstriction, an influx of inflammatory cells and the release of proteolytic enzymes, and fibroblast recruitments with resultant fibroplasia.

Lily Intoxication

Species from the genera *Lilium* and *Hemerocallis* have been implicated in feline AKI of varying severity. Although neither the toxic principle nor a toxic dose has been clearly established, a report suggests that the aqueous fraction of the flowers and leaves of these plants is toxic and that ingestion of a single flower can cause clinically apparent AKI.[11] Pancreatitis has been implicated as a complicating factor in experimental models, as well as clinically and at the time of necropsy,[12] but whether pancreatitis precedes, is a consequence of, or occurs independently of AKI has yet to be determined. Early reports of lily intoxication portrayed a poor prognosis.[12,13] However, more recent studies suggest that azotemia develops infrequently secondary to lily exposure.[14,15] In the authors' experience, AKI secondary to lily intoxication that results in anuria carries a poor prognosis.

Pyelonephritis

In the authors' experience, the most commonly cited differential diagnosis for AKI (alone or superimposed on

BOX 50-1   List of Etiologies for Feline Acute Kidney Injury

Nephrotoxins

Antimicrobial Agents
Aminoglycosides
Aztreonam
Carbapenems
Cephalosporins
Penicillins
Polymyxins
Quinolones
Rifampin
Sulfonamides
Tetracyclines
Vancomycin

Antifungal Agents
Amphotericin B

Antineoplastic Drugs
Cisplatin and carboplatin
Doxorubicin
Methotrexate

Antiviral Agents
Acyclovir
Foscarnet

Antiprotozoal Agents
Dapsone
Pentamidine
Sulfadiazine
Thiacetarsamide
Trimethoprim-sulfamethoxazole

Immunosuppressive Drugs
Azathioprine
Calcineurin inhibitors (e.g. cyclosporine, tacrolimus)
Interleukin-2

Miscellaneous Therapeutic Agents
Acetaminophen
Allopurinol
Angiotensin-enzyme converting inhibitors
Antidepressants
Apomorphine
Cimetidine
Deferoxamine
Dextran-40
Diuretics
e-Aminocaproic acid
Ethylenediaminetetraacetic acid
Lipid-lowering drugs
Lithium
Methoxyflurane

Nonsteroidal anti-inflammatory drugs
Penicillamine
Phosphorus-containing urinary acidifiers
Streptokinase
Tricyclic antidepressants
Vitamin D analogs

Endogenous compounds
Hemoglobin
Myoglobin (e.g. trauma/rhabdomyolysis)

Heavy Metals
Antimony
Arsenic
Bismuth salts
Cadmium
Chromium
Copper
Gold
Lead
Mercury
Nickel
Silver
Thallium
Uranium

Organic Compounds
Carbon tetrachloride and other chlorinated hydrocarbons
Chloroform
Ethylene glycol
Herbicides
Pesticides
Solvents

Miscellaneous Nontherapeutic Agents
Bee venom
Diphosphonate
Calcium antagonists
Gallium nitrate
Illicit drugs
Lilies
Mushrooms
Radiocontrast agents
Snake venom
Sodium fluoride
Superphosphate fertilizer
Vitamin D-containing rodenticides

Continued

BOX 50-1 List of Etiologies for Feline Acute Kidney Injury—cont'd

Non-Nephrotoxic Insults

Decreased Cardiac Output/Ischemia
Volume depletion
Congestive heart failure
Arrhythmia
Cardiac arrest
Cardiac tamponade
Fluid overload
Deep anesthesia
Extensive surgery
Renal vessel thrombosis
Hyperviscosity/polycythemia
Hepatorenal syndrome

Infectious
Bacterial/fungal pyelonephritis
Leptospirosis
Feline infectious peritonitis
Bacterial endocarditis

Immune-Mediated/Inflammatory
Acute glomerulonephritis
Systemic lupus erythematosus
Renal transplant rejection
Vasculitis
Systemic inflammatory response syndrome
Sepsis
Disseminated intravascular coagulation

Obstructive
Ureteral obstruction
Urethral obstruction

Miscellaneous
Lymphoma
Blood transfusion reaction
Heatstroke/hyperthermia
Malignant hypertension
Neoplasia
Hypercalcemia

pre-existing chronic kidney disease [CKD]) is pyelonephritis. A definitive diagnosis of pyelonephritis requires identification of bacteria within the urine collected by pyelocentesis, but this procedure is rarely performed due to the associated risks of uroretroperitoneum, uroperitoneum, or urosepsis. Therefore, this diagnosis is frequently made based on the ultrasonographic appearance of the renal pelves with or without a positive bacterial culture of urine obtained by cystocentesis. The use of renal pelvic dimensions for the diagnosis of pyelonephritis is problematic for several reasons. First, there appears to be a large overlap in renal pelvic dimensions among healthy cats and cats with a variety of renal diseases, including pyelonephritis.[16] Second, the association between renal pelvic dilation and pyelonephritis was largely shaped by an experimental study in which pyelonephritis was induced in cats by ligation of the ureter and intravenous injection of *Escherichia coli*.[17] Finally, in other species (particularly humans), imaging criteria for pyelonephritis do not typically include the degree of renal pelvic dilation that is accepted as supportive for this disorder in veterinary medicine.[18] For these reasons, despite its ubiquity as a presumptive diagnosis for AKI, the true incidence and importance of this disease in the feline population are currently unknown.

Leptospirosis

Although feline AKI is not frequently associated with leptospirosis, there have been reports of acute azotemia associated with positive microscopic agglutination titers for specific *Leptospira* spp. serogroups.[19] Furthermore, serologic surveys have demonstrated exposure among a significant proportion of domestic cats.[20,21] This data, along with the fact that cats frequently prey on rodents which serve as reservoirs for many pathogenic leptospires, suggest the role of leptospirosis as an emerging cause of feline AKI should be re-examined.[22]

EPIDEMIOLOGY

Epidemiologic data characterizing feline AKI is lacking. The information available is limited to case series and anecdotal reports from referral centers with high caseloads. Furthermore, epidemiologic data likely varies, depending on the underlying etiology of AKI. For example, the patient population susceptible to unilateral ureteral obstructions resulting in uremic complications (i.e., typically middle-aged to older cats with underlying CKD) is likely different from the population at greatest risk for AKI secondary to lily exposure (i.e., young, curious cats). Lastly, the limited data that is available characterizing feline AKI has been generated from single institutions with limited patient and client demographics and geographic range. Therefore, generalizations regarding epidemiologic characteristics of feline AKI should be interpreted with caution.

In addition to the difficulties inherent in characterization of a syndrome with broad etiologic and epidemiologic characteristics, the lack of a standard definition for AKI and the wide spectrum of injury (ranging from clinically undetectable, subcellular damage to fulminant, excretory failure) has

Table 50-1	International Renal Interest Society Grading Scheme for Acute Kidney Injury	
Grade[†]	**Creatinine**	**Clinical Description**
Stage I	<1.6 mg/dL (<140 µmol/L)	Nonazotemic AKI Documented AKI: Historical, clinical, laboratory, or imaging evidence of AKI; clinical oliguria/anuria; volume responsiveness* *and/or* Progressive *nonazotemic* increase in serum creatinine ≥0.3 mg/dL (≥26.4 µmol/L) within 48 hours Measured oliguria (<1 mL/kg/hr) or anuria over 6 hours
Stage II	1.7-2.5 mg/dL (141-220 µmol/L)	Mild AKI Documented AKI and static or progressive azotemia Progressive azotemic increase in serum creatinine ≥0.3 mg/dL (≥26.4 µmol/L) within 48 hours, or volume responsiveness* Measured oliguria (<1 mL/kg/hr) or anuria over 6 hours
Stage III Stage IV Stage V	2.6-5.0 mg/dL (221-439 µmol/L) 5.1-10.0 mg/dL (440-880 µmol/L) >10.0 mg/dL (>880 µmol/L)	Moderate to severe AKI Documented AKI and increasing severities of azotemia and functional failure

AKI, Acute kidney injury.
*Volume responsive is an increase in urine production to >1 mL/kg/hr over 6 hours and/or decrease in serum creatinine to baseline over 48 hours.
[†]Each stage of AKI is further substaged on the basis of current urine production as oliguric or nonoliguric and on the requirement for renal replacement therapy.

hindered progress in understanding the scope of this disease. Recent standardization of the definition and stratification of severity of AKI in human medicine has not only allowed for more applicable epidemiologic studies but has allowed for the extraction of more clinically meaningful results from various clinical trials. The two most widely accepted schemes for defining and classifying human AKI are the Risk Injury Failure End-Stage Kidney Disease (RIFLE) scheme and the Acute Kidney Injury Network (AKIN), the latter of which was developed by modification of the former, with the intent to improve the sensitivity of detection of AKI.[23,24] Both sets of criteria appear to perform equally well when both sensitivity for detection of AKI and predictive ability for adverse outcomes are evaluated; therefore, these schemes have become accepted within the human nephrology community as the standard means of defining AKI for epidemiologic characterization. Based on several obstacles preventing application of these schemes to the feline population, Cowgill recently proposed a veterinary staging scheme designed for application to the veterinary population (Table 50-1).[25] This proposed scheme has yet to be validated for clinical utility in cats.

HISTORY, CLINICAL SIGNS, AND PHYSICAL EXAMINATION

Common historical findings include lethargy, vomiting, diarrhea, and anorexia, but these signs are nonspecific and may be the result of a variety of extra-renal diseases. Oliguria, anuria, or polyuria may be reported. When a patient is polyuric, compensatory polydipsia may be present, or water intake may be reduced due to anorexia. When patients are severely affected, reports of seizures, syncope, and dyspnea may overshadow more classic presenting signs associated with AKI.

Physical examination yields few findings specific to AKI, aside from enlarged, painful kidneys. Renomegaly and renal angina are inconsistently present, however, and for some cases in which underlying CKD is present concurrently, the kidneys are small. Dehydration is a common finding at the time of initial presentation, especially in those cats with AKI superimposed on CKD. However, inaccurate assessment of hydration status by physical examination parameters is common, and many euhydrated and overhydrated patients are erroneously categorized as dehydrated. Other findings may include halitosis, scleral injection, bradycardia, cutaneous bruising, peripheral edema, melena, and diarrhea. Oral mucosa ulceration and necrosis are common in patients with severe uremia. These findings may be due to the phenomenon of either uremic calciphylaxis or uremic stomatitis. Although the anatomic distribution and histologic lesions vary between these two processes, the gross appearance may be similar (i.e., ulceration).[26,27] Further work is warranted to better characterize these lesions because appropriate treatment may vary. Many of the aforementioned physical examination findings may be secondary to uremia, the primary disease process resulting in AKI (e.g., disseminated intravascular coagulation, vasculitis), or concurrent extra-renal organ injury (e.g., pancreatitis). Hypothermia is a frequent finding, and in the absence of circulatory shock, is thought to be associated with alteration of the hypothalamic thermoregulatory set point secondary to the influence of uremia.[28] Normothermia or hyperthermia may be suggestive of an infectious, inflammatory, or immune-mediated etiology.

A diagnostic dilemma often associated with the initial evaluation of the feline patient is the determination whether there is an underlying chronic component to AKI. The presence of underlying CKD can have serious implications in determining a patient's prognosis and potential for renal recovery and can influence a cat owner's willingness to pursue the intensive treatment often necessary to maximize the likelihood of a positive outcome. Clinicopathologic data characterizing prior renal function is frequently not available, however, making subtle historical and physical examination findings vital in assessing the likelihood of underlying CKD. Body fat and muscle condition can provide insight into the chronicity of renal or extra-renal disease. Careful palpation of the kidneys can aid in assessment of renal size and shape (e.g., small size or irregular contours of kidneys are often detected in association with CKD). A more sensitive means of assessing these characteristics is visualization with radiography or ultrasonography. Although the use of imaging, clinicopathologic techniques, and (rarely) renal histopathology can be helpful for cases in which underlying CKD is not readily apparent, many feline AKI cases with an underlying chronic component can be identified by a thorough questioning of the owner and physical examination.

DIAGNOSIS

Because most cases of feline AKI are manifested as a severe decline in renal excretory function, diagnosis is typically made based on a single evaluation or serial evaluations of creatinine and/or urea concentration in whole blood, serum, or plasma. Therefore, the diagnostic techniques discussed in the following sections are employed to determine the etiology, appropriate treatment options, and prognosis of the already identified AKI.

Laboratory Tests

Although changes in the complete blood count are often nonspecific in AKI, subtle changes in various components of the erythron and leukon can be useful for gaining insight into the chronicity, etiology, and prognosis. Although the presence of anemia can be due to a multitude of causes, this abnormality has important implications for both determination of chronicity and planning for treatment options, such as hemodialysis. Although anemia can be a complication of both acute and CKD, it is more frequently encountered and is more frequently severe (i.e., hematocrit less than 20%) in cases with an underlying chronic component. A moderate to severely anemic cat will almost assuredly require a red blood cell (RBC) transfusion during an extended course of treatment, given the need for serial blood sampling. Therefore, the availability of donor blood products, as well as blood typing and crossmatching capabilities, should be determined near

the time of initial presentation. Although the leukon frequently displays abnormalities consistent with a stress or inflammatory response, changes such as the presence of a left shift (circulating band neutrophils) may indicate more clinically significant inflammation, such as systemic inflammatory response syndrome (with or without concurrent sepsis).

The serum or plasma biochemistry panel may provide insight into extra-renal manifestations or consequences of AKI, as well as the presence of multisystemic disease. The severity of azotemia depends on the etiology and duration of AKI. The ratio of blood urea nitrogen to creatinine can be high from gastrointestinal (GI) bleeding or dehydration, or it can be low in early stages of AKI. The degree of hyperphosphatemia typically mirrors that of hypercreatinemia with few exceptions (e.g., acute ethylene glycol intoxication, juvenile growing animal, refeeding syndrome). Ionized calcium concentrations are normal or low, provided that hypercalcemia is not the cause of the AKI. Ethylene glycol intoxication causes a profound ionized hypocalcemia, due to both severe hyperphosphatemia and chelation of calcium by oxalate. The anion gap is usually high secondary to retained organic and inorganic acids, but it can be normal early in the course of disease, or if hypoalbuminemia is present. A high anion gap without (or prior to) the presence of azotemia is supportive of intoxication in cases of suspected ethylene glycol exposure. The anion gap is calculated by the formula*:

$$\text{Anion gap} = (Na^+ + K^+) - (HCO_3^- + Cl^-)$$

The normal anion gap is approximately 13 to 27 mEq/L.

The urinalysis can provide information regarding the etiology and severity of AKI. Care must be taken, however, to examine urine shortly after collection to avoid artifactual changes in biochemical and cellular composition. The urine specific gravity is frequently isosthenuric (1.007 to 1.015) in cases of intrinsic failure. A urine dipstick may reveal any combination of glucosuria (without hyperglycemia), proteinuria, bilirubinuria, and hemoglobinuria, depending on the underlying etiology. Care must be taken to obtain a thorough history, however, as administration of various medications (e.g., ascorbic acid, cephalexin, enrofloxacin) can interfere with the results of certain assays aimed at detecting glucosuria.[29,30] Proteinuria is frequently present, but qualitative (dipstick) and quantitative (urine protein:creatinine ratio) severity can vary within a specific etiology. Dipstick assessment of proteinuria has limited value in cats, due to discordance with urine protein:creatinine ratios.[31] The urine pH is usually acidic, unless there is a concurrent bacterial urinary tract infection (UTI). Careful microscopic assessment of urine sediment may disclose pyuria (suggestive of nephritis), dysmorphic RBCs (suggestive of glomerular disease, an uncommon diagnosis in the cat), or casts (most frequently granular, but red and white blood cell casts are uncommonly observed). In human medicine, eosinouria has historically

---

*Na^+, Sodium; K^+, potassium; HCO_3^-, bicarbonate; Cl^-, chloride.

been associated with acute interstitial nephritis (secondary to a drug reaction). However, more recent publications have shown that this finding lacks the satisfactory test characteristics to make it useful in the identification of this specific etiology.[32] Calcium oxalate crystals present in large numbers are supportive of ethylene glycol intoxication, although a few oxalate crystals may be present in the urine of healthy patients. Crystalluria is a common *in vitro* artifact that is secondary to prolonged storage of urine prior to analysis.[33] An in-house variation of a Romanowsky stain is frequently useful for detailed assessment of red and white blood cell morphology, as well as for the identification of bacteria. A bacterial urine culture is important to confirm the presence of a UTI and to guide antimicrobial therapy.

Imaging

Survey abdominal radiographs may show a normal renal silhouette or renomegaly, but hydronephrosis cannot be detected by radiography. Uroliths may be apparent, provided their size is above the limit of detection (typically 3 to 4 mm in diameter). Although radiography and ultrasonography are typically complementary (ureteral calculi that may be obscured by gas or ingesta during ultrasonography frequently can be detected by radiography), ultrasonography often provides more information.

In cases of AKI without an underlying chronic component, abdominal ultrasonography usually shows normal or enlarged kidneys with normal parenchymal architecture. Because many (especially geriatric) patients with AKI have underlying CKD, ultrasonographic changes (such as decreased corticomedullary definition, cysts, infarcts, small size, and irregular renal contour) are significant, and they should be considered important factors in formulating a long-term prognosis. The presence of ultrasonographic changes consistent with CKD does not preclude the possibility of a superimposed acute injury and, thus, the potential for at least partial renal recovery. Likewise, normal ultrasonographic renal architecture does not rule out the possibility of CKD. Perirenal fluid is commonly seen with a variety of etiologies of AKI and can also be seen secondary to volume overload. Aspiration and analysis of the perirenal fluid is typically unrewarding, because the fluid can be viscous, resulting in an inability to collect a sufficient volume for analysis.[34] A renal ultrasonographic finding described as subcapsular hypoechoic thickening has been described in cats undergoing fine-needle aspiration (FNA) or needle biopsy of the kidney. The presence of renal subcapsular hypoechoic thickening has a reasonably high positive predictive value for the identification of renal lymphoma (80.9%), but the negative predictive value (66.7%) does not allow for lymphoma to be ruled out in the absence of this finding.[35]

Ultrasonography of the renal pelves and ureters is the most practical tool for diagnosing ureteral obstructions. The renal pelvic diameter should always be measured in the transverse plane from the tip of the renal papilla to the most proximal aspect of the ureter (Figure 50-1A), because this

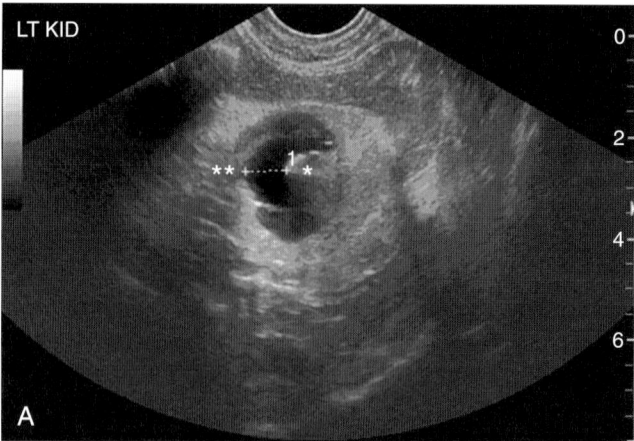

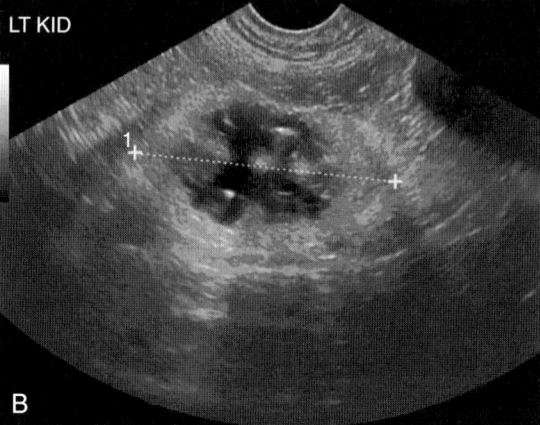

Figure 50-1: A, The renal pelvic diameter measured in the transverse plane. The calipers measure a renal pelvic diameter of 0.83 cm from the tip of the renal papilla (*) to the most proximal portion of the ureter (**). **B,** The same kidney viewed in the sagittal plane. Note the irregularity of the renal pelvic margin.

convention allows consistent methodology in evaluation of serial ultrasound studies. Measurement of the renal pelvic diameter in the sagittal plane can be problematic because the periphery of the renal pelvis can be uneven when evaluated from this view (see Figure 50-1B). In a recent study of both dogs and cats, a renal pelvic width equal to or exceeding 13 mm (0.5 inches) had 100% specificity for identification of renal outflow obstruction.[16] Serial examinations are occasionally necessary in patients where a ureteral obstruction is strongly suspected, but the initial renal pelvic diameter is not supportive of obstruction. The documentation of an increasing renal pelvic width over hours to days is strongly supportive of an acute ureteral obstruction.

Occasionally, an intravenous (IV) pyelogram can aid in the identification of pelvic, ureteral, and cystic disease processes, especially obstructive renal lesions that are not readily apparent with survey radiography or ultrasound. In addition, it can provide information regarding renal function in the contralateral kidney. For example, if uptake of radiocontrast is not detectable in the renal parenchyma or collecting system, the likelihood of a substantial glomerular filtration rate

(GFR) in that kidney is low. If the GFR in an obstructed kidney is below a certain threshold, historically identified with a serum creatinine concentration greater than 3.5 mg/dL (267 µmmol/L),[36] an IV pyelogram will result in inadequate study quality due to poor uptake of contrast. Antegrade pyelography may be a better choice for detection of obstructive ureteral lesions, because this technique does not rely on an adequate GFR for proper distribution of contrast material.[37] Computed tomography (CT) or magnetic resonance imaging can add information about renal architecture and better characterize obstruction. These techniques also eliminate the problems associated with superimposition of soft tissue and bone, as well as shadowing artifact encountered when the overlying GI tract is filled with gas. With the recently increased availability of high-speed image acquisition on many CT platforms, this technique is likely to become the standard means of acquiring images from contrast studies.

Other Diagnostic Modalities

Measurement of GFR (e.g., via iohexol clearance, endogenous creatinine clearance, or scintigraphy) has limited applicability in the initial identification of clinical AKI, because the degree of impairment in GFR is almost always detectable by surrogate markers, such as serum or plasma creatinine concentration. Typically, following a diagnosis of AKI with serum or plasma creatinine and urea concentrations, no additional tests are useful in confirming that renal impairment is present or further characterizing the degree of impairment. Although more advanced procedures (e.g., nuclear scintigraphy, contrast-enhanced CT) may provide information characterizing the GFR of each individual kidney, these techniques can be expensive and are not readily available.

Cytology of tissue acquired by FNA has limited utility in cases of AKI but can aid in detection of an infiltrative etiology. Cases of feline lymphosarcoma are frequently diagnosed based on percutaneous FNA of the kidney. Occasionally, false-negative results are obtained from cytologic analysis, and histopathology is necessary to confirm the diagnosis. Diagnosis of glomerular amyloidosis and feline infectious peritonitis requires special cytologic techniques (e.g., Congo red staining or coronavirus immunocytochemistry, respectively), and these diagnostic techniques have not been rigorously assessed. The risk of bleeding secondary to FNA of the kidneys is low, but possible, especially when platelet dysfunction is present.

Histopathologic samples can be obtained by percutaneous, ultrasonographically-guided needle biopsy, laparoscopy, or surgical wedge biopsy. Histopathology may confirm a suspected etiology (e.g., ethylene glycol intoxication, renal lymphosarcoma) or it may disclose nonspecific findings. When AKI cannot be distinguished from end-stage CKD clinically, histopathology (particularly Masson's trichrome stain) can aid in assessment of the severity of fibrosis and provide insight into the potential for renal recovery. The risk of significant hemorrhage secondary to percutaneous renal biopsy is high in cats due to the small size of their kidneys. This risk is intensified when uremia is severe and platelet dysfunction in present.[38]

THERAPY

Treatment of AKI is primarily aimed at addressing the underlying cause (if it can be identified and treated) and supportive measures to minimize the clinical sequelae of uremia (Table 50-2). There are no pharmacologic options available that reliably result in improvement of renal excretory and regulatory function. When treatable causes of AKI have been addressed and conventional medical therapy is insufficient for controlling the consequences of uremia, renal replacement therapy (e.g., intermittent hemodialysis, continuous renal replacement therapy, peritoneal dialysis, or renal transplantation) should be considered.

Addressing the Underlying Cause

There are few etiologies of AKI that can be addressed with a specific maneuver that directly results in improved excretory renal function. Fortunately, one of the most common causes of feline AKI, ureteral obstruction, can be addressed surgically or (in select cases) endoscopically. Restoration of ureteral patency can be achieved with the surgical removal of ureteroliths (ureterotomy) or, in cases in which concern for reobstruction exists, the placement of ureteral stents specifically sized for the feline patient. Potential exists, however, for stent encrustation, obstruction, and/or migration. Additionally, in some cases, the presence of a ureteral stricture prevents stent placement. An alternative to ureteral stents is placement of a SC ureteral bypass device.[39] This device consists of a nephrostomy tube and a cystostomy tube, both of which are tunneled SC and connected to a SC port (Figure 50-2). This device allows for aspiration of urine, as well as flushing of the entire device to maintain patency and perform positive contrast radiographic studies.

Traditionally, ureteral obstructions have been addressed surgically, but a recent study describing treatment of AKI with intermittent hemodialysis documented spontaneous resolution of ureteral obstruction in cats supported with hemodialysis alone. In this study, eight of 13 cats with ureteral obstructions that were not treated surgically survived longer than 365 days following hospital discharge.[40] This data is in contrast to a previous study that documented a lower success rate for medical management of cats with ureteral obstruction. The latter study, however, described cats with ureteral obstructions secondary to ureteral calculi, whereas the former study did not differentiate between obstructive disease caused by calculi versus alternative causes (e.g., stricture, spasm, edema, etc.).[41] Based on the results of these two studies, the authors do not recommend withholding surgery from cats with severe AKI secondary to ureteral calculi but consider supportive care (either with conventional methods or with renal replacement therapy) an option when

Table 50-2	Indications, Doses, Adverse Effects, and Comments for Drugs Frequently Used in Cases of Acute Kidney Injury			
Drug	**Indication**	**Dosage**	**Adverse Effects**	**Comments**
Furosemide	Fluid overload, oliguria/anuria, hyperkalemia	2 to 5 mg/kg IV bolus, may be repeated three to five times; 0.5 to 1 mg/kg/hr CRI if urine production increased following bolus	Ototoxicity; volume depletion (unlikely if patient is monitored)	Results are frequently not satisfactory in cases of severe AKI but adverse effects minimal, so use in anuric AKI
Regular insulin	Hyperkalemia	0.5 units/kg IV or IM, may be repeated every 4 to 6 hours, provided hypoglycemia is avoided	Hypoglycemia	Hypokalemic effect modest and transient; IV dextrose must be administered concurrent with and following insulin administration
Dextrose	Hyperkalemia; avoidance of hypoglycemia following insulin administration	IV bolus of 2 g/unit of insulin administered; bolus followed by CRI (the dextrose concentration and administration rate is dependent on serial blood glucose concentrations, patient's fluid status, and accessibility of central line)	Hyperglycemia, hyperosmolarity, hyponatremia, phlebitis with high dextrose concentrations	Dextrose should be diluted to avoid phlebitis; frequent changes in dextrose CRI frequently necessary based on serial blood glucose measurements
Calcium gluconate (10%)	Hyperkalemia; symptomatic hypocalcemia	0.5 to 1.5 mL/kg of 10% solution or 50 to 150 mg/kg IV slowly, to effect, while monitoring ECG; may be repeated	Worsening bradycardia and ECG changes; hypercalcemia; soft tissue mineralization	ECG should be monitored during administration; will not affect extracellular potassium concentration; effective in rapidly normalizing ECG but results transient; administration of large volumes may contribute to soft tissue mineralization
Sodium bicarbonate	Severe acidemia	$\frac{1}{4}$ to $\frac{1}{3}$ of the base deficit over 30 to 60 minutes, followed by an additional $\frac{1}{4}$ over the next 4 to 6 hours; additional dosing based on serial blood gas analyses	Paradoxical central nervous system acidosis, hypernatremia, fluid overload, hypochloremia; may cause or exacerbate hypokalemia if patient is polyuric; may exacerbate hypocalcemia	Requires close monitoring of blood gases and electrolytes for effective treatment and avoidance of adverse effects
Albuterol (inhaled)	Hyperkalemia	Four puffs; 90 microgram actuation via Aerokat device; repeated every 1 to 4 hours as necessary	Tachycardia, tremors, hyperexcitability	Adverse effects are uncommon at this dose; effects observed within 1 to 2 hours but may require multiple doses; effects can be sustained (several hours); only recommended for peracute hyperkalemia
Sodium polystyrene sulfonate	Hyperkalemia	2 g/kg per day PO or via feeding tube, divided into three to four doses per day; dose can be adjusted to effect	Hypernatremia, constipation, colonic necrosis	Rarely used except in chronic dialysis patients

AKI, Acute kidney injury; *CRI,* continuous rate infusion; *ECG,* electrocardiogram; *IM,* intramuscularly; *IV,* intravenously; *PO, per os* (orally).

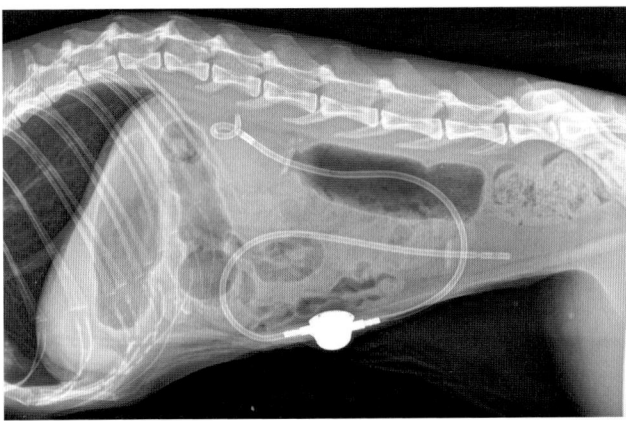

Figure 50-2: This lateral radiograph depicts proper placement of a subcutaneous ureteral bypass device. The locking loop pigtail catheter is secured in the right renal pelvis and the cuffed, fenestrated catheter allows urine drainage through the apex of the bladder. The two catheters are connected by a titanium access port.

ureteral calculi are not documented by radiography or ultrasonography.

Fluid Therapy

The goal of parenteral fluid therapy is to restore (the resuscitative phase) and maintain normal fluid balance among all body compartments. To ensure adequate tissue perfusion, extracellular fluid deficits should be corrected with a balanced polyionic solution. Colloidal support may also be considered to reduce the total amount of fluid administered if oliguria or anuria is suspected to be secondary to severe deficits in renal perfusion, although no benefit over crystalloid therapy has been documented in human or veterinary medicine.[42] Historically, synthetic colloids have been considered to have a volumetric equivalence ratio of 1:4 compared to crystalloids.[43] However, evidence suggests that the true, overall volume-sparing benefit of colloids is far less.[44] Furthermore, evidence compiled in multiple meta-analyses in humans suggests that synthetic colloidal solutions may have a deleterious effect not only on renal function, but overall survival, especially in septic patients.[45,46] For these reasons, it is the authors' opinion that colloids should be used with caution and only be considered in the resuscitative phase of fluid therapy. In the resuscitative phase, goal-directed therapy to restore surrogate markers of perfusion (e.g., blood pressure, venous lactate concentration, venous oxygen saturation) should be employed with endpoints set to be reached within 24 hours. If oliguria or anuria is present and persists despite achievement of normal surrogate markers of perfusion, additional fluid administration should be withheld to avoid fluid overload. Avoidance of fluid overload (typically defined as fluid accumulation greater than 10% of baseline body weight) is essential, because there is ample evidence documenting the association between fluid overload and worse clinical outcomes in both humans[47-50] and, more recently, dogs.[51]

The benefits of a restrictive fluid administration plan are becoming evident not only in AKI, but in a variety of disease states. In humans with AKI, avoidance of fluid overload is associated with a reduced risk of mortality. Furthermore, in disease states frequently encountered concurrently with AKI, such as acute lung injury, a restrictive fluid plan was associated with improved oxygenation parameters and increased numbers of ventilator-free and intensive care unit–free days.[52] In patients undergoing various abdominal surgeries, complications were significantly reduced with restrictive fluid regimens.[53]

Aggressive fluid therapy resulting in volume loading frequently has the effect of decreasing serum or plasma creatinine concentrations. Although historically, aggressive fluid therapy has been lauded as an effective means of diuresing uremic toxins, the relationship between this treatment strategy and effect is more complex. A recent human study demonstrates that changes in serum creatinine concentrations were directly proportional to the degree of fluid accumulation in patients with AKI, suggesting that changes in serum creatinine concentrations are directly related to changes in the volume of distribution of creatinine.[54] Therefore, changes in serum creatinine concentration associated with administration of fluid products beyond that which is necessary to restore normal renal perfusion (when affected by volume deficits) is likely a result of dilution of this creatinine, rather than increased renal excretion.

Maintenance fluid administration (both the volume and composition) should be guided by the volume and composition of urine produced, as well as ongoing sensible losses (e.g., from vomitus, diarrhea, and yield from gastric suction) and insensible loss (e.g., from respiration, formed stools). Many oliguric or anuric patients require no parenteral fluid therapy, because the obligatory fluid load that accompanies such treatments as parenteral or enteral nutrition administration (canned foods are typically composed of 80% to 90% water), IV antibiotics (frequently diluted), and IV catheter flushes sufficiently replace that which is lost from sensible and insensible routes. Insensible losses have been estimated to range between 12 and 29 mL/kg/day[55,56] and are dependent on a variety of factors, such as patient activity level, underlying disease process, and body temperature. Careful attention must be given to serial changes in the patient's body weight, because peracute fluctuations in weight are most likely due to changes in fluid balance rather than changes in lean muscle or fat content. High maintenance fluid rates have been historically advocated for patients producing urine, based on the rationale that high volume fluid administration beyond that which is necessary to restore normal volume status will improve GFR. However, there is no evidence supporting this claim and, in the author's experience, this practice is often futile in restoring GFR and frequently results in fluid overload. Fluid overload with concurrent oliguria or anuria is a clear indication for dialysis.

Monitoring fluid status to avoid volume overload is an ongoing process that must be repeated frequently. Efforts should be made to adhere to objective monitoring parameters (e.g., body weight, venous lactate concentration, urine production) of fluid status, because subjective parameters (e.g., skin turgor, saliva production) are inaccurate and often affected by variables other than hydration status. Body weight should be measured two to six times daily to assess for trends in fluid accumulation or deficit. Central venous pressure measurement has traditionally been recommended as a surrogate marker of cardiac preload and, thus, fluid status. However, a thorough understanding of the limitations of this technique is necessary for appropriate interpretation, because the correlation between central venous pressure and blood volume (as well as the clinical manifestations of fluid overload) is poor.[57,58]

Diuretics

The use of diuretics in the treatment of AKI is a controversial topic in both human and veterinary medicine.[59,60] Many of the benefits of the most commonly used diuretics in veterinary AKI, furosemide and mannitol, have only been theorized or demonstrated in experimental models of AKI. In fact, there is little or no clinical evidence in human or veterinary medicine that diuretics improve outcome in established AKI. It has been postulated that the ability to respond to diuretics is a marker of less severe renal injury associated with a better prognosis. However, an increase in urine output after diuretic administration does not necessarily coincide with an increase in uremic solute excretion and, therefore, does not preclude the need for renal replacement therapy if severe uremia or acid-base and electrolyte abnormalities persist. In veterinary medicine, because renal replacement therapies are not readily available, diuretic administration plays a large role in volume management. Conversion from an oliguric or anuric state to normal urine production or polyuria may enhance the clinician's ability to prevent or manage fluid overload and thus allow administration of necessary medications and nutrition that would otherwise contribute to fluid overload.

No class of diuretics has been proven to be superior to another. However, the use of loop diuretics predominates in both human and veterinary AKI patients due to the relatively high efficacy and safety margin of these drugs, compared to the osmotic diuretics. There are several potential adverse effects associated with the administration of mannitol. Mannitol is typically administered in concentrations ranging from 20% to 25%, which correspond to osmolalities of 1100 to 1373 mOsm/L, and this high osmolality can contribute to fluid overload by promoting water movement from the intracellular to extracellular space. Furthermore, administration of mannitol has been associated with the development of a renal tubular morphologic lesion called *osmotic nephrosis*.[61] This lesion is characterized by swelling and vacuolization of the renal tubules and resultant renal tubular dysfunction and obstruction. Cumulative doses of approximately 200 g/person/day have been associated with this lesion, but when baseline renal function is normal, the toxic dose appears to be significantly higher.[62] When extrapolating a dose of 200 g

for a 70 kg (154 lb) human to that for a 5 kg (11 lb) feline patient, the g/kg cumulative dosage frequently found in many veterinary textbooks (0.25 to 1 g/kg bolus a variable number of times, followed by 1 to 2 mg/kg/min as a constant rate infusion) reaches the human nephrotoxic dose. For these reasons, the author does not recommend the use of mannitol as a diuretic for AKI.

Acid-Base Balance

Metabolic acidosis is a frequent complication in AKI of varying severity and is due to the damaged nephron's inability to excrete hydrogen ions and reabsorb bicarbonate ions, as well as lactic acidosis secondary to compromised tissue perfusion (i.e., either volume deficit or excess). Once perfusion has been restored, provision of supplemental alkali, usually in the form of parenteral sodium bicarbonate, should be considered if severe acidemia (pH less than 7.2; bicarbonate less than 12 mmol/L) persists. The bicarbonate dosage can be calculated from the formula:

$$0.3 \times \text{body weight (kg)} \times \text{base deficit} = \text{bicarbonate (mEq)},$$

where the base deficit = 24 mEq/L − patient bicarbonate concentration.

One-fourth to one-third of the dose is typically given IV as a slow bolus, and an additional one-fourth is typically given over the next 4 to 6 hours. Although the preceding formula provides a framework for estimating appropriate bicarbonate dosing, the osmolality of readily available formulations of bicarbonate must be taken into account when formulating and dosing this drug. For example, the most commonly used concentration of sodium bicarbonate is 8.4% (2000 mOsm/L). The osmole load administered with this formulation is considerable, and volumes necessary to correct acid-base derangements may easily result in hypernatremia. Therefore, an alternative strategy for administration of this medication is dilution with sterile water and IV administration at the desired maintenance parenteral fluid rate (provided the patient is not anuric or severely polyuric). In the authors' experience, this practice allows for gradual (over 24 hours) correction of acidemia and avoidance of rapid administration of a large solute load. In cases of oliguria or anuria, it is difficult to provide supplementary, parenteral alkali without provoking solute and fluid perturbations. In these cases, hemodialysis is indicated to correct acid-base derangements. With this treatment modality, provision of bicarbonate is accomplished by diffusion of the anion across the dialysis membrane, without concurrent administration of a sodium or fluid load.

Whether provided by IV injection or by hemodialysis, administration of bicarbonate to a hypoventilating patient or rapid administration of large loads of bicarbonate can further increase the partial pressure of carbon dioxide and can lead to paradoxical central nervous system acidosis.[63,64] This phenomenon is due to the ability of carbon dioxide to diffuse across the blood-brain barrier, whereas the charged bicarbonate molecule diffuses across this barrier less readily.

Despite the potential benefits, multiple routes, and relative ease of bicarbonate administration, it is important to note that, as with diuretic therapy, there is no evidence in the form of randomized controlled trials supporting supplementation of alkali in human AKI.[65]

Electrolyte Balance

Hyperkalemia can be an immediately life-threatening complication of AKI and is secondary to a decline in renal excretory function. Excitable cells become refractory to repolarization, thus resulting in decreased conduction of both cardiac and neuromuscular tissue. Typical electrocardiographic changes include bradycardia; tall T waves; shortened QT intervals; wide QRS complexes; and small, wide, or absent P waves. However, electrocardiographic abnormalities are variable and difficult to predict based on the degree of hyperkalemia. Concurrent acidemia and hypocalcemia likely potentiate the effect of hyperkalemia on cardiac conduction. Therefore, addressing these abnormalities may mitigate the adverse effects of hyperkalemia. Severe hyperkalemia can lead to a ventricular fibrillation or standstill. There are a variety of pharmacologic treatments available for severe hyperkalemia, but these therapies act to translocate potassium to the intracellular space or increase the resting membrane potential to allow repolarization of excitable cells, rather than enhance excretion of potassium. The efficacy of these treatments is typically modest and transient. Only provision of renal replacement therapy or restoration of native renal excretory function can significantly reduce the potassium burden in fulminant AKI.

Expansion of the extracellular space with a non-potassium containing fluid (e.g., 0.9% sodium chloride) may be sufficient to at least partially correct hyperkalemia. This maneuver should be implemented in cases of suspected volume depletion, but should be used with caution or not at all if a patient is anuric or has volume overload. Despite recent evidence supporting the use of balanced (potassium-containing) crystalloids for the treatment of feline urethral obstruction, this practice is not recommended in the case of intrinsic parenchymal injury (renal azotemia). Drobatz and Cole were unable to demonstrate a difference in the rate of decline of blood potassium concentrations among cats treated with 0.9% sodium chloride and Normosol-R following restoration of urethral patency.[66] Results of this study should not be extrapolated to feline patients with intrinsic AKI, because these patients are not provided with an excretory route for potassium. Therefore, provision of a fluid with potassium of 5 mEq/L is far less effective at diluting the extracellular potassium concentration than a fluid that contains no potassium.

Administration of regular insulin is a common pharmacologic treatment for hyperkalemia. Insulin upregulates synthesis of subunits of the sodium/potassium adenosine triphosphatase (Na^+/K^+-ATPase) pump, recruits the pump to the plasma cell membrane, and activates those pumps already

located in the plasma membrane to stimulate intracellular translocation of potassium.[67] The potassium lowering effect of regular insulin may be observed as early as 15 minutes following administration,[68-70] but the effect is typically modest (decline of 1 to 2 mmol/L) and transient (redosing is frequently necessary within 3 to 4 hours). A potentially catastrophic adverse effect associated with regular insulin administration is hypoglycemia, so dextrose must be administered concurrently with regular insulin. If fluid overload is not present, the administration of a continuous rate infusion of dextrose following the initial bolus is recommended. Frequent assessment of blood glucose concentration is imperative, as dextrose is metabolized more rapidly than insulin, and redosing of dextrose is often required.

Calcium salts are frequently administered IV to increase the threshold potential of polarized cells,[71] thus allowing depolarization at high extracellular potassium concentrations. The membrane stabilizing effects of calcium salts are rapid and dramatic; however, the beneficial effects are even more transient than those of regular insulin. Readministration is typically necessary within 1 hour.[72] The patient should be monitored with an electrocardiogram during administration to identify worsening bradycardia, a shortened QT interval, a widened T wave, or alterations in the ST amplitude. If any of these changes are recognized, the calcium infusion should be discontinued. Calcium gluconate is favored over calcium chloride due to the severe extravasation injuries that can occur with calcium chloride administration. Calcium gluconate can also cause extravasation injuries (albeit less severe), so care must be taken to ensure IV catheter patency prior to administration. Lastly, theoretical concerns regarding promotion of calcium-phosphorus/phosphate precipitation and soft tissue mineralization exist with repeated administration of calcium salts.

The beta-2 agonist drug, albuterol, which is administered by the inhalant route, is frequently used by the authors as a first-line treatment for emergent hyperkalemia, having an effect within 15 to 30 minutes and lasting 2 to 3 hours. Beta-2 agonists exert a hypokalemic effect by activating membrane bound Na^+/K^+-ATPase pumps. Nebulized albuterol, in combination with IV insulin with or without IV calcium gluconate, is considered the treatment of choice in human medicine;[73] and with the development of masks and spacers designed specifically for cats, controlled drug delivery via the inhalant route is possible. The use of inhaled albuterol eliminates many of the adverse effects associated with systemic administration of beta-agonist drugs and experimental studies have demonstrated a large margin of safety[74,75] with doses that have been anecdotally recognized as effective. Inhaled albuterol does not contribute to the volume loading that many other medications entail.

Sodium polystyrene sulfonate is a cation exchange resin that is administered orally through an enteral feeding tube, or by colonic enema, and is the one treatment other than renal replacement therapy that removes potassium from the body. Within the GI lumen, sodium polystyrene sulfonate exchanges sodium ions for potassium ions. Administration via enema or use of formulations containing sorbitol increases the risk of colonic necrosis and perforation in human patients. In cases where hyperkalemia cannot be controlled with the most aggressive therapy (i.e., renal replacement therapy), the use of sodium polystyrene sulfonate can be beneficial, especially in the interdialytic period. A lag period of 1 to 3 days following initiation of therapy should be allowed before the maximum effect of a particular dose can be determined.

Historically, sodium bicarbonate was thought to promote intracellular translocation of potassium via exchange of hydrogen ions. However, recent evidence suggests that the hypokalemic effects of sodium bicarbonate may be a result of the promotion of kaliuresis,[76] and is likely independent of a change in blood pH.[77] Kaliuresis, however, may be difficult to achieve in a patient with injured or compromised function of the majority of nephrons. Nonetheless, correction of acidemia may mitigate the deleterious effects of hyperkalemia on cardiac conduction. Loop diuretics can promote kaliuresis in the distal nephron by promoting tubular flow. Although conversion from an oliguric state to one of increased urine production assists in management of electrolyte excesses (such as hyperkalemia), the authors have treated several patients whose hyperkalemia persisted despite resumption of urine production. Furthermore, loop diuretics are not a reliable means of increasing urine production in cases of anuric AKI. For these reasons, sodium bicarbonate and furosemide are not recommended as stand-alone treatments for emergent hyperkalemic AKI.

Although ionized hypocalcemia occurs frequently in AKI, clinical signs (e.g., tetany) associated with this problem are rare. Ionized calcium concentrations should be assessed and continuously monitored however, regardless of whether supplemental calcium salts are being administered, because ionized calcium concentrations may influence the tendency for cardiac arrhythmias. When manifestations of hypocalcemia (e.g., neurologic complications, arrhythmias) do occur, the minimum dose of supplemental calcium that controls clinical signs should be used to minimize precipitation with phosphorus. As with the treatment of hyperkalemia, the electrocardiogram should be monitored closely during infusion.

Additional electrolyte abnormalities may be present or develop during the course of disease, the most common of which are hyponatremia and hyperphosphatemia. Hyponatremia may be the result of GI or urinary losses, with or without the contribution of decreased excretion of free water. Hyponatremia, if severe (less than 120 mmol/L), may result in neurologic sequelae. In critically ill human patients, hyponatremia has been identified as a poor prognostic indicator.[78,79] However, this association has not been made in cats. Hyponatremia is frequently encountered in the authors' practices and is putatively associated with the profound natriuresis that typically accompanies recovery phase polyuria (especially in cases in which ureteral patency is re-established following an obstruction) or aggressive water supplementation via enteral feeding tubes. This phenomenon has been documented in a cat administered both enteral water via

esophagostomy tube and a cat administered 5% dextrose in water SC.[80] If fluid is being lost in sufficient volumes to require enteral or parenteral replacement, care should be taken to either investigate the electrolyte composition of the lost fluid or to closely monitor the patient's blood electrolyte concentrations so that the appropriate replacement fluid composition is administered.

Hyperphosphatemia contributes to acidosis and renal secondary hyperparathyroidism.[81] However, the use of phosphate-binding drugs has not been shown to improve outcome in human or feline cases of AKI. Furthermore, administration of aluminum hydroxide (the most commonly used phosphate-binding drug in veterinary medicine) may result in acute aluminum intoxication, which manifests as encephalopathy, a condition which may not be readily recognizable in a patient severely affected with AKI.[82] Therefore, aluminum-containing phosphate-binding drugs should be used with caution in AKI. The authors recommend withholding phosphate-binding drugs during the initial phase of diagnostic investigation and therapy and considering administration of these drugs only when the patient's overall status is stable.

Nutritional Support

Nutritional support is an important but often overlooked component of supportive care for AKI. Nutritional support may be precluded by the need to restrict nonessential potassium loading and administration of enteral or parenteral fluids (e.g., anuria). Enteral feeding is the preferred method of nutrient delivery but is often limited by vomiting and ileus. For those patients that are not vomiting, esophageal, gastric, and jejunal feeding devices can be used. If vomiting cannot be controlled, partial or total parenteral nutrition should be considered. Administration of parenteral nutrition can pose difficult challenges in regulating plasma osmolality and electrolyte concentrations. Furthermore, this route of nutritional provision necessitates a dedicated central line and increases the risk of septic complications.[83,84] In patients that are anuric or oliguric, total or partial parenteral nutrition may constitute a relative contraindication unless there is a method of excess fluid and solute removal (e.g., renal replacement therapies).

The optimal dietary composition for veterinary AKI patients has not been determined. The authors are unaware of any particular diet that is appropriate in all scenarios of AKI. Rather, individual patients should be evaluated for the following factors, because each may influence the choice of diet to be fed: the requirement of a liquid diet for tube delivery, the availability of renal replacement to assist in mitigating the obligatory volume load, the electrolyte balance, and the availability of assisted feeding (e.g., esophagostomy or gastrostomy tube). Human guidelines do not support protein restriction for patients with AKI.[85,86] Furthermore, some disease states associated with AKI promote a hypercatabolic state and, therefore, may result in greater protein requirements than the established maintenance requirements.

Patients treated with dialysis may actually require more protein than patients with extra-renal disease, due to loss of amino acids in dialysate/filtrate. Protein restriction for the purpose of restricting the generation of uremic solutes has traditionally been advocated in veterinary medicine. However, a negative protein balance may hinder renal repair/recovery. Therefore, prescription diets marketed for feline patients with CKD may not be appropriate for feline patients with AKI.

Patients that are prone to volume overload and have feeding tubes in place should be fed the most calorically dense diet that will pass through the tube to minimize the amount of fluid administered. Some commercially-available recovery diets have caloric contents of approximately 2 kcal/mL and easily pass through most 14 French feeding tubes. Most other commercial diets (including prescription renal diets) must be diluted and blended with water in order to achieve a consistency that will pass through a feeding tube. Many patients with AKI are hyponatremic due to GI and renal losses; administration of large volumes of hypotonic enteral fluid in the form of a diluted renal diet may exacerbate hyponatremia and cause severe neurologic sequelae. Recovery diets typically have a high protein and potassium content, the latter of which may be problematic in hyperkalemic patients. The same problem exists for most feline prescription renal diets as well.

Based on the complexity associated with choosing a proper commercial diet and ensuring adequate provision of appropriate amounts of minerals, vitamins, and essential amino and fatty acids, as well as the difficulty in formulating and preparing custom home- or hospital-cooked diets, the authors typically administer recovery diets through feeding tubes as a first-line option for nutritional management. Hyperkalemia, if present, is addressed with polystyrene sodium sulfonate and renal replacement therapy, if the latter is available.

Renal Replacement Therapy/Dialysis

Extracorporeal renal replacement therapy (intermittent hemodialysis and continuous renal replacement therapy) is being used with increasing frequency for control of acid-base, electrolyte, and fluid imbalances, as well as the uremic manifestations of AKI. Because details regarding the use of this treatment modality are beyond the scope of this chapter, the reader is referred to publications describing the technical aspects, although a few factors particular to treating cats are mentioned later.[87-90] Extracorporeal renal replacement therapy is the most efficient means of managing uremic, acid-base, electrolyte, and fluid-related sequelae of AKI. In fulminant cases, available pharmacologic therapies are, at best, incompletely effective at reversing the aforementioned complications, and their effects are transient.

One of the greatest determinants of the ease of application of extracorporeal renal replacement therapy is the size and associated blood volume of the patient. Therefore, treatment of the feline patient poses some important problems regarding blood volume regulation and RBC transfusion requirements. First, the size of the extracorporeal circuit determines the amount of blood that must circulate outside of the patient's body during the treatment. The smallest circuits currently used in veterinary medicine are approximately 60 mL. In a typical 5 kg (11 lb) cat with a normal RBC concentration, removal of this volume of RBCs should not contribute greatly to overall cardiovascular instability. However, removal of this volume of blood can be catastrophic in a smaller patient (e.g., 2.5 kg [5.5 lb]) that is anemic. Second, the chemical composition of some of the available hollow fiber membranes affects the tendency for blood to clot or to adhere to the fibers. If a large volume of the patient's blood remains within the fibers following attempts to return blood to the patient at the end of the treatment, significant blood loss accompanies each treatment. For these reasons, the authors recommend that any institution providing extracorporeal renal replacement therapies for cats have access to a plentiful donor RBC supply. Lastly, the extracorporeal circuits must be primed with either a crystalloid, colloid, or blood product prior to treatment. The priming solution represents a volume load obligatory to commencement of treatment. Therefore, ultrafiltration (plasma water removal) of *at least* the extracorporeal circuit must be achieved to maintain a neutral fluid balance throughout the treatment, unless the clinician plans to discard the blood present in the circuit following completion of the treatment. Ultrafiltration of any volume of plasma water may be difficult in patients that are hemodynamically unstable.

Additional Treatment Considerations

Antiemetic therapy is recommended for all patients with severe AKI, regardless of whether they are vomiting. It is beyond the scope of this chapter to discuss antiemetic options in detail, but the authors prefer the use of 5-HT3 antagonists or neurokinin-1 antagonists, because the former was found to be superior to metoclopramide in prevention of vomiting and nausea in uremic human patients.[91]

The use of antisecretory drugs (e.g., histamine-2 (H2) receptor antagonists, proton pump inhibitors) has historically been recommended for patients with AKI. Although uremic gastritis and stress-related mucosal disease are concerns in human AKI patients, gastric acid output and intragastric pH are not compatible with a hypersecretory state.[92] Nonetheless, due to the high incidence of hemorrhage from the GI tract in human AKI patients (presumably related to a combination of uremic injury and stress-related mucosal disease) and its association with mortality,[93] antisecretory drugs should be considered in high-risk patients. A recent meta-analysis showed superiority of proton pump inhibitors versus H2 receptor antagonists in the prevention of stress-related mucosal bleeding.[94] These results, in combination with the potential for accumulation of H2 receptor antagonists in patients with diminished renal function, favor the use of proton pump inhibitors. Sucralfate is frequently used for gastroprotection, but human data shows that even short-term administration of this drug to patients with AKI can result in toxic aluminum concentrations.[95,96]

Dopamine is a pharmacologic treatment for AKI that has fallen out of favor with both human and veterinary nephrologists. Dopamine was initially advocated for its perceived augmentation of renal blood flow. Its benefit in cats, however, was doubted as it was originally thought that cats did not possess renal dopamine receptors, a concept supported by the absence of changes in urine output, sodium excretion, or GFR in cats administered a low-dose dopamine infusion.[97] However, a putative dopamine receptor (DA-1) has been identified in the feline renal cortex.[98] Regardless of this recent discovery, the evidence available assessing the effect of dopamine on the feline kidney, when infused via the IV and intra-arterial routes, suggests that an increase in renal blood flow is not due to the renal effects of dopamine, but rather to the systemic cardiovascular effects.[99] Furthermore, the observed increase in urine flow is likely due to a combination of these systemic effects and an alteration in renal tubular function.[99] Fenoldopam is a drug that has received recent interest as a pharmacologic treatment option for feline AKI, because the feline DA-1 receptors show higher affinity for this drug versus dopamine.[98] Although a prolonged infusion of fenoldopam increased creatinine clearance and urine output in healthy cats,[100] the authors are unaware of any evidence of efficacy in conversion from an oliguric or anuric state in clinical cases of feline AKI. The authors do not recommend this drug as a first-line treatment, because the expense, undetermined efficacy, and unknown pharmacokinetic properties in feline AKI are major drawbacks to its use.

PROGNOSIS

There is sparse information available regarding the prognosis for feline AKI. One study of 32 cats documented a 53% survival rate, with approximately 50% of survivors left with CKD, although obstructive etiologies of AKI were excluded from analysis.[101] Another study assessed survival in cats with AKI treated with intermittent hemodialysis, documenting a 50% survival rate at the time of discharge, a 48% survival rate at 30 days following discharge, and a 38% survival rate at 365 days following discharge.[40] Considering that patients treated with dialysis are more likely to have a greater severity of renal dysfunction and more complications associated with AKI, it can be deduced that dialysis offers a survival benefit in these cases.

References

1. Payen D, Legrand M: Can we identify prerenal physiology and does it matter? *Contrib Nephrol* 174:22–32, 2011.
2. Uchino S, Bellomo R, Bagshaw SM, et al: Transient azotaemia is associated with a high risk of death in hospitalized patients. *Nephrol Dial Transplant* 25:1833–1839, 2010.
3. Capelouto CC, Saltzman B: The pathophysiology of ureteral obstruction. *J Endourol* 7:93–103, 1993.
4. Kochin EJ, Gregory CR, Wisner ER, et al: Evaluation of a method of ureteroneocystostomy in cats. *J Am Vet Med Assoc* 202:257–260, 1993.
5. Mathews K: Ureters. In Tobias KM, Johnston SA, editors: *Veterinary surgery small animal*, ed 1, Philadelphia, 2012, Saunders, pp 1962–1977.
6. Kyles AE, Hardie EM, Wooden BG, et al: Clinical, clinicopathologic, radiographic, and ultrasonographic abnormalities in cats with ureteral calculi: 163 cases (1984-2002). *J Am Vet Med Assoc* 226:932–936, 2005.
7. Westropp JL, Ruby AL, Bailiff NL, et al: Dried solidified blood calculi in the urinary tract of cats. *J Vet Intern Med* 20:828–834, 2006.
8. Zaid MS, Berent AC, Weisse C, et al: Feline ureteral strictures: 10 cases (2007-2009). *J Vet Intern Med* 25:222–229, 2011.
9. Steinhaus J, Berent A, Weiss C, et al: Circumcaval ureters in twenty-one cats. *J Vet Intern Med* 27:731, 2013.
10. Vaughan ED, Jr, Marion D, Poppas DP, et al: Pathophysiology of unilateral ureteral obstruction: studies from Charlottesville to New York. *J Urol* 172:2563–2569, 2004.
11. Rumbeiha WK, Francis JA, Fitzgerald SD, et al: A comprehensive study of Easter lily poisoning in cats. *J Vet Diagn Invest* 16:527–541, 2004.
12. Langston CE: Acute renal failure caused by lily ingestion in six cats. *J Am Vet Med Assoc* 220:49–52, 2002.
13. Hall JO: Nephrotoxicity of Easter lily (*Lilium longiflorum*) when ingested by the cat. *J Vet Intern Med* 6:121, 1992. (Abstract).
14. Bennett AJ, Reineke EL: Outcome following gastrointestinal tract decontamination and intravenous fluid diuresis in cats with known lily ingestion: 25 cases (2001-2010). *J Am Vet Med Assoc* 242:1110–1116, 2013.
15. Slater MR, Gwaltney-Brant S: Exposure circumstances and outcomes of 48 households with 57 cats exposed to toxic lily species. *J Am Anim Hosp Assoc* 47:386–390, 2011.
16. D'Anjou MA, Bedard A, Dunn ME: Clinical significance of renal pelvic dilatation on ultrasound in dogs and cats. *Vet Radiol Ultrasound* 52:88–94, 2011.
17. Kelly DF, Lucke VM, McCullagh KG: Experimental pyelonephritis in the cat. 1. Gross and histological changes. *J Comp Pathol* 89:125–139, 1979.
18. Rollino C, Beltrame G, Ferro M, et al: Acute pyelonephritis in adults: a case series of 223 patients. *Nephrol Dial Transplant* 27:3488–3493, 2012.
19. Arbour J, Blais MC, Carioto L, et al: Clinical leptospirosis in three cats (2001-2009). *J Am Anim Hosp Assoc* 48:256–260, 2012.
20. Lapointe C, Plamondon I, Dunn M: Feline leptospirosis serosurvey from a Quebec referral hospital. *Can Vet J* 54:497–499, 2013.
21. Markovich JE, Ross L, McCobb E: The prevalence of leptospiral antibodies in free roaming cats in Worcester County, Massachusetts. *J Vet Intern Med* 26:688–689, 2012.
22. Hartmann K, Egberink H, Pennisi MG, et al: Leptospira species infection in cats: ABCD guidelines on prevention and management. *J Feline Med Surg* 15:576–581, 2013.
23. Bellomo R, Ronco C, Kellum JA, et al: Acute renal failure—definition, outcome measures, animal models, fluid therapy and information technology needs: the Second International Consensus Conference of the Acute Dialysis Quality Initiative (ADQI) Group. *Crit Care* 8:R204–R212, 2004.
24. Mehta RL, Kellum JA, Shah SV, et al: Acute Kidney Injury Network: report of an initiative to improve outcomes in acute kidney injury. *Crit Care* 11:R31, 2007.
25. Cowgill LD, Langston CE: Acute kidney disease. In Bartges JW, Polzin DJ, editors: *Nephrology and urology of small animals*, Ames, IA, 2011, Wiley-Blackwell, pp 472–523.
26. Sowers KM, Hayden MR: Calcific uremic arteriolopathy: pathophysiology, reactive

oxygen species and therapeutic approaches. *Oxid Med Cell Longev* 3:109–121, 2010.

27. Antoniades DZ, Markopoulos AK, Andreadis D, et al: Ulcerative uremic stomatitis associated with untreated chronic renal failure: report of a case and review of the literature. *Oral Surg Oral Med Oral Pathol Oral Radiol Endod* 101:608–613, 2006.

28. Ash SR: An explanation for uremic hypothermia. *Int J Artif Organs* 14:67–69, 1991.

29. Rotblatt MD, Koda-Kimble MA: Review of drug interference with urine glucose tests. *Diabetes Care* 10:103–110, 1987.

30. Rees CA, Boothe DM: Evaluation of the effect of cephalexin and enrofloxacin on clinical laboratory measurements of urine glucose in dogs. *J Am Vet Med Assoc* 224:1455–1458, 2004.

31. Syme HM: Proteinuria in cats. Prognostic marker or mediator? *J Feline Med Surg* 11:211–218, 2009.

32. Perazella MA, Markowitz GS: Drug-induced acute interstitial nephritis. *Nat Rev Nephrol* 6:461–470, 2010.

33. Sturgess C, Hesford A, Owen H, et al: An investigation into the effects of storage on the diagnosis of crystalluria in cats. *J Feline Med Surg* 3:81–85, 2001.

34. Holloway A, O'Brien R: Perirenal effusion in dogs and cats with acute renal failure. *Vet Radiol Ultrasound* 48:574–579, 2007.

35. Valdes-Martinez A, Cianciolo R, Mai W: Association between renal hypoechoic subcapsular thickening and lymphosarcoma in cats. *Vet Radiol Ultrasound* 48:357–360, 2007.

36. Biery DN: Upper urinary tract. In O'Brien TR, editor: *Radiographic diagnosis of abdominal disorders in dogs and cats*, Davis, 1981, Covell Park Vet, pp 481–542.

37. Adin CA, Herrgesell EJ, Nyland TG, et al: Antegrade pyelography for suspected ureteral obstruction in cats: 11 cases (1995-2001). *J Am Vet Med Assoc* 222:1576–1581, 2003.

38. Vaden SL, Levine JF, Lees GE, et al: Renal biopsy: a retrospective study of methods and complications in 283 dogs and 65 cats. *J Vet Intern Med* 19:794–801, 2005.

39. Berent A, Weisse C, Wright M, et al: The use of a subcutaneous ureteral bypass device for ureteral obstructions in cats. *Vet Surg* 39:E30, 2010.

40. Eatroff AE, Langston CE, Chalhoub S, et al: Long-term outcome of cats and dogs with acute kidney injury treated with intermittent hemodialysis: 135 cases (1997-2010). *J Am Vet Med Assoc* 241:1471–1478, 2012.

41. Kyles AE, Hardie EM, Wooden BG, et al: Management and outcome of cats with ureteral calculi: 153 cases (1984-2002). *J Am Vet Med Assoc* 226:937–944, 2005.

42. Finfer S, Bellomo R, Boyce N, et al: A comparison of albumin and saline for fluid resuscitation in the intensive care unit. *N Engl J Med* 350:2247–2256, 2004.

43. Hughes D, Boag A: Fluid therapy with macromolecular plasma volume expanders. In Dibartola S, editor: *Fluid, electrolyte, and acid-base disorders in small animal practice*, ed 4, St Louis, 2012, Elsevier, pp 647–664.

44. Hartog CS, Bauer M, Reinhart K: The efficacy and safety of colloid resuscitation in the critically ill. *Anesth Analg* 112:156–164, 2011.

45. Zarychanski R, Abou-Setta AM, Turgeon AF, et al: Association of hydroxyethyl starch administration with mortality and acute kidney injury in critically ill patients requiring volume resuscitation: a systematic review and meta-analysis. *JAMA* 309:678–688, 2013.

46. Serpa Neto A, Veelo DP, Peireira VG, et al: Fluid resuscitation with hydroxyethyl starches in patients with sepsis is associated with an increased incidence of acute kidney injury and use of renal replacement therapy: a systematic review and meta-analysis of the literature. *J Crit Care* 29(1):185.e1–7, 2013.

47. Modem V, Thompson M, Gollhofer D, et al: Timing of continuous renal replacement therapy and mortality in critically ill children. *Crit Care Med* 42(4):943–953, 2014.

48. Sutherland SM, Zappitelli M, Alexander SR, et al: Fluid overload and mortality in children receiving continuous renal replacement therapy: the prospective pediatric continuous renal replacement therapy registry. *Am J Kidney Dis* 55:316–325, 2010.

49. Bouchard J, Soroko SB, Chertow GM, et al: Fluid accumulation, survival and recovery of kidney function in critically ill patients with acute kidney injury. *Kidney Int* 76:422–427, 2009.

50. Heung M, Wolfgram DF, Kommareddi M, et al: Fluid overload at initiation of renal replacement therapy is associated with lack of renal recovery in patients with acute kidney injury. *Nephrol Dial Transplant* 27:956–961, 2012.

51. Mobley A, Sullivan L: Retrospective determination of fluid overload in critically ill dogs. *J Vet Emerg Crit Care* 22:2012.

52. Wiedemann HP, Wheeler AP, Bernard GR, et al: Comparison of two fluid-management strategies in acute lung injury. *N Engl J Med* 354:2564–2575, 2006.

53. Bundgaard-Nielsen M, Secher NH, Kehlet H: "Liberal" vs. "restrictive" perioperative fluid therapy—a critical assessment of the evidence. *Acta Anaesthesiol Scand* 53:843–851, 2009.

54. Macedo E, Bouchard J, Soroko SH, et al: Fluid accumulation, recognition and staging of acute kidney injury in critically-ill patients. *J Crit Care* 14:R82, 2010.

55. Hamlin R, Tashjian R: Water and electrolyte intake and output of feces in healthy cats. *Vet Med Small Anim Clin* 59:746, 1964.

56. Thrall B, Miller L: Water turnover in cats fed dry rations. *Feline Pract* 6:10, 1976.

57. Marik P, Barram M, Vahid B: Does central venous pressure predict fluid responsiveness? A systemic review of the literature and the tale of seven mares. *Chest* 134:172–178, 2008.

58. Reems MM, Aumann M: Central venous pressure: principles, measurement, and interpretation. *Compend Contin Educ Vet* 34:E1, 2012.

59. Bagshaw SM, Bellomo R, Kellum JA: Oliguria, volume overload, and loop diuretics. *Crit Care Med* 36:S172–S178, 2008.

60. Bagshaw SM, Delaney A, Haase M, et al: Loop diuretics in the management of acute renal failure: a systematic review and meta-analysis. *Crit Care Resusc* 9:60–68, 2007.

61. Dickenmann M, Oettl T, Mihatsch MJ: Osmotic nephrosis: acute kidney injury with accumulation of proximal tubular lysosomes due to administration of exogenous solutes. *Am J Kidney Dis* 51:491–503, 2008.

62. Dorman HR, Sondheimer JH, Cadnapaphornchai P: Mannitol-induced acute renal failure. *Medicine (Baltimore)* 69:153–159, 1990.

63. Kindig NB, Sherrill DS, Shapiro JI, et al: Extracorporeal bicarbonate space after bicarbonate or a bicarbonate-carbonate mixture in acidotic dogs. *J Appl Physiol (1985)* 67:2331–2334, 1989.

64. Shapiro JI, Whalen M, Kucera R, et al: Brain pH responses to sodium bicarbonate and Carbicarb during systemic acidosis. *Am J Physiol* 256:H1316–H1321, 1989.

65. Hewitt J, Uniacke M, Hansi NK, et al: Sodium bicarbonate supplements for treating acute kidney injury. *Cochrane Database Syst Rev* (6):CD009204, 2012.

66. Drobatz K, Cole S: The influence of crystalloid type on acid-base and electrolyte status of cats with urethral obstruction. *J Vet Emerg Crit Care* 18:355–361, 2008.

67. Sweeney G, Klip A: Regulation of the Na$^+$/K$^+$-ATPase by insulin: why and how? *Mol Cell Biochem* 182:121–133, 1998.

68. Li Q, Zhou MT, Wang Y, et al: Effect of insulin on hyperkalemia during anhepatic stage of liver transplantation. *World J Gastroenterol* 10:2427–2429, 2004.

69. Allon M, Copkney C: Albuterol and insulin for treatment of hyperkalemia in hemodialysis patients. *Kidney Int* 38:869–872, 1990.

70. Allon M, Shanklin N: Effect of bicarbonate administration on plasma potassium in dialysis patients: interactions with insulin and albuterol. *Am J Kidney Dis* 28:508–514, 1996.

71. Bisogno JL, Langley A, Von Dreele MM: Effect of calcium to reverse the electrocardiographic effects of hyperkalemia in the isolated rat heart: a prospective, dose-response study. *Crit Care Med* 22:697–704, 1994.

72. Weisberg LS: Management of severe hyperkalemia. *Crit Care Med* 36:3246–3251, 2008.

73. Mahoney BA, Smith WA, Lo DS, et al: Emergency interventions for hyperkalemia. *Cochrane Database Syst Rev* (2):CD003235, 2005.

74. Leemans J, Kirschvink N, Bernaerts F, et al: A pilot study comparing the antispasmodic effects of inhaled salmeterol, salbutamol and ipratropium bromide using different aerosol devices on muscarinic bronchoconstriction in healthy cats. *Vet J* 180:236–245, 2009.

75. Reinero CR, Delgado C, Spinka C, et al: Enantiomer-specific effects of albuterol on airway inflammation in healthy and asthmatic cats. *Int Arch Allergy Immunol* 150:43–50, 2009.

76. Carlisle EJ, Donnelly SM, Ethier JH, et al: Modulation of the secretion of potassium by

accompanying anions in humans. *Kidney Int* 39:1206–1212, 1991.

77. Fraley DS, Adler S: Correction of hyperkalemia by bicarbonate despite constant blood pH. *Kidney Int* 12:354–360, 1977.

78. Funk GC, Lindner G, Druml W, et al: Incidence and prognosis of dysnatremias present on ICU admission. *Intensive Care Med* 36:304–311, 2010.

79. Stelfox HT, Ahmed SB, Khandwala F, et al: The epidemiology of intensive care unit-acquired hyponatraemia and hypernatraemia in medical-surgical intensive care units. *Crit Care* 12:R162, 2008.

80. Lee JY, Rozanski E, Anastasio M, et al: Iatrogenic water intoxication in two cats. *J Vet Emerg Crit Care* 23:53–57, 2013.

81. Druml W, Schwarzenhofer M, Apsner R, et al: Fat soluble vitamins in patients with acute renal failure. *Miner Electrolyte Metab* 24:220–226, 1998.

82. Segev G, Bandt C, Francey T, et al: Aluminum toxicity following administration of aluminum-based phosphate binders in two dogs with renal failure. *J Vet Intern Med* 22:1432–1435, 2008.

83. Wylie MC, Graham DA, Potter-Bynoe G, et al: Risk factors for central line-associated bloodstream infection in pediatric intensive care units. *Infect Control Hosp Epidemiol* 31:1049–1056, 2010.

84. Peter JV, Moran JL, Phillips-Hughes J: A metaanalysis of treatment outcomes of early enteral versus early parenteral nutrition in hospitalized patients. *Crit Care Med* 33:213–220, discussion 260–261, 2005.

85. Fiaccadori E, Cremaschi E: Nutritional assessment and support in acute kidney injury. *Curr Opin Crit Care* 15:474–480, 2009.

86. Gervasio JM, Garmon WP, Holowatyj M: Nutrition support in acute kidney injury. *Nutr Clin Pract* 26:374–381, 2011.

87. Langston C: Hemodialysis. In Bartges J, Polzin D, editors: *Nephrology and urology of small animals*, Ames, IA, 2011, Blackwell, pp 354–400.

88. Bloom CA, Labato MA: Intermittent hemodialysis for small animals. *Vet Clin North Am Small Anim Pract* 41:115–133, 2011.

89. Acierno MJ: Continuous renal replacement therapy. In Bartges JW, Polzin DJ, editors: *Nephrology and urology of small animals*, Ames, IA, 2011, Wiley-Blackwell, pp 286–292.

90. Acierno MJ: Continuous renal replacement therapy in dogs and cats. *Vet Clin North Am Small Anim Pract* 41:135–146, 2011.

91. Ljutic D, Perkovic D, Rumboldt Z, et al: Comparison of ondansetron with metoclopramide in the symptomatic relief of uremia-induced nausea and vomiting. *Kidney Blood Press Res* 25:61–64, 2002.

92. Wesdorp RI, Falcao HA, Banks PB, et al: Gastrin and gastric acid secretion in renal failure. *Am J Surg* 141:334–338, 1981.

93. Fiaccadori E, Maggiore U, Clima B, et al: Incidence, risk factors, and prognosis of gastrointestinal hemorrhage complicating acute renal failure. *Kidney Int* 59:1510–1519, 2001.

94. Barkun AN, Bardou M, Pham CQ, et al: Proton pump inhibitors vs. histamine 2 receptor antagonists for stress-related mucosal bleeding prophylaxis in critically ill patients: a meta-analysis. *Am J Gastroenterol* 107:507–520, quiz 521, 2012.

95. Thorburn K, Samuel M, Smith EA, et al: Aluminum accumulation in critically ill children on sucralfate therapy. *Pediatr Crit Care Med* 2:247–249, 2001.

96. Mulla H, Peek G, Upton D, et al: Plasma aluminum levels during sucralfate prophylaxis for stress ulceration in critically ill patients on continuous venovenous hemofiltraiton: a randomized, controlled trial. *Crit Care Med* 29:267–271, 2001.

97. Wohl JS, Schwartz DD, Flournoy WS, et al: Renal hemodynamic and diuretic effects of low-dose dopamine in the cat. *Seventh International Veterinary Emergency and Critical Care Symposium* 14–24, 2000.

98. Flournoy WS, Wohl JS, Albrecht-Schmitt TJ, et al: Pharmacologic identification of putative D1 dopamine receptors in feline kidneys. *J Vet Pharmacol Ther* 26:283–290, 2003.

99. Wassermann K, Huss R, Kullmann R: Dopamine-induced diuresis in the cat without changes in renal hemodynamics. *Naunyn Schmiedebergs Arch Pharmacol* 312:77–83, 1980.

100. Simmons JP, Wohl JS, Schwartz DD, et al: Diuretic effects of fenoldopam in healthy cats. *J Vet Emerg Crit Care* 16:96–103, 2006.

101. Worwag S, Langston CE: Acute intrinsic renal failure in cats: 32 cats (1997-2004). *J Am Vet Med Assoc* 232:728–732, 2008.

Update on Feline Urolithiasis

Amanda Callens and Joseph W. Bartges

ETIOPATHOGENESIS

Urolithiasis refers to the condition of uroliths (stones) located anywhere in the urinary system. Urolith formation is not a specific disease but results from underlying disorders that promote precipitation of minerals in urine. These factors include genetic, environmental, and nutritional influences. Urolith formation, dissolution, and prevention involve complex physiochemical processes. Major factors include: (1) urine supersaturation resulting in crystal formation (nucleation); (2) the effect of inhibitors of mineral nucleation, crystal aggregation, and crystal growth; (3) crystalloid complexors; (4) effects of promoters of crystal aggregation and growth; (5) effects of noncrystalline matrix; and (6) sufficient urine retention time or slowed transit for the process to occur.[1] Urolith formation begins with microscopic crystalluria, and if conditions are favorable, microscopic crystals aggregate to form uroliths.

The important driving force behind urolith formation is supersaturation of urine with calculogenic substances. The initial phase of urolith formation involves an increase in supersaturation of the urine followed by precipitation of calculogenic substances. The initial phase is called *nucleation* and involves the formation of a crystalline nidus. Growth of this nidus depends on the ability of the crystal to remain in the urine, urine pH, duration of urine supersaturation, and presence of other risk factors, such as infection.[2]

Uroliths may pass through the urinary tract without intervention, spontaneously dissolve depending on composition, grow in size and/or number, or become inactive. Urolith behavior and repercussions associated with urolithiasis will often determine the action needed for diagnostics or treatment.

LOCATION OF UROLITHS AND CLINICAL SIGNS

Cystoliths and Urethroliths

Feline lower urinary tract disease has many causes, including crystal-related disease. There are many minerals that may precipitate to form uroliths, but more than 80% of uroliths in cats are caused by magnesium ammonium phosphate (struvite) or calcium oxalate monohydrate or dihydrate.[3] Urethral plugs occur only in male cats. They occur in approximately 20% of male cats with lower urinary tract obstruction.[4] These plugs contain at least 45% matrix and variable amounts of mineral. The most common mineral type found in urethral plugs is magnesium ammonium phosphate (struvite). Matrix components include mucoproteins, serum proteins, cellular debris, and viral particles. In male cats, urethral crystalline matrix plugs may represent an intermediate phase between inflammatory disease of the lower urinary tract and urolith formation.[5]

Clinical signs of lower urinary tract uroliths include dysuria, inappropriate urination, pollakiuria, and hematuria. Presence of cystoliths may be unassociated with clinical signs. Urethral obstruction may occur; the predominant clinical sign is stranguria without the passing of urine. Total obstruction is often preceded by pollakiuria, vocalization during urination, inappropriate urination, and hematuria. In severe and prolonged cases, cats can become uremic, and signs, such as extreme lethargy and vomiting, can occur. Diagnosis of urethral obstruction includes a history of stranguria without urine passage and palpation of a large, firm urinary bladder. Care must be taken in palpating these patients because the urinary bladder may have been distended for a long period of time, and palpation may result in bladder tear or rupture and uroabdomen.

Nephrolithiasis and Ureterolithiasis

Upper urinary tract uroliths account for a small percentage of uroliths in cats. These stones may be found incidentally on radiographs taken for other reasons because they are frequently not associated with clinical signs. Clinical signs when present include vomiting, anorexia, lethargy, and hematuria; occasionally nonlocalizing pain is found on abdominal palpation.[6] A large kidney may be palpated due to hydronephrosis secondary to ureteral obstruction.

Biochemical abnormalities associated with upper urinary tract stones include hyperkalemia, hypercalcemia, hyperphosphatemia, anemia, azotemia, and leukocytosis.[6] On urinalysis, hematuria, pyuria, proteinuria, and crystalluria may be noted. Urine culture and sensitivity testing are imperative because an estimated one-third of cats with upper urinary tract stones have a concurrent urinary tract infection (UTI).[7]

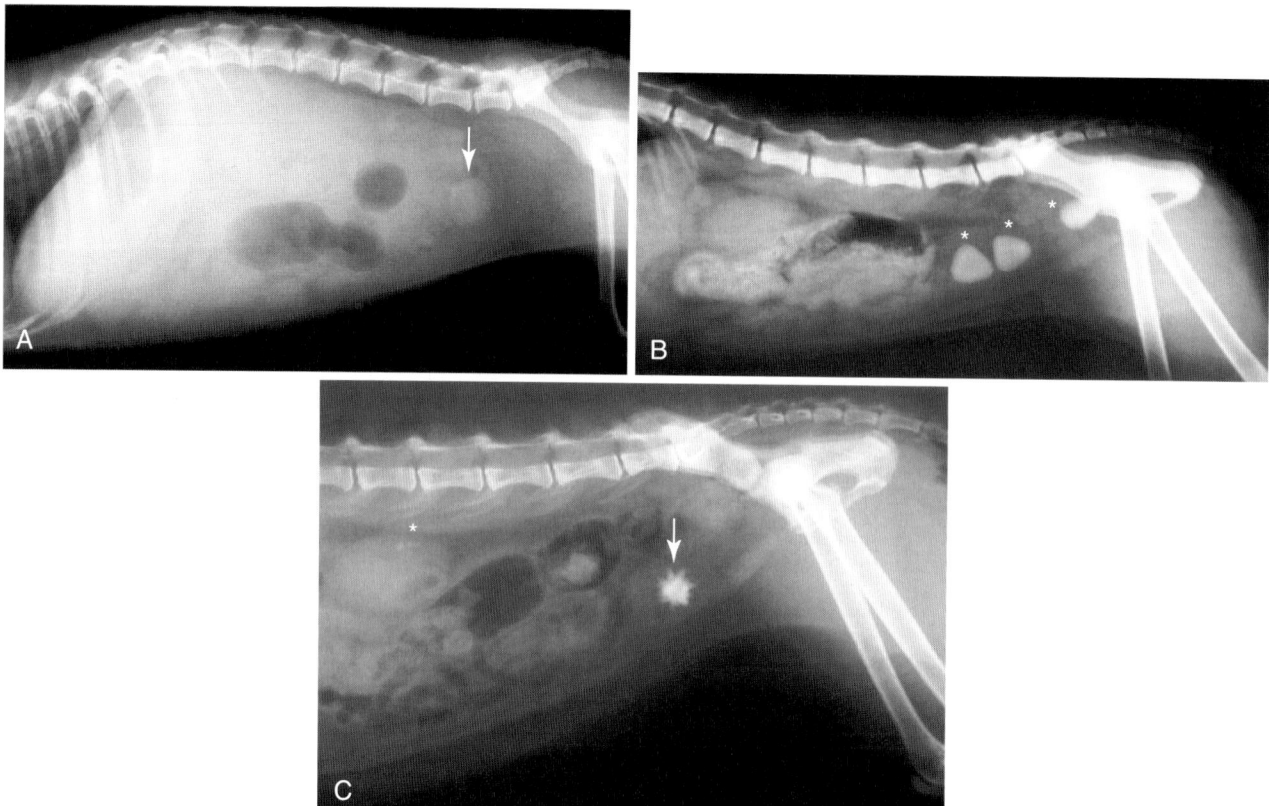

Figure 51-1: Radiographical Appearance of Struvite and Calcium Oxalate Uroliths. A, Lateral abdominal radiograph of a 4-year-old, castrated, male, domestic shorthair cat showing a single round radiopaque sterile struvite urocystolith (*white arrow*). **B,** Lateral abdominal radiograph of a 16-week-old, female, domestic shorthair cat showing three radiopaque infection-induced struvite urocystoliths; two are pyramidal shaped, and one is oblong (*asterisks*). **C,** Lateral abdominal radiograph of an 8-year-old, castrated, male, domestic shorthair cat showing one calcium oxalate dehydrate urocystolith (*arrow*). Renal mineralization is also present (*asterisk*).

DIAGNOSIS OF UROLITHS

Imaging is the most definitive diagnostic tool for detection of uroliths. Abdominal radiography is generally the first diagnostic imaging modality used to detect radiopaque uroliths (Figure 51-1). Ultrasonography can be used to detect uroliths, including those that are radiolucent (Figure 51-2); however, it is less useful in determining mineral content, quantitating uroliths, and identifying location of uroliths.[8] With double-contrast cystography (Figure 51-3) the bladder is distended with air and a small amount of positive contrast medium is injected into the bladder through a urethral catheter to form a puddle. Then the patient is rotated to coat the bladder mucosa so that uroliths can be visualized as radiolucent filling defects in the positive contrast puddle.[9] These abdominal imaging techniques are used to verify the presence of uroliths and location, number, size, shape, and density.

In patients with suspected urinary tract disorders, urinalysis is an important part of diagnostic evaluation. Crystalluria can be an important finding (Figure 51-4). Crystals do not confirm the presence of uroliths, but they do suggest crystalline oversaturation.[3] Temperature change due to elapsed time between urine collection and urinalysis can cause crystals to form in urine, resulting in a false-positive crystalluria.[10] Therefore, in patients with suspected urolithiasis, freshly collected urine should be evaluated.[11]

Urine specific gravity and pH can help assess the chemical environment in the urinary bladder. The chemical environment of the urine determines urolith formation and can suggest which type of urolith is present. A high urine specific gravity suggests an increase in concentration of calculi precursors.[1] Calcium oxalate, purines, and cystine uroliths form typically in urine with a pH less than 7.0, whereas struvite calculi form typically in urine with a pH greater than 7.0.[11]

Urine culture and sensitivity testing is indicated because UTIs may occur secondarily in patients with urolithiasis.[12] Factors contributing to this include mucosal damage induced by the stones, incomplete urine voiding, or microorganism entrapment in the stone.

When uroliths are found, it is important to obtain a blood biochemical profile. Blood biochemical results can sometimes suggest presence of underlying diseases, such as hypercalcemia, that can predispose patients to urolith formation.[13] Because calculi occasionally cause obstruction, electrolyte, mineral, creatinine, and blood urea nitrogen concentrations should be monitored. Urate calculi may be caused by underlying liver disease, particularly congenital vascular anomalies;

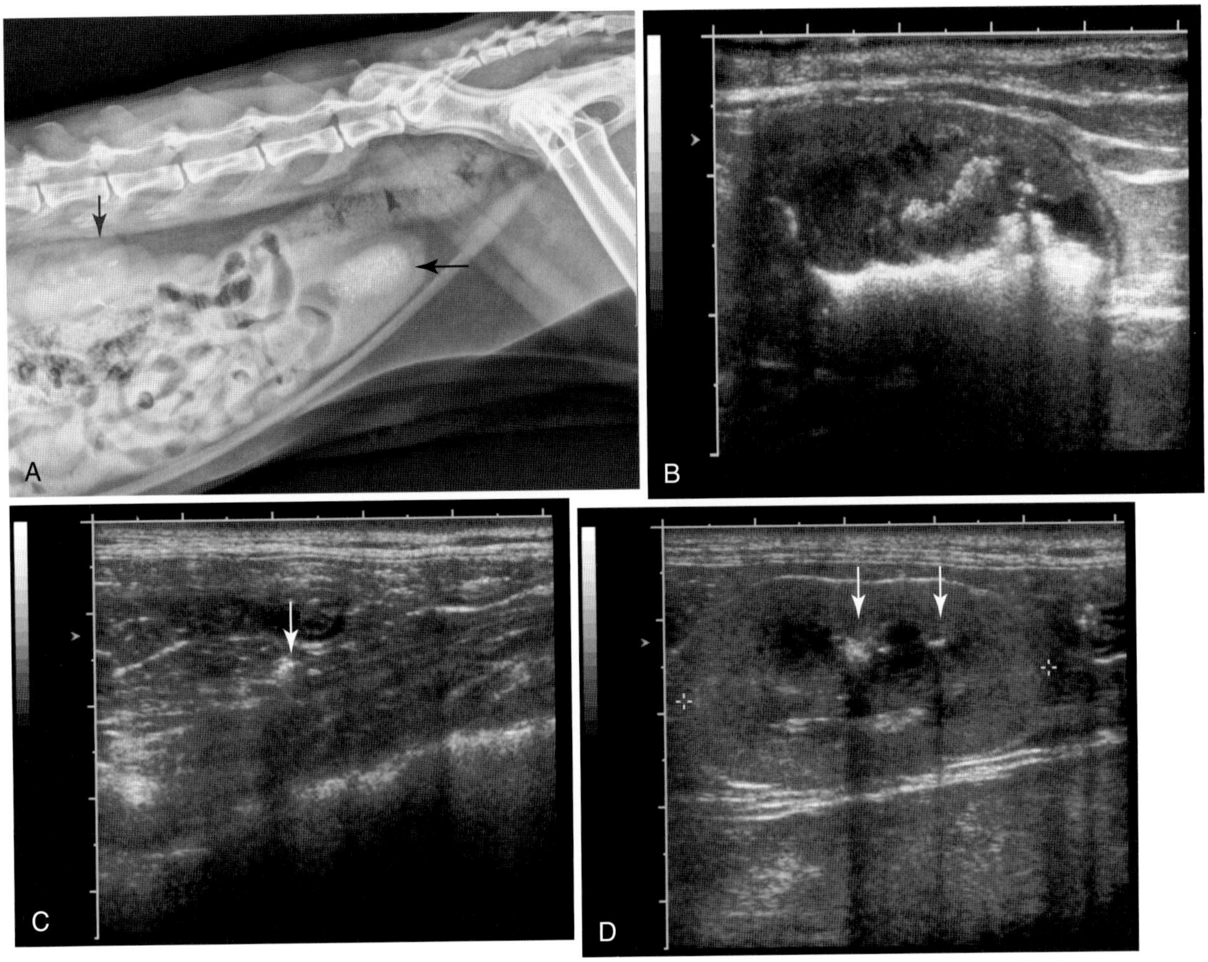

Figure 51-2: Images from a 14-Year-Old, Castrated, Male, Domestic Shorthair Cat with Urolithiasis. A, Nephroureteroliths (*red arrow*) and urocystoliths (*black arrow*) on lateral abdominal radiograph. **B,** Urocystoliths appear as shadowing hyperechoic objects on ultrasonographic image of the urinary bladder. **C,** Ureterolith (*white arrow*) in left proximal ureter. **D,** Nephroliths (*white arrows*) in left kidney on ultrasonographic image.

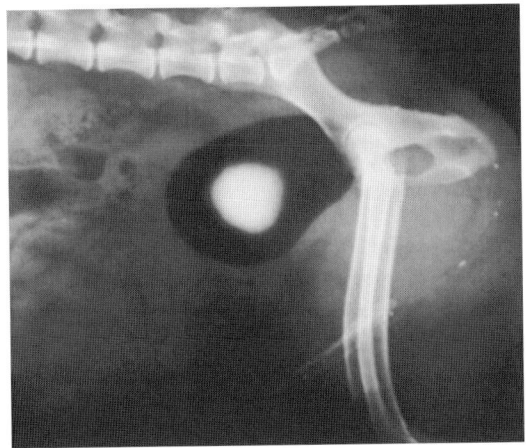

Figure 51-3: Double Contrast Cystogram.

therefore, hepatic function should be determined in patients with suspected or confirmed urate uroliths.

DESCRIPTION OF UROLITHS

Determining the composition of uroliths is essential to prevent recurrence. Although many types of uroliths have a characteristic appearance, guessing composition by appearance is unreliable and subject to error.[14] All removed or voided uroliths should be analyzed to determine mineral composition, which aids in developing a successful treatment and prevention plan. Analysis results report the chemical makeup of the different components of the urolith. In cases of recurrence, uroliths should be resubmitted because mineral composition can change from one episode to another.[14]

A urolith is composed primarily of one or more minerals in combination with small quantities of organic matrix. The composition of uroliths may be mixed with uneven mixtures of minerals throughout the stone or minerals deposited in

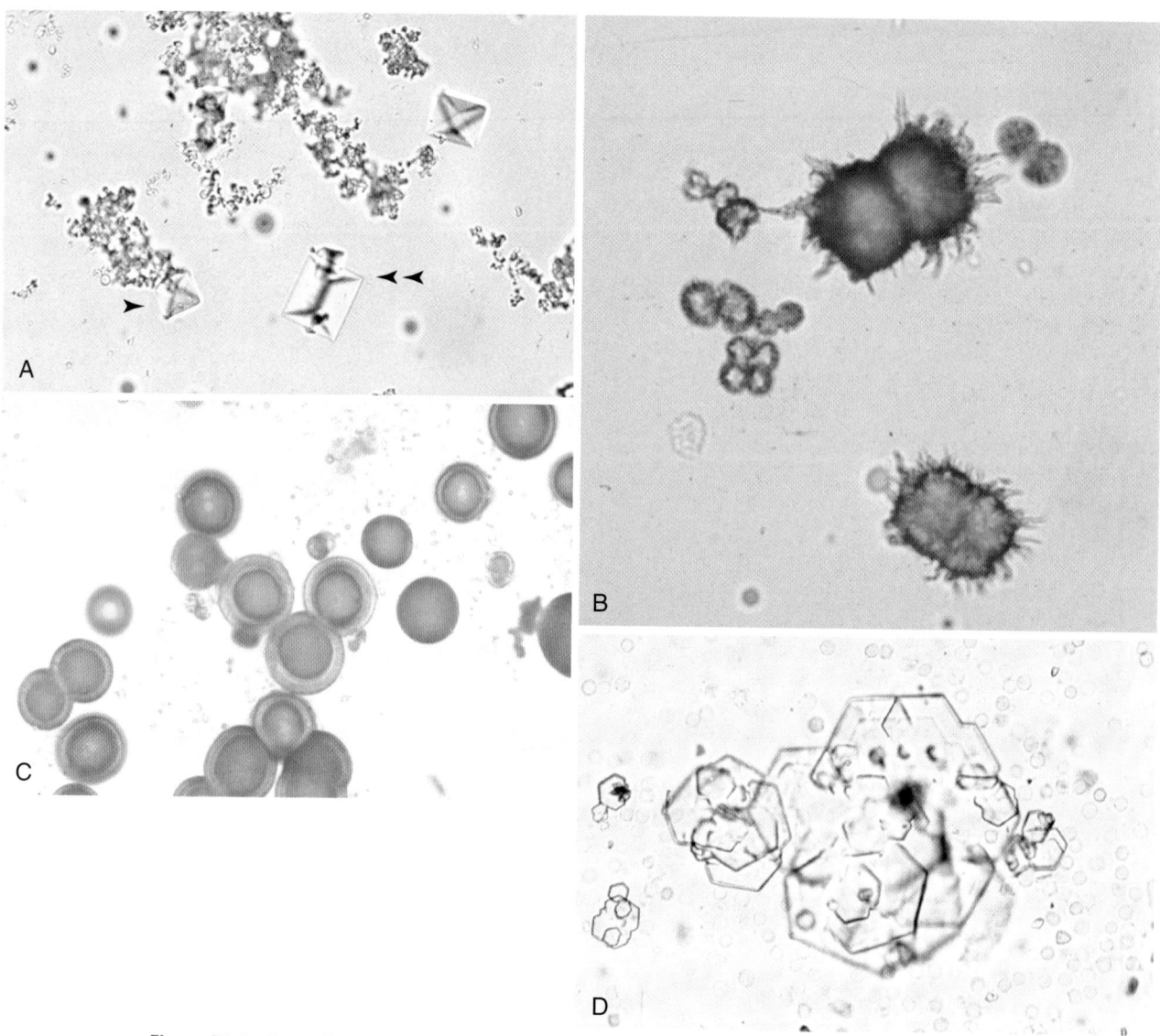

Figure 51-4: Crystalluria. A, Struvite (*double arrowhead*) and calcium oxalate (*single arrowhead*) crystals in a urine sample collected from a 6-year-old, castrated, male, domestic shorthair cat. **B,** Ammonium urate crystals in a urine sample collected from a 1.5-year-old, castrated, male, domestic shorthair cat. **C,** Xanthine crystals in a urine sample collected from a 2-year-old, castrated, male domestic shorthair cat. **D,** Cystine crystals in a urine sample collected from a 1-year-old, castrated, male, domestic shorthair cat.

layers. The different layers of stone are the nidus, stone, shell, and surface crystals. The nidus is the area of obvious initiation of stone growth. The stone refers to the major portion of the urolith. The shell is the material that surrounds the body of the stone, and the surface crystals are an incomplete coating of the outer surface of the stone.[12] A urolith may be defined as a single mineral type, as mixed if the composition consists of more than one mineral type, or as a compound stone if there are mineral layers.

MANAGEMENT OF UROLITHS

Uroliths may result in urethral obstruction. Often urethral obstruction is associated with azotemia, hyperkalemia, meta-

bolic acidosis, and dehydration. Treatment for urethral obstruction involves relieving the obstruction and correcting the metabolic imbalances as quickly as possible. If urethral obstructions are recurrent, perineal urethrostomy may be considered; however, this procedure is associated with increased risk of lower urinary tract disease and bacterial UTIs.[15]

The treatment of obstructive ureteroliths is only necessary when they become problematic. Indications for intervention include recurrent UTIs despite appropriate treatment, hydronephrosis, decreased renal function, pain, or progressive azotemia. Management of upper urinary tract uroliths poses unique problems because most upper urinary tract stones are calcium oxalate, which have no dissolution potential. Also, ureteral surgery in cats is associated with risk, including irreparable damage to the ureters and kidneys.[16] Determining when benefits of ureteral and renal surgery outweigh the risks is difficult. Initial noninvasive methods for cats with renal dysfunction and ureterolithiasis are designed to correct biochemical imbalances and restore fluid volume and may promote migration of the stones into the urinary bladder.[16] More invasive intervention is often determined by the rate of progressive renal dysfunction, presence of discomfort in the patient, and risk associated with the interventional method. Further information on urinary diversion techniques can be found in Chapter 88.

Surgical Treatment

Detection of calculi does not necessarily warrant surgical intervention; however, obstruction of urine outflow, an increase in size and/or number of calculi, persistent clinical signs, and a lack of response to therapy are indications for calculi removal.[12] Surgery is required in patients with nondissolvable calculi and clinical signs. Traditional open surgical options are available for treatment of urolithiasis, including cystotomy and nephrotomy. Nephrotomy has been associated with complications and decrease in glomerular filtration rate even in healthy animals.[17]

Minimally Invasive Techniques

There are several minimally invasive treatment options for retrieval of bladder and urethral stones. These include voiding urohydropropulsion, transurethral cystoscopic stone removal with or without use of laser lithotripsy, and minilaparotomy-assisted cystoscopic stone removal, also called percutaneous cystolithotomy.

In catheter-assisted retrieval or voiding urohydropropulsion of calculi, the patient is sedated or anesthetized, the bladder is filled with sterile crystalloid solution, and a catheter is passed into the urinary bladder transurethrally. In cats, a 3.5 Fr or 5 Fr catheter is used, depending on patient size. During catheter retrieval, the contents of the bladder are aspirated while the bladder is agitated by palpating and manipulating it or rotating the patient's body. This is difficult in most cats due to the limiting size of the urethra, especially in male cats. With voiding urohydropropulsion, the patient is held vertically while the distended bladder is manually expressed (Figure 51-5).[18] In male cats, uroliths up to approximately 1 mm in size may be retrieved whereas in most females, uroliths up to approximately 5 mm in size may be retrieved. These methods are used to eliminate small calculi and to collect them for analysis to plan further treatment. These techniques will not be successful, however, if a feline patient presents with urethral obstruction, as this situation indicates that there is at least one urolith that is too large to pass through the urethra.

Interventional techniques for urolithiasis require endoscopy, fluoroscopy, and/or ultrasonography to perform minimally invasive diagnostic and therapeutic procedures. These modalities are used to visualize, guide, and gain access to the

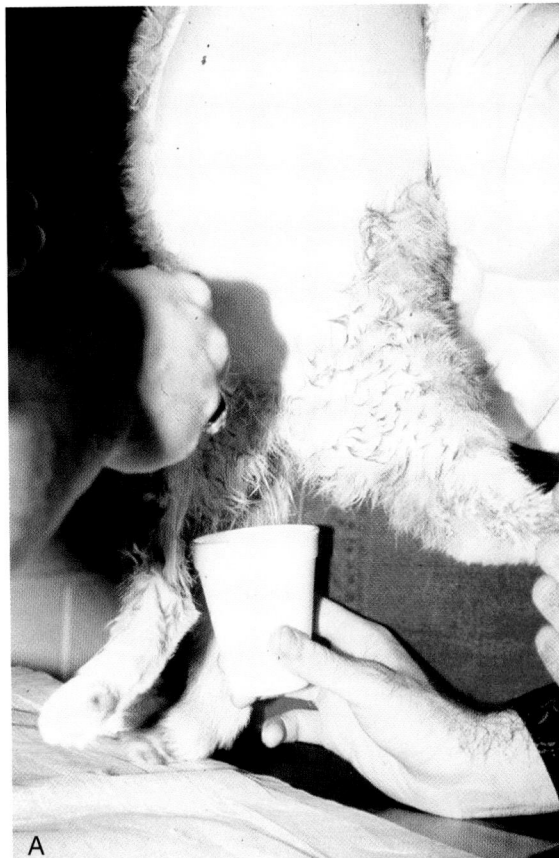

Figure 51-5: Voiding Urohydropropulsion. In voiding urohydropropulsion, the cat is held in a vertical position after the urinary bladder is distended by infusion of fluid through a transurethral catheter **A,** The transurethral catheter is removed and the urinary bladder is gently agitated by grasping it through the abdominal wall. **B,** The urinary bladder is gently compressed inducing micturition and voiding of the urocystoliths.

urogenital tract. Interventional techniques are appealing due to their minimally invasive nature, shorter anesthesia times, reduced perioperative morbidity and mortality, and quicker recovery times.[19] Disadvantages to these techniques include their technically challenging nature, the need for specialized equipment, and the need for appropriate training.

Percutaneous cystolithotomy is a procedure where the bladder is temporarily fastened to the incised linea alba and

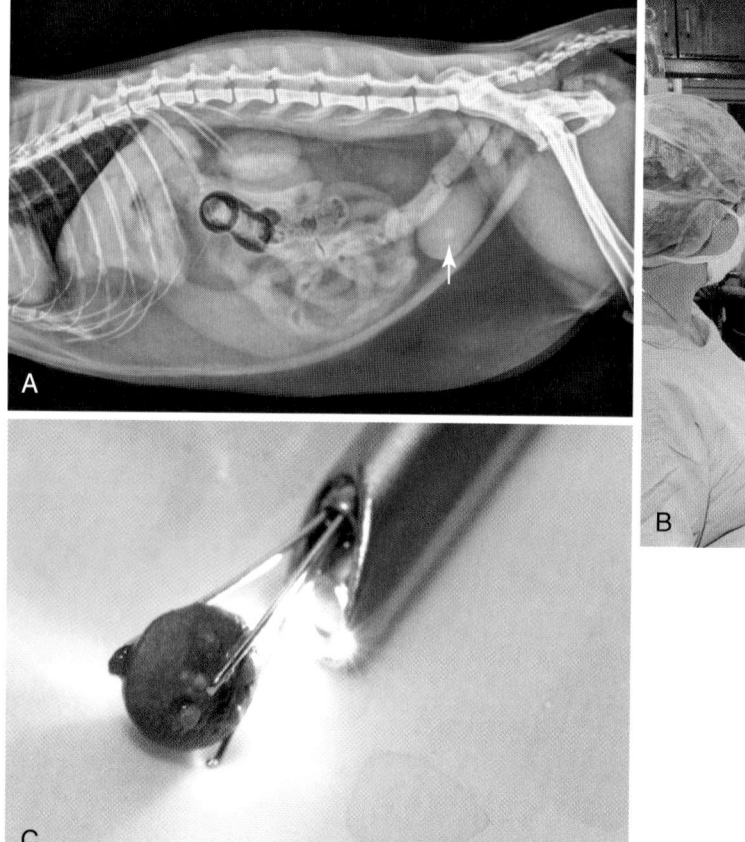

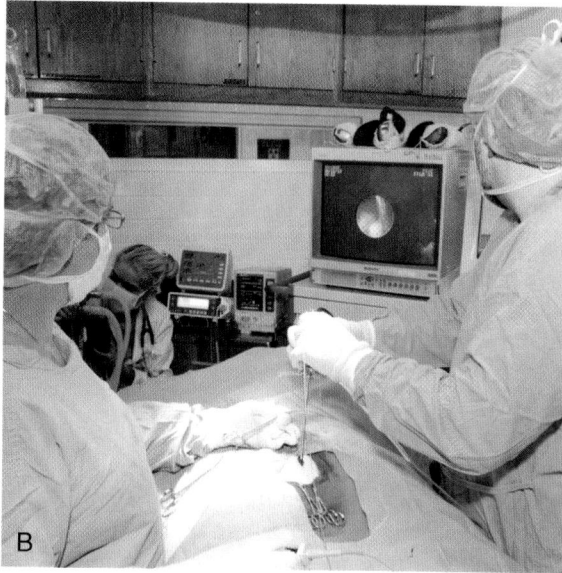

Figure 51-6: Minilaparotomy-Assisted Cystotomy. A, Lateral abdominal radiograph of an 8-year-old, castrated, male, domestic shorthair cat with a single urocystolith (*white arrow*). **B,** The urinary bladder is grasped through a small incision and tacked to the body wall. A stab incision is made through the bladder wall and a rigid cystoscope is inserted. Urocystoliths are retrieved using retrieval devices. Cystoscopy provides magnification and better visualization. The urocystolith being grasped with four-prong Nitinol graspers is projected on the endoscopic monitor. **C,** Urocystolith retrieved via the procedure.

allows for cystoscopic stone removal through a stab incision in the urinary bladder (Figure 51-6).[20] This method is an effective, safe, and efficient means for managing urocystoliths.[20] Cystoscopy produces magnified images of the fluid-distended urinary bladder, allowing identification of abnormalities such as strictures, masses, and calculi.[21,22] This is the minimally invasive procedure of choice for male cats because the diameter of the male cat urethra limits insertion of a cystoscope with an operating channel. Cystoscopic techniques are more efficient than surgical procedures, decreasing the risk of trauma and abdominal contamination.[21,22]

In transurethral cystoscopy, a cystoscope is inserted into the urethra and passed into the urinary bladder. This procedure is preferred for use in female cats because it is less invasive than other diagnostic and treatment methods. If calculi are small enough, they can be removed using stone retrieval devices, such as stone baskets and graspers. For larger calculi, lithotripsy may be used if available (Figure 51-7).[22] Lithotripsy uses a laser fiber that is passed through the operating channel on the cystoscope. The fiber emits light at an infrared wavelength to fragment calculi.[23] The resulting fragments are removed transurethrally. This procedure is possible only in female cats due to the limiting size of the male cat urethra and inability to insert a large enough scope with an operating channel.

Medical Management

Struvite

Magnesium ammonium phosphate hexahydrate crystals or uroliths are more commonly referred to as struvite. For struvite formation, the urine must be oversaturated with magnesium, ammonium, and phosphate ions.[12] Increased urine concentrations of magnesium, ammonium, and phosphate may be a result of a UTI with a urease-producing organism or without the presence of an infection. When no organisms are present, uroliths are termed sterile struvite, and when organisms are present, uroliths are termed infection-induced struvite.

Sterile Struvite Uroliths. Sterile struvite uroliths form in equal frequency in male and female cats and more commonly in cats 1 to 8 years of age.[12] Alkaluria, concentrated urine,

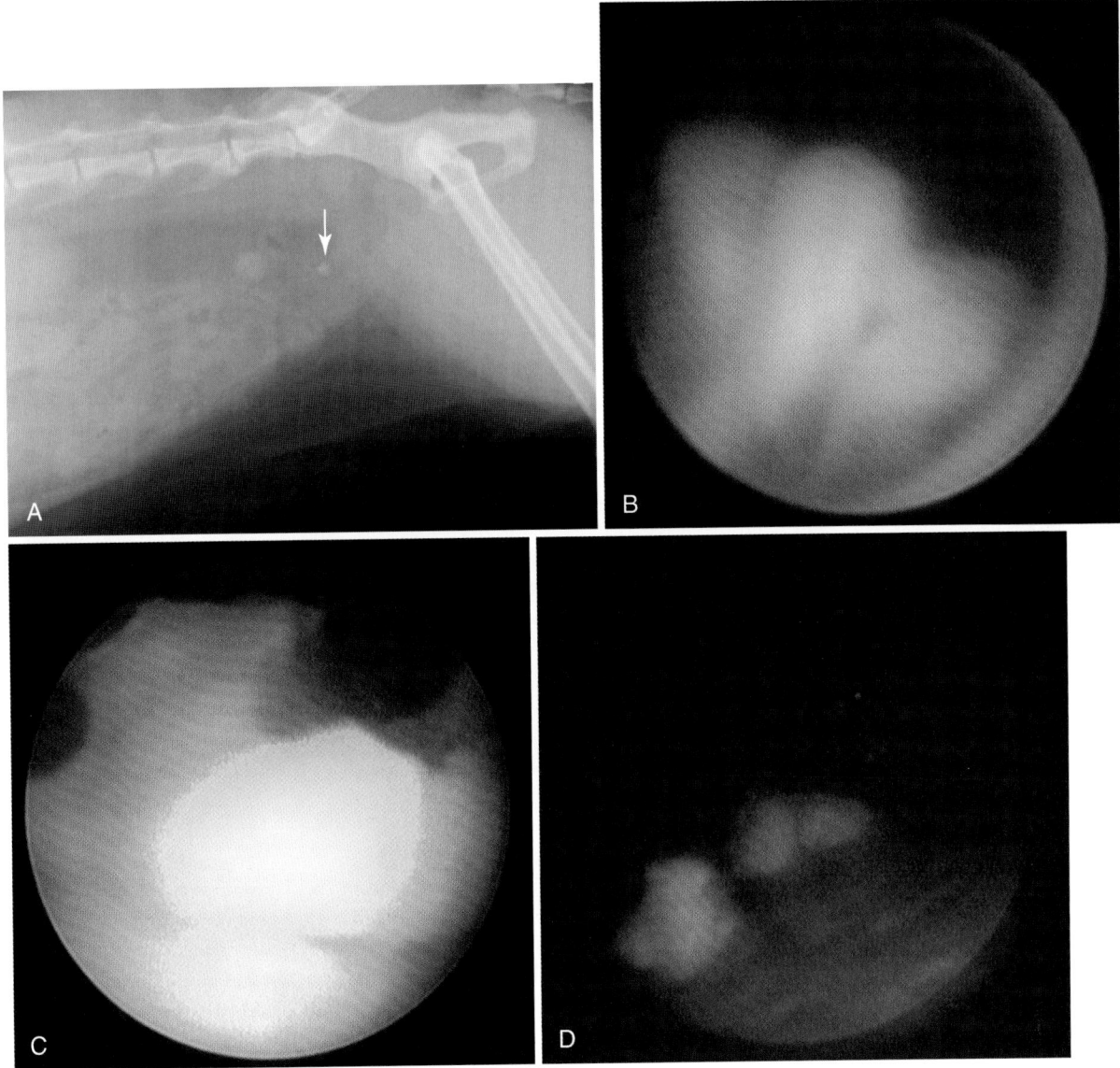

Figure 51-7: Transurethral Cystoscopy and Holmium:YAG (Ho:YAG) Laser Lithotripsy of a Calcium Oxalate Urocystolith in a 10-Year-Old, Spayed, Female, Domestic Shorthair Cat. **A,** Lateral abdominal radiograph showing a urocystolith (*white arrow*). **B,** Appearance of the urocystolith by cystoscopic imaging. **C,** Using a Ho:YAG laser, the urocystolith is fragmented into smaller pieces. The green light is the aiming beam. **D,** Urocystolith fragments retrieved following Ho:YAG laser lithotripsy of the urocystolith.

and increased urinary concentrations of magnesium, ammonium ion, and phosphate are risk factors for sterile struvite urolith formation. Sterile struvite uroliths are amenable to medical dissolution. Dissolution involves feeding a diet low in magnesium, phosphate, and protein that also induces an acidic and dilute urine.[24] Prevention of sterile struvite stones involves inducing an acidic urine pH, decreasing urine specific gravity, and decreasing urine concentrations of magnesium, ammonium, and phosphorus.[25,26] Increased water consumption can decrease risk of urolithiasis formation by decreasing the concentration of calculogenic substances in the urine. Commercial diets are available that promote these factors.

Infection-Induced Struvite Uroliths. Infection-induced struvite uroliths occur most commonly in very young or older

cats. The driving force behind these stones is production of an enzyme, urease, by microbial organisms (most commonly *Staphylococcus* spp., but occasionally *Enterococcus* spp. or *Proteus* spp.). Diet has minimal influence on infection-induced struvite urolith formation. There is dissolution potential for infection-induced struvite stones by feeding a dissolution diet and administering appropriate antimicrobials based on urine culture and sensitivity testing.[24] Both the diet and antimicrobials should be administered throughout the dissolution process and for two additional weeks following radiographical documentation of urolith dissolution. When infection-induced uroliths form, bacteria are trapped in the stone's matrix, and as the stone dissolves, these bacteria are released into the urine. Without antimicrobial therapy, the bacteria can thrive and cease the dissolution process. If dissolution is not successful, the cause may be inappropriate antimicrobial selection, a nontherapeutic level of antimicrobials, inappropriate diet, or poor client compliance. Prevention of infection-induced struvite uroliths does not require a diet change because the driving force for this urolith is the bacterial infection. Prevention is focused on infection prevention and early treatment of UTIs.[27]

Calcium Oxalate

Calcium oxalate urolith formation occurs when urine is oversaturated with calcium and oxalic acid. Formation of these uroliths is complex and incompletely understood. There are metabolic factors known to increase the likelihood of calcium oxalate urolith formation. These include hypercalcemia, hypercalciuria, and metabolic acidosis.

Hypercalcemia is associated with an increased risk of calcium oxalate formation in cats due to development of hypercalciuria. Hypercalciuria can result from increased gastrointestinal (GI) absorption of calcium, impaired renal reabsorption of calcium, or excessive skeletal resorption of calcium.[26] Metabolic acidosis results in hypercalciuria due to increased bone turnover, resulting in increased serum ionized calcium concentrations and therefore increased calcium excretion into the urinary tract. Crystalline inhibitor function is also altered with acidic urine. Urinary citrate concentrations are decreased with a low urine pH via increased proximal tubular resorption of citrate.[26] Calcium oxalate is less soluble in acidic urine when compared with alkaline urine.[25] The metabolic end-product of ascorbic acid (vitamin C) and numerous amino acids derived from dietary sources is oxalic acid. When combined with sodium and potassium ions, oxalic acid forms soluble salts; however, when combined with calcium ions, insoluble salts are formed. Increased concentrations of oxalic acid may promote calcium oxalate formation. There is an increased risk for calcium oxalate urolith formation when there is decreased urine volume.

There are no current medical protocols that promote dissolution of calcium oxalate uroliths. Therefore, the only method of stone resolution is physical removal. Once stones are detected, nutritional and/or medical protocols should be considered to prevent further urolith growth or to prevent recurrence in the case of urolith removal. Calcium oxalate urolith recurrence is significant in patients where stone prevention protocols are not used.[28] Metabolic factors known to increase calcium oxalate formation should be altered when possible, including decreasing urine calcium and oxalic acid concentrations, increasing concentrations of calcium oxalate inhibitors, inducing alkaluria, and promoting a dilute urine specific gravity.[12,26]

Increasing urine volume is imperative in calcium oxalate urolith prevention. Urine concentrations of calculogenic compounds decrease with increased urine volume. An increase in water consumption decreases urine concentrations and increases urine transit time and urine voiding frequency, decreasing the amount of time that the calculogenic substances reside in the urinary tract. Increasing water intake is the easiest way to decrease urine concentrations, and in cats

the most direct way of doing this is to feed a canned diet. A specific gravity of 1.030 or lower is the goal in these patients. In cats that refuse to eat canned food, adding flavoring to drinking water, using running water fountains or purified water, and adding water to dry food are methods that can be used to increase water consumption. Some diets contain sodium chloride to induce diuresis and increase water consumption.

Use caution when considering diet changes in cats with calcium oxalate urolithiasis. Consumption of acidifying diets is a risk factor for calcium oxalate stone formation.[29] Potassium citrate is often included medically or in diets used for calcium oxalate prevention. In urine, soluble complexes are formed when citric acid combines with calcium. This decreases ionic calcium concentrations.[30] Citric acid also directly inhibits calcium and oxalate nucleation of crystals. Supplemental citrate, when oxidized, produces bicarbonate, resulting in urine alkalization. Dietary phosphorus should not be restricted in patients with calcium oxalate urolithiasis. Decreased dietary phosphorus may increase vitamin D_3 production, which promotes calcium absorption and hypercalciuria.

Purines

Urates. Urate uroliths are observed occasionally in cats. Most occur in cats less than four years of age. Urate uroliths can occur as a result of liver dysfunction in association with portal vascular anomalies.[31] Affected cats are often less than one year of age. They can also occur in the absence of liver disease, termed idiopathic urate urolithiasis. Purine uroliths include ammonium acid urate, xanthine, and uric acid monohydrate. Purine-rich diets and animal proteins are the major sources of exogenous purines in veterinary patients. Endogenous purines are synthesized in the liver. Supersaturation of urine with uric acid is required for urate urolith formation. Hyperuricosuria is promoted by increased renal excretion, excess production of uric acid, or decreased resorption of uric acid. In cats, urate urolithiasis has been linked to renal tubular resorption defects and portal vascular anomalies. It is likely that a defective purine metabolism is a cause of hyperuricosuria in cats with idiopathic urate urolithiasis.[26] Urine pH is an important physiological factor for promoting urate crystalluria. When urine pH is greater than 5.5, uric acid is converted into urate. Urate uroliths are more likely to form in urine supersaturated with uric acid and a low urine pH.[32] Cats with urate stones may have elevated liver enzymes on biochemical analysis or abnormal values on liver function tests. Urate uroliths are often radiolucent and may require contrast cystography or ultrasonography for detection.

Medical protocols to promote ammonium urate dissolution in cats have not been developed. However, dissolution using a low purine diet and allopurinol (a xanthine oxidase inhibitor) has been successful in some cats.[32]

Prevention of recurrence is accomplished by treating underlying causes, such as ameroid constrictor placement for extrahepatic portovascular anomalies. For cats with idiopathic urate uroliths, dietary modification is the primary treatment. Diets restricted in purines and promoting alkaline urine should be fed. Xanthine oxidase inhibitors in cats can cause side effects, including GI upset, leukopenia, thrombocytopenia, hepatitis, and kidney failure. Therefore, their use is reserved for highly recurrent disease.[32]

Xanthine. Xanthine uroliths have been reported rarely in cats (0.14% of uroliths analyzed at the Minnesota Urolith Center). They are composed typically of pure xanthine, and they have been reported to occur in cats less than 5 years of age with approximately even distribution between males and females. Often, xanthine uroliths occur in multiple numbers but are less than 5 mm in size; they are radiolucent. In one unpublished study (J.W. Bartges, personal communication, 2014), urinary uric acid excretion was similar between eight xanthine urolith-forming cats and healthy cats (2.09 ± 0.8 mg/kg/day versus 1.46 ± 0.56 mg/kg/day); however, urinary xanthine excretion (2.46 ± 1.17 mg/kg/day) and urinary hypoxanthine excretion (0.65 ± 0.17 mg/kg/day) were higher in the urolith-forming cats (neither are detectable in urine from healthy cats). No medical dissolution protocol for feline xanthine uroliths exists. Prevention involves feeding a protein-restricted, alkalinizing diet. Without preventative measures, xanthine uroliths often recur within 3 to 12 months following removal. In an unpublished observational study (J.W. Bartges, personal communication, 2014), 10 cats with quantitative analysis confirmation of xanthine uroliths have been consuming the protein-restricted alkalinizing diet and followed for at least 2 years; only one has had recurrence to date.

Xanthine is a product of purine metabolism and is converted to uric acid by the enzyme xanthine oxidase.[33] Hereditary xanthinuria is a rarely recognized disorder of humans characterized by a deficiency of xanthine oxidase.[34] As a consequence, abnormal quantities of xanthine are excreted in urine as a major end-product of purine metabolism. Because xanthine is the least soluble of the purines naturally excreted in urine, xanthinuria may be associated with formation of uroliths. The precise metabolic abnormality has not been identified in cats; however, a familial or congenital defect in xanthine oxidase activity is likely.

Cystine

Cystine uroliths occur rarely in cats, accounting for less than 0.2% of uroliths analyzed by the Minnesota Urolith Center; most occur in middle-aged and older cats. The pathogenesis of cystine urolith formation in cats is unknown but is likely to be a heritable proximal tubulopathy.[35] No medical dissolution protocol exists for feline cystine uroliths. In addition to increasing urine volume, cystine solubility increases exponentially above a pH of 7.2.[26] Feeding a low-protein, alkalinizing diet that induces diuresis appears logical for management. Potassium citrate may be administered to induce alkaluria. Thiol-containing drug therapy, such as 2-mercaptoproprionyl-glycine and D-penicillamine, has not been evaluated in cats.

References

1. Bartges JW: Urinary saturation testing. In Bartges J, Polzin DJ, editors: *Nephrolgy and urology of small animals*, West Sussex, UK, 2011, Wiley-Blackwell, pp 75–85.
2. Elliott DA: Nutrition management of the lower urinary tract conditions. In Ettinger S, Feldman E, editors: *Textbook of veterinary internal medicine*, St Louis, 2010, Saunders, pp 696–701.
3. Osborne CA, Lulich JP, Kruger JM, et al: Analysis of 451,891 canine uroliths, feline uroliths, and feline urethral plugs from 1981 to 2007: perspectives from the Minnesota Urolith Center. *Vet Clin North Am Small Anim Pract* 39:183–197, 2009.
4. Kruger JM, Osborne CA, Goyal SM, et al: Clinical evaluation of cats with lower urinary tract disease. *J Am Vet Med Assoc* 199:211–216, 1991.
5. Osborne CA, Lulich JP, Kruger JM, et al: Feline urethral plugs. Etiology and pathophysiology. *Vet Clin North Am Small Anim Pract* 26:233–253, 1996.
6. Kyles AE, Hardie EM, Wooden BG, et al: Clinical, clinicopathologic, radiographic, and ultrasonographic abnormalities in cats with ureteral calculi: 163 cases (1984-2002). *J Am Vet Med Assoc* 226:932–936, 2005.
7. Markovich J, Labato M: Medical management of nephroliths and ureteroliths. In Bonagura JD, Twedt DC, editors: *Kirk's current veterinary therapy*, St Louis, 2014, Elsevier, pp 892–896.
8. Hecht S, Henry GA: Ultrasonography of the urinary tract. In Bartges J, Polzin DJ, editors: *Nephrology and urology of small animals*, Ames, 2011, Wiley-Blackwell, pp 128–145.
9. Feeney DA, Anderson KL: Radiographic imaging in urinary tract disease. In Bartges J, Polzin DJ, editors: *Nephrology and urology of small animals*, West Sussex, UK, 2011, Wiley-Blackwell, pp 97–127.
10. Sturgess CP, Hesford A, Owen H, et al: An investigation into the effects of storage on the diagnosis of crystalluria in cats. *J Feline Med Surg* 3:81–85, 2001.
11. Langston C, Gisselman K, Palma D, et al: Diagnosis of urolithiasis. *Compend Contin Educ Vet* 30:447–450, 452–444, 2008.
12. Lulich JP, Osborne CA, Albasan H: Canine and feline urolithiasis: diagnosis, treatment, and prevention. In Bartges J, Polzin DJ, editors: *Nephrology and urology of small animals*, West Sussex UK, 2011, Wiley-Blackwell, pp 687–706.
13. Gisselman K, Langston CE, Douglas P, et al: Calcium oxalate urolithiasis. *Compend Contin Educ Vet* 31:496–502, 2009.
14. Koehler LA, Osborne CA, Buettner MT, et al: Canine uroliths: frequently asked questions and their answers. *Vet Clin North Am Small Anim Pract* 39:161–181, 2009.
15. McLoughlin MA: Complications of lower urinary tract surgery in small animals. *Vet Clin North Am Small Anim Pract* 41:889–913, 2011.
16. Kyles AE, Hardie EM, Wooden BG, et al: Management and outcome of cats with ureteral calculi: 153 cases (1984-2002). *J Am Vet Med Assoc* 226:937–944, 2005.
17. King MD, Waldron DR, Barber DL, et al: Effect of nephrotomy on renal function and morphology in normal cats. *Vet Surg* 35:749–758, 2006.
18. Lulich JP, Osborne CA: Voiding urohydropropulsion. In Bartges J, Polzin DJ, editors: *Nephrology and urology of small animals*, West Sussex, UK, 2011, Wiley-Blackwell, pp 375–378.
19. Berent A, Weisse C: Interventional strategies for urinary disease. In Bonagura JD, Tweardy DJ, editors: *Kirk's current veterinary therapy*, St Louis, 2014, Elsevier, pp 884–892.
20. Bartges J, Sura P, Callens A: Minilaparotomy-assisted cystoscopy for urocystoliths. In Bonagura JD, Twedt DC, editors: *Kirk's current veterinary therapy*, St Louis, 2014, Elsevier, pp 906–909.
21. Rawlings C: Diagnostic rigid endoscopy: otoscopy, rhinoscopy, and cystoscopy. *Vet Clin North Am Small Anim Pract* 39:849–868, 2009.
22. Rawlings C: Surgical views: endoscopic removal of urinary calculi. *Compend Contin Educ Vet* 31:476–484, 2009.

23. Adams LG, Berent AC, Moore GE, et al: Use of laser lithotripsy for fragmentation of uroliths in dogs: 73 cases (2005-2006). *J Am Vet Med Assoc* 232:1680–1687, 2008.

24. Osborne CA, Lulich JP, Kruger JM, et al: Medical dissolution of feline struvite urocystoliths. *J Am Vet Med Assoc* 196:1053–1063, 1990.

25. Bartges JW, Kirk CA, Cox SK, et al: Influence of acidifying or alkalinizing diets on bone mineral density and urine relative supersaturation with calcium oxalate and struvite in healthy cats. *Am J Vet Res* 74:1347–1352, 2013.

26. Bartges JW, Kirk CA: Nutrition and lower urinary tract disease in cats. *Vet Clin North Am Small Anim Pract* 36:1361–1376, 2006.

27. Pressler B, Bartges JW: Urinary tract infection. In Ettinger SJ, Feldman EC, editors: *Textbook of small animal internal medicine*, ed 7, St Louis, 2010, Elsevier Saunders, pp 2036–2047.

28. Lulich JP, Osborne CA, Lekcharoensuk C, et al: Effects of diet on urine composition of cats with calcium oxalate urolithiasis. *J Am Anim Hosp Assoc* 40:185–191, 2004.

29. Kirk CA, Ling GV, Franti CE, et al: Evaluation of factors associated with development of calcium oxalate urolithiasis in cats. *J Am Vet Med Assoc* 207:1429–1434, 1995.

30. Pak CY, Fuller C, Sakhaee K, et al: Long-term treatment of calcium nephrolithiasis with potassium citrate. *J Urol* 134:11–19, 1985.

31. Bartges JW, Cornelius LM, Osborne CA: Ammonium urate uroliths in dogs with portosystemic shunts. In Bonagura JD, editor: *Current veterinary therapy XIII*, Philadelphia, 1999, Saunders, pp 872–874.

32. Gnanandarajah J, Lulich JP, Albasan H, et al: Purine uroliths. In August J, editor: *Consultations in feline internal medicine*, St Louis, 2010, Saunders, pp 499–508.

33. Bartges JW, Osborne CA, Lulich JP, et al: Canine urate urolithiasis. Etiopathogenesis, diagnosis, and management. *Vet Clin North Am Small Anim Pract* 29:161–191, 1999.

34. Holmes EWJ, Mason DHJ, Goldstein LI, et al: Xanthine oxidase deficiency: Studies of a previously unreported case. *Clin Chem* 20:1076–1079, 1974.

35. DiBartola SP, Chew DJ, Horton ML: Cystinuria in a cat. *J Am Vet Med Assoc* 198:102–104, 1991.

Urinary Tract Infection

Shelly Olin and Joseph W. Bartges

ETIOLOGY AND EPIDEMIOLOGY

Urinary tract infection (UTI) occurs when there is compromise of host defense mechanisms and a virulent microbe adheres, multiplies, and persists in a portion of the urinary tract. Host defenses include normal micturition, anatomical structures, the mucosal barrier, properties of urine, and systemic immunocompetence (Box 52-1). Most commonly, UTIs are caused by bacteria, but fungi and viruses also may infect the urinary tract. UTIs may involve more than one anatomic location, and the infection should be categorized as upper urinary tract (i.e., kidneys and ureters) versus lower urinary tract (i.e., bladder, urethra, and vagina).

Bacterial UTI is uncommon in young cats with lower urinary tract disease, but bacterial UTI is an important problem in geriatric cats.[1,2] Older cats may be at increased risk for development of bacterial UTI because of diminished urinary tract defenses. Whether impaired defenses are intrinsic to the aging process or secondary to disorders that are common in geriatric cats is unknown. It seems reasonable to hypothesize that comorbidities of older cats (e.g., chronic kidney disease [CKD], diabetes mellitus, and hyperthyroidism) impair normal defense mechanisms.

PATHOGENESIS

The majority of bacterial UTIs occur as a consequence of ascending migration of pathogens through the genital tract and urethra to the bladder, ureters, and one or both kidneys. Rectal, perineal, and genital bacteria serve as the principal reservoirs for infection.[3,4]

The upper urinary tract is most commonly infected by ascending microbes rather than through hematogenous routes. Renal cortical tissue appears to be more resistant to infection than medullary tissue. Most hematogenous bacteria do not reach the renal medulla, because circulating blood must pass through glomerular capillaries located in the cortex before reaching the medulla. However, urinary tract obstruction or trauma can increase risk of hematogenous seeding of the urinary tract by interfering with renal microcirculation.[5]

Microbial Isolates

The bacteria that most commonly cause UTIs are similar in dogs and cats. *Escherichia coli* infections are most common, accounting for one-third to one-half of all positive urine cultures.[6,7] Gram-positive cocci are the second major group of uropathogens; *Staphylococcus* spp., *Streptococcus* spp., and *Enterococcus* spp. account for one-fourth to one-third of isolates recovered.[6,7] Cats may be infected with a unique strain of *Staphylococcus, Staphylococcus felis,* and commercial phenotypic identification systems may not differentiate between *S. felis* and other coagulase-negative *Staphylococcus* spp.[8,9] One study found that *S. felis* was the third most common UTI isolate based on 16S ribosomal DNA sequencing (*n* = 25 out of 106, 19.8% of bacterial isolates cultured), suggesting *S. felis* is the most common staphylococcal species causing UTI in cats.[8]

Bacteria that cause the remaining one-fourth to one-third of bacterial UTI in dogs and cats include *Proteus, Klebsiella, Pasteurella, Pseudomonas, Corynebacterium,* and several other rarely reported genera.[6,7] The role of *Mycoplasma* spp. and *Ureaplasma* spp. in UTIs in cats is unclear. *Mycoplasma* spp. are isolated from urine of dogs with clinical signs referable to the lower urinary tract in less than 5% of samples; whether or not *Mycoplasma* spp. are associated with urinary tract disease in cats is disputed.[6,10-12] Similar to infections in dogs, a single bacterial pathogen is isolated from approximately 75% of bacterial UTIs in cats, 20% of UTIs are caused by two coinfecting species, and approximately 5% are caused by three species.[6,13,14]

Microbial Virulence Factors

The establishment of UTI depends on the virulence and number of microbes and their interaction with host defenses. In addition to gaining access to the urinary tract, microbes must adhere to and colonize the uroepithelial surface. Not all microbes, particularly bacteria, are pathogenic. For example, of the more than several hundred serotypes of *E. coli*, fewer than 20 account for most bacterial UTIs.

E. coli is the most common bacterial uropathogen in humans, dogs, and cats, and its virulence (uropathogenicity) has been studied extensively.[15-19] The ability to adhere to the uroepithelium via adhesions is one of the major determinants of pathogenicity for uropathogenic *E. coli.*[16] Numerous virulence factor encoding genes have been identified in canine and feline uropathogenic *E. coli* strains, including adhesins, toxins, siderophores, and polysaccharide coatings (Box 52-2).[17-19] Less is known about the uropathogenicity of other pathogens.

BOX 52-1 Normal Host Defenses against Urinary Tract Infection

I. Normal micturition
   A. Adequate urine volume
   B. Frequent voiding
   C. Complete voiding
II. Anatomic structures
   A. Urethral high pressure zones
   B. Surface characteristics of uroepithelium
   C. Urethral peristalsis
   D. Prostatic secretions (antibacterial fraction, immunoglobulins)
   E. Urethral length
   F. Ureterovesical flap valves
   G. Ureteral peristalsis
   H. Glomerular mesangial cells
   I. Extensive renal blood supply and flow
III. Mucosal defense barriers
   A. Antibody production
   B. Surface glycosaminoglycan layer
   C. Intrinsic mucosal antimicrobial properties
   D. Exfoliation of urothelial cells
   E. Commensal microbes of distal urogenital tract
IV. Urine antimicrobial properties
   A. Extreme urine pH (high or low)
   B. Hyperosmolality
   C. High urea concentration
   D. Organic acids
   E. Low-molecular weight carbohydrates
   F. Tamm-Horsfall mucoproteins
V. Systemic immunocompetence

Adapted from Osborne CA, Lees GE: Bacterial infections of the canine and feline urinary tract. In Osborne CA, Finco DR, editors: *Canine and feline nephrology and urology,* Baltimore, 1995, Williams & Wilkins, pp 759-797.

CLINICAL SIGNS

Bacterial UTIs may be symptomatic or asymptomatic. Bacterial infection of the lower urinary tract is usually associated with clinical signs that are similar to other diseases of the lower urinary tract. These signs include, but are not limited to, pollakiuria, dysuria, stranguria, hematuria, and inappropriate urination. Bacterial infection of the kidneys may be associated with hematuria; if septicemia develops, the cat may be systemically ill. In addition, upper UTI may cause recurrent lower UTI.

DIAGNOSIS

Urinalysis

Urinalysis should be performed as a routine part of a minimum database in older or ill cats. A complete urinalysis involves

BOX 52-2 Selected Factors That May Enhance the Virulence (Uropathogenicity) of Bacteria Causing Urinary Tract Infections

I. *Escherichia coli*
   A. Adhesive fimbriae (pili)
      1. Proteinaceous filamentous organelles that protrude from the bacterium surface
      2. Specific types of fimbriae (p-fimbriae) enhance the ability of a bacterium to remain adherent to uroepithelium despite cleansing action of urinary system (e.g., adhesins: P, S, F1C, type I fimbriae)
   B. Toxins
      1. Hemolysin
         a) Increases amount of free iron available for bacterial growth
         b) May cause tissue damage
      2. Cytotoxic necrotizing factor-1
   C. Siderophores (iron-chelating system)
      1. Aerobactin
         a) Iron-binding protein
         b) Facilitates bacterial growth
   D. R-plasmids
      1. Promote resistance to antimicrobial agents (e.g., extended spectrum beta-lactamases)
      2. For example, extended spectrum beta-lactamases
   E. Polysaccharides
      1. Certain O (somatic) antigens
         a) Outer polysaccharide portion of bacterial envelope
         b) Protect against complement-mediated killing
         c) Indirect marker of virulence (human studies)
      2. Certain K (capsular) antigens
         a) Capsule surrounds bacterium
         b) May inhibit phagocytosis and complement-mediated bactericidal activity
         c) Increased resistance to inflammation favors persistence of bacteria in tissue
II. *Proteus* spp., *Staphylococcus* spp., and some *Klebsiella* spp.
   A. Adherence factors
   B. Urease activity
      1. Bacterial enzyme that hydrolyzes urea to ammonia
      2. Ammonia directly injures uroepithelium
      3. Urease promotes production of magnesium ammonium phosphatase uroliths, which serve as niduses for infection
   C. R-plasmids
III. *Pseudomonas* spp.
   A. Heavy mucoid polysaccharide capsule prevents antibody adherence
   B. R-plasmids

determining urine specific gravity (USG) using a refractometer, biochemical analysis using colorimetric test pads on urine dipsticks, and microscopic sediment examination. Cystocentesis is the preferred method of urine collection when evaluating a patient for a UTI. With UTI, the USG is variable depending on whether the infection involves the upper urinary tract or an associated disease. Dipstick analysis often, but not always, reveals hematuria and proteinuria. Leukocyte esterase (white blood cells) and nitrite (bacteria) test pads are not reliable and should not be used as indicators of bacterial UTI in cats.[20]

Examination of urine sediment should be a routine part of a complete urinalysis. Significant numbers of white blood cells (>5 per high power field), along with hematuria and proteinuria, in a properly collected urine sample suggest inflammation. Detection of significant bacteriuria in samples with pyuria indicates active inflammation associated with an infection. Rod-shaped bacteria may be identified in unstained preparations of urine sediment if more than 10,000 bacteria/mL are present but may not be consistently detected if present in fewer numbers. Cocci are difficult to detect in urine sediment if their numbers are less than 100,000 bacteria/mL. Bacteria are more difficult to identify in dilute urine, making a diagnosis of UTI challenging in the face of polyuria. Failure to detect bacteria on examination of urine sediment does not exclude their presence or rule out a UTI. On the other hand, bacterial UTI may exist without concurrent inflammation if host defenses are compromised (e.g., feline leukemia virus infection).[13,21] Urine sediment may be stained with Wright stain, Gram stain, or new methylene blue to aid in detection of bacteria. Although detection of bacteria in urine sediment suggests bacterial UTI, infection should be verified by urine culture.

Urine Culture

A positive urine culture from a cystocentesis sample is the gold standard for diagnosing bacterial UTI. A quantitative urine culture includes isolation and identification of the organism and determination of the number of bacteria (colony-forming units [CFUs] per unit volume). Quantitation of bacteria enables interpretation of the significance of its presence in a urine sample. Caution should be exercised when interpreting quantitative urine cultures obtained by midstream voiding or manual expression of urine; voided urine samples may be contaminated from the urethra, vagina, or environment. Urine collected from nonresorbable cat litter is the least desirable sample for culture.

Sample processing immediately after urine collection provides optimal results. If immediate processing (within 30 minutes) is not possible, then the sample may be stored in a sterile, dry, transparent container (e.g., a serum red top tube), and the sample should be refrigerated. Culture of refrigerated urine is the most accurate when performed within 24 hours.

Additional Testing

Most cats with bacterial UTI have complicated infections; therefore, other laboratory testing and imaging studies are often required. In addition to urinalysis and urine culture, a minimum database includes complete blood count and biochemical profile with electrolytes. Other logical choices are thyroid hormone and retroviral testing, as well as abdominal radiographs and sonography.

DIFFERENTIAL DIAGNOSES

Differential diagnoses for bacterial infection of the lower urinary tract in cats include urolithiasis, idiopathic cystitis, neoplasia, and behavioral disorders (Figure 52-1). Upper urinary tract signs, including renomegaly, renal pain, hematuria, or renal failure, may be caused by UTI or many other primary renal disorders. Causes of renal failure are many, and often it is impossible to determine the role, if any, that bacterial UTI plays in the development or progression of CKD in cats. If renomegaly is present, differential diagnoses should include feline infectious peritonitis, neoplasia (most notably lymphosarcoma), hydronephrosis due to ureteral obstruction, and polycystic kidney disease.

TREATMENT

Antimicrobial Selection

Antimicrobial drugs are the cornerstone of treatment for UTI. The antimicrobial agent selected should be (1) easy to administer, (2) associated with few, if any, adverse effects, (3) inexpensive, and (4) able to attain urine concentrations (and tissue concentrations in the event of kidney or prostatic infection) that exceed the minimum inhibitory concentration (MIC) for the uropathogen by at least fourfold. In most cases

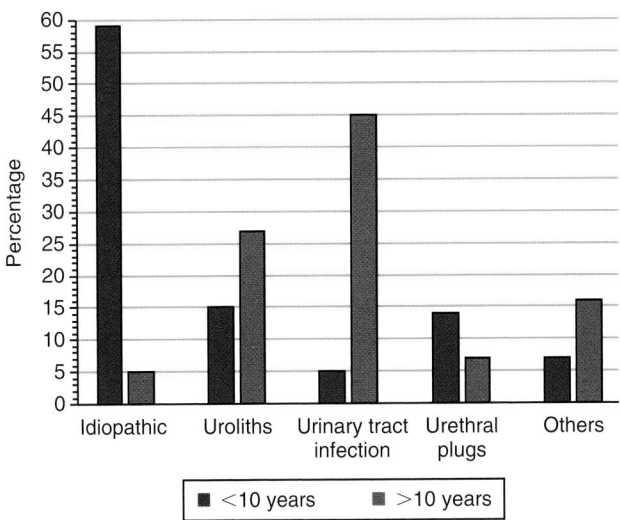

Figure 52-1: Causes of lower urinary tract signs in cats.

the antimicrobial agent chosen should be based on susceptibility testing of the uropathogen.

Overuse and misuse of antimicrobial drugs may result in the emergence of resistant organisms, a situation that has implications for successful treatment of infections in the patient as well as overall veterinary and human health. Patients with uncomplicated UTI and those with clinical signs severe enough to merit therapy prior to results of urine culture and sensitivity testing should receive a broad-spectrum antimicrobial that has excellent urine penetration. Suggested first-line antimicrobials for uncomplicated UTIs include amoxicillin, cephalexin, or trimethoprim-sulfonamide (Table 52-1). Unfortunately, many veterinarians choose to avoid these drugs because they require more than twice-per-day dosing, bacteria are more likely to be resistant to these drugs than second-line agents, or the frequency of adverse effects are higher than with other antimicrobials. Nevertheless, the use of potentiated beta-lactams (i.e., amoxicillin/clavulanate), fluoroquinolones, or extended release cephalexin (i.e., cefovecin) is inappropriate for most uncomplicated UTIs and should be reserved for complicated or resistant infections (Table 52-2).

Table 52-1	Summary of First-Line Antimicrobial Options for Urinary Tract Infections in the Cat
Infection	**First-Line Drug Options**
Uncomplicated UTI	Amoxicillin, trimethoprim-sulfonamide
Complicated	Guided by culture and susceptibility testing, but consider amoxicillin or trimethoprim-sulfonamide initially
Subclinical bacteriuria	Antimicrobial therapy not recommended unless high risk for ascending infection; if so, treat as per complicated UTI
Pyelonephritis	Start with a fluoroquinolone with reassessment based on culture and susceptibility testing

Adapted from Weese J, Blondeau JM, Boothe D, et al: Antimicrobial use guidelines for treatment of urinary tract disease in dogs and cats: antimicrobial guidelines Working Group of the International Society for Companion Animal Infectious Diseases, *Vet Med Int* Article ID 263768:1-9, 2011. *UTI*, Urinary tract infection.

Table 52-2	Antimicrobial Treatment Options for Urinary Tract Infection in Cats	
Drug	**Dosage**	**Comments**
Amikacin	10 to 14 mg/kg every 24 h, IV/IM/SC	Not recommended for routine use but may be useful for treatment of multidrug-resistant organisms. Potentially nephrotoxic. Avoid in animals with renal insufficiency.
Amoxicillin	11 to 15 mg/kg every 8 h, PO	Good first-line option. Excreted in urine predominantly in active form if normal renal function is present. Ineffective against beta-lactamase–producing bacteria.
Amoxicillin/ clavulanate	12.5 to 25 mg/kg every 12 h, PO (dose based on combination of amoxicillin + clavulanate)	Not established whether there is any advantage over amoxicillin alone.
Ampicillin		Not recommended because of poor oral bioavailability. Amoxicillin is preferred.
Cefovecin	8 mg/kg single SC injection. Can be repeated once after 7 to 14 days.	Should only be used in situations where oral treatment is problematic. Enterococci are resistant. Pharmacokinetic data are available to support its use in cats with a duration of 21 days. The long duration of excretion in the urine makes it difficult to interpret post-treatment culture results.
Cefpodoxime proxetil	5 to 10 mg/kg every 24 h, PO	Enterococci are resistant.
Ceftiofur	2.2 mg/kg every 24 h, SC	Enterococci are resistant.
Cephalexin, Cefadroxil	12 to 25 mg/kg every 12 h, PO	Enterococci are resistant. Resistance may be common in *Enterobacteriaceae* in some regions.
Chloramphenicol	12.5 to 20 mg/kg every 12 h, PO	Reserved for multidrug-resistant infections with few other options. Myelosuppression can occur, particularly with long-term therapy. Avoid contact by humans because of rare idiosyncratic aplastic anemia.
Ciprofloxacin	30 mg/kg every 24 h, PO	Sometimes used because of lower cost than enrofloxacin. Lower and more variable oral bioavailability than enrofloxacin, marbofloxacin, and orbifloxacin. Difficult to justify over approved fluoroquinolones. Dosing recommendations are empirical.

Table 52-2 Antimicrobial Treatment Options for Urinary Tract Infection in Cats—cont'd

Drug	Dosage	Comments
Doxycycline	3 to 5 mg/kg every 12 h, PO	Highly metabolized and excreted through intestinal tract, so urine levels may be low. Not recommended for routine use.
Enrofloxacin	5 mg/kg every 24 h, PO	Excreted in urine predominantly in active form. Reserve for documented resistant UTIs. Limited efficacy against enterococci. Associated with risk of retinopathy in cats. Do not exceed 5 mg/kg/day.
Imipenem-cilastatin	5 mg/kg every 6 to 8 h, IV/IM	Reserve for treatment of multidrug-resistant infections, particularly those caused by *Enterobacteriaceae* or *Pseudomonas aeruginosa*. Recommend consultation with a urinary or infectious disease veterinary specialist or veterinary pharmacologist prior to use.
Marbofloxacin	2.7 to 5.5 mg/kg every 24 h, PO	Excreted in urine predominantly in active form. Reserve for documented resistant infections, but good first-line choice for pyelonephritis. Limited efficacy against enterococci.
Meropenem	8.5 mg/kg every 12 h, SC or every 8 h, IV	Reserve for treatment of multidrug-resistant infections, particularly those caused by *Enterobacteriaceae* or *Pseudomonas aeruginosa*. Recommend consultation with a urinary or infectious disease veterinary specialist or veterinary pharmacologist prior to use.
Nitrofurantoin	4.4 to 5 mg/kg every 8 h, PO	Good second-line option for simple uncomplicated infection, particularly when multidrug-resistant pathogens are involved.
Orbifloxacin	Tablets: 2.5 to 7.5 mg/kg every 24 h, PO Oral suspension: 7.5 mg/kg every 24 h, PO	Excreted in urine predominantly in active form.
Pradofloxacin	5 mg/kg every 24 h, PO*	
Trimethoprim-sulfadiazine	15 mg/kg every 12 h, PO Note: Dosing is based on total trimethoprim + sulfadiazine concentration	Good first-line option. Concerns regarding idiosyncratic and immune-mediated adverse effects in some patients, especially with prolonged therapy. Adverse effects in cats include anorexia, leukopenia, anemias, and, potentially, hepatoxicity.

Adapted from Weese J, Blondeau JM, Boothe D, et al: Antimicrobial use guidelines for treatment of urinary tract disease in dogs and cats: antimicrobial guidelines Working Group of the International Society for Companion Animal Infectious Diseases, *Vet Med Int* Article ID 263768:1-9, 2011.
IM, Intramuscularly; *IV*, intravenously; *PO, per os* (by mouth, orally); *SC*, subcutaneously; *UTI*, urinary tract infection.
*Dose extrapolated from previous studies.[24]

The use of fluoroquinolones for empiric treatment of bacterial UTI is particularly discouraged because of the inherent resistance of many gram-positive organisms to this class of antimicrobials and the developing resistance of many gram-negative organisms, including *E. coli*, to this class of drugs.[22] Studies have found variable cross-resistance among different generations of fluoroquinolones, except pradofloxacin (Veraflox, Bayer). Once fluoroquinolone resistance has developed, a later generation of drug may not be beneficial.[23] *In vitro*, pradofloxacin, a third-generation fluoroquinolone, outperformed other fluoroquinolones in terms of potency and efficacy; enrofloxacin was the least potent second only to ciprofloxacin. Molecular alterations of pradofloxacin allow increased bactericidal activity and decreased propensity for antimicrobial resistance.[22-24] These features make pradofloxacin an attractive choice for susceptible fluoroquinolone-naïve isolates or pathogens with reduced fluoroquinolone susceptibility.[23,25] Currently, pradofloxacin is only licensed for feline skin infections in the United States, whereas the European license includes a wide range of indications for both dogs and cats. One prospective clinical trial ($n = 78$) found pradofloxacin was effective and well tolerated for feline bacterial UTI.[25] In experimental studies, cats treated with six to 10 times the recommended dose did not experience retinal toxicity.[26]

Uncomplicated Infection

Uncomplicated bacterial UTIs are lower tract infections where no underlying structural, neurological, or functional abnormality is identified. Uncomplicated UTIs are usually successfully treated with a 10- to 14-day course of an appropriate antimicrobial agent. If the proper antimicrobial is chosen and administered at the appropriate dosage and frequency, clinical signs should resolve within 48 hours. Additionally, results of a complete urinalysis should improve within this same time frame. If possible, a urine culture should be performed 5 to 7 days after cessation of antimicrobial therapy. Uncomplicated infections are rare in cats because of their inherent resistance to bacterial UTIs, so there is typically a predisposing cause.

Complicated Infection

Many cats have identifiable predisposing causes for bacterial UTI (e.g., CKD, diabetes mellitus, etc.) and should be considered to have a complicated bacterial UTI. Antimicrobials are usually administered for 4 to 6 weeks. Urine should be evaluated in the first week of treatment for response to therapy and prior to discontinuing therapy. After antimicrobial therapy, prophylactic antibiotic treatment may be necessary in order to control bacterial UTI that are difficult to eradicate or are frequently recurrent (see later).

Recurrent Infection

Relapse

A *relapse* is defined as recurrence of a bacterial UTI due to the same organism. Relapses usually occur within days to weeks of discontinuing antimicrobial therapy and are due to failure to eradicate the organism. Possible causes include poor owner compliance, use of an inappropriate antimicrobial agent, or administering an appropriate antimicrobial agent at an inappropriate dosage, frequency, or duration. Alternatively, the organism may be deep-seated in the urinary tract, such as chronic pyelonephritis. Uropathogenic *E. coli* may remain quiescent within the host bladder epithelial cells for a period of time before recrudescence. A urine culture should be evaluated prior to reinstituting antimicrobial therapy. Additionally, further diagnostic evaluation for predisposing causes or a nidus of infection is indicated.

Refractory

A refractory infection is similar to a relapsing infection, but there is a persistently positive culture during treatment despite *in vitro* susceptibility to an antimicrobial. Bacteriuria is not eliminated during or after treatment.[29]

Reinfection

Reinfection is defined as a recurrence caused by a different organism than was initially present. Reinfections usually occur at a later time (weeks to months) after cessation of antimicrobial therapy. Although predisposing risk factors may be present, some animals that become reinfected may not have identifiable risk factors. If reinfections are infrequent, each episode may be treated as an uncomplicated bacterial UTI. However, if reinfections occur at a frequency of more than three episodes per year, then animals should be treated as having a complicated bacterial UTI. Additionally, prophylactic antimicrobial therapy may be indicated.

There are no good studies evaluating prophylactic antimicrobial therapy in animals with frequent reinfections. Before prophylactic treatment is undertaken, urine culture and susceptibility testing should be done to ensure that the bacterial UTI has been eradicated. For long-term prophylaxis, a drug that is excreted in high concentration in urine and unlikely to cause adverse effects is selected. Often a fluoroquinolone, cephalosporin, or beta-lactam antimicrobial is chosen. The antimicrobial agent is administered at approximately one-third of the therapeutic daily dose immediately after the patient has voided, at a time when the drug and its metabolites will be retained in the urinary tract for 6 to 8 hours (typically at night). The drug is given for a minimum of 6 months. Urine samples, preferably collected by cystocentesis (not by catheterization because this may induce bacterial UTI), are collected every 4 to 8 weeks for urinalysis and quantitative urine culture. If the sample is free of infection, then prophylactic treatment is continued. If bacterial UTI is identified, active (break-through) infection is treated as a complicated bacterial UTI prior to returning to a prophylactic strategy. If a break-through bacterial UTI does not occur after 6 months of prophylactic antimicrobial therapy, then treatment may be discontinued and the patient should be monitored for reinfection.

Superinfection

A superinfection occurs when a second bacterial organism is isolated while an animal is receiving antimicrobial therapy. Oftentimes, this organism displays a high degree of antimicrobial resistance. A bacterial UTI that occurs in an animal with an indwelling catheter that is receiving antimicrobial therapy is an example of a superinfection.

Asymptomatic Bacteriuria

Asymptomatic bacteriuria is a common and often benign finding in healthy women. Risk factors include pregnancy, diabetes mellitus, spinal cord injury, indwelling urinary catheter, and being an elderly nursing home resident. Women with asymptomatic bacteriuria have more frequent symptomatic episodes, but antimicrobial treatment does not decrease the number of episodes. A benefit to treatment has not been found with clinical trials in humans, and potential complications of treatment include adverse drug reactions and the development of antimicrobial resistance.[27] In one veterinary study, approximately 10% to 15% of cats presented for hyperthyroidism, diabetes mellitus, or CKD had asymptomatic bacteriuria.[28] There are no prospective studies comparing clinical outcomes in cats with and without antimicrobial treatment for asymptomatic bacteriuria. Treatment is not recommended for asymptomatic bacteriuria, unless there is high risk for ascending or systemic infection (e.g., immunocompromised patients, CKD, etc.).[29]

Ancillary Therapies

A number of strategies have been used in humans to prevent recurrent bacterial UTI, including cranberry extracts, D-mannose, methenamine hippurate, and gastrointestinal (GI) probiotics. Randomized controlled trials are required to support the efficacy and safety of these therapies in veterinary species before they can be recommended for common clinical use.[29]

Proanthocyanidin, the "active ingredient" in cranberry, alters the genotypic or phenotypic expression of fimbriae, which subsequently inhibits *E. coli* adherence to human bladder and vaginal epithelial cells. In meta-analysis ($n = 1049$), humans supplemented with cranberry products had fewer UTI episodes over a 12-month period compared to placebo.[30] There are few veterinary studies in healthy dogs and no feline studies.[31,32] Additionally, quality and potency is variable among over-the-counter products; ideally each formulation would be tested in the species of interest. The consensus of the Antimicrobial Guidelines Working Group of the International Society for Companion Animal Infectious Diseases is that there is insufficient evidence to support use of cranberry extract to prevent recurrent UTIs in dogs and cats.[29]

D-mannose anecdotally is used to prevent recurrent UTI, but there are no studies of clinical efficacy in veterinary patients. The D-mannose sugar competitively binds to mannose-fimbriae on certain *E. coli* strains, which inhibits adhesion to the uroepithelium. There is little data available for other bacteria that may express mannose fimbriae. In a small unblinded randomized clinical trial ($n = 308$) over 6 months, women that received D-mannose had a significantly reduced episodes of recurrent UTI compared to placebo.[33]

Methenamine hippurate is a urinary antiseptic that is converted to formaldehyde in an acidic environment (urine pH < 5.5). Methenamine is poorly tolerated by feline patients. Gastrointestinal upset is the most commonly reported adverse event. Studies of safety, efficacy, and appropriate dosing are lacking.

The GI microbiome has immunomodulatory effects throughout the body, and alteration of the microbiome is thought to impact the immune response in distant locations. Additionally, the GI microbiome may impact the vaginal microflora. Alterations of vaginal microflora may play a role in establishment of UTI. For example, women with recurrent UTI often have depletion of vaginal *Lactobacillus* spp., whereas increased vaginal colonization with *Lactobacillus* spp. is associated with reduced numbers of recurrent UTI.[34] Probiotics on the market vary by bacterial species, potency (number of CFUs), and viability. Prospective studies are needed to evaluate the role of probiotics for lower urinary tract disease in veterinary species.

PREVENTION

Iatrogenic Infection

Normal host defense mechanisms are effective in preventing bacterial UTIs; however, they are not impenetrable. Normal host defenses may be overwhelmed if large quantities of a virulent uropathogen are introduced into the urinary tract during diagnostic and therapeutic procedures. Iatrogenic bacterial UTI is a common complication of indwelling urinary catheters, especially if an open-ended system is used.

In a clinical study, infection developed in 52% of dogs and cats with indwelling urinary catheters; risk of infection increased with duration of catheterization.[35] Use of indwelling urinary catheters during diuresis or corticosteroid administration is particularly dangerous. The risk of infection is further compounded if the patient has pre-existing urinary tract disease.

Iatrogenic bacterial UTIs may be prevented by (1) avoiding indiscriminate use of urinary catheters, (2) using a closed system of collection when indwelling urinary catheters are used, (3) being cautious about use of indwelling urinary catheters when patients are undergoing diuresis, (4) avoiding indwelling catheters in patients that are immunosuppressed or receiving immunosuppressive medications such as glucocorticoids, (5) using antimicrobials appropriately with urinary catheterization, and (6) using diagnostic and therapeutic techniques that minimize trauma and microbial contamination of the urinary tract. Although it seems logical to administer antimicrobial agents while an indwelling urinary catheter is inserted in an effort to decrease iatrogenic infection, the practice is strongly discouraged. Concomitant oral or parenteral administration of antimicrobial agents during indwelling urethral catheterization reduces the frequency of developing a bacterial UTI; however, it promotes development of UTI caused by multidrug-resistant bacteria.[35]

It is not necessary to treat bacteriuria associated with an indwelling catheter if there is no clinical or cytological evidence of infection. There is no evidence to support routine urine culture or culture of the urinary catheter tip following removal in asymptomatic patients; such cultures do not predict the development of catheter-associated infection.[29] In contrast, urine culture is always indicated for a patient with clinical signs of UTI, fever of undetermined origin, or abnormal urine cytology (i.e., hematuria, pyuria). If the patient develops new clinical signs or fever after a urinary catheter has been placed, then, ideally, the urine catheter is removed and a cystocentesis is performed to provide a sample for culture once the bladder fills. Alternatively, the original urinary catheter is replaced and a urine sample is collected through the second catheter. It is less ideal to sample the urine through the original catheter, and a sample from the collection bag should never be used.[29]

For patients that develop a catheter-associated UTI, treatment is more likely to be successful if the catheter can be removed. The infection may be treated as uncomplicated if there is not a history of recurrent infection and there are no relevant comorbidities. Otherwise, the infection should be treated as complicated with 4 to 6 weeks of an appropriate antimicrobial based on the culture and sensitivity.[29]

Eradication of Underlying Cause(s)

Although antimicrobial agents are the cornerstone of treatment of bacterial UTI, they should be used in a logical fashion. A bacterial UTI occurs in association with compromise of host defense mechanisms, which may be transient or permanent. Transient compromise often results in development of a simple of uncomplicated UTI; however, permanent compromise results in development of complicated UTI. Evaluation for and correction or control of the compromise(s) in host defense mechanisms is important in treating UTI, especially with recurrent UTI.

NONBACTERIAL URINARY TRACT INFECTION

Fungal

Fungal UTI is rare in cats. Funguria may be due to primary infections of the lower urinary tract, or secondary to shedding of fungal elements into the urine in animals with systemic infections. Diagnosis of fungal UTI most commonly occurs by identification of fungal elements during routine or concentrated urine sediment examination; clinical signs are indistinguishable from bacterial UTI or other causes of lower urinary tract disease.

Primary fungal UTI is most commonly due to *Candida* spp., a commensal inhabitant of the genital mucosa, upper respiratory tract, and GI tract in cats.[36,37] *Candida albicans* is the most commonly identified species, followed by *Candida glabrata* and *Candida tropicalis*. Other ubiquitous fungi may also occasionally cause primary fungal UTI, including *Aspergillus* spp. and *Cryptococcus* spp. As with bacterial UTI, fungal UTI occurs due to temporary or permanent breaches in local or systemic immunity of the lower urinary tract. In the two largest retrospective studies of fungal UTI in dogs and cats, the most commonly identified concurrent diseases were diabetes mellitus, lower urinary tract neoplasia (particularly transitional cell carcinoma), and urinary tract stomata, including perineal urethrostomy or cystotomy tubes.[36,37] Additional conditions, which may predispose to development of fungal (and particularly candidal) UTIs, include antimicrobial or corticosteroids administered within 1 month, nonurogenital neoplasia, and noncandidal urogenital diseases.

Treatment of animals with fungal UTI involves correction or control of the predisposing cause or causes and administration of antifungal drugs. Fluconazole is recommended as initial treatment in most patients because of its high margin of safety, sensitivity of most strains of *Candida* spp. to the drug, and excretion of active drug into urine in high concentrations. *Candida* spp. other than *C. albicans* are more likely to be resistant to fluconazole, and antifungal sensitivity testing is recommended to determine if a higher dose of fluconazole is appropriate or if another drug should be used. Although amphotericin B is renally excreted and achieves high concentration in urine, it is not often used because it is parenterally administered and nephrotoxic. Other commonly used antifungal drugs, including itraconazole and ketoconazole, are not renally excreted in active form.

Primary fungal UTIs should always be treated as complicated infections, with a minimum of 6 to 8 weeks of antifungal therapy and regular monitoring during and after cessation of therapy. Infections that fail to respond completely to fluconazole should be recultured and antifungal sensitivity testing performed. Some susceptible isolates may respond to intravesicular administration of 1% clotrimazole or amphotericin B.[38-40] Urinary alkalinization has historically been proposed as adjunctive therapy in patients with fungal UTI, because increased urine pH may inhibit fungal growth. However, this is not currently favored for treatment of fungal UTI in people and is of questionable efficacy in veterinary patients.

Secondary fungal UTI occurs due to shedding of organisms into urine in patients with systemic infections. *Cryptococcus* spp. are the most common in cats.[41] These patients should be treated with standard antifungal agents recommended for systemic infections.

Viral

Although viruses are associated with urinary tract disease in humans, their role in urinary tract disease in dogs and cats is unknown. Viral infection of the lower urinary tract may be a cause of lower urinary tract disease in cats.[42]

References

1. Lekcharoensuk C, Osborne CA, Lulich JP: Epidemiologic study of risk factors for lower urinary tract diseases in cats. *J Am Vet Med Assoc* 218:1429–1435, 2001.
2. Bartges JW, Barsanti JA: Bacterial urinary tract infections in cats. In Bonagura JD, editor: *Current veterinary therapy XIII*, Philadelphia, 2001, Saunders, pp 880–882.
3. Johnson JR, Kaster N, Kuskowski MA, et al: Identification of urovirulence traits in *Escherichia coli* by comparison of urinary and rectal E. coli isolates from dogs with urinary tract infection. *J Clin Microbiol* 41:337–345, 2003.
4. Osborne CA, Caywood DD, Johnston GR, et al: Perineal urethrostomy versus dietary management in prevention of recurrent lower urinary tract disease. *J Small Anim Pract* 32:296–305, 1991.
5. Bartges JW, Finco DR, Polzin DJ, et al: Pathophysiology of urethral obstruction. *Vet Clin North Am Small Anim Pract* 26:255–264, 1996.
6. Ling GV, Norris CR, Franti CE, et al: Interrelations of organism prevalence, specimen collection method, and host age, sex, and breed among 8,354 canine urinary tract infections (1969-1995). *J Vet Intern Med* 15:341–347, 2001.
7. Barsanti JA: Genitourinary infections. In Greene CE, editor: *Infectious diseases of the dog and cat*, ed 4, St Louis, 2012, Elsevier/Saunders, pp 1013–1031.
8. Litster A, Moss SM, Honnery M, et al: Prevalence of bacterial species in cats with clinical signs of lower urinary tract disease: recognition of *Staphylococcus felis* as a possible feline urinary tract pathogen. *Vet Microbiol* 121:182–188, 2007.
9. Litster A, Thompson M, Moss S, et al: Feline bacterial urinary tract infections: an update on an evolving clinical problem. *Vet J* 187:18–22, 2011.
10. Jang SS, Ling GV, Yamamoto R, et al: Mycoplasma as a cause of canine urinary tract infection. *J Am Vet Med Assoc* 185:45–47, 1984.
11. Ulgen M, Cetin C, Senturk S, et al: Urinary tract infections due to *Mycoplasma canis* in dogs. *J Vet Med A Physiol Pathol Clin Med* 53:379–382, 2006.
12. Abou N, Houwers DJ, van Dongen AM: PCR-based detection reveals no causative role

CHAPTER 52 Urinary Tract Infection 517

for *Mycoplasma* and *Ureaplasma* in feline lower urinary tract disease. *Vet Microbiol* 116:246–247, 2006.

13. Bartges JW, Blanco L: Bacterial urinary tract infections in cats. *Compend Stand Care* 3:1–5, 2001.

14. Davidson AP, Ling GV, Stevens F, et al: Urinary tract infection in cats: a retrospective study (1977-1989). *California Vet* 46:32–34, 1992.

15. Oluoch AO, Kim CH, Weisiger RM, et al: Nonenteric *Escherichia coli* isolates from dogs: 674 cases (1990-1998). *J Am Vet Med Assoc* 218:381–384, 2001.

16. Ghanbarpour R: Detection of β-lactamase and urovirulence genes in *Escherichia coli* serogroups isolated from urinary tract infection in cats. *Comp Clin Pathol* 22:591–596, 2013.

17. Siqueira AK: Virulence factors in *Escherichia coli* strains isolated from urinary tract infection and pyometra cases and from feces of healthy dogs. *Res Vet Sci* 86:206–210, 2009.

18. Senior DF, deMan P, Svanborg C: Serotype, hemolysin production, and adherence characteristics of strains of *Escherichia coli* causing urinary tract infection in dogs. *Am J Vet Res* 53:494–498, 1992.

19. Yuri K, Nakata K, Katae H, et al: Serotypes and virulence factors of *Escherichia coli* strains isolated from dogs and cats. *J Vet Med Sci* 61:37–40, 1999.

20. Vail DM, Allen TA, Weiser G: Applicability of leukocyte esterase test strip in detection of canine pyuria. *J Am Vet Med Assoc* 189:1451–1453, 1986.

21. Barsanti JA, Brown J, Marks A, et al: Relationship of lower urinary tract signs to seropositivity for feline immunodeficiency virus in cats. *J Vet Intern Med* 10:34–38, 1996.

22. Boone D, Smaha T, Carpenter M, et al: Antimicrobial resistance and pharmacodynamics of canine and feline pathogenic *E. coli* in the United States. *J Am Anim Hosp Assoc* 48:379–389, 2012.

23. Liu X, Booth DM, Jin Y, et al: *In vitro* potency and efficacy favor later generation fluoroqui-nolones for treatment of canine and feline *Escherichia coli* uropathogens in the United States. *World J Microbiol Biotechnol* 29:347–354, 2013.

24. Lees P: Pharmacokinetics, pharmacodynamics and therapeutics of pradofloxacin in the dog and cat. *J Vet Pharmacol Ther* 36:209–221, 2013.

25. Litster A, Moss S, Honnery M, et al: Clinical efficacy and palatability of pradofloxacin 2.5% oral suspension for the treatment of bacterial lower urinary tract infections in cats. *J Vet Intern Med* 21:990–995, 2007.

26. Messias A, Gekeler F, Wegener A, et al: Retinal safety of a new fluoroquinolones, pradofloxacin, in cats: assessment with electroretinography. *Doc Ophthalmol* 116:177–191, 2008.

27. Nicolle LE: Asymptomatic bacteriuria: review and discussion of the IDSA guidelines. *Int J Antimicrob Agents* 28:S42–S48, 2006.

28. Litster AL, Moss S, Platell J, et al: Urinary tract infections in cats with hyperthyroidism, diabetes mellitus and chronic kidney disease. *J Feline Med Surg* 9:124–132, 2009.

29. Weese J, Blondeau JM, Boothe D, et al: Antimicrobial use guidelines for treatment of urinary tract disease in dogs and cats: antimicrobial guidelines Working Group of the International Society for Companion Animal Infectious Diseases. *Vet Med Int* Article ID 263768:1-9 2011.

30. Gupta K, Chou M, Howell A, et al: Cranberry products inhibit adherence of p-fimbriated *Escherichia coli* to primary cultured bladder and vaginal epithelial cells. *J Urol* 177:2357–2360, 2007.

31. Howell AB, Griffin DW, Whalen MO, et al: Inhibition of p-fimbriated *Escherichia coli* adhesion in an innovational ex-vivo model in dogs receiving a bioactive cranberry tablet (Crananidin). *J Vet Intern Med* 24:660, 2010. (Abstract).

32. Smee N, Grauer GF, Schermerhorn T: Investigations into the effect of cranberry extract on bacterial adhesion to canine uroepithelial cells. *J Vet Intern Med* 25:722–723, 2011. (Abstract).

33. Kranjcec B, Papes D, Altrac S, et al: D-mannose powder for prophylaxis of recurrent urinary tract infections in women: a randomized clinical trial. *World J Urol* 32(1):79–84, 2014.

34. Petricevic L, Unger FM, Viernstein H, et al: Randomized, double-blind, placebo-controlled study of oral lactobacilli to improve the vaginal flora of postmenopausal women. *Eur J Obstet Gynecol Reprod Biol* 141:54–57, 2008.

35. Barsanti JA, Blue J, Edmunds J: Urinary tract infection due to indwelling bladder catheters in dogs and cats. *J Am Vet Med Assoc* 187:384–388, 1985.

36. Jin Y, Lin D: Fungal urinary tract infections in the dog and cat: a retrospective study (2001-2004). *J Am Anim Hosp Assoc* 41:373–381, 2005.

37. Pressler BM, Vaden SL, Lane IF, et al: *Candida* spp. urinary tract infections in 13 dogs and seven cats: predisposing factors, treatment, and outcome. *J Am Anim Hosp Assoc* 39:263–270, 2003.

38. Forward ZA, Legendre AM, Khalsa HD: Use of intermittent bladder infusion with clotrimazole for treatment of candiduria in a dog. *J Am Vet Med Assoc* 220:1496–1498, 1474–1495, 2002.

39. Toll J, Ashe CM, Trepanier LA: Intravesical administration of clotrimazole for treatment of candiduria in a cat with diabetes mellitus. *J Am Vet Med Assoc* 223:1156–1158, 1129, 2003.

40. Pressler BM: Urinary tract infections—fungal. In Polzin DJ, Bartges JW, editors: *Nephrology and urology of small animals*, Ames, IA, 2011, Blackwell, pp 717–724.

41. Gerds-Grogan S, Dayrell-Hart B: Feline cryptococcosis: a retrospective evaluation. *J Am Anim Hosp Assoc* 33:118–122, 1997.

42. Kruger JM, Osborne CA, Venta PJ, et al: Viral infections of the feline urinary tract. *Vet Clin North Am Small Anim Pract* 26(2):281–296, 1996.

Feline Idiopathic Cystitis

Jodi L. Westropp and C.A.Tony Buffington

Signs referable to the lower urinary tract (LUT) are among the most common reasons cats are presented to veterinarians for care. These signs can include stranguria, hematuria, periuria, dysuria, or a combination of these. Differentials the clinician should consider for these clinical signs include urolithiasis, urinary tract infection (UTI), neoplasia of the urinary tract, and anatomical abnormalities of the LUT. When no underlying cause can be diagnosed, the disease is often referred to as feline idiopathic (interstitial) cystitis (FIC). The name for this group of diseases has gone through several changes over the years. In 1984, Osborne and colleagues[1] recommended that replacement of the then commonly used term "feline urologic syndrome (FUS)", "would be of considerable value because it would help to eliminate the stereotypical approach to treatment and prevention of feline urological syndrome that is currently in vogue." They "suggest that the term FUS be substituted with descriptive terms pertaining to the site (urethra, bladder, and so on), causes (bacteria, parasites, neoplasms, metabolic disturbances, idiopathic forms, and so on), morphologic changes (inflammation, neoplasia, and so on), and pathophysiologic mechanisms (obstructive uropathy, reflex dyssynergia, and so on) whenever possible. In this fashion, the same terminology and approach to diagnosis and treatment used for other species (dogs, humans, and so on) will more likely be used for cats."

This recommendation is at least as important today as it was when it was originally written, and repeated 12 years later in 1996.[2] Unfortunately, the 1984 chapter was subtitled, "Feline Lower Urinary Tract Disease with Heterogeneous Causes," which appears to have had the unintended consequence of replacement of one acronym, "FUS," with another "FLUTD." Such terms should likely be retired, as the most research now suggests that these signs might reflect a disease affecting the bladder or LUT and *not* a problem intrinsic to the LUT itself.

Researchers and clinicians are now looking beyond the bladder and considering the whole individual when evaluating these cases. This change came as the result of studies using cats with severe, recurrent LUT signs (LUTS) (and variable comorbidities) as a model of a chronic pain syndrome in humans called interstitial cystitis (IC). As in veterinary medicine, the names to describe the human syndrome are also in flux and include painful bladder syndrome/IC, bladder hypersensitivity syndrome, and bladder pain syndrome.

Names such as FUS or FLUTD to describe recurrent LUTS may therefore be oversimplified and focused on the end organ, rather than the current understanding of this disease. A name like "Pandora syndrome" for some of these cats has been proposed, for at least two reasons. First, it does not identify any specific cause or organ, and second, it seems to capture the dismay and dispute associated with the identification of so many problems outside the organ of interest of any particular subspecialty.[3]

Clinical research on IC has certainly expanded and identified genetic[4] and epigenetic influences,[5] documented that the time course of the appearance of comorbid disorders often occurs before the LUTS,[6] and shown again how much systemic involvement occurs in most patients.[7] Similar to humans, evidence has accumulated that additional problems outside the LUT are commonly present in cats.[3] This evidence has led to reconsideration of the cause(s) of the syndrome in these individuals, as well as to considerable debate about the most appropriate name, diagnostic approach, and treatment recommendations. Regardless of the name used for this "syndrome," the clinician must take a "global" approach when obtaining a history, performing the physical examinations, and considering pertinent diagnostics and therapeutics to manage the clinical signs of the patient. However, to avoid confusion for this chapter, the authors shall still refer to this syndrome as FIC because it was what was used at the time the results were published.

RISK FACTORS FOR FELINE INTERSTITIAL CYSTITIS

Cats with FIC can be presented for an initial occurrence of clinical signs and may not return for care because of a presumed improvement in the condition, or can return with recurrent signs of disease. Both sexes appear to be affected equally. Although FIC can be obstructive or nonobstructive in its presentation, urethral obstruction is far more common in male cats, with no difference reported between intact and castrated males.[8] In addition to genetic and possible early adverse life events, other risk factors for FIC have been reported, which include excessive body weight, decreased activity, multicat households, and indoor housing.[9] Environmental stressors such as conflict with another cat in the household have also been identified as risk factors.[10]

HISTOPATHOLOGY

Histologically, FIC can be classified in two different forms, nonulcerative (type I) and ulcerative (type II). Cats with FIC almost always present with the nonulcerative form; however, the classic Hunner's ulcers seen in humans (type II) have been described rarely in cats.[11] It is possible that the etiopathogenesis of these two forms of FIC are different. In humans with IC, those with Hunner's ulcers (about 10% of patients) have more mononuclear cellular infiltrates in the perineural and perivascular areas of the bladder and can show urothelial spongiosis and detachment.[12] These patients also generally are older and appear to respond to cystectomy. In contrast, the more common nonulcerative subtype (about 90% of patients) lacks the inflammatory cellular infiltrates and might be associated with neuroendocrine abnormalities (see the following discussion). It has been shown in research on the bladder of cats with chronic FIC that histopathologic changes are generally nonspecific and may include an intact or damaged urothelium with submucosal edema, dilation of submucosal blood vessels with marginated neutrophils, submucosal hemorrhage, and sometimes increased mast cell density.[13] Histopathologic abnormalities are usually not specific for FIC, and lesions present are not pathognomonic for the disease. Therefore, bladder biopsies are not routinely recommended for cats suspected to have FIC.

RESEARCH ON INFECTIOUS EITOLOGY FOR FELINE INTERSTITIAL CYSTITIS

The role of viruses has been and continues to be evaluated in cats that present with FIC.[14,15] The feline caliciviruses (FCVs), FCV-U1 and FCV-U2, have been the most studied. Feline calicivirus viruria was detected in cats described as having FLUTD and in cats with upper respiratory infections; however, its etiologic significance was not ascertained.[16] Serological results suggested increased FCV exposure in cats with FLUTD, as compared with controls. A weak association between seropositivity for *Bartonella* spp. and FIC has also been reported.[17] What, if any, relationship these infectious agents play in the etiopathogenesis of LUTS in FIC thus remains unknown at this time, and to the authors' knowledge their role(s), if any, in the systemic manifestations of the syndrome have not been reported.

Although microorganisms in the LUT might not commonly cause FIC or IC, this does not mean that microbes have no association with LUTS. A report of 134 cats in Norway evaluated for LUTS found bacteriuria exceeding 10^3 colony-forming units (CFU)/mL in 44 (33%) cats, and exceeding 10^4 CFU/mL in 33 (25%), either alone or with variable combinations of crystals and uroliths.[18] These results suggested a prevalence of bacteriuria higher than reported previously, which the authors speculated might have resulted from differences between cases diagnosed at primary and tertiary care facilities. However, it may represent geographical differences in UTI distribution. In humans, one study found evidence of UTI within the past 2 years in 38% of the painful bladder syndrome/IC patients studied, although,[7] "…the infection domain was not associated with any increased symptoms." It also has been speculated that intrinsic abnormalities of the LUT make it more vulnerable to microbial colonization,[19] which might be consistent with the observation of increased risk for bacterial UTI in patients with FIC and IC.

BLADDER AND SYSTEMATIC ABNORMALITIES IN FELINE INTERSTITIAL CYSTITIS

It has been proposed that the urothelial cells themselves can be targets of various stimuli, including adenosine triphosphate and nitric oxide, which could potentiate inflammation and exacerbate clinical signs.[20] The urothelial cells themselves can be targets of these mediators and potentiate this inflammation. The bladder (and nonbladder) sensory neurons in cats with FIC exhibit an increased excitability to physical and chemical stimuli as compared with unaffected cats.[21] Sympathoneural-epithelial interactions appear to play an important role in permeability. Birder and colleagues[22] have shown that application of norepinephrine to urinary bladder strips induced the release of nitric oxide from the urinary bladder epithelium. Application of capsaicin resulted in the release of nitric oxide from epithelium, as well as nervous tissue in the urinary bladder. In light of reports that nitric oxide may increase permeability in the urothelium[23,24] (and elsewhere[25,26]), these results suggest that some of the sympathetically mediated alterations in permeability may be mediated by norepinephrine via this mechanism.

In humans presenting with LUTS, urodynamic evaluations are often performed to rule out other urinary tract diseases, such as overactive bladder, that could account for the clinical signs. Although a decrease in bladder compliance has been found in cats with FIC, no evidence of spontaneous bladder contractions (overactive bladder) was noted in female cats with FIC when cystometrograms were evaluated.[27] However, increased urethral closure pressures were noted in FIC cats compared with healthy cats, despite a lack of clinical signs at the time the studies were performed.

A variety of abnormalities have been identified in dorsal root ganglion cell bodies of both bladder-identified and non-bladder neurons from cats with FIC.[21] Cells from affected cats were 30% larger, expressed altered neuropeptide profiles, and exhibited slowly desensitizing, capsaicin-induced currents related to increased protein kinase C-mediated phosphorylation of the transient receptor potential vanilloid-1 receptor. Similar findings were observed in dorsal root ganglion cells throughout the lumbosacral (L4-S3) spinal cord, suggesting widespread abnormalities of sensory neuron function.

Clinical signs of FIC can wax and wane, and appear to be exacerbated by internal and external stressors. In the brain, significant increases in tyrosine hydroxylase (TH) immunoreactivity, the rate-limiting enzyme of catecholamine synthesis, have been identified in the pontine locus coeruleus[28] and the paraventricular nucleus of the hypothalamus[29] of cats with FIC. Moreover, chronic stress can increase TH activity in the locus coeruleus,[30] with accompanying increases in autonomic outflow.[31] The locus coeruleus contains the largest number of noradrenergic neurons; it is the most important source of norepinephrine in the feline (and human) central nervous system. It is involved in such global brain functions as vigilance, arousal, and analgesia, and appears to mediate visceral responses to stress.[32] The increased TH immunoreactivity observed in the locus coeruleus of cats with FIC may provide a clue to the observation that clinical signs of FIC in cats follow a waxing-and-waning course and can be aggravated by environmental stressors.[33,34]

The acoustic startle response is a brainstem reflex in response to unexpected loud stimuli that is amplified in cats with FIC. The acoustic startle response in cats with FIC is greatest and most different from that of healthy cats during stressful situations, but is still greater in cats with FIC than in healthy cats, even when adapted to enriched housing conditions.[35]

Enhanced stimulus-induced local norepinephrine release from the bladder[36] could lead to a functional desensitization of the central alpha-2 adrenoceptors in cats with FIC.[37] In the brainstem (particularly the area of the locus coeruleus), α-2 agonists inhibit norepinephrine release, whereas in the spinal cord they inhibit transmission of nociceptive input to the brain.[38] A functional desensitization of α-2 adrenergic receptors in affected cats also has been identified by evaluating their response to the selective α-2 adrenergic receptor agonist, medetomidine, in both *in vivo* and *in vitro* studies.[36,37]

In addition to the sympathetic nervous system, abnormalities in the hypothalamic-pituitary-adrenal axis (HPA) have also been observed in cats with FIC. After a high dose (125 μg) of synthetic adrenocorticotropic hormone was administered, cats with FIC had significantly decreased serum cortisol responses as compared with healthy cats.[39] Although no obvious adrenal abnormalities were identified by histopathology, morphometric analysis revealed that the areas consisting of the zonae fasciculata and reticularis were significantly smaller in sections of glands from cats with FIC than in glands from healthy cats. Therefore, it appears that although the sympathoneural system is fully activated in this disorder, the adrenocortical component of the HPA axis is not.

EPIGENETIC STUDIES

Recent research suggests that one mechanism underlying the sensitization of the stress response system involves a process called epigenetic modulation of gene expression (Figure 53-1).[40] Epigenetic modulation of gene expression is a prominent candidate mechanism for the exaggerated stress responsiveness found in cats with FIC because it has been shown to occur in the offspring of pregnant females exposed to stressors, and to result in long-term neuroendocrine abnormalities.[41] Importantly, research in both rodents[42] and cats[33,37,43] has demonstrated that effective environmental enrichment can mitigate many of the effects of early life adversity.

COMORBIDITIES

A study of healthy cats and cats with FIC found that environmental stressors resulted in increased number of sickness

The role of the environment

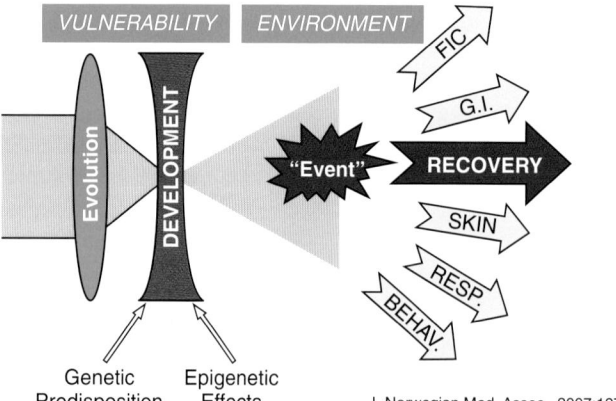

J. Norwegian Med. Assoc.. 2007;127:3228-31

Figure 53-1: Hypothesis for Epigenetic and Environmental Influences in Cats. Depending on conditions, developmental trajectories may be modified by variable combinations of genetic predispositions and epigenetic events during the period of development. The environment can further modify the cat's trajectory. Many cats also experience "events" during early life, such as infection or trauma from which most recover. In a subset, however, recovery does not occur, and these may go on to develop a variety of adverse outcomes. (Adapted from Kirkengen AL, Ulvestad E: Heavy burdens and complex disease—an integrated perspective. *Tidsskr Nor Lægeforen* 2007;127:3228–3231.)

FIC, Feline idiopathic (interstitial) cystitis; *GI,* gastrointestinal.

behaviors (e.g., vomiting, lethargy, and anorexia) in cats with FIC when the results were controlled for other factors.[44] Further, cats with FIC have a variable combination of comorbid disorders[9,45-47] such as behavioral, endocrine, cardiovascular, and gastrointestinal problems. Therefore, it is imperative that a complete physical examination and detailed environmental history be evaluated in these cats and that the examination does not focus entirely on the bladder. Most humans with IC also suffer from variable combinations of comorbid disorders that affect a variety of other body systems. That patients with FIC and IC have variable combinations of other comorbid disorders raises the question of the extent to which a different etiology affects each organ versus the extent to which some common disorder affects all organs, which then respond in their own characteristic ways.

CLINICAL IMPLICATIONS OF RESEARCH

Based on the evidence available to date, some cats evaluated for chronic LUTS might instead have a "Pandora syndrome." Given the comorbid disorders sometimes found in cats with various chronic disorders, other presentations of the syndrome seem likely. Based on these observations, and on the current limited understanding of the many factors potentially involved, a reasonable diagnostic strategy for cats with chronic clinical signs referable to a particular organ system might be to conduct a comprehensive investigation of the animal's history, environment, and other organ system function. Additional supportive data might include evidence of early adverse experience (e.g., orphaned or abandoned), presence of related signs in family members, waxing-and-waning of signs related to environmental threat, and the absence of evidence for an alternative cause. Evidence for the presence of these additional factors would support a diagnosis of "Pandora syndrome," whereas evidence of absence of these factors would argue for an organ-specific disorder.

APPROACH TO THE PATIENT

Diagnostic Biomarkers

When choosing the appropriate diagnostic tests for a cat that presents with LUTS, several factors must be considered, including the number of episodes that the cat has had, the severity of the cat's clinical signs, and how much the owner is willing or able to spend. No well-accepted diagnostic test for FIC currently exists. In humans, various markers such as antiproliferative factor and heparin-binding epidermal growth factor[48] have been investigated, but these are not clinically available. Similarly, biomarkers in cats have also been investigated. A decrease in trefoil factor 2 has been documented in both obstructed and nonobstructed cats with FIC. The researchers suggested that this reflects an impaired ability for bladder repair and immune response, as well as a greater susceptibility to inflammation.[49] The same group of researchers also reported that fibronectin concentrations were increased in the urine of cats with FIC.[50] Fibronectin is involved in cell adhesion and migration, wound healing, and clot stabilization. These biomarkers may be altered because of the secondary changes that occur in the bladder, particularly when urethral obstruction is present.

In humans and cats, findings suggest the potential usefulness of infrared microspectroscopy as a serum biomarker in the diagnosis of FIC.[51] Differences in the intermediate compounds of tryptophan and its metabolites were found in cats (and humans) with IC. These data were analyzed in cats that had been diagnosed with FIC, but may not have had clinical signs at the time of sampling. This test was still able to differentiate FIC from control cats. Interestingly, the kynurenine pathway for tryptophan metabolism appears to play a role in the pathobiology of a variety of altered mood states. However, the specificity of this diagnostic test must be evaluated further, and it is not available for commercial use at this time. Therefore, FIC currently remains a diagnosis of exclusion.

Diagnostic Tests

Because approximately 20% of cats that present with LUTS have cystic calculi, abdominal radiography is recommended; abdominal ultrasonography of cats with urethral obstruction generally is not as helpful because the urethra cannot be imaged well. If a cat presents with a urethral obstruction, abdominal radiographs should be obtained before decompressive cystocentesis, as long as the cat is stable. A urinalysis and urine bacterial culture should be evaluated at least once, but most young, otherwise healthy cats do not have a true bacterial cystitis. However, aerobic bacterial urine cultures should be evaluated in cats with LUTS that have had previous urethral catheterizations or a perineal urethrostomy, as these procedures increase the incidence of bacterial UTIs. Advanced diagnostic tests such as contrast cystourethrography, abdominal ultrasonography, and even cystoscopy can be performed for recurrent cases to be certain that no other disease that could account for the clinical signs is present. A diagnostic algorithm for assessing cats with LUTS is presented in Figure 53-2.

INITIAL MANAGEMENT

Although some cases of presumed FIC may appear to resolve quickly and not recur, the clinician should be aware that the patient's environmental needs are likely not being met. In addition to environmental alteration (see also the following discussion), analgesic therapy for initial management of LUTS should be provided. Providing analgesia with narcotics such as oral transmucosal buprenorphine (0.01 mg/kg every 8 to 12 hours), butorphanol (0.2 mg/kg subcutaneously [SC] or orally [PO] every 8 to 12 hours), or a fentanyl patch can be used, depending on the severity of the pain. Nonsteroidal anti-inflammatory drugs have also been described for this disease, with variable results. Because of the risk for

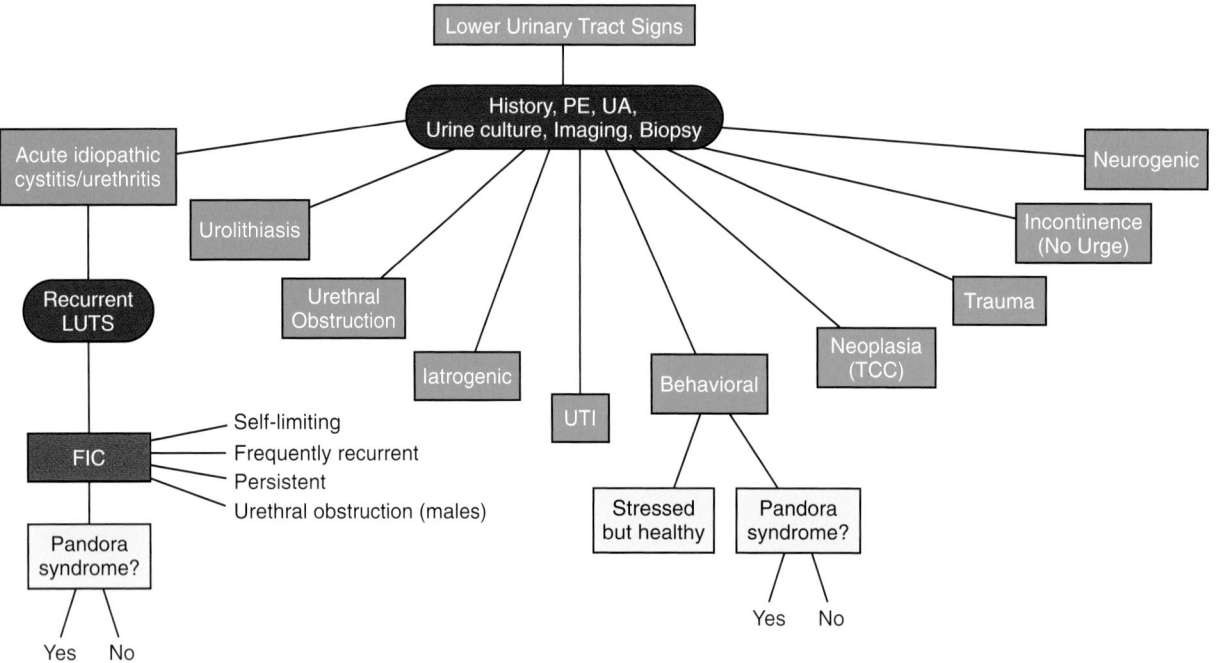

Figure 53-2: A diagnostic algorithm for assessing cats with lower urinary tract signs. *FIC,* Feline idiopathic (interstitial) cystitis; *LUTS,* lower urinary tract signs; *PE,* physical examination; *TCC,* transitional cell carcinoma; *UA,* urinalysis; *UTI,* urinary tract infection.

dehydration-associated reductions in blood flow to the kidneys and the potential for acute kidney injury, these medications might increase the risk for adverse outcomes. Further, they have not been found to benefit humans with IC and are not routinely recommended.

CHRONIC MANAGEMENT

Environmental Alterations

No cure is currently available for cats with FIC; treatment options are aimed at clinical recovery, keeping the cat's clinical signs to a minimum, and increasing the disease-free survival. After the diagnosis of FIC is made, a thorough environmental history, as well as notation of all other comorbidities present, must be obtained so that the clinician can establish that all the environmental needs of the cat have been met. A nurse/technician-based program, in which a staff member works with these patients as often as necessary, can help ensure that owners understand the disease process enough to feel comfortable with managing their cat's disease.

Following a staged approach to therapy that begins with client education and multimodal environmental modifications (MEMO) seems beneficial in many cats with FIC. The MEMO approach to therapy involves obtaining a thorough environmental history, including but not limited to the topics presented in Box 53-1. A detailed client history form as well as additional client and veterinarian resources can be found online at http://indoorpet.osu.edu. Guidelines for meeting the environmental needs of cats have been published by the American Association of Feline Practitioners and the International Society of Feline Medicine.[52]

The owner should complete the questionnaire for all cats in the household. The clinician can then review the list and identify issues that may be contributing to the cat's clinical signs. After the questionnaire is completed, the technician can review it with the owner and agree on helpful modifications.[53,54] Initially, only one or two changes should be recommended so as not to overwhelm the owner or the cat. Proper litter box management should be followed, and a structured MEMO plan should be provided. The goal is to make sure the environmental needs of the cat are met. Based on previous findings, in which catecholamine concentrations decreased and clinical signs improved after environmental modifications, MEMO therapy was found to be successful in most cats with FIC followed over a 1-year period.[43]

As a part of the MEMO therapy, dietary modifications may be warranted and should be discussed with clients. Increasing water intake by feeding canned food, or other methods, such as broths or automatic water dispensers, may or may not be beneficial for cats with FIC. Some hypothesize that added water might help dilute the potential "noxious" stimulants in the urine such as urea and potassium chloride. Potassium chloride has been used as a diagnostic probe for IC in human patients[55] because it has been speculated, but never demonstrated, that the urine potassium concentration plays a role in the pathophysiology of IC. For some cats, canned food or added dietary moisture in the forms described earlier may be a form of environmental enrichment, which might have a positive effect on the cat's clinical signs. Efforts to acidify the urine using dry foods have no proven value in the treatment of cats with FIC; however, if pronounced struvite crystalluria is present in an obstructed male cat, a diet formulated for struvite dissolution may be warranted.

1. Where was the cat was obtained?
2. Number of cats in the household
   - Is intercat conflict an issue?
   - Number and type of other pets?
   - Number of family members?
5. Size and type of the household dwelling
6. Litter boxes
   - Number of litter boxes?
   - How often are they cleaned?
   - How often are they changed?
   - Location in the house?
   - Type of litter used?
   - Depth of litter preferred by the cat?
7. Feeding
   - Type of food (including brand, canned vs dry)?
   - Location of bowls?
   - Food preferences?
   - Is competition for food present in the household?
8. Play and rest activity
   - Preferred toys?
   - Is there space in the house available for play?
   - Preferred type of play?
9. Indoor or outdoor housing status
10. Resting or hiding areas preferred
11. Changes in household
12. Behavioral concerns
    - Aggression?
    - Fear?
    - Nervousness?
    - Separation anxiety?
13. Other sickness behaviors or diseases present

Finally, obesity may be a risk factor for FIC, and implementing an obesity therapy program may be of benefit.[56] All of the cat's needs and concurrent diseases, if present, must be considered when making dietary and environmental recommendations.

Pheromones

Pheromones are fatty acids that transmit highly specific information among animals of the same species. Although the exact mechanisms of action are unknown, pheromones reportedly induce changes in the limbic system and hypothalamus that alter the emotional state of the animal. Feliway (Ceva Animal Health, St. Louis, Missouri) is the synthetic F3 fraction of the naturally occurring feline facial pheromone. Treatment with this pheromone has been reported to reduce the amount of anxiety experienced by cats in unfamiliar circumstances, a response that may or may not[57] be helpful for FIC cats and others that experience anxiety-related problems.[58] In a pilot study evaluating Feliway in cats with FIC, a decrease in the number of days that clinical signs were exhibited was reported, although this finding was not significant ($p = 0.06$).[59] Feliway can be purchased as a spray formulation or a room diffuser. The spray can be used in areas such as where the litter box is kept, or sprayed in cat carriers 10 to 15 minutes before transporting the cat. Room diffusers can be placed in designated rooms for cats, which may help decrease anxiety and clinical signs of FIC.

Drug Therapy

A variety of drugs has been tried in cats with FIC, but prospective, randomized, properly masked, placebo-controlled studies are lacking to confirm clinical efficacy. If MEMO (and possible pheromone) therapy fails to control signs, medications can be considered. These drugs should not be used for cats on initial presentation for care of LUTS, but should be considered only for cats if their environmental needs have been addressed and should not be stopped abruptly.

Amitriptyline (2.5 to 7.5 mg/cat PO every 24 hours), a tricyclic antidepressant (TCA), was evaluated in an open, non–placebo-controlled trial. It appeared to reduce clinical signs in some cats with severe, refractory FIC.[60] This drug, or clomipramine, another TCA (0.25 to 0.5 mg/kg PO every 24 hours), may need to be administered for at least one week or longer before a beneficial effect may be noted. If no improvements are noted, or medicating the cat is too stressful (for owner or cat), these drugs should be tapered over a period of 1 to 2 weeks. Side effects of the TCAs can include sedation, lethargy, weight gain, and urine retention. Because of the possibility of urine retention, it is advised to monitor the cat for urolithiasis if clinical signs redevelop after receiving this class of drugs for an extended period. Fluoxetine (0.5 to 1 mg/kg PO every 24 hours) is a selective serotonin reuptake inhibitor (SSRI). It has been shown to decrease signs of urine marking in cats.[61] This drug should also not be abruptly stopped. SSRI side effects can include behavior changes such as anxiety, and sleep disturbances. Many drugs used for FIC are considered "off-label," and owner consent should be obtained before therapy.

Pentosan polysulfate sodium is a semisynthetic carbohydrate derivative similar to glycosaminoglycans that is also approved for humans with IC. A multicentered, placebo-controlled, masked study in cats reported no significant differences when comparing pentosan polysulfate sodium to placebo.[62] However, all groups had clinical benefit, suggesting a strong "placebo" effect. All medication was provided to the cat in a food treat; the authors of this study hypothesized that improving the interaction and environmental needs of the cat may inadvertently have contributed to the positive outcomes noted in all groups. Similar findings were reported in two other studies evaluating glycosaminoglycan therapy in cats with FIC.[63,64]

MANAGING THE CAT WITH CHRONIC FELINE INTERSTITIAL CYSTITIS

The clinician and owner must understand that FIC is not limited to abnormalities related solely to the bladder. Because FIC can be a chronic condition in some cats, excellent owner communication in conjunction with MEMO therapy, meeting the environmental needs of the cat, and possibly pharmacological agents may be beneficial for managing chronic FIC. Some cats may retain their underlying predisposition for this disorder and, if exposed to a significant stressor, clinical signs can recur. Analgesics can be used short term if the cat is presented with recurrent clinical signs. Continual work with the owner and cat can yield positive results, and encouragement to reinforce these behaviors during successes can be beneficial, as is the case with any chronic medical condition.

SUMMARY

The terminology used to describe what is currently referred to as FIC certainly must be addressed as research progresses and a better understanding of the underlying pathophysiology of this disease is gained. This is important because, by not focusing on a bladder etiology for the clinical signs, a "global" treatment approach can be implemented by the clinician in appropriate circumstances. Early intervention may help prevent an initial episode from progressing to a chronic disease. Further, gaining a better understanding of this disease (and what to call it) may help pet food companies tailor prescription diets to a specific LUT disorder, such as struvite or calcium oxalate urolithiasis, and help them tailor marketing campaigns while using more accurate terminology when referring to the many diseases that affect the LUT in cats.

References

1. Osborne CA, Johnston GR, Polzin DJ, et al: Redefinition of the feline urologic syndrome: feline lower urinary tract disease with heterogeneous causes. *Vet Clin North Am Small Anim Pract* 134:409–438, 1984.
2. Osborne CA, Kruger JM, Lulich JP: Feline lower urinary tract disorders: definition of terms and concepts. *Vet Clin North Am Small Anim Pract* 20:169–179, 1996.
3. Buffington CA: Idiopathic cystitis in domestic cats—beyond the lower urinary tract. *J Vet Intern Med* 25:784–796, 2011.
4. Dimitrakov J, Guthrie D: Genetics and phenotyping of urological chronic pelvic pain syndrome. *J Urol* 181:1550–1557, 2009.
5. Buffington CA: Developmental influences on medically unexplained symptoms. *Psychother Psychosom* 78:139–144, 2009.
6. Warren JW, Howard FM, Cross RK, et al: Antecedent nonbladder syndromes in case-control study of interstitial cystitis/painful bladder syndrome. *Urology* 73:52–57, 2009.
7. Nickel JC, Shoskes D, Irvine-Bird K: Clinical phenotyping of women with interstitial cystitis/painful bladder syndrome: a key to classification and potentially improved management. *J Urol* 182:155–160, 2009.
8. Hostutler RA, Chew DJ, DiBartola SP: Recent concepts in feline lower urinary tract disease. *Vet Clin North Am Small Anim Pract* 35:147–170, vii, 2005.
9. Buffington CA: External and internal influences on disease risk in cats. *J Am Vet Med Assoc* 220:994–1002, 2002.
10. Buffington CA, Westropp JL, Chew DJ, et al: Risk factors associated with clinical signs of lower urinary tract disease in indoor-housed cats. *J Am Vet Med Assoc* 228:722–725, 2006.
11. Clasper M: A case of interstitial cystitis and Hunner's ulcer in a domestic shorthaired cat. *N Z Vet J* 38:158–160, 1990.
12. Peeker R, Fall M: Toward a precise definition of interstitial cystitis: further evidence of differences in classic and nonulcer disease. *J Urol* 167:2470–2472, 2002.
13. Buffington CA, Chew DJ, Woodworth BE: Animal model of human disease—feline interstitial cystitis. *Comparat Pathol Bull* 29, 1997.
14. Fabricant CG, King JM, Gaskin JM, et al: Isolation of a virus from a female cat with urolithiasis. *J Am Vet Med Assoc* 158:200–201, 1971.
15. Kruger JM, Osborne CA, Goyal SM, et al: Clinical evaluation of cats with lower urinary tract disease. *J Am Vet Med Assoc* 199:211–216, 1991.
16. Kruger JM, Osborne CA: The role of viruses in feline lower urinary tract disease. *J Vet Intern Med* 4:71–78, 1990.
17. Sykes JE, Westropp JL, Kasten RW, et al: Association between Bartonella species infection and disease in pet cats as determined using serology and culture. *J Feline Med Surg* 12:631–636, 2010.
18. Eggertsdottir AV, Lund HS, Krontveit R, et al: Bacteriuria in cats with feline lower urinary tract disease: a clinical study of 134 cases in Norway. *J Feline Med Surg* 9:458–465, 2007.
19. Keay SK, Warren JW: Is interstitial cystitis an infectious disease? *Int J Antimicrob Agents* 19:480–483, 2002.
20. Birder LA, Barrick S, Roppolo JR, et al: Feline interstitial cystitis results in mechanical hypersensitivity and altered ATP release from bladder Urothelium. *Am J Physiol Renal Physiol* 285:F423–F429, 2003.
21. Sculptoreanu A, de Groat WC, Buffington CA, et al: Abnormal excitability in capsaicin-responsive DRG neurons from cats with feline interstitial cystitis. *Exp Neurol* 193:437–443, 2005.
22. Birder LA, Nealen ML, Kiss S, et al: Beta-adrenoceptor agonists stimulate endothelial nitric oxide synthase in rat urinary bladder urothelial cells. *J Neurosci* 22:8063–8070, 2002.
23. Jezernik K, Romih R, Mannherz HG, et al: Immunohistochemical detection of apoptosis, proliferation and inducible nitric oxide synthase in rat urothelium damaged by cyclophosphamide treatment. *Cell Biol Int* 27:863–869, 2003.
24. Oter S, Korkmaz A, Oztas E, et al: Inducible nitric oxide synthase inhibition in cyclophosphamide induced hemorrhagic cystitis in rats. *Urol Res* 32:185–189, 2004.
25. Kubes P: Nitric oxide modulates epithelial permeability in the feline small intestine. *Am J Physiol* 262:G1138–G1142, 1992.
26. Cals-Grierson MM, Ormerod AD: Nitric oxide function in the skin. *Nitric Oxide* 10:179–193, 2004.
27. Wu CH, Buffington CA, Fraser MO, et al: Urodynamic evaluation of female cats with idiopathic cystitis. *Am J Vet Res* 72:578–582, 2011.
28. Reche AJ, Buffington CA: Increased tyrosine hydroxylase immunoreactivity in the locus coeruleus of cats with interstitial cystitis. *J Urol* 159:1045, 1998.
29. Welk KA, Buffington CA: *Effect of interstitial cystitis on central neuropeptide in receptor immunoreactivity in cats*, Columbus, 2003, Thesis, Department of Human Anatomy, The Ohio State University.
30. Sands SA, Strong R, Corbitt J, et al: Effects of acute restraint stress on tyrosine hydroxylase mRNA expression in locus coeruleus of Wistar and Wistar-Kyoto rats. *Brain Res Mol Brain Res* 75:1–7, 2000.
31. Goldstein DS: *Catecholamines, and cardiovascular disease*, New York, 1995, Oxford, pp 234–266.
32. Valentino RJ, Miselis RR, Pavcovich LA: Pontine regulation of pelvic viscera: pharmacological target for pelvic visceral dysfunctions. *Trends Pharmacol Sci* 20:253–260, 1999.
33. Westropp JL, Kass PH, Buffington CA: Evaluation of the effects of stress in cats with idiopathic cystitis. *Am J Vet Res* 67:731–736, 2006.

34. Buffington CA, Pacak K: Increased plasma norepinephrine concentration in cats with interstitial cystitis. *J Urol* 165:2051–2054, 2001.

35. Hague DW, Stella JL, Buffington CA: Effects of interstitial cystitis on the acoustic startle reflex in cats. *Am J Vet Res* 74:144–147, 2013.

36. Buffington CA, Teng B, Somogyi GT: Norepinephrine content and adrenoceptor function in the bladder of cats with feline interstitial cystitis. *J Urol* 167:1876–1880, 2002.

37. Westropp JL, Kass PH, Buffington CA: *In vivo* evaluation of alpha(2)-adrenoceptors in cats with idiopathic cystitis. *Am J Vet Res* 68:203–207, 2007.

38. Stevens CW, Brenner GM: Spinal administration of adrenergic agents produces analgesia in amphibians. *Eur J Pharmacol* 316:205–210, 1996.

39. Westropp JL, Welk K, Buffington CA: Small adrenal glands in cats with feline interstitial cystitis. *J Urol* 170(6):2494–2497, 2003.

40. Jensen P: Transgenerational epigenetic effects on animal behaviour. *Prog Biophys Mol Biol* 113:447–454, 2013.

41. Reynolds RM, Labad J, Buss C, et al: Transmitting biological effects of stress *in utero*: implications for mother and offspring. *Psychoneuroendocrinology* 38:1843–1849, 2013.

42. Russo SJ, Murrough JW, Han MH, et al: Neurobiology of resilience. *Nat Neurosci* 15:1475–1484, 2012.

43. Buffington CA, Westropp JL, Chew DJ, et al: Clinical evaluation of multimodal environmental modification (MEMO) in the management of cats with idiopathic cystitis. *J Feline Med Surg* 8:261–268, 2006.

44. Stella JL, Lord LK, Buffington CA: Sickness behaviors in response to unusual external events in healthy cats and cats with feline interstitial cystitis. *J Am Vet Med Assoc* 238:67–73, 2011.

45. Buffington CA: Comorbidity of interstitial cystitis with other unexplained clinical conditions. *J Urol* 172:1242–1248, 2004.

46. Buffington CA, Westropp JL, Chew DJ: A case-control study of indoor-housed cats with lower urinary tract signs. *J Am Vet Med Assoc* 228:722–725, 2006.

47. Freeman LM, Brown DJ, Smith FW, et al: Magnesium status and the effect of magnesium supplementation in feline hypertrophic cardiomyopathy. *Can J Vet Res* 61:227–231, 1997.

48. Erickson DR, Xie SX, Bhavanandan VP, et al: A comparison of multiple urine markers for interstitial cystitis. *J Urol* 167:2461–2469, 2002.

49. Lemberger SI, Dorsch R, Hauck SM, et al: Decrease of Trefoil factor 2 in cats with feline idiopathic cystitis. *BJU Int* 107:670–677, 2011.

50. Lemberger SI, Deeg CA, Hauck SM, et al: Comparison of urine protein profiles in cats without urinary tract disease and cats with idiopathic cystitis, bacterial urinary tract infection, or urolithiasis. *Am J Vet Res* 72:1407–1415, 2011.

51. Rubio-Diaz DE, Pozza ME, Dimitrakov J, et al: A candidate serum biomarker for bladder pain syndrome/interstitial cystitis. *Analyst* 134:1133–1137, 2009.

52. Ellis SL, Rodan I, Carney HC, et al: AAFP and ISFM feline environmental needs guidelines. *J Feline Med Surg* 15:219–230, 2013.

53. Herron ME, Buffington CA: Environmental enrichment for indoor cats. *Compend Contin Educ Vet* 32:E4, 2010.

54. Herron ME, Buffington CA: Environmental enrichment for indoor cats: implementing enrichment. *Compend Contin Educ Vet* 34:E3, 2012.

55. Parsons CL, Greenberger M, Gabal L, et al: The role of urinary potassium in the pathogenesis and diagnosis of interstitial cystitis. *J Urol* 159:1862–1867, 1998.

56. Michel K, Scherk M: From problem to success: feline weight loss programs that work. *J Feline Med Surg* 14:327–336, 2012.

57. Frank D, Beauchamp G, Palestrini C: Systematic review of the use of pheromones for treatment of undesirable behavior in cats and dogs. *J Am Vet Med Assoc* 236:1308–1316, 2010.

58. Griffith CA, Steigerwald ES, Buffington CA: Effects of a synthetic facial pheromone on behavior of cats. *J Am Vet Med Assoc* 217:1154–1156, 2000.

59. Gunn-Moore DA, Cameron ME: A pilot study using synthetic feline facial pheromone for the management of feline idiopathic cystitis. *J Feline Med Surg* 6:133–138, 2004.

60. Chew DJ, Buffington CA, Kendall MS, et al: Amitriptyline treatment for severe recurrent idiopathic cystitis in cats. *J Am Vet Med Assoc* 213:1282–1286, 1998.

61. Hart BL, Cliff KD, Tynes VV, et al: Control of urine marking by use of long-term treatment with fluoxetine or clomipramine in cats. *J Am Vet Med Assoc* 226:378–382, 2005.

62. Chew DJ, Bartges JW, Adams LG, et al: Randomized, placebo-controlled clinical trial of pentosan polysulfate sodium for treatment of feline interstitial (idipathic) cystitis. *J Vet Intern Med* 23:690, 2009.

63. Gunn-Moore DA, Shenoy CM: Oral glucosamine and the management of feline idiopathic cystitis. *J Feline Med Surg* 6:219–225, 2004.

64. Wallius BM, Tidholm AE: Use of pentosan polysulphate in cats with idiopathic, nonobstructive lower urinary tract disease: a double-blind, randomised, placebo-controlled trial. *J Feline Med Surg* 11:409–412, 2009.

Antony S. Moore, MVSc

Squamous Cell Carcinoma in Cats

Suzanne Murphy

Stratified squamous epithelium forms most of the skin; lines the oral cavity, tongue, and esophagus; and forms the nail beds and foot pads. Squamous cell carcinoma (SCC) accounts for 15% of feline skin tumors and at least 70% of feline oral malignant tumors.[1] SCC is seen in older cats with a median age of 10 to 12 years. The underlying causes of SCC are related to the site involved. Tumor behavior and appropriate treatment choices vary according to the anatomic area involved, and for these reasons this chapter separately considers oral SCC, cutaneous SCC, and SCC of other sites.

ORAL SQUAMOUS CELL CARCINOMA

Oral cancer accounts for 3% to 10% of all feline tumors, and SCC is the most common cancer at this site.[2,3] Cats can present with various signs, including pain, excess salivation, oral bleeding, anorexia, loose teeth (especially with otherwise good dentition), dysphagia, inability to eat or groom properly, weight loss, and halitosis. Often an inflamed, ulcerated abnormal area can be appreciated in the mouth (Figure 54-1). Differential diagnoses include eosinophilic granuloma, lymphocytic-plasmacytic stomatitis, severe periodontal disease, and other oral tumors.[3]

Behavior

Feline oral SCC is an extremely locally aggressive disease that can arise on any mucosal surface within the oral cavity. It is often not identified until the disease is advanced, partly due to the difficulty of examining conscious cats' mouths and partly because it can commonly arise in the sublingual area. If it involves the gingiva, it frequently extends into the bone. If managed conservatively, it usually leads to death or euthanasia a median of 33 days after biopsy due to progressive local disease.[4] Unfortunately, even with treatment including radical surgery, radiation therapy, and adjunctive chemotherapy, rates of survival for longer than 1 year are typically less than 10%, much the same as they are with conservative treatment.[4,5]

The occurrence of metastatic disease is often reported as low, although in 49 cats with advanced disease (identified as a primary tumor 2 cm^3 to 74.5 cm^3 in size), 31% had metastatic disease in the submandibular lymph nodes and 10% had evidence of possible thoracic metastasis.[6]

Etiology

In humans, papillomaviruses are thought to cause approximately 25% of oral SCCs, whereas 75% are caused by other carcinogens, such as tobacco and alcohol.[7] An epidemiological case control study of 148 cats examined the effect of various external factors, including dietary tuna intake and high canned food intake on the relative risk (RR) of developing oral SCC. Environmental tobacco smoke (ETS) and flea collar–derived pesticides, which the cat might ingest through grooming its coat, were also included. Feeding canned food was associated with an RR of 3.6, and feeding canned tuna was associated with an RR of 4.7. Environmental tobacco smoke was associated with a statistically nonsignificant increase in risk, with the suggestion of a greater risk in cats exposed for 5 years or longer and those living with more than one smoker.[8] In a subset of these cats, increased tumor protein p53 expression was seen in cats exposed to ETS.[9] Nicotine and cotinine are found in significant levels in the urine of cats exposed to ETS, supporting findings that cats are taking up carcinogens from tobacco, even if the effect of this uptake is unclear.[10]

The controversial role of papillomaviruses in the carcinogenesis of SCC is discussed later.

Diagnosis and Staging

Oral tumors are frequently inflamed, infected, or necrotic. Therefore, fine-needle aspiration (FNA) is not a useful technique to achieve a diagnosis. A large intraoral biopsy should be performed using a blade or punch biopsy technique that should be angled deep into the lesion to avoid sampling only the inflammation. Any bleeding can be controlled by

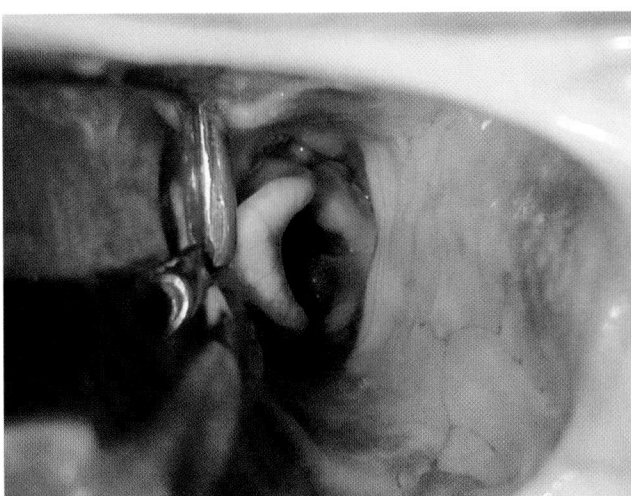

Figure 54-1: A laryngeal squamous cell carcinoma (SCC).

electrocautery or by digital pressure. The biopsy should not be taken using electrocautery because any neoplastic cells at the edge of the sample will be destroyed by this technique and tissue architecture may also be distorted. Intraoral radiographs can be used as part of clinical staging and to help delineate the extent of surgical margins, although it should be remembered that radiographs underestimate the extent of bone lysis. Thoracic radiographs can be taken at the same time to evaluate for lung metastasis, although this is an unusual event. Cross-sectional imaging may be more valuable than survey radiographs to evaluate local and distant tumor extent, although there are no reported studies describing the use of magnetic resonance imaging. The one small study looking at computed tomography (CT) in cats with oral SCC could not identify lymph node metastasis with any reliability, although the number of "events" (metastases) in the study was low.[3]

Positron emission tomography (PET) has also been used with 2-[^{18}F]-fluoro-2-deoxy-D-glucose (^{18}F-FDG) in a series of 12 cats with oral SCC in combination with CT to aid stereotactic radiotherapy planning. The hypothesis was that, as in human head and neck cancers, PET would improve on CT by delineating metabolically active areas of tumor within the planned radiotherapy field and by identifying areas that would have been missed if radiotherapy had been planned by CT alone.[11] The same group of cats were evaluated to see if PET contributed to staging by identifying lymph nodes with increased uptake of ^{18}F-FDG, which would be suspicious for metastasis where CT had not identified an abnormality. Two metastatic lesions were identified with PET which were equivocal on CT.[12] Although this technique has practical limitations at the moment, it may be more widely used in the future.

Staging is defined by the World Health Organization (WHO) TNM system where *T* refers to the size and invasiveness of the primary tumor, *N* refers to whether or not the draining lymph node is affected, and *M* refers to whether or not distant metastasis have been identified. This system was adapted from human medicine and published over 30 years ago for use in domestic animals (Table 54-1).

Table 54-1	World Health Organization Classification for Canine or Feline Oral Tumors
Stage	**Clinical Description**

T: Primary Tumor

Tis	Tumor *in situ*
T1	Tumor less than 2 cm maximum diameter
a	Without evidence of bone invasion
b	With evidence of bone invasion
T2	Tumor 2 to 4 cm maximum diameter
a	Without evidence of bone invasion
b	With evidence of bone invasion
T3	Tumor over 4 cm maximum diameter
a	Without evidence of bone invasion
b	With evidence of bone invasion

N: Regional Lymph Nodes

N0	No evidence of regional lymph node involvement
N1	Moveable ipsilateral nodes
a	Nodes not considered to contain growth*
b	Nodes considered to contain growth*
N2	Moveable contralateral or bilateral nodes
a	Nodes not considered to contain growth*
b	Nodes considered to contain growth*
N3	Fixed nodes

M: Distant Metastasis

M0	No evidence of distant metastasis
M1	Distant metastasis detected—specify site(s)

TNM System Stage Grouping

Stage	Primary Tumor (T)	Regional Nodes (N)	Metastasis (M)
I	T1	N0, N1a, N2a	M0
II	T2	N0, N1a, N2a	M0
III	T3	N0, N1a, N2a	M0
	Any T	N1b	M0
IV	Any T	N2b, N3	M0
	Any T	Any N	M0

*(−), Histologically negative; (+), histologically positive.

Treatment Options

Treatment options depend on the location of the tumor in the oral cavity. Surgery as sole therapy is limited to tumors of the mandible and maxilla and small tumors of the tongue. Partial glossectomy is feasible in cats, although in practice many patients are not candidates for surgery because they have sublingual tumors and acceptable surgical margins are unachievable. *Major glossectomy*, defined as removing the entire free portion of the tongue or more than 75% of the tongue, is not an option for cats because it compromises quality of life profoundly by interfering with swallowing.[13] The biggest study of surgical intervention examined the outcome for 42 cats treated with partial or complete unilateral or bilateral rostral mandibulectomy.[14] Half of the cats (21 out of 42) had SCC, including eight with stage T3 tumors. Twelve cats were treated with unilateral mandibulectomy, five cats were treated with rostral bilateral mandibulectomy, and four cats had greater than 50% of one side of the mandible removed. Even then, margins were incomplete in nine cases, and the median survival time (MST) for all 21 cats was 217 days. It should also be noted that three of eight local recurrences occurred in cats that had complete margins assessed by histopathology. Of the cats in the study, 72% were dysphagic immediately after surgery, and 12% never ate again. Despite this, 83% of owners were happy with their decision to treat. Tumor location is important because it dictates the extent of resection feasible. For example, cats with rostral tumors in the aforementioned study had an MST of 911 days.

External beam radiotherapy alone is not a durable treatment option for SCC regardless of site or protocol. Tumors respond initially but rapidly recur.[15] An accelerated protocol giving once daily fractions of 4.8 Gy to a total dose of 48 Gy to 21 cats staged T1N0M0 to T3N0M0 gave an MST of 174 days, with T1-staged cats having a median progression-free survival of 590 days.[16] Similarly, a protocol using 14 fractions of 3.5 Gy in 9 days gave an MST of 86 days,[17] and a palliative five-fraction protocol of 4 Gy per day gave an MST of 120 days.[18] A group of 12 cats that underwent stereotactic radiotherapy had an MST of 106 days.[19] Etanidazole has been used as a radiosensitizer, and although the majority of cats

achieved a clinical response, the MST (112 days) was not greatly improved.[20]

Tonsillar SCC is quite uncommon in cats; and few studies address this site specifically. In dogs, tonsillar SCC is considered the most aggressive variant, but a small study implied that cats with tonsillar SCC responded well to radiation therapy. In that study, the MST was nearly 2 years, whereas cats with SCC from other oral sites lived a median of less than 5 months when treated in the same way.[21]

Strontium-90 is a radioactive isotope producing beta radiation. Strontium-90 plesiotherapy has been tested in two cases of oral SCC. It is applied directly to a lesion using an ophthalmic applicator designed for use in humans that incorporates a disc impregnated with the isotope. The disc is touched to the lesion for a calculated length of time, depending on the dose of radiation to be administered. The results were not clear-cut, because multiple treatments were used and recurrence was a feature in one cat.[22] Strontium-90 has been used as sole therapy in a case of extensive but superficial SCC of the ventral surface of the tongue. This has been extremely successful, with the cat alive and well over 2 years after treatment (S. Verganti, unpublished data).

Small studies using various cytotoxic drugs together with external beam radiotherapy have also showed relatively small improvement in survival times. The cytotoxic drugs used and radiotherapy protocols are described in Table 54-2.

Mitoxantrone was used as sole therapy in 32 cats and gave one complete remission (CR) for 60 days and three partial responses for up to 60 days, with similar results reported using doxorubicin and cyclophosphamide.[23]

Oral SCC is known to express cyclooxygenase (COX)-2 to a varying degree. In one study, COX-1 was more obviously expressed in the neoplastic tissue than the normal adjacent

Table 54-2 **Outcome of Studies Using Cytotoxic Drugs Together with External Beam Radiotherapy to Treat Oral Squamous Cell Carcinoma**

Study	Number of Cats	External Beam Radiotherapy Protocol	Medical Protocol	Outcome
Ogilvie et al.[23]	11	44-65 Gy in 10-15 fractions	Mitoxantrone at varying doses	73% CR DFI: 170 days
Jones et al.[24]	8	Six fractions of 6 Gy	Gemcitabine given at 25 mg/m² twice weekly	25% CR 50% PR MST: 111.5 days
Fidel et al.[21]	31	14 fractions of 3.5 Gy given within a 9-day period	Carboplatin given at 90-100 mg/m² on day 1 and day 4.5	MST for all cats 163 days Cats with tumors of tonsil or cheek were long-term survivors with a mean survival of 724 days
Marconato et al.[25]	6	Two fractions daily, 5 consecutive days to 48 Gy	Bleomycin, piroxicam, and thalidomide given to all cases	50% CR for 759 days, 458 days, and 362 days for these three cats Two died of other causes, one 51 days in CR, the other 82 days in CR One cat had metastases after 144 days

CR, Complete remission; *DFI,* disease-free interval; *Gy,* Gray; *MST,* median survival time; *PR,* partial response.

tissue.[26] There are no published clinical trials looking at response to nonsteroidal anti-inflammatory drugs (NSAIDs) alone, although overall survival in a United Kingdom general practice study was better when NSAIDs were given.[4]

Prognostic Indicators

Various potential prognostic markers have been evaluated, including histopathologic grading, mitotic index (MI), tumor proliferation marker Ki67 score, epidermal growth factor receptor (EGFR) status, and microvascular density (MVD, a morphologic measure of vascularization).[2,19,27,28] In one study by Bergkvist and colleagues, a lower than median Ki67 score in the cohort studied correlated with increased survival time.[2] In this study, the cats were divided into early and late euthanasia groups. The Ki67 score was significantly correlated with survival time in the later euthanasia group. Low Ki67 expression was defined as expression below the median level (54.6%). High Ki67 expression was defined as expression at or above the median level. A high score was significantly associated with a poor survival time. In another study, Ki67, MI, MVD, and EGFR expression were not significantly correlated with prognosis.[27] However, in this study, there was a wide variety of treatments given to this small cohort of cats, which may have confounded the study, and in contrast to the Bergkvist and colleagues study, the median survival was 10½ days.

In a small study of cats treated with stereotactic radiotherapy, those with higher MVD had shorter MST compared to patients with a lower MVD.[19] The fact that tumors have been identified with EGFR expression in several studies may present an opportunity for therapeutic intervention in the future.[2,27,28]

CUTANEOUS SQUAMOUS CELL CARCINOMA

Cutaneous SCC can be divided into two distinct presentations. The rare multicentric squamous Bowenoid *in situ* carcinoma (BISC) is seen on the trunk and limbs of older cats, unrelated to pigmentation. Solar-induced SCC is far more common and is seen almost exclusively on the head. Fur and pigmented skin are physical barriers to the effects of the sun, therefore cutaneous SCCs are found on nonpigmented, sparsely haired areas such as the pinnae, eyelids, and nasal planum of white or white-patched cats (Figure 54-2). Long-haired breeds, Siamese, and similarly marked cats are protected. It is common to see multiple lesions on the same cat at different stages of development from actinic change to carcinoma *in situ* to higher stage disease involving all vulnerable areas, because all of the skin has been exposed to the same ultraviolet (UV) light damage over a similar length of time. The lesions appear as non-healing scabby areas of erythema. The owner often believes the cat has been in a fight and has a wound. However, the lesion ulcerates and develops into a crater without healing. Ears often become thickened and curl before scabbing.

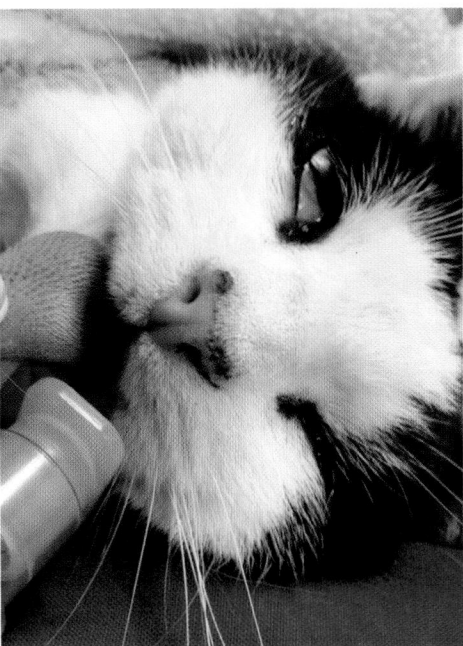

Figure 54-2: Typical appearance of squamous cell carcinoma of the nasal planum.

In contrast, BISC appears as multiple superficial areas of well-demarcated crusty erythematous plaques, which may be melanotic. The lesions are distributed on both haired and less-haired sites and in variably pigmented skin but usually are not identified on the head.

Etiology

The cause of most cutaneous SCCs is thought to be chronic exposure to UV light. In humans, betapapillomaviruses are hypothesized to be cofactors in conjunction with UV light as a cause of cutaneous SCC.[29] Various studies have investigated the presence of papillomaviruses in feline SCC from different sites with varying results, which is described in Table 54-3.

Papillomaviruses are small double-stranded DNA viruses. Thirty different genera exist. Papillomaviruses tend to be host specific. *Felis domesticus* papillomavirus type 1 (FDPV1), *F. domesticus* papillomavirus type 2 (FDPV2), and *Felis catus* papillomavirus type 3 (FCaPV3)[34] have been identified in affected cats, but sequences related to bovine and human papillomaviruses have also been found associated with lesions of varying histologic type affecting cats.[35] The significance of the presence of papillomaviruses is further complicated by the fact that normal feline skin can harbor these viruses.[30] It is not known whether papillomaviruses predispose cats to SCC, or whether the damaged tumor tissue is a good medium for papillomaviruses to colonize *after* SCC has arisen.[29] Lesions of BISC have been more commonly documented as associated with papillomavirus infection than other forms of SCC, most clearly with FDPV2.[30]

There is evidence that papillomaviruses induce a percentage of oral SCCs in humans. In human oral SCCs, increased expression of p16 protein is indicative of papillomavirus

Table 54-3	Papillomaviruses Identified in Feline Squamous Cell Carcinoma		
Study	**Viruses Identified**	**Way Identified**	**Number of Tumor Sites Investigated**
Munday et al.[30]	72% UV light–protected lesions FDPV2	PCR	45 UV light exposed (42% PV positive)
			25 UV light protected (76% PV positive)
O'Neill et al.[31]	50% FDPV2	PCR	12 BISC (58% PV positive)
	50% most consistent with HPV		39 cutaneous SCC (23% positive)
			35 non-cutaneous SCC (5% positive)
Anis et al.[32]	70% FDPV2	L1 gene characterization	5/10 samples were cutaneous SCC
	30% HPV		3/10 samples were carcinoma *in situ*
			1/10 samples was dysplastic skin
			1/10 samples was oral SCC
			All were PV positive
Munday et al.[7]	FDPV2 in 27 out of 33	PCR	All nasal planum SCC
	FDPV-MY2 in 6 out of 33		Virus found in 63% cases
	Some lesions had two viruses identified		
	FDPV-MY2 is now sequenced as FCaPV3[31]		
Ravens et al.[33]	FDPV2	Fluorescence *in situ* hybridization	Unusual case of BISC that progressed and developed metastatic SCC

BISC, Bowenoid *in situ* carcinoma; *FDPV2, felis domesticus* papillomavirus type 2; *FDPV-MY2, felis domesticus* papillomavirus; *HPV,* human papillomavirus; *PCR,* polymerase chain reaction; *PV,* papillomavirus; *SCC,* squamous cell carcinoma; *UV,* ultraviolet.

etiology and increased p16 may indicate loss of normal tumor-suppressor functions of the retinoblastoma protein.[30] In cats, two studies have detected papillomavirus DNA in low percentages of oral SCCs, but this finding is of unknown significance.[31,36] Immunohistochemistry has identified p16 in BISC and some supposedly solar-induced SCCs but not in oral SCC.[7,30]

Diagnosis and Behavior

For both types of cutaneous SCC, reliable ways of achieving a diagnosis include a punch biopsy, an excisional biopsy, or an incisional biopsy. Fine-needle aspiration is unsatisfactory due to the possibility of sampling inflammation and secondary infection. In cases of suspected solar-induced SCC, multiple areas may need to be biopsied to achieve a diagnosis. Some areas might be dysplastic, but others may be cancerous. Cutaneous SCC is slow to metastasize. The tumor may spread to draining lymph nodes and lungs. Therefore, staging cutaneous SCC would involve thoracic radiographs and investigation of local lymph nodes with FNA biopsy. In practical terms, the size of the primary tumor and its location are probably more important for prognosis than the low risk of metastatic disease. Staging should be discussed with the owner if the discovery of metastatic disease would significantly alter the treatment plan, particularly if the treatment is expensive and time-consuming or cosmetically challenging. For cases of BISC, the lesions have not breached the basement membrane (by definition), so metastatic disease is not a problem. However, up to 17% of cases do progress into higher stage SCC, and some cases have invasive lesions

concurrently. However, only one reported case developed distant metastasis, and that cat had been treated with prednisone.[33] Staging is defined by the WHO TNM system, which is described in Table 54-4.

Treatment Options

The treatment options for the two types of cutaneous SCC vary. For BISC, the options are usually surgical, where very superficial surgical techniques with narrow margins can often effect a cure. If there are too many lesions to be dealt with surgically or they are in a difficult-to-treat location, imiquimod, an immunomodulator with both antitumor and antiviral effects, can be used. Imiquimod has been used as a 5% cream preparation for the treatment of actinic keratosis, basal cell carcinoma, and genital warts in humans. In a study of 12 cats with BISC, all cats responded to treatment with this preparation. Nine cats developed new lesions during the study, which then responded to treatment.[37] Treatment was carried out either daily or three times weekly for most cats, with equal effect. Erythema and skin flaking were noted as adverse events in three cases, and neutropenia and elevated serum alanine aminotransferase activity were noted in one cat, which resolved with temporary cessation of treatment.[37]

Imiquimod has been used for one case of solar-induced SCC of the pinna and has been used for solar keratosis in humans.[38,39] However, there are many treatment options available for solar-induced cutaneous SCC, and choice of therapy depends on the site and stage of the primary tumor, together with the facilities available locally. Surgery,

Table 54-4	World Health Organization Classification for Canine or Feline Tumors of Epidermal or Dermal Origin (Excluding Lymphoma or Mast Cell Tumors)
Stage	**Clinical Description**

T: Primary Tumor

Tis	Preinvasive carcinoma (carcinoma *in situ*)
T0	No evidence of tumor
T1	Tumor less than 2 cm maximum diameter, superficial or exophytic
T2	Tumor 2 to 5 cm maximum diameter, or with minimal invasion, irrespective of size
T3	Tumor over 5 cm maximum diameter, or with invasion of the subcutis, irrespective of size
T4	Tumor invading other structures, such as fascia muscle bone or cartilage

N: Regional Lymph Nodes

N0	No evidence of regional lymph node involvement
N1	Moveable ipsilateral nodes
a	Nodes not considered to contain growth*
b	Nodes considered to contain growth*
N2	Moveable contralateral or bilateral nodes
a	Nodes not considered to contain growth*
b	Nodes considered to contain growth*
N3	Fixed nodes

M: Distant Metastasis

M0	No evidence of distant metastasis
M1	Distant metastasis detected—specify site(s) (including lymph nodes beyond the region in which the primary is situated)

*(−), Histologically negative; (+), histologically positive.

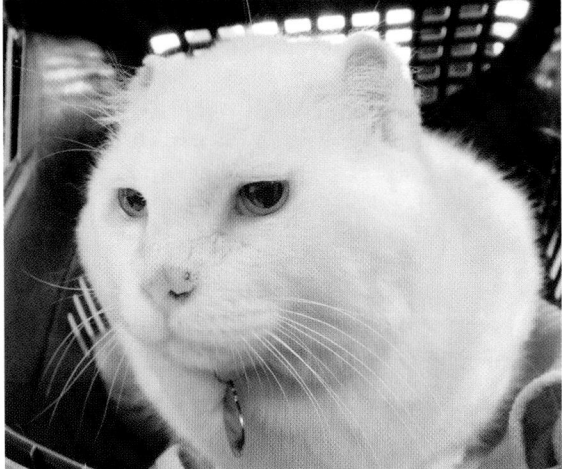

Figure 54-3: A cat that has undergone bilateral pinnectomy. Note the developing lesion on the nasal planum.

photodynamic therapy (PDT), cryotherapy, diathermy, plesiotherapy, and external beam radiation have all been used with varying success.

For tumors involving the pinnae, surgery is usually the treatment of choice. A 1-cm margin of normal tissue is recommended to give the best chance of complete surgical margins. To improve skin healing, the edges of the skin should be opposed to hide the cartilage. The best way of achieving this is to remove the pinnae with a V-shape technique (Figure 54-3). For eyelid SCC, surgery with a 4- to 5-mm clear margin is recommended.[40] This often means a full eyelid resection. The lower lid can be replaced with a lip to lid graft to fill the deficit, but adequate resection of the upper lid while maintaining function is more challenging. In one study, five cats with lower lid lesions resected with clean margins had median disease-free periods of 319 days (range: 95 to 1510 days).[41] In another study of five cats (with six eyelids treated overall), all cats were alive and disease-free more than 12 months later.[42]

For tumors of the nasal planum, treatment options depend on the stage of the primary tumor. More infiltrative tumors (stage T3 or T4) can only be successfully treated with surgery or external beam radiotherapy. The most successful way to treat these tumors is to remove the neoplastic tissue with a 5-mm margin from the normal tissue.[40] Nosectomy can be cosmetically challenging, although functionally most cats do well. More superficial lesions (stage Tis,* T1, or T2) can be treated successfully with PDT, cryosurgery, strontium-90 plesiotherapy, surgery, or external beam radiotherapy.[43-51]

Photodynamic therapy involves the use of a photosensitizer, which is preferentially taken up by tumor cells. This substance is activated by light of a specific wavelength and kills tumor cells with little bystander effect. Topical treatment of a photosensitizing cream, 5-aminolaevulinic acid, gave an 85% remission rate in one study of 55 cats but a 51% recurrence rate with a disease-free interval of 157 days.[43] In one report of 61 cats, the use of intravenous photosensitizers gave a 49% remission rate (61% controlled at 1 year); and in another report of 18 cats, there was a 100% remission rate (75% controlled at 1 year).[44] The limiting factor is the ability of the light to penetrate into the tumor, with superficial tumors responding better in all three studies.

Cryosurgery has been used with mixed outcomes, probably because the surgical margins cannot be properly assessed. Again, it is a treatment best restricted to superficial (stage T1 and T2) tumors. A median disease-free interval (DFI) of 254 days was reported in a study of 11 cats with lesions on the pinnae and nasal planum.[45] In another study, 102 cats were treated with a median remission time of 26.7 months overall, with SCC of the ear and eyelids responding most successfully. In this study, 17 out of 102 cats experienced recurrence a median of 6.6 months after treatment.[46]

---

*Tumor *in situ*.

In a study from New Zealand, 34 cats with lesions affecting 50% or less of the nasal planum were treated with curettage and diathermy using a three-cycle technique. Sixteen of these cats had only actinic change, nine had carcinoma *in situ,* and the other seven had frank SCC. Median follow-up was 18 months, and 94% of cats were disease-free at 1 year.[47]

Strontium-90 plesiotherapy is a very successful, cosmetically-sparing treatment but is only useful for stage Tis, T1, and T2 lesions because the beta radiation penetrates only a few millimeters. In one study, 13 out of 15 cats treated went into CR with an MST of 692 days. The two cats that did not initially respond were successfully treated with a second course.[48] Another study of 49 cats showed CR in 88% with an MST of 1071 days.[49]

External beam radiotherapy has also been used as sole therapy. Orthovoltage, megavoltage, electron, and proton beam irradiation have all been used for nasal planum SCC with similar outcomes, again with tumors staged as T1 responding better than higher-staged masses. Cats with T1 SCC had an 85% chance of being alive for 1 year in comparison to cats with T3 SCC, which had a 45% chance of being alive at 1 year.[50] In another study, 16 out of 17 cats, staged T2b (six cats), T1b (five cats), and T1a and T2a (three cats each), responded for a median DFI of 414 days. For this study, electrons were used to achieve a total dose of 48 Gy, which was given in 10 fractions of 4.8 Gy each on 5 consecutive days.[51] Boron capture neutron therapy has been reported in three cats with partial tumor control.[52]

There are few reports of using cytotoxic drugs, either alone or in combination with radiotherapy, to treat cutaneous SCC. In a small study, advanced (one stage T2, two stage T3, and three stage T4) tumors of the nasal planum were treated with intralesional carboplatin and orthovoltage radiotherapy. All six cats had a complete response with time to progression ranging from 52 to 562 days; four of the six were still in CR at the end of the study.[53] Intralesional carboplatin suspended in a sesame seed oil emulsion was used alone to treat 23 cats; 73% achieved CR with 55% progression-free at 1 year.[54] Seven of nine cats treated with electrochemotherapy using intralesional bleomycin had a CR lasting up to 3 years.[55]

Immunohistochemistry has identified COX-2 in cutaneous as well as oral SCC, although the role of COX-2 is yet to be understood.[56] Human actinic keratosis is treated with COX-2 inhibitors and therefore these drugs may be useful in veterinary medicine, but studies are lacking.[57]

Prognostic Indicators

Prognostic markers have been evaluated to help predict outcome for cutaneous SCCs, including Ki67 score, EGFR positivity, and p16 immunostaining. A high Ki67 score was associated with a durable response to radiotherapy in a study of 17 cats.[51] In another study, EGFR status was investigated in 19 formalin-fixed biopsy specimens by immunohistochemistry. Tumors identified as EGFR-positive had a poorer outcome with decreased DFI and survival time.[58] Intense p16 immunostaining was associated with increased survival of cats with nasal planum SCC.[7]

SQUAMOUS CELL CARCINOMA IN OTHER SITES

Squamous cell carcinoma has been identified in case reports affecting various organs, including the renal pelvis,[59] the cornealimbus of the eye,[60] the uterine stump of a spayed cat,[61] lungs, and esophagus.[62] However, the most common other sites affected by SCC are the digits. Squamous cell carcinoma was the most commonly identified malignant tumor in a pathology-based audit and was associated with an MST of 73 days, although this was based on data from only seven cats.[63] In this study, multiple digits on the front paws or both the front and hind paws were affected in four out of 15 cats.

SUMMARY

Most cases of SCC have a low risk of metastasis but need to be identified promptly for the best chance of cure. This is particularly true of oral SCC and cutaneous SCC of the eyelid and nasal planum where treatment options, and cosmetic and functional outcome, are heavily dependent on the site and stage of the primary tumor at diagnosis. Oral SCCs are frustrating to treat, because they are frequently identified late in the course of disease or in a site where there is no possibility of definitive treatment. Novel approaches are desperately needed to improve outcomes for these cats. In contrast, cutaneous SCC is very often curable.

References

1. Liptak JM, Withrow SJ: Cancer of the gastrointestinal tract. In Withrow SJ, Vail DM, editors: *Withrow & MacEwen's small animal clinical oncology,* ed 5, St Louis, 2013, Saunders/Elsevier, p 381.
2. Bergkvist GT, Argyle DJ, Morrison L, et al: Expression of epidermal growth factor receptor (EGFR) and Ki67 in feline oral squamous cell carcinomas (FOSCC). *Vet Comp Oncol* 9:106–117, 2011.
3. Gendler A, Lewis JR, Reetz JA, et al: Computed tomographic features of oral squamous cell carcinoma in cats: 18 cases (2002-2008). *J Am Vet Med Assoc* 236:319–325, 2010.
4. Hayes AM, Adams VJ, Scase TJ, et al: Survival of 54 cats with oral squamous cell carcinoma in United Kingdom general practice. *J Small Anim Pract* 48:394–399, 2007.
5. Moore AS, Ogilvie GK: Tumors of the alimentary tract. In Ogilvie GK, Moore AS, editors: *Feline oncology,* ed 1, Trenton, NJ, 2001, Veterinary Learning Systems, pp 271–291.
6. Soltero-Rivera MM, Krick EL, Reiter AM, et al: Prevalence of regional and distant metastasis in cats with advanced oral squamous cell carcinoma: 49 cases (2005-2011). *J Feline Med Surg* 16:164–169, 2014.
7. Munday JS, French AF, Gibson IR, et al: The presence of p16 CDKN2A protein immunostaining within feline nasal planum squamous

cell carcinomas is associated with an increased survival time and the presence of papillomaviral DNA. *Vet Pathol* 50:269–273, 2013.

8. Bertone ER, Snyder LA, Moore AS: Environmental and lifestyle risk factors for oral squamous cell carcinoma in domestic cats. *J Vet Intern Med* 17:557–562, 2003.

9. Snyder LA, Bertone ER, Jakowski RM, et al: p53 expression and environmental tobacco smoke exposure in feline oral squamous cell carcinoma. *Vet Pathol* 41:209–214, 2004.

10. McNiel EA, Carmella SG, Heath LA, et al: Urinary biomarkers to assess exposure of cats to environmental tobacco smoke. *Am J Vet Res* 68:349–353, 2007.

11. Yoshikawa H, Randall EK, Kraft SL, et al: Comparison between 2-(18) F-fluoro-2-deoxy-D-glucose positron emission tomography and contrast-enhanced computed tomography for measuring gross tumor volume in cats with oral squamous cell carcinoma. *Vet Radiol Ultrasound* 54:307–313, 2013.

12. Randall EK, Kraft SL, Yoshikawa H, et al: Evaluation of ¹⁸F-FDG PET/CT as a diagnostic imaging and staging tool for feline oral squamous cell carcinoma. *Vet Comp Oncol* 2013. [Epub ahead of print].

13. Liptak JM, Lascelles BDX: Oral tumors. In Kudnig S, Seguin B, editors: *Veterinary surgical oncology*, ed 1, Ames, IA, 2012, Wiley Blackwell, p 164.

14. Northrup NC, Selting KA, Rassnick KM, et al: Outcomes of cats with oral tumors treated with mandibulectomy: 42 cases. *J Am Anim Hosp Assoc* 42:350–360, 2006.

15. Bregazzi VS, LaRue SM, Powers BE, et al: Response of feline oral squamous cell carcinoma to palliative radiation therapy. *Vet Radiol Ultrasound* 42:77–79, 2001.

16. Poirier VJ, Kaser-Hotz B, Vail DM, et al: Efficacy and toxicity of an accelerated hypofractionated radiation therapy protocol in cats with oral squamous cell carcinoma. *Vet Radiol Ultrasound* 54:81–88, 2013.

17. Fidel JL, Sellon RK, Houston RK, et al: A nine-day accelerated radiation protocol for feline squamous cell carcinoma. *Vet Radiol Ultrasound* 48:482–485, 2007.

18. McDonald C, Looper J, Greene S: Response rate and duration associated with a 4Gy 5 fraction palliative radiation protocol. *Vet Radiol Ultrasound* 53:358–364, 2012.

19. Yoshikawa H, Ehrhart EJ, Charles JB, et al: Assessment of predictive molecular variables in feline oral squamous cell carcinoma treated with stereotactic radiation therapy. *Vet Comp Oncol* 2013. [Epub ahead of print].

20. Evans SM, LaCreta F, Helfand S, et al: Technique, pharmacokinetics, toxicity, and efficacy of intratumoral etanidazole and radiotherapy for treatment of spontaneous feline oral squamous cell carcinoma. *Int J Radiat Oncol Biol Phys* 20:703–708, 1991.

21. Fidel J, Lyons J, Tripp C, et al: Treatment of oral squamous cell carcinoma with accelerated radiation therapy and concomitant carboplatin in cats. *J Vet Intern Med* 25:504–510, 2011.

22. Nagata K, Selting KA, Cook CR, et al: 90Sr therapy for oral squamous cell carcinoma in two cats. *Vet Radiol Ultrasound* 52:114–117, 2011.

23. Ogilvie GK, Moore AS, Obradovich JE, et al: Toxicoses and efficacy associated with administration of mitoxantrone to cats with malignant tumors. *J Am Vet Med Assoc* 202:1839–1844, 1993.

24. Jones PD, de Lorimier LP, Kitchell BE, et al: Gemcitabine as a radiosensitizer for nonresectable feline oral squamous cell carcinoma. *J Am Anim Hosp Assoc* 39:463–467, 2003.

25. Marconato L, Buchholz J, Keller M, et al: Multimodal therapeutic approach and interdisciplinary challenge for the treatment of unresectable head and neck squamous cell carcinoma in six cats: a pilot study. *Vet Comp Oncol* 11:101–112, 2013.

26. Hayes A, Scase T, Miller J, et al: COX-1 and COX-2 expression in feline oral squamous cell carcinoma. *J Comp Pathol* 135:93–99, 2006.

27. Yoshikawa H, Ehrhart EJ, Charles JB, et al: Immunohistochemical characterization of feline oral squamous cell carcinoma. *Am J Vet Res* 73:1801–1806, 2012.

28. Looper JS, Malarkey DE, Ruslander D, et al: Epidermal growth factor receptor expression in feline oral squamous cell carcinomas. *Vet Comp Oncol* 4:33–40, 2006.

29. Munday JS, Kiupel M: Papillomavirus-associated cutaneous neoplasia in mammals. *Vet Pathol* 47:254–264, 2010.

30. Munday JS, Gibson I, French AF: Papillomaviral DNA and increased p16CDKN2A protein are frequently present within feline cutaneous squamous cell carcinomas in ultraviolet-protected skin. *Vet Dermatol* 22:360–366, 2011.

31. O'Neill SH, Newkirk KM, Anis EA, et al: Detection of human papillomavirus DNA in feline premalignant and invasive squamous cell carcinoma. *Vet Dermatol* 22:68–74, 2011.

32. Anis EA, O'Neill SH, Newkirk KM, et al: Molecular characterization of the L1 gene of papillomaviruses in epithelial lesions of cats and comparative analysis with corresponding gene sequences of human and feline papillomaviruses. *Am J Vet Res* 71:1457–1461, 2010.

33. Ravens PA, Vogelnest LJ, Tong LJ, et al: Papillomavirus-associated multicentric squamous cell carcinoma in situ in a cat: an unusually extensive and progressive case with subsequent metastasis. *Vet Dermatol* 24:642–645, 2013.

34. Munday JS, Dunowska M, Hills SF, et al: Genomic characterization of *Felis catus* papillomavirus-3: a novel papillomavirus detected in a feline Bowenoid in situ carcinoma. *Vet Microbiol* 165:319–325, 2013.

35. Egberink H, Thiry E, Möstl K, et al: Feline viral papillomatosis: ABCD guidelines on prevention and management. *J Feline Med Surg* 15:560–562, 2013.

36. Munday JS, Howe L, French A, et al: Detection of papillomaviral DNA sequences in a feline oral squamous cell carcinoma. *Res Vet Sci* 86:359–361, 2009.

37. Gill VL, Bergman PJ, Baer KE, et al: Use of imiquimod 5% cream (Aldara) in cats with multicentric squamous cell carcinoma *in situ*: 12 cases (2002-2005). *Vet Comp Oncol* 6:55–64, 2008.

38. Peters-Kennedy J, Scott DW, Miller WH, Jr: Apparent clinical resolution of pinnal actinic keratoses and squamous cell carcinoma in a cat using topical imiquimod 5% cream. *J Feline Med Surg* 10:593–599, 2008.

39. Samrao A, Cockerell CJ: Pharmacotherapeutic management of actinic keratosis: focus on newer topical agents. *Am J Clin Dermatol* 14:273–277, 2013.

40. Ayres SA, Liptak JM: Head and neck tumors. In Kudnig S, Seguin B, editors: *Veterinary surgical oncology*, ed 1, Ames, IA, 2012, Wiley Blackwell, pp 87–94.

41. Schmidt K, Bertani C, Martano M, et al: Reconstruction of the lower eyelid by third eyelid lateral advancement and local transposition cutaneous flap after "en bloc" resection of squamous cell carcinoma in 5 cats. *Vet Surg* 34:78–82, 2005.

42. Hunt GB: Use of the lip-to-lid flap for replacement of the lower eyelid in five cats. *Vet Surg* 35:284–286, 2006.

43. Bexfield NH, Stell AJ, Gear RN, et al: Photodynamic therapy of superficial nasal planum squamous cell carcinomas in cats: 55 cases. *J Vet Intern Med* 22:1385–1389, 2008.

44. Buchholz J, Wergin M, Walt H, et al: Photodynamic therapy of feline cutaneous squamous cell carcinoma using a newly developed liposomal photosensitizer: preliminary results concerning drug safety and efficacy. *J Vet Intern Med* 21:770–775, 2007.

45. Lana SE, Ogilvie GK, Withrow SJ, et al: Feline cutaneous squamous cell carcinoma of the nasal planum and the pinnae: 61cases. *J Am Hosp Assoc* 33:329–332, 1997.

46. Clarke RE: Cryosurgical treatment of feline cutaneous squamous cell carcinoma. *Aust Vet Pract* 21:148–153, 1991.

47. Jarrett RH, Norman EJ, Gibson IR, et al: Curettage and diathermy: a treatment for feline nasal planum actinic dysplasia and superficial squamous cell carcinoma. *J Small Anim Pract* 54:92–98, 2013.

48. Goodfellow M, Hayes A, Murphy S, et al: A retrospective study of (90) strontium plesiotherapy for feline squamous cell carcinoma of the nasal planum. *J Feline Med Surg* 8:169–176, 2006.

49. Hammond GM, Gordon IK, Theon AP, et al: Evaluation of strontium Sr 90 for the treatment of superficial squamous cell carcinoma of the nasal planum in cats: 49 cases (1990-2006). *J Am Vet Med Assoc* 231:736–741, 2007.

50. Théon AP, Madewell BR, Shearn VI, et al: Prognostic factors associated with radiotherapy of squamous cell carcinoma of the nasal plane in cats. *J Am Vet Med Assoc* 206:991–996, 1995.

51. Melzer K, Guscetti F, Rohrer Bley C, et al: Ki67 reactivity in nasal and periocular squamous cell carcinomas in cats treated with electron beam radiation therapy. *J Vet Intern Med* 20:676–681, 2006.

52. Trivillin VA, Heber EM, Rao M, et al: Boron neutron capture therapy (BNCT) for the treatment of spontaneous nasal planum squamous

cell carcinoma in felines. *Radiat Environ Biophys* 47:147–155, 2008.

53. de Vos JP, Burm AG, Focker BP: Results from the treatment of advanced stage squamous cell carcinoma of the nasal planum in cats, using a combination of intralesional carboplatin and superficial radiotherapy: a pilot study. *Vet Comp Oncol* 2:75–81, 2004.

54. Théon AP, VanVechten MK, Madewell BR: Intratumoral administration of carboplatin for treatment of squamous cell carcinomas of the nasal plane in cats. *Am J Vet Res* 57:205–211, 1996.

55. Spugnini EP, Vincenzi B, Citro G, et al: Electrochemotherapy for the treatment of squamous cell carcinoma in cats: a preliminary report. *Vet J* 179:117–120, 2009.

56. Bardagí M, Fondevila D, Ferrer L: Immunohistochemical detection of COX-2 in feline and canine actinic keratoses and cutaneous squamous cell carcinoma. *J Comp Pathol* 146:11–17, 2012.

57. Zhan H, Zheng H: The role of topical cyclooxygenase-2 inhibitors in skin cancer: treatment and prevention. *Am J Clin Dermatol* 8:195–200, 2007.

58. Sabattini S, Marconato L, Zoff A, et al: Epidermal growth factor receptor expression is predictive of poor prognosis in feline cutaneous squamous cell carcinoma. *J Feline Med Surg* 12:760–768, 2010.

59. Gómez Selgas A, Scase TJ, Foale RD: Unilateral squamous cell carcinoma of the renal pelvis with hydronephrosis in a cat. *J Feline Med Surg* 16:183–188, 2014.

60. Scurrell EJ, Lewin G, Solomons M, et al: Corneolimbal squamous cell carcinoma with intra-ocular invasion in two cats. *Vet Ophthalmol* 16:151–154, 2013.

61. Hayashi A, Tanaka H, Tajima T, et al: A spayed female cat with squamous cell carcinoma in the uterine remnant. *J Vet Med Sci* 75:391–393, 2013.

62. Berube D, Scott-Moncrieff JC, Rohleder J, et al: Primary esophageal squamous cell carcinoma in a cat. *J Am Anim Hosp Assoc* 45:291–295, 2009.

63. Wobeser BK, Kidney BA, Powers BE, et al: Diagnoses and clinical outcomes associated with surgically amputated feline digits submitted to multiple veterinary diagnostic laboratories. *Vet Pathol* 44:362–365, 2007.

Plasma Cell Disorders

Paul Mellor

In classical terms, a plasma cell is a terminally differentiated B lymphocyte, and a myeloma cell is its neoplastically transformed progeny. These are simplistic definitions, for plasma cell disorders (PCDs) are a complex group comprising a diverse spectrum of benign conditions to cancers known as myeloma-related disorders (MRDs).[1]

Multiple myeloma (MM) is the primogenitor of the PCD. First reported in humans in 1844, it is a cancer that has become synonymous with skeletal involvement.[2] A multistep transformation model had been hypothesized for the development of myeloma in humans. The myeloma cell is believed to be derived from a somatically mutated and isotype-switched, postgerminal center B cell corresponding to a long-lived plasma cell.[3] Intramedullary plasma cells develop karyotypic instability and form immortalized clone(s). As clone numbers increase, a premalignant bone marrow MRD becomes evident. As clonal cells evolve, there is morphological transition with concomitant cancerous myeloma features, the development of multiple myeloma and eventual extension of extramedullary metastases.[4]

Historical diagnostic criteria applied in human patients emphasizing the centrality of bone involvement were widely adopted in the diagnosis of feline myeloma.

Numerous other disorders of plasma cells, both neoplastic and nonneoplastic, have been recognized over time. Three disorders in particular provide further illustration of the historical background to PCD, namely; extramedullary plasmacytoma (EMP), monoclonal gammopathy of undetermined significance (MGUS), and immunoglobulin amyloidosis (IA).

Extramedullary plasmacytomas are tumors of plasma cells arising in soft tissues and not involving the bone marrow. In humans, they are considered rare tumors constituting approximately 5% of all MRDs; they can progress to MM in a small proportion of people.[5]

Blurred diagnostic distinctions occur not only among different MRDs but also among nonneoplastic, preneoplastic, and neoplastic PCDs. Kyle[6] introduced the term "monoclonal gammopathy of undetermined significance (MGUS)" in 1978 after observing that a proportion of asymptomatic human patients with a monoclonal protein and no discernible neoplasia have a higher risk of going on to develop MRD such as MM, Waldenström's macroglobulinemia, and IA.

In 1971, it was established that the amyloid fibrils of primary amyloidosis were comprised of immunoglobulin (Ig) light chains.[7] Note that biopsies from patients with IA typi-cally show significant abnormal protein deposition (amyloid), but the appearance of plasma cells is either not evident or low in density within the tissue of interest and elsewhere such as bone marrow. In general historical terms, IA has perhaps more often been considered within the context of the protein conformation diseases (see Pathology of Protein Deposition Diseases) and less in relation to MRD.

The first authors to describe a case of feline myeloma were Holzworth and Meier in 1957.[8] Since then, over 130 cats with a variety of MRDs have been described in the form of case studies or small case series.[9-61] Many have been reported through the prism of myeloma as defined in humans. However it appears that extramedullary involvement may be more common in cats and that the diagnostic criteria for myeloma should be reviewed.[1,62] The largest peer-reviewed case series thus far describes 26 cats.[1,62]

EPIDEMIOLOGY

In three large series of feline neoplasms, MRD accounted for 0.0012% ($n = 3248$),[14] 0.0025% ($n = 395$),[18] and up to 0.9% ($n = 1491$)[46] of all malignancies. For comparison, MRDs account for just over 1% of all tumors in dogs and in humans.[63] Within the subset of hematological neoplasia, MRDs account for 1.9% ($n = 670$) of affected cats, and 10% of affected humans.[46,64]

Reported sex distributions in feline MRD are 50% female: 50% male in one study, and 44% female: 56% male in another.[1,46] For comparison, in humans, myeloma is more common in males (61%).[65]

In the cat, the majority of MRD cases have been reported in domestic shorthair cats and in older cats (reported medians of 12 to 14 years with a range from 4 to 18 years).[1,46]

ETIOLOGY

The etiology of feline MRDs is relatively unexplored. In one study, the entire medical record was obtained for all reported cats and specifically assessed for evidence of historic or concurrent chronic antigenic stimulation. Only two of 24 cats had evidence of chronic inflammation.[1] In the same study, the entire vaccination history of all patients was examined, with no indication of an association with MRD.[1]

Overall, 37 cases of feline MRD have been assessed for feline infectious peritonitis (FIP), including feline coronavirus serology which was either negative or low-titer. The presence of feline leukemia virus was examined in 47 cases by either p27 antigen enzyme-linked immunosorbent assay (ELISA) or direct immunofluorescence assay, and only a single test in a single case was positive.[59] Similarly, the ELISA test for the antibody to feline immunodeficiency virus was carried out in 44 cats revealing two cases with single-test positive results.[50,56] A role of chronic infection in the establishment of some feline MRDs should not be ruled out. For example, infection of susceptible mice with Abelson murine leukemia virus and other retroviral constructs hastens the development of plasma cell neoplasia.[66] In human MRD patients, most have no definable etiology. However, connections to MRD have been reported for ionizing radiation,[67] petroleum-related products,[68] medicinal mineral oil,[69] Epstein-Barr virus in isolation or in combination with human immunodeficiency virus,[70,71] as well as hereditary factors.[72]

CLINICAL FEATURES

Cats with MRD may be free of clinical signs at the time of presentation, and diagnostic investigations may be mounted as a result of incidental findings on a routine blood analysis. Nonspecific clinical signs described in feline myeloma include lethargy, weakness, reduced appetite, vomiting, and diarrhea.[1] Alternatively, a number of common clinical manifestations arise which may be pathogenetically summarized as:

(i) focal problems attributable to local cellular infiltration of plasma cells or myeloma cells (an infiltrative lesion or mass development) such as bone lysis, organomegaly, or mass.
(ii) focal problems attributable to the consequences of clonal plasma cell protein production (i.e., focal light chain amyloid or Ig deposition).
(iii) systemic problems attributable to the consequences of plasma cell protein production (e.g., renal insufficiency, reciprocal humoral immunoparesis, coagulopathy, hyperviscosity, amyloidosis, or Ig deposition diseases).
(iv) systemic problems attributable to damage arising from widespread local cellular infiltration of myeloma cells (e.g., hypercalcemia from widespread osteolysis).

The following clinical features are commonly ascribed to myeloma: anemia, renal dysfunction, hypercalcemia, intramedullary involvement, extramedullary involvement, hyperviscosity, neurological signs, coagulopathy, immunosuppression, and other clinical signs.

Anemia

A nonregenerative, normocytic normochromic anemia is common in feline MRD (46% to 75% in the larger case series).[1,48] The pathogenesis of anemia can be multifactorial, including altered bone marrow microenvironment, myelophthisis, hypoerythropoietinemia in association with myeloma-related renal dysfunction, blood loss due to coagulopathies, and immune-mediated hemolytic anemia.[73,74]

Renal Dysfunction

Renal insufficiency affected 21% to 25% of feline MRD cases in the two largest case series, the pathogenesis of which can be multifactorial.[1,48] An interstitial nephritis arises from the development of light chain casts.[75] Myeloma-associated hypercalcemia and hyperviscosity can induce renal failure. Renal IA has been reported.[17] A report consistent with noncongophilic Ig deposition disease causing renal failure has recently been described.[76] Proteinuria has been reported, and this can arise through intercurrent glomerulonephropathy.[1] Medication usage (e.g., bisphosphonates, nonsteroidal antiinflammatory drugs, some chemotherapeutics) can exacerbate the renal failure.

Hypercalcemia

Hypercalcemia has been reported in 8% to 20% of feline MRD cases.[1,48] Neoplasia induced bone lysis is a key pathogenetic mechanism.[77] Elevated parathyroid hormone-related peptide is likely to be a mechanism in some cases of feline MRD as has been reported in feline lymphoma.[78] Ideally, ionized calcium should be measured since this is the functionally active element within plasma.

Intramedullary Involvement

Bone pain due to osteolysis has been a key feature in the historical understanding of MM in humans. However, in contrast, it may not be as common a feature in feline MRD.[1] In one feline MRD series, lameness was reported in 16% of cases, but none of the patients with reported lameness had radiographic evidence for bone lysis.[1] In other reports, lameness and/or skeletal pain and radiographic evidence for bone lysis have been described.[11,48] Assessing bone pain poses difficulties in cats, and it is likely underestimated by both owners and clinicians.

Extramedullary Involvement

Extramedullary involvement is frequently apparent at the time of initial presentation in feline MRD.[1] This is in contrast to humans, where extramedullary involvement is rarely a presenting feature, and instead is usually associated with metastatic progression from the intramedullary compartment.[79] The spleen, liver, and skin are commonly affected organs in cats, but a wide range of organ systems either singly or in combination with multiorgan involvement (including bone marrow) have been reported.[1,48]

Hyperviscosity

The risk of hyperviscosity syndrome (HVS) rises with increasing levels of serum monoclonal protein. It also increases with certain types of monoclonal protein (e.g., most commonly with IgM, but also IgA, and some subclasses of IgG).[80] Hyperviscosity syndrome can cause neurological signs, visual changes including blindness due to retinal hemorrhage or detachment, renal failure, hypertrophic cardiomyopathy, cardiac failure, thromboembolic disease, and bleeding diathesis.[13,19,24,28,31,56,59]

Neurological Signs

Central neurological signs have been reported in 13% of cats with MRD.[1] A wide range of neurological signs have been reported including behavioral changes, seizures, tremors, ataxia, and paresis.[24-27,31,32,46,58] The pathogenesis of most neurological signs is attributed to tumor mass effect, be that intracranial, spinal cord, or nerve compression. Hyperviscosity, hypercalcemia, meningeal involvement, and peripheral neuropathies have also been reported as potential causes for the neurologic signs.

Coagulopathy

Serum monoclonal proteins interfere with coagulation cascade, endothelial, and platelet function. Hyperviscosity and reduced capillary flow exacerbate clotting problems. Both bleeding and thrombotic problems can be observed.[81] Bleeding disorders including epistaxis, oral bleeding, melena, hyphema, and retinal hemorrhages have been reported in feline MRD.[1,29,48,56]

Immunosuppression

Numerous mechanisms for reduced cellular and humoral immunity have been described in human myeloma patients. These include numerical and functional abnormalities of dendritic cells, T cells, and Natural killer cells. Reciprocal humoral immunoparesis (reduced levels of polyclonal Igs as a result of the high serum monoclonal protein level) predisposes patients to infection by encapsulated bacteria, in particular organisms associated with pneumonia.[82] Many myeloma therapies worsen this immunosuppression. Infections are the principal cause of death and a leading cause of morbidity in human myeloma patients.[83] Immunosuppression and infection are likely under-recognized in feline patients. Severe or fatal infections have been reported in a few individual feline MRD cases (e.g., respiratory tract infection, sepsis, severe fungal infections, and pyothorax).[17,19,24,36,48,58]

Other Clinical Signs

A diversity of other signs have been reported in association with feline MRD, including constipation in a case with small intestinal plasma cell masses,[27] iridal color change with intraocular involvement,[45] pleural effusion,[28,30,36] facial edema,[19] lymphadenomegaly,[48] glaucoma with iridal involvement,[35] and chronic nasal discharge with sinonasal involvement.[53]

DIAGNOSTIC INVESTIGATIONS

Initial investigations will follow the presenting features of PCD patients who, as previously stated, may display protean clinical signs. The route to diagnosis is typically achieved through the following two pathways: discovery of hyperglobulemia and investigation of a lesion or mass.

Discovery of Hyperglobulinemia

The appropriate next stage test is serum protein electrophoresis (SPE, see Clinical Pathology of Gammopathies). Regardless of whether the globulin rise is poly- or monoclonal, where there are "significantly" elevated globulins or where progressive elevations over time have been demonstrated, these patients should have their clinical history and examination reviewed. Efforts to localize and identify possible lesion(s) associated with the hyperglobulinemia are indicated. Where SPE indicates a monoclonal protein, biopsy of soft tissue lesions (particularly of the liver, spleen, or skin masses), skeletal lesions, and/or bone marrow sampling, including aspirate(s) and core trephine(s) are warranted.

Investigation of a Lesion or Mass

The lesion may be macroscopically visible or an imaging discovery such as organomegaly or a skeletal lesion. Usually the lesion of interest will be sampled, although individual clinical judgment will be used where a surrogate sampling site associated with a lower risk of morbidity is necessary or desirable. Diagnosis is initiated by a tentative cytological or histopathological report of plasma cell lesions and/or amyloid. In the case of the former, it is essential to demonstrate the presence or absence of plasma cell clonality in the tissue of interest (see Achieving a Pathological Diagnosis in Myeloma-Related Disorders). In the case of amyloid like lesions, amyloid typing confirms the diagnosis of IA.

Once a PCD is suspected, patients should have any outstanding clinical issues re-evaluated. For example, is hyperviscosity suspected? Hyperviscosity syndrome is a clinical diagnosis based on demonstration of an elevated serum monoclonal protein in conjunction with appropriate clinical signs, in particular ophthalmic signs. While viscosity can be measured in serum, plasma, or whole blood, it is not typically used for diagnosis, and instead has been used for monitoring of patients undergoing plasmapheresis.[84] In the event of suspected HVS, are concurrent neurological signs or cardiovascular problems such as heart murmurs in association with hypertrophic cardiomyopathy present? If water intake and/or urine output are thought to be abnormal, then have renal function, calcium status, and urinalysis been assessed? If pallor is present, has any anemia been characterized? If bleeding has been reported, has coagulation been assessed? Could bone pain be a possibility in the patient, with or without imaging evidence of bone lesions? What is the confidence level that a lesion is solitary, or is there evidence for multifocal

Table 55-1	Investigations That Can Be Indicated in the Diagnosis of Plasma Cell Disorders
Tests	**What to Look for**
Ophthalmological examination	Retinal hemorrhage, retinal vessel distension and tortuosity, aneurysms
Blood pressure	Appropriate ocular signs in the absence of hypertension is consistent with hyperviscosity syndrome
Hematology	Anemia, thrombocytopenia, plasma cells in peripheral blood
Biochemistry	Hyperglobulinemia, azotemia, hypercalcemia, liver function
Rule out FIP	Coronavirus titers, alpha-1 acid glycoprotein along with other aspects of the clinical picture, plus tissue analysis
Serum gammopathy	Serum protein electrophoresis and immunoelectrophoresis or immunofixation—allowing quantification of the paraprotein concentration as well as the identity of the Ig type
Immunoglobulin profile	IgA, IgG and IgM quantification
FeLV antigen and FIV antibody	Confirm positive test results with a second assay
Microbiology—blood and/or other cultures	Where intercurrent infection is clinically suspected in these immunosuppressed patients
Blood viscosity	Can be considered for monitoring (e.g., in patients undergoing plasmapheresis)
Urinalysis	Microscopy (white blood cell count), bacterial culture
Urine Ig light chains	Urine protein electrophoresis or immunofixation
Urine protein:creatinine ratio	A high UPC combined with evidence of urine Ig light chains is highly suggestive of renal amyloidosis
Survey skeletal radiographs	Lytic lesions, osteoporosis, compression fractures, osteosclerotic lesions
Survey abdominal radiographs	Organ enlargement/masses
Abdominal ultrasonography	Enlargement/distortion of normal organ architecture (in particular of the liver/spleen) or the presence of masses
Magnetic resonance imaging	MRI is recommended (over computed tomography) in suspected myeloma patients with normal conventional radiography findings, as well as in patients with an apparently solitary plasmacytoma (of bone or extramedullary)[90]
Coagulation profiles prior to biopsy	Thrombocytopathia and altered coagulation times as a result of hyperglobulinemia
Cytology	Bone marrow aspirate, fine-needle aspirates of abnormal organs, masses on the liver or spleen; B cell immunomorphology
Histopathology	Bone marrow core, tissue biopsy of abnormal organs/masses; B cell immunomorphology, amyloid
Immunohistochemistry or immunocytochemistry	Indication of clonality; expression of a single light or heavy chain type
Polymerase chain reaction	Indication of clonality[151]

FeLV, feline leukemia virus; *FIP,* feline infectious peritonitis; *FIV,* feline immunodeficiency virus; *Ig,* immunoglobulin; *UPC,* urine protein:creatinine ratio; *MRI,* magnetic resonance imaging

involvement? Are additional imaging studies indicated? A description of some of the tests that may be considered in feline MRD is given in Table 55-1.

CLINICAL PATHOLOGY OF GAMMOPATHIES

Hyperglobulinemias (or gammopathies) can broadly be divided into polyclonal and monoclonal protein increases. Polyclonal globulin increases are associated with reactive or inflammatory plasma cell disorders and these patients are generally not considered to have a MRD. Monoclonal proteins (also known as M-proteins or myeloma proteins and a subset of the paraproteins) are Igs typically of normal structure and charge but present in excessive quantity, and they are a hallmark of MRD.[85] Standard high-resolution agarose gel SPE has been reported to identify a monoclonal protein in 82% of human patients with MM.[86] However, low levels of monoclonal protein can be concealed within the beta or gamma regions of a routine SPE trace. Over time electrophoretic tests have improved (e.g., capillary zone electrophoresis). Furthermore, a combination of tests are used to increase the diagnostic accuracy for PCD.[87] Serum protein electrophoresis will detect monoclonal levels as low as 500 mg/L, immunofixation as low as 150 mg/L, but the latest nephelometric immunoassays for serum immunoglobulin free light chains (SFLC) are capable of detecting less than 1 mg/L. Quantification of SFLC is now recommended in all human MRD patients for the purposes of diagnosis, prognosis, and monitoring.[88] Note that even where standard electrophoresis methodologies do detect a quantitative abnormality, they cannot always reliably identify a monoclonal protein and differentiate it from, for example, a restricted oligoclonal gammopathy. Therefore, immunofixation electrophoresis is used as the confirmatory gold standard test for the presence of a monoclonal protein and to distinguish its heavy and light chain type. A 24-hour urine collection for urine protein electrophoresis, protein quantification, and immunofixation are additional tests frequently used in the investigation of monoclonal gammopathies in humans.[89]

Although most cases of hyperglobulinemia can be commonly assigned to either a poly- or a monoclonal gammopathy, it is not universally dichotomous. Human patients with biclonal and triclonal gammopathies have been described, most with a confirmed lymphoproliferative neoplasm, but some were of undetermined significance, and others had non-hematological diseases.[90,91]

In the cat, cases of hyperglobulinemia are typically further assessed by standard agarose gel electrophoresis. Use of capillary zone electrophoresis and immunoelectrophoresis (but not immunofixation) have recently been described in feline MRD.[18,21]

Most cases of feline hyperglobulinemia have a polyclonal gammopathy. The underlying cause of a polyclonal gammopathy is a diverse range of disorders with a reactive or inflammatory plasma cell component.[93]

Monoclonal gammopathies in cats are most commonly associated MRD and/or lymphoma.[1,19,26,36,48] Monoclonal gammopathies have been reported in rare cases of FIP, lymphocytic-plasmacytic stomatitis, and anaplasmosis.[19,40,92-94] However, the stringency of diagnosis in these latter reports is relatively uncertain (where described, it is based on histopathology or hematopathology only and no further confirmatory tests). Furthermore, there is a possibility of ascertainment bias and coincidental association.[95] Note that biclonal paraproteinemias have been reported in feline MRD.[1,12,38]

The evolved complexity, precision of analysis, and interpretation of gammopathies seen in human patients have not been available in the cat. Some reports in the feline literature of monoclonal and biclonal gammopathies in association with MRD may be incorrect in the absence of immunofixation electrophoresis and confirmation of a clonal MRD within the tissue of interest. Furthermore, there are four cases reported in the feline literature to have MRD on the basis of routine histopathology, with no demonstration of tissue clonality but instead having a polyclonal gammopathy.[26,58,62] They

may be cases of MRD intercurrent with another disease process inducing the polyclonal gammopathy, but it is more probable that they are misdiagnoses, reflecting reactive or inflammatory plasma cell lesions. They are not considered further in this review.

PATHOLOGY OF PLASMA CELLS AND PLASMA CELL DISORDERS

Cellular Morphology

The key morphological features of a mature plasma cell (also known as a terminally differentiated plasma cell, Marschalko cell, or plasmacyte) are as follows: intensely basophilic cytoplasm due to the high ribonucleoprotein content, an acroplasm (or pale perinuclear "hof", a focal area of clearing) representing a prominent Golgi apparatus, an eccentric nuclear position, and "cartwheel" chromatin arrangement. Variations in plasma cell morphology have been clearly defined in humans. Plasmacytoid is a descriptor for (1) any nonspecific variation of mature plasma cell characteristics, and (2) plasma cell type appearance of cells of non-B cell origin. Lympho-plasmacytoid cells have a mixed lymphocyte and mature plasma cell appearance with typically less basophilic cytoplasm. Flame cells and/or thesaurocytes have red to violaceous coloration of the cytoplasm attributed to the accumulation of high carbohydrate content Ig within the endoplasmic reticulum cisternae.[96] Mott cells contain multiple cytoplasmic Russell bodies (Ig inclusions).[97] Proplasmacytes are larger than mature plasma cells with greater anisocytosis, asynchronous nuclear and cytoplasmic maturation, and indistinct or small nucleoli.[98] Plasmablasts are larger than mature plasma cells with greater anisocytosis, a narrow rim of cytoplasm, less distinct or inapparent perinuclear hof, high N : C ratio, a large and immature round to ovoid eccentric nucleus with anisokaryosis, and one or more prominent nucleoli.[98] Binucleate, trinucleate, and multinucleate giant myeloma cells may also be observed.[99]

In the feline MRD literature, many histopathologic and cytopathologic reports of feline MRD simply describe the neoplasia as comprising of plasma cells. Other reports have provided greater detail and virtually all of the morphological descriptors used in human myeloma have been used in the cat including mature (Marschalko-type) plasma cells,[64] plasmacytoid,[14,25,39] lympho-plasmacytoid,[23,50,59] flame cells,[48] Russell bodies,[64] Mott cells,[53] proplasmacytes,[64] plasmablasts,[64] and giant multinucleated myeloma cells.[78,94] Cytopathological and histopathological examples of these cells may be seen at the *Veterinary Myeloma Website*.[100]

Achieving a Pathological Diagnosis in Myeloma-Related Disorders

Taken in isolation, the examination of a single plasmacytoid cell or even groups of plasma cells does not allow the cytopathologist or histopathologist to define that these cells are myeloma cells (that is to say, neoplastically transformed).

Progressive morphologic changes within plasma cells (with ultimately the development of plasmablastic features) have clearly been correlated with accumulating cytogenetic aberrations and progressive clinical disease.[101,102] Yet these morphologic changes do not take place uniformly. Diverse populations of plasma cell morphology may be seen within a single biopsy. Therefore, a *provisional diagnosis* of a MRD is achieved through synthesis of multiple observations including lesional and perilesional tissue and cellular changes, density of plasma cells, as well as the above plasma cell morphological features and the relative proportions between these cells. In soft tissues, the presence of mass-related changes allows greater confidence in the provisional diagnosis. Within bone marrow, although near complete effacement of the marrow cavity by plasma cells is occasionally observed, it is more common to see varying degrees of plasma cell density and a cut off of 10% or greater infiltration is required for diagnosis.[103]

The demonstration of monoclonality in the tissue of interest remains the gold standard for the pathological component of diagnosis of this hematopoietic neoplasia (e.g., patients can have concurrent MGUS and an unrelated round cell tumor misinterpreted as a MRD). The demonstration of polyclonality within the tissue of interest implies a reactive or inflammatory plasma cell population. Clonality may be investigated via a number of techniques. Immunohistochemistry and immunocytochemistry allow the surrogate demonstration of clonality when expression of a single Ig light chain only is revealed, and this is the most common technique in veterinary medicine. Alternative techniques include flow cytometry, molecular biological tests such as polymerase chain reaction and Southern blot, and an array of cytogenetic and epigenetic tests.[89,104-108] In practical terms, the confirmed presence of IA can also be used as a surrogate marker of clonality, but there should be an awareness that in rare patients there may be discordant results.[109,110]

In some of the published feline MRD series, there have been arguably insufficiently stringent inclusion criteria, with some individual patients diagnosed with MRD on the basis of histopathology alone, with no serum or urine protein electrophoresis carried out, and no other assessment of clonality.[26,36,48] In the practice of veterinary medicine, there is often a pragmatic clinical supposition of a MRD if routine hematoxylin and eosin (H&E) stained pathology or cytopathology provide a morphological diagnosis consistent with a MRD and this is combined with an indirect indication of clonality (i.e., the detection of a monoclonal protein in serum or urine). However, the importance of clonal confirmation in the tissue of interest in cases of feline MRD has been reported. In one study, 34 histopathological samples with an original diagnosis of MRD made by a diversity of board-certified pathologists in various institutions and laboratories were subjected to review by an independent panel of board-certified pathologists who examined H&E stained sections along with additional histochemical and immunohistochemical stained sections. Only 56% (*n* = 19) of the cases were eventually shown to be clonal MRD by light chain

restriction.[64] Some of the excluded feline cases were not of B cell origin despite a plasmacytoid appearance (instead proving to be histiocytic neoplasms or mast cell tumors). Cellular morphology is linked to function, and other non-B lymphoid cells that have high demand for protein production (e.g., not Ig) may have a plasmacytoid appearance. Further examples include plasmacytoid dendritic cells, histiocytes, salivary gland duct luminal cells, and myoepithelial cells.[110-114]

Pathological Classification and Grading

In human patients, there is no internationally accepted standard for the morphologic categorization of MRD, but a key feature of most reported systems is the division into well-differentiated, intermediate-grade, or poorly differentiated tumors, depending on the proportions of cell types from mature plasma cells to poorly differentiated plasmablastic cells. Tumor grading has prognostic significance.[115,116] There is generally good agreement between cytologic and histologic categorization of tumors.[64,98]

Only two case series with clonally confirmed MRD have presented tumor morphologic classification systems in the cat.[41,64] In the largest case series of feline MRD thus far, tumors were classified as well-differentiated (less than 15% plasmablasts, with the remainder being mature myeloma cells, proplasmacytes, or lymphocytes), intermediate-grade (15% to 49% plasmablasts), or poorly differentiated (greater than 50% plasmablasts). A correlation between morphology and survival was proved with statistical significance. Cats with well-differentiated tumors had increased median survival time relative to those with poorly differentiated tumors (254 versus 14 days [Figure 55-1]).[64]

PATHOLOGY OF PROTEIN DEPOSITION DISEASES—AMYLOIDOSIS AND MONOCLONAL IMMUNOGLOBULIN DEPOSITION DISEASE

Amyloidosis is a subset of the protein conformation diseases that share a common pathophysiological mechanism, proteotoxicity. This occurs through both the direct cellular toxic effect of amyloid precursors, as well as damage to organ structure and function via massive deposition of amyloid fibrils in extracellular spaces. Biopsies must show amyloid deposition confirmed by Congo-red staining and apple-green birefringence under polarizing light microscopy. The amyloid must then be typed, which historically has been achieved through histochemical assessment or immunohistochemistry, although more recently it has been supplanted by laser microdissection with mass spectrometry (LMD/MS).[117] Typing allows precise categorization of the amyloid. Numerous amyloidogenic proteins have been discovered, but only a single group is relevant to the MRD—the IA.[118] Historically, IA diseases have largely been considered separately from MRD. Even in recent times, IA is described by some authors as a nonproliferative and nonneoplastic PCD.[119] However, current work confirms shared aspects of pathogenesis in terms of the

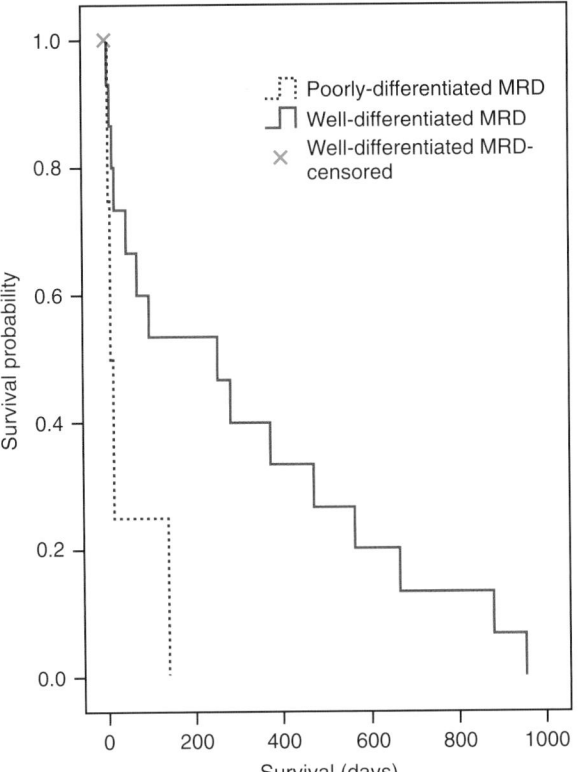

Figure 55-1: Kaplan-Meier survival curves for poorly differentiated myeloma-related disorders (MRD) versus well-differentiated MRD.[64] (Redrawn from Mellor PJ, Haugland S, Smith KC, Powell RM, Archer J, Scase TJ, et al. Histopathologic, immunohistochemical, and cytologic analysis of feline myeloma-related disorders: further evidence for primary extramedullary development in the cat. Vet Pathol Online. 2008;45(2):159–73.)

underlying cytogenetic aberrations, as well as outcomes in subsets of human patients, with the suggestion that IA be considered as low-proliferative, neoplastic MRD.[120,121]

In feline PCD, amyloidosis confirmed by light microscopy has been reported, but confirmation of amyloid type (to Ig) has been inconsistent. Both systemic and local forms of IA have been suspected in the cat.[46,48,70,71,79,81,94] Precise amyloid typing in cats (including immunohistochemistry and LMD/MS) can be conducted with assistance from human medical laboratories (Paul Mellor, unpublished observations).

Monoclonal immunoglobulin deposition diseases (MIDD) are rare in humans. They are characterized by the deposition of monoclonal Ig molecules in basement membranes and in contrast to amyloidosis, the deposits are nonfibrillar and Congo-red negative.[122] Noncongophilic Ig deposition has been described in the cat, but MIDD has not yet been described in the feline literature.[76]

FELINE PLASMA CELL DISORDER—EXISTING DIAGNOSES IN THE PUBLISHED LITERATURE

The existing feline literature outlines a diversity of PCD presentations. Plasma cell disorders are described with sometimes confusing terminology and diagnostic criteria, and

where this is relevant it is highlighted later. Table 55-2 outlines a range of existing diagnoses and diagnostic criteria for PCD in cats.

Polyclonal Plasma Cell Disorders

Reactive plasmacytosis and a plethora of inflammatory diseases contain lesser or greater numbers of polyclonal plasma or plasmacytoid cells, particularly in the feline species. Plasma cell pododermatitis, nasal plasma cell dermatitis, and plasma cell stomatitis-pharyngitis are inflammatory plasma cell disorders in the cat.[123-127] Some cats present with a combination of the aforementioned disorders.[128,129] An accompanying polyclonal gammopathy has been reported in some cases across all three disorders.[130] No infectious etiology has been demonstrated and an immune-mediated pathogenesis is suspected.[131] Only in two cats have possible connections to a MRD been construed. In a single report of feline stomatitis, a monoclonal protein was demonstrated in serum and urine. However, the validity of this report is questionable with no proof or disproof of clonality within the tissue biopsy, and no exclusion of intercurrent MRD in alternate locations.[93] In the second case, a cat with pododermatitis was reported to have subsequently developed systemic amyloidosis. There was no typing of the amyloidosis (to confirm Ig origin) and no exclusion of intercurrent MRD in alternate locations.[123]

Plasma cell granulomas (more commonly known as inflammatory pseudotumor in the cat or inflammatory myofibroblastic tumor) contain polyclonal plasma cells but are clinically and pathologically readily distinguishable from other PCDs and MRDs.[132,133]

Monoclonal Plasma Cell Disorders

Monoclonal Gammopathy of Undetermined Significance, Benign Monoclonal Gammopathy, and Smoldering Myeloma

Monoclonal gammoptahy of undetermined significance describes the finding of a serum monoclonal protein without clinical or investigational evidence for myeloma (see Table 55-2 for diagnostic criteria). The proportion of healthy people with MGUS increases with age. In long-term follow-up studies of MGUS in humans, approximately 75% of patients do not evolve into classical MM.[8,134] These patients can be described as having had a benign monoclonal gammopathy at point of death only and where death was due to nonmyeloma-related causes. However, despite the fact that most MGUS patients do not within their lifespan develop overt symptoms of myeloma, most or all are expected to have a clonal plasma cell disorder. In cytogenetic studies alone, plasma cell clone(s) have been demonstrated in 77% of human patients with MGUS.[135] All human myeloma patients are believed to progress from MGUS, through smoldering myeloma (asymptomatic myeloma), and to myeloma (see Table 55-2 for diagnostic criteria).

Monoclonal gammopathy of undetermined significance was first reported in a cat in 1977, although the stringency

Table 55-2   **Traditional Diagnostic Scheme for Plasma Cell Disorders, with Alternate Diagnostic Names and Summarized Diagnostic Criteria**

Principal Name (Alternate Names in Italics)	Diagnostic Criteria Typically Applied in Cats
Plasma cell disorders	
Plasma cell pododermatitis *(Plasmacytic pododermatitis)*	Clinical signs with histopathology/cytology, +/– polyclonal gammopathy; note demonstration of polyclonality within the tissue is desirable for academic confirmation
Nasal plasma cell dermatitis	As above
Plasma cell stomatitis-pharyngitis *(Plasma cell stomatitis, lympho-plasmacytic stomatitis)*	As above
Monoclonal gammopathy of undetermined significance *(monoclonal gammopathy of unknown/uncertain significance, monoclonal gammopathy unassociated/ unattributed, paraproteinemia, monoclonal gammopathy, benign monoclonal gammopathy, monoclonal hypergammaglobulinemia)*	SPE monoclonal protein without initial evidence of clinical signs, nor hematologic or biochemical abnormalities, nor radiographic evidence for bone lytic lesions, and <10% marrow plasma cell content[48]
Preneoplasmic plasma cell disorder	
Smoldering myeloma *(Indolent myeloma, asymptomatic myeloma)*	Not formally described in feline literature; however, at least one reported feline case would be consistent with the description[48]
Malignant plasma cell disorders—Myeloma-related disorders	
Multiple myeloma *(Plasma cell sarcoma, plasma cell tumor, plasma cell myeloma, reticulum cell myeloma, Kahler's disease, myelomatosis)*	Variable criteria used historically; typical example—at least two of the following criteria: (1) monoclonal gammopathy, (2) radiographic evidence of osteolysis, (3) Bence Jones proteinuria, (4) >5% marrow plasma cells[26]
Symptomatic multiple myeloma	Not reported in the feline literature
Nonsecretory & oligo-secretory myeloma	Not adequately reported in the feline literature
Solitary extramedullary plasmacytoma *(soft tissue plasmacytoma, nonosseous* plasmacytoma, cutaneous, noncutaneous)	Variable criteria used historically; typical example—neoplastic plasma cell formation in soft tissue without primary evidence of bone marrow involvement[1]
Multiple solitary extramedullary plasmacytoma	Strict criteria are undefined in the feline literature
Solitary plasmacytoma of bone	Inadequately stringent diagnostic criteria in the feline literature[44]
Multiple solitary plasmacytoma of bone	Not reported in the feline literature
Immunoglobulin M macroglobulinemia *(Waldenström's macroglobulinemia, lymphoplasmacytic lymphoma, immunocytoma)*	Strict criteria are undefined in the feline literature[59]
Immunoglobulin secreting lymphoma	Based on morphological description (histopathology/cytopathology) only
Osteosclerotic myeloma *(POEMS syndrome, multicentric Castleman disease, Crowe-Fukase syndrome, Takatsuki syndrome)*	Not reported in the feline literature
Plasma cell leukemia *(Myeloma with leukemic overspill)*	Variable criteria used historically; typical example—peripheral blood plasma cells >20% or $>2 \times 10^9$ cells/L[49]
Low proliferative clonal plasma cell disorders as protein deposition diseases	
Immunoglobulin amyloidosis	Inadequately stringent diagnostic criteria in the feline literature

POEMS, polyneuropathy, organomegaly, endocrinopathy, monoclonal gammopathy, and skin changes; *SPE*, serum protein electrophoresis.

of exclusion of MRD is not known as details of the clinical investigations are lacking in this earlier paper.[40] Feline MGUS has been reported in a 4-year-old cat with monoclonal gammopathy, with no evidence of clinical signs, nor other abnormalities (hematologic, biochemical, radiographic evidence for lytic lesions, ultrasonographic evidence for lesions, light chain proteinuria) and less than 10% marrow plasma cell content. This cat developed myeloma at 9 years of age.[48] The details of progression are not documented in the report, but the expectation is that this cat will have evolved from MGUS though to smoldering myeloma and ultimately myeloma.

Multiple Myeloma

Classical cases of MM have been described in the cat, with marked bone marrow plasma cell infiltration, radiographic evidence for bone lysis, and a monoclonal protein detectable in serum and/or urine.[1,26,28,29,32,40,48,54] Diagnostic criteria are given in Table 55-2. However, there has been some confusion in earlier literature regarding the diagnostic criteria of MM in cats. For example, cats have been reported as having MM despite pathological evidence of the *absence* of bone marrow infiltration, and instead having extramedullary involvement.[36,46] In general, across the feline literature, given the historical diagnostic criteria, there will likely have been a tendency to a reporting bias towards MM cases that involved radiographic bone lesions. Examining the literature prior to 2005, 75 cases of all types of MRD had been described, of which 36 provided clinical details of investigations (mainly in the form of case reports or small case series). Of these, 22 cases were explicitly described as MM, of which only 6 (27%) had radiographically evident bone lesions—a notably low proportion in comparison to humans—in whom 80% of MM cases have radiographically detectable osteolysis.[136] Then in 2005, two larger clinical case series of MM were published. In one series from a single institution, 58.3% of MM cases had radiographically evident bone lesions.[48] In another series from a single veterinary practice with an orthopedic bias, the proportion was 71.4%.[26] However, in 2006, in a multidepartmental, multicenter clinical case series, the authors proposed that feline MRD cases infrequently (8%) present with radiographic bone lesions, with some additional statistical support for this hypothesis.[1] The conclusions that can be drawn are limited by the retrospective nature of all of these studies, the failure to obtain complete skeletal survey radiographs in all cases, and the imperfect comparisons made. However, given the pre-existing literature and the authors' findings, it is probable that fewer feline MRD cases have classical radiographically detectable osteolysis compared to human patients.

Extramedullary Plasmacytoma

Soft tissue involvement can arise by metastatic extension from intramedullary myeloma via the hematogenous route, by direct extension from skeletal disease (arising from a focal marrow lesion broaching cortical bone with adjacent soft tissue infiltration), and by infiltration of traumatized areas (including sites of subcutaneous injection, intravenous catheter placement, surgery, and pathological fracture).[137-139] However, a primary (true) EMP is a monoclonal plasma cell neoplasm that arises *de novo* in soft tissue without evidence for concurrent bone marrow involvement (see Table 55-2). There is evidence that extramedullary tissue may be a more common primary site of myeloma cell development than the intramedullary compartment in the cat.[1,64]

There have been pathological reports of cutaneous masses in feline MRD,[14,39,41] but relatively few with accompanying comprehensive clinical investigations that allow a diagnosis of cutaneous extramedullary plasmacytoma (CEMP—see Table 55-2). Some feline CEMPs have been apparently solitary masses, not associated with systemic signs or hyperglobulinemia and where surgical excision resulted in prolonged survival.[1] This is similar to the biologic behavior typically shown in other species, where CEMPs are usually nonsecretory, have a benign course, and surgical excision is curative.[79,140] Rarely, CEMPs show a malignant course with progression to myeloma in either humans or the dog.[79,141] By contrast, a number of feline MRD reports exist where cats with cutaneous plasma cell neoplasms exhibited systemic signs, had a demonstrable monoclonal protein, were affected by multi-organ plasma cell infiltration, and experienced rapid tumor development.[1,15,19,27,49]

Noncutaneous extramedullary plasmacytoma (NCEMP) appears to be common in the cat, comprising 50% of those MRD cases that had both bone marrow and abdominal organ sampling carried out in one series.[1] Occasional feline NCEMP reports have described isolated tumors showing localized signs, without evidence for systemic involvement or hyperglobulinemia (e.g., within the uveal tract or sinonasal cavities).[35,45,53] However, the majority of feline NCEMP feline cases have had signs of systemic illness, an accompanying monoclonal protein, and later metastatic or multisite development.[1,27,42,48,56,61] Typically, the liver and/or spleen were infiltrated. Other locations have included the kidneys, gastrointestinal tract, lymph nodes, stomach, epidura, orbit, and retroperitoneal space. In the largest clinical series of confirmed feline MRD, the hypothesis that cats with MRD commonly present with extramedullary involvement in contrast to human patients with MRD was demonstrated (67% versus 5% respectively, $p < 0.001$).[1]

Nonsecretory Myeloma

A single cat with a pathological diagnosis of uveal and mandibular lymph node plasma cell neoplasia along with immunohistochemically confirmed cellular cytoplasmic IgG expression, did not have a monoclonal gammopathy as assessed by serum protein electrophoresis alone, but further serum or urine studies for a monoclonal protein were not carried out.[45] More stringent diagnostic criteria are necessary for a tentative diagnosis of nonsecretory myeloma (see Table 55-2). Less than 3% of human patients diagnosed with a MRD are described as having nonsecretory myeloma.[142] Immunohistochemical studies demonstrate the presence of cytoplasmic monoclonal proteins within the plasma cells of most of these patients, (e.g., Ig synthesis is intact).[143] In humans, true nonsecretory myeloma patients have no detectable monoclonal protein in serum or urine by any of the aforementioned methods (including SFLC).[103,144]

Solitary Plasmacytoma of Bone

Solitary plasmacytoma of bone (SPB) patients present with a single lesion of monoclonal plasma cells in bone but with no evidence of myeloma cells elsewhere. Typically, these patients present with localized signs (e.g., bone pain in association with the lesion), although some patients will have a painless bony deformity, neurological signs in association with compression, or lesion(s) discovered as an incidental finding during radiographic surveys for other purposes. Solitary plasmacytoma of bone is a rare MRD. Clinical evolution from SPB to MM is recognized, although a key feature of SBP patients is the slow natural time course of disease progression. As diagnostic testing methodology has advanced, the diagnostic criteria for SPB have changed. For example, many more SPB patients have been discovered with monoclonal proteins with the advent of more sensitive techniques for assessment. Patients thought to be affected with SPB have instead been reclassified as MM through magnetic resonance imaging (MRI) discovery of additional bone lesions not apparent on standard skeletal radiographic survey.[145] Current diagnostic criteria for SBP are given in Table 55-2. Two feline cases of SBP have been reported.[44] Both cats presented with single spinal lesions causing neurological signs. Both were treated, and prolonged remissions for several years were achieved with radiotherapy in one case and chemotherapy in the other.

Immunoglobulin M Macroglobulinemia

In humans, Waldenström macroglobulinemia is the most common subset of the comparatively rare IgM macroglobulinemias. It has rarely been reported in cats.[40,60] A feline case providing greater investigational detail including postmortem findings, was found to have IgM-secreting lympho-plasmacytoid cells in the liver only and no evidence of bone marrow infiltration.[59]

Immunoglobulin-Secreting Lymphoma

Some patients present with either risk factors for the development of, or actual clinical signs of MRD dysfunction (e.g., gammopathy or amyloidosis), but they lack typical plasma cell or plasmacytoid cell characteristics (as assessed by routine cytopathology, histopathology, immunocyto- or immunohistochemistry, flow cytometry, etc.) instead being classified as lymphoma.

Several feline cases have been described in the literature as having Ig-secreting lymphoma (but with limited pathological descriptions ranging from lymphoid cells to lympho-plasmacytic cells).[19,33,34,40,50,146]

Plasma Cell Leukemia

Plasma cell leukemia (PCL) is a rare and aggressive MRD characterized by the presence of circulating plasma cells (see Table 55-2). Note that nonneoplastic conditions, such as severe sepsis, can occasionally result in transient elevations of circulating plasma cells.[147] Therefore, demonstration of monoclonality is required as per other MRDs (e.g., by flow cytometry, immunocytochemistry, cell block preparations for immunohistochemistry, or molecular techniques). It is classified as either primary PCL when it presents "*de novo*" in patients with no previous history of MRD or as secondary when it is observed as a leukemic transformation of a preexisting progressive MRD. Primary PCL is a distinct clinicpathological entity with different cytogenetic and molecular findings.[147] Plasma cell leukemia has been reported in three cats, of which two case reports provide good clinical description of secondary PCL.[49,55]

A SUGGESTED RECLASSIFICATION OF PLASMA CELL DISORDER

From the earlier sections, it can be seen that the PCDs form a complex set of disorders. Indeed in humans, there are additional disorders involving plasma cell pathology and gammopathies that have yet to be described in the feline literature. In the past two decades, there has been a move to classify human patients into a new category: "Symptomatic Multiple Myeloma." This new diagnosis accommodates patients with either intramedullary or extramedullary disease, or both (see Table 55-2). Symptomatic multiple myeloma also accords significance to whether patients are displaying signs of myeloma-related end organ damage. There may be value in recategorizing MRDs in veterinary medicine, employing a system that potentially facilitates greater consistency in diagnostic investigation and classification. The proposed system retains a central role for pathological diagnosis, but with an altered, more patient-centric focus explicitly incorporating a broader range of myeloma-related clinical problems. A system that incorporates other lymphoproliferative disorders into MRD when they have protein-related functional disorders (e.g., lymphoma patients producing a monoclonal protein, or patients with IA or MIDD). Ultimately, this system is a combined diagnosis and risk stratification system. This last point in particular is of assistance when there are indistinct boundaries between traditional MRD diagnostic categories which may be observed in patients of any species. Patients may be asymptomatic with low cellular proliferation (benign monoclonal gammopathy at time of death), clinically affected with low cellular proliferation (immunoglobulin amyloidosis), or clinically affected with high cellular proliferation (multiple myeloma). Furthermore, clonal plasma cells can show widely varying biological behavior within the same patient over the course of a lifetime.

In the proposed new system, a plasma cell disorder may be subcategorized as a myeloma-related disorder typically by combining (i) cytopathology or histopathology with (ii) a demonstration of clonality in the tissue of interest and (iii) evidence of clinical problems attributable to the MRD. Therefore, the distinguishing feature of a MRD is a judgment regarding the transition to neoplastic behavior (Table 55-3)

Table 55-3	Mellor's Classification Scheme for Myeloma-Related Disorders				
Area	**Pathology**	**Protein— Serum/Urine Monoclonal**	**Problems—MRD Attributable**	**Mellor's Classification Based on Location and Rate of Progression Risk**	**Traditional Example(s)**
Single site	Amyloid positive and predominant pathology, typically with minimal plasma cell content	Usually negative, but low positive possible	None	**Solitary** MRD—**slow** rate of progression risk	Primary cutaneous immunoglobulin amyloidosis
Single site	Plasma cells (WD or Int) and/or amyloid positive (local single site only); no MIDD	Negative, low positive or positive	None	**Solitary** MRD— **moderate** rate of progression risk	CEMP or NCEMP or IgM macroglobulinaemia or SBP or amyloidoma
Single site	Plasma cells (WD or Int) and/or amyloid positive (local single site only); no MIDD	As above	Yes (but no vital organ failure)	**Solitary** MRD—**high** rate of progression risk	As above
Single site	As above but plasma cells PD or WD or Int grade if accompanied by vital organ failure (see signs)	As above	Yes (up to and including vital organ failure)	**Solitary** MRD—**very high** rate of progression risk	As above
No clearly defined lesion	Marrow negative; no soft tissue lesion. No amyloid; no MIDD	Low positive or positive	None	**Multifocal suspected** MRD—**slow** rate of progression risk	MGUS
Lesion(s) may/may not be clearly defined	Marrow negative; or marrow positive, but no other organs, or soft tissue infiltration is uncertain (e.g., liver with sinusoidal plasma cells); no amyloid; no MIDD	Positive with recent evidence for accelerating levels	None	**Multifocal suspected** MRD—**moderate** rate of progression risk	Smoldering myeloma
Two or more lesions	Plasma cells (WD or Int) at ≥2 marrow sites, ≥2 soft tissue sites, or marrow plus soft tissue site(s) and/or amyloid positive (internal organ(s)) and/or MIDD-positive	Usually positive (but can be negative in nonsecretory myeloma, amyloidosis and MIDD cases)	Yes (but no vital organ failure)	**Multifocal** MRD—**high** rate of progression risk	MM, EMP, combined intra- & extramedullary myeloma, IgM macroglobulinaemia, systemic Ig amyloidosis, MIDD

Continued

Table 55-3 **Mellor's Classification Scheme for Myeloma-Related Disorders—cont'd**

Area	Pathology	Protein— Serum/Urine Monoclonal	Problems—MRD Attributable	Mellor's Classification Based on Location and Rate of Progression Risk	Traditional Example(s)
Two or more lesions	As earlier but plasma cells PD, WD, or Int grade if accompanied by vital organ failure (see signs)	As above	Yes (up to and including vital organ failure)	**Multifocal** MRD— **very high** rate of progression risk	As above
Blood	Blood positive for plasma cells or other Ig secreting leukemic cells (≥5%)	Usually positive	Yes (up to and including vital organ failure)	**Multifocal** MRD— **very high** rate of progression risk	Plasma cell leukaemia and Ig secreting leukaemias (primary or secondary)
Two or more lesions	Amyloid positive and predominant pathology, typically with minimal plasma cell content; bone marrow usually negative, but can be positive (any grade)	Usually positive	Yes—including vital organ failure	**Multifocal** MRD— **very high** rate of progression risk	Systemic Ig amyloidosis
Two or more lesions	Monoclonal Ig deposition—usually both kidneys—but with minimal intralesional plasma cell content; other organs can be affected by Ig deposition; plasma cell infiltration of bone marrow and/or soft tissues can be positive or negative (and any grade)	Usually positive	Yes—including vital organ failure	**Multifocal** MRD— **very high** rate of progression risk	MIDD

This is a novel combined diagnostic and staging scheme based around "APPP" (Area, Pathology, Protein, Problems), allowing patients to be broadly stratified according to their "rate of progression risk". This new system is designed to facilitate greater consistency in diagnostic investigation, clarify classification, and assist in therapeutic decision making.

Notes:

In the pathology column; WD = well-differentiated grade, Int = intermediate grade, PD = poorly differentiated grade tumours. Marrow negative implies <10% plasma cells in bone marrow, where (a) marrow has been successfully sampled at preferably two separate anatomic sites and (b) preferably at least one aspirate and one trephine biopsies have been obtained. Marrow positive implies ≥10% plasma cells in bone marrow obtained by any sampling technique. Amyloid must be demonstrated to be of immunoglobulin origin. MIDD—deposits must be shown not to be amyloid.

In the protein column: "Usually negative" or "usually positive" refers to the absence or presence of a monoclonal spike by standard protein electrophoresis of serum or urine. "Low positive" refers to the presence of a small monoclonal spike as detected by either examination of the original densitometer trace in standard protein electrophoresis or other more sensitive assessment techniques (see text for details), when the total serum globulin level is only slightly elevated or within normal limits.

In the problems column: refer to text for the description of key MRD attributable problems arising from organ damage or tissue impairment (systemic, multifocal or local). Vital organ failure (e.g., of the kidneys or liver) may have a chronic or acute-on-chronic presentation. Vital organ failure does not always include simple visceral organ capsular compromise leading to capsular rupture and hemorrhage (e.g., an infiltrated spleen).

CEMP, cutaneous extramedullary plasmacytoma; EMP, extramedullary plasmacytoma; Ig, immunoglobulin; MGUS, monoclonal gammopathy of undetermined significance; MIDD, monoclonal immunoglobulin deposition diseases; MM, multiple myeloma; MRD, myeloma-related disorders; NCEMP, noncutaneous extramedullary plasmacytoma; SBP, solitary plasmacytoma of bone.

that results in accompanying local or systemic clinically relevant problems. A tentative diagnosis of "suspected MRD" can be achieved in the absence of cellular evidence of plasma cell infiltration or IA through confident demonstration of a serum and/or urine monoclonal protein (preferably by immunofixation) and with no alternate diagnosis for the monoclonal protein evident. Suspected MRD is a preneoplastic categorization in a proportion of patients. Examples include MGUS and smoldering myeloma. In the event of patient death due to unrelated causes, these conditions may never have progressed to displaying neoplastic behavior (in terms of evident pathological damage or clinical relevant problems attributable to a MRD). Nevertheless they are clonal disorders, and the rationale for the ongoing monitoring of these patients is contingent upon the known risk of the development of overt neoplasia.

In summary, the proposed new system categorizes patients according to whether the disease is apparently solitary or multifocal, examines pathological grade, and describes disease effects of monoclonal protein production and/or deposition, as well as any key clinically relevant problems seen in the patient. This assessment may be summarized to the mnemonic; "APPP" (Area, Pathology, Protein, Problems). From this, patients can be stratified according to their "rate of progression risk":

Area (or anatomic location) defines the location(s) of affected areas. Either:

(a) multifocal lesions (a single osteolytic lesion plus a separate bone marrow site [not associated with clinical or imaging evidence of a lesion] showing greater than 10% plasma cell content, ideally in both sites), two or more osteolytic lesions with proof of plasma cell infiltration in at least one lesion, combined intramedullary and extramedullary biopsy confirmed lesions, or two or more biopsy confirmed extramedullary lesions,

(b) apparently solitary lesion (with qualification as to the imaging and/or other investigational techniques used to assess the absence of lesions), or

(c) no definite lesion (e.g., no imaging evidence for lesions and marrow with less than 10% plasma cell content with qualification as to the technique used such as two-site aspiration and trephine).

Pathology assesses cellular pathology and where appropriate, assigns a pathological grade: (a) well differentiated, (b) intermediate, or (c) poorly differentiated (plasmablastic). It may be that a biopsied lesion has low plasma cell content (e.g., in some localized amyloid lesions or MGUS) or very minimal plasma cell content (systemic amyloidosis).

Protein production or deposition include: (a) monoclonal protein (serum or urine) and Ig type, (b) IA, (c) MIDD, or (d) monoclonal protein not detected (with qualification as to the technique used to assess for monoclonal protein).

Key MRD attributable problems arise from related organ damage or tissue impairment. These may comprise the following:

(a) Key systemic or multifocal problems. While other pathogenetic mechanisms of disease may be present, the

systemic problems should be principally attributable to myeloma or IA and include, but are not limited to: renal failure, HVS, coagulopathy, anemia, and hypercalcemia. Multifocal organ problems include multiple osteolytic lesions or multifocal soft tissue organ disruption or impairment.

(b) Key localized problems such as solitary osteolysis, solitary organ disruption, or focal compressive signs resulting in organ damage or impairment.

(c) No key problems. The patient is either apparently asymptomatic or has limited clinical signs (not including the key local or systemic MRD attributable problems earlier).

The final consideration is an overall "rate of progression risk" based on the earlier and natural behavior of the MRD allowing a tentative "global" categorization of the risk of progression of morbidity (see Table 55-3). In veterinary medicine this will be a crude stratification estimate, but the system should prove adaptable to additional diagnostic and stratification criteria over time (e.g., "APPPO", where the inclusion of "O" for "other" allows consideration of independent prognostic features such as serum albumin, beta-2 microglobulin, cytogenetics, etc., as used in humans).[148] Case examples of the diagnostic approach are given in Table 55-4. By stratifying patients in this way—according to the evolutionary stage of their disease—this new system should prove useful in aiding clinical decision making with respect to therapy (see Table 55-3).

TREATMENT AND OUTCOME

Treatment of polyclonal PCDs is not reported here. There is a paucity of systematic data regarding the treatment of feline MRDs. Treatment of suspected and confirmed MRD is dictated by the risk stratification suggested earlier.

Solitary Lesions

From the earlier sections concerning diagnostics, it should be clear that apparently solitary lesions should be examined skeptically and with a sound knowledge of the diversity of diagnostic presentations available in MRDs, and a planned, sensible sufficiency of investigative tests. In general, many solitary lesions can be controlled with local therapy (with exceptions—seen further in this section and in Table 55-3). However, all owners should be informed that in general, there remain levels of risk of progression of disease following local therapy for a solitary MRD lesion.

In cases where the rate of progression risk is slow (see Table 55-3), such as localized amyloidosis, excisional biopsy is indicated. This can result in long-term remission or cure.[35]

In cases where the rate of progression risk is moderate (see Table 55-3), such as solitary EMP, surgical excision may be considered for the purposes of diagnostic confirmation and therapy where appropriate. Statistically significant survival

Table 55-4	Case Examples of the Working Diagnostic Approach to Patients with MRD as Categorized by APPP Methodology and Mellor's Classification

Example 1

	Area	*Pathology*	*Protein— Serum/Urine Monoclonal*	*Problems—MRD Attributable*
Notes:	Single skin lesion	Cutaneous plasma cell lesion—well-differentiated grade; contains intralesional amyloid	Low positive	None
Qualifications	Complete skeletal survey radiography negative, abdominal sonography negative	Immunohistochemistry confirms clonality (IgG, lambda) Amyloid Ig confirmed by LMD/MS Bone marrow negative on two-site assessment using both trephine and aspirate; liver Tru-Cut biopsy negative for amyloid	SPE only UPE negative	No relevant clinical signs; no key hematologic or serum biochemical problems
Classification (Mellor's and Traditional)		**Apparently solitary MRD— moderate rate of progression risk**, (CEMP with intralesional amyloid)		

Example 2

	Area	*Pathology*	*Protein— Serum/Urine Monoclonal*	*Problems—MRD Attributable*
Notes:	1) Suspected splenomegaly 2) Osteolysis	1) Splenic aspirate cytology—plasma cell lesion—well-differentiated grade 2) Bone marrow sample—borderline (around 8%-10% plasma cell content)	Monoclonal protein	Yes
Qualifications	Clinical exam, sonography and radiography-suspected moderate splenomegaly. Complete skeletal survey radiography—single vertebral osteolytic lesion. MRI spine—multiple vertebral osteolytic lesions	Immunocytochemistry confirms splenic aspirate clonality Bone marrow Vertebral osteolytic lesions—suboptimal sample acquisition, borderline positive for plasma cell content; difficult locations—so not repeated Humerus (nonlesioned site)—aspirate & trephine. Borderline positive	SPE and UPE positive	Anemia. Probable spinal pain with multiple osteolytic lesions
Classification (Mellor's and Traditional)		**Probable* multifocal MRD—high rate of progression risk**, (probable combined intramedullary and extramedullary myeloma)		

In the first example, the patient presents with a skin mass; in the second the patient presents with an abdominal mass and is subsequently discovered to have osteolysis at imaging.

*Probable—on the basis that pathology was confirmed at a single site only, but there is a high risk of multisite involvement given the imaging lesions.

APPP, Area, Pathology, Protein, Problems; *CEMP,* cutaneous extramedullary plasmacytoma; *IgG,* immunoglobulin G; *LMD/MS,* laser microdissection with mass spectrometry; *MRD,* myeloma-related disorders; *MRI,* magnetic resonance imaging; *SPE,* serum protein electrophoresis; *UPE,* urine protein electrophoresis.

benefit for selected cats receiving surgery has been demonstrated when compared to cats that received no therapy or glucocorticoids alone.[1,64] A variety of surgical therapies including cutaneous mass excision, splenectomy, and enucleation have been reported across the feline literature, and generally positive responses have been documented in appropriately selected cases. For example, in a typical clinical decision-making process, a solitary plasmacytoma of the spleen might be suspected on the basis of a discovered serum/urine monoclonal protein along with sonographic evidence for splenic structural changes, cytopathological indications of well differentiated plasma cells, and no radiographic evidence for bone lesions (based on a complete skeletal survey). Further testing could include additional splenic aspirates for immunocytochemistry or flow cytometry or polymerase chain reaction for antigen receptor rearrangements as well as further imaging (e.g., MRI or fluorodeoxyglucose positron emission tomography scans and concurrent bone marrow aspirate and trephine). If there are no further involved sites identified, then splenectomy would follow. This paradigm follows the current best evidence in human patients—that truly localized EMP at accessible sites should be completely surgically excised.[79] However, in areas of poor surgical access (e.g., the upper respiratory or digestive tract), radiotherapy alone is the treatment of choice.[79] Solitary visceral organs that are diffusely infiltrated and cannot be safely excised or irradiated (e.g., hepatic plasmacytoma with diffuse hepatic infiltration) may be treated with chemotherapy as per other myeloma cases (see Multifocal Lesions).

Solitary plasmacytoma of bone (confirmed) is classified as moderate for rate of progression risk. It may also be optimally treated by local megavoltage radiotherapy.[44]

Solitary MRD in the high-risk progression category (e.g., EMP with a pathology grade of a poorly differentiated tumor—see Table 55-3), should be approached with caution with regard to local therapy alone. There should be suspicion of the possibility of undiagnosed lesions and/or more rapid transition to multifocal myeloma. Risks of local therapy should be considered with respect to the potential morbidity to the patient versus any potential therapeutic gain.

Multifocal Lesions

Monoclonal gammopathy of undetermined significance is an example of an assumed multifocal, suspected MRD with risk of slow progression, and where monitoring alone is appropriate. Extrapolating from current data in humans, smoldering myeloma should be monitored only, although further trials for early stage therapies are underway.[149] In multifocal disease where the rate of progression risk is high (see Table 55-3), systemic chemotherapy is appropriate. Where the rate of progression risk is classed as "very high" and the MRD is accompanied by organ failure, then chemotherapeutic options and dosages should be considered carefully.

In the feline literature, many individual reports describe the usage of a wide range of options from no therapy to the use of steroids alone, or more commonly, combination chemotherapy protocols including melphalan and prednisolone (the most commonly used combination); COP (cyclophosphamide, vincristine, prednisolone); or permutations that have included dexamethasone, chlorambucil, lomustine, and L-asparaginase. Across the literature, generally positive responses to chemotherapy have been documented. However, caution must be employed in the usage of melphalan in cats. A typical historical regime has been the administration of a 2 mg tablet every four days (equating to approximately 8 mg/m^2 for a 4 kg [9 lb] cat). However, myelosuppression may be cumulative, and in some individuals this has resulted in severe illness accompanied by marked neutropenia. Recompounding of chemotherapeutics is recommended to allow for accurate dosing. Both a qualitative description and a statistical assessment of the effect of treatment on survival have been published in only one series of feline MRD, which showed significant survival benefit in those cats receiving combination chemotherapy versus cats that received no therapy or glucocorticoids alone.[1,64] Novel therapies such as low dose dexamethasone alone, thalidomide and derivatives, and other newer generation antimyeloma drugs might be appropriate to try in appropriately selected cats with relapse, but there is no data at this time.

There is a lack of data on the treatment of confirmed cases of feline systemic IA. In humans, therapy directed against the plasma cell clone as per treatments employed for myeloma has resulted in improved outcomes for patients with systemic IA.[150]

Adjunctive and Supportive Therapies

Myeloma-related disorder complications including hypercalcemia, renal failure, anemia, bone lysis, bone pain, pathological fractures or bone collapse, hyperviscosity syndrome, coagulopathy, thromboembolic disease, and infections may be managed with an array of adjunct therapies. There is a paucity of data in feline MRD. Reports have described the use of plasmapheresis to alleviate congestive heart failure resultant from HVS in three cats.[13] The use of bisphosphonates to control hypercalcemia or bone-related signs has not been described in the cat, but could be appropriate in selected cases. Effective management of bleeding, embolic disease, and infections has not been described in detail in the cat, but awareness should facilitate treatment.

Monitoring

In the slow to moderate progression of suspected MRDs (MGUS and smoldering myeloma), owners should be appraised of the clinical signs of myeloma, extramedullary plasmacytoma, or amyloidosis that may develop over time. Laboratory testing of total globulin, and/or quantification of serum, and/or urine monoclonal protein should be considered at 3- to 6-month intervals, or more frequently if there is suspicion of more rapidly progressing disease. New bone lesions or visceral organomegaly can occasionally develop in the absence of a rising monoclonal protein, so in the event of appropriate clinical suspicion, further imaging may be conducted. Further assessments (e.g., serum biochemistry or hematopathology) are useful in the detection of impending organ failure or increasing peripheral blood plasma cell content with respect to the development of secondary leukemia.

In patients with a secretory MRD that are undergoing combination chemotherapy, some improvement in clinical signs can often be expected within days and usually by 2 to 4 weeks. In one study, of feline MRD patients responding to chemotherapy, half achieved normoglobulinemia within this time period.[1]

Prognosis

The outlook with regard to the initial response to combination chemotherapy in feline MRD is good. In one study, 85% responded (reduced clinical signs and concomitant decreases in serum globulin levels).[1] A return to good quality of life can be expected in most of these patients.

The long-term prognosis is however invariably grave. Cats that received no treatment or glucocorticoids alone had a median survival time (MST) of less than 1.5 months. This was statistically worse than for cats receiving combination chemotherapy (MST 9.4 months). The subgroup of responders to chemotherapy (those that improved clinically and had reduced globulinemia) had a median survival of 12.4 months.

References

1. Mellor PJ, Haugland S, Murphy S, et al: Myeloma-related disorders in cats commonly present as extramedullary neoplasms in contrast to myeloma in human patients: 24 cases with clinical follow-up. *J Vet Intern Med* 20(6):1376–1383, 2006.
2. Solly S: Remarks on the pathology of mollities ossium with cases. *Med Chir Trans* 27:435–461, 1844.
3. Seidl S, Kaufmann H, Drach J: New insights into the pathophysiology of multiple myeloma. *Lancet Oncol* 4(9):557–564, 2003.
4. Hallek M, Bergsagel PL, Anderson KC: Multiple myeloma: increasing evidence for a multistep transformation process. *Blood* 91(1):3–21, 1998.
5. Kapadia SB, Desai U, Cheng VS: Extramedullary plasmacytoma of the head and neck. A clinicopathologic study of 20 cases. *Medicine* 61(5):317–329, 1982.
6. Kyle RA: Monoclonal gammopathy of undetermined significance. Natural history in 241 cases. *Am J Med* 64(5):814–826, 1978.
7. Alexiou C, Kau RJ, Dietzfelbinger H, et al: Extramedullary plasmacytoma. *Cancer* 85(11):2305–2314, 1999.
8. Holzworth J, Meier H: Reticulum cell myeloma in a cat. *Cornell Vet* 47(2):302–316, 1957.
9. Glenner GG, Terry W, Harada M, et al: Amyloid fibril proteins: proof of homology with immunoglobulin light chains by sequence analyses. *Science* 172(3988):1150–1151, 1971.
10. Woodruff RK, Whittle JM, Malpas JS: Solitary plasmacytoma. I: Extramedullary soft tissue plasmacytoma. *Cancer* 43(6):2340–2343, 1979.
11. Appel SL, Moens NMM, Abrams-Ogg ACG, et al: Multiple myeloma with central nervous system involvement in a cat. *J Am Vet Med Assoc* 233(5):743–747, 2008.
12. Bienzle D, Silverstein DC, Chaffin K: Multiple myeloma in cats: variable presentation with different immunoglobulin isotypes in two cats. *Vet Pathol* 37(4):364–369, 2000.
13. Boyle TE, Holowaychuk MK, Adams AK, et al: Treatment of three cats with hyperviscosity syndrome and congestive heart failure using plasmapheresis. *J Am Anim Hosp Assoc* 47(1):50–55, 2011.
14. Breuer W, Colbatzky F, Platz S, et al: Immunoglobulin-producing tumours in dogs and cats. *J Comp Pathol* 109(3):203–216, 1993.
15. Carothers MA, Johnson GC, DiBartola SP, et al: Extramedullary plasmacytoma and immunoglobulin-associated amyloidosis in a cat. *J Am Vet Med Assoc* 195(11):1593–1597, 1989.
16. Carpenter JL, Andrews LK, Holzworth J: Tumours and tumour like lesions. In *Diseases of the cat: medicine and surgery*, Philadelphia, 1987, Saunders, pp 406–596.
17. Drazner FH: Multiple myeloma in the cat. *Compend Contin Educ Pract Vet* 4:206–216, 1982.
18. Dunbar MD, Lyles S: Hemophagocytic syndrome in a cat with multiple myeloma. *Vet Clin Pathol* 42(1):55–60, 2013.
19. Dust A, Norris AM, Valli VEO: Cutaneous lymphosarcoma with IgG monoclonal gammopathy, serum hyperviscosity and hypercalcemia in a cat. *Can Vet J* 23(8):235–239, 1982.
20. Engle GC, Brodey RS: A retrospective study of 395 feline neoplasms. *J Am Anim Hosp Assoc* 5(1):21–31, 1969.
21. Facchini RV, Bertazzolo W, Zuliani D, et al: Detection of biclonal gammopathy by capillary zone electrophoresis in a cat and a dog with plasma cell neoplasia. *Vet Clin Pathol* 39(4):440–446, 2010.
22. Fan TM, Kitchell BE, Dhaliwal RS, et al: Hematological toxicity and therapeutic efficacy of lomustine in 20 tumor-bearing cats: critical assessment of a practical dosing regimen. *J Am Anim Hosp Assoc* 38(4):357–363, 2002.
23. Farrow BR, Penny R: Multiple myeloma in a cat. *J Am Vet Med Assoc* 158(5):606–611, 1971.
24. Forrester SD, Greco DS, Relford RL: Serum hyperviscosity syndrome associated with multiple myeloma in two cats. *J Am Vet Med Assoc* 200(1):79–82, 1992.
25. Greenberg MJ, Schatzberg SJ, DeLahunta A, et al: Intracerebral plasma cell tumor in a cat: a case report and literature review. *J Vet Intern Med* 18(4):581–585, 2004.
26. Hanna F: Multiple myelomas in cats. *J Feline Med Surg* 7(5):275–287, 2005.
27. Harbison ML: Plasma cell myeloma and plasmacytoma. In *Diseases of the cat—medicine and surgery*, Philadelphia, 1987, Saunders, pp 442–444.
28. Hawkins EC, Feldman BF, Blanchard PC: Immunoglobulin A myeloma in a cat with pleural effusion and serum hyperviscosity. *J Am Vet Med Assoc* 188(8):876–878, 1986.
29. Hay LE: Multiple myeloma in a cat. *Aust Vet Pract* 8(1):45–48, 1978.
30. Hickford FH, Stokol T, vanGessel YA, et al: Monoclonal immunoglobulin G cryoglobulinemia and multiple myeloma in a domestic shorthair cat. *J Am Vet Med Assoc* 217(7):1029–1033, 1007–1008, 2000.
31. Hribernik TN, Barta O, Gaunt SD, et al: Serum hyperviscosity syndrome associated with IgG myeloma in a cat. *J Am Vet Med Assoc* 181(2):169–170, 1982.
32. Jacobs T: Multiple myeloma in a cat with paraparesis. *Feline Pract [Internet]* 22(4):28–32, 1994 <http://agris.fao.org/agris-search/search/display.do?f=1995/US/US95176.xml;US9516155> (Accessed November 28, 2013.)
33. Kagawa Y, Yamashita T, Maetani S, et al: Cutaneous lymphoplasmacytic lymphoma with systemic metastasis in a cat. *J Vet Med Sci* 73(9):1221–1224, 2011.
34. Kehoe JM, Hurvitz AI, Capra JD: Characterization of three feline paraproteins. *J Immunol* 109(3):511–516, 1972.
35. Kershaw O, Linek J, Linke RP, et al: Intraocular ALλ amyloidoma with plasma cell neoplasia in a cat. *Vet Ophthalmol* 14(Suppl 1):88–92, 2011.
36. King AJ, Davies DR, Irwin PJ: Feline multiple myeloma: literature review and four case reports. *Aust Vet Pract* 32(4):146–151, 2002.
37. Kyriazidou A, Brown PJ, Lucke VM: Immunohistochemical staining of neoplastic and inflammatory plasma cell lesions in feline tissues. *J Comp Pathol* 100(3):337–341, 1989.

38. Larsen AE, Carpenter JL: Hepatic plasmacytoma and biclonal gammopathy in a cat. *J Am Vet Med Assoc* 205(5):708–710, 1994.

39. Lucke VM: Primary cutaneous plasmacytomas in the dog and cat. *J Small Anim Pract* 28(1):49–55, 1987.

40. MacEwen EG, Hurvitz AI: Diagnosis and management of monoclonal gammopathies. *Vet Clin North Am* 7(1):119–132, 1977.

41. Majzoub M, Breuer W, Platz SJ, et al: Histopathologic and immunophenotypic characterization of extramedullary plasmacytomas in nine cats. *Vet Pathol* 40(3):249–253, 2003.

42. Mandel NS, Esplin DG: A retroperitoneal extramedullary plasmacytoma in a cat with a monoclonal gammopathy. *J Am Anim Hosp Assoc* 30(6):603–605, 1994 <http://agris.fao.org/agris-search/search/display.do?f=1996/US/US96248.xml;US9555014> (Accessed November 28, 2013.)

43. McDonald WJ, Burton SA, Fuentealba IC: Plasma cell myeloma producing an immunoglobulin A paraprotein in a cat. *Can Vet J* 35(3):157, 1994.

44. Mellor P, Polton G, Brearley M, et al: Solitary plasmacytoma of bone in two successfully treated cats. *J Feline Med Surg* 9(1):72–77, 2007.

45. Michau TM, Proulx DR, Rushton SD, et al: Intraocular extramedullary plasmacytoma in a cat. *Vet Ophthalmol* 6(2):177–181, 2003.

46. Mills JN, Eger CE, Robinson WF, et al: A case of multiple myeloma in a cat. *J Am Anim Hosp Assoc* 18(1):1982.

47. Mitcham SA, McGillivray SR, Haines DM: Plasma cell sarcoma in a cat. *Can Vet J* 26(3):98–100, 1985.

48. Patel RT, Caceres A, French AF, et al: Multiple myeloma in 16 cats: a retrospective study. *Vet Clin Pathol* 34(4):341–352, 2005.

49. Radhakrishnan A, Risbon RE, Patel RT, et al: Progression of a solitary, malignant cutaneous plasma-cell tumour to multiple myeloma in a cat. *Vet Comp Oncol* 2(1):36–42, 2004.

50. Rosenberg M, Hohenhaus A, Matus R: Monoclonal gammopathy and lymphoma in a cat infected with FIV. *J Am Anim Hosp Assoc* 27:335–337, 1991.

51. Rowland PH, Linke RP: Immunohistochemical characterization of lambda light-chain-derived amyloid in one feline and five canine plasma cell tumors. *Vet Pathol* 31(3):390–393, 1994.

52. Saar C, Saar U, Opitz M, et al: Paraproteinemic reticuloses in the cat. Report on a case of plasma cell reticulosis and a case of macroglobulinemia. *Berl Münch Tierärztl Wochenschr* 86(1):11–15, 1973.

53. Schöniger S, Bridger N, Allenspach K, et al: Sinonasal plasmacytoma in a cat. *J Vet Diagn Invest* 19(5):573–577, 2007.

54. Sheafor SE, Gamblin RM, Couto CG: Hypercalcemia in two cats with multiple myeloma. *J Am Anim Hosp Assoc* 32(6):503–508, 1996.

55. Takeuchi Y, Iizuka H, Kanemitsu H, et al: Myeloma-related disorder with leukaemic progression in a cat. *J Feline Med Surg* 12(12):982–987, 2010.

56. Ward DA, McEntee MF, Weddle DL: Orbital plasmacytoma in a cat. *J Small Anim Pract* 38(12):576–578, 1997.

57. Webb J, Chary P, Northrup N, et al: Erythrophagocytic multiple myeloma in a cat. *Vet Clin Pathol* 37(3):302–307, 2008.

58. Weber NA, Tebeau CS: An unusual presentation of multiple myeloma in two cats. *J Am Anim Hosp Assoc* 34(6):477–483, 1998.

59. Williams DA, Goldschmidt MH: Hyperviscosity syndrome with IgM monoclonal gammopathy and hepatic plasmacytoid lymphosarcoma in a cat. *J Small Anim Pract* 23(6):311–323, 1982.

60. Yamada T, Ogura A, Inoue J, et al: A case of feline macroglobulinemia. *Nihon Juigaku Zasshi* 45(3):395–399, 1983.

61. Zikes CD, Spielman B, Shapiro W, et al: Gastric extramedullary plasmacytoma in a cat. *J Vet Intern Med* 12(5):381–383, 1998.

62. Eastman CA: Plasma cell tumours in a cat. *Feline Pract* 24:26–30, 1996.

63. Mukaratirwa S: Feline nasal and paranasal sinus tumours: clinicopathological study, histomorphological description and diagnostic immunohistochemistry of 123 cases. *J Feline Med Surg* 3(4):235–245, 2001.

64. Mellor PJ, Haugland S, Smith KC, et al: Histopathologic, immunohistochemical, and cytologic analysis of feline myeloma-related disorders: further evidence for primary extramedullary development in the cat. *Vet Pathol* 45(2):159–173, 2008.

65. Priester WA, McKay FW: The occurrence of tumors in domestic animals. *Natl Cancer Inst Monogr* 54:1–210, 1980.

66. Potter M: Neoplastic development in plasma cells. *Immunol Rev* 194:177–195, 2003.

67. Ichimaru M, Ishimaru T, Mikami M, et al: Multiple myeloma among atomic bomb survivors in Hiroshima and Nagasaki, 1950-76: relationship to radiation dose absorbed by marrow. *J Natl Cancer Inst* 69(2):323–328, 1982.

68. Speer SA, Semenza JC, Kurosaki T, et al: Risk factors for acute myeloid leukemia and multiple myeloma: a combination of GIS and case-control studies. *J Environ Health* 64(7):9–16, quiz 35–36, 2002.

69. Doody MM, Linet MS, Glass AG, et al: Leukemia, lymphoma, and multiple myeloma following selected medical conditions. *Cancer Causes Control* 3(5):449–456, 1992.

70. Aguilera NS, Kapadia SB, Nalesnik MA, et al: Extramedullary plasmacytoma of the head and neck: use of paraffin sections to assess clonality with in situ hybridization, growth fraction, and the presence of Epstein-Barr virus. *Mod Pathol* 8(5):503–508, 1995.

71. Dong HY, Scadden DT, de Leval L, et al: Plasmablastic lymphoma in HIV-positive patients: an aggressive Epstein-Barr virus-associated extramedullary plasmacytic neoplasm. *Am J Surg Pathol* 29(12):1633–1641, 2005.

72. Grosbois B, Jego P, Attal M, et al: Familial multiple myeloma: report of fifteen families. *Br J Haematol* 105(3):768–770, 1999.

73. Munshi NC, Anderson KC: Plasma cell neoplasms. In *DeVita, Hellman, and Rosenberg's Cancer: principles & practice of oncology*, ed 8, Philadelphia, 2008, Lippincott Williams & Wilkins, pp 2305–2342.

74. Friedland M, Schaefer P: Myelomatosis and hemolytic anemia. Hemolytic anemia, a rare complication of multiple myeloma, is successfully managed by splenectomy. *R I Med J* 62(12):469–471, 1979.

75. Solomon A, Weiss DT, Kattine AA: Nephrotoxic potential of Bence Jones proteins. *N Engl J Med* 324(26):1845–1851, 1991.

76. Cavana P, Capucchio MT, Bovero A, et al: Noncongophilic fibrillary glomerulonephritis in a cat. *Vet Pathol* 45(3):347–351, 2008.

77. Oyajobi BO: Multiple myeloma/hypercalcemia. *Arthritis Res Ther* 9(Suppl 1):S4, 2007.

78. Bolliger AP, Graham PA, Richard V, et al: Detection of parathyroid hormone-related protein in cats with humoral hypercalcemia of malignancy. *Vet Clin Pathol* 31(1):3–8, 2002.

79. Soutar R, Lucraft H, Jackson G, et al: Guidelines on the diagnosis and management of solitary plasmacytoma of bone and solitary extramedullary plasmacytoma. *Br J Haematol* 124(6):717–726, 2004.

80. Kwaan HC: Hyperviscosity in plasma cell dyscrasias. *Clin Hemorheol Microcirc* 55(1):75–83, 2013.

81. Coppola A, Tufano A, Di Capua M, et al: Bleeding and thrombosis in multiple myeloma and related plasma cell disorders. *Semin Thromb Hemost* 37(8):929–945, 2011.

82. Nucci M, Anaissie E: Infections in patients with multiple myeloma in the era of high-dose therapy and novel agents. *Clin Infect Dis* 49(8):1211–1225, 2009.

83. Paradisi F, Corti G, Cinelli R: Infections in multiple myeloma. *Infect Dis Clin North Am* 15(2):373–384, vii–viii, 2001.

84. Stone MJ, Bogen SA: Role of plasmapheresis in Waldenström's macroglobulinemia. *Clin Lymphoma Myeloma Leuk* 13(2):238–240, 2013.

85. Kyle RA: The monoclonal gammopathies. *Clin Chem* 40(11):2154–2161, 1994.

86. Kyle RA: Sequence of testing for monoclonal gammopathies. *Arch Pathol Lab Med* 123(2):114–118, 1999.

87. Vermeersch P, Van Hoovels L, Delforge M, et al: Diagnostic performance of serum free light chain measurement in patients suspected of a monoclonal B-cell disorder. *Br J Haematol* 143(4):496–502, 2008.

88. Dispenzieri A, Kyle R, Merlini G, et al: International Myeloma Working Group guidelines for serum-free light chain analysis in multiple myeloma and related disorders. *Leukemia* 23(2):215–224, 2009.

89. Dimopoulos M, Kyle R, Fermand JP, et al: Consensus recommendations for standard investigative workup: report of the

International Myeloma Workshop Consensus Panel 3. *Blood* 117(18):4701–4705, 2011.

90. Grosbois B, Jégo P, de Rosa H, et al: Triclonal gammopathy and malignant immunoproliferative syndrome. *Rev Méd Interne* 18(6):470–473, 1997.

91. Kyle RA, Robinson RA, Katzmann JA: The clinical aspects of biclonal gammopathies. Review of 57 cases. *Am J Med* 71(6):999–1008, 1981.

92. Taylor SS, Tappin SW, Dodkin SJ, et al: Serum protein electrophoresis in 155 cats. *J Feline Med Surg* 12(8):643–653, 2010.

93. Lyon KF: Feline lymphoplasmacytic stomatitis associated with monoclonal gammopathy and Bence-Jones proteinuria. *J Vet Dent* 11(1):25–27, 1994.

94. Tarello W: Microscopic and clinical evidence for Anaplasma (Ehrlichia) phagocytophilum infection in Italian cats. *Vet Rec* 156(24):772–774, 2005.

95. Bida JP, Kyle RA, Therneau TM, et al: Disease associations with monoclonal gammopathy of undetermined significance: a population-based study of 17,398 patients. *Mayo Clin Proc* 84(8):685–693, 2009.

96. Maldonado JE, Bayrd ED, Brown AL, Jr: The flaming cell in multiple myeloma. A light and electron microscopy study. *Am J Clin Pathol* 44(6):605–612, 1965.

97. Alanen A, Pira U, Lassila O, et al: Mott cells are plasma cells defective in immunoglobulin secretion. *Eur J Immunol* 15(3):235–242, 1985.

98. Wutke K, Várbíró M, Rüdiger KD, et al: Cytological and histological classification of multiple myeloma. *Haematologia (Budap)* 14(3):315–329, 1981.

99. Di Guglielmo R: Unusual morphologic and humoral conditions in the field of plasmocytoms and M-dysproteinemia. *Acta Med Scand Suppl* 445:206–211, 1966.

100. Mellor PJ: Veterinary Myeloma Website <http://www.vin.com/Projects/Myeloma/M07711.htm>. (Accessed October 24, 2015.)

101. Garand R, Avet-Loiseau H, Accard F, et al: t(11;14) and t(4;14) translocations correlated with mature lymphoplasmacytoid and immature morphology, respectively, in multiple myeloma. *Leukemia* 17(10):2032–2035, 2003.

102. Weh HJ, Bartl R, Seeger D, et al: Correlations between karyotype and cytologic findings in multiple myeloma. *Leukemia* 9(12):2119–2122, 1995.

103. International Myeloma Working Group: IMWG criteria for the diagnosis of myeloma and guidelines for the diagnostic work-up of myeloma <http://myeloma.org/ArticlePage.action?articleId=2970>. (Accessed October 24, 2015.)

104. Chesi M, Kuehl WM, Bergsagel PL: Recurrent immunoglobulin gene translocations identify distinct molecular subtypes of myeloma. *Ann Oncol* 11(Suppl 1):131–135, 2000.

105. Chi J, Ballabio E, Chen XH, et al: MicroRNA expression in multiple myeloma is associated with genetic subtype, isotype and survival. *Biol Direct* 6:23, 2011.

106. Kosmas C, Stamatopoulos K, Stavroyianni N, et al: Molecular analysis of immunoglobulin genes in multiple myeloma. *Leuk Lymphoma* 33(3–4):253–265, 1999.

107. Kumar S, Kimlinger T, Morice W: Immunophenotyping in multiple myeloma and related plasma cell disorders. *Best Pract Res Clin Haematol* 23(3):433–451, 2010.

108. Nadiminti K, Zhan F, Tricot G: Cytogenetics and chromosomal abnormalities in multiple myeloma-a review. *Clon Transgen* 2(114):2, 2013.

109. Hoshii Y, Kiyama M, Cui D, et al: Immunohistochemical study of immunoglobulin light chain amyloidosis with antibodies to the immunoglobulin light chain variable region. *Pathol Int* 56(6):324–330, 2006.

110. Kaul E, Pilichowska M, Vullaganti M, et al: Twists and turns of determining amyloid type and amyloid-related organ damage: discordance and clinical skepticism in the era of proteomic typing. *Amyloid* 21(1):62–65, 2014.

111. Kuwabara H, Uda H, Miyabe K, et al: Malignant plasmacytoid myoepithelioma of the palate: histological observations compared to benign predominant plasmacytoid myoepithelial cells in pleomorphic adenoma of the palate. *Ultrastruct Pathol* 22(2):153–160, 1998.

112. Ogawa Y, Kishino M, Atsumi Y, et al: Plasmacytoid cells in salivary-gland pleomorphic adenomas: evidence of luminal cell differentiation. *Virchows Arch* 443(5):625–634, 2003.

113. Soumelis V, Liu Y-J: From plasmacytoid to dendritic cell: morphological and functional switches during plasmacytoid pre-dendritic cell differentiation. *Eur J Immunol* 36(9):2286–2292, 2006.

114. Vital C, Vital A, Lagueny A, et al: Subacute inflammatory polyneuropathy: two cases with plasmacytoid histiocytes in the endoneurium. *Ultrastruct Pathol* 22(5):377–383, 1998.

115. Carter A, Hocherman I, Linn S, et al: Prognostic significance of plasma cell morphology in multiple myeloma. *Cancer* 60(5):1060–1065, 1987.

116. Greipp PR, Raymond NM, Kyle RA, et al: Multiple myeloma: significance of plasmablastic subtype in morphological classification. *Blood* 65(2):305–310, 1985.

117. Rosenzweig M, Landau H: Light chain (AL) amyloidosis: update on diagnosis and management. *J Hematol Oncol* 4(1):1–8, 2011.

118. Cohen AD, Comenzo RL: Systemic light-chain amyloidosis: advances in diagnosis, prognosis, and therapy. *Hematology Am Soc Hematol Educ Program* 2010(1):287–294, 2010.

119. Gertz MA: Immunoglobulin light chain amyloidosis: 2013 update on diagnosis, prognosis, and treatment. *Am J Hematol* 88(5):416–425, 2013.

120. Dinner S, Witteles W, Witteles R, et al: The prognostic value of diagnosing concurrent multiple myeloma in immunoglobulin light chain amyloidosis. *Br J Haematol* 161(3):367–372, 2013.

121. Kourelis TV, Kumar SK, Gertz MA, et al: Coexistent multiple myeloma or increased bone marrow plasma cells define equally high-risk populations in patients with immunoglobulin light chain amyloidosis. *J Clin Oncol* 31(34):4319–4324, 2013.

122. Nasr SH, Valeri AM, Cornell LD, et al: Renal monoclonal immunoglobulin deposition disease: a report of 64 patients from a single institution. *Clin J Am Soc Nephrol* 7(2):231–239, 2012.

123. Dias Pereira P, Faustino AMR: Feline plasma cell pododermatitis: a study of 8 cases. *Vet Dermatol* 14(6):333–337, 2003.

124. Taylor JE, Schmeitzel LP: Plasma cell pododermatitis with chronic footpad hemorrhage in two cats. *J Am Vet Med Assoc* 197(3):375–377, 1990.

125. Bensignor E, Merven F: Nasal plasma cell dermatitis in cats. *Vet Dermatol* 22(3):286, 2011.

126. Declercq J, De Bosschere H: Nasal swelling due to plasma cell infiltrate in a cat without plasma cell pododermatitis. *Vet Dermatol* 21(4):412–414, 2010.

127. White SD, Rosychuk RA, Janik TA, et al: Plasma cell stomatitis-pharyngitis in cats: 40 cases (1973-1991). *J Am Vet Med Assoc* 200(9):1377–1380, 1992.

128. Declercq J, De Man M: Plasma cell pododermatitis and nasal swelling. *Vlaams Diergeneeskd Tijdschr* 71:277–281, 2002.

129. Scott DW: Feline dermatology 1979-1982: introspective retrospections. *J Am Anim Hosp Assoc* 20:537–564, 1984.

130. Gruffydd-Jones TJ, Orr CM, Lucke VM: Foot pad swelling and ulceration in cats: a report of five cases. *J Small Anim Pract* 21(7):381–389, 1980.

131. Bettenay SV, Lappin MR, Mueller RS: An immunohistochemical and polymerase chain reaction evaluation of feline plasmacytic pododermatitis. *Vet Pathol* 44(1):80–83, 2007.

132. Patnana M, Sevrukov AB, Elsayes KM, et al: Inflammatory pseudotumor: the great mimicker. *AJR Am J Roentgenol* 198(3):W217–W227, 2012.

133. Van der Woerdt A: Orbital inflammatory disease and pseudotumor in dogs and cats. *Vet Clin North Am Small Anim Pract* 38(2):389–401, 2008.

134. Kyle RA: "Benign" monoclonal gammopathy—after 20 to 35 years of follow-up. *Mayo Clin Proc* 68(1):26–36, 1993.

135. Schmidt-Hieber M, Gutiérrez ML, Pérez-Andrés M, et al: Cytogenetic profiles in multiple myeloma and monoclonal gammopathy of undetermined significance: a study in highly purified aberrant plasma cells. *Haematologica* 98(2):279–287, 2013.

136. International Myeloma Working Group: Criteria for the classification of monoclonal gammopathies, multiple myeloma and related disorders: a report of the International Myeloma Working Group. *Br J Haematol* 121(5):749–757, 2003.

137. De Larrea CF, Rosiñol L, Cibeira MT, et al: Extensive soft-tissue involvement by plasmablastic myeloma arising from displaced humeral fractures. *Eur J Haematol* 85(5):448–451, 2010.

138. Rosenblum MD, Bredeson CN, Chang CC, et al: Subcutaneous plasmacytomas with tropism to sites of previous trauma in a multiple myeloma patient treated with an autologous bone marrow transplant. *Am J Hematol* 72(4):274–277, 2003.

139. Bladé J, Larrea CF, de Rosiñol L, et al: Soft-tissue plasmacytomas in multiple myeloma: incidence, mechanisms of extramedullary spread, and treatment approach. *J Clin Oncol* 29(28):3805–3812, 2011.

140. Clark GN, Berg H, Engler SJ, et al: Extramedullary plasmacytomas in dogs: results of surgical excision in 131 cases. *J Am Anim Hosp Assoc* 28:105–111, 1992.

141. Lester SJ, Mesfin GM: A solitary plasmacytoma in a dog with progression to a disseminated myeloma. *Can Vet J* 21(10):284–286, 1980.

142. Lonial S, Kaufman JL: Non-secretory myeloma: a clinician's guide. *Oncology (Williston Park, N.Y.)* 27(9):924–928, 930, 2013.

143. Turesson I, Grubb A: Non-secretory or low-secretory myeloma with intracellular kappa chains. Report of six cases and review of the literature. *Acta Med Scand* 204(6):445–451, 1978.

144. Drayson M, Tang LX, Drew R, et al: Serum free light-chain measurements for identifying and monitoring patients with nonsecretory multiple myeloma. *Blood* 97(9):2900–2902, 2001.

145. Dimopoulos MA, Moulopoulos LA, Maniatis A, et al: Solitary plasmacytoma of bone and asymptomatic multiple myeloma. *Blood* 96(6):2037–2044, 2000.

146. Brockley LK, Heading KL, Jardine JE, et al: Polyostotic lymphoma with multiple pathological fractures in a six-month-old cat. *J Feline Med Surg* 14(4):285–291, 2012.

147. Fernández de Larrea C, Kyle RA, Durie BGM, et al: Plasma cell leukemia: consensus statement on diagnostic requirements, response criteria and treatment recommendations by the International Myeloma Working Group. *Leukemia* 27(4):780–791, 2013.

148. Kyle R, Rajkumar S: Criteria for diagnosis, staging, risk stratification and response assessment of multiple myeloma. *Leukemia* 23(1):3–9, 2009.

149. Rajkumar SV, Lacy MQ, Kyle RA: Monoclonal gammopathy of undetermined significance and smoldering multiple myeloma. *Blood Rev* 21(5):255–265, 2007.

150. Merlini G, Seldin DC, Gertz MA: Amyloidosis: pathogenesis and new therapeutic options. *J Clin Oncol* 29(14):1924–1933, 2011.

151. Werner JA, Woo JC, Vernau W, et al: Characterization of feline immunoglobulin heavy chain variable region genes for the molecular diagnosis of B-cell neoplasia. *Vet Pathol* 42(5):596–607, 2005.

Feline Soft Tissue Sarcomas

Katherine A. Skorupski

PATHOGENESIS AND EPIDEMIOLOGY

Soft tissue sarcomas in cats may occur spontaneously or may be induced by vaccinations or other injections. An association between vaccination and sarcoma development in cats was first proposed in 1991 by veterinary pathologists at the University of Pennsylvania who noted an increase in the number of vaccine reaction and soft tissue sarcoma submissions from cats.[1,2] This discovery followed enactment of a law requiring rabies vaccination of cats in Pennsylvania, as well as the development and marketing of injectable killed vaccines for rabies and feline leukemia virus (FeLV). Subsequent epidemiologic studies have confirmed this association between the injection of vaccines and sarcoma development at the site of administration.[3,4] The reported prevalence of these tumors varies somewhat by study but is estimated to be approximately one in 10,000 vaccinated cats.[5,6] The time between vaccination and tumor detection is highly variable, but it can range from 4 weeks to 10 years with a median time to development of 11 months.[3,7] Initial studies suggested that rabies and FeLV vaccines were most responsible for tumor development in cats, but follow-up studies have shown that up to one-third of cases may be related to vaccination for feline rhinotracheitis, calicivirus, and panleukopenia.[2,8-10]

Inflammation incited by vaccination appears to play a lead role in sarcoma development in cats.[2-6] The pathogenesis of vaccine-associated sarcomas is believed to be through malignant transformation of fibroblasts and myofibroblasts driven by the body's inflammatory and immunologic reaction to vaccination. Inflammatory responses to vaccines involve several growth factors including platelet-derived growth factor, epidermal growth factor, and transforming growth factor-β (TGF-β); and these are known to drive myofibroblast cell division and contribute to malignant transformation. This theory is supported by the presence of a significant inflammatory component often visible in and around these tumors as well as positive staining for these growth factors in vaccine-associated sarcomas but not in spontaneous sarcomas.[7-9] Vaccine adjuvants, including aluminum hydroxide, are believed to contribute significantly to the exuberant inflammatory reaction that leads to tumor development in cats postvaccination.[4] Macrophages containing blue-gray material have been identified within some tumors, and ultrastructural studies have proven that this material is aluminum adjuvant.[8,9] Further evidence that cats may be predisposed to overzealous inflammatory responses leading to neoplasia can be found in the existence of feline ocular sarcomas that occur following trauma to the eye or after chronic uveitis.[11] Mutations resulting in overexpression of tumor protein p53 have also been documented in vaccine-associated sarcomas and are theorized to play a pivotal role in the malignant transformation of fibroblasts following vaccination.[12-14] p53 is a tumor suppressor gene that plays a major role in regulation of the cell cycle, and cells lacking functional p53 progress through the cell cycle unregulated, leading to neoplasia.

There is evidence that suggests that nonvaccine injections and implants can also induce sarcomas in cats. Two studies have identified an association between injection with long-acting corticosteroids and sarcoma development.[4,15] In addition, individual reports exist describing tumors that developed after injection with meloxicam; after injection with lufenuron; and around nonabsorbable suture material, an identifying microchip, a retained surgical sponge, and a subcutaneous access port.[16-22] However, these allegations have not been confirmed through rigorous epidemiologic study.

Spontaneous (nonvaccine–associated) soft tissue sarcomas in cats are most commonly recognized in the oral cavity, on the head, lower extremities, or digits. Although there may be clues in the histologic appearance and location of a tumor, it is not always possible to definitively determine whether a sarcoma is spontaneous or vaccine-associated, especially when a full vaccination history is not available. However, differentiating spontaneous and vaccine-associated sarcomas is not usually clinically important, because the recommended diagnostic and therapeutic approaches do not differ significantly between them.

PATHOLOGY AND BIOLOGIC BEHAVIOR

The most common histologic type of vaccine-associated soft tissue sarcoma is fibrosarcoma, representing approximately half of tumors. Other tissue types described include

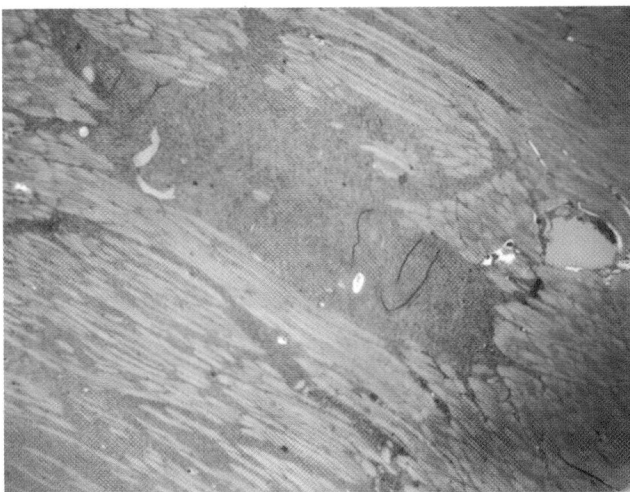

Figure 56-1: Histology of a vaccine-associated sarcoma demonstrating the presence of infiltrative tendrils at the periphery of the tumor. Normal surrounding muscle tissue appears pink and tumor tissue appears purple in this hematoxylin and eosin–stained tissue sample. (Image courtesy of Dr. Michael Kent, MAS, DVM, DACVIM, DACVR, University of California, Davis.)

malignant fibrous histiocytoma, extraskeletal osteosarcoma, rhabdomyosarcoma, chondrosarcoma, and undifferentiated sarcoma.[8,9,23-25] The histologic appearance of vaccine-associated sarcoma varies by type, but common features include the presence of multinucleated giant cells, associated lymphofollicular inflammation, and/or macrophages containing blue-gray adjuvant material.[8,9,23] When compared histologically to soft tissue sarcomas in nonvaccine sites, vaccine-associated sarcomas were found to be more often located in the hypodermis, be poorly differentiated, be of higher grade, have higher mitotic rates, have larger areas of necrosis, and have more peri-tumoral lymphocytic inflammation.[23-25] The distribution of tumor grade varies by study, but between 28% and 51% of vaccine-associated sarcomas are reported to be high grade.[23,26]

Feline sarcomas are highly locally invasive as demonstrated by visible tumor tendrils infiltrating surrounding tissues on imaging studies and in histopathologic samples (Figure 56-1). These tendrils may track between tissues planes and extend significant distances beyond palpable tumor. Distant metastasis, usually to lung, occurs in approximately 25% of cats with vaccine-associated sarcomas at some point in the course of the disease.[27-31] Although data is limited, metastasis appears to be more likely to occur in cats with histologically high-grade (grade III) tumors.[32]

DIAGNOSTIC EVALUATION

Most cats are brought to the clinic after the owner notices a swelling or mass under the skin. Feline sarcomas, particularly large ones, may have a cystic component that can be mistaken by owners for an abscess or seroma.[23] Although recent

vaccination may be reported, this is not always the case, because there may be a significant lag between vaccination and tumor development. For this reason, lack of recent vaccination cannot rule out vaccine as a potential etiology. The Vaccine-Associated Feline Sarcoma Task Force (VAFSTF) was formed in 1996 to develop policies to increase awareness and decrease the impact of these tumors on pet cats.[33] The VAFSTF recommended that veterinarians use the "3-2-1 rule" to aid in the diagnosis of subcutaneous masses in cats with known vaccination history and to help differentiate sarcomas from vaccine reactions. This rule recommends biopsy of all masses present in vaccine sites 3 months after vaccination or larger than 2 cm in diameter at any time point or increasing in size 1 month after vaccination.[33]

Biopsy is preferred over fine-needle aspiration, because the inflammatory component of tumors can mask the diagnosis of neoplasia in aspirate samples.[34] Incisional rather than excisional biopsy is recommended because of the extremely wide surgical margins necessary for successful removal of vaccine-associated sarcomas. Further, studies have shown that the first surgery is the best chance of successful removal. A small excisional biopsy followed by a large re-excision is known to result in poorer patient outcome than a single large resection.[27,35] Thoracic radiographs are recommended prior to instituting therapy to screen for pulmonary metastasis.

TREATMENT

Surgery

Wide excision is recommended as the first step in treatment of both vaccine and nonvaccine–associated soft tissue sarcomas. Advanced imaging with computed tomography or magnetic resonance imaging is recommended for surgical planning due to the highly invasive nature of these tumors and their small, infiltrative tendrils that may not be palpable but can often be seen with advanced imaging.[36,37] Palpation alone has been shown to significantly underestimate the surgical margins necessary for complete excision.

When vaccine-associated sarcomas were first recognized, a recommendation for surgery was made to plan removal of 2 to 3 cm of tissue around palpable tumor; however, recurrence rates were very high when that guideline was used.[27,33,37] A recent study found a recurrence rate of only 14% after surgery utilizing a guideline recommending the removal of 5 cm from lateral margins around the tumor and two fascial planes deep.[30] Depending on the tumor location, removal of this amount of tissue may require resection of large amounts of muscle tissue and/or bone and require significant reconstruction of the surgical defect (Figure 56-2). In the interscapular location, removal of portions of the scapulae and/or dorsal spinous processes is commonly required. In flank locations, body wall resection may be necessary; and on limbs, amputation is frequently the best way to assure complete removal of the sarcoma. Resection should be performed *en bloc* without incising tissue that is potentially contaminated with tumor. Care should be taken to position scars along

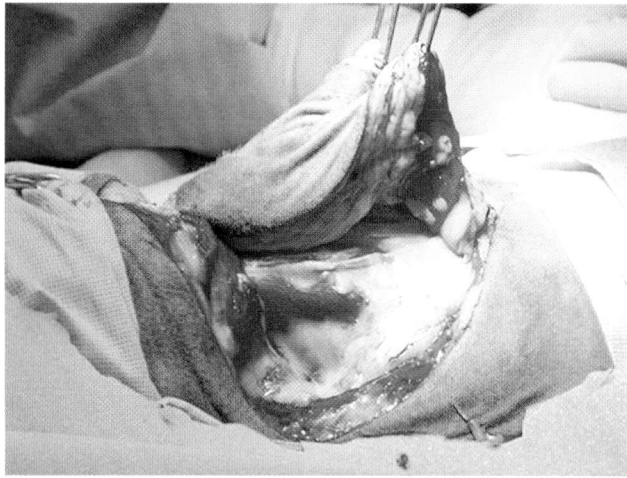

Figure 56-2: Intraoperative photograph of a cat undergoing en bloc resection of a vaccine-associated sarcoma in the caudal interscapular area. The cat's head is located to the left in the photograph, and the scapulae can be seen protruding just caudal to the most cranial portion of the surgical defect. (Image courtesy of Dr. Michael Kent, MAS, DVM, DACVIM, DACVR, University of California, Davis.)

planes that can be easily irradiated postoperatively if needed. Surgical drains should be avoided if at all possible. If they cannot be avoided, drains should be placed so that they exit through the main incision instead of through distant dissected tissue, which may encourage tracking of microscopic tumor tissue away from the central surgical field. Drain position can significantly affect radiation planning, expanding the radiation field considerably (and possible risk of complications) if drains exit through distant tissue. Ideally, the surgeon should be experienced in aggressive resection and reconstruction. This is emphasized by one study that showed cats that had surgery performed by experienced specialist surgeons had longer local control of their sarcomas than cats treated surgically by referring veterinarians.[27]

A thorough surgical margin evaluation should be requested when the tissue sample is submitted to a pathology laboratory. Unfortunately, even when surgical margins are reported by the pathologist to be free of tumor tissue, sarcoma recurrence is reported to occur in 31% to 42% of affected cats.[31,35] The reason for this unclear but may be due to the existence of small projecting tendrils at the edge of the submitted tissue that are not included in the sections prepared by the pathology laboratory. Methodical labeling of resected tissue by the surgeon prior to submission to the pathologist may improve the reliability of the margin evaluation. This labeling should include staining of cut surfaces with multiple colors of tissue ink that correlate to a written description. If the surgeon is concerned about completeness of excision in a particular region, that location should be marked with suture material and a special evaluation of that tissue requested.

Outcome in cats treated with surgery alone has improved with the implementation of guidelines recommending wider

surgical margins. Survival after surgery alone was first reported to result in median disease-free interval (DFI) and survival times of less than 1 year.[27,35] In 2005, Dillon and colleagues reported a median survival time of 608 days in 42 cats treated with surgery at a referral institution; and in 2011, Phelps and colleagues reported a median survival time of 901 days after surgery aimed at removing 5 cm margins.[30,38] Neither of these studies reported median DFI in the study population as a whole.

Radiation

Except in cases of distal limb tumors where amputation results in wide surgical margins, irradiation should be considered as an adjunct to surgical excision of vaccine-associated sarcomas. Treatment with photons, electrons, both, or brachytherapy have been described. Dosing of external beam radiation varies by publication, but total delivered doses range from 48 to 63 Gy administered in 16 to 21 fractions of 3.0 to 4.0 Gy.[26,28,29,39-41] There has been some debate as to whether radiation therapy is best administered before or after surgery for vaccine-associated sarcomas. Most publications suggest that there is no significant difference in patient outcome depending on timing of radiation, but one publication found that cats undergoing preoperative radiation had a poorer survival time (median of 310 days) compared to cats undergoing postoperative radiation (median of 705 days).[41] Other studies have shown that cats with larger sarcomas had shorter survival times than cats with smaller tumors.[30,38] This led the authors of the comparative study to suggest that there may have been selection bias where cats with larger tumors were more likely to be prescribed preoperative radiation in an attempt to shrink the tumor and make it easier to excise. Prospective evaluation comparing preoperative and postoperative radiation is necessary to further explore this aspect of therapy.

Chemotherapy

Chemotherapy may be used in cats with vaccine-associated sarcomas as an adjunct to surgery and radiation therapy, after surgery when radiation is not feasible, or as palliative treatment of bulky tumors when neither surgery nor radiation are feasible. The role of chemotherapy after aggressive local therapy remains unclear because outcome with and without chemotherapy has not been directly compared. Most publications report the use of chemotherapy in combination with surgery and radiation, making it difficult to separately evaluate the role of chemotherapy in delaying or preventing recurrence or extending survival times.[28,29,31,39,40] Although chemotherapy would be expected to reduce the risk of metastasis in cats with sarcomas, it is difficult to prove this benefit without a large-scale prospective study due to the fact that only approximately one in four cats with these tumors will develop metastasis.[28,31]

Doxorubicin, alone or in combination with cyclophosphamide, has been used in the treatment of feline sarcomas and is associated with a 50% response rate for a median of 125 days in cats with measureable disease.[42] Doxorubicin and liposome-encapsulated doxorubicin have been used postoperatively in cats with vaccine-associated sarcomas and resulted in a median DFI of 388 days, which was significantly improved from the 93-day median DFI in a control group of cats that had surgery alone.[43] In contrast, another study showed no difference in recurrence rate, metastasis, or survival between cats treated with surgery alone versus surgery and doxorubicin chemotherapy.[44] Doxorubicin has also been used in many studies in combination with surgery and radiation, but it is difficult to determine what role treatment with chemotherapy played in patient outcome.[28,29,31,39,40]

Carboplatin, ifosfamide, and lomustine have also been used to treat vaccine-associated sarcomas in cats. In a phase I study of carboplatin, four of 24 (17%) cats with sarcomas achieved partial remission as a result of treatment.[45] Carboplatin has also been used in the adjuvant setting after surgery and radiation therapy, however it is difficult to ascertain its effect in this setting.[31] Ifosfamide treatment in cats with vaccine-associated sarcomas was associated with a 41% response rate and a median response duration of 70 days in 27 cats with nonresectable, recurrent, or metastatic tumors.[46] Lomustine treatment in a similar population of 28 cats with measurable disease resulted in a 25% response rate and median response duration of 83 days.[47] The role of chemotherapy in the treatment of feline sarcomas remains unclear, however there is evidence that cats with high-grade tumors are at higher risk for distant metastasis.[32] Systemic chemotherapy may delay or prevent metastasis in this population and should, therefore, be considered in cats with high-grade tumors.

Electrochemotherapy

Electrochemotherapy, the use of electric pulses to increase cell permeability to chemotherapy, has been reported in the treatment of feline sarcomas.[48-50] Bleomycin and cisplatin are the most commonly used chemotherapeutics, and this modality has been applied to treat tumors alone and in combination with surgical resection. Tumor regressions have been reported, and a recent study of electrochemotherapy for incompletely excised fibrosarcomas documented longer DFI in cats treated with surgery and electrochemotherapy compared to cats treated with surgery alone.[48,50] Further study into the role of postoperative electrochemotherapy in cats with vaccine-associated sarcomas is warranted. For more on electrochemotherapy, see Chapter 58.

Immunotherapy

Immunotherapy in the form of feline interleukin-2, provided either as magnetic DNA or in a recombinant canarypox virus, has been studied in a small number of cats with vaccine-associated sarcoma.[51,52] Treatment timing, frequency, and delivery varied in these studies, but both administered the treatment in or around the tumor or tumor bed in an attempt to stimulate an immune reaction against cancer cells. The study administering magnetic DNA used magnetofection to introduce the DNA into patient tissues and was conducted as a phase I dose-finding and safety study. Further study into the efficacy of this delivery method is necessary.[52] Cats treated with the canarypox virus formulation were found to be significantly less likely to develop tumor recurrence after surgery and radiation therapy than controls (28% versus 61%).[51] This formulation has been licensed for distribution in Europe and is intended for the treatment of cats with fibrosarcomas between 2 and 5 cm in diameter without metastasis in addition to surgery and radiation therapy.[53]

Combination Therapy

There are many published studies describing outcome in cats treated with a combination of surgery and radiation therapy with or without chemotherapy.* Although results differ among studies, DFIs and survival times have generally increased since this tumor was first recognized (Table 56-1). This is hypothesized to be due to increased awareness of the existence and invasive behavior of vaccine-associated sarcomas, improved availability and quality of preoperative imaging modalities, increased numbers of surgeons trained in the resection of these highly invasive tumors, and increased availability of highly accurate radiation planning software and delivery systems. The most recent literature suggests that cats treated aggressively may enjoy prolonged DFI in the realm of 2 to 3 years and that some cats may be cured.† The main cause of treatment failure is local recurrence, which is reported to occur in up to 42% of cats treated with surgery and radiation therapy.[28,29,31,39] Metastasis may also occur in about 25% of cats with a median time to metastasis of approximately 300 days.[27-31]

PROGNOSIS AND PROGNOSTIC FACTORS

Outcome in cats with soft tissue sarcomas is highly dependent on whether adequate local control is achieved. In some cats, this may be possible with surgery alone, but many require treatment with surgery and radiation to achieve long-term tumor control. Factors that have been shown to be associated with outcome in cats with vaccine-associated sarcomas include tumor location, tumor size, training of the surgeon performing tumor resection, number of surgeries performed before definitive tumor resection, surgical margins, tumor grade, and anemia.[26-32,35,38,40] For example, consider the following:

- Cats with tumors located on limbs had a longer DFI than cats with tumors in truncal locations (median of 325 days versus 66 days, respectively).[27]
- Cats with tumor diameter less than 2 cm had a median survival time of 643 days compared to 558 days for cats

---

*†26,28,29,31,39,40,41.

Table 56-1	Summary of Publications Reporting Outcome in Cats with Vaccine-Associated Sarcoma Treated with Surgery and Curative-Intent Radiation Therapy with or without Chemotherapy			
Reference	**Publication Year**	**Number of Cats**	**Median Disease-Free Interval**	**Median Survival Time**
Cronin et al.[28]	1998	33	398 days	600 days
Cohen et al.[29]	2001	78	405 days	730 days
Bregazzi et al.[39]	2001	25	661 days	701 days
Kobayashi et al.[31]	2002	92	584 days	NR
Hahn et al.[40]	2007	71	234 days	771 days
Mayer et al.[41]	2009	24	NR	310 days
Mayer et al.[41]	2009	55	NR	705 days
Eckstein et al.[26]	2009	46	1110 days	1290 days

NR, Not reported.

with tumors between 2 and 5 cm and 394 days for cats with tumors larger than 5 cm.[38]

- Cats undergoing excision at a referral institution had a longer DFI (median of 274 days) than cats undergoing surgery by a referring veterinarian (median of 66 days).[27]
- Cats undergoing a single surgery had a median DFI of 469 days compared to 345 days in cats undergoing more than one surgery.[29]
- Cats with tumor cells visible at the surgical margin had a median DFI of 112 days compared to 700 days for cats with clean margins.[28]
- Three of three cats with grade III tumors developed metastasis in one study compared to 16% of cats with grade I or II tumors.[32]
- One study found that cats with a packed cell volume (PCV) less than 25% had a median survival of 308 days after surgery and radiation therapy, compared to 760 days in cats with a higher PCV.[41]
- Tumor expression of p53 has also been shown to predict patient outcome. In one study, cats whose tumors had cytoplasmic staining with an antibody against p53 had a shorter time to tumor recurrence (median of 135 days) than cats with nuclear staining (median of 325 days).[12]

PREVENTION AND RISK REDUCTION

Because vaccine-associated sarcomas in cats can be expensive and frustrating to treat, it is important to also focus on prevention in at-risk cats. Recommendations from the VAFSTF and others include vaccinating as infrequently as possible while still providing adequate infectious disease protection.[33] This includes giving vaccinations approved for 3-year administration no more frequently than that and avoiding FeLV vaccination in indoor cats that are not exposed to cats that

may carry the virus. Administering more than one vaccine per injection site has been shown to increase the risk of tumor development and should be avoided.[4] The VAFSTF guidelines also included a recommendation to use nonadjuvanted vaccines when available under the assumption that these carry less risk of inciting tumor development than their adjuvanted counterparts. To date, limited epidemiologic data exists comparing risk between adjuvanted and nonadjuvanted vaccines, but one recent study compared tumor development after inactivated, recombinant, and modified-live vaccines.[15] The authors found that cats with sarcomas in the rear limb region were significantly less likely to have received recombinant vaccines than inactivated ones suggesting that nonadjuvanted vaccines may, in fact, be safer. In contrast, there was no difference found among the types of vaccines administered in interscapular sites. In both locations, sarcomas were documented to occur in sites where recombinant and modified-live vaccines were given, indicating that these vaccines are not without risk. Further study is still necessary to determine how to best reduce the risk of tumor development after vaccination in cats.

To maximize the chance that a vaccine-associated sarcoma will arise in a location where surgery may be curative, vaccinations should be administered subcutaneously and as distally as possible on the limbs or on the tail.[10,54] Tumors in these locations can often be treated effectively through amputation without the need for radiation therapy. The VAFSTF also recommended against vaccinating in the interscapular space and, instead, recommended uniform guidelines for placement of individual vaccines on the limbs. Rabies vaccines should be injected in the distal right hindlimb, FeLV in the distal left hindlimb, and other vaccines in the right forelimb. As a result of these recommendations, a shift in tumor location has been documented with decreasing frequency of tumors in the interscapular region and lateral thorax and increasing frequency of tumors on the limbs and

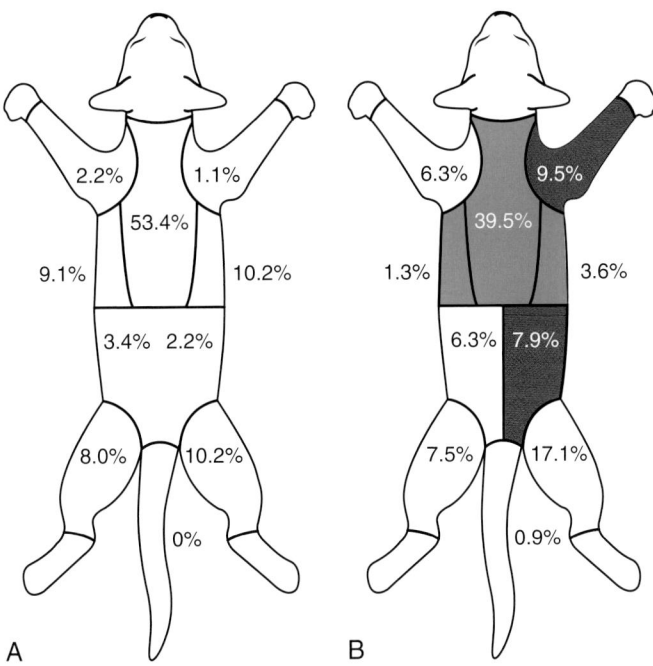

Figure 56-3: Change in location of vaccine-associated sarcoma diagnoses in cats over time. **A,** This drawing identifies the frequency of tumors diagnosed in each location between 1990 and 1996. **B,** This drawing identifies the frequency of tumors diagnosed between 1996 and 2006. *Red color* marks locations that had a significant increase in tumor frequency over time, and *blue color* marks locations that had a significant decrease in tumor frequency over time. (Shaw SC, Kent MS, Gordon IK, et al: Temporal changes in characteristics of injection-site sarcomas in cats: 392 cases (1990-2006). *J Am Vet Med Assoc* 234:376-380, 2009; image courtesy of Dr. Steve Shaw, DVM, DACVIM, Sage Centers for Veterinary Specialty and Emergency Care, Campbell, CA.)

lateral abdomen (Figure 56-3).[10] The increasing number of sarcomas located on the lateral abdomens of cats is theorized to be due to placement of vaccine injections intended for pelvic limbs below skin that is mobile and covers the lateral abdomen in a crouching cat. Care should be taken to vaccinate cats as distally on the limb as possible to avoid this phenomenon, which can result in tumors that are difficult to fully excise. Current recommendations for feline vaccinations and an update on risk reduction strategies for injection site sarcomas can be found in the 2013 American Association of Feline Practitioners Feline Vaccination Advisory Panel Report, available at http://www.catvets.com.

SUMMARY

Sarcomas in cats often occur secondary to vaccine administration, and these tumors are highly invasive into surrounding tissues. Optimal therapy consists of extremely wide surgical excision, if possible, or surgical excision followed by adjuvant radiation therapy. Cats treated aggressively frequently enjoy long survival times after treatment. Veterinarians can play a pivotal role in reducing the incidence and impact of vaccine-associated sarcomas by choosing vaccination protocols cautiously and by administering vaccines in sites most amenable to surgery.

References

1. Hendrick MJ, Goldschmidt MH: Do injection site reactions induce fibrosarcomas in cats? *J Am Vet Med Assoc* 199:968, 1991.
2. Hendrick MJ, Goldschmidt MH, Shofer FS, et al: Postvaccinal sarcomas in the cat: epidemiology and electron probe microanalytical identification of aluminum. *Cancer Res* 52:5391–5394, 1992.
3. Kass PH, Barnes WG, Spangler WL, et al: Epidemiologic evidence for a causal relation between vaccination and fibrosarcoma tumorigenesis in cats. *J Am Vet Med Assoc* 203:396–405, 1993.
4. Kass PH, Spangler WL, Hendrick MJ, et al: Multicenter case-control study of risk factors associated with development of vaccine-associated sarcomas in cats. *J Am Vet Med Assoc* 223:1283–1292, 2003.
5. Gobar GM, Kass PH: World wide web-based survey of vaccination practices, postvaccinal reactions, and vaccine site-associated sarcomas in cats. *J Am Vet Med Assoc* 220:1477–1482, 2002.
6. Coyne MJ, Reeves NC, Rosen DK: Estimated prevalence of injection-site sarcomas in cats during 1992. *J Am Vet Med Assoc* 210:249–251, 1997.
7. Hendrick MJ: Historical review and current knowledge of risk factors involved in feline vaccine-associated sarcomas. *J Am Vet Med Assoc* 213:1422–1423, 1998.

8. Hendrick MJ, Books JJ: Postvaccinal sarcomas in the cat: histology and immunohistochemistry. *Vet Pathol* 31:126–129, 1994.

9. Hendrick MJ, Shofer FS, Goldschmidt MH, et al: Comparison of fibrosarcomas that developed at vaccination sites and at nonvaccination sites in cats: 239 cases (1991-1992). *J Am Vet Med Assoc* 205:1425–1429, 1994.

10. Shaw SC, Kent MS, Gordon IK, et al: Temporal changes in characteristics of injection-site sarcomas in cats: 392 cases (1990-2006). *J Am Vet Med Assoc* 234:376–380, 2009.

11. Dubielzig RR, Everitt J, Shadduck JA, et al: Clinical and morphologic features of posttraumatic ocular sarcomas in cats. *Vet Pathol* 27:62–65, 1990.

12. Hershey AE, Dubielzig RR, Padilla ML, et al: Aberrant p53 expression in feline vaccine-associated sarcomas and correlation with prognosis. *Vet Pathol* 42:805–811, 2005.

13. Nambiar PR, Haines DM, Ellis JA, et al: Mutational analysis of tumor suppressor gene p53 in feline vaccine site-associated sarcomas. *Am J Vet Res* 10:1277–1281, 2000.

14. Nambiar PR, Jackson ML, Ellis JA, et al: Immunohistochemical detection of tumor suppressor gene p53 protein in feline injection site-associated sarcomas. *Vet Pathol* 38:236–238, 2001.

15. Srivastav A, Kass PH, McGill LD, et al: Comparative vaccine-specific and other injectable-specific risks of injection-site sarcomas in cats. *J Am Vet Med Assoc* 241:595–602, 2012.

16. Carminato A, Vascellari M, Marchioro W, et al: Microchip-associated fibrosarcoma in a cat. *Vet Dermatol* 22:565–569, 2011.

17. Buracco P, Martano M, Morello E, et al: Vaccine-associated-like fibrosarcoma at the site of a deep nonabsorbable suture in a cat. *Vet J* 163:105–107, 2002.

18. Esplin DG, Bigelow M, McGill LD, et al: Fibrosarcoma at the site of lufenuron injection in a cat. *Vet Cancer Soc Newsletter* 23:8, 1999.

19. Munday JS, Banyay K, Aberdein D, et al: Development of an injection site sarcoma shortly after meloxicam injection in an unvaccinated cat. *J Feline Med Surg* 13:988–991, 2011.

20. McLeland SM, Imhoff DJ, Thomas M, et al: Subcutaneous fluid port-associated soft tissue sarcoma in a cat. *J Feline Med Surg* 15:917–920, 2013.

21. Haddad JL, Goldschmidt MH, Patel RT: Fibrosarcoma arising at the site of a retained surgical sponge in a cat. *Vet Clin Pathol* 39:241–246, 2010.

22. Daly MK, Saba CF, Crochik SS, et al: Fibrosarcoma adjacent to the site of microchip implantation in a cat. *J Feline Med Surg* 10:202–205, 2008.

23. Couto SS, Griffery SM, Duarte PC, et al: Feline vaccine-associated fibrosarcoma: morphologic distinctions. *Vet Pathol* 39:33–41, 2002.

24. Doddy FD, Glickman LT, Glickman NE, et al: Feline fibrosarcomas at vaccination sites and non-vaccination sites. *J Comp Pathol* 114:165–174, 1996.

25. Abertein D, Munday JS, Dyer CB, et al: Comparison of the histology and immunohistochemistry of vaccination-site and non-vaccination-site sarcomas from cats in New Zealand. *N Z Vet J* 55:203–207, 2007.

26. Eckstein C, Guscetti F, Roos M, et al: A retrospective analysis of radiation therapy for the treatment of feline vaccine-associated sarcoma. *Vet Comp Oncol* 7:54–68, 2009.

27. Hershey AE, Sorenmo KU, Hendrick MJ, et al: Prognosis for presumed feline injection-site sarcoma after excision: 61 cases (1986-1996). *J Am Vet Med Assoc* 216:58–61, 2000.

28. Cronin K, Page RL, Spodnick G, et al: Radiation therapy and surgery for fibrosarcoma in 33 cats. *Vet Radiol Ultrasound* 39:51–56, 1998.

29. Cohen M, Wright JC, Brawner WR, et al: Use of surgery and electron beam irradiation, with or without chemotherapy, for treatment of vaccine-associated sarcomas in cats: 78 cases (1996-2000). *J Am Vet Med Assoc* 219:1582–1589, 2001.

30. Phelps HA, Kuntz CA, Milner RJ, et al: Radical excision with five-centimeter margins for the treatment of feline injection-site sarcomas: 91 cases (1998-2001). *J Am Vet Med Assoc* 239:97–106, 2011.

31. Kobayashi T, Hauck ML, Dodge R, et al: Preoperative radiotherapy for vaccine associated sarcoma in 92 cats. *Vet Radiol Ultrasound* 43:473–479, 2002.

32. Romanelli G, Marconato L, Olivero D, et al: Analysis of prognostic factors associated with injection-site sarcomas in cats: 57 cases (2001-2007). *J Am Vet Med Assoc* 232:1193–1199, 2008.

33. Romatowski J: Recommendations of the Vaccine-Associated Feline Sarcoma Task Force. *J Am Vet Med Assoc* 210:890, 1997.

34. Borjesson D: Cytology of sarcomas. *Vet Cancer Soc Newsletter* 23:2, 1999.

35. Davidson EB, Gregory CR, Kass PH: Surgical excision of soft tissue fibrosarcomas in cats. *Vet Surg* 26:265–269, 1997.

36. McEntee MC, Samii VF, Madewell BR, et al: Contrast-enhanced computed tomography for treatment planning of feline vaccine-associated sarcomas; preliminary findings. In *Proceedings of the 19th Annual Meeting of the Veterinary Cancer Society*, 1999, p 62.

37. Travetti O, di Giancamillo M, Stefanello D, et al: Computed tomography characteristics of fibrosarcoma—a histologic subtype of feline injection-site sarcoma. *J Feline Med Surg* 15:488–493, 2013.

38. Dillon CJ, Mauldin GN, Baer KE: Outcome following surgical removal of nonvisceral soft tissue sarcomas in cats: 42 cases (1992-2000). *J Am Vet Med Assoc* 227:1955–1957, 2005.

39. Bregazzi VS, LaRue SM, McNiel E, et al: Treatment with a combination of doxorubicin, surgery, and radiation versus surgery and radiation alone for cats with vaccine-associated sarcomas: 25 cases (1995-2000). *J Am Vet Med Assoc* 218:547–550, 2001.

40. Hahn KA, Endicott MM, King GK, et al: Evaluation of radiotherapy alone or in combination with doxorubicin chemotherapy for the treatment of cats with incompletely excised soft tissue sarcomas: 71 cases (1989-1999). *J Am Vet Med Assoc* 231:742–745, 2007.

41. Mayer MN, Treuil PL, LaRue SM: Radiotherapy and surgery for feline soft tissue sarcoma. *Vet Radiol Ultrasound* 50:669–672, 2009.

42. Barber LG, Sorenmo KU, Cronin KL, et al: Combined doxorubicin and cyclophosphamide chemotherapy for nonresectable feline fibrosarcoma. *J Am Anim Hosp Assoc* 36:416–421, 2000.

43. Piorier VJ, Thamm DH, Kurzman ID, et al: Liposome-encapsulated doxorubicin (Doxil) and doxorubicin in the treatment of vaccine-associated sarcoma in cats. *J Vet Intern Med* 16:726–731, 2002.

44. Martano M, Morello E, Ughetto M, et al: Surgery alone versus surgery and doxorubicin for the treatment of feline injection-site sarcomas: a report on 69 cases. *Vet J* 170:84–90, 2005.

45. Kisseberth WC, Vail DM, Yaissle J, et al: Phase I clinical evaluation of carboplatin in tumor-bearing cats: a Veterinary Cooperative Oncology Group study. *J Vet Intern Med* 22:83–88, 2008.

46. Rassnick KM, Rodriguez CO, Khanna C, et al: Results of a phase II clinical trial on the use of ifosfamide for treatment of cats with vaccine-associated sarcomas. *Am J Vet Res* 67:517–523, 2006.

47. Saba CF, Vail DM, Thamm DH: Phase II clinical evaluation of lomustine chemotherapy for feline vaccine-associated sarcoma. *Vet Comp Oncol* 10:283–291, 2012.

48. Mir LM, Devauchelle P, Quintin-Colonna F, et al: First clinical trial of cat soft-tissue sarcomas treatment by electrochemotherapy. *Br J Cancer* 76:1617–1622, 1997.

49. Spugnini EP, Baldi A, Vincenzi B, et al: Intraoperative versus postoperative electrochemotherapy in high grade soft tissue sarcomas: a preliminary study in a spontaneous feline model. *Cancer Chemother Pharmacol* 59:375–381, 2007.

50. Spugnini EP, Renaud SM, Bugloni S, et al: Electrochemotherapy with cisplatin enhances local control after surgical ablation of fibrosarcoma in cats: an approach to improve the therapeutic index of highly toxic chemotherapy drugs. *J Transl Med* 9:152, 2011.

51. Jourdier TM, Moste C, Bonnet MC, et al: Local immunotherapy of spontaneous feline fibrosarcomas using recombinant poxviruses expressing interleukin 2 (IL2). *Gene Ther* 10:2126–2132, 2003.

52. Jahnke A, Hirschberger J, Fischer C, et al: Intra-tumoral gene delivery of feIL-2, feIFN-gamma and feGM-CSF using magnetofection as a neoadjuvant treatment option for feline fibrosarcomas: a phase-I study. *J Vet Med A Physiol Pathol Clin Med* 54:599–606, 2007.

53. European Medicines Agency. Oncept IL-2. European Medicines Agency (website): <http://www.ema.europa.eu/ema/index.jsp?curl=pages/medicines/veterinary/medicines/002562/vet_med_000273.jsp&mid=WC0b01ac058001fa1c>, Accessed June 13, 2015.

54. Hendricks CG, Levy JK, Tucker SJ, et al: Tail vaccination in cats: a pilot study. *J Feline Med Surg* 16:275–280, 2014.

A Review and Update on Gastrointestinal Lymphoma in Cats

Erika L. Krick and Karin U. Sorenmo

HISTORY, RISK FACTORS, ETIOLOGY, AND EPIDEMIOLOGY

Lymphoma is the most common gastrointestinal (GI) malignancy in cats.[1] Our understanding of this subgroup of feline lymphoma has evolved over the past few decades and parallels the changing epidemiology of feline leukemia virus (FeLV)–associated lymphomas as well as an increased recognition of the histologic and biologic diversity of this disease.[2-4] The early publications on lymphomas in cats reported a strong causal association with FeLV, and it was reported that up to 70% of cats with lymphoma tested positive for FeLV.[5] In these studies, the prevalence of FeLV infection varied significantly according to anatomic location; younger cats with mediastinal lymphoma were commonly infected with FeLV, whereas older cats with GI lymphoma were more often FeLV-negative.[6,7] Lymphoma is also a common malignancy associated with feline immunodeficiency virus (FIV) infection. However compared to FeLV, the risk associated with FIV infection is significantly lower with only a fivefold versus sixtyfold increased risk for lymphoma associated with FIV versus FeLV, respectively.[8]

The prevalence of FeLV infection has decreased substantially since the 1980s, and the majority of cats with lymphomas diagnosed today are FeLV-negative.[2] Despite the decline in FeLV infection and therefore a decrease in FeLV-associated lymphoma, the overall incidence of lymphoma has not gone down, rather the opposite has occurred. A study from the University of California—Davis spanning over two decades (1980s and 1990s) reported that the incidence of lymphoma doubled during that time period, but less than 2% of the cases diagnosed in the latter years were FeLV-positive.[2] A significant rise in the number of cats diagnosed with GI lymphoma contributed to this increase. This shift may be due to a combination of factors including but not limited to increased awareness, more routine use of endoscopic and surgical biopsies that allows for the necessary histopathologic and molecular confirmation, changes in owner attitudes, and an overall increase in cats being seen at referral hospitals. Nevertheless, it is plausible that other factors, including dietary and environmental as well as other unrecognized influences, contribute to this increase.

The etiology of GI lymphomas in cats is incompletely understood. Many researchers have hypothesized that chronic antigenic stimulation from diet or ingested environmental carcinogens (including exposure to tobacco smoke residue due to grooming) may lead to an expansion of reactive or inflammatory lymphocytes, resulting in tumorigenic mutations and subsequent clonal expansion.[9-11] Thus, lymphoma may represent the end-stage of a histopathologic continuum spanning from inflammatory bowel disease (IBD) to malignant lymphoma. This pathogenesis is biologically plausible, especially in cats with small cell lymphoma (SCL; see the definition in Table 57-1) and supported by clinical and histopathologic evidence. For example, the clinical signs are usually chronic with slow progression, some cats have evidence of concurrent multifocal inflammation and lymphoma throughout the intestines, the IBD diagnosis may precede the lymphoma diagnosis, and some cases require molecular or clonality assays to differentiate between the two conditions.[9]

HISTOPATHOLOGY AND BIOLOGIC BEHAVIOR

Gastrointestinal lymphoma in cats represents a histologically and biologically diverse disease characterized by distinct morphological characteristics and a wide range in outcome.[3] The earlier literature on feline lymphoma did not differentiate among cell types or histological features, so all cases were grouped together and treated as if one disease. The outcome data from these studies, however, suggested that this indeed was a heterogeneous disease with differing responses to treatment. The clinical importance of distinguishing between large cell lymphoma (LCL) and SCL became apparent with a hallmark publication in 1999 where cats with GI SCL were treated with chlorambucil and prednisone, whereas cats with LCL received standard cyclophosphamide, vincristine, prednisone (COP)–based protocols.[4] The results showed that cats with SCL lived significantly longer than cats with LCL, despite receiving a less aggressive protocol. Several follow-up studies reported similar results, and today chlorambucil and prednisone protocols have become standard of care for GI SCL (see later).[9,12-14] This histologic and biologic diversity has been recognized in people with lymphoma for decades

Table 57-1	Simplified Summary of the Classification and Characteristics of Feline Gastrointestinal Lymphoma*				
Lymphoma Type/Size	**Histology and World Health Organization Classification**	**Cytology**	**T Cell versus B cell**	**Location**	**Biological Behavior**
Small to intermediate <2× RBC	Low MI Mucosal (no invasion through lamina propria, epitheliotropism diffuse/multifocal) WHO: EATCL type II	Monomorphic population of small cells; need biopsy ± PARR for diagnosis	T cells	Small intestines	Indolent
Large cell >2× RBC	High MI Includes LGL lymphoma[†] Transmural mass WHO: EATCL type I	Predominantly large/blastic cells; can be diagnostic	T cells	Small intestines	Aggressive
Large cell >2× RBC	High MI Large cells WHO: Diffuse, large B cells Centroblastic	Large or blastic cells; can be diagnostic	B cells	Stomach/small intestines Ileo-cecal-colic junction	Aggressive

EATCL, Enteropathy-associated T cell lymphoma; *LGL*, large granular lymphocyte; *MI*, mitotic index; *PARR*, polymerase chain reaction for antigen receptor rearrangement; *RBC*, red blood cell; *WHO*, World Health Organization.
*Note the exception regarding size and behavior for small cell transmural EATCL type 1 discussed in the text.
[†]Very aggressive.

and has prompted the creation of classification schemes, such as the National Cancer Institute Working Formulation (NCI-WF) followed by the Revised European-American Lymphoma system.[15,16] In 2000, Valli and colleagues[3] used the NCI-WF system to characterize and classify 602 cases of feline lymphoma. Similar to people and other domestic animals, a long list of histologic subtypes were described. These subtypes were grouped into three main categories using the same criteria as described in the original NCI-WF: (1) low grade, (2) intermediate grade, and (3) high-grade. No attempt to correlate outcome with grade was made in this study. However, most of the subtypes included in the low-grade categories were SCLs, and most of the high grade lymphomas were blastic or LCL (Figures 57-1 and 57-2). Today the World Health Organization (WHO) classification system is used to characterize and grade feline lymphoma. Similar to the limitations associated with the NCI-WF system, little is known about the association among WHO subtypes, grade, and outcome. A recent study, however, provides some clarification and clinical direction.[11] Using the WHO classification scheme, the authors in this study showed that feline GI lymphomas fall into one of three main categories[11]:

1. Enteropathy-associated T cell lymphoma (EATCL) type II is the predominant type and consists of small to intermediate T lymphocytes originating from mucosa-associated lymphoid tissue, various degrees of epitheliotropism are common, and the malignant lymphocytes typically do not invade into the submucosa.
2. EATCL type I includes cases with transmural infiltrates of malignant T lymphocytes of variable cell size. Large cell types are, however, more common than small cells (11 out

of 19 versus eight out of 19, respectively). Large granular lymphocyte (LGL) lymphomas are included in this category.
3. Diffuse large B cell lymphoma, also characterized by transmural involvement.

Cats with mucosal, (predominantly small cell) T cell lymphoma (type II) had a significantly longer survival than cats with transmural (predominantly large cell) T cell lymphomas (type I), with a survival of 29 months versus 1½ months, respectively. Survival was also shorter in cats with large B cell lymphoma.[11] These results validate the practice of using the term *small cell* to imply indolent behavior and *large cell* to imply aggressive behavior and, thus, simplifies treatment decisions in cats with GI lymphomas (see Table 57-1). A notable exception to this simplified approach is the relatively rare subset of cases with SCL with transmural involvement. According to the WHO, these are included in the subtype EATCL type I and have a shorter survival.[11] Full-thickness biopsies are required to identify these cases, and it may be difficult or impossible for the clinician to recognize these EATCL type I SCLs in cases diagnosed by endoscopic biopsies. The size classification scheme is based on the size of the lymphocytes compared to red blood cells (RBCs). Small lymphocytes are 1 to 1.5 times RBC, intermediate lymphocytes are 1.5 to 2 times RBC, and large lymphocytes are greater than 2 times RBC. The behavior of the intermediate cell size lymphomas have not been well characterized and, thus, continue to pose therapeutic challenges in terms of choosing the right protocol. However, according to a recent publication on the use of the WHO classification scheme, most of these intermediate cell lymphomas fall into the subtype EATCL type II and as such have an indolent behavior.[11]

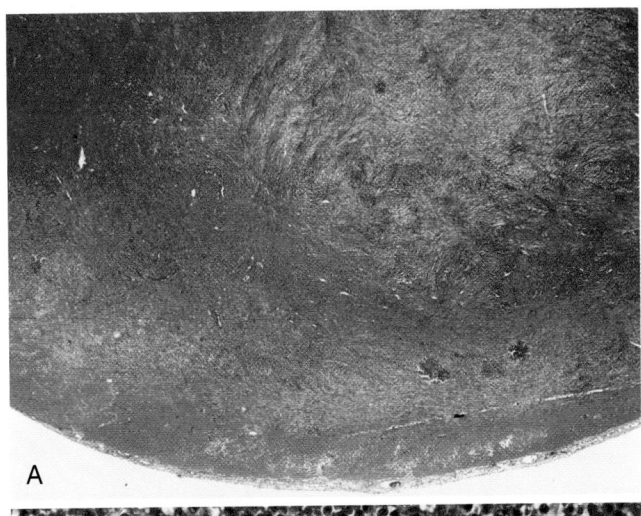

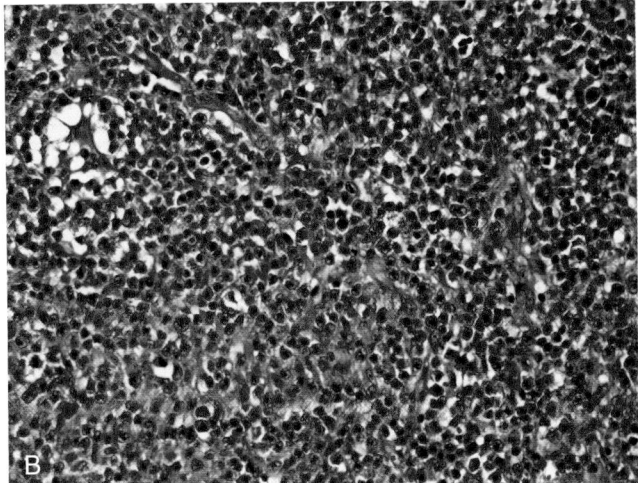

Figure 57-1: A, The wall of the small intestine is expanded and effaced by sheets of neoplastic lymphocytes. (Small intestine, hematoxylin and eosin [H&E], magnification ×2.) **B,** The individual cells are large (nuclei equal two times the diameter of a red blood cell) with round-oval, irregularly shaped nuclei and prominent central nucleoli. Mitotic figures are numerous, often more than 10 in a single high-power field. (Small intestine, H&E, magnification ×40.) (**A** and **B,** Courtesy of Amy Durham, VMD, DACVP, University of Pennsylvania.)

Anatomic location within the GI tract and distribution/ extent of disease within the intestinal wall also correlate with cell type and prognosis. In general, lymphoma is predominantly a small intestinal disease, with the jejunum affected more commonly than the duodenum in cases with SCL.[1,3,11] In addition to the small intestine, the gastric mucosa and the ileo-cecal-colic junction are also involved in large B cell lymphomas. Colonic involvement is relatively rare in both cell types. The superficial layers of the small intestines are most often affected in cases with SCL.[11] Many show various degrees of epitheliotropism, and extension through the lamina propria (transmural involvement) can occur but is more common in cases with LCLs. LCLs are typically larger transmural masses and can be B cell or T cell lymphomas.[11]

The information regarding the relative prevalence of GI SCL versus GI LCL is inconsistent and potentially misleading. Most of the papers describing the histopathologic features of GI lymphomas were biopsy-based case series and do

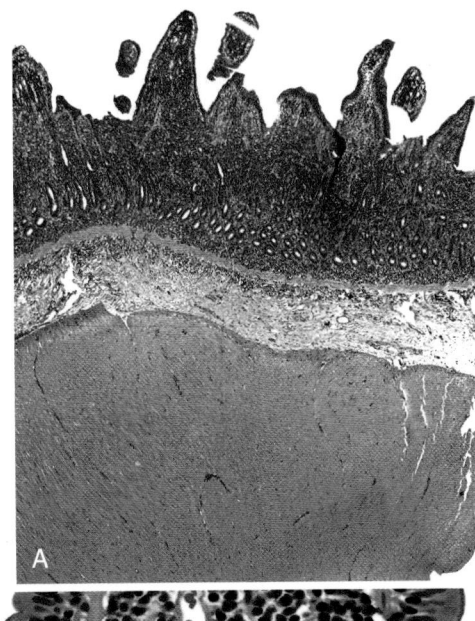

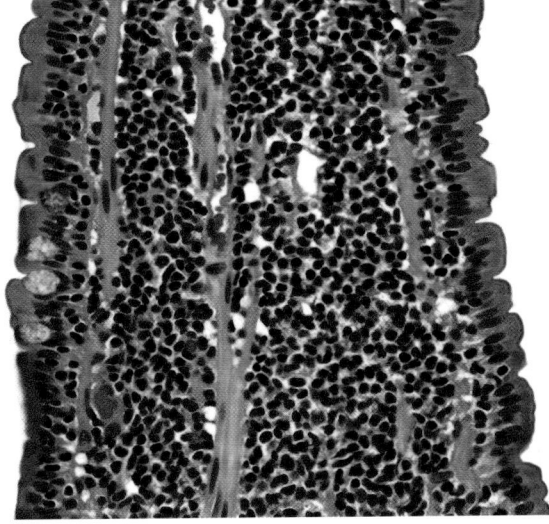

Figure 57-2: A, Neoplastic cells expand the lamina propria, widen the villi, and separate crypts. Cells extend beyond the muscularis mucosae and infiltrate the submucosa. (Small intestine, hematoxylin and eosin [H&E], magnification ×2.) **B,** The neoplastic lymphocytes are small (nuclei equal one times the diameter of a red blood cell) with scant cytoplasm and hyperchromatic, round-oval nuclei with occasional sharp indentations. These cells colonize the mucosal epithelium. Mitoses are rare. (Small intestine, H&E, magnification ×40.) (**A** and **B,** Courtesy of Amy Durham, VMD, DACVP, University of Pennsylvania.)

not include cats diagnosed and treated based on cytological diagnosis alone, thus overestimating the relative incidence of SCL. A more recent study where both histopathology- and cytology-based diagnoses were included suggests that LCL is still the most common lymphoma cell type in the GI tract, and only 28% of all cases were SCL.[17]

CLINICAL SIGNS, DIAGNOSTIC TESTS, AND STAGING

Common clinical signs of cats with GI lymphoma include lethargy, poor appetite, weight loss, vomiting, and/or diarrhea. Although the clinical signs are similar between cats with LCL and SCL, the chronicity and severity are often different. Cats with LCL tend to have more severe and faster onset of clinical signs, whereas cats with SCL often have less severe clinical signs with an indolent history. Cats with GI SCL are more likely to have diffuse intestinal thickening, whereas cats with GI LCL tend to have discrete GI masses and more significant lymphadenopathy compared to cats with SCL, and often have a palpable abdominal mass. Abdominal ultrasound changes found in cats with SCL are often similar to changes found in cats with IBD, and thickening of the muscularis layer has been associated with SCL rather than IBD in one study.[18] A more recent prospective study, however, found no difference in the thickness of the muscularis layer between cats with SCL and IBD, although both groups of cats had increased thickness of this layer compared to healthy cats.[19] Loss of intestinal wall layering has been documented in cats with GI lymphoma.[20] The success of cytology or biopsy in making a definitive diagnosis depends on the type of lymphoma (see Table 57-1). If there is a clinical suspicion of lymphoma but cytology results are not diagnostic, biopsy should be considered.

Both endoscopic and full-thickness biopsy samples have been used to diagnose GI lymphoma (particularly SCL) in cats, and there are advantages and disadvantages to both techniques. Endoscopy is less invasive and costly than open or laparoscopic abdominal exploratory surgery. However, the size of the samples is smaller, and affected areas can be missed in cases with focal or patchy disease and in cases where the mucosa is not involved.[9] Furthermore, it can be difficult to access the jejunum, which is the most common small intestinal site for SCL.[1,3,11] Full-thickness intestinal biopsies were compared to endoscopic biopsies in a prospective study by Evans and colleagues[21] and showed that SCL was more commonly diagnosed using full-thickness versus endoscopic biopsy samples. When only the duodenal samples were compared, the difference in the histopathological results (SCL versus IBD) from endoscopic and full-thickness biopsy techniques was statistically significant. Non-GI samples, including mesenteric lymph node biopsies can also be obtained during abdominal exploratory surgery. Although there is a risk of dehiscence associated with full-thickness biopsies, a recent retrospective study reported a low incidence of complications in the perioperative period following full-thickness GI biopsies in cats with lymphoma.[22] The risk of postsurgical complications after discharge from the hospital remains undocumented.

Differentiating between IBD and SCL can be challenging when based on histopathology alone. Immunohistochemistry and/or polymerase chain reaction for antigen receptor rearrangement (PARR) can be used in addition to the clinical picture to increase the chances of distinguishing between the two conditions. Cytology slides and formalin-fixed tissue can be used for PARR testing. Most cats with SCL have T cell lymphoma, but the lymphocyte population in IBD is also predominantly T cells.[11,23] Therefore, evaluation of the lymphocyte population for clonality may be a more useful test to

use when attempting to distinguish between these two diseases.[24] Clonal populations can be detected with PARR to confirm the clinical suspicion of lymphoma. Unfortunately, the sensitivity for detecting a clonal lymphocyte population in cats with GI lymphoma using PARR is 78% for T cell lymphoma and 50% for B cell lymphoma.[11,25] It is important, therefore, to examine the entire clinical picture and not rely on just one diagnostic test.

A modified staging system for feline lymphoma that specifically addresses GI lesions has been developed.[26] The accuracy of this staging system in predicting outcome is controversial, and more information will be presented later in this chapter during the discussion of prognostic factors. According to this staging system, cats with resectable GI lesions are considered Stage 2 (of 5), whereas cats with unresectable lesions are considered Stage 3. This definition introduces subjectivity into the staging and does not necessarily take size into account, because specific anatomic location is often considered a factor when assessing the resectability of an intestinal mass. Furthermore, cats with SCL are likely to have diffuse intestinal involvement and thus non-resectable disease, whereas cats with LCL may be more likely to have solitary, possibly resectable masses and therefore be assigned to a lower stage category. It is worth noting that the current staging system for feline lymphoma was published in 1986. Given that more recent studies have not found this staging system to carry prognostic significance,[26-32] the changing anatomic distribution of feline lymphoma,[2] and the fact that surgery is infrequently performed as part of routine treatment for GI lymphoma, there is an essential need for a revised and more accurate staging system for feline lymphoma

SUBTYPES AND TREATMENT RECOMMENDATIONS

Several distinct varieties of lymphoma have been documented in the GI tract of cats. These subtypes vary in their cellular morphology, clinical behavior, and recommended treatment plan (Figures 57-3 and 57-4).

Large Cell Lymphoma

Large cell lymphoma has been recognized the longest, and much of the early literature, especially from the FeLV era, is exclusively about this variant. However, many of the publications from the 1980s and 1990s do not specify cell type and likely include both SCL and LCL. The response rates and outcome reported in these studies are generally much better than what has been more recently reported and is likely due to the inclusion of cats with SCL.

Several studies of cats with LCL include cats with GI involvement, but the majority of these studies are retrospective and contain relatively small numbers of cats with GI lymphoma (Table 57-2). More recently, however, results from two prospective studies on feline lymphoma were published.[30,33] Both of these included both GI and non-GI cases.

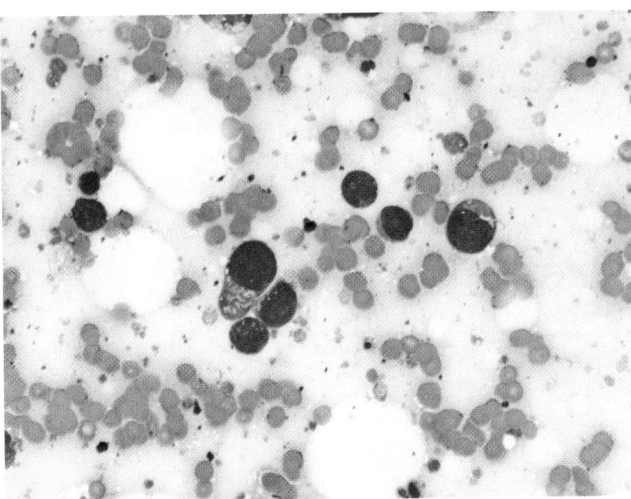

Figure 57-3: Cat, intestinal mass: **Large cell lymphoma** (LCL; 40× objective). The neoplastic lymphocytes are large (12 to 18 μm in diameter), and they contain small discrete intracytoplasmic vacuoles. This cytological appearance is most commonly associated with LCL of intestinal origin in cats. (Courtesy of Roberta DiTerlizzi, DVM, DACVP, Clinical Pathology, University of Pennsylvania.)

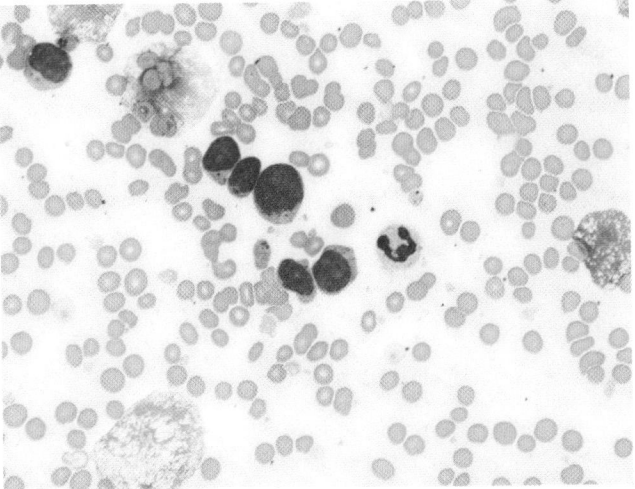

Figure 57-4: Cat, intestinal mass: **Granulated lymphocytic lymphoma** (40× objective). The neoplastic lymphocytes are large (12 to 16 μm in diameter), and they contain small fine magenta intracytoplasmic granules, which is a characteristic of this variant of lymphoma. (Courtesy of Roberta DiTerlizzi, DVM, DACVP, Clinical Pathology, University of Pennsylvania.)

No difference in survival between cases with GI or non-GI lymphoma was reported in either of these two studies. These findings were confirmed by a later large retrospective study on predominantly large and intermediate cell lymphoma (*n* = 96).[34]

Only two studies specifically report on the use of COP-based chemotherapy or cyclophosphamide, doxorubicin, vincristine, prednisone (CHOP)–based chemotherapy in feline GI lymphoma. Both of these small, retrospective studies were published over 15 years ago, but they remain the only studies reporting on CHOP or COP chemotherapy specifically for cats with GI lymphoma.[29,35] The response rates were 39% (COP) and 95% (CHOP). However, the former study required responses to last for at least 4 weeks, whereas there was no such requirement for the latter study. Median complete remission duration was 213 and 276 days, and median overall survival was 50 and 280 days, respectively. These survival figures may be misleading because three of 28 cats were noted to have SCL in the COP-treated cats,[35] and no distinction between LCL and SCL was made in the CHOP-treated cats.[29] Based on these results, one might conclude that CHOP-based chemotherapy is superior to COP; however, it is important to note that information about cell type was not included in the latter study.

Whether COP is superior to CHOP in treating GI LCL cannot be answered by dissecting and comparing data from nonrandomized and retrospective studies; only a well-designed, adequately powered prospective randomized study can settle this controversy.

The standard COP and CHOP protocols contain vincristine, which has well-documented activity in lymphoma but is also associated with significant GI toxicity. This can be particularly problematic in GI lymphoma where the patients' primary clinical signs include vomiting, diarrhea, ileus, anorexia, and malaise. A randomized study showed that vinblastine-based COP was significantly better tolerated than the standard vincristine-based COP while maintaining efficacy.[33] This modified COP approach may be a reasonable option for cats that do not tolerate vincristine or have significant GI clinical signs due to lymphoma.

The efficacy of doxorubicin in treating cats with high-grade lymphoma is lower than reported in dogs with lymphoma; in cats treated with single agent doxorubicin, response rates of 26% and 32% were reported.[36,37] Nevertheless, doxorubicin may still have a role in feline lymphoma. A prospective randomized study (all anatomic sites including GI) showed that cats treated with doxorubicin-based maintenance chemotherapy after COP induction had significantly longer remission than cats randomized to receive COP maintenance chemotherapy (281 versus 83 days).[31] Doxorubicin maintenance was also tolerated better than COP in this study.

Radiation therapy alone or in combination with chemotherapy has been evaluated in cats with lymphoma. One retrospective study examined the effect of half body radiation therapy with or without chemotherapy in cats with hematologic malignancies.[38] Of the six cats in this study with GI lymphoma and measurable disease at the time of radiation therapy treatment, three had a complete response. All of these cats eventually died of progressive lymphoma with a survival time range of 18 to 1201 days. The variety of tumor types and chemotherapy protocols in this study makes it difficult to make significant conclusions about the efficacy and tolerability of this treatment for cats with GI lymphoma; however, a prospective pilot study focused on cats with GI and multicentric abdominal lymphoma provides additional information.[39] All eight cats in that study received a 6-week CHOP chemotherapy protocol followed by abdominal cavity irradiation. Only cats in complete remission after the CHOP protocol received radiation therapy. Treatment-related

Table 57-2 | **Reported Response Rates, Remission Duration, and Survival Times for Cats Treated with Cyclophosphamide, Vincristine, Prednisone and Cyclophosphamide, Doxorubicin, Vincristine, Prednisone Chemotherapy Protocols**

Protocol	Number of Cats	Response Rate	Median Response Duration (days)	Median Survival (days)	Comments
COP[35] Retrospective	28 (GI only)	32% CR 7% PR	213 CR 260, 149 PR	50 All cats	Mixed cell types
CHOP[29] Retrospective	21 (GI only)	38% CR 57% PR	276.5* CR 75.3 PR	290.5* CR 220.5 PR 280 All cats	No cell type distinction
COP then COP or doxorubicin[31] PRT	38 (mixed locations)	47% CR after COP induction	83 COP maintenance 281 Doxorubicin maintenance	Not reported	No cell type distinction
CHOP[48] Retrospective	61 (13 abdominal)	80% CR 3.3% PR	112 CR	187 CR 116 All cats	Mixed cell types
COP[32] Retrospective	61 (11 GI)	75.4% CR 13.1% PR 63.6% CR for GI	251 CR 245 CR GI	266 All cats 191 For GI	No cell type distinction
CHOP[49] Retrospective	38 (16 GI)	47% CR 37% PR	654 CR 114 PR 156 All cats	654 CR 122 PR 210 All cats	Mixed cell types
CHOP[47] Retrospective	61 (13 GI)	43% CR	Not reported	62 All cats	Large cell only
CHOP[30] Prospect	23 (5 GI)	74% CR 17% PR	264 CR 23 PR	296 CR 47 PR 242 All cats	No cell type distinction
COP[33] (vincristine arm reported) PRT	40 (17 GI)	11% CR 56% PR	48 All cats (PFS)	139 All cats	Mixed cell types
COP[34] Retrospective	114 (57 GI)	47.4% Clinical response	364 Responders 65.5 All cats (PFS)	581 Responders 108 All cats	Mixed cell types

CHOP, Cyclophosphamide, doxorubicin, vincristine, prednisone; *COP*, cyclophosphamide, vincristine, prednisone; *CR*, complete response; *GI*, gastrointestinal; *PFS*, progression free survival; *PR*, partial response; *PRT*, prospective randomized trial.
*Response duration and survival times converted from weeks to days by the authors.

toxicities were mild, and at the time of writing, five cats remained in remission at least 266 days after treatment. All of these cats responded to CHOP chemotherapy, however, which likely biased the study population toward cats that had treatment-responsive lymphoma.

A relatively rare subtype of GI lymphoma in cats is LGL lymphoma (see Figure 57-4). The LGL lymphomas are characterized by an aggressive biologic behavior and progress quickly to terminal stages. The cells are distinguished from other lymphoma cells based on the presence of azurophilic intracytoplasmic granules, and they may be large or small. Studies have suggested natural killer cell or cytotoxic T cell origin for the majority of cells in this lymphoma subtype,[40-42] with the most recent report confirming cytotoxic T cell origin for most LGL lymphomas in cats.[40] Several studies have reported that LGL lymphoma most commonly affects the

intestines and abdominal lymph nodes.[41-43] Neutrophilia, elevated liver enzymes, hypoalbuminemia, and hyperbilirubinemia are also frequently noted.[40,44,45] Relatively few studies report on treatment of these cats. Survival times of less than 3 months are commonly reported; however, the majority of cats in these studies did not receive cytotoxic therapy.[40,43-45] One paper specifically reports on the outcome of chemotherapy treatment with COP-based and CHOP-based protocols in 23 cats with LGL lymphoma, and the median survival time was 57 days, with one complete response and six partial responses.[44]

Small Cell Lymphoma

The standard of care treatment for this type of lymphoma in cats is combination therapy with prednisone or prednisolone

Table 57-3	Published Chemotherapy Protocols for Treating Small Cell Gastrointestinal Lymphoma in Cats				
Number of Cats	Prednis(ol)one Schedule	Chlorambucil Schedule	Response Rate	Remission Duration (days)	Survival (days)
50[4]	Prednisolone 10 mg PO every 24 h	15 mg/m^2 PO every 24 h × 4 days every 3 weeks	69% CR (only response assessed)	488 CR*	518*
41[12]	Prednisone 5 to 10 mg every 12 to 24 h	2 mg PO every 48 to 72 h	CR 56% PR 39%	897 CR 428 PR	704
17[13]	Prednisolone 3 mg/kg PO every 24 h until CR, then 1 to 2 mg/kg every 24 h	15 mg/m^2 PO every 24 h × 4 days every 3 weeks	76% CR (only response assessed)	576*	454*
28[14]	Both, ranged from 1 mg/kg every 48 h to 2 mg/kg every 24 h × 1 week, then all tapered to 1 mg/kg PO every 48 h	20 mg/m^2 PO every 2 weeks	96% Clinical remission	786	Not reported

CR, Complete response; PO, per os (orally); PR, partial response.
*Remission duration and survival times converted from months to days by the authors.

and chlorambucil.[4,12-14] Both drugs are administered orally. Several different prednisone or prednisolone and chlorambucil protocols have been published (Table 57-3). Myelosuppression and GI toxicity have been reported with chlorambucil, but these toxicities are generally mild to moderate.[4,13,14] Other toxicities, such as myoclonus and seizures, have been reported.[46] Idiosyncratic hepatocellular enzyme elevation related to chlorambucil administration in cats has been documented by the authors; therefore, the authors have incorporated monitoring of liver enzymes into prednisone or prednisolone and chlorambucil protocol for cats with SCL at their institution. This liver enzyme elevation is reversible with drug withdrawal but often recurs when treatment is restarted, so alternate therapies are considered for cats that have experienced this side effect.

According to one study, 78% of cats with SCL are cobalamin deficient at diagnosis, so measurement of serum cobalamin is recommended as part of routine staging for these cats, and supplementation is recommended where indicated.[12]

RESPONSE ASSESSMENT

Assessing response to therapy in cats with GI lymphoma remains challenging. Currently, there is no standard method for assessing response in cats with GI lymphoma. Most studies of both GI LCL and GI SCL are retrospective and use different methods, which add to the difficulty in comparing the outcome of different treatment protocols.

Most cats are ill at the time of their lymphoma diagnosis, and resolution or improvement in clinical signs can provide helpful information but can be subjective. Unfortunately, clinical signs associated with progressive lymphoma are often similar to clinical chemotherapy toxicity, so it may not be accurate to rely solely on clinical parameters.

Objective criteria, such as palpation or measurements of masses and/or enlarged lymph nodes, in combination with clinical findings, are often used when making decisions in cats with LCL. For cats with discrete masses or diffuse intestinal wall thickening, imaging can be performed to repeat measurements of these lesions. Abdominal ultrasound is most commonly used for these assessments, and provides an objective measurement of tumor size or intestinal wall thickening and layering. Cats with SCL can, however, be difficult to assess using ultrasound. The lesions visible with abdominal imaging in these patients are often subtle, consisting of mild to moderate intestinal thickening, loss of layering, and lymphadenopathy, with no one focal mass lesion to measure in more than one dimension. Many of these cats also have concomitant IBD and associated intestinal thickening and lymphadenopathy. Therefore, the traditional objective response criteria are not useful and cannot be applied to these cats. As a result, subjective criteria based on changes in clinical signs are heavily relied upon when assessing response for cats with GI SCL. In fact, assessment of response based solely on clinical improvement has been associated with outcome in cats with SCL.[4,12,13]

Body weight has also been examined in cats with GI lymphoma as a surrogate marker for response to treatment. Although body weight is a clinical parameter, it is a simple objective measurement that is part of a routine physical examination and thus does not incur increased patient stress or cost when performed at each visit. Both baseline weight and body condition score are prognostic factors for cats with lymphoma, and weight changes over time have been associated with survival in cats with LCL. This suggests that body weight and body condition may be promising surrogate markers for response to and tolerance of treatment.[47-49] In addition to body weight and body condition scoring, one paper proposes a specific scoring system for fat and muscle mass for cats with lymphoma.[47] Both fat and muscle mass were scored on a four-point scale assessing specific anatomic locations: ribs and abdominal fat pad for fat mass and temporal muscles, hindlimbs, and scapulae for muscle mass. Fat mass was reduced in 60% of cats, whereas muscle mass was reduced in 91% of cats. These findings also emphasize the importance of supportive care of cats undergoing induction chemotherapy as well as serial monitoring of body weight and other body condition parameters.

PROGNOSTIC FACTORS

Long-documented prognostic factors for feline lymphoma include FeLV infection status, anatomic location, substage, and response to therapy.[28-30,32,36,50,51] None of the reported prognostic factors for lymphoma in cats are specific to the GI location, so this portion of the chapter focuses on those factors that are clinically applicable to feline GI lymphoma. One of the most significant prognostic factors for lymphoma in cats is the cell type, specifically SCL or LCL. Higher response rates and longer progression free and overall survival are reported for SCL versus LCL (see Tables 57-2 and 57-3).

Few prognostic factors have been specifically documented for cats with GI SCL. Lethargy has been specifically associated with a decreased likelihood of response and shorter response duration.[4,13] Vomiting and anorexia have also been associated with a significantly decreased likelihood of response, shorter response duration, and shorter survival.[4] Low serum cobalamin was associated with shorter remission duration on univariate, but not multivariate, analysis in one study.[12]

The effect of stage on prognosis (using the modified feline lymphoma staging system) has been inconsistently documented. Clinical stage was prognostic for response to treatment and survival in older studies,[26,28] but more recent retrospective and prospective studies have not confirmed this association.[27,29-32]

Cats that have experienced complete or partial responses to chemotherapy have improved outcomes compared to cats that do not respond as well, as would be expected. One paper describing treatment of cats with GI lymphoma found response to treatment as the only factor associated with remission duration.[29] A recent paper describing the outcome with COP chemotherapy in a large number of cats with lymphoma (not all GI) found specifically that the response after the first cycle of treatment was significantly associated with survival time (see Table 57-2).[34] This paper was the first to provide data regarding a specific time point for response assessment and indicates that protocol changes may be reasonable early in the course of treatment for cats that are not responding.

Immunophenotype is a strong prognostic factor in canine lymphoma, with T cell being associated with a worse prognosis. This association has not been documented in cats, but it needs to be analyzed in the context of cell size. As noted earlier, SCL tends to be T cell in origin and associated with a significantly better prognosis than LCL (regardless of phenotype).[11] Further studies are needed to determine whether there is a difference in outcome between cats with B cell or T cell LCL.

Several studies have documented increased feline-specific acute phase proteins in cats with cancer, including lymphoma, and it is possible that these levels may have an impact on disease staging and prognosis in the future.[52-54] Cats with elevated serum amyloid A associated with a variety of neoplastic and nonneoplastic diseases were found to have a shorter survival compared to cats with nonelevated values.[52] In a study including a large number of cats with varied tumor types, cats with cancer had higher serum alpha-1 acid glycoprotein levels compared to healthy cats. No significant differences were found among the cats with cancer according to tumor type, although cats with round-cell tumors (mostly lymphoma) had the highest mean value.[53] Serum alpha-1 acid glycoprotein was higher in nine cats with lymphoma compared to 25 healthy controls, but serial measurements in the cats with lymphoma did not show any correlation between serum levels and tumor response or survival time.[54] These studies demonstrate an association between cancer and increased acute phase proteins in cats, and more research is needed to determine how to use this information in the clinical setting.

RESCUE PROTOCOLS

A great majority of cats treated for their lymphoma, especially those with LCL or LGL, will relapse and require rescue therapy. The information regarding the efficacy of rescue therapies in feline lymphoma is sparse, with only two publications with the specific purpose of evaluating response to rescue chemotherapy. Both studies were retrospective and included cats with both LCL and SCL. Contrary to what one might have expected, both studies reported significantly better response durations in cats with SCL compared to LCL, even though the drugs used, doxorubicin and lomustine, are both traditionally used to treat large cell, aggressive lymphomas in dogs and thus a better response in cats with LCL might have been expected.

The first study describes the outcomes in cats treated with doxorubicin or a doxorubicin-based rescue protocol; objective responses (i.e., partial responses or complete responses) were noted in five out of 23 cats.[55] All of the responders had small to intermediate cell lymphoma, and none had LCL.

The second study evaluated lomustine (CCNU) in cats with relapsed lymphoma. In that study, both objective and subjective measurements (such as palpation, improvements in blood work, and clinical signs noted by the owners) were used to determine progression free survival.[56] It is therefore feasible that the slow progression associated with SCL and the relative tolerability of CCNU might contribute to the improvements noted in this particular study.

In addition, two of the studies evaluating the efficacy of chlorambucil in cats with SCL also included information about rescue and response to rescue with cyclophosphamide in cats that failed chlorambucil. Both reported significant benefit. All seven cats treated with rescue cyclophosphamide responded in one paper; response rates or duration were not reported in the other paper but the authors stated that "rescue extended the life of some of the cats."[4,14]

One study reported on the efficacy of abdominal radiation therapy in relapsed lymphoma in 11 cats.[57] Both SCL and LCL cases were included. Responses were reported in 10 out of 11 cats, and no significant difference was found between cell types. The median survival after radiation therapy was 214 days, which is substantially longer than reported with any of the published rescue chemotherapy protocols. One must be careful when interpreting these results; only a few cats were evaluated, and all of the cats had either complete or partial responses to previous chemotherapy. Nevertheless, the results are intriguing and warrant further investigation.

In the authors' experience, relapses that occur after completion of a protocol or during a maintenance phase of a protocol may be reversed by simply restarting the original protocol or intensifying the current protocol. Intensification can be achieved by either shortening treatment intervals or delivering drugs concurrently. COP is often administered as a sequential protocol—COP(s)—during which vincristine and cyclophosphamide are administered sequentially on an alternating week basis.[28,34] A more intense version, COP(c), is achieved when vincristine and cyclophosphamide are given concurrently in the same week, similar to the original Cotter protocol.[58] In the authors' experience, cats that tolerate COP(s) may tolerate COP(c) and respond favorably to this relatively simple adjustment and intensification of COP.

L-asparaginase has a long and well-established history in lymphoma therapy and is often used in addition to COP-based or CHOP-based chemotherapy in cats.[28-30,33-35,49-51] L-asparaginase has been reported to have a 30% response rate in untreated lymphomas but does not represent a rescue protocol by itself, because there are limits to how often it can

be administered with efficacy, and the duration of the benefit is typically relatively short.[59] However, it can be particularly useful in a patient that needs chemotherapy due to rapidly progressing disease but also needs more time to recover from the previous chemotherapy administration. L-asparaginase is well tolerated and can help to "tide over" until the patient becomes ready for the next rescue protocol.

As reflected from the preceding information, there are no publications that report on effective rescue protocols in cats with relapsed GI LCL. And this group of cats is the subset where the need is the greatest; many cats with LCL do not respond to COP-based or CHOP-based induction, and the median response duration is relatively short in the ones that do. Despite the lack of published evidence, many oncologists, including the authors, offer rescue chemotherapy in cats with LCL and use similar protocols as those published in relapsed canine lymphomas. Some adjustments in dosing and scheduling may be required when using these "dog protocols" in cats and may be a practice best performed under supervision by trained oncologists.

Most cats with relapsing LCL progress and become resistant to all attempts at rescue relatively quickly. It is important to prepare owners for this outcome and to establish an agreement that the goal of therapy is to prolong a good quality life for the cat. Continuing therapy in a debilitated sick cat with little hope of achieving benefit and risk of increasing nausea, anorexia, and malaise is not consistent with that goal. Discontinuing treatment is difficult for both the clinician and owner, but sometimes a break from chemotherapy can provide the cat a period with reasonable quality of life despite living with progressive lymphoma. It is crucial that supportive medications, such as antiemetics and appetite stimulants, and adequate hydration are maintained during this period to alleviate disease-related discomfort.

Figure 57-5 provides the authors' algorithm for approaching chemotherapy rescue therapy and decisions. Rescue

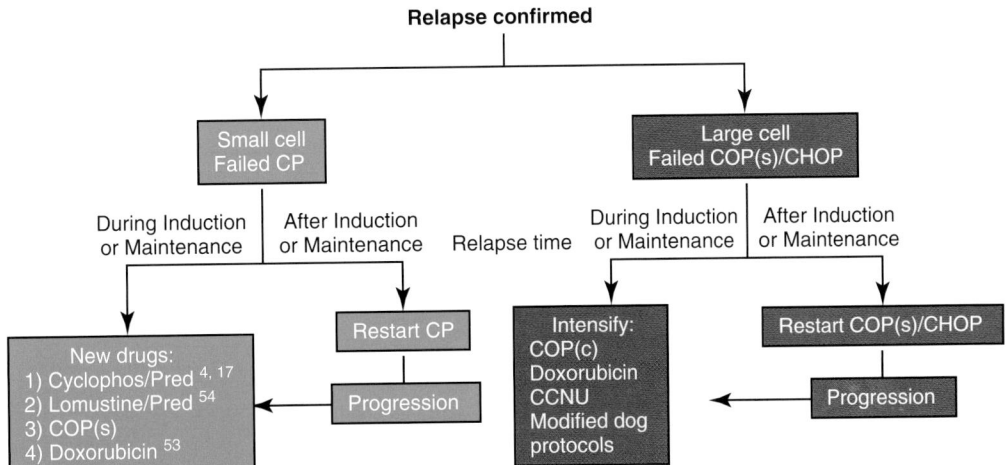

Figure 57-5: Treatment decision algorithm for rescue chemotherapy for cats with gastrointestinal lymphoma. *CCNU*, Lomustine; *CHOP*, cyclophosphamide, doxorubicin, vincristine, prednis(ol)one; *COP*, cyclophosphamide, vincristine, prednisone; *COP(c)*, vincristine and cyclophosphamide are given concurrently in the same week; *COP(s)*, vincristine and cyclophosphamide are administered sequentially on an alternating week basis; *CP*, chlorambucil and prednis(ol)one; *Cyclophos*, cyclophosphamide; *Pred*, prednis(ol)one.

abdominal radiation therapy has not been included in this algorithm. The data is promising, but it is important to note that this study involved cases at their first relapse, which may be a more aggressive step than most clinicians feel comfortable with when other drug choices are available. Additional studies need to be performed to evaluate safety and provide guidelines regarding appropriate patient selection for this type of rescue therapy.

THE FUTURE

As knowledge about feline GI lymphoma has increased, new challenges have emerged in the diagnosis, staging, and treatment of this disease. Further evaluation of less common lymphoma subtypes, such as intermediate cell lymphoma, would result in more accurate prognostic estimates and treatment recommendations for these patients. Although most cats with SCL have a favorable prognosis with standard treat-

ment, the response rate and survival of cats with LCL remains poor. An updated staging system that could predict outcome for cats with LCL combined with a clinically useful and accurate method for measuring response that involves standardized clinical and objective assessments are essential for our understanding of the disease as well as evaluating novel treatment strategies. Understanding the role of body weight and body condition score in prognosis and response assessment is emerging, and future studies to elucidate the underlying mechanisms and potentially target the mediators of cachexia are needed. Controlled, randomized trials are needed to determine the optimal chemotherapy protocol for feline lymphoma, and treatment strategies with a two-pronged approach of eliminating disease while providing adequate supportive care to the patient are particularly important for cats with GI lymphoma. It is well documented that response to therapy in cats with lymphoma is associated with longer survival times; therefore, one of the future challenges is to develop strategies that increase the response rate.

References

1. Risetto K, Villamil JA, Selting KA, et al: Recent trends in feline intestinal neoplasia: an epidemiological study of 1,129 cases in the veterinary medical database from 1964 to 2004. *J Am Anim Hosp Assoc* 47:28–36, 2011.
2. Louwerens M, London CA, Pedersen NC, et al: Feline lymphoma in the post-feline leukemia virus era. *J Vet Intern Med* 19:329–335, 2005.
3. Valli VE, Jacobs RM, Norris A, et al: The histological classification of 602 cases of feline lymphoproliferative disease using the National Cancer Institute working formulation. *J Vet Diagn Invest* 12(4):295–306, 2000.
4. Fondacaro JV, Richter KP, Carpenter JL: Feline gastrointestinal lymphoma: 67 cases (1988-1996). *Eur J Comp Gastroenterol* 4(2):5–11, 1999.
5. Hardy WD, Jr, McClelland AJ, Zuckerman EE, et al: Development of virus non producer lymphosarcomas in pet cats exposed to FeLV. *Nature* 288:90, 1980.
6. Hardy WD, Jr, Zuckerman EE, MacEwen EG, et al: A feline leukemia virus-and sarcoma virus-induced tumor-specific antigen. *Nature* 270:249–251, 1977.
7. Hardy WD, Jr: Hematopoietic tumors of cats. *J Am Anim Hosp Assoc* 17:921–940, 1981.
8. Shelton GH, Grant CK, Cotter SM, et al: Feline immunodeficiency virus and feline leukemia virus infections and their relationships to lymphoid malignancies in cats: a retrospective study. *J Acquir Immune Def Syndrome* 3:623–630, 1990.
9. Kiupel M, Scedley RC, Pfent C, et al: Diagnostic algorithm to differentiate lymphoma from inflammation in feline small intestinal biopsy samples. *Vet Pathol* 48:212–222, 2011.
10. Bertone ER, Snyder LA, Moore AS: Environmental tobacco smoke and risk of malignant lymphoma in pet cats. *Am J Epidemiol* 156:268–273, 2002.

11. Moore PF, Rodriguez-Bertos A, Kass PH: Feline gastrointestinal lymphoma: mucosal architecture, immunophenotype, and molecular clonality. *Vet Pathol* 49:658–668, 2012.
12. Kiselow MA, Rassnick KM, McDonough SP, et al: Outcome of cats with low-grade lymphocytic lymphoma: 41 cases (1995-2005). *J Am Vet Med Assoc* 232:405–410, 2008.
13. Lingard AE, Briscoe K, Beatty JA, et al: Low-grade alimentary lymphoma: clinicopathological findings and response to treatment in 17 cases. *J Feline Med Surg* 11:692–700, 2009.
14. Stein TJ, Pellin M, Steinberg H, et al: Treatment of feline gastrointestinal small cell lymphoma with chlorambucil and glucocorticoids. *J Am Anim Hosp Assoc* 246:413–417, 2010.
15. National Cancer Institute: National Cancer Institute sponsored study of classifications of non-Hodgkin's lymphomas: summary and description of a working formulation for clinical usage. The Non-Hodgkin's Lymphoma Pathologic Classification Project. *Cancer* 9:2112–2135, 1982.
16. Harris N, Jaffe E, Stein H, et al: A revised European-American classification of lymphoid neoplasma: a proposal for the international lymphoma study group. *Blood* 84:1361–1392, 1994.
17. Russel KJ, Beatty JA, Dhand N, et al: Feline low-grade alimentary lymphoma, how common is it? *J Feline Med Surg* 14(12):910–912, 2012.
18. Zwingenberger AL, Marks SL, Baker TW, et al: Ultrasonographic evaluation of the muscularis propria in cats with diffuse small intestinal lymphoma or inflammatory bowel disease. *J Vet Intern Med* 24:289–292, 2010.
19. Daniaux LA, Laurenson MP, Marks SL, et al: Ultrasonographic thickening of the muscularis propria in feline small intestinal small cell T cell lymphoma and inflammatory bowel disease. *J Feline Med Surg* 16(2):89–90, 2014.

20. Grooters AM, Biller DS, Ward H, et al: Ultrasonographic appearance of feline alimentary lymphoma. *Vet Radiol Ultrasound* 35:468–472, 1994.
21. Evans SE, Bonczynski JJ, Broussard JD, et al: Comparison of endoscopic and full-thickness biopsy specimens for diagnosis of inflammatory bowel disease and alimentary tract lymphoma in cats. *J Am Vet Med Assoc* 229:1447–1450, 2006.
22. Smith AL, Wilson AP, Hardie RJ, et al: Perioperative complications after full-thickness gastrointestinal surgery in cats with alimentary lymphoma. *Vet Surg* 40:849–852, 2011.
23. Carreras JK, Goldschmidt M, Lamb M, et al: Feline epitheliotropic intestinal malignant lymphomas: 10 cases (1997-2000). *J Vet Intern Med* 17:326–331, 2003.
24. Avery AC: Molecular diagnostics of hematologic malignancies in small animals. *Vet Clin Small Anim* 42:97–110, 2012.
25. Moore PF, Woo JC, Vernau W, et al: Characterization of feline T cell receptor gamma (TCRG) variable region genes for the molecular diagnosis of feline intestinal T cell lymphoma. *Vet Immunol Immunopathol* 106:167–178, 2005.
26. Mooney SC, Hayes AA: Lymphoma in the cat: an approach to diagnosis and management. *Semin Vet Med Surg (Small Animal)* 1:51–57, 1986.
27. Vail DM, Moore AS, Ogilvie GK, et al: Feline lymphoma (145 cases): Proliferation indices, CD3 immunoreactivity and their association with prognosis in 90 cats receiving therapy. *J Vet Intern Med* 12:349–354, 1998.
28. Mooney SC, Hayes AA, MacEwen EG, et al: Treatment and prognostic factors in lymphoma in cats: 103 cases (1977-1981). *J Am Vet Med Assoc* 194:696–699, 1989.
29. Zwahlen CH, Lucroy MD, Kraegel SA, et al: Results of chemotherapy for cats with

alimentary malignant lymphoma: 21 cases (1993-1997). *J Am Vet Med Assoc* 213:1144–1149, 1998.

30. Simon D, Eberle N, Laacke-Singer L, et al: Combination chemotherapy in feline lymphoma: treatment outcome, tolerability, and duration in 23 cats. *J Vet Intern Med* 22:394–400, 2008.

31. Moore AS, Cotter SM, Frimberger AE, et al: A comparison of Doxorubicin and COP for maintenance of remission in cats with lymphoma. *J Vet Intern Med* 10:372–375, 1996.

32. Teske E, van Straten G, van Noort R, et al: Chemotherapy with cyclophosphamide, vincristine, and prednisolone (COP) in cats with malignant lymphoma: new results with an old protocol. *J Vet Intern Med* 16:179–186, 2002.

33. Krick EL, Cohen RB, Gregor TP, et al: Prospective clinical trial to compare vincristine and vinblastine in a COP-based protocol for lymphoma in cats. *J Vet Intern Med* 27:134–140, 2013.

34. Waite AHK, Jackson K, Gregor TP, et al: Retrospective study of 114 cases of feline lymphoma treated with a weekly COP-based protocol: 1998-2008. *J Am Vet Med Assoc* 242:1104–1109, 2013.

35. Mahoney OM, Moore AS, Cotter SM, et al: Alimentary lymphoma in cats: 28 cases (1988-1993). *J Am Vet Med Assoc* 207:1593–1598, 1995.

36. Kristal O, Lana SE, Ogilvie GK, et al: Single agent chemotherapy with doxorubicin for feline lymphoma: a retrospective study of 19 cases (1994-1997). *J Vet Intern Med* 15:125–130, 2001.

37. Peaston AE, Maddison JE: Efficacy of doxorubicin as an induction agent for cats with lymphosarcoma. *Aust Vet J* 77:422–424, 1999.

38. Husbands BD, McNiel EA, Modiano JF: Initial evaluation of safety of wide-field irradiation in the treatment of hematopoietic neoplasia in the cat. *Vet Radiol Ultrasound* 51:688–698, 2010.

39. Williams LE, Pruitt AF, Thrall DE: Chemotherapy followed by abdominal cavity irradiation for feline lymphoblastic lymphoma. *Vet Radiol Ultrasound* 51:681–687, 2010.

40. Roccabianca P, Vernau W, Caniatti M, et al: Feline large granular lymphocyte (LGL) lymphoma with secondary leukemia: primary intestinal origin with predominance of a CD3/CD8(alpha)(alpha) phenotype. *Vet Pathol* 43:15–28, 2006.

41. Endo Y, Cho KW, Nishigaki K, et al: Clinicopathological and immunological characteristics of six cats with granular lymphocyte tumors. *Comp Immunol Microbiol Infect Dis* 21:27–42, 1998.

42. Darbes J, Majzoub M, Breuer W, et al: Large granular lymphocyte leukemia/lymphoma in six cats. *Vet Pathol* 35:370–379, 1998.

43. McEntee MF, Horton S, Blue J, et al: Granulated round cell tumor of cats. *Vet Pathol* 30:195–203, 1993.

44. Krick E, Little L, Patel R, et al: Description of clinical and pathologic findings, treatment and outcome of feline large granular lymphoma (1996-2004). *Vet Comp Oncol* 6:102–110, 2008.

45. Wellman ML, Hammer AS, DiBartola SP, et al: Lymphoma involving large granular lymphocytes in cats: 11 cases (1982-1991). *J Am Vet Med Assoc* 201:1265–1269, 1992.

46. Benitah N, de Lorimier LP, Gaspar M, et al: Chlorambucil-induced myoclonus in a cat with lymphoma. *J Am Anim Hosp Assoc* 39:283–287, 2003.

47. Baez JL, Michel KE, Sorenmo K, et al: A prospective investigation of the prevalence and prognostic significance of weight loss and changes in body condition in feline cancer patients. *J Feline Med Surg* 9:411–417, 2007.

48. Krick EL, Moore RH, Cohen RB, et al: Prognostic significance of weight changes during treatment of feline lymphoma. *J Feline Med Surg* 13:976–983, 2011.

49. Hadden AG, Cotter SM, Rand W, et al: Efficacy and toxicosis of VELCAP-C treatment of lymphoma in cats. *J Vet Intern Med* 22:153–157, 2008.

50. Malik R, Gabor LJ, Foster SF, et al: Therapy for Australian cats with lymphosarcoma. *Aust Vet J* 79:808–817, 2001.

51. Milner RJ, Peyton J, Cooke K, et al: Response rates and survival times for cats with lymphoma treated with the University of Wisconsin-Madison chemotherapy protocol: 38 cases (1996-2003). *J Am Vet Med Assoc* 227:1118–1122, 2005.

52. Tamamoto T, Ohno K, Takahashi M, et al: Serum amyloid A as a prognostic marker in cats with various diseases. *J Vet Diagn Invest* 25:428–432, 2013.

53. Correa SS, Mauldin GN, Mauldin GE, et al: Serum alpha 1-acid glycoprotein concentration in cats with lymphoma. *J Am Anim Hosp Assoc* 37:153–158, 2001.

54. Selting KA, Ogilvie GK, Lana SE, et al: Serum alpha 1-acid glycoprotein concentrations in healthy and tumor-bearing cats. *J Vet Intern Med* 14:503–506, 2000.

55. Oberthaler KT, Mauldin E, McManus PM, et al: Rescue therapy with doxorubicin-based chemotherapy for relapsing or refractory lymphoma: a retrospective study of 23 cases. *J Feline Med Surg* 11:259–265, 2009.

56. Dutelle AL, Bulman-Fleming JC, Lewis CA, et al: Evaluation of lomustine as a rescue agent for cats with resistant lymphoma. *J Feline Med Surg* 10:694–700, 2012.

57. Parshley DL, LaRue SM, Kitchell B, et al: Abdominal irradiation as a rescue therapy for feline gastrointestinal lymphoma: a retrospective study of 11 cats (2001-2008). *J Feline Med Surg* 13:63–68, 2011.

58. Cotter SM: Treatment of lymphoma and leukemia with cyclophosphamide, vincristine, and prednisone: II. Treatment of cats. *J Am Anim Hosp Assoc* 19:166–171, 1983.

59. LeBlanc AK, Cox SK, Kirk CA, et al: Effects of L-asparaginase on plasma amino acid profiles and tumor burden in cats with lymphoma. *J Vet Intern Med* 21:760–763, 2007.

Electrochemotherapy in Feline Oncology

Enrico P. Spugnini

Electrochemotherapy (ECT) is a local, high-efficiency treatment that combines chemotherapy agents with high voltage (in excess of 1000 V/cm), short (100 µs) square or biphasic electric pulses.[1] Electric pulses increase cellular permeability and improve the delivery of lipophobic chemotherapy agents (such as cisplatin and bleomycin) within the cytoplasm of cancer cells (Figure 58-1). This new anticancer strategy increases the local efficacy of these drugs, therefore decreasing the chemotherapy dosages needed and their side effects.[2,3] Electrochemotherapy, with high voltage direct current electric field (1300 V/cm) and a short duration (100 µs or 50 + 50 µs in case of biphasic pulses), significantly enhances the cytotoxicity of the lipophobic drug bleomycin, through single- and double-strain DNA breaks.[4,5] Preclinical and clinical studies have demonstrated the high antitumor efficiency of ECT as well as the other advantages of this therapy, such as requirements of low drug concentration (secondary to membrane proteins rearrangement; Figure 58-2) and low systemic toxicity.[6-8]

FUNDAMENTALS OF ELECTROCHEMOTHERAPY

The application of short, intensive electric fields having appropriate waveforms leads to the creation of aqueous pathways (electropores) in the cell membrane, a phenomenon known as *electroporation*. This transient alteration of the membrane stability allows molecules, ions, and water to freely pass from the outside to the inside of the cytoplasm and vice versa.[9] The electroporation is reversible if the membrane returns to the normal state after the end of the field exposure, which occurs when the cell is able to pump the calcium ions outside the membrane and sequester them within the endoplasmic or the sarcoplasmic reticulum.[9,10] Otherwise, the pores cannot be resealed, the process becomes irreversible, and it leads to cell death through calcium-mediated activation of the apoptotic or necrotic pathways.[10]

The short field exposure must be considered as a complex stress applied on the cell assembly.[11] In order to allow a better understanding, electroporation can be conveniently divided into five phases: induction, expansion, stabilization, resealing, and memory effect.[12] These phases happen within microseconds, milliseconds, milliseconds, seconds, and hours, respectively. As a simple illustration, the cell can be seen as surrounded by a conducting medium and having a conducting cytoplasm with the two compartments separated by a lipid bilayer that is the cell membrane.

Over the years, electroporation has shown to be an effective and practical way to deliver drugs or other molecules, such as gene constructs, into cells. Factors that influence the efficacy of ECT are: (1) electrode size, shape, and composition; (2) electrical field strength; (3) pulse duration; (4) pulse shape; (5) total number of applied pulses; and (6) pulse frequency.[9,10,13] Currently available electroporators used in veterinary oncology are:

- Cliniporator (Igea, Italy): Used for the treatment of cancer in dogs
- Onkodisruptor (developed by the authors and produced by Biopulse, Italy): Used in dogs, cats, exotic animals, and horses
- ELECTRO vet S13 (Beta Tech, France): Used in horses
  Figure 58-3 shows examples of the square and biphasic pulses currently adopted in veterinary oncology.

ELECTROCHEMOTHERAPY FOR FELINE SOFT TISSUE SARCOMA

The first ECT study was devised as a treatment for cats with recurring soft tissue sarcoma after radiation therapy and surgical excision.[14] Patients were randomized to receive either bleomycin alone or combined with the implant of interleukin-1 secreting cells, followed by the delivery of eight single square pulses at the voltage of 1300 V/cm. A control group, consisting of untreated animals whose owners declined further treatments, was included as well. Objective responses were limited to just one partial remission, which could be a consequence of the previous treatments that could have elicited chemoresistance or of massive fibrosis secondary to the treatment at the tumor site that prevented a correct evaluation of tumor response.[15] After this pilot study, two phase I/II studies were conducted in companion animals to assess the efficacy of ECT as first-line treatment in pets with inoperable carcinomas and sarcomas, including several feline soft tissue sarcomas. In the first study, pets were treated with intralesional cisplatin coupled with square electric pulses, whereas in the second one, tumors were treated using trains of biphasic pulses associated with intralesional bleomycin; the second technique allowed shorter treatment times, thus reducing patient morbidity while maintaining efficacy.[16,17] The overall

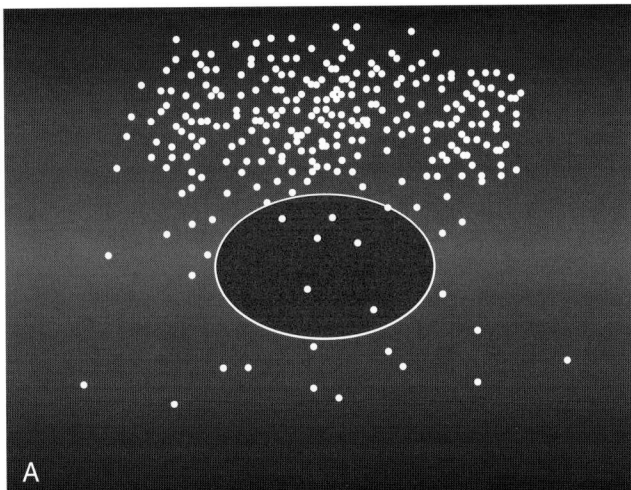

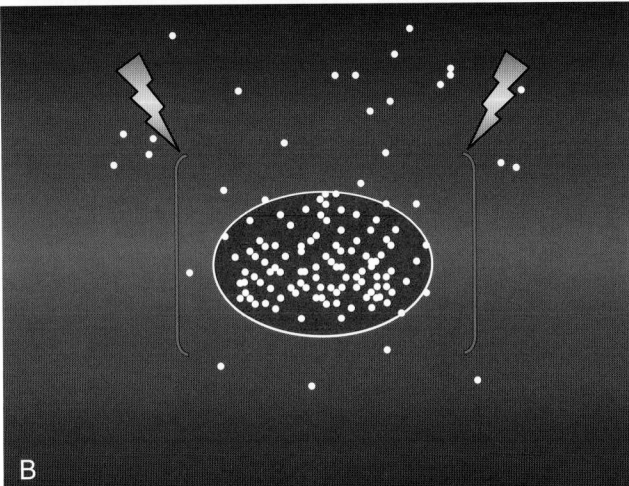

Figure 58-1: A schematic representation of the different uptakes of lipophobic chemotherapy molecules *(white dots)* by tumor cells in absence of electroporation **(A)** and following the application of permeabilizing pulses **(B).** (Modified from Spugnini EP, Citro G, D'Avino A, et al: Potential role of electrochemotherapy for the treatment of soft tissue sarcoma: first insights from preclinical studies in animals. *Int J Biochem Cell Biol* 40:159, 2008.)

response rate in both investigations was almost 80%. These studies pointed out the requirement of dedicated electrodes for the therapy of large solid tumors and the obstacle represented by the connective tissue to a smooth permeabilization, particularly in mesenchymal tumors.[17] This latter factor may be the explanation (i.e., massive fibrosis mimicking tumor growth) for the poor results in a previous study and suggest that using this modality for postsurgical recurrences may not be as effective as using ECT as a first-line therapy. After this preliminary phase, several studies have been performed to develop specific ECT protocols in cats with soft tissue sarcomas aimed at overcoming tumor electric impedance. The easiest strategy has been to remove the tumor mass and to follow immediately with adjuvant ECT.

ADJUVANT ELECTROCHEMOTHERAPY FOR THE TREATMENT OF SOFT TISSUE SARCOMAS

A large study recruited 72 cats with injection-site sarcomas to evaluate and compare the efficacy of intraoperative versus postoperative ECT versus surgery alone.[18] Cats were assigned to two different ECT cohorts on the basis of tumor behavior: (1) cats with bulky (greater than 5 cm diameter) or rapidly growing sarcomas were assigned to the intraoperative ECT cohort, where ECT was performed immediately after tumor removal, whereas (2) cats with smaller (less than 5 cm diameter) or slowly growing sarcomas were treated 2 weeks postoperatively.[18] Electroporation was performed using eight biphasic pulses lasting 50 + 50 μs with 800 V/cm (for intraoperative ECT) or 1300 V/cm voltage (in case of postoperative ECT) and 1 Hz frequency. Treatment was delivered using needle array or caliper electrodes; for the latter, adherence was maximized using an electroconductive gel (Figure 58-4). To increase the probability of homogeneous distribution of bleomycin following multiple chemotherapy injections in the tumor bed, the cats were pretreated with 300

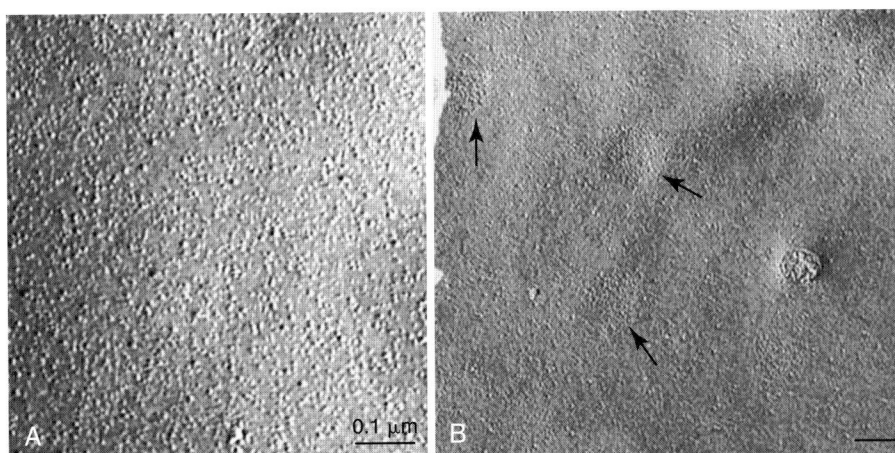

Figure 58-2: Ultrastructural modifications induced by electroporation in M14 amelanotic melanoma murine xenografts. **A,** Untreated tumor. **B,** Tumor after electroporation. Note the clustering of transmembrane proteins *(arrows)*. (Modified from Spugnini EP, Arancia G, Porrello A, et al: Ultrastructural modifications of cell membranes induced by "electroporation" on melanoma xenografts. *Microsc Res Tech* 70:1041, 2007.)

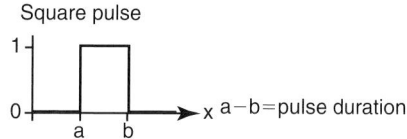

Square pulse

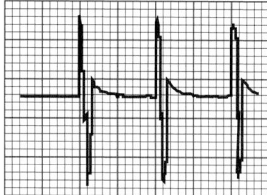

Biphasic pulses delivered as a train of waveforms

Figure 58-3: A schematic representation of square *(top)* and biphasic pulses *(bottom)* currently used in veterinary oncology as part of electrochemotherapy protocols.

International Units of hyaluronidase 5 minutes before the local chemotherapy to dissolve remaining connective tissue after tumor removal. A second ECT session was performed 1 week later in both treatment groups. Median time to recurrence was 12 and 19 months for the two ECT cohorts, whereas the control group recurred within a median of 4 months, as has been reported previously.[19] This study identified two prognostic factors for cats treated with ECT: (1) previous treatments and (2) tumor size. More specifically, for the macroscopic disease phase, cats with treatment fields smaller than 25 cm[2] had a longer remission time than cats with tumor beds greater than 25 cm[2] (median 16 and 5 months, respectively). Although the number of pretreated patients was too low to reach statistical significance, in the microscopic (postoperative) disease phase, cats that had no previous treatment fared much better than pretreated patients (median remissions of 33 and 5 months, respectively). Finally, cats in the microscopic ECT cohort with tumor fields smaller than 10 cm[2] had longer remissions (46 months) than those having larger areas (10 months). The side effects of adjuvant ECT were confined to local inflammation and occasional wound dehiscence in three cats.

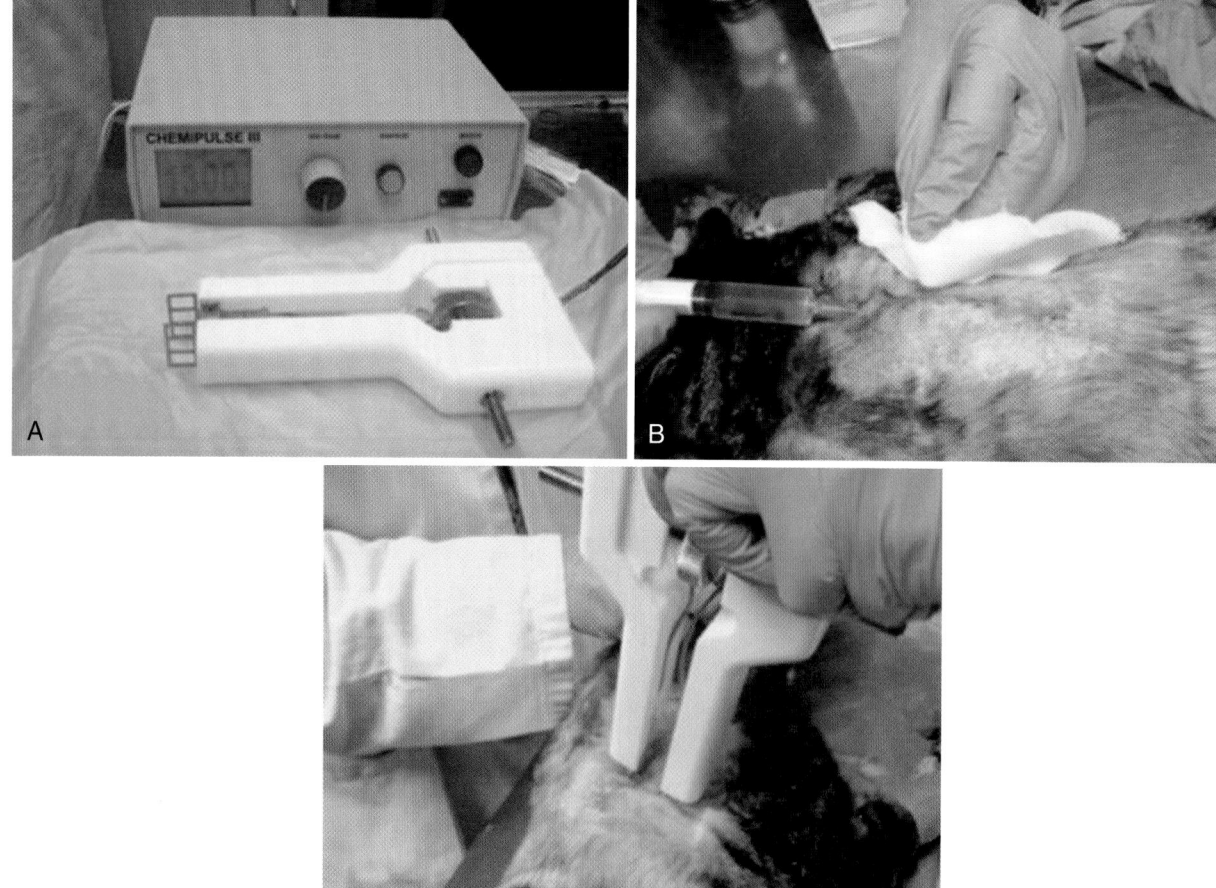

Figure 58-4: A session of postoperative electrochemotherapy in a cat after the removal of a soft tissue sarcoma. **A,** A second generation electroporator with autoclavable caliper electrodes. **B,** The local injection of chemotherapy agent in the tumor bed. **C,** The application of permeabilizing pulses with caliper electrodes.

Electrochemotherapy may not be suitable for treatment of patients that have received previous radiotherapy at the treatment site. Radiation recall is a cancer treatment complication involving redness, resembling severe sunburn, that can occur within a previously radiated area following the administration of several chemotherapy agents, including doxorubicin, bleomycin, or cisplatin.[20] One cat treated with surgery and ECT with cisplatin following full-course adjuvant radiation therapy experienced a severe radiation recall.[20] The systemic use of cisplatin is contraindicated in cats due to acute fatal pulmonary toxicity; however, a locally injected cisplatin-based ECT protocol was used to treat 64 cats with sarcomas, matched against a control group of 14 cats treated with surgery alone.[21] This report showed a high control rate (70%) in the treatment group without systemic toxicities. The disease control was greater in the cats receiving ECT (disease-free interval of 666 days versus 180 in the control group), and there were no systemic toxicities observed. Local inflammation was seen in three cats and skin burns (1 cm long and 1 mm wide) secondary to electrode application were seen in seven cats. The lack of systemic side effects in cats treated with local injection of cisplatin (an otherwise lethal drug in cats) was presumably due to the rapid shifting of the drug within the target cells after ECT and implies that a broader use of this technique may be possible in the future, increasing the choices of drugs available for ECT. There has been a low incidence of distant metastases (less than 2%) reported in patients treated with this modality, which is lower than that reported for cats treated with surgery alone.[22] The reasons for this are speculative but include possible immune modulation following tumor apoptotic death.[18,21,23]

FELINE LYMPHOMA

Lymphoma is a systemic disease, and therefore localized therapy usually only has a palliative role. Bleomycin-based ECT has been investigated for the local control of lymphoma. Three cats (one with retrobulbar, one with cervical, and one with nasal lymphoma) achieved a complete remission for 635, 180, and 730 days, respectively.[24] Two of these cats developed lymphoma at different sites, and one had local recurrence that was unresponsive to further ECT treatment. Overall, the treatment was well tolerated, and side effects were limited to transient local inflammation and discomfort (especially for sensitive locations, such as the retrobulbar space). The two cats that had this mild complication recovered within 48 hours without the need for any therapy. These results imply ECT may have a palliative role for treatment of advanced localized lymphoma.

FELINE HEAD AND NECK CARCINOMA

Feline actinic squamous cell carcinoma (SCC) of the nasal planum is very common in regions with high levels of solar radiation and where cats are allowed outside during daylight hours. There is often a long period between tumor induction (following solar dermatitis) and tumor progression, and the local control of these neoplasms poses a significant challenge in veterinary medicine as a consequence of the advanced stage of this disease by the time of patient referral. Bleomycin ECT with biphasic pulses has been used to treat SCC of the nasal planum in cats.[25] The treatment resulted in a total response rate (complete and partial responses) of 100% with 77% complete responders. Side effects were limited to transient erythema, swelling, and focal inflammation. More recently, ECT has been described for the treatment of advanced head and neck carcinoma in cats (not including cats with oral SCC). In this report, a cohort of cats treated with intravenous (IV) bleomycin followed by electroporation was matched against a cohort of cats treated with IV bleomycin alone. Electrochemotherapy resulted in increased local control with 90% complete responders, whereas the controls had a response rate of 30%. Median time to recurrence in the ECT group was 60 weeks versus 2 weeks in the control group; this difference was statistically significant.[26] A cat with advanced nasal SCC treated with ECT is shown in Figure 58-5.

ELECTROCHEMOTHERAPY IN UNCOMMON FELINE TUMORS

The first case of an unusual tumor treated with ECT was a thoracic hemangiopericytoma in a cat that was treated with adjuvant bleomycin-based electroporation, obtaining local control in excess of 2 years.[27] A cat with appendicular ganglioneuroblastoma was also treated with ECT using local application of bleomycin as a first choice drug and then ECT with cisplatin as a rescue, resulting in prolonged tumor control and limb preservation.[28] Finally, a cat with a bilateral facial rhabdomyosarcoma was treated with cisplatin-based adjuvant ECT, achieving tumor control in excess of 1 year.[29]

CURRENTLY ADOPTED ELECTROCHEMOTHERAPY PROTOCOLS IN FELINE ONCOLOGY

Current protocols involve premedication with sedatives, such as butorphanol, medetomidine, and ketamine, as per manufacturers' directions. After sedation, the level of anesthesia is increased by using IV drugs such as propofol or thiopental. For intraoperative ECT, the cat is anesthetized with isoflurane. When the desired level of sedation and analgesia is reached, a systemic or intralesional dose of anticancer agent is delivered (after local administration of hyaluronidase). The decision between the local or systemic administration of the anticancer drug is based on the systemic toxicities and the degree of tumor infiltration in the deeper tissue layers. For local administration, the drug dose is calculated as mg/cm², whereas for systemic administration, the drug dose is

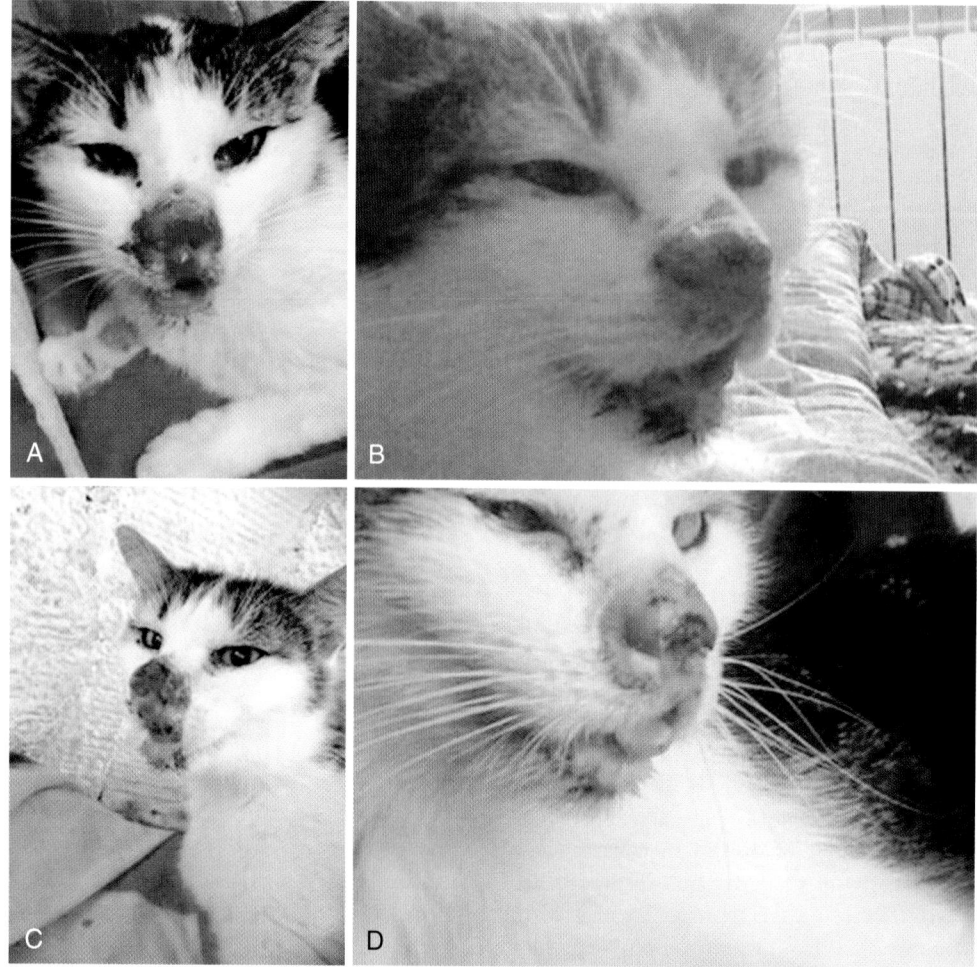

Figure 58-5: Electrochemotherapy (ECT) for the treatment of advanced actinic squamous cell carcinoma in a cat. **A,** Patient at presentation. **B,** Patient after the first session of ECT. Note the local necrosis and inflammation. **C,** Patient after second session of ECT; a large eschar at the tumor site causes stertorous respiration. **D,** Patient after the eschar has dislodged; most of the nasal planum appears in an advanced stage of healing.

calculated in mg/m². Five minutes after the chemotherapy is administered, permeabilizing pulses are delivered using electrodes inserted into or adhered to the surface of the tumor or the exposed tumor bed. Adherence of the external electrodes to the lesion is maximized using an electroconductive gel. The two currently adopted waveforms are square and biphasic, with biphasic being the more frequently used. In the author's standard protocol, a train of eight biphasic pulses lasting 50 + 50 μs each, with 1 μs interpulse intervals, are delivered in bursts of 1300 V/cm (800 V/cm for intraoperative ECT), 1 Hz frequency, by means of caliper or needle array electrodes. The treatment is repeated after 1 or 2 weeks for a total of two times in case of adjuvant ECT, or until a complete response is reached or tumor progression is documented, for measurable tumors treated as first line with ECT.

SUMMARY

Electrochemotherapy is a novel anticancer therapy that is gaining popularity due to its consistent efficacy, ease of administration, minimal toxicity, and low cost. Electrochemotherapy may be particularly applicable in the palliative and compassionate treatment of tumors occurring in colony cats due to the financial constraint of the associations that take care of them. For localized (nonmetastatic) solid tumors in privately owned cats, although surgery remains the cornerstone of treatment, ECT is becoming more common as a first adjuvant option due to the limited number of sessions that are required, without the need for overnight hospitalization. Ongoing and future studies will help determine the usefulness of ECT in treatment of the more aggressive forms of feline cancer.

References

1. Spugnini EP, Citro G, D'Avino A, et al: Potential role of electrochemotherapy for the treatment of soft tissue sarcoma: first insights from preclinical studies in animals. *Int J Biochem Cell Biol* 40:159–163, 2008.

2. Shankayi Z, Firoozabadi SM: Antitumor efficiency of electrochemotherapy by high and low frequencies and repetitive therapy in the treatment of invasive ductal carcinoma in BALB/c mice. *Cell J* 14:110–115, 2012.

3. Spugnini EP, Fanciulli M, Citro G, et al: Preclinical models in electrochemotherapy: the role of veterinary patients. *Future Oncol* 8:829–837, 2012.

4. Tounekti O, Pron G, Belehradek J, Jr, et al: Bleomycin, an apoptosis-mimetic drug that induces two types of cell death depending on the number of molecules internalized. *Cancer Res* 53:5462–5469, 1993.

5. Pron G, Mahrour N, Orlowski S, et al: Internalisation of the bleomycin molecules responsible for bleomycin toxicity: a receptor-mediated endocytosis mechanism. *Biochem Pharmacol* 57:45–56, 1999.

6. Tounekti O, Kenani A, Foray N, et al: The ratio of single- to double-strand DNA breaks and their absolute values determine cell death pathway. *Br J Cancer* 84:1272–1279, 2001.

7. Sersa G, Miklavcic D, Cemazar M, et al: Electrochemotherapy in treatment of tumours. *Eur J Surg Oncol* 34:232–240, 2008.

8. Spugnini EP, Arancia G, Porrello A, et al: Ultrastructural modifications of cell membranes induced by "electroporation" on melanoma xenografts. *Microsc Res Tech* 70:1041–1050, 2007.

9. Dotsinky I, Mudrov N, Mudrov T: Technical aspects of the electrochemotherapy. In Spugnini EP, Baldi A, editors: *Electroporation in laboratory and clinical investigations*, ed 1, New York, 2012, Nova Science, p 45.

10. Gissel H, Raphael C, Gehl J: Electroporation and cellular physiology. In Kee SJ, Gehl J, Lee EW, editors: *Clinical aspects of electroporation*, ed 1, New York, 2011, Springer, p 9.

11. Vernhes MC, Cabanes PA, Teissie J: Chinese hamster ovary cells sensitivity to localized electrical stresses. *Bioelectrochem Bioenerg* 48:17–25, 1999.

12. Teissie J, Golzio M, Rols MP: Mechanisms of cell membrane electropermeabilization: a minireview of our present (lack of?) knowledge. *Biochim Biophys Acta* 1724(3):270–280, 2005.

13. Porrello A, Giansanti A: Mathematical-physical modeling and biomedical optimization of cell electropermeabilization: an overview. In Spugnini EP, Baldi A, editors: *Electroporation in laboratory and clinical investigations*, ed 1, New York, 2012, Nova Science, p 1.

14. Mir LM, Devauchelle P, Quintin-Colonna F, et al: First clinical trial of cat soft-tissue sarcomas treatment by electrochemotherapy. *Br J Cancer* 76:1617–1622, 1997.

15. Mocellin S, Rossi CR, Brandes A, et al: Adult soft tissue sarcomas: conventional therapies and molecularly targeted approaches. *Cancer Treat Rev* 32:9–27, 2006.

16. Tozon N, Sersa G, Cemazar M: Electrochemotherapy: potentiation of local antitumour effectiveness of cisplatin in dogs and cats. *Anticancer Res* 21:2483–2488, 2001.

17. Spugnini EP, Porrello A: Potentiation of chemotherapy in companion animals with spontaneous large neoplasms by application of biphasic electric pulses. *J Exp Clin Cancer Res* 22:571–580, 2003.

18. Spugnini EP, Baldi A, Vincenzi B, et al: Intraoperative versus postoperative electrochemotherapy in high grade soft tissue sarcomas: a preliminary study in a spontaneous feline model. *Cancer Chemother Pharmacol* 59:375–381, 2007.

19. Hershey AE, Sorenmo KU, Hendrick MJ, et al: Prognosis for presumed feline vaccine-associated sarcoma after excision: 61 cases (1986-1996). *J Am Vet Med Assoc* 216:58–61, 2000.

20. Spugnini EP, Dotsinsky I, Mudrov N, et al: Electrochemotherapy-induced radiation recall in a cat. *In Vivo* 22:751–753, 2008.

21. Spugnini EP, Renaud SM, Buglioni S, et al: Electrochemotherapy with cisplatin enhances local control after surgical ablation of fibrosarcoma in cats: an approach to improve the therapeutic index of highly toxic chemotherapy drugs. *J Transl Med* 9:152, 2011.

22. Romanelli G, Marconato L, Olivero D, et al: Analysis of prognostic factors associated with injection-site sarcomas in cats: 57 cases (2001-2007). *J Am Vet Med Assoc* 232:1193–1199, 2008.

23. Spugnini EP, Baldi F, Mellone P, et al: Patterns of tumor response in canine and feline cancer patients treated with electrochemotherapy: preclinical data for the standardization of this treatment in pets and humans. *J Transl Med* 5:48, 2007.

24. Spugnini EP, Citro G, Mellone P, et al: Electrochemotherapy for localized lymphoma: a preliminary study in companion animals. *J Exp Clin Cancer Res* 26:343–346, 2007.

25. Spugnini EP, Vincenzi B, Citro G, et al: Electrochemotherapy for the treatment of squamous cell carcinoma in cats: a preliminary report. *Vet J* 179:117–120, 2009.

26. Spugnini EP: Electroporation enhances bleomycin efficacy in cats with advanced head and neck carcinoma. In *Proceedings of the Second World Veterinary Cancer Congress*, Paris, 2012, p 34.

27. Baldi A, Spugnini EP: Thoracic haemangiopericytoma in a cat. *Vet Rec* 159:598–600, 2006.

28. Spugnini EP, Citro G, Dotsinsky I, et al: Ganglioneuroblastoma in a cat: a rare neoplasm treated with electrochemotherapy. *Vet J* 178:291–293, 2008.

29. Spugnini EP, Filipponi M, Romani L, et al: Electrochemotherapy treatment for bilateral pleomorphic rhabdomyosarcoma in a cat. *J Small Anim Pract* 51:330–332, 2010.

Feline Mammary Carcinoma

Beth Overley-Adamson and Jennifer Baez

EPIDEMIOLOGY AND RISK FACTORS

Epidemiology

After skin and hematopoietic tumors, mammary tumors are the third most common tumor type in female domestic cats and account for 17% of feline tumors.[1-3] The reported incidence is 25.4 per 100,000 female cats per year, although geographical variation is likely because of different neutering and care practices.[1,4,5] Mammary tumors are most common in middle-aged to older female cats, with a mean age at diagnosis of 10 to 12 years.[1,6,7] Breed has been variably considered as a risk factor for cats. Siamese and domestic shorthair cats are reported to be at increased risk, and Siamese are reported to be significantly younger than other breeds when diagnosed with mammary tumors.[3,8,9]

Risk Factors

The most significant risk factor is exposure to endogenous female hormones, as in other species. Female cats are at significantly increased risk of mammary tumors, and sexually intact cats have a sevenfold higher risk than spayed cats.[10-12] Similar to what has been found in dogs, prolonged exposure to ovarian hormones increases risk of mammary tumor development, and ovariohysterectomy (OVH) performed during the first year of a cat's life significantly reduces its risk. In one study, cats spayed before 6 months of age had 9% risk, and those spayed between 6 and 12 months of age had 14% risk of mammary carcinoma development compared with intact cats.[10] Put differently, risk reductions of 91% and 86% were noted in cats that underwent OVH before 6 months and between 6 and 12 months of age, respectively. Minimal to no risk reduction was observed for cats spayed after 1 year of age.

Prolonged use of exogenous hormones (e.g., megestrol acetate, medroxyprogesterone acetate) to prevent pregnancy, treat skin diseases, or control aggression has also been implicated in mammary tumor development in cats. Studies have shown that progestins induce changes in mammary gland tissues, with fibroepithelial hyperplasia as the most common glandular change associated with short-term use of these drugs.[13,14] In one study, cats treated with progestins had a relative risk of mammary tumor development of 3.4 compared with those that did not receive progestin treatment.[12]

Also, while most mammary tumors occur in female cats, approximately 3% occur in male cats, many of whom have a history of exposure to exogenous progestins.[3,13,15] In one study, 36% (eight of 22) male cats had a history of progestin administration.[15]

RELEVANT ANATOMY

Queens have four pairs of mammary glands that include two pairs of thoracic glands and two pairs of abdominal glands.[16] Rarely, additional mammary glands may occur in the inguinal region.[17] Reports indicate that the thoracic glands drain cranially to the axillary lymph nodes, while the abdominal glands drain caudally to the superficial inguinal lymph nodes.[17] However, it is also known that the central glands (the second thoracic and first abdominal glands) occasionally drain bidirectionally, and the thoracic and first pair of abdominal glands may also drain to the cranial sternal lymph node.[17,18] These drainage patterns should be considered both for staging and treatment planning (Figure 59-1).

TUMOR BIOLOGY

Histopathological Features

Eighty-five to 95% of feline mammary tumors are malignant; however, benign lesions do occur.[19] Hyperplastic and dysplastic lesions include fibroepithelial hyperplasia, lobular hyperplasia, and mammary duct ectasia.[19,20] Most common in the cat is a hormone-associated condition called fibroepithelial hyperplasia (also called fibroadenomatous change and hypertrophy), which can be induced by exogenous progestin administration in both female and male cats, or by luteal progesterone in pregnant cats.[21] In contrast to malignant lesions of the mammary gland, benign lesions—such as fibroepithelial hyperplasia—usually appear in younger, intact cats. Unlike benign and malignant tumors, however, fibroepithelial hyperplasia usually regresses at the end of pregnancy or when progestin use ends.[19,20] Other benign lesions of the feline mammary gland include adenoma, ductal adenoma, fibroadenoma, and intraductal papillary adenoma.[19]

Most malignant feline mammary lesions are simple epithelial tumors, but sarcomas and other nonepithelial tumor types, such as mast cell tumors or lymphoma, arise on

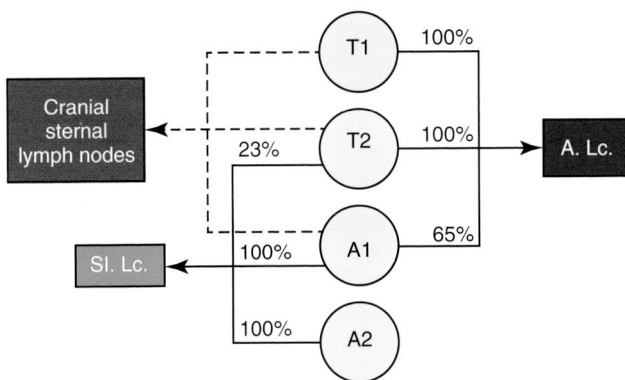

Figure 59-1: Drainage Patterns of Mammary Gland Lymphatics in Cats. *A. Lc.*, Axillary lymph center; *Sl. Lc.*, superficial inguinal lymph center. (From Raharison F, Sautet J: Lymph drainage of the mammary glands in female cats. *J Morphol* 267:292-299, 2006.) T, thoracic; A, abdominal

occasion.[19,22,23] Most feline mammary carcinomas (FMCs) develop from the luminal epithelium of the ducts and alveoli.[19] Mixed tumors involving both luminal and myoepithelial cells are rare.[24,25] Feline mammary carcinomas can be of tubulopapillary, solid, cribriform, or anaplastic types.[19,24,25] Less common forms include lipid-rich carcinoma, mucinous carcinoma, spindle cell carcinoma, and carcinoma with squamous differentiation.[16,19,24,25] Inflammatory mammary carcinoma has been reported but appears much less frequently than in the dog.[26]

Hormones

Risk of mammary tumor development in cats appears to be determined mostly by exposure to female sex hormones, but the precise role these hormones play in tumorigenesis is unknown.[27] Across mammalian species, female hormones are necessary for mammary gland development, and it is known that these hormones can act as mitogens that induce proliferation of the ductal epithelium.[28,29] Reports from other species have shown that estrogen and its metabolites may have direct genotoxic effects on mammary tissue, and that progesterone increases mammary gland production of growth hormone and growth hormone receptors that have been implicated in mammary tumorigenesis.[28-31] It is likely that both hormonal exposure and growth factor pathways play a role in feline mammary tumor development as in other species, but other factors are likely to contribute as well.

Comparative Data

Studies have shown that hormone receptor expression is less frequent in FMCs in contrast to canine or human breast cancers.[32-35] In human breast cancers, estrogen receptors (ERs) and progesterone receptors (PRs) are expressed in about 70% to 80% of cases, whereas 15% to 20% are negative for both ER and PR.[36] In contrast, few FMCs express ERs (7% to 22%) and PRs (approximately 33%).[32-34,37] Therefore, comparative studies have focused on the subset of human

breast cancers that are hormone-negative. These human hormone-negative tumors are often additionally negative for human epidermal growth factor receptor 2 (HER2) expression. These tumors comprise a particularly aggressive subset of human breast cancers known as triple negative breast cancer (TNBC).[38] In addition to hormone receptor evaluation, comparative studies have evaluated HER2 expression in FMCs, and, although results have been highly variable[39] among studies, the feline studies that have used the Food and Drug Administration-approved human assay HercepTest have reported HER2 expression rates similar to those in humans (16% to 17%).[38,40] One of these studies reported that 58% of the assessed FMCs were triple negative cancers similar to human TNBC; therefore, FMCs may be a valuable comparative model to evaluate treatment therapies for an aggressive human breast cancer subtype that currently lacks effective targeted therapies.[38]

Another study tested FMCs for mammalian target of rapamycin (mTOR) overexpression.[41] Mammalian target of rapamycin overexpression in human hormone-independent breast cancers, such as TNBC, forms the basis for the development of the mTOR inhibitor rapamycin. The feline study evaluated 58 FMCs and six FMC cell lines by Western blot analysis.[41] Results showed that 53% of the feline tumors were triple negative (ER, PR, and HER2 negative), and those that expressed mTOR were more likely to be triple negative samples, which further supports the possibility of feline mammary carcinoma as a useful comparative model for future evaluation of targeted treatments.

Finally, it is well known that BRCA1 and BRCA2 mutations can increase the risk of breast cancer in women. BRCA1 and BRCA2 genes produce tumor suppressor proteins involved with DNA repair. Dysfunctional BRCA1 and BRCA2 genes increase the risk of breast and ovarian cancers and account for 5% to 10% of breast cancers in humans.[42] One study tested FMCs for BRCA1 and BRCA2 mutations but found no mutations or allelic losses in these genes.[38] However, the sample size may have been too small.[38] Also, BRCA1 and BRCA2 dysfunction could arise through other pathways, such as mutations in different parts of the gene or epigenetic gene silencing.[38] More testing will need to be done to clarify the role of BRCA1 and BRCA2 in feline tumors.

CLINICAL DATA

History and Presentation

Patient history often includes chronic progestin use, intact reproductive status, or late ovariectomy. Tumors generally arise as round, discrete masses within the mammary glands, and 60% of cats have more than one tumor at presentation.[8] The associated nipples may be swollen and may exude clear or tan fluid. Larger tumors may appear inflamed or ulcerated secondary to trauma or from tumor necrosis, although true inflammatory mammary carcinomas are rare in cats.[26] Patients may also present with swelling, edema, and discomfort secondary to tumor thrombi lodged in the femoral arteries and from decreased venous return from the femoral veins.[43] Unfortunately, physical examination findings are not specific for benign or malignant disease; however, nipple association, tumor ulceration, or the presence of enlarged lymph nodes—particularly in an older patient—would lead one to suspect malignancy.

Diagnosis and Staging

Diagnosis can be obtained by cytology or biopsy. Because chain mastectomy is usually the recommended surgery for FMCs, malignancy should be established before definitive treatment by incisional biopsy or cytology.[43] Staging is imperative for all patients with malignant tumors and most particularly for those with larger tumors (greater than 2 to 3 cm in diameter) or high-grade tumors. The most common sites of metastasis include the regional lymph nodes (axillary, inguinal), lungs, pleura, and liver.[44] Staging diagnostics should include a thorough physical examination, complete blood count, serum biochemistries, urinalysis, cytological and/or histological assessment of all masses, lymph node evaluation via palpation and cytology or biopsy, and either three-view thoracic radiographs or thoracic computed tomography (CT) scan. The CT scan is the preferred thoracic staging modality for patients that will undergo extensive surgical treatment because it is a more sensitive test. An abdominal ultrasound is also recommended to assess general health and to check for hepatic, renal, splenic, and nodal metastasis.

Feline mammary carcinomas are categorized with a four-stage system based on tumor size, regional lymph node metastasis, and systemic metastasis.[19,45] Stage I tumors are less than 2 cm in diameter and have no evidence of tumor spread. Stage II tumors are larger (2 to 3 cm in diameter) and have no evidence of tumor spread. Stage III tumors are tumors with positive regional lymph nodes or tumors of increased size (greater than 3 cm in diameter) regardless of lymph node status. Stage IV tumors have distant metastatic disease and can be of any size or lymph node state (Table 59-1).

PROGNOSTIC FACTORS

Clinical Factors

Prognosis is guarded for most cats, and death is usually caused by clinical effects secondary to progression of local disease (disease within the mammary chain) or metastatic spread to vital organs. On average, the time from tumor diagnosis until death is about 10 to 12 months,[46] but the prognostic factors outlined earlier can adjust outcome expectations for individual cases.

Tumor size has been the most consistent prognostic factor among studies. Patients with stage I FMCs (those with less than 8 cm³ in volume or 2 cm in diameter and no evidence of metastasis) have reported median survival times (MSTs) greater than 2 years with surgery alone.[46,47] Cats with FMCs greater than 27 cm³ in volume or 3 cm in diameter have reported MSTs of 4 to 12 months.[47-49] Median survival times for cats with 2- to 3-cm diameter tumors are more variable among studies, but one larger study reported the MST as 24 months (Table 59-2).[47-49]

Lymph node status also affects prognosis, and FMCs with positive regional lymph nodes have significantly worse outcomes.[47-50] In one study of 92 cats with FMC, all those with lymph node metastasis (stage III) died within 9 months of diagnosis (Figure 59-2).[51]

Clinical stage at presentation has also been shown to be prognostic, with median survival times for cats with stage I, II, III, and IV disease reported to be 29, 12.5, 9, and 1 month(s), respectively (see Table 59-2).[9]

Table 59-1 Staging of Feline Mammary Cancers

Stage	Tumor Size	Lymph Node Status	Metastasis
Stage I	T1 <2 cm	N0	M0
Stage II	T2 2-3 cm	N0	M0
Stage III	T1 or T2	N1 (positive)	M0
	T3 >3 cm	N0 or N1	M0
Stage IV	Any	Any	M1

From McNeill CJ, Sorenmo KU, Shofer FS, et al: Evaluation of adjuvant doxorubicin-based chemotherapy for the treatment of feline mammary carcinoma, *J Vet Intern Med* 23:123-129, 2009.

Table 59-2 Prognostic Factors for Feline Mammary Tumors

Factor	Details
Tumor size	Diameter <3 cm—MST 21-24 months Diameter >3 cm—MST 4-12 months
Clinical stage	Stage I—MST 29 months Stage II—MST 12.5 months Stage III—MST 9 months Stage IV—MST 1 month
Surgical extent	Radical mastectomy reduces recurrence rate compared with conservative mastectomy or lumpectomy
Histopathological grade	Well-differentiated—100% survival at 1 year postsurgery Poorly differentiated—0% survival at 1 year postsurgery
Mitotic index	<2 mitotic figures per high-power field are associated with longer survival times

MST, median survival time.

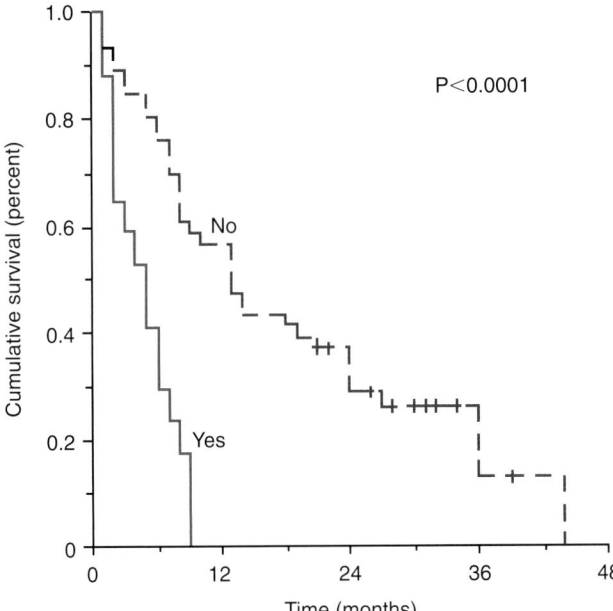

Figure 59-2: Kaplan-Meier Survival Curves According to Lymph Node Status. Queens with lymph node metastasis (positive nodes) on clinical presentation (*n* = 17, continuous line) showed shorter overall survival time compared with queens with negative nodes (*n* = 47, dashed line). (From Seixas, F, Palmeira, C, Pires, MA, et al: Grade is an independent prognostic factor for feline mammary carcinomas: a clinicopathologic and survival analysis. *Vet J.* 187:65-71, 2011.)

Histological Factors

A grading system similar to that used in dogs and humans has been applied to FMCs and has been shown to be prognostic both for survival and disease-free interval (DFI).[51-53] Tumor grading is based upon a system that scores for tubule formation, nuclear pleomorphism, and mitotic count. In one study, the death rate at 1 year postsurgery for cats with well-differentiated mammary carcinoma was 0%, whereas the rate was 100% at 1 year in patients with poorly differentiated tumors (see Table 59-2).[52] Another study correlated tumor grade with both DFI and overall survival.[51] In that study, the tumor-related death rate at 1 year was 0% for grade 1, 30% for grade 2, and 90% for grade 3 tumors. Progression-free survival rates at 1 year were 100% with grade 1 tumors, 50% with grade 2 tumors, and 6% with grade 3 tumors. Median overall survival for cats with grade 3 tumors was 6 months and 36 months for those with grade 1 tumors; grade correlated strongly with patient age (younger cats had more grade 1 tumors) and tumor size (larger tumors tended to be higher grade).[51] Lymphatic invasion, vascular invasion, lymph node metastasis, and mitotic index have all been shown to correlate with survival time.[51,52] Several other factors have been evaluated (Ki67, argyrophilic nucleolar organizer region, proliferating cell nuclear antigen, hormone receptors, HER2 overexpression, cyclooxygenase-2 expression, AKT expres-

sion), but these have yet to find utility in routine clinical practice.[54-64]

TREATMENT

Surgery

Surgery should be the primary treatment recommendation for FMCs without distant metastatic disease, and the recommended surgical procedure should be either a unilateral or staged bilateral chain mastectomy depending on the extent of disease.[45,47] There is a high rate of locoregional recurrence with more conservative treatment.[45] Studies have shown that chain mastectomy significantly improves disease-free survival and reduces the need for recurrent surgeries.[47] Although overall survival time has not been shown to be significantly improved with chain mastectomy, overall survival is considered the more subjective metric, because it varies based on the owner's perception of the patient's quality of life and on the owner's willingness to euthanize when the patient is suffering. Both for quality-of-life purposes and according to principles of cancer treatment, given the aggressive nature of this disease and the known lymphatic drainage pathways for FMC, the recommendation for a chain mastectomy makes sense.[64] Furthermore, for tumors that are fixed, portions of the body wall and the muscular fascia should be removed in *en bloc* resections.[65] Bilateral chain mastectomy is usually performed in two stages unless the surgeon believes there is adequate tissue to attempt a bilateral chain mastectomy all at once. With these larger surgeries, associated lymph nodes are also removed and should be separately evaluated histologically. Because lymph node involvement significantly changes the prognosis for these cats, efforts should be made to assess the draining lymph nodes via cytology or histopathology. Ultrasound guidance can also be used to identify lymph nodes, and lymph node mapping has been described in the cat.[66,67]

Systemic Treatment

The current literature supports the recommendation that small (less than 2 cm diameter), low-grade tumors with negative staging that are treated with adequate surgery need no adjunctive treatment for long-term survival.[45,47] However, standard-of-care treatment recommendations for FMCs have not yet been formulated.

Hormonal and targeted therapies that are currently used in human medicine are not commonly used in feline medicine and have not been well evaluated in feline patients, in part because the laboratory testing of FMCs for estrogen receptors, progesterone receptors, or HER2 overexpression is not routine. Also, because it has been recognized that many FMCs are negative for these molecular markers, it is unlikely that the use of these targeted therapies will become common in feline practice. Most treatment studies to date instead have focused on the use of traditional chemotherapeutics.

Doxorubicin has been the most studied chemotherapy agent for the treatment of FMC. In the macroscopic disease setting for stage III and IV FMCs, doxorubicin-based treatment resulted in objective tumor responses in about 50% of cases reported.[53,68,69] These studies have provided the rationale to test doxorubicin-based protocols in the postoperative setting as well, as it would be assumed that the response rate of tumors in the microscopic or adjuvant setting would be as good as or better than that of the macroscopic or gross tumor state. Table 59-3 summarizes prognostic factors, guidelines for systemic therapy based on these factors, and strength of supporting evidence.

Unfortunately, studies have yet to show clear benefit from adjunctive treatment. This may be because there is no benefit, but it is more likely that further evaluation is needed to make an accurate determination. Currently, there are no prospective, randomized treatment studies to guide recommendations. One study of 23 cats with stage III or less FMC showed a MST of 460 days with surgery and a protocol that used doxorubicin and meloxicam; however, no control group was used for comparison and so no conclusions can be drawn

about the benefits of one treatment versus the other.[70] Another study of 67 cats with stage III or less FMC reported an MST of 448 days; however, this study also lacked a control group.[71] A third report used a contemporaneous control population in a multi-institutional, retrospective study that included 73 cats with stage III or less FMC, and this study found no significant differences in survival between those treated with an adjuvant doxorubicin-based protocol and those that were not.[45] However, there was a subgroup of cats treated with chain mastectomy and adjuvant doxorubicin-based chemotherapy that survived significantly longer than those treated with chain mastectomy alone (1998 versus 414 days) (Table 59-4).[45] The conclusion reached was that not all FMC patients will benefit from chemotherapy treatment, but certain subsets might. To test this, prospective randomized trials are needed. Although these data can make treatment recommendations confusing at this time, it seems most appropriate to recommend chain mastectomy for local disease control and adjunctive doxorubicin-based treatment for larger tumors, histologically or clinically high-grade tumors, and those with positive lymph nodes.

Table 59-3	Prognostic Factors and Indications for Adjuvant Chemotherapy with Level of Supporting Evidence in Cats with Malignant Mammary Tumors				
Tumor Size	**Lymph Node Involvement**	**Histopathologic Parameters**	**Indication for Chemotherapy −(No) or +(Yes)**		**Evidence Level***
<2 cm/8 cm^3	Negative	Carcinoma	−		−1
			− +[†]		+3
2-3 cm/8-27 cm^3	Negative	Carcinoma	−		−3
			+[†]		+3
>3 cm/27 cm^3	Negative	Carcinoma	+		1, 2, 3
Any	Positive	Carcinoma	+		2, 3, 5

From Sorenmo KU, Worley DR, Goldschmidt MH: Tumors of the mammary gland. In *Withrow and MacEwen's small animal clinical oncology*, ed 5, St Louis, 2013, Elsevier/Saunders, pp 550.
*Evidence level 1: prospective randomized trial; level 2: prospective, nonrandomized trial; level 3: retrospective study; level 5: extrapolation from human breast cancer studies. Minus (supports chemotherapy), Plus (against chemotherapy).
[†]Vascular invasion and high grade were found to be independent negative prognostic factors in multivariate analysis.

Table 59-4	Analysis of Effect of Surgery vs Surgery Plus Chemotherapy on Survival Times for Feline Mammary Carcinoma						
Surgical Procedure	**SURGERY ALONE**			**SURGERY + ADJUVANT DOXORUBICIN-BASED CHEMOTHERAPY**			**P-Value**
	No. of Cats	**ST (Days)**	**95% CI**	**No. of Cats**	**ST (Days)**	**95% CI**	
Local	24	1406	454-NR	16	729	496-NR	0.47
Radical	13	414	203-NR	20	892	616-1998	0.16
Radical unilateral	10	414	266-NR	8	1998	NR	0.03
Radical bilateral	3	NR	67-NR	12	761	476-1751	0.90

From McNeill CJ, Sorenmo KU, Shofer FS, et al: Evaluation of adjuvant doxorubicin-based chemotherapy for the treatment of feline mammary carcinoma. *J Vet Intern Med* 23:123-129, 2009.
Results shown are median number of days with 95% confidence intervals (CI). *P* < 0.05 considered statistically significant.
NR, median survival time not reached (more than half the cats were censored at study end); *ST*, survival time.

References

1. Dorn CR, Taylor DO, Frye FL, et al: Survey of animal neoplasms in Alameda and Contra Costa Counties, California. I. Methodology and description of cases. *J Natl Cancer Inst* 40:295–305, 1968.
2. Dorn CR, Taylor DO, Schneider R, et al: Survey of animal neoplasms in Alameda and Contra Costa Counties, California. II. Cancer morbidity in dogs and cats from Alameda County. *J Natl Cancer Inst* 40:307–318, 1968.
3. Hayes HM, Jr, Milne KL, Mandell CP: Epidemiological features of feline mammary carcinoma. *Vet Rec* 108:476–479, 1981.
4. Vascellari M, Baioni E, Ru G, et al: Animal tumour registry of two provinces in northern Italy: incidence of spontaneous tumours in dogs and cats. *BMC Vet Res* 5:39, 2009.
5. Egenvall A, Bonnett BN, Haggstrom J, et al: Morbidity of insured Swedish cats during 1999-2006 by age, breed, sex, and diagnosis. *J Feline Med Surg* 12:948–959, 2010.
6. Johnston SD, Kustritz MVR, Olson PNS: Disorders of the mammary gland of the queen. In Johnston SD, Kustritz MVR, Olson PNS, editors: *Canine and feline theriogenology*, Philadelphia, 2001, Saunders, pp 474–485.
7. Kustritz MV: Determining the optimal age for gonadectomy of dogs and cats. *J Am Vet Med Assoc* 231:1665–1675, 2007.
8. Hayes AA, Mooney S: Feline mammary tumors. *Vet Clin North Am Small Anim Pract* 15:513–520, 1985.
9. Ito T, Kadosawa T, Mochizuki M, et al: Prognosis of malignant mammary tumor in 53 cats. *J Vet Med Sci* 58:723–726, 1996.
10. Overley B, Shofer FS, Goldschmidt MH, et al: Association between ovariohysterectomy and feline mammary carcinoma. *J Vet Intern Med* 19:560–563, 2005.
11. Misdorp W: Progestagens and mammary tumours in dogs and cats. *Acta Endocrinol (Copenh)* 125(Suppl 1):27–31, 1991.
12. Misdorp W, Romijn A, Hart AA: Feline mammary tumors: a case-control study of hormonal factors. *Anticancer Res* 11:1793–1797, 1991.
13. Weijer K, Head KW, Misdorp W, et al: Feline malignant mammary tumors. I. Morphology and biology: some comparisons with human and canine mammary carcinomas. *J Natl Cancer Inst* 49:1697–1704, 1972.
14. Loretti AP, Ilha MR, Ordas J, et al: Clinical, pathological and immunohistochemical study of feline mammary fibroepithelial hyperplasia following a single injection of depot medroxyprogesterone acetate. *J Feline Med Surg* 7:43–52, 2005.
15. Skorupski KA, Overley B, Shofer FS, et al: Clinical characteristics of mammary carcinoma in male cats. *J Vet Intern Med* 19:52–55, 2005.
16. Silver IA: The anatomy of the mammary gland of the dog and cat. *J Small Anim Pract* 7:689–696, 1966.
17. Raharison F, Sautet J: Lymph drainage of the mammary glands in female cats. *J Morphol* 267:292–299, 2006.
18. Raharison F, Sautet J: The topography of the lymph vessels of mammary glands in female cats. *Anat Histol Embryol* 36:442–452, 2007.
19. Hayden DW, Nielsen SW: Feline mammary tumours. *J Small Anim Pract* 12:687–698, 1971.
20. Misdorp W, Else R, Hellmen E, et al: *Histological classification of mammary tumors of the dog and the cat*, Washington, DC, 1999, American Registry of Pathology.
21. Hayden DW, Barnes DM, Johnson KH: Morphologic changes in the mammary gland of megestrol acetate-treated and untreated cats: a retrospective study. *Vet Pathol* 26:104–113, 1989.
22. Withrow SJ, Vail DM, Page R: *Withrow and MacEwen's small animal clinical oncology* (Kindle Location 31795). Elsevier Health Sciences 2013. Kindle Edition.
23. Zappulli V, Caliari D, Rasotto R, et al: Proposed classification of the feline "complex" mammary tumors as ductal and intraductal papillary mammary tumors. *Vet Pathol* 50:1070–1077, 2013.
24. Seixas F, Palmeira C, Pires MA, et al: Are complex carcinoma of the feline mammary gland and other invasive mammary carcinoma identical tumours? Comparison of clinicopathologic features, DNA ploidy and follow-up. *Res Vet Sci* 84:428–433, 2008.
25. Seixas F, Pires MA, Lopes CA: Complex carcinomas of the mammary gland in cats: pathological and immunohistochemical features. *Vet J* 176:210–215, 2008.
26. Perez-Alenza MD, Jimenez A, Nieto AI, et al: First description of feline inflammatory mammary carcinoma: clinicopathological and immunohistochemical characteristics of three cases. *Breast Cancer Res* 6:R300–R307, 2004.
27. Withrow SJ, Vail DM, Page R: *Withrow and MacEwen's small animal clinical oncology* (Kindle Location 31718). Elsevier Health Sciences 2013. Kindle Edition.
28. Russo J, Russo IH: The role of estrogen in the initiation of breast cancer. *J Steroid Biochem Mol Biol* 102:89–96, 2006.
29. Okoh V, Deoraj A, Roy D: Estrogen-induced reactive oxygen species-mediated signalings contribute to breast cancer. *Biochim Biophys Acta* 1815:115–133, 2011.
30. Mol JA, Lantinga-van Leeuwen IS, van Garderen E, et al: Mammary growth hormone and tumorigenesis—lessons from the dog. *Vet Q* 21:111–115, 1999.
31. van Garderen E, Schalken JA: Morphogenic and tumorigenic potentials of the mammary growth hormone/growth hormone receptor system. *Mol Cell Endocrinol* 197:153–165, 2002.
32. Rutteman GR, Blankenstein MA, Minke J, et al: Steroid receptors in mammary tumours of the cat. *Acta Endocrinol (Copenh)* 125(Suppl 1):32–37, 1991.
33. Millanta F, Calandrella M, Bari G, et al: Comparison of steroid receptor expression in normal, dysplastic, and neoplastic canine and feline mammary tissues. *Res Vet Sci* 79:225–232, 2005.
34. de las Mulas JM, van Niel M, Millán Y, et al: Immunohistochemical analysis of estrogen receptors in feline mammary gland benign and malignant lesions: comparison with biochemical assay. *Domest Anim Endocrinol* 18:111–125, 2000.
35. Mulas JMD, Van Niel M, Millán Y, et al: Progesterone receptors in normal, dysplastic and tumourous feline mammary glands. Comparison with oestrogen receptors status. *Res Vet Sci* 72:153–161, 2002.
36. Zafrani B, Aubriot MH, Mouret E, et al: High sensitivity and specificity of immunohistochemistry for the detection of hormone receptors in breast carcinoma: comparison with biochemical determination in a prospective study of 793 cases. *Histopathology* 37:536–545, 2000.
37. Hamilton JM, Else RW, Forshaw P: Oestrogen receptors in feline mammary carcinoma. *Vet Rec* 99:477–479, 1976.
38. Wiese DA, Thaiwong T, Yuzbasiyan-Gurkan V, et al: Feline mammary basal-like adenocarcinoma: a potential model for human triple-negative breast cancer (TNBC) with basal-like subtype. *BMC Cancer* 13:403, 2013.
39. Rasotto R, Caliari D, Castagnaro M, et al: An immunohistochemical study of HER-2 expression in feline mammary tumours. *J Comp Pathol* 144:170–179, 2011.
40. Ordas J, Millan Y, Dios R, et al: Proto-oncogene HER2 in normal, dysplastic and tumorous feline mammary glands: an immunohistochemical and chromogenic in situ hybridization study. *BMC Cancer* 7:179–184, 2007.
41. Maniscalco L, Millan Y, Lussich S, et al: Activation of mammalian target of rapamycin (mTOR) in triple negative feline mammary carcinomas. *BMC Vet Res* 9:80, 2013.
42. Campeau PM, Foulkes WD, Tischkowitz MD: Hereditary breast cancer: new genetic developments, new therapeutic avenues. *Hum Genet* 124:31–42, 2008.
43. Giménez F, Hecht S, Craig LE, et al: Early detection, aggressive therapy: optimizing the management of feline mammary masses. *J Feline Med Surg* 12:214–224, 2010.
44. Hahn KA, Adams WH: Feline mammary neoplasia: biological behavior, diagnosis, and treatment alternatives. *Feline Pract* 25:5–11, 1997.
45. McNeill CJ, Sorenmo KU, Shofer FS, et al: Evaluation of adjuvant doxorubicin-based chemotherapy for the treatment of feline mammary carcinoma. *J Vet Intern Med* 23:123–129, 2009.
46. Lana SE, Rutteman GR, Withrow SJ: Tumors of the mammary gland. In Withrow SJ, Vail DM, editors: *Small animal clinical oncology*, St Louis, 2007, Elsevier, pp 619–636.
47. MacEwen EG, Hayes AA, Harvey HJ, et al: Prognostic factors for feline mammary tumors. *J Am Vet Med Assoc* 185:201–204, 1984.
48. Ito T, Kadosawa T, Mochizuki M, et al: Prognosis of malignant mammary tumor in 53 cats. *J Vet Med Sci* 58:723–726, 1996.

49. Viste JR, Myers SL, Singh B, et al: Feline mammary adenocarcinoma: tumor size as a prognostic indicator. *Can Vet J* 43:33–37, 2002.

50. Weijer K, Hart AA: Prognostic factors in feline mammary carcinoma. *J Natl Cancer Inst* 70:709–710, 1983.

51. Seixas F, Palmeira C, Pires MA, et al: Grade is an independent prognostic factor for feline mammary carcinomas: a clinicopathological and survival analysis. *Vet J* 187:65–71, 2011.

52. Castagnaro M, Casalone C, Bozzetta E, et al: Tumour grading and the one-year post-surgical prognosis in feline mammary carcinomas. *J Comp Pathol* 119:263–275, 1998.

53. Jeglum KA, deGuzman E, Young KM: Chemotherapy of advanced mammary adenocarcinoma in 14 cats. *J Am Vet Med Assoc* 187:157–160, 1985.

54. Millanta F, Lazzeri G, Mazzei M, et al: MIB-1 labeling index in feline dysplastic and neoplastic mammary lesions and its relationship with postsurgical prognosis. *Vet Pathol* 39:120–126, 2002.

55. Birner P, Oberhuber G, Stani J, et al, Austrian Breast & Colorectal Cancer Study Group: Evaluation of the United States Food and Drug Administration-approved scoring and test system of HER2 protein expression in breast cancer. *Clin Cancer Res* 7:1669–1675, 2001.

56. Preziosi R, Sarli G, Benazzi C, et al: Multiparametric survival analysis of histological stage and proliferative activity in feline mammary carcinomas. *Res Vet Sci* 73:53–60, 2002.

57. Dias Pereira P, Carvalheira J, Gartner F: Cell proliferation in feline normal, hyperplastic and neoplastic mammary tissue—an immunohistochemical study. *Vet J* 168:180–185, 2004.

58. Castagnaro M, Casalone C, Ru G, et al: Argyrophilic nucleolar organiser regions (AgNORs) count as indicator of post-surgical prognosis in feline mammary carcinomas. *Res Vet Sci* 64:97–100, 1998.

59. Millanta F, Calandrella M, Citi S, et al: Over-expression of HER-2 in feline invasive mammary carcinomas: an immunohistochemical survey and evaluation of its prognostic potential. *Vet Pathol* 42:30–34, 2005.

60. Millanta F, Citi S, Della Santa D, et al: COX-2 expression in canine and feline invasive mammary carcinomas: correlation with clinicopathological features and prognostic molecular markers. *Breast Cancer Res Treat* 98:115–120, 2006.

61. Millanta F, Silvestri G, Vaselli C, et al: The role of vascular endothelial growth factor and its receptor Flk-1/KDR in promoting tumour angiogenesis in feline and canine mammary carcinomas: a preliminary study of autocrine and paracrine loops. *Res Vet Sci* 81:350–357, 2006.

62. Maniscalco L, Iussich S, de las Mulas JM, et al: Activation of AKT in feline mammary carcinoma: a new prognostic factor for feline mammary tumours. *Vet J Med* 25:297–302, 2011.

63. Preziosi R, Sarli G, Benazzi C, et al: Detection of proliferating cell nuclear antigen (PCNA) in canine and feline mammary tumours. *J Comp Pathol* 113:301–313, 1995.

64. Morris J: Mammary tumors in the cat: size matters, so early intervention saves lives. *J Feline Med Surg* 15:391, 2013.

65. Withrow SJ, Vail DM, Page R: *Withrow and MacEwen's small animal clinical oncology* (Kindle Locations 31857-31858). Elsevier Health Sciences 2013. Kindle Edition.

66. Wong JH, Cagle LA, Morton DL: Lymphatic drainage of skin to a sentinel lymph node in a feline model. *Ann Surg* 214:637–641, 1991.

67. Patsikas MN, Papadopoulou PL, Charitanti A, et al: Computed tomography and radiographic indirect lymphography for visualization of mammary lymphatic vessels and the sentinel lymph node in normal cats. *Vet Radiol Ultrasound* 51:299–304, 2010.

68. Mauldin GN, Matus RE, Patnaik AK, et al: Efficacy and toxicity of doxorubicin and cyclophosphamide used in the treatment of selected malignant tumors in 23 cats. *J Vet Intern Med* 2:60–65, 1988.

69. Stolwijk JA, Minke JM, Rutteman GR, et al: Feline mammary carcinomas as a model for human breast cancer. II. Comparison of *in vivo* and *in vitro* adriamycin sensitivity. *Anticancer Res* 9:1045–1048, 1989.

70. Borrego JF, Cartagena JC, Engel J: Treatment of feline mammary tumours using chemotherapy, surgery and a COX-2 inhibitor drug (meloxicam): a retrospective study of 23 cases (2002-2007). *Vet Comp Oncol* 7:213–221, 2009.

71. Novosad CA, Bergman PJ, O'Brien M, et al: Retrospective evaluation of adjunctive doxorubicin for the treatment of feline mammary gland adenocarcinoma: 67 cases. *J Am Anim Hosp Assoc* 42:110–120, 2006.

Vascular Access Ports in Cats

Alane Kosanovich Cahalane

A vascular access port (VAP) is an implantable medical device that allows repeated percutaneous access to blood vessels, first developed for delivery of chemotherapeutic drugs to human cancer patients.[1-3] In veterinary medicine, VAPs have been used in both clinical and research settings for blood sampling as well as drug delivery.[4-9] The design of the veterinary VAP is much the same as those used in human medical fields, consisting of an injection port and catheter tubing, with specialized Huber point needles for port access. Due to the simplicity of placement and the versatility of VAPs, their use is becoming more common in veterinary settings. Potential benefits of permanent central venous access through a subcutaneously (SC) implanted system include decreased rates of bacterial infection and reduced discomfort when compared to traditional intravenous (IV) catheter placement. Importantly, in chemotherapy patients that require repeated venipuncture or IV catheterization, VAPs may help to maintain vessel patency, reduce incidence of phlebitis, and minimize the risk of drug extravasation.[4,5] Vascular access ports have been successfully used in a number of animal species, including pigs, ferrets, rabbits, dogs, and cats.[4-10]

Vascular access ports are available in various sizes for use in veterinary medicine. In cats, 4 or 5 Fr catheter tubing and a small- or medium-sized port are usually chosen. The port base is composed of either a titanium or plastic (polyoxymethylene) base with a self-sealing, centralized silicone hub or septum. The hub is designed to withstand repeated punctures without damage to the silicone, using a specialized Huber point needle. The titanium or plastic port base has pre-existing holes for suture placement. A single adaptor protrudes from the side of the port base for connection to catheter tubing (Figure 60-1). Various port and catheter sizes as well as manufacturer information are shown in Table 60-1. Variations on basic VAPs include dual-chamber and low-profile ports, as well as Groshong catheters. Groshong catheter tubing (Bard Access Systems, Salt Lake City, UT) contains a three-way valve that allows infusion and withdrawal but closes when flow is not present, preventing unintentional flow of blood or air through the tubing and minimizing the risk of clot occlusion. Reports of the use of alternative port and catheter configurations in veterinary patients are not currently available.

The silicone or polyurethane catheter tubing is radiopaque, flexible, and smooth with a single tapered opening for vessel lumen access at one end. The vessel end of the catheter tubing has depth markings to ensure that the correct length of tubing is placed into the vessel. The remainder of the catheter tubing can be cut to achieve custom length for an individual patient prior to attachment to the port base adaptor. Once the catheter tubing is attached to the base, a locking device is slid over the connection to lock it in place (Figure 60-2).

The Huber point needle (Figure 60-3) has a curved, tapered tip, which parts the port hub without the risk of tearing or core sampling of the silicone. Huber needles are available in 19-, 20-, and 22-gauge and in 0.75- and 1-inch lengths. The female Luer end can be connected and locked to syringes, caps, and extension tubing. Huber needles with attached extension lines are also available and can be sourced from the same manufacturers as the VAPs.

Do not use standard hypodermic needles to puncture the silicone septum, because irreversible damage to the septum may occur. In an emergency situation where Huber needles are not available and another venous site cannot be accessed, the tip of a hypodermic needle can be manually curved toward the bevel using a sterile hemostat. Although curving the needle may prevent core sampling of the septum, this technique is not recommended for routine use.

CLINICAL USES

Vascular access ports provide permanent, SC access to the central venous system via the jugular or femoral vein. Clinical uses include repeated drug injections, such as chemotherapeutic medications, sedation for radiation therapy, IV fluid therapy, long-term antibiotic treatment, or parenteral nutrition. VAPs can also be used for repeated blood withdrawal, such as serial blood testing in patients being treated for neoplasia or renal disease. A recent study also evaluated the use of VAPs for obtaining whole blood from donor cats for transfusion.[8] In addition, although there may be few clinically relevant settings, arterially placed VAPs have been successfully used in research settings for monitoring systemic blood pressure.[11]

The decision to place a VAP is dependent on the disease process, treatment plan, owner willingness, and patient status. General anesthesia is usually required for placement. Contraindications for port placement include disseminated intravascular coagulation, bacteremia, septicemia, or endotoxemia.[12]

Table 60-1	Vascular Access Port Manufacturers			
Manufacturer	**Port Name**	**Port Material**	**Port Diameter**	**Catheter Sizes and Material**
Norfolk Vet Products*	CompanionPort	Titanium	Le Grande: 24.3 mm Le Port: 21 mm Le Petite: 19 mm	7.0 Fr silicone 5.0 Fr silicone 4.0 Fr silicone
Cook Medical	Vital Port	Titanium	Standard: 30 mm Petite: 24.1 mm Mini: 19 mm	6.5 Fr silicone 6.5 Fr silicone 5.0 Fr silicone
Smiths Medical*	Port-a-Cath, Preclinical MiniPort, P.A.S Port Elite	Titanium		3 to 9 Fr polyurethane or silicone
Bard Access Systems*	PowerPort	Titanium or plastic	13 different port designs, wide range of sizes	8 Fr polyurethane catheter 9.6 Fr silicone catheter 8 Fr Groshong catheter

*Manufacturer of vascular access ports specifically for veterinary use.

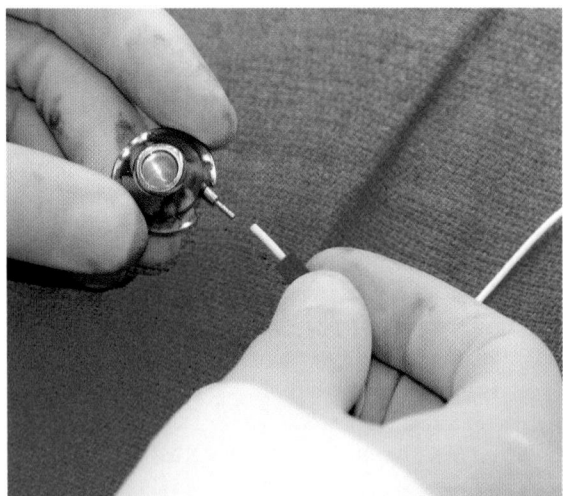

Figure 60-1: Components of the vascular access port system: port hub, catheter tubing, and blue locking sleeve. (Courtesy of James A. Flanders.)

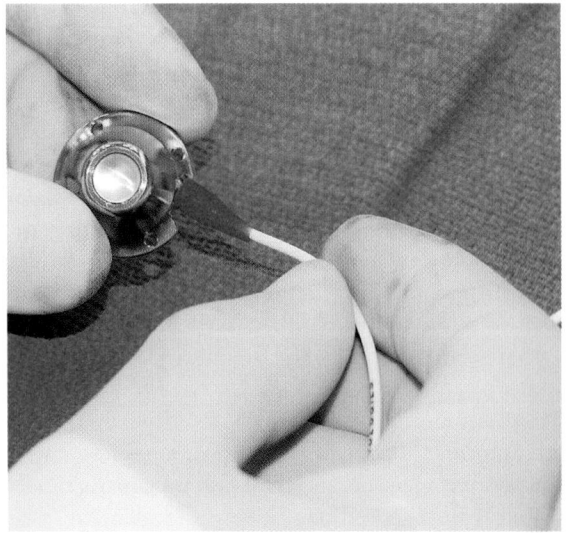

Figure 60-2: Assembled vascular access port prior to surgical placement. (Courtesy of James A. Flanders.)

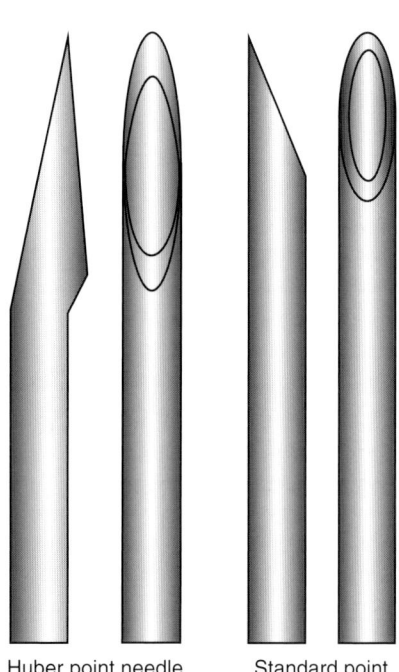

Huber point needle   Standard point

Figure 60-3: Schematic drawings of Huber point needle and standard point needle. Note the curved end of the Huber point that prevents core sampling of the silicone hub. (Courtesy of Norfolk Vet Products.)

VASCULAR ACCESS PORT PLACEMENT

A surgical approach is required to place the port base. Catheter insertion can be performed using a minimally invasive Seldinger technique or via surgical approach to the jugular or femoral vein. All ports and tubing should be inspected and tested prior to placement.

Jugular Vein Vascular Access Port Placement

For jugular port implantation, the anesthetized patient is placed in lateral recumbency, and a wide region (including

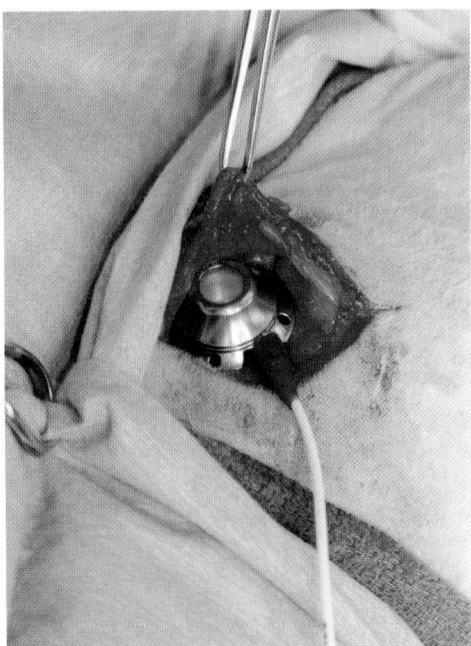

Figure 60-4: Intraoperative photograph of a port being placed into the subcutaneous pocket. (Courtesy of James A. Flanders.)

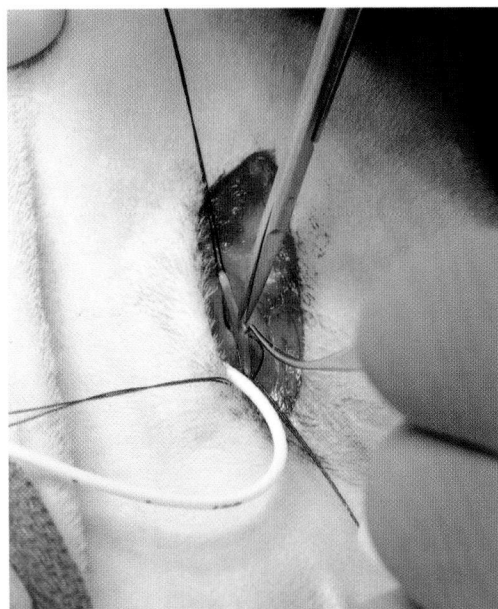

Figure 60-5: Isolated femoral vein prior to venotomy for surgical vascular access port placement. (Courtesy of James A. Flanders.)

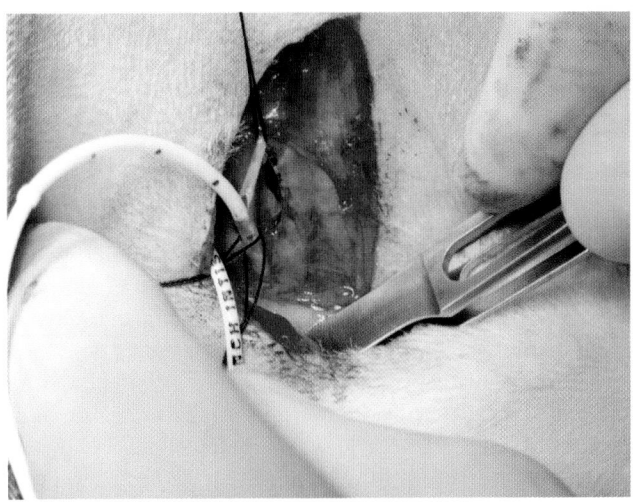

Figure 60-6: Catheter insertion into femoral vein. (Courtesy of James A. Flanders.)

the jugular furrow, epaxial musculature, and dorsal scapula) is clipped and sterilely prepared for both catheter insertion and port placement. The length of required catheter tubing is measured based on preoperative radiographs and estimated intraoperatively. Intraoperative fluoroscopy is helpful to document the correct level of insertion of the catheter tubing but is not required for successful VAP placement. A 3- to 5-cm skin incision is made over the dorsolateral cervical musculature. A SC pocket is made, exposing the underlying muscular fascia (Figure 60-4). The pocket should be made large enough to house the entire port hub and positioned such that the skin incision is cranial or caudal to the port itself and not directly overlying it. The port hub must be firmly attached to the muscular or fascial layer, deep to SC fat, using monofilament, non-absorbable suture material. Suturing to the SC fat increases the risk of port migration. Sutures may be preplaced through all predrilled port hub attachment holes and then tied, or placed and tied sequentially. The connector should be pointed toward the catheter tubing and in general, tight turns and kinks should be avoided. If necessary, use absorbable, interrupted sutures to close dead space within the port pocket to prevent seroma formation.

In a surgical approach, a longitudinal skin incision, 1 to 3 cm in length, is made directly over the jugular vein—separate from the port hub incision. Careful dissection is used to isolate and free approximately 2 cm of vessel from the surrounding tissue. Stay sutures (the author prefers 3-0 silk) are placed at the cranial and caudal aspects of the vein segment and are used to partially and temporarily occlude blood flow. Using vascular or ophthalmic forceps to stabilize the vein, iris scissors or a #11 blade is used to make a small incision (0.2 cm) into the vein (Figure 60-5). The catheter tubing is inserted into the vessel in the direction of blood

flow for central access (Figure 60-6). If enlargement of the venotomy site is required, fine scissors are used to extend it longitudinally, taking care not to sever the vessel. Once the catheter tubing is advanced to its desired length, the stay sutures are carefully ligated around the catheter. The catheter is flushed with sterile saline to ensure that the ligatures have not caused lumen occlusion. Have a scrubbed assistant place gentle tension on the stay sutures to provide temporary venous occlusion during venotomy and catheter insertion. This technique helps prevent backflow of blood into the surgical site.

For a minimally invasive (Seldinger) approach,[13] an 18-gauge needle connected to a syringe of sterile, heparinized saline (100 units/mL) is inserted directly into the vessel. Blood is drawn to ensure that the needle is within the vessel lumen, and then the needle is flushed and the syringe removed. A guide wire is passed through the needle to the level of the right atrium in the jugular vein, and the needle removed. A vessel dilator and peel-away sheath introducer is passed over the guide wire and inserted into the vessel. Once within the vessel lumen, the vessel dilator and wire are removed, leaving the sheath introducer in place. The catheter tubing is passed through the sheath introducer to the pre-measured length. Radiography or fluoroscopy can be used to document the level of the catheter tubing within the cranial vena cava, approaching but not entering the right atrium. The handles of the peel-away introducer are then grasped and pulled, removing the sheath from the vessel. A tunneling device is passed from the port site to exit at the venipuncture site, and the catheter end is passed SC to be connected to the port as previously described.

Regardless of the method of placement of the catheter, the port end of the catheter tubing can be cut to a desired length to minimize excess and tunneled SC to the port hub site, using a small hemostat or tunneling device. The catheter tubing is slid over the full length of the port connection adapter, and the locking device is slid over the connection to secure it. Subcutaneous tissue is apposed using monofilament, absorbable suture, and skin is closed routinely over the jugular and port hub sites.

Femoral Vascular Access Port Placement

For VAP placement into the left femoral vein, the patient is placed in right lateral recumbency, and the entire limb and lateral body wall are clipped and prepared. The procedure for creation of a SC pocket, port base attachment, and femoral venotomy or Seldinger catheter placement are as described earlier for the jugular vein. The SC pocket that will house the injection port may be placed over the left iliac wing or caudal portion of the left thoracic wall (Figure 60-7). Following catheter placement into the femoral vein, catheter tubing is tunneled SC from the inguinal region to the port base site on the ipsilateral side of the patient. Excess catheter tubing can be looped in the SC tissue near the port to help prevent temporary occlusion related to patient position during VAP use.

An Elizabethan collar should be used postoperatively to prevent self-mutilation or irritation. Ice-packing the incisions for 24 hours postoperatively may help prevent seroma formation. Should a seroma develop, warm-packing should be initiated. Standard protocol for skin suture removal should be followed as necessary.

VASCULAR ACCESS PORT USE

For each use of the VAP, appropriate hand hygiene must be used, and the port site must be aseptically prepared. The use of sterile gloves and a mask is recommended with each use.

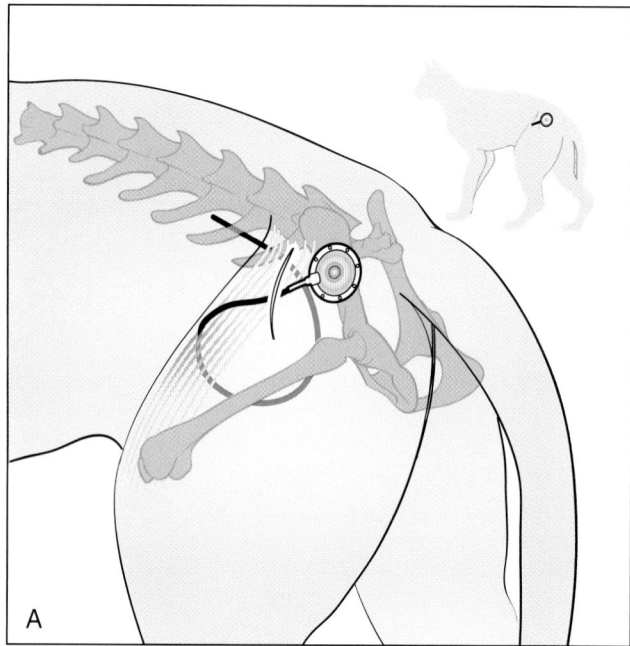

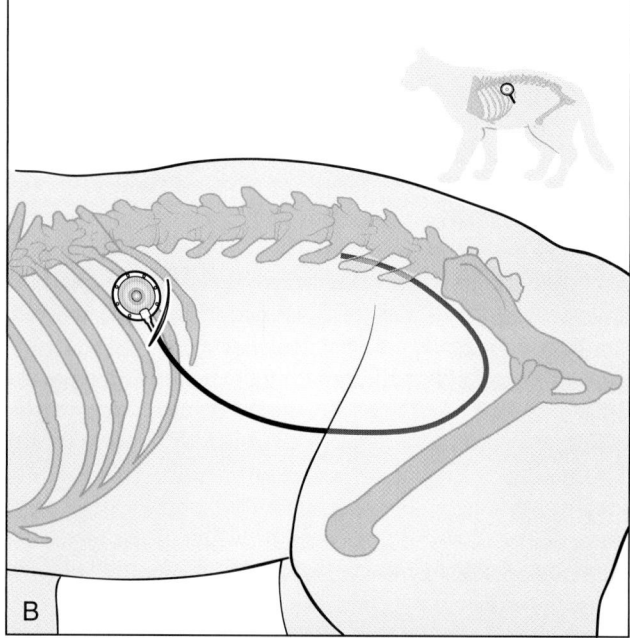

Figure 60-7: **A,** Schematic drawing of port location over the iliac wing. **B,** Schematic drawing of port location over the caudal thorax. (Courtesy of Kenneth M. Rassnick.)

The skin over the port should be prepped using a chlorhexidine-based or povidone-iodine–based solution. As with any surgical preparation, the skin should be swiped in a circular direction starting at the center and radiating outwardly. A minimum of three separate swabs should be used.

Following sterile preparation, the following steps are followed to access the port for infusion[14]:

1. The port is stabilized between the user's gloved thumb and index finger (Figure 60-8). The center of the port, defined by the center point between the thumb and index finger, is visualized and palpated.

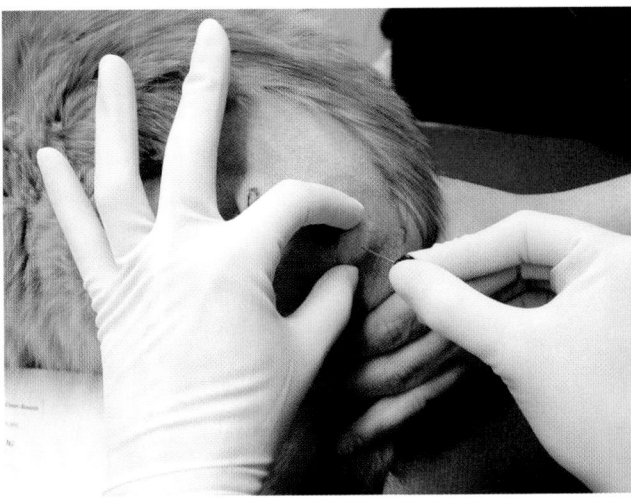

Figure 60-8: Femoral vascular access port in a cat receiving chemotherapy. Note the port is stabilized in the user's gloved hand, between the thumb and index finger. (Courtesy of Kenneth M. Rassnick.)

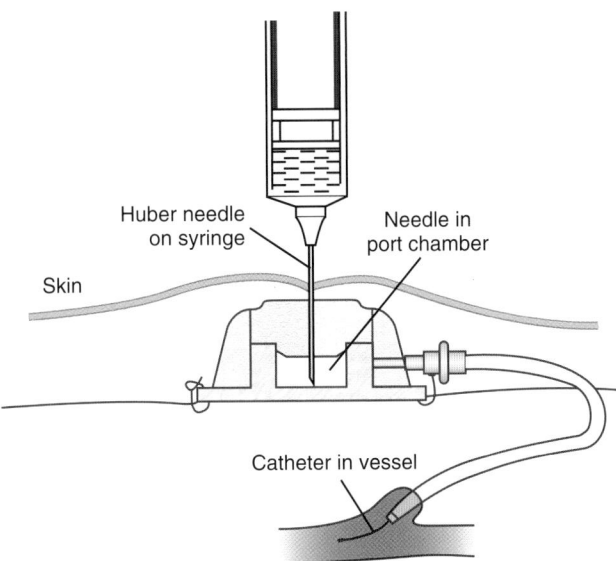

Figure 60-9: Schematic drawing of Huber point needle insertion into the vascular access port hub. (Courtesy of Norfolk Vet Products.)

2. The Huber needle is inserted with firm, consistent pressure at a 90-degree angle to the skin. The needle is advanced until a firm "click" is felt, corresponding to the needle contacting the base of the port (Figure 60-9). Failure to insert the needle to the base of the hub could result in SC leakage of the contents to be injected or blood being withdrawn. Tilting or maneuvering the needle once it is inside the port could damage the port septum.

3. A 10-mL or larger syringe is attached to the Huber point needle and aspirated to withdraw the lock solution from the previous use. Smaller syringes create increased pressure and may damage the port or catheter tubing. At least 1 mL of blood should be withdrawn to confirm VAP patency and proper placement of the needle.

Table 60-2	Approximate Fill Volumes of CompanionPort Ports including 12 Inches of Catheter Tubing
Description of Port and Catheter Tubing	**Approximate Fill Volume**
Small (Le Petite) port with 12 in. of 4 Fr catheter tubing	0.20 mL
Medium (Le Port) port with 12 in. of 5 Fr catheter tubing	0.40 mL
Large (Le Grande) port with 12 in. of 7 Fr catheter tubing	1.23 mL

Courtesy of Norfolk Vet Products.

4. Discard the first 1 mL of blood.
   a. For infusion, a new syringe of sterile saline is attached, and the saline is slowly infused, using a gentle pulsatile motion. The treatment infusion is then given, followed by another sterile saline flush.
   b. For blood sampling or donation, a new, empty syringe is attached and the sample collected, followed by another sterile saline flush.

5. A heparinized saline lock with a suggested concentration of 100 units/mL is used to minimize the risk of clot formation within the catheter tubing. Approximate fill volumes are listed in Table 60-2.

6. For removal of the Huber point needle, the port is supported with the user's thumb and index finger to prevent excessive tension on its connection to the body wall.

POTENTIAL COMPLICATIONS

A troubleshooting guide to VAP use can be found in Table 60-3. Reported complications associated with VAP use and placement include obstruction, infection, disconnection of the port from the catheter tubing, catheter breakage, seroma formation, and port hub migration.[15,16] A recent case report describes the development of pyothorax related to migration of a VAP catheter fragment that had embolized through the pulmonary circulation in a human patient.[17] In a review of 172 cases (46 cats, and 126 dogs), major complications (defined as permanent loss of VAP patency, catheter breakage, suture breakage, infection, and incision dehiscence) occurred in 10.5% of patients (Table 60-4).[5] Minor complications, defined as difficulty accessing the VAP, seroma formation, and temporary loss of VAP patency, occurred in 20.9% of patients. Femoral VAPs were associated with a 17.20 times higher rate of minor complications compared to jugular VAPs. Due to high motion in the catheter region, seroma formation may be more likely to occur in patients with femoral vein VAPs than with jugular VAPs.

One study evaluating the use of VAPs for blood sampling in 14 healthy cats found significant differences in potassium,

Table 60-3   Troubleshooting Guide to Vascular Access Port Use

Problem	Sign	Possible Causes	Possible Solution
Difficulty flushing or aspirating the VAP	Resistance or inability to flush Slow gravity infusions Blood is slow to withdraw from port or cannot be withdrawn	Huber needle may not be fully inserted Catheter tubing may be occluded by vessel wall, clot or fibrin sleeve, or catheter may be kinked	Make sure needle is fully inserted to the base of the port hub; rotate, or remove and reinsert needle, but do not tilt or bend Change patient position Using a 10 mL syringe, flush with heparinized saline, alternating between flushing and aspirating Use fibrinolytic agent if necessary
Pain over the VAP site	Pain reaction from patient during palpation Redness, swelling, heat, or discharge from port site	Port site may be infected Needle may have been withdrawn from port, causing subcutaneous drug or fluid injection	Check patient temperature and CBC for other signs of infection If discharge is present, evaluate cytology and/or bacterial culture

CBC, Complete blood count; *VAP*, vascular access port.

Table 60-4   Overview of Vascular Access Port–Related Complications Reported in 46 Cats

Vascular Access Port–Related Complications	Number of Cats
Major Complications (10%)	
Permanent loss of VAP patency	4
Inadvertent catheter removal	3
Catheter breakage	0
Suture breakage	0
Infection	0
Incision dehiscence	0
Minor Complications (21%)	
Difficulty accessing the VAP	0
Seroma formation	1
Temporary loss of VAP patency	9

Culp WT, Mayhew PD, Reese MS, et al.: Complications associated with use of subcutaneous vascular access ports in cats and dogs undergoing fractionated radiotherapy: 172 cases (1996-2007), *J Am Vet Med Assoc* 236:1322-1327, 2010.
VAP, Vascular access port.

Table 60-5   Dosing of Fibrinolytic Agents

Drug	Dosage	Infusion
Tissue plasminogen activator*	2 mg/cat	In 2 mL 0.9% NaCL, injected into port
Streptokinase[†]	90,000 IU/cat	Injected into port

*Cathflo Activase, Genentech Inc, San Francisco, CA.
[†]Streptase, Hoechst Marion Roussel—distributed by Astra USA.
IU, International units.

In this study, no differences in albumin and potassium levels were seen. Despite a level of presumptive hemolysis, red blood cell morphology does not appear to be affected in port samples. Similarly, white blood cell counts do not appear to be affected.

The most commonly reported complication in both human and veterinary VAP patients is occlusion, particularly the loss of sampling ability.[4,9,17] Vascular access port catheter tubing may become completely or partially obstructed, even when the user adheres to heparin-locking techniques. Thrombus formation within the catheter may occur. In addition, VAP catheter tubing may develop a fibrin sheath at the open end, presumably related to endothelial trauma and inflammation. The fibrin sheath may result in the ability to flush but not withdraw from the VAP. Occlusion can be treated using fibrinolytic agents, such as streptokinase or, preferably, tissue plasminogen activator (Table 60-5). However, these drugs have the potential to produce life-threatening side effects, and extreme caution is recommended if their use is to be considered. The use of drugs that inhibit platelet aggregation, such as clopidogrel, has been suggested as a prophylactic measure in patients with VAPs, but clinical studies have yet to be performed. Although larger catheter tubing may be less susceptible to thrombus obstruction, it may also result in

total protein, and albumin concentrations between VAP and venipuncture samples.[18] The difference in these variables is likely related to hemolysis from the port samples. However, this study evaluated only samples obtained 10 weeks after port placement. Another study evaluating the use of VAPs for feline blood donation compared samples obtained conventionally and via port, every 6 to 8 weeks for 6 months.[9]

increased endothelial trauma and therefore increased risk of fibrin sheath formation. Further studies are indicated to determine the best method of catheter size selection and thrombus prophylaxis.

Infection can occur in the immediate postoperative period or late in the course of VAP usage. Sterile skin preparation prior to VAP use is critical for prevention of infection. Patients with VAP-related infections may have fever, lethargy, swelling around the port site, or other generalized signs of sepsis. VAP removal is indicated if port- or catheter-related infection is suspected or confirmed or if bacteremia or sepsis is present. Antibiotic therapy based on culture and sensitivity is best, but broad-spectrum coverage may be indicated to improve clinical status before culture can be obtained at surgery.

If VAP removal is required, an approach is made through the previous incision. Sharp and blunt dissections are used to access the port through the fibrous capsule surrounding it. The catheter tubing is removed, and pressure is placed at the vessel site for a minimum of 15 minutes to prevent backflow of blood. Alternatively, the vessel may be ligated.

Overall, client satisfaction with VAPs is high.[4] Owner concerns related to clinical veterinary patients with femoral VAPs included appearance of the port, perceived discomfort related to the VAP, and VAP dysfunction. Therefore, educating clients about the appearance of the port and potential complications is important prior to VAP placement.

SUMMARY

VAPs can provide safe, reliable central venous access in small animal patients. The jugular site is most commonly used and may result in fewer VAP-related complications; however, the femoral vein may be used in patients that require radiation therapy or surgery of the head or neck or that have behavior issues that may prohibit safe manipulation of the head and neck region. Placement technique should be based on surgeon preference and experience; both surgical and minimally invasive techniques are feasible. Care of the VAP is simple; however, use of a heparinized saline flush and strict aseptic technique are critical to successful, long-term maintenance.

References

1. Dalton MJ: The vascular access port: a subcutaneously implanted drug delivery depot. *Lab Anim* 14:21–30, 1985.
2. Lokich JJ, Bothe A, Benotti P, et al: Complications and management of implanted venous access catheters. *J Clin Oncol* 3:710–717, 1985.
3. Gyves JW, Ensminger WD, Niederhuber JE, et al: A totally implanted injection port system for blood sampling and chemotherapy administration. *J Am Med Assoc* 251:2538–2541, 1984.
4. Cahalane AK, Rassnick KM, Flanders JA: Use of vascular access ports in femoral veins of dogs and cats with cancer. *J Am Vet Med Assoc* 231:1354–1360, 2007.
5. Culp WT, Mayhew PD, Reese MS, et al: Complications associated with use of subcutaneous vascular access ports in cats and dogs undergoing fractionated radiotherapy: 172 cases (1996-2007). *J Am Vet Med Assoc* 236:1322–1327, 2010.
6. Perry-Clark LM, Meunier LD: Vascular access ports for chronic serial infusion and blood sampling in New Zealand white rabbits. *Lab Anim Sci* 41:495–497, 1991.
7. Webb AI, Bliss JM, Herbst LH: Use of vascular access ports in the cat. *Lab Anim Sci* 44:491–494, 1994.

8. Aubert I, Abrams-Ogg AC, Sylvestre AM, et al: The use of vascular access ports for blood collection in feline blood donors. *Can J Vet Res* 75:25–34, 2011.
9. Morrison JA, Lauer SK, Baldwin CJ, et al: Evaluation of the use of subcutaneous implantable vascular access ports in feline blood donors. *J Am Vet Med Assoc* 230:855–861, 2007.
10. Rassnick KM, Gould WJ, III, Flanders JA: Use of a vascular access system for administration of chemotherapeutic agents to a ferret with lymphoma. *J Am Vet Med Assoc* 206:500–504, 1995.
11. Zwijnenberg RJ, del Rio CL, Cobb RM, et al: Evaluation of oscillometric and vascular access port arterial blood pressure measurement techniques versus implanted telemetry in anesthetized cats. *Am J Vet Res* 72:1015–1021, 2011.
12. Kock HJ, Pietsch M, Krause U, et al: Implantable vascular access systems: experience in 1500 patients with totally implanted central venous port systems. *World J Surg* 22:12–16, 1998.
13. Valentini F, Fassone F, Pozzebon A, et al: Use of totally implantable vascular access port with mini-invasive Seldinger technique in 12 dogs undergoing chemotherapy. *Res Vet Sci* 94:152–157, 2013.

14. Norfolk Vet Products: *CompanionPort Accessing and Maintenance Guide*. <http://www.norfolkvetproducts.com/PDF'S/Companion Port%20accessing%20guide.pdf>, (Accessed June 1, 2015.)
15. Sariego J, Bootorabi B, Matsumoto T: Major long-term complications in 1,422 permanent venous access devices. *Am J Surg* 165:249–251, 1993.
16. Mayer MN, Grier CK, Yoshikawa H, et al: Complications associated with the use of vascular access ports in dogs receiving external beam radiation therapy. *J Am Vet Med Assoc* 233:96–103, 2008.
17. Oduntan O, Turner J: Empyema thoracis due to intrapleural migration of retained vascular catheter. *Ann Thorac Surg* 95:123–125, 2013.
18. Henry CJ, Russell LE, Tyler JW, et al: Comparison of hematologic and biochemical values for blood samples obtained via jugular venipuncture and via vascular access ports in cats. *J Am Vet Med Assoc* 220:482–485, 2002.

P. Jane Armstrong, DVM and Angela Witzel, DVM

Feeding the Senior and Geriatric Cat

Amy K. Farcas and Kathryn E. Michel

The discussion of optimal nutrition for the older cat presents a number of challenges. Without question, aging is associated with biological changes that affect the structure and function of tissues and organs. Over a lifetime, there is an increase in cellular degeneration and a decrease in cellular regeneration. There are also numerous diseases whose incidence increases with aging. Questions arise with regard to what criteria are used to define old age in a cat and where to draw the line between changes associated with aging (e.g., osteoarthritis) and disease. Ultimately, dietary recommendations for older cats come down to how we parse life stage nutrition from therapeutic nutrition. Are there aspects of feline aging where we have sufficient evidence to make blanket nutritional recommendations? When should we treat each patient as an individual? This chapter explores our current understanding of nutritionally relevant biological alterations that likely occur in aging cats, approaches for assessing the needs of individual patients, and general dietary recommendations.

LIFE STAGE NUTRITION

In 2009, the American Association of Feline Practitioners issued guidelines on the care of senior cats. While acknowledging that the rate of aging will vary among individuals, they established three categories of older cats: mature (7 to 10 years), senior (11 to 14 years), and geriatric (15 years or more).[1] Subsequently, these designations have been increasingly adopted and serve as the basis for the terminology used in this chapter.

The rationale for life stage appropriate nutrition is scientifically sound based on distinct nutritional requirements for feline growth and adult maintenance that have been established for decades.[2] Investigations of aging humans have identified a handful of micronutrients with dietary recommendations for people over 70 years of age that differ from those established for intake in younger adults.[3] It is likely that continued research in this area will lead to further refinements in the dietary recommendations for geriatric humans.

At present, analogous studies in feline nutrition are not available or are only in preliminary stages. Consequently, the National Research Council's (NRC's) Nutrient Requirements of Dogs and Cats does not include specific life stage nutritional recommendations for older cats (or dogs),[2] nor does the Association of American Feed Control Officials (AAFCO) provide nutrient profiles for the manufacture of commercial cat foods beyond growth/reproduction and adult maintenance, a matter that is discussed further in the Senior Diets section.[4]

AGING AND AGE-RELATED DISEASE

The statement "age is not a disease" is pervasive throughout veterinary medicine, as well as the reminder that older patients are at increased risk of developing well-described age-related diseases. Thus, the question: Is age a disease or not?

It can be argued that this assertion would be more accurate if stated as: Age is not a disease as long as there is absence of undiagnosed or untreated age-related diseases. Examples of these age-related diseases include overweight and underweight conditions, degenerative joint diseases, chronic kidney disease (CKD), hyperthyroidism, and cognitive impairment.

It can also be reasonably argued that at some point, age becomes a disease; progressing from benign loss of function as a normal physiologic change to age-related disease. Some outcomes of this "physiologic degeneration" include the effect of aging on nutrient digestion and absorption, body weight, muscle mass, metabolism, nervous and immune systems, kidneys, and joints. Undiagnosed or untreated age-related diseases may be partly responsible for the difference between cats that "look their age" or older and those that don't, with those that don't being either free of, or appropriately treated for, their age-related disease. Recognition of this as a possibility should cause veterinarians to aggressively screen for and treat age-related disease (most of which have at least some

Static to increased maintenance energy requirement
Overall weight loss
Loss of lean body mass
    Higher rate of protein turnover
Loss of fat mass
No change in proportions of lean/fat mass
Decreased food intake
Metabolic hormonal changes
    Insulin resistance
    Increased insulin concentration
    Increased leptin concentration
    Increased adiponectin concentration

Decreased digestive capacity for protein
Decreased digestive capacity for fat
Decreased overall digestive capacity for dry matter
Altered gut bacterial populations
No change in bone mineral density
No change in mineral absorption

Changes in Digestive Capacity

Aging cats also appear to experience a decline in some digestive capabilities (Box 61-2),[15,17] which is apparently due to altered gastrointestinal (GI) function, the specifics of which have not been investigated. When young, mature, and old cats were compared, mature cats had the highest digestive capacity for dry matter, protein, fat, and starch, and the old cats had the lowest.[18]

In addition, there are changes in GI bacterial populations, usually demonstrating an unfavorable shift, with decreases in *Lactobacillus* spp. and *Bifidobacteria* spp., and increases in *Clostridium perfringens*, compared to younger cats.[19]

Fat digestion is noted to have the most significant decline in senior cats.[20] Incidence of low digestive capacity for fat increases with age, affecting 10% to 15% of cats 7 to 12 years of age and one-third of cats over 12 years of age.[20] Peachey and colleagues[21] reported significantly lower digestive capacity for fat and energy and a trend for decreased digestive capacity for protein in 11-year-old, compared with 3-year-old, cats. The decrease in digestive capacity for fat with aging has led pet food manufacturers to formulate diets intended for these cats with decreased fat concentrations, although it may be more reasonable to increase the fat concentration of these diets to allow these cats to consume enough calories to maintain their body weight. Because feline MER does not greatly change with age or may actually increase[8] but digestive efficiency decreases, older cats are more likely to be underweight than obese.[6]

In addition to decreases in digestive capacity for fat, that for protein also declines in senior cats.[18,20] This decreased capacity for protein digestion affects 20% of cats over 14 years of age;[7] these cats digest only 77% or less dietary protein (normal range of 85% to 90%).[7] This decreased digestive capacity for protein, in addition to increased protein turnover discussed earlier, suggests that senior cats should be fed ample dietary protein to allow maintenance of lean body mass. The degree of increase needed will be influenced by the protein quality of the diet fed.[16,22] For practical purposes, Laflamme suggested that commercial diets providing cats with about 34% of calories as protein would be expected to maintain proper protein turnover.[23,24] This recommendation, however, is based on data from younger cats.[25]

Bone mineral density in cats was found not to be affected by age.[26] Mineral absorption in old cats compared to mature and young cats appears to be unaltered,[18] indicating that

potential for nutritional management), resulting in improved care, quality of life, and longevity.

Weight Loss and Changes in Body Composition

Perhaps the best described of several features of physiologic alterations in aging cats is an overall decline in body weight without changes in body composition (Box 61-1).[5] Obesity in cats is common, particularly between 5 to 12 years of age,[5-7] but this should not be seen as cause for instituting caloric restriction in all aging cats. Many senior cats begin their senior years obese but lose fat mass as they age.[7] Cats tend to gain body weight steadily between 1 to 9 years, and then after 9 years, body weight generally begins to decrease.[7] Contrary to most other species, including dogs, cats do not appear to exhibit an age-related decline in maintenance energy requirement (MER).[8,9] In fact, there appears to be an increased MER in cats older than 11 to 12 years.[10,11] The increase in MER with age may have several causes, including a relatively constant low level of physical activity throughout adult life, lack of body composition changes,[5,12] and higher rate of protein turnover. Unchanging body composition can be both cause and effect of this increase in MER. It is causal in the sense that loss of metabolically active muscle mass in other species is thought to contribute to a decline in energy requirement. Lack of change in body composition is also an effect of unchanged MER. With MER increasing and intake often remaining static,[13-15] body fat is metabolized to meet the cat's energy needs. At the same time, protein turnover increases in older animals (data are available for dogs and are presumed to also apply to cats),[16] often causing a matching loss of muscle mass (see Chapter 95). Thus, the cat loses weight as it ages, but this weight loss involves both lean and fat mass such that the overall body composition does not change dramatically. This decline in body weight is relevant to veterinary care, because cats that died of cancer, CKD, or hyperthyroidism were reported to have lost weight for $2\frac{1}{2}$ years before death;[7] cats dying of other causes lost weight over a longer period.[7]

although macronutrient composition merits alteration in diets for senior cats, mineral composition may not. There has not been much work completed with respect to vitamin utilization in older cats. One study showed that older cats with GI disease were significantly more likely to have low serum cobalamin concentrations compared to younger cats with GI disease, but it is not possible to sort out the effects of GI disease versus aging from this study.[27]

In addition to alterations in digestion, older cats exhibited altered metabolic responses to food compared to younger cats. Aging is associated with peripheral insulin resistance in cats, with higher concentrations of insulin, leptin, and adiponectin in lean 8- to 9-year-old cats than in lean 1-year-old cats.[28]

Oxidative Damage

The free radical theory of aging[29] postulates that reactive oxygen species, most of which are a result of mitochondrial respiration, produce the cellular damage that manifests as aging.[30] The overall antioxidant status of an individual, and that of individual tissues and cells, can affect the aging process. One long-term study reported that cats 7- to 17-years-old fed a diet fortified with vitamin E, beta carotene, omega-3 and omega-6 fatty acids, and inulin lived significantly longer than cats fed a control diet.[31] However, it is not possible to determine whether the effect was caused by antioxidants, fatty acids, or dietary fiber.

Cognitive Dysfunction

The frequency of behavioral problems in cats increases with advancing age.[32] Many of these problems can be related to decline in cognitive function, resulting from the aging process specific to the brain (Box 61-3). It is known that in aging dogs, there is an increase in brain production of reactive oxygen species;[33] it is presumed that the same occurs in cats. The very high metabolic rate and high concentration of polyunsaturated fatty acids present in brain tissue make the brain particularly sensitive to oxidative damage. Although there are insufficient data to determine age-of-onset of impairments resulting from oxidative damage, learning impairments were evident in 8- to 9-year-old cats compared to 2- to 4-year-old cats, suggesting that cognitive deficits precede clinical signs.[33,34]

Nutritional and dietary interventions can improve antioxidant defense, thereby reducing the negative effects of free radicals.[33] In dogs, cognitive benefits of dietary manipulations are enhanced by environmental enrichment; the same is expected to be true in cats. Therapeutic diets aimed at improving cognitive function of cats have not yet been developed. Also in dogs, there has been some success in treating cognitive dysfunction with dietary supplements containing phosphatidylserine, a phospholipid component of cell membranes.[35] Although labeled for use in cats, there are no published studies of the efficacy of phosphatidylserine supplements in treating feline cognitive dysfunction. Dietary

BOX 61-3 Cognitive Changes in Aging Cats[32,33]

Possible Manifestations of Central Nervous System Aging
Decreased visual and auditory ability
Heightened sensitivity to environmental change
Decreased ability to adapt to environmental change
Changes in eating habits
Changes in elimination patterns
Aggression
Alterations in the sleep-wake cycle
Changes in ability to perform tasks
Memory deficits
Alterations in motor function and sleep patterns

Brain Pathology Reported in Senior Cats
Loss of neurons
Cerebral atrophy
Widening of sulci
Increases in ventricular size
Microhemorrhage
Amyloid plaque deposition
Infarcts
Decreases in the number of dendrites per neuron
Axonal degeneration
Decreased cholinergic tone within the brain

supplementation with S-adenosyl-L-methionine is also marketed to improve cognitive dysfunction with one study in aged cats showing improved learning capacity.[36] The most benefit was seen in the least cognitively impaired subjects, suggesting that this supplement may be most effective in earlier stages of the disease.

Immune System Dysfunction

Like the brain, the immune system of cats also sees changes with age. The immune system of old cats is sensitive to alterations in nutrition. It was shown that feeding healthy old cats below their energy and nutrient requirements for 4 days caused variation in several immune-related parameters of varying clinical significance.[37] The short time frame in which nutrition can affect the immune system highlights the importance of assessing each individual's nutrition needs and aiming to provide them.

Degenerative Joint Disease

Although significant work has been done with respect to the role of nutrition in prevention and treatment of arthritis in dogs, much less has been performed in cats.[38] Although up to 92% of cats are affected radiographically by the disease,[39,40] a much smaller proportion of cats are examined or treated for it.[40] The prevalence and severity of degenerative joint disease is strongly associated with age.[39] Given the nature of cats to hide illness, it is not surprising that a radiographically evident abnormality would go undetected, but this emphasizes the need for proactive management to ensure that cats are screened and managed appropriately. Despite the average cat's attempt to hide development of arthritic changes, these changes are evident when studied objectively—arthritic cats are more active when their pain is controlled.[41] In addition, when specifically assessed for joint pain, physical examination was able to detect pain in a majority of radiographically affected joints.[42] Radiographic evaluation may underdetect degenerative joint disease as assessed by gross examination of joint surfaces at necropsy.[43] These findings emphasize the importance of maintaining older cats at an appropriate weight and ensuring that they receive adequate amounts of exercise so that they can remain mobile and maintain appropriate muscle mass.[44]

Because there are limited options for uncomplicated pain control in cats, dietary therapy or dietary supplements are an attractive alternative. Indeed, diets specifically formulated for cats with joint disease do exist. A study of one of these diets fortified with long-chain omega-3 polyunsaturated fatty acids, green-lipped mussel extract, glucosamine and chondroitin resulted in increased activity in cats clinically affected by degenerative joint disease when compared to the control group, although there was no difference between groups with respect to subjective improvement in clinical signs.[45] Despite some published data that variably demonstrate improvement or no change in measures of canine degenerative joint disease with glucosamine, chondroitin, long-chain omega-3 polyunsaturated fatty acids, green-lipped mussel extract, turmeric, and other supplements, there are no published data regarding response of cats to any of these supplements. A safety study of a supplement containing glucosamine, chondroitin, and manganese found minimal change in hematologic, hemostatic, and biochemical parameters in cats at twice the labeled dose.[46]

Chronic Kidney Disease

Chronic kidney disease is the clinical manifestation of loss of function of individual nephrons over time. Because renal tubular epithelial cells are so metabolically active, there is similarity to the brain and immune system in terms of susceptibility to oxidative damage, which may contribute to this loss of nephrons.[47] Historically, veterinarians recommended low-protein and low-phosphorus diets to delay this loss; however, this approach has been shown to have no bearing on the onset of disease.[48,49] Once CKD is diagnosed, these strategies are reasonable if correctly applied. These strategies, particularly protein restriction, may actually be detrimental to an older cat with a relatively higher protein requirement, because it may increase its rate of loss of muscle mass. One argument commonly proposed in support of this strategy is that it "may help in case the cat develops chronic kidney disease." However, this proposes that a potentially detrimental diet be fed in order to manage a disease that the cat does

not have. Reduction of dietary sodium for senior diets is also advocated by some to avoid contribution to hypertension. However, sodium intake has not been shown to have significant effects on systemic blood pressure.[50] Although a lower-sodium diet that meets a cat's sodium requirement is not contraindicated in healthy senior cats, limiting diet choices to one that includes reduction in sodium may exclude more appropriate diets from consideration.

NUTRITIONAL ASSESSMENT OF SENIOR AND GERIATRIC FELINE PATIENTS

Given that there is a lack of clearly defined nutritional requirements for aged cats, much variation in the feline population in the rate and impact of aging, and the potential for concurrent disease, dietary recommendations for senior and geriatric cats are best made on an individual basis. Nutritional assessment is the first step in this process and involves evaluation of the patient, its diet, and its feeding management by performing a dietary history and physical examination, including body and muscle condition scoring. Nutritional assessment is both an essential part of the initial evaluation of any patient and a critical component of the ongoing management and supervision of that patient's care and medical treatment, in particular any dietary recommendations that have been made. There are routine steps that comprise the basic nutritional screening that all patients should undergo. However, additional considerations arise when evaluating senior and geriatric cats as well as patients exhibiting nutritional risk factors.

Taking a Dietary History

Changes in appetite, food preferences, and feeding behavior may signal physiologic changes associated with aging, such as changes in sensory perception, cognitive function, or altering energy requirement. They can also be signs associated with underlying disease. A dietary history will provide essential information about the patient's diet and feeding management that will permit the clinician to be able to assess the adequacy of nutrient intake, the suitability of feeding practices, and whether any dietary modification is indicated. A properly done dietary history will give an accurate picture of the foods that the patient routinely consumes as well as any nutritional risk factors exhibited by the patient or presented by the patient's diet, feeding management, or environment. Ideally, the person who is most responsible for feeding the patient should be questioned; however, it is important to find out who else resides in the household or has regular contact with the cat, including other pets. The patient's caregiver should be questioned about all foods that it receives (including treats, table foods, dietary supplements, and foods used to deliver medications) and should be asked whether the information reflects what is typical for this pet. If changes have occurred, the time frame in which those have taken place should be established.

BOX 61-4 Nutritional Risk Factors of Particular Significance for Senior and Geriatric Cats

Altered appetite or food preferences
Altered feeding behaviors
Altered gastrointestinal function
Perceived or documented changes in body or muscle condition or body weight
Previous or ongoing medical conditions, including dental disease
Currently receiving medications and/or dietary supplements

In addition to particulars about the patient's diet, the history should also include information regarding appetite, documented or perceived changes in body weight or condition, level of physical activity, and occurrence of any GI signs. Again, it is important to document whether the information reflects what is typical for the cat, or if this is not the case, the time frame over which changes have occurred. Box 61-4 lists some risk factors of special significance for senior and geriatric cats that should be considered. Forms are available that can be used as an aid in collecting and recording a comprehensive dietary history.[51]

Physical Examination Findings

Changes in body weight and condition are often gradual, occurring over an extended period of time and consequently may be overlooked by the patient's caregiver. Documenting and recording the patient's weight using an accurate scale at every office visit is critical, because it may provide early evidence of changes in body weight, permitting timely and possibly more effective intervention. This is of particular significance for older cats given the evidence that a greater proportion of cats older than 11 years of age are underweight and the association of weight loss with mortality in cats with certain conditions (i.e., CKD, hyperthyroidism, and cancer).[5-7]

Evaluation of body condition is a chief consideration in the nutritional assessment of a patient. Body condition scoring, while subjective, is simple to learn and requires no special equipment. The body condition scoring systems that have been published for cats are principally based on characterization of body silhouette and palpation of body fat. These systems are useful, particularly for identification of patients that have an overweight body condition; however, they may misclassify some malnourished patients that have experienced muscle wasting while still retaining excessive adipose tissue. Therefore, the process of body condition assessment should include not only the standard evaluation of body silhouette and evaluation of subcutaneous fat, but also a separate evaluation of muscle mass. This can be accomplished by palpation of skeletal muscle over the axial skeleton and other bony prominences. There are a variety of resources, including body and muscle condition scoring charts, available in the Global Nutrition Toolkit found on the World Small

Animal Veterinary Association website (http://www.wsava.org/nutrition-toolkit).[51]

Other aspects of the physical examination that should be taken into consideration include hair coat quality, skin condition, and clinical signs that may indicate specific micronutrient deficiencies (e.g., neck ventroflexion and other neurological signs due to thiamin deficiency).

Assessing the Diet

The adequacy of the patient's overall dietary intake should be evaluated for calories, essential nutrients, and suitability for any conditions amenable to nutritional intervention. Beware of making assumptions about the adequacy and suitability of a diet simply because it is a complete and balanced commercial cat food. Regulations give pet food manufacturers considerable leeway in the formulation of complete and balanced feline diets. Although this is not a drawback for a cat without special nutritional concerns, an individual older cat may benefit from a more calorically-dense food or a specific macronutrient profile that may be found in only a subset of commercially available products (see Senior Diets).

Senior cats are at risk of consuming insufficient calories for a number of reasons. The cat's voluntary intake may decrease because of changes in olfaction or taste, presence of dental disease, or as a consequence of an untreated underlying condition. If the diet has been changed, the cat may find it less appealing, or the new diet may be of lower caloric density than what was previously fed. The patient's caloric intake should be estimated from the dietary history and compared to an estimate of the patient's MER. For patients experiencing weight loss, this exercise helps to detect whether insufficient voluntary intake is contributing to the problem. If the cat is receiving a home-prepared diet or foods that are not nutritionally balanced, the proportion that is contributed to the cat's daily calorie intake should be investigated. Even if the cat is consuming adequate calories, it may not be getting sufficient protein or other essential nutrients if unbalanced foods are providing a substantial proportion of the daily calorie intake.

Assessing the Feeding Management

The dietary history provides key information about the patient's feeding management and environment, including the frequency, timing, and location of meals as well the presence of other pets and potential sources of environmental stress. Older cats may be less resilient and less able to cope with changes in routine, conflict, or competition among pets for food, or something as simple as feeding in a location difficult to access due to increasing osteoarthritis.

For the aged cat that is exhibiting reduced food intake, careful review of its feeding management may reveal one or more aspects that can be modified with beneficial results. For example, feeding more frequent smaller meals may improve overall intake. Warming food slightly can improve aroma, which may be beneficial in cases where olfaction is suspected to be impaired. In particular, if it is necessary to introduce a new diet, care should be taken to avoid doing so at times of illness or stress, and the introduction should be done gradually over days or even weeks. Initially offering the new diet and old diets side by side may improve success.

Ongoing Assessment

Patients with identified nutritional risk factors and, in particular, patients for which any modifications in diet or feeding management have been prescribed must have a plan in place for continued monitoring. The patient should have rechecks scheduled as appropriate for monitoring body weight and condition, appetite and diet acceptance, and any indicated diagnostic testing. Following up with the patient's caregiver to inquire about concerns and perceptions regarding the dietary plan and the patient's response as well as assessing adherence is equally as important for success as evaluation of the patient.

SENIOR DIETS

Although there are specific sets of nutrient requirements determined by the AAFCO and NRC for growth, reproduction, and adult maintenance in cats, there is no specific set of requirements for senior cats. Senior diets, then, are simply modifications of adult maintenance diets. A recent survey on senior cat diets reported a wide variation in caloric density and concentrations of protein, fat, crude fiber, sodium, and phosphorus (Table 61-1).[52] In this study, senior diets ranged from lower to higher than a typical adult maintenance diet for all variables reported. Thus, the term *senior diet* is not nutritionally descriptive and is interchangeable with *adult maintenance diet* with regard to assessment of the nutrient

composition of a diet. Individual manufacturers are free to apply their own perspective to formulation of senior diets; some may make senior diets more energy-dense, whereas others may do the opposite. Some may increase protein compared to an adult maintenance formulation, whereas others may decrease it, and so on.

MAKING INDIVIDUALIZED RECOMMENDATIONS FOR OLDER CATS

Best practice for making diet recommendations for a senior cat is to perform a complete nutritional assessment,[53] and then consider how diet may impact parameters of concern. Once this has been addressed, a diet is chosen based on its concentration of nutrients that affect the parameters of most concern, weighing the evidence for each strategy employed. The recommendation should also include a plan for monitoring response to the diet change.

In order to choose one diet among several, comparisons must be made on an energy basis—meaning the proportion of calories from protein, fat, and carbohydrates, or the amount of specific nutrients per calorie. This allows direct comparison of diets. In contrast, comparing on an "as-fed" or dry matter basis allows the amounts of water ("as-fed" only), fiber, and ash in each diet to variably affect the concentrations of other nutrients. Board-certified veterinary clinical nutritionists can be consulted as needed for more complex cases. This evidence-based, individualized approach is key to providing senior cats with dietary recommendations that meet their needs. Simply put, there is a reasonable amount of evidence to suggest that cats should be maintained at an ideal body weight and that they should be provided with ample calories and protein to allow maintenance of lean body mass in addition to immune status (Figure 61-1). Theoretically, this maintenance of lean

Table 61-1	Diets Marketed for Senior Cats Have Marked Variation in Caloric Density and Concentrations of Protein, Fat, Crude Fiber, Sodium, and Phosphorus		
Nutrient	**AAFCO Adult Minimum***	**Representative Adult Diet†**	**Median Nutrient Content in Senior Diets (Range)**
Kilocalories (kcal)			
per cup (*n* = 13)	—	412	388 (326-499)
per can (*n* = 14)	—		162 (146-191)
Protein (g/100 kcal)	6.5	9.0	9.2 (7.9-11.3)
Fat (g/100 kcal)	2.3	3.6	4.2 (3.5-9.4)
Sodium (mg/100 kcal)	50	150	106 (64-346)
Phosphorus (mg/100 kcal)	130	336	257 (111-606)
Crude fiber (g/100 kcal)	—	0.4	0.9 (0.3-2.1)

Used with permission: Hutchinson D, Freeman LM: Optimal nutrition for older cats. *Compendium on Continuing Education for Veterinarians,* 33(5), 2011.
AAFCO, Association of American Feed Control Officials.
*AAFCO: *Official publication*. Oxford, IN, 2010, AAFCO.
†Purina Cat Chow Complete Formula, Nestlé Purina PetCare.

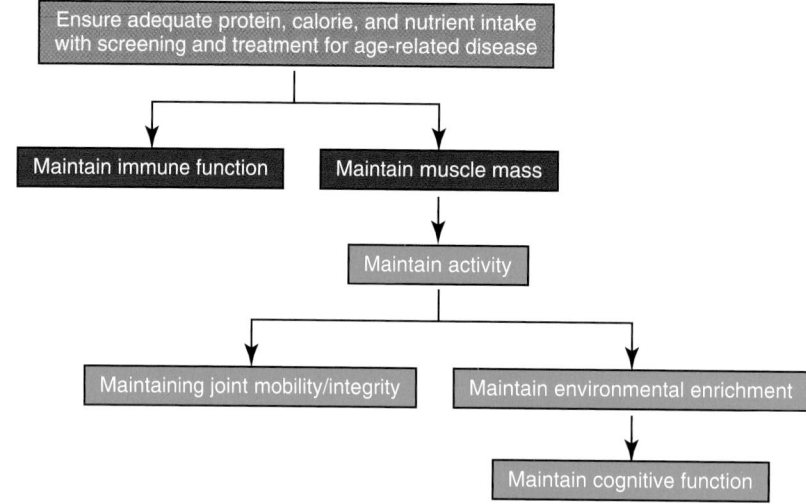

Figure 61-1: The importance of ensuring proper nutrition for older cats is illustrated by highlighting potential nutritional effects on major aspects of health and quality of life.

body mass could contribute to maintaining mobility and strength, which may affect the onset of clinical signs of degenerative joint disease. This maintenance of activity may also help to maintain the cat's cognitive abilities. Providing a complete and balanced diet that meets requirements for adult maintenance with respect to vitamin and mineral concentration appears to be adequate for most senior cats.

There is no significant evidence in cats to support the use of many possible strategies to delay the aging process. However, this does not mean that their use cannot be considered—only that these strategies should not drive diet recommendations, particularly at the expense of strategies that do have evidence to support their use. Addition of

omega-3 fatty acids, antioxidants, and chondroprotectants may have a somewhat protective effect against the progression of physiologic aging changes, and they do not appear to be inherently unsafe (although there are few safety studies in cats to support this). Addition of these ingredients as either dietary components or as dietary supplements is not unreasonable as long as their potential benefit is considered to outweigh potential risks.

For cats whose assessment reveals one or more age-related diseases, appropriate nutritional management of these should be prioritized, while other strategies, such as maintaining body weight and muscle mass should still be incorporated as appropriate.

References

1. Pittari J, Rodan I, Beekman G, et al: American Association of Feline Practitioners senior care guidelines. *J Feline Med Surg* 11:763–778, 2009.
2. National Research Council: *Nutrient requirements of dogs and cats*, Washington DC, 2006, National Academies Press.
3. Otten JJ, Hellwig JP, Meyers LD, editors: *Dietary reference intakes: the essential guide to nutrient requirements*, Washington DC, 2006, National Academies Press. <http://www.nap.edu/catalog/11537.html>. (Accessed June 1, 2015).
4. Association of American Feed Control Officials (AAFCO): *Official publication*, Oxford IN, 2013, AAFCO.
5. Harper EJ: Changing perspectives on aging and energy requirements: aging, body weight and body composition in humans, dogs and cats. *J Nutr* 128:2627S–2631S, 1998.
6. Armstrong PJ, Lund EM: Changes in body composition and energy balance with aging. *Vet Clin Nutr* 3:83–96, 1996.
7. Perez-Camargo G: What is new in the old? *Compend Contin Educ Pract Vet* 26:5–10, 2004.
8. Peachey SE, Harper EJ, Dawson JM: Effect of ageing on resting energy expenditure in cats. *Vet Rec* 144:420, 1999.
9. Fahey GC, Jr, Barry KA, Swanson KS: Age-related changes in nutrient utilization by companion animals. *Annu Rev Nutr* 28:425–445, 2008.
10. Laflamme DP: Nutritional care for aging cats and dogs. *Vet Clin North Am Small Anim Pract* 42:769–791, vii, 2012.
11. Cupp C, Perez-Camargo G, Patil A, et al: Long-term food consumption and body weight changes in a controlled population of geriatric cats. *Compend Contin Educ Pract Vet* 26:60, 2004 (Abstract).
12. Harper EJ: Changing perspectives on aging and energy requirements: aging and energy intakes in humans, dogs and cats. *J Nutr* 128:2623S–2626S, 1998.
13. Burger IH: Energy needs of companion animals: matching food intakes to require-

ments throughout the life cycle. *J Nutr* 124:2584S–2593S, 1994.
14. Peachey SE, Harper EJ: Aging does not influence feeding behavior in cats. *J Nutr* 132:1735S–1739S, 2002.
15. Taylor EJ, Adams C, Neville R: Some nutritional aspects of ageing in dogs and cats. *Proc Nutr Soc* 54:645–656, 1995.
16. Wannemacher RW, Jr, McCoy JR: Determination of optimal dietary protein requirements of young and old dogs. *J Nutr* 88:66–74, 1966.
17. Harper EJ: Changing perspectives on aging and energy requirements: aging and digestive function in humans, dogs and cats. *J Nutr* 128:2632S–2635S, 1998.
18. Teshima E, Brunetto MA, Vasconcellos RS, et al: Nutrient digestibility, but not mineral absorption, is age-dependent in cats. *J Anim Physiol Anim Nutr (Berl)* 94:e251–e258, 2010.
19. Patil AR: Effect of age on fecal microflora in cats. *Compend Contin Educ Pract Vet* 26:60, 2004 (Abstract).

20. Patil AR, Cupp C, Perez-Camargo G: Incidence of impaired nutrient digestibility in aging cats. *Compend Contin Educ Pract Vet* 26:72, 2004 (Abstract).

21. Peachey SE, Dawson JM, Harper EJ: The effect of ageing on nutrient digestibility by cats fed beef tallow-, sunflower oil- or olive oil-enriched diets. *Growth Dev Aging* 63:61–70, 1999.

22. Burkholder WJ: Age-related changes to nutritional requirements and digestive function in adult dogs and cats. *J Am Vet Med Assoc* 215:625–629, 1999.

23. Laflamme DP: Nutrition for aging cats and dogs and the importance of body condition. *Vet Clin North Am Small Anim Pract* 35(3):713–742, 2005.

24. Hannah S, Laflamme D: Effect of dietary protein on nitrogen balance and lean body mass in cats. *Vet Clin Nutr* 3:30, 1996 (Abstract).

25. Laflamme DP, Hannah SS: Discrepancy between use of lean body mass or nitrogen balance to determine protein requirements for adult cats. *J Feline Med Surg* 15:691–697, 2013.

26. Perez-Camargo G, Patil AR, Cupp CJ: Body composition changes in aging cats. *Compend Contin Educ Pract Vet* 26:71, 2004 (Abstract).

27. Williams DA, Steiner JM, Ruaux CG: Older cats with gastrointestnal disease are more likely to be cobalamin deficient. *Compend Contin Educ Pract Vet* 26:62, 2004 (Abstract).

28. Hoenig M, Jordan ET, Glushka J, et al: Effect of macronutrients, age, and obesity on 6- and 24-h postprandial glucose metabolism in cats. *Am J Physiol Regul Integr Comp Physiol* 301: R1798–R1807, 2011.

29. Harman D: Aging: a theory based on free radical and radiation chemistry. *J Gerontol* 11:298–300, 1956.

30. Zicker SC, Wedekind KJ, Jewell DE: Antioxidants in veterinary nutrition. *Vet Clin North Am Small Anim Pract* 36:1183–1198, v, 2006.

31. Cupp C, Jean-Philippe C, Kerr W, et al: Effect of nutritional interventions on longevity of senior Cats. *Int J Appl Res Vet Med* 4:34–50, 2006.

32. Gunn-Moore D, Moffat K, Christie LA, et al: Cognitive dysfunction and the neurobiology of ageing in cats. *J Small Anim Pract* 48:546–553, 2007.

33. Landsberg GM, Nichol J, Araujo JA: Cognitive dysfunction syndrome: a disease of canine and feline brain aging. *Vet Clin North Am Small Anim Pract* 42:749–768, vii, 2012.

34. Landsberg GM, Denenberg S, Araujo JA: Cognitive dysfunction in cats: a syndrome we used to dismiss as 'old age'. *J Feline Med Surg* 12:837–848, 2010.

35. Heath SE, Barabas S, Craze PG: Nutritional supplementation in cases of canine cognitive dysfunction—a clinical trial. *Appl Anim Behav Sci* 105:284–296, 2007.

36. Araujo JA, Faubert ML, Brooks ML, et al: NOVIFIT(NoviSAMe) tablets improve executive function in aged dogs and cats: implications for treatment of cognitive dysfunction syndrome. *Intl J Appl Resin Vet Med* 10:90, 2012.

37. Freitag KA, Saker KE, Thomas E, et al: Acute starvation and subsequent refeeding affect lymphocyte subsets and proliferation in cats. *J Nutr* 130:2444–2449, 2000.

38. Lascelles BD: Feline degenerative joint disease. *Vet Surg* 39:2–13, 2010.

39. Lascelles BD, Henry JB, 3rd, Brown J, et al: Cross-sectional study of the prevalence of radiographic degenerative joint disease in domesticated cats. *Vet Surg* 39:535–544, 2010.

40. Hardie EM, Roe SC, Martin FR: Radiographic evidence of degenerative joint disease in geriatric cats: 100 cases (1994-1997). *J Am Vet Med Assoc* 220:628–632, 2002.

41. Lascelles BD, Hansen BD, Roe S, et al: Evaluation of client-specific outcome measures and activity monitoring to measure pain relief in cats with osteoarthritis. *J Vet Intern Med* 21:410–416, 2007.

42. Lascelles BD, Dong YH, Marcellin-Little DJ, et al: Relationship of orthopedic examination, goniometric measurements, and radiographic signs of degenerative joint disease in cats. *BMC Vet Res* 8:10, 2012.

43. Freire M, Robertson I, Bondell HD, et al: Radiographic evaluation of feline appendicular degenerative joint disease vs. macroscopic appearance of articular cartilage. *Vet Radiol Ultrasound* 52:239–247, 2011.

44. Rychel JK: Diagnosis and treatment of osteoarthritis. *Top Companion Anim Med* 25:20–25, 2010.

45. Lascelles BD, DePuy V, Thomson A, et al: Evaluation of a therapeutic diet for feline degenerative joint disease. *J Vet Intern Med* 24:487–495, 2010.

46. McNamara PS, Barr SC, Erb HN, et al: Hematologic, hemostatic, and biochemical effects in cats receiving an oral chondroprotective agent for 30 days. *Vet Ther* 1:108–117, 2000.

47. Brown SA: Oxidative stress and chronic kidney disease. *Vet Clin North Am Small Anim Pract* 38:157–166, vi, 2008.

48. Finco DR, Brown SA, Crowell WA, et al: Effects of aging and dietary protein intake on uninephrectomized geriatric dogs. *Am J Vet Res* 55:1282–1290, 1994.

49. Bovee KC: Mythology of protein restriction for dogs with reduced renal function. *Compend Contin Educ Vet* 21:15–20, 1999.

50. Chandler ML: Pet food safety: sodium in pet foods. *Top Companion Anim Med* 23:148–153, 2008.

51. World Small Animal Veterinary Association Global Nutrition Committee: Global nutrition toolkit. <http://wsava.org/nutrition-toolkit>. (Accessed June 1, 2015).

52. Hutchinson D, Freeman LM: Focus on nutrition—optimal nutrition for older cats. *Compend Contin Educ Vet* 33:E1–E3, 2011.

53. Baldwin K, Bartges J, Buffington T, et al: AAHA nutritional assessment guidelines for dogs and cats. *J Am Anim Hosp Assoc* 46:285–296, 2010.

The Unique Metabolic Adaptations and Nutrient Requirements of the Cat

Beth Hamper

The domestic cat is believed to have evolved from the African wildcat *Felis sylvestris libyca* between 4000 and 10,000 years ago.[1,2] Cats belong to the order Carnivora, meaning "flesh eating," and the family Felidae. The felids diverged from the other carnivorous groups early in the evolutionary tree.[3] Other members of the order Carnivora include canids, bears, pandas, weasels, raccoons, and hyenas. There is a wide diversity of feeding patterns within this order. Canids and bears are considered omnivores, whereas pandas are strict herbivores. All felids are meat eaters, or strict carnivores. This specialized and exclusive meat diet has led to unique metabolic and nutritional adaptations not seen in canids or other members of the order Carnivora. The goal of this chapter is to review the research regarding the unique metabolic adaptations of the cat and provide a review of their subsequent unique requirements.[3,4] Some highlights of this research in feline nutrition and metabolism include the following:

- A limited ability to downregulate enzymes of nitrogen catabolism and urea cycle enzymes
- A strict requirement for the amino acid arginine, which can lead to life-threatening consequences if lacking in the diet for longer than 24 hours
- Limited synthesis of taurine from cysteine
- Limited capabilities in handling carbohydrates in the diet
- Limited synthesis of vitamin A from beta-carotenes
- Limited synthesis of niacin from the amino acid tryptophan
- High level of gluconeogenesis from proteins and fats

Arginine, taurine, niacin, and vitamin A are abundant in an all-flesh diet, along with high levels of protein and amino acids and very limited carbohydrates.

ANATOMY AND PHYSIOLOGY

Cats have fewer teeth than dogs. They have the same number of incisors, canine, and carnassial teeth but fewer premolar and molar teeth with fissured surfaces. Their dentition is more specialized for shearing flesh rather than grinding it. Both dogs and cats lack salivary amylase, which is the enzyme that is involved in early starch digestion.[4] Because cats are smaller than most dogs and evolved to eat small, frequent meals throughout the day, their absolute stomach capacity is smaller than that of dogs. The maximum stomach capacity

of both the dog and cat is typically 45 to 90 mL/kg body weight.[5]

Relative intestinal length is determined by the ratio of intestinal length to body length. Intestinal length is one of the factors that influences the amount of time for digestion and absorption to occur. Cats have a shorter intestinal length than dogs and other omnivores and herbivores. In the cat, this ratio is 4:1 compared with 6:1 in dogs.[4] In herbivorous species, this ratio is much higher due to the lower digestibility of their foodstuffs (e.g., 12:1 in the horse, 20:1 in the ox, and 27:1 in the sheep).[4] Because of this shorter intestinal length and time for digestion, cats need diets with higher digestibility compared to dogs.

Cobalamin, or vitamin B_{12}, requires binding to intrinsic factor for its absorption and uptake in the ileum. Most mammals manufacture and secrete intrinsic factor from both the stomach and pancreas. In the cat, intrinsic factor is produced only in the pancreas.[5]

Researchers are beginning to uncover the role of the gut microbiome in metabolism and immune function as well as the consequences for health. The human gastrointestinal (GI) microbiome contains approximately 10^{14} microorganisms, which is 10 times the number of human cells.[6] The metabolic functions of the microbiome within the GI tract include production of metabolites, such as short-chain fatty acids used as an energy source for colonocytes; degradation of potentially toxic compounds; enhanced metabolism of amino acids and nondigestible carbohydrates; and synthesis of vitamins and lipids.[7] A previous study in clinically healthy cats demonstrated that cats have larger numbers of bacteria in their proximal small intestine compared to dogs. The total bacterial counts from duodenal cultures in cats ranged from 10^5 to 10^8 colony-forming unit (CFU)/mL, compared to a maximum of 10^4 CFU/mL in dogs.[8] Higher bacterial levels in the small intestine may be another adaption to a carnivorous diet. Further research examining the environment effect of diet on the gut microbiome is warranted. See Chapter 8 for more on the gut microbiome.

FEEDING BEHAVIOR

In the wild, cats hunt small prey, such as mice, rats, rabbits, birds, frogs, reptiles, and insects. Predatory behavior is a strong drive in the cat and will even take precedence over feeding. Cats will stop eating a meal to kill prey and then go back to eating the original meal rather than the freshly killed item.[9]

Mice are a common prey species for the cat with a caloric density of approximately 30 kcal per mouse. The small size and low caloric density of their prey dictates that cats need to eat many small meals throughout the day to meet their energy and nutritional requirements. Cats prefer to ingest freshly killed prey rather than carrion.[10] Domestic cats will have seven to 20 small meals per day if given free access to food.

Previous work has demonstrated that domestic cats are able to regulate macronutrient intake when given a variety of wet and/or dry foods. The macronutrient target intake for cats is approximately 52% total energy as protein, 36% total energy as fat, and up to 12% total energy as carbohydrate.[11,12] This closely matches the nutrient profile of feral cats that target 52% total energy from protein, 46% total energy from fat, and only 2% from carbohydrate.[13]

Smell, taste, and texture all play important roles in the cat's dietary preferences. The most abundant taste receptors (neurons of the facial nerve) are those for amino acids, particularly those amino acids that are described as sweet.[14] These include proline, cysteine, ornithine, lysine, histidine, and alanine. Cats reject bitter-tasting amino acids, such as arginine, isoleucine, phenylalanine, and tryptophan. The second most abundant taste receptors are for acidic foods. These receptors are stimulated by phosphoric acid, carboxylic acids, and nucleotide dipeptides and tripeptides.[14] Cats avoid monophosphate nucleotides, which accumulate in tissues after death. This may be why cats dislike carrion. Cats do not have functional taste receptors for sucrose or other sugars.[14,15] Temperature is also important, with cats preferring food at body or room temperature. Cats generally reject foods at temperatures colder than 15°C (59°F) or warmer than 50°C (122°F).[16] Food preferences are strongly correlated with the amount of protein in the diet, particularly animal protein. Liver, blood, and red meat are highly palatable to cats. Other than protein, fat has been shown to be palatable to cats. Fats applied to the outside of dry kibble are positive flavor enhancers, but it is believed that the positive influence of fat is more related to textural changes rather than flavor. Despite this, cats do show a strong aversion to medium-chain fatty acids.[3] Cats generally select moist foods similar in water content to animal tissue, compared to dry, extruded diets. However, cats that have been fed exclusively dry foods for an extended period of time can develop a strong preference for eating only dry foods.[17]

Food preferences in offspring are influenced by the diet of the queen during pregnancy and lactation. Particularly important to later food preferences and choices are the flavors and textures kittens experience between 1 and 6 months of age.[16] Owners should be encouraged to feed kittens a variety of flavors and textures at this stage with the hope that it will lead to more flexibility in the adult.

Stressful situations can result in learned aversions to new or novel foods; therefore, starting a new therapeutic diet in hospitalized cats is inadvisable. Some animals, like rodents, have a keen ability to detect dietary deficiencies and avoid foods that lack essential nutrients. Cats are intermediate in their ability to avoid foods that can result in deficiencies over a long period of time; for example, cats will consistently eat taurine-free diets despite development of cardiac, reproductive, and retinal diseases.

SPECIFIC NUTRIENTS

Water
Water is the single most important nutrient in sustaining life, yet frequently the least discussed. Water serves multiple functions including serving as the solvent wherein the vast majority of intracellular and extracellular chemical processes occur.[4] Water is the major component of body tissues and fluids, facilitates the transport of oxygen and nutrients via the blood, and is needed for normal digestion, thermoregulation, and excretion of urine and feces.[4]

The cat evolved as a desert animal with the ability to highly concentrate its urine under low environmental water conditions (i.e., specific gravity up to 1.080-1.085).[18] Water balance in dogs and cats comes from water content of food, water derived from metabolism, environmental losses, and drinking. The amount of water in food varies greatly, from 7% to 10% in dry extruded diets and up to 80% in canned diets. Dogs adjust their water intake in response to changes in the water content of their diet. Unlike dogs, cats do not adjust their water intake based on the water content of their diets. When fed a dry food, cats replace only half their total daily water intake with drinking, in comparison to being fed a canned diet.[19] Studies have shown that dry diets are a risk factor for feline lower urinary tract disease.[20] Consumption of canned foods leads to increased water consumption and diuresis, which results in lower supersaturation of stone-forming minerals.[21] Canned diets have also been found to result in lower energy intake and body weight in cats; thus, canned diets may help promote weight loss.[22]

Protein and Amino Acids
Protein
Dietary protein is required for two reasons. The first is for amino acids that the animal cannot synthesize, which are called the *essential amino acids*. The second is for nitrogen and carbon skeletons used for the synthesis of nonessential amino acids and other necessary compounds containing nitrogen (i.e., purines, pyrimidines, heme, hormones, and neurotransmitters). Both essential and nonessential amino acids become part of the amino acid pool for protein synthesis in the tissues. The essential amino acids for both dogs and cats are arginine, histidine, isoleucine, leucine, lysine, methionine, phenylalanine, threonine, tryptophan, and valine.[4] Although dogs are able to synthesize the amino acid taurine from cysteine, the synthesis of taurine in strict carnivores (i.e., cats)

is very limited, making it an absolute dietary requirement. Determination of protein requirements in adult dogs and cats has been based on maintaining nitrogen balance or nitrogen intake equal to nitrogen losses in feces and urine. However, a study using maintenance of lean body tissues as the determinant for protein requirement rather than nitrogen balance found significantly higher protein requirements for cats (5.2 g/kg body weight versus the current Association of American Feed Control Officials recommendation of 3.5 to 3.9 grams of protein per kilogram body weight).[23] It seems that nitrogen balance is an inadequate marker for determining optimal protein requirements and that veterinarians may not be recommending optimal dietary protein levels for cats. In the wild, cats have been found to tolerate high levels of protein in their diet. Average protein levels in feral cat diets as expressed on a dry matter basis are 63%, which is higher than any current commercial cat food.[13]

The dietary protein requirement for the kitten is approximately 1.5 times the dietary protein requirement for the puppy. In contrast, adult cats require two times more protein than adult dogs and four times more protein than an omnivore, such as the rat (Table 62-1).[4,24] The increased protein requirement in the cat is not for increased levels of essential amino acids but rather a dietary source of nitrogen. Excess nitrogen from proteins and other sources is removed by way of the urea cycle in the liver. Most omnivorous species, when given a low-protein diet, conserve amino acids by decreasing enzyme levels involved in amino acid catabolism. Omnivorous species can also conserve amino acids and nitrogen when given low-protein diets by altering the activity of the urea cycle enzymes. Cats are not able to downregulate enzymes for both amino acid catabolism and the urea cycle despite being fed low-protein diets.[25] Therefore, cats cannot conserve nitrogen when given low-protein diets and will begin to catabolize protein sources within the body (i.e.,

muscle) to supply tissue needs. Endogenous urinary nitrogen losses in animals fed protein-free diets have been found to be 360 mg nitrogen/kg in cats, compared with 210 mg nitrogen/kg in dogs, 128 mg nitrogen/kg in rats, and 62 mg nitrogen/kg in humans, illustrating this lack of enzyme adaptation in the cat.[4]

Protein is also continually used for gluconeogenesis in the cat. Because of the very limited number of carbohydrates cats ingest in the feral diet, they are very efficient at synthesizing glucose from proteins by gluconeogenesis. In other species, gluconeogenesis occurs several hours after a meal, whereas in cats, it occurs immediately after a meal and is permanently active to maintain blood glucose levels. The benefit of these adaptations is the immediate ability to catabolize high levels of protein without developing hyperammonemia and the rapid ability to make glucose from protein for energy through gluconeogensis.[26]

Arginine

Arginine is a key intermediate in the urea cycle. The urea cycle is a group of reactions involved in the excretion of nitrogen via urea. A single meal without the amino acid arginine can result in life-threatening effects in the cat. Arginine-deficient cats develop emesis, hypersalivation, hyperactivity, and hyperesthesia—eventually leading to death as a result of ammonia intoxication.[27] These dramatic results were found to be due to the cat's inability to synthesize arginine from other dietary precursors. In many mammals, arginine can be synthesized from ornithine and citrulline in the intestine. The cat has lost this ability because of the lack of two enzymes in the pathway, pyrroline-5-carboxylate synthase and ornithine aminotransferase. Overnight food deprivation results in a low concentration of plasma arginine and urea cycle intermediates. When the cat eats a meal with protein that includes arginine, dietary arginine replenishes liver levels for urea cycle function with subsequent disposal of nitrogen and ammonia. If arginine is missing from the meal, the cat cannot replenish its urea cycle intermediates and severe hyperammonemia develops.[26] Animal tissue is high in arginine content, making its *de novo* synthesis unnecessary in carnivores on all-meat diets. Also, depletion of urea cycle intermediates after a meal results in conserving nitrogen needed for synthesis of disposable amino acids.

Methionine and Cysteine

The dietary requirement for the sulfur amino acids, methionine and cysteine, is higher in cats than in other mammals.[4] Methionine can be converted to cysteine; therefore, the sulfur amino acid requirement can be met with either methionine alone or methionine and cysteine. Methionine serves as a methyl group donor important for DNA and RNA synthesis and is a component of many proteins. Cysteine plays an important structural role in proteins and is a major constituent of hair. Cysteine is also the precursor for glutathione, a major antioxidant in mammalian systems and a precursor for the synthesis of felinine. Felinine, a branched-chain amino acid found in the urine of domestic cats, is believed to

| | **Table 62-1** | **Minimum Crude Protein Requirements in Carnivores and Omnivores (Percentage on a Dry Matter Basis)** |

Animal Type	Recommended Crude Protein Requirement for Growth	Recommended Crude Protein Requirement for Maintenance
Carnivore (mink)	32% to 38%	21.8% to 26%
Carnivore (cat)	22.5%	20%
Omnivore (dog)	17.5% to 22.5%	10.0%
Omnivore (rat)	16.6%	5.5%

Nutrient requirements of mink and foxes, ed 2, Washington DC, 1982, National Academy Press, p 33; *Nutrient requirements of dogs and cats*, Washington DC, 2006, National Academy Press, pp 357-369; *Nutrient requirements of laboratory animals*, Washington DC, 1995, National Academy Press, p 13.

function as a pheromone and is important in territorial marking. It can be found in the urine of cats as young as 2 months of age with levels being highest in intact male cats (0.4 to 8 g/L of urine).[28] Felinine concentrations in females are only 20% to 25% of that in intact males. The high requirement for sulfur amino acids in cats has been attributed to their need to synthesize felinine, high glutathione requirement, and dense haircoat.[3]

Taurine

Taurine is a beta-sulfonic amino acid that is not used in protein synthesis but is found as a free amino acid in tissues. The highest concentrations of taurine are found in the heart, muscle, brain, and retina. Taurine serves numerous important functions, including osmoregulation, calcium channel modulation, antioxidant activity, and bile acid conjugation.[29] Many mammals are able to use either glycine or taurine for bile acid conjugation. Cats and dogs are only able to use taurine to conjugate bile acids. Whereas dogs are able to synthesize sufficient taurine from cysteine, cat taurine synthesis is negligible due to low activity of two enzymes in the pathway.[26] Taurine deficiency may be due to:

- Inadequate dietary supply
- Loss of taurine in the enterohepatic circulation associated with increases in bacterial flora that degrade taurine
- Loss of taurine in a diet due to processing effects

Taurine deficiency in the cat is well documented, resulting in dilated cardiomyopathy, central retinal degeneration, and reproductive failure.[30] As taurine is abundant in animal tissue, the need to synthesize taurine would not be necessary in the cat's normal required metabolic pathways.

Fat and Fatty Acids

The essential or required fatty acids in cats as in other mammals include linoleic acid (18:2n-6), and linolenic acid (18:3n-3).[31] Most mammals can convert linoleic acid (n-6) and linolenic acid (n-3) to their respective longer-chain derivatives, arachidonic acid, eicosapentaenoic acid (EPA), and docosahexaenoic acid (DHA), through the delta-6-desaturase enzyme.

Arachidonic acid is a precursor for eicosanoid synthesis and is an abundant component of cell membranes. Cats are unique in that they have low delta-6-desaturase activity. Initially, it was believed that cats lacked any delta-6-desaturase activity and thus had an absolute requirement for arachidonic acid as well as linoleic acid. Further studies have shown that cats may have an alternative pathway for arachidonic acid synthesis. For example, they are able to synthesize sufficient quantities for maintenance, but females have an absolute requirement for arachidonic acid during reproduction, and kittens have an absolute requirement during early growth.[31] Similarly, for the n-3 fatty acids EPA and DHA, cats have limited synthesis from the precursor α-linolenic acid. High levels of DHA are required for neural and retinal tissue development in kittens, so DHA becomes conditionally essential for cats at this life stage.

Carbohydrates

The diet of feral cats is very low in carbohydrates.[13] As with protein, cats have evolved several unique adaptations to metabolism of carbohydrates, compared with omnivores or herbivores. These include the following:

- An absence of glucokinase activity in the liver
- Lower levels of amylase and the disaccharides sucrase and lactase in the pancreas and intestine
- Little adaptation in amylase activity with increased carbohydrate diets
- High levels of gluconeogenesis from proteins and fats

Cats have no dietary requirement for carbohydrates but do have a dietary requirement for energy. As long as their diet contains fats and gluconeogenic proteins, they are able to synthesize glucose and energy sufficient for maintenance. One study demonstrated that lactating dogs given a carbohydrate-free diet became hypoglycemic, with a low survival rate among the puppies.[32] It is probable that although cats have no absolute carbohydrate requirement, queens with some carbohydrate in the diet are better able to support lactation and nursing kittens.

Mammals have up to four isoenzymes in the liver that catalyze the conversion of glucose to glucose-6-phosphate, the first step in glucose utilization. The hexokinase responsible for operating under high glucose loads is hexokinase D, or glucokinase. The cat does not have glucokinase activity, in line with a diet containing low levels of carbohydrates.[33] In contrast, enzyme levels involved in gluconeogenesis (e.g., pyruvate carboxylase, fructose 1,6-bisphosphate, and glucose-6-phosphatase) are much higher in the feline than canine liver.[33] It was previously believed that cats do not express fructokinase activity because high-sucrose diets resulted in fructosuria and fructosemia. It has since been found that cats do have fructokinase enzyme activity in their liver, producing frucose-1-phosphate.[28] Fructose-1-phosphate is then catalyzed to dihydroxyacetone and glyceraldehyde by way of the enzyme aldolase. It is believed that fructose intolerance in humans is due to a defect in this enzyme. The level of aldose activity has not been analyzed in the cat, but low levels would support their low tolerance for elevated levels of fructose with resulting fructosuria.

Amylase activity, the enzyme responsible for hydrolysis of starch to glucose, is low in cats compared to dogs. The cat lacks salivary amylase, with pancreatic amylase levels only 5% of those found in dogs and intestinal values only 10% of those found in dogs.[34] The activity of the sugar transporters in the intestine is also not adaptable to higher levels of carbohydrate in the diet, compared to the dog. Compared with other species, cats have much lower levels of maltase, isomaltase, and sucrase activity in the small intestinal mucosa.[35]

Lactase activity is high in newborn kittens but rapidly declines at weaning, as has been found in other mammals. Compared to puppies, however, kittens exhibit a more rapid decrease in lactase.[35] Despite limited enzymatic breakdown of sugars, once absorbed, the digestibility of all the sugars, with the exception of lactose, is between 98% and

100%.[35] Apparent protein digestibility was found to be reduced in diets containing lactose or sucrose by 4% to 5% compared with the carbohydrate-free diet.[36] This is believed to be due to the accelerated rate of passage of the food resulting from the osmotic effects of the soluble sugars and increased bacterial carbohydrate fermentation with increased bacterial nitrogen fixation. There has been much speculation recently regarding high-carbohydrate diets and the increasing incidence of obesity and diabetes mellitus in cats. Dry foods can contain up to 40% carbohydrate on a dry matter basis. Long-term studies are needed to fully evaluate relative risks of moderate to high carbohydrate feeding in the cat.

Vitamins

The cat has several unique vitamin requirements, both quantitatively and qualitatively different from those of other mammals, including the following:

- An absolute requirement for preformed vitamin A
- An increased tolerance for high levels of vitamin A in the diet
- An absolute requirement for niacin
- A four times higher requirement for thiamine, pyridoxine, and folate, compared to the dog

Vitamin A

Cats are able to absorb carotenoids but cannot efficiently convert these to the active form of vitamin A because they lack the enzyme 15,15′-dioxygenase.[26,37] Carotenoids are vitamin A precursors synthesized in plant lipids. Preformed vitamin A occurs naturally only in animal tissues where high levels occur within the viscera. It would therefore be redundant to convert carotenoids when the preformed vitamin is already present in the wild diet.

Vitamin A, being lipid soluble, can become toxic if given in large doses. Vitamin A toxicity occurs in cats given all-liver diets or given high dosages of vitamin A supplements. Chronic hypervitaminosis A in cats is characterized by the formation of exostoses on the cervical vertebrae, causing ankylosis, deformity, and crippling.[38] Unlike humans, cats transport vitamin A primarily as retinyl esters rather than retinol and are able to excrete large amounts of retinyl esters in the urine.[39] Cats are also able to store higher concentrations of vitamin A in their livers compared with humans, rats, and dogs. A small amount is also stored in the kidneys.[4] Because animal viscera can be high in vitamin A content, increased storage and the ability to excrete large amounts in the urine would be protective mechanisms for minimizing vitamin A toxicity.

Vitamin D

For most mammals, vitamin D is conditionally essential as it can be synthesized during ultraviolet (UV) radiation to the skin, converting the precursor 7-dehydrocholesterol to previtamin D. Cats and dogs are unable to use this conversion pathway. This is not due to a thick hair coat inhibiting UV penetration of the skin, but rather to high levels of an enzyme in an alternative pathway that converts 7-dehydrocholesterol to cholesterol rather than previtamin D.[4] Insofar as the carnivorous wild diet has adequate amounts of vitamin D abundant in animal tissue, pathways for synthesis would be unnecessary.

Niacin (Vitamin B₃)

Niacin can be endogenously synthesized from the amino acid tryptophan, but the efficiency of this conversion varies among mammals. Rats are able to do this conversion very well, whereas cats are able to synthesize only negligible amounts of niacin. This is due to the high activity of an enzyme at a branching point in the pathway. The enzyme, picolinic carboxylase, dominates this branching point in the cat and directs it to the production of acetyl coenzyme A (CoA) and rather than niacin synthesis.[26] Because muscle tissue is well supplied with niacin, *de novo* synthesis is unnecessary in the wild diet, and the production of acetyl CoA for adenosine triphosphate production would be energetically advantageous.

Pyridoxine (Vitamin B₆)

One of the major biological functions of pyridoxine is to serve as a coenzyme in transamination reactions or amino group transfers from amino acids.[40] Cats have high transaminase activity because of their constant state of gluconeogenesis. Therefore, they have a high pyridoxine requirement, approximately four times higher than that of the dog.

Thiamine (Vitamin B₁)

Thiamine is one of the water-soluble B vitamins that is required for the formation of the coenzyme thiamin pyrophosphate. Thiamin pyrophosphate serves as a coenzyme in decarboxylation reactions in both carbohydrate and amino acid catabolism. Cats require four times as much thiamine in their diet compared to dogs, secondary to their high level of amino acid catabolism and gluconeogenesis. Thiamin pyrophosphate is also a coenzyme in the branched-chain alpha-keto acid dehydrogenase complex, which is involved in the catabolism of leucine, isoleucine, and valine.

Thiamine deficiency can be seen in cats fed raw or undercooked fish diets. Certain raw fish contain thiaminase enzymes, resulting in destruction of thiamin.[41] Sulfites, which have been used for pet food preservation, also cause destruction of thiamine, resulting in deficiency.[42] Thiaminase enzymes have also been found in certain species of *Clostridium* spp. and *Bacillus* spp. bacteria. Bacterial production of thiaminase has been found in the contents of ruminant animals, resulting in neurological deficits.[43] Cats have greater numbers of bacteria within their intestinal tract compared to dogs.[8] Whether there are thiaminase bacteria within these populations, resulting in a higher requirement for thiamine in the cat, is unknown at this time. Clinical signs of thiamine deficiency include anorexia, weight loss, and depression, progressing to neurological signs of dilated pupils, ataxia, weakness, seizures, and eventually death.

Folate

Folate, similar to the other B vitamins, is an important coenzyme in several metabolic pathways. Folate is used in metabolic reactions involving one-carbon transfers. It is important in amino acid metabolism, DNA synthesis, and protein synthesis.[40] Specifically, folate is involved in histidine catabolism, interconversion of the amino acids serine and glycine, and methionine catabolism. Cats have a fourfold greater requirement for folate compared to dogs due to higher amino acid catabolic activity.

SUMMARY

The unique nutritional requirements of cats reflect their adaptation to an all-meat diet. Their high protein requirement reflects their high level of gluconeogenic activity and amino acid catabolism and their inability to downregulate the nitrogen catabolic enzyme pathways. Their unique requirement for arginine, taurine, vitamin A, vitamin D, and niacin are due to adaptations in their enzyme systems secondary to deletion or downregulation of enzymes for synthesis of nutrients found abundantly in their wild diet.

References

1. Driscoll CA, Menotti-Raymond M, Roca AL, et al: The Near Eastern origin of cat domestication. *Science* 317:519–523, 2007.
2. O'Brien SJ, Yukhi N: Comparative genome organization of the major histocompatibility complex: lessons from the Felidae. *Immunol Rev* 167:133–144, 1999.
3. MacDonald ML, Rogers QR, Morris J: Nutrition of the domestic cat, a mammalian carnivore. *Annu Rev Nutr* 4:521–562, 1984.
4. National Research Council Ad Hoc Committee on Dog and Cat Nutrition: *Nutrient requirements of dogs and cats*, Washington DC, 2006, National Academies Press.
5. Saker KE, Remillard RL: Critical care nutrition and enteral-assisted feeding. In Hand MS, Thatcher CD, Remilliard RL, et al, editors: *Small animal clinical nutrition*, ed 5, Topeka, KS, 2010, Mark Morris Institute, pp 439–476.
6. Turnbaugh PJ, Ley RE, Hamady M, et al: The human microbiome project. *Nature* 449:804–810, 2007.
7. Verberkmoes NC, Russell AL, Shah M, et al: Shotgun metaproteomics of the human distal gut microbiota. *ISME J* 3:179–189, 2009.
8. Johnston K, Lamport A, Batt RM: An unexpected bacterial-flora in the proximal small-intestine of normal cats. *Vet Rec* 132:362–363, 1993.
9. Adamec RE: Interaction of hunger and preying in domestic cat *(Felis catus)*—an adaptive hierarchy. *Behav Biol* 18:263–272, 1976.
10. Kane E: Feeding behavior of the cat. In Rivers JPW, et al, editors: *Waltham Symposium nutrition of the dog and cat*, Cambridge, 1989, Cambridge University Press, pp 147–158.
11. Hewson-Hughes AK, Hewson-Hughes VL, Miller AT, et al: Geometric analysis of macronutrient selection in the adult domestic cat, *Felis catus. J Exp Biol* 214:1039–1051, 2011.
12. Hewson-Hughes AK, Hewson-Hughes VL, Colyer A, et al: Consistent proportional macronutrient intake selected by adult domestic cats *(Felis catus)* despite variations in macronutrient and moisture content of foods offered. *J Comp Physiol [B]* 183:525–536, 2013.
13. Plantinga EA, Bosch G, Hendriks WH: Estimation of the dietary nutrient profile of free-roaming feral cats: possible implications for nutrition of domestic cats. *Br J Nutr* 106: S35–S48, 2011.
14. Bradshaw JW, Goodwin D, Legrand-Defrétin V, et al: Food selection by the domestic cat, an obligate carnivore. *Comp Biochem Physiol A Physiol* 114:205–209, 1996.
15. Li X, Li W, Wang H, et al: Cats lack a sweet taste receptor. *J Nutr* 136:1932S–1934S, 2006.
16. Zaghini G, Biagi G: Nutritional peculiarities and diet palatability in the cat. *Vet Res Commun* 29:39–44, 2005.
17. Hamper BA, Rohrbach B, Kirk CA, et al: Effects of early experience on food acceptance in a colony of adult research cats: a preliminary study. *J Vet Behav-Clin Appl Res* 7:27–32, 2012.
18. DiBartola SP: Clinical approach and laboratory evaluation of renal disease. In Ettinger SJ, Feldman EC, editors: *Textbook of veterinary internal medicine*, vol 2, Philadelphia, 2000, Saunders/Elsevier, p 1604.
19. Anderson R: Water-balance in the dog and cat. *J Small Anim Pract* 23:588–598, 1982.
20. Jones BR, Sanson RL, Morris RS: Elucidating the risk factors of feline lower urinary tract disease. *N Z Vet J* 45:100–108, 1997.
21. Buckley CMF, Hawthorne A, Colyer A, et al: Effect of dietary water intake on urinary output, specific gravity and relative supersaturation for calcium oxalate and struvite in the cat. *Br J Nutr* 106:S128–S130, 2011.
22. Wei A, Fascetti AJ, Villaverde C, et al: Effect of water content in a canned food on voluntary food intake and body weight in cats. *Am J Vet Res* 72:918–923, 2011.
23. Laflamme D, Hannah S: Discrepancy between use of lean body mass or nitrogen balance to determine protein requirements for adult cats. *J Feline Med Surg* 15:691–697, 2013.
24. National Research Council Subcommittee on Laboratory Animal Nutrition: *Nutrient requirements of laboratory animals*, Washington DC, 1995, National Academy of Sciences. <http://site.ebrary.com/id/10072063>. (Accessed August 30, 2014.)
25. Rogers QR, Morris JG, Freedland RA: Lack of hepatic enzymatic adaptation to low and high levels of dietary-protein in adult cats. *Enzyme* 22:348–356, 1977.
26. Morris JG: Idiosyncratic nutrient requirements of cats appear to be diet-induced evolutionary adaptations. *Nutr Res Rev* 15:153–168, 2002.
27. Morris JG, Rogers QR: Arginine: an essential amino acid for the cat. *J Nutr* 108:1944–1953, 1978.
28. Springer N, Lindbloom-Hawley S, Schermerhorn T: Tissue expression of ketohexokinase in cats. *Res Vet Sci* 87:115–117, 2009.
29. Huxtable RJ: Physiological actions of taurine. *Physiol Rev* 72:101–163, 1992.
30. Markwell PJ, Earle KE: Taurine—an essential nutrient for the cat—a brief review of the biochemistry of its requirement and the clinical consequences of deficiency. *Nutr Res* 15:53–58, 1995.
31. Bauer JE: Metabolic basis for the essential nature of fatty acids and the unique dietary fatty acid requirements of cats. *J Am Vet Med Assoc* 229:1729–1732, 2006.
32. Romsos DR, Palmer HJ, Muiruri KL, et al: Influence of a low carbohydrate diet on performance of pregnant and lactating dogs. *J Nutr* 111:678–689, 1981.
33. Washizu T, Tanaka A, Sako T, et al: Comparison of the activities of enzymes related to glycolysis and gluconeogenesis in the liver of dogs and cats. *Res Vet Sci* 67:205–206, 1999.
34. Kienzle E: Carbohydrate-metabolism of the cat. 1. Activity of amylase in the gastrointestinal tract of the cat. *J Anim Physiol Anim Nutr* 69:92–101, 1993.
35. Kienzle E: Carbohydrate-metabolism of the cat. 3. Digestion of sugars. *J Anim Physiol Anim Nutr* 69:203–210, 1993.
36. Kienzle E: Effect of carbohydrates on digestion in the cat. *J Nutr* 124:2568S–2571S, 1994.
37. Green AS, Tang G, Lango J, et al: Domestic cats convert [H-2(8)]-beta-carotene to [H-2(4)]-retinol following a single oral dose. *J Anim Physiol Anim Nutr* 96:689–700, 2012.
38. Polizopoulou ZS, Kazakos G, Patsikas MN, et al: Hypervitaminosis A in the cat: a case report and review of the literature. *J Feline Med Surg* 7:363–368, 2005.
39. Raila J, Mathews U, Schweigert FJ: Plasma transport and tissue distribution of beta-carotene, vitamin A and retinol-binding

protein in domestic cats. *Comp Biochem Physiol A Mol Amp Integr Physiol* 130:849–856, 2001.

40. Stipanuk MH: *Biochemical, physiological, and molecular aspects of human nutrition*, ed 2, St Louis, 2006, Saunders/Elsevier, pp 694–712.

41. Lonsdale D: Review of the biochemistry, metabolism and clinical benefits of thiamin(e) and its derivatives. *Evid Based Complement Alternat Med* 3:49–59, 2006.

42. Studdert V, Labuc R: Thiamin deficiency in cats and dogs associated with feeding meat preserved with sulfur-dioxide. *Aust Vet J* 68:54–57, 1991.

43. Edwin EE, Jackman R: Ruminant thiamine requirement in perspective. *Vet Res Commun* 5:237–250, 1982.

Cats and Carbohydrates: How Much Should We Feed?

Claudia A. Kirk

The nutritional requirements of the domestic cat exemplify evolutionary adaptation to a strict carnivorous diet and predatory lifestyle. These adaptations limit the rate and amount of carbohydrate utilization in the cat compared to omnivorous species. High carbohydrate intake and carbohydrate excess have been implicated in certain health disorders, but evidence for a cause and effect relationship is lacking. The feral domestic cat *(Felis domesticus)* eats a wide variety of prey, including small mammals, birds, insects, and reptiles. Because this prey-directed diet is composed exclusively of animal tissues, the typical composition of the natural diet is limited in carbohydrates. The primary sources of carbohydrates in the diet of adult feral cats are tissue glycogen and the gut contents of the prey. As the cat became domesticated, the nutritional profile of the diet changed to include larger proportions of carbohydrates from milk products, sugars, grains, and other vegetable matter. In contrast to a whole rat carcass (carbohydrate 1.18% dry matter; 0.18 g/100 kcal),[1] commercial cat foods provide up to fiftyfold the amount of carbohydrates. Dry cat foods commonly provide 30% to 40% metabolizable energy (ME) (33% to 45% dry matter, 8 to 10 g/100 kcal) as carbohydrate. The divergence of nutritional profiles of commercial cat foods from that of the cat's natural diet has led to debate regarding the impact of high carbohydrate feeding in this obligate carnivore with concerns that these levels represent carbohydrate excess.

While definitions for carbohydrate content of cat foods are not standardized, many current publications suggest these classifications: high (greater than 50% ME), moderate (26 to 50% ME), low (5% to 25% ME), and ultralow (less than 5% ME).[2] This definition of carbohydrate level refers to the content of simple carbohydrates (digestible starches and sugar) in foods as opposed to complex carbohydrates such as fibers or resistant starches, that are largely undigested. This discussion will focus on digestible (simple) carbohydrates.

Carbohydrates are included in commercial feline foods as a readily available energy substrate, a source of dietary fiber, or for functional properties in the processing of foods. Gums, mucilage, and starch serve as gelling agents in canned foods, starch aids expansion and kibble structure in dry extruded diets, and simple sugars reduce water activity to help preserve semimoist foods and treats. The proportion of carbohydrates in commercial foods varies, with lower levels typically found in canned foods, and moderate to high levels in dry foods. Most domestic cats consume increased carbohydrate levels compared to their wild or feral counterparts, which derive approximately 2% ME from carbohydrates.[3]

Despite the nutritional adequacy of modern commercial cat foods, consumption of high dietary carbohydrate levels are suggested to alter energy metabolism, promote insulin resistance, and contribute to increased risk for obesity, diabetes mellitus, and other health disorders.[4] Many studies have been published evaluating the impact of various dietary carbohydrate levels on changes in body weight, impact on plasma glucose and insulin concentrations, insulin sensitivity, and biomarkers for disease risk.*

While the majority of studies do not support a direct cause and effect relationship between higher carbohydrate intake and increased risk for obesity or diabetes, the diversity of study designs, animal populations, feeding methods, and diet variables allow for alternate interpretations of study findings.* Because changes in dietary carbohydrate content require changes in the proportion of protein and/or fat, it is difficult to isolate the effect of carbohydrates from that of increased or decreased fat and protein. The question remains, are some levels or sources of carbohydrates deleterious to the health of the cat?

FELINE CARBOHYDRATE METABOLISM

Feline Requirement for Carbohydrates

Adult cats have evolved on a diet that is high in protein and low in carbohydrates. Nursing kittens consume up to 20% of their energy in the form of lactose, while the natural diet of adult cats is less than 5% dry matter carbohydrate.[5] Like most mammals, adult cats do not have a dietary requirement for carbohydrates, although maximum lactation performance and minimization of weight loss are enhanced

---

*American College of Veterinary Internal Medicine Consensus Statement: The role of dietary carbohydrate in causing and managing feline obesity and diabetes mellitus. American College of Veterinary Internal Medicine Forum 2011.

by higher carbohydrate intake in lactating queens.[6] It is clear that kittens greater than 8 weeks of age have no dietary carbohydrate need if adequate protein is supplied to support gluconeogenesis.

Carbohydrate requirements in nursing neonatal kittens have not been reported. Association of American Feed Control Officials (AAFCO) feeding studies were conducted in kittens fed two raw meat formulations compared to a low-carbohydrate canned food. Health parameters and growth rates in kittens fed 0%, 3.9%, or 7.3% dry matter carbohydrate were similar among female kittens and highest in male kittens consuming the 0% dry matter carbohydrate diet.[7]

Physiologic Adaptations of Carbohydrate Metabolism

Several metabolic adaptations in carbohydrate metabolism differentiate the cat from more omnivorous species. Cats, like all other mammals, require metabolic glucose to support cellular requirements for adenosine triphosphate production in the glucose-requiring tissues like nervous tissue, red blood cells, renal medulla, and active reproductive tissues. Efficient metabolism of protein via hepatic gluconeogenesis sustains blood glucose levels in the absence of dietary carbohydrate.

Several physiological changes in cats attest to their adaptation to low-carbohydrate diets. The cat's ability to rapidly digest and absorb sugars and other carbohydrates is reduced through elimination, reduction, or lack of adaptation of glucose-metabolizing enzymes.[8] Cats lack salivary amylase, which is designed to initiate the digestion of starches and, in one study, cats were found to have pancreatic amylase levels that are 5% of the levels in dogs.[9] Brush border disaccharidase activity is 40% that of canine activity.[10] Disaccharidases, amylase, and intestinal sugar transporters in cats are nonadaptive to changes in dietary carbohydrate levels.[8-12]

Enzymatic changes within the liver reflect the cat's evolutionary adaptation to a diet low in carbohydrates, especially simple sugars like glucose and fructose. The cat has low levels of hepatic glucokinase, which limits efficient metabolism of large glucose loads following dietary intake.[8,11] Reports of limited fructose utilization resulting in fructosemia and fructosuria, following high sucrose or fructose intake, have implied there is a lack of active fructokinase in the liver of cats.[13] Interestingly, however, the feline liver demonstrates fructokinase distribution similar to other animals and higher activity of hexokinase compared to canine liver.[14,15] Therefore, altered enzyme activities do not necessarily limit total capacity for hepatic glucose uptake in cats as other pathways may be active; however, the rate of hepatic glucose disposal appears to be slowed.

Hepatic protein catabolic enzymes appear to be constitutively active in cats and provide continuous carbon skeletons (ketoacids) for gluconeogenesis or oxidation. This adaptation facilitates ongoing gluconeogenesis to sustain blood glucose levels during consumption of a low-carbohydrate diet.[8,16]

Digestion and Utilization of Carbohydrates

The aforementioned metabolic adaptations have led many to suggest poor carbohydrate utilization by the cat and a state of adaptive insulin resistance described as *the carnivore connection*.[3] Yet cats readily digest, absorb, and use many types and levels of dietary carbohydrates. Carbohydrate digestion in commercial foods is reported to be greater than 90% for starches and greater than 94% for most sugars, although some studies have reported values as low as 36% for uncooked potato starch.[13,16,17,18] While microbial fermentation of undigested starches in the colon likely overestimates apparent carbohydrate digestibility compared to true carbohydrate digestibility, the difference is not so great as to discount the high digestibility and intestinal uptake of carbohydrates. Lactose digestion declines in kittens with weaning in association with a decrease in intestinal lactase production and downregulation of sugar transporters.[12] Kittens tolerate up to 6 grams lactose/kg body weight (BW) during nursing[5] while adult cats can consume up to 1.3 g/kg BW of lactose/day without adverse gastrointestinal (GI) signs.[13] Starch intake up to 5 g/kg BW/day is readily digested and was suggested by Kienzle[18] as an upper limit for the cat, while de-Oliveira and colleagues demonstrated excellent starch digestibility (up to 6.7 g/kg BW/day) in adult cats.[19]

Experimental feeding studies using uncooked starches and high levels of sugars demonstrate limited capacity for rapid absorption or utilization of these ingredients in cats.[13,14,17,19,20] Carbohydrate digestibility varies based on starch or sugar source, processing, particle size (fine grinding versus coarse meal), and the diet matrix. Thus, defining a level of carbohydrate excess is specific to many ingredient and processing criteria along with specificity of effect.

CARBOHYDRATE EXCESS

While cats do not require dietary carbohydrates, identifying a level of carbohydrate excess is not straightforward. Definition of carbohydrate excess presumes negative health effects from consumption above a defined level. When maximum capacity for carbohydrate digestion is exceeded, excessive fermentation and osmotic effects of undigested sugars in the GI tract lead to bloating, gas production, discomfort, and diarrhea. Lactose consumption above 1.3 g/kg BW/day and above 5 g/kg BW/day for simple sugars and certain starches represents a maximum intake for some adult cats without increasing blood biomarkers of altered carbohydrate metabolism and urinary loss of various monosaccharides.[13,18] Most cats, however, tolerate complex starches in the food matrix at levels of at least 6.7 g/kg BW/day with no observable adverse effect.[19]

Excess dietary carbohydrate may also be practically defined as the amount of carbohydrate added to a food that will imbalance the nutrient profile by limiting the additions of other ingredients and diluting nutrient content. Based on AAFCO nutrient guidelines[21] for adult cats, diets containing carbohydrates of approximately 60% (dry matter or ME) or greater risk unbalancing an adult feline diet. Lesser carbohydrate amounts would impact the diet of kittens due to their higher protein requirements, suggesting an approximate practical carbohydrate maximum for kittens of 40% ME or 51% dry matter.[20] Foods with marginal nutrient concentration or bioavailability may be altered by levels of carbohydrates lower than this maximum, depending on carbohydrate source and the impact of altered nutrient digestion. Protein digestibility is sometimes reduced by high carbohydrate feeding, while the availability of certain minerals (e.g., phosphorus and magnesium) may actually increase with increased carbohydrate feeding.[22]

Carbohydrate Intake and Relationship to Disease

Carbohydrate source and levels of intake may influence metabolic function or disease parameters. Dietary carbohydrates (primarily in the form of sugars) have resulted in changes in water balance, glucose metabolism, secretion of gut incretins, and adipokines.[1-4] While changes are observed in various metabolic pathways, evidence does not support carbohydrate excess as a factor, but more likely reflects adaptive changes to altered nutrient profiles.

Carbohydrates and Urinary Tract Disorders

High-sugar diets may alter urinary tract health by exceeding the renal threshold for monosaccharides and disaccharides, resulting in increased water loss by osmotic diuresis. Glycosuria was demonstrated in cats fed simple sugars between 11% and 40% dry matter while cooked starches up to 40% dry matter had no effect on renal glucose excretion or postprandial blood glucose levels in healthy cats.[13] Renal histologic changes were noted in the kidney of one cat fed high sucrose levels (36.1% dry matter, 7.2 g/kg BW).[13]

The impact of carbohydrate intake on urinary tract disease was reported in an epidemiologic study by Lekcharoensuk and colleagues.[23] Cats fed increased carbohydrates in canned diets (mean 7.84 g/100 kcal ME) compared to the referent group (0.52 to 4.15 g/100 kcal ME) were at increased risk of calcium oxalate urolithiasis. The level of carbohydrate intake had no influence on struvite urolithiases.

Ocular Effects of Carbohydrates

One cat fed 39% galactose developed cataracts that resolved with diet discontinuation.[5,13] Similar findings have been reported for other species but at higher levels of galactose. Thus, 5.6 g/kg BW of galactose intake is clearly in excess, but the threshold for galactose toxicity in cats is unknown.

Role in Satiety

While there is data in dogs to support the use of fiber in promoting satiety, there is little data regarding the role of carbohydrates in appetitive behaviors in cats.[6,7] However, feeding a diet high in complex carbohydrates to obese pet cats at 0.94 g/100 kcal (4.5% dry matter) versus 10.2 g/100 kcal (31.3% dry matter) failed to demonstrate differences in owner satisfaction with appetitive behaviors or weight loss plan.[24]

Role in Obesity

Numerous laboratory and epidemiological studies have been published evaluating the impact of diet profile on rate of weight gain and loss, impact of neutering, energy requirements, glucose levels, and insulin response in healthy cats.* While the results are not uniformly consistent, the majority of studies suggest excess energy consumption, neutering, and limited exercise are the greatest risk factors for obesity. Most studies also support the effect of weight loss (obesity reduction) on improved insulin sensitivity in obese cats.* Epidemiologic studies suggest that high-carbohydrate, low-fat dry foods do not favor the development of obesity, but that feeding energy-dense, high-fat, dry foods in caloric excess does.[25] There may also be some benefit to feeding high-protein, low-carbohydrate food. There appears to be an energetic benefit to feeding high-protein diets for maintenance of lean body mass due to the thermic effect of proteins.[8] While one study evaluating the impact of high-protein diets on energy expenditure in cats did not find a benefit with regard to metabolic rate, it did determine that cats on high-protein diets retained more muscle mass during weight loss.[9]

Therapeutic low-carbohydrate diets and a moderate-carbohydrate, high-fiber diet have been compared to a maintenance high-carbohydrate diet for the management of diabetes mellitus.[26] In five cats, a reduction of postprandial glycemia and insulin levels along with increased nonesterified fatty acids were observed. While the study is limited by the small numbers of cats, the findings suggest low carbohydrate intake and fiber fortification were beneficial as independent factors in improving glycemic regulation. Similar to this observation, mean plasma glucose concentrations were higher in cats fed 12.1 g carbohydrate/100 kcal compared to 8.3 g/100 kcal or 3.2 g/100 kcal (estimated ME of 48%, 33%, or 12.8%, respectively).[27]

Increases in dietary fat and carbohydrate levels in rats and people are suggested to alter the gut microbiome toward lower numbers of Bacteroidetes bacteria and higher numbers of Firmicutes, a pattern termed *obese microbiota* because of improved energy extraction from the diet in this microbial environment.[28-29] Diet is known to influence the microbial population of the feline intestine, but the influence of carbohydrates on an *obese microbiome* in cats has not been described.

While most studies suggest a limited role for carbohydrates in obesity causation, the aforementioned studies suggest carbohydrates in excess of 12.1 g/100 kcal (48% ME) may be inappropriate in obese cats at risk for insulin resistance and impaired glucose tolerance.

---

*American College of Veterinary Internal Medicine Consensus Statement: The role of dietary carbohydrate in causing and managing feline obesity and diabetes mellitus. American College of Veterinary Internal Medicine Forum 2011.

Role in Diabetes Mellitus

Low- to moderate-carbohydrate diets are beneficial in the management of feline diabetes mellitus. Utilizing the cat's innate metabolic adaptations to provide a steady source of glucose from the liver via gluconeogenesis and avoiding postprandial fluctuations in glucose absorption appear to be beneficial in managing diabetic cats.

Sustained hyperglycemia by intravenous (IV) glucose infusion contributes to glucose toxicity of feline beta cells, leading to decreased glucose sensing, impaired insulin secretion, hydropic degeneration, and beta cell death.[29] In addition to glucose toxicity, chronic hyperglycemia leads to chronic stimulation of insulin secretion from beta cells. In people, carbohydrate intolerance, insulin resistance, and hypersecretion of insulin increase the risk of beta cell exhaustion, pancreatic amyloid accumulation, and overt type 2 diabetes mellitus (T2DM). A similar relationship to high carbohydrate feeding has been suggested to occur in the cat and to contribute to the development of diabetes mellitus, although evidence to support this hypothesis is lacking.

Creation of sustained hyperglycemia of 29 mmol/L (522 mg/dL) by IV glucose infusion results in transient diabetes mellitus in the healthy cat.[30] Lower levels of sustained hyperglycemia (17 mmol/L [310 mg/dL]) did not result in glucose toxicity.[30] Postprandial elevation of blood glucose in nonstressed healthy cats is unlikely to reach such levels. Dietary carbohydrate intake across a range of available carbohydrate sources providing 1 g/kg of available carbohydrate was not associated with significant increases in plasma glucose in healthy cats.[31] Dietary carbohydrate ingestion resulted in minimal postprandial blood glucose change when diabetic cats were allowed eat free choice.[32] In normal cats fed once daily, mean plasma glucose levels increased from 8 or more hours postprandially (6.2 mmol/L [112 mg/dL]) and remained elevated up to 12 hours following the rise (4.7 mmol/L [85 mg/dL]).[27,33,34] Further study is needed to assess the relationship of these findings to cats that are fed meals twice daily, fed free choice, or that are obese and insulin resistant.

In diabetic cats treated with long-acting insulin and fed low-carbohydrate foods, several studies have documented improved glucose regulation and insulin sensitivity, but the rate of diabetic remission (becoming noninsulin dependent) varies.[35,36] Higher rates of diabetic remission appear to correlate most closely with control of obesity, but improved blood glucose regulation and reversal of glucose toxicity with a low-carbohydrate diet may contribute to the positive outcome. While diabetic regulation was similar using diets with carbohydrate levels of 3.5 g/100 kcal (12% ME) and 7.6 g/100 kcal (26% ME), remission rates were higher in cats eating the lower carbohydrate level.[35] In a study by Hall and colleagues[36] comparing diets with carbohydrate levels of 1.1 g/100 kcal and 7.9 g/100 kcal, a reduction in serum fructosamine levels was observed when feeding the lower carbohydrate diet, but no differences in other parameters of glucose regulation or remission rates were noted. At present, an upper limit of carbohydrate intake for the treatment of diabetic cats has not been established. From experience and study results to date, it would appear diabetic regulation may benefit from feeding carbohydrate levels below 20% ME or 25% dry matter. Feeding diets with moderate carbohydrate levels, however, especially when supplemented with fiber, provides similar glycemic control.[35] A level of carbohydrate excess for the diabetic cat remains uncertain but would appear to be above 8.3 g/100 kcal in low-fiber foods and possibly higher in fiber-fortified foods.

SUMMARY

Diet composition is known to alter metabolic processes, health, and disease risk in many species. The domestic cat has adapted to a low-carbohydrate diet (less than 2% ME) with resulting limitations on carbohydrate utilization and rate of glucose disposal compared to more omnivorous species. Cats have no dietary requirement for carbohydrates, yet commercial diets commonly provide levels of carbohydrates well above the evolutionary nutritional profile. It has been suggested that high carbohydrate levels, especially those in dry foods, predispose all cats to disorders including glucose intolerance, insulin resistance, obesity, and T2DM. To date, solid evidence to support these hypotheses has not been satisfactorily demonstrated to the majority of experts in the field.

Review of current studies suggests cats have a rate-limiting capacity to digest or use large amounts of simple sugars but tolerate a wide range of starches and complex carbohydrates. Carbohydrate excess is evident for certain simple sugars at levels over 1.3 g/kg BW/day (6.5% ME), with maximum intake of rapidly available starches limited to 4 g/kg BW/day (20% ME). Practical limits based on formulation constraints suggest an approximate maximum of 60% ME carbohydrate in adult diets and a maximum of 40% ME carbohydrate in diets for kittens, as higher carbohydrate levels would limit protein inclusion, creating a nutritionally deficient diet.

High carbohydrate intake does not appear to increase the risk for obesity. Energy excess, low energy expenditure, neutering, and high fat intake have the highest association with obesity development in cats. Evidence supports the conclusion that high-carbohydrate foods can contribute to glucose intolerance in cats with ongoing insulin resistance (obesity) or diabetes. This population of cats often benefits from low carbohydrate feeding. Remission rates for T2DM in cats may increase when low-carbohydrate foods are fed, along with insulin administration, to improve glycemic control. Suggested limits on dietary carbohydrate for cats with T2DM are 20% ME (25% dry matter, 5.8 g/100 kcal ME) in low-fiber foods. Higher levels of carbohydrate combined with dietary fiber provide acceptable diabetic control and remission rates, but an upper limit that would constitute carbohydrate excess has yet to be defined.

References

1. Vondruska JF: The effect of a rat carcass diet on the urinary pH of the cat. *Comp Anim Prac* 1:5–9, 1987.
2. Rucinsky R, Cook A, Haley S, et al: AAHA diabetes management guidelines. *J Am Anim Hosp Assoc* 46:215–224, 2010.
3. Platinga EA, Bosch G, Hendriks WH: Estimation of dietary nutrient profiles of free-roaming feral cats: possible implications for nutrition of domestic cats. *Brit J Nutr* 106:S35–S48, 2011.
4. Zoran DL: The carnivore connection to nutrition in cats. *J Am Vet Med Assoc* 221:1559-1567, 2002.
5. Meyer H: Lactose intake of carnivores. *Wien Tierarztl Monatsschr* 79:236–441, 1992.
6. Piechota T, Rogers QR, Morris JG: Nitrogen requirement of cats during gestation and lactation. *Nut Res* 15:1535-1546, 1995.
7. Hamper BA: Nutritional Adequacy and Performance of Raw Food Diets in Kittens. PhD dissertation, University of Tennessee Knoxville. 2012; 67-78.
8. MacDonald ML, Rogers QR: Nutrition of the domestic cat, a mammalian carnivore. *Ann Rev Nutr* 4:521-562, 1984.
9. Kienzle E: Carbohydrate metabolism of the cat 1. Activity of amylase in the gastrointestinal tract of the cat. *J Am Physio Anim Nutr* 69:92–101, 1993.
10. Kienzle E: Carbohydrate metabolism of the cat 4. Activity of maltase, isomaltase, sucrose, and lactase in the gastrointestinal-tract in relation to age and diet. *J Am Physio Anim Nutr* 70:289–296, 1993.
11. Baker DH, Czarnecki-Maulden GL: Comparative nutrition of cats and dogs. *Ann Rev Nutr* 11:239–263, 1991.
12. Buddington RK, Diamond J: Ontogenetic development of nutrient transporters in cat intestine. *Am J Phys Soc* 263(5):G605–G616, 1992.
13. Kienzle E: Carbohydrate metabolism of the cat 3. Digestion of sugars. *J Anim Physio Anim Nutr* 69:203–210, 1993.
14. Kienzle E: Effect of carbohydrates on digestion in the cat. *J Nutr* 124:2568S–2571S, 1994.

15. Tanaka A, Inoue A, Takeguchi T, et al: Comparison of expression of glucokinase gene and activities of enzymes related to glucose metabolism in livers between dog and cat. *Vet Res Comm* 29(6):477–485, 2005.
16. Washizu T, Tanaka A, Sako T, et al: Comparison of the activities of enzymes related to glycolysis and gluconeogenesis in the liver of dogs and cats. *Res Vet Sci* 67(2):205–206, 1999.
17. Morris JG, Trudell J, Pencovic T: Carbohydrate digestion by the domestic cat (Felis catus). *Br J Nutr* 37(3):365–373, 1997.
18. Kienzle E: Carbohydrate metabolism of the cat 2. Digestion of starch. *J Anim Physio Anim Nutr* 69:102–114, 1993.
19. de Oliveira LD, Carciofi AC, Oliveira MCC, et al: Effects of six carbohydrate sources on diet digestibility and postprandial glucose and insulin responses in cats. *J Anim Sci* 86(9):2237–2246, 2008.
20. Kienzle E: Investigations on intestinal and intermediary metabolism of carbohydrates in the domestic cat (felis catus). *Der Tierarztlichen Hochschule* 1989:219–222, 1989.
21. Association of American Feed Control Officials: 2011 Official Publication-Association of American Feed Control Officials. Association of American Feed Control Officials. 2011.
22. National Research Council (US): *Ad Hoc Committee on Dog, and Cat Nutrition. Nutrient requirements of dogs and cats*, 2006, National Academy Press.
23. Lekcharoensuk C, Osborne CA, Lulich JP, et al: Association between dietary factors and feline calcium oxalate and magnesium ammonium phosphate uroliths. *J Am Vet Med Assoc* 219:1228–1237, 2001.
24. Cline M, Witzel A, Moyers T, et al: Comparison of high fiber and low carbohydrate diets on owner perceived satiety of cats during weight loss. *Am J Anim Vet Sci* 7:218–225, 2012.
25. Lund EM, Armstrong PJ, Kirk CA, et al: Prevalence and risk factors for obesity in adult cats from private US veterinary practices. *Intern J Appl Res Vet Med* 3(2):88–96, 2005.
26. Mimura K, Mori A, Lee P, et al: Impact of commercially available diabetic prescription

diets on short-term post-prandial serum glucose, insulin, triglyceride and free fatty acids concentrations of obese cats. *J Vet Med Sci* 75:929–937, 2013.
27. Hewson-Hughes AK, Gilham MS, Upton S, et al: The effect of dietary starch level on postprandial glucose and insulin concentration in cats and dogs. *Brit J Nutr* 106:S105–S109, 2011.
28. Turnbaugh PJ, Ley RE, Mahowald MA, et al: An obesity-associated gut microbiome with increased capacity for energy harvest. *Nature* 444(7122):1027–1131, 2006.
29. Turnbaugh PJ, Bäckhed F, Fulton L, et al: Diet-induced obesity is linked to marked but reversible alterations in the mouse distal gut microbiome. *Cell Host Microbe* 3(4):213, 2008.
30. Link KRJ, Rand JS: Glucose toxicity in cats (abstract). *J Vet Intern Med* 10:185, 1996 (abstract).
31. Cave NJ, Monroe JA, Bridges JP: Dietary variables that predict glycemic response to whole foods in cats. *Compend Contin Educ Vet* 30:57, 2008 (abstract).
32. Martin GJW, Rand JS: Food intake and blood glucose in normal and diabetic cats fed ad libitum. *J Feline Med Surg* 1(4):241–251, 1999.
33. Mori A, Sako T, Lee P, et al: Comparison of three commercially available prescription diet regimens on short-term post-prandial serum glucose and insulin concentrations in healthy cats. *Vet Res Comm* 33(7):669–680, 2009.
34. Coradini MA, Rand JS, Morton JM, et al: Delayed gastric emptying may contribute to prolonged postprandial hyperglycemia in meal-fed cats. *J Vet Intern Med* 20:726–727, 2006 (abstract).
35. Bennett N, Greco DS, Peterson ME, et al: Comparison of a low carbohydrate–low fiber diet and a moderate carbohydrate–high fiber diet in the management of feline diabetes mellitus. *J Feline Med Surg* 8(2):73–84, 2006.
36. Hall TD, Mahony O, Rozanski EA, et al: Effects of diet on glucose control in cats with diabetes mellitus treated with twice daily insulin glargine. *J Feline Med Surg* 11:125–130, 2009.

Current Concepts in Preventing and Managing Obesity

Angela Witzel

PREVALENCE AND RISK FACTORS

The incidence of human obesity has reached epidemic proportions worldwide. The rate of obesity in the United States population in 2008 was more than 30%, with approximately 10% of the population having elevated fasting blood glucose indicative of diabetes mellitus.[1] Obesity in cats has similar prevalence patterns and health consequences and should receive the same attention from practitioners as other chronic diseases. Cats are typically considered overweight at 10% to 20% above their ideal body weight and obese if their weight exceeds the ideal weight by 20% to 30%.[2,3] Although more studies are needed to conclude this, the number of obese cats may be on the rise in developed countries. In the 1970s, a study by Anderson[4] reported that 6.5% to 12% of cats were overweight or obese. More recent studies report approximately 25% to 40% of cats as being overweight or obese.[5-7] Whereas researchers in New Zealand did not detect a change in obesity prevalence between 1993 and 2008, a door-to-door evaluation of cats revealed that 67% of cats were overweight and 27% were obese.[8] The higher rate of overweight cats in this study could be attributed to having trained researchers evaluating body composition, rather than relying on owner perceptions or general practice evaluations.

The prevalence of feline obesity increases at middle age (5 to 11 years), is often associated with gonadectomy, and is more common in male cats.[7] Several studies in cats suggest that weight gain after spaying or neutering is a combination of increased food intake and slower metabolic rate.[9,10] Neutered male and spayed female cats need approximately 25% to 30% fewer calories to maintain their weight following surgery.[11,12] Activity level does not appear to change significantly following castration.[9] Although it seems intuitive that feeding patterns (e.g., *ad libitum*) would influence the prevalence of obesity, study results have been mixed.[8,13-14]

Genetics may also play a role in the development of obesity. Syndromic obesity secondary to genetic mutations such as Prader-Willi syndrome and leptin receptor deficiencies in humans is rare. Although there appears to be widespread genetic predispositions to being overweight or obese, current human evidence suggests excess energy provided *in utero* and in early child development has a greater impact on obesity development.[15] A study using selective breeding of overweight colony cats provides evidence that inheritance plays a part in obesity development in domestic felids.[16]

HEALTH RISKS OF OBESITY

In human patients, obesity is associated with numerous pathologies, including coronary heart disease, hypertension, dyslipidemias, and type 2 diabetes mellitus. Certain cancers (e.g., breast, ovarian, and prostate), respiratory diseases, osteoarthritis, and reproductive disorders also occur more commonly in conjunction with obesity.[17-20] Many of the same chronic health problems observed in obese humans can be found in obese cats, including diabetes mellitus, neoplasia, dental disease, dermatologic diseases, and lower urinary tract disease.[21] Obese cats are also almost five times more likely to have lameness that requires veterinary care.[21] In addition to the ailments mentioned here, obesity impairs a veterinarian's ability to perform thorough physical examinations of the abdomen and lymph nodes and can make routine diagnostic testing more difficult (e.g., blood collection and urinary cystocentesis are more challenging in obese cats). These factors may lead to delayed detection of serious illness in obese cats.

ADIPOSE TISSUE PATHOLOGY

Another consequence of obesity that likely impacts overall health in cats is increased levels of systemic inflammation. It is thought that hypoxia within adipose tissue is a main factor for inducing inflammation. Obese humans and rodents have been shown to have reduced adipose tissue blood flow. In addition, oxygen can only diffuse through about 120 μm of tissue, and adipocytes can be as large as 150 μm. Obese mice also appear to have reduced angiogenesis and increased vasoconstriction.[22] Chronic inflammatory states result in overproduction of reactive oxygen species and systemic oxidative stress (Figure 64-1). High levels of oxidative stress are thought to be a key link among obesity, vascular abnormalities, and the elevated risk of atherosclerosis and cardiovascular disease in humans.[23]

A variety of endocrine, paracrine, and autocrine signals are released from cells within adipose tissues. These signals are referred to as adipokines.[24] The metabolic role of most

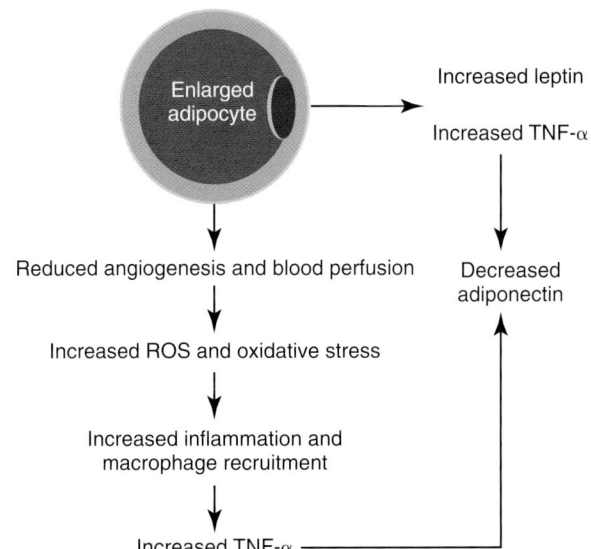

Figure 64-1: Adipocyte Inflammation. With obesity, adipocytes enlarge and have reduced angiogenesis and perfusion. As a result of hypoxia, increased reactive oxygen species and oxidative stress are produced. This leads to elevated inflammatory mediators in the tissue and the recruitment of macrophages, which increase the inflammatory cytokine, tumor necrosis factor-alpha (TNF-α). TNF-α also suppresses production of adiponectin, an anti-inflammatory adipokine. Enlarged adipocytes also release more leptin and TNF-α. *ROS,* reactive oxygen species.

adipokines is complex and incompletely understood. Leptin, adiponectin, and tumor necrosis factor-α (TNF-α) are some of the most intensely studied adipokines. Leptin was the first adipokine identified, and its primary function is to regulate body fat mass through appetite control and increased energy metabolism. Leptin correlates positively with body fat mass in both humans and cats, is able to cross the blood-brain barrier where it inhibits neurotransmitters that increase appetite and lower energy expenditure, and stimulates neurons that decrease appetite and increase in energy expenditure.[25-31] As evidenced by the high prevalence of obesity in both humans and pets, leptin is sometimes unable to effectively regulate appetite and energy expenditure; this is termed "leptin resistance."[32] The consequences of leptin resistance were demonstrated in a clinical study in which leptin had to be administered at a dose 20 to 30 times higher than normal physiological levels to induce significant weight loss in obese human subjects.[33] Similar to humans, obese cats tend to have high levels of serum leptin and may also develop resistance to the metabolic effects of leptin.[26,27] These studies suggest that despite higher concentrations, leptin has an impaired ability to maintain ideal body weight in overweight and obese cats.

One of the most metabolically important adipokines is adiponectin. Although adiponectin is released from adipocytes, higher levels of body fat actually lower its serum concentration. Therefore, overweight individuals have lower circulating levels of adiponectin than lean individuals.[34] The reason for this paradoxical relationship is not clear. Adipocyte

size and insulin sensitivity may affect adiponectin production. As adipocytes swell in size, they become more insulin resistant and secrete less adiponectin *in vitro.*[35] In addition, hormones such as testosterone and inflammatory cytokines such as TNF-α negatively impact adiponectin production.[36,37] Although adiponectin influences metabolism in many ways, perhaps it is best known for its anti-inflammatory and insulin-sensitizing effects. Prospective and longitudinal studies in people demonstrate that lower adiponectin levels are closely associated with insulin resistance, diabetes mellitus, and cardiovascular disease.[38-41]

Tumor necrosis factor-α is an inflammatory cytokine expressed by a variety of cells, including macrophages, mast cells, neuronal cells, fibroblasts, and adipocytes. Although there are species differences, TNF-α secretion from adipose tissue can have significant effects on insulin sensitivity. In human beings, adipose TNF-α primarily acts locally through paracrine and autocrine actions.[42,43] Mice and dogs tend to release adipose TNF-α into the systemic circulation.[44,45] The circulation patterns of TNF-α derived from adipose tissue are not well understood in cats, but messenger ribonucleic acid expression within fat increases with obesity.[46] One of the primary actions of adipose TNF-α is induction of localized insulin resistance. Tumor necrosis factor-α downregulates genes responsible for insulin-mediated glucose uptake into cells.[47-49] In addition to inhibiting glucose entry into cells, TNF-α decreases uptake of free fatty acids (FFAs) into adipocytes and promotes lipolysis and release of FFA into circulation.[42,50,51] As a result, FFA levels increase in circulation and negatively affect insulin sensitivity in peripheral tissues. In addition to directly influencing insulin sensitivity of adipose tissue, TNF-α can alter secretion of other adipokines involved in glucose metabolism. In particular, TNF-α inversely correlates with adiponectin and may alter its gene expression.[42,50,52,53] In summary, TNF-α secreted from adipose tissue plays an important role in glucose and lipid metabolism at both the local and systemic levels and is a key component in inflammation associated with obesity.

PREVENTION OF OBESITY

Owner education is key to obesity prevention. It is important for veterinarians to perform a nutritional assessment and make dietary recommendations at every visit. A good time to discuss obesity prevention is when kittens are spayed or neutered. Many cats need their food intake reduced by 10% to 20% following surgery, and most sexually altered indoor house cats only need to eat about 1.0 to 1.2 times their resting energy requirements (see Treatment) to maintain an ideal body weight. Cats that are spayed or neutered at a young age (less than 12 weeks) can be allowed to continue their current feeding strategy until they are approximately 5 to 6 months old. Once they have reached about 75% of their adult body weight, the kitten may need to have portions monitored closely to prevent excessive weight gain. It is also recommended to have owners measure their cat's food portion, rather than allowing the bowl to always be full. Veterinarians should describe to owners how a cat with ideal body condition looks and feels: an hourglass figure from above, no fat within the inguinal fat pad (although hanging skin is often present), and bony prominences easy to feel, but not protruding. Environmental enrichment is also an important part of obesity prevention so that cats do not overeat out of stress or boredom (see Role of Exercise and Enrichment).

Most indoor cats need about 185 to 300 kcal/day to maintain ideal body weight. Commercial cat foods can vary widely in caloric density. Many grain-free and low-carbohydrate diets can exceed 600 kcal per cup. Therefore, a 9 lb (4 kg) cat may only need about one-third cup of dry food for the entire day. Beginning in 2015, the kilocalorie content per cup is required by Association of American Feed Control Officials on pet food labels and this should help owners and veterinarians to better assess caloric intake. Weight loss in cats can be challenging due to the low-energy intake required, difficulty in promoting exercise, and negative behaviors associated with hunger. Therefore, prevention of obesity is critical, and educating cat owners about what cats should look like and adjusting food intake if they notice weight gain is a necessity.

DIAGNOSIS OF OBESITY

Recognizing obesity in cats is the first step to successful management. Often pet owners and even veterinarians have misconstrued ideas of what an "ideal" body composition for a cat should be. The most precise way to diagnose obesity is via quantitative analysis. The gold standard for quantitative analysis of body composition is via desiccation and chemical analysis of tissues from euthanized or deceased animals. Outside of a research setting, this is not a realistic method to employ; however, it has been used to validate other noninvasive quantitative methods, including radioisotope total body water analysis, dual energy X-ray absorptiometry (DEXA), bioelectrical impedance analysis, and morphometric measurements.[54-56]

Although some methods of quantitative analysis tend to be more objective and accurate than others, body condition scoring is the most commonly used method for estimating body composition in clinical practice. Multiple scales exist, but much of the published research describes the nine-point body condition score (BCS) system (Figure 64-2), which has been validated by DEXA.[57] Each unit increase on the scale is associated with a change of approximately 5% body fat (BF) where an ideal score of 5/9 equates to 20% to 25% BF and 9/9 equals 40% to 45% BF. Another widely used scale is a five-point system where 2.5/5 to 3/5 is considered ideal for most mature cats, based on life stage, lifestyle, and intended use.[3] A major drawback of both scales is an inability to accurately predict % BF in animals with more than 45% BF. A body fat index (BFI) system has recently been developed and validated for overweight cats up to 65% BF (Figure 64-3).[58] Although more validation is needed, morphometric measure-

ments can also be used to assess obesity in cats that are already overweight or obese.[58] Whether one uses the nine-point BCS, BFI system, or morphometric measurements, being familiar with how a patient's assessment equates to percentages of body fat can allow for estimations of ideal body weight for energy calculations and help owners grasp the degree of obesity their cat suffers from (Table 64-1). For example, if a cat weighs 4 lb (9 kg) and has a body condition score of 9/9 (body fat greater than 45%) and a BFI of 60 (approximately 60% BF), one can roughly assume that if 60% of the cat is fat mass then, 40% is lean mass.

$$9.0 \text{ kg} \times 0.4 = 3.6 \text{ kg of lean tissue (60\% BF)}$$

In order to estimate a body weight with the desired 20% BF, one assumes that the lean tissue makes up 80% of the ideal body weight: 3.6 kg/0.8 = 4.5 kg. This can be summarized by the equation: [Current body weight × (100 − % BF)]/0.8 = ideal body weight. Table 64-2 also provides a quick reference for determining ideal body weight from an estimate of body fat percentage.

TREATMENT

The basic premise of weight loss is simple: calorie expenditure should exceed calorie intake. However, practical issues such as owner compliance, multiple-animal households, and dietary restrictions can make weight loss challenging. One must also try to avoid protein and nutrient deficiencies when caloric intake is restricted. What follows is an outline of steps to consider when designing a weight loss plan.

Diet History

By taking a thorough history before prescribing a weight loss strategy, the clinician addresses issues early and minimizes owner frustration. Questions to ask include the following:
- What diet makes up the majority of your cat's food? Diet brand, texture, flavor?
- How much of this food do you feed each day?
- How is the food measured or is it fed *ad libitum*?
- How many times per day do you feed your cat?
- Does your cat get other sources of food or treats? If so, what are they and how much is given?
- Does your cat have access to another pet's food?
- What challenges do you anticipate if we change your cat's diet or restrict food intake?

Getting an accurate diet history can be challenging; sometimes it is not possible to assess how much food a cat is eating (e.g., *ad libitum* feeding or outdoor scavenging). However, having a sense for whether a cat is grossly overfed versus eating an appropriate amount of food may better guide your initial weight loss recommendations. Diet history forms, such as the one provided by the World Small Animal Veterinary Association Global Nutrition Committee (Box 64-1), are helpful.

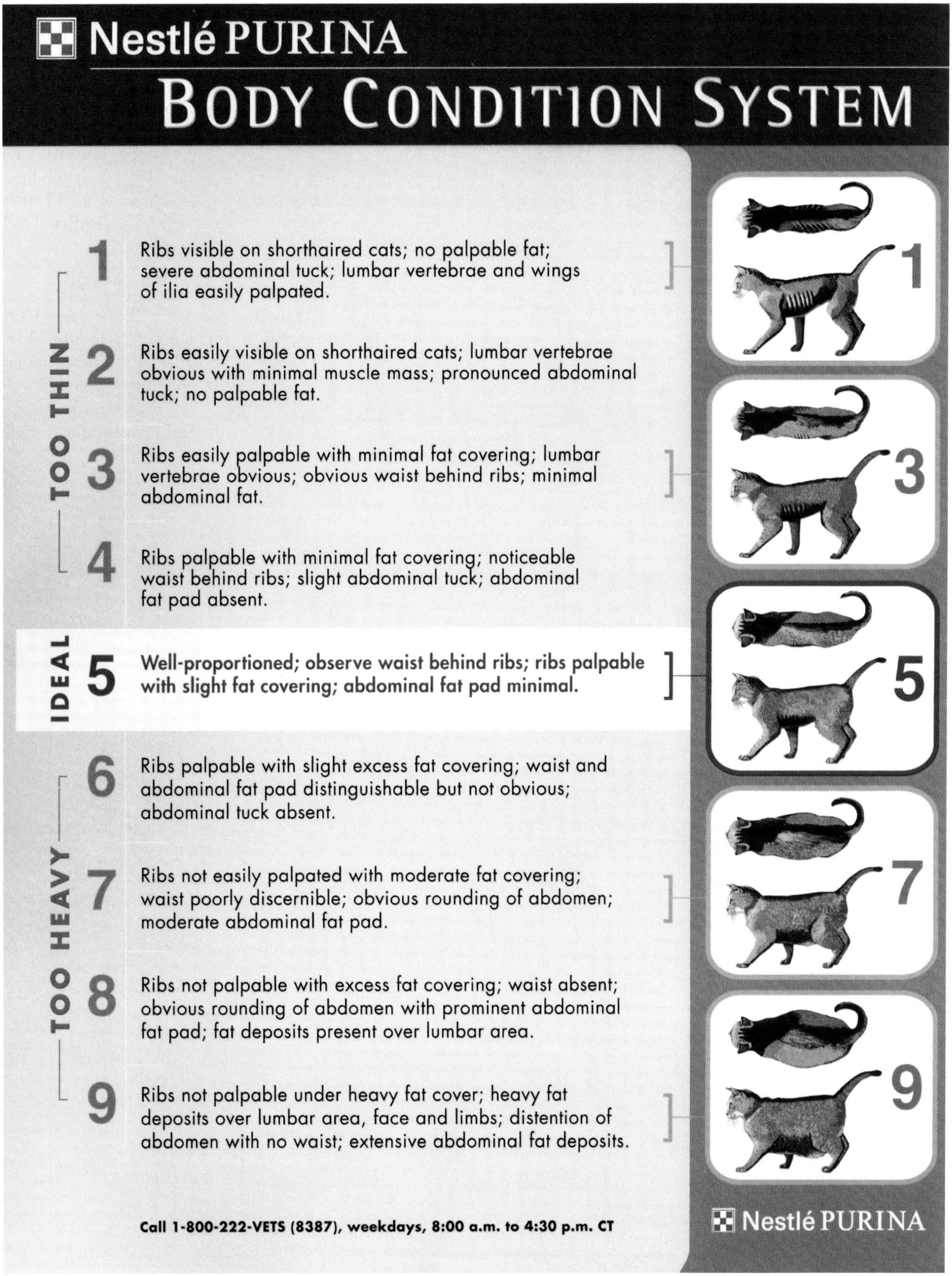

☒ Nestlé PURINA

BODY CONDITION SYSTEM

TOO THIN

1 Ribs visible on shorthaired cats; no palpable fat; severe abdominal tuck; lumbar vertebrae and wings of ilia easily palpated.

2 Ribs easily visible on shorthaired cats; lumbar vertebrae obvious with minimal muscle mass; pronounced abdominal tuck; no palpable fat.

3 Ribs easily palpable with minimal fat covering; lumbar vertebrae obvious; obvious waist behind ribs; minimal abdominal fat.

4 Ribs palpable with minimal fat covering; noticeable waist behind ribs; slight abdominal tuck; abdominal fat pad absent.

IDEAL

5 Well-proportioned; observe waist behind ribs; ribs palpable with slight fat covering; abdominal fat pad minimal.

TOO HEAVY

6 Ribs palpable with slight excess fat covering; waist and abdominal fat pad distinguishable but not obvious; abdominal tuck absent.

7 Ribs not easily palpated with moderate fat covering; waist poorly discernible; obvious rounding of abdomen; moderate abdominal fat pad.

8 Ribs not palpable with excess fat covering; waist absent; obvious rounding of abdomen with prominent abdominal fat pad; fat deposits present over lumbar area.

9 Ribs not palpable under heavy fat cover; heavy fat deposits over lumbar area, face and limbs; distention of abdomen with no waist; extensive abdominal fat deposits.

Call 1-800-222-VETS (8387), weekdays, 8:00 a.m. to 4:30 p.m. CT

☒ Nestlé PURINA

Figure 64-2: Nine-Point Body Condition Scoring System. (Courtesy of Nestlé Purina.)

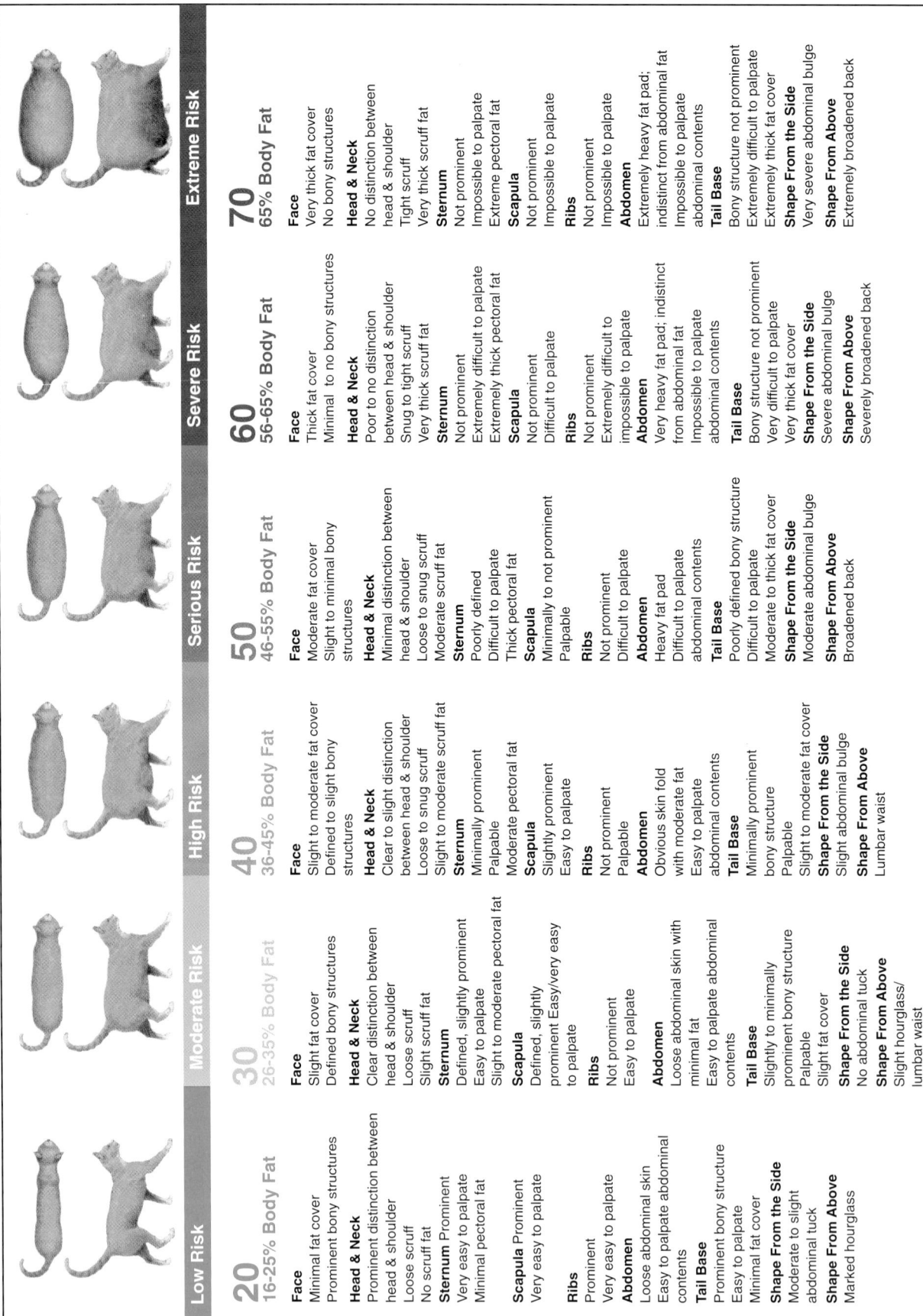

	Low Risk **20** 16-25% Body Fat	Moderate Risk **30** 26-35% Body Fat	High Risk **40** 36-45% Body Fat	Serious Risk **50** 46-55% Body Fat	Severe Risk **60** 56-65% Body Fat	Extreme Risk **70** 65% Body Fat
Face	Minimal fat cover; Prominent bony structures	Slight fat cover; Defined bony structures	Slight to moderate fat cover; Defined to slight bony structures	Moderate fat cover; Slight to minimal bony structures	Thick fat cover; Minimal to no bony structures	Very thick fat cover; No bony structures
Head & Neck	Prominent distinction between head & shoulder; Loose scruff; No scruff fat	Clear distinction between head & shoulder; Loose scruff; Slight scruff fat	Clear to slight distinction between head & shoulder; Loose to snug scruff; Slight to moderate scruff fat	Minimal distinction between head & shoulder; Loose to snug scruff; Moderate scruff fat	Poor to no distinction between head & shoulder; Snug to tight scruff; Very thick scruff fat	No distinction between head & shoulder; Tight scruff; Very thick scruff fat
Sternum	Prominent; Very easy to palpate; Minimal pectoral fat	Defined, slightly prominent; Easy to palpate; Slight to moderate pectoral fat	Minimally prominent; Palpable; Moderate pectoral fat	Poorly defined; Difficult to palpate; Thick pectoral fat	Not prominent; Extremely difficult to palpate; Extremely thick pectoral fat	Not prominent; Impossible to palpate; Extreme pectoral fat
Scapula	Prominent; Very easy to palpate	Defined, slightly prominent; Easy/very easy to palpate	Slightly prominent; Easy to palpate	Minimally to not prominent; Palpable	Not prominent; Difficult to palpate	Not prominent; Impossible to palpate
Ribs	Prominent; Very easy to palpate	Not prominent; Easy to palpate	Not prominent; Palpable	Not prominent; Difficult to palpate	Not prominent; Extremely difficult to impossible to palpate	Not prominent; Impossible to palpate
Abdomen	Loose abdominal skin; Easy to palpate abdominal contents	Loose abdominal skin with minimal fat; Easy to palpate abdominal contents	Obvious skin fold with moderate fat; Easy to palpate abdominal contents	Heavy fat pad; Difficult to palpate abdominal contents	Very heavy fat pad; indistinct from abdominal fat; Impossible to palpate abdominal contents	Extremely heavy fat pad; indistinct from abdominal fat; Impossible to palpate abdominal contents
Tail Base	Prominent bony structure; Easy to palpate; Minimal fat cover	Slightly to minimally prominent bony structure; Palpable; Slight fat cover	Minimally prominent bony structure; Palpable; Slight to moderate fat cover	Poorly defined bony structure; Difficult to palpate; Moderate to thick fat cover	Bony structure not prominent; Very difficult to palpate; Very thick fat cover	Bony structure not prominent; Extremely difficult to palpate; Extremely thick fat cover
Shape From the Side	Moderate to slight abdominal tuck	No abdominal tuck	Slight abdominal bulge	Moderate abdominal bulge	Severe abdominal bulge	Very severe abdominal bulge
Shape From Above	Marked hourglass	Slight hourglass/lumbar waist	Lumbar waist	Broadened back	Severely broadened back	Extremely broadened back

Figure 64-3: Body Fat Index. Descriptions of the Body Fat Index (BFI) system. One can mark assessments in each category and count which columns have the most descriptions to assign a BFI. (Courtesy of Hills Pet Nutrition.)

5-Point Scale	9-Point Scale	Body Fat Index	% Body Fat
1	1	—	≤5
2	2	—	6-9
	3	—	10-14
3	4	20	15-19
	5		20-24
4	6	30	25-29
	7		30-34
5	8	40	35-39
	9		40-44
—		50	45-54
		60	55-64

Table 64-1 Comparison of Composition Assessment Methods with Their Respective Body Fat Percentages

BOX 64-1 Veterinary Nutrition Resources

American College of Veterinary Nutrition:
http://www.acvn.org.
European Society of Veterinary and Comparative Nutrition:
http://www.esvcn.eu.
World Small Animal Veterinary Association Global Nutrition
Committee Toolkit: http://www.wsava.org/nutrition-toolkit.

Estimating Desired Caloric Intake

Obesity occurs when energy intake exceeds energy output. Energy output can also be called the daily energy requirement (DER). It comprises several components, but the resting energy requirement (RER) and the exercise energy requirement (EER) are the two largest contributors. The RER is the energy needed to maintain normal metabolic functions (e.g., blood flow, cellular metabolism, and respiration) and is closely correlated with lean body mass. The RER typically accounts for 60% to 80% of the total DER. The EER is the energy exerted through muscular activity and exercise and accounts for roughly 10% to 20% of DER in inactive humans. Compared with lean mass, fat mass contributes little to the RER. Therefore, estimations of RER should be based on ideal rather than current weight using the following formula:

$$RER = 70 \times (\text{body weight}_{kg}^{0.75})$$

If a scientific calculator is not available (although most smartphones and computer calculators have an x^y function key), the linear equation achieves similar results in animals that weigh more than 2 kg (4.4 lb) and less than 30 kg (66 lb):

$$RER = (30 \times \text{body weight}_{kg}) + 70$$

BOX 64-2 Weight Loss Case Example

A 7-year-old, male, castrated domestic shorthair cat weighing 7 kg (15.4 lb) with a body condition score of 9/9, a body fat index of 40, and estimated percentage of body fat of 40% arrives at your clinic for a weight loss program. First, you must estimate his ideal weight so you can calculate energy needs. You do not have a history of this cat's weight at around 1 year of age, and the owner says he has always been a little heavy. Therefore, you calculate his ideal weight with the formula: [Current body weight × (100 − % fat)]/0.8 = ideal body weight. This equals 5.25 kg (11.5 lb).

Next, resting energy requirement (RER) is calculated based on ideal weight (5.25 kg): $70 \times (5.25_{kg}^{0.75})$ = 242 kcal/day. You decide to feed at 0.8 × RER: 242 × 0.8 = 194 kcal/day = daily energy requirement for weight loss.

Two weeks later, the patient returns weighing 6.75 kg. To calculate the rate of weight loss, you take the amount lost (0.25 kg) and divide by the initial weight (0.25 kg/7 kg = 0.035 × 100 = 3.5%). Next, divide by the number of weeks you are assessing (3.5%/2 weeks = 1.8% weight loss per week).

The DER needed to achieve weight loss is then estimated using the RER. The result is the total number of calories that should be fed in a 24-hour period. For cats, it is typically recommended to feed 80% of their RER at ideal weight for weight loss (DER = 0.8 × RER). Careful monitoring of patients should occur during any weight loss program. Because cats need to eat small volumes of food, weighing portions with a kitchen scale is more accurate and allows greater flexibility in calorie adjustment than relying on measuring cups.[59] The goal is to achieve 1% to 2% loss of body weight per week. Although the formulas given here are useful for initial estimations, many cats require further restriction to achieve weight loss. Reducing energy by 10% of calories every 2 weeks until adequate weight loss is achieved may be necessary.

It is not uncommon for patients to have their rate of weight loss slow down several months into a weight loss plan. If a cat is losing at 0.5% per week after being on a plan for a while, this is still a desirable rate. However, if weight loss slows to less than 0.5% per week, further restricting calories by 10% to 20% may be needed. Cats can safely eat as little as 60% of their ideal weight RER without concern for hepatic lipidosis.[60] A case example is provided in Box 64-2.

Choosing an Appropriate Diet

Weight loss diets for cats typically fall into two categories: over-the-counter light and lean products or therapeutic weight loss diets (available by veterinary prescription only). Although over-the-counter products may be sufficient in animals that are mildly overweight, therapeutic weight loss diets are recommended for moderate to substantial weight loss. Owners often ask if they can simply reduce the amount fed of the animal's current diet. Switching to a diet designed

Table 64-2	Chart Depicting Ideal Body Weight Values (lb) Based on Current Body Weight and Estimated Body Fat Percentages					
Current Weight (lb)	20% BF	30% BF	40% BF	50% BF	60% BF	70% BF
8	8	7.0	6.0	5.0	4.0	3.0
9	9	7.9	6.8	5.6	4.5	3.4
10	10	8.8	7.5	6.3	5.0	3.8
11	11	9.6	8.3	6.9	5.5	4.1
12	12	10.5	9.0	7.5	6.0	4.5
13	13	11.4	9.8	8.1	6.5	4.9
14	14	12.3	10.5	8.8	7.0	5.3
15	15	13.1	11.3	9.4	7.5	5.6
16	16	14.0	12.0	10.0	8.0	6.0
17	17	14.9	12.8	10.6	8.5	6.4
18	18	15.8	13.5	11.3	9.0	6.8
19	19	16.6	14.3	11.9	9.5	7.1
20	20	17.5	15.0	12.5	10.0	7.5
21	21	18.4	15.8	13.1	10.5	7.9
22	22	19.3	16.5	13.8	11.0	8.3
23	23	20.1	17.3	14.4	11.5	8.6
24	24	21.0	18.0	15.0	12.0	9.0
25	25	21.9	18.8	15.6	12.5	9.4
26	26	22.8	19.5	16.3	13.0	9.8
27	27	23.6	20.3	16.9	13.5	10.1
28	28	24.5	21.0	17.5	14.0	10.5
29	29	25.4	21.8	18.1	14.5	10.9
30	30	26.3	22.5	18.8	15.0	11.3
31	31	27.1	23.3	19.4	15.5	11.6
32	32	28.0	24.0	20.0	16.0	12.0
33	33	28.9	24.8	20.6	16.5	12.4
34	34	29.8	25.5	21.3	17.0	12.8
35	35	30.6	26.3	21.9	17.5	13.1

For example, a cat with a current weight of 12 lb and 30% body fat would have an estimated ideal body weight of 10.5 lb.
Courtesy Hill's Pet Nutrition. *BF,* body fat.

for weight loss is a more desirable approach. Maintenance foods are balanced to provide adequate amounts of nutrients when standard feeding guidelines are followed. When the amount of a maintenance diet is significantly reduced below feeding recommendations, deficiencies in protein and other nutrients can occur. Diets formulated for weight loss are balanced to provide both adequate nutrients and energy restriction. In addition, carnitine supplementation may aid in weight loss and fatty acid oxidation, and most therapeutic weight loss diets have increased levels of carnitine.[61,62] Car-

nitine may also help prevent the development of hepatic lipidosis.[63] In cases in which the diet cannot be changed because of medical conditions, the quantity of the current diet can be reduced, but review of total intake should be performed to ensure adequate nutrient intake, and consultation with a veterinary nutritionist may be warranted (Box 64-1).

In recent years, there has been much debate about the most appropriate diets for feline weight control (see Chapter 63). Cats are strict carnivores and naturally consume high-protein and high-fat diets with few carbohydrates. Therefore, some veterinarians are advocating low-carbohydrate weight loss diets for cats instead of more traditional high-fiber weight loss diets. Dietary protein is a potent stimulator for the release of satiety hormones. Prescription diets currently marketed for feline weight loss all contain similar levels of protein but vary in their fat and carbohydrate content. Studies have shown that low-carbohydrate diets have beneficial effects on insulin sensitivity and diabetic control.[64] However, a study evaluating only weight loss in cats did not detect any differences between low-carbohydrate and high-fiber diets.[65] Although canned diets appear to reduce voluntary food intake in cats,[66] a comparison of low-carbohydrate versus high-fiber canned diets with similar protein levels showed no difference in owner-perceived satiety.[67] In summary, cats should ideally be placed on a canned diet designed for weight loss and calorie restriction. The diet should contain sufficient levels of protein (ideally more than 100 g protein/1000 kcal) and other nutrients to avoid muscle wasting or vitamin and mineral deficiencies. If a cat eats only dry food, owner compliance may be better if a lower-caloric-density high-fiber weight loss diet, rather than a calorie-dense, low-carbohydrate dry food is used.

Role of Exercise and Enrichment

Increasing physical activity is an intuitive part of any weight loss program, and some creativity may be needed when trying to increase the physical activity levels of cats. Indoor cats lead more sedentary lives than outdoor cats, and special efforts must be made to increase their activity. Owners can begin by changing the cat's environment; window hammocks, platforms, and cat furniture provide more vertical space for cats to explore. Barriers such as baby gates force cats to exert more effort while moving around the house. Meals can be served on surfaces that require cats to climb. Toys that hide kibble and require effort to extract it can occupy some cats (Figure 64-4). In addition, owner interaction in the form of play can be very effective. Even increasing play or exercise for just 10 minutes per day can be highly effective in promoting weight loss.

Troubleshooting

To be effective long term, weight loss plans must work for an owner's lifestyle and preserve the human-animal bond. Therefore, it is important to address owner concerns and design appropriate plans for the household. For example, many cat owners in multicat households struggle when some cats are thin and like to graze on food all day and another is obese. In these cases, the thin cats might be able to jump onto surfaces (such as a clothes dryer) that the obese cat cannot. One could also cut a hole in a large plastic container or cardboard box that is big enough for thin cats but too small for the larger cat and place food inside the container (Figure 64-5). In addition, collar or microchip systems are available that work with specialized crates or feeders to allow only animals with the collar or microchip to enter.

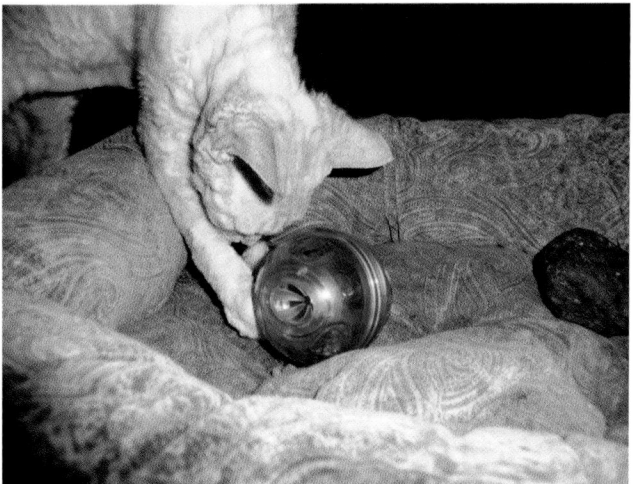

Figure 64-4: Treat Dispensing Toys. An example of a treat-dispensing toy ball. Overweight cats are often reluctant to play with toys, so providing food in a toy encourages play and provides a more engaging method of accessing food. (Photo courtesy of Steve Dale.)

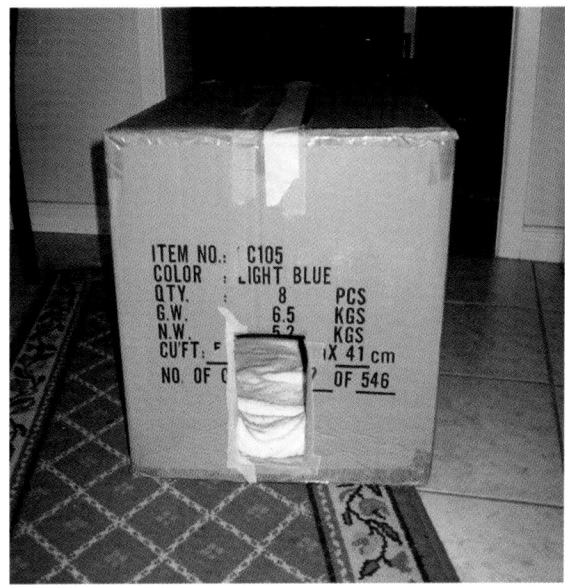

Figure 64-5: Example of Size-Restricted Food Access. Restricting a cat's access to food in a multicat household can be challenging. If other cats are thin and require *ad libitum* feeding, one can cut a hole in a large cardboard box that is big enough for the thin cat, but too small for the overweight cat to enter. Food for the thin cat can be placed in the box. (Photo courtesy of Berga MacGillivray.)

Begging behavior is a common problem with cats on restricted-calorie diets. Owners should be reassured that their cat is receiving all of the nutrients it needs. Dividing food into smaller, more frequent meals may help. It is also important to offer a social or environmental substitute for food. Owners could hide bits of food around the house for the cat to find or play with or hide food in treat-dispensing toys. It can also be helpful to disassociate the owner from meals by using automated feeders. Feeding in rooms that are infrequently used (e.g., spare bedroom or bathroom) can also decrease unwanted behaviors in frequently trafficked rooms such as the kitchen.

Acceptance of a new diet can be especially challenging in cats. Very gradual changes are recommended for finicky cats. Owners may need to very slowly add a higher proportion of the new food over a 2- to 4-week period. For example, feed 10% of the new diet, 90% of the old diet for 3 to 4 days, then try 20% new diet, 80% old diet for 3 to 4 days, etc. Cats often have very strong texture preferences, so it may be especially difficult to get an exclusively dry-food eater to accept a canned diet and vice versa. If human foods or home-made diets are desired, then owners should consult with a veterinary nutritionist (Box 64-1).

Maintaining after Weight Loss

Obese cats that have lost weight usually require lifelong calorie restriction. Once a cat reaches its ideal body weight, one can try increasing caloric intake by 10% to 20% (depending on rate of weight loss) and checking weight in 1 month to look for gains or continued losses. It is essential for owners to continue regular weight rechecks over the next 3 to 4 months to determine the number of calories needed to achieve weight maintenance.

SUMMARY

For many veterinarians, overweight cats present a frustrating challenge. It is important to remember that even partial weight loss is beneficial for health. If a cat can reduce from 50% to 35% BF, it will dramatically reduce the risk of diabetes and joint disease. Educating owners about the morbidities associated with obesity and listening to their concerns will improve success. It is critical to design weight loss plans that work for the owner's household and lifestyle. Rechecking weight monthly is perhaps the most important aspect of any weight loss program. These visits provide accountability, encouragement, and troubleshooting. Cats can lose weight, and using a team approach with the owner is the key to success.

References

1. World Health Organization: World Health Statistics 2013. <http://www.who.int/gho/publications/world_health_statistics/2013/>, 2013 (Accessed December 5, 2014.)
2. Toll P, Yamka R, Schoenherr W, et al: Obesity. In Hand M, Thatcher C, Remillard R, et al, editors: Small animal clinical nutrition, ed 5, Topeka, 2010, Mark Morris Institute, pp 501–544.
3. Toll P, Burkholder W, et al: Obesity. In Hand M, Thatcher C, Remillard R, editors: Small animal clinical nutrition, ed 4, Topeka, 2000, Mark Morris Institute, pp 401–430.
4. Anderson RS: Obesity in the dog and cat. Vet Annu 14:182–186, 1973.
5. Courcier EA, O'Higgins R, Mellor DJ, et al: Prevalence and risk factors for feline obesity in a first opinion practice in Glasgow, Scotland. J Feline Med Surg 12:746–753, 2010.
6. Colliard L, Paragon B, Lemuet B, et al: Prevalence and risk factors for obesity in an urban population of healthy cats. J Feline Med Surg 11:135–140, 2009.
7. Lund E, Armstrong P, Kirk C, et al: Prevalence and risk factors for obesity in adult cats from private US veterinary practices. Intern J Appl Res Vet Med 3:88–96, 2005.
8. Cave N, Allan F, Schokkenbroek S, et al: A cross-sectional study to compare changes in the prevalence and risk factors for feline obesity between 1993 and 2007 in New Zealand. Prev Vet Med 107:121–133, 2012.
9. Kanchuk ML, Backus RC, Calvert CC, et al: Weight gain in gonadectomized normal and lipoprotein lipase-deficient male domestic cats results from increased food intake and not decreased energy expenditure. J Nutr 133: 1866–1874, 2003.
10. Fettman MJ, Stanton CA, Banks LL, et al: Effects of neutering on bodyweight, metabolic rate and glucose tolerance of domestic cats. Res Vet Sci 62:131–136, 1997.
11. Mitsuhashi Y, Chamberlin AJ, Bigley KE, et al: Maintenance energy requirement determination of cats after spaying. Br J Nutr 106:S135–S138, 2011.
12. Russell K, Sabin R, Holt S, et al: Influence of feeding regimen on body condition in the cat. J Small Anim Pract 41:12–17, 2000.
13. Allan FJ, Pfeiffer DU, Jones BR, et al: A cross-sectional study of risk factors for obesity in cats in New Zealand. Prev Vet Med 46:183–196, 2000.
14. Scarlett J, Donoghue S, Saidla J, et al: Overweight cats: prevalence and risk factors. Int J Obes Relat Metab Disord 8:S22–S28, 1994.
15. Savona-Ventura C, Savona-Ventura S: The inheritance of obesity. Best Pract Res Clin Obstet Gynaecol 29:300–308, 2015.
16. Haring T, Wichert B, Dolf G, et al: Segregation analysis of overweight body condition in an experimental cat population. J Hered 102:S28–S31, 2011.
17. ten Hacken NHT: Physical inactivity and obesity: relation to asthma and chronic obstructive pulmonary disease? Proc Am Thorac Soc 6:663–667, 2009.
18. Fulop T, Tessier D, Carpentier A: The metabolic syndrome. Pathol Biol 54:375–386, 2006.
19. Teucher B, Rohrmann S, Kaaks R: Obesity: focus on all-cause mortality and cancer. Maturitas 65:112–116, 2010.
20. Guh D, Zhang W, Bansback N, et al: The incidence of co-morbidities related to obesity and overweight: a systematic review and meta-analysis. BMC Public Health 9:88, 2009.
21. Scarlett J, Donoghue S: Associations between body condition and disease in cats. J Am Vet Med Assoc 212:1725–1731, 1998.
22. Ye J, Gimble J: Regulation of stem cell differentiation in adipose tissue by chronic inflammation. Clin Exp Pharmacol Physiol 38:872–878, 2011.
23. Alfadda AA, Sallam RM: Reactive oxygen species in health and disease. J Biomed Biotechnol 936486, 2012.
24. Fain JN, Tagele BM, Cheema P, et al: Release of 12 adipokines by adipose tissue, nonfat cells, and fat cells from obese women. Obesity 18:890–896, 2010.
25. Zhang F, Chen Y, Heiman M, et al: Leptin: structure, function and biology. Vitam Horm 71:345–372, 2005.
26. Appleton DJ, Rand JS, Sunvold GD: Plasma leptin concentrations in cats: reference range, effect of weight gain and relationship with adiposity as measured by dual energy X-ray absorptiometry. J Feline Med Surg 2:191–199, 2000.
27. Backus RC, Havel PJ, Gingerich RL, et al: Relationship between serum leptin immunoreactivity and body fat mass as estimated by use of a novel gas-phase Fourier transform infrared spectroscopy deuterium dilution method in cats. Am J Vet Res 61:796–801, 2000.
28. Martin LJM, Siliart B, Dumon HJW, et al: Spontaneous hormonal variations in male cats following gonadectomy. J Feline Med Surg 8:309–314, 2006.
29. Hoenig M, Thomaseth K, Waldron M, et al: Insulin sensitivity, fat distribution, and adipocytokine response to different diets in lean and obese cats before and after weight loss. Am J Physiol Regul Integr Comp Physiol 292:R227–R234, 2007.

30. Oswal A, Yeo GSH: The leptin melanocortin pathway and the control of body weight: lessons from human and murine genetics. *Obes Rev* 8:293–306, 2007.

31. Horvath TL: Synaptic plasticity in energy balance regulation. *Obesity* 14:228S–233S, 2006.

32. Shimizu H, Oh-I S, Okada S, et al: Leptin resistance and obesity. *Endocrine J* 54:17–26, 2007.

33. Heymsfield SB, Greenberg AS, Fujioka K, et al: Recombinant leptin for weight loss in obese and lean adults: a randomized, controlled, dose-escalation trial. *JAMA* 282:1568–1575, 1999.

34. Arita Y, Kihara S, Ouchi N, et al: Paradoxical decrease of an adipose-specific protein, adiponectin, in obesity. *Biochem Biophysical Res Commun* 257:79–83, 1999.

35. Waki H, Yamauchi T, Kamon J, et al: Generation of globular fragment of adiponectin by leukocyte elastase secreted by monocytic cell line THP-1. *Endocrinology* 146:790–796, 2005.

36. Swarbrick M, Havel P: Physiological, pharmacological, and nutritional regulation of circulating adiponectin concentrations in humans. *Metab Syndr Relat Disord* 6:87–102, 2008.

37. Iwaki M, Matsuda M, Maeda N, et al: Induction of adiponectin, a fat-derived antidiabetic and antiatherogenic factor, by nuclear receptors. *Diabetes* 52:1655–1663, 2003.

38. Côté M, Cartier A, Reuwer AQ, et al: Adiponectin and risk of coronary heart disease in apparently healthy men and women (from the EPIC-Norfolk Prospective Population Study). *Am J Cardiol* 108:367–373, 2011.

39. Lindsay RS, Funahashi T, Hanson RL, et al: Adiponectin and development of type 2 diabetes in the Pima Indian population. *Lancet* 360:57–58, 2002.

40. Yamamoto Y, Hirose H, Saito I, et al: Adiponectin, an adipocyte-derived protein, predicts future insulin resistance: two-year follow-up study in Japanese population. *J Clin Endocrinol Metab* 89:87–90, 2004.

41. Snehalatha C, Mukesh B, Simon M, et al: Plasma adiponectin is an independent predictor of type 2 diabetes in Asian Indians. *Diabetes Care* 26:3226–3229, 2003.

42. Ryden M, Arner P: Tumour necrosis factor-alpha in human adipose tissue—from signalling mechanisms to clinical implications. *J Internal Med* 262:431–438, 2007.

43. Mohamed-Ali V, Goodrick S, Rawesh A, et al: Subcutaneous adipose tissue releases interleukin-6, but not tumor necrosis factor-alpha, in vivo. *J Clin Endocrinol Metab* 82:4196–4200, 1997.

44. Hotamisligil GS, Shargill NS, Spiegelman BM: Adipose expression of tumor necrosis factor-alpha: direct role in obesity-linked insulin resistance. *Science* 259:87–91, 1993.

45. German AJ, Hervera M, Hunter L, et al: Improvement in insulin resistance and reduction in plasma inflammatory adipokines after weight loss in obese dogs. *Domest Anim Endocrinol* 37:214–226, 2009.

46. Hoenig M, McGoldrick JB, deBeer M, et al: Activity and tissue-specific expression of lipases and tumor-necrosis factor [alpha] in lean and obese cats. *Domest Anim Endocrinol* 30:333–344, 2006.

47. Stephens JM, Lee J, Pilch PF: Tumor necrosis factor-alpha-induced insulin resistance in 3T3-L1 adipocytes is accompanied by a loss of insulin receptor substrate-1 and GLUT4 expression without a loss of insulin receptor-mediated signal transduction. *J Biol Chem* 272:971–976, 1997.

48. Qi C, Pekala PH: Tumor necrosis factor-alpha induced insulin resistance in adipocytes. *Proc Soc Exp Biol Med* 223:128–135, 2000.

49. Peraldi P, Xu M, Spiegelman BM: Thiazolidinediones block tumor necrosis factor-alpha induced inhibition of insulin signaling. *J Clin Invest* 100:1863–1869, 1997.

50. Cawthorn WP, Sethi JK: TNF-[alpha] and adipocyte biology. *FEBS Lett* 582:117–131, 2008.

51. Memon RA, Feingold KR, Moser AH, et al: Regulation of fatty acid transport protein and fatty acid translocase mRNA levels by endotoxin and cytokines. *Am J Physiol* 274:E210–E217, 1998.

52. Kita A, Yamasaki H, Kuwahara H, et al: Identification of the promoter region required for human adiponectin gene transcription: Association with CCAAT/enhancer binding protein-[beta] and tumor necrosis factor-[alpha]. *Biochem Biophys Res Commun* 331:484–490, 2005.

53. Kim KY, Kim JK, Jeon JH, et al: c-Jun N-terminal kinase is involved in the suppression of adiponectin expression by TNF-alpha in 3T3-L1 adipocytes. *Biochem Biophys Res Commun* 327:460–467, 2005.

54. Mawby DI, Bartges JW, d'Avignon A, et al: Comparison of various methods for estimating body fat in dogs. *J Am Anim Hosp Assoc* 40:109–114, 2004.

55. Speakman J, Booles D, Butterwick R: Validation of predictive equations for use of deuterium oxide dilution to determine body composition of dogs and cats. *Intern J Obesity* 25:439–447, 2001.

56. Burkholder W: Dissertation: Body composition of dogs and cats determined by carcass composition analyis, deuterium oxide dilution, subjective and objective morphometry, and bioelectrical impedance. Virginia Polytechnic Institute and State University, 1994.

57. Laflamme D: Development and validation of a body condition score system for cats: a clinical tool. *Feline Pract* 25:13–18, 1997.

58. Witzel A, Kirk CA, Toll P, et al: A morphometric method and body fat index system for improved estimation of body composition in overweight and obese cats. *J Am Vet Med Assoc* 244:1285–1290, 2014.

59. German AJ, Holden SL, Mason SL, et al: Imprecision when using measuring cups to weigh out extruded dry kibbled food. *J Anim Physiol Anim Nutr (Berl)* 95:368–373, 2011.

60. Biourge V, Groff J, Munn R, et al: Experimental induction of hepatic lipidosis in cats. *Am J Vet Res* 55:1291–1302, 1994.

61. Center SA, Harte J, Watrous D, et al: The clinical and metabolic effects of rapid weight loss in obese pet cats and the influence of supplemental oral L-carnitine. *J Vet Intern Med* 14:598–608, 2000.

62. Center SA, Warner KL, Randolph JF, et al: Influence of dietary supplementation with l-carnitine on metabolic rate, fatty acid oxidation, body condition, and weight loss in overweight cats. *Am J Vet Res* 73:1002–1015, 2012.

63. Ibrahim WH, Bailey N, Sunvold GD, et al: Effects of carnitine and taurine on fatty acid metabolism and lipid accumulation in the liver of cats during weight gain and weight loss. *Am J Vet Res* 64:1265–1277, 2003.

64. Bennett N, Greco DS, Peterson ME, et al: Comparison of a low carbohydrate-low fiber diet and a moderate carbohydrate-high fiber diet in the management of feline diabetes mellitus. *J Feline Med Surg* 8:73–84, 2006.

65. Michel KE, Bader A, Shofer FS, et al: Impact of time-limited feeding and dietary carbohydrate content on weight loss in group-housed cats. *J Feline Med Surg* 7:349–355, 2005.

66. Wei A, Fascetti A, Villaverde C, et al: Effect of water content in canned food on voluntary food intake and body weights in cats. *Am J Vet Res* 72:918–923, 2011.

67. Cline M, Witzel A, Moyers T, et al: Comparison of high fiber and low carbohydrate diets on owner-perceived satiety of cats during weight loss. *Am J Anim Vet Sci* 7:218–225, 2012.

Current Feeding Practices of Cat Owners

Martha G. Cline

The majority of cat owners feed nutritionally complete and balanced commercial pet foods. A survey of feeding practices from the United States and Australia including 469 cat owners found that 98.8% of cats consumed at least half of their intake from commercial foods.[1] Twenty-nine percent of cats received at least half of their diet from canned foods and 13.1% of cats were provided noncommercial foods (i.e., table scraps, leftovers, or home-made foods) as part of their main diet. Data from this study was collected in 2004, prior to the large-scale pet food recall in 2007 involving the illegal adulteration of pet foods with melamine. Since this recall, there appears to be a growing interest in alternative feeding practices that can range from simply providing a more natural commercial product to providing home-prepared cooked or raw-meat based foods.

The provision of vegan or vegetarian, raw meat-based diets (RMBDs), or home-cooked diets is an area of controversy for owners and veterinarians. It is the responsibility of the veterinarian to inform cat owners of the risks involved with feeding these types of diets and the level of appropriateness for each pet. There are also a growing number of pet foods that are marketed as all natural, grain-free, byproduct-free, or organic. Many of these types of food are made due to consumer demand and do not reflect a known benefit to the animal. It is important for the veterinarian to understand marketing strategies used by the pet food industry and definitions behind popular claims. The inclusion of high levels of carbohydrates in commercial cat foods has also received much attention and debate among veterinarians and the public. A detailed discussion of the use of carbohydrates in commercial cat foods and their potential impact on health and disease in domestic cats can be found in Chapter 63.

CATS AS OBLIGATE CARNIVORES

Cats are obligate carnivores and require nutrients found in meat sources (see Chapter 62). Cats have a high protein requirement due to the lack of adaptation of urea cycle enzymes and regulation of aminotransferases for nitrogen metabolism.[2,3] The protein requirement of adult cats to maintain lean body mass (LBM) is now thought to be higher than the current 2006 National Research Council (NRC) (50 grams/1000 kcal metabolizable energy [ME]) and Association of American Feed Control Officials (AAFCO) (65 grams/1000 kcal ME) guidelines which are

based on studies determining nitrogen balance.[4,5] Adult cats fed a high protein diet (95 grams/1000 kcal) for 2 months gained LBM, while cats fed both a moderate (73 grams/1000 kcal) and a low (56 grams/1000 kcal) protein diet lost LBM.[6] Cats in all dietary groups were able to maintain nitrogen balance by the end of the study. The researchers concluded that while current recommendations are sufficient to maintain nitrogen balance, a higher amount of protein is needed to maintain LBM (7.8 g/kg^{75}).

Cats have a dietary requirement for taurine, which is found in high amounts in animal tissues. This is the result of a low rate of hepatic synthesis due to low enzyme activities in the synthetic pathway, microbial degradation in the intestinal lumen, and the exclusive use of taurine to conjugate bile acids.[3,7,8] Cats cannot convert beta-carotene, the precursor of vitamin A found in plants, to retinol which must be provided in the diet.[3,9] The synthesis of arachidonic acid, found in animal tissues, from linoleic acid is limited in cats due to low amounts of hepatic Δ-6 desaturase.[10] Niacin, found in abundance in animal tissues as nicotinamide adenine dinucleotide and nicotinamide adenine dinucleotide phosphate coenzymes, cannot be synthesized sufficiently from tryptophan in the cat as in other species.[3] These are just some of the unique nutritional requirements making the cat an obligate carnivore.

NATURAL, ORGANIC, GRAIN-FREE, AND BYPRODUCT-FREE PET FOODS

According to AAFCO guidelines, a natural ingredient or product is derived solely from plant, animal, or mined sources.[5] The ingredient or product can still be physically or heat processed, rendered, purified, extracted, hydrolyzed, fermented, or undergo enzymolysis. In the author's experience, many pet owners are under the impression that labeling a pet food product as natural reflects minimal processing, which it may not. A natural product cannot however be chemically synthesized or contain any chemically synthesized additives or preservatives. A pet food that does not bear an *all natural* claim may be using vitamins, minerals, additives, or preservatives that have been chemically synthesized, while protein, fat, and carbohydrate ingredients will come from natural sources. Organic ingredients must be produced and handled in compliance with the requirements of the United States Department of Agriculture National Organic Program.[5]

Terms such as premium, holistic, or gourmet have no legal definition or regulation in the pet food industry.

Grain-free cat diets are also readily available to consumers. To the author's knowledge, there are no studies demonstrating a benefit of a grain-free diet when compared to diets that contain grain. These types of diet may be used because the consumer is attempting to avoid potential grain allergens. The most common types of food-related allergens reported in the cat include beef, dairy products, and fish.[11] It is possible that some cats may demonstrate food intolerance or allergy to grain-based products, and when documented, these ingredients should be avoided. It is important to note that grain-free diets often still contain carbohydrate, which may ultimately be what the consumer is trying to avoid.

Animal-based byproducts used in pet foods are primarily organ meats and may contain high quality protein and fat with natural sources of vitamins and minerals. The AAFCO definition of meat byproducts is the nonrendered, clean parts, other than meat, derived from slaughtered mammals including, but not limited to, lungs, spleen, kidneys, brain, liver, blood, bone, partially defatted low-temperature fatty tissue, stomachs, and intestines freed from their contents.[5] Byproducts do not include hair, horns, teeth, and hoofs. Poultry byproduct can include feet, necks, and undeveloped eggs, while excluding feathers. Many owners have misconceptions about byproducts, and their definitions should be discussed when these concerns arise. Commonly used pet food terms and definitions are provided in Table 65-1.

VEGAN AND VEGETARIAN DIETS

Given the unique nutritional requirements of cats as obligate carnivores, vegan and vegetarian diets are generally not recommended. However, veterinarians will encounter owners wanting to feed vegan or vegetarian diets. It is important to recognize why owners may be making these decisions and to know how to ensure they are meeting their cat's nutritional needs. Results of a telephone survey indicated the primary reason owners choose to feed a vegetarian diet was due to ethical concerns.[12] Other reasons cited included the perception that conventional cat foods are unwholesome and purported health benefits of a vegetarian diet, including a decreased risk of cancer and healthier hair coat. For these reasons, it may be difficult for veterinarians to persuade owners feeding vegetarian or vegan diets to change. Choosing a reputable commercial product or working with a board certified veterinary nutritionist is advised.

Two commercial vegan diets labeled to be nutritionally complete and balanced when compared to AAFCO nutrient profile for adult maintenance in cats have been independently evaluated.[13] Investigators found that both diets contained multiple deficiencies, including less than the AAFCO minimums for methionine, taurine, arachidonic acid, and pyridoxine. One diet, labeled for all life stages (adult maintenance including growth and reproduction) was found to be deficient in crude protein, lysine, methionine, taurine, arachidonic acid,

Table 65-1	Commonly Used Pet Food Terminology
Term	**AAFCO Definition**
Natural	A feed or ingredient derived solely from plant, animal, or mined sources; can either be unprocessed or subject to physical processing, including heat processing, rendering, purification, extraction, hydrolysis, enzymolysis, or fermentation; cannot undergo chemical synthetic processing or contain chemically synthetic additives or processing aids
Organic	Must be produced or handled in compliance with the requirements of the USDA National Organic Program
Byproduct	Meat: nonrendered, clean parts, other than meat from the slaughter of mammals, including lungs, spleen, kidneys, brain, liver, blood, bone, partially defatted low temperature fatty tissue, and stomachs and intestines freed of their contents; does not include hair, horns, teeth, and hoofs Poultry: ground, rendered, clean parts of the carcass from slaughter, including necks, feet, undeveloped eggs, and intestines; exclusive of feathers
Meal	An ingredient which has been ground or otherwise reduced in particle size
Human-grade	No legal definition, may be considered false and misleading by AAFCO*
Premium	Not an official feed term
Holistic	Not an official feed term
Gourmet	Not an official feed term

*Association of American Feed Control Officials Labeling & Labeling Requirements. <http://petfood.aafco.org/labelinglabelingrequirements.aspx#human_grade> (Accessed August 31, 2014.)
AAFCO, Association of American Feed Control Officials; *USDA*, United States Department of Agriculture.
Source: *Association of American Feed Control Officials: 2013 Official publication.* Association of American Feed Control Officials, Inc, 2013.

BOX 65-1 Nutrients of Concern Typically Derived From Meat Sources That Must be Addressed for Cats on a Vegetarian or Vegan Diet

Total protein intake
Taurine
Arachadonic acid
Vitamin A
Vitamin B_{12} (cobalamin)
Niacin

---

calcium, phosphorus, vitamin A, niacin, pyridoxine, and vitamin B_{12} when compared to AAFCO nutrient profiles for growth and reproduction in cats. Based on this information, veterinarians should encourage owners feeding a vegan or vegetarian commercial diet to use products that have undergone both nutrient laboratory analysis and feeding trials before use rather than diets that have simply been formulated to meet the nutrient requirements.

Several nutrients are of particular concern for cats on vegan or vegetarian diets (Box 65-1). Whole blood taurine and serum cobalamin concentrations were measured in 17 cats fed a commercial vegetarian diet, vegetarian food prepared with a commercially available supplement, or a combination of the two for greater than 1 year.[12] Serum cobalamin concentrations were within the reference range for all cats. Whole blood taurine concentrations were below the reference range in three cats, but above the point of clinical deficiency (200 nmol/L), suggesting that their intake of taurine was marginal. Cats fed meat-free diets should be regularly evaluated by a veterinarian to monitor for signs of nutrient deficiency. The author recommends annual evaluation of complete blood count, biochemistry panel, urinalysis, whole blood taurine, and serum cobalamin levels, especially for those cats fed home-prepared diets. As part of their regular physical exam, special attention should be given to the patient's muscle condition score, skin, and hair coat to monitor for subtle signs of inadequate protein or essential fatty acid intake. Owners providing home-prepared vegetarian or vegan diets should be offered referral to a board-certified veterinary nutritionist (or person with equivalent training) for nutritional evaluation of their cat's diet and to ensure proper supplementation of essential nutrients.

HOME-PREPARED DIETS

Home-prepared diets can provide complete and balanced nutrition when formulated and prepared properly. These types of diets can contain cooked or raw ingredients or a combination of both. The two areas of controversy surrounding home-prepared diets are the nutritional adequacy and the safety of RMBDs, both of which have led to considerable debate in the public forum.

Motivations Behind Home-Prepared Diets

A variety of reasons exist for why owners choose to home prepare their pet's food. This may stem from distrust or concerns regarding commercial pet food products; to avoid additives, preservatives, or potential contaminants; to offer a more natural or organic diet; as a way to strengthen the human-animal bond; out of habit to feed finicky eaters; or to manage a medical condition.[14,15] A home-prepared diet may be recommended by a veterinarian for a variety of reasons, including a food trial to rule out possible food allergy or intolerance, poor appetite for commercial therapeutic foods, or due to concurrent medical conditions where no commercial diet is available. For example, there are currently no commercial food options for a cat with advanced chronic kidney disease and concurrent food allergy; therefore, a home-prepared diet may be recommended.

It may be a challenge for some cats to accept a home-prepared diet if they have consumed commercial pet food for a long period of time. This can be due to sensitivities related to the hedonic aspects of their food, including odor, form, texture, and palatability.[16,17] Dietary preferences can be influenced in the cat as early as the prenatal period.[18] The author recommends a trial period using recommended ingredients to test the cat's acceptance and level of tolerance of new ingredients prior to formulation of a home-prepared diet.

Impact on Health

Few studies are available evaluating the health impact of home-prepared diets in cats. A recent study evaluating the oral health of 6371 cats found a higher probability of an oral health problem in cats eating a home-prepared diet when compared to cats eating a commercial canned or dry food or a home-prepared diet in combination with a commercial food.[19] The investigators reported cats fed a home-prepared diet had a significantly higher probability of an oral health problem (56%) compared to cats fed a dry commercial diet (24%). Many owners will report a benefit of smaller stool volumes, less fecal odor, and improved gastrointestinal (GI) health for pets fed home-prepared cooked or raw meat-based diets.[14] One study investigated the impact of a commercial raw beef-based diet fed raw or cooked in the microwave to at least 160°F on total tract energy and macronutrient digestibility in cats.[20] The investigators found no difference in dry matter, organic matter, crude protein, fat, and gross energy digestibility between the cooked and raw diets, and both diets had an overall high digestibility.

Nutritional imbalance of home-prepared diets, raw or cooked, can lead to a variety of clinical manifestations. Nutritional secondary hyperparathyroidism has been reported in a number of cats manifesting as spontaneous fracture, muscle twitching, or seizures.[21] Figure 65-1 depicts a case of a 6-month-old Serval kitten kept as a house pet with diffuse osteopenia and pathologic vertebral fracture of L5 due to nutritional secondary hyperparathyroidism after consuming a diet exclusively of raw chicken breast meat. Other cases of

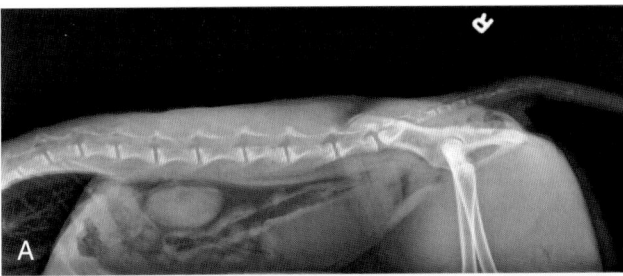
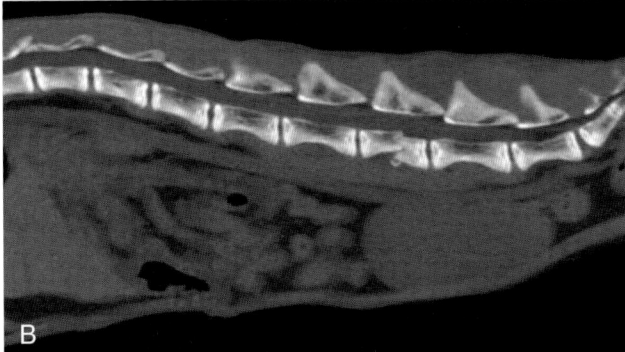
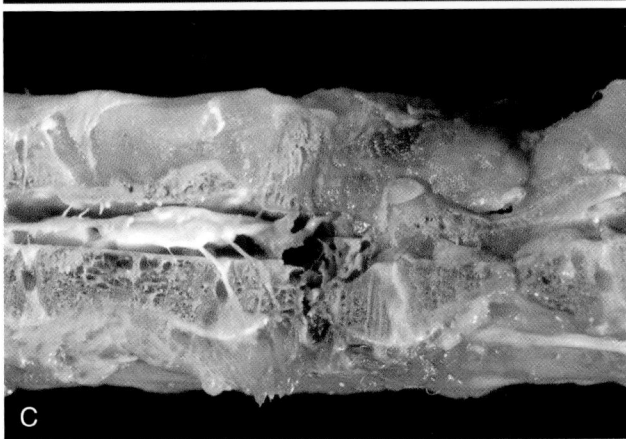

Figure 65-1: Lateral spinal radiograph **(A)**, computed tomography scan **(B)**, and necropsy photo **(C)** of spinal cord from a six-month-old female spayed Serval kitten with a pathologic fracture of L5 and diffuse osteopenia from nutritional secondary hyperparathyroidism. This kitten had consumed a diet consisting solely of chicken breast meat since it was adopted. (Images copyright University of Tennessee College of Veterinary Medicine, Knoxville.)

clinical disease associated with deficient diets are documented in the veterinary literature. Metabolic osteopathy with extensive new bone formation from hypervitaminosis A was reported in a 9-year-old, male castrated, domestic shorthair cat fed a home-prepared diet of raw pork liver.[22] Pansteatitis secondary to vitamin E deficiency in the face of high polyunsaturated consumption has also occurred in cats consuming home-prepared diets of pig brains or oily fish such as sardines, anchovies, and mackerel.[23] Four RMBDs (beef, bison, elk, and horse) for exotic and domestic cats were found to have essential fatty acid deficiencies.[24] Clinical cases of nutritional imbalances are considered to be rare in veterinary medicine due to the availability of complete and balanced commercial products. However, with the growing popularity of home-prepared diets, cooked or raw, and the susceptibility of veterinary patients to these nutrient imbalances, a diet history is recommended with all veterinary patients presenting for evaluation.

Nutritional Assessment of Home-Prepared Diets

Owners may obtain published recipes from a variety of sources, including the Internet, pet magazines, and books written by veterinarians and nonveterinarian with varying levels of nutritional training. Several studies[25-28] have evaluated the nutrition adequacy of home-prepared diets in companion animals. However, only one of these studies[28] has evaluated diets specifically for cats. Twenty-eight diets promoted for use in cats with chronic kidney disease were evaluated and found to have deficiencies below the NRC nutrient recommended allowances for crude protein (42.9%), choline (82.1%), selenium (32.1%), zinc (67.9%), and calcium (25%).[28] An evaluation of 200 published home-prepared recipes for adult maintenance in dogs written by veterinarians (64.5%) and nonveterinarians (35.5%) revealed at least one essential nutrient deficiency according to NRC or AAFCO guidelines in the majority of diets (95%), and 83.5% of recipes had multiple deficiencies.[25] Unfortunately, many published recipes for companion animals for both health and disease are nutritionally inadequate.

When evaluating home-prepared diets for cats, it is important to first identify the presence of essential nutrients, including protein, fat, minerals, trace minerals, and vitamins. An animal-based protein source and supplemental taurine is recommended. Cats do not have a nutritional requirement for carbohydrates, and home-prepared diets can be formulated without their inclusion. Carbohydrates can provide energy and serve as a source of dietary fiber, both soluble and insoluble, to optimize intestinal health.[14] Some cats may benefit from the use of carbohydrates during lactation,[29] for the inclusion of fiber, or if restriction of protein or fat is needed. If carbohydrates are used, a ratio of 1:1 or 1:2 protein to carbohydrate is recommended.[15] A source of linoleic acid should be provided by a specific vegetable oil such as corn or canola oil but can also be provided by some animal fats. Animal-based fat is specifically required to provide arachidonic acid. A source of macro (i.e., calcium, phosphorus) and trace (i.e., zinc, copper, selenium) minerals should be present as well as a source of both water-soluble and fat-soluble vitamins.

Ingredient amounts should be specific and include both weight (grams or ounces) and common measurements where appropriate (e.g., 140 grams [1 cup of chopped or diced] boneless, skinless, roasted chicken breast). Descriptions of ingredients should not be vague (e.g., chicken or beef) but should contain descriptions of types of cuts and/or fat percentages (e.g., chicken thigh without bone or skin or 90% lean ground beef). The recipe should indicate if the ingredient should be measured prior to or following cooking. Many feline vitamin and mineral supplements are inadequate to balance home-prepared diets unless specifically formulated to do so. Human vitamin and mineral supplements have varying formulations, some of which may be harmful to companion animals (e.g., high levels of vitamin D, poorly bioavailable forms of copper); therefore, specific supplements should be recommended in a recipe. Ingredient substitutions can be made, but the proportions of carbohydrate, protein, and fat should be maintained. Clients should be instructed to follow any recipe meticulously and to consult with their veterinarian before making any adjustments.

The author recommends that home-prepared diets be obtained or evaluated by a board-certified veterinary nutritionist or a veterinarian with advanced training in nutrition able to recognize and minimize health risks through formulation and preparation. A directory of diplomats is available through the American College of Veterinary Nutrition (http://www.acvn.org) and the European Society of Veterinary and Comparative Nutrition (http://www.esvcn.eu).

RAW MEAT-BASED DIETS

In the United States and Australia, raw food or bones were reported to be fed at least daily as part of the main meal in 9.6% of cats, and another 0.9% of cats received raw meat or bones as a treat or snack at least once weekly.[1] *Biologically appropriate raw food* or *bone and raw food* (BARF) diets came to popularity in the early 1990s with the publications of several highly publicized raw feeding guidelines.[30-32] To date, there is limited data available on the health impacts of RMBDs in cats. Much of the scientific literature surrounding cats and RMBD concerns nutritional adequacy and digestibility. Further studies are needed to investigate many of the claims that are often cited by advocates of RMBDs. An extensive review of the literature surrounding RBMDs in veterinary medicine has recently been published by Freeman and colleagues.[33]

Nutritional Adequacy of Raw Meat-Based Diets

Raw meat-based diets are available commercially or can be home-prepared. These diets will include uncooked meat ingredients from a variety of animal species that include skeletal muscles, internal organs, bones, egg, or in some cases unpasteurized milk.[33] Commercial RMBDs come in a variety of forms, including fresh, frozen, or freeze dried. These diets can be nutritionally complete and balanced, formulated to meet AAFCO recommendations, and may have even undergone feeding trials to evaluate their nutritional adequacy. Some RMBDs will be labeled for intermittent or supplemental feeding only, indicating they are not nutritionally complete and balanced. Carbohydrate-based premixes containing vitamins and minerals intended to be mixed with raw meat provided by the owner are also available. Owners should be instructed to review the AAFCO statement on any com-

mercial food to ensure it is complete and balanced for their pet's appropriate life stage.

In order to mimic the natural diet of wildcats, the use of whole prey may be advocated. In one study, whole 1- to 3-day-old chicks and adult ground chicken were found to meet macronutrient requirements but were deficient in some mineral requirements, including manganese, copper, potassium, and sodium compared to AAFCO requirements for domesticated cats.[34] These diets were not evaluated for vitamin content. The authors of this study suggested a need to monitor whole-prey composition and to adjust the diet for potential nutrient deficiencies if necessary.

Potential Benefits of Raw Meat-Based Diets

Owners may choose to feed a RMBD to their cats due to anecdotal health benefits and to provide a more natural or ancestral diet. Many of these benefits remain unproven, although the body of scientific evidence surrounding RMBDs in cats is small. Cats in the wild will consume a variety of small prey to support survival and reproduction, and some owners will choose to mimic this type of diet closely. However, this same type of diet may not be optimal for domestic cats expected to live long and healthy lives, as they have been moved indoors and reproductively altered. As previously demonstrated,[34] some whole-prey animals may not be nutritionally adequate for long-term feeding in adult cats. As well, the diet of prey animals (e.g., mice and chicks) sold for pet consumption may not be naturally based, so their nutrient profile may differ from wild prey.

Several authors[30,32] have cited that heat processing foods will alter or destroy nutrients and essential enzymes needed for digestion, making these types of diets inappropriate for companion animals. Heat processing through canning or extrusion of dry foods can result in physical changes to proteins and amino acids such as denaturation and the loss of secondary and tertiary protein structure. The Maillard reaction, responsible for the browning of foods during heat processing, accounts for significant losses in amino acids and may have harmful biologic effects.[35] To counter the losses of amino acids from Maillard reactions, pet food manufacturers must ensure their formulations maintain the nutrition adequacy of the diet. However, heat processing may improve the digestibility of animal proteins through collagen breakdown and plant-based proteins through denaturing of antinutritional factors such as trypsin and chymotrypsin inhibitors.[33]

Several studies have demonstrated a high digestibility of RMBDs fed to both exotic and domestic cats when compared to extruded diets.[20,24,36,37] One study[37] reported a significantly higher digestibility for crude protein but not fat, energy, or dry matter, while another study[20] reported significantly higher digestibility for energy, crude protein, fat, dry matter, and organic matter of the RMBD when compared to an extruded dry diet. The differences in these studies may be related to the composition of the specific dry extruded diets used. The high digestibility of these diets can result in decreased fecal output, which is perceived as a benefit by some owners.[37] Enhanced immune function is also cited as a benefit of consuming a RMBD. Domestic cats consuming a RMBD had a significant increase in lymphocyte and immunoglobulin production when compared to cats eating a commercial cooked moist diet.[38] Cats in this study shed *Salmonella* spp. in their feces, and it is unclear if their immune response is related to a higher exposure to potentially pathologic microbes, changes in intestinal microflora, or the nutritional differences in the diet. Additionally, no significant differences between the RMBD groups and the cooked diet group were found in feline herpesvirus-specific titers following vaccination or parameters of innate immune response, including oxidative burst and phagocytosis. The author concludes that additional studies are needed to evaluate cell-mediated immunity, secretory immunoglobulin A levels, and microbiome changes in animals consuming a RMBD compared to a heat-processed commercial pet food.

The Safety of Raw Meat-Based Diets

In addition to the nutritional imbalances that can occur with home-prepared RMBDs, the potential for pathogen contamination and the health risk to the animals consuming these foods as well as the people and other in-contact animals are concerns. These concerns have led organizations such as the American Veterinary Medical Association, the American Animal Hospital Association, and the Canadian Veterinary Medication Association to discourage the use of RMBDs.[39-41] Bones included in RMBDs also present a health risk, as they can cause obstruction or perforation of the GI tract and can damage teeth. Bone foreign bodies were present in the esophagus of two of 33 cats presenting to a referral practice for evaluation of esophageal disease.[42]

A number of studies have documented the presence of bacterial contamination in both commercial and home-prepared RMBDs for dogs and cats.[43-48] A recent study by the United States Food and Drug Administration (FDA) found that out of 196 commercial RMBDs, 15 (7.7%) were positive for *Salmonella*, and 32 (16%) positive for *Listeria monocytogenes*.[43] *L. monocytogenes* is of a particular public health concern due to its high mortality rate (20-30%), with over 90% of people infected requiring hospitalization.[43] Another study examining 25 commercial raw canine and feline RMBDs found *Clostridium perfringens* in 20% of diets, *Escherichia coli* in 64%, *Salmonella spp.* in 20%, *Clostridium difficile* in 4%, and *Staphylococcus aureus* in 4% based on bacterial culture.[45] *Salmonella spp.* contamination is found in raw meats sold for human consumption at reported rates of up to 44% in nonorganic chicken and 4% in beef and pork; therefore, it is not surprising to find *Salmonella* contamination in RMBDs for animal consumption.[49,50] Consuming a RMBD is a risk factor for *Toxoplasma gondii* infection in cats, as demonstrated in studies in multiple countries.[51-53] Once fed a RMBD containing *Salmonella*, cats can shed bacteria in their feces.[33,48] Septicemic salmonellosis in two cats resulting in death after being fed a diet containing uncooked beef has

been reported.[54] In one of the cases, *Salmonella newport* was isolated and found to be identical to the bacteria isolated in the diet.

Clinical Recommendations and Resources

No studies are currently available on the number of cats or people exposed to RMBDs or animals consuming RMBDs that have become sick as a result of their exposure. The potential for human and animal disease with both commercial and home-prepared RMBDs is well documented. Food utensils, feeding bowls, litter boxes, additional areas of possible fecal contamination, the RMBD itself, and cats with bacteria present in their mouths or on their coats secondary to grooming habits are all sources of potential pathogen exposure for people. Further research is needed on the potential health consequences of contamination from RMBDs for both people and animals. The risk of pathogen contamination is particularly a concern among elderly, young, pregnant, lactating, or immunocompromised pets and people. Policies to protect veterinary staff and hospitalized animals from pathogens shed in feces are recommended when treating an animal consuming a RMBD. Veterinarians should discuss the risks associated with RMBDs with their clients and document these conversations in the medical record. Several resources are available to help veterinarians discuss with clients the selection of commercial pet food products and tools for navigating nutritional information about cats on the Internet (Box 65-2). Recommendations for selecting commercial cat foods are summarized in Box 65-3. Manufacturers of pet foods should be able to provide reasonable answers to each of the questions provided. If they are unable to answer these questions, the client should be advised to avoid the company. The FDA also has resources available on safe handling tips for pet food and treats and recommendations to owners who choose to feed a RMBD (see Box 65-4). The owners should be advised that even with thorough cleaning, contamination

---

BOX 65-2 Resources to Help Pet Owners With the Selection of Commercial Pet Food Products and Tools for Navigating Nutritional Information About Cats on the Internet

Baldwin K, Bartges J, Buffington T, et al: AAHA nutritional assessment guidelines for dogs and cats. *J Am Anim Hosp Assoc* 46:285-296, 2010. <https://www.aahanet.org/Library/NutritionalAsmt.aspx> (Accessed July 23, 2015.)

World Small Animal Veterinary Association Global Nutrition Committee. The savvy cat owner's guide: nutrition on the internet. http://www.wsava.org/sites/default/files/nutrition on the internet cats.pdf. Accessed July 23, 2015.

World Small Animal Veterinary Association Global Nutrition Committee: Recommendations on selecting pet foods. <http://www.wsava.org/sites/default/files/Recommendations on Selecting Pet Foods.pdf.> (Accessed July 23, 2015.)

BOX 65-3 Recommendations for Selecting Commercial Pet Foods

1. Does the company employ a full-time qualified nutritionist, and can they provide their name and qualifications? Nutritionist qualifications include those with either a PhD in animal nutrition or board certification by the American College of Veterinary Nutrition or the European College of Veterinary Comparative Nutrition.
2. Who formulates the company's diets and what are their credentials?
3. Are the company's diets tested using AAFCO feeding trials or by formulation to meet AAFCO nutrient profiles? If the diets are formulated, is the finished product analyzed to ensure it meets the AAFCO nutrient profiles?
4. Where are the diets produced and manufactured?
5. What specific quality control measures does the company employ to assure the consistency and quality of its ingredients and end-products?
6. Can the company provide a complete nutrient analysis for a specific dog or cat food beyond a guaranteed analysis? Ideally, it should be able to provide the amount of all AAFCO-required nutrients on an energy basis (gram or milligram per 100 or 1000 kilocalories) or dry matter percentage.
7. What kind of product research has the company conducted? Are the results of these studies published in peer-reviewed journals?

AAFCO, Association of American Feed Control Officials.
Adapted from: World Small Animal Veterinary Association Global Nutrition Committee: Recommendations on selecting pet foods. <http://www.wsava.org/sites/default/files/Recommendations on Selecting Pet Foods.pdf.> (Accessed July 23, 2015.)

BOX 65-4 United States Food and Drug Administration's Recommendations for Handling Raw Meat-Based Diets

After handling a RMBD, wash hands thoroughly for at least 20 seconds with soap and hot water.
RMBDs should be frozen until ready to use.
Thaw RMBDs in the refrigerator or microwave (not countertop or sink).
RMBDs should be separate from other foods.
All surfaces, bowls, utensils, and any items that come into contact with a RMBD should be thoroughly washed with soap and hot water, and then disinfected.
Cover and refrigerate or toss out leftover RMBDs.
Plastic or nonporous cutting boards should be washed in the dishwasher after each use.

RMBD, raw meat-based diet.
Source: Food and Drug Administration: Tips for safe handling of pet food and treats. <http://www.fda.gov/AnimalVeterinary/ResourcesforYou/AnimalHealthLiteracy/ucm369141.htm> (Accessed July 23, 2015.)

of harmful bacteria may remain on food preparation surfaces, utensils, and food bowls. Forty-two percent and 67%, respectively, of plastic and stainless steel food bowls remained contaminated with *Salmonella* following experimental exposure after a warm water rinse and scrub followed by a 5-minute immersion in 10% bleach solution or washing in a dishwasher at 85 °C (185 °F) respectively.[55] The author strongly recommends consultation with a board-certified veterinary nutritionist or individual with similar training for owners wanting to home prepare any diet, whether raw or cooked.

References

1. Laflamme DP, Abood SK, Fascetti AJ, et al: Pet feeding practices of dog and cat owners in the United States and Australia. *J Am Vet Med Assoc* 232:687–694, 2008.
2. Rogers QR, Morris JG, Freedland RA: Lack of hepatic enzymatic adaptation to low and high levels of dietary protein in the adult cat. *Enzyme* 22:348–356, 1977.
3. Morris JG: Idiosyncratic nutrient requirements of cats appear to be diet-induced evolutionary adaptations. *Nutr Res Rev* 15:153–168, 2002.
4. National Research Council Ad Hoc Committee on Dog and Cats: *Nutrient requirements of dogs and cats,* Washington, DC, 2006, National Academies Press.
5. *Association of American Feed Control Officials: 2013 Official publication.* Champaign, IL, Association of American Feed Control Officials, 2013.
6. Laflamme DP, Hannah SS: Discrepancy between use of lean body mass or nitrogen balance to determine protein requirements for adult cats. *J Feline Med Surg* 15:691–697, 2013.
7. Rentschler LA, Hirschberger LL, Stipanuk MH: Response of the kitten to dietary taurine depletion: effects on renal reabsorption, bile acid conjugation and activities of enzymes involved in taurine synthesis. *Comp Biochem Physiol B* 84:319–325, 1986.
8. Morris JG, Rogers QR, Kim SW, et al: Dietary taurine requirement of cats is determined by microbial degradation of taurine in the gut. *Adv Exp Med Biol* 359:59–70, 1994.
9. Zoran DL: The carnivore connection to nutrition in cats. *J Am Vet Med Assoc* 221:1559–1567, 2002.
10. Pawlosky R, Barnes A, Salem N, Jr: Essential fatty acid metabolism in the feline: relationship between liver and brain production of long-chain polyunsaturated fatty acids. *J Lipid Res* 35:2032–2040, 1994.
11. Verlinden A, Hesta M, Millet S, et al: Food allergy in dogs and cats: a review. *Crit Rev Food Sci Nutr* 46:259–273, 2006.
12. Wakefield LA, Shofer FS, Michel KE: Evaluation of cats fed vegetarian diets and attitudes of their caregivers. *J Am Vet Med Assoc* 229:70–73, 2006.
13. Gray CM, Sellon RK, Freeman LM: Nutritional adequacy of two vegan diets for cats. *J Am Vet Med Assoc* 225:1670–1675, 2004.
14. Weeth LP: Focus on nutrition: home-prepared diets for dogs and cats. *Compend Contin Educ Vet* 35:E1–E3, 2013.
15. Remillard RL: Homemade diets: attributes, pitfalls, and a call for action. *Top Companion Anim Med* 23:137–142, 2008.
16. Bradshaw JW, Goodwin D, Legrand-Defrétin V, et al: Food selection by the domestic cat, an obligate carnivore. *Comp Biochem Physiol A Physiol* 114:205–209, 1996.
17. Zoran DL, Buffington CAT: Effects of nutrition choices and lifestyle changes on the well-being of cats, a carnivore that has moved indoors. *J Am Vet Med Assoc* 239:596–606, 2011.
18. Hepper PG, Wells DL, Millsopp S, et al: Prenatal and early sucking influences on dietary

preference in newborn, weaning, and young adult cats. *Chem Senses* 37:755–766, 2012.

19. Buckley C, Colyer A, Skrzywanek M, et al: The impact of home-prepared diets and home oral hygiene on oral health in cats and dogs. *Br J Nutr* 106(Suppl):S124–S127, 2011.

20. Kerr KR, Vester Boler BM, Morris CL, et al: Apparent total tract energy and macronutrient digestibility and fecal fermentative end-product concentrations of domestic cats fed extruded, raw beef-based, and cooked beef-based diets. *J Anim Sci* 90:515–522, 2012.

21. Tomsa K, Glaus T, Hauser B, et al: Nutritional secondary hyperparathyroidism in six cats. *J Small Anim Pract* 40:533–539, 1999.

22. Polizopoulou ZS, Kazakos G, Patsikas MN, et al: Hypervitaminosis A in the cat: a case report and review of the literature. *J Feline Med Surg* 7:363–368, 2005.

23. Niza MMRE, Vilela CL, Ferreira LMA: Feline pansteatitis revisited: hazards of unbalanced home-made diets. *J Feline Med Surg* 5:271–277, 2003.

24. Kerr KR, Beloshapka AN, Morris CL, et al: Evaluation of four raw meat diets using domestic cats, captive exotic felids, and cecectomized roosters. *J Anim Sci* 91:225–237, 2013.

25. Stockman J, Fascetti AJ, Kass PH, et al: Evaluation of recipes of home-prepared maintenance diets for dogs. *J Am Vet Med Assoc* 242:1500–1505, 2013.

26. Streiff EL, Zwischenberger B, Butterwick RF, et al: A comparison of the nutritional adequacy of home-prepared and commercial diets for dogs. *J Nutr* 132:1698S–1700S, 2002.

27. Heinze CR, Gomez FC, Freeman LM: Assessment of commercial diets and recipes for home-prepared diets recommended for dogs with cancer. *J Am Vet Med Assoc* 241:1453–1460, 2012.

28. Larsen JA, Parks EM, Heinze CR, et al: Evaluation of recipes for home-prepared diets for dogs and cats with chronic kidney disease. *J Am Vet Med Assoc* 240:532–538, 2012.

29. Piechota TR, Rogers QR, Morris JG: Nitrogen requirement of cats during gestation and lactation. *Nutr Res* 15:1535–1546, 1995.

30. Billinghurst I: *Give your dog a bone: the practical commonsense way to feed dogs for a long healthy life*, Alexandria, NSW, Australia, 1993, Bridge Printery Ian Billinghurst.

31. Schultze K: *Natural nutrition for dogs and cats: the ultimate diet*, Carlsbad, 1998, CA, Hay House Inc.

32. Volhard W, Brown K: *The holistic guide for a healthy dog*, New York, 1995, Howell Book House.

33. Freeman LM, Chandler ML, Hamper BA, et al: Current knowledge about the risks and benefits of raw meat-based diets for dogs and cats. *J Am Vet Med Assoc* 243:1549–1558, 2013.

34. Kerr KR, Morris CL, Burke SL, et al: Apparent total tract macronutrient and energy digestibility of 1- to 3-day-old whole chicks, adult ground chicken, and extruded and canned chicken-based diets in African wildcats (Felis silvestris lybica). *Zoo Biol* 32:510–517, 2013.

35. Friedman M: Biological effects of Maillard browning products that may affect acrylamide safety in food: biological effects of Maillard products. *Adv Exp Med Biol* 561:135–156, 2005.

36. Crissey SD, Swanson JA, Lintzenich BA, et al: Use of a raw meat-based diet or a dry kibble diet for sand cats (Felis margarita). *J Anim Sci* 75:2154–2160, 1997.

37. Vester BM, Burke SL, Liu KJ, et al: Influence of feeding raw or extruded feline diets on nutrient digestibility and nitrogen metabolism of African wildcats (Felis lybica). *Zoo Biol* 29:676–686, 2010.

38. Hamper BA: Nutritional adequacy and performance of raw food diets in kittens. PhD diss., University of Tennessee, 2012. <http://trace.tennessee.edu/utk_graddiss/1389>. (Accessed July 23, 2015.)

39. American Veterinary Medical Association: Policy on raw or undercooked animal-source protein in cat and dog diets. <https://www.avma.org/About/Governance/Documents/2012S_Resolution5_raw_food.pdf>. (Accessed July 23, 2015.)

40. American Animal Hospital Association: Raw protein diet position statement. <https://www.aahanet.org/library/Raw_Food_Diet.aspx>. (Accessed July 23, 2015.)

41. Canadian Veterinary Medical Association and Public Health Agency of Canada Joint Position Statement: Raw Food Diets for Pets. <http://www.canadianveterinarians.net/documents/raw-food-diets-for-pets>. (Accessed July 23, 2015.)

42. Frowde PE, Battersby IA, Whitley NT, et al: Oesophageal disease in 33 cats. *J Feline Med Surg* 13:564–569, 2011.

43. U.S. Food and Drug Administration: Animal health literacy—get the facts! Raw pet food diets can be dangerous to you and your pet.

<http://www.fda.gov/AnimalVeterinary/ResourcesforYou/AnimalHealthLiteracy/ucm373757.htm#The_Pet_Food_Study>. (Accessed July 23, 2015.)

44. Strohmeyer RA, Morley PS, Hyatt DR, et al: Evaluation of bacterial and protozoal contamination of commercially available raw meat diets for dogs. *J Am Vet Med Assoc* 228:537–542, 2006.

45. Weese JS, Rousseau J, Arroyo L: Bacteriological evaluation of commercial canine and feline raw diets. *Can Vet J* 46:513–516, 2005.

46. Joffe DJ, Schlesinger DP: Preliminary assessment of the risk of Salmonella infection in dogs fed raw chicken diets. *Can Vet J* 43:441–442, 2002.

47. Mehlenbacher S, Churchill J, Olsen KE, et al: Availability, brands, labelling and Salmonella contamination of raw pet food in the Minneapolis/St. Paul area. *Zoonoses Public Health* 59:513–520, 2012.

48. Clyde VL, Ramsay EC, Bemis DA: Fecal shedding of Salmonella in exotic felids. *J Zoo Wildl Med* 28:148–152, 1997.

49. Cui S, Ge B, Zheng J, et al: Prevalence and antimicrobial resistance of Campylobacter spp. and Salmonella serovars in organic chickens from Maryland retail stores. *Appl Environ Microbiol* 71:4108–4111, 2005.

50. Mollenkopf DF, Kleinhenz KE, Funk JA, et al: Salmonella enterica and Escherichia coli harboring blaCMY in retail beef and pork products. *Foodborne Pathog Dis* 8:333–336, 2011.

51. Opsteegh M, Haveman R, Swart AN, et al: Seroprevalence and risk factors for Toxoplasma gondii infection in domestic cats in The Netherlands. *Prev Vet Med* 104:317–326, 2012.

52. Jokelainen P, Simola O, Rantanen E, et al: Feline toxoplasmosis in Finland: cross-sectional epidemiological study and case series study. *J Vet Diagn Invest* 24:1115–1124, 2012.

53. Besné-Mérida A, Figueroa-Castillo JA, Martínez-Maya JJ, et al: Prevalence of antibodies against Toxoplasma gondii in domestic cats from Mexico City. *Vet Parasitol* 157:310–313, 2008.

54. Stiver SL, Frazier KS, Mauel MJ, et al: Septicemic salmonellosis in two cats fed a raw-meat diet. *J Am Anim Hosp Assoc* 39:538–542, 2003.

55. Weese JS, Rousseau J: Survival of *Salmonella copenhagen* in food bowls following contamination with experimentally inoculated raw meat: Effects of time, cleaning, and disinfection. *Can Vet J* 47:887–889, 2006.

Critical Care Nutrition

Daniel L. Chan

IMPORTANCE OF NUTRITION DURING CRITICAL ILLNESS

Compared with other animals, cats have several metabolic adaptations that impact their ability to maintain homeostasis in the face of injury, disease, and food deprivation. For example, cats have a higher requirement for protein and certain amino acids compared with other species.[1] Critical illness induces further metabolic alterations in cats that put them at even higher risk for the development of malnutrition and experiencing its deleterious effects. Similar to other species, diseased and injured cats respond differently to inadequate nutritional intake compared with healthy cats. During periods of nutrient deprivation, a healthy animal primarily loses glycogen and fat (simple starvation). However, sick or traumatized patients catabolize lean body mass when they are not provided with sufficient calories (stressed starvation). During the initial stages of fasting in the healthy state, glycogen stores are used as the primary source of energy. Within days, a metabolic shift occurs toward the preferential use of stored fat deposits, sparing catabolic effects on lean muscle tissue. In diseased states, the inflammatory response triggers alterations in cytokines and hormone concentrations and rapidly shifts metabolism toward a catabolic state.[2,3]

There are alterations in lipid, carbohydrate, and protein metabolism that can affect the animal's nutritional status and the outcome of the condition. The metabolic changes documented in critically ill cats include lower circulating concentration of insulin and higher concentrations of glucose, lactate, cortisol, glucagon, norepinephrine, and nonesterified fatty acids.[4,5] Glycogen stores are quickly depleted, especially in strict carnivores such as the cat, and this leads to an early mobilization of amino acids from muscle stores (upregulation of proteolysis). Because cats undergo continuous gluconeogenesis, the mobilization of amino acids from muscles is more pronounced than that observed in other species. Unlike other species, cats do not downregulate gluconeogenesis or proteolysis in the face of low protein intake.[6] With continued lack of food intake, energy is almost completely derived from accelerated proteolysis, which in itself is an energy-consuming process. Thus, these animals may preserve fat deposits in the face of lean muscle tissue losses. These shifts in metabolism commonly result in significant negative nitrogen and energy balance. The consequences of continued lean body mass losses include negative effects on wound healing, immune function, strength (both skeletal and respiratory), and ultimately on overall prognosis.[7] The metabolic derangements that occur in critically ill cats and the deleterious effects of malnutrition make the provision of nutritional support to hospitalized cats an essential and vital part of the therapeutic approach.

INDICATIONS FOR NUTRITIONAL SUPPORT

In cats, inadequate calorie intake is commonly due to a loss of appetite (hyporexia), an inability to eat, or results from persistent vomiting that accompanies many diseases processes. Appetite suppression may be instigated directly by inflammatory cytokines (e.g., interleukin [IL]-1β, IL-6, tumor necrosis factor-alpha) or secondarily by pathologic processes (e.g., nausea, pyrexia, pain, and/or ileus).[8] Because malnutrition can occur quickly in these animals, it is important to provide nutritional support by either enteral or parenteral means if oral intake is not adequate. Identification of overt malnutrition in cats can be challenging, because there are no established criteria of malnutrition in companion animals. As detectable impairment of immune function (e.g., decreased lymphocyte counts, reduced CD4/CD8) can be demonstrated in healthy cats subjected to acute starvation by day 4, nutritional support should be considered in any ill cat with inadequate food intake for more than 3 days.[9] The need to implement a nutritional intervention becomes more urgent when a cat has not fed for more than 5 days, because this increases the risk for the development of hepatic lipidosis.

There are many goals of nutritional support, but two important objectives are to treat malnutrition when it is present and to prevent malnutrition in animals at risk. Whenever possible, the enteral route should be used, because it is the safest, most convenient, and most physiologically sound method of nutritional support.[10] However, when patients are unable to tolerate enteral feeding (e.g., vomiting or diarrhea, intestinal cramping, nausea, discomfort from feeding, decreased mentation, risk of aspiration) or unable to use nutrients administered enterally (e.g., severe inflammatory bowel disease, intestinal lymphoma), parenteral nutrition (PN) should be considered. Ensuring the successful nutritional management of critically ill patients involves selecting the right patient, making an appropriate nutritional assessment, and implementing a feasible nutritional plan (Figure 66-1).

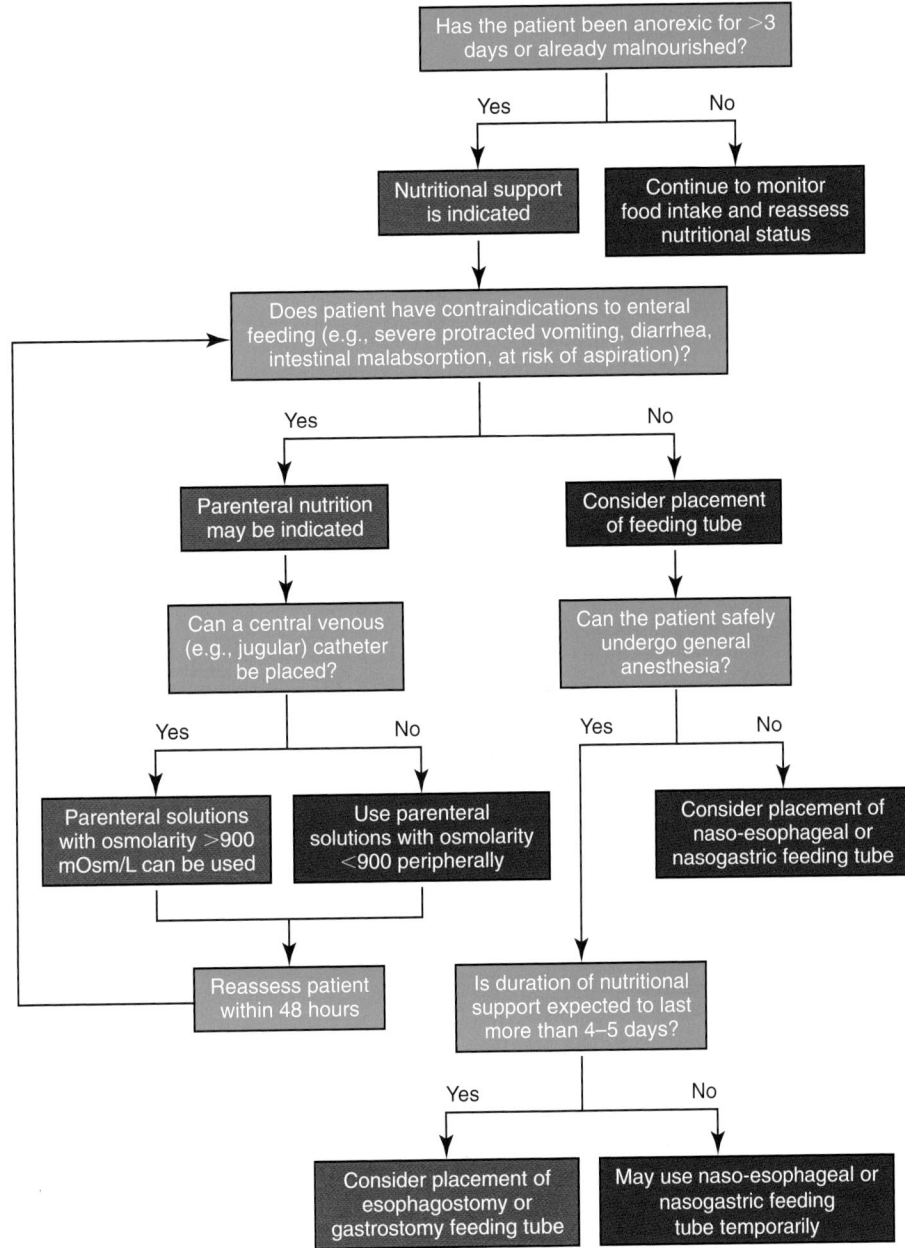

Figure 66-1: Algorithm for assessing need for nutritional support and route of feeding.

NUTRITIONAL ASSESSMENT

As with any medical intervention, there are risks of complications when initiating nutritional interventions. Minimizing such risks depends on patient selection and patient assessment. The first step in designing a nutritional strategy is to conduct a *nutritional assessment*. This involves taking into consideration the patient's life stage, history, clinical signs, underlying condition, and presence of organ dysfunction. By performing a thorough nutritional assessment, clinicians can identify malnourished patients that require immediate nutritional support, as well as patients that require nutritional support because they are at high risk for developing malnutrition.[11] Nutritional assessment guidelines have been published by the World Small Animal Veterinary Association (http://www.wsava.org/guidelines/global-nutrition-guidelines) and the American Animal Hospital Association (https://www.aahanet.org/Library/NutritionalAsmt.aspx).

Purported indicators of overt malnutrition include recent weight loss of at least 10% of body weight, poor hair coat quality, muscle wasting, signs of poor wound healing, hypoalbuminemia, lymphopenia, and coagulopathies (e.g., as a result of vitamin K deficiency).[12] However, these abnormalities are not specific to malnutrition and are not present early in the process. In addition, fluid shifts may mask weight loss in critically ill patients. Factors that predispose a patient to malnutrition include anorexia lasting longer than 3 days, serious underlying disease (e.g., trauma, sepsis, peritonitis, pancreatitis, and gastrointestinal [GI] surgery), and large protein losses (e.g., protracted vomiting, diarrhea, or draining wounds).[12,13] Nutritional assessment also identifies factors that can impact the nutritional plan (e.g., cardiovascular instability, electrolyte abnormalities, hyperglycemia, and hypertriglyceridemia) or concurrent conditions (e.g., renal or hepatic disease) that will impact the nutritional plan. A main priority of nutritional support centers on avoidance of metabolic complications. Identification of abnormalities via nutritional assessment may prompt alterations to the nutritional plan. For example, cats with uremia may not tolerate high protein diets. Appropriate laboratory analysis should be performed in all patients to assess these parameters. Before implementation of any nutritional plan, the patient must be cardiovascularly stable, with major electrolyte, fluid, and acid-base abnormalities corrected.

GOALS OF NUTRITIONAL SUPPORT

Even in patients with severe malnutrition, the immediate goals of therapy should focus on fluid resuscitation, cardiovascular stabilization, and identification of the primary disease process. As steps are made to address the primary disease, formulation of a nutritional plan should strive to prevent (or correct) overt nutritional deficiencies and imbalances. By providing adequate energy substrates, protein, essential fatty acids, and micronutrients, the body can support wound healing, immune function, and tissue repair. A major goal of nutritional support is to minimize metabolic derangements and catabolism of lean body tissue. During hospitalization, repletion of body weight is not a priority, because this will only occur when the animal is recovering from a state of critical illness. The ultimate goal of nutritional support is to have the patient eating adequate amounts of food in its own environment.

NUTRITIONAL PLAN

Proper diagnosis and treatment of the underlying disease are the keys to the success of nutritional support. Based on the nutritional assessment, a plan is formulated to meet energy and other nutritional requirements of the patient. The anticipated duration of nutritional support should be determined and factored into the plan. This largely depends on clinical familiarity with the specific disease process and sound clinical judgment. For example, a cat diagnosed with idiopathic hepatic lipidosis is likely to require long-term nutritional support (several weeks) and to benefit from tube feeding. Conversely, cats with minor injuries are unlikely to require feeding tubes for nutritional management. For each patient, the best route of nutrition should be determined—enteral versus parenteral. This decision should be based on the underlying disease and the patient's clinical signs. Important factors to consider include the urgency of commencing nutritional support (e.g., cat is showing overt signs of malnutrition or is at high risk of developing malnutrition, or has serious under-

lying disease expected to take several weeks to recover) and whether there are any contraindications to a particular mode of nutritional support (e.g., cats with protracted vomiting will not tolerate oral or esophageal feeding; cats with oral or pharyngeal disease may benefit from gastric tube feeding). Whenever possible, the enteral route should be considered as the first choice (see Figure 66-1). If enteral feedings are not tolerated or the GI tract or parts of the GI tract must be bypassed, PN should be instituted. In cases where only a portion of the cat's nutritional needs can be met enterally (e.g., minimal tolerance for small volumes of enteral feeding), supplemental PN has been demonstrated to be beneficial.[14,15] The various alterations in metabolic pathways that occur following injury and food deprivation suggest that nutritional support should be introduced gradually and reach target levels in 48 to 72 hours.[4,5]

CALCULATING NUTRITIONAL REQUIREMENTS

The resting energy requirement (RER) of an animal represents the energy requirement of a normal but fed animal at rest in a thermoneutral environment. The precise energy requirement of ill animals is unknown, so the RER is used as an initial estimate of a critically ill patient's energy requirements. The RER is calculated using the following formula:

$$RER = 70 \times (\text{body weight in kg})^{0.75}$$

or alternatively, a close approximation can be obtained by using:

$$RER = (30 \times \text{body weight in kg}) + 70$$

Previously, the RER was then multiplied by an illness factor between 1.0 and 2.0 to account for increases in metabolism associated with different conditions and injuries. Recently, there has been less emphasis on these subjective illness factors and current recommendations are to use more conservative energy estimates (i.e., RER) to avoid overfeeding.[10,12] Overfeeding can result in metabolic and GI complications, hepatic dysfunction, increased carbon dioxide production, and weakened respiratory muscles. Of the metabolic complications, the development of hyperglycemia is most common and possibly the most detrimental. In two recent studies evaluating PN in cats, the application of illness factors greater than 1.0 was associated with higher complication rates and even perhaps higher mortality rates.[16,17]

It should be emphasized that animals receiving nutritional support should be closely monitored for tolerance of nutritional support, and energy targets may require adjustments. Although hospitalized cats should be typically fed at least 75% RER to be considered adequately supported, there are cases where the patient will only tolerate a smaller percentage of RER, because greater amounts result in further complications (e.g., vomiting, regurgitation). This approach is termed *hypocaloric nutrition* or *trophic nutritional support* when this is delivered enterally. Feeding a minimal of 30% to 50% RER may provide sufficient benefits, such as a reduction of the risk for developing hepatic liposis; however, currently there is no data to support this claim. Continual decline in body weight or body condition should prompt the clinician to reassess and perhaps modify the nutritional plan (e.g., increasing the number of calories provided by 25%).

Although definitive studies determining the actual nutritional requirements of critically ill cats have not been performed, general recommendations can be made. Currently, it is generally accepted that cats should be supported with 6 or more grams of protein per 100 kcal (25% to 35% of total energy requirements). This goal is typically met through the use of commercial diets formulated for recovery or convalescence, which tend to have a relatively high fat and protein content. Patients with protein intolerance (e.g., hepatic encephalopathy, severe azotemia) should receive reduced amounts of protein (i.e., 4 grams of protein per 100 kcal).[12]

ENTERAL NUTRITION

The enteral route of nutritional support is the preferable route, primarily because it is safer and less expensive than PN, and it helps to maintain intestinal structure and function. Even with the use of feeding tubes, patients can easily be discharged for home care with good owner compliance. The majority of complications with feeding tubes include tube occlusion and localized irritation at the tube exit site. Occasionally, more serious complications can occur, and they include infection at the exit site or, rarely, complete tube dislodgment that could result in peritonitis if the tube is a gastrostomy or jejunostomy tube. Complications can be avoided by using the appropriate tube, proper food selection and preparation, and careful monitoring and owner education.

Although the enteral route should be used if at all possible, there are contraindications to its use. Contraindications include persistent vomiting and severe malabsorptive conditions or comatose cats. If the enteral route is chosen for nutritional support, the next step is selecting the type of feeding tube to be used (Table 66-1). Feeding tubes commonly used in cats include naso-esophageal, esophagostomy, gastrostomy, and jejunostomy tubes. With nonsurgically placed feeding tubes, such as naso-esophageal or esophagostomy tubes, confirmation of correct placement via radiology or fluoroscopy is highly recommended. Additionally, proper placement of these feeding tubes within the esophagus may be confirmed by achieving negative pressure with suction or by use of an end tidal CO_2 monitor that would detect CO_2 if the tube was incorrectly placed in the trachea (Figure 66-2).

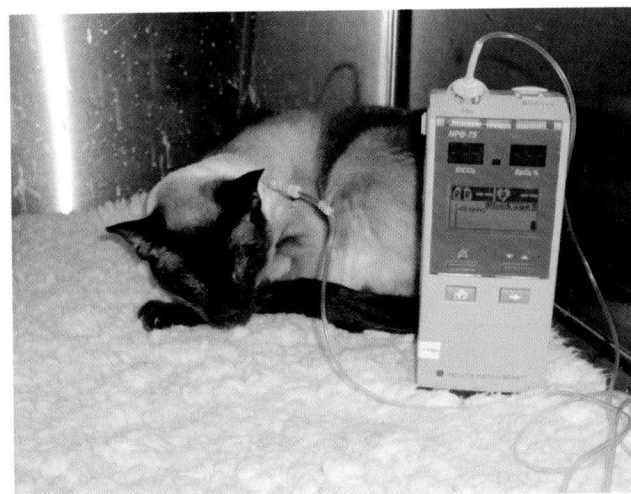

Figure 66-2: End tidal CO_2 monitor being used to confirm proper placement of esophagostomy tube within the esophagus.

Table 66-1	Types of Feeding Tubes		
Feeding Tube	**Typical Duration of Use**	**Advantages**	**Disadvantages**
Naso-esophageal	Short-term (less than 5 days)	Inexpensive Easy to place No anesthesia required	Must use complete liquid diet Prone to being dislodged
Esophagostomy	Extended (weeks to months)	Inexpensive Simple to place Can accommodate high-calorie semiliquid diets	Requires brief anesthesia Prone to becoming obstructed Incision can become inflamed or infected
Gastrostomy	Extended (weeks to months)	Can accommodate high-calorie semiliquid diets	Requires general anesthesia for placement Endoscopic placement requires special equipment Tube displacement may result in peritonitis
Jejunostomy	Long-term (weeks)	Can bypass upper gastrointestinal tract	Requires general anesthesia Requires laparotomy and special expertise for placement Requires complete liquid diet Tube displacement may result in peritonitis

Preferably, more than one method should be employed to confirm proper placement of the tube.

Based on the type of feeding tube chosen and the disease process being treated, an appropriate diet should be selected. For most critically ill cats, an energy-dense, high-protein, and high-fat commercial feline diet is preferred. However, the choice of diet may also depend upon the animal's clinical parameters and laboratory results. The use of specially designed diets for other species (e.g., dogs, humans) is not suitable for cats, because they often do not meet unique nutritional needs of cats (see Chapter 62).

The amount of food is then calculated, and a specific feeding plan is devised (Box 66-1). Generally, feedings are administered every 4 to 6 hours, and feeding tubes should be flushed with 5 to 10 mL of water after each feeding to minimize clogging of the tube. By the time of discharge, the number of feedings should be reduced to three to four times per day to facilitate owner compliance. Commercially-available veterinary liquid diets should be used for naso-esophageal and jejunostomy tube feedings due to the small bore sizes of these catheters (typically less than 5 Fr). Typical canned recovery diets are usually unsuitable for small bore tubes because of the tendency of these diets to clog the tubes. In the event that a feeding tube becomes clogged, a recent *in vitro* study reported that a mixture of pancreatic enzymes and bicarbonate solution was the most effective means of dissolving enteral diet clots.[18] Jejunostomy tubes are primarily for in-hospital use, because they require administration of a liquid diet by continuous rate infusion and this technique also requires more vigilant monitoring. Esophagostomy and gastrostomy tubes are generally larger (greater than 14 Fr) and allow for more calorically dense, blenderized diets to be administered. This decreases the volume of food necessary for each feeding. These tubes can be used for long-term enteral feeding. Placement of esophagostomy tubes requires minimal equipment, is a straightforward technique, and enables effective nutritional support. Complications associated with esophagostomy tubes are minimal, and client compliance and satisfaction are very good. Detailed stepwise instructions are listed in Box 66-2 and Figure 66-3.

The maximum safe volume of food to administer per feeding to a cat likely depends on a combination of factors, including underlying disease and individual variation. A volume of 5 to 10 mL/kg per individual feeding is generally well tolerated, but this may vary with the individual patient. In cats that are generally healthy but cannot consume food orally (e.g., symphyseal jaw fractures), larger volumes of food per feeding (15 to 20 mL/kg) may be tolerated but this volume must be given slowly over 15 to 20 minutes to allow for gastric accommodation, or vomiting will occur. Because

---

BOX 66-1 Formulating an Enteral Nutritional Plan

1. Calculate patient's resting energy requirement (RER):
   RER = $70 \times$ (current body weight in kg)$^{0.75}$
   = _____ kcal/day
   or
   RER = $(30 \times$ current body weight in kg$) + 70$
   = _____ kcal/day
2. Select diet to use based on type of tube used:
   - For naso-esophageal tubes: Use liquid diets designed for cats (typically 1 kcal/mL)
   - For esophageal tubes: Tube greater than 14 Fr; can use blenderized diets
   - For gastrostomy tubes: Blenderized diets
   - For jejunostomy tubes: Use liquid diets designed for cats
3. Product selected: _____
   Contains: _____ kcal/mL
4. Total amount to be administered per day:
   kcal required per day ÷ kcal/mL in diet = _____ mL of diet mixture/day
5. Feeding schedule:
   50% of total requirement on day 1 = _____ mL/day
   Total requirement on day 2 = _____ mL/day
   Divide total daily amounts into four to six feedings = _____ feedings/day
6. Calculate volume per feeding:
   Total mL/day ÷ Number of feedings/day
   = _____ mL/feeding (day 1)
   = _____ mL/feeding (day 2)

Diet Options

Esophagostomy and Gastrostomy Tubes

Eukanuba Maximum Calorie (Canned)
Supplies 2.1 kcal/mL straight from can but needs to be diluted further for feeding tubes
   1 can + 50 mL water = 1.6 kcal/mL
   1 can + 25 mL water = 1.8 kcal/mL

Hill's a/d (Canned)
Supplies 1.3 kcal/mL straight from can but needs to be diluted further for feeding tubes
   1 can + 50 mL water = 1.0 kcal/mL
   1 can + 25 mL water = 1.1 kcal/mL

Royal Canin Canine/Feline Recovery RS
Supplies 1 kcal/mL straight from can but needs to be diluted further for feeding tubes
   1 can + 25 mL water = 0.9 kcal/mL

Naso-esophageal and Jejunostomy Tubes

Veterinary Liquid Diets
CliniCare Canine/Feline liquid diet (1 kcal/mL) (Abbott Animal Health)
CliniCare RF Feline Liquid diet (1 kcal/mL) (Abbott Animal Health)

1. Proper placement of an esophagostomy feeding tube requires the distal tip to be placed in the distal esophagus at the level no further than the ninth intercostal space. This may require premeasuring the tube. Rather than cutting the distal tip and creating a sharp edge, the exit hole should be elongated using a small blade.

2. The patient should be anesthetized and preferably intubated. While in right lateral recumbency, the left side of the neck should be clipped and a routine surgical scrub should be performed (see Figure 66-3A).

3. A curved Rochester Carmalt clamp is placed into the mouth and down the esophagus to the midcervical region. The jugular vein should be identified and avoided.

4. The tip of the Rochester Carmalt clamp is then pushed dorsally, elevating the esophagus toward the skin.

5. The tip of the Rochester Carmalt clamp is palpated over the skin to confirm its location, and an incision is made through the skin onto the tip of the Rochester Carmalt in the esophagus. The mucosa of the esophagus is relatively more difficult to incise than the skin (see Figure 66-3B-C).

6. The tip of the instrument is then forced through the incision, which can be slightly enlarged with the blade to allow opening of the tips of the Rochester Carmalt clamp and placement of the esophagostomy tube within the tips (see Figure 66-3D).

7. The Rochester Carmalt clamp is then clamped closed and pulled from the oral cavity (see Figure 66-3E).

8. Disengage the tips of the Rochester Carmalt clamp, and curl the tip of the esophagostomy back into the mouth and feed into esophagus. As the curled tube is pushed into the esophagus, the proximal end is gently pulled simultaneously. This will result in subtle "flip" as the tube is redirected within the esophagus. The tube should easily slide back and forth a few millimeters, confirming that the tube has straightened (see Figure 66-3F-G).

9. Visually inspect the oropharynx to confirm that the tube is no longer present within the oropharynx.

10. The incision site should be briefly rescrubbed before a purse-string suture is placed followed by a Chinese finger trap suture, further securing the tube in place (see Figure 66-3H).

11. A light wrap is applied to the neck.

12. Correct placement should be confirmed with either radiography or fluoroscopy (see Figure 66-3I).

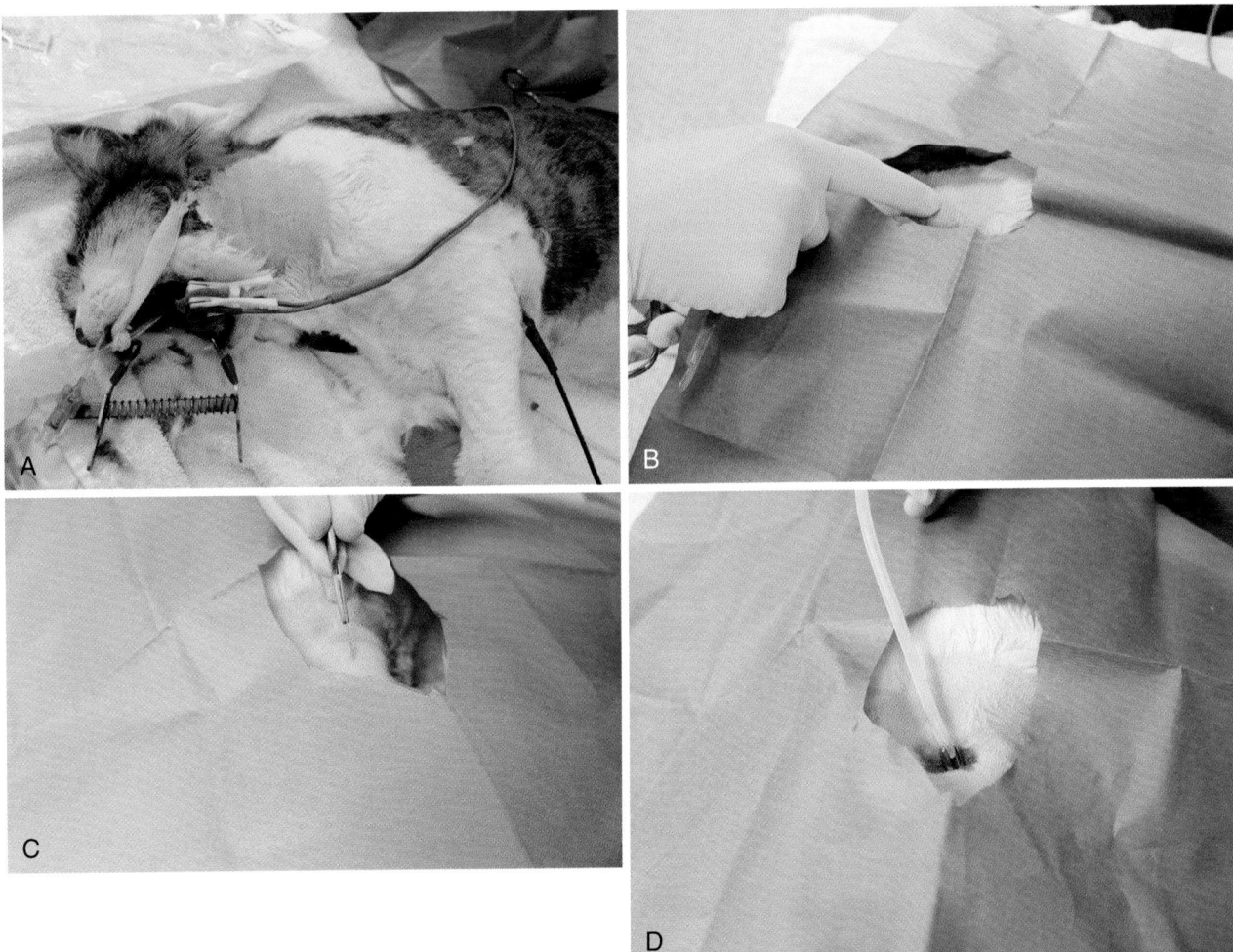

Figure 66-3: Placement of esophagostomy tube. **A,** Cat is anesthetized and placed in right lateral recumbency; the neck is clipped and aseptically prepared. **B,** A Rochester Carmalt clamp is placed within the esophagus, and the tip of the instrument is palpated through the skin. **C,** An incision is made directly over the palpated tip of the instrument until the tip of the clamp comes through the incision. **D,** The tip of the esophagostomy tube is clamped with the Rochester Carmalt clamp.

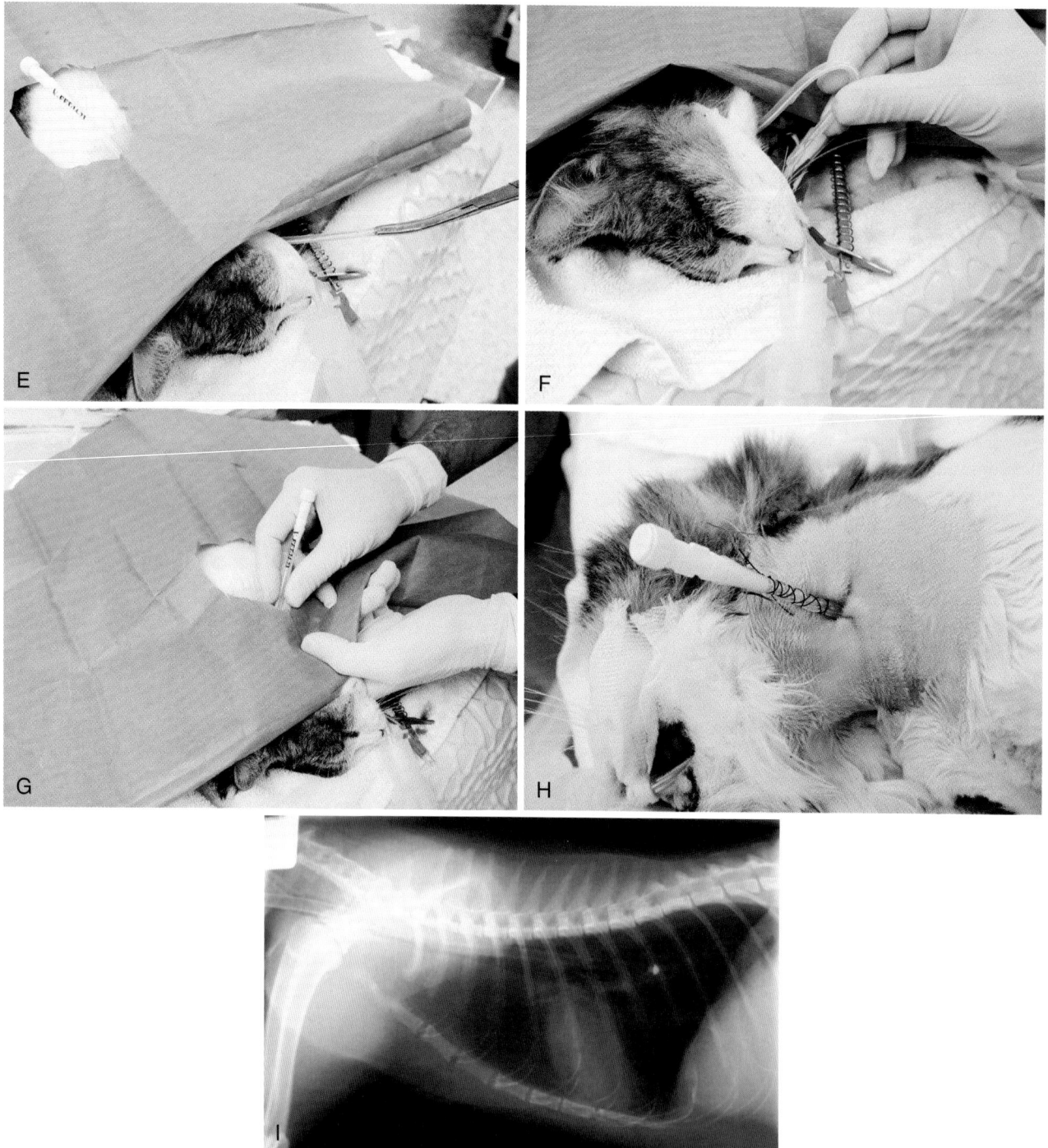

Figure 66-3, cont'd: **E,** The clamped tube is pulled through the mouth. **F,** The tube is curled back into the pharynx. **G,** The curled tube is pushed back into the pharynx while slightly pulling at the distal end to straighten the tube within the esophagus. **H,** A purse-string suture is placed around the incision and a Chinese finger trap suture is applied to the tube. Care should be exercised so that the purse-string suture is not too loose or too tight, because either can increase risk of stoma complications, such as infections. **I,** Radiograph of cat with esophagostomy tube in place, demonstrating ideal placement of tube within the esophagus.

enteral diets are mostly composed of water (most canned food are already greater than 75% water), the amounts of fluids administered parenterally should be adjusted accordingly to avoid volume overload. Prevention of premature removal of tubes can be accomplished by wrapping the tube securely, or alternatively, using a proprietary Velcro-fastened collar (http://www.kittykollar.com). Care should be taken to avoid wrapping it too tightly, because this could lead to patient discomfort and even compromise proper respiration.

PARENTERAL NUTRITION

Parenteral nutrition is more expensive than enteral nutrition and is only recommended for in-hospital use. True indications for PN include intractable vomiting, severe malabsorptive disorders, and severe ileus. Although not technically true indications, patients that are comatose or recumbent could be fed parenterally. Examples of cases that may require PN include severe inflammatory bowel disease, diffuse intestinal lymphoma, and acute necrotizing pancreatitis. In the initial management stages of these disorders, therapies directed at the underlying etiology may take time to have an effect, and therefore PN may allow nutrient delivery until GI function normalizes.

Terminology for PN in the veterinary literature can be confusing and inconsistent. Therefore, this chapter uses newer recommendations when describing PN, namely, central parenteral nutrition (CPN) when PN admixtures are administered via central intravenous (IV) catheters and peripheral parenteral nutrition (PPN), when the PN admixture is administered via a peripheral catheter.[15] Parenteral nutrition admixtures are typically composed of solutions of amino acids, dextrose, and lipids. Technically speaking, cats do not have a carbohydrate requirement, but meeting all of a cat's energy requirements with lipid and protein alone without exceeding recommended upper limits would be difficult. As a result of a high glucose concentration, cats on CPN become hyperglycemic and may require insulin therapy. Due to the high osmolarity of the CPN solution (usually 1100 to 1500 mOsm/L), it must be administered through a central venous (jugular) catheter. Peripheral parenteral nutrition is formulated so that it can be administered through a peripheral catheter but, because it is more dilute, it can only meet a portion of the patient's energy requirements (40% to 70%). The lower osmolarity of the solution makes it possible to be administered through a large peripheral vein (e.g., the femoral vein in cats), which is more feasible in practice. Because PPN only provides a portion of the patient's requirements, it is intended for short-term use in a nondebilitated patient with average nutritional requirements. Regardless of the exact form of PN, IV nutrition requires a dedicated catheter that is placed using aseptic technique. Long catheters composed of silicone, polyurethane, or tetrafluoroethylene are recommended for use with PN to reduce the risk of thrombophlebitis. Multilumen catheters (Figure 66-4) are often recommended for PN, because they can remain in place for

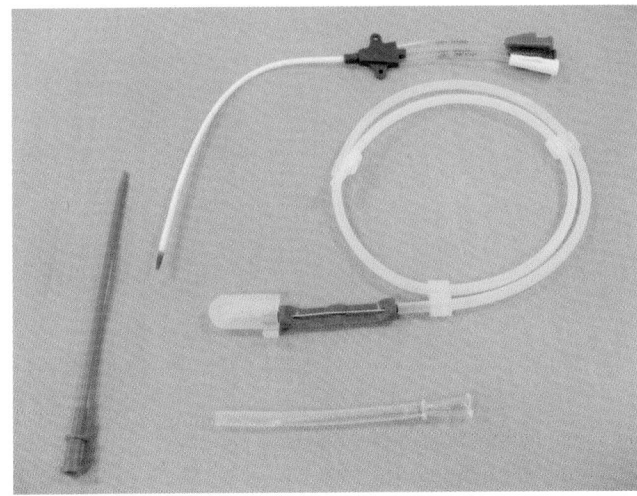

Figure 66-4: Example of triple lumen catheter that can be used for administration of parenteral nutrition.

longer periods of time as compared to normal jugular catheters and provide other ports for blood sampling and administration of additional fluids and IV medications. Most PN solutions are composed of a carbohydrate source (dextrose), a protein source (amino acids), and a fat source (lipids). Vitamins and trace metals can also be added.

Formulation of CPN and PPN solutions can be individualized to each patient according to the worksheets in Boxes 66-3 and 66-4. The CPN and PPN solutions must be mixed sterilely; in most cases, it is easiest to have a local human hospital or human home healthcare company formulate them.

Alternatively, commercial ready-to-use preparations of glucose and amino acids are available for peripheral use, but these provide less than 50% of required calories (when administered at maintenance fluid rate) and should only be used for short-term or interim nutritional support. As with enteral nutrition, PN should be instituted gradually over 48 to 72 hours. With both CPN and PPN, the animal's catheter and lines must be handled with aseptic technique to avoid complications. Adjust other IV fluids accordingly for the amount of fluid being administered in the PN to avoid volume overload.

MONITORING AND REASSESSMENT

Body weights should be monitored daily in all hospitalized cats, but especially those receiving enteral nutrition or PN. However, the clinician should take into account fluid shifts in evaluating changes in body weight. For this reason, body condition scoring is important as well, especially in determining those cats that have muscle wasting. The use of the RER as the patient's caloric requirement is merely a starting point. The number of calories provided may need to be increased to keep up with the patient's changing needs, which is typically by 25% if nutritional support is well tolerated. In patients unable to tolerate the prescribed amounts, the clinician should consider reducing amounts of enteral feedings and supplementing the nutritional plan with PN. This strategy of

BOX 66-3 Calculation of Central Parenteral Nutrition in Cats

1. Calculate resting energy requirement (RER):
   RER = 70 × (current body weight in kg)$^{0.75}$ = _____ kcal/day
   or
   RER = (30 × current body weight in kg) + 70
   = _____ kcal/day
2. Protein requirements for cats:

Standard	6 g/100 kcal
Reduced (hepatic/renal disease)	3 to 4 g/100 kcal
Increased (excessive protein losses)	6 to 8 g/100 kcal

   (RER ÷ 100) × _____ g protein/100 kcal = _____ g protein required/day
3. Volume of nutrient solutions required:
   a. 8.5% amino acid solution = 0.085 g protein/mL
      _____ g protein required/day ÷ 0.085 g/mL =
      _____ mL/day of amino acids
   b. Nonprotein calories:
      The calories supplied by protein (4 kcal/g) are subtracted from the RER to get total nonprotein calories needed.
      _____ g protein required/day × 4 kcal/g = _____ kcal provided by protein
      RER − kcal provided by protein = _____ total nonprotein kcal/day required
   c. Nonprotein calories are usually provided as a 70:30 mixture of lipid and dextrose:
      20% lipid solution = 2 kcal/mL
      To supply 50% of nonprotein calories:
      _____ lipid kcal required ÷ 2 kcal/mL = _____ mL of lipid
      50% of dextrose solution = 1.7 kcal/mL
      To supply 50% of nonprotein calories:
      _____ dextrose kcal required ÷ 1.7 kcal/mL
      = _____ mL of dextrose
4. Total daily requirements:
   _____ mL of 8.5% amino acid solution
   _____ mL of 20% lipid
   _____ mL of 50% dextrose
   _____ Total mL of central parenteral nutrition solution to be administered over 24 hours

BOX 66-4 Calculation of Peripheral Parenteral Nutrition in Cats

1. Calculate resting energy requirement (RER):
   RER = 70 × (current body weight in kg)$^{0.75}$
      = _____ kcal/day
   or
   RER = (30 × current body weight in kg) + 70
      = _____ kcal/day
2. Calculate the targeted energy requirement to be delivered peripherally (PER).
   Plan to supply 50% of the RER with peripheral parenteral nutrition (PPN):
   PER = RER × 0.50 = _____ kcal/day
3. Proportion of nutrient requirements according to body weight:
   (Note: For animals ≤3 kg, the formulation exceeds maintenance fluid requirements.)
   a. Cats (3 to 5 kg):
      PER × 0.20 = _____ kcal/day carbohydrate required
      PER × 0.20 = _____ kcal/day protein required
      PER × 0.60 = _____ kcal/day lipid required
   b. Cats (6 to 10 kg):
      PER × 0.25 = _____ kcal/day carbohydrate required
      PER × 0.25 = _____ kcal/day protein required
      PER × 0.50 = _____ kcal/day lipid required
4. Volumes of nutrient solutions required:
   a. 5% dextrose solution = 0.17 kcal/mL
      _____ kcal carbohydrate required/day ÷ 0.17 kcal/mL = _____ mL/day dextrose
   b. 8.5% amino acid solution = 0.34 kcal/mL
      _____ kcal protein required/day ÷ 0.34 kcal/mL = _____ mL/day amino acids
   c. 20% lipid solution = 2 kcal/mL
      _____ kcal lipid required/day ÷ 2 kcal/mL
      = _____ mL/day lipid
      = _____ total mL of PPN to be administered over 24 hours

combining enteral nutrition with PN, while not overfeeding, has been associated with positive results.[14,15]

As previously mentioned, the incidence of metabolic complications in cats receiving PN can be high. In a recent study, 84% of cats developed hyperglycemia within the first 96 hours of PN therapy.[15] Specific guidelines for instituting insulin therapy in non-diabetic cats receiving PN have not been published, although the practice has been reported.[15,19] In the study by Queau and colleagues, 35% of non-diabetic cats required insulin therapy.[15] Other studies have reported a decreased need for insulin therapy in cats,[17] and this may

be related to lower energy targets (i.e., close to RER) rather than more generous targets (e.g., 130% of RER) reported in the Queau and colleagues study.[15] This may be an important point, because avoidance of hyperglycemia in critically ill cats may be prudent because there is growing evidence that the development of this abnormality in cats may be detrimental.[16,17] In the event of cats developing hyperglycemia or hyperlipidemia, the author transiently decreases the rate of infusion by 50% and reassesses after 6 hours. If these abnormalities persist, the author reformulates the parenteral admixture to include reduced amounts of dextrose or lipids. Other nutritional requirements depend upon the patient's underlying disease, clinical signs, and laboratory parameters.

Metabolic complications of enteral nutritional support include electrolyte disturbances, hyperglycemia, volume overload, and GI signs (e.g., vomiting, diarrhea, cramping, bloating). Rarely, feeding a chronically debilitated and severely malnourished cat results in a condition known as *refeeding syndrome*. In most cases, severe hypophosphatemia results in muscle weakness and hemolysis. However, it can also result in severe neurological impairment, hypoventilation, cardiac failure, and even death.[20,21] The major shifts in electrolytes observed in refeeding syndrome relate to the resurgence of insulin following administration of carbohydrates. In severe malnourished states, insulin levels are extremely low and adenosine triphosphatase (ATP) synthesis is minimal. Following administration of carbohydrates, insulin instigates electrolyte shifts and cellular processes, such as synthesis of ATP, until phosphorus is depleted. This results in the clinical manifestations of refeeding syndrome.[20] The time frame for development of electrolyte shifts following refeeding may be 2 to 5 days. For this reason, patients deemed to be at risk for refeeding syndrome should have electrolytes checked daily. Strategies to decrease risk of the development of refeeding syndrome include very gradual and conservative provision of nutrition and very low amounts of carbohydrates.[20] However, a recent report highlights the possibility of refeeding syndrome even when such precautions are undertaken.[22] Correction of fluid and electrolyte imbalances should take priority over nutritional support in such extreme malnourished cases.

Monitoring parameters for patients receiving enteral nutrition include body weight, serum electrolytes, tube patency, appearance of tube exit site, GI signs (e.g., vomiting, regurgitation, diarrhea), and signs of volume overload or aspiration pneumonia.

Possible complications with PN include sepsis, mechanical complications of the catheter and lines, thrombophlebitis, and metabolic disturbances, such as hyperglycemia, electrolyte shifts, hyperammonemia, and hypertriglyceridemia. Avoiding serious consequences of complications associated with PN requires early identification of problems and prompt action. Frequent monitoring of vital signs, catheter exit sites, and routine biochemistry panels may alert the clinician of developing problems.

With continual reassessment, the clinician can determine when to transition the patient from assisted feeding to voluntary consumption of food. The discontinuation of nutritional support should only begin when the patient can consume approximately its RER without much coaxing. In patients receiving CPN, transitioning to enteral nutrition should occur over the course of at least 12 to 24 hours, depending on patient tolerance of enteral nutrition.

PHARMACOLOGICAL AGENTS IN NUTRITIONAL SUPPORT

Because critically ill animals are often hyporexic or anorexic, the temptation exists to use appetite stimulants to increase food intake. Unfortunately, appetite stimulants are generally unreliable and seldom result in adequate food intake in critically ill cats.[23] Although there have been some positive results with the use of appetite stimulants in cats with stable chronic kidney disease (CKD),[24] pharmacological stimulation of appetite in critically ill cats is often short-lived and only delays true nutritional support. Loss of appetite is simply a symptom and not a disease process itself; therefore, the use of pharmacological agents to treat this symptom without addressing the underlying condition is ill-advised. The author does not believe in the use of appetite stimulants in hospitalized patients when more effective measures of nutritional support, such as placement of feeding tubes, are more appropriate. For example, a uremic cat with CKD that is inappetent should be treated with fluid therapy and antiemetics rather than with appetite stimulants. An argument could be made that such a cat could be treated for its uremia for a few days and reassessed for the need of further nutritional interventions (i.e., placement of feeding tube). Appetite stimulants may be considered in animals that are managed as outpatients (i.e., not sick enough to be hospitalized or with stable conditions) or in recovering animals, because the primary reason for loss of appetite should ideally be addressed by this time. As with many drugs, appetite stimulants also have adverse effects, such as behavioral changes (associated with cyproheptadine), sedation, and severe hepatotoxicity (associated with oral diazepam), and therefore they should be used with caution or completely avoided. Mirtazapine is a tetracyclic antidepressant that appears to have some antiemetic and appetite stimulating effects.[24] There is very limited information regarding the use of this agent in cats. Recently, there have been studies evaluating the use of mirtazapine as an appetite stimulant in cats with CKD.[24] Mirtazapine also relies on glucuronidation for clearance, and therefore, this agent should be used with caution in cats with hepatic disease.[25] The aforementioned study in cats with CKD reported a consistent increase in alanine transferase activity whenever one of the cats was treated with mirtazapine.[24] Moreover, adverse effects associated with mirtazapine include sedation, hypotension, excitability, dysphoria, and vocalization,[25,26] although these were not noted in cats recently evaluated with CKD.[24]

FUTURE DIRECTION IN CRITICAL CARE NUTRITION

The current state of veterinary critical care nutrition revolves around proper recognition of animals requiring nutritional support and implementing strategies to best provide nutritional therapies. Important areas needing further evaluation in critically ill cats include the optimal composition and caloric target of nutritional support and strategies to minimize complications and optimize outcome. Studies implicating poor clinical outcome in the development of hyperglycemia in critically ill people led to more vigilant monitoring and stricter control of blood glucose, with obvious implications for nutritional support. Evidence of a similar relationship in cats is mounting although further studies are warranted.[15,16] Until studies demonstrate otherwise, efforts to reduce the incidence of hyperglycemia in critically ill cats, especially those being administered nutritional support, should be strongly pursued.

SUMMARY

Critically ill cats are often not regarded as being in urgent need of nutritional support given their more pressing problems. However, the severity of their injuries, altered metabolic condition, and necessity of frequent fasting (e.g., for diagnostic or surgical procedures) place these patients at high risk of becoming malnourished during their hospitalization. The unique metabolic peculiarities of cats make them particularly prone to energy and protein catabolism, and nutritional support in this species may be more pertinent during critical illness. Proper identification of patients in need of nutritional support and careful planning and execution of a nutrition plan can be key factors in the successful recovery of these patients. In the future, the use of immunemodulating nutrients may play a bigger role in modulating disease in critically ill cats.

References

1. MacDonald ML, Rogers QR, Morris JG: Nutrition of the domestic cat, a mammalian carnivore. *Annu Rev Nutr* 4:521–562, 1984.
2. Mitchel KE: Nitrogen metabolism in critical care patients. *Vet Clin Nutr* (Suppl):20–22, 1998.
3. Sakurai Y, Zhang X, Wolfe RR: Short-term effects of tumor necrosis factor on energy and substrate metabolism in dogs. *J Clin Invest* 91:2437–2445, 1993.
4. Brown B, Mauldin GE, Armstrong J, et al: Metabolic and hormonal alterations in cats with hepatic lipidosis. *J Vet Intern Med* 14:20, 2000.
5. Chan DL, Freeman LM, Rozanski EA, et al: Alterations in carbohydrate metabolism in critically ill cats. *J Vet Emerg Crit Care* 16:S7, 2006.
6. Rogers QR, Morris JG, Freedland RA: Lack of hepatic enzymatic adaptation to low and high levels of dietary protein in the adult cat. *Enzyme* 22:348, 1977.
7. Remillard RL: Nutritional support in critical care patients. *Vet Clin North Am Small Anim Pract* 32:1145–1164, 2002.
8. Perbone S, Inui A: Anorexia in cancer: role of feeding-regulatory peptides. *Philos Trans R Soc Lond B Biol Sci* 361:1281, 2006.
9. Freitag KA, Saker KE, Thomas E, et al: Acute starvation and subsequent refeeding affect lymphocyte subsets and proliferation in cats. *J Nutr* 130:2444–2449, 2000.
10. Freeman LM, Chan DL: Total parenteral nutrition. In DiBartola SP, editor: *Fluid, electrolyte, and acid-base disorders in small animal practice,* ed 3, St Louis, 2006, Elsevier, p 584.
11. Buffington T, Holloway C, Abood A: Nutritional assessment. Part 1. In Buffington T, Holloway C, Abood S, editors: *Manual of veterinary dietetics,* St Louis, 2004, Saunders/Elsevier.
12. Chan DL: Nutritional requirements of the critically ill patient. *Clin Tech Small Anim Pract* 19:1, 2004.
13. Thatcher CD: Nutritional needs of critically ill patients. *Compend Contin Educ Pract Vet* 18(12):1303–1311, 1996.
14. Chan DL, Freeman LM, Labato MA, et al: Retrospective evaluation of partial parenteral nutrition in dogs and cats. *J Vet Intern Med* 16(4):440–445, 2002.
15. Queau Y, Larsen JA, Kass PH, et al: Factors associated with adverse outcomes during parenteral nutrition administration in dogs and cats. *J Vet Intern Med* 25(3):446–452, 2011.
16. Pyle SC, Marks SL, Kass PH: Evaluation of complications and prognostic factors associated with administration of total parenteral nutrition in cats: 75 cases (1994-2001). *J Am Vet Med Assoc* 255:242, 2004.
17. Crabb SE, Chan DL, Freeman LM: Retrospective evaluation of total parenteral nutrition in cats: 40 cases (1991-2003). *J Vet Emerg Crit Care* 16:S21, 2006.
18. Parker VJ, Freeman LM: Comparison of various solutions to dissolve critical care diet clots. *J Vet Emerg Crit Care* 23(3):344–347, 2013.
19. Lippert AC, Fulton RB, Parr AM: A retrospective study of the use of total parenteral nutrition in dogs and cats. *J Vet Intern Med* 7(1):52–64, 1993.
20. Justin RB, Hoenhaus AE: Hypophosphatemia associated with enteral alimentation in cats. *J Vet Intern Med* 9:228, 1995.
21. Armitage-Chan EA, O'Toole T, Chan DL: Management of prolonged food deprivation, hypothermia and refeeding syndrome in a cat. *J Vet Emerg Crit Care* 16:S41, 2006.
22. Brenner K, KuKanich KS, Smee NM: Refeeding syndrome in a cat with hepatic lipidosis. *J Feline Med Surg* 13(8):614–617, 2011.
23. Delaney SJ: Management of anorexia in dogs and cats. *Vet Clin North Am Small Anim Pract* 36:1243, 2006.
24. Quimby JM, Lunn KF: Mirtazapine as an appetite stimulant and anti-emetic in cats with chronic kidney disease: a masked placebo-controlled crossover clinical trial. *Vet J* 197(3):651–655, 2013.
25. Plumb DC: *Plumb's veterinary drug handbook,* ed 7, Ames, IA, 2011, Wiley Blackwell.
26. Quimby JM, Gustafson DL, Samber BJ, et al: Studies on the pharmacokinetics and pharmacodynamics of mirtazapine in healthy young cats. *J Vet Pharm Ther* 34(4):388–396, 2011.

Brian A. DiGangi, DVM and Brenda Griffin, DVM

Evidence-Based Feline Medicine: Principles and Practicalities

Rachel Dean

WHAT IS EVIDENCE-BASED MEDICINE?

The Centre for Evidence-Based Veterinary Medicine (CEVM) at the University of Nottingham states:

Evidence-based veterinary medicine is the use of the best relevant evidence in conjunction with clinical expertise to make the best possible decision about a veterinary patient. The circumstances of each patient, and the circumstances and values of the owner/carer must also be considered when making an evidence-based decision.

It is very important to consider the whole definition and not just focus on the evidence itself. For evidence-based decision making to be possible in feline practice, a clinician needs to be aware of the most up-to-date evidence available relative to the disease that presents with each patient. A good evidence-based clinician will then apply the evidence to the clinical situation at hand, which is unique every time due to the individual nature of each cat and its owner. Evidence-based feline medicine, therefore, involves not only the evidence and the clinician but also the feline patient and its owner.

Evidence-based veterinary medicine (EVM) does not mean there is a set of rules that must be followed in every patient. Variable therapeutic options arise because the way in which the evidence is applied may differ from one case to the next as each patient has a unique clinical state and setting. It is possible that two cats presenting with the same condition may be treated in very different ways despite the evidence being the same in each case. This is because treatment decisions may vary based upon the owners' or care-givers' particular circumstances and values, as well as the circumstances surrounding the individual cats. For example, the treatment of a hyperthyroid cat in a single-cat household belonging to a devoted owner may be very different from the treatment choices for a hyperthyroid cat in a rescue shelter. The evidence available to the feline clinician regarding "best treatment" remains the same, but the treatment choices for each case may differ based upon financial resources, time available for treatment and monitoring, demeanor of the cat, and the treatment preferences of each owner.

ORIGINS AND HISTORY OF EVIDENCE-BASED VETERINARY MEDICINE

Evidence-based veterinary medicine evolved from evidence-based medicine (EBM), which has been a great success in human health care since the mid-1980s. There are many excellent resources now available to medical professionals to enable them to make evidence-based decisions and create evidence-based guidelines to direct clinical care (Box 67-1). The veterinary profession can use this framework to develop resources and promote the use of evidence in veterinary practice.

The concept of EVM was first mentioned in the literature on veterinary medicine in 1998[1] and the *Handbook of Evidence-Based Veterinary Medicine* was published in 2003.[2] The Evidence-Based Veterinary Medicine Association was founded in 2004 to improve the coordination and communication among individuals by promoting research, teaching, and clinical application of EVM to practice.[3] In 2009, the CEVM at the University of Nottingham in the United Kingdom was established and is the only dedicated multidisciplinary research group working in this field.[4] The CEVM has adapted a number of EBM methodologies to the veterinary profession and more research groups, professional organizations, and practitioners are now becoming involved in EVM. There is also a small but increasing number of articles being published about the teaching, methodologies, and delivery of EVM to practitioners.[5-8]

WHY DO WE NEED EVIDENCE-BASED FELINE MEDICINE?

Feline medicine and surgery are rapidly expanding areas of the veterinary profession. Over the last 10 to 15 years, the amount of clinical research (i.e., evidence) concerning the health of cats has exponentially increased. Currently it remains unclear how many feline clinicians are aware of and follow the principles of EVM and how much of this evidence has been translated into clinical practice and improved care for feline patients. It is important that feline clinicians acknowledge the importance of EVM and use the principles to promote the best interests of their feline patients and clients. Applying EVM to feline practice is challenging; this chapter will outline the steps of EVM and highlight the challenges that may be encountered at each step.

WHAT IS EVIDENCE?

There are many different types of evidence available to feline clinicians from systematic reviews and individual research papers to textbooks and expert opinion. Each type of evidence has its weaknesses and strengths, and these must be recognized by the clinician before incorporating the evidence into clinical decision making. Some aspects of feline practice have a larger body of good-quality evidence in the form of scientific research papers (e.g., the use of renal diets and their effect on life expectancy of cats with chronic kidney disease),[8-10] while others have almost no evidence available other than expert opinion (e.g., the best way of treating a cat bite abscess).

Feline clinicians commonly rely on textbooks and expert opinion; however, these evidence sources often vary in terms of their quality and always include bias that reflects the authors' experience, opinion, and interpretation of the evidence. Care must be taken when applying expert opinion to practice. For example, the opinion of a feline urologist working in a tertiary referral hospital may have high relevance to the caseload at that hospital, but it may not necessarily be relevant to the caseload seen by a primary-care clinician in feline practice. Understanding that many traditional sources of information are outdated is also an important step in understanding the limitations of the evidence sources clinicians rely on.

GETTING STARTED

The first step in being a good evidence-based clinician is to pause and consider the basis for one's current clinical decision making. Decisions may be based on what was learned in veterinary school, what has seemed to work for the last 20 years, what experts in the field promote, or what feline textbooks recommend. Alternatively, decisions may be based on the most recent published evidence.

It is important to consider the scientific basis for the decisions that are made each day in clinical practice, as well as clinicians' own internal biases. One must accept that procedures performed many times or prescribed treatments that appear to be successful may in fact be outdated or proven ineffective. It is essential to recognize that one clinician's experiences and successes may not reflect that of the rest of the profession. Acknowledging the many areas of uncertainty in feline practice and the relative lack of evidence in others is a key to being a good evidence-based clinician. Uncertainty and a need for change can be a challenge to some clinicians, and this can be one of the biggest barriers to practicing EVM.

The next step is to identify what skills are needed to become a more evidence-based clinical decision maker. Some of these skills are now being taught in veterinary curricula,[11,12] but many veterinary graduates did not receive training in these areas. It can be easy to dismiss EVM as a theoretical academic framework for decision making, but feline practitioners who make clinical decisions every day are in the best position to elicit change by incorporating evidence into their daily practice.

THE STEPS OF EVIDENCE-BASED FELINE MEDICINE

There are five steps to the EVM cycle[13] (Figure 67-1): ask, acquire, appraise, apply, and assess.

Step One: Ask

There are many questions feline clinicians face each day that may or may not have an evidence base. The first step in EVM is to capture clear, relevant questions that are important to clinicians. Important issues for one feline practitioner may be very different from another. They may consider areas of practice where there is a clinical problem (e.g., wound breakdown in feline spays) or where there is a difference of

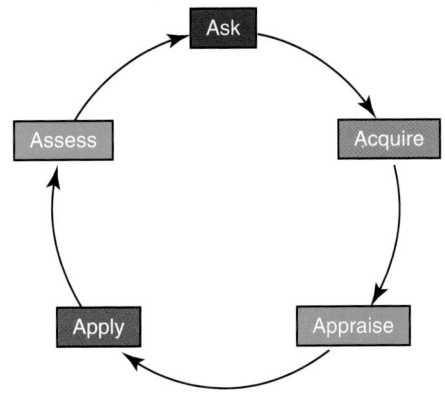

Figure 67-1: The Cycle of Evidence-Based Veterinary Medicine

opinion among colleagues (e.g., the use of nonsteroidal anti-inflammatory drugs in elderly cats).

Clinical Questions

Structuring clinical questions using the PICO format ensures that the question is clear, targeted, and that only relevant evidence is identified.[13] The acronym PICO stands for:

P—the **P**atient group, **P**roblem, or **P**opulation of interest
I—the **I**ntervention or action or test of **I**nterest
C—a **C**omparator of interest
O—the **O**utcome of interest for the patient group and clinician

The PICO format was initially designed to encompass questions about treatment interventions but can be adapted to questions about diagnostic tests, risk factors for diseases, and many other clinical areas of interest. A PICO question can be very broad or very specific depending on the subject of interest (Box 67-2). A broad clinical question will generally lead to a larger body of literature that needs to be appraised than a more specific question would. It is important to ensure that the four parts of the PICO question accurately describe the subject of interest because this will form the basis of the search strategy to follow.

Types of Study

Ideally, well-designed, high-quality research studies should be used to answer the clinical questions. The type of question being asked dictates the type of research studies (or study design) that is needed to answer the question (Table 67-1). It is important that feline clinicians are familiar with different study types to ensure that the right type of evidence is identified (Table 67-2).

Descriptive studies, such as case series and case reports, are commonplace in the feline literature. These studies can be very useful in describing techniques used and the outcomes of treatment for an individual or a number of cats. However, they are of limited use in answering clinical questions because they do not compare one group with another and cannot be used as good evidence for describing treatment success, disease frequency, or risk factors for disease.

BOX 67-2 Examples of PICO Questions

The topic of interest may be the role of prescription diets in disease management of cats.

A broad PICO question may be:
1. In cats, do prescription diets compared to nonprescription diets improve clinical outcomes?

More specific PICO questions may be:
2. In cats with chronic kidney disease, do renal prescription diets compared to normal diets improve clinical signs in affected cats?
3. In cats with hyperthyroidism, do iodine-restricted diets compared to nonrestricted diets improve life expectancy of affected cats?

	Question 1	Question 2	Question 3
P	Cats	Cats with chronic kidney disease	Cats with hyperthyroidism
I	Prescription diets	Renal prescription diets	Iodine-restricted diet
C	Nonprescription diets	Normal diet	Nonrestricted diet
O	Clinical outcomes	Clinical signs	Life expectancy

PICO, Patient, Problem, or Population; Intervention or Interest; Comparator; Outcome.

Table 67-1	Types of PICO Questions and the Study Designs That Best Answer Each Question
Focus of PICO Question	**Best Study Design(s) to Answer the Question**
Efficacy of treatment or intervention	Randomized controlled clinical trial*
Risk factors for disease	Cohort study; most useful for common diseases Case control study; most useful for rare diseases Cross-sectional studies; most useful for static risk factors (e.g., age and breed)
Diagnosis	Diagnostic validation studies
Prognosis	Cohort study
Incidence of disease	Cohort study
Prevalence of disease	Cross-sectional studies

*When a good randomized controlled clinical trial is lacking, well-designed cohort studies may provide useful evidence in assessing treatment efficacy. However, these cohort studies are more subject to bias, and care must be taken when interpreting the results and applying them to practice.
PICO, Patient, Problem, or Population; Intervention or Interest; Comparator; Outcome.

Table 67-2	Basic Descriptions of Study Types	
Type of Study	**Category of Study**	**Basic Description**
Randomized controlled trial (RCT)	Interventional	A prospective clinical trial that has at least one *control* group and one treatment group. The control group may receive nothing or a placebo (negatively controlled or placebo-controlled RCT) or a comparator/standard therapy (positively controlled RCT). The initial population of diseased cats are *randomly* allocated to a treatment or control group. The effect of treatment can be assessed and compared between the treatment and control groups. Ideally, the assessors who measure the treatment outcomes and those administering treatments should be unaware of the treatment allocation (blinded).
Cohort study	Observational	A population of cats of interest is studied over time for a defined period. Cats are included that will have different exposures during the period of the study. At the end of the period of time, the outcome of interest (often the presence or absence of disease) is measured in all cats. It can then be determined if there is an association between certain exposures and the outcome of interest by comparing the frequency of the outcome in the exposed and unexposed individuals. The incidence of disease over time within the population of cats studied can also be measured.
Case control study	Observational	Cats are included because they have disease (cases) or because they do not have disease (controls). The exposure of cats to certain risk factors of interest is retrospectively identified for cases and controls. The presence or absence of association between risk factors and disease can then be identified.
Cross-sectional study	Observational	The presence of disease in individuals within a specific population of cats is gathered at a single point in time. The prevalence of a disease in a population can then be calculated. Certain static risk factors, such as sex and breed, can be compared between the diseased and nondiseased groups.

For further information about study designs, please refer to a general epidemiology text.

In an ideal world there would be more than one study to answer each clinical question that can be synthesized into a systematic review. A systematic review is a high-level summary of primary research on a particular research question that attempts to identify, select, synthesize, and appraise all high-quality research evidence relevant to that question to find an answer. A systematic review will have a distinct section describing the methods used to identify the primary research articles (including the search terms and databases used to find them) as well as a description of how the studies were appraised. This is different from narrative reviews such as those found in textbooks, review articles, and at the start of scientific papers because these types of reviews do not contain the methods used to find the research papers cited.

Recently a database of veterinary systematic reviews, VetSRev (http://webapps.nottingham.ac.uk/refbase), was established. There are currently only a small number of systematic reviews concerning cats but as the amount of literature increases and more researchers undertake systematic

reviews, more will be available to clinicians. Other types of evidence syntheses, such as critically appraised topics and Best BETs for Vets (https://bestbetsforvets.org), which generally cover more specific questions, are available in feline medicine.[14,15]

Other Clinical Questions That Drive Research

It is important to recognize that feline practitioners are not the only ones who have questions about diseases in cats; cat owners also have an interest in the evidence available to aid clinical decision making but are rarely involved in the prioritization and design of clinical research. In human health care, organizations such as the James Lind Alliance (http://www.lindalliance.org) have a role in identifying and prioritizing research questions of interest to both clinicians and patients and use the information gathered to guide and inform agencies that fund research. In the future, increased involvement of veterinarians and pet owners will improve the relevance of research projects to clinical practice.

Step Two: Acquire

Searching for and acquiring evidence to answer clinical questions is the next step in EVM. Many papers are published every week on various aspects of feline medicine that may be relevant to clinical practice. To be able to search effectively for the evidence most relevant to the question at hand, good databases and effective search strategies are required.

Electronic Databases for Searching for Evidence

A variety of search engines and databases are available to search for evidence, and the Centre for Agriculture and Biosciences International (CABI) and MEDLINE have been shown to be the most useful databases for the veterinary literature.[16] Although abstracts are frequently available free of charge, it is unwise to base clinical decisions on abstracts alone, as these do not always reflect the content of the full scientific report.[17,18] Therefore, it is necessary to obtain the entire paper so the quality of the science can be appraised. Unfortunately, accessing original research can be difficult and costly, and this can be a significant challenge for practitioners wishing to undertake EVM. The increase in the number of veterinary journals that are able to publish articles as open access (http://www.jisc.ac.uk/open-access) means that, rather than paying for a physical copy of the research, it is freely available online.

If this trend continues, it will mean more feline research becomes readily available for practitioners to read and to use in clinical decision making. For most journals, the peer-review process for open-access articles is the same as for subscription-only articles.

In addition to searching for individual articles, it is advisable to include VetSRev in any literature search. Other resources on evidence syntheses such as BestBETS for VETs[15] and the critically appraised topics produced by Banfield Applied Research and Knowledge (BARK)[18] may also be helpful when searching for evidence.

Effective Search Strategies

Learning how to formulate effective search strategies to find evidence relevant to feline practice is one of the key skills of EVM. It is important to use both thesaurus and keyword searching when using bibliographic databases. Thesaurus terms enable a searcher to find articles indexed to a particular subject by information specialists who administer the databases. Different databases use different thesaurus terms, and advice on how to use them is commonly given on their websites. It is important also to use keyword searching because it is possible that some articles relevant to the clinical question may not be identified by a thesaurus term but would be via keyword searching and vice versa.

The PICO questions can be used to generate search terms, although it is often not necessary to use terms relating to the outcome. Boolean operators such as "AND" and "OR" can be used to formulate the search strategy.

Once the search has been undertaken, it is important to look at all of the citations in the output from the database and decide if they are relevant to the clinical question. In general, the title and abstract are enough to establish if a paper is relevant, but sometimes the whole manuscript is required. If the search strategy has been well formulated and the clinical question is specific, this is not a time-consuming process. To maximize the limited time available to read and appraise evidence, it is important that only the evidence pertaining to the clinical question at hand is reviewed.

Despite the exponential increase in feline clinical research over the last 20 years, there is still a lack of primary research evidence for many common clinical questions. In these circumstances, other forms of evidence, such as textbooks, websites, and expert opinion can be sought. It is important to appraise these types of evidence critically in a way similar to primary research studies. Areas of feline medicine where there are important "evidence gaps" need to be identified so that future research can be targeted to answer these questions.

Step Three: Appraise

The systematic critical appraisal of evidence is one of the cornerstones of EVM, and some basic skills are required to differentiate "good" science from "bad" science. All types of evidence, from systematic reviews to expert opinion, can be critically appraised. In good-quality journals, to ensure that well-designed and well-reported studies are published, the peer-review process is rigorous. However, the peer-review process does not guarantee quality and, just because an article is published, the reader cannot be assured that it represents "good" science. For example, a randomized controlled trial (the best form of evidence for treatment efficacy) may be available to assess a certain treatment; however, if it is poorly designed and/or executed, it may provide weaker evidence than a well-designed cohort study. The impact factor of a journal does not necessarily give an indication of quality (e.g., a high-impact-factor journal may still contain poor-quality science, and a low-impact-factor journal may contain some science of excellent quality). The impact factors are based on how frequently the papers published in the journal are cited by other articles, so care must be taken if the reader is using impact factors alone to indicate quality.

It is important that a study is reported well to appraise the study critically. There are many guidelines available to enable researchers to report their studies effectively, such as Equator Network (http://www.equator-network.org). However, it would appear that not all editors of veterinary journals are aware of these guidelines, and it is unknown how many authors know about them.[19] Veterinary editors, reviewers, and authors need to be aware of reporting guidelines if the quality of the published literature in feline medicine is to be improved.

There are a number of critical appraisal tools available to enable the reader to assess the quality of evidence.[20-22] Critical appraisal tools, in the form of discrete lists of questions, enable a reader to appraise evidence in a systematic way and identify biases and errors in the study that may influence the reliability of the results. Because each study design is different, a slightly different checklist would ideally be tailored to

BOX 67-3 Basic Critical Appraisal Questions That Can Apply to All Study Types

Introduction
- Are the study aims clearly stated?

The aim of the study should be given at the end of the introduction of any scientific study. It is important that this is clear, so the reader knows what has been done and to ensure that the paper is relevant to the clinical question and therefore worth reading.

Methods
- Is the study design suitable for the study aims?

The methods should clearly explain the study design because particular study types answer different types of questions (see Table 67-1).
- What population was studied?

The method should include a description of the specific population of cats that was studied. This information is used to determine if the study subjects are similar enough to the clinician's own clinical population to make the results of the study being appraised relevant to practice.
- Was the sample size justified?

Somewhere in the text it should be stated that a sample size or power calculation was performed to establish how many animals need to be included to yield statistically significant results. The sample size or power calculation dictates what p value should be used to state significance in the results.
- What measurements were used?

When undertaking clinical research, it is important to use valid and reliable measurements when assessing outcomes and factors that may affect outcomes. All measurements need to be clinically useful, relevant, and repeatable.
- Are the statistical methods clearly described?

The statistical methods used should also be described in enough detail to enable the reader to repeat them if the data

were made available. Statistics can be very complicated, and clinicians do not need to understand all of the detail to believe the results. However, the authors need to clearly state what they did to get the results that are presented.

Results
- Are the basic information and data provided about the cats in the study clear?

Is the population well described in terms of demographic information and disease status at the start and the end of the study? Is it possible to establish what happened to the cats before any statistics were undertaken? The basic data should be clear and easy to understand and should consist of both numbers and percentages.
- Are all cats accounted for within the study? Did any adverse events occur?

It is important that all animals are accounted for at the end of the study and it is known what happened to all of them. This includes adverse events and deaths as well as treatment successes.
- What are the main findings of the study?

It is very important that the key results relevant to the aim are identified. Only results that generate a p value that was stated in the methods should be classified as significant. Statistical calculations that yield significant results but involve fewer numbers of cats than stated in the sample size or power calculation should be interpreted with care.
- What, if any, are the implications of the results of this study for practice?

This question should be asked after reading every study to establish if a change in current practice is needed.

appraise each type of study. The sections on methods and results in an article tell the clinician what was done and what was found, so most critical appraisal tools focus on these parts of the paper. Box 67-3 contains a general critical appraisal checklist that can be used for all types of studies.

Step Four: Apply

Once the evidence relating to a specific question has been identified and appraised, it then needs to be applied to existing practice. To do this, clinicians need to be aware of the evidence, believe it, implement it, and adhere to it. It may be that current practice is in line with the current evidence so nothing needs to change, or that current practice differs from what a good appraisal of the evidence suggests is optimal. The application of evidence to practice can be a challenge because it is difficult to change practice policy and alter the opinions and habits of fellow colleagues.

There are many organizations in the medical field that have tried to address the issue of delivering evidence to practicing clinicians (see Box 67-1). In fact, the implementation of science has an entire journal dedicated to the topic, *Implementation Science* (http://www.implementationscience .com). The extent to which feline clinicians integrate evidence with their expertise is unknown, and identifying the best ways of delivering science to feline clinicians to enable them to incorporate it in decision making has not yet been determined.

There are now some evidence-based guidelines available in veterinary medicine, such as the Reassessment Campaign on Veterinary Resuscitation guidelines for cats and dogs (http://www.acvecc-recover.org/).

It should be emphasized that guidelines are not rulebooks; each practice should evaluate such guidelines and apply them to their local setting as they see fit. The actual application of guidelines is likely to differ from one practice to the next.

BOX 67-4 Example of the Five Steps in the Evidence-Based Veterinary Medicine Cycle

Step One: Ask

In cats with chronic kidney disease (CKD), does a renal prescription diet compared to a normal diet improve survival time of affected cats?

This PICO question is about efficacy of an intervention (diet) on survival time. Hence the type of evidence that is needed to answer this question would ideally be a systematic review of randomized controlled trials (RCTs) involving cats with naturally occurring CKD. These are rarely available in feline medicine, so the next best evidence would be individual RCTs. If no RCTs are available, the next best evidence would be a cohort study.

Step Two: Acquire

In cats with CKD, does a renal prescription diet compared to a normal diet improve survival time of affected cats?

Both CABI and MEDLINE could be searched and would provide good coverage of the clinical veterinary literature. Both keywords and medical subject headings (MeSH) and thesaurus terms could be used. Suggested search terms could include:

For "cats": cat, cats, feline, felines, felis
For "chronic kidney disease": chronic renal failure, chronic renal disease, chronic renal insufficiency, chronic kidney failure, chronic kidney disease, chronic kidney insufficiency
For "diet": renal diet, kidney diet, prescription diet, therapeutic diet

At the point of publication of this chapter, this search finds three relevant studies: two randomized and controlled trials[9,10] and one cohort study.[8]

Step Three: Appraise

In cats with CKD, does a renal prescription diet compared to a normal diet improve survival time of affected cats?

Randomized controlled trials are the best form of evidence for assessing treatment efficacy. A cohort study can also provide weak evidence of treatment efficacy.

Different definitions for CKD and end-stage renal failure or death were used in the studies, which makes comparing the results difficult.

All three studies identified were small with no sample size calculation, so were likely to be underpowered. The statistical methods were described in all three papers, but the basic data was not always shown clearly. Some cats died during the study periods, not all of kidney disease.

All three studies demonstrated an improved survival time and clinical status in the cats given a prescription renal diet compared to a nonprescription diet.

Step Four: Apply

In cats with CKD, does a renal prescription diet compared to a normal diet improve survival time of affected cats?

The evidence found suggests that a renal prescription diet will improve the survival of cats with CKD.

The first step in applying this evidence to practice could be a "journal club" to critically appraise the evidence found, so all members of the practice are aware of current evidence. This could be followed by a practice meeting that reviews current policy and actions on the use of prescription diets in CKD patients. After a discussion, how the evidence can be applied can be formulated. The treatment priorities of all owners of newly identified feline patients with CKD can then be identified and a diet prescribed for the appropriate cases.

Step Five: Assess

In cats with CKD, does a renal prescription diet compared to a normal diet improve survival time of affected cats?

A small internal audit could be conducted on the survival times of cats prescribed a renal diet. Alternatively, the rate at which diets are given to cats with CKD before and after the evaluation of the evidence could be undertaken.

CABI, Centre for Agriculture and Biosciences International; *PICO,* Patient, Problem, or Population; Intervention or Interest; Comparator; Outcome.

Step Five: Assess

To assess the effects of applying evidence and changing practice, one must be able to monitor the effects of a change. This assessment process often includes some form of clinical audit. According to the National Institute for Clinical Excellence (http://www.nice.org.uk), an audit is "a quality improvement process that seeks to improve patient care and outcomes through systematic review of care against explicit criteria and the implementation of change." The clinical audit process involves:

1. Assessing how a procedure is conducted
2. Evaluating specific outcomes, which can be positive, negative, or unchanged
3. Implementing a change
4. Reassessing the effect of the change on the outcome of interest

A good assessment of the application of evidence to practice should generate more clinical PICO questions that continue to drive the EVM cycle. An example of the EVM cycle is given in Box 67-4.

THE FUTURE OF EVIDENCE-BASED FELINE MEDICINE

All researchers, clinicians, and pet owners who are passionate about promoting the health and welfare of cats through EVM have a role to play in its advancement. It is not possible for one individual or one group of individuals to make EVM a reality. Both clinical and nonclinical researchers working within the sphere of feline practice should consider involving clinicians and cat owners in the design and reporting of research. The involvement of clinicians and cat owners will ensure that the research produced is both applicable and available to the people who can elicit change. Reporting guidelines can be used by researchers to facilitate the publication of research in a transparent format that enables critical appraisal by the reader. Targeting open-access journals to publish scientific findings will also increase the availability of the results to clinicians, further stimulating the EVM cycle.

Editors and reviewers of scientific journals can also promote the use of reporting guidelines by advising authors during the submission and review of scientific manuscripts.

Editors and producers of scientific journals are also well placed to increase the amount of literature that is available through open access. Increasing the evidence available to clinicians is vital to facilitate evidence-based feline medicine.

Clinicians and cat owners are the decision makers in feline practice and therefore they hold the key to implementing evidence and changing practice. Only by recognizing the need to get involved in research and by using good-quality evidence in decision making can improved health and welfare of cats become a reality.

References

1. Malycincz G: Evidence-based veterinary medicine. *Vet Record* 143(22):619, 1998.
2. Cockcroft PD, Holmes MA: *Handbook of evidence-based veterinary medicine*, Oxford, 2003, Blackwell.
3. Evidence-Based Veterinary Medicine Association. <http://ebvma.org/home/index.php>. (Accessed June 11, 2015.)
4. Centre for Evidence-Based Veterinary Medicine. <http://www.nottingham.ac.uk/cevm/index.aspx>. (Accessed June 11, 2015.)
5. Schmidt PL: Evidence-based veterinary medicine: evolution, revolution, or repackaging of veterinary practice? *Vet Clin North Am Small Anim Pract* 37(3):409–417, 2007.
6. Slater MR: Epidemiological research and evidence based medicine: how do they fit and for whom. *Prev Vet Med* 97(3/4):157–164, 2010.
7. Olivry T, Mueller RS: The International Task Force on Canine Atopic Dermatitis: Evidence-based veterinary dermatology: a systematic review of the pharmacotherapy of canine atopic dermatitis. *Vet Dermatol* 14(3):121–146, 2003.
8. Elliot J, Rawlings JM, Markwell PJ, et al: Survival of cats with naturally occurring chronic

renal failure: effect of dietary management. *J Small Anim Pract* 41:235–242, 2000.
9. Ross SJ, Osborne CA, Kirk CA, et al: Clinical evaluation of dietary modification for treatment of spontaneous chronic kidney disease in cats. *J Am Vet Med Assoc* 229:949–957, 2006.
10. Harte JG, Markwell PJ, Moraillon RM, et al: Dietary management of naturally occurring chronic renal failure in cats. *J Nutr* 124:2660S–2662S, 1994.
11. Steele M, Crabb NP, Moore LJ, et al: Online tools for teaching evidence-based veterinary medicine. *J Vet Med Educ* 40(3):272–277, 2013.
12. Hardin LE, Robertson S: Learning evidence-based veterinary medicine through development of a critically appraised topic. *J Vet Med Educ* 33(3):474–478, 2006.
13. Heneghan C, Badenoch D: *Evidence-based medicine toolkit*, ed 2, Malden, 2006, Blackwell.
14. Banfield Applied Research and Knowledge (BARK) Critically appraised topics (CATs). <www.banfield.com/veterinaryprofessionals/resources/research/cats>. (Accessed October 25, 2015.)

15. BestBETs for Vets. <www.bestbetsforvets.org>. (Accessed October 25, 2015.)
16. Grindlay DJC, Brennan ML, Dean RS: Searching the veterinary literature: a comparison of the coverage of veterinary journals in 9 bibliographic databases. *J Vet Med Educ* 39(4):404–412, 2012.
17. Berwanger O, Rodrigo R, Finkelszstejn A, et al: The quality of reporting trail abstracts is suboptimal: survey of major general medical journals. *J Clin Epidemiol* 62:387–392, 2009.
18. Pitkin RM, Branaghan MA, Burmeister LF, et al: Accuracy of data in abstracts of published research articles. *JAMA* 281(12):1110–1111, 1999.
19. A survey of the awareness, knowledge, policies and views of veterinary journal Editors-in-Chief on reporting guidelines for publication of research. *BMC Vet Res* 10:10, 2014.
20. Dean R: How to read a paper and appraise the evidence. *In Pract* 35(5):282–285, 2013.
21. Crombie IK: *The pocket guide to critical appraisal*, London, 2009, BMJ.
22. Greenhalgh T: *How to read a paper—the basics of evidence based medicine*, ed 4, London, 2003, BMJ.

Lost Cats: Epidemiology and Best Practices for Identification and Recovery

Brenda Griffin

> *Collar and ID tag: $*
> *Microchip: $$*
> *Helping an owner finding their lost cat: Priceless!*

Losing a pet cat is a common occurrence. According to one large survey of cat owners, 15% of respondents reported losing their cat within the previous 5 years, and approximately one-quarter of these were never found by their owners.[1] Current estimates suggest that there are 74 million owned cats in the United States, with one or more cats residing in approximately 30% of all households.[2] Hypothetically extrapolating from these data, one could surmise that somewhere in the neighborhood of 15% of 74 million owned cats in the United States, or *11 million cats*, may become lost within a 5-year time frame. Further, one could then assume that 2.75 million of these cats will not be recovered.

The fates of lost cats that are not found or otherwise reunited with their owners vary. Some are taken in by other owners. Some are admitted to animal shelters. Some become part of the population of free-roaming community cats, and some succumb to trauma or predation. In all cases, however, an owner is left without his or her cat, a heartbreaking scenario for anyone who experiences this.

The term *community cat* refers to any unowned free-roaming cat, including unsocialized feral cats, as well as socialized strays, some of which were no doubt previously owned pet cats.[3] To what extent lost cats contribute to the population of free-roaming community cats is unknown, but stray cats do comprise a significant proportion of this population. In many communities in the United States, the number of community cats is believed to rival that of owned cats.[4] Not surprisingly, cats currently outnumber dogs entering animal shelters in the United States. An estimated 3 to 4 million cats enter shelters annually, and tragically, approximately 70% of them are euthanized.[5,6] Common sense dictates that a significant number of these are lost cats, yet return-to-owner rates at United States animal shelters are dismally low. In fact, national estimates indicate that less than 2% of cats entering shelters are claimed by their owners, whereas as many as 15% to 19% of lost dogs are claimed.[7]

This problem is not unique to the United States. For example, in Canada, approximately 120,000 cats are admitted to shelters annually. Less than 5% of these are returned to their owners (compared with 25% to 30% of dogs), and 41% of these cats are euthanized.[8] In the United Kingdom, large numbers of cats also enter shelters, exceeding the capacity of many available organizations, and likewise very few of these (1.4%) are reunited with owners.[9] Even in countries where very few dogs enter animal shelters, such as Sweden, substantial numbers of stray cats must be cared for by available agencies. Indeed, these issues are global in nature, and efforts to reduce the numbers of lost cats are important regardless of geographic location.

The use of collars with identification (ID) tags as a visually obvious form of ID is extremely valuable although overlooked by many cat owners.[10-12] In two studies of lost pets, only 14% of cats were wearing any visual ID such as an ID tag or rabies tag at the time they were lost, whereas 43% of dogs had ID when lost. Not surprisingly, the reunification rate for cats in these studies was much lower than that for dogs, 53% and 71% respectively.[10,13]

Cats wearing collars are more likely to be identified as owned and not mistaken for strays (Figure 68-1). When cats are wearing ID tags, people that find them can contact the owner directly. Studies indicate that many people that find lost animals do not take them to an animal shelter because they fear that they may be euthanized.[10,14] In this case, a lost cat would not have an opportunity to be reclaimed by the owner through an animal shelter; however, the provision of an ID tag would enable the finder to contact the owner.

Identification is important not only for cats that are allowed outside by their owners but also for those that are kept strictly indoors. Indoor cats require ID in case they escape. In one study of lost cats, their owners described 40% of the cats as exclusively indoor cats.[10] Reasons commonly cited by cat owners for not using ID collars include that their cats do not go outside and that their cats do not get lost. Another common reason is related to the collar itself. Many cat owners perceive that their cat would not tolerate wearing

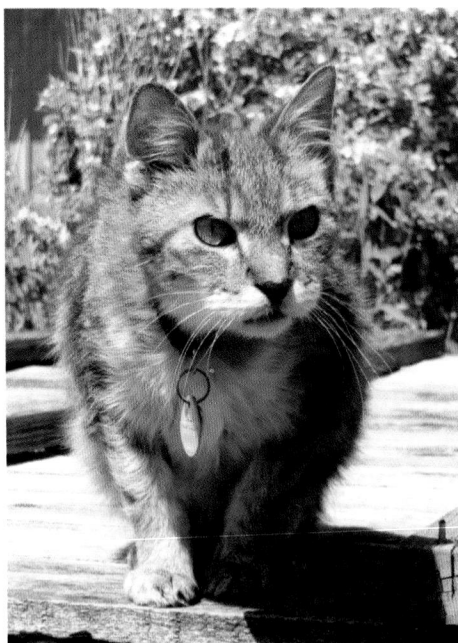

Figure 68-1: Cats with identification collars are instantly recognized as owned pets and not mistaken as strays. Visual identification is the best and most effective method. When a cat is lost, it enhances the odds of cat-owner reunification dramatically.

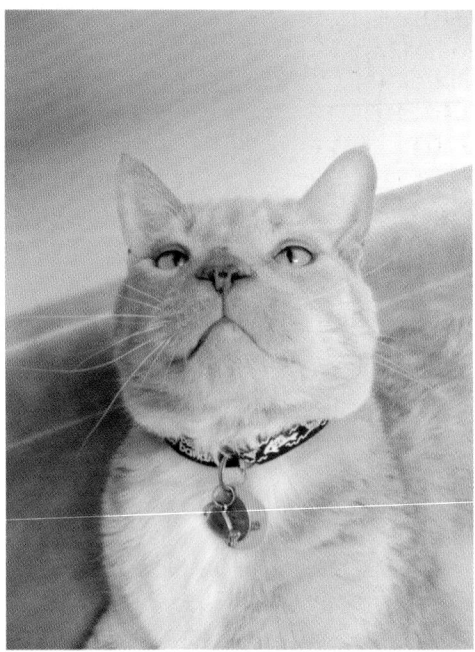

Figure 68-2: Most cats can wear collars safely and comfortably. Owners should be instructed on proper fit and educated about the propensity for many cats to remove their collars periodically, making it necessary for the owner to find it and put it back on them.

a collar and/or that wearing a collar could threaten the safety of their cat, fearing a collar-related injury.[11]

Although microchips have been available in the United States since the 1980s, only a small percentage (e.g., less than 5%) of the pet population is microchipped.[15] Common reasons cited by cat owners for not using microchip ID are similar to those for not using ID collars (indoor only and do not get lost). In addition, the expense associated with microchipping is also a significant concern for many owners.[11]

Ironically, even though many owners do not provide ID for their cats, surveys indicate that most pet owners acknowledge that ID is very important for their pets.[12] In one study, investigators collaborated with animal shelters and veterinary clinics to provide ID collars and tags at the time of adoption or office visit and conducted telephone interviews with owners 6 to 8 weeks later. The follow-up interviews revealed that 73% of veterinary clients and 89% of adopters, respectively, reported that their pets were wearing the ID collars.[16] This illustrates the importance of proactively ensuring that cats are outfitted with ID collars—once this crucial step is taken, owners may be more likely to comply with keeping ID on their cats.

Given the large number of lost pets and the low rate of reunification, the fact that so few owned cats wear ID collars and that even fewer have been microchipped are disturbing information because these forms of ID greatly enhance the odds of reunification when a cat is lost. Studies clearly demonstrate that visual ID improves the odds of pet-owner reunification.[10,13] Moreover, the provision of permanent ID in the form of a microchip represents an important backup, further improving the odds of pet-owner reunification

because collars and tags can be lost. In one study, cats entering animal shelters with microchips were 20 times more likely to be returned to their owners, compared with cats without them.[17] Given the large numbers of owners that lose their cats each year, the potential effect of improving ID and recovery of companion cats is enormous.

VISUAL IDENTIFICATION

Pet Cats: Collars and Identification Tags

Commercially available cat collars with an ID tag affixed are an excellent form of ID for cats (Figure 68-2). Contrary to popular belief, most cats can wear collars reliably, safely, and comfortably, despite common owner perceptions to the contrary. In one study, more than 500 pet cats were fitted with collars and ID tags and followed for 6 months.[11] Approximately three-quarters of the cats successfully wore their collars throughout the study period.

A notable barrier to the use of ID tags is the perception that collars are potentially dangerous. Cat owners commonly express concern that a collar may catch on something and harm their cat. In the aforementioned study,[11] many cats tolerated their collars better than their owners expected they would, with 59% of owners indicating as much. Although uncommon, collars did pose some degree of danger to cats in this study: 3.3% of the study cats got their collars caught on an object, in their mouths, or on their own forelimbs. Fortunately, none of the cats in the study were seriously injured because of collar wearing. However, the incidents involving collars being caught in the cats' mouths were very concerning because the cats could have been injured if not readily discovered by their owners. In the study, the median interval to a collar being caught in the mouth was only 5 days. This suggests that cats should be watched very closely for the first few days after collar application to ensure that the collar is fitted correctly and that the cat is adjusting to wearing it without problems. For cats that experience such an event, owners should be advised to check the fit of the collar carefully or to remove the collar and select a different type of collar instead. If the collar is reapplied, owners should be available to monitor the cat closely for several days to ensure that the cat is wearing the collar safely. Certainly, for some individual cats, not using a collar may be the best response, given the serious nature of this complication. That being said, for most cats the potential benefits of wearing an ID collar are likely to outweigh the potential risks significantly.

The best type of collar is not known, and to date, studies have not demonstrated the safety of one particular collar type over another. In the aforementioned study, cats were assigned randomly to one of three different nylon collar types, including regular buckle collars, breakaway buckle collars, and elastic stretch collars; however, no collar performed statistically better compared with another.[11] Irrespective of collar type, slightly more than one-third of the cats got their collars off during the study, requiring owners to reapply them. Regular plastic buckle collars stayed on better than breakaway buckle or elastic stretch collars did on the study cats; however, the owner's willingness to replace a collar repeatedly if it did come off was more important for success than collar type. Indeed, keeping a collar on a cat may require some effort by the owner. Some cats show more of a propensity to remove their collars than others do. Outfitting cats with collars in kittenhood may be helpful so that they become used to wearing them from an early age. Careful fitting using the "two-finger rule" (i.e., fitting the collar such that one can comfortably place two fingers between the strap and the cat's neck), monitoring, and patience in replacing the collar during the cat's adjustment period are all keys to success.

Without data to support a recommendation for the best type of cat collar, one must rely on clinical judgment until additional studies are conducted or other new information becomes available. Historically, breakaway collars have been commonly recommended and were presumed to be safer for cats because they are designed to break away if caught on something and to prevent the cat from becoming entrapped. In the aforementioned study, however, the authors note that in all instances where an owner reported that a breakaway collar was caught on either an object or on the cat's foot or mouth, the collar failed to break away as the design intended.[11] Whether this is typical of all breakaway collars is unknown, but it certainly provides additional insight for consideration.

In the author's opinion, the best type of collar is one that the cat wears comfortably and reliably and that the owner is comfortable with the cat wearing. This may vary depending on the individual cat's conformation, personality, and prefer-

ences, as well as the owner's biases. With any collar type, it is crucial to educate owners about the importance of periodically checking the fit of the collar and adjusting it as needed. If clients know that it is normal and expected that a cat might periodically remove the collar, then they may be more comfortable reapplying it when this happens.[11] The author's personal cats typically wear soft, slightly stretchy band-style collars with Velcro closures (Beastie Bands, Twin Cat, http://www.beastiebands.com).

Community Cats: Ear Tipping for Identification

Increasingly, trap-neuter-return is being used as a means of reducing birthrates and improving welfare of community cats. Ear tipping is a standard practice for ID of community cats that have been trapped, neutered, and returned to their site of capture. The procedure involves removal of the tip of one of the pinna at the time of surgical sterilization, which is the accepted global standard for indicating that a free-roaming community cat has been neutered (Figure 68-3). Ear notching is not recommended because torn earflaps are a frequent occurrence in cats because of fighting and are easily mistaken for surgically notched ears (Figure 68-4).[3,18]

Ear tipping is a humane procedure that provides a safe, permanent form of ID for community cats. In the United States, removal of the left ear tip is widely used; however, some organizations identify cats by removing the right ear tip, or by removing the tip on one side or the other, depending on the sex of the cat.[18] Consistency with the standard in a given community is the best practice.[18] A simple procedure for ear tipping is described in Box 68-1.

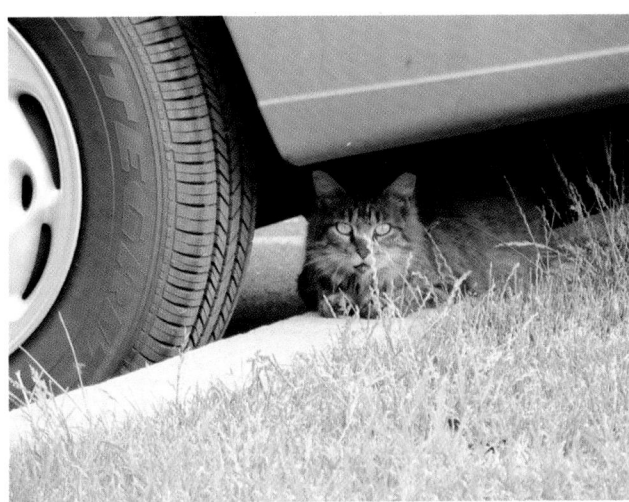

Figure 68-3: Community cat with a tipped ear: The cropped left ear tip identifies the cat as neutered. Note the tipped ear's distinctive straight edge, which is the key to this universally recognizable symbol.

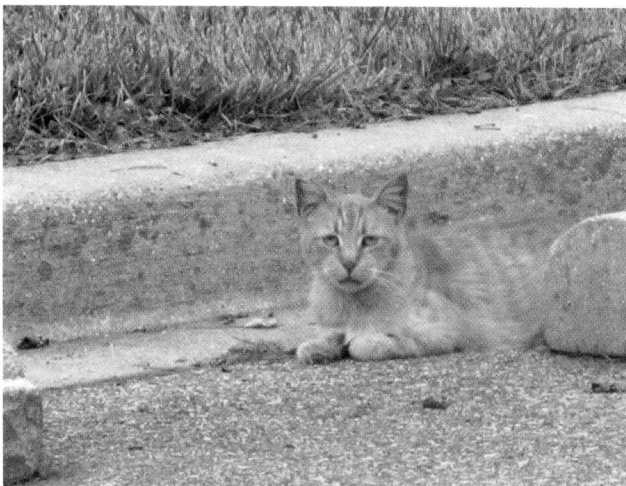

Figure 68-4: The margin of the left ear tip appears irregular. It is impossible to know if this is the result of injury or surgical ear notching. For this reason, ear tipping, rather than notching, serves as the standard universal symbol for neutered community cats.

BOX 68-1 Ear Tipping Procedure Performed Under General Anesthesia for Community Cat Identification[18]

Use a pair of straight scissors and straight hemostatic forceps to create the desired visual effect. Following removal of the ear tip, the ear margin should have a distinct straight edge that is easy to recognize from a distance (Figure 68-3).

- A straight hemostat is placed perpendicular to the long axis of the pinna, exposing proportionately approximately one-third of the distal earflap.
- Sterile scissors are used to remove the tip by cutting distally along the edge of the instrument.
- The hemostat is left in place while the cat undergoes surgery, and it is removed during recovery. Gluing or suturing the ear margin is neither necessary nor recommended.

LESS OBVIOUS FORMS OF IDENTIFICATION

Microchips

Microchips have been used for animal ID for decades. These tiny devices, which are about the size of a grain of rice, are easily implanted in subcutaneous tissue using a large-gauge hypodermic needle. Some newer microchips (called mini chips) are even smaller. The implantation procedure is simple and only rarely requires sedation.[11] Moreover, most cats readily tolerate microchip insertion just as they generally tolerate injection of a vaccine. Although the application needles are large (e.g., 12- to 15-gauge), they are very sharp and well polished, making insertion relatively smooth and atraumatic. In the United States, microchips are typically implanted in the subcutaneous tissue over the midline of the dorsal shoulders or lower neck.[15,19,20] The technique for implanting a microchip is described in Box 68-2.

BOX 68-2 Procedure for Implanting a Microchip[20]

1. Perform a systematic scan of the entire cat to ensure that no pre-existing microchip is present. The scanner should indicate, "No ID found."
2. Verify the code of the microchip before implantation by scanning it within its applicator and cross-referencing the number on the product packaging.
3. Do not clip the hair coat or use antiseptic solution on the implantation site because these procedures are neither necessary nor recommended.
4. Remove the cap from the applicator needle. Avoid holding the needle downward because it may be possible for the microchip to fall out.
5. If the patient is awake, provide gentle restraint as needed. Many feline patients will allow microchip administration with no resistance while eating a treat such as canned cat food.
6. Tent the skin over the dorsal shoulder blades and insert the needle, burying it to the hub.
7. Depress the plunger completely, and then deliberately turn the needle 90° to one side before withdrawing it. (Note: Turning the needle before withdrawal helps to dislodge the microchip from the applicator tip, preventing it from accidentally being withdrawn from the injection site along with the needle. This process does not increase patient discomfort.)
8. Inspect the injection site as the needle is removed. Apply gentle pressure to oppose the skin at the insertion site.
9. Scan the cat and recheck the radiofrequency identification device code.
10. Discard the applicator needle in the appropriate sharps disposal.
11. Complete the registration process. Enter the microchip number and animal and owner information in the microchip registry. In addition, record the same information in the shelter or hospital's database as a backup.
12. Attach the corresponding tag (if available) to the cat's collar.
13. Encourage rest and avoid stimulating physical activity for 24 hours following microchip insertion. The goal is to prevent migration by encouraging adherence to the subcutaneous tissue in the initial hours following placement.

Microchips, also known as radiofrequency identification devices (RFIDs), rely on bar code technology. When activated by a low-power radiofrequency scanner, they emit a unique, preprogrammed ID number. The number must be linked to a registry with a database containing the animal's identity and owner contact information. Unlike visual means of pet ID, both an effective scanner and registry system are required for positive ID via microchip. Microchips should not be used in place of visual ID, but when used in conjunction with ID collars, they provide an important form of backup ID. This is especially true given the propensity of many cats to remove or lose their collars periodically. Another advantage of microchips is that they cannot be removed readily or altered, making them a permanent form of ID.

Over the last two decades, microchips of varying radiofrequencies (125, 128, and 134.2 kHz) have been sold in the United States, each with its own registry and database.[15] Market competition and intentional incompatibility among different manufacturers' microchips, scanners, and registries have resulted in controversies and lawsuits. The 125 kHz chips have been the most widely used by far, but all three radiofrequencies continue to be marketed and used. This has created problematic situations because scanners do not necessarily read all available radiofrequencies, and thus, in some instances, available scanners are not able to detect the presence of some microchips. Further, it can be difficult to ascertain which registry to contact when a microchip is identified. It is important to recognize the serious implications of these issues. Failure to detect a microchip and/or inaccessible or inaccurate owner registration may result in failure to reunify a pet and owner or, even worse, euthanasia of a beloved pet in an animal shelter.

This lack of a national standard for microchip ID of companion animals is unique to the United States. In contrast, the International Organization for Standardization (ISO) standard is the accepted standard in nearly every country of the world where microchips are used for pet ID.[15] In countries that embrace this standard, only 134.2 kHz microchips are used for RFID of companion animals, and registration is centralized, improving the effectiveness of the system.

Currently, there are efforts to standardize microchipping in the United States. These efforts are endorsed by numerous organizations including the American Veterinary Medical Association (AVMA), the American Animal Hospital Association (AAHA), the American Association of Feline Practitioners (AAFP), the Humane Society of the United States, and the American Society for the Prevention of Cruelty to Animals. As a part of these efforts, some companies have developed and distributed universal scanners (also known as "global scanners" or "forward and backward reading scanners") capable of reading all of the currently available microchip radiofrequencies.[15] Widespread availability of universal scanners will make it possible to transition safely to the use of 134.2 kHz (ISO) microchips, thus adopting the microchip standard used in the rest of the world.

Efforts in the United States have also focused on improving, updating, and centralizing microchip registries. In pursuit of this goal, the AAHA developed and implemented a web-based search engine for pet microchip ID numbers (http://www.petmicrochiplookup.org) as an attempt to centralize microchip registries functionally by linking existing national databases. The search engine, which is called the Universal Pet Microchip Lookup Tool, allows users to enter a microchip code and directs them to participating microchip registries associated with that microchip's number and manu-

facturer. The site does not provide registration information and only provides information linking to microchip databases that operate in the United States. Another issue surrounding registration is that a substantial proportion of owner contact information may become obsolete within a short time frame if the database is not updated regularly to ensure that consumer information is current and correct. A study involving 53 animal shelters revealed that 63.5% of cats entering shelters with a microchip were successfully returned to their owners.[17] In the cases in which microchipped cats were not reunified with their owners, the main reasons included incorrect owner contact information, unregistered microchips, or microchips registered in a database other than those of the manufacturer.

The United States is also the only country in which microchip implantation and microchip registration are not always integrated processes.[15] In other words, microchips are not always registered at the time of implantation. Instead, in some instances, owners are given the corresponding paperwork and instructed to register the microchip. If they fail to do so, the microchip is in effect rendered useless. To ensure that microchips are always registered, both animal shelters and veterinarians must always register them at the time of implantation.[17] This will maximize their effectiveness, increasing the likelihood of reuniting pets with their families.

The variety of available radiofrequencies of microchips in the United States has prompted studies to evaluate the reliability of available scanners for detection of the various microchips.[19,21] Important information gleaned from these studies has been used to enhance scanning procedures to optimize the detection of microchips. It is important to recognize that no scanner performs with 100% sensitivity for all microchips. Universal scanners tend to have the highest sensitivity for 134.2 kHz (ISO) microchips, but slightly lower for 125 and 128 kHz microchips. In a study of 7700 animals admitted to shelters, 13% of the animals scanned more than once were found to have microchips on subsequent scans that were undetected on initial scanning.[17] Therefore, scanning more than one time and using proper technique are crucial to success. Box 68-3 contains detailed recommendations for scanning to maximize detection of microchips. As the market continues to evolve, available microchips and scanners will vary. The AVMA maintains detailed information about microchips on its website, including a listing of commonly used microchips and scanners.[15]

Unfortunately, much work remains to standardize microchipping effectively in the United States. To maximize the potential benefits of microchips, standardization as well as widespread acceptance and use by animal shelters, veterinarians, and pet owners will be required. Nonetheless, even with the limitations of the current system, microchips clearly afford pets with a significant benefit by providing them with a greater degree of protection should they become lost.[17]

Besides the lack of standardized technology and a centralized registry database, other reported barriers to the use of microchips include cost, fear of lack of information privacy, safety concerns, religious beliefs, and simply the lack of

BOX 68-3 Microchip Scanning Technique[17,19,21]

General Instructions

Scanners and batteries: Use a universal (global) scanner (i.e., one that will read all microchip frequencies that are currently in use in one's country). Always ensure that the scanner batteries are well charged because weak batteries are a leading cause of scanner failure. If the scanner freezes, remove and replace the batteries before proceeding. Although microchip migration is rare, it does occur; therefore, careful, systematic scanning of the entire animal is essential. Finally, because it is possible to miss a microchip on an initial scan, repeat scanning is always recommended.

Preventing Scanner Interference

Do not scan cats in carriers, cages, or traps because of the high likelihood of scanner interference and the difficulty in performing a thorough scan under these conditions. Position the cat on an examination table for scanning. If present, remove collars or anything covering the cat prior to scanning. Towels or newspapers should be placed under the cat if scanning on a stainless steel surface. Extra care should be taken with obese cats.

Before proceeding, pass the scanner over a test chip to verify proper functioning.

1. *Scanner orientation:* The scanner should be held parallel to the cat. Rocking the scanner slightly from side to side will maximize the potential for optimal chip orientation and successful detection. The button on the scanner should be depressed continuously during the entire scanning procedure. Scanning multiple times in slightly different orientations each time will maximize the scanner's potential to detect a microchip.
2. *Scanning distance:* The scanner should be held in contact with the cat during scanning such that it is lightly touching the hair coat.

3. *Scanner speed:* The scanner should not be advanced any faster than 0.15 m (0.5 feet) per second. Scanning slowly is crucial because universal scanners must cycle through various modes to read all possible chip frequencies.
4. *Areas of animal to scan:* The standard implant site is midway between the shoulder blades, and scanning should begin over this area (A). If a microchip is not detected here, scanning should proceed systematically down the back and on the sides, neck, and shoulders, continuing distally and taking care to include the cranial and caudal aspects of the limbs, all the way down to the elbows in the front and the hindquarters in the rear (B).

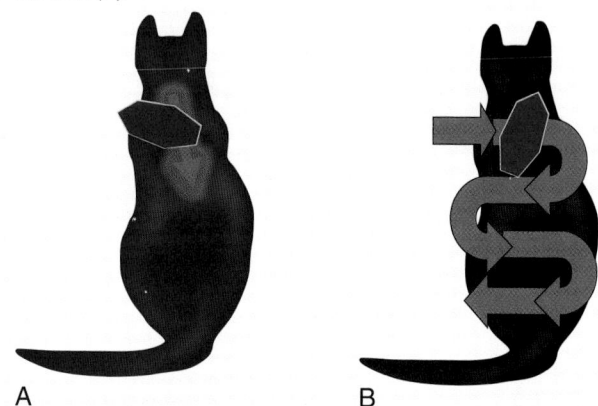

A   B

5. *Scanning pattern:* The scanner should be moved over the scanning areas in an S-shaped pattern in a transverse direction (from side to side, B). If no microchip is detected, the scanner should be rotated 90° and then the S-shaped pattern should be repeated in a longitudinal direction (e.g., long ways) ON BOTH SIDES of the cat (C, D). This pattern of scanning will maximize the ability of the scanner to detect the microchip, regardless of its orientation. Always scan the entire cat.

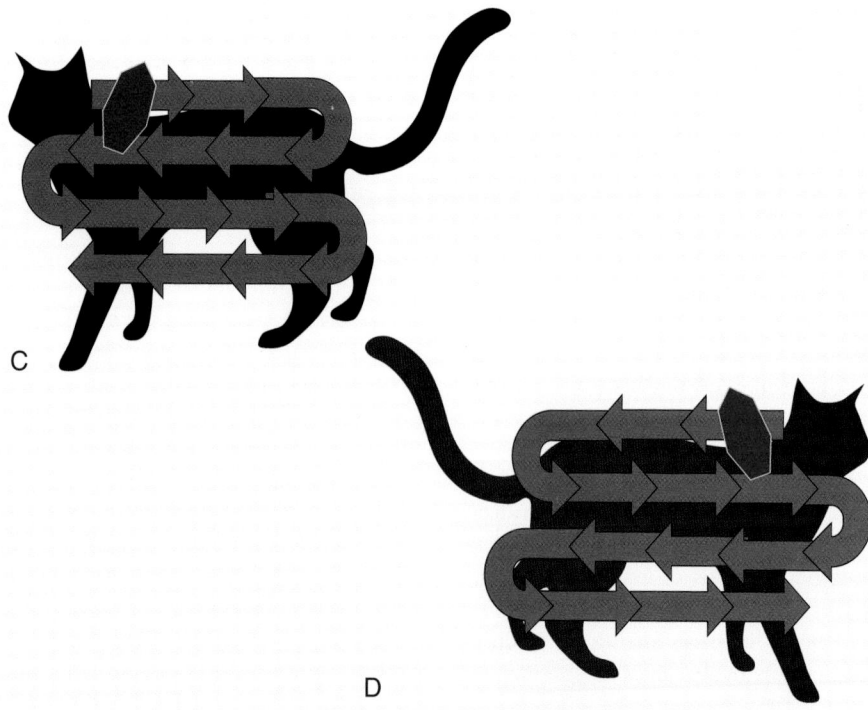

C

D

awareness of their availability and benefits.[10-14] Migration of the microchip has also been cited as a potential concern.

Over the past few years, several highly publicized studies of microchip-induced tumors in laboratory mice triggered concern in the animal community about the safety of microchipping.[15] In cats, chronic inflammation has been associated with fibrosarcoma formation as observed in postvaccinal sarcomas and ocular post-traumatic sarcomas. One case report suggests the possibility of a microchip-associated sarcoma in a cat.[22] The tumor and microchip were excised and approximately 1 year after excision, and the cat was reportedly healthy with no sign of recurrence. As with any injection site in a cat, microchip injection sites should be monitored carefully, and owners should always be instructed to look for swelling at the site. Latency between trauma and the development of injection-site neoplasia is often several years, making it difficult to determine the underlying etiology with certainty. Using standard vaccination sites, as well as standard microchip insertion sites, may help investigators to correlate events better.

Fortunately, the number of adverse events associated with microchipping is extremely low. According to the British Small Animal Veterinary Association, which has collected data for nearly two decades, during which time millions of pets have been microchipped in the United Kingdom, serious adverse events are exceedingly rare.[15] With a well-documented record for safety, there is widespread agreement among experts that the use of microchips for pet ID should not be discouraged. Veterinarians should check microchip sites annually and report any adverse reactions.

An additional safety concern of note involves injury to the animal related to improper microchip implantation. One case report describes acute tetraparesis in a cat following forceful restraint and microchip insertion by the cat's owners.[23] Fortunately, the cat recovered following surgical removal of the microchip from the spinal canal, but this report underscores the importance of proper injection technique by trained personnel.

Presumably, because of such safety concerns, some state boards have lobbied to make microchipping a veterinary-only procedure. It is important to recognize that widespread use of microchipping is necessary to maximize the benefit of this technology for all companion animals. In recognition of this, animal shelters, breeders, and owners are allowed to implant microchips in their own animals in many jurisdictions. This serves to ensure that animals in their care can benefit from this technology whenever possible.

Finally, the potential for microchips to migrate from their site of implantation has also been cited as a concern.[15,17] When chips are found at sites other than the standard implantation site, which in the United States is the region of the dorsal shoulders or lower neck, the microchip is believed to have migrated. Theoretically, migration may result in microchips being located virtually anywhere in the subcutaneous tissue of the animal's body. If migration occurred frequently, it would make detection of microchips less likely, negating the benefit of the device. Fortunately, two studies have demonstrated that migration is an infrequent occurrence. In one study of 7700 dogs and cats entering shelters, migration was reported in only 1.6% of the animals.[17] In a study of more than 500 cats, only 0.6% of microchips were determined to have migrated from their original implantation sites 6 months later.[11] The lateral elbow and shoulder are common locations for migration.[15] Some clinicians have suggested that physical activity following implantation may be responsible for migration before the microchip has adhered to the subcutaneous tissue. Given this possible explanation, it seems prudent to keep animals quiet, so that the animal can avoid physical activity for 24 hours following the procedure.

Although microchips are generally considered a permanent form of ID, it is possible for them to fail. Fortunately, this is considered even rarer than migration, based on available data. For example, in the aforementioned study, only one cat had a microchip that was not functional at the end of the study.[11] Its presence was confirmed by radiography, yet it could not be detected using a scanner. The cause of such microchip failure is unknown, although damage or trauma to the microchip is likely the culprit. If a nonfunctional chip is present, removal is not recommended, but a second microchip should be implanted to identify the animal. Although previously believed to render microchips nonfunctional, a study of 53 veterinary patients with microchips undergoing magnetic resonance imaging (MRI) revealed that MRI did not interfere with the functionality of any of the microchips in the patients.[24] Although migration and failure are rare occurrences, routine scanning of cats at preventive health care visits is prudent and provides an important opportunity to ensure that microchips remain functional and are present in the expected location (Figure 68-5). At the same time, owners should be reminded to update their contact information as needed in the microchip registry.[11,15]

A logistical concern of note occasionally arises when a pet with a pre-existing 125 kHz microchip is required to have a 134.2 kHz (ISO) chip for travel to another country. It is not problematic to implant a second microchip because both will function normally and could be detected separately.[15] However, it is crucial in this case for the owner to register both chips because either one could be detected upon scanning should the pet be lost.

Tattoos

Tattooing is an uncommon means of primary ID for pet cats and is not recommended for such. This is because compared with other methods of ID, tattooing is associated with numerous disadvantages, which make it both impractical and ineffective for this purpose. Tattooing requires heavy sedation or general anesthesia, as well as special equipment including multiple needles, which should be properly disinfected between patients to prevent transmission of blood-borne viruses or other infections. Once applied, tattoos are often difficult to read because of hair growth, fading, and distortions that occur over time. Finally, there are no standards for tattoo placement, and tattoo registries are not

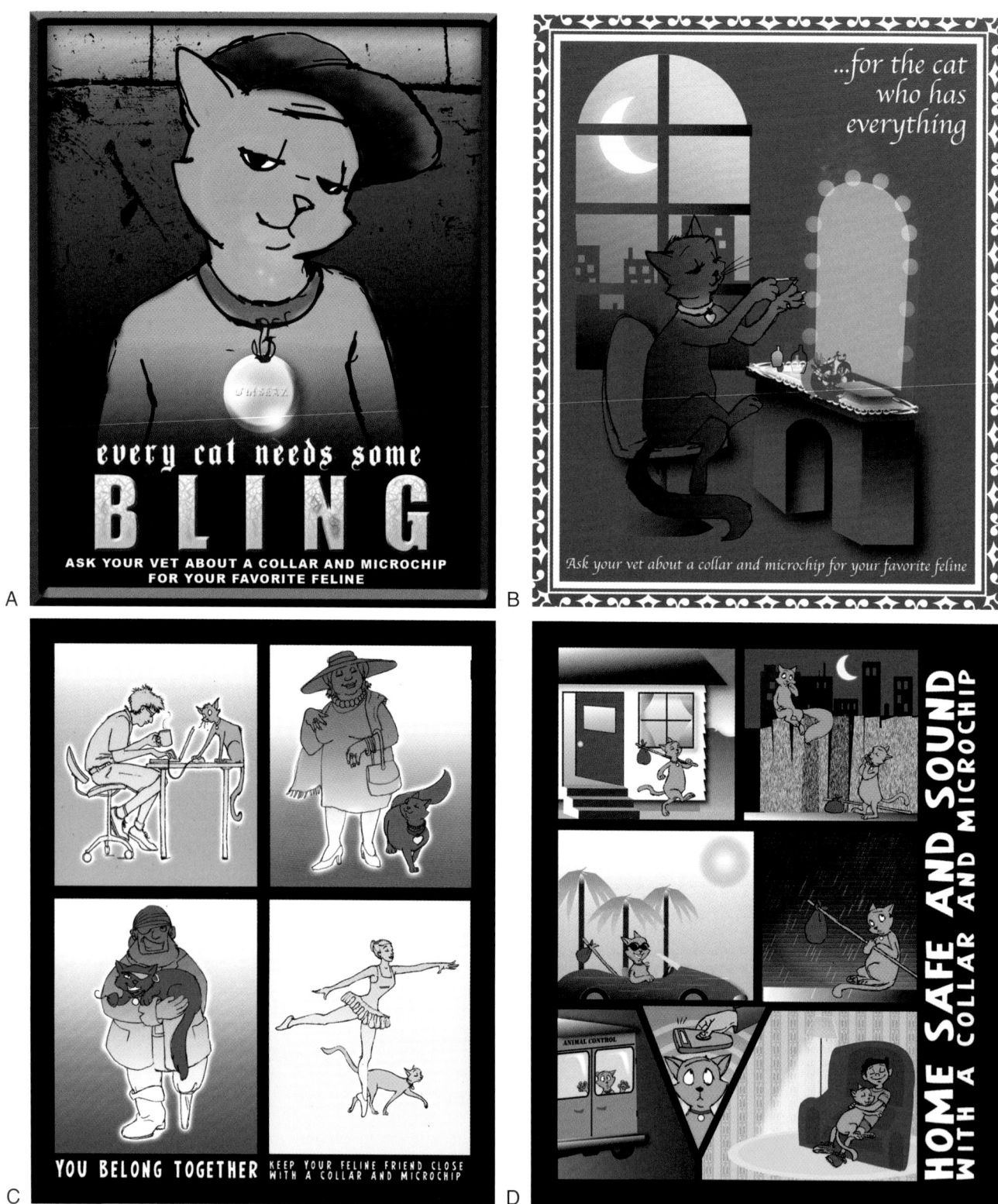

Figure 68-5: Sample educational posters relating the importance and benefits of identification collars and microchips to cat owners. (Courtesy of Brenda Griffin.)

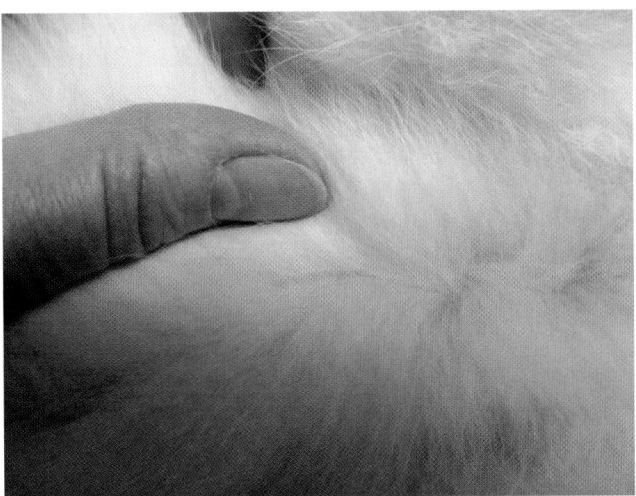

Figure 68-6: Line tattoo on the ventral abdomen of a cat: A simple green line is the recommended standard mark to identify spayed or neutered pet cats.

widely available, making tattoos of little use as a primary means of ID.[25,26]

In contrast, tattooing is a very useful and practical means of identifying animals as neutered. It is strongly recommended as a means of "marking" pet cats at the time of spay or neuter surgery.[18,27] Because it can be difficult to determine the reproductive status of stray cats that are presented with little or no history, a tattoo may ultimately prevent a cat from undergoing unnecessary exploratory surgery. Simple tattoo techniques, which do not require special needles or instrumentation, have been developed for this purpose.[18] A small line is created on the ventral abdomen and its presence is meant to indicate that the animal has been surgically sterilized (Figure 68-6). Examination for a ventral midline scar ("spay scar") is a standard practice to determine sterilization status of females. Thus the presence of a tattoo in this area would be easily discovered and could verify that surgical sterilization had been performed.[28] Because neutered tomcats are sometimes mistaken for queens, placement of a ventral midline tattoo at the time of neutering is also recommended for them.[18] National guidelines for spay and neuter programs recommend the use of tattoos for this purpose.[27,28] Box 68-4 describes a simple procedure for marking cats at the time of spay or neuter surgery. The time and cost of incorporating this tattoo technique into spay and neuter procedures are negligible; however, the value of providing a permanent mark to indicate a cat's sterilization status is extremely valuable.

ENHANCING IDENTIFICATION AND RECOVERY

Plain and simple, the provision of ID is an essential component of wellness care for cats. In fact, the AAFP strongly supports the use of ID collars and microchips for cats.[29] Leadership from both veterinary and animal shelter personnel will serve to maximize the benefit of these lifesaving tools.

Green tattoo paste (Ketchum Manufacturing, Inc., Brockville, Ontario, Canada) is used to create a simple line on the ventral abdomen to mark the animal at the time of surgery.
- A separate superficial skin incision (0.5 to 1.0 cm) is made through the dermis.
- A tiny drop of paste is applied directly into this incision using the edge of a paper strip. A sterility indicator strip from the surgery pack may be conveniently used for this purpose.
- The skin edges are slightly inverted, and a drop of tissue adhesive is applied on top of the skin for closure.

Room for Improvement

Although many veterinary clinics do recommend pet ID, a survey of 1086 clinics in the southeastern Unites States demonstrated that many veterinarians are less likely to recommend ID collars and microchips for cats compared to dogs, including cats that spend time outdoors.[30] Investigators noted that for the clinics surveyed that recommended microchips, they reported that only a small number of clients elected the procedure. In addition, microchip scanning was only occasionally performed by some clinics, usually in response to a client's request, and 38% of clinics did not have universal scanners.[30]

In animal shelters, practices surrounding pet ID and microchip scanning vary tremendously from community to community and agency to agency. Over the past decade, there has been a growing trend for shelters to microchip pets before adoption; however, the provision of ID collars is unfortunately an uncommon practice. Although microchip scanning is considered an industry standard,[31,32] the use of universal scanners and proper scanning protocols are frequently inconsistent.

Striving for Best Practices

The pet ID and recovery systems that are most effective will require widespread acceptance and support by animal shelters, veterinarians, and cat owners. Pet ID is an important part of responsible ownership. Notably, it is especially crucial in times of disaster. The Federal Emergency Management Agency strongly recommends the provision of ID collars and microchips as a standard protocol for pets during disaster response.

Fortunately, it is not difficult to find inspiration to improve current practices. The Internet is filled with powerful documentaries of lost animals that are reunited with their owners because of accurate ID. In some cases, reunification occurs over extremely long distances (i.e., hundreds or even thousands of miles) or long after the pet has been lost (i.e., months or years later).

What Can Veterinarians Do?

Improving pet ID and recovery is an important goal for veterinarians. In addition to being "good medicine," it is also "good business" because keeping pets safely in their homes improves the odds that they will remain patients in the practice. By removing barriers, clearly explaining risks and benefits, and making pet ID convenient and readily available, veterinarians can ensure that their patients receive the potentially lifesaving benefits of these tools. Studies have demonstrated that many owners, even well-educated people, do not think to put a collar on their cats but are willing to do so once educated, and that making microchips widely available and affordable may increase compliance.[11] Boxes 68-5 and

---

BOX 68-5 Recommendations for Veterinary Practices (Figure 68-7)

- Recognize that both visual and permanent identification are essential components of a comprehensive preventive medical plan for cats and that the potential benefits far exceed any potential adverse effects.
  - Recognize that this holds true even for indoor cats.
- Place client-education handouts and posters in waiting areas and examination rooms. See Box 68-6 for a sample handout and Figure 68-7 for sample posters.
- Lead by example.
  - Ensure that any cats residing at the veterinary clinic wear identification (ID) collars and have microchips.
  - For education and media materials, use images in which cats are clearly wearing ID collars.
- Prioritize time for pet identification in wellness visits.
- Include "lack of an ID collar" or "lack of a microchip" on medical problem lists and address them in medical plans.
- For cats without identification:
  - Remove barriers—let clients know it is safe and good medicine.
  - Paint the picture so the client understands the risks—no one plans to lose their cat (i.e., accidents, disasters, and everyday life).
  - Assure them that collars and microchips are safe.
    - Empathize and self-disclose—tell them that your cats wear collars.
  - Let them know that microchips are not a "gimmick."
    - Relate real-life experiences where pets that were lost were recovered because of a microchip.
  - Let them know the procedure is not going to be highly stressful or painful for their cat (i.e., implanting microchips is quick, easy, and minimally stressful and does not require use of excessive restraint or sedation).
  - Provide collars and tags for purchase or as a part of a preventive health care package.
    - Point out that visual ID is the easiest method for pet reunification.
    - Instruct owners on proper collar application, beginning in kittenhood whenever possible.
    - Explain that they will need to monitor the collar—educate owners that collars do come off and need to be put back on and adjusted periodically.
    - Consider purchasing a tag engraver and display it in the reception area.
      - Engrave ID tags for client pets.
      - Engrave the back of the rabies tag with the client's phone number.

- If no engraver is available, offer tags that do not require engraving such as Rescue Tags (Campbell Pet Products, Brush Prairie, Washington).
- Consider using free Get Me Home Tags (Merial, USA, http://www.getmehome.com/).
- Use tags that are provided with microchips.
  - Provide microchips for purchase.
    - Offer microchipping during kitten visits, wellness examinations, boarding, and elective procedures such as spay or neuter surgery.
    - Offer "microchip only" appointments.
    - Periodically offer microchip clinics (higher volume, lower cost).
    - Participate in American Veterinary Medical Association's Check the Chip Day on August 15 each year.
    - NEVER separate the microchip implantation process from the registration process with a national microchip registry—collect the information and process the registration for the client.
    - Educate owners that any inflammatory reaction theoretically can contribute to tumor formation, especially in cats, but this remains extremely rare.
    - Follow American Association of Feline Practitioners guidelines for vaccine placement.
- For cats with identification:
  - Perform an annual tag checkup—is the tag legible? Is the information correct? Is the collar fitted properly?
  - Perform an annual chip checkup (Figure 68-7).
    - Scan cats at the time of the annual wellness examination.
    - Make sure the microchip is still in place and functional.
    - Remind owners to update their information in the registry.
- Identify all cats as neutered at the time of spay or neuter surgery.
  - Apply line tattoos to all tame cats at the time of spay or neuter surgery.
  - Ear tip all community cats at the time of trap-neuter-return.
  - Note: These can literally be lifesaving marks because neutered cats are more likely to be allowed to live in outdoor colonies or to be rehomed if tame.
- Provide advice for owners who have lost a cat (Box 68-8).

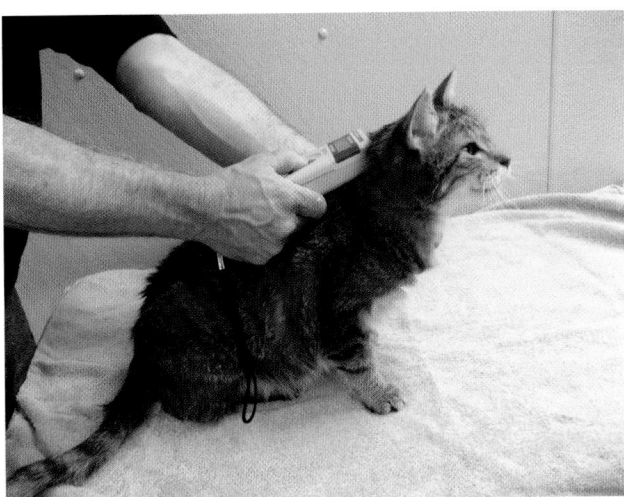

Figure 68-7: Scanning for a microchip during an annual chip checkup: The initial pass of the scanner is directed over the standard implantation site, with the scanner held parallel and in close contact with the cat. In addition to ensuring that the microchip is in place and functional, steps should be taken to ensure that it is registered with the owner's current contact information.

68-6 contain a list of recommendations and best veterinary practices for cat ID and recovery.

What Can Shelters Do?

Improving pet ID and recovery is also an important goal for animal shelters. Lost-and-found pet matching programs have the potential to improve return-to-owner rates at shelters, and implementation of widespread tagging and microchipping programs have the potential to significantly reduce the number of stray cats admitted to shelters and living in communities.[16] Box 68-7 contains a list of recommendations and best sheltering practices for cat ID and recovery.

Advice for Owners Who Have Lost Their Cat

Studies have evaluated search methods used by owners to find their lost cat, as well as search methods used by finders of lost cats to locate their owners.[10,14] Knowledge gleaned from these studies can be used to shape optimal recommendations to increase the odds of successful reunification. Studies reveal that many cats do return home on their own in time.[1,10] This is comforting to know; however, it also creates a potentially dangerous situation because many people do not actively search for their missing cat right away, believing that the cat will return. Consequently, fewer people visit local shelters, and if they do, it is typically beyond the period for legal holding (Figure 68-7). In other words, if a lost cat has been taken to an area animal shelter as a stray, most shelters will hold that animal in accordance with local ordinances to allow the owner a chance to claim. The required legal holding period is usually only a few days; however, many cat owners either do not visit the local shelter or delay visiting for several days to look for their lost cat. In either case, the owner may have missed a vital opportunity to claim their cat. Another

Every Pet Needs Identification

Each year, it is estimated that as many as one million pets will be lost and not recovered. Providing pets with both an identification tag and a microchip is good medicine. It is a proactive, preventive measure to greatly enhance the odds of reunification should the pets become lost.

Why Both a Collar and a Microchip?

Think of it as a safety belt and an airbag. A collar with a tag serves as a visible form of identification and clearly indicates to anyone who finds your pet that you are the owner. The microchip is a very important backup form of identification. If the collar and tag are lost and your pet ends up in an animal shelter or veterinary clinic, the "invisible" microchip can be detected with a scanner.

Special Considerations for Cats

My Cat Is an Indoor Cat—Why Identification?

As diligent as we all are, accidents and natural disasters happen, and there is no guarantee that indoor-only cats will not accidentally get out or escape and become lost. Indeed, almost half of owners who have lost a cat report they never expected their cat to get outside. Cats that are unaccustomed to being outdoors may have a particularly difficult time returning home.

I've Heard That Cats Can't Wear Collars

Most cats will reliably wear collars safely and comfortably. Select a collar and fit it so that you can comfortably place two fingers between the strap and your cat's neck. Be prepared to monitor your cat to ensure that the collar remains correctly fitted and in place. Many cats remove their own collars periodically, so be prepared to put it back on if this happens. It is best to start kittens out with collars as soon as possible so they learn to wear them from an early age. Check the collar each week and adjust it as your kitten grows.

common scenario is for an owner to call the agency rather than visiting in person. Given the large numbers of cats admitted to shelters and the variability of cat coat color and pattern descriptions used by cat owners and shelter staff, it can be extremely problematic to match a lost cat and owner by telephone.

The fact that most cats are found close to home is also important when considering best practices to optimize the odds of reunification.[10] Searching the neighborhood can be highly rewarding, and certain key search tips may improve the odds of finding the pet. Importantly, posting signs in the neighborhood is one of the most effective methods used by owners for finding a pet cat.[10] It is also important to note that people that find a pet cat without ID tags often report it to the local shelter, although they may not take the cat to the shelter. They may also place an advertisement in a local newspaper or online, or place signs in the neighborhood. When geriatric cats go missing, many owners may not search

BOX 68-7 Recommendations for Animal Shelters

- Check for visual identification (ID) at the time of admission.
  - Create a protocol detailing the action steps to follow if an ID collar, rabies tag, or license tag is present.
  - Create a protocol detailing the action steps to follow if an ear tip is present.
- Require the use of universal scanners so that microchips of all frequencies can be detected (125, 128, and 134.2 kHz).
- Provide universal scanners, extra batteries, and test microchips at all admission areas and in all transport vehicles (i.e., animal control trucks).
- Train all personnel including animal control officers, shelter staff, and others on proper microchip scanning technique. (See Box 68-3.)
- Schedule regular battery changes, and use high-quality batteries for scanners.
- Scan all cats at intake, including those relinquished by their owners.
  - In some instances, cats will belong to someone else, which may be discovered through microchip scanning.
- For cats that are too fractious to scan at intake, allow 24 hours for acclimation to see if the cat will accept handling. Cats that remain too fractious to handle should be sedated for scanning.
  - It is crucial to recognize that socialized house cats may remain in an agitated state for a prolonged period if highly stressed at intake. It should not be assumed that such cats are feral, and thus all cats should be scanned regardless of behavior status.[34]
- Scan cats at multiple checkpoints.
  - Scan in the field for immediate reunification with owner whenever possible.
  - Scan as part of the intake examination upon entry to the shelter.
  - Scan at the time of medical examination.
  - Scan at the time of spay or neuter surgery.
  - Scan at the time of adoption or transfer.
  - Scan before euthanasia.
    - Cats that are too fractious to handle should be sedated and thoroughly scanned for a microchip using a global scanner before euthanasia.

- Create a protocol detailing the action steps to follow when a microchip is detected.
  - Use the American Animal Hospital Association Microchip Lookup Tool (http://www.petmicrochiplookup.org) to find out which registry has the information associated with the microchip.
  - Consider contacting more than one registry if the manufacturer's registry does not have current registration information for a microchip.
  - Always contact the microchip registry for owner-surrendered animals and stray animals because the person surrendering the animal may not be the actual or original owner.
- Because owners and shelter staff often describe cat coat colors and patterns differently, post intake photographs online to improve lost pet matching and enable owners to look for their pet even if they are unable physically to come to the shelter.
- Send home all adopted cats with ID collars and microchips.
- Send home all reclaimed cats with ID collars and microchips.
- Register all microchips before the cat leaves the shelter because many owners will neglect to do so following adoption, making the microchip an ineffective means of identification.
- Apply line tattoos to all tame cats at the time of spay or neuter surgery.
- Ear tip all community cats at the time of trap-neuter-return.
- Provide advice for owners who have lost a cat. (See Box 68-8.)
- Ask people that find a cat to search for the owner or have volunteers search.
  - Educate them that geriatric cats and neutered cats are more likely to be owned and are usually lost close to home.
  - Ask them to speak with neighbors and post fliers in the area where the cat was found.

for them because of the widely purported myth that older cats "wander off to die" at the end of life[33] (Figure 68-8); on the contrary, when a cat goes missing, it is most likely because the cat's routine was disrupted (i.e., the cat was let out by accident or was chased by a dog or was otherwise disturbed or frightened). The owner may mourn at home, never imagining that their beloved cat is hiding nearby or is at a neighbor's home or local shelter. Finally, and not surprisingly, studies indicate that neutered cats are more likely to be recovered, which is another benefit of spaying or neutering to share with clients.[10] Box 68-8 contains advice for cat owners who have lost a cat.

SUMMARY

Given that many pet cats are lost and not recovered, veterinarians have a unique opportunity to develop proactive pet ID protocols as a part of every wellness plan for feline patients. Veterinarians can play a key role in educating owners about the value of pet ID, and thus overcoming the barriers that prevent some owners from providing their pets with ID collars and microchips. By offering sound advice on search methods when a client loses a pet, veterinarians will enhance the odds of a happy reunion. At the same time, community animal sheltering agencies can also play a vital

BOX 68-8 Advice for Looking for a Lost Cat

- Act quickly and immediately.
  - The more time that passes, the less likely you will be to find your beloved cat.
  - Ask friends and family for help and begin your search right away.
- Look nearby.
  - Cats become frightened by something unusual that disrupted their routine and may be hiding under a deck or in a crawlspace nearby, or they may have climbed a tree and cannot get down from it. Indoor cats that escape may be especially frightened and may be difficult to coax out of their hiding place.
  - Choose a quiet time of the day such as early morning or near dusk. Call to the cat, shake a bag of cat food or treats, or pop the lid on a can of cat food. Sometimes, the cat may remain too scared to come out, but it might begin to vocalize and you will be able to locate it as it calls to you.
  - Repeat this procedure every morning and evening.
  - Personally notify neighbors and ask them to be on the lookout for your cat.
    - Talk to children and retirees in your neighborhood. They may be the most likely to have seen your cat.
  - Post signs in the neighborhood. Include a photo, the date your cat went missing, and a telephone number.
    - Consider offering a reward.
    - Fliers can also be posted at neighborhood stores, pet departments, and at your veterinary clinic.
  - Alert and visit local animal shelters.
    - Visit the shelter in person on a daily basis is possible.
    - Leave behind a flier with the cat's picture.
    - Note: Providing clients with a list of local agencies may be extremely helpful to them.
  - Advertise that your cat is lost and look for "found-pet" advertisements.
    - Include an advertisement in local newspapers and on Craig's list, or other local resources if applicable.
  - For more information and tips for finding a lost cat, visit: http://www.missingpetpartnership.org.

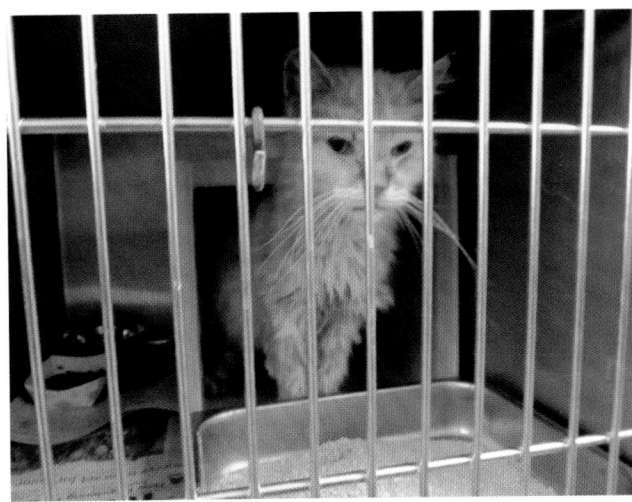

Figure 68-8: This stray geriatric cat was admitted to an animal shelter without an ID collar or microchip. Unfortunately, many owners do not think to look for their missing cat at local shelters. When no owner came forward to claim the cat during the legally required 5-day holding period, the cat was euthanized.

role in improving ID and recovery of pets using visual and microchip ID, scanning all animals using universal scanners and proper technique, and implementing effective lost-and-found pet matching programs.

Amid numerous competing priorities of a busy veterinary clinic or animal shelter, it may seem difficult, mundane, or perhaps impractical to devote time to convince a reluctant owner to use an ID collar for their cat. Weighing the potential lifesaving benefit of something so simple, however, gives pause for thought—just ask anyone who has lost his or her cat.

ACKNOWLEDGMENT

The author acknowledges the work of all of the investigators, their assistants, and students who have contributed to the current body of knowledge on pet ID and recovery, and especially Dr. Linda Lord whose steadfast passion and leadership for improving recovery of lost pets must be recognized.

References

1. Weiss E, Slater M, Lord L: Frequency of lost dogs and cats in the United States and the methods used to locate them. *Animals* 2:301–315, 2012.
2. U.S. Pet Ownership & Demographics Sourcebook (2012): *AVMA: Center for Information Management*, U.S. Pet Ownership & Demographics Sourcebook, Schaumburg, IL, 2012.
3. Griffin B: Care and control of community cats. In Little SE, editor: *The cat: clinical medicine and management*, St Louis, 2011, Elsevier, pp 1290–1309.
4. Levy JK, Crawford PC: Humane strategies for controlling feral cat populations. *J Am Vet Med Assoc* 225:1354–1360, 2004.
5. American Society for the Prevention of Cruelty to Animals: Pet Statistics. <http://www.aspca.org/about-us/faq/pet-statistics>, 2014 (Accessed April 30, 2015.)
6. Humane Society of the United States: U.S. shelter and adoption estimates. <http://www.humanesociety.org/issues/pet_overpopulation/facts/overpopulation_estimates.html>, 2013 (Accessed April 30, 2015.)
7. National Council on Pet Population Study and Policy: The Shelter Statistics Survey. <http://www.petpopulation.org/statsurvey.html>, 1994 (Accessed April 30, 2015.)
8. Canadian Federation of Humane Societies: Animal Shelter Statistics. <http://cfhs.ca/athome/shelter_animal_statistics>, 2012 (Accessed April 30, 2015.)
9. Stavisky J, Brennan ML, Downes M, et al: Demographics and economic burden of un-owned cats and dogs in the UK: results of a 2010 census. *BMC Vet Res* 8:163, 2012.

10. Lord LK, Wittum TE, Ferketich AK, et al: Search and identification methods that owners use to find a lost cat. *J Am Vet Med Assoc* 230:217–220, 2007.

11. Lord LK, Griffin B, Slater MR, et al: Evaluation of collars and microchips for visual and permanent identification of pet cats. *J Am Vet Med Assoc* 237:387–394, 2010.

12. Slater M, Weiss E, Lord L: Current use of and attitudes towards identification in cats and dogs in veterinary clinics in Oklahoma City, USA. *Animal Welfare* 21:51–57, 2012.

13. Lord LK, Wittum TE, Ferketich AK, et al: Search and identification methods that owners use to find a lost dog. *J Am Vet Med Assoc* 230:211–216, 2007.

14. Lord LK, Wittum TE, Ferketich AK, et al: Search methods that people use to find owners of lost pets. *J Am Vet Med Assoc* 230:1835–1840, 2007.

15. American Veterinary Medical Association: Microchipping of animals. <https://www.avma.org/KB/Resources/Reference/Pages/Microchipping-of-Animals-Backgrounder.aspx>, 2013 (Accessed April 30, 2015.)

16. Weiss E, Slater MR, Lord LK: Retention of provided identification for dogs and cats seen in veterinary clinics and adopted from shelters in Oklahoma City, OK, USA. *Prevent Vet Med* 101:265–269, 2011.

17. Lord LK, Ingwersen W, Gray JL, et al: Characterization of animals with microchips entering animal shelters. *J Am Vet Med Assoc* 235:160–167, 2009.

18. Griffin B, DiGangi B, Bohling M: A review of neutering cats. In August JR, editor: *Consultations in feline internal medicine VI*, St Louis, 2010, Elsevier/Saunders, pp 776–790.

19. Lord LK, Pennell ML, Ingwersen W, et al: Sensitivity of commercial scanners to microchips of various frequencies implanted in dogs and cats. *J Am Vet Med Assoc* 233:1729–1735, 2008.

20. Griffin B: Care of the cat in the shelter. In Miller L, Zawistowski S, editors: *Shelter medicine for veterinarians and staff*, ed 2, Ames, 2013, Blackwell, pp 145–184.

21. Lord LK, Pennell ML, Ingwersen W, et al: In vitro sensitivity of commercial scanners to microchips of various frequencies. *J Am Vet Med Assoc* 233:1723–1728, 2008.

22. Carminato A, Vascellari M, Marchioro W, et al: Microchip-associated fibrosarcoma in a cat. *Vet Dermatol* 22:565–569, 2011.

23. Platt S, Wieczorek L, Dennis R, et al: Spinal cord injury resulting from incorrect microchip placement in a cat. *J Feline Med Surg* 9:157–160, 2007.

24. Haifley KA, Hecht S: Functionality of implanted microchips following magnetic resonance imaging. *J Am Vet Med Assoc* 240(5):577–579, 2012.

25. Griffin B, Baker HJ: Domestic cats as laboratory animals. In Fox JG, editor: *Laboratory animal medicine*, San Diego, 2002, Harcourt Academic, pp 459–482.

26. Griffin B: Population wellness: keeping cats physically and behaviorally healthy. In Little SE, editor: *The cat: clinical medicine and management*, St Louis, 2011, Elsevier, pp 1312–1353.

27. Looney A, Bohling M, Bushby P, et al: The Association of Shelter Veterinarian's Veterinary Medical Guidelines for Spay-Neuter Programs. *J Am Vet Med Assoc* 233(1):74–86, 2008.

28. Griffin B: Diagnostic usefulness of and clinical syndromes associated with reproductive hormones. In August JR, editor: *Consultations in feline internal medicine*, vol 5, St Louis, 2006, Elsevier Saunders, pp 217–226.

29. American Association of Feline Practitioners Position Statement Identification of Cats. <http://www.catvets.com/guidelines/position-statements/identification-cats>, 2007 (Accessed April 30, 2015.)

30. Dingman PA, Levy JK, Rockey LE, et al: Use of visual and permanent identification for pets by veterinary clinics. *Vet J* 201:46–50, 2014.

31. Association of Shelter Veterinarians. Guidelines for Standards of Care in Animal Shelters. <http://sheltervet.org/wp-content/uploads/2012/08/Shelter-Standards-Oct2011-wForward.pdf>, 2010 (Accessed April 30, 2015.)

32. Griffin B: Wellness. In Miller L, Hurley KF, editors: *Infectious disease management in animal shelters*, Ames, 2009, Blackwell, pp 17–38.

33. Griffin B: Keeping golden years golden: recognizing and responding to the unique needs of senior shelter cats. *Animal Shelter* Sept-Oct:54–57, 2013.

34. Griffin B: Scaredy cat or feral cat? *Animal Shelter* Nov/Dec:57–61, 2009.

Clinical Management of Large-Scale Cruelty Cases

Melinda D. Merck

INTRODUCTION

Large-scale feline cruelty cases typically arise from investigations involving individual hoarders, rescue organizations, sanctuaries, or breeders. These cases involve the crime scene, animal processing at the scene and temporary shelter, animal removal and transport, sheltering, and final animal disposition. The veterinarian plays a role in the planning of the operation, at the crime scene, the temporary shelter, and the hospital receiving cats for more advanced treatment. The clinical management of these cases is different from traditional shelter medicine or feline practice. To act and respond appropriately, the veterinarian must have an understanding of all aspects of the operation. These are legal cases requiring certain types of documentation and procedures. The organization of the entire operation should be conducted similar to disaster response using the Incident Command System—where the medical management on scene and at the temporary shelter is incorporated into this reporting structure with direct communication to the lead investigator.[1] Extensive planning is needed, anticipating the number of cats, age ranges, known or likely medical issues, and socialization status. Decisions must be made considering practicality, stress on the animals, costs, resources, future animal placement, and any legal impact. The goal is a successful outcome for the individual cat and the criminal case.

Supplies

Supplies needed for on-scene and shelter medical operations need to be planned very early in the investigation. All team leaders should be involved in this planning, including those from the medical, forensic evidence, and shelter branches, with a supply list compiled for each branch (Table 69-1). Arrangements should be made to obtain supplies during the case response for items that were not anticipated or depleted due to use.

Color Code System

The use of color codes is important for large-scale cases to implement a visual system of communication at the scene, from scene to the shelter, within the shelter, and for forensic examinations. The colors are used to designate triage categories, initial cat temperament, and other conditions that determine placement and housing within the shelter. In addition, this system serves to establish the examination sequence. The assignment of color categories may vary with each case based on the availability of the color devices used (Table 69-2). Colored duct tape is easily used and readily purchased at home improvement, hardware, office supply, and general merchandise stores. Colored flagging tape may also be used but poses a risk of animal ingestion and can be difficult to remove from transport carriers or cages. A piece of the appropriate colored duct tape is placed on the animal identification (ID) label located on the transport carrier or cage; some animals may have more than one color assigned (Figure 69-1). The primary use of the color system is at the scene, but some colors may continue to be used within the sheltering system. The color system and their assigned categories should be posted at the scene, within each forensic examination area, and at multiple areas within the shelter.

VETERINARY MEDICAL TEAMS

Critical Triage Team

The purpose of the critical triage team, comprised of veterinarians with or without veterinary technicians, is to identify any animals in need of urgent care. The critical triage team assesses animals after the initial scene walk-through is complete and as the physical evidence, animal ID, and animal removal teams begin their work. Any critically ill or injured animals should have priority for ID assignment and removal from the scene. Provisions for an on-site critical examination area should be made, such as a mobile veterinary clinic, trailer, tent, or one of the buildings within the scene itself. Cats requiring more extensive diagnostics or treatment should be transported to a local veterinary hospital.

Forensic Examination Teams

The forensic examination teams are responsible for examination of all the animals. These teams are comprised of a veterinarian, scribe, and animal handler. It is important that all animals are examined in a timely fashion, within 72 hours, to ensure the examination evidence is representative of the

Table 69-1	Large-Scale Cruelty Case Medical Supply List		
Medical Supplies		**Quantity**	**Check**
Examinations			
Alcohol			
Animal shampoo			
Antibiotics—injectable, ophthalmic, oral, topical			
Bandage scissors			
Bath mats for examination table surface			
Blood collection tubes—lavender top, serum separator			
Body warming equipment			
Canine nail trimmers			
Canned cat food			
Centrifuge for blood/urine/fecal samples			
Clipper blade cleaner, cooling spray			
Controlled drug log			
Cordless clippers			
Cotton balls			
Cotton tip applicators			
Dewormer medications (roundworms, hookworms, tapeworms, *Coccidia, Giardia*)			
Digital thermometers			
Ear cleaner			
Euthanasia solution			
Examination forms and diagram			
Examination gowns			
Eye wash solution			
Fecal loops			
Fecal sample cups			
Fecal solution for centrifugation			
Fecal tubes with plastic caps for centrifuge			
Feline nail trimmers			
Feliway spray			
Flea treatment—oral, topical			
Fluids 1 L for subcutaneous administration (e.g., lactated Ringer's solution)			
Fluorescein stain			
Frosted microscope slides			
Gloves—small, medium, large—nitrile only			
Glucometer licensed for animal use			
Grooming tools—dematting comb, brush, flea comb			
Hematocrit centrifuge machine, tubes, clay, reader			
Immersion oil			
Intravenous catheters (22-, 25-, and 18-gauge)			

Table 69-1	Large-Scale Cruelty Case Medical Supply List—cont'd		
Medical Supplies		Quantity	Check
Intravenous lines (72-inch)—for subcutaneous fluid administration, 10 to 15 drops/mL			
Lubricating jelly			
Laboratory forms			
Laboratory test log			
Microscope			
Microscope cover slips			
Milk replacer for kittens			
Necropsy equipment			
Ophthalmoscope and otoscope			
Patient-side test kits (feline leukemia virus, feline immunodeficiency virus, parvovirus)			
Protective coverings for sleeves			
Rabies vaccination certificates			
Sedatives and reversal agents			
Stethoscopes			
Surgical blades for skin scrapings			
Towels			
Universal microchip scanner			
Urine chemistry sticks			
Urine centrifugation tubes			
Vaccines			
Weigh scales			
Animal First Aid			
Burn relief gel pack			
Bandage scissors			
Bandaging materials			
Chlorhexidine scrub			
Chlorhexidine solution			
Cotton roll			
Dextrose 50% injectable			
Forceps			
Hemostats			
Hydrogen peroxide, 3%			
Nonadhesive pads			
Porous tape			
Scalpel blade holder			
Suture materials			
Vitamin B injectable			

Continued

Table 69-1	Large-Scale Cruelty Case Medical Supply List—cont'd

Medical Supplies	Quantity	Check
Crash Cart List		
22-, 25-, and 18-gauge catheters		
Allergic reaction medications		
Cardiac arrest medications		
Endotracheal tubes		
Laryngoscope		
High-calorie nutritional supplement		
Shock medications		
Needles and Syringes		
18-gauge needles		
1-mL syringes with 25-gauge needles		
1-mL syringes without needles		
22-gauge needles		
25-mL syringes without needles		
3-mL syringes with 22-gauge needles		
3-mL syringes with 25-gauge needles		
3-mL syringes without needles for oral medications		
3-mL syringes without needles for injectable medications		
6-mL syringes without needles		

Table 69-2	Color Code System	
Color	**Indication**	**Notes**
Red	Bite case	Has bitten a human
Yellow	Handle with caution	Exhibited shyness, fear, or aggression; intended for handlers to be cautious, especially at shelter intake
Pink	Pregnant	Suspected at the scene or confirmed on examination
Green	Infectious	Suspected at the scene or confirmed on examination
Blue	Priority examination	As determined by the forensic examination teams
Orange	First general examination	Examined after blue priority examinations are complete
Black	Emergency	To be transported to off-site veterinary facility

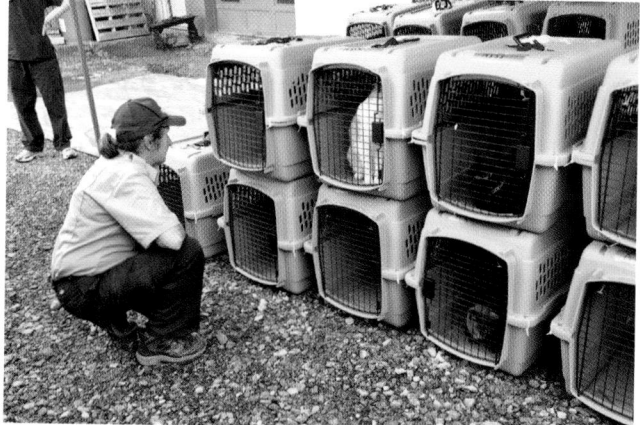

Figure 69-1: Yellow, blue, and green flagging tapes are attached to each carrier to designate initial animal triage categories.

animal's condition at the original scene and any health issues are addressed as quickly as possible. The examination and treatment process should be complete and efficient. These teams usually work best when the scribe, who must be familiar with medical terminology, fills out the examination form as the veterinarian dictates the findings. The creation of special laboratory and treatment teams can improve efficiency and free the veterinarian to focus on examination and documentation. It is preferable to have one team designated to examine the more severe medical cases and animals that may require sedation to handle. This team should have ample medical supplies, controlled drugs, and the most secure examination area.

CRIME SCENE EVALUATION

There are several assessments that must be made at the crime scene that directly impact handling of the cats throughout the operation and have important legal ramifications. These evaluations may be conducted by veterinarians along with case investigators. It is critical that the veterinary teams, off-site hospitals, and sheltering operations take this into consideration. The assessment should include information about the cats and current housing conditions along with medications and supplies present. The most important consideration, and most overlooked, is the evaluation and continuous monitoring of stressors on the cats.

It is important to document any obvious medical, husbandry, or behavioral care needs at the scene. This includes the presence of neonates, nursing queens, chronic medical conditions, infectious diseases, and potential zoonotic diseases. Any records present should be assessed for pertinent information, including intake date, medical history, and individual cat names. Any medications, supplies, and supplements should be documented, noting any prescriptions for individual cats, the date prescribed, expiration dates, the original amount and quantity remaining, and the prescribing veterinarian's information. The medications and supplies should be assessed for indicators of current or past medical issues.

The general housing of the cats should be assessed and documented with photography and mapping. This assessment is an important consideration for housing decisions at the sheltering site. Special note should be taken of the number of cats in a room or cage and natural groupings or obvious social bonds. The flow of people and animals within and between housing areas should be documented, with special focus on the potential for fomite transmission of pathogens. The type and brand of food offered should be recorded as well as the number of feeding stations and the number of cats that have access to each one. The availability and potability of water sources should be assessed. The litter boxes should be evaluated, including the type of litter, the amount of urine and feces, the type of litter box, and the number of cats with access to each litter box. Samples of diarrhea should be taken for individual cats and representative samples for group housing situations. Any unsanitary living conditions should be noted and consideration given to the effects of such conditions on the respiratory tracts, eyes, fur, and skin of the cats.

SCENE RESPONSE

Stress Management

The effect of stress on cats has been well documented.[2] In large-scale cases, stress can come from crowding, prolonged confinement, isolation, lack of environmental enrichment, an unsanitary environment, poor food and water resources, and untreated medical conditions. Every consideration should be made to minimize stress during removal, transport, sheltering, and examination of the cats. Physical handling of the cats and change of environment are additional but necessary stressors in these cases that carry a risk of exacerbating any pre-existing medical conditions. It is not unusual for these large groups of cats to be subclinical disease carriers that have reached a state of homeostasis that when disrupted results in new outbreaks. In addition, many of these cases involve animals that lack proper socialization and/or have been under severe emotional stress. They may exhibit aggression (due to fear or pain), or they may be completely unable to interact. Some cats may exhibit subtle behavioral clues of extreme distress. It is the initial handling at the scene that can set the animal up for success or failure more so than any setbacks that may occur during examination or sheltering.

Resistance to handling and restraint is almost always the result of fear, anxiety, or pain, which is compounded when force is used. If possible, it is preferable to take several hours to remove a cat from the scene rather than forcefully remove it, which can reinforce the animal's fear and behavioral response. It is important to recognize that these cats may have reactions to novel stimuli different from those raised as pets in private homes. Therefore, any negative behavioral designations assigned at the scene should be considered temporary and only for the purpose of cautionary handling. The key to successful handling of animals involves the accurate appraisal of behavior, an adequate number of staff, and the appropriate equipment; proper training in each of these areas being the most important aspect.

Transportation

Transportation of cats from the scene to the sheltering site should be done in such a manner to minimize stress on the animals and to maintain compliance with applicable laws and regulations. Considerations should be given to the environmental conditions and the time required to load the vehicle (which directly affects the first animals loaded). The spacing of the animal transport carriers within the transport unit should be planned to provide adequate ventilation for the cats inside. Individual transport carriers should be of sturdy construction, put together properly to prevent animal escape or injury, have adequate ventilation, and consist of a design that allows stacking of carriers. Special areas may need to be designated at the offloading area for animals requiring immediate veterinary care or assessment upon arrival to the shelter, especially neonates. Planning for animal carrier placement based on infectious disease status is difficult and usually unnecessary as in most cases there has been ongoing exposure among animals due to their living conditions.

Sheltering

For large-scale cat cruelty cases, there is rarely an existing animal shelter that can house all of the animals at one location. This requires creating a temporary shelter, which follows the same principles used for animal disaster sheltering, with the primary difference that the animals are evidence in a criminal case. Protocols must be in place for monitoring, treatment, daily assessment, and progress documentation, including change of medical or behavioral status. There should be a shelter mapping system to identify and track the location of every animal, including when animals are moved. It is important to have the veterinarian's input on the initial design and any adjustments made based on the crime scene assessment or forensic examinations. The shelter should be designed to be flexible based on changing medical or behavioral conditions of the animals. Shelter design should take into account the number of cats, special housing needs, ease of handling, infectious disease, temperature control, airflow, foot traffic, noise levels, animal stress, and environmental enrichment. Continued assessment and reassessment of cat behavior and temperament should be conducted, with changes made to address any issues noted. Any final behavior or temperament designations should only be assigned after the cats have had time to adjust to their new environment and recover from all stressors, which may take several days to weeks.

Consideration should be given to the original housing, grouping, and social bonds of the cats at the scene. Often these cases involve group housing or free-roaming shelter settings, and the temporary shelter results in isolation of cats into individual cages. Although this can be another stressor on the cats, it can be offset (at least for the short term) by the positive change to a sanitary environment and the elimination of competition for resources of space, litter, food, and water. Cats should be paired or group-housed whenever possible and practical to reduce stress. Shy or feral cats are often less stressed when paired with another cat. Wire cages are especially amenable to alteration, creating a "double-wide" space for this purpose. Environmental enrichment is important to incorporate into the sheltering design and protocols. This includes soft bedding, boxes, or small carriers to hide in, toys, treats, and catnip. It is critical to offer canned food, especially for cats with upper respiratory or dental disease, to assess and stimulate appetite, and for further enrichment. It is important to minimize changing of bedding and other items within the cages, which can create additional stress.[3] The use of synthetic pheromones (e.g., Feliway, Ceva Animal Health) may be effective in stress reduction when sprayed on bedding and through the use of plug-in diffusers.[4,5]

Whenever possible, the same persons should care for the same cats to help reduce stress, enhance opportunities for socialization, and decrease risk for injuries. Assessments and monitoring may be improved when performed by personnel familiar with individual cats.

Creating separate sections in housing areas should be carefully considered, because they can create more stress on the cats and complicate management of the shelter. These separations are often based on infectious diseases, zoonotic diseases, critical medical observation, bite quarantine, reproductive status, and special needs (such as those cats that are difficult to handle, pregnant, neonates, or nursing). Decisions for separate housing areas must be done with consideration of the crime scene assessment. Most of these cases involve cats that have previously been exposed to each other either through housing design or fomite transmission; therefore, separation based on infectious disease is neither necessary nor recommended. In large open shelters, separate areas can be created by hanging tarps or clear plastic sheets that are open at the ceiling for airflow. Other considerations for housing of cats include lighting, number of separate rooms, secure areas, and airflow. Cats are more stressed when at ground level, so every effort should be made to elevate the housing.[3]

EXAMINATION, DIAGNOSTICS, AND TREATMENT

In the planning stages, it is important to develop medical protocols, including those for examinations, diagnostic testing, and all treatments. Planning should include what tests will be conducted at the shelter and what outside laboratories will be used. Because this is a legal case, the use of standard examination forms that are developed specifically for these types of cases is recommended (Box 69-1). These forms should be structured to prompt and guide the veterinarian through a complete examination.

Examination of the Cat

Photographic ID of the cat can be performed by one of the forensic examination team members, or a separate floating photographer may support multiple examination teams. The photographs should begin with the case information, including the case number, date, and animal ID written on a card or dry erase board. This first picture with the case and animal information may be taken with or without the animal in the photo, and all photographs following this initial picture should only be of that animal. General photos should be taken showing the entire body of the cat: right and left sides, front (facial), hind (rear), dorsal, and ventral (if possible or appropriate) views. Photographs, with and without a photo scale, should be taken of any obvious lesions, abnormal physical findings, and any evidence found on the body.[6]

It is important that each veterinarian use the same examination form (see Box 69-1). It is the responsibility of the scribe to ensure that the entire form is complete, and it is the veterinarian's responsibility to review it for accuracy. In

BOX 69-1 Live Animal Examination Form

AGENCY: _____ Animal ID #_____

CASE #: _____ MICROCHIP: Y N #_____

DATE: _____ DOCTOR: _____ TIME: Start   Finish

BREED:_____COLOR: _____SEX: _____AGE EST:_____

TEMPERAMENT: _____ WT (lbs.): _____

BCS: (1) Emaciated (2) Very Thin (3) Thin (4) Lean (5) Ideal (6) Mildly overweight (7) Overweight (8) Obese (9) Morbidly obese

T:_____MM/CRT:_____HYD:_____

EENM: _____

H/L: _____

ABD/PERINEUM: _____

U/G: _____

M/S: _____

SKIN: _____

FEET/TAIL: _____

PARASITES: _____

APPETITE: _____

COMMENTS: _____

SAMPLES TAKEN: _____ ON SCENE TESTS: _____

PARASITE TX: _____ VACCS: _____

OTHER DIAGNOSTICS REQUIRED: _____

EUTH: Y N REASON: _____ APPVD BY: _____

TX INSTRUCTIONS: _____

ABD, abdomen; *APPVD*, approved; *BCS*, body condition score; *CRT*, capillary refill time; *EENM*, eyes, ears, nose, mouth; *EST*, estimated; *EUTH*, euthanasia; *H/L*, heart and lung auscultation; *HYD*, hydration; *ID*, identification; *MM*, mucous membranes; *M/S*, musculoskeletal; *T*, temperature; *TX*, treatment; *U/G*, urogenital; *VACCS*, vaccinations; *WT*, weight.

addition, the veterinary teams should use consistent terminology and abbreviations, which may be posted in the exam areas. Breed descriptions should be done carefully. Unless the breed is known, it is often best to use "breed-type" or predominant "breed-mix." The body condition score (BCS) to be used should be posted in each examination area so that the veterinarians can refer to it. The age or estimated age of a cat should only be documented if supported by examination findings, such as dentition or ocular changes. It is preferable to use designations of *neonatal, juvenile, adult,* or *geriatric* with documentation of the basis for the determination. After the examination is complete, a check mark should be placed on the animal's ID marker to create a visual indication that the animal has been examined. Any color-coded markers should be assessed and removed or changed based on the examination; those that may impact shelter operations should be communicated to the shelter manager.

Medical Protocols

The standard medical protocols enacted depend on the known existing conditions and diseases within the population, the expected length of stay in the temporary shelter, and the

expected disposition of the cats; however, a variety of infectious diseases (including respiratory, enteric, and dermatologic pathogens) should be expected.[7] Depending on the legal process, the cats may be adopted directly from the shelter, placed at another animal facility within or outside the area, placed in foster homes, or euthanized. These potential scenarios and outcomes may be fluid and will dictate what protocols are most appropriate for the cats at any given time. The medical protocols should be implemented during the forensic examination process.

Vaccination and Deworming

Standard vaccination protocols should follow the American Association of Feline Practitioners (AAFP) recommendations for shelter-housed cats.[8] Vaccinations should be given at the time of intake to the temporary shelter and should include feline herpesvirus type 1, feline calicivirus, feline panleukopenia, and rabies. Vaccination for feline leukemia virus (FeLV) may be considered based on viral test results and group housing.

A majority of intensively housed cats will harbor at least one enteropathogen, often of zoonotic significance; the presence of such pathogens is not limited to cats with clinical signs of illness.[9] Therefore, routine deworming for roundworms, hookworms, and tapeworms should be part of the standard medical protocol. Fecal testing is not necessary unless there is unresolved diarrhea after deworming, or it is otherwise dictated based on clinical illness. Coccidiosis is a common finding in large-scale cat cruelty cases; it is found in up to 23% of cats with diarrhea and 33% of clinically healthy cats.[9] Based on observed diarrhea findings at the scene, within the temporary shelter, or diagnostic test results, it may be reasonable to treat all cats for coccidiosis. Ponazuril is an effective treatment for coccidiosis and is easily administered to large numbers of cats, given orally once daily at 15 to 30 mg/kg for 1 to 3 days and repeated if necessary in 1 week.[3,10] The stressors the cats have been exposed to along with dietary changes at the temporary shelter can contribute to diarrhea. In addition, many cats from these cases may harbor other enteropathogens, such as *Tritrichomonas*, *Giardia*, or *Cryptosporidium* species, as well as feline enteric coronavirus, which may or may not be a cause of refractory diarrhea.[9,11] Any additional testing and interpretation should be conducted as discussed later in this chapter.

Diagnostic Testing

All diagnostic testing decisions for the cat population should be done with consideration for the goals of the operation; the legal impact; the health of the individual cat and the general population; the stress on the cat; the expected time length for housing; the future placement of the cats and the placing agency's responsibilities; the financial and personnel resources; and clinical relevance. For each test considered, both the test itself and the action to be taken based on its result must be appropriate and reasonable. In a large-scale case, tests that may be recommended or conducted in private or shelter medicine practice may not be appropriate or reasonable. The goal is not to cure all animals and eliminate all pathogens prior to the cat leaving the temporary shelter, rather it is to immediately identify and address any important medical issues, improve overall physical and mental health, and address any obvious zoonotic issues. This should be a clear and constant guidepost for decisions made. It cannot and should not be the expectation to test and treat for everything. As with any shelter situation, these cats may be asymptomatic carriers of a variety of pathogens. Testing can result in information that is not currently relevant to the health of the animal yet force decisions for unnecessary and inappropriate actions for that individual animal or the general population.

For large-scale cruelty cases, it is recommended to test cats for FeLV and feline immunodeficiency virus (FIV) based on the guidelines established by the AAFP.[12] Depending on the test results and the original housing at the crime scene (i.e., pre-existing exposure), changes in the housing location within the temporary shelter may or may not be recommended. Cats that appear ill without a grossly apparent cause should have routine laboratory work analyzed, including a full biochemistry profile, complete blood count, and urinalysis. Such documentation is especially important in legal cases.

Euthanasia

Protocols for euthanasia, necropsy examinations, and the storage of deceased animals should also be determined in advance. Because the animals are evidence and also to remain sensitive to the case responders and public sentiment, the criteria and parameters for euthanasia decisions should be discussed with the lead investigator and prosecutor prior to the day of seizure. The decision for euthanasia should first be agreed upon by the examining veterinarian and the case lead veterinarian. The lead veterinarian should obtain permission from the lead investigator to perform euthanasia according to the agreed upon parameters. Another factor to address in the planning phase is the use and storage of controlled drugs, including euthanasia solution and sedatives. A controlled drug log must be maintained according to applicable laws.

COMMON MEDICAL FINDINGS

Many of the cats may have obvious medical needs. Regardless of the presence or absence of clinical signs, it should be expected that most of the cats are likely carrying multiple different pathogens.[13] These may or may not become clinically relevant, depending on the individual cat and the stressors placed on it.

Upper Respiratory Tract Disease

The most common medical finding is upper respiratory tract disease (URTD). This may vary from mild to severe with secondary pneumonia, ulcerations of the nasal or oral area, nasopharyngeal polyps, and ocular involvement (Figure 69-2). Mild cases may not need to be treated while being closely monitored for disease progression; most cases will resolve within 7 to 10 days.[14] The more severe cases typically involve secondary bacterial infection, regardless of the primary pathogen, which should be treated aggressively.

Considerations for choices of medication should include the availability of personnel and their ability to administer

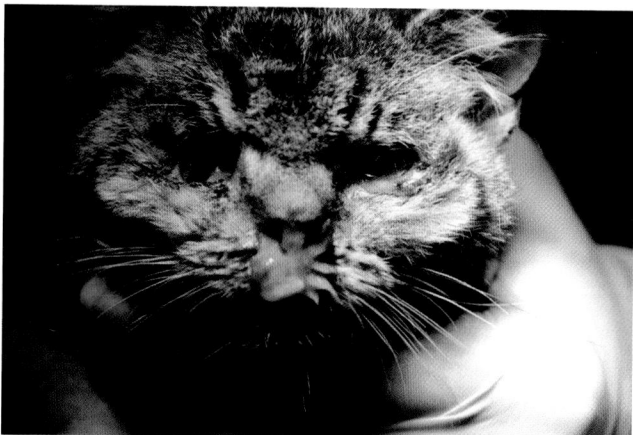

Figure 69-2: Severe upper respiratory tract disease in a cat with significant nasal and ocular involvement, including loss of the right eye.

medication, the possibility of administering medication through canned food or treats, dosing intervals, possibility of multiple pathogens, and risk of side effects. Stress reduction plays the single greatest role in the remission and prevention of URTD in cats;[14] therefore, particular attention should be given to providing an enriched environment as a component of the treatment plan.

Dermatologic Disease

Skin and fur conditions are quite common in large-scale cruelty cases. The cats often have urine and/or fecal staining of fur, especially on the feet, usually with associated dermatitis. Other issues related to the feet include contact pododermatitis, plasma cell pododermatitis, and overgrown or embedded claws (Figure 69-3). Cat bite abscesses are not uncommon. Severe matting may be seen on longhaired cats with fecal soiling or impaction in the perineal area with associated dermatitis (Figures 69-4 and 69-5). In addition to fleas and associated dermatitis, there may be other external parasites, such as *Cheyletiella*, lice, and demodectic or sarcoptic mange. Stress can cause alopecia due to overgrooming or self-mutilation (Figure 69-6). Less commonly, cases of

Streptococcus canis have been reported in intensively housed cats, often manifesting with skin ulceration and necrotizing fasciitis (Figure 69-7).[15]

Dermatophytosis may be seen in some cats but rarely is a widespread issue within the population. Cats may be mechanical carriers and never develop clinical lesions themselves; such cats are seldom clinically relevant to the case, the individual animals, or the general population. For these reasons, dermatophyte testing is not routinely recommended on intake of cats or for those without dermatologic lesions. Rather, the focus should be on diagnosing and treating cats with suspicious lesions and enacting precautions for handling and cleaning. Housing placement within the shelter for cats suspected or diagnosed with dermatophytosis should be based on the considerations previously discussed.

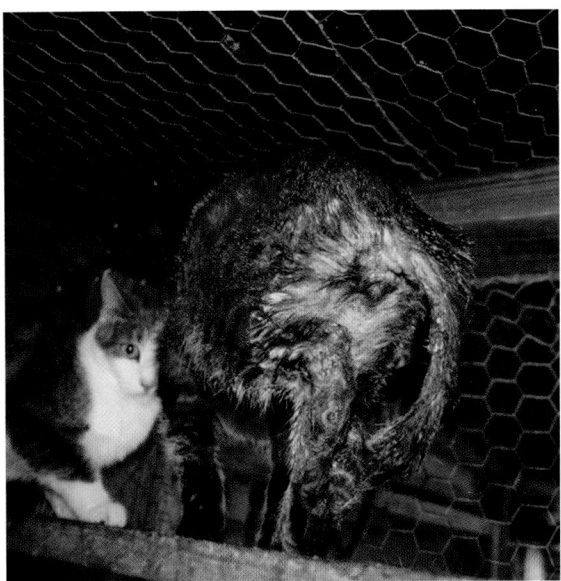

Figure 69-5: Severe skin ulceration and dermatitis on the perineum and lower legs from chronic fecal contact.

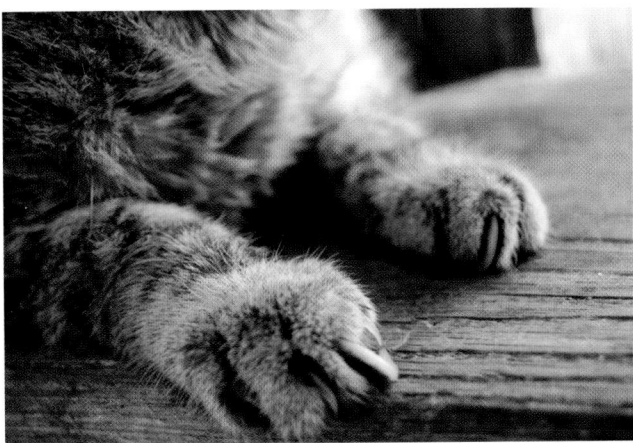

Figure 69-3: Severely overgrown and embedded claws.

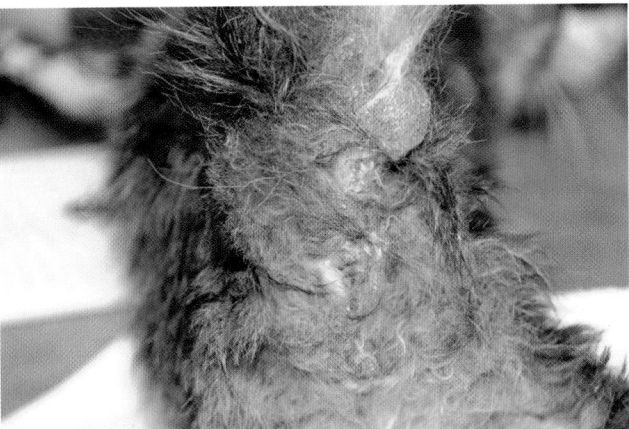

Figure 69-4: Severe fecal soiling and matting on the perineal area and hind legs.

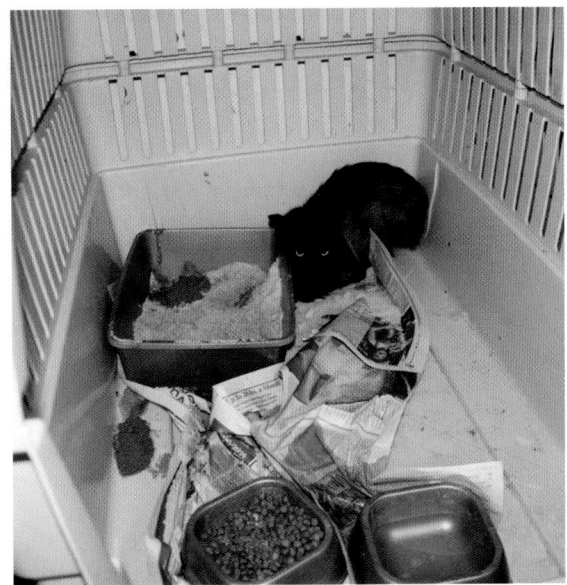

Figure 69-6: Severe alopecia due to stress-induced overgrooming.

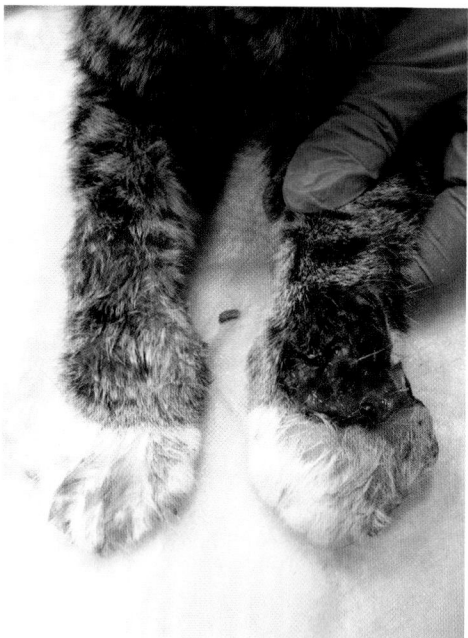

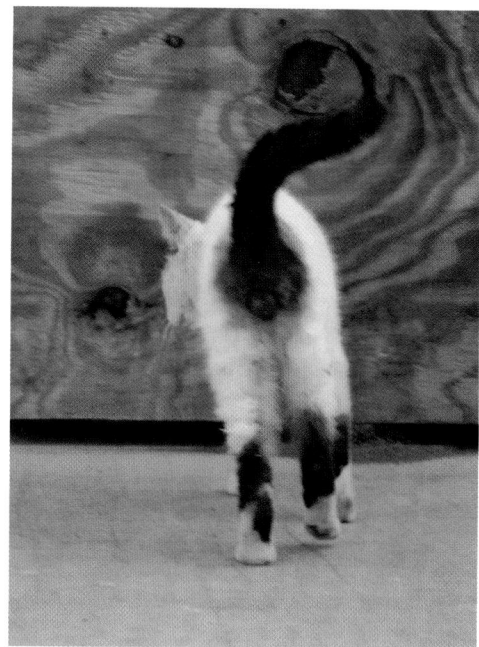

Figure 69-7: Ulcerations on the dorsal aspect of the front left paw as a result of infection with *Streptococcus canis*. (Courtesy of Dr. Brian DiGangi.)

Figure 69-9: Rectal prolapse due to chronic diarrhea.

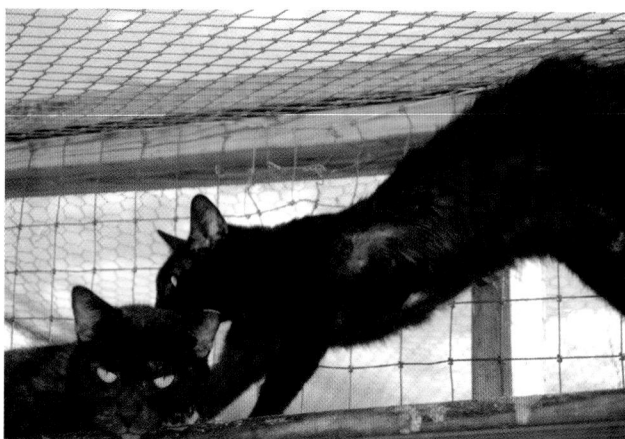

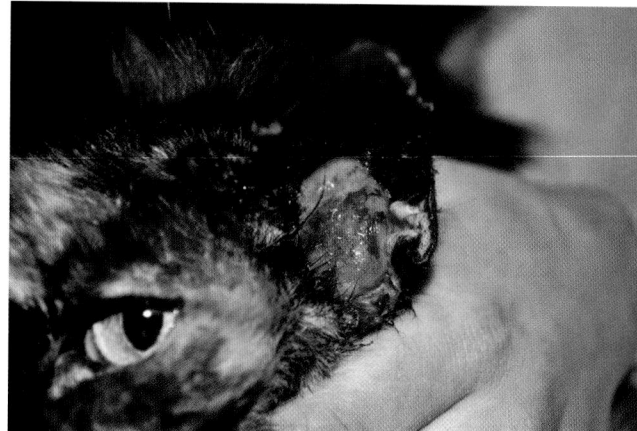

Figure 69-8: Red coat changes along with healing wound on the left hemithorax.

Figure 69-10: Large nasopharyngeal polyp protruding out of the external ear canal.

A variety of clinical abnormalities of the skin result from nutritional deficiencies, including starvation. A common finding is a sparse, dry, dull, and brittle hair coat with hairs that epilate easily. Seborrhea sicca and patchy alopecia may be seen. Loss of hair occurs due to anagen and/or telogen defluxion. In the anagen or growth phase of the hair cycle, there can be loss and/or abnormal growth of hair, resulting in broken hair shafts. With telogen defluxion, there is widespread loss of hair in the quiescent phase of the hair cycle due to large numbers of hair follicles being synchronized in this phase. Loss of normal hair color and hair keratinization abnormalities can occur. In cats, decreased melanin deposition due to amino acid deficiencies results in a reddish cast to the hairs, sometimes called *red coat* (Figure 69-8). Erythema or crusting in areas of friction or stretching, such as

in the distal extremities, may be found. Other common findings include decubital ulcers, poor wound healing, and secondary bacterial or yeast skin infections.[16]

Other Medical Conditions

There are numerous other medical findings that may be seen or develop in these cases:
- Mild to severe anemia associated with severe flea infestation, *Mycoplasma haemofelis* (feline infectious anemia), FeLV, FIV, chronic disease, or malnutrition
- Feline panleukopenia, especially in young kittens
- Exposure to *Salmonella* spp. from living in unsanitary conditions
- Rectal prolapse in cats with chronic diarrhea (Figure 69-9)
- Ear mites, bacterial otitis, nasopharyngeal polyps, and aural hematomas (Figures 69-10 and 69-11)

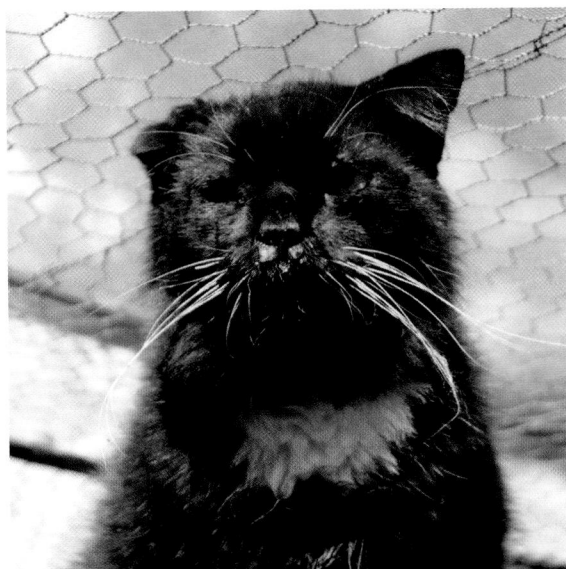

Figure 69-11: Cat with nasal discharge and hematoma of the right pinna.

- Oral lesions, including ulcerations associated with URTD, stomatitis, and dental disease
- Urinary tract issues (e.g., urinary tract infection, idiopathic cystitis, nephroliths, uroliths, crystalluria, and vaginitis) are often the reason the cat was presented to the original shelter or sanctuary

The clinician should be cognizant of the possibility for these and other underlying medical issues that may be primary or secondary to other medical conditions, malnutrition, dehydration, stress, and/or an unsanitary environment. Often, the investigation findings may provide information on pre-existing conditions through intake paperwork or hospital records. These underlying issues may only be detected with routine blood work and urinalysis; affected cats may require further diagnostic testing, imaging, or hospitalization.

SUMMARY

The clinical management of large-scale feline cruelty cases starts at the scene and continues to the temporary housing in a shelter or hospital. It is critical that veterinarians understand the importance of the role they play as part of the investigative team and the requirements for documentation in a legal case. The veterinarian may become involved in these cases directly at the scene and shelter or by receiving a patient into the hospital. By the very nature of large-scale cruelty cases, the cats will have a wide range of issues associated with high volume housing and long-term neglect. It is important to be mindful that this will be a fluid situation requiring a process of continuous assessment of the animal's health and behavior to detect early signs of developing issues and initiate treatment. The simple actions of providing appropriate housing, food, routine medical treatments on intake, and overall stress reduction will often result in rapid improvement of cat health. There is a greater chance of recovery—even for the most severely affected cats—when both physical and mental needs are addressed.

References

1. Merck MD, LeCouteur RA: Special considerations in animal cruelty cases. In Merck MD, editor: *Veterinary forensics: animal cruelty investigations*, ed 2, Ames, IA, 2013, Wiley, pp 69–96.
2. Griffin B, Hume KR: Recognition and management of stress in housed cats. In August JR, editor: *Consultations in feline internal medicine*, ed 5, St Louis, 2006, Elsevier/Saunders, pp 717–734.
3. Griffin B: Feline care in the animal shelter. In Miller L, Zawitowski S, editors: *Shelter medicine for veterinarians and staff*, ed 2, Ames, IA, 2013, Wiley, pp 145–184.
4. Griffith C, Steigerwald E, Buffington C: Effects of a synthetic facial pheromone on behavior of cats. *J Am Vet Med Assoc* 217:1154–1156, 2000.
5. Kronen PW, Ludders JW, Hollis NE, et al: A synthetic fraction of feline facial pheromones calms but does not reduce struggling in cats before venous catheterization. *Vet Anaesth Analg* 33:258–265, 2006.
6. Merck MD: Crime scene investigation. In Merck MD, editor: *Veterinary forensics: animal cruelty investigations*, ed 2, Ames, IA, 2013, Wiley, pp 17–35.
7. Polak KC, Levy JK, Crawford PC: Prevalence of infectious diseases in large scale cat hoarding responses. *J Vet Intern Med* 27:729, 2013.
8. Scherk MA, Ford RB, Gaskell RM, et al: 2013 AAFP Feline Vaccination Advisory Panel Report. *J Feline Med Surg* 15:785–808, 2013.
9. Andersen LA, Levy JK, McManus JK, et al: Prevalence of enteropathogens in four management models for unowned cats in the southeast United States. *J Vet Intern Med* 25:709, 2011.
10. Litster A, Hall K, Nichols J: Clinical trial to assess the efficacy of ponazuril for the treatment of Coccidiosis in dogs and cats. *J Vet Intern Med* 27:725–726, 2013.
11. Sabshin SJ, Levy JK, Tupler T, et al: Enteropathogens identified in cats entering a Florida animal shelter with normal feces or diarrhea. *J Am Vet Med Assoc* 241:331–337, 2012.
12. Levy C, Crawford C, Hartmann K, et al: 2008 American Association of Feline Practitioners retrovirus management guidelines. *J Feline Med Surg* 10:300–316, 2008.
13. McManus CM, Levy JK, Andersen LA, et al: Prevalence of upper respiratory pathogens in four models for unowned cats in the southeast United States. *J Vet Intern Med* 25:705, 2011.
14. Hurley KF: Feline infectious respiratory disease. In *Proceedings North Am Vet Conf*, 2011, pp 1377–1381.
15. Pesavento PA, Bannasch MJ, Bachmann R, et al: Fatal *Streptococcus canis* infections in intensively housed shelter cats. *Vet Pathol Online* 44:218–221, 2007.
16. Merck MD, Miller DM, Reisman RW: Neglect. In Merck MD, editor: *Veterinary forensics: animal cruelty investigations*, ed 2, Ames, IA, 2013, Wiley, pp 207–232.

Strategies for Infectious Disease Management in Shelter Cats

Brian A. DiGangi

The animal shelter environment is an ideal setting for the introduction, transmission, and maintenance of a variety of infectious diseases. For the feline population of a shelter, the most prevalent and significant diseases almost universally include feline panleukopenia virus (FPV), feline herpesvirus type 1 (FHV-1, also known as *feline viral rhinotracheitis*), and feline calicivirus (FCV). Indeed, in many sheltering facilities, disease caused by FHV-1 and FCV is considered endemic.[1] In contrast to the pet cat population, these diseases present a constant and serious threat to the health and welfare of cats living in shelters.

The incidence of upper respiratory disease in the shelter setting has been reported to range from 26% to 44% with prevalence of FHV-1 and FCV as high as 38% and 36%, respectively.[2-4] The role of stress in the development and severity of these infections cannot be overemphasized, particularly in the case of FHV-1. The shelter environment often presents a constant variety of stressors that threaten both physical and mental health (e.g., inadequate cat housing, frequent introduction of new cats, housing in close association with other species, and inadequate nutrition and medical care).[5] Some common shelter characteristics, including high housing density, poor biosecurity, and frequent changes in housing conditions, have all been associated with increased shedding of respiratory pathogens and associated clinical disease.[6-9] These same factors can also contribute to outbreaks of FPV. Recognition and mitigation of these factors are critical to protect the behavioral and physical health of shelter cats and have a measurable impact on immune function.[5,10] Given its particular association with stress and intensive housing conditions,[6,11] FHV-1 is frequently the major contributor to clinical respiratory disease in shelter cats.[4,12] In contrast, FCV often emerges episodically, owing to the existence of numerous strains for which cross-protection is often poor.[1]

Infection with *Bordetella bronchiseptica*, *Chlamydophila felis*, and *Mycoplasma* species are also frequently identified in shelter cats, commonly concurrent with viral respiratory infection.[4,7,9,11,12] With constraints of time, space, money, and compromised welfare at play, euthanasia of affected cats is not an unusual management response to disease associated with these pathogens. Similarly, outbreaks of FPV are frequently reported in shelters in the United States and, although rarely indicated or necessary to humanely control

the spread of disease, complete depopulation may be carried out in response to the presence of infected cats in a given population.[13-15]

Fortunately, environmental enrichment is inexpensive and easily attainable (see Chapters 73 and 93), and vaccination against these diseases is readily available and highly effective. In the event of a disease outbreak, vaccination, along with other strategies for assessing the immune response and mitigating the risk of infection, are recommended in order to minimize the morbidity and mortality associated with these diseases in shelter cats.[16] This chapter focuses on the development of immunization protocols and the use of immunity-related risk factor analysis and antibody titer assessment as means of protecting cats from serious disease in the shelter setting.

IMMUNIZATION PROTOCOLS

With the advancement of shelter medicine, scientific research and analyses of best practices have provided new evidence that serve as the foundation for current professional recommendations for immunization of shelter cats. The high likelihood of disease exposure and infection in these settings as compared to that of most privately owned household pets justifies the need for protocols customized for population-level care. High stress levels, high-density housing, endemic disease, constant turnover of individual cats, inadequate housing facilities, poor biosecurity protocols, lack of proper isolation, and lack of veterinary oversight are frequently contributors to the elevated risk of disease exposure in the shelter setting.[17] Many of these factors are inherent in the design of the sheltering system and facility itself. Fortunately, there is much room for improvement through good management practices, including adjusting vaccination practices to comply with the latest scientific evidence. Adhering to such guidelines and best practices will maximize the chances that *vaccination* will lead to *immunization*.

Core Vaccines

Similar to that for privately-owned pet cats, vaccination against FPV, FHV-1, and FCV is considered essential for cats housed in shelters.[17] In one community in the southeastern United States, antibody titer assessment of more than 300 cats at the time of shelter intake suggested a lack of protection against FPV, FHV-1, and FCV in 60%, 89%, and 63% of cats, respectively. Although 70% of cats protected against FPV were neutered prior to admission, no single historical or clinical finding was predictive of protection against all three pathogens.[18] Such findings provide additional evidence of the need for widespread vaccination against these pathogens in shelter populations. In addition to vaccination against FPV, FHV-1, and FCV, rabies vaccination should be administered to all cats prior to adoption or release into the community where the disease is endemic or where required by law.[17]

Although vaccination against each of these pathogens is universally recommended, it is important to have accurate expectations of their impact on population health. Proper vaccination against FPV and rabies produces complete or sterilizing immunity and prevents the development of clinical signs associated with infection. In contrast, vaccination against FHV-1 and FCV induces partial immunity, reducing the severity and duration of clinical signs, but it does not prevent infection.[19-21]

Noncore Vaccines

Vaccinations that may be considered in select circumstances include those against feline leukemia virus (FeLV), *B. bronchiseptica*, *C. felis*, and multivalent calicivirus. An appreciation for the basic tenets of FeLV transmission is important when deciding whether or not vaccination is indicated in a given facility. Because FeLV is easily inactivated by common disinfectants and is not spread by indirect contact, individually housed shelter cats are at low risk for acquiring this disease in the shelter setting, and vaccination is considered optional. For many of these shelters, resources that might be devoted to vaccination are better used for retroviral testing or other veterinary expenses. However, the risk of direct contact and virus transmission increases in cat shelters that use group housing (including foster homes), have high turnover of cats from multiple sources, co-house cats with unknown disease status, or have unusually long lengths of stay (i.e., months to years). In those settings, vaccination against FeLV may be warranted.[17,22,23] Age-related susceptibility to progressive FeLV infection may also influence the specific vaccination protocol employed.[23] For example, a shelter may choose to selectively administer FeLV vaccinations to kittens less than 20 weeks of age that will be in group housing after completion of their initial vaccination series.

B. bronchiseptica and *C. felis* have been identified as components of upper respiratory tract disease in many shelters, although usually to a lesser extent than the viral pathogens.[4,12] Vaccination may be helpful in reducing severity of illness in shelters where laboratory testing (e.g., testing of nasopharyngeal samples with polymerase chain reaction or bacterial culture) has confirmed their presence. Other indications for vaccination against *B. bronchiseptica* include bordetellosis in the shelter's canine population and regular direct or indirect contact between cats and shelter dogs, rabbits, or guinea pigs.[17,22,24-27] Interestingly, a recent study reported decreased clinical illness after challenge with *B. bronchiseptica* when cats were vaccinated against FHV-1 and FCV, emphasizing the importance of the nonspecific immune response in combating respiratory disease.[28]

The wide genetic diversity of FCV strains and reports of virulent systemic calicivirus infections in different populations of cats have led to renewed interest in improving FCV vaccines.[29-32] An inactivated, multivalent FCV vaccine has been developed to provide broader cross-protection against different strains of FCV. Although efficacious, protection against challenge was only demonstrated 1 week after administration of two vaccinations given 3 to 4 weeks apart.[33,34] As with any inactivated vaccine, full protection should not be expected sooner than 7 to 14 days after the second vaccination,[17,35] which may limit practical application in the shelter setting. Shelters experiencing disease attributed to FCV in fully vaccinated cats, those using group housing, or those with increased length of stay (i.e., months to years) may experience some benefit from the inclusion of multivalent FCV products in their vaccination protocols in an attempt to provide broader cross-protection against FCV strains, including those that may lead to virulent systemic disease.[17,33,34]

Vaccination against feline immunodeficiency virus (FIV), feline infectious peritonitis (FIP), and dermatophytosis (which is not currently available in the United States or Canada) are not recommended in the shelter setting, because they are considered to be of limited benefit for shelter cats.[17,22,36] In the case of FIV, the threat of transmission in the shelter setting is low because direct contact, such as a bite wound, is generally required.[23] Furthermore, as an inactivated vaccine, the onset of protection may occur too late to be of benefit in the shelter setting.[37] In addition, vaccination against FIV can lead to future false-positive diagnostic test results.[38] Current evidence suggests that vaccination in attempt to prevent or treat dermatophytosis is ineffective,[39,40] and vaccination against FIP has variable efficacy and does not consistently confer protection against challenge.[41,42] For all of these reasons, administration of these products is a poor use of limited shelter resources in most situations.

Table 70-1 summarizes current recommendations regarding vaccination of cats in the shelter environment.

Type of Vaccination

In the shelter setting, use of modified-live virus (MLV) products whenever available is considered the standard of care.[17,22,36] Several scientific studies have demonstrated the ability of MLV products to rapidly induce immunologic protection against challenge, to provide protective immunity after a single vaccination, and to overcome interference from maternal-derived antibodies (MDAs) more effectively than inactivated products.[47-52] When inactivated products are used, careful consideration should be given to the time required to develop protective immunity and the risk of disease exposure. In most shelters, disease exposure is likely to occur prior to

| Table 70-1 | Vaccination Recommendations for Shelter-Housed Cats |

	TIMING OF VACCINATION	
Vaccination	**Kittens** **(4-20 Weeks of Age)***	**Adults** **(>20 Weeks of Age)**
Feline panleukopenia virus[†,‡]	On or before intake to shelter; repeat every 2 weeks until 18 to 20 weeks of age	On or before intake to shelter; may repeat once in 2 to 3 weeks
Feline herpesvirus type 1 (feline viral rhinotracheitis)[‡]	On or before intake to shelter; repeat every 2 weeks until 18 to 20 weeks of age	On or before intake to shelter; may repeat once in 2 to 3 weeks
Feline calicivirus[‡]	On or before intake to shelter; repeat every 2 weeks until 18 to 20 weeks of age	On or before intake to shelter; may repeat in 2 to 3 weeks
Rabies[§]	Administer one dose prior to leaving the facility in accordance with local regulations	
Feline leukemia virus[‖]	Consider use at the time of intake if cats are group housed; begin as early as 8 weeks of age; repeat once in 2 to 4 weeks Complete primary vaccination series prior to group housing Testing prior to vaccination is recommended	
Bordetella bronchiseptica[‡]	Consider use when clinical signs and laboratory testing are consistent with endemic disease, outbreak, or other risk factors are present (see text); administer a single dose at intake beginning at 4 weeks of age	
Chlamydophila felis[¶]	Consider use when clinical signs and laboratory testing are consistent with endemic disease or outbreak; administer a single dose at intake beginning at 9 weeks of age; repeat once in 3 to 4 weeks	
Multivalent calicivirus[§]	Consider use when clinical signs or laboratory testing are consistent with disease in fully vaccinated adults; administer a single dose at intake beginning at 4 weeks of age; repeat once in 2 weeks	
Feline infectious peritonitis	Not recommended for use in the shelter setting	
Feline immunodeficiency virus	Not recommended for use in the shelter setting	
Dermatophytosis	Not recommended for use	

Scherk MA, Ford RB, Gaskell RM, et al: 2013 AAFP feline vaccination advisory panel report. *J Feline Med Surg* 15:785-808, 2013; Griffin B: Wellness. In Miller L, Hurley K, editors: *Infectious disease management in animal shelters,* Ames, IA, 2009, Wiley-Blackwell, pp 17-38; Griffin B: Feline care in the animal shelter. In Miller L, Zawistowski S, editors: *Shelter medicine for veterinarians and staff,* ed 2, Ames, IA, 2013, Wiley-Blackwell, pp 145-184; Ford RB: 2012 Vaccines and vaccination: the facts and the fiction. In *Proceedings Florida Veterinary Medical Association 83rd Annual Conference.* <http://www.fvmace .org/FVMA_83rd_Annual_Conference/Proceedings/2012%20VACCINES%20&%20VACCINATION%20The%20FACTS%20vs%20The%20FICTION.html>, 2012 (Accessed June 3, 2015).
*Kitten age can be estimated by dentition or body weight[43-46]
[†]If an intranasal product is utilized, simultaneous vaccination with an injectable product is recommended.
[‡]Modified-live virus (MLV) product
[§]Inactivated vaccine product
[‖]Inactivated or recombinant vaccine product
[¶]Inactivated or MLV vaccine product

the onset of protection, thus negating any potential benefits of an inactivated vaccine.

In the case of FPV, FHV-1, and FCV, both parenteral and intranasal products are available. Both types of products have been shown to be effective against clinical challenge.[51-54] In fact, there is some evidence that protection against upper respiratory disease may occur more quickly with intranasal than with parenteral vaccination.[3] However, the ability of intranasal products to induce sterilizing immunity against FPV quickly enough to provide protection in the high-risk shelter environment has been called into question.[21,22,55] For

this reason, when intranasal vaccination is used, vaccination protocols should also include administration of a parenteral MLV FPV vaccine.[21,22] There is no evidence that concurrent use of intranasal and parenteral vaccines will result in decreased efficacy and some evidence that there may be an added protective benefit.[3]

Mild, self-limiting clinical signs of upper respiratory disease may be seen 1 or more days following administration of intranasal products.[22,56] In many shelters, such signs could inadvertently lead to population management decisions that compromise the care of individual cats mistakenly identified as harboring disease. Even though they do not represent a health risk to the population (and in fact may serve to protect the population through herd immunity), such cats may be transferred to isolation areas for observation or treatment, exposing them to clinically ill animals and unnecessarily increasing their length of stay in the shelter. In some facilities, cats with clinical signs of upper respiratory infection may be euthanized. Intranasal vaccination does have the benefit of stimulating local immunity against FHV-1 and FCV (i.e., immunoglobulin [Ig] A and IgM)[53] and is therefore not subject to interference from MDA. This quality may make intranasal vaccination especially useful in kittens less than 20 weeks of age. Each of these considerations must be taken into account when choosing a specific vaccine product for an individual shelter's cat population.

Timing of Vaccination

The timing of vaccine administration in the shelter setting is a crucial component of ensuring successful immunization against common disease threats. As discussed earlier, many cats entering the shelter population are known to be at risk for infection with common pathogens based on the absence of protective antibody titers. In addition, MLV vaccines against FPV, FHV-1, and FCV have been shown to induce immunity rapidly after administration, with protection against challenge demonstrated in as few as 3 days for FPV and 4 days for FHV-1.[52,53] Development of protective antibody titers was reported 7 days after vaccination with an MLV FCV vaccine (Table 70-2).[48] It is important to note that the assessment of vaccine efficacy is often limited to measurement of the adaptive immune system response (i.e., antibody titer measurement); however, stimulation of the innate immune system is responsible for immediate host defense and is essential for ensuring the effectiveness of the adaptive response.[58] For these reasons, vaccination immediately at or before the time of intake to the shelter environment—even if the animal is within a legal holding period—is universally recommended.[17,22,36] Delays in vaccination of even just a few hours could be clinically significant in the high-risk environment of an animal shelter.

Vaccine Handling and Administration

In order to accomplish the goal of vaccination immediately on or before shelter intake, shelter staff members should be trained on proper handling and administration of vaccine products. Vaccine products should be administered in accordance with the American Association of Feline Practitioners' vaccination site recommendations (namely, subcutaneously as distal on the limb as possible) to improve the odds of definitive treatment in the event of an injection site sarcoma.[17] Complete tumor removal may be more feasible when tumors arise in such locations.[17] In the context of a shelter, where minimizing stress and timely vaccination are of the utmost importance, using low-stress handling techniques and administering the vaccination in any site that is easily accessible should take priority over specific administration locations. In cases where alternate vaccination sites are used, it is particularly important that the injection location is documented in the medical record. Box 70-1 reviews practical guidelines for handling and administration of vaccine products.

Vaccination of Kittens

In the absence of vaccination, the primary means of pathogen protection for young kittens is through MDA, yet individual levels of MDA can vary widely even within a single litter, necessitating the institution of initial vaccination as early as 4 weeks of age in kittens housed in a shelter environment.[17,21,22,35,36] Accordingly, the rate at which MDA declines and can no longer confer protection is also variable. Maternal-derived antibody interference with immunization has been reported up to 20 weeks of age for FPV and 17 weeks of age for FHV-1 and FCV.[47,60] The unpredictability of MDA protection and the high risk of disease exposure in the shelter

Table 70-2	Fastest Reported Time to Efficacy after a Single Vaccination against Feline Panleukopenia, Feline Herpesvirus Type 1, or Feline Calicivirus			
Pathogen	**Time to Protection**	**Determination of Efficacy**	**Type of Vaccine**	**Route**
Feline panleukopenia	3 days[52]	Challenge	MLV	Parenteral
	7 days[48]	Antibody titer	MLV	Parenteral
	7 days[49]	Antibody titer	MLV	IN, Parenteral
	7 days[57]	Challenge	MLV	Parenteral
	10 days[48]	Antibody titer	IA	Parenteral
Feline herpesvirus type 1	4 days[53]	Challenge	MLV	IN
	14 days[48]	Antibody titer	MLV, IA	Parenteral
Feline calicivirus	1 day[48]	Antibody titer	IA	Parenteral
	7 days[48]	Antibody titer	MLV	Parenteral

IA, Inactivated; *IN,* intranasal; *MLV,* modified-live virus.

BOX 70-1 Practical Guidelines for Handling and Administration of Vaccine Products[59]

Storage and Handling
- Unload shipments of vaccine products within 1 hour of arrival.
  - Ensure shipping container is intact, packaging is sealed, and ice packs are cold; reject product if any of these parameters are not met.
- Store vaccines in the refrigerator at 35° to 45° F (2° to 7° C).
  - Place a thermometer in each refrigerator and regularly monitor temperature fluctuations.
- When transporting vaccines to another location for administration, place products in a cooler with frozen ice packs.
  - Protect from temperature extremes and replace ice packs as needed.

Administration
- Do not use expired vaccine products.
- Gently shake multidose vials before drawing up vaccine product.
- Discard vials if rubber stopper is damaged.
- Reconstitute single-dose vials with supplied diluent.
  - Do not interchange diluent from different products or substitute diluent with another product or solution without manufacturer authorization.

- Administer reconstituted vaccines within 60 minutes of preparation.
- Do not clean administration site with alcohol prior to vaccination.
  - Alcohol is only an effective disinfectant when applied to surfaces free from organic contamination and allowed at least 30 seconds of contact time; the odor is offensive to many cats.
- Do not split supplied dose between multiple animals.
- Readminister vaccine if misinjection, including partial injection, occurs.
- Administer products according to standard site recommendations.
  - Products containing FPV, FHV-1, and FCV should be given distal to the right elbow.
  - Products containing FeLV should be given distal to the left stifle.
  - Rabies vaccines should be given distal to the right stifle.

Scherk MA, Ford RB, Gaskell RM, et al: 2013 AAFP feline vaccination advisory panel report. *J Feline Med Surg* 15:785-808, 2013; Richards JR, Elstron TH, Ford RB, et al: The 2006 American Association of Feline Practitioners feline vaccine advisory panel report. *J Am Vet Med Assoc* 229:1405-1441, 2006; DiGangi BA: Proper handling and use of vaccines in animal shelters, *Maddie's Fund.* <http://www.maddiesfund.org/Maddies_Institute/Articles/Proper_Use_and_Handling_of_Vaccines_in_Animal_Shelters.html>, April 2012 (Accessed June 3, 2015).
FCV, Feline calicivirus; *FeLV,* feline leukemia virus; *FHV-1,* feline herpesvirus type 1; *FPV,* feline panleukopenia virus.

environment justify extending the traditional vaccination protocol through 18 or 20 weeks of age.[17,22,36] Decreasing the intervaccination interval for kittens and adult cats that are receiving their first vaccination to 2 weeks is also recommended in the shelter environment and may enhance immune response particularly in the face of low levels of MDA.[17,22,35,36] There is no evidence that vaccination at intervals less than 14 days apart provides any additional protective benefit, and this practice is not recommended.[17,35] Similarly, vaccination at less than 4 weeks of age with a MLV product containing panleukopenia virus is generally not recommended to minimize the risk of cerebellar hypoplasia.[17,61] All cats should be assumed to be naïve to previous vaccination unless accompanied by verifiable, written documentation of appropriate vaccine administration.

Health Status

One additional consideration when designing an immunization protocol for shelter cats is the need for vaccination regardless of health status. Standard recommendations for privately owned cats that are clinically ill, pregnant, or lactating advise practitioners to postpone vaccination until these conditions are resolved.[17] This is due to the fact that vaccine products are not labeled (and therefore have not been evaluated for efficacy) in such situations. In the case of MLV FPV

vaccination of a queen in early pregnancy, deleterious effects on developing fetuses have been documented,[61] but these are rare occurrences and there is no evidence that vaccination in the face of these conditions will not be effective. To the contrary, vaccination remains effective and is essential to protect both the individual cats and the shelter population as a whole against infectious disease outbreaks. In the case of vaccination against FHV-1 and FCV, vaccination during pregnancy may serve to enhance protection for both the queen and the offspring through the provision of higher levels of MDA and reduce the risk of clinical illness or death from upper respiratory disease.[17] The risk-to-benefit ratio in the shelter setting lies in favor of vaccination of each of these groups of patients, regardless of health status.[22,36]

IMMUNITY-RELATED RISK FACTORS

Appreciation of the known risk factors for infection can help the shelter medicine practitioner develop customized strategies for combating common infectious diseases in their own facility. Risk factors for disease are commonly categorized according to the epidemiologic triad: the environment (e.g., population density, biosecurity protocols, animal segregation), the host (e.g., stress, nutritional status, concurrent disease), and the infectious agent (e.g., virulence, dose, incubation period). Recognizing and mitigating such risks are crucial to the development of a comprehensive disease prevention protocol; however, host-related factors are often most relevant when it comes to clinical decision making for an individual patient.

Immunity-related individual animal risk factors include vaccination status, the presence or absence of MDA, and the likelihood of natural exposure to the agent of concern.[62] Such risk factors are commonly assessed through two basic mechanisms: evaluation of clinical and physical examination findings correlated with infection and assessment of levels of antibody titers against a given disease. In the case of diseases where protective levels of antibody titers are known to equate to sterilizing immunity against infection (e.g., FPV), such evidence is usually considered a strong indication of the degree of risk. Thus, cats with protective titers are considered to be at low risk of infection, whereas those without are considered to be at high risk. It is important to note that regardless of the presence or absence of protective antibody titers, kittens less than 5 months of age must always be regarded as high risk (see discussion of MDA earlier). Furthermore, the presence or absence of protective antibody titers does not always correlate to risk level depending on the disease in question. Notably, in the face of diseases where antibodies play a lesser role in combating infection (e.g., FHV-1 and FCV), titer assessment may not be particularly useful, and evaluation of individual clinical factors should be given greater weight.

Clinical Findings

Several scientific studies have evaluated risk factors for infection with FPV, FHV-1, and FCV. In the case of FPV, clinical factors associated with an increased risk of disease include age of less than 1 year and having an incomplete vaccination history.[63] Furthermore, the likelihood of infection and death from FPV increases with decreasing age.[64] Factors such as young age, a recent visit to a boarding facility, lapses in vaccination history, living in a research colony, and living with dogs with respiratory disease were all found to increase the risk of clinical disease caused by both FHV-1 and FCV.[8] One study suggested that cats that come into contact with cats outside of their home may be at greater risk for FHV-1 infection.[65] Specifically regarding animal shelter populations, it has been demonstrated that increasing length of stay is correlated with clinical signs of upper respiratory infection. This effect was greatest in populations of kittens less than or equal to 6 months of age.[2] As previously noted, environmental features are also important determinants of disease caused by FHV-1 and FCV in animal shelters. For example, cats housed in shelters with separate designated areas for admissions and isolation were at lower risk for development of clinical disease than those in facilities that did not have a system for segregation of new intakes and clinically ill cats.[66] Factors such as stress, housing density, and biosecurity and husbandry protocols also warrant consideration when assessing the risk of clinical disease in an animal shelter.

Protective Antibody Titers

Evaluation of nine different clinical and historical findings in more than 300 cats admitted to one animal shelter revealed that being neutered was the only factor significantly associated with protective levels of antibody titers against FPV.[18] This relationship, likely the result of previous veterinary care that included vaccination before or at the time of surgical sterilization, emphasizes the ability of FPV vaccination to induce long-lasting immunity.

Although less predictive of protection against clinical disease than for FPV, protective levels of antibody titers against FHV-1 have been correlated with increasing age and being neutered. Similarly, increasing age and being relinquished by an owner (versus being found as a stray) were associated with greater odds of protective antibody titers against FCV.[18]

In the absence of other information (e.g., complete medical records), consideration of these individual animal risk factors can assist the clinician in the assessment of an animal's likelihood of prior vaccination and risk for infection during a disease outbreak. They can also be used to guide management decisions, such as where to house a particular cat in the shelter and whether or not to send a patient off-site to an adoption event or spay-neuter clinic. Table 70-3 summarizes some of the known individual animal risk factors for FPV, FHV-1, and FCV.

ANTIBODY TITER ASSESSMENT

Assessment of individual animal titer levels has become a key component of disease outbreak response in shelter populations.[16,67,68] Titer assessment can indeed be a useful tool in the development of an outbreak response plan; however, the shelter medicine practitioner must be familiar with the appropriate uses of this tool as well as its limitations.

Antibody titer evaluation can provide evidence of previous infection or vaccination against the agent of concern. Such information allows the practitioner to predict the likelihood of protection in the face of disease exposure. In particular, titers against FPV in patients without clinical signs of disease have been used in the assessment of individual animal risk during disease outbreaks in animal shelters. In these cases, the presence of a high titer against FPV is presumed to predict little to no risk of disease for that individual.[68] Armed with such information, evidence-based management decisions can be made to minimize the impact of the disease outbreak (see Evidence-based Outbreak Response).

It is important to recognize that although an antibody titer labeled as "protective" is thought to be sufficient to prevent disease when challenged by an infectious dose of a given virus, the precise numerical value considered protective varies by laboratory and methodology. In addition, the presence of high antibody titers does not ensure protection against disease and absence does not indicate susceptibility in every case. The method of antibody measurement (i.e.,

Table 70-3   **Risk Factors for Increased Risk of Disease Caused by Feline Panleukopenia, Feline Herpesvirus Type 1, and Feline Calicivirus**

Pathogen	Parameter Associated with Clinical Disease	Parameter Associated with Absence of Protective Antibody Titers
Feline panleukopenia virus	Less than 1 year of age Incomplete vaccination history	Sexually intact
Feline herpesvirus type 1 and feline calicivirus	Young age Incomplete vaccination history Living in a research colony Living with dogs with respiratory disease Contact with cats outside of the home Increased shelter length of stay	Young age Sexually intact Entered shelter as stray (for feline calicivirus only)

Edinboro CH, Janowitz LK, Guptill-Yoran L, et al: A clinical trial of intranasal and subcutaneous vaccines to prevent upper respiratory infection in cats at an animal shelter. *Feline Pract* 27:7-11, 13, 1999; Binns SH, Dawson S, Speakman AJ, et al: A study of feline upper respiratory tract disease with reference to prevalence and risk factors for infection with feline calicivirus and feline herpesvirus. *J Feline Med Surg* 2:123-133, 2000; DiGangi BA, Levy JK, Griffin B, et al: Prevalence of serum antibody titers against feline panleukopenia virus, feline herpesvirus 1, and feline calicivirus in cats entering a Florida animal shelter. *J Am Vet Med Assoc* 241:1320-1325, 2012; Kruse BD, Unterer S, Horlacher K, et al: Prognostic factors in cats with feline panleukopenia. *J Vet Intern Med* 24: 1271-1276, 2010; Cave TA, Thompson H, Reid SWJ, et al: Kitten mortality in the United Kingdom: a retrospective analysis of 274 histopathological examinations (1986 to 2000). *Vet Rec* 151:497-501, 2002; Sykes JE, Anderson GA, Studdert VP, et al: Prevalence of feline Chlamydia psittaci and feline herpesvirus 1 in cats with upper respiratory tract disease. *J Vet Intern Med* 13:153-162, 1999; Edwards DS, Coyne K, Dawson S, et al: Risk factors for time to diagnosis of feline upper respiratory tract disease in UK animal adoption shelters. *Prev Vet Med* 87:327-339, 2008.

serum neutralization, hemagglutination inhibition, enzyme-linked immunosorbent assay [ELISA], immunofluorescent antibody), the type of infection (i.e., extracellular, intracellular), and the type of antibody measured (i.e., IgG, IgA, IgM) all influence the degree of correlation between a titer value and protection against disease.[35] Despite these limitations, studies have demonstrated that the presence of serum antibody titers can be a useful measure of protection against FPV infection and correlate with a reduction in clinical signs of disease from FHV-1 and FCV in vaccinated cats.[54,69-71]

The development of several commercially available, point-of-care, serum or plasma antibody titer assessment test kits for dogs and cats has heightened awareness of the utility of antibody titer assessment and made such measurement feasible and cost effective in the shelter setting (Figure 70-1). These point-of-care test kits also carry the additional advantage of providing immediate results. The practitioner is cautioned to ensure the accuracy of the methodology chosen for clinical use and to use such kits strictly according to manufacturer instructions. Independent evaluations have demonstrated variability in the accuracy of such kits for the detection of antibodies against FPV.[72,73] In addition, kits designed for the detection of canine parvovirus antibodies in serum or plasma are unable to detect those against FPV.[72]

EVIDENCE-BASED OUTBREAK RESPONSE

An infectious disease outbreak can be defined as an increase in the frequency and/or severity of disease within a population. The development of a comprehensive outbreak response plan is discussed in depth elsewhere. However, six core response measures for animal shelters have been identified (Figure 70-2)[16,67]:

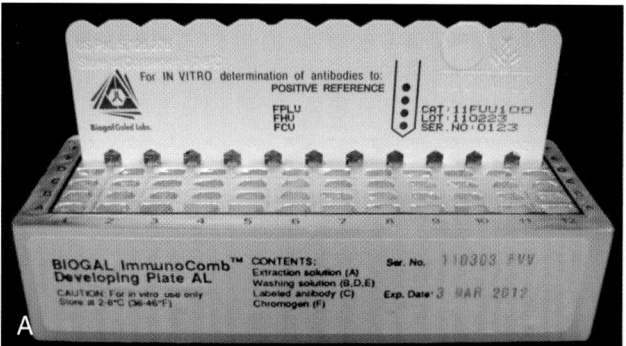

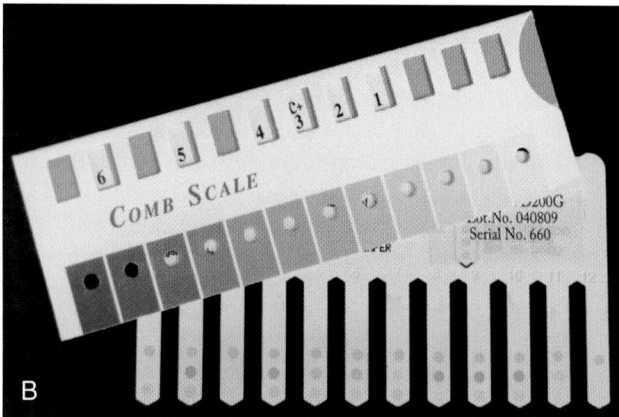

Figure 70-1: A, A commercially available, point-of-care test kit for antibodies against feline panleukopenia virus, feline herpesvirus type 1, and feline calicivirus (ImmunoComb Feline VacciCheck, Biogal Galed Labs, Kibbutz Galed, Israel). **B,** A 12-toothed comb with antigen test spots is moved through wells of the developing plate at timed intervals. Results are displayed as gray color tones and are compared with a comb scale for interpretation. (From DiGangi BA, Gray LK, Levy JK, et al: Detection of protective antibody titers against feline panleukopenia virus, feline herpesvirus-1, and feline calicivirus in cats entering Florida animal shelters using a point-of-care ELISA. *J Feline Med Surg* 13:912-918, 2011.)

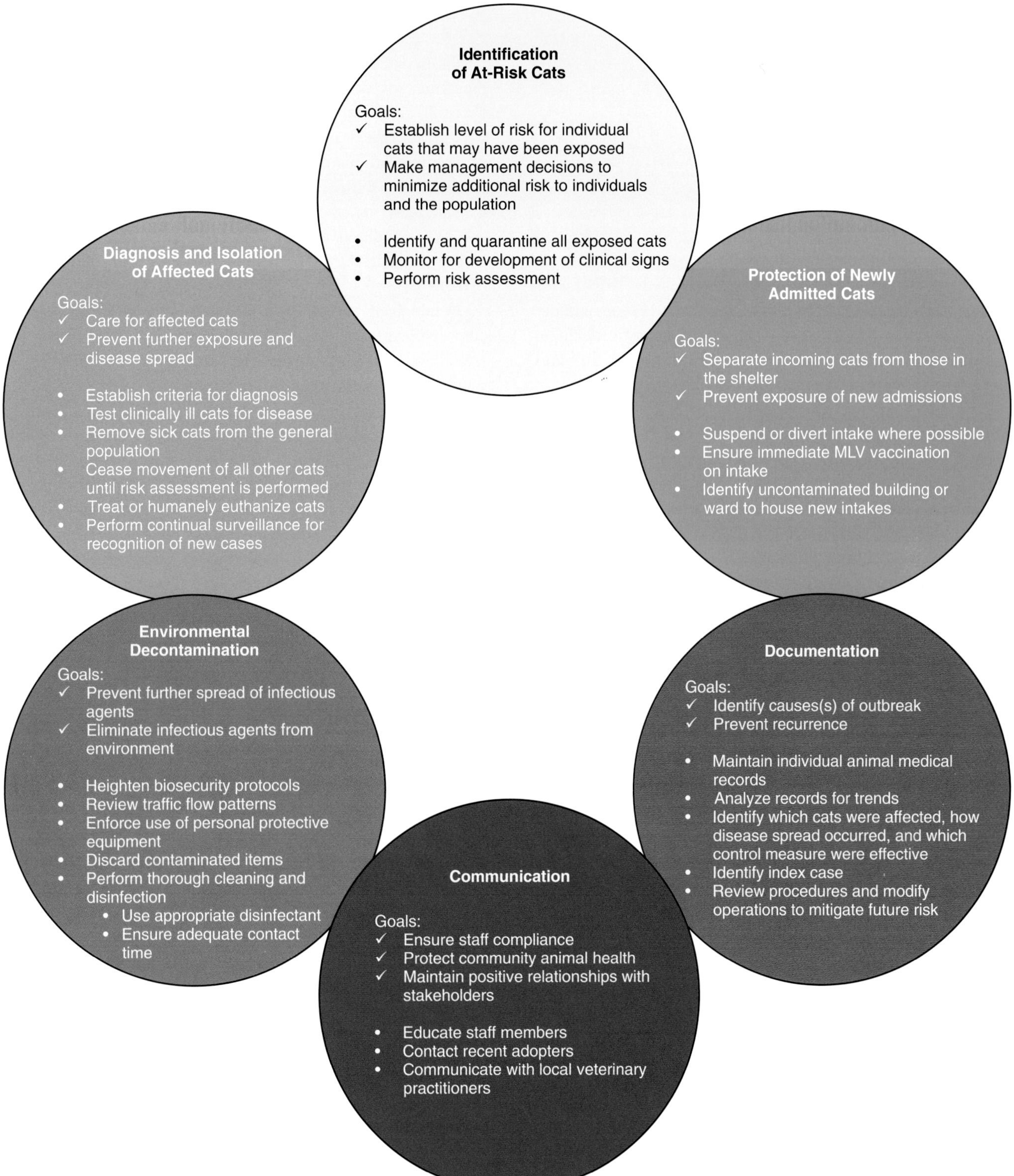

Identification of At-Risk Cats

Goals:
✓ Establish level of risk for individual cats that may have been exposed
✓ Make management decisions to minimize additional risk to individuals and the population

- Identify and quarantine all exposed cats
- Monitor for development of clinical signs
- Perform risk assessment

Diagnosis and Isolation of Affected Cats

Goals:
✓ Care for affected cats
✓ Prevent further exposure and disease spread

- Establish criteria for diagnosis
- Test clinically ill cats for disease
- Remove sick cats from the general population
- Cease movement of all other cats until risk assessment is performed
- Treat or humanely euthanize cats
- Perform continual surveillance for recognition of new cases

Protection of Newly Admitted Cats

Goals:
✓ Separate incoming cats from those in the shelter
✓ Prevent exposure of new admissions

- Suspend or divert intake where possible
- Ensure immediate MLV vaccination on intake
- Identify uncontaminated building or ward to house new intakes

Environmental Decontamination

Goals:
✓ Prevent further spread of infectious agents
✓ Eliminate infectious agents from environment

- Heighten biosecurity protocols
- Review traffic flow patterns
- Enforce use of personal protective equipment
- Discard contaminated items
- Perform thorough cleaning and disinfection
  - Use appropriate disinfectant
  - Ensure adequate contact time

Documentation

Goals:
✓ Identify causes(s) of outbreak
✓ Prevent recurrence

- Maintain individual animal medical records
- Analyze records for trends
- Identify which cats were affected, how disease spread occurred, and which control measure were effective
- Identify index case
- Review procedures and modify operations to mitigate future risk

Communication

Goals:
✓ Ensure staff compliance
✓ Protect community animal health
✓ Maintain positive relationships with stakeholders

- Educate staff members
- Contact recent adopters
- Communicate with local veterinary practitioners

Figure 70-2: Core response measures for infectious disease outbreaks in animal shelters. Note that most response measures will occur simultaneously and at multiple times throughout the response. *MLV,* Modified-live virus. (Adapted from Hurley KF: Outbreak management. In Miller L, Hurley K, editors: *Infectious disease management in animal shelters,* Ames, IA, 2009, Wiley-Blackwell, pp 39-48.)

1. Diagnosis and isolation of diseased animals
2. Identification and management of exposed and at-risk animals
3. Environmental decontamination
4. Protection of newly admitted animals
5. Documentation
6. Communication with staff members, stakeholders, adopters, and the public

Immune strategies that play a role in these core response measures include vaccination of all individuals on intake and identification of animals at risk for disease through risk factor assessment, including antibody titer evaluation. Risk factor analysis has been used in the human medical field for a variety of disease states to aid in clinical and diagnostic decision making and is particularly helpful in limiting morbidity and mortality during an outbreak in the shelter setting.[74-76]

Parameters such as the proximity to a known infected animal, the dose of infectious agent to which an animal is exposed, and vaccination history including age at the time of vaccination are some important considerations in individual animal risk assessment.[16] For diseases for which antibody titers correlate with protection against illness (e.g., FPV), assessment of serum antibody titers can also be factored into the decision-making algorithm. In turn, identification of animal factors that are reliably associated with the presence of protective antibody titers could greatly enhance individual risk assessment and animal management during an outbreak. For example, because being neutered prior to shelter admission is correlated with the presence of protective levels of antibodies against FPV, asymptomatic cats that are neutered could be presumed to be at low risk of disease if exposed during an outbreak without the need for direct antibody titer assessment. Such animals could be selectively directed toward adoption or transferred out of the shelter system rather than held in quarantine or euthanized.[77] Although this method of risk assessment is practiced on a regular basis and is supported by clinical experience, its scientific validity has not yet been demonstrated in the setting of a disease outbreak in an animal shelter.

In the case of a suspected outbreak of FPV, the first response step is to establish a definitive diagnosis in one or more affected cats. In the shelter setting, this is most commonly done through confirmation of clinical signs of disease (e.g., diarrhea, vomiting, peracute death) in combination with positive fecal antigen test results.[78] It is noteworthy that canine parvovirus fecal ELISAs are an accurate means of detecting FPV infection in cats[79,80]; however, weak false-positive test results may be seen up to 14 days after administration of an MLV FPV vaccine.[14,79] Neutropenia (i.e., <2500/μL or 1 to 2 neutrophils per 40× field) and, in the case of necropsy findings, segmental hyperemia of the jejunum and ileum, are also strongly suggestive of FPV infection.[20] Once a diagnosis has been obtained, infected cats must be removed from the general population and thorough decontamination of the environment must be undertaken.

The appropriate management steps are often less clear in the case of cats that are asymptomatic, yet have been exposed to cats diagnosed with FPV. As the initial step in risk analysis, age, neuter status prior to admission, and vaccination history should be assessed and used to infer the most likely level of risk for each individual cat (Figure 70-3). Cats less than 20 weeks of age should be considered at high risk for disease regardless of neuter status or vaccination history, whereas those 20 weeks of age or older and neutered prior to admission should be considered at low risk for disease regardless of vaccination history. Sexually intact adult cats (i.e., ≥20 weeks of age) with an unknown or inadequate shelter vaccination history (i.e., vaccinated ≤7 days prior to FPV exposure) can be considered at high risk for disease. Those that were well vaccinated (i.e., more than 7 days previously) at the time of FPV exposure can be considered at low risk for disease.

When antibody titer testing is available and feasible, adult cats determined to be of high risk can be further characterized based on test results. Although it would be ideal to measure antibody titers on all cats, this is often not feasible and prioritizing testing to those considered to be at the highest risk may best direct limited resources. Those found to have protective antibody titers can be moved to a low-risk category and can safely be selected for adoption or transfer out of the shelter. Those with inadequate antibody titers can be maintained as high risk and prioritized for further observation (i.e., quarantine on-site or in an appropriate foster home) or selected for euthanasia. Such cats should remain in a period of quarantine until expiration of the disease incubation period—14 days for FPV—in the absence of clinical signs or re-exposure to infected cats. Should re-exposure occur, the quarantine period must start anew.

It is important to remember that antibody titer testing is only useful in this sense when dealing with pathogens for which vaccination and the presence of high levels of antibodies equate to sterilizing immunity. For the feline population, this is generally limited to FPV. In addition, in the shelter environment, it is not usually a good use of resources to measure antibody titers in symptomatic animals, those in which a definitive diagnosis has been made, or those that may have circulating MDA (i.e., <20 weeks of age). Symptomatic animals should always be isolated from asymptomatic animals for treatment or humane euthanasia; knowledge of antibody titers in these animals is not likely to impact treatment or management decisions. Finally, in the midst of an outbreak, regardless of risk status, all exposed cats should be vaccinated with a MLV FPV vaccine if they have not received one within the previous 14 days; cats less than 20 weeks of age should receive regular boosters every 2 weeks until they are 20 weeks of age or older.

SUMMARY

Recent advances in the field of shelter medicine have resulted in the development of improved disease management strategies specifically tailored to these unique environments. By employing the latest techniques in vaccination strategies, assessing individual animal risk for disease, and using new tools for antibody titer assessment, the practitioner can create scientifically sound, yet practical approaches to the prevention and treatment of common diseases of shelter cats.

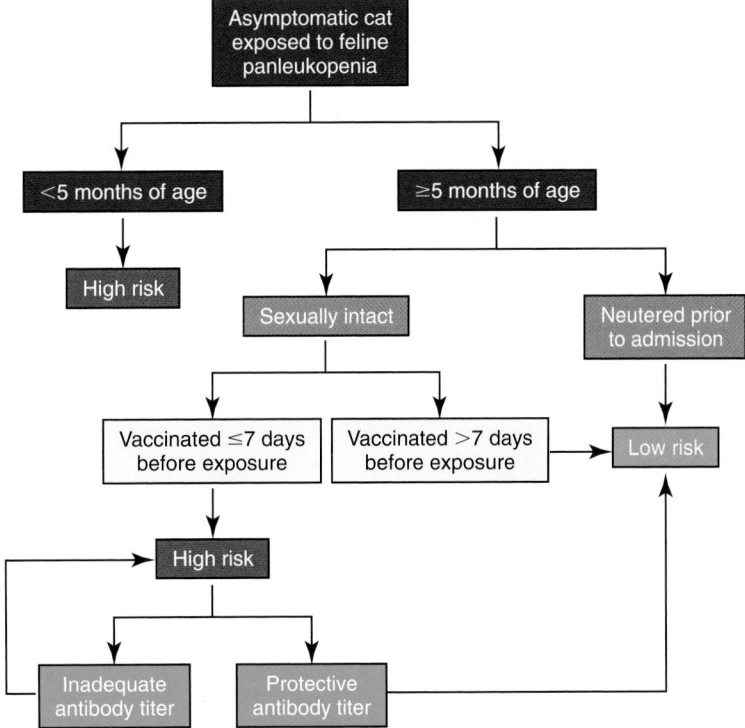

Figure 70-3: Risk assessment algorithm for asymptomatic, exposed cats during a feline panleukopenia (FPV) outbreak in an animal shelter. Cats found to be at high risk can be placed in quarantine; those found to be at low risk can safely be adopted or transferred out of the shelter system. Regardless of risk status, all exposed cats should be vaccinated with a modified-live virus FPV vaccine if they have not received one within the previous 14 days; cats less than 20 weeks of age should receive regular boosters every 2 weeks until 20 weeks of age or older.

References

1. Scarlett JM: Feline upper respiratory disease. In Hurley K, Miller LA, editors: *Infectious disease management in animal shelters*, Ames, IA, 2009, Wiley-Blackwell, pp 125–146.

2. Dinnage JD, Scarlett JM, Richards JR: Descriptive epidemiology of feline upper respiratory tract disease in an animal shelter. *J Feline Med Surg* 11:816–825, 2009.

3. Edinboro CH, Janowitz LK, Guptill-Yoran L, et al: A clinical trial of intranasal and subcutaneous vaccines to prevent upper respiratory infection in cats at an animal shelter. *Feline Pract* 27:7–11, 13, 1999.

4. Bannasch MJ, Foley JE: Epidemiologic evaluation of multiple respiratory pathogens in cats in animal shelters. *J Feline Med Surg* 7:109–119, 2005.

5. Newbury S, Blinn MK, Bushby PA, et al: Guidelines for standards of care in animal shelters: The Association of Shelter Veterinarians, 2010. <http://www.sheltervet.org/assets/docs/shelter-standards-oct2011-wforward.pdf>, (Accessed June 3, 2015.)

6. Gaskell RM, Povey RC: Experimental induction of feline viral rhinotracheitis virus re-excretion in FVR-recovered cats. *Vet Rec* 12:128–133, 1977.

7. Binns SH, Dawson S, Speakman AJ, et al: Prevalence and risk factors for feline *Bordetella bronchiseptica* infection. *Vet Rec* 144:575–580, 1999.

8. Binns SH, Dawson S, Speakman AJ, et al: A study of feline upper respiratory tract disease with reference to prevalence and risk factors for infection with feline calicivirus and feline herpesvirus. *J Feline Med Surg* 2:123–133, 2000.

9. Helps CR, Lait P, Damhuis A, et al: Factors associated with upper respiratory tract disease caused by feline herpesvirus, feline calicivirus, *Chlamydophila felis* and *Bordetella bronchiseptica* in cats: experience from 218 European catteries. *Vet Rec* 156:669–673, 2005.

10. Gourkow N, LaVoy A, Dean GA, et al: Associations of behavior with secretory immunoglobulin A and cortisol in domestic cats during their first week in an animal shelter. *Appl Anim Behav Sci* 150:55–64, 2014.

11. Gaskell R, Dawson S, Radford A: Feline respiratory disease. In Greene CE, editor: *Infectious diseases of the dog and cat*, ed 3, St Louis, 2006, Saunders, pp 145–154.

12. Veir JK, Ruch-Gallie R, Spindel ME, et al: Prevalence of selected infectious organisms and comparison of two anatomic sampling

sites in shelter cats with upper respiratory disease. *J Feline Med Surg* 10:551–557, 2008.

13. King R: Everett euthanizes cats, closes feline shelter to stem disease outbreak, *HeraldNet.* <http://www.heraldnet.com/article/20100927/NEWS01/709279847>, (Accessed June 3, 2015.)

14. Patterson EV, Reese MJ, Tucker SJ, et al: Effect of vaccination on parvovirus antigen testing in kittens. *J Am Vet Med Assoc* 230:359–363, 2007.

15. Pappas ML: Panleukopenia fears, *Nuvo.* <http://www.nuvo.net/indianapolis/panleukopenia-fears/Content?oid=1229350>, (Accessed June 3, 2015.)

16. Hurley KF: Outbreak Management. In Miller L, Hurley K, editors: *Infectious disease management in animal shelters*, Ames, IA, 2009, Wiley-Blackwell, pp 39–48.

17. Scherk MA, Ford RB, Gaskell RM, et al: 2013 AAFP feline vaccination advisory panel report. *J Feline Med Surg* 15:785–808, 2013.

18. DiGangi BA, Levy JK, Griffin B, et al: Prevalence of serum antibody titers against feline panleukopenia virus, feline herpesvirus 1, and feline calicivirus in cats entering a Florida animal shelter. *J Am Vet Med Assoc* 241:1320–1325, 2012.

19. Gaskell RM: Feline respiratory disease. In Greene CE, editor: *Infectious diseases of the dog and cat*, ed 3, St Louis, 2006, Saunders, pp 145–154.

20. Greene CE, Addie DD: Feline parvovirus infections. In Greene CE, editor: *Infectious diseases of the dog and cat*, ed 3, St Louis, 2006, Saunders, pp 78–88.

21. Richards JR, Elstron TH, Ford RB, et al: The 2006 American Association of Feline Practitioners feline vaccine advisory panel report. *J Am Vet Med Assoc* 229:1405–1441, 2006.

22. Griffin B: Wellness. In Miller L, Hurley K, editors: *Infectious disease management in animal shelters*, Ames, IA, 2009, Wiley-Blackwell, pp 17–38.

23. Levy J, Crawford C, Hartmann K, et al: 2008 American Association of Feline Practitioners' feline retrovirus management guidelines. *J Feline Med Surg* 10:300–316, 2008.

24. Egberdink H, Addie D, Belak S, et al: *Bordetella bronchiseptica* infection in cats. ABCD guidelines on prevention and management. *J Feline Med Surg* 11:610–614, 2009.

25. Lennox A: Respiratory disease and pasteurellosis. In Quesenberry KE, Carpenter JW, editors: *Ferrets, rabbits, and rodents clinical medicine and surgery*, ed 3, St Louis, 2012, Elsevier, pp 205–216.

26. Hawkins MG, Bishop CR: Disease problems of guinea pigs. In Quesenberry KE, Carpenter JW, editors: *Ferrets, rabbits, and rodents clinical medicine and surgery*, ed 3, St Louis, 2012, Elsevier, pp 295–310.

27. Rougier S, Galland D, Boucher S, et al: Epidemiology and susceptibility of pathogenic bacteria responsible for upper respiratory tract infections in pet rabbits. *Vet Microbiol* 15:192–198, 2006.

28. Bradley A, Kinyon J, Frana T, et al: Efficacy of intranasal administration of a modified live feline herpesvirus 1 and feline calicivirus vaccine against disease caused by *Bordetella bronchiseptica* after experimental challenge. *J Vet Intern Med* 26:1121–1125, 2012.

29. Coyne KP, Christley RM, Pybus OG, et al: Large-scale spatial and temporal genetic diversity of feline calicivirus. *J Virol* 86:11356–11357, 2012.

30. Hurley KE, Pesavento PA, Pedersen NC, et al: An outbreak of virulent systemic feline calicivirus disease. *J Am Vet Med Assoc* 224:241–249, 2004.

31. Reynolds BS, Poulet H, Pingret JL, et al: A nosocomial outbreak of feline calicivirus associated virulent systemic disease in France. *J Feline Med Surg* 11:633–644, 2009.

32. Battilani M, Vaccari F, Carelle MS, et al: Virulent feline calicivirus disease in a shelter in Italy: a case description. *Res Vet Sci* 95:283–290, 2013.

33. Huang C, Hess J, Gill M, et al: A dual-strain feline calicivirus vaccine stimulates broader cross-neutralization antibodies than a single-strain vaccine and lessens clinical signs in vaccinated cats when challenged with a homologous feline calicivirus strain associated with virulent systemic disease. *J Feline Med Surg* 12:129–137, 2010.

34. Poulet H, Jas D, Lemeter C, et al: Efficacy of a bivalent inactivated non-adjuvanted feline calicivirus vaccine: relation between in vitro cross-neutralization and heterologous protection in vivo. *Vaccine* 26:3647–3654, 2008.

35. Greene CE, Levy JK: Immunoprophylaxis. In Greene CE, editor: *Infectious diseases of the dog and cat*, ed 4, St Louis, 2012, Elsevier, pp 1163–1206.

36. Griffin B: Feline care in the animal shelter. In Miller L, Zawistowski S, editors: *Shelter medicine for veterinarians and staff*, ed 2, Ames, IA, 2013, Wiley-Blackwell, pp 145–184.

37. Pu R, Coleman J, Coisman J, et al: Dual-subtype FIV vaccine (Fel-O-Vax FIV) protection against a heterologous subtype B FIV isolate. *J Feline Med Surg* 7:65–70, 2005.

38. Levy JK, Crawford PC, Slater MR: Effect of vaccination against feline immunodeficiency virus on results of serologic testing in cats. *J Am Vet Med Assoc* 225:1558–1561, 2004.

39. Deboar DJ, Moriello KA: The immune response to *Microsporum canis* induced by a fungal cell wall vaccine. *Vet Dermatol* 5:47–55, 1994.

40. Deboar DJ, Moriello KA, Blum JL, et al: Safety and immunologic effects after inoculation of inactivated and combined live-inactivated dermatophytosis vaccines in cats. *Am J Vet Res* 63:1532–1537, 2002.

41. Gerber JD, Ingersoll JD, Gast AM, et al: Protection against feline infectious peritonitis by intranasal inoculation of a temperature-sensitive FIPV vaccine. *Vaccine* 8:536–542, 1990.

42. Fehr D, Holznagel E, Bolla S, et al: Placebo-controlled evaluation of a modified life virus vaccine against feline infectious peritonitis: safety and efficacy under field conditions. *Vaccine* 15:1101–1109, 1997.

43. Ford RB: 2012 Vaccines and vaccination: the facts and the fiction. In *Proceedings Florida Veterinary Medical Association 83rd Annual Conference*. <http://www.fvmace.org/FVMA_83rd_Annual_Conference/Proceedings/2012%20VACCINES%20&%20VACCINATION%20The%20FACTS%20vs%20The%20FICTION.html>, (Accessed June 3, 2015.)

44. How to determine a cat's or dog's age, *The Humane Society of the United States: Animal Sheltering*. <http://www.animalsheltering.org/resources/magazine/may_jun_1996/how_to_determine_age.html>, (Accessed June 3, 2015.)

45. DiGangi BA: Aging kittens. <https://vetmed-sacs.sites.medinfo.ufl.edu/files/2014/01/Aging-Kittens.pdf>, (Accessed June 3, 2015.)

46. Graves J, DiGangi BA, Levy JK: Assessment of body weight for age determination in kittens. In *Proceedings Maddie's Shelter Medicine Conference*, Orlando, FL, 2012.

47. DiGangi BA, Levy JK, Griffin B, et al: Effects of maternally-derived antibodies on serologic responses to vaccination in kittens. *J Feline Med Surg* 14:118–123, 2012.

48. Lappin MR: Feline panleukopenia virus, feline herpesvirus-1 and feline calicivirus antibody responses in seronegative specific pathogen-free kittens after parenteral administration of an inactivated FVRCP vaccine or a modified live FVRCP vaccine. *J Feline Med Surg* 14:161–164, 2012.

49. Lappin MR, Veir J, Hawley J: Feline panleukopenia virus, feline herpesvirus-1, and feline calicivirus antibody responses in seronegative specific pathogen-free cats after a single administration of two different modified live FVRCP vaccines. *J Feline Med Surg* 11:159–162, 2009.

50. Lappin MR, Jensen WA: Panleukopenia antibody responses following a single inoculation with one of five FVRCP vaccines. *J Vet Intern Med* 21:578, 2007. (Abstract).

51. Lappin MR, Sebring RW, Porter M, et al: Effects of a single dose of an intranasal feline herpesvirus 1, calicivirus, and panleukopenia vaccine on clinical signs and virus shedding after challenge with virulent feline herpesvirus 1. *J Feline Med Surg* 8:158–163, 2006.

52. Brun A, Chappuis G, Precausta P, et al: Immunisation against panleukopenia: early development of immunity. *Comp Immunol Microbiol Infect Dis* 1:335–339, 1979.

53. Cocker FM, Newby TJ, Gaskell RM, et al: Responses of cats to nasal vaccination with a live, modified feline herpesvirus type 1. *Res Vet Sci* 41:323–330, 1986.

54. Lappin MR, Andrews J, Simpson D, et al: Use of serologic tests to predict resistance to feline herpesvirus 1, feline calicivirus, and feline parvovirus infection in cats. *J Am Vet Med Assoc* 220:38–42, 2002.

55. Schultz RD: A commentary on parvovirus vaccination. *J Feline Med Surg* 11:163–164, 2009.

56. Heska Corporation: *HESKA feline UltraNasal FVRCP vaccine*, product insert, 2004.

57. Jas D, Aeberle C, Lacombe V, et al: Onset of immunity in kittens after vaccination with a non-adjuvanted vaccine against feline panleucopenia, feline calicivirus and feline herpesvirus. *Vet J* 182:86–93, 2008.

58. Medzhitov R, Janeway CA: Innate immunity: impact on the adaptive immune response. *Curr Opin Immunol* 9:4–9, 1997.

59. DiGangi BA: Proper handling and use of vaccines in animal shelters, *Maddie's Fund*. <http://www.maddiesfund.org/Maddies_Institute/Articles/Proper_Use_and_Handling_of_Vaccines_in_Animal_Shelters.html>, (Accessed June 3, 2015.)

60. Jakel V, Cussler K, Hanschmann KM, et al: Vaccination against feline panleukopenia: implications from a field study in kittens. *BMC Vet Res* 21:62, 2012.

61. Sharp NG, Davis BJ, Guy JS, et al: Hydranencephaly and cerebellar hypoplasia in two kittens attributed to intrauterine parvovirus infection. *J Comp Pathol* 121:39–53, 1999.

62. Hurley KF: Feline infectious disease control in shelters. *Vet Clin North Am Small Anim Pract* 35:21–37, 2005.

63. Kruse BD, Unterer S, Horlacher K, et al: Prognostic factors in cats with feline panleukopenia. *J Vet Intern Med* 24:1271–1276, 2010.

64. Cave TA, Thompson H, Reid SWJ, et al: Kitten mortality in the United Kingdom: a retrospective analysis of 274 histopathological examinations (1986 to 2000). *Vet Rec* 151:497–501, 2002.

65. Sykes JE, Anderson GA, Studdert VP, et al: Prevalence of feline Chlamydia psittaci and feline herpesvirus 1 in cats with upper respiratory tract disease. *J Vet Intern Med* 13:153–162, 1999.

66. Edwards DS, Coyne K, Dawson S, et al: Risk factors for time to diagnosis of feline upper respiratory tract disease in UK animal adoption shelters. *Prev Vet Med* 87:327–339, 2008.

67. O'Quin J: Outbreak management. In Miller L, Zawistowski S, editors: *Shelter medicine for veterinarians and staff*, ed 2, Ames, IA, 2013, Wiley-Blackwell, pp 349–367.

68. Larson LJ, Newbury S, Schultz RD: Canine and feline vaccinations and immunology. In Miller L, Hurley K, editors: *Infectious disease management in animal shelters*, Ames, IA, 2009, Wiley-Blackwell, pp 61–82.

69. Scott FW, Csiza CK, Gillespie JH: Maternally derived immunity to feline panleukopenia. *J Am Vet Med Assoc* 156:439–453, 1970.

70. Lappin MR, Jensen W, Andrews J: Prediction of resistance to panleukopenia, herpesvirus 1 and calicivirus utilizing serology. *J Vet Intern Med* 14:364, 2000. (Abstract).

71. Scott FW, Geissinger CM: Long-term immunity in cats vaccinated with an inactivated trivalent vaccine. *Am J Vet Res* 60:652–658, 1999.

72. DiGangi BA, Gray LK, Levy JK, et al: Detection of protective antibody titers against feline panleukopenia, feline herpesvirus-1, and feline calicivirus in shelter cats using a point-of-care ELISA. *J Feline Med Surg* 13:912–918, 2011.

73. Mende K, Stuetzer B, Truyen U, et al: Evaluation of an in-house dot enzyme-linked immunosorbent assay to detect antibodies against feline panleukopenia virus. *J Feline Med Surg* 4:2014.

74. Antman EM, Cohen M, Bernink PJ, et al: The TIMI risk score for unstable angina/non-ST elevation MI: A method for prognostication and therapeutic decision making. *JAMA* 284:835–842, 2000.

75. Mann CD, Neal CP, Metcalfe MS, et al: Clinical risk score predicts yield of staging laparoscopy in patients with colorectal liver metastases. *Br J Surg* 94:855–859, 2007.

76. Singh M, Gersh BJ, Li S, et al: Mayo Clinic risk score for percutaneous coronary intervention predicts in-hospital mortality in patients undergoing coronary artery bypass graft surgery. *Circulation* 117:356–362, 2008.

77. DiGangi BA: An evidence-based approach to the control of feline panleukopenia, feline herpesvirus-1, and feline calicivirus in shelter cats, *Master of Science thesis*, Gainesville, University of Florida, 2011. <http://ufdc.ufl.edu/UFE0042943/00001>, (Accessed October 5, 2014.)

78. Tuzio H: Feline panleukopenia. In Miller L, Hurley K, editors: *Infectious disease management in animal shelters*, Ames, IA, 2009, Wiley-Blackwell, pp 183–196.

79. Neuerer FF, Horlacher K, Truyen U, et al: Comparison of different in-house test systems to detect parvovirus in faeces of cats. *J Feline Med Surg* 10:247–251, 2008.

80. Abd-Eldaim M, Beall MJ, Kennedy MA: Detection of feline panleukopenia virus using a commercial ELISA for canine parvovirus. *Vet Ther* 10:E1–E6, 2009.

Foster Care Programs in Animal Shelters

Stephanie Janeczko

Foster care is an integral component of modern animal sheltering services. Some animal shelters use foster care programs as a means of protecting animal health and well-being while effectively extending their capacity for care and ultimately increasing the number of animals they can serve and save. Other organizations use foster care as a primary means of providing care for all of the animals they serve, negating the need for a physical facility to house animals. Instead, these foster-based organizations coordinate the placement of animals in networks of private homes that provide daily animal care and assist with permanent placement of animals in accordance with the organization's policies and procedures.

Foster care programs are especially crucial for cats. This is because the demand for sheltering services for cats far exceeds the available capacity in most communities in the United States. More than three million cats enter American and Canadian shelters each year, and many communities are experiencing an increase in feline admissions compared to dogs.[1-4] Indeed, feline intake is often twice that of dogs, especially in northeastern states and Canada.[4-9] These high admission rates can rapidly overwhelm an organization's capacity to provide humane care for cats. As a result, cats in animal shelters often experience high-density housing and inadequate husbandry and medical care. This not only compromises welfare but may ultimately reduce the odds of adoption. Foster care programs are an important tool for effectively addressing these challenges. When properly designed and implemented, these programs enable shelters to provide a higher level of care for a greater number of animals than would typically be possible if operations were limited to a physical facility.

In addition, foster care provides numerous benefits for the animals themselves as well as the organizations that implement these programs. By using a network of off-site housing locations, a shelter can provide better care for animals both in and out of the shelter. Animals placed in foster homes benefit from being housed in environments that are typically more appropriate for their behavioral needs and that have a lower risk of exposure to infectious diseases. Foster caregivers are often able to provide a greater level of individual animal attention and treatment than is possible in a busy shelter, increasing the feasibility and success of assessing, treating, and managing medical and behavioral conditions. Observations reported by the foster caregiver may provide a more accurate picture of a cat's health and/or behavior than could be expected in an adoptive home. These observations may

lead to a more informed assessment and help shelters to better plan for appropriate care and placement options for the cat.

At the same time, cats and kittens remaining in the shelter facility experience a less crowded environment and reduced exposure to infectious disease. If crowding is indeed reduced, staff and volunteers will be able to devote more time to each animal, resulting in better overall care and less stress for animals and staff alike. This can positively affect staff morale as well as the public's perception of the sheltering organization.

Because of the tremendous benefits associated with them, every organization that provides sheltering services for cats should consider developing a foster program. The first step is to establish specific goals for the program that will be influenced by the shelter's mission, admission policy, available resources, as well as the populations served (both human and animal). Common goals are listed in Box 71-1. These goals will guide what type(s) of foster care program(s) will be created. They will also shape the policies and protocols to help it operate in a way that is most likely to achieve those goals. Establishing specific goals may also determine what data and metrics need to be recorded in order to assess the program's effectiveness. Ultimately, the success or failure of a foster care program depends upon management and oversight practices, selection of cats, caregiver recruitment and training, and the development and implementation of cat care protocols.

TYPES OF PROGRAMS

There are several different types of foster care programs. All programs place animals in private homes for a period of time, but that may be the only thing they have in common. A description of several kinds of programs follows.

Traditional Foster Programs

Traditional foster programs focus on providing temporary housing and care for cats and kittens that cannot, or should not, remain in the shelter environment. The need for temporary housing outside of the shelter environment may be the result of individual characteristics of the cat (e.g., being too young for adoption) or having needs (e.g., illness, injury, or behavior problem) that can be better addressed in foster care. Foster care placement may also be sought for healthy cats and

BOX 71-1 Potential Goals of Foster Care Programs

Increase live release rate and lifesaving capacity

Reduce stress for cats

Minimize exposure to infectious diseases

Socialize young kittens

Enhance ability to assess and treat animals (for medical and/or behavioral problems)

Expand sheltering capacity

Prevent or alleviate overcrowding

Reduce shelter length of stay

Provide end-of-life hospice care

Improve staff and volunteer morale

Meet community expectations for animal care

Facilitate adoptions (e.g., foster-to-adopt programs)

Assist owners in transition

Prevent relinquishment/decrease shelter intake (e.g., during emergency or provide crisis care)

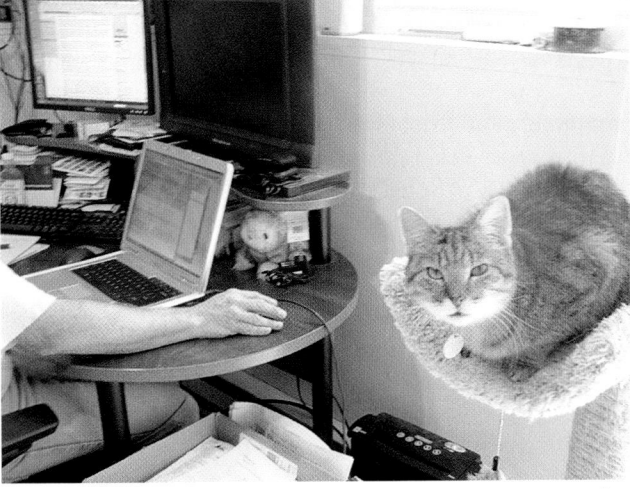

Figure 71-1: Foster programs may place cats in office settings rather than home environments. This alternate housing can be particularly beneficial for stressed cats or for long-term residents but must be balanced with the risk of infectious disease transmission. (Courtesy of Dr. Brenda Griffin.)

kittens based on the shelter's needs, such as a requirement to provide long-term housing for legal cases (when permitted in the jurisdiction), to alleviate crowding in busy summer months, or to have enough animals to send to a large adoption event. Cats and kittens placed in traditional programs are often relatively young, need placement for a relatively short period of time, and are considered to be good candidates for adoption following completion of foster care. These cats are typically healthy or have a minor ailment that is readily treatable. Although most programs place animals in a home with a foster caregiver, some include alternate housing, such as in a staff member's pet-friendly office at the shelter (Figure 71-1). Selection criteria for traditional foster care programs are discussed in detail in the following sections.

Special Treatment and Recovery Foster Programs

Some foster care programs focus on the treatment and recovery of animals with special needs requiring care beyond that typically provided by the shelter, which is often made possible through restricted donations. Animals entering these programs have treatable medical and/or behavioral problems that would generally preclude their placement in a traditional foster program. Because funding is typically limited, it is critical that all cases go through a selection process to ensure that the cats or kittens selected are good candidates for the program. Candidates should have a good long-term prognosis without significant underlying or ongoing medical and/or behavioral problems, be friendly and easy to handle, and be easily adopted following recovery. The financial cost, recovery time, overall prognosis, and need for any ongoing follow-up care must be evaluated when treatment options are being considered. Many organizations use the images and stories of animals cared for through these lifesaving programs to generate positive media coverage and fundraise for the care of future animals, creating a sustainable source of income to rehabilitate animals that would otherwise likely be euthanized. These programs are often maintained in parallel with a traditional foster program.

Foster-to-Adopt

The term *foster-to-adopt* typically refers to those programs that place cats into the care of a private individual temporarily, with the understanding and intention that ownership and responsibility of the animal will be transferred to that caregiver through adoption in the future. Generally adoption at the time of placement into foster care is not possible for one or more reasons. These may be legal (e.g., restrictions such as legal holding periods for stray cats or ongoing investigation of an animal abuse case) or the result of internal policies of the shelter (e.g., a requirement for spay/neuter before adoption). Many animals in foster-to-adopt placements are undergoing treatment (e.g., for an upper respiratory infection). Foster-to-adopt placement can reduce the length of stay in the shelter and provide an enriched, less stressful environment while securing an adoptive home for the cat until the restrictions are no longer applicable. The term *foster-to-adopt* is also used by some shelters that allow interested adopters to bring a cat into their home on a trial basis (often 30 days or less) before formalizing the commitment to adopt.

This term can also be used to describe specific programs (such as "Adoption Ambassadors") that permit and encourage foster caregivers or "Ambassadors" to find permanent adoptive homes for the animals in their care.[10] Animals placed into these programs are fully ready for adoption, having been evaluated medically and behaviorally, spayed or neutered, and received all necessary preventive healthcare. Foster caregivers are trained in advance on the shelter's policies and procedures regarding the adoption process, as well as on strategies for marketing the animals in their care. They are then empowered to find a new home for the animal, likely reaching potential adopters who would not otherwise go to an animal shelter to adopt a pet.[10] Because these animals are placed into foster homes "ready to adopt," the adoption process can be completed remotely, allowing a seamless transition from foster care to a permanent home and avoiding unnecessary delays at the shelter.

Foster-to-Surrender

Some shelters have incorporated "foster-to-surrender" programs to provide humane care and improve the chances of a successful live outcome for animals arriving at the shelter in a condition that would generally preclude adoption.[11,12] These programs vary widely among different organizations with regard to program size and eligibility criteria. They may provide care for either stray or owner-relinquished cats, but only as a means to improve their health and/or behavior so that they may be rehomed. Foster-to-surrender programs are not a mechanism by which free veterinary care is provided to pets that will ultimately be retained by their owners. Underage kittens and stray cats too ill for immediate adoption typically represent most of the cats placed into foster-to-surrender programs.

Individuals bringing a cat or cats to the shelter may be asked to keep the cat(s) until they are ready for adoption if the animal(s) meet the criteria for inclusion in the program. For example, a good Samaritan that brings a litter of 5-week-old kittens to the shelter would be asked if she or he is willing to care for the kittens for a few weeks until they are old enough to be made available for adoption. The individual becomes a foster volunteer for the animal shelter, providing necessary care for the cat(s) in his or her home. The shelter generally provides all needed supplies and any required veterinary care until the cat(s) can be made available for adoption. The request to temporarily foster animals that are presented to the shelter for relinquishment is often well-received by individuals, who become active participants in addressing the welfare of those animals. Foster-to-surrender programs improve feline health and welfare and can have an immediate positive impact on live release rates, because they find alternate placement—often at little cost to the shelter—for cats that would otherwise be at risk for euthanasia. These programs may also help create understanding in the community of the challenges faced by the shelter in caring for and attempting to rehome cats. Furthermore, it is not uncommon for the person surrendering or fostering to find placement for the cat(s) without returning them to the shelter.

Intake Prevention Foster Programs

Many organizations have proactive programs that provide support to pet owners in a community in order to help keep pets in their homes and prevent relinquishment to the shelter. Various types of support may be offered to qualified individuals and can include subsidized medical care or spay/neuter services, behavioral counseling and training, housing advice (e.g., landlord-tenant conflict), food banks, and temporary housing through boarding or foster care. This approach can be financially beneficial to the shelter because providing these services may be less costly than admitting, housing, and rehoming. In addition, feline health and welfare is improved by keeping the cat in its home, strengthening the human-animal bond, and providing support for owners in the community. Lastly, this approach reduces population density stress for already sheltered cats. At the same time, preventing the admission of this cat to the shelter is beneficial to the cats already at the shelter for the reasons previously discussed.

Intake prevention programs may be a part of an animal shelter's operations or may be run by separate organizations that partner with shelters and rescue groups to provide these services. These stand-alone organizations are typically established as nonprofit legal entities with a focus on providing temporary care for animals at risk of displacement due to a very specific set of circumstances, such as deployment of military personnel[13] or following significant natural disasters.[14] A variety of models have been used; some serving simply as a network or database to connect owners in need with volunteer foster homes in their community without any screening, monitoring, or support, whereas others are intimately involved in matching pets to prospective homes and provide ongoing support for animals and humans involved.

Emergency and Crisis Foster Programs

Another need met by foster care is temporary housing to assist during a personal emergency (e.g., domestic violence, military deployment) or following a disaster (e.g., house fire, flooding, wildfires, tornados, etc.). The goal is to return the cat to the owners once the crisis is resolved or has been controlled. Long-term stays in foster care may be necessary and, unfortunately, a proportion of these pet owners may be unable to make appropriate arrangements, necessitating relinquishment of the pet(s) to the organization.

Therefore, it is important that a written agreement exists between the shelter and the pet owner outlining the length of time care will be provided, how medical care will be provided and paid for, what options may exist for pet visitation, and a transfer of ownership of the pet to the shelter if the owner is unable to make alternate arrangements or fails to make contact with the shelter after the agreed upon time has passed. Strict confidentiality is critical when shelters provide such care for pet owners who have been victims of domestic violence.

Hospice Care

A few shelters may have a sufficient network of foster homes and adequate resources to place cats with foster caregivers for hospice care. Candidates include cats with serious medical problems that would be ineligible for adoption, or those with terminal conditions for which only palliative care is possible. Hospice placement is only an option if their condition may be managed in such a way as to preserve a good quality of life until euthanasia is warranted. These cats are likely to be elderly, stay for long periods, need a high level of ongoing treatment, and ultimately leave foster care via euthanasia rather than adoption. As a result, there is a need for a greater level of veterinary care and a more significant allocation of resources on a per-cat basis than that typically required for traditional foster programs. Highly skilled, emotionally grounded foster caregivers willing to provide long-term care, help assess of quality of life, and aid in deciding when humane euthanasia is appropriate are needed to make hospice foster programs feasible.

Foster Networks

Some sheltering organizations do not have animal housing facilities but rely instead entirely on foster homes for housing the animals in their care. This is a common model for rescue groups, including breed-specific organizations, those that focus on providing care for and rehoming special needs animals, and organizations that provide temporary housing for owned pets in need. The benefits of providing care and rehoming through a network of foster homes instead of at a central housing facility are increasingly recognized; some sheltering organizations have chosen to rely solely on this model even when building a central facility would have been possible.

Admission criteria differs among organizations, depending on their mission, available resources, and target populations. Significant variability may be seen among organizations that appear, on the surface, to be quite similar. As a result, it is difficult to provide a description of the cats most often cared for and rehomed through foster networks. In many cases, these cats will be similar to those placed in traditional programs (i.e., young and either healthy or easily treated cats that are good candidates for adoption). However, other programs may select cats with specific medical and/or behavioral problems, such as retrovirus-infected cats. As with other types of foster care programs, it is critical that clear selection criteria exist for the placement of cats into foster networks. Veterinarians working with these programs must be familiar with their goals and target population(s) so that they can provide effective advice.

SELECTION OF ANIMALS FOR FOSTER CARE

Most organizations have many more cats and kittens that would benefit from foster placement than they have available homes. A clear process by which eligibility for foster care is determined as well as thorough assessment and planning is necessary to maximize the productive use of this precious, limited resource. Selection criteria must be established that not only determine whether or not a cat may be a candidate, but also prioritize which cats to send to foster care when space needs to be rationed. The overarching goal of every animal welfare organization is to help as many animals as possible, thus efficient use of foster care is critical in achieving this goal. Considerations for cat selection are summarized in Box 71-2. These include the age, personality, and health of

---

BOX 71-2 Factors to Consider in Selection of Cats for Foster Care

Need for foster care
Availability of a suitable foster home
Skill set, training, and expertise of foster homes
Expected length of stay in foster care
Physical health findings
Behavioral health findings
Prognosis for recovery
Ability to provide adequate veterinary care
Cost to shelter (including supplies and staff time)
Likelihood of adoption at end of foster care
Risk of disease spread to other animals
Risk of zoonotic disease transmission

---

the individual cat; the makeup of the shelter population; resources necessary for the cat's care; the type of foster home required (including the skill set of the caregiver); the expected length of stay in foster care; and likely outcomes.

A staff person should begin with determining why foster care is necessary or highly desirable for a particular animal. Cats that are not thriving or that can be expected to do poorly in the shelter environment take a high priority for foster placement. All information regarding the cat's health and behavior should be reviewed, including all history available from previous owners. This information helps the staff member evaluate whether or not the cat is likely to maintain or improve its health in the shelter and if the organization has the ability to provide for that cat's needs (e.g., veterinary care) should it be placed in foster care. When sufficient resources are available to meet the cat's needs, a determination must also be made as to the prognosis for recovery. Risks to people and/or other animals, including the potential for transmission of infectious diseases to other animals and humans as well as the risk of environmental contamination, must be evaluated for both the shelter and any potential foster homes.

The likelihood of adoption once the cat or kitten is returned from foster care must be critically evaluated. The adoptability assessment for a particular cat will be very specific to the community in which the shelter is located and may vary with time of year. A unique breed or coat color, having been previously declawed, or young age (e.g., kittens) may be characteristics that are highly desirable within a particular community. Highly desirable cats are better candidates for placement when capacity in foster care is limited because they are more easily adopted, thus allowing a more efficient use of limited resources. This is especially true during times of the year when a large surplus of adoptable cats leads to increased competition for adoptive homes. That is not to say, however, that less adoptable cats will be ineligible for foster care; they may still be candidates during certain times of the year (e.g., quieter winter months with few kittens) or with creative marketing campaigns. However, it is important that the shelter balance the expected length of time a cat will wait for an adoptive home with the relative proportions of more easily adopted and more challenging-to-adopt cats in order to maximize the organization's lifesaving capacity.

The shelter should estimate how long the cat will need to remain in foster care. This is important not only in identifying a suitable foster home but also for planning purposes. Knowing the approximate date of return to the shelter for preadoption care (e.g., spay or neuter surgery) and/or adoption allows the organization to evaluate its capacity to provide services in a timely fashion and to humanely care for that cat. Foster placement will only be successful when a plan is in place for ultimate disposition and how to achieve this in a timely, humane fashion. When shelters fail to plan for the return of animals from foster care, the results can be disastrous if arrangements have not been made to ensure adequate staffing and sufficient housing or to allow for alternate models of placement (i.e., foster-to-adopt). With indiscriminate fostering, there is a significant risk that cats will linger for prolonged periods of time or that the organization may slip into warehousing of animals through its foster care program in order to alleviate an immediate capacity concern at the shelter.[15]

A determination must be made if a suitable foster home is available that can accept the cat(s). This requires careful matching of the animal's physical, behavioral, and environmental needs to the particular home and a caregiver with the necessary skills and training for the cat(s). For example, placing a large litter of neonatal orphan kittens with a novice foster caregiver is likely to have a poor outcome for all involved. Even if a foster caregiver with the necessary training and skills is available, consideration should be given as to whether or not placement of a particular cat in that home is the most appropriate decision in the context of the ongoing operations of the shelter. The highly experienced foster caregiver who takes an older, somewhat fractious cat with a chronic medical condition will not be available to take the litter of neonatal orphans requiring bottle feeding for several weeks. When continual intake of cats requiring foster care is likely to occur (such as with preweaning kittens arriving in the spring and summer months), shelters should consider these needs when prioritizing placement.

Algorithms can be very helpful to guide staff or volunteers in making consistent, judicious decisions regarding foster care placement (Figure 71-2). Common reasons for placement in traditional foster care programs are discussed in greater detail in the following sections.

Age-Related Reasons: Too Young for Adoption

Perhaps the most common reason for placement in a foster care program is that a kitten is too young to be considered for adoption. The age at which a kitten may be made available for adoption depends on the shelter's policies and any applicable laws, such as those requiring sterilization prior to

adoption. Even in states where legal restrictions do not exist, many shelters have a policy against the adoption of intact animals. If kittens are housed in the shelter until spay/neuter surgery can be performed or they reach a legally adoptable age (typically 6 to 8 weeks old), the population will rapidly exceed nearly any organization's capacity for care, particularly during seasons of high intake (such as spring and summer months).

There are also serious health and behavioral concerns that preclude holding young kittens in the shelter environment for any significant period of time. Shelters should work to develop procedures that allow for foster placement immediately or within 48 hours of arrival (Figure 71-3).[15-17] Orphaned neonates and underage kittens have substantial health and behavioral needs, including frequent feeding, monitoring, and socialization. Foster caregivers are generally better able to provide this care, particularly the daily handling and consistent positive interactions that are necessary for adequate socialization. Kittens in foster homes also have a greatly reduced risk of infectious disease, including upper respiratory infections and panleukopenia. When placed in a foster home following vaccination, they may be able to mount an adequate immune response before disease exposure occurs, particularly if they will be returned to the shelter at a later date.

Medical Reasons for Foster Care

A variety of medical conditions may be adequately managed in a foster care setting, including those for which treatment may be impossible or ill advised in the shelter environment (Figure 71-4). Some organizations will only place cats with these medical conditions in foster care if they can be fully cured, whereas others may consider foster placement for cats with chronic conditions that may be more easily managed in a less stressful environment and/or with a higher level of monitoring (e.g., diabetes mellitus). Cats may also be placed in foster care following surgery if they have specific recovery needs that cannot be provided in the shelter, such as ongoing physical therapy following orthopedic procedures. Postoperative foster care may also be beneficial for cats that will not be available for adoption until they have fully healed. See the Hospice Care section for a discussion of foster care for cats with serious and/or terminal medical conditions.

Animals with infectious diseases (e.g., upper respiratory infections or dermatophytosis) may be better treated in foster care, especially for organizations with insufficient isolation areas within the shelter. However, the decision to place infected cats in foster situations should be made only after careful consideration of the risks and benefits and with full disclosure to the caregiver.

Behavioral Reasons for Foster Care

Placement in foster care can be particularly helpful in evaluating a cat's behavior, reducing its stress, and providing treatment for any known or subsequently identified behavioral problems. Cats or kittens may be placed in foster care for a

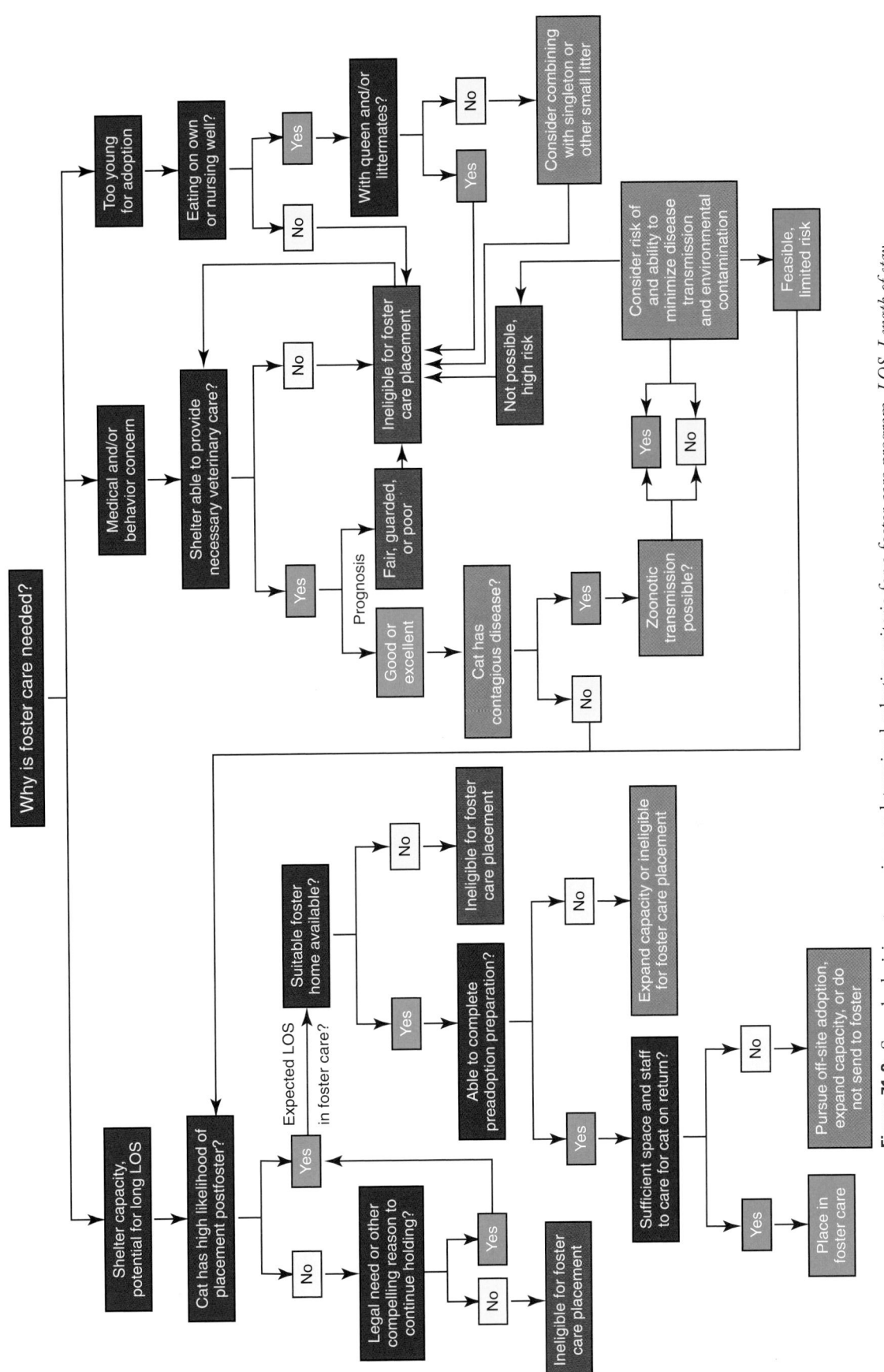

Figure 71-2: Sample decision tree using predetermined selection criteria for a foster care program. *LOS, Length of stay.*

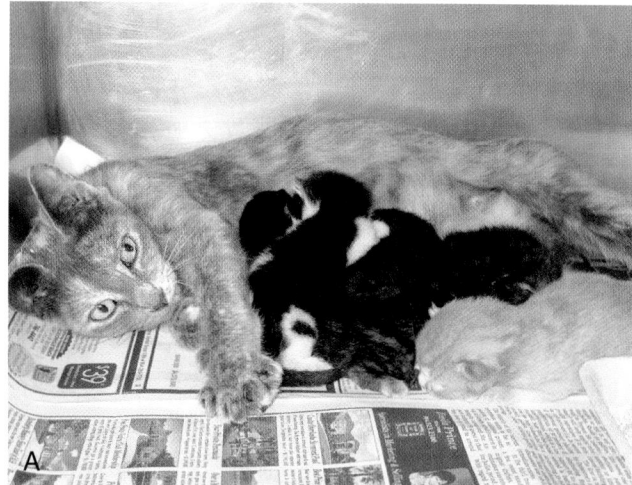

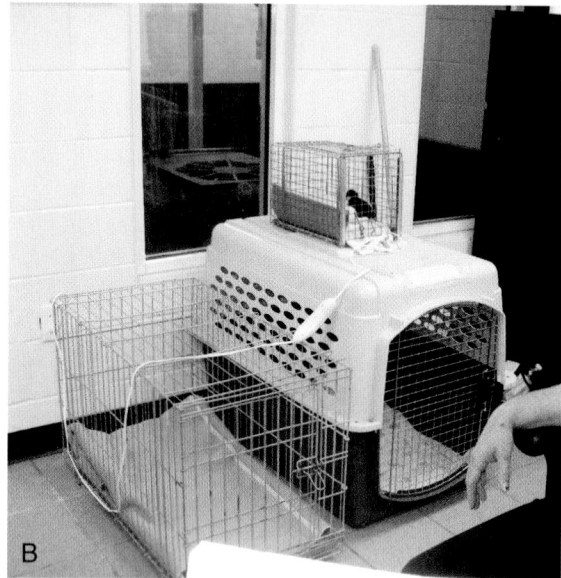

Figure 71-3: A, Neonatal kittens with a queen in a typical cage in an animal shelter. Housing young kittens in the shelter poses substantial challenges in protecting animal health and meeting behavioral needs. **B,** Temporary holding area for newly admitted preweaning kittens behind the shelter's admission desk. In this case, the shelter transferred kittens to foster care within 1 hour of arrival at the shelter, negating the need to house them in the shelter and substantially reducing the risk of disease exposure.

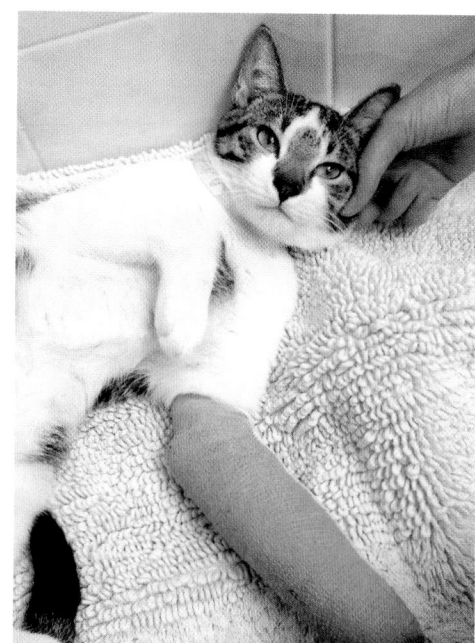

Figure 71-4: Shelters may be able to conservatively manage animals with traumatic injuries in foster care. This 7-month-old domestic shorthair cat was presented to the shelter with a mid-diaphyseal fracture of the left radius. Resources were not available for surgical repair of the fracture. Following appropriate immobilization of the limb and analgesia the cat was released to a foster caregiver and reexamined on a weekly basis until the fracture had fully healed. (Photo courtesy of Christina Trovato and Animal Care Centers of NYC.)

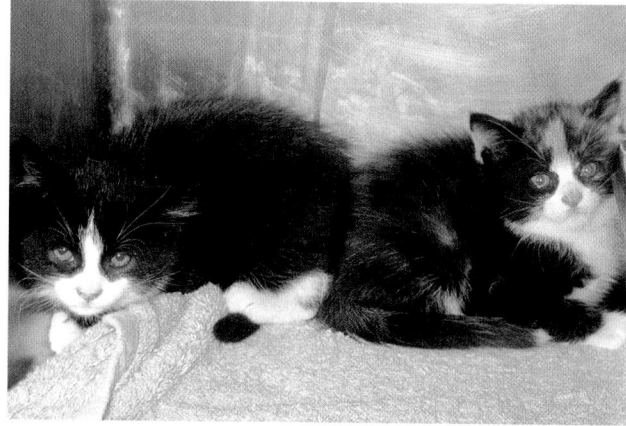

Figure 71-5: These kittens displayed fearful behavior whenever handled by staff at the shelter. Adequate socialization for kittens such as these can best be accomplished in foster care given the time-consuming and labor-intensive nature of the process.

number of reasons related to behavior, including the need to provide adequate socialization for young kittens, for observation in a less stressful, homelike setting, or for the assessment and management of a particular behavioral problem.

The placement of young kittens born to poorly socialized or feral queens is particularly important. Socializing or "taming" feral kittens is a time-consuming, labor-intensive process that can rarely be accomplished in the shelter environment (Figure 71-5). The critical socialization period for cats lasts from approximately 2 to 7 weeks of age; thus, there is often a very small window of time to provide the level of socialization to humans and environmental variety that will be necessary for these kittens to be successfully placed in a typical adoptive home.[18] Because the process of socializing older kittens (e.g., more than 8 weeks of age) takes consider-

ably longer and is likely to be less successful than efforts targeted at kittens still within their critical socialization period, many shelters limit foster care resources to younger kittens only.

Placement in foster care for behavioral observation can be tremendously valuable for some cats. Cats may show extreme fear or aggressive behavior when introduced to the unfamiliar shelter environment. Although many will acclimate over a period of several hours to several days, some cats may require 2 weeks or longer to fully adjust and show their normal or typical behaviors.[19] When cats fail to adapt over a relatively short time period, prolonged housing in the highly stressful shelter environment is inhumane and may be dangerous to staff and volunteers; alternate housing must be arranged.[17] In a less stressful, less threatening environment, many of these cats will show acceptable behaviors that make them suitable for placement in a home, thereby increasing their chances of adoption, particularly when direct adoption without return to the shelter is possible (Figure 71-6).

Insight into the cat's behavior, personality, and habits is valuable information that may be obtained from observations in a foster home, especially when a prior behavioral history is not available (e.g., stray cats). This information can be used in determining what type of placement would be the best match for a particular cat, as well as what support may be needed following adoption or transfer to another animal welfare organization.

Preventing Crowding

Foster care may be used as a means to provide additional capacity for cats and/or kittens when an organization does not want, or is unable, to house them in the shelter before they are adopted, transferred, or returned to an owner. In many communities, intake of adult cats remains relatively constant throughout the year, but intake of kittens increases

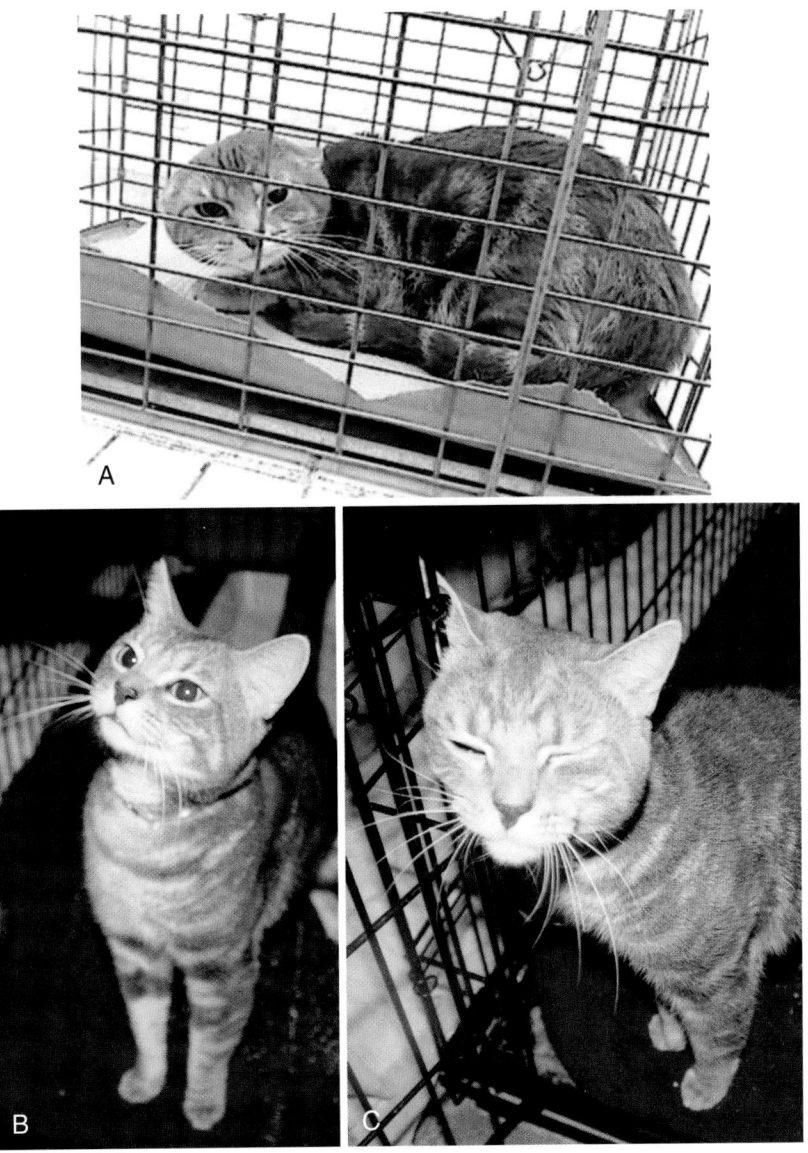

Figure 71-6: Some cats will remain profoundly stressed and continue to exhibit aggressive behaviors in the shelter setting. **A,** This photograph was taken of an adult intact male domestic shorthair cat at an animal shelter at the time of the intake examination. Very limited handling was possible due to the aggressive behaviors displayed at that time. Note the dilated pupils, flattened ears, and crouched body posture. **B** and **C,** The cat was placed in foster care for observation. After less than 48 hours in the lower-stress environment, the cat was much more relaxed, displaying affiliative behaviors and approaching the caregiver to solicit attention when the cage door was opened.

dramatically in the spring and summer months. Subsequent high-density housing and crowding increase the risk for inadequate housing, significant stress, and infectious disease outbreaks and may reduce chances for live release. A similar situation may also occur when an organization unexpectedly receives a large number of animals, such as from a hoarding case or following a disaster, that overwhelms capacity and risks displacing cats and kittens that otherwise would be shelter-housed and be made available for adoption.

Foster care may also be used to expand housing capacity for animals whose adoptability changes throughout the year. For example, many shelters see a higher rate and more rapid adoption of kittens than adult cats. In these cases, healthy adult cats can be expected to stay in the shelter for longer periods when many kittens are available. Rather than holding the adult cats for extended periods of time in the shelter, they may be placed in foster care—where they remain available and are promoted for adoption. When there is less competition (i.e., fewer kittens available), the cat may be returned to the shelter for adoption. This can provide the individual cat with enriched housing in a lower-stress environment than would otherwise be possible and helps reduce the population density in the shelter. This type of placement must be evaluated in the overall use of foster care to save as many lives as possible.

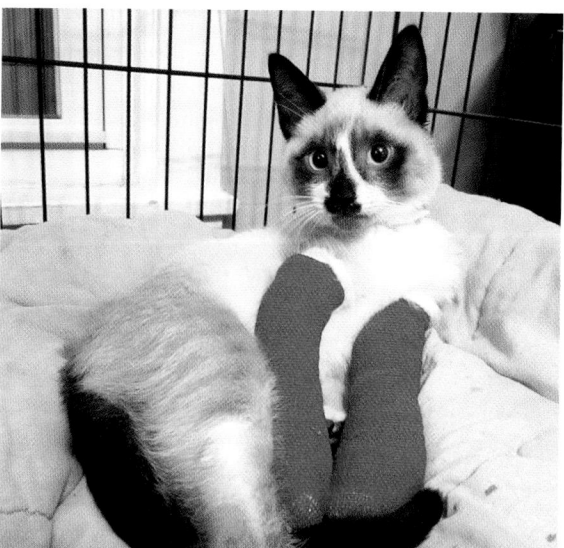

Figure 71-7: This kitten suffered bilateral radius and ulna fractures and a fractured hard palate following a fall from a seventh floor apartment window. After approximately 48 hours of intensive care, the kitten was discharged to a veterinarian who volunteered as a foster caregiver for the organization. This allowed the kitten to receive the necessary ongoing care for its injuries according to a management plan that was financially feasible for the shelter once hospitalization was no longer necessary.

MANAGEMENT AND OVERSIGHT

Although there are many benefits to well-run foster programs, poorly run programs can have disastrous effects on the animals, people, and organizations involved. When organizations fail to provide the necessary structure and oversight, systemic problems may result. These include, but are not limited to, inconsistent or inadequate animal care, unapproved adoptions occurring without an organization's knowledge or outside existing procedures, frequent loss or high turnover rates of volunteers, and increased financial costs arising from unanticipated or unapproved incidents (e.g., bills for private emergency care). A thorough risk assessment should be completed when the foster program is initiated and then reviewed periodically. All organizations must be aware of the applicable laws and regulations pertaining to animals in their care, develop policies and protocols that are in compliance, and ensure that foster caregivers adhere to these requirements. Careful attention must be given to caregiver recruitment, training, supervision, monitoring, and retention. See the available resources regarding management of volunteer programs in animal shelters;[20,21] a full discussion of this important topic exceeds the scope of this chapter.

Caregiver Recruitment and Retention

Volunteers are the foundation of most foster programs. Passive acceptance of volunteers who self-identify and seek out the opportunity to provide foster care for an animal shelter is common but rarely adequate to meet a program's needs. Ongoing active recruitment is generally necessary to meet the need for foster homes. Shelters may consider a variety of ways to recruit potential foster volunteers, such as through the organization's website, social media, local media outlets, mass emails, personal phone calls, distribution of promotional materials for the program, and personal referrals by other volunteers.

Shelters often choose to target groups or populations who may have a particular interest in fostering and/or have special skills or resources that would be especially useful in caring for some or all of the cats that are candidates for foster care (Figure 71-7). These may include professionals, such as veterinarians, veterinary technicians, or animal behaviorists. Some universities allow students to keep pets (most frequently cats) with them on campus, and at least two regional colleges have foster programs that specifically pair students with animals in need from the local community.[22] A few shelters have had great success placing cats in foster care through prison programs.[23] Senior citizens/retirees, families with small children, military homes, and members of the general public may all be considered as well. In some instances, an individual or family may be unable to make the long-term commitment to responsible pet ownership but is able to provide temporary care for a foster animal. Virtually any appropriately screened individual can foster cats for an animal shelter if they are provided with the requisite training, mentorship, and resources and are matched with appropriate cats and/or kittens.

Animals must be matched with an appropriate foster home—not just on the basis of the animal's physical, behavioral, and environmental needs, but also the skill set of the caregiver. Proactive, preplanned strategies for matching animals with foster caregivers are preferred, because they facilitate timely placement more efficiently and reduce unproductive waiting time in the shelter. This type of structured matching system is sometimes referred to as a *Foster On Deck* system.[24] One or more people, typically the foster program coordinator, maintains an active listing of all available foster caregivers by skill level and in order of when they would next be assigned a matching foster animal. Caregivers are notified when they are "next in line" for foster placement so that they can make the necessary preparations to be able to accept the animal(s) on the same day they are notified of a match.

Volunteer foster homes may also become temporarily or permanently unavailable due to changes in a caregiver's interests, capacity, or time constraints or environmental contamination with contagious pathogens. The risk of burnout and subsequent loss of a foster home is increased if caregivers do not take breaks, if their capacity for care is exceeded (i.e., crowding in the foster home), if they are matched with animals requiring care that is extensive or beyond their training and abilities, or if they have negative experiences with the animals or program personnel. Placing limits on the total amount of time and number of animals that can be fostered as well as instituting mandatory "rest periods" between foster animals may be beneficial. Volunteer recognition should be emphasized.

It is important to realize that even with proactive efforts aimed at retention, every program will face some level of caregiver attrition. This may result from a change in the volunteers' circumstances, whereby they no longer have sufficient time, financial resources, or space within their homes to continue fostering animals. One of the most common reasons for previous caregivers dropping out of a program is "foster failure." This term refers to the adoption of the foster animal by its caregiver. It is not surprising that people often choose to adopt an animal they have fostered because of the emotional bond that is forged and because they have experienced seeing that animal fit their lifestyle and home. However, not every caregiver who adopts their foster animal will leave the program, and many individuals continue to volunteer for the organization.

Training, Supervision, and Monitoring

It is crucial to have a staff member who is at least partially (and ideally, completely) dedicated to the oversight and administration of the program. This person is typically responsible for placement of animals and communication and coordination with approved caregivers, providing support, answering questions, and ensuring regular follow-up so that all necessary veterinary care is provided at appropriate times. The staff member is also responsible for scheduling and managing the return of foster animals to the shelter (or their adoption). This individual is typically responsible for monitoring caregivers and their adherence to shelter policies, as well as having oversight of the number of animals in foster care, average length of stay, and any health or behavior

problems. Ideally, he or she will also be involved in the recruitment, approval, and training of the volunteer caregivers.

Potential foster caregivers should be thoroughly screened before being accepted by the shelter as volunteers. Candidates are typically asked to complete a volunteer application and may be required to interview with the foster coordinator or other staff member to ascertain whether the individual and organization are a good match for one another. Following acceptance in the program, caregivers should undergo orientation and receive training before any animal is placed in their care. A foster care manual that has been developed in consultation with a veterinarian should be provided so that information on animal care, shelter policies, required forms and documentation, and emergency procedures are readily accessible. Contact information for relevant shelter personnel should also be included. Several examples of foster care manuals may be accessed online.[25-27]

Some shelters involve experienced foster caregivers in the training process for new volunteers and/or use them as mentors to provide support and advice to less experienced individuals. This can facilitate the management of a large foster care program with a small number of paid staff by effectively delegating less complicated or sensitive tasks (Figure 71-8).

The foster caregivers should be in regular communication with the organization whenever they have animals in their care. Prescheduling follow-up appointments for necessary preventive healthcare and continued monitoring of an animal's condition help to streamline the process and ensure that appointments are not forgotten. Caregivers should record observations regularly as discussed in the Care of Foster Cats During Placement section.

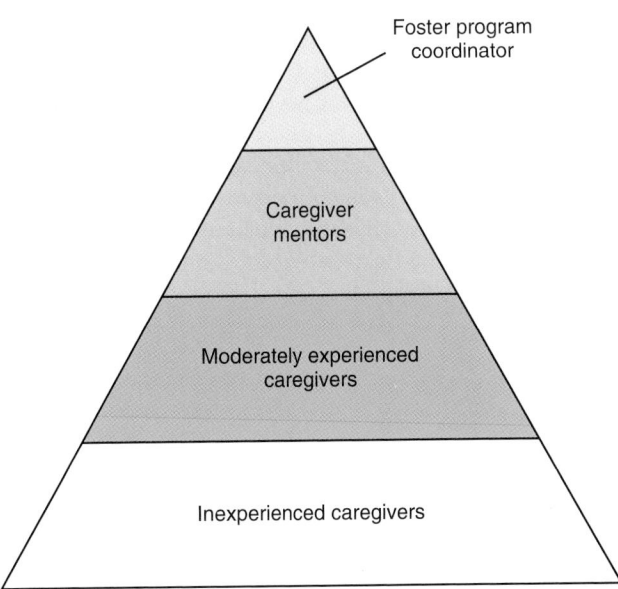

Figure 71-8: Example caregiver, mentor, and program hierarchy for foster care programs. Many shelters use experienced caregivers to provide training and support for those with less experience. In this example, inexperienced and moderately experienced caregivers would be assigned to a caregiver mentor, who in turn would be assigned to the foster program coordinator.

Open communication between staff and volunteers is critical not only for animal health and well-being but also for caregiver satisfaction with the program. Poor communication can easily create misunderstandings that may rapidly escalate and could ultimately result in loss of that foster caregiver from the program. Unmet expectations as to the level or extent of medical care that will be provided, the organization's responsibility to reimburse for medical bills or other ancillary care costs, and adoption and euthanasia decisions may all become potential problems if not agreed upon in advance. Written policies and protocols, appropriate training of caregivers, and ongoing communication with the foster coordinator can help address any problems to preserve and even strengthen the relationship.

Risk Assessment and Legal Considerations

Shelters must be aware of and adhere to all legal requirements pertaining to the placement of animals in foster homes. These vary by jurisdiction. For instance, there may be requirements for foster homes to be registered and/or inspected, and certain states require that each individual foster home be licensed as an affiliate of the shelter. Shelters must also be aware of all applicable laws that pertain to keeping pets in a home. Examples include pet limit laws that restrict the number of animals that may be present in a private citizen's home (but that often exclude preweaned animals), pet licensing laws, or mandatory spay/neuter requirements. Some jurisdictions have specific exemptions for animals in temporary custody of an individual through foster placement that may completely exclude the animal(s) from these legal requirements altogether or for a certain period of time.

Shelters that allow employees to foster animals in their homes must also be aware of the potential for labor law violations. In the United States, the federal Fair Labor Standards Act (FLSA) outlines various rights under the law, such as minimum wage and overtime pay. Under the FLSA, employees (unless exempt) must be paid for all time considered to be hours worked, including additional overtime pay if necessary. Although public and nonprofit employees may volunteer their services to an organization they work for, these services cannot be considered part of regular job duties and/or performed during working hours (even if the employee is thought to be "working off the clock").[28]

The Supreme Court has previously held that the FLSA must be applied to all employees regardless of their intent in performing the work due to concern that exempting volunteers could create a situation whereby employees who were truly working might be coerced into claiming that work was voluntary when it was not.[29] As a result, it is likely that the regular job activities of most shelter employees whose job descriptions include various aspects of animal care would be considered too similar to foster care activities to permit them to volunteer their time caring for animals in their homes as volunteers. Employers who permit such practices could be liable for unpaid overtime. Individual organizations should seek legal counsel to determine how such regulations

may impact them and what steps, if any, should be taken to reduce risk.

Irrespective of any legal requirements, animal shelters should have thorough written documentation for every foster home. This includes an application as well as a written agreement and/or contract that clearly outlines all expectations, rights, responsibilities, and limitations for the foster caregiver and the organization.[30] Sample forms are shown in Appendices A and B.

ANIMAL CARE IN FOSTER PROGRAMS

Environment and Home Considerations

One of the greatest benefits of foster care is the provision of a homelike environment. However, foster housing arrangements vary tremendously, depending on the health and behavior of the individual animals, reasons for foster placement, the presence of other animals (foster or owned), and available space with the foster home. Regardless, the environment provided for cats and kittens within the foster home must be conducive to maintaining physical and emotional health. Appropriate segregation should be maintained between pets in the home and foster animals for at least an initial period of time. In some instances, allowing contact between owned pets and foster animals in a controlled environment may be particularly desirable. For example, bold and friendly kittens may greatly benefit from early socialization with a well-behaved, cat-friendly dog in the home. When multiple animals are being fostered that have not otherwise been exposed to one another in the same household or enclosure at the shelter, separation should be maintained for an established period of time (typically 14 days) to minimize the risk of disease transmission by a cat incubating an infectious disease. If multiple animals will be allowed to comingle in a foster home, this should be planned in advance to mitigate risk. Species and prey-predator status (if applicable), age, health status, and behavior should also be considered when determining what degree and type of separation are most appropriate.[17]

The ideal housing setup within a foster home varies from animal to animal, and strict confinement may not be necessary in all instances. Increased biosecurity is important for cats with contagious disease, as well as for kittens if there is a risk of infectious disease exposure within the home. Well-vaccinated, clinically normal cats housed in foster care are at lower risk of becoming infected by or shedding infectious agents, particularly after a quarantine period, and can often be housed in an entire room or portion of the house. Cats likely to stay in foster long-term, hospice cases, and those placed through foster-to-adopt arrangements are often best served by being gradually integrated into the household.

Caregivers must be trained in methods (frequency, thoroughness) and materials used for appropriate sanitation. This is especially critical for foster homes that house young kittens or cats with contagious disease. The potential for contamination is increased when foster homes are crowded and/or

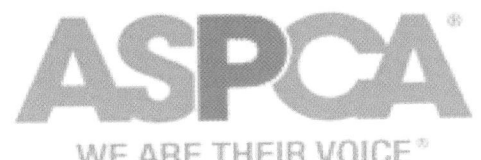

424 East 92nd Street
New York, New York 10128
212.876.7700

Cat Foster Care Application

Name:	Occupation:
Address: Apt #:	Employer: Phone:
City: State: Zip:	Address:
Phone:	City: State: Zip:
E-mail:	
Living Accommodations: Rent Own Other:	Does your lease allow pets? Yes No
Where will your foster animals stay?	Do you have screens on windows? Yes No
How many children at home?_____Ages?_____	
	Do you have transportation? Yes No
Do you currently have other pets? Yes No	How much time can you devote to foster care:
How many?_____ Breeds:_____	Do you: Work Go to school Are at home
Sexes:_____ Ages:_____	Is it: F/T P/T
Are they neutered/spayed? Yes No	What is your schedule/availability?
Name/address of current vet:	
	Have you had pets in the past? Yes No
	Dogs Cats
How do you keep them separated?	Where are they now?

What kind of Cat(s) or kitten(s) would you like to foster?

[ ] Injured Adult Cat   [ ] Ill Adult Cat   [ ] Injured Kitten(s)   [ ] Ill Kitten(s)   [ ] Mother with Kittens

[ ] Litter of Orphaned Kittens   [ ] Pregnant Cat   [ ] Adult Kitty Cat Camp   [ ] Shy Adult Cat   [ ] Shy Kitten(s)

[ ] Fospice Cat   [ ] Young Under Weight Kitten(s)

How did you hear about the Foster Care Program?	Does anyone in the household have allergies? Yes No
	If so how will you cope?
Why do you want to foster?	What pet supplies do you have?
When would you like to start?	Have you taken other foster care or training classes?

FOR OFFICE USE ONLY:

Recommendations: Date of Foster Class:

Appendix A

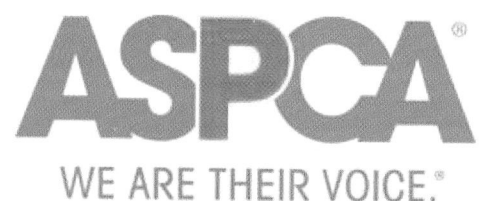

WE ARE THEIR VOICE.®

AMERICAN SOCIETY FOR THE PREVENTION OF CRUELTY TO ANIMALS

FOSTER CARE VOLUNTEER AGREEMENT

My signature below indicates that I have read, understand, and agree to the following:

1) Prior to the fostering of any ASPCA animal, I must have attended the initial Foster Orientation class and, if fostering a dog, I must also have attended the required Dog Foster class.

2) I have read and agree to abide by all applicable ASPCA policies and procedures.

3) I have offered my time and services to the ASPCA freely and voluntarily, and I understand that I will not receive any compensation for my volunteer work with the ASPCA.

4) I am a volunteer and not an employee, agent, independent contractor, or representative of the ASPCA and I shall not hold myself out as having any other relationship with the ASPCA, other than as a volunteer. This Foster Care Volunteer Agreement (the "Agreement") does not constitute a partnership, joint venture, agency, employee/employer, or any other similar relationship between me and the ASPCA.

5) I agree to be supervised by the ASPCA's Foster Care Staff, including Ben Li 'Gon or his designee, and will directly report to that person with any problems that arise.

6) I authorize the ASPCA to seek emergency medical treatment for me in case of accident, injury, or illness. If I am injured while acting as an unpaid member of the volunteer staff, I may be covered by the ASPCA's liability insurance.

7) I agree that the ASPCA may take photographs or video of me, or permit others to take photos or video of me, while I am volunteering for the ASPCA and that the ASPCA may use or authorize the use of the photographs or video of me in any way it deems appropriate to support its mission, including for fundraising purposes.

8) I understand that the ASPCA may discontinue my participation in the volunteer program at any time, with or without cause or notice, in its sole discretion, including if I fail to abide by the terms of this Agreement or am otherwise unable to meet the foster care program requirements.

9) No promises regarding volunteer work or any duration of service have been made to me and I understand that no such promise is binding on the ASPCA unless made by the ASPCA in writing.

10) I understand and agree that my volunteer position is contingent upon, among other things, my signing and agreeing to abide by this Agreement.

11) I agree that I may receive from the ASPCA the animal(s) listed in Exhibit A (the "Animal(s)") for foster care. I acknowledge that all foster placements are subject to the approval of and are at the sole discretion of ASPCA management.

12) I agree to provide the Animal(s) with good care, including, but not limited to, adequate food, water, shelter, grooming, training and medication when required. I agree to follow all additional oral and/or written instructions from the ASPCA and to comply with any training from foster care/volunteer or medical staff, if any. In addition, I agree to adhere to all federal, state and local animal laws, including but not limited to the New York City Anti-Tethering Law, if the Animal(s) will be kept within New York City.

13) I understand that as between me and the ASPCA, the Animal(s) shall remain the sole property of the ASPCA.

14) I agree that the Animal(s) shall be retuned immediately to the ASPCA (a) upon request by the ASPCA, (b) if I am no longer able to care for the Animal(s) adequately, or (c) if I am relocating outside of the New York City metropolitan area. In addition, I agree that should the Animal(s) require extensive veterinary medical treatment, the ASPCA may request immediate return of the Animal(s).

15) I agree to notify the ASPCA in the event any change occurs in my address or telephone number provided to the ASPCA below or as later provided to the ASPCA in writing.

16) Agents of the ASPCA will be allowed to inspect the premises in which the Animal(s) will be maintained or are maintained, from time to time, for the purpose of determining the suitability of those premises for the care and maintenance of the Animal(s). The premises must be kept in suitable condition for the Animal(s). I shall not cause or maintain any condition on the premises that presents any danger to the Animal(s).

Appendix B

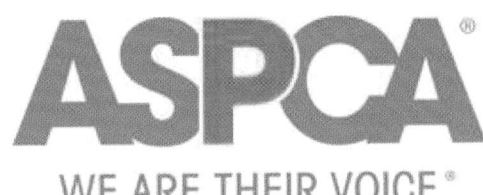

17) I agree to keep the Animal(s) indoors at all times unless the Animal(s) is securely on a leash. I agree that if I have other animals in my home, they will be kept up to date on all of their shots and vaccinations. I further agree that I will keep any other animals in my home separated from the Animal(s) that I will foster if requested by the ASPCA. If permitted by the ASPCA, introduction of the Animal to other animals in my home must take place only under my supervision. I agree that the ASPCA is not responsible if the Animal injures or otherwise harms any other animal.

18) I understand and acknowledge that I do not have any right or authority to keep the Animal(s) or to place the Animal(s) in other homes or place the Animal(s) with other individuals unless permission is given in writing in advance by the Senior Manager, Intake for the ASPCA.

19) The ASPCA has provided me with emergency contact information for certain ASPCA employees (the "Emergency Contacts"). If an Animal I am fostering requires emergency veterinary care, I agree to contact an Emergency Contact before seeking emergency veterinary care for an Animal. I agree to bring the Animal to the ASPCA Adoption Center or to the ASPCA Animal Hospital if instructed to do so by the Emergency Contact. In the event that the Animal(s) becomes ill during foster care, I will, at the request of the ASPCA, supply the ASPCA with any and all veterinary medical documentation from her/his veterinarian(s) that has been generated while I fostered the Animal. Notwithstanding the generality of the foregoing, I agree not to allow any veterinarian to provide any treatments that are not necessary or advisable for veterinary medical reasons. Specifically, I will not allow a veterinarian to alter in any way the appearance of any Animal, including declawing and/or cropping of ears or tails, or to devocalize any Animal.

20) I acknowledge and agree that the ASPCA may determine that an Animal has become so ill as to warrant humane euthanasia. Unless otherwise authorized by the ASCPA, only an ASPCA veterinarian may euthanize an Animal. I agree that I will <u>NOT</u> allow the Animal to be euthanized other than by the ASPCA unless otherwise authorized by the ASPCA and that determinations of euthanasia are in the sole discretion of the ASPCA.

21) I acknowledge receipt from the ASPCA of the Animal(s) described on Exhibit A on the date specified on Exhibit A and in accepting to foster the Animal(s) on my premises, I acknowledge and affirm my understanding that this Animal(s) has been deemed by the ASPCA as presently unsuitable for adoption for behavioral and/or medical reasons. I further acknowledge my understanding that such behavioral reasons may include, but not be limited to, the Animal(s)' propensity to bite, scratch, or otherwise attack individual(s). Such aggressive behavior may result in the Animal(s) biting, scratching, or otherwise physically attacking me, other animal(s) in my care or custody (if any), and/or any third party that encounters the Animal(s), including children, which may lead to these people or animals becoming cut, scratched, maimed, killed, or otherwise injured or harmed. In addition, the Animal(s) may destroy any physical property that may belong to me or to a third party. Any harm that I, my personnel, other animal(s) in my care or custody, and/or any third party that encounters the Animal may sustain, may be irreparable.

22) I hereby agree to release, indemnify and hold harmless the ASPCA, its officers, directors, employees, and agents from any and all claims, damages, and liability arising from or related to my activities as an ASPCA volunteer under this agreement or for any negligent act or omission by the ASPCA, its officers, directors, employees, and agents which cause, in whole or in part, any damages to me. In connection with my activities as an ASPCA volunteer, I further agree to release, hold harmless, and indemnify the ASPCA, its officers, directors, employees and agents, from any and all claims, damages and liability arising from my riding as a passenger in any motor vehicle owned or leased by the ASPCA and operated by an employee or authorized agent of the ASPCA.

I HAVE READ THIS AGREEMENT CAREFULLY AND FULLY UNDERSTAND ITS CONTENTS. I AM AWARE THAT THIS IS A WAIVER AND RELEASE OF LIABILITY AND INDEMNITY AGREEMENT, AND AN ENFORCEABLE CONTRACT BETWEEN ME AND THE ASPCA, AND I SIGN OF MY OWN FREE WILL.

Signature:	Date:
Print Name:	
Current Street Address:	
Current Telephone Number(s):	
Current Email Address(es):	

Appendix B, cont'd

maintain animals in unsanitary conditions. Contamination with environmentally resilient pathogens (such as feline parvovirus, dermatophytes, and various intestinal parasites) is of particular concern. Such contamination can lead to exposure of other animals or people in the home and may result in loss of that foster home for a period of time. Environmental decontamination may be especially challenging, because homes are seldom designed with sturdy, nonporous materials that can be adequately cleaned and disinfected or that caregivers are willing to dispose of and replace (e.g., furniture, carpeting). For this reason, prevention of environmental contamination is critical, particularly in the first 2 weeks following placement in a foster home.

Regardless of whether the primary enclosure is a crate, kennel, or an entire room (e.g., spare bathroom), it should be readily cleaned and disinfected. Regular hygiene to maintain a sanitary and pleasant environment cannot be overemphasized, including regular cleaning of litter boxes and food and water bowls. Cats should be provided with an environment that allows for and encourages a natural repertoire of feline behaviors. This includes having comfortable bedding, vertical space to allow for climbing and perching on elevated surfaces, a place to hide, toys to hunt, materials to scratch, and opportunities for exploration and exercise (Figure 71-9). An enriched environment that provides the cat with choice and variety is critical in meeting behavioral needs.[17] At a minimum, any enclosure should be of sufficient size to permit adequate separation of functional spaces, as well as to give the cat the ability to make normal postural adjustments. At least 2 feet of triangulated space between the litter box, bedding, and food and water bowls should be provided.[17] Foster caregivers should be careful to thoroughly assess the environment that the cat(s) will have access to in order to ensure that obvious hazards are not present, such as poisonous household plants, toxic substances, or small spaces where the cat could become trapped or hide. The area should be warm and quiet with sufficient ventilation. Fresh air and daylight are ideal when possible (Figure 71-10). Foster caregivers must be prepared to provide every cat with positive social interactions on a daily basis.

Care of Foster Cats Before Placement

A complete medical and behavioral assessment should be performed prior to placement in foster care. This is necessary to determine whether the animal is a good candidate for the program, to determine if the organization has the ability to provide for medical and behavioral needs, and to appropriately match candidate animals with available foster homes.

Shelters have an obligation to provide necessary care for animals in foster care, including treatment and monitoring of any medical or behavioral health problems. Placing an animal in foster care without a clear plan of how adequate veterinary care will be provided is inappropriate. For this reason, medical or behavioral conditions that require a moderate investment of resources may qualify an animal for placement in foster care at one shelter but disqualify that animal from foster placement at another shelter. See the Selection of Animals for Foster Care section for more information on determining a cat's eligibility for foster care.

Examination
A thorough physical examination should be performed, ideally by a veterinarian, of every cat prior to placement in foster care. Shelter staff can be trained to perform a basic

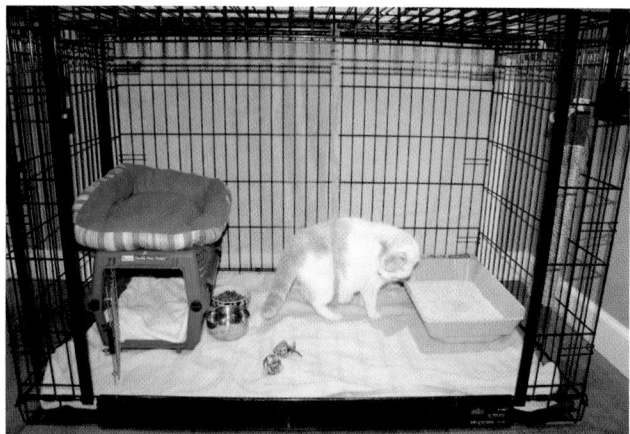

Figure 71-9: An appropriate primary enclosure suitable for temporary housing can be created for most cats and kittens using a dog crate. The cat carrier provides a place for the cat to hide, as well as to perch on top, and the soft bedding is secured to the top of the carrier with Velcro to prevent it from falling off. There is adequate separation of food and water bowls from the litter box, and the cage contains toys and a scratching post. This enclosure was located in a warm, quiet area not accessed by other animals in the household where the cat could be allowed out for exercise and exploration each day until confinement was no longer necessary. All items and materials shown in this set up can be cleaned and disinfected, laundered, or disposed. The crate in this photograph measures 49 inches (124.5 cm) long × 30 inches (76.2 cm) wide × 32 inches (81.3 cm) high and contains two doors; the large door on the long axis of the crate has been opened to more clearly show the layout.

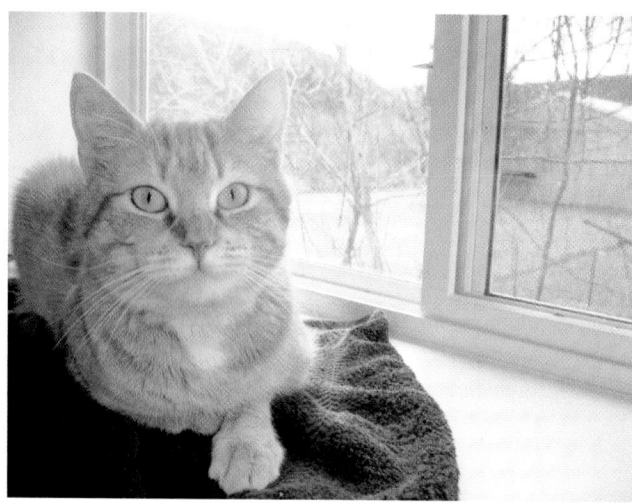

Figure 71-10: A window provides fresh air, natural light, and visual stimulation for a cat in foster care (Courtesy of Dr. Brian DiGangi.)

assessment of the animal's physical condition and to identify abnormalities that require further evaluation and/or treatment when veterinary examination is not feasible.[16,17] All cats and kittens should be carefully evaluated for signs of infectious disease, especially those common to a shelter environment (e.g., diarrhea, upper respiratory tract infections, dermatophytosis). Attempts should be made to estimate a cat's age as precisely as possible. Such information is particularly important for kittens in determining necessary medical and preventive care and what parameters should be monitored in the foster environment, as well as estimating how long the kitten(s) is/are likely to spend in foster care. Sex and reproductive status of the cat must also be determined, especially if cats will be placed in foster homes where they will be co-housed with other cats. Pregnancy detection in female cats of unknown reproductive status should be considered; this is critical if cats will not be spayed prior to placement in foster care and may be achieved through careful physical examination, hormonal assays, imaging, or some combination thereof. All findings, results of diagnostic testing, and all treatments should be recorded in the cat's medical record. This information should be provided to the foster caregiver.

When abnormalities are identified, veterinary advice should be sought regarding management, diagnostic testing, and treatment. A realistic assessment must be made as to the shelter's ability to provide adequate ongoing medical care for ill or injured cats and kittens, including repeated veterinary assessments and all necessary medications and supplies. If an organization is unable to ensure that sufficient care will be provided, placement of the animal(s) into foster care is inappropriate unless the caregiver is fully informed and is able and willing to provide for this veterinary care at their own expense. Placement of cats with signs of infectious disease in foster care should be carefully considered, particularly if the cat is infected with potentially zoonotic pathogens.

Behavioral Evaluation

Shelters should collect as much information regarding a cat's behavior from as many sources as possible. This includes any available behavioral history, observations of the cat's behavior by staff and volunteers in the shelter, and the results of a structured assessment (if one was performed).[17] Combining information provides the shelter with the most comprehensive picture of the cat's unique needs for housing, handling, and behavioral modification; this can be shared with the foster caregiver and used to develop a plan for behavioral care. These needs should also be considered in light of a realistic assessment of the shelter's resources, the suitability of available foster homes, and the likelihood of adoption before making a decision to place any particular animal in foster care.

It is important to recognize, however, that cats are often highly stressed in a shelter environment and may show fearful, withdrawn, or aggressive behaviors as a result. This behavior can be in stark contrast to what was reported by a previous owner and to the behavior the cat may exhibit in a homelike environment outside of the shelter. It has been

reported that defensively aggressive behavior seen in socialized pet cats housed in a boarding facility was rarely predictive of aggressive behavior in the home.[19] Because cats take a variable and possibly prolonged amount of time to acclimate and begin showing affiliative and social behavior, it is reasonable to provide information regarding the cat's behavior in the shelter to a foster caregiver as part of a larger discussion on ways to manage that animal's emotional state.

Vaccination

Vaccination at, or before, the time of intake to the shelter is a significant component of shelter preventive healthcare protocols and a standard of care in animal shelters.[16,17,31] Foster homes often fall into an intermediate category for disease exposure that is somewhere between the higher risk of a shelter setting and the lower risk experienced in a typical pet household. Just as no single protocol will be appropriate for all animal shelters in all situations, vaccination protocols should be developed by individual shelters, in consultation with a veterinarian, for animals placed in foster care. However, because caregivers may handle multiple foster animals concurrently or sequentially, it is generally most appropriate to vaccinate cats and kittens being placed into foster care according to the same protocol used for those animals that will remain in the shelter environment.

Parasite Control

Internal and external parasites are not uncommon in shelter cats and may cause a spectrum of clinical signs ranging from subclinical infections to serious disease. Because parasite eggs, larvae, or oocysts are often highly resilient within the environment, a foster home can become contaminated and ultimately require exclusion of part or all of that home from being used for other cats. Shelters could be held liable if a person contracts disease from a foster animal that was not treated by the shelter for common parasites with zoonotic potential (e.g., hookworms, roundworms). All cats and kittens 2 weeks of age and older should be treated with a broad-spectrum anthelmintic prior to release from the shelter into foster care. The author prefers to also administer an anticoccidial treatment, such as ponazuril (Marquis, Bayer Animal Health; 50 mg/kg orally once daily for 1 to 3 days,[32] repeated in 7 days if necessary) to all young kittens prior to placement in foster care to reduce the risk of environmental contamination.

Consideration must also be given to the treatment of common ectoparasites, particularly ear mites and fleas. Both are easily transmitted and can quickly contaminate an environment. A wide variety of ectoparasiticides are available for this purpose.[16,33-35]

Retrovirus Testing

Screening of all cats for feline leukemia virus and/or feline immunodeficiency virus at the time of intake to an animal shelter is considered optional but ideal.[16,36] However, all cats being placed in foster care should be routinely tested for both pathogens, particularly if the cat will be going to an environment where it may come into contact with other cats. Retrovirus screening prior to placement is also strongly recommended for cats being placed in households without other animals in order to identify cats requiring additional veterinary care, as well as those that may be poor candidates for treatment and/or placement in foster care due to their overall condition and prognosis. Retrovirus-positive cats, even when subclinically infected, are often difficult to adopt. As such, many shelters do not make these cats available for adoption or limit which infected cats may be made available for adoption based on their general health, behavior, appearance, or other considerations. For shelters that foster and adopt retrovirus-positive cats, knowledge of a cat's status is also an important consideration when determining appropriate placement of a particular cat or kitten into foster care. Infected cats should be placed as the sole animal in the home, in a home with similarly infected cats, or in a home that will be willing and able to ensure adequate separation between infected and uninfected cats.

Care of Foster Cats During Placement

Veterinary Care

Timely and appropriate veterinary care, including routine preventive care and examination, diagnosis, and treatment for any health problems existing at the time of or that arise subsequent to placement, is a requirement for all animals in foster programs. A plan should be in place regarding when, where, and how veterinary care will be provided for all known and anticipated healthcare needs; foster caregivers should be trained in, understand, and be provided with clear written documentation regarding this plan.

Policies and procedures should be created as to whether or not veterinary care can be arranged by caregivers independently, to what extent the organization will provide treatment for an animal with various conditions, and what the financial responsibilities of the shelter and caregiver are in such cases. Failure to develop these policies and to adequately communicate them with foster caregivers can diminish the success or even jeopardize the existence of a foster care program. Although shelters have an obligation to provide all necessary medical care to animals in foster care, it is common for organizations to establish policies that restrict where and/or what level of care may be obtained and at what cost without prior approval. Shelters with sufficient veterinary support that are able to provide all necessary care in-house often do not permit foster caregivers to seek private veterinary care and/or will not provide reimbursement for care provided outside the shelter. Other shelters may permit foster caregivers to arrange for veterinary care at specific facilities. If caregivers are permitted to seek private veterinary services, it is important that financial limitations are agreed upon in advance and that a process exists to obtain all necessary information regarding the care provided so that it can be added to the shelter's permanent record. A simple form can often be used to capture basic information, and copies of medical records can be requested as needed (see Appendix C).

Monitoring

Caregivers should monitor foster animals' general health and behavior. Regular assessment of appetite, water consumption, urination and defecation, energy level, behavior, and any clinical signs of illness should be recorded on a daily basis. The level of detail that is necessary for each individual animal depends, in part, on that animal's condition and reason for foster care. Neonatal and underage kittens must be weighed frequently on a kitchen/postage scale to ensure adequate growth and be assessed regularly to ensure that each kitten is meeting expected developmental milestones. Young kittens must be handled multiple times each day and be exposed to people, animals, and novel stimuli under safe and favorable circumstances during their critical socialization period to facilitate normal behavioral development.[18] Animals that have health or behavioral concerns and those recovering from surgery should be monitored and provided with all necessary treatments according to a standard protocol, if appropriate, or a specific plan tailored to the individual animal (e.g., what to monitor, how often, and what action to take) that is communicated verbally and in writing to the foster caregiver.

Caregivers should be provided with training and instructions as to what actions should be taken when abnormalities are noted, including whether or not reassessment by the shelter and/or emergency medical care is indicated. Written documentation of the animals' condition should be reviewed by shelter staff periodically, each time an animal is scheduled for routine preventive healthcare, and whenever abnormalities or concerns are noted by the foster caregiver. This information can be captured in a simple log kept for each animal or, preferably, through completion of standardized templates. This information is valuable in assessing an animal's condition, as well as for determining likely options for placement. All information provided by the foster caregiver should be added to the shelter's permanent medical record for that individual cat on a regular basis.

Emergency Care

Clear arrangements must be made for emergency veterinary care should the need arise. Emergencies may be more or less likely depending on the population of cats and kittens sent to foster care. Neonatal mortality rates can approach 30%,[37] and significant mortality may be seen in very young nursing kittens placed in foster care (particularly when orphaned). As such, a higher rate of emergency visits should be anticipated for this population; this should be explained in advance to foster caregivers.

Shelters should train foster volunteers, as well as staff, on the appropriate procedures to follow in the event of an emergency, including who (if anyone) to contact, where animals should be presented for veterinary attention, and any limitations on treatment and diagnostics that may exist. It is important to provide clear, written direction as to when euthanasia may be authorized in the event of an emergency and who can authorize it, especially if animals are sent to foster care while they are still within a legal holding period.

Private Veterinary Care Form

To be completed by the foster volunteer:

Caregiver name: _____

**Foster Animal
Name and ID#:** _____

**Veterinary Clinic Address
and Phone Number:** _____

_____

Date of exam: _____ **Reason for visit:** _____

To be completed by the veterinarian:

Exam findings, including current weight: _____

_____

_____

Diagnostic tests performed & results: _____

_____

Treatments administered/medications prescribed: _____

_____

Follow-up recommended: _____

_____

_____   _____

Name and license number: **Signature:**

Owned Pets of Foster Caregivers

The introduction and co-housing of foster animals and owned pets in a household can be highly beneficial for the foster animals but may result in physical and/or behavioral health problems in the owned pet that require veterinary attention and treatment. Shelters should take proactive measures to limit the likelihood of such problems arising as well as their potential liability should they occur. Prior to animal placement, caregivers should be informed of and receive thorough written policies and procedures clarifying expectations regarding each party's responsibilities in the event that an owner's pets become ill or injured. Serious consideration should be given to the risk of disease transmission when placing cats with known or suspected infectious diseases or a high likelihood of exposure to such pathogens.

Similarly, foster volunteers must be appropriately trained and provided with written documentation regarding potential risks and recommended biosecurity measures, including separation of foster animals from owned pets and sanitation procedures. General recommendations, including current vaccinations and regular preventive treatment for internal and external parasites, may be made by the shelter for pets owned by foster volunteers. Volunteers should be provided with information on the standard preventive medical protocols used for foster animals, a complete listing of any known medical problems or treatments prescribed for the specific animal(s) in their care, and information about any disease concerns in the larger shelter population. Shelters may consider requiring documentation of certain types of medical care as part of the application process and a prerequisite to placing foster animals in the home; such decisions should be made following a thorough risk assessment.

Veterinarians should be aware that pets seen in their practices may have direct or indirect contact with shelter animals if owners are volunteering as foster caregivers. This information is critical in determining potential exposure and disease risk. Fostering shelter cats has specifically been recognized as a practice that increases the risk of infectious disease in resident cats, but this risk is manageable and can be limited with appropriate precautions and veterinary care. Current guidelines recommend that veterinarians reassess risk factors for exposure at least once a year so that any necessary modifications in vaccination protocols can be made.[31] Knowledge of this potential source of exposure and the indirect impact of stress-induced immunosuppression is also necessary in formulating appropriate differential diagnoses and treatment plans for clinically ill patients.

OUTCOMES FOR FOSTER ANIMALS

Foster care programs are most effective when detailed outcome-oriented plans are in place.[15] This requires a holistic approach to the needs of each individual animal in foster care, as well as an overview of the entire program and shelter operations. Shelters need to ensure that sufficient resources are available and that ongoing veterinary care can be provided in a timely fashion without unduly prolonging an animal's length of stay in foster care, or worse yet, in the shelter upon return by the foster caregiver. Programs must be monitored carefully to ensure that the number of animals in foster care does not overwhelm the shelter's resources, including their ability to accept animals returning from foster care. This is particularly true for organizations that place large numbers of underage kittens in foster care until they are 8 weeks of age, because returns from foster care can increase intake by hundreds or even thousands of kittens during peak season.

With the exception of hospice cases, animals are usually placed in foster care with the intention that they will ultimately be adopted once the conditions that required foster care have been sufficiently resolved. Foster care represents an investment of time and resources for the shelter as well as for the foster caregiver, who often makes a significant emotional and sometimes financial commitment as well. Clarifying expectations regarding the extent of care that a shelter may be able to provide for an individual animal, as well as what criteria are used in determining an animal's eligibility for adoption or other placement, well in advance of an emotional situation is necessary to minimize the possibility for conflict. Caregivers often develop a strong bond with the animals in their care and may have high expectations regarding the level of care and commitment to adoption that should be provided by the shelter. All shelters should have a written protocol regarding euthanasia of animals in foster care, as well as those that have been returned from foster care. This information should be clearly communicated with foster volunteers during initial training and prior to placement of any animal(s) in their care. This will also help with the recruitment and retention of appropriate individuals who best match a specific shelter's program and help staff determine which cats or kittens are suitable candidates for a specific foster caregiver.

SUMMARY

Foster care programs play a critical role in improving animal welfare and increasing the lifesaving capacity of sheltering organizations. Many foster programs target animals that are at risk for poor welfare and/or euthanasia due to their young age, treatable diseases, or behavioral concerns that are not manageable in a traditional shelter environment but can be successfully addressed in the homelike setting provided through foster care. As a result, these programs enhance an organization's ability to provide appropriate care and treatment or to modify behavior. Adequate supervision, resources, and monitoring are necessary to ensure that programs run according to plan. Careful consideration must be given to the policies and procedures by which animals are selected for, placed into, and cared for in foster homes. An understanding of these increasingly popular programs is beneficial for all veterinarians, including those working in animal shelters as well as in private practice.

References

1. American Society for the Prevention of Cruelty to Animals (ASPCA): *Pet statistics, ASPCA: about us.* <http://www.aspca.org/about-us/faq/pet-statistics>. (Accessed June 3, 2015.)

2. Lord LK, Wittum TE, Ferketich AK, et al: Demographic trends for animal care and control agencies in Ohio from 1996 to 2004. *J Am Vet Med Assoc* 229:48–54, 2006.

3. Morris KN, Wolf JL, Gies DL: Trends in intake and outcome data for animal shelters in Colorado, 2000 to 2007. *J Am Vet Med Assoc* 238:329–336, 2011.

4. Canadian Federation of Humane Societies: *Cats in Canada: a comprehensive report on the cat overpopulation crisis.* <http://cfhs.ca/files/cfhs_catreport_english_1.pdf>. (Accessed June 3, 2015.)

5. Animal Care and Control Team Philly: *City of Philadelphia, animal care & control intakes.* <http://www.acctphilly.org/wp-content/uploads/2011/01/Animal-Care-and-Control-7-Year-Intakes1.pdf>. (Accessed June 3, 2015.)

6. Animal Care & Control of New York City: *intake and outcome totals of dogs.* <http://nycacc.org/pdfs/stats/2014/01Jan/intake-outcome-2014-dogs_v15.pdf>. (Accessed June 3, 2015.)

7. Animal Care & Control of New York City: *intake and outcome totals of cats.* <http://nycacc.org/pdfs/stats/2014/01Jan/intake-outcome-2014-cats-v15.pdf>. (Accessed June 3, 2015.)

8. New Jersey Department of Health and Senior Services Infectious and Zoonotic Disease Program: *2010 Animal intake and disposition survey.* <http://www.state.nj.us/health/cd/documents/animaldisp10.pdf>. (Accessed June 3, 2015.)

9. Weiss E, Patronek G, Slater M, et al: Community partnering as a tool for improving live release rate in animal shelters in the United States. *J Appl Anim Welf Sci* 16:221–238, 2013.

10. American Society for the Prevention of Cruelty to Animals (ASPCA): *Adoption ambassadors, ASPCA professional.* <http://www.aspcapro.org/ambassadors>. (Accessed June 3, 2015.)

11. American Society for the Prevention of Cruelty to Animals (ASPCA): *A foster-to-surrender program for puppies and kittens, ASPCA professional.* <http://www.aspcapro.org/resource/saving-lives-foster-care-safety-net/foster-surrender-program-puppies-and-kittens>. (Accessed June 3, 2015.)

12. American Society for the Prevention of Cruelty to Animals (ASPCA): *Foster to surrender: decreasing kitten euthanasia, ASPCA professional.* <http://www.aspcapro.org/webinar/2013-03-28-000000/foster-surrender-decreasing-kitten-euthanasia>. (Accessed June 3, 2015.)

13. Dogs on Deployment: *Welcome to dogs on deployment, dogs on deployment.* <http://www.dogsondeployment.org/index.php>. (Accessed June 3, 2015.)

14. Cammisa H: *Foster a sandy pet.* <http://fosterasandypet.ning.com/>. (Accessed June 3, 2015.)

15. Smith-Blackmore M, Newbury S: Foster care. In Miller L, Zawistowski S, editors: *Shelter medicine for veterinarians and staff,* ed 2, Ames, IA, 2013, Wiley-Blackwell, pp 495–516.

16. Griffin B: Feline care in the animal shelter. In Miller L, Zawistowski S, editors: *Shelter medicine for veterinarians and staff,* ed 2, Ames, IA, 2013, Wiley-Blackwell, pp 145–184.

17. Newbury S, Blinn MK, Bushby PA, et al: *Guidelines for standards of care in animal shelters, the association of shelter veterinarians.* <http://www.sheltervet.org/assets/docs/shelter-standards-oct2011-wforward.pdf>. (Accessed June 3, 2015.)

18. Radosta L: Feline behavioral development. In Peterson ME, Kutzler MA, editors: *Small animal pediatrics: the first 12 months of life,* ed 1, St Louis, MO, 2011, Elsevier/Saunders, pp 88–96.

19. Kessler MR, Turner DC: Stress and adaptations of cats *(Felis silvestris catus)* housed singly, in pairs and in groups in boarding catteries. *Anim Welf* 6:243–254, 1997.

20. McFarland B: *Volunteer management for animal care organizations,* ed 2, Washington DC, 2005, Humane Society Press.

21. Chesne B, Horn S: *Operational guide: volunteer management, american humane association.* <http://www.americanhumane.org/assets/pdfs/animals/operational-guides/op-guide-volunteermanagement.pdf>. (Accessed June 3, 2015.)

22. Nitopi S, Hake C: *Introducing a pet-friendly resident hall program at Penn State.* <http://www.personal.psu.edu/san5111/blogs/stephanie_nitopis_technical_writing/Recommendation%20Report.pdf>. (Accessed June 3, 2015.)

23. Peterson N: The power of purr: improving lives with prison-based cat fostering programs. *Animal Sheltering* 32–36, 2013.

24. Newbury S: The foster on deck system at the ARL of Boston. *Animal Sheltering* 24–26, 2011.

25. San Francisco Society for the Prevention of Cruelty to Animals: *Foster care program: foster kitten manual.* <https://www.sfspca.org/sites/default/files/sfspca_foster_kitten_manual.pdf>. (Accessed June 3, 2015.)

26. *Seattle animal shelter 2009 cat foster manual.* <http://aspcapro.org/sites/default/files/foster_cat_manual_seattle.pdf>. (Accessed June 3, 2015.)

27. Animal Care and Control Team (ACCT) powered by the PSPCA: *Cat foster care manual.* <http://www.animalsheltering.org/resources/sample/philadephia-spca-cat-foster-manual.pdf>. (Accessed June 3, 2015.)

28. United States Department of Labor: *elaws: Fair Labor Standards Act advisor: volunteers, United States Department of Labor.* <http://www.dol.gov/elaws/esa/flsa/docs/volunteers.asp>. (Accessed June 3, 2015.)

29. Dunn LE: "Protection" of volunteers under federal employment law: discouraging voluntarism. *Fordham Law Rev* 61:450–472, 1992.

30. McBride J: Legal issues for shelters. In Miller L, Zawistowski S, editors: *Shelter medicine for veterinarians and staff,* ed 2, Ames, IA, 2013, Wiley-Blackwell, pp 59–79.

31. Scherk MA, Ford RB, Gaskell RM, et al: 2013 AAFP feline vaccination advisory panel report. *J Feline Med Surg* 15:785–808, 2013.

32. Litster A, Nichols J, Hall K, et al: Use of ponazuril paste to treat coccidiosis in shelter-housed cats and dogs. *Vet Parasitol* 202:319–325, 2014.

33. Companion Animal Parasite Council (CAPC): *Current advice on parasite control: ectoparasites—fleas, CAPC.* <http://www.capcvet.org/capc-recommendations/fleas>. (Accessed June 3, 2015.)

34. Siak M, Burrows M: Flea control in cats: new concepts and the current armoury. *J Feline Med Surg* 15:31–40, 2013.

35. Beugnet F, Franc M: Insecticide and acaricide molecules and/or combinations to prevent pet infestation by ectoparasites. *Trends Parasitol* 28:267–279, 2012.

36. Levy JK, Crawford C, Harmann K, et al: 2008 American Association of Feline Practitioners' feline retrovirus management guidelines. *J Feline Med Surg* 10:300–316, 2008.

37. Root MV, Johnston OD, Olson PN: Estrous length, pregnancy rate, gestation and parturition lengths, litter size, and juvenile mortality in the domestic cat. *J Am Anim Hosp Assoc* 31:429–433, 1995.

Kitten Nurseries: A Practical Guide

Jennifer Broadhurst

With the arrival of spring each year, animal shelters know that they will soon face the overwhelming influx of kittens, many orphaned and under the age of 8 weeks. In the past, these young kittens were generally considered unadoptable because of the intensive amount of care needed to keep them nourished and healthy until they are old enough for adoption. Because these kittens would not survive without constant care, euthanasia was often considered the most viable and humane course of action, even in well-resourced animal shelters, including those with robust foster programs. This is because preweaning-age kittens require more time and resources than shelters can provide to properly care for them, particularly orphaned kittens under the age of 4 weeks, when round-the-clock care is necessary. In addition, several other factors confound successful care in the shelter setting. Young kittens are highly susceptible to infectious disease, particularly when orphaned and too young for vaccination. Kittens also need proper socialization to become appealing as pets. For the majority of shelters, the two items most needed to raise healthy kittens to adoption age, resources and time, are constantly in short supply. Yet despite these challenges, creative programs aimed at increasing live-release rates are emerging. One such innovative program is the development of kitten nurseries. A well-run nursery provides for the physical needs of the kittens, minimizes exposure to infectious diseases, and supports proper social and emotional development by providing opportunities for healthy social contact and play with both people and other kittens (Figure 72-1).

Shelter and other organization leaders associated with animal care must decide how great the need for a nursery is and how well it will serve the community. In communities where large numbers of kittens are euthanized annually and the sheltering agencies are looking for solutions, a kitten nursery may be a good fit. The establishment of such a program in one large city in the Southeastern United States resulted in the doubling of kitten adoptions and a nearly 75% reduction in euthanasia over a 2-year period (Box 72-1).

Kitten nurseries save lives, but they require planning, funding, good protocols, and a network of dedicated staff and volunteers to succeed. Creating a successful kitten nursery takes commitment and resources from the shelter, local affiliates, and community. Protocols governing care of kittens, cleanliness of the nursery, and methods of controlling infectious diseases are other critical elements. This chapter discusses the following keys to establishing a successful nursery:

- Planning the nursery
- Setting up the nursery
- Biosecurity
- Neonatal care
- Medical care and protocol development
- Training staff and volunteers
  Further resources are provided in Box 72-2.

PLANNING THE NURSERY

Before establishing a nursery program, many questions must be answered, such as the following:
- Where will the nursery be located?
- How long will it be open each year?
- How many kittens can be properly cared for at any given time?
- How prevalent are different infectious diseases in the area?
- Who will work in the nursery: permanent, temporary, or volunteer staff?
- What equipment is needed?
- Will the community support this project?
- How will it be funded?

Adequate time must be set aside to plan carefully for the nursery to optimize the chances for success.

The availability of physical space is one of the first determinations. A separate building with multiple small rooms is ideal. The primary reason for maintaining a separate facility is to prevent the spread of infectious diseases within such a vulnerable population. In addition, it allows volunteer staff to enter and leave the nursery without accessing the main shelter building. If a separate physical location is not an option, the ability to isolate the nursery from the main shelter is necessary. The chosen location will also affect the number of kittens housed and staff required, as well as the daily routines and medical protocols.

When considering space requirements, it is important to determine how the kittens will be grouped as they enter the nursery; the author's recommendations follow. Because few shelters have the resources to run a 24-hour kitten nursery, unweaned orphaned kittens may be cared for best in skilled foster homes. Therefore, the importance of planning for a strong foster care program to complement the available on-site nursery care cannot be overestimated. Ideally, qualified foster homes prepared to care for the unweaned orphaned

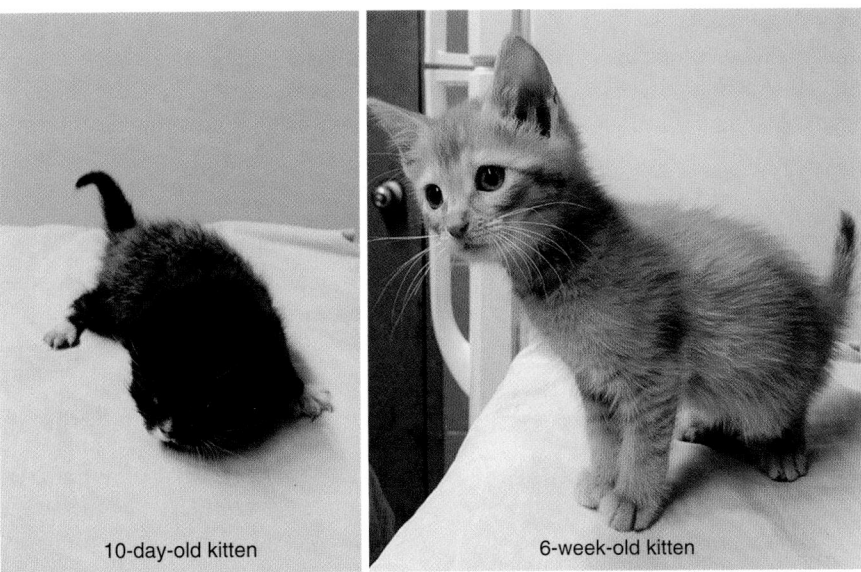

10-day-old kitten
6-week-old kitten

Figure 72-1: These kittens, less than 4 weeks apart in age, show major differences in physical abilities and awareness.

BOX 72-1 Kitten Nursery Case Study

The Jacksonville Humane Society (JHS), a private, limited-admission, no-kill facility, partnered with the City of Jacksonville's Animal Care and Protective Services and First Coast No More Homeless Pets, a private spay-neuter facility, to establish a kitten nursery at JHS in 2012. The first year, the nursery was open April to August and resulted in a modest increase in the intake of kittens under the age of 8 weeks (Figure 72-2). However, the learning curve for caring for these kittens and increasing their chances of survival, especially around the issues of controlling infectious diseases, was steep. The kitten mortality at the nursery in 2012 was 26% compared with 10% in 2011, when JHS exclusively used foster homes. During the time the nursery was closed from the end of August 2012 until reopening April 2013, protocols were revised based upon the experiences and observations of that first year. The result was increased kitten intake and adoptions and decreased death and euthanasia rates.

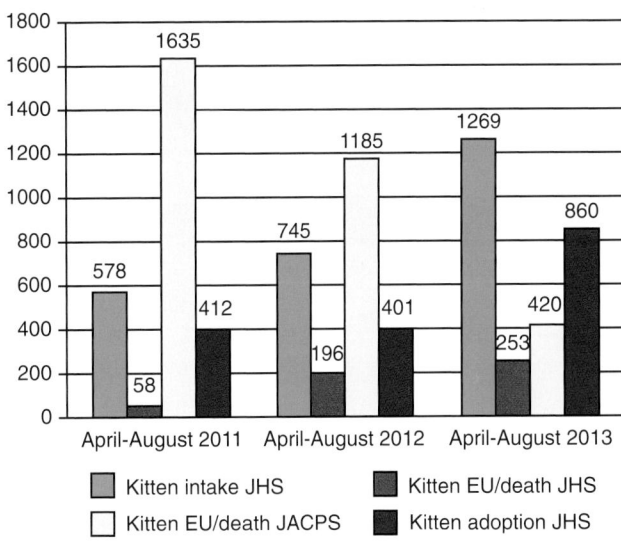

Kitten Population Dynamics

Figure 72-2: Jacksonville Humane Society Kitten Population Dynamics, 2011-2013. *EU,* Euthanasia; *JACPS,* Jacksonville Animal Care and Protective Services; *JHS,* Jacksonville Humane Society.

kittens and those not thriving in the nursery should be identified before the nursery is opened. For more information on foster homes, see Chapter 71.

When planning the nursery, shelter management should examine statistics from previous years for both kitten-intake and euthanasia rates to decide what time frame each year presents the greatest need. The time of the greatest influx of kittens will vary based on geographic location, but, typically, it lasts from February to late September in the Northern Hemisphere.[1] Some shelters may determine a nursery is required for 3 or 4 months each year; others for 6 months; and some year-round. Staffing requirements, necessary resources, and medical expenses will all be dependent upon how long the nursery is operational.

Staffing the nursery will involve most likely a combination of permanent and part-time personnel, seasonal help, and volunteers. At least one permanent, full-time staff member should be assigned to the nursery, but funding for additional staff hours during peak kitten-intake season should be identified. Kitten nurseries generally rely heavily on volunteer participation. Consistency and communication with nursery volunteers are necessary for success. It is essential that at least one staff member be present at all times to ensure facility consistency and adherence to procedures, and to relay important information to veterinary and management staff.

Participation and commitment are the foundations of a successful kitten nursery. The shelter management, governing board, and community must be dedicated to the establishment and longevity of the nursery. Management and board members must be willing to allocate the funding, staff, physical space, and equipment needed. They must be part of educating the community about the nursery, including its needs and its benefits. In addition, they must work to secure community partnerships, recruit volunteers, apply for grants, and host fundraising events. Fundraising efforts can help offset expenses and raise community awareness. The community itself also plays a critical role. In addition to being the source of volunteers and foster homes, it must support the nursery with donations and by adopting nursery graduates. Local rescue groups and city or county animal welfare organizations are good sources for community partnerships that may enhance or increase available resources. For example, such partnerships may provide joint staff and volunteers, increase the pool of available foster homes, or provide assistance with funding or fundraising. These partnerships also allow larger (e.g., citywide, countywide, or regional) adoption events, and partners may take kittens from the nursery program directly into their own adoption facilities.

The importance of planning cannot be overemphasized. Many questions will and should arise as planning advances; the more time spent planning, the better the chances are that the nursery will succeed in the long term.

SETTING UP THE NURSERY

By far, the most significant threat to all kittens is exposure to infectious disease; therefore, the primary focus of any nursery setup must be to minimize this threat, and as stated previously, the best practice for nursery design is to have multiple small rooms, which allow for isolation and quarantine. In addition to protecting the kittens against the spread of infectious disease, the nursery must also provide for physical and emotional needs and promote proper social development. The plan described in this chapter is based on a four-room model that houses kittens 4 weeks of age and older and those kittens of any age with a nursing mother.

Kittens residing in the nursery are divided into two groups: (1) nursing kittens under 4 weeks of age with a mother or surrogate and (2) kittens between 4 and 8 weeks of age that are eating on their own (see Figure 72-1). As previously mentioned, most shelters do not have the resources for around-the-clock nurseries. Instead, foster care is used to house kittens less than 4 weeks of age without a mother, as well as kittens that are not thriving in the nursery environment. The younger group of kittens (less than 4 weeks of age) is completely dependent upon the nursing mother and the care she provides. The second group comprising 4- to 8-week-old kittens has achieved some level of independence (i.e., they can eat and use a litter box on their own), but they are not quite ready for adoption. In some cases shelters may elect to sterilize and adopt out healthy kittens as early as 6 to 7 weeks of age. In other instances local animal ordinances restrict the adoption age. For example, adopting kittens younger than 8 weeks of age may not be permitted in some locales. The developmental characteristics of kittens by age are described in Table 72-1 (see also Box 72-2).

Kittens live in their assigned room for 2 to 4 weeks, and then "graduate" to the adoption area. This design allows for an "all in-all out" setup, whereby each week, newly admitted kittens are kept together in one room and essentially quarantined for at least 2 weeks before leaving that room. By using this four-room approach, a room is emptied and can be cleaned and disinfected before it is needed again for a week of new arrivals. This system facilitates infectious disease control greatly by reducing contact among new groups of kittens. When handled appropriately, kittens with mild illnesses (e.g., mild upper respiratory infection (URI), diarrhea, or ear mites) can be treated in their cage. In contrast, when kittens are moved from cage to cage or from ward to ward for reasons such as age or illness, the risk of a catastrophic disease outbreak increases greatly.

In addition to facilitating infectious disease control, grouping kittens by intake week helps to ensure that the nursery's capacity for care is not exceeded, because each room is equipped to house a predetermined number of kittens. Determining the appropriate number will depend on the available housing and staffing as well as the kitten adoption rates. There is no specifically recommended number of kittens per room or cage; the number is dependent on the size of the cages, the number of cages in the room, and how many kittens can be cared for properly in the nursery, which varies depending on the skill of the care-givers and resources of the organization. Regulating the number of kittens entering the nursery not only prevents staff and volunteers from becoming overwhelmed but also helps to ensure quality care, which in turn will improve kitten health and well-being. Common sense dictates that an overcrowded nursery must be avoided.

Table 72-1	Kitten Development 0 through 6 Weeks[3,4,7,21]		
Age	**Weight (g)**	**Body Temperature °F (°C)**	**Physical and Behavioral Milestones**
Birth-Week 1	90–110	96–98 (35.5–36.5)	Unable to thermoregulate; eyes and ears closed; purrs at day 2; responds to sound at day 5
Week 2	230–320	96–98 (35.5–36.5)	Eyes and ears open; increased strength and motor skills; may hiss at unfamiliar smells; explores environment; forms relationships with littermates
Week 3	300–425	99 (37)	Starting to thermoregulate; rudimentary walking; improved vision; deciduous incisors erupt; weaning begins; voluntary elimination may begin; litter box can be introduced; social play starts
Week 4	370–530	100.5 (38)	Improved thermoregulation; may start avoiding heat sources in the nest box; good hearing and vision; improving coordination; deciduous canine teeth erupt; weaning underway; beginning to interact with people and animals in environment
Week 5	440–635	100.5 (38)	Deciduous premolars erupt; weaning almost complete but nursing continues; can eat dry kitten food; running; playing; using the litter box; grooming
Week 6	510–740	100.5 (38)	Full control of elimination and litter box usage; eating solid food and may be teething; deciduous teeth still emerging; engaging in complex play with littermates and hiding behavior; able to cope with regular handling by people

For ease of management and operation, each room should be identically equipped and identified by a dominant color (e.g., blue room and green room). Recommended supplies and equipment for each room are shown in Table 72-2. Each room, as well as nonhousing areas such as workspaces, laundry, and storage, should be color coordinated by painting at least one wall of each room in its assigned color and using spray paint or colored tape to color-code supplies and equipment (Figure 72-3). Any item that might serve as a fomite (i.e., anything that can be moved) should be color-coded, including signage, food containers, litter containers, watering cans, trash cans, laundry baskets, brooms, dustpans, mops, and bottles of disinfectant. This system helps to control the spread of infectious disease by giving staff and volunteers a visual reference to make sure that everything that belongs in a room stays in that room. Educating staff and volunteers on the rationale behind the color-coding system is important for compliance and ultimately success. With this model, staffing will be needed for approximately 10 hours per day, 7 days per week.

In contrast to the model described herein, some shelters elect to design a nursery facility based on housing kittens according to age groups. In this case, there is often an increased risk of infectious disease, which results from the constant introduction of new kittens to a room. This type of arrangement focuses on meeting the physical and social needs of the different age groups (e.g., nursing moms with litters, unweaned orphaned kittens up to 4 weeks of age, and 4- to 8-week-old kittens transitioning to solid foods).

Shelters that consider housing kittens of less than 4 weeks of age must consider the expense of a 24-hour, 7-days-per-week operation because orphaned and unweaned neonates are a fragile population requiring continuous care, frequent examinations, and supervision. In addition, employees and volunteers trained in the care of neonates must be available and assigned to work exclusively with this age group.

BIOSECURITY

Even the healthiest, most resilient kittens can quickly succumb to infectious disease. Every action within the nursery (e.g., feeding, cleaning, and staff members entering and exiting the rooms) must be performed in such a manner as to minimize the risk of pathogen entry and spread.

Each room in the nursery should contain a bound or electronic copy of all husbandry protocols. Protocols should contain detailed systematic instructions on cleaning and disinfecting everything within the room. The order of task completion should be included along with details such as how to change bedding or measure out the proper amount of food. Explanations of why certain steps are performed, as well as how to perform them, will help improve compliance. For example, rolling up the edge of newspaper placed in the bottom of the cage will help prevent litter and other debris from being spread throughout the nursery, thus enhancing biosecurity and easing the cleaning burden. Without this

Table 72-2	Minimum Equipment Needs for a Kitten Nursery
Category	**Suggested Supplies and Equipment**
General	Protocol book (bound or electronic)
	Microwave
	Refrigerator
	Cat toys
	Digital pediatric scale
	Records binder with daily care cards
	Containers for food and litter
	Nonclumping litter
	Medical supplies
Housing	Double-sided enclosures
	Commercially available cat den (available through distributors such as Tomahawk Live Trap, Hazelhurst, Wisconsin, and ACES Animal Care, Boulder, Colorado)
	Blankets, towels, fleeces
	Disposable litter boxes
Feeding	Dry kitten food
	Canned kitten food
	Kitten milk replacer
	Small double-sided bowls
	Small bowls for canned food
	Spoons
	Bottles
Cleaning	Disinfectant
	Spray bottles
	Paper towels
	Gowns and gloves
	Alcohol gel hand sanitizer (60%-68% alcohol)
	Broom and dustpan
	Mop and bucket
	Trash can
	Trash bags
	Laundry basket

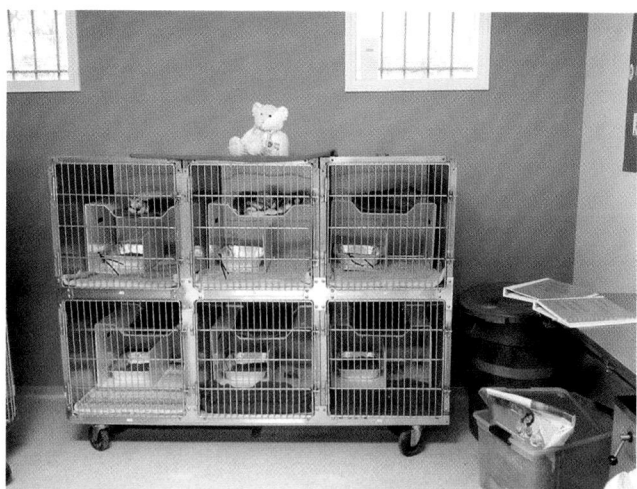

Figure 72-3: Color-coded rooms reduce opportunities for cross-contamination.

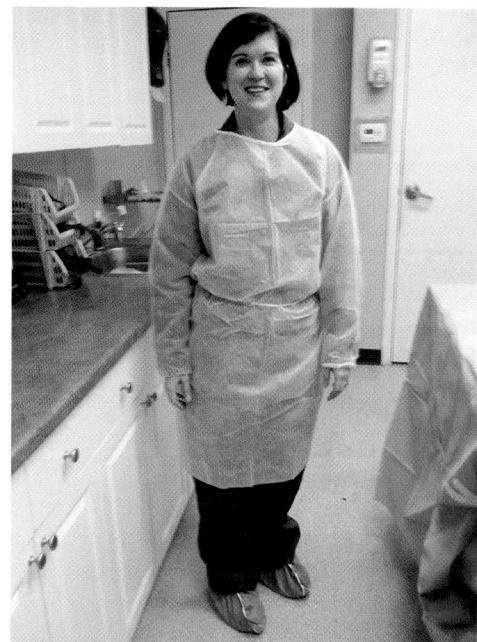

Figure 72-4: Personal protective equipment in the form of gowns, gloves, and booties are often needed to prevent the spread of infectious disease.

explanation, some staff members might not see the benefits of this extra step.

Personal Protective Equipment

Most commonly, personal protective equipment (PPE) in kitten nurseries is limited to the use of gowns and gloves (Figure 72-4). Typically, one reusable gown or smock is assigned to each cage in the nursery and is stored directly above or below the assigned cage. Reusable gowns should be laundered or discarded daily. Staff or volunteers wear the assigned gowns when cleaning, feeding, and socializing the kittens in that cage. Single-use disposable gowns are available but are often cost prohibitive. Similarly, single-use disposable

gloves should be worn when working within one cage and discarded when that work is complete. Staff and volunteers should be well trained in the indications for donning and discarding PPE. These practices may seem impractical for some nurseries, but allowing any contact among items in individual rooms invites the spread of infectious disease.

Establishing Order of Care

To minimize the risk of disease spread, a specific order of care should be established; cleaning and feeding should progress from the healthiest kittens to those with mild illnesses

Table 72-3	Example of Color-Coded Health Status Tags	
Color Tag	**Clinical Signs**
Red: currently undergoing treatment	Anorexia at last meal Weight loss Diarrhea Dehydration Listlessness Vomiting (more than one time) Bleeding Weakness Neurologic deficits
Yellow: medical evaluation required	Sneezing, wheezing, nasal discharge, and/or coughing Ocular discharge Mild lethargy or depression Unthrifty Lack of weight gain Loose stool Occasional vomiting Decreased appetite Difficulty urinating or defecating Limping Unusual behavior
Green	Apparently healthy

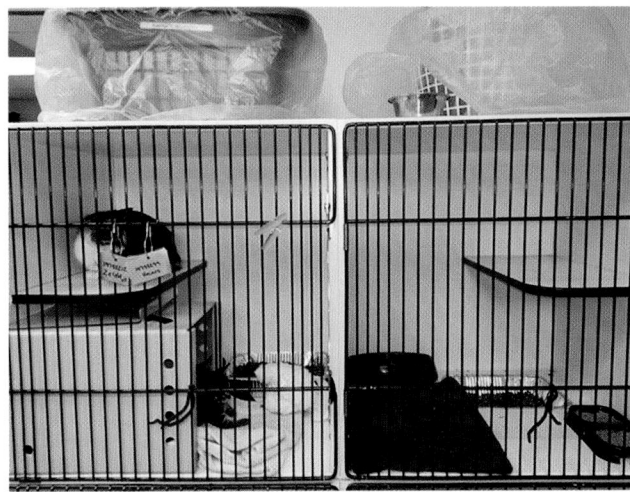

Figure 72-5: The green clothespin on the cage indicates the health status of the occupants.

and then to those more seriously ill. Color-coding of individual kittens and/or cages is a practical way of maintaining proper order of care by conveying the health status. For example, green tags indicate kittens that were healthy on intake; yellow tags indicate a need for medical evaluation; and red tags indicate kittens currently undergoing treatment for an illness (Table 72-3). Health-status coding is best accomplished with a visual signal, such as a laminated care card, clip, or clothespin (Figure 72-5).

Cleaning and Disinfection

Within the nursery, one of the most important allies in fighting potential pathogens is an effective disinfectant. Disinfectants considered for use should be researched for required concentration, contact time, efficacy against the pathogens of interest, and staff and animal safety. The feline respiratory tract is sensitive, but in the kitten, it is especially sensitive and easily irritated, so the disinfectant must be effective against the pathogens targeted but nonirritating and nontoxic. The author prefers accelerated hydrogen peroxide as the disinfectant of choice in kitten nurseries. At proper dilutions, products such as Accel (Virox Technologies) are effective against common pathogens of interest (e.g., calicivirus and panleukopenia) with a contact time of 1 to 5 minutes. They are also effective against dermatophytes with a 10-minute contact time.[2]

All cages undergo deep cleaning before housing any kittens and between housing different groups of kittens. Deep cleaning is also recommended whenever a cage is heavily soiled. Deep cleaning involves emptying the cage of all contents before cleaning and disinfection. Kittens that may be residing in the cage must be moved to a clean carrier until the cage is cleaned and the disinfectant has thoroughly dried. Nursery protocols should include descriptions of what cage contents to discard, what to clean or launder, and how to do so safely.

Spot cleaning of cages must be done daily. Spot cleaning involves performing light tasks, such as scooping the litter box while the kittens remain in the cage. Kittens housed in double-sided cages can be moved to one side while the other is being cleaned. Alternatively, a cat den or hiding box (Figure 72-6) can be used to contain the kittens in smaller cages during the spot cleaning process. As with any other task that involves interacting with the kittens or the cage, the staff member or volunteer must wear appropriate PPE for the task. Nursery protocols should dictate the specific tasks to be completed during spot cleaning; however, at a minimum, bowls should be cleaned if required, food and water refreshed, litter boxes scooped or emptied, and the bedding straightened or replaced if soiled. All bedding, toys, and newspapers may remain in place during spot cleaning if they are not soiled. The use of disposable litter boxes is recommended because of the difficulty of disinfecting plastic litter boxes effectively. Depending on the type of disposable litter box, they can be used for a few days by being scooped or emptied (if not soiled) before replacing.

General cleaning protocols should also be described, and instructions for cleaning transport carriers, food and water dishes, litter boxes, and dirty laundry should be included. Bottle-feeding equipment for orphans must be cleaned after each feeding. Each bottle and nipple must be washed with soapy water until all residues are gone, and disinfected according to manufacturer's instructions for proper dilution and contact time. Regardless of the product chosen, thorough

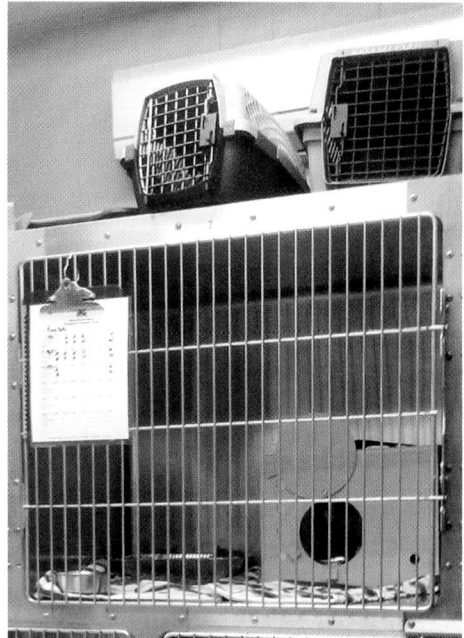

Figure 72-6: A feral cat den can be used to confine kittens during spot cleaning.

rinsing with freshwater and drying before use are highly recommended.

KITTEN CARE (BIRTH THROUGH 8 WEEKS)

In addition to protecting kittens from infectious diseases, other less obvious yet critical elements are required to ensure the successful rearing of kittens. These include preventing hypothermia, providing adequate nutrition, keeping kittens clean, and providing opportunities for socialization with other kittens and with humans. For litters of kittens with nursing mothers, care is much easier because most queens will provide warmth, nutrition, and regular grooming, while teaching the kittens important social skills. Nonetheless, the queens and kittens in the nursery still need to be provided with routine daily care and monitoring. A nursing queen that will accept a new litter when hers becomes weaned can also be used to assist with kitten care. This will not be successful with every queen, but some will accept a new litter. Queens that are indifferent to their current litter will not be the best candidates. Nursing queens that are attentive and taking care of their kittens until they are ready to wean are better candidates. The new kittens should be introduced as soon as the current litter is weaned. The new litter should be rubbed on the queen, her kittens if they are still available, or her bedding to give them a familiar scent. The kittens should be warm, as the foster queen may avoid hypothermic kittens. The foster queen can be gently persuaded to first lie with the new kittens and then to nurse them. The queen and kittens should be monitored for the first hour and then closely for the next 24 to 48 hours. If the queen hisses at the new kittens, tries to

get away, pushes the kittens away, or will not feed them, the kittens must be taken away for bottle-feeding.

Preventing Hypothermia

Because kittens cannot regulate their body temperature for the first 4 weeks of life, care must be taken to help maintain body warmth. Kittens need a steady environmental temperature of 86 to 90 °F (30 to 32 °C) for the first week of life. This temperature can be lowered gradually to 75 °F (24 °C) over the next 3 weeks.[3] When maintaining such temperatures in the nursery room is not possible or practical, a warm microclimate can be created within each cage through the use of a towel-covered heated disk (e.g., Snuggle Safe®, Lenric) or a rice-filled sock that has been warmed in a microwave. One area of the cage floor must be free from heating devices to allow kittens to self-regulate their temperature as much as possible by moving to cooler areas. Creating a nesting area out of rolled up fleece or a towel will also allow kittens to comingle comfortably for warmth. The nest area should be created in such a way that the kittens can crawl in and out of the nest at will.

External heat sources should be provided until kittens are 4 to 6 weeks of age. Even though kittens more than 4 weeks old may start avoiding the warmed bed, they will still seek out a warm spot when the room is cool. Finally, in addition to the social benefits, pairing up singleton kittens of similar age will help prevent hypothermia.

Ensuring Adequate Nutrition

Ensuring adequate nutrition is another key element in kitten care. Daily weight gain is an indication that the diet is meeting nutritional needs; ideally, kittens should be weighed at the same time each day. This practice ensures that weight is monitored, and it provides a means for calculating the amount of food needed at each feeding. Kittens should gain about 10 to 15 g (0.35 to 0.53 oz) per day and 50 to 100 g (1.8 to 3.5 oz) per week.[4] It is important to remember that the younger the kittens are, the more accustomed they are to ingesting small amounts at frequent intervals (i.e., through frequent nursing on the queen). This frequency of intake accommodates the small volume of a kitten's stomach and aids in digestion. If kittens need to be bottle-fed, milk replacer should be warmed to 101.5 °F (38.6 °C) to approximate maternal body temperature.[3] In general, kittens need to nurse from the queen or be fed milk replacer until 4 weeks of age, at which time they can start transitioning to gruel (i.e., canned food mixed with water or kitten milk replacer); by 6 weeks of age, kittens should be eating canned food, as well as dry kitten kibble.[5]

Kitten weight should be monitored daily to ensure that they are thriving. If a kitten does not gain weight within a 24-hour period, it should be fed more frequently and monitored more closely. If a kitten loses weight, it should receive a veterinary examination and be closely monitored to ensure that it is eating. For any kitten not thriving, consideration should be given to moving the kitten out of the nursery into a private foster home for more intensive care.

In addition to weight gain or loss, kittens should also be monitored for genital suckling. Genital suckling is common in orphaned kittens and can be a sign of inadequate nutrition or a need to suckle that is not being fulfilled (e.g., kittens fed via naso-esophageal tube). It can also cause permanent urethral damage to the kitten being suckled. Any kittens with this behavior should be separated, and urination should be monitored closely.

Keeping Kittens Clean

Maintaining a hygienic state is another element that is essential to the physical health of kittens. Orphaned, unweaned kittens should be wiped down with a damp, warm washcloth to simulate cleaning by the queen. This activity keeps the kitten's fur clean and provides socialization. For the older kittens, bathing will be a regular occurrence in the kitten nursery setting. Most weaning kittens are messy eaters. They will walk through their food, and this is another potential cause of hypothermia. Volunteers and staff must be trained to bathe kittens safely without risking hypothermia by using tepid water, making the procedure quick, and ensuring thorough drying. Towels and cage bedding should be prewarmed in the dryer for use after bathing. Use of protective equipment by staff, such as long sleeves and/or gloves, is recommended to minimize cat scratches and bites. Although alternative methods of handling may be preferred for adults, gently holding kittens up to 8 weeks of age by the scruff during the bathing process may help them relax and allow for easier handling.[6]

Socialization

Kittens should be well socialized for successful adoption. Kittens naturally socialize with their mother and littermates, but many orphaned kittens lose that critical interspecies socialization component of their development. Pairing single, similar-age kittens together may help them develop the social skills needed to be well-adjusted young cats. Kittens start to play and explore at about 4 weeks of age.[7] At this stage, toys should be provided for mental and physical stimulation. Pipe cleaners and cardboard rolls from toilet paper and paper towels are appropriate play items, in addition to safe commercial kitten toys, and such items are inexpensive and disposable, which makes their use feasible in the nursery setting. If the nursery cages do not have shelves to make extra room for play and napping, a commercially available cat den, kitten crib, or small platform bed can be added to the cage (Figure 72-7).

Kittens also need hands-on socialization time with humans, especially before 9 weeks of age. In the nursery setting, this activity is best done as in-cage socialization with nursery care-givers. Additional activities and interactions should be designed to support the behaviors and needs appropriate for each stage of development (Table 72-1).

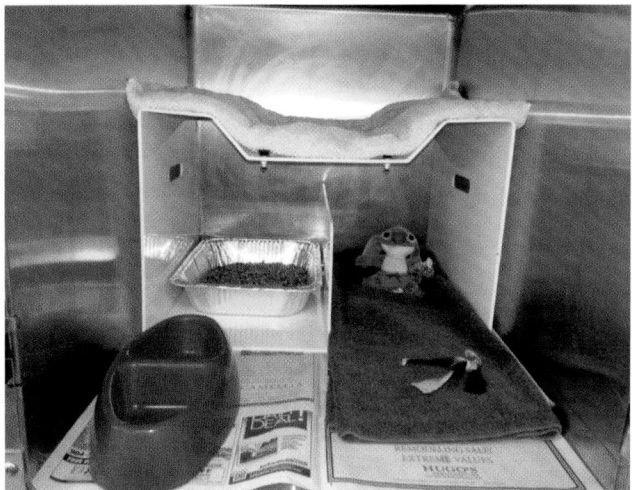

Figure 72-7: Adding an elevated bed or feral cat den lets kittens develop their play skills.

Staff and volunteers must be well trained in appropriate handling of cats and kittens.[8] Because the feline stress response is intimately linked to disease susceptibility, stress reduction is an essential component of daily care. The nursery should provide a predictable, nurturing environment, which is free of loud noises and aversive stimulation, and volunteers and staff should use gentle and quiet handling techniques.

Establishing a Daily Routine

A routine is extremely important for consistency of care, behavioral development, and stress reduction. Kittens should be on a regular feeding and cleaning schedule. This also helps ensure that staff and volunteers do not forget any of the daily care duties. Schedules should be posted in each room with space for staff and volunteers to check off each item as completed. Table 72-4 shows a sample daily schedule.

MEDICAL CARE AND PROTOCOL DEVELOPMENT

Young kittens are vulnerable to infectious disease because of their immature immune system and maternal antibody interference with vaccination.[9] Medical protocols should be developed by or with the help of an experienced shelter veterinarian. Protocols for kitten nurseries may vary based on the geographical location of the nursery, infectious diseases prevalent in that area, design of the nursery, and the ability of the shelter to isolate and treat highly contagious diseases. Protocols should also include provisions for animal care, including humane euthanasia if isolation and disease treatment are not possible.

Nursery intake protocols should include provisions for animal identification (ID), vaccination, internal and external parasite control, initial physical examination, and screening for infectious diseases. Intake staff should be trained to recognize and initiate treatment protocols for common medical conditions. Such conditions include flea infestation, fleabite

Table 72-4	**Sample Daily Care Schedule**
Shift	**Tasks**
8:00 AM to noon	Feed in all areas (complete by 10:00 AM)
	Stock supplies for the day (food, newspaper, bedding, litter, etc.) from the clean room
	Clean kennels, sweep, mop, and take out trash from kitten housing rooms
	Clean dishes, crates, and laundry
	Fill the sinks in the clean room with detergent solution, disinfectant, and fresh water
Noon to 4:00 PM	Weigh all kittens
	Clean kennels, sweep, mop, and take out trash from kitten housing rooms
	Clean dishes, crates, and laundry
	Take trash out to dumpster
	Socialize kittens
4:00 PM to 8:00 PM	Medicate in all areas (start after 6:00 PM)
	Refeed all areas (start after 6:00 PM)
	Sweep, mop, and take out trash in the kitchen, bathrooms, work room, and clean room
	Clean dishes, crates, and laundry
	Empty remaining formula, mush, etc.

anemia, ear mites, intestinal parasites, URI, conjunctivitis, diarrhea, and failure to thrive.

In addition to sound intake protocols, nursery staff and volunteers need to observe kitten health daily. This task should include monitoring of appetite, urination, defecation, signs of illness, and changes in body weight. Tracking the kittens' health and progress is most easily accomplished with individual monitoring sheets, which are kept in a binder in each room (Figure 72-8). Keeping individual monitoring sheets on the cage front may seem more practical, but soiling and destruction are common given the nursery population. To assist with ongoing health monitoring, each room should post a schedule for daily veterinary checks and the handling of any emergencies that arise. Record keeping in a kitten nursery presents unique challenges because of the high volume and frequency of medical needs (e.g., frequent examinations, vaccination boosters, deworming). For this reason, commercially available shelter-management software programs are recommended to ensure that critical care provisions are not missed. Such software makes it easy to keep medical records current and schedule reminders for care.

Intake Protocols

Intake protocols define the required steps for initial preventive health care and treatment. Intake staff, as well as nursery staff, must be trained to do a basic physical examination to identify any medical concerns. This is important for color-coding the kitten for cleaning order within each nursery room (see Establishing Order of Care), for identifying common illnesses such as URI and conjunctivitis, and for identifying any animals needing immediate veterinary attention. Kittens should receive a routine Wood's lamp screening as part of their intake exam to identify any suspected cases of ringworm immediately.[10]

Upon intake, all kittens under 4 weeks of age should receive routine deworming with the antiparasitic pyrantel pamoate and the antiprotozoal ponazuril (Box 72-3). If fleas are present, kittens need a quick bath with warm soapy water, taking care to prevent hypothermia. Fleas should then be manually removed.[11] Intake staff could be trained to estimate the age of incoming kittens based on the general guideline that they gain an average of 10 to 15 g/day (averaging 0.45 kg/month) and using the developmental guidelines shown in Table 72-1.[4]

All kittens 4 weeks of age or older and weighing at least 0.45 kg (1 lb) should receive routine deworming with pyrantel pamoate and ponazuril, a routine topical flea preventative treatment such as selamectin dosed by body weight,[11] and an initial vaccination with a modified live vaccine containing feline panleukopenia virus, feline herpesvirus type 1, and feline calicivirus. Booster vaccinations should be administered every 2 weeks until 16 to 20 weeks of age while the kitten is in the sheltering environment.[12] More information on vaccination protocols for shelter cats can be found in Chapter 70.

Some shelters may consider giving nitenpyram (Capstar, Novartis) if fleas are visible and the kitten meets minimum weight requirements. Praziquantel may also be administered if the kitten has tapeworms. Shelters should screen for feline retrovirus infection before combining unrelated kittens and ideally before adoption, although this is not an absolute necessity for individually housed kittens or individually housed litters of kittens.[13]

All cats and kittens entering the shelter, including those in the kitten nursery, should have a photograph taken on intake and individual ID established. This is essential for accuracy of medical records. For litters of kittens too small for ID bands or microchips, alternate ID methods include placing different colored dots or numbers in the pinna with a permanent marker. Each kitten should be assigned an individual ID number on intake. Cage cards help track the individual ID numbers and will be important for maintaining accurate medical records and tracking daily weight.[14]

Dermatophytosis

The number of dermatophytosis cases varies, often by season and by shelter location. An increase in prevalence of the disease usually coincides with "kitten season," and for shelters in areas such as the Southeastern United States, it is a constant challenge.[10] Regardless of the geographical location of a kitten nursery, young kittens often enter the shelter infected

Location _____

Name _____ Pet ID Number _____ Type of feeding: mush, wet & dry

	Sun		Mon		Tues		Wed		Thu		Fri		Sat	
	8 AM	4 PM	8 AM	4 PM	8 AM	4 PM	8 AM	4 PM	8 AM	4 PM	8 AM	4 PM	8 AM	4 PM
Medications/treatments— please initial when given														

Attitude—quiet or active

Water consumption +/−

Food consumption +/−

Feces +/− and normal Y or N

Urine +/−

Vomiting +/− and # times/day

Sneezing or eye discharge +/−

Weight in lb and oz	Sunday	Monday	Tuesday	Wednesday	Thursday	Friday	Saturday

Figure 72-8: Individual Monitoring Sheet.

BOX 72-3 Intake Treatments for Kittens*

4 weeks of age (kittens under 1 lb/0.45 kg)
  Pyrantel pamoate (10 mg/kg, by mouth [PO]), repeat in 2 weeks
  Ponazuril (20 mg/kg, PO), repeat in 2 weeks
4–8 weeks of age (kittens at least 1 lb/0.45 kg)
  Pyrantel pamoate (10 mg/kg, PO), repeat in 2 weeks
  Ponazuril (20 mg/kg, PO), repeat in 2 weeks
  Praziquantel if fleas present (according to product directions)
  First vaccination: Feline herpesvirus, feline calicivirus, and feline panleukopenia virus
  Selamectin (Revolution, Zoetis; according to product directions, for kittens 8 weeks of age and older)
8 weeks of age and older
  Pyrantel pamoate (10 mg/kg, PO), repeat in 2 weeks
  Ponazuril (20 mg/kg, PO), repeat in 2 weeks
  Praziquantel, if fleas are present (according to product directions)
  First vaccination: Feline herpesvirus, feline calicivirus, and feline panleukopenia virus
  Feline leukemia virus and feline immunodeficiency virus test
  Selamectin (Revolution, Zoetis; according to product directions, for kittens 8 weeks of age and older)
  Nitenpyram (Capstar, Novartis Animal Health; according to product directions) if visible fleas are present

*All cats and kittens receive a Wood's lamp screening with their initial intake exam.

---

with ringworm. Intake staff must be trained to carry out the next steps for any cats or kittens with a positive Wood's lamp examination at intake or those with clinical signs consistent with infection (e.g., focal areas of alopecia or crusts).

Staff handling ringworm suspects should wear a gown and gloves and take precautions to avoid contamination of surfaces such as an examination table. To avoid contamination of work surfaces, disposable drapes are a useful option, followed by disinfection with a product effective against dermatophyte spores such as accelerated hydrogen peroxide or diluted bleach (for more information, see Chapter 31). Confirmation of a diagnosis of ringworm requires direct microscopic examination of fluorescing hairs and a fungal culture.[10]

All shelters, particularly those with a kitten nursery, should develop formal, written protocols dealing with ringworm-infected cats in their care. These protocols must address diagnosis, isolation, treatment, cleaning protocols, and releasing the cats or kittens for adoption.

Feline Panleukopenia

Panleukopenia can be a devastating disease in a kitten nursery. Strict isolation of the kittens in the nursery and sound protocols help minimize the spread of panleukopenia, but even these steps will not completely prevent isolated cases from occurring in kittens exposed before admission and kittens asymptomatic on intake.

Panleukopenia diagnosis can be made using a fecal enzyme-linked immunosorbent assay test for canine parvovirus (e.g., SNAP Parvo Test, IDEXX Laboratories) and is suspected in patients with leukopenia.[15] Because sudden death can occur in kittens that appeared healthy the day before, any kitten found dead in its cage should be tested for panleukopenia. Sound written medical, vaccination, isolation, and cleaning protocols that address diagnosis, isolation, treatment, cleaning protocols, and the decision to euthanize help minimize the potential for spread of the disease. Staff and volunteers must understand the importance of adhering to the protocols. Infected kittens, as well as their cagemates, must be removed from the nursery and placed into a strict isolation area for treatment, transferred to a veterinary clinic for treatment, or humanely euthanized. The potentially exposed kittens in the room must be quarantined for 14 days.[15]

Common Illnesses

Many kittens will be admitted into the facility in poor body condition, heavily parasitized, and suffering from mild illnesses. Even though this chapter cannot cover all of the common ailments seen in kittens and recommended treatment options, it is important to mention that there should be nursery protocols in place for diagnosis, treatment, and prevention of the common illnesses seen in the local kitten population, such as flea infestation, fleabite anemia, ear mites, intestinal parasites, URI, and diarrhea.

No matter how good the nursery care is, some kittens in the nursery and in foster care will suffer from failure to thrive. These previously healthy kittens stop gaining weight and rapidly decompensate, often with hypothermia and hypoglycemia. The cause is not completely clear, but it has been linked to birth defects, environmental stresses, malnutrition, sepsis, and, of course, infectious diseases. Neonatal sepsis is particularly common in the first 3 weeks of life.[16] Some signs of sepsis include reluctance to nurse, weakness, vocalization, diarrhea, cyanosis, and cold extremities.[17] Kittens with sepsis may have decreased urine output, and they will need fluid and antibiotic therapy and may require oxygen therapy.[18] Given the limitations of many shelters, humane euthanasia may be chosen for a kitten with suspected sepsis.

The hypothermic kitten should be warmed up slowly over a 2- to 3-hour period, dehydration should be corrected, and antibiotics started if sepsis is suspected.[19] Kittens should not be fed until they are normothermic. The staff and volunteers should know who to contact in the case of an emergency and how to start treatment in the meantime. Even with intensive veterinary care, these kittens often do not survive because early identification of the underlying cause and intensive care are required.

TRAINING THE STAFF AND VOLUNTEERS

Abandoned kittens are often underweight, heavily parasitized, and suffering from untreated illness when admitted to

Table 72-5	Suggested Content for Kitten Care Handbooks
Chapter	**Suggested Content**
Kitten care	Maintaining warmth, feeding, urination and defecation, weight gain, physical and behavioral milestones, socialization, and bathing
Medical needs	Signs of illness, fecal monitoring guide, hydration assessment, common illnesses, intake protocols, vaccination protocols, and treatment protocols
Sanitation	Order of cleaning, daily cleaning protocols, spot cleaning, deep cleaning, end-of-day cleaning, laundry, toys, food and water dishes, and personal protective equipment
Daily routine	Schedule for feeding, cleaning, medicating, and socializing

an animal shelter, which makes their care in the nursery even more challenging. Only good protocols and practices strictly followed by everyone entering the nursery will afford these kittens the opportunity to flourish and survive. Therefore, all persons involved with the nursery will need some level of training.

Good training involves a variety of teaching techniques, including short seminars, guided tours, hands-on practice, and shadowing. Nursery staff members are often lay volunteers. These persons may have little knowledge or understanding of caring for young kittens. Training for both staff and volunteers should cover explanations of the practices and protocols as well as the reasons to promote compliance. Dedicating time to learning the protocols and practicing the basic steps described in a kitten care handbook (Table 72-5) is often a good use of seminar time. Depending upon individual roles, hands-on training might include learning to draw blood, performing fecal examination, appropriately dosing medications based on charts provided, administering medications, and making entries into medical records. In one form or another, training must cover every step and procedure for caring, cleaning, socializing, handling, and feeding kittens from the time of intake until adoption.

No matter how good and engaging the training program may be, trainees will not recall everything. If relying heavily on volunteers, one to two permanent staff members should be on each shift to supervise, ensure consistency, and relay important information to shelter decision makers. A detailed and thorough handbook is also essential (see Table 72-5). All those involved in the kitten nursery should receive (or have access to) the nursery protocols.

EFFECTIVE ADOPTION PROGRAMS

In the midst of developing protocols and intensive health monitoring, it is important not to lose sight of the end goal of the kitten nursery: all of these kittens need homes. Shelters with nurseries will need creativity for effective adoption programs. Kittens should be made available for adoption as soon as possible because they are often the most desirable to adopters when they are between 6 and 8 weeks of age. Because they should be spayed or neutered before adoption, the increased volume of kitten surgery requires planning, as well. Marketing the nursery and adoption program (e.g., calling kittens "graduates"), having creatively named adoption specials (e.g., Free Feline Fridays or Two Purr One), considering a fee-waived adoption program, and using adoption space at local pet supply stores are all successful tactics for many organizations. High-quality photographs, kitten biographies, and videos posted on the organization's website and social media outlets will help spread the word. Media partnerships with local television, radio stations, and newspapers often result in free publicity. Establishing partnerships with other community animal welfare organizations can often draw in more potential adopters, eliminate competition among agencies, strengthen community relationships, and pool operational funds.

SUMMARY

Kitten nurseries may not eliminate the enormous cat overpopulation problem, but they can succeed in making major reductions in kitten euthanasia in a community. It is important to note that despite a shelter's best efforts and well-established protocols, some kittens will be lost. Estimated kitten loss during the first 12 weeks of life is anywhere from 15% to 40%, from causes such as congenital anomalies, malnutrition, trauma, and infectious diseases.[20] Thoughtful facility design and careful protocol development can minimize such losses. For most shelters, there is a learning curve with starting a kitten nursery, and with increased kitten intake, particularly from multiple sources, there will be increased kitten loss. A well-managed nursery should strive for a 10% to 15% kitten-loss rate and should not have greater than 20% kitten loss.

A successful kitten nursery will require an investment in funds, time, staff, and community commitment, but can result in thousands of lives saved each year. Results have shown that instead of overburdening facilities with unadopted kittens, shelters with nurseries find rising adoption rates and improved morale. People want to adopt kittens. Shelter nursery programs can help.

References

1. Griffin B: Prolific cats: the estrous cycle. *Compendium* 23(12):1049–1057, 2001.
2. Moriello KA: Hondzo H: Efficacy of disinfectants containing accelerated hydrogen peroxide against conidial arthrospores and isolated infective species of *Microsporum canis* and *Trichophyton* sp. *Vet Dermatol* 25:191–194, e48, 2014.
3. Peterson M: Care of the orphaned puppy and kitten. In Peterson ME, Kutzler MA, editors: *Small animal pediatrics, the first 12 months of life*, St Louis, 2011, Elsevier Saunders, pp 67–72.
4. Prendergast H: Nutritional requirements and feeding of growing puppies and kittens. In Peterson ME, Kutzler MA, editors: *Small animal pediatrics, the first 12 months of life*, St Louis, 2011, Elsevier Saunders, pp 58–66.
5. Case LP, Fahey GC, Jr: Nutritional challenges for shelter animals. In Miller L, Zawistowski S, editors: *Shelter medicine for veterinarians and staff*, Oxford, 2004, Blackwell, pp 79–93.
6. Rodan I, Sundahl E, Carney H, et al: AAFP and ISFM feline-friendly handling guidelines. *J Feline Med Surg* 13:364–375, 2011.
7. Radosta L: Feline behavioral development. In Peterson ME, Kutzler MA, editors: *Small animal pediatrics, the first 12 months of life*, St Louis, 2011, Elsevier Saunders, pp 88–96.
8. Overall KL, Rodan I, Beaver BV, et al: Feline behavior guidelines from the American Association of Feline Practitioners. *J Am Vet Med Assoc* 227:70–84, 2005.
9. Larson LJ, Newbury S, Schultz RD: Canine and feline vaccinations and immunology. In Miller L, Hurley K, editors: *Infectious disease management in animal shelters*, Ames, 2009, Wiley-Blackwell, pp 61–82.
10. Moriello K, Newbury S, Diesel A: Dermatophytosis. In Miller L, Hurley K, editors: *Infectious disease management in animal shelters*, Ames, 2009, Wiley-Blackwell, pp 243–273.
11. Moriello K, Newbury S, Diesel A: Ectoparasites. In Miller L, Hurley K, editors: *Infectious disease management in animal shelters*, Ames, 2009, Wiley-Blackwell, pp 275–298.
12. Scherk MA, Ford RB, Gaskell RM, et al: AAFP feline vaccination advisory panel report. *J Feline Med Surg* 15:785–808, 2013.
13. Levy J, Crawford C, Hartmann K, et al: American association of feline practitioners' feline retrovirus management guidelines. *J Feline Med Surg* 10(3):300–316, 2008.
14. Association of Shelter Veterinarians Website. Guidelines for Standards of Care in Animal Shelters, <http://www.sheltervet.org/wp-content/uploads/2011/08/Shelter-Standards-Oct2011-wForward.pdf>, 2010, (Accessed April 30, 2015.)
15. Tuzio H: Feline panleukopenia. In Miller L, Hurley K, editors: *Infectious disease management in animal shelters*, Ames, 2009, Wiley-Blackwell, pp 183–196.
16. Daniels J, Spencer E: Bacterial infections. In Peterson ME, Kutzler MA, editors: *Small animal pediatrics, the first 12 months of life*, St Louis, 2011, Elsevier Saunders, pp 113–118.
17. Fitzgerald K, Newquist K: Husbandry of the neonate. In Peterson ME, Kutzler MA, editors: *Small animal pediatrics, the first 12 months of life*, St Louis, 2011, Elsevier Saunders, pp 44–52.
18. McMichael M: Emergency and critical care issues. In Peterson ME, Kutzler MA, editors: *Small animal pediatrics, the first 12 months of life*, St Louis, 2011, Elsevier Saunders, pp 73–81.
19. Little S: Feline pediatrics: how to treat the small and the sick. *Compendium* 33:E1–E6, 2011.
20. Peterson M: Neonatal mortality. In Peterson ME, Kutzler MA, editors: *Small animal pediatrics, the first 12 months of life*, St Louis, 2011, Elsevier Saunders, pp 82–87.
21. Krebsbach S: Maddie's Institute: from helpless newborn to skilled acrobat: feline development and the orphaned kitten, <http://www.maddiesfund.org/Maddies_Institute/Articles/From_Helpless_Newborn.html>, 2013, (Accessed November 14, 2014.)

Environmental Strategies to Promote Health and Wellness

Judith L. Stella and C.A. Tony Buffington

States of health and wellness result from complex interactions between individuals and environments. Even definitions of the terms "health" and "wellness" are complex, and sometimes controversial. In 1946, the World Health Organization defined health as "a state of complete physical, mental, and social well-being and not merely the absence of disease or infirmity."[1] Although comprehensive, this definition has been controversial because it is not clear what "complete" means or how to establish and maintain these states.

Although this definition was intended to apply to human beings, much of it seems relevant for the health and welfare of animals in our care. Health at least means absence of disease or infirmity and could include sufficient physical, mental, and social well-being to preclude suffering. In fact, animal welfare has been defined as "... how an animal is coping with the conditions in which it lives. An animal is in a good state of welfare if (as indicated by scientific evidence) it is healthy, comfortable, well nourished, safe, able to express innate behavior, and if it is not suffering from unpleasant states, such as pain, fear, and distress. Good animal welfare requires disease prevention and appropriate veterinary treatment, shelter, management and nutrition, humane handling, and humane slaughter or killing."[2]

We infer the presence or absence of health and the welfare of individual animals by observing them; we infer physical health by the absence of problems with form or function and the presence of species-typical form and function, moderate body condition score, activity, food intake, and elimination. We infer mental and social well-being from the animal's behavior and interactions with its surroundings and other animals. Although the World Health Organization definition of health seems to imply the simultaneous presence of good welfare, the converse is not always the case. Even in the absence of health, humans and animals appear to have the capacity to sustain acceptable welfare with appropriate care and conditions. Research has resulted in a paradigm shift in the understanding of these relationships. Studies have identified new individual factors that influence health and welfare, including the effects of inhabiting environments far removed from the animal's natural history, and the central role of the interactions between humans and animals for the health and well-being of each. This chapter will focus on the influence of the external environment on the health and welfare of domestic cats (*Felis silvestris catus*) confined in cages or their owners' home and how we can improve cats' health and welfare through effective environmental enrichment.

ENVIRONMENTAL EFFECTS ON HEALTH AND WELFARE

Exposing animals to situations that exceed their homeostatic coping abilities can result in activation of the stress response system (SRS). Activation of the SRS results in behavioral and physiological (neural, endocrine, and immune) responses that can be subsumed under the umbrella of a "psycho-neuro-endocrine-immune" (PNEI) super-system that mediates interactions between the external and internal environments and ultimately influences behavior.[3] In a review,[4] the eminent neuroscientist Bruce McEwen pointed out that "The brain is the key organ of the stress response for three principal reasons: (a) The brain interprets what is threatening and therefore stressful; (b) it determines and regulates behavioral and physiological stress responses, the latter through the autonomic, immune, neuroendocrine, and metabolic systems that may result in successful adaptation or lead to... disease; and (c) the brain is a target of stress and undergoes structural and functional remodeling and significant changes in gene expression that affect its function."

The SRS can be activated peripherally by internal factors, such as infection or inflammation ("bottom up"), or centrally by perception of an external threat ("top down"). External environmental threats may be: (1) physical (e.g., blood loss, heat, cold, or noise), (2) psychological (e.g., learned responses to previously experienced adverse events), and (3) social (e.g., predation, territorial disputes). These threats also can be categorized as either acute (single, infrequent, time limited) or chronic (frequent, recurrent, prolonged).

Most sensory input from the internal and external environments that reaches areas of the higher or conscious brain (the vast majority being excluded by the brainstem) is received in the thalamus and then forwarded to the cortex for further processing before transmission to the motor systems. Threatening information also can be transferred directly to the amygdala, hippocampus, and hypothalamus to activate the SRS.

Activation of the SRS by either internal or external stimuli can result in initiation of variable combinations of peripheral neural, hormonal, and immune responses. The pattern of activation depends both upon the nature of the threat and individual animal factors.[5] Increased SRS activity is common in animals confined in unenriched environments.[6] This can complicate interpretation of diagnostic procedures by influencing the cat's temperature, heart and respiratory rates, and blood pressure,[7] and may play a role in predisposing, precipitating, or perpetuating a variety of chronic diseases in cats.[8]

The Nervous System

Animals collect a constant stream of new information through their sensory systems (olfactory, gustatory, auditory, tactile, visual, and pheromonal) when they interact with their environments. A primary function of the epithelium is to "sense" the local environment and communicate input to neighboring epithelial and sensory nerve cells.[9-11] Sensory nerve cells in turn transmit information concerning the state of the environment to the spinal cord and then to the brain. Negative sensory input from the periphery stimulates, among other things, release of corticotrophin-releasing factor (CRF) from the hypothalamus, which in turn can activate the SRS.[12,13] Activation of the SRS can increase autonomic, particularly sympathetic, outflow, which in turn can increase epithelial permeability acutely and result in epithelial damage if chronic. External threats also can sensitize the acoustic startle response, a brainstem reflex that responds to unexpected loud stimuli. Increased startle responsiveness, which has been shown to result from both fear and anxiety mediated by higher brain structures,[14] may explain the "hypervigilance" observed in some cats housed in threatening environments. Activation of the SRS also can increase plasma catecholamine concentrations.[15,16] Moreover, these may increase further as exposure to stressors goes on,[16] possibly due to desensitization of alpha-2 adrenergic receptors.[17,18]

The Endocrine System

Concentrations of CRF[19,20] and adrenocorticotropic hormone (ACTH)[21] increase in response to stress, whereas plasma glucocorticoid concentrations may increase, decrease, or remain unchanged.[22] Decreased glucocorticoid responsiveness to ACTH stimulation suggests the presence of mild primary adrenocortical insufficiency or decreased adrenocortical reserve. For example, the adrenocortical response to ACTH stimulation is reduced in cats with feline idiopathic (interstitial) cystitis (FIC), and they often have small adrenal glands[13] (possibly due to adverse developmental and early life influences on the developing adrenal cortex).[19,23] Decreased adrenocortical responsiveness to activation of the SRS results in a relative predominance of sympathetic to hypothalamic-pituitary-adrenal activity,[24] suggesting a decrease in glucocorticoid-mediated restraint of sympathoneural outflow.[25] This abnormality has been found in cats with FIC[13,19] and may occur in cats with other chronic syndromes as well.

The Immune System

Vasodilation and vascular leakage in the general absence of any significant mononuclear or polymorphonuclear infiltrate suggest the presence of neurogenic inflammation and are the most common histological findings in the bladder of cats with FIC.[26] Increased numbers of mast cells have been observed in biopsy specimens from cats with FIC,[27] which is likely to be a nonspecific, neurally mediated result of activation of the SRS that can occur in a variety of tissues.[28]

Chronic psychosocial stress also is well known to stimulate low-grade systemic inflammation,[29] which can result in the expression of sickness behaviors.[30] Sickness behaviors refer to variable combinations of vomiting, diarrhea, decreased food and water intake, fever, lethargy, somnolence, enhanced pain-like behaviors, as well as decreased general activity, body care activities (grooming), and social interactions. They reflect efforts to promote recovery by inhibiting metabolically expensive (e.g., foraging) or dangerous (e.g., exposure to predators) activities during sickness or threat.

Sickness behaviors can result from peripheral or central immune activation.[6,16,31] In cats with FIC, the authors found that external stressors were associated with significantly increased risks for centrally mediated sickness behaviors, including decreases in food intake and elimination, and increases in elimination outside the litter box.[32] The authors also observed sickness behaviors similar to those reported previously in healthy cats housed in a caging environment designed to model initial exposure to a veterinary or shelter facility.[33] Thus, some of the most commonly observed abnormalities in client-owned cats, "finicky" eating and litter box problems, can occur after exposure to external threats in caged cats. Both cats with FIC and healthy cats were similarly affected, suggesting that clinicians include environmental threat in the differential diagnosis of cats presented for these signs.

Behavior

In addition to sickness behaviors, a variety of other behavioral abnormalities have been observed in the response of cats exposed to threats. The authors have identified increased nervous and fearful behaviors,[34,35] as well as "doglike" behaviors (e.g., following the owners around the house, incessant demands for attention) in some cats with FIC.[36] Although nervous and fearful behaviors are common responses to threat, doglike behavior in cats might suggest dysregulated attachment as a consequence of some adverse early life experience.[37] Importantly, the authors also have observed resolution of these behaviors in both laboratory[32] and clinical[35] studies in response to multimodal environmental modification.

Integration: The Psycho-Neuro-Endocrine-Immune "Super-system"

The components of the PNEI systems interconnect to create an emergent "super-system," the properties of which may not be explainable by evaluation of any one component of the underlying systems.[38] This super-system represents the interface between the external and internal environments that permits organisms to act in the world, avoiding threats and exploiting opportunities. When the system perceives threat, it activates the SRS to attempt to cope with the challenge. Although acute activation of the SRS has high survival value, persistent activation can lead to wear and tear on the system and ultimately to disease,[39] the particular manifestations of which may depend on the familial (genetic, epigenetic, environmental) vulnerabilities of the individual.[40] As McEwen concludes,[4] "A major challenge for future research and practice is to harness the capacity of the brain and body to show plasticity in situations where adversity has left its mark."

PHYSIOLOGICAL AND BEHAVIORAL CHANGES ASSOCIATED WITH STRESS IN THE VETERINARY CLINIC

Veterinary care-givers have long conflated "fractious" (difficult to control, unruly) with fearful (afraid for one's safety) behaviors displayed by cats. Perceived threats activate the SRS, which can result in variable combinations of freezing, flight, or fight behaviors to reduce the cat's risk of injury or death from the threat. Although people know that they are only trying to help the cat, their actions can seem like mortal threats from the cat's point of view.

A variety of physiological parameters also can change when cats are exposed to potentially threatening environments. Reported changes include alterations in urine pH, blood pressure, heart rate, respiratory rate, and body temperature. Although many pathological processes can result in alterations in these parameters, results suggest that activation of the SRS should be considered when alternative explanations are unlikely or excluded during evaluation of the patient. For example, in 1996, Buffington and Chew[41] provided a case report of a cat that produced acidic urine (pH 6.2) in the home environment, whereas alkaline urine (pH 8) was observed during evaluation at the hospital. After excluding a variety of alternative explanations, stress-induced respiratory alkalosis associated with automobile transport to the hospital was presumed to be the cause of the alkaline urine.

In an early study of the presence of a "white-coat" effect, Belew and colleagues[42] used radiotelemetry to measure systolic, mean, and diastolic blood pressure as well as heart rate of six healthy, conscious cats in a research colony while undisturbed in their cages and while subjected to simulated visits to a veterinarian's office (Figure 73-1). Although all values measured during the simulated office visit were statistically significantly greater than those measured in the home cage, marked heterogeneity occurred in the pattern and magnitude of the increases in blood pressure, which ranged from 75 to 227 mm Hg. Variation in response to the simulated veterinary visit also was observed among cats and among visits by the same cat. The magnitude of the white-coat effect tended to decrease, but did not disappear, over time.

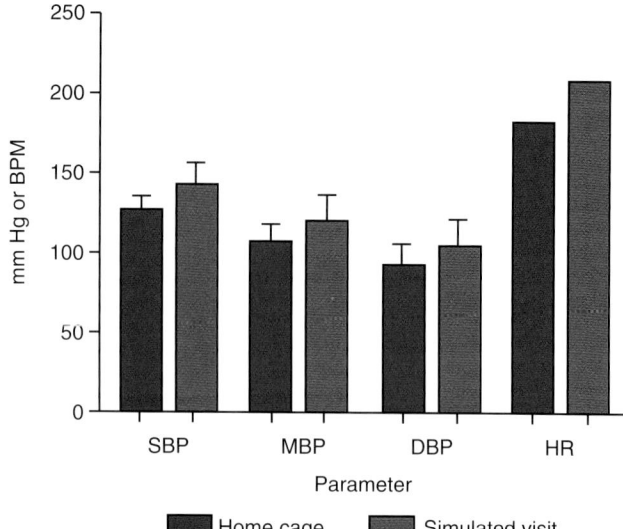

Figure 73-1: Values for Cardiovascular Parameters in Normal Cats (*n* = 6) during a Simulated Clinic Visit (Mean + Standard Deviation). *HR*, Heart rate; *DBP*, diastolic blood pressure; *MBP*, mean blood pressure; *SBP*, systolic blood pressure. (Adapted from Belew AM, Barlett T, Brown SA: Evaluation of the white-coat effect in cats. *J Vet Intern Med* 13:134-142, 1999.)

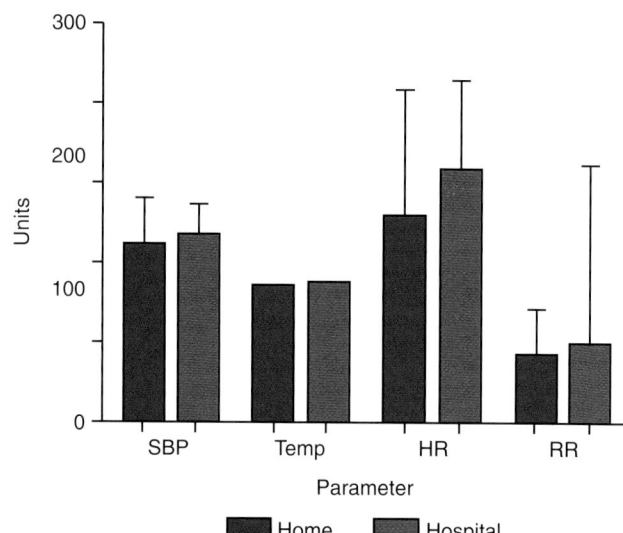

Figure 73-2: Values for physiological parameters in normal cats (*n* = 30) at home or at a veterinary hospital (median + range). Units are mm Hg for systolic blood pressure (*SBP*), degrees Fahrenheit for temperature (*Temp*), beats per minute for heart rate (*HR*), and breaths per minute for respiratory rate (*RR*). (Adapted from Quimby JM, Smith ML, Lunn KF: Evaluation of the effects of hospital visit stress on physiologic parameters in the cat. *J Feline Med Surg* 13:733-737, 2011.)

Furthermore, Quimby and colleagues[43] compared physiological parameter data gathered from 30 cats in their home environment with those gathered in a veterinary hospital (Figure 73-2). Although they found significant differences in blood pressure, heart rate, and respiratory rate between the home and veterinary hospital, large individual differences for blood pressure and temperature were observed. In contrast, the increases in heart and respiratory rates were more consistent among the cats between the two environments. As they concluded, "This information may help practitioners recognize that physiologic abnormalities can sometimes be due to transportation or environmental stress rather than medical illness."

In the authors' experience, observed behavioral and measured physiological parameters seem roughly concordant. One important exception occurs when cats are immobile in a cage as they may be resting or they may be engaged in freezing behavior. In addition to other observations, respiratory rate provides one useful physiological parameter to differentiate resting (slow respiratory rate) from freezing (rapid respiratory rate) behaviors.

ENVIRONMENTAL ENRICHMENT

David Shepherdson defined environmental enrichment as "a concept which describes how the environments of captive animals can be changed for the benefit of the inhabitants. Behavioral opportunities that may arise or increase as a result of environmental enrichment can be appropriately described as behavioral enrichment."[44] The goals of environmental enrichment are to (1) increase behavioral diversity, (2) reduce the frequency of abnormal behaviors, (3) increase the range or number of normal behavior patterns, (4) increase positive utilization of the environment, and (5) increase the ability to cope with challenges in a more "normal" way.[44]

The effects of environmental enrichment have been studied in a variety of species and have been found to decrease sickness behaviors,[32] obesity,[45] anxiety,[46] and tumor growth,[47] and to improve learning, cognitive function,[48] and resistance to environmental challenges.[49] Mechanisms underlying the beneficial effects of environmental enrichment are an active area of research, which has identified changes at the molecular, cellular, organ, cognitive, and behavioral levels of organization.

Environmental enrichment is a dynamic process of making changes to structures in the environment and husbandry practices with the goal of increasing behavioral choices for animals to promote species-appropriate behaviors and abilities, thus enhancing animal welfare.[44] The connection between environmental enrichment for captive animals and domestic cats may not be apparent until one considers that cats confined in homes or in cages in veterinary hospitals, shelters, and research facilities live in spaces much smaller than their natural home range.[50] Cats kept in these environments live akin to zoo animals and, as with zoo animals, environmental quality can exert important salutary effects on their health and welfare.[51] Relatively few published studies of environmental enrichment specific to cats have been published.[52] Several published guidelines for care of cats are better thought of as general recommendations, because much of what is in them was based on expert opinion rather than scientific studies.[53,54] This is an area in need of further scientific

evaluation. The following sections will elaborate on what is known and best current recommendations.

The authors have coined the term *multimodal environmental modification* (MEMO) to describe the process of evaluating and modifying the environment of cats to improve their health and well-being. All aspects of the evaluation are applicable to cats in cages or in homes because cats have a finite number of responses to the environment. In addition, cats will need the same environmental conditions regardless of the housing system (e.g., cage in hospital or shelter or indoor housed in a home). The goals of MEMO are those of environmental enrichment in general and are intended to create and sustain a perception of control and predictability about the surroundings that permits cats to thrive. When cats perceive their environments to be safe and predictable, they become easier to work with, which reduces risk of injury to staff, improves workflow and patient welfare, and promotes faster recovery and discharge to home.

THE MULTIMODAL ENVIRONMENTAL MODIFICATION PROCESS

Evaluating the Cat

The first step in the MEMO process is assessment of the cat(s) because, if all are healthy and well, no further action may be needed for the present time. People can learn something about cats' health and wellness just by watching how they behave. Cats that enjoy good health and welfare generally explore and interact with their surroundings in a relaxed and confident way. In contrast, cats suffering poor health or welfare tend not to engage in these behaviors. Table 73-1 describes some positive and negative indicators of behavioral health and welfare in cats. Although behaviors associated with good welfare are similar among cats, those associated with poor welfare can vary widely and occur for many reasons. For example, a cat may be feeling threatened, fearful, or anxious for some reason, or may be sick or in pain. These differences can be difficult to sort out.

Changes in the cat's behavior such as the presence or increase in aggressive, agonistic, avoidant, or sickness behaviors can be indications that something may be wrong in the cat's environment. Additionally for cats in cages, resting in litter pans and the condition of the cage can signal an environmental problem. Resting in the litter pan, although "common" in some environments, is not "normal" for cats in cages. In the authors' experience, this behavior often indicates a failure to cope with the environment, typically occurring when cats want to hide, but are not provided with an appropriate opportunity to do so, when they are sick, or when they are cold or otherwise struggling to cope with the environment. In addition, the condition of the cage may indicate a failure to cope. For example, a cage that does not look like a cat has been housed in it after several hours indicates the cat is exhibiting freezing behavior indicative of the negative affective states of fear or anxiety. By contrast, a cage that shows disuse or looks destroyed indicates a cat that may be

Table 73-1	Behavioral Assessment of Cat Health and Welfare	
Behavior	**Positive Indicators**	**Negative Indicators**
Activity	Moves around the home smoothly and confidently Jumps fluidly Relaxed body at rest Positive interactions with human care-taker Enjoys being petted or handled	Reluctant to move, difficulty getting up from a lying position Limps, cannot jump as high as usual Trembles or shakes Seeks more affection Avoids being held, picked up, handled, or petted Restless Gets up and lies down repetitively Hides Growls, hisses, bites, or scratches when approached
Daily habits	Seeks social interaction Usual and cat-appropriate eating, sleeping, and drinking patterns Usual litter box use	Withdraws from social interaction Changes (usually decreases) in eating, sleeping, or drinking Stops using the litter box Urinates frequently
Facial expression	Relaxed face Calm gaze Pupils appropriate size for light conditions Ears erect Breathes quietly when at rest	Grimaces, furrowed brow, vacant stare Looks glazed, wide-eyed, or sleepy Pupils enlarged Ears flattened Pants when at rest
Grooming	Gentle, relaxed grooming of entire body	Does not groom or grooms less, looks unkempt Licks, bites, or scratches any particular areas of the body
Posture	Generally lays on side in relaxed position	Lays with feet tucked underneath Arches back or tucks in abdomen
Vocalizing	"Happy" meowing Purring	Decreased normal vocalizations Plaintive meowing Yowling Hissing Growling

attempting to hide (especially if no hide box has been offered) or a cat that is frustrated and is trying to escape, both of which suggest the cat is experiencing a negative affective state.

The presence of any of these behaviors warrants investigation of the environment and closer monitoring of the cat to identify and resolve the problems. Any sudden changes in a cat's behavior, particularly a negative change, should lead to an increase in monitoring of the individual and attempts to determine if the new behavior resulted from threatening external events. For example, increases in sickness behaviors have been shown in response to unusual external events in research colony-housed cats as well as owned cats placed in a cage environment.[32,33] Therefore, it is important for caretakers to observe, monitor, and record sickness behaviors, which can include variable combinations of anorexia or decreased food intake; decreased or no eliminations in a 24-hour period; eliminating out of the litter pan; vomiting of food, hair, or bile; and diarrhea. In addition, pet cats generally are not aggressive toward or avoidant of human contact, so the presence of aggressive or hiding behaviors may indicate significant fear or pain.

Evaluating the Environment

The environmental needs of cats are similar whether they are confined to a home or to a cage in a veterinary hospital, shelter, research, or boarding facility. Aspects of the macroenvironment (the room), the microenvironment (the individual cage or restricted area of the cat), predictability and control of the environment, and the quality of the social environment (including the human-cat relationship as well as interactions with conspecifics and other animals in the environment [e.g., dogs]) all influence cats' perception of threat. The authors will now discuss aspects of the environment that may impact the behavior and welfare of confined cats and the best scientific recommendations available at this time. Table 73-2 provides a summary.

Macroenvironmental factors that can be stressful to cats include lighting, sound, odor, and temperature.[55] These environmental factors will affect cats differently depending on whether they are housed in cages or areas where they are unable to control or move away from a factor they find aversive.

Table 73-2   Evaluating the Environment*

Factors	Aspects	Recommendations	Things to Avoid	Enrichment	References
Light	Light-dark cycle	Natural light (H, C)	Inconsistency (C, H)		55
	Intensity (lux)	Less than 400 lux at 1 m from the floor (C)	Less than 400 lux at 1 m from the floor for extended periods of time (C)		
Sound	Sound intensity	Less than 60 dB (C)	Less than 60 dB (C, H)	Quiet music (C, H)	55, 32, 33
	Source	Soundproof or quiet cat rooms; housing away from dog areas (C)	Barking dogs, anthropogenic noise (e.g., loud talking, radios) (C)	Recordings for cats or classical music (C, H)	32, 33
	Unpredictability	Turn off overhead paging systems, cell phones, etc. (C)	Any loud unexpected noises throughout the cat housing area (C, H)		32
Temperature	Range (ambient room temperature)	Near 80 F (26.7 C) (C)	Less than 72 F (22.2 C) (C)	Bedding (e.g., blankets, towels, shredded paper), boxes to allow behavioral thermoregulation (C, H)	53, 55, 57
Odor	Source	Minimize potentially aversive odors to the extent possible (C)	Chemical cleaners, perfume, dog odor, alcohol hand rubs, cigarette smells, laundry detergent, etc. (C)	Spray catnip, herbs (mint), prey smells, other natural odors (C, H)	55, 56
Food	Presentation	Provide wet and dry in separate bowls; place in rear half of cage; offer diet change as a choice; offer small, frequent meals (C, H)	Sudden change of diet; mixing of diets (C, H)	Novel or special foods as treats (e.g., tuna); food puzzle toys; using food to train cat; tossing kibble to encourage hunting/chase behavior (C, H)	32, 33, 58, 59, 60, 61, 62, 63, 64, 65, 93
Water	Presentation	Large bowls (C) or running water (H)	Small, narrow containers; bowls that can be easily spilled (C, H)	Fountains, running water in a sink or tub (H)	
Litter	Type of litter	Clumping litter is thought to be preferred by most cats (C, H)	Small amounts of litter, infrequent scooping (at least twice a day for caged cats); any changes in type of litter should be offered as a choice (C, H)	Make sure the litter is deep; cats like to dig and cover their eliminations (C, H)	66, 67, 68, 69, 70
Litter container	Size	At least twice the length of the cat (C, H)	Small, shallow containers (C, H)	One study reported cats preferred even larger containers (C, H)	66
	Type	Most cats prefer uncovered containers (C, H)	Offer a choice (H)		67
	Number	The general rule is one litter container per cat plus one (H)	Too few pans for the number of cats, placement in the same area or in a row, placement near appliances or where the cat can be trapped by other cats (H)		68, 69, 70

Continued

Table 73-2	Evaluating the Environment—cont'd			
Factors	**Aspects**	**Recommendations**	**Things to Avoid**	**Enrichment**	**References**
Bedding	Size	Make sure it is large enough to offer comfort to the cat (C)	Washing daily (C)	Clean bedding infused with pleasing odors such as catnip (C, H)	74
Flooring	Substrate	Nonslip, solid (not slatted), warm (C)	Bare stainless steel (C)	Cover floors with mats, newspaper, or bedding (C)	
Hide	Size	A box of some type large enough for the cat to rest comfortably inside (C, H)	Not providing an opportunity to hide (C, H)	Cardboard box (C, H) or towel hanging over the cage door if cage is too small for a hiding place or one cannot be provided for some other reason (e.g., IV catheter) (C)	33,71,72, 73
Perch		Perches built into cage wall or a box that the cat can sit atop (C), elevated resting areas (H)	Placing cats in cages at floor level (C), providing no opportunity to elevate (H)	Perches, cardboard box, upper tier (C); ladders, cat tree, window shelf, furniture (H)	71
Other		Opportunities for other species-typical behaviors are recommended for longer stays in a cage (C) and always in homes (H)	Placing too many items in a small cage (C); barren home (H)	Scratching opportunities (hung on the door or a cardboard box), toys (be sure to rotate every day or two) (C, H), supervised time outdoors (H)	77
Space		Be sure each cat has its own resources (C, H)	Providing too few resources (C, H)		74, 75, 76
Predictability		Maintain a husbandry, feeding, and treatment schedule that will allow the cat to predict when things will happen (C, H)	Unpredictability (C, H)		79, 94, 95
Control		Allow the cat to maintain some control over its environment and interactions with care-takers (C, H)	Forced interactions; allow the cat to choose when/if it interacts with people (C, H)	Enriched environments that allow the cat to move away from perceived threats (C, H)	94, 95

Category	Item				References
Care-taker	Consistency	To the extent possible, care-takers should be consistent so the cat becomes familiar with him/her (C, H)	Multiple care-takers (C, H)	Care-takers and technical staff treating cats can play with cats, provide food treats, brush, pet, etc. (C)	79, 80, 81, 82, 83, 84
	Other	Spot clean cages whenever possible, especially in the first 24-48 h of confinement as this is the most stressful time for cat (C)			33
Low stress handling		All interactions with cats should use LSH techniques (C, H)	Force, punishment (C, H)		80, 81, 82, 86, 87, 88, 96, 97, 98
Red flags: If any of these are observed, assess the environment and provide additional resources or enrichment	Resting in litter pan			Provide hide box or cover cage door (C)	
	Sickness behaviors	Investigate the environment to determine reason (C, H)	Implementing any changes until the source of stress is identified and removed (C, H)		
	Cage condition	No use or disuse	No use is typically due to fear, whereas disuse can be either frustration and attempts to escape the cage environment or an attempt to hide if no opportunity for that behavior is provided (C)	Provide hide box, toys, other enrichment (C)	
	Aggressive behavior	Fear or dislike of other cats (C, H)	Introduction of a new cat (C, H)	Provide hiding opportunity, move to quieter area, move to an area away from other cats (C, H)	
	Sudden change in behavior	Could be due to improvement in condition or acclimation to environment or to worsening of condition or lack of ability to adapt to environment (C, H)	Implementing any changes until the source of stress is identified and removed (C, H)	Provide what is missing in the environment after assessment (C, H)	

IV, Intravenous; *LSH*, low stress handling.
*Aspects pertaining particularly to the home are indicated with an H, those more important to a cage environment are indicated with a C, and factors equally relevant to cats regardless of housing are indicated with both H and C.

Cats are more sensitive to light brightness than humans are; this should be considered in housing facilities because light intensity can affect cat welfare. The authors are not aware of light intensity recommendations for confined cats, but the general recommendation for rodent housing is less than 400 lux at 1 m from the floor (light meters can be obtained as free smartphone applications). In addition, light is an environmental cue that allows confined cats to become accustomed to daily activities. Lights in hospital wards and other areas where cats are confined should be controlled by a timer that provides a predictable light-dark cycle from day to day if natural light cannot be provided. If a timer is not possible, then manually controlling the light-dark cycle is an acceptable alternative. The authors recommend that lights *not* be turned on and off each time someone enters or exits the housing room or hospital ward.

The auditory frequency range of cats (and most species) exceeds that of humans, making assessment of the welfare implications of high frequency noise difficult. Housing areas and hospital wards should aim to minimize noise levels to less than 60 dB, a quiet conversational level (dB meters can be obtained as free smartphone applications). This recommendation is based on observations of cats successfully maintained in environments in this range.[32,33] This level is still well above sound pressure levels in nature, which range from 20 to 37 dB in savannah habitats to 27 to 40 dB in the rain forest. Speaking in quiet voices when in the presence of cats, conducting conversations outside of the cat housing areas whenever possible, housing barking dogs as far from cats as possible, closing cage and room doors quietly, and avoiding sudden and unexpected noises that can be especially disturbing to cats (such as telephones, radios, equipment alarms, door bells) will help minimize the stress associated with noise.

Cats depend more on olfactory cues (macro-osmotic) than humans do. Therefore, aversive odors can be an additional source of chronic stress for confined animals (including hospitalized cats), although cats appear to habituate to some odors rather quickly.[56] Odors the authors have observed to be objectionable to cats include dogs (a natural predator), other cats, alcohol (from hand sanitizers), cigarettes, cleaning chemicals (including laundry detergent), some perfumes, and citrus scents. This may be more important to cats in cages because they are less able to move away from aversive odors than are cats in the home.

Finally, cats prefer a warmer ambient temperature than many other species. The thermoneutral zone for domestic cats is between 30 and 38 °C (85 and 100 °F).[57] Most cat-housing areas and veterinary hospital ward rooms are not this warm. Most homes, veterinary hospitals, and laboratory housing for cats are maintained closer to 18 to 26 °C (64 to 79 °F),[53] so the authors recommend providing bedding that allows cats to behaviorally thermoregulate. If using towels, make sure they are large enough for the cat to get under or to make a nest. Shredded paper in a box can also be used. If providing an additional heat source (e.g., heating pad or microwaveable heat pads for pets, such as Snuggle Safe ([Lenric C21 Ltd.,

West Sussex, United Kingdom]), be sure the cat can move away from the heat source to another comfortable resting area if it chooses.

Microenvironmental (caging) factors that can be sources of stress for cats include food (type and presentation), elimination facilities (litter pan), hiding and perching opportunities, and outlets for expression of species typical behaviors. The type and presentation as well as the availability of these features of the environment can be either a source of stress or enrichment (Figure 73-3A and 73-3B).

Free-living cats, as opportunistic predators of small prey, typically eat frequent small meals throughout the day, spending a large portion of their day engaged in food acquisition. Commercial dry cat food is of a different composition and texture than the "wild" diet, and provision of one or two large meals a day in a bowl requires minimal effort on the cat's part to feed itself. Together, this may lead to under- or over-eating and boredom in the confined cat. Cats with free access to food usually prefer to eat several small meals throughout the day as opposed to one or two large meals, and most will hunt for prey when given the option.[58] Although free access to food may allow for frequent feeding sessions, this feeding

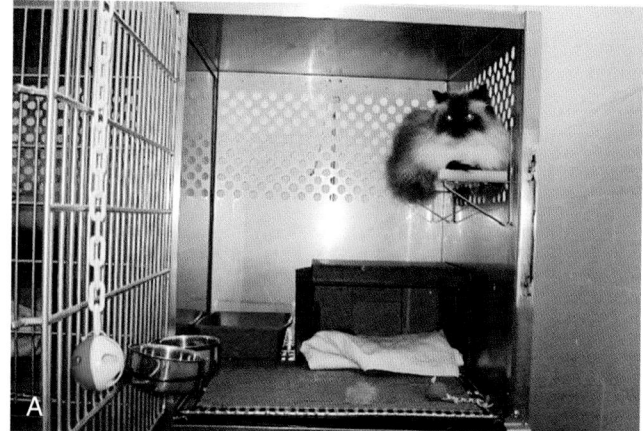
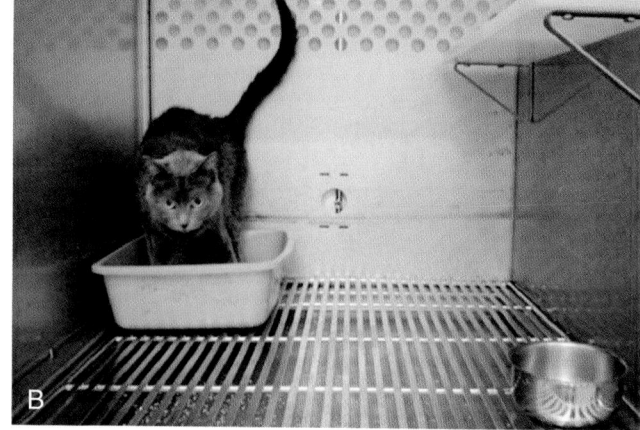

Figure 73-3: A, Enriched cage that provides a hide box, perching area, toys, bedding, food, water, and litter pan as well as a rubber mat to cover the stainless steel slatted floor. **B,** Unenriched cage that has no hide box, bedding, toys, or floor covering. Note that the cat is standing in the litter pan, indicating that she finds the flooring aversive.

strategy still does not allow the cat the opportunity to express natural predatory instincts[59] and may contribute to development of obesity and other health problems.[60] Meeting nutrient needs in ways that best mimic cats' natural feeding preferences can provide mental and physical enrichment. For example, care-takers can accommodate cats' natural predatory habits and increase their daily activity by offering food in puzzle toys, such as balls or other devices designed specifically for cats to release dry food or treats when physically manipulated.[61] Because cats evolved as solitary hunters,[59] separate feeding stations for each cat out of sight of the others facilitates "solitary" feeding and reduces the risk of conflict over resources.

Although available evidence confirms that currently available commercial diets adequately meet the nutritional needs of domestic cats[62,63] (with the possible exception of protein[64]), cats sometimes display strong food preferences based on foods encountered early in life, although these usually can be modified by later experience. Some cats also develop decreased preference for foods that have formed a large part of their diet in the past, the so-called monotony effect, and display preferences for novel food.[65] Although some owners perceive their cats to be "finicky" eaters, evidence suggests that food refusal is a common feline response to environmental threat.[32,33] Therefore, care-takers should offer the same food to hospitalized cats that is eaten at home whenever possible; when feeding both dry and canned food, offer them in separate bowls and provide fresh food at least twice a day. Double-sided bowls are an acceptable option if only one type of food (wet or dry) is offered or if each compartment contains one type of food with water offered in a separate bowl.

Cats also seem to have preferences for water that can be investigated. Water-related factors to consider include freshness, taste, movement (e.g., water fountains, dripping faucets, or aquarium pump-bubbled air into a bowl), and shape of container (some cats seem to resent having their vibrissae touch the sides of the container when drinking).

Elimination facilities are another microenvironmental factor of importance to cats. Many types of litter pans and litters are available, so the type chosen often depends on the resources available to the care-taker and individual cat preference.[66,67] Several important points should be kept in mind when assessing elimination resources. First, provide a litter pan that is big enough for the cat (preferably 1.5 times the length of the cat). Secondly, for group-housed cats, provide a litter pan for each cat (or cat group) plus one additional pan, all out of sight of each other.[68]

Covered litter pans may trap odors and prevent the cat from having a safe vantage point for the approach of other animals during elimination, making them a less desirable option for many cats. The litter container should be placed in a quiet area that will permit the cat to use it without being disturbed by other animals, humans, or machinery (e.g., washing machine, refrigerator) that could come on unexpectedly and disrupt the normal elimination behavior sequence. Placing litter pans in quiet, convenient locations could help improve conditions for eliminative behavior. Litter pans should be cleaned with mild dish soap at least weekly so that some smell familiar to the cat remains.

Finally, the type of litter is important as well. Most cats display a preference for unscented and finely particulate litter material,[69] making clumping litter a desirable option. Cats prefer to dig (without hitting the bottom of the litter pan) and then bury their eliminations, so it is important that the litter is deep enough. If different litters are provided, the authors find it preferable to offer them in separate litter pans because individual preferences for litter type have been documented.[70] At least daily (although twice daily is recommended by some) scooping of eliminations from the container is recommended. Cats housed in veterinary facilities should be offered the same litter the cat uses at home, whenever possible.

For caged cats, placement of food, water, and shelter (hide box) in the back half of the cage and the litter pan in the front half of the cage allows them to better use the space provided. Cats eat, drink, and hide more often than they eliminate, and fearful cats tend to spend most of the time in the back of their cages. Placing the resources used most frequently where the cat spends most of its time increases the likelihood of use, and placing the litter container in the front of the cage decreases the likelihood that cats will rest in it (Figure 73-4).

The physical environment should include opportunities for hiding, climbing, scratching, and resting. Results from several studies indicate that hiding is a highly motivated behavior in cats.[33,71-73] Cats may have a need to hide that allows them to partially isolate themselves from unfamiliar conspecifics and humans when confronted with a threatening environment. Not providing cats the opportunity to hide is likely to increase their level of distress and in turn decrease their overall welfare, so all efforts should be made to meet this need both in the home and in the veterinary hospital. Cardboard boxes work well, are inexpensive, and are disposable. Cats will use the boxes to keep warm, escape threats, and scratch and perch on. Place the box in the back half of the cage with the opening facing the side, not the front, of the cage. Cat carriers also work well.

Cats seem to prefer soft resting substrates, such as pillows or fleece beds[74] in warm areas, such as safely heated beds or sunny windows. Because most cats prefer familiar bedding, change it only when it is soiled rather than daily. Even in a hospital setting, the authors recommend spot cleaning of cages. This is perceived as less threatening to the cat, eliminates the need for removing the cat from the cage for cleaning, and leaves familiar odors in the cage environment. Care-takers of multicat households or group-caged cats need to provide enough space to permit each cat to keep a social distance of 1 to 3 m,[75] horizontally as well as vertically, in spaces shared with other cats. Although some cats rest together, allogroom, and rub each other, most cats use common resting, perching, and hiding locations at different times of the day.[76] Hence, caretakers of more than one cat need to provide safe, comfortable, and private locations for each cat to avoid creating competition for scarce resources.

Reducing our feline patient's stress: The right way to set up a cage

1. **Select a top cage.** Cats feel safer when they are close to one's level. Top cages also help one avoid leaning over the patient, which can be threatening to cats.

2. **Cover the bottom of the cage completely.** Bare metal is cold, loud, and uncomfortable. Use cage pads to completely cover the bottom of the cage.

3. **A hiding box (or the cat's carrier)** gives patients both a place to hide in and a place to rest on.

4. **Bowls.** Put food and water bowls close to the opening of the hiding box, and as far away from the litter box as possible without interfering with access to the hiding box.

5. **Litter box.** Put the litter box in front of the hiding box and away from bowls. Use a generous amount of litter, enough for the cat to paw without "hitting bottom".

6. **Cover the cage door.** Place a cage pad over the cage door when your patient arrives in the ward to reduce stressful stimulation. Apply 10 sprays of Feliway* onto the pad, wait ~30 seconds for the alcohol to dissipate, then place the pad over the lower 2/3 of the cage to block their view, and so you can still observe them. Binder clips are available if the pad slips.

7. **Enrichment.** Feel free to add personal items from home, toys, and catnip as one sees fit so patients can enjoy their stay as much as possible!

*NEVER SPRAY FELIWAY SPRAY DIRECTLY ONTO THE CAT OR INTO THE CAGE WHILE THE CAT IS IN IT.

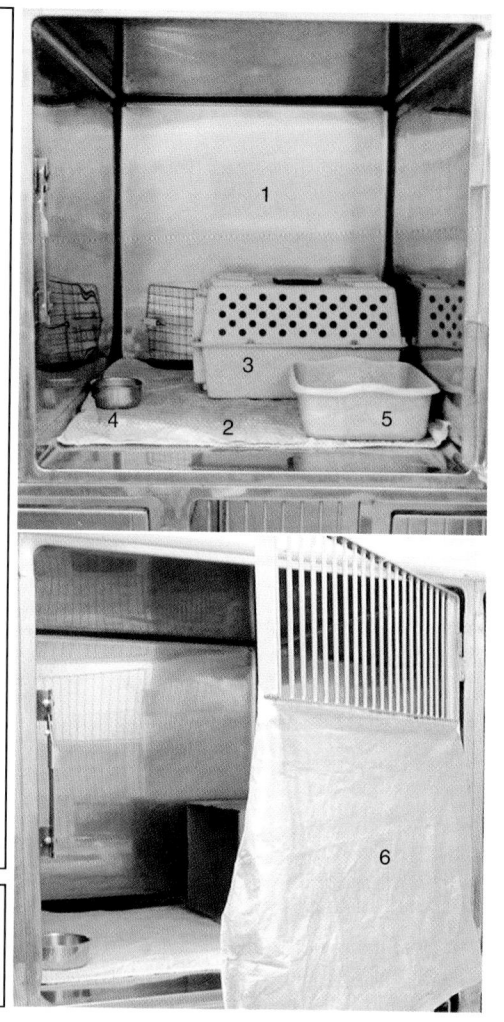

Figure 73-4: How to Set Up a Cage to Minimize Cat Distress. (Courtesy of The Ohio State University, College of Veterinary Medicine.)

Cats are a prey as well as a predator species, so climbing for observation and safe vantage is an important feline behavior. Cats seem to prefer to monitor their surroundings from elevated vantage points and appear to welcome provision of climbing frames, hammocks, platforms, raised walkways, shelves, or window seats.[71] Understanding this behavioral need permits care-takers to perceive the cat's climbing proclivity as natural and to enjoy providing acceptable opportunities for cats to climb.

Scratching and marking are species-typical behaviors of cats. Thus, providing appealing, appropriate objects to confined cats permits them to express these behaviors. Scratching behavior maintains claw health and leaves both visual and pheromonal territorial marks.[77] Different types and textures of scratching materials should be offered to permit the cat to express its preferences.

Other enrichments that can be offered include toys (rotated often to prevent habituation and boredom), music (played softly; less than 60 dB), catnip or grasses, food treats, supervised time outdoors, or if caged, playtime out of the cage with other cats (if they like other cats and being out of their cage), and extra attention from a familiar, dedicated person, such as brushing or playing.

Although guidelines for minimum cage size have been published,[53,54] true minimum requirements based on scientific evidence of diminished welfare when housed in a smaller cage have not been established for cats in either short- or long-term cage confinement. There has been much discussion

in the shelter community that cats require more than 0.56 m²
of floor space (6 square feet), but little scientific investigation
to make reliable recommendations. Studies conducted in
the authors' laboratory found that the quality of the environment was more relevant to the cat than the size of the cage
during both short and long periods of cage confinement.[32,33]
A study investigating the behavior of cats housed in cages
providing 1.1 m² (11.8 square feet) of floor space found no
improvements in sickness behaviors or adaptation to the
environment in the first 48 hours compared with cats housed
in cages half that size.[78] Although there must be a lower
limit to the size of cage a cat can be housed in and expected
to have reasonably good welfare, at this time the authors'
recommendations are to use a cage that is large enough to
comfortably provide the furnishings discussed earlier. For cats
housed in cages for longer periods of time in a shelter or
research facility, time to exercise out of the cage each day in
a play area is an option that worked well in the authors'
research colony (Figures 73-5).

The quality of human-cat interactions is another important aspect of the environment that needs to be investigated
to ensure the health and welfare of cats. Primates are a natural
predator of cats, and human beings are often the dominant
animate feature of many cats' environment. Repeated interactions between the cat and human occur, eventually allowing
each to make predictions about the other's behavior. The
quality (positive or negative) of the resulting human-animal
relationship likely determines the quality of the cat's (and the
owner's) life. Moreover, the human mostly determines the
number and nature of interactions and hence the quality of
the relationship. When put into the context of environmental
enrichment, human contact can meet the criteria that traditional environmental enrichment aims to meet: the identification and provision of the appropriate stimuli necessary for
the physiological and psychological well-being of captive
animals.[44] As with all other aspects of confinement, control
and predictability of care-taker behavior are of great importance to how the animal perceives humans. For example,
Hemsworth and colleagues[79] showed that intermittent
unpredictable negative handling of pigs (in a ratio of one
negative for every six positive exposures) led to pigs that were
as fearful toward humans and chronically stressed as were
pigs handled negatively all the time.

Research has identified the most aversive human behaviors toward animals to include hits, slaps, shouting, and fast
speed of movement. By contrast, positive interactive behaviors included pats, strokes, resting the hand on the animal,
talking to the animal, and slow deliberate movement.[80,81]
Avoiding punishment behaviors may be even more important
in cats than in other animal species with which humans
interact. Possibly because of their heritage as a relatively solitary species, cats do not appear to have developed some
behaviors typical of interactions among members of more
gregarious species. As with other animals, use of a soft voice
(and avoiding sounds that resemble hissing), indirect eye
contact (to avoid predatory gazing), displaying slow blinks
and movements, and letting the cat initiate and control the

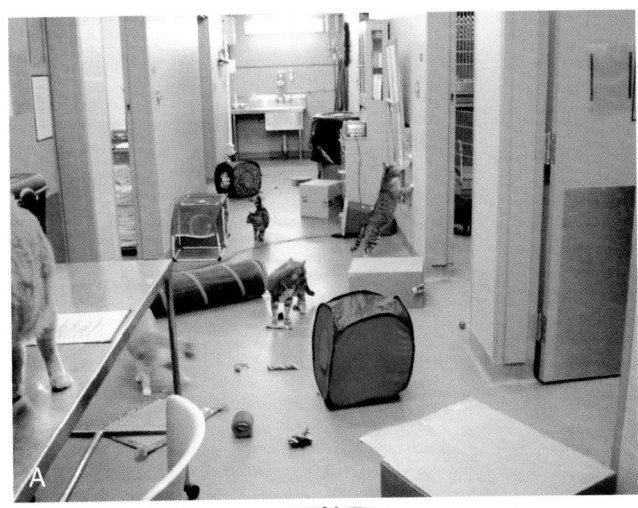

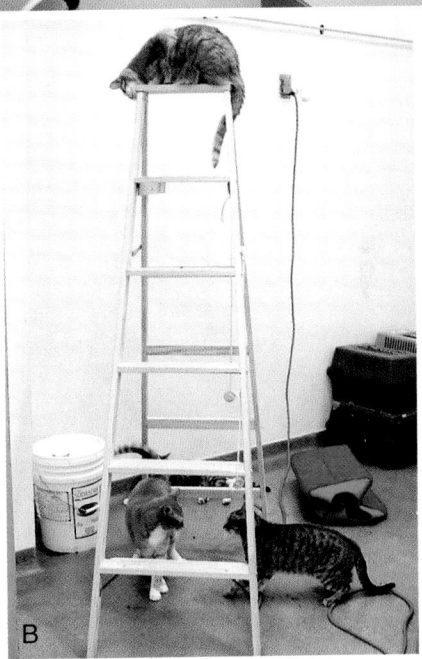

Figure 73-5: **A** and **B,** Research colony cats engaging in free play
time. Cats had access to boxes, tunnels, cubes, vertical and horizontal
scratching items, climbing opportunities, toys, classical music, and
interaction with conspecifics. A familiar care-taker supervised them
while cleaning litter pans and providing treats in their cages for
when they were returned to them. They received additional interaction, play, brushing, etc. from the familiar care-taker. All cats were
allowed to interact as desired; cage doors were opened, and they
could either come out to play or not as they wished.

extent of contact during initial interaction[82] reduce the probability of creating a perception of threat in the cat.

In effective cat management, a friendly, familiar person
appears to be crucial. Cats adapt more quickly and easily to
new environments when they see the same friendly person
each day. Studies have shown that animals can easily learn to
discriminate between two people.[83,84] If animals are able to
recognize and discriminate among the humans they regularly
come in contact with, then these same persons can become
predictors of salient events (food, pain) in animals' lives. This
is a classical conditioning response, in which the person
becomes the conditioned stimulus or predictor of the salient
event, and can be used to improve the animals' welfare. Wild

felids are considered sensitive to the captive environment, resulting in large numbers of abnormal behaviors and decreased reproductive success. Studies have shown this can be ameliorated by improved keeper-cat relationships. Mellon[84] found a positive correlation between the quality of interactions with the keeper and increased reproductive success in small captive felids. In addition, Wielebnowski and colleagues[85] found a negative correlation between fecal cortisol levels and the amount of time the primary keeper spent with clouded leopards and a positive correlation between fecal cortisol and the number of keepers. The interpretation of these results was that a higher number of keepers prevented the animals from forming and maintaining a predictable relationship with any keeper, thus increasing the stress of captivity.[85]

Given time constraints in many environments, the quality of human-animal interactions may be more important than the quantity of interactions. When a familiar person takes some time to pet, talk to, and offer food treats daily, the cat is more likely to respond positively when that person enters the room. The person also becomes familiar with the usual affect and behavior of the cat, and so can quickly recognize any changes in behavior that may signal a change in health or welfare. This is true in home environments as well as in more confined situations. The more threatening the environment, the more important a familiar person becomes to the cat's well-being. This may be of particular value for hospitalized patients. In fact, some feline practitioners "prescribe" daily nonmedical attention (petting, grooming, etc.) by a friendly human to enhance the welfare and recovery of their hospitalized patients. A Welfare Screening Checklist (Box 73-1) has been provided as an aid in applying the information discussed earlier in veterinary practice or the home environment.

LOW STRESS HANDLING

As stated earlier, cats are both a predator and a prey species. As such, they will use their teeth and claws to defend themselves when they feel threatened if they cannot run or hide. Even though one may have only the best intentions when performing husbandry and medical procedures, cats often perceive them as threatening. The use of low stress handling is important to both the handler and the cat. Cats are much easier (and more fun) to work with when they look forward to being handled. During husbandry this may be accomplished by letting the cat out of its cage during cleaning for some fun and exercise or by training the cat to sit on a perch by rewarding this behavior with food treats and praise. Cats can be offered high-value food, such as baby food or tuna, or be gently restrained using clipnosis[86] or a towel[87,88] during medical examinations and treatments, as well as for nail trimming and other grooming procedures. Having a familiar person handle the cat whenever possible or be present during threatening procedures also helps minimize the stress associated with the procedure. It is important to remember that

"less is more" when handling cats, both fewer people and less restraint. Cats should never be yelled at or punished because they can only perceive such behaviors as threatening. Proper evaluation of the level of distress the cat is experiencing will aid in identifying the proper tool to use; information presented in Figure 73-6 can be used as a guideline.

CONSPECIFIC SOCIAL INTERACTIONS

Free-living domestic cats tend to live in small groups consisting of related females and their young. Females will pool their kittens into crèche groups allowing all the young to be alloparented. In contrast, males are more solitary, tending to live on the margins of the group. Male cats typically hunt by themselves in larger home ranges and do not provide food to the female or offspring. In a study of households with two cats,[72] some 50% of time was spent out of one another's sight, even though they were most often within 1 to 3 m of each other. Cats thus may be unusually susceptible to health and welfare effects of indoor restriction and multicat households because of their relatively independent nature.

Additionally, cats do not appear to develop conflict resolution strategies to the extent that more gregarious species do, so they may attempt to circumvent agonistic encounters by avoiding others or decreasing their activity.[76] Cats prefer to have separate food and water sources, litter containers, and resting areas to avoid competition for resources, and to avoid unwanted interactions. Unrelated cats housed together in groups also appear to spend less time interacting with conspecifics than related ones do.[89] Published guidelines for introducing new cats into a home or group living system are available.[90]

When cats' perception of safety becomes threatened, they appear to respond in an attempt to restore "control." During such responses, some cats become aggressive, some become withdrawn, and some become ill. Conflict among cats can develop because of threats from other animals (including humans) or from cats outside the cage or house. With a little practice, one can recognize the signs of conflict; in this way, care-takers can act to reduce the intensity of the conflict by providing additional resources, including sanctuaries (e.g., a dedicated cat area, such as a spare room or "catio") or hiding or perching places. Of course some conflict within a group is normal, regardless of species. The goal is to reduce unhealthy conflict to attain a manageable level for the cats involved.

IMPLEMENTING CHANGE IN THE HOME ENVIRONMENT

The authors begin implementing changes by first reviewing each cat's basic needs systems: space, food and water, elimination areas, social contact, and body care and activity, using an extended evaluation questionnaire with the client (http://indoorpet.osu.edu/veterinarians/environmental-enrichment-resources-and-references).[91]

BOX 73-1 Welfare Screening Checklist

Cat Factors	Parameter	Description	Check (√) if Present
Behavioral	Position in cage	Front half, rear half, in litter pan, in hide box, on perch	
	Body posture	≥3 (Figure 73-6)	
	Behaviors indicative of negative affective state	*Fear, anxiety*: licks lips (nonappetitive), averts gaze, trembles, freezes, flattens body, feigns sleep, hides, attempts to hide, attempts to flee	
		Defensive aggression: hisses, growls, spits, tail twitches, ears flick, scratches, bites, crouched body, lunge	
	Behaviors indicative of positive affective state	*Affiliative*: approach, tail up, rub, meow, make eye contact, play, solicit attention, roll, knead	
		Maintenance: groom, rest, sleep, eat, drink, use litter pan	
Physiological	Respiratory rate	Increased	
	Pupil diameter	Increased	
	Paws	"Sweaty," leave marks on cage	
	Hair coat	Excessive shedding	
	Face	Flushing	
Cage Factors			
Intake	Food	Ate less than 50% of the offered food	
	Water	Did not drink	
Elimination	Urine	Urine deposited out of the litter pan	
	No urine	Did not urinate	
	Feces	Feces deposited out of the litter pan	
	No feces	Did not defecate	
Other sickness behaviors	Lower GI signs	Feces soft or diarrhea	
	Upper GI signs	Vomited hair, food, bile, or foreign material	
Cage	Resources moved	Food, water bowls, litter box, cage paper rearranged in cage	
Room Factors			
Sounds	Intensity	Loud (greater than 60 dB) machinery, other animals, humans or electronic (radio, television, etc.)	
Smells	Type, intensity	Other animals, cigarettes, cleaning products, perfumes, etc.	
Lights	Type, predictability	Unpredictably turned on and off when entering or exiting room, no consistent light-dark cycle	
Activity	Type, predictability	Unpredictable arrival or departure of humans (including care-takers) or other animals; inconsistent care-givers or caregiving	

GI, Gastrointestinal.

First, the authors thank the client for completing the form. Next, the authors identify any rows marked "Don't Know" and clarify the intended meaning for the client to get an answer. The authors then praise the owner for all "Yes" answers and explore the importance of any "No" answers. The authors' objective is never to "blame" the client for any deficiencies but to identify areas of improvement in the basic needs systems that the client believes are changeable.

If the presence of factors that can be changed to enrich the cat's environment are identified, a number of potential "solutions" can be found within each area. The authors present options to clients, saying something like, "These are things that have worked for other clients. They might work for you or stimulate your thinking about something that you can do in your setting". The reasons for this "menu-based" approach include (1) avoiding offering unworkable solutions, which are met with "yes, but..." by the client, (2) acknowledging the client's greater understanding of their home environment, and (3) creating "buy-in" to enhance adherence.

Once clients understand the benefits of change and have agreed on a goal, a set of clear objectives that are well defined, measurable, realistic, and time driven are developed. The

Score	Body Postures	Head Postures	Handling Procedures Counter Conditioning (CC)/Food[a]	Handling Procedures Level of restraint[b]	Handling Procedures Handling tools
1 Relaxed	**Activity** – sleeping or resting, alert or active, may be playing **Body** – lying on side, on belly or sitting; if standing or moving, back horizontal **Breathing** – slow to normal **Legs** – bent, hind legs may be laid out; when standing extended **Tail** – extended or loosely wrapped; up or loosely down when standing.	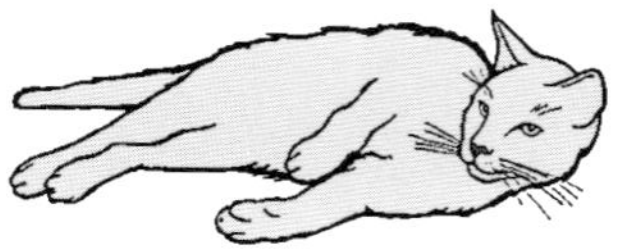 **Head** – laid on surface or over body, some movement **Eyes** – closed to open, pupils slit to normal size **Ears** – normal to forward **Whiskers** – normal to forward **Sounds** –none, purr	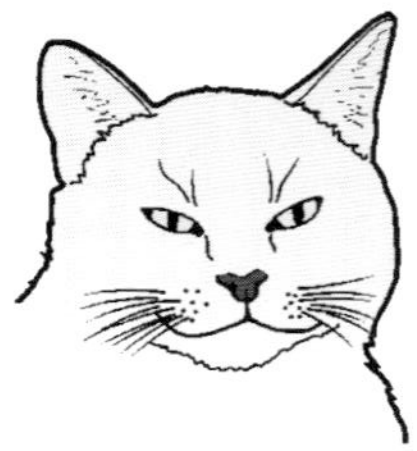 +++	Light	Food, Pheromones, Carrier
2 Alert	**Activity** – resting, awake, or actively exploring **Body** – lying on belly or sitting; if standing or moving the back is horizontal **Breathing** – normal **Legs** – bent; when standing extended **Tail** – on body or curved back; up or tense downwards when standing; may be twitching	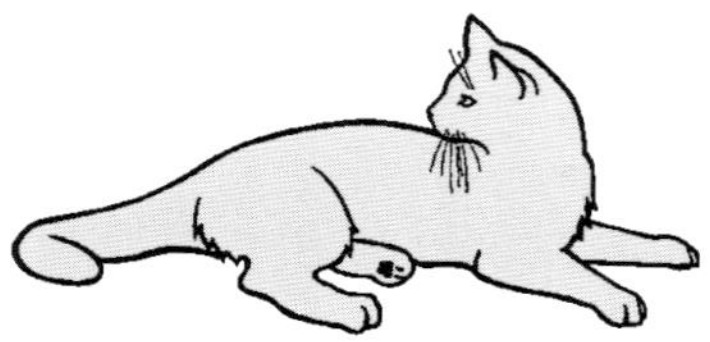 **Head** – over the body, some movement **Eyes** – open normally, pupils normal **Ears** – normal or erected to front or back **Whiskers** – normal to forward **Sounds** – none or meow	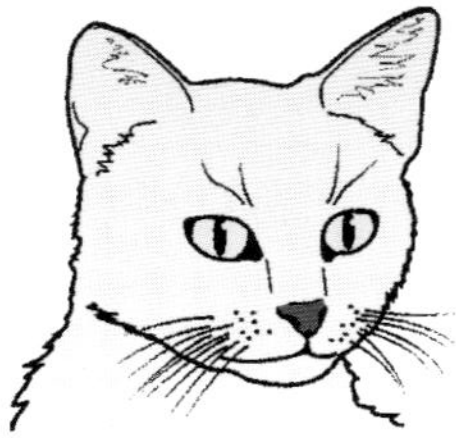 +++	Light	Food, Pheromones, Clipnosis, Calming Cap, Carrier
3 Tense	**Activity** – resting or alert, may be actively exploring, trying to escape **Body** – lying on belly or sitting; if standing or moving the back of the body is lower than the front ("slinking") **Breathing** – normal **Legs** – bent, hind legs bent and front legs extended when standing **Tail** – close to body; tense downwards or curled forward, may be twitching when standing.	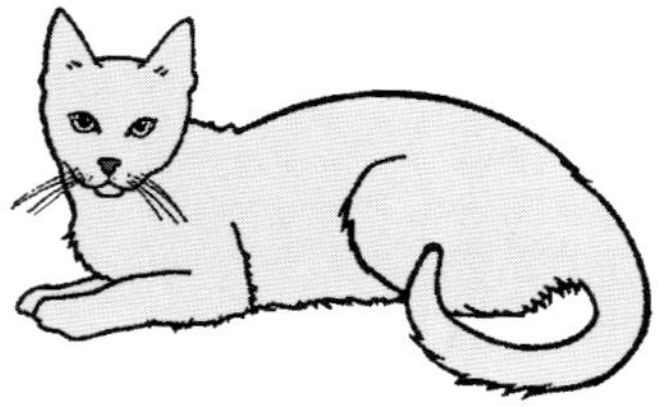 **Head** – over the body or pressed to body, little or no movement **Eyes** – wide open or pressed together, pupils normal to partially dilated **Ears** – erected to front or back **Whiskers** – normal to forward **Sounds** – none, meow, or plaintive meow	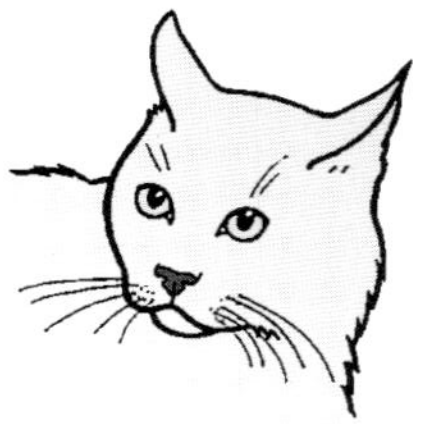 ++	Intermediate/chemical	Food, Pheromones, Clipnosis, Towel, Calming Cap, Thunder Shirt, Carrier

[a]Assuming the cat can eat. Cats with increasing levels of distress often will not eat even highly palatable food.

[b]If the pet struggles in response to restraint for longer than 3 seconds, stop, reposition, and try again. Wait until the pet has relaxed, and preferably has started eating, before beginning the procedure. If after two to three attempts the patient does not relax and/or becomes fractious, stop and consider whether the procedure is essential. If it is nonessential, send the animal home and create a plan for a more successful visit the following day.

Figure 73-6: Low stress handling for cats. This table summarizes, but does not replace, recommendations for low stress handling. It assumes a relatively healthy cat and a relatively inexperienced handler. The goal of low stress handling is to choose the least stressful handling procedure for the cat after determining its current stress score and to do everything possible to ensure that the patient's stress score improves (becomes lower) during interactions with it. (From Herron ME, Shreyer T: The pet-friendly veterinary practice: a guide for practitioners. *Vet Clin N Am Small Anim Pract* 44:451–481, 2014.)

Score	Body Postures	Head Postures	Counter Conditioning (CC)/Food[a]	Level of restraint[b]	Handling tools
4 Anxious	**Activity** – alert, may be actively trying to escape **Body** – lying on belly or sitting; if standing or moving the back of the body is lower than the front **Breathing** – normal or fast **Legs** – under body, bent when standing **Tail** – close to the body; may be curled forward close to body when standing. Tip may move up and down or side to side.	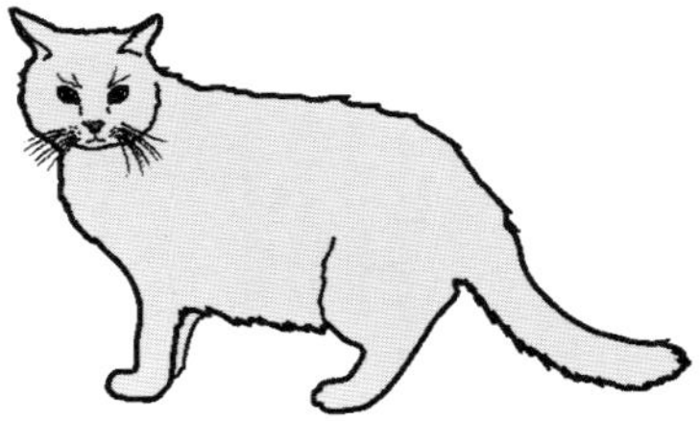 **Head** – on the plane of the body, little or no movement **Eyes** – wide open, pupils dilated **Ears** – partially flattened **Whiskers** – normal to forward or back **Sounds** – none, plaintive meow, growling, yowling	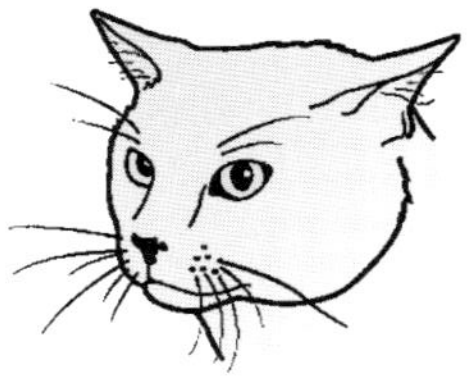 +	Firm/ chemical	Food, Pheromones, "Burrito" wrap, Muzzle, Carrier
5 Fearful	**Activity** – motionless, alert, or crawling **Body** – lying on belly or crouched directly on top of all paws, may be shaking; if standing the whole body is near to the ground, may be shaking **Breathing** – fast **Legs** – bent; when standing bent near to surface **Tail** – close to the body; curled forward close to the body when standing.	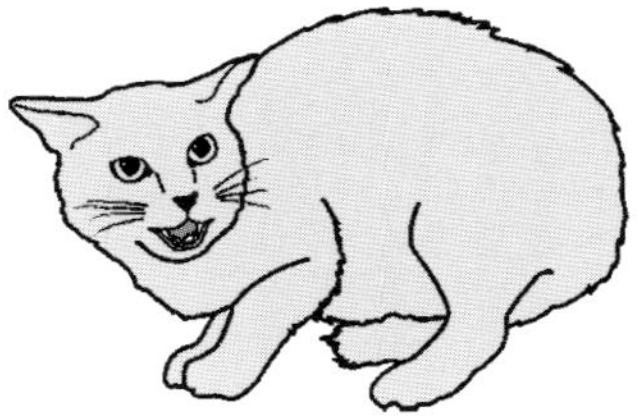 **Head** – near to surface motionless **Eyes** – fully open, pupils fully dilated **Ears** – fully flattened **Whiskers** – back **Sounds** – none, plaintive meow, growling, yowling	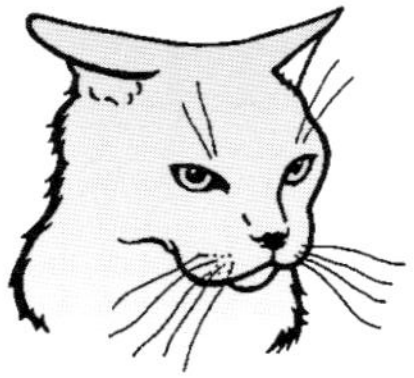 –	Chemical	Pheromones, Muzzle, EZ nabber, Towel, Carrier
6 Terrified	**Activity** – motionless alert **Body** – crouched directly on top of all paws, shaking. Hair on back and tail bushy. **Breathing** – fast **Legs** – stiff or bent to increase apparent size **Tail** – close to body	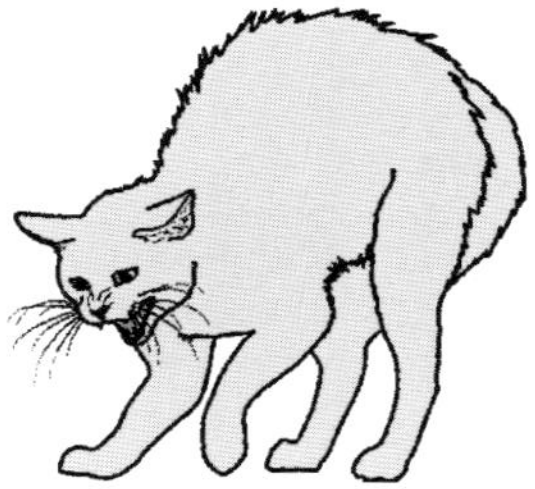 **Head** – lower than the body **Eyes** – fully opened, pupils fully dilated **Ears** – fully flattened, back on head **Whiskers** – back **Sounds** – none, plaintive meow, growling, yowling, hissing	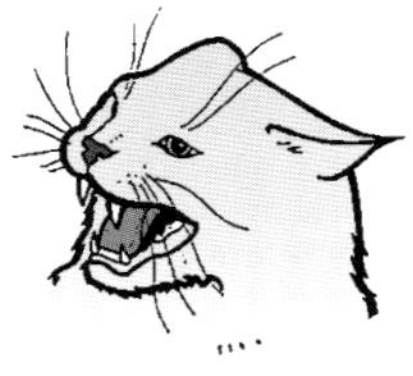 –	Chemical	Pheromones, Muzzle, EZ nabber, Towel, Carrier

[a]Assuming the cat can eat. Cats with increasing levels of distress often will not eat even highly palatable food.
[b]If the pet struggles in response to restraint for longer than 3 seconds, stop, reposition, and try again. Wait until the pet has relaxed, and preferably has started eating, before beginning the procedure. If after two to three attempts the patient does not relax and/or becomes fractious, stop and consider whether the procedure is essential. If it is essential, make a plan for chemical restraint; if it is nonessential, send the animal home and create a plan for a more successful visit the following day.

Figure 73-6: cont'd

authors recommend use of a simple process called "SMARTR" goals for writing down goals to help to assure that they are clearly communicated, well defined, and agreed upon by all involved in the change.[57]

SMARTR goals are Specific, Measureable, Action-oriented, Realistic, Time-Driven/Timely, and Rewarded. A number of factors can be used to enhance the success of SMARTR plans. These include writing goals in positive terms, ensuring that the SMARTR goals are the *client's* goals rather than one's own, posting the plan in a prominent place so clients and others in the household can stay focused, and staying flexible as situations change when life circumstances change. If a SMARTR plan becomes unrealistic, it must be changed. The key is to be clear on the objective to be achieved and willing to change tactics to match changing situations by making another SMARTR plan as necessary to achieve and sustain success.

One of the critical keys to any successful MEMO program is to follow the client's progress, providing praise for success and coaching for setbacks, as appropriate. The authors tell clients what the follow-up schedule is and ask them to agree to a preferred method (telephone, email) and time to be contacted by a technician familiar with the case. The first contact with the client occurs within a week after initial recommendations are made, with follow-up evaluations (whether by telephone or office appointment) at roughly 3 to 6 weeks, 3 months, 6 months, and 1 year, depending on progress and circumstances. This allows the authors to monitor the patient's progress, make adjustments as needed, and continue to support and motivate the client. It also helps alert the authors when the owner is becoming frustrated or having problems with the plan so that the authors can provide encouragement or suggestions to help to keep them on the plan and to praise their successes.[57]

SUMMARY

Many confined cats appear to tolerate relatively barren housing environments. However, the authors are concerned more with optimizing the environments of confined cats than with identifying minimum requirements for survival. Cats have a variety of unique behaviors and needs, so the authors encourage caretakers to set up the cats in their care for success by providing a diverse, enriched environment free from physical, psychological, and social stressors. The authors' current approach to implementation of MEMO in homes is to let the client identify the most appropriate intervention for their particular situation and then to help them create and implement an effective plan for change.[92] How this approach and its value are communicated, both verbally and nonverbally, is directly related to the prognosis for success. The effectiveness of environmental enrichment efforts ultimately depend on parameters of the cat, the housing situation, the care-taker, and the quality and dedication of the veterinary team overseeing and supporting the efforts.

References

1. Awofeso N: Re-defining "Health." World Health Organization Bulletin Board. <http://www.who.int/bulletin/bulletin_board/83/ustun11051/en>, 2005 (Accessed July 5, 2015).
2. World Organization for Animal Health. Terrestrial Animal Health Code. <http://www.oie.int/en/international-standard-setting/terrestrial-code>, 2014 (Accessed July 5, 2015).
3. McEwen BS: Brain on stress: how the social environment gets under the skin. *Proc Natl Acad Sci U S A* 109(Suppl 2):17180–17185, 2012.
4. McEwen BS: The brain on stress: toward an integrative approach to brain, body, and behavior. *Perspect Psychol Sci* 8:673–675, 2013.
5. Pacak K, Palkovits M: Stressor specificity of central neuroendocrine responses: implications for stress-related disorders. *Endocr Rev* 22:502–548, 2001.
6. Carlstead K, Brown JL, Strawn W: Behavioral and physiological correlates of stress in laboratory cats. *Appl Anim Behav Sci* 38:143–158, 1993.
7. Belew AM, Barlett T, Brown SA: Evaluation of the white-coat effect in cats. *J Vet Intern Med* 13:134–142, 1999.
8. Buffington CAT, Westropp JL, Chew DJ: From FUS to Pandora syndrome. *J Feline Med Surg* 16:385–394, 2014.
9. Paus R, Theoharides TC, Arck PC: Neuroimmunoendocrine circuitry of the "brain-skin connection." *Trends Immunol* 27:32–39, 2006.
10. Funakoshi K, Nakano M, Atobe Y, et al: Differential development of TRPV1-expressing sensory nerves in peripheral organs. *Cell Tissue Res* 323:27–41, 2006.
11. Birder LA: Urinary bladder urothelium: molecular sensors of chemical/thermal/mechanical stimuli. *Vascul Pharmacol* 45:221–226, 2006.
12. Kovacs KJ: CRH: The link between hormonal, metabolic and behavioral responses to stress. *J Chem Neuroanat* 54:25–33, 2013.
13. Buffington CAT: Comorbidity of interstitial cystitis with other unexplained clinical conditions. *J Urol* 172:1242–1248, 2004.
14. Davis M: Neural systems involved in fear and anxiety measured with fear-potentiated startle. *Am Psychol* 61:741–756, 2006.
15. Buffington CAT, Pacak K: Increased plasma norepinephrine concentration in cats with interstitial cystitis. *J Urol* 165:2051–2054, 2001.
16. Westropp JL, Kass PH, Buffington CAT: Evaluation of the effects of stress in cats with idiopathic cystitis. *Am J Vet Res* 67:731–736, 2006.
17. Westropp JL, Kass PH, Buffington CAT: *In vivo* evaluation of the alpha(2)-adrenoceptors in cats with idiopathic cystitis. *Am J Vet Res* 68:203–207, 2007.
18. Buffington CAT, Teng BY, Somogyi GT: Norepinephrine content and adrenoceptor function in the bladder of cats with feline interstitial cystitis. *J Urol* 167:1876–1880, 2002.
19. Westropp JL, Buffington CAT: Cerebrospinal fluid corticotrophin releasing factor and catecholamine concentrations in healthy cats and cats with interstitial cystitis. In *Proceedings: Research insights into interstitial cystitis: a basic and clinical science symposium*, Alexandria, 2003, Virginia, p 74.
20. Welk KA, Buffington CAT: Effect of interstitial cystitis on central neuropeptide and receptor immunoreactivity in cats. In *Research insights into interstitial cystitis: a basic and clinical science symposium*, Alexandria, 2003, Virginia, p 74.
21. Westropp JL, Buffington CAT: Effect of a corticotropin releasing factor (CRF) antagonist on hypothalamic-pituitary-adrenal activation in response to CRF in cats with interstitial cystitis. In *Research insights into interstitial cystitis: a basic and clinical science symposium*, Alexandria, 2003, Virginia, p 74.
22. Raison CL, Miller AH: When not enough is too much: the role of insufficient glucocorticoid signaling in the pathophysiology of stress-related disorders. *Am J Psychiatry* 160:1554–1565, 2003.
23. Westropp JL, Welk KA, Buffington CAT: Small adrenal glands in cats with feline

interstitial cystitis. *J Urol* 170:2494–2497, 2003.

24. Schommer NC, Hellhammer DH, Kirschbaum C: Dissociation between reactivity of the hypothalamus-pituitary-adrenal axis and the sympathetic-adrenal-medullary system to repeated psychosocial stress. *Psychosom Med* 65:450–460, 2003.

25. Kvetnansky R, Fukuhara K, Pacak K, et al: Endogenous glucocorticoids restrain catecholamine synthesis and release at rest and during immobilization stress in rats. *Endocrinology* 133:1411–1419, 1993.

26. Buffington CAT, Chew DJ, Woodworth BE, et al: Idiopathic cystitis in cats: an animal model of interstitial cystitis. In Sant GR, editor: *Interstitial cystitis*, Philadelphia, 1997, Lippincott-Raven, pp 25–31.

27. Buffington CAT, Chew DJ, Woodworth BE: Animal model of human disease—feline interstitial cystitis. *Comp Path Bull* 29:3–6, 1997.

28. Theoharides TC, Cochrane DE: Critical role of mast cells in inflammatory diseases and the effect of acute stress. *J Neuroimmunol* 146:1–12, 2004.

29. Rohleder N: Stimulation of systemic low-grade inflammation by psychosocial stress. *Psychosom Med* 76:181–189, 2014.

30. Dantzer R, O'Connor JC, Freund GG, et al: From inflammation to sickness and depression: when the immune system subjugates the brain. *Nat Rev Neurosci* 9:46–56, 2008.

31. Carlstead K, Shepherdson DS: Alleviating stress in zoos with environmental enrichment. In Moberg GP, Mench JA, editors: *The biology of animal stress: basic principles and implications for animal welfare*, New York, 2000, CABI Publishing, pp 337–354.

32. Stella JL, Lord LK, Buffington CAT: Sickness behaviors in response to unusual external events in healthy cats and cats with feline interstitial cystitis. *J Am Vet Med Assoc* 238:67–73, 2011.

33. Stella J, Croney C, Buffington T: Environmental factors that affect the behavior and welfare of domestic cats (*Felis silvestris catus*) housed in cages. *Appl Anim Behav Sci* 160:94–105, 2014.

34. Buffington CAT, Westropp JL, Chew DJ, et al: A case-control study of indoor-housed cats with lower urinary tract signs. *J Am Vet Med Assoc* 228:722–725, 2006.

35. Buffington CAT, Westropp JL, Chew DJ, et al: Clinical evaluation of multimodal environmental modification (MEMO) in the management of cats with idiopathic cystitis. *J Feline Med Surg* 8:261–268, 2006.

36. Buffington CAT, unpublished observations.

37. Schore AN: Back to basics: attachment, affect regulation, and the developing right brain: linking developmental neuroscience to pediatrics. *Pediatr Rev* 26:204–217, 2005.

38. Anderson NB: Levels of analysis in health science—a framework for integrating sociobehavioral and biomedical research. *Neuroimmunomodulation* 840:563–576, 1998.

39. Peters A, McEwen BS: Special issue: allostasis and allostatic load introduction. *Physiol Behav* 106:1–4, 2012.

40. Chelimsky G, Heller E, Buffington CA, et al: Co-morbidities of interstitial cystitis. *Front Neurosci* 6:114, 2012.

41. Buffington CA, Chew DJ: Intermittent alkaline urine in a cat fed an acidifying diet. *J Am Vet Med Assoc* 209:103–104, 1996.

42. Belew AM, Barlett T, Brown SA: Evaluation of the white-coat effect in cats. *J Vet Intern Med* 13:134–142, 1999.

43. Quimby JM, Smith ML, Lunn KF: Evaluation of the effects of hospital visit stress on physiologic parameters in the cat. *J Feline Med Surg* 13:733–737, 2011.

44. Young R: *Environmental enrichment for captive animals*, Oxford, 2003, Blackwell.

45. Cao L, Choi EY, Liu X, et al: White to brown fat phenotypic switch induced by genetic and environmental activation of a hypothalamic-adipocyte axis. *Cell Metab* 14:324–338, 2011.

46. Benaroya-milshtein N, Hollander N, Apter A, et al: Environmental enrichment in mice decreases anxiety, attenuates stress responses and enhances natural killer cell activity. *Eur J Neurosci* 20:1341–1347, 2004.

47. Cao L, During MJ: What is the brain-cancer connection? *Annu Rev Neurosci* 35:331–345, 2012.

48. Pham T, Soderstrom S, Winblad B, et al: Effects of environmental enrichment on cognitive function and hippocampal NGF in non-handled rats. *Behav Brain Res* 103:63–70, 1999.

49. Gross A, Richter S, Engel K, et al: Cage-induced stereotypies, perseveration and the effects of environmental enrichment in laboratory mice. *Behav Brain Res* 234:61–68, 2012.

50. Turner DC: Social organisation and behavioral ecology of free-roaming domestic cats. In Turner DC, Batson P, editors: *The domestic cat: the biology of its behavior*, ed 3, Cambridge, 2014, Cambridge University Press.

51. Buffington CAT: External and internal influences on disease risk in cats. *J Am Vet Med Assoc* 220:994–1002, 2002.

52. Rochlitz I: Recommendations for the housing of cats in the home, in catteries and animal shelters, in laboratories and in veterinary surgeries. *J Feline Med Surg* 1:181–191, 1999.

53. NRC, National Research Council: *Guide for the Care and Use of Laboratory Animals*, Washington, DC, 2013, National Academy Press.

54. Association of Shelter Veterinarians, Guidelines for Standards of Care in Animal Shelters. <http://www.sheltervet.org/assets/docs/shelter-standards-oct2011-wforward.pdf>, 2014 (Accessed June 3, 2015).

55. Morgan KN, Tromborg CT: Sources of stress in captivity. *Appl Anim Behav Sci* 102:262–302, 2007.

56. Ellis SLH, Wells DL: The influence of olfactory stimulation on the behaviour of cats housed in a rescue shelter. *Appl Anim Behav Sci* 123:56–62, 2010.

57. NRC, National Research Council: *Nutrient requirements for dogs and cats*, Washington, DC, 2006, National Academy Press, p 2006.

58. Bradshaw JWS, Thorne CJ: Feeding behaviour. In Thorne CJ, editor: *Waltham book of dog and cat behaviour*, Oxford, 1992, Pergamon, pp 115–129.

59. Morris JG: Idiosyncratic nutrient requirements of cats appear to be diet-induced evolutionary adaptations. *Nutr Res Rev* 15:153–168, 2002.

60. Kienzle E, Bergler R: Human-animal relationship of owners of normal and overweight cats. *J Nutr* 136:1947S–1950S, 2006.

61. Ellis SL: Environmental enrichment: practical strategies for improving feline welfare. *J Feline Med Surg* 11:901–912, 2009.

62. Hoyumpa Vogt A, Rodan I, Brown M, et al: AAFP-AAHA: feline life stage guidelines. *J Feline Med Surg* 12:43–54, 2010.

63. Hewson-Hughes AK, Hewson-Hughes VL, Colyer A, et al: Consistent proportional macronutrient intake selected by adult domestic cats (*Felis catus*) despite variations in macronutrient and moisture content of foods offered. *J Comp Physiol [B]* 183:525–536, 2013.

64. Laflamme DP, Hannah SS: Discrepancy between use of lean body mass or nitrogen balance to determine protein requirements for adult cats. *J Feline Med Surg* 15:691–697, 2013.

65. Bradshaw JW: The evolutionary basis for the feeding behavior of domestic dogs (*Canis familiaris*) and cats (*Felis catus*). *J Nutr* 136:1927S–1931S, 2006.

66. Guy NC, Hopson M, Vanderstichel R: Litterbox size preference in domestic cats (*Felis catus*). *J Vet Behav Clin Appl Res* 9:78–82, 2014.

67. Grigg EK, Pick L, Nibblett B: Litter box preference in domestic cats: covered versus uncovered. *J Feline Med Surg* 15:280–284, 2013.

68. Neilson J: Thinking outside the box: feline elimination. *J Feline Med Surg* 6:5–11, 2004.

69. Horwitz DF: Behavioral and environmental factors associated with elimination behavior problems in cats: a retrospective study. *Appl Anim Behav Sci* 52:129–137, 1997.

70. Borchelt PL: Cat elimination behavior problems. *Vet Clin North Am Small Anim Pract* 21:257–264, 1991.

71. Roclitz I: Feline welfare issues. In Turner DC, Bateson P, editors: *The domestic cat: the biology of its behavior*, ed 2, Cambridge, 2000, Cambridge University Press, pp 207–226.

72. Gourkow N, Fraser D: The effect of housing and handling practices on the welfare, behaviour and selection of domestic cats (*Felis sylvestris catus*) by adopters in an animal shelter. *Anim Welf* 15:371–377, 2006.

73. Kry K, Casey R: The effect of hiding enrichment on stress levels and behaviour of domestic cats (*Felis sylvestris catus*) in a shelter setting and the implications for adoption potential. *Anim Welf* 16:375–383, 2007.

74. Crouse SJ, Atwill ER, Lagana M, et al: Soft surfaces: a factor in feline psychological well-being. *Contemp Top Lab Anim Sci* 34:94–97, 1995.

75. Barry KJ, Crowell-Davis SL: Gender differences in the social behavior of the neutered indoor-only domestic cat. *Appl Anim Behav Sci* 64:193–211, 1999.

76. Bernstein PL, Strack M: A game of cat and house: spatial patterns and behavior of 14

domestic cats (*Felis catus*) in the home. *Anthrozoos* 9:25–39, 1996.

77. Landsberg GM, Hunthausen W, Ackerman L: Feline destructive behaviors. In Landsberg GM, Hunthausen W, Ackerman L, editors: *Handbook of behavior problems of the dog and cat*, ed 2, Philadelphia, 2003, Elsevier, pp 341–347.

78. Stella J: Environmental factors that affect the behavior and welfare of domestic cats (*Felis silvestris catus*) housed in cages, PhD Thesis, 2013.

79. Hemsworth PH, Barnett JL, Hansen C: The influence of inconsistent handling by humans on the behaviour, growth and corticosteroids of young pigs. *Appl Anim Behav Sci* 17:245–252, 1987.

80. Coleman GJ, Hemsworth PH, Hay M: Predicting stockperson behaviour towards pigs from attitudinal and job-related variables and empathy. *Appl Anim Behav Sci* 58:63–75, 1998.

81. Pajor EA, Rushen J, de Passillé AMB: Aversion learning techniques to evaluate dairy cattle handling practices. *Appl Anim Behav Sci* 69:89–102, 2000.

82. Turner DC: The ethology of the human-cat relationship. *Schweiz Arch Tierheilkd* 133:63–70, 1991.

83. Davis H, Taylor A: Discrimination between individual humans by domestic fowl (*Gallus gallus domesticus*). *Br Poult Sci* 42:276–279, 2011.

84. Mellen JD: Factors influencing reproductive success in small captive exotic felids (*Felis spp.*): a multiple regression analysis. *Zoo Biol* 10:95–110, 1991.

85. Wielebnowski NC, Fletchall N, Carlstead K, et al: Noninvasive assessment of adrenal activity associated with husbandry and behavioral factors in the North American clouded leopard population. *Zoo Biol* 21:77–98, 2002.

86. Pozza ME, Stella JL, Chappuis-Gagnon AC, et al: Pinch-induced behavioral inhibition ("clipnosis") in domestic cats. *J Feline Med Surg* 10:82–87, 2008.

87. Herron ME, Shreyer T: The pet-friendly veterinary practice: a guide for practitioners. *Vet Clin North Am Small Anim Pract* 44:451–481, 2014.

88. Yin S: *Low stress handling, restraint and behavior modification of dogs and cats: techniques for developing patients who love their visits*, Davis, 2009, Cattle Dog Publishing.

89. Bradshaw JWS, Hall SL: Affiliative behaviour of related and unrelated pairs of cats in catteries: a preliminary report. *Appl Anim Behav Sci* 63:251–255, 1999.

90. Bohnenkamp G: *From the cat's point of view*, San Francisco, 1991, Perfect Paws.

91. Herron ME, Buffington CA: Environmental enrichment for indoor cats: implementing enrichment. *Compend Contin Educ Vet* 34:E3, 2012.

92. Buffington T: Cat Mastery, iBook. <https://itunes.apple.com/us/book/catmastery/id859588058?mt=11>, 2014. (Accessed November 9, 2014).

93. McMillan FD: Stress-induced and emotional eating in animals: a review of the experimental evidence and implications for companion animal obesity. *J Vet Behav* 8:376–385, 2013.

94. Weiss JM: Effects of coping behavior in different warning signal conditions on stress pathology in rats. *J Comp Physiol Psychol* 77:1–13, 1971.

95. Weiss JM: Psychological factors in stress and disease. *Sci Am* 226:104–113, 1972.

96. Anseeuw E, Apker C, Ayscue C, et al: Handling cats humanely in the veterinary hospital. *J Vet Behav Clin Appl Res* 1:84–88, 2006.

97. Rodan I: Understanding feline behavior and application for appropriate handling and management. *Top Companion Anim Med* 25:178–188, 2010.

98. Rodan I, Sundahl E, Carney H, et al: AAFP and ISFM feline-friendly handling guidelines. *J Feline Med Surg* 13:364–375, 2011.

Population Structure and Genetic Testing in Cats

Leslie A. Lyons

Genetic testing is a key component for state-of-the-art healthcare. Since the 1960s, direct DNA disease-causing variant testing has been performed on newborn humans for rapid detection of inborn errors of metabolism.[1] Each state in the United States and various countries worldwide tailor their now more extensive newborn DNA screening programs to detect the common disease-causing variants found in their region's most predominant ethnic groups. The same high standard of healthcare is available for companion animals, including cats, with breeds being analogous to human ethnic groups and races. Dozens of DNA disease-causing variants have been identified in cats that are pertinent to specific breeds. Because controlled breeding is routine in pedigreed cats, the potential for a higher standard of healthcare is even greater than in humans as genetic testing can be used to prevent the mating of individual cats that might produce unhealthy or undesired offspring.

An excellent example of proper genetic management of health concerns within a breed is the control of two different lysosomal storage diseases (gangliosidoses) in Korat cats. Korats are a specific color variant of street cats from Thailand.[2,3] Korats come in one color, solid blue, but they are from a diverse population of cats that have recessive variants for brown *(TYRP1: b)* and the Siamese-points variant *(TYR: c^s)*. Because Korats are derived from streets cats, their foundation seems to have had significant genetic variety. Breeders did their best to avoid producing Siamese-pointed and brown variant cats just by using pedigree analyses; they learned not to breed carriers together. However, in the early 1970s, a Siamese cat with a progressive neurologic motor disability was shown to have extensive neuronal degeneration caused by the accumulation of GM1 ganglioside in its tissues.[4] The presentation was suggested to have autosomal recessive inheritance and was one of the first cat models for a human inborn error of metabolism.[5] Korats, which come from the same street population of Thai cats as the Siamese, also presented with the same disease. A second type of gangliosidosis, beta-hexosaminidase deficiency, was later recognized in Korats demonstrating neurologic deficiencies due to GM2 ganglioside accumulation in the lysosomes.[6] Until the DNA disease-causing variants were discovered for these traits, Siamese and Korat breeders managed these diseases in their populations (like their undesired color variants) by pedigree analyses, trying their best to not breed together two

carriers of an undesired trait. However, the Siamese breed has historically been a very popular breed and present since the inception of the cat fancy, whereas the Korat was accepted in the 1960s and has had a small breed population size.[7-9] Siamese breeders eradicated gangliosidoses from the breed by strong selection against specific family lines, because the breed population was large and the disease variant was rare. Thus, the population could withstand this minor genetic reduction. However, the Korat breeders have used pedigree analyses and genetic testing to maintain the undesired variants (chocolate, Siamese points, GM1 and GM2) by not breeding carrier cats together. Korats now have minimal, if any, disease presentation and have actually a higher level of overall genetic diversity than many cat breeds, including the Siamese.[10] This is the perfect scenario, where genetic testing is used wisely to slowly eliminate undesired variants but maintain genetic diversity at the same time.

Whole genome sequencing of individual patients is becoming routine in human medicine and is likely to become a part of routine healthcare management within one's lifetime.[11] Hence, the novel disease-causing variants that cause children to have what appear to be sporadic and random health issues and dysmorphologies may be readily detected, providing a reason for their devastating congenital defects. Similarly, whole genome sequencing of individual cats has been initiated, suggesting the possibility of routine use for feline health management in the future. This chapter reviews the breeds and races of domestic cats and the pertinent genetic disease-causing variants that should be monitored for their healthcare. The current power and limitations of whole genome sequencing of individual patients is presented, as well as concerns with genetic counseling and management of breeding programs. A description of genetic terminology is found in Box 74-1.

GENETIC STRUCTURE OF THE CAT POPULATION

The earliest archeological evidence for cat associations with humans has been dated from 3000 to 6000 BC in Cyprus,[12-14] Egypt,[15] and China.[16] Whether cats migrated to these different regions with trade and agriculture or if regional wildcats were independently domesticated in different parts of the Old World remains an unresolved mystery. Since these early

BOX 74-1 Genes, Loci, and Alleles

A gene for a trait is made up of DNA, which produces a protein that gives rise (directly or indirectly) to the trait of interest. A *locus* refers to the place on the chromosome, within the DNA sequence, that the gene is localized. For example, it was known there was a region in the cat genome that controlled when the yellow and black pigment would be turned on and off during the production of a hair. That locus is known as *agouti*. A given DNA sequence for a gene is called an *allele*. The normal allele for *agouti* was defined as "A^+", and the variant was defined as "*a.*" Lowercase letters imply recessive alleles; uppercase letters imply dominant alleles. Thus, to get a non-agouti (solid color) cat, it must have two copies of the variant allele, "*aa.*" Once it is learned what protein was produced by the given gene at a specific locus, the gene name is then redefined after a function of the protein. *Agouti* is defined by the gene termed *agouti-signaling protein*, which is abbreviated to *ASIP*. In cats, *ASIP* has two alleles, A^+ and *a*. Alleles, loci, and gene names are written in italics, but the actual protein is written in normal font. The wild-type allele is designated by a superscript +, which can be an allele with any inheritance pattern. Additional alleles at a gene can be indicated by other superscript letters that help define the effect. For *Agouti*, the A^{Pbe} allele indicates that this is the agouti allele from the leopard cat *(Prionailurus bengalensis [Pbe])* that is found in the Bengal cat breed.

times, cats have continued their friendship and symbiotic relationship with humans, providing vermin control while gaining low energy expenditure for meals.[12,17-19]

As trade and exploration opened new opportunities and resources for humans, the cat expanded its territory around the world as people's constant but often inconspicuous companion.[20,21] However, similar to the formation of human ethnic groups and races, complete panmictic (random) worldwide breeding has not been possible for the cat, because it is limited by natural boundaries, few founders, and sporadic migrations. Thus, disease-causing variants and allele frequencies differ among cat populations, thereby forming races and breeds. Genetic studies of worldwide feral cat populations and breeds have shed light on the population structure of domestic cats,[10] providing important clues to their genetic identity and genetic health management.

Genetic Races of Domestic Cats

The domestic cat likely derived from one or more subspecies of wildcat *(Felis silvestris)*.[22] At least one domestication event for the cat was very likely to have taken place in the Near East;[23] however, independent domestications may be plausible due to the significant genetic distinction of cats in the Far East and the archeological find in China that associates cats with humans in an ancient agricultural site.[16] Different domestication events from many, and perhaps different, subspecies of wildcats implies high genetic diversity for the

founding population(s) of domestic cats. Such diversity should support health and the ability to adapt to different niches and physiological insults. Without archeological samples with sufficient DNA to analyze, only the present day populations of cats can be examined to evaluate genetic diversity and population differentiations. This genetic data can allow the potential extrapolation back to the number and different sites of cat domestication. Regardless of the cat's ancient history, the present day feline populations are the concern of owners, breeders, and veterinarians.

Worldwide cat populations have been genetically examined to define the differences that may be important for genetic-based health management.[10] Different genetic markers, such as mitochondrial DNA (mtDNA),[24] short tandem repeats (STRs, or microsatellites),[10,25] and single-nucleotide polymorphisms (SNPs),[26] all have different "genetic clocks" and examine different time points in domestic cat history and evolution.[23,27] The combined analysis of these different markers paints a picture of the present geographical demarcations and genetic distinction of cat populations. To date, several published studies have examined breeds, but only one has extensively examined feral cat populations.[10] This study of feral cats has been expanded to include additional worldwide populations, refining the genetic races of feral cat populations (Figure 74-1). The DNA variants used for population studies are usually random DNA variants that are not important to health or physical appearance. However, one can infer that other genetic variants (such as those causing specific phenotypes, diseases, or health concerns) would have similar frequencies in the genetically similar populations.

Knowledge of the genetic similarities among cats in a particular geographic region can help prioritize differential diagnoses, particularly in the case of rare conditions. For example, gangliosidosis, a rare genetic condition documented in feral Japanese domestic shorthair cats,[28-30] might be highly prioritized in sick cats from the region with compatible clinical signs of the disease. Cats from the United Kingdom share genetic composition with cats in the United States and Canada, and those in Australia, Kenya, and the Americas show similarities to their European counterparts. As such, veterinarians in Australia need to be cognizant of health concerns documented in cats in both the United States and Europe. However, founder effects and perhaps different selection pressures do make cat populations different that were historically similar. Feral cats in Turkey and Australia have different frequencies of blood type B as compared to other regions of the world.[31-33] Cats in Italy seem to be a conglomerate of individuals from the Mediterranean and other regions of the world. Despite these geographically distant relationships, cats in close proximity can have different genetic origins, such as those seen in the Iberian Peninsula and France. The Pyrenees mountain chain has apparently been an ecological barrier to cats; and like other species,[34] cats of Portugal and Spain appear to be genetically different from the remaining European continental cats.

Overall, 11 different groupings, clusters, or races of cats can be genetically defined from the various locations that

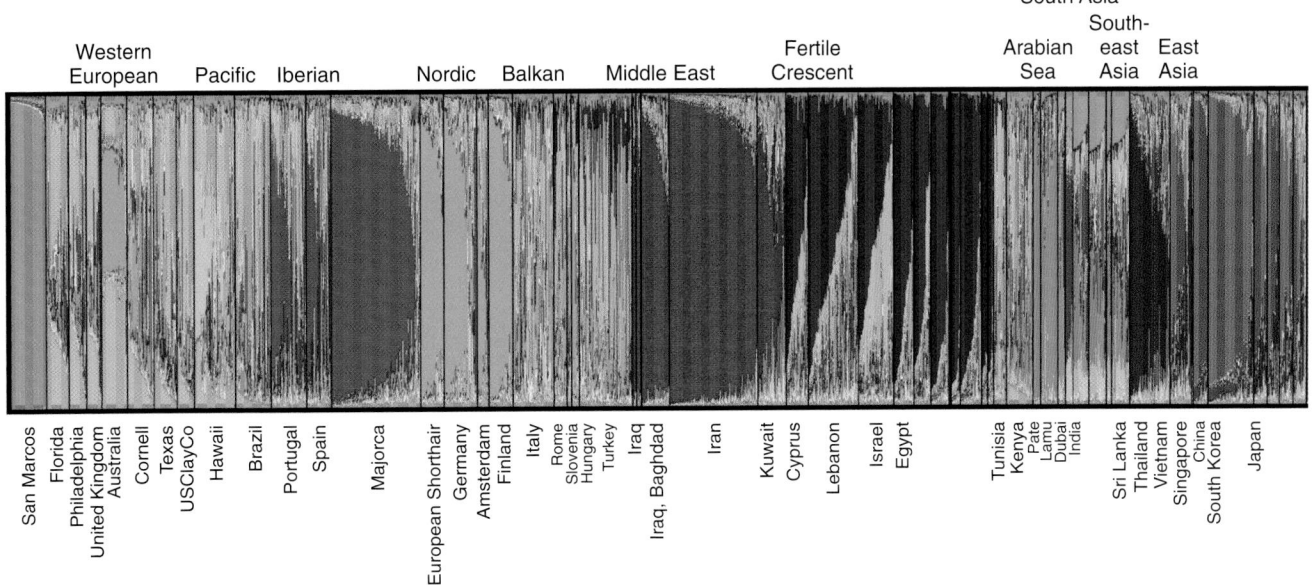

Figure 74-1: Genetic Structuring of World Cat Populations. The figure presents individual cats and their contributions from different genetic groupings based on microsatellite analyses. Cats with similar genetic contributions are grouped in the figure. After the analysis, the groups are labeled with the country of origin of each cat *(bottom labels)* and the group depicted with a color. For example, the cats from Majorca are genetically similar to cats from Spain and Portugal *(dark pink)* but different from other world populations. Some island populations are very distinct (such as San Marcos Island), whereas others are genetically similar to related continental areas (such as Cyprus). Some areas are a conglomerate of cats, such as the cats designated as the Balkans, which includes cats from Italy and Turkey. Cats in Kenya are a mixture of cats from colonial importations. Eleven groupings are significantly distinct *(top labels)*, suggesting 11 worldwide races of cats. (Courtesy of Razib Khan and Erica Creighton, USClayCo, Clay County, Missouri.)

have been sampled. Some island populations appear to have similar genetic signatures to the associated mainland (e.g., Majorca and Iberia), whereas others are more distinct (e.g., San Marcos Island off the coast of California). Distinct island populations are likely unique when cat migrations are very limited or forbidden, such as the case of San Marcos Island. In addition, this island is small and likely had a limited founding population. Thus, the lack of continued gene flow and limited founders have led to a genetically unique and likely highly inbred population of cats. For the development of cat breeds, in general, specific cats from a given race have been used as the founders of a given pedigreed breed.

Genetic Distinction of Domestic Cat Breeds

Genetically, breeds of cats are similar to ethnic groups of humans. Studies have shown that cat breeds were developed from western European, Mediterranean, Arabian, and southeast Asian populations (Figure 74-2).[10] Ongoing studies may suggest that breeds like the Norwegian Forest cat can now be refined to more specific populations, such as the northern European/Nordic race of cats. Thus, cat breeds share health concerns and genetic traits in common with their races of origin. The same types of genetic analyses that were used to compare feral, randomly bred populations of cats have also been used to compare different cat breeds (Table 74-1). More than three dozen breeds have been genotyped with the same genetic markers as the cat races and compared genetically

using allele frequencies of the markers. Approximately 24 breeds appear to be genetically distinct, whereas the remaining breeds are derived from a specific breed family, such as the Persian, Siamese, or Burmese families. These "parent" breeds have been bred to produce slightly different cat groups that are often declared a different breed, but are different by perhaps only one genetic variant. For example, the Persian family is composed of the Persian, Exotic Shorthair, Selkirk Rex, Scottish Fold, and British Shorthair breeds (see Figure 74-2).[35] Exotic Shorthairs are different from Persians by having short hair,[36,37] Selkirk Rex differ by having curly hair,[35,38] and Scottish Fold differ by having folded ears.[39,40] Each difference is caused by a single gene variant, which is not truly sufficient to affect the overall genetic constitution of the breed.

Although the definition of cat breeds is arbitrary and of no major consequence, the health of the new and derived breeds can be significantly impacted by the individuals used to found and propagate the new breed. Selkirk Rex and Scottish Folds are new derivatives of Persians that have historically been riddled with polycystic kidney disease (PKD).[41-45] Thus, each derivative breed should be monitored for the same health and genetic conditions found in the parent breed. Breeds produced from Burmese parentage may be at risk of craniofacial defects,[46,47] feline orofacial pain syndrome,[48,49] hypokalemia,[50] and diabetes mellitus.[51,52] Those associated with Abyssinians, such as the Ocicat and Singapura, may be at risk of progressive retinal atrophies and pyruvate kinase

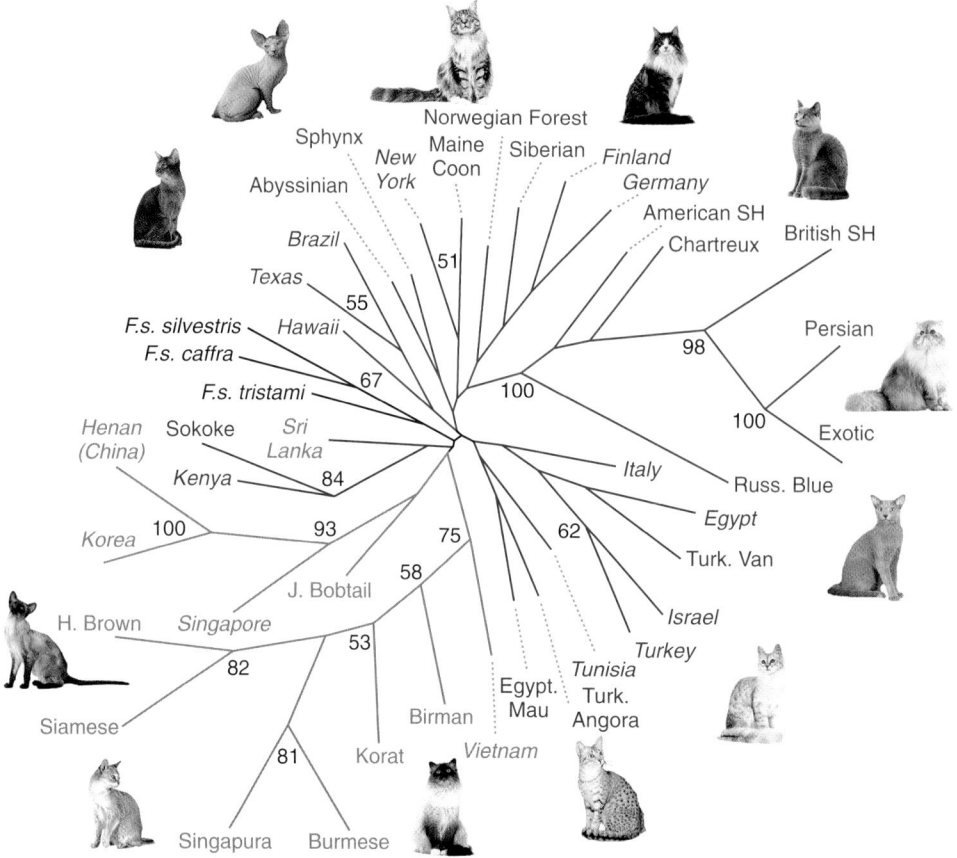

Figure 74-2: Genetic Tree of Cat Breeds and Populations. The phylogenetic tree was constructed using a genetic calculation termed *Cavalli-Sforza's chord distance.* Bootstrap values (a type of significance value) above 50% are presented at the base of the relationship branches (nodes); the higher the value, the more confidence in the relationship. Asian *(green)*, Western European *(red)*, East African *(purple)*, Mediterranean basin *(blue)*, and wildcat *(black)* populations form strongly supported monophyletic (one branch point) branches. European and African wildcats are closely related, whereas short branches of most of the other populations indicate close relationships of these breeds and populations. Random-bred populations are indicated in italics; breeds are in standard font. *F.s.*, *Felis silvestris; H. Brown,* Havana Brown; *J. Bobtail,* Japanese Bobtail; *SH,* Shorthair. (Cat photographs courtesy of Royal Canin and Richard Katris—Chanan Photography. Reprinted with permission. Lipinski MJ, Froenicke L, Baysac KC, et al: The ascent of cat breeds: genetic evaluations of breeds and worldwide random-bred populations. *Genomics* 91:12-21, 2008.)

Table 74-1	Genetic Families of Domestic Cat Breeds	
Breed/Family	**Place Founded**	**Derived Breed/Grouping***
Abyssinian	Founder: India?	Somali
American Bobtail	Natural variant	United States—random bred cats
American Curl	Natural variant	United States—random bred cats
American Shorthair	Founder: United States	American Wirehair
American Wirehair	Natural variant	American Shorthair
Australian Mist	Cross-breed hybrid	Burmese derived
Balinese	Variant	Colorpoint, Havana Brown, Javanese, Oriental, Siamese
Bengal	Species hybrid	Leopard cat × Egyptian Mau and Abyssinian
Birman	Founder: Southeast Asia	
Bombay	Variant	Burmese, Singapura, Tonkinese
British Shorthair	Founder: Europe	Scottish Fold

Table 74-1	Genetic Families of Domestic Cat Breeds—cont'd	
Breed/Family	**Place Founded**	**Derived Breed/Grouping***
Burmese	Founder: Southeast Asia	Bombay, Singapura, Tonkinese
Burmilla	Cross-breed hybrid	Burmese, Persian
Chartreux	Founder: Europe	
Colorpoint Shorthair	Variant	Balinese, Havana Brown, Javanese, Oriental, Siamese
Cornish Rex	Natural variant	United Kingdom—random bred cats
Devon Rex	Natural variant	United Kingdom—random bred cats, Sphynx
Egyptian Mau	Founder: Mediterranean	
European	Founder: Europe	
Exotic	Variant	Persian
Havana Brown	Variant	Balinese, Colorpoint, Javanese, Oriental, Siamese
Japanese Bobtail	Founder	
Javanese	Variant	Balinese, Colorpoint, Havana Brown, Oriental, Siamese
Korat	Founder: Southeast Asia	
Kurilean Bobtail	Natural variant	Eastern Russia, Kuril Islands
LaPerm	Natural variant	United States—random bred cats
Maine Coon	Founder: United States	
Manx	Natural variant	United Kingdom—random bred cats
Munchkin	Natural variant	United States—random bred cats
Norwegian Forest	Founder: Europe	
Ocicat	Cross-breed hybrid	Siamese × Abyssinian
Oriental	Variant	Balinese, Colorpoint, Havana Brown, Javanese, Siamese
Persian	Founder: Europe	Exotic Shorthair
Peterbald	Natural variant	Russian—random bred cats, Don Sphynx
Pixie-bob	Cross-breed hybrid	Manx, Japanese Bobtail, United States—random bred cats
Ragdoll	Founder: United States	United States—random bred cats
Russian Blue	Founder: Europe	
Savannah	Species hybrid	Serval × domestic cat
Scottish Fold	Natural variant	United Kingdom—random bred cats, British Shorthair, Persian
Selkirk Rex	Natural variant	United States—random bred cats, Persian
Siamese	Founder: Southeast Asia	Balinese, Havana Brown, Javanese, Colorpoint, Oriental
Siberian	Founder: Europe	Russian—random bred cats
Singapura	Variant	Bombay, Burmese, Tonkinese
Sokoke	Founder: Arabian Sea	African—random bred cats
Somali	Variant	Abyssinian
Sphynx	Natural variant	Devon Rex
Tonkinese	Variant	Bombay, Burmese, Singapura
Turkish Angora	Founder: Mediterranean	
Turkish Van	Founder: Mediterranean	

*Modified from genetic studies based on 29 tetranucleotide short tandem repeat markers, 39 dinucleotide short tandem repeat markers, and unpublished data (LA Lyons, 2014).

deficiency.[53-55] The demonstrated genetic relationships need to override the folklore of cat breed development. Singapura breeders may not want to admit to the relationship with Abyssinians; however, the genetic signal is clear and strong. British Shorthairs have nearly lost their independent genetic signal and now appear to be a color variant of Persians/Exotic Shorthairs. Like many breeds in Europe that were nearly decimated in population size as a result of the world wars, the British Shorthair had to use other breeds for outcrossing to produce a viable population. However, a consequence is that PKD has become a valid concern in this breed.

GENETIC TESTING IN DOMESTIC CATS

Disease-causing Variants for Simple Traits and Diseases

Inherited diseases arise in cats, especially pedigreed cats; and in some cases, the genetic defects associated with the diseases are known and testable by DNA analyses. If a veterinarian uses the results of DNA testing along with other diagnostic tests, a definitive diagnosis and a more efficient treatment plan can be developed for the patient, and the production of other cats with the same disease may be prevented by providing genetic counseling to the breeder. In a growing number of cases, DNA tests may provide the definitive answer as to why a cat has a health problem and what exactly is causing the disease. To date, more than 40 genes with approximately 70 DNA variants have been documented to cause phenotypic, disease, or blood type variations in the domestic cat (Tables 74-2 to 74-4).[56-58] The mode of inheritance is presented for each trait and disease so that inheritance patterns can be considered in deciding future breeding practices and determining if other cats in the cattery or household may be

at risk for the same disease. Since 2010, 12 new genes causing cat phenotypes and health issues have been identified at a rate of three to four new disease-causing variants per year. The clinical descriptions and phenotypes of each of these diseases and traits have been curated at the Online Mendelian Inheritance in Animals website (http://omia.angis.org.au/home), which is an invaluable resource for comparison of the phenotypes across 2216 animal species.[59] The 26 genes in Table 74-2 are often under positive selection in cats, particularly breeds, and are mainly aesthetic traits; however, some cause secondary health concerns, such as *Tailless*, the disease-causing variant defining Manx cats. By considering the breed relationships in Table 74-1, genetic health concerns across cat populations can be inferred using the genetic disease tests that are listed in Table 74-3. Polycystic kidney disease was identified as a Persian cat disease; however, any breeder using Persians in a breeding program should be aware that the PKD DNA test will be appropriate in any cross-breed cats. The PKD test applies to any breed that is using Persians to modify facial structure, including American and British Shorthairs. Breeders should be sharing with their veterinarians the true genetic contributions to their lines so that the veterinarian can make proper recommendations and diagnostics for healthcare. Breed-based genetic tests are available as commercial services from a wealth of companies and veterinary programs around the world (Table 74-5).

Two of the most commonly used disease genetic tests in cats are those for PKD and hypertrophic cardiomyopathy (HCM). These two diseases are in very popular breeds worldwide, the Persian breed family and Maine Coon cats, respectively. Both diseases can cause early death in a cat and can lead to long-term medical treatment if detected early. The frequencies of the disease-causing variants are significant, historically greater than 30% for PKD in Persians[41,44,45,60] and

Table 74-2	The Phenotypic Traits of the Domestic Cat				
Disease/Trait (Alleles) OMIA Entry*	**MOI†**	**Phenotype**	**Gene**	**Gene Name**	**Disease-causing Variant**
Agouti (A+, a)[84] 000201-9685	AR	Banded fur to solid	*ASIP*	Agouti-signaling protein	c.122_123delCA
Brown (B+, b, b^l)[85,86] 001249-9685	AR	Brown, light brown color variants	*TYRP1*	Tyrosinase-related protein	b = −5IVS6, b^l = c.298C>T
Color (C+, C^b, C^s, c)[86-88] 000202-9685	AR	Burmese, Siamese color pattern, full albino	*TYR*	Tyrosinase	c^b = c.715G>T, c^s = c.940G>A, c = c.975delC
Dilution (D+, d)[89] 000206-9685	AR	Black to grey/blue, orange to cream	*MLPH*	Melanophilin	c.83delT
Dwarfism 000299-9685	AD	Shortening of long bones	Unknown	Unknown	Unknown
Extension (E+, e)— Amber[90] 001199-9685	AR	Brown/red color variant	*MC1R*	Melanocortin receptor 1	c.250G>A

| Table 74-2 | The Phenotypic Traits of the Domestic Cat—cont'd | | | | |

Disease/Trait (Alleles) OMIA Entry*	MOI†	Phenotype	Gene	Gene Name	Disease-causing Variant
Fold (Fd, fd+) 000319-9685	AD	Ventral ear fold	Unpublished	Unpublished	Unpublished
Gloves (G+, g)[73] 001580-9685	AR	White feet	KIT	KIT	c.1035_1036delinsCA
Hairless (Hr+, hr)	AR	Atrichia	KRT71	Keratin 71	c.816+1G>A
Inhibitor (I, i+) 001583-9685	AD	Absence of phaeomelanin	Unknown	Unknown	Unknown
Japanese Bobtail (J, j+)	AD	Kinked tail	Unknown	Unknown	Unknown
Kurl (K, k+) 000244-9685	AD	Rostral curled pinnea	Unknown	Unknown	Unknown
LaPerm 000245-9685	AD	Curly hair coat	Unknown	Unknown	Unknown
Longhair (L+, l)[36,37] 000439-9685	AR	Long fur	FGF5	Fibroblast growth factor 5	c.356_367insT, c.406C>T, c.474delT, c.475A>C
Manx (M, m+)[66] 000975-9685	AD	Absence/short tail	TBOX	T-box	c.998delT, c.1169delC, and c.1199delC, c.998_1014dup17delGCC
Orange (O, o+)	X-linked	Change in pigment hue	Unknown	Unknown	Unknown
Peterbald 001201-9685	AD	Hairless, brush coat	Unknown	Unknown	Unknown
Polydactyla (Pd, pd+)[91] 000810-9685	AD	Extra toes	SHH	Sonic hedgehog	c.479A>G, c.257G>C, c.481A>T
Rexing (R+, r)[92] 001684-9685	AR	Curly hair coat	LPAR6	Lysophosphatidic acid receptor 6	c.250_253delTTTG
Rexing (Re+, re)[93] 001581-9685	AR	Curly hair coat	KRT71	Keratin 71	c.1108-4_1184del, c.1184_1185insAGTTGGAG, c.1196insT
Rexing (R^S, r^s+)[38] 001712-9685	AD	Curly hair coat	KRT71	Keratin 71	c.445-1G>C
Spotting (S, s+)[72] 000214-9685	Co-D	Bicolor/van white	KIT	KIT	7125ins FERV1 element
Tabby (T^M, t^b)[94] 001429-9685	AR	Blotched/classic pattern	TAQPEP	Transmembrane aminopeptidase Q	S59X, T139N, D228N, W841X
Ticked (T^a, t) 001484-9685	AD	No tabby pattern	Unknown	Unknown	Unknown
White (W, w+)[72] 000209-9685	AD	Loss of pigmentation	KIT	KIT	FERV1 LTR ins
Wide-band	AR?	Length of pheomelanin band in hair	Unknown	Unknown	Unknown

*Online Mendelian Inheritance in Animals (OMIA; http://omia.angis.org.au/home/) entries provide links to citations and clinical descriptions of the phenotypes and the diseases. Presented citations are for the causative variant discovery. A superscript plus sign (+) implies the wild-type allele when known.

†Mode of inheritance (MOI) of the nonwild-type variant. In reference to the variant allele, *AD* implies autosomal dominant, *AR* implies autosomal recessive, and *Co-D* implies codominant.

Table 74-3 Inherited Diseases of Domestic Cats for Which a Commercial DNA Test Is Available

Disease/Trait (Alleles) OMIA Entry*	MOI[†]	Phenotype	Gene	Gene Name	Disease-causing Variant
AB Blood Type (A+, b)[95] 000119-9685	AR	Determines Type B	CMAH	Cytidine monophospho-N-acetylneuraminic acid hydroxylase	c.1del-53_70, c.139G>A
Craniofacial Defect	AR	Craniofacial Defect	Unpublished	Unpublished	Unpublished
Gangliosidosis 1[96] 000402-9685	AR	Lipid storage disorder (GM1)	GLB1	Galactosidase, beta 1	c.1457G>C
Gangliosidosis 2[97] 01462-0985	AR	Lipid storage disorder (GM2)	HEXB	Hexominidase B	c.1356del-1_8, c.1356_1362delGTTCTCA
Gangliosidosis 2[98] 01462-0985	AR	Lipid storage disorder (GM2)	HEXB	Hexominidase B	c.39delC
Glycogen Storage Disease IV[99] 000420-9685	AR	Glycogen storage disorder (GSD)	GBE1	Glycogen branching enzyme 1	IVS11+1552_IVS12-1339 del6.2kb ins334 bp
Hypertrophic Cardiomyopathy[83] 000515-9685	AD	Cardiac disease (HCM)	MYBPC	Myosin binding protein C	c.93G>C
Hypertrophic Cardiomyopathy[100] 000515-9685	AD	Cardiac disease (HCM)	MYBPC	Myosin binding protein C	c.2460C>T
Hypokalemia[50] 001759-9685	AR	Potassium deficiency (HK)	WNK4	WNK lysine deficient protein kinase 4	c.2899C>T
Progressive Retinal Atropy[54] 001244-9685	AR	Late onset blindness (rdAC)	CEP290	Centrosomal protein 290kDa	IVS50 + 9T>G
Progressive Retinal Atropy[53] 000881-9685	AD	Early onset blindness (rdy)	CRX	Cone-rod homeobox	c.546delC
Polycystic Kidney Disease[62] 000807-9685	AD	Kidney cysts (PKD)	PKD1	Polycystin 1	c.10063C>A
Pyruvate Kinase Def.[55] 000844-9685	AR	Hemopathy (PK deficiency)	PKLR	pyruvate kinase, liver, RBC	c.693+304G>A
Spinal Muscular Atrophy[101] 000939-9685	AR	Muscular atrophy (SMA)	LIX1-LNPEP	limb expression 1 homolog—leucyl/cystinyl aminopeptidase	Partial gene deletions

*Online Mendelian Inheritance in Animals (OMIA; http://omia.angis.org.au/home/) entries provide links to citations and clinical descriptions of the phenotypes and the diseases. Presented citations are for the causative variant discovery.
[†]Mode of inheritance (MOI) of the nonwild-type variant. Not all transcripts for a given gene may have been discovered or well documented in the cat; disease-causing variants presented as interpreted from original publication. A superscript plus sign (+) implies the wild-type allele when known. In reference to the variant allele, AD implies autosomal dominant, AR implies autosomal recessive, and Co-D implies codominant.

HCM in Maine Coons.[61] Because these frequencies are high and not specific to particular breeding lines or regions of the world, a slow eradication of the disease-causing variants would maintain the present genetic variation in the populations. Both disease-causing variants have an autosomal dominant mode of inheritance, implying that at least one parent also had the disease and at least 50% of offspring are at risk for the disease. For a dominant trait, an affected individual can have one or two copies of the disease-causing variant. However, in the case of PKD, the homozygote individual does not survive gestation as the disease-causing variant is lethal *in utero*.[62] Thus, all PKD affected cats have only one

Table 74-4	Uncommon Disease-causing Variants for Inherited Domestic Cat Diseases*		
Disease/OMIA Entry[†]	**OMIA Entry**	**Gene**	**Disease-causing Variant**[‡]
11b-hydroxylase Def. (Congenital Adrenal Hypoplasia)[102]	001661-9685	CYP11B1	Exon 7 G>A
Dihydropyrimidinase Deficiency[103]	001776-9685	DPYS	c.1303G>A
Factor XII Deficiency[104]	000364-9685	FXII	c.1321delC
Fibrodysplasia Ossificans Progressiva	000388-9685	Unpublished	Unpublished
Gangliosidosis 1[29]	000402-9685	GLB1	c.1448G>C
Gangliosidosis 2[105]	001462-9685	HEXB	c.1467_1491inv
Gangliosidosis 2[106]	001462-9685	HEXB	c.667C>T
Gangliosidosis 2[99]	001427-9685	GM2A	c.390_393GGTC
Hemophilia B[107]	000438-9685	F9	c.247G>A, c.1014C>T
Hyperoxaluria[108]	000821-9685	GRHPR	G>A I4 acceptor site
Hypothyroidism	000536-9685	Unpublished	Unpublished
Lipoprotein Lipase Deficiency[109]	001210-9685	LPL	c.1234G>A
Mucolipidosis II[110]	001248-9685	GNPTAB	c.2655C>T
Mannosidosis, alpha[111]	000625-9685	LAMAN	c.1748_1751delCCAG
Mucopolysaccharidosis I[112]	000664-9685	IDUA	c.1107_1109delCGA; c.1108_1110GAC
Mucopolysaccharidosis VI[113]	000666-9685	ARSB	c.1427T>C
Mucopolysaccharidosis VI[114, 115]	000666-9685	ARSB	c.1558G>A
Mucopolysaccharidosis VII[116]	000667-9685	GUSB	c.1052A>G
Muscular Dystrophy[117]	001081-9685	DMD	900bp del M promoter-exon 1
Niemann-Pick C[118]	000725-9685	NPC	c.2864G>C
Polydactyly[91]	000810-9685	SHH	c.479A>G, c.257G>C, c.481A>T
Porphyria (congenital erythropoietic)[119§]	001175-9685	UROS	c.140C>T, c.331G>A
Porphyria (acute intermittent)[120§]	001493-9685	HMBS	c.842_844delGAG, c.189dupT, c.250G>A, c.445C>T
Vitamin D Resistant Rickets[121]	000837-9685	CYP27B1	c.223G>A, c.731delG
Vitamin D Resistant Rickets[122]	000837-9685	CYP27B1	c.637G>T

*The presented conditions are not prevalent in breeds or populations but may have been established into research colonies.
[†]Online Mendelian Inheritance in Animals (OMIA; http://omia.angis.org.au/home/) entries provide links to citations and clinical descriptions of the phenotypes and the diseases. Presented citations are for the causative variant discovery.
[‡]Not all transcripts for a given gene may have been discovered or well documented in the cat; disease-causing variants presented as interpreted from original publication.
§A variety of disease-causing variants have been identified but not published for porphyrias in domestic cats. Contact PennGen at the University of Pennsylvania for additional information on porphyrias.

copy of the disease-causing variant, and offspring have a 50% chance of inheriting the disease. If the cat has the PKD disease-causing variant, the cat will get kidney cysts. Thus, an early genetic test can be used to select breeding cats free of the disease, prior to the kitten's maturity. However, the DNA test will not predict severity of disease. Some cats progress quickly, have severe kidney cysts, and die an early death from chronic kidney disease. Most cats have small cysts, never have renal compromise, and die of other causes. Thus, the genetic

test must be used with clinical diagnostics, such as ultrasound and blood chemistries, to develop a health management plan for a PKD-positive cat.

Hypertrophic cardiomyopathy is a more complex situation. Cats can have one or two copies of the DNA disease-causing variant; however, cats with two copies are more likely to progress to cardiac failure at a faster rate than cats with one copy of the DNA disease-causing variant.[63] Some cats progress very slowly to disease and after years of echocardiograms,

Table 74-5 Domestic Cat DNA Testing Laboratories

Laboratory and Webpage	Region	University Research Affiliate	DNA Profile	CAT TEST* Disease	CAT TEST* Coat Color	Blood Type	Coat Type
Animal DNA Testing www.animalsdna.com	Australia		Yes	8	4	Yes	Longhair
Animal Health Trust www.aht.org.uk	United Kingdom	Animal Health Trust	Yes	PKD	No	No	No
Antagene Immeuble Le Meltem www.antagene.com	France		Yes	4	Siamese/ Burmese color	Yes	No
BioAxis DNA Research Centre Ltd. www.dnares.in	India		Yes	PKD	No	No	No
DNA Diagnostics Center www.dnacenter.com	US		No	PKD	No	No	No
GENINDEXE www.genindexe.com	France		Yes	7	5	Yes	No
Genoscoper www.genoscoper.com	Finland		Yes	7	Yes	Yes	Longhair
Gribbles www.gribblesvets.com	Australia		No	PKD	No	No	No
IDEXX www.idexx.ca	Canada		No	PK Def.	No	No	No
Laboklin www.laboklin.de/	Germany		Yes	9	5	Yes	Longhair
Langford Veterinary Services Langfordvets.co.uk	United Kingdom	Bristol University	Yes	10	8	Yes	Longhair
PennGen† research.vet.upenn.edu/penngen†	United States	University of Pennsylvania	No	PK Def. GSD	No	No	No
PROGENUS S.A. www.progenus.be	Belgium		Yes	7	6	No	Longhair
Van Haeringen Laboratory www.vhlgenetics.com	Netherlands		Yes	10	6	Yes	Longhair
Veterinary Cardiac Genetics Lab www.ncstatevets.org/genetics/submitdna	United States	Washington State University	No	HCM	No	No	No
Veterinary Genetics Lab www.vgl.ucdavis.edu	United States	University of California, Davis	Yes	14	All	Yes	All
VetGen www.vetgen.com	United States	Michigan State University	Yes	No	Brown dilute	No	Longhair
Vetogene www.vetogene.com	Italy	University of Milan	Yes	5	No	Yes	Longhair

GSD, Glycogen storage diseases; *HCM*, hypertrophic cardiomyopathy; *PK Def.*, pyruvate kinase deficiency; *PKD*, polycystic kidney disease.
*Tests reference to those listed in Tables 74-2 and 74-3. If a laboratory offers only one or two tests, those tests are listed; otherwise the number of tests they offer for cats is presented. PKD and the HCMs are the most popular cat test offerings.
†PennGen also offers genetic and biochemical tests for diseases that are not of concern to the cat breeds.

show slow progression and no clinical signs of disease. Slow progressing or nonprogressing cats likely have some other genetic variants that support cardiac function and override the disease-causing variant. However, genetic counseling should be the same for these individuals. Slow or nonprogressing cats have the disease-causing variant, and the risk for their offspring cannot be predicted. The offspring, with a different genetic background, may very well be a cat with fast progressing disease. Thus, like PKD, the HCM disease-causing variant should be balanced with other good attributes of breeding cats and considered for slow eradication from a breed. A common suggestion is to replace an affected breeding cat with the first negative "clear" cat that can be produced—provided that the new cat is healthy in other regards.

Additional DNA disease-causing variants have been identified in domestic cats that are not of significant consequence to breeds (see Table 74-4). Note that some types of gangliosidosis are breed-specific, whereas others were found in random domestic shorthair cats. If similar conditions are suspected in cats, many research laboratories will generally consider testing for the known disease-causing variant as a noncommercial service to support the diagnosis. In fact, if a DNA test is not positive for a disease trait (such as PKD), and PKD is determined to be present by ultrasound or a cat is negative for the known GM disease-causing variants but a cat clearly has ganglioside accumulation, many research-based DNA testing services will continue analysis of the entire gene to determine if new disease-causing variants can be identified and are causative for the conditions. These positive interactions among veterinarians, breeders, and researchers often lead to the ascertainment of new disease models and eventually causative disease-causing variants that lead to new genetic tests.

Many disease-causing variants that have been identified in domestic cat breeds control the phenotypes that dictate the aesthetic value of our pets. Knowledge and understanding of the mode of inheritance and the effect of the phenotypic alleles can support cat health indirectly through population management. Breeders can be counseled on breeding schemes that will produce more desirable color and fur type varieties in a manner that will produce fewer cats overall. If a breeder has more desired cats and fewer excess cats, more time, energy, and precious funds can be designated to their healthcare. Importantly, the reduction of cattery size inherently reduces stress and stress-associated health issues, such as upper respiratory tract diseases, urinary tract diseases, and feline infectious peritonitis.[64,65] Thus, the correct genetic management of a simple coat color trait may indirectly improve the health of the entire cattery.

Several desired genetic disease-causing variants are associated with health concerns and are now documented. The disease-causing variants for taillessness *(Tailless: T)* have been identified.[66] Continued studies of the Manx breed and other background genetics may now elucidate why some Manx cats have lameness, constipation, or incontinence as a secondary impact of improper vertebral development. The discovery of the *Tailless* disease-causing variants has also

revealed that Japanese Bobtail cats do not have disease-causing variants in the same gene as the Manx and that the Pixie-bob breed has genetic contributions from both the Manx and Japanese Bobtail breeds.[67] The genetic disease-causing variant for Scottish Fold has been identified but as of this writing is yet to be published. Once this disease-causing variant is revealed, studies to understand the development of osteochondroplasia can be initiated.[68-71] Coat color patterns displaying white (such as the *Gloves* in Birmans, dominant *White*, and *Spotting* traits) are caused by disease-causing variants in the gene called *KIT*.[72,73] Dominant *White* is associated with deafness but *Spotting*, which causes the bicolor and high white patterns, is not associated with deafness.[74-76] Now that the major causative gene for dominant *White* in known, deaf versus nondeaf cats and blue-eyed versus odd-eyed versus nonblue-eyed cats can be genetically compared to decipher other genetic disease-causing variants that may influence these additional plieotrophic traits. Genetic testing for dominant *White* and *Spotting* will indicate the presence of one or two copies of the *White* disease-causing variant or if a cat is a compound heterozygote in the *KIT* gene, having one copy of the *White* disease-causing variant and one copy of the *Spotting* disease-causing variant.[72] This information should be correlated to see if a specific genotype may be more predictive of deafness risk. Thus, research has demonstrated the cause of deafness for an all-white cat, but the more important aspect to decipher is what causes the deafness and can we identify DNA variants associated with deafness risk.

The Future: Whole Genome Sequencing for Feline Healthcare

Genetic testing has been a part of modern human healthcare since the national implementation of the DNA disease-causing variant test for phenylketonuria in the 1960s.[1] Rapid detection of inborn errors of metabolism in infants allows rapid intervention and the prevention of devastating consequences, such as permanent mental retardation and early death.[77,78] Newborn screening programs are mostly routine, with the United States testing for a wealth of different diseases, depending on the ethnic representations in the region.[79] Most people do not realize that they were tested for a battery of genetic diseases through blood samples collected shortly after birth.[11] Such testing is now commercially available to the public through several companies that specialize in the detection of single gene trait disease-causing variants as well as analysis of genetic ancestry, such as 23andMe (http://www.23andme.com), FamilyTreeDNA (http://www.familytreedna.com), and the Genographic Project (http://genographic.nationalgeographic.com). Similar offerings are available for domestic cats. Many laboratories, such as the Veterinary Genetics Laboratory at the University of California, Davis (http://www.vgl.ucdavis.edu), offer both a majority of the genetic tests important for cat breeds as well as a cat ancestry test that can determine a nonpedigreed cat's race and potential breed. In humans and hopefully cats, the future of individual healthcare will rely on the individual's personal genome.[80]

A result of the Human Genome Project has been the development of rapid and cost effective means to sequence the entire genome of an individual in less than 1 month. Currently costing approximately $10,000 USD, technological advancements should reduce that cost to approximately $1000 USD per individual.[81] Whole genome sequencing is becoming the standard of healthcare for genetic profiling of cancers and newborns with congenital abnormalities at specialty hospitals around the world.[80,82] With more than 100,000 individual human genomes sequenced, the database of normal and detrimental genetic disease-causing variants is well defined.[77] For cats, whole genome sequencing is being used to investigate diseases and traits that are known to be heritable, but sufficient individuals are not yet available for genetic analysis of families or population-based association studies. As the feline genetic database grows, sporadic and idiopathic conditions will slowly be attributed to specific individual genetic causes, leading to highly specific personalized medicine for our companion animals.

Genetic Counseling in Veterinary Medicine

Veterinarians are expected to obtain, understand, and interpret DNA results and provide "genetic counseling." However, because a majority of the cat population does not represent pedigreed cats, breeders are not generally the largest portion of clientele in a standard veterinary practice. Genetic testing in random bred cats is currently rather minimal and occurs primarily for rare and orphan diseases, such as mucopolysaccharidoses or porphyrias. With regard to genetic testing, what pertains to cats likely pertains to other domestic animals, including dogs, cattle, and horses. Genetics courses are a standard prerequisite for veterinary school admission; and for the past 10 to 15 years, many veterinary schools in the United States have formally added genetics into their curriculum. At a minimum, different modes of inheritance are reviewed and graduate veterinarians should be able to provide minimal genetic counseling as a result. The *mode of inheritance* (i.e., autosomal, sex-linked, recessive, dominant), *incomplete penetrance, variable expression, age of onset,* and *risk* are terms the modern veterinarian should come to know, understand, and hopefully embrace.

Genetic counseling can be structured into three distinct processes. The initial process is the procedure conducted by the veterinarian to obtain a diagnosis for a clinical presentation. Collection of the patient's signalment and history should include considerations of the cat's breed and the general health of its lineage, including parents, siblings, and offspring. Thus, the veterinarian may be looking for clues to a possible genetic cause for a condition by asking if this clinical presentation has been documented in the breed or noticed in any close relatives. Any early presentation of a disease that normally affects older cats, such mediastinal lymphoma, may indicate a potential genetic influence. Bilateral presentation, such as vessel attenuation in both eyes in normotensive cats,

is a hallmark for heritable disease, such as retinal degeneration. At this time, the veterinarian and client will need to discuss if a DNA-based diagnostic test, such as a DNA test for PKD, is more warranted, perhaps in lieu of or prior to additional more costly diagnostics, such as ultrasound examinations. Considerations such as what happens if the DNA test is positive or negative need to be considered and discussed. Handy access to charts of available DNA tests and available commercial testing laboratories will be a benefit to the process (see Tables 74-2 to 74-5). In some cases, accuracy of the test may need to be considered. DNA testing can be performed by a variety of techniques to assay for the DNA variant of interest; generally they all include some manner of polymerase chain reaction and even whole genome sequencing. A plethora of laboratories are also available for testing. The reputation, customer service, and association with active researchers interested in cat genetics are important factors to consider when selecting a commercial service (see Table 74-5). A good laboratory reputation and a close involvement with researchers are good indicators of test accuracy.

Once a DNA test is obtained on a cat, test interpretation and prognosis need to be considered. This is a major secondary step in genetic counseling. The client and the veterinarian need to recognize that the current DNA tests for cats do not predict severity of disease. In the case of PKD, many mildly affected cats will never develop kidney disease and will die of causes not related to PKD, whereas others develop end-stage kidney disease within a few years and have an early death attributed to the disease. Thus, ultrasound imaging is an important diagnostic in the cat's healthcare management for PKD. Another important example is HCM in Maine Coon cats.[83] The presence of the genetic disease-causing variant clearly confers risk, but the extent of the risk is nebulous.[63] Thus, genetic tests should be used as tools for the veterinarian and the owner, supporting the overall picture of a given cat's healthcare plan. In the case of PKD, ultrasound and/or serum creatinine levels should be used to monitor disease progression in PKD-positive cats. Echocardiographic monitoring remains the standard for HCM patients, although early detection cardiac biomarkers are being explored. Genetic testing should be used to enhance (not replace) interactions among the patient, client, and veterinarian.

The third step in genetic counseling is communication with the client, which hopefully is a long-lasting interaction over the healthcare management of the cats. Directed (active) versus nondirected (passive) counseling is a concept that should be considered. Most veterinarians want to provide "directed" counseling. For example, "Your cat has PKD. You should never breed the cat again and should spay or neuter the cat." Directed counseling is unacceptable in human medicine, and if the "big picture" is considered, directed counseling should also be nonstandard in veterinary medicine. The "big picture" pertains to not only the cat itself but also the breed population and the livelihood of the breeder. Thus, a more passive, nondirected approach where all the information regarding the patient's health and likely information regarding the owner's breeding program will need to be considered. As noted with the gangliosidoses in the Korat breed, a passive approach led to a slow eradication of the disease variant in the population, without the production of unhealthy cats, but with maintenance of high genetic diversity in the breed population—the "big picture." In individual cases, the veterinarian caused no harm to the patient or the breed, likely kept the breeder as a client, the client developed a healthier breeding program, and the veterinarian and breeder improved the overall health of the breed.

Genetics is not going to solve every health problem, even the ones with highly heritable influences. Interpretations and the determination of risk may be difficult for many conditions. As determined by sequencing of thousands of humans, each individual (human or cat) has several severe disease-causing variants in their genome that should render them unfit—we should all have some major health problem! It is important for veterinarians and pet owners to recognize that it is not yet understood how all the approximately 21,000 genes of the body interact and therefore the overall health of an individual cannot be predicted based on the presence or absence of a single disease-causing variant. Thus, in genetic counseling, one should consider all the good things as well as the bad things that a cat has to determine future breeding and population management strategies. The present health condition of the cat should be the primary concern, but temperament, reproductive success, resistance to other health problems, and aesthetic qualities should also be considered. By understanding the mode of inheritance, diseases and undesirable traits can be slowly removed from the feline population. Veterinarians play a vital role in human public health. So too with cats, the health of the individual and the health of the population both need to be considered in health management plans.

SUMMARY

Understanding the relationship of cats to their race of origin and breed family can be predictive for selected health threats. Currently, most genetic tests focus on diseases and abnormalities that are prevalent in a specific breed. When presented with clinical conditions that can have a variety of causes, such as kidney disease, genetic testing can provide definitive answers for many health concerns and also predict risk for certain other diseases. As more genetic tests become available in the domestic cat (like humans), personalized medicine will become available, individualizing healthcare to a greater extent. Technology and competition will reduce the costs of genetic testing in cats, making it feasible to perform large batteries of genetic tests and eventually whole genome sequencing, the ultimate in personalized, predictive, preventive, and participatory (so-called "P4") healthcare. Veterinarians will have more predictive powers for health concerns and will be able to implement proper interventions at an earlier stage in the disease process. As genetic data become more readily available, veterinarians will be able to play a larger role and provide earlier intervention into healthcare management of individual cats and their populations. Genetic counseling will continue to become an important aspect of veterinary medicine, bringing together the tests of the individual into consideration with the genetic diversity and health of the entire breed population. As humans continue to live longer and higher quality lives, so too will their furry companion felines.

References

1. Brosco JP, Paul DB: The political history of PKU: reflections on 50 years of newborn screening. *Pediatrics* 132:987–989, 2013.
2. Morris D: *Cat breeds of the world*, New York, 1999, Penguin Books.
3. Morris D: *Cat breeds of the world: a complete illustrated encyclopedia*, New York, 1999, Viking Penguin, pp 10–12.
4. Baker HJ, Jr, Lindsey JR, McKhann GM, et al: Neuronal GM1 gangliosidosis in a Siamese cat with beta-galactosidase deficiency. *Science* 174:838–839, 1971.
5. Baker HJ, Lindsey JR: Animal model: feline GM1 gangliosidosis. *Am J Pathol* 74:649–652, 1974.
6. Neuwelt EA, Johnson WG, Blank NK, et al: Characterization of a new model of GM2-gangliosidosis (Sandhoff's disease) in Korat cats. *J Clin Invest* 76:482–490, 1985.
7. CFA: *The Cat Fanciers' Association cat encyclopedia*, New York, 1993, Simon & Schuster, pp 128–136.
8. CFA: *The Cat Fanciers' Association complete cat book*, ed 1, New York, 2004, Harper Collins.
9. CFA: Cat Fanciers' Association registration totals by color and breed—2003, and 1/1/58 to 12/31/03. *Cat Fanciers' Almanac* 20:72–86, 2004.
10. Lipinski MJ, Froenicke L, Baysac KC, et al: The ascent of cat breeds: genetic evaluations of breeds and worldwide random-bred populations. *Genomics* 91:12–21, 2008.
11. Roberts JS, Dolinoy DC, Tarini BA: Emerging issues in public health genomics. *Annu Rev Genomics Hum Genet* 15:461–480, 2014.
12. Vigne JD: The origins of animal domestication and husbandry: a major change in the history of humanity and the biosphere. *C R Biol* 334:171–181, 2011.
13. Vigne JD, Briois F, Zazzo A, et al: First wave of cultivators spread to Cyprus at least 10,600 y ago. *Proc Natl Acad Sci U S A* 109:8445–8449, 2012.
14. Vigne JD, Guilaine J, Debue K, et al: Early taming of the cat in Cyprus. *Science* 304:259, 2004.
15. Malek J: *The cat in ancient Egypt*, Philadelphia, 1993, University of Pennsylvania.
16. Hu Y, Hu S, Wang W, et al: Earliest evidence for commensal processes of cat domestication. *Proc Natl Acad Sci U S A* 111:116–120, 2014.
17. Clutton-Brock J: *A natural history of domesticated mammals*, London, 1987, Cambridge University Press, British Museum.
18. Driscoll CA, Clutton-Brock J, Kitchener AC, et al: The taming of the cat. Genetic and archaeological findings hint that wildcats became housecats earlier—and in a different place—than previously thought. *Sci Am* 300:68–75, 2009.
19. Tresset A, Vigne JD: Last hunter-gatherers and first farmers of Europe. *C R Biol* 334:182–189, 2011.
20. Todd NB: Cats and commerce. *Sci Am* 237:100–107, 1997.
21. Todd NB: An ecological, behavioral genetic model for the domestication of the cat. *Carnivore* 1:52–60, 1978.
22. Nowell K, Jackson P: *Wild cats status survey and conservation action plan*, Gland, 1996, IUCN.

23. Driscoll CA, Menotti-Raymond M, Roca AL, et al: The Near Eastern origin of cat domestication. *Science* 317:519–523, 2007.

24. Grahn RA, Kurushima JD, Billings NC, et al: Feline non-repetitive mitochondrial DNA control region database for forensic evidence. *Forensic Sci Int Genet* 5:33–42, 2011.

25. Menotti-Raymond M, David VA, Pflueger SM, et al: Patterns of molecular genetic variation among cat breeds. *Genomics* 91:1–11, 2008.

26. Kurushima JD, Lipinski MJ, Gandolfi B, et al: Variation of cats under domestication: genetic assignment of domestic cats to breeds and worldwide random-bred populations. *Anim Genet* 44:311–324, 2013.

27. Driscoll CA, Menotti-Raymond M, Nelson G, et al: Genomic microsatellites as evolutionary chronometers: a test in wild cats. *Genome Res* 12:414–423, 2012.

28. Yamato O, Matsunaga S, Takata K, et al: GM2-gangliosidosis variant 0 (Sandhoff-like disease) in a family of Japanese domestic cats. *Vet Rec* 155:739–744, 2004.

29. Uddin MM, Hossain MA, Rahman MM, et al: Identification of Bangladeshi domestic cats with GM1 gangliosidosis caused by the c.1448G>C mutation of the feline *GLB1* gene: case study. *J Vet Med Sci* 75:395–397, 2013.

30. Hasegawa D, Yamato O, Kobayashi M, et al: Clinical and molecular analysis of GM2 gangliosidosis in two apparent littermate kittens of the Japanese domestic cat. *J Feline Med Surg* 9:232–237, 2007.

31. Arikan S, Gurkan M, Ozaytekin E, et al: Frequencies of blood type A, B and AB in non-pedigree domestic cats in Turkey. *J Small Anim Pract* 47:10–13, 2006.

32. Giger U, Bucheler J, Patterson DF: Frequency and inheritance of A and B blood types in feline breeds of the United States. *J Hered* 82:15–20, 1991.

33. Malik R, Griffin DL, White JD, et al: The prevalence of feline A/B blood types in the Sydney region. *Aust Vet J* 83:38–44, 2005.

34. Martin-Burriel I, Rodellar C, Canon J, et al: Genetic diversity, structure, and breed relationships in Iberian cattle. *J Anim Sci* 89:893–906, 2011.

35. Filler S, Alhaddad H, Gandolfi B, et al: Selkirk Rex: morphological and genetic characterization of a new cat breed. *J Hered* 103:727–733, 2012.

36. Kehler JS, David VA, Schaffer AA, et al: Four independent mutations in the feline *fibroblast growth factor 5* gene determine the long-haired phenotype in domestic cats. *J Hered* 98:555–566, 2007.

37. Drogemuller C, Rufenacht S, Wichert B, et al: Mutations within the *FGF5* gene are associated with hair length in cats. *Anim Genet* 38:218–221, 2007.

38. Gandolfi B, Alhaddad H, Joslin SE, et al: A splice variant in *KRT71* is associated with curly coat phenotype of Selkirk Rex cats. *Sci Rep* 3:2013, 2000.

39. Todd NB: Folded-ear cats: further observations. *Carn Genet News* 2:64–65, 1972.

40. Dyte C, Turner P: Further data on folded-ear cats. *Carn Genet News* 2:112, 1973.

41. Cannon MJ, MacKay AD, Barr FJ, et al: Prevalence of polycystic kidney disease in Persian cats in the United Kingdom. *Vet Rec* 149:409–411, 2001.

42. Biller DS, DiBartola SP, Eaton KA, et al: Inheritance of polycystic kidney disease in Persian cats. *J Hered* 87:1–5, 1996.

43. Biller D, Chew D, DiBartola S: Polycystic kidney disease in a family of Persian cats. *J Am Vet Med Assoc* 196:1288–1290, 1990.

44. Barthez PY, Rivier P, Begon D: Prevalence of polycystic kidney disease in Persian and Persian related cats in France. *J Feline Med Surg* 5:345–347, 2003.

45. Barrs VR, Gunew M, Foster SF, et al: Prevalence of autosomal dominant polycystic kidney disease in Persian cats and related-breeds in Sydney and Brisbane. *Aust Vet J* 79:257–259, 2001.

46. Zook BC: Encephalocele and other congenital craniofacial anomalies in Burmese cats. *Vet Med Small Anim Clin* 78:695–701, 1983.

47. Noden DM, Evans HE: Inherited homeotic midfacial malformations in Burmese cats. *J Craniofac Genet Dev Biol Suppl* 2:249–266, 1986.

48. Rusbridge C, Heath S, Gunn-Moore DA, et al: Feline orofacial pain syndrome (FOPS): a retrospective study of 113 cases. *J Feline Med Surg* 12:498–508, 2010.

49. Heath S, Rusbridge C, Johnson N, et al: Orofacial pain syndrome in cats. *Vet Rec* 149:660, 2001.

50. Gandolfi B, Gruffydd-Jones TJ, Malik R, et al: First *WNK4*-hypokalemia animal model identified by genome-wide association in Burmese cats. *PLoS ONE* 7:e53173, 2012.

51. Rand JS, Bobbermien LM, Hendrikz JK, et al: Over representation of Burmese cats with diabetes mellitus. *Aust Vet J* 75:402–405, 1997.

52. O'Leary CA, Duffy DL, Gething MA, et al: Investigation of diabetes mellitus in Burmese cats as an inherited trait: a preliminary study. *N Z Vet J* 61:354–358, 2013.

53. Menotti-Raymond M, Deckman K, David V, et al: Mutation discovered in a feline model of human congenital retinal blinding disease. *Invest Ophthalmol Vis Sci* 51:2852–2859, 2010.

54. Menotti-Raymond M, David VA, Schaffer AA, et al: Mutation in *CEP290* discovered for cat model of human retinal degeneration. *J Hered* 98:211–220, 2007.

55. Grahn RA, Grahn JC, Penedo MC, et al: Erythrocyte pyruvate kinase deficiency mutation identified in multiple breeds of domestic cats. *BMC Vet Res* 8:207, 2012.

56. Lyons LA: Genetic testing in domestic cats. In August JR, editor: *Consultations in feline internal medicine*, pp 794–803 St. Louis, 2010, Saunders Elsevier.

57. Lyons LA: Feline genetics: clinical applications and genetic testing. *Top Companion Anim Med* 25:203–212, 2010.

58. Lyons LA: Genetic testing in domestic cats. *Mol Cell Probes* 26:224–230, 2012.

59. Nicholas F: Online Mendelian Inheritance in Animals (OMIA), *The University of Sydney: Faculty of Veterinary Science* <http://omia.angis.org.au/home/>. (Accessed June 4, 2015.)

60. Eaton KA, Biller DS, DiBartola SP, et al: Autosomal dominant polycystic kidney disease in Persian and Persian-cross cats. *Vet Pathol* 34:117–126, 1997.

61. Fries R, Heaney AM, Meurs KM: Prevalence of the *myosin-binding protein C* mutation in Maine coon cats. *J Vet Intern Med* 22:893–896, 2008.

62. Lyons LA, Biller DS, Erdman CA, et al: Feline polycystic kidney disease mutation identified in *PKD1*. *J Am Soc Nephrol* 15:2548–2555, 2004.

63. Longeri M, Ferrari P, Knafelz P, et al: *Myosin-binding protein C* DNA variants in domestic cats (A31P, A74T, R820W) and their association with hypertrophic cardiomyopathy. *J Vet Intern Med* 27:275–285, 2013.

64. Pedersen NC, Allen CE, Lyons LA: Pathogenesis of feline enteric coronavirus infection. *J Feline Med Surg* 10:529–541, 2008.

65. Stella J, Croney C, Buffington T: Effects of stressors on the behavior and physiology of domestic cats. *Appl Anim Behav Sci* 143:157–163, 2013.

66. Buckingham KJ, McMillin MJ, Brassil MM, et al: Multiple mutant *T* alleles cause haploinsufficiency of Brachyury and short tails in Manx cats. *Mamm Genome* 24:400–408, 2013.

67. Pollard RE, Koehne AL, Peterson CB, et al: Japanese Bobtail: vertebral morphology and genetic characterization of an established cat breed. *J Feline Med Surg* 2014. [Epub ahead of print].

68. Takanosu M, Takanosu T, Suzuki H, et al: Incomplete dominant osteochondrodysplasia in heterozygous Scottish Fold cats. *J Small Anim Pract* 49:197–199, 2008.

69. Simon D: Osteochondrodystrophy in the Scottish Fold cat. *Tierarztliche Praxis Ausgabe Kleintiere Heimtiere* 28:107–110, 2000.

70. Malik R, Allan G, Howlett C, et al: Osteochondrodysplasia in Scottish Fold cats. *Aust Vet J* 77:85–92, 1999.

71. Chang J, Jung J, Oh S, et al: Osteochondrodysplasia in three Scottish Fold cats. *J Vet Sci* 8:307–309, 2007.

72. David VA, Menotti-Raymond M, Wallace AC, et al: Endogenous retrovirus insertion in the *KIT* oncogene determines *White* and white *Spotting* in domestic cats. *G3 (Bethesda)* 4:1881–1891, 2014.

73. Montague MJ, Li G, Gandolfi B, et al: Comparative analysis of the domestic cat genome reveals genetic signatures underlying feline biology and domestication. *Proc Natl Acad Sci U S A* 111:17230–17235, 2014.

74. Wilson TG, Kane F: Congenital deafness in white cats. *Acta Otolaryngolica* 50:269–275, discussion 75–7, 1959.

75. Bergsma DR, Brown KS: White fur, blue eyes, and deafness in the domestic cat. *J Hered* 62:171–185, 1971.

76. Bamber RC: Correlation between white coat colour, blue eyes, and deafness in cats. *J Genetics* 27:407–413, 1933.

77. Torjesen I: Genomes of 100,000 people will be sequenced to create an open access research resource. *BMJ* 347:f6690, 2013.

78. Roach JC, Glusman G, Smit AF, et al: Analysis of genetic inheritance in a family quartet by whole-genome sequencing. *Science* 328:636–639, 2010.

79. Hoffmann GF, Lindner M, Loeber JG: 50 years of newborn screening. *J Inherit Metab Dis* 37:163–164, 2014.

80. Rabbani B, Tekin M, Mahdieh N: The promise of whole-exome sequencing in medical genetics. *J Hum Genet* 59:5–15, 2014.

81. Hayden EC: Technology: the $1,000 genome. *Nature* 507:294–295, 2014.

82. Saunders CJ, Miller NA, Soden SE, et al: Rapid whole-genome sequencing for genetic disease diagnosis in neonatal intensive care units. *Sci Transl Med* 4:154ra35, 2012.

83. Meurs KM, Sanchez X, David RM, et al: A *cardiac myosin binding protein C* mutation in the Maine Coon cat with familial hypertrophic cardiomyopathy. *Hum Mol Genet* 14:3587–3593, 2005.

84. Eizirik E, Yuhki N, Johnson WE, et al: Molecular genetics and evolution of melanism in the cat family. *Curr Biol* 13:448–453, 2003.

85. Lyons LA, Foe IT, Rah HC, et al: Chocolate coated cats: *TYRP1* mutations for brown color in domestic cats. *Mamm Genome* 16:356–366, 2005.

86. Schmidt-Kuntzel A, Eizirik E, O'Brien SJ, et al: *Tyrosinase and tyrosinase related protein 1* alleles specify domestic cat coat color phenotypes of the albino and Brown loci. *J Hered* 96:289–301, 2005.

87. Imes DL, Geary LA, Grahn RA, et al: Albinism in the domestic cat (*Felis catus*) is associated with a *tyrosinase (TYR)* mutation. *Anim Genet* 37:175–178, 2006.

88. Lyons LA, Imes DL, Rah HC, et al: *Tyrosinase* mutations associated with Siamese and Burmese patterns in the domestic cat (*Felis catus*). *Anim Genet* 36:119–126, 2005.

89. Ishida Y, David VA, Eizirik E, et al: A homozygous single-base deletion in *MLPH* causes the dilute coat color phenotype in the domestic cat. *Genomics* 88:698–705, 2006.

90. Peterschmitt M, Grain F, Arnaud B, et al: Mutation in the *melanocortin 1 receptor* is associated with amber colour in the Norwegian Forest cat. *Anim Genet* 40:547–552, 2009.

91. Lettice LA, Hill AE, Devenney PS, et al: Point mutations in a distant *sonic hedgehog* cis-regulator generate a variable regulatory output responsible for preaxial polydactyly. *Hum Mol Genet* 17:978–985, 2008.

92. Gandolfi B, Alhaddad H, Affolter VK, et al: To the root of the curl: a signature of a recent selective sweep identifies a mutation that defines the Cornish Rex cat breed. *PLoS ONE* 8:e67105, 2013.

93. Gandolfi B, Outerbridge C, Beresford L, et al: The naked truth: Sphynx and Devon Rex cat breed mutations in *KRT71*. *Mamm Genome* 21:509–515, 2010.

94. Kaelin CB, Xu X, Hong LZ, et al: Specifying and sustaining pigmentation patterns in domestic and wild cats. *Science* 337:1536–1541, 2012.

95. Bighignoli B, Niini T, Grahn RA, et al: *Cytidine monophospho-N-acetylneuraminic acid hydroxylase (CMAH)* mutations associated with the domestic cat AB blood group. *BMC Genet* 8:27, 2007.

96. De Maria R, Divari S, Bo S, et al: Beta-galactosidase deficiency in a Korat cat: a new form of feline GM1-gangliosidosis. *Acta Neuropathol (Berl)* 96:307–314, 1998.

97. Bradbury AM, Morrison NE, Hwang M, et al: Neurodegenerative lysosomal storage disease in European Burmese cats with hexosaminidase beta-subunit deficiency. *Mol Genet Metab* 97:53–59, 2009.

98. Muldoon LL, Neuwelt EA, Pagel MA, et al: Characterization of the molecular defect in a feline model for type II GM2-gangliosidosis (Sandhoff disease). *Am J Pathol* 144:1109–1118, 1994.

99. Martin DR, Cox NR, Morrison NE, et al: Mutation of the GM2 activator protein in a feline model of GM2 gangliosidosis. *Acta Neuropathol* 110:443–450, 2005.

100. Meurs KM, Norgard MM, Ederer MM, et al: A substitution mutation in the *myosin binding protein C* gene in ragdoll hypertrophic cardiomyopathy. *Genomics* 90:261–264, 2007.

101. Fyfe JC, Menotti-Raymond M, David VA, et al: An approximately 140-kb deletion associated with feline spinal muscular atrophy implies an essential *LIX1* function for motor neuron survival. *Genome Res* 16:1084–1090, 2006.

102. Owens SL, Downey ME, Pressler BM, et al: Congenital adrenal hyperplasia associated with mutation in an *11 beta-hydroxylase-like* gene in a cat. *J Vet Intern Med* 26:1221–1226, 2012.

103. Chang HS, Shibata T, Arai S, et al: Dihydropyrimidinase deficiency: the first feline case of dihydropyrimidinuria with clinical and molecular findings. *JIMD Rep* 6:21–26, 2012.

104. Bender DE, Kloos MT, Pontius JU, et al: Molecular characterization of cat *Factor XII* gene and identification of a mutation causing factor XII deficiency in a domestic shorthair cat colony. *Vet Pathol* 52:312–320, 2015.

105. Martin DR, Krum BK, Varadarajan GS, et al: An inversion of 25 base pairs causes feline GM2 gangliosidosis variant. *Exp Neurol* 187:30–37, 2004.

106. Kanae Y, Endoh D, Yamato O, et al: Nonsense mutation of feline *beta-hexosaminidase beta-subunit (HEXB)* gene causing Sandhoff disease in a family of Japanese domestic cats. *Res Vet Sci* 82:54–60, 2007.

107. Goree M, Catalfamo JL, Aber S, et al: Characterization of the mutations causing hemophilia B in 2 domestic cats. *J Vet Intern Med* 19:200–204, 2005.

108. Goldstein R, Narala S, Sabet N, et al: Primary hyperoxaluria in cats caused by a mutation in the feline *GRHPR* gene. *J Hered* 100:S2–S7, 2009.

109. Ginzinger DG, Lewis ME, Ma Y, et al: A mutation in the *lipoprotein lipase* gene is the molecular basis of chylomicronemia in a colony of domestic cats. *J Clin Invest* 97:1257–1266, 1996.

110. Mazrier H, Van Hoeven M, Wang P, et al: Inheritance, biochemical abnormalities, and clinical features of feline mucolipidosis II: the first animal model of human I-cell disease. *J Hered* 94:363–373, 2003.

111. Berg T, Tollersrud OK, Walkley SU, et al: Purification of feline lysosomal alpha-mannosidase, determination of its cDNA sequence and identification of a mutation causing alpha-mannosidosis in Persian cats. *Biochem J* 328(Pt 3):863–870, 1997.

112. He X, Li CM, Simonaro CM, et al: Identification and characterization of the molecular lesion causing mucopolysaccharidosis type I in cats. *Mol Genet Metab* 67:106–112, 1999.

113. Yogalingam G, Litjens T, Bielicki J, et al: Feline mucopolysaccharidosis type VI. Characterization of recombinant N-acetylgalactosamine 4-sulfatase and identification of a mutation causing the disease. *J Biol Chem* 271:27259–27265, 1996.

114. Yogalingam G, Hopwood JJ, Crawley A, et al: Mild feline mucopolysaccharidosis type VI. Identification of an *N-acetylgalactosamine-4-sulfatase* mutation causing instability and increased specific activity. *J Biol Chem* 273:13421–13429, 1998.

115. Crawley AC, Yogalingam G, Muller VJ, et al: Two mutations within a feline mucopolysaccharidosis type VI colony cause three different clinical phenotypes. *J Clin Invest* 101:109–119, 1998.

116. Fyfe JC, Kurzhals RL, Lassaline ME, et al: Molecular basis of feline beta-glucuronidase deficiency: an animal model of mucopolysaccharidosis VII. *Genomics* 58:121–128, 1999.

117. Winand NJ, Edwards M, Pradhan D, et al: Deletion of the dystrophin muscle promoter in feline muscular dystrophy. *Neuromuscul Disord* 4:433–445, 1994.

118. Somers K, Royals M, Carstea E, et al: Mutation analysis of feline Niemann-Pick C1 disease. *Mol Genet Metab* 79:99–103, 2003.

119. Clavero S, Bishop DF, Giger U, et al: Feline congenital erythropoietic porphyria: two homozygous *UROS* missense mutations cause the enzyme deficiency and porphyrin accumulation. *Mol Med* 16:381–388, 2010.

120. Clavero S, Bishop DF, Haskins ME, et al: Feline acute intermittent porphyria: a phenocopy masquerading as an erythropoietic porphyria due to dominant and recessive *hydroxymethylbilane synthase* mutations. *Hum Mol Genet* 19:584–596, 2010.

121. Geisen V, Weber K, Hartmann K: Vitamin D-dependent hereditary rickets type I in a cat. *J Vet Intern Med* 23:196–199, 2009.

122. Grahn RA, Ellis MR, Grahn JC, et al: A novel *CYP27B1* mutation causes a feline vitamin D-dependent rickets type IA. *J Feline Med Surg* 14:587–590, 2012.

Anesthetic-Related Morbidity and Mortality in Cats

Sheilah A. Robertson

"What are the risks of anesthesia in cats today?" Until recently this was a question to which one did not have an accurate answer. The data generated by the Confidential Enquiry into Perioperative Small Animal Fatalities (CEPSAF), a multicenter prospective cohort study conducted in the United Kingdom between 2002 and 2004, currently provides the most comprehensive information regarding feline mortality.[1] In veterinary medicine, there is no mandatory reporting or investigation of anesthetic-related deaths as there is in human medicine, and previous animal studies have been difficult to interpret due to study design (e.g., retrospective versus prospective data collection and sample size limitations), patient population (e.g., general practice versus referral centers and university hospitals), anesthetic drugs used (which have changed over time), and variation in anesthetic management among clinics and among countries. In addition, the definition of mortality has not been precisely given, and it has been difficult to differentiate between a perianesthetic death, which could have resulted from surgical error or the patient's health status, from one that was directly caused by anesthesia alone.

The CEPSAF study recorded patient outcome (alive, dead, or euthanized) after premedication and within 48 hours of the end of the procedure and calculated specific risks of anesthetic-related death. Anesthetic- or sedation-related death was defined as "death where surgical or pre-existing medical causes did not solely cause death." This study has generated risk factors for the different companion animal species (dog, cat, rabbit, and "other small animals") and paves the way for improving anesthetic management and decreasing mortality in small animal practice.[1-4]

Practitioners are also interested in patient morbidity data. This is more difficult to obtain, because there is no uniformly accepted definition of morbidity or organized reporting system for perioperative "mishaps" related to veterinary anesthesia. In human medicine, one proposed definition of morbidity is "any complication, excluding death, occurring during the perioperative period," and these have been classified into "minor," "intermediate," and "major" groupings.[5]

FELINE PERIOPERATIVE MORTALITY

Historically, perioperative mortality rates for cats have ranged from 0.1% to 5.8%, but as previously mentioned, the studies that provide such data are fraught with problems.[6] The first prospective multicenter cohort study of small animal anesthetic mortality was conducted in the United Kingdom in the mid-1980s and reported the risk of anesthetic-related death in cats to be 0.29%.[7] The CEPSAF study included 79,178 cats and was performed to see if mortality rates had dropped in the intervening time and to investigate the impact of newer anesthetics and monitoring modalities. The *overall* risk of death, that of *healthy* cats and dogs, and that of *sick* cats and dogs were compared (Table 75-1). "Healthy" (ASA 1 and 2) and "sick" (ASA 3 to 5) classifications were based on the American Society of Anesthesiologists (ASA) classification scheme.[8] In this study, cats had a higher mortality rate than dogs, but of note is the fact that cats classified as *healthy* were twice as likely to die compared to dogs in this category. A single-center study in France reported a mortality rate of 0.19% for healthy cats (ASA 1 and 2) and 4.6% for sick cats (ASA 3 to 5), which was not statistically significantly different than the data for dogs at this clinic, although the authors stated that cat mortality tended to be higher than dog mortality.[9]

Regardless of the study, these numbers compare poorly to data for humans where the mortality rate solely attributable to anesthesia in developed countries declined from approximately 0.03% prior to the 1970s to less than 0.005% in the 1990s to 2000s.[10]

When Do Most Deaths Occur?

Analysis of the results of the CEPSAF study reveals that most deaths, regardless of species, occur postoperatively. In cats, 61% of all deaths occur during this time (Table 75-2). The most critical time appears to be in the *first 3 hours* after the end of anesthesia, which is when 62% of all postanesthetic deaths occur compared to 8.5% in the 3- to 6-hour time frame.[4] Cats may be vulnerable during this time because they are usually transitioned from 100% oxygen to room air at a time when they are cold and begin shivering, which increases oxygen demand. This can be especially detrimental in sick cats and those with cardiac disease. Monitoring equipment is often removed during this time and cats are extubated, leading to the possibility of airway obstruction (see Special Topics in Feline Anesthesia). In addition, this is when cats regain consciousness and may become aware of pain, the consequences of which include tachycardia and

Table 75-1	Mortality Rates in Dogs and Cats Derived from the Confidential Enquiry into Perioperative Small Animal Fatalities		
Mortality	**Dogs**	**Cats**	
Overall	0.17%	0.24%	
Healthy (ASA 1-2)	0.054%	0.112%	
Sick (ASA 3-5)	1.33%	1.40%	

Brodbelt DC, Blissitt KJ, Hammond RA, et al: The risk of death: the Confidential Enquiry into Perioperative Small Animal Fatalities. *Vet Anaesth Analg* 35:365-373, 2008.
ASA, American Society of Anesthesiologists classification.

Table 75-2	Time of Death in Dogs and Cats Derived from the Confidential Enquiry into Perioperative Small Animal Fatalities*		
Time of Death	**Dog**	**Cat**	
After premedication	1%	1%	
Induction	6%	8%	
Maintenance	46%	30%	
Postoperative	47%	61%	
Total	100%	100%	

Brodbelt DC, Blissitt KJ, Hammond RA, et al: The risk of death: the Confidential Enquiry into Perioperative Small Animal Fatalities. *Vet Anaesth Analg* 35:365-373, 2008.
*Reported as percentage of total deaths.

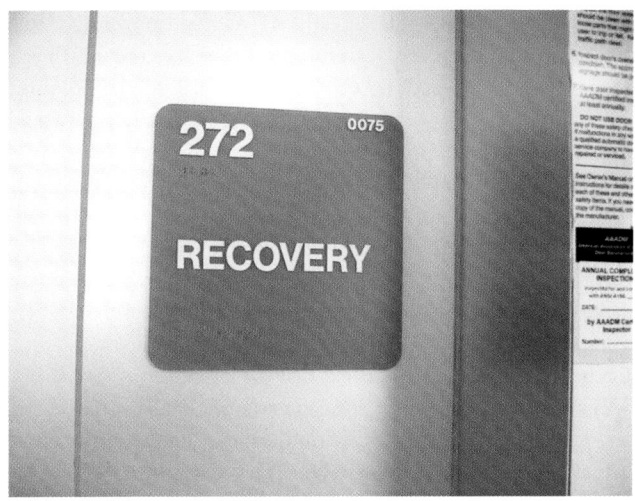

Figure 75-1: Continuous observation in a designated recovery area during the first 3 hours after the end of a procedure is recommended, because this is when most deaths occur.

Table 75-3	Cause of Death in 79,178 Cats Based on Data from the Confidential Enquiry into Perioperative Small Animal Fatalities*	
Cause of Death	**Percentage of Total**	
Cardiovascular	6%	
Respiratory	9%	
Either cardiovascular or respiratory	57%	
Neurologic	5%	
Renal	3%	
Unknown	20%	

Brodbelt DC, Blissitt KJ, Hammond RA, et al: The risk of death: the Confidential Enquiry into Perioperative Small Animal Fatalities. *Vet Anaesth Analg* 35:365-373, 2008.
*Reported as percentage of total deaths.

hypertension, and defensive behaviors can further reduce our ability to monitor the patient. A large proportion of deaths (20%) during the postoperative period were classified as being of "unknown cause," suggesting that cats were not closely observed or monitored during this time. Clear identification of a high risk period should lead one to rethink how one uses resources and staff. Increased vigilance and oversight of cats by trained staff during the first 3 postanesthetic hours could reduce the risk of death (Figure 75-1).

What Are the Causes of Death?

An independent panel reviewed details of each anesthetic death reported in the CEPSAF study and tried to ascertain a cause. Death was most commonly attributed to a combination of cardiovascular and respiratory causes followed by respiratory, cardiovascular, neurologic, and renal causes alone. In 20% of cases, a cause of death could not be determined with any certainty (Table 75-3).[4]

Risk Factors

Overall, the risk associated with anesthesia for cats in the CEPSAF study was significantly higher than for dogs.[1] Of particular interest is data showing that the risk in "healthy cats" is greater than in "healthy dogs," but mortality was similar in both species if they were classified as being "sick." A greater mortality rate in cats compared to dogs has been reported in other studies.[6,9] A number of specific risk factors for feline morbidity and mortality were identified or implicated from the CEPSAF data, including the impact of overall health status, subclinical disease, body weight, age, hypothermia, intravenous (IV) fluid use, anesthetic drugs and techniques, monitoring procedures, and duration of anesthesia.

Health Status. The correlation between health status and postoperative outcome is documented in several veterinary species and in humans. Cats with a higher ASA status carry a greater risk for anesthesia-related morbidity and mortality.[1,11] Therefore, careful attention to preanesthetic assessment, stabilization, choice of anesthetic techniques, monitoring, and postanesthetic care are especially important in patients with compromised health.

Subclinical Disease. One reason for the higher risk in "healthy" cats reported in the CEPSAF study may be the presence of subclinical cardiac disease. In "overtly" or "apparently" healthy cats, the prevalence of cardiomyopathy may be as high as 15%.[12,13] Thus, a cat may be misclassified when using the ASA system. Detection of a heart murmur is not a reliable indicator of cardiac disease in cats. In one study, only 53% of cats that were considered healthy based on history and physical examination—except for the presence of a heart murmur on auscultation—had echocardiographic evidence of disease.[14] There may be a higher level of suspicion in certain breeds. For example, in a population of Sphynx cats, 34.2% had abnormal findings on echocardiography and were diagnosed with congenital heart disease, hypertrophic cardiomyopathy, or mitral valve dysplasia.[15] Because cats with cardiac disease can appear clinically healthy and may or may not have a heart murmur, it is difficult to know how one can detect patients at risk during anesthesia due to compromised cardiac function without preanesthetic screening with echocardiography or cardiac biomarker testing.

Other reasons for misclassifying a cat's physical status may include difficulty in interpreting physiologic parameters during the preoperative examination or complete inability to conduct a full clinical examination. One study documented a significant difference in systolic blood pressure, heart rate, and respiratory rate between cats examined in their home versus in a veterinary hospital; therefore, it is important to consider the impact of stress during clinical examinations.[16] Not all veterinary clinics are feline friendly, and not all veterinarians and staff are trained in feline-friendly handling and nursing care.[17,18] Without good feline handling skills, physical examination of cats may be cursory and postoperative monitoring may be minimal, with a detrimental outcome.

Body Weight. Cats that weigh less than 2 kg (4.4 lbs) are at high risk for anesthetic-related mortality with more than 15 times greater odds of death as compared to cats weighing 2 to 6 kg (4.4 to 13.2 lbs) (Figure 75-2). The large surface area–to-body weight ratio of smaller cats may predispose them to hypothermia and its associated complications.

At the other end of the spectrum, obese cats were also at risk; this may be related to a greater risk for respiratory compromise (i.e., airway obstruction and reduced diaphragmatic excursions due to abdominal and thoracic fat, especially when placed in dorsal recumbency). Obese cats are also likely to have reduced cardiovascular reserves; cardiac work is increased due to the requirement for increased cardiac output as body fat increases.[19] Relative anesthetic overdose may be another contributing factor when injectable drugs are based on current body weight rather than on lean or ideal body weight. Adipose tissue may act as a depot for inhalant anesthetic agents and delay recovery.

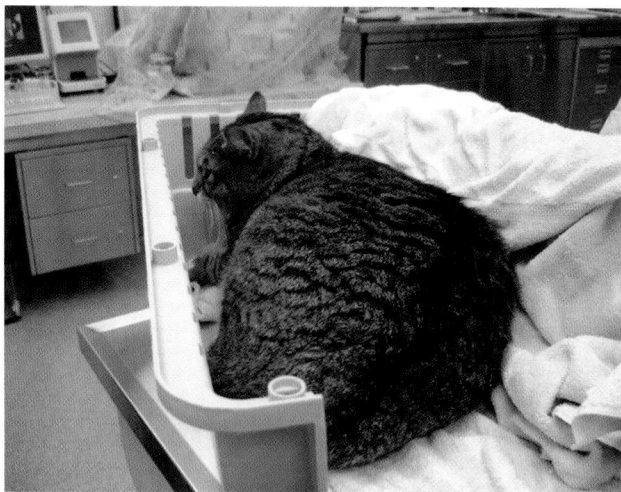

Figure 75-2: Cats less than 2 kg (4.4 lbs) and those that are overweight or obese carry a high risk of anesthetic-related mortality.

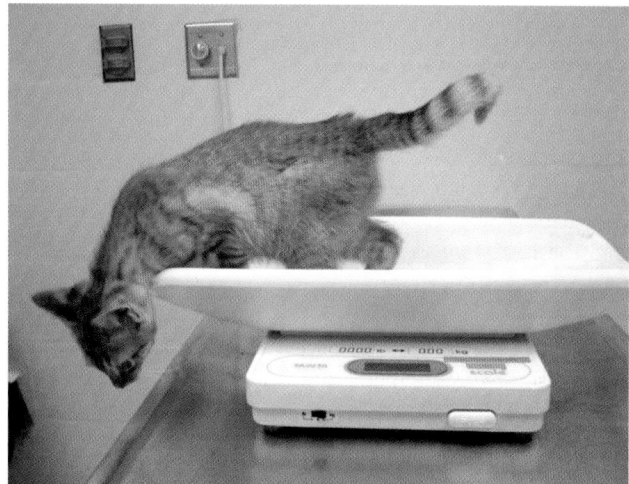

Figure 75-3: Estimates or inaccurate measurement of body weight increases the risk of relative drug overdoses.

Animal size is also related to the risk of hypothermia.[20,21] Without active warming strategies, rectal temperature in animals weighing less than 10 kg (22 lbs) can fall as much as 3.4 to 6.3 °C (6.1 to 11.3 °F) during a 1- to 2-hour period compared to a 1.5 °C (2.7 °F) drop in animals greater than 30 kg (66 lbs). The small size of cats may also lead to more problems with IV catheter placement, intubation, and monitoring. In addition, if cats are not accurately weighed, it is likely that relative drug overdoses occur (Figure 75-3). The CEPSAF study revealed that body weight is estimated approximately 20% of the time.[4]

Age. The CEPSAF study is the first to find a correlation between age and anesthetic risk in cats. Older patients carry a higher anesthetic risk; cats older than 12 years are twice as likely to die compared to cats aged 6 months to 5 years. This increased risk was independent from the ASA status and may be a result of decreased respiratory and cardiovascular reserve, decreased thermoregulatory ability, and decreased anesthetic requirements. The age-related decrease in inhalant anesthetic requirements is documented in humans[22] and dogs.[23] Although such changes are not reported in cats, age-related changes similar to those in humans are found in cat brains.[24]

Routine health screening is important in cats of all ages; however, findings that may be significant to anesthetic risk management have been described in cats more than 10 years of age.[25] Cats more than 10 years of age had higher blood pressure values, heart rates, urine protein:creatinine ratios, serum urea and bilirubin concentrations, and lower body condition scores, hematocrit, albumin and total calcium concentrations compared to cats aged between 6 and 10 years. With up to 30% of animals seen by practitioners classified as "senior," age-related sensitivity to anesthesia is a significant factor to consider. The American Association of Feline Practitioners (AAFP) has published guidelines for the care of senior cats that include a section on anesthesia.[26]

Hypothermia. Hypothermia increases intraoperative bleeding, increases the risk of postoperative wound infection, results in shivering and increased oxygen consumption in the recovery period, slows metabolism of drugs, delays recovery, decreases perfusion, and increases catecholamine release leading to cardiac complications.[27-29] In addition, shivering can contribute to pain and discomfort at the operative site; in humans, hypothermia is reported to be extremely unpleasant in the recovery period. Brodbelt and colleagues[1] reported that patient temperature was infrequently monitored during anesthesia (1% to 2% of cases) and only in 11% to 15% of cats after the procedure.

A retrospective study of 275 cats by Redondo and colleagues[29] provides insight into the prevalence of post-anesthetic hypothermia. In this study, both rectal and esophageal temperatures were recorded and classified as follows: hyperthermia (greater than 39.5 °C [103.1 °F]; two cats), normothermia (38.5 to 39.5 °C [101.3 to 103.1 °F]; five cats), slight hypothermia (38.5 to 36.5 °C [101.3 to 97.7 °F]; 73 cats), moderate hypothermia (36.5 to 34.0 °C [97.7 to 93.2 °F]; 166 cats), and severe hypothermia (less than 34.0 °C [93.2 °F]; 29 cats). In 96.7% of cats, the temperature at the end of anesthesia was below their baseline value. The main predictors of temperature at the end of the procedure were the cat's basal temperature, duration of anesthesia, reason for anesthesia, severity of the procedure, and ASA status. The magnitude of hypothermia also correlated with outcome with reported mortality rates of 0% (hyperthermia and normothermia), 2.73% (slight hypothermia), 1.20% (moderate hypothermia), and 6.89% (severe hypothermia). Time to extubation was also affected by temperature with severely hypothermic cats taking twice as long to reach this stage compared to normothermic cats,[29] a phenomenon also reported in dogs.[28]

There are many strategies that can be initiated to prevent and minimize heat loss in cats.[30] These include active warming techniques that provide external heat beginning at or before the time of premedication, avoiding contact with cold surfaces, avoiding the use of cold preparation solutions (especially alcohol), and using passive techniques, such as jackets,

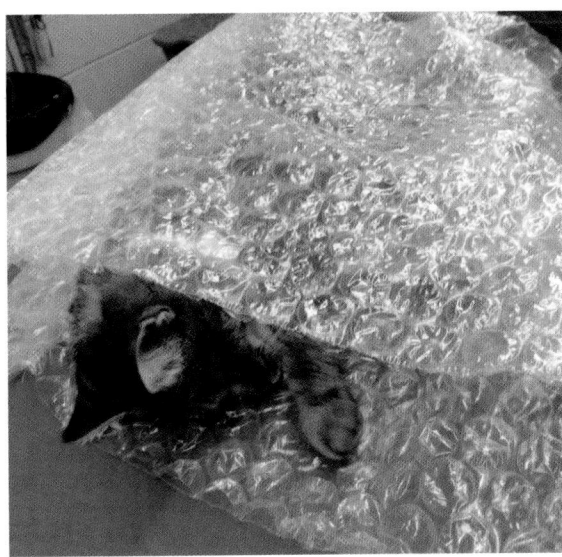

Figure 75-4: Bubble wrap can be used as a passive warming technique to reduce hypothermia.

blankets, and "bubble wrap" (Figure 75-4). Active warming is highly effective; after 90 minutes of anesthesia, cats that were placed under forced-air warming blankets had mean body temperatures 0.9 °C (1.6 °F) higher than those receiving no active warming.[31]

Intravenous Fluids. Surprisingly, the use of IV fluids increased the risk of dying by fourfold in both healthy and sick cats.[1] Although confounding factors (i.e., those cats receiving IV fluids may have been at greater anesthetic risk to begin with) should be taken into account, these findings should make one reconsider fluid therapy protocols in anesthetized cats. The difference in blood volume between dogs and cats may be overlooked when delivering fluids to feline patients. The blood volume of cats is approximately 60 mL/kg body weight compared to 80 to 90 mL/kg in dogs.[32] Historically, intraoperative fluid rates of 10 mL/kg/hour were recommended with little evidence to support such rates. The 2013 American Animal Hospital Association and AAFP Fluid Therapy Guidelines for Dogs and Cats are much more conservative with 3 mL/kg/hour as a suggested starting rate when using crystalloid fluids in cats.[33]

Even if lower rates are used, inaccurate administration and resultant fluid overload must be avoided. The use of infusion or syringe pumps (Figure 75-5A) or a Buretrol (see Figure 75-5B) is advised in cats to ensure accurate volume delivery and to prevent accidental delivery (i.e., drip inadvertently set fully open). When using a Buretrol, only the volume of fluids to be given over 1 hour should be put in the chamber at a time so that administration is limited, even in the case of incorrect drip rate setting. With the knowledge that apparently healthy cats may have underlying and undiagnosed cardiac disease, it is possible that vascular overload in the face of impaired pumping ability contributes to mortality.

Anesthetic Drugs and Techniques. Unlike dogs, no specific anesthetic drug or technique (e.g., mask induction) was implicated in cat mortality. Reduced odds of mortality were

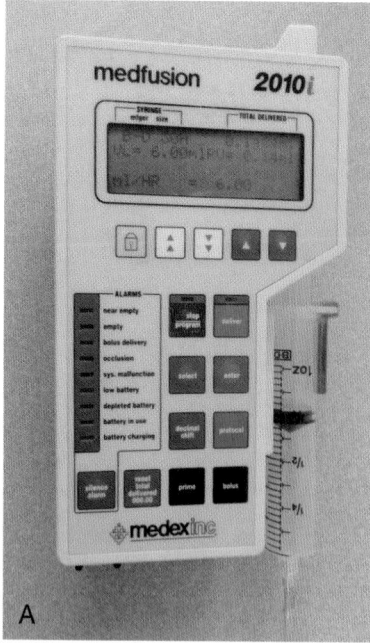

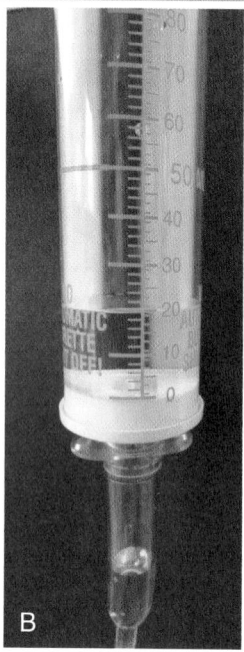

Figure 75-5: Administration of intravenous fluids has been associated with increased anesthetic-related mortality. The American Animal Hospital Association/American Association of Feline Practitioners Fluid Therapy Guidelines for Dogs and Cats recommend a starting rate of 3 mL/kg/hour, and the fluids should be accurately delivered using a syringe pump **(A)** or a Buretrol **(B). B,** A Buretrol containing 20 mL of crystalloid fluid; this is the volume of fluid to be administered over 1 hour for a 5 kg cat at a rate of 4 mL/kg/hour and is an additional safety measure. Once this volume is delivered, fluid administration ceases. (Courtesy of Docsinnovent, Ltd. London.)

found when acepromazine, benzodiazepines, and opioid combinations were used as premedicants compared to when no preinduction sedation was used, but these relationships were not statistically significant.[1] Nevertheless, sedation makes handling of cats easier, reduces stress, and decreases the dose of induction and maintenance agents and is highly

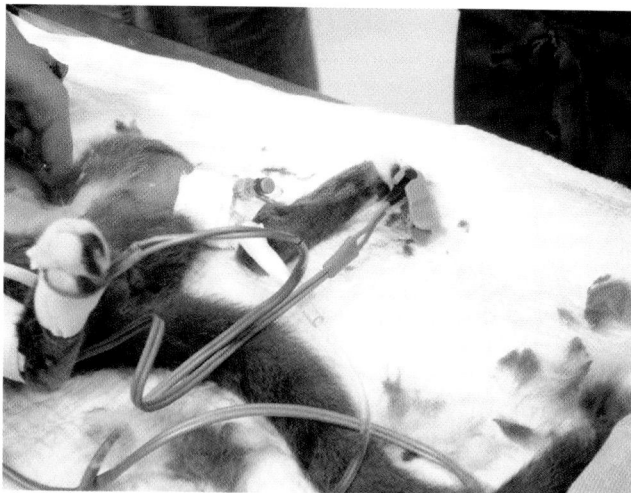

Figure 75-6: The recommended site for placement of a pulse oximeter probe in the cat is the hind paw.

recommended. The alpha$_2$-adrenergic agonist, medetomidine, was not associated with an increased risk, whereas in previous studies, xylazine was implicated.[7,11] There is evidence, at least in dogs, that xylazine sensitizes the heart to ventricular arrhythmias,[34] whereas the newer and more selective alpha$_2$-adrenergic agonist drugs do not. There is no data on dexmedetomidine, but there is no reason to think it would act differently from medetomidine.

Monitoring. A monitor can be described as an instrument or device used for observing, checking, or keeping a continuous record. The verb *to monitor* means to observe and check the progress or quality of something over a period of time. Monitors extend the human senses but do not replace them. As such, a monitor can only warn the user of an adverse event, it cannot intervene. Such response remains a vital function of the person in charge of a patient's anesthetic event. It is imperative that practitioners understand the data that the monitors display and what to do when an abnormality arises. Much of the reduction in anesthetic patient mortality in the human arena is a result of better anesthetic drugs, equipment, and monitoring devices, yet an intraoperative incident still occurs in one out of 10 patients;[5] these are primarily due to human error. Dyson showed the value of trained personnel in veterinary medicine; the presence of a technician whose primary focus was anesthetic management of the patient significantly reduced the odds of a complication occurring.[11]

The study by Brodbelt and colleagues[1] is the first time that the value of monitoring has been shown to save lives in veterinary medicine. Monitoring the pulse and using a pulse oximeter significantly reduced mortality. It is well worth investing time in learning how best to use a pulse oximeter in cats; one study indicated that the best site for probe placement in cats is the rear paw[35] (Figure 75-6). This is an ideal site when performing dental surgery or if a cat is not intubated but receiving oxygen via face mask. A common cause of interference with the light-emitting diode of the probe and sensor is fluorescent and operating room lights; therefore, it is recommended to cover the probe with a gauze sponge.

Duration of Anesthesia. An increase in duration of the procedure contributes to mortality. An anesthetic period of greater than 90 minutes increases the odds of mortality more than three times as compared to procedures less than 30 minutes in duration. Based on this data, every effort should be made to ensure procedures are done as quickly as possible and no "wasted" anesthesia time occurs because of poor scheduling or planning—in other words, efficiency is key to a good outcome. When possible, diagnostic (e.g., imaging, endoscopy, and so on) and surgical procedures should be performed during separate anesthetic events.

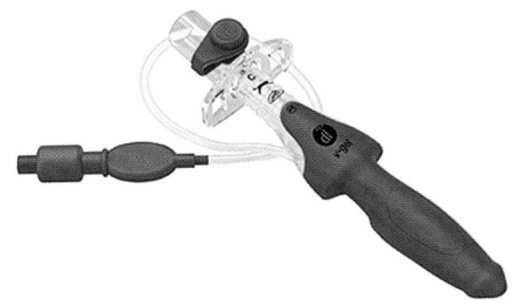

Figure 75-7: Supraglottic airway device, the Cat v-gel (Docsinnovent Ltd., London).

SPECIAL TOPICS IN FELINE ANESTHESIA

Airway Management

Brodbelt and colleagues[1] reported that 63% of cats that died were intubated compared to 48% of cats that were not. For short procedures (less than 30 minutes), intubation increased the risk of death. Respiratory obstruction as a cause of death has been reported more frequently in cats than in dogs, indicating that close attention to the airway in this species is important.[1,7,11]

Respiratory problems were most common in the postoperative period, suggesting airway trauma and edema may be involved. Tracheal injury related to intubation is well documented in cats[36-39] as is damage to the larynx.[40] Approximately 70% to 75% of tracheal rupture reports are related to the cat having undergone a dental procedure, with presenting signs of subcutaneous emphysema, coughing, gagging, and varying degrees of dyspnea occurring 4 hours to 12 days after the procedure.

These data indicate that great care should be taken when placing an endotracheal tube (ETT) in a cat; the propensity of cats to have laryngospasm may play a role. Intubation should be performed under the correct plane of anesthesia (not too light) and with direct visualization (through use of a laryngoscope). The use of topical local anesthetics (e.g., lidocaine) applied to the arytenoids and vocal cords, in correctly metered doses (if given by aerosolized spray), are recommended; however, these can negatively affect the laryngeal mucosa.[41] Patience is required, and the tube should only be advanced when the vocal cords are open. Distal tracheal tears are associated with a poor outcome.[36] Therefore, the length of the ETT should be measured against the cat prior to insertion, and the tip of the tube should not extend beyond the point of the shoulder.

Hardie and colleagues[36] documented that tracheal tears occur directly over the ETT cuff as a result of overinflation. One theory is that cuffs are overinflated for dental procedures due to a fear of aspiration. Larger tears are more difficult to repair or medically manage; therefore, the choice of ETT should be made with care. Tubes with low-volume, high-pressure cuffs and those with high-volume, low-pressure cuffs are available; the latter have a longer cuff, so they should be used with caution. The cuff should only be inflated if necessary; the seal can be tested by closing the pop-off valve and

squeezing the reservoir bag. Air is added in small increments to the cuff until there is no leak at 15 cm H_2O. A small (3 mL) syringe should be used to prevent overinflation, and the use of water soluble gel on the cuff will improve the airway seal, even at low cuff inflation pressures.[42] To avoid these risks, consideration should be given to using noncuffed ETTs (with or without pharyngeal packs), oxygen masks, laryngeal mask airways, or supraglottic airway devices (SGADs) as alternatives to cuffed ETTs. For short procedures (less than 30 minutes), an oxygen mask will usually suffice; however, in brachycephalic cats, establishing an airway is always advisable.

Laryngeal mask airways have not been designed specifically for cats; however, one SGAD (Cat v-gel, Docsinnovent Ltd., London) has been designed to conform to the shape of the feline larynx and pharynx and has recently been evaluated (Figure 75-7).[43,44] This device is comprised of a soft, dedicated, noninflatable cuff that rests over the laryngeal inlet and a dorsal pressure adjuster that can be inflated to depress the cuff over the laryngeal opening. The SGAD can be inserted without the use of local anesthetics. The time to obtain a clinically acceptable capnograph (end tidal carbon dioxide) reading was shorter when a SGAD was used compared to an ETT (median time 44 seconds and 109 seconds, respectively), suggesting that the airway can be more rapidly secured using the former technique. There was less stridor in the immediate recovery period after use of a SGAD compared to an ETT.[44] In spontaneously breathing cats, there was no difference in the measured isoflurane concentration at the mouth when ETTs and SGADs were compared, but there is currently no data on inhalant anesthetic leakage when positive pressure ventilation is used.[44]

Postanesthetic Blindness

There are reports of cats being temporarily or permanently blind with or without other neurological abnormalities following anesthesia[45,46] (Figure 75-8). The purpose of anesthesia in the majority of these cases was for dental or oral endoscopy procedures, but blindness and neurologic deficits are also reported following resuscitation after cardiac arrest. Most cats undergoing endoscopy and dental procedures had spring-loaded mouth gags inserted, often to full extension, for variable periods of time (45 minutes to 5.5 hours), although

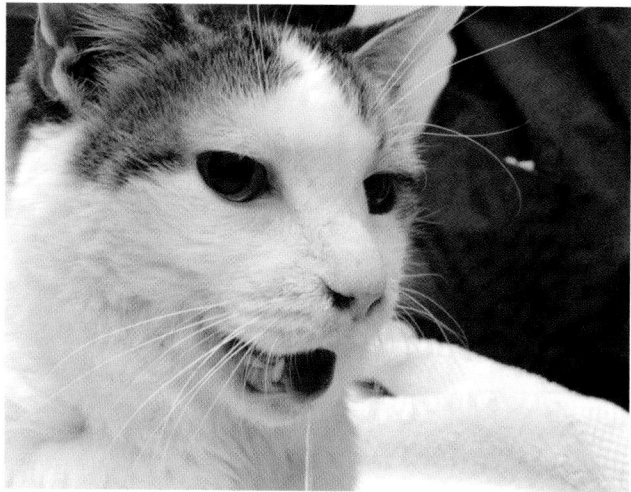

Figure 75-8: This cat underwent a prolonged dental procedure with a spring-loaded mouth gag inserted to keep the mouth in an open position. Immediately after anesthesia, the cat was blind, ataxic, and had difficulty swallowing.

there was no association between length of anesthesia and severity of clinical signs. In one report, three out of 20 cats exhibited cortical blindness only, and the other 17 had cortical blindness along with ataxia, head tilt, proprioceptive deficits, and abnormal mentation.[46] Of those that had a known outcome, 70% regained sufficient vision to adequately navigate their surroundings, three cats that remained blind were reported to adapt well, 59% of cats with neurologic deficits made a full recovery, and one cat was euthanized. Based on cadaver dissection[46] and evaluation of maxillary blood flow,[47] the cause of these postanesthetic deficits in cats that underwent endoscopy or dental procedures is presumed to be cerebral ischemia due to impaired blood flow in the maxillary artery (the primary cerebral blood supply in cats) when the mouth is held open. Additional studies using magnetic resonance angiography, computed tomography, electroretinography, and brainstem auditory-evoked potentials demonstrate that indicators of cerebral blood flow can be diminished in some cats when their mouth is open.[47] To prevent these adverse events, spring-loaded mouth gags should be opened just enough to perform the procedure, or replaced with a mouth gag made by cutting a short length from a tuberculin syringe or needle cap and inserting the canine teeth into either end, again opening the mouth only as wide as needed (Figure 75-9). Removing the gag and closing the mouth at 10 to 15 minute intervals are advisable.

SUMMARY

Although feline anesthetic-related mortality has decreased over the past two decades, there is still room for improvement, and some key factors to focus on have been identified (Table 75-4):

- It should be recognized that cats may have underlying cardiac disease that will not be apparent from the history and physical examination.

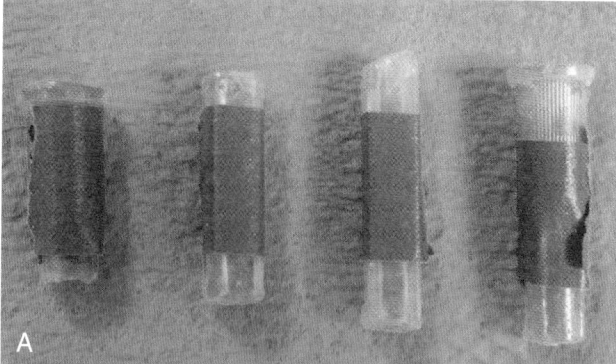

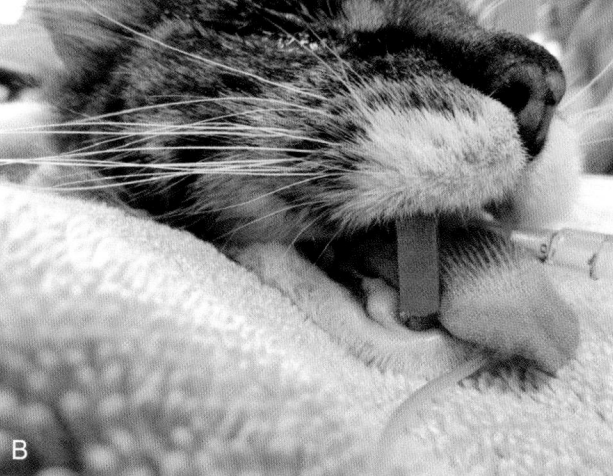

Figure 75-9: A, A mouth gag constructed by cutting a short length of a tuberculin syringe or needle cap. These can be filled with nontoxic Silly Putty or dental wax to prevent the canine teeth from slipping out. **B,** This homemade device may place less tension on the jaw, reducing the risk of complications, such as postanesthetic cortical blindness, as compared to spring-loaded devices.

- Care should be taken to carefully assess and stabilize older cats and those with a higher ASA status before administering anesthesia.
- Unintentional hypothermia is common, and steps should be taken early in the anesthetic process to prevent or mitigate heat loss.
- The association between fluid therapy and poor outcomes should prompt reassessment of fluid administration rates in anesthetized cats.
- Respiratory compromise is an important cause of morbidity and mortality in cats; airway management protocols should be re-evaluated.

Because most deaths occur in the first 3 hours after the end of a procedure, the recovery area should be well staffed, and cats should be continuously observed during this time. More attention should be given to monitoring and support during this period, including providing warmth and assessing pain.

Perhaps one of the biggest mistakes practitioners can make in clinical medicine is *not to learn* from previous mistakes. Based on how the aviation industry has dealt with "critical incidents," the medical profession is also seeing the benefits of standard operating procedures, checklists, clinical

Table 75-4	Key Factors Related to Mortality and Morbidity and Methods to Mitigate Them
Factor	**Solution**
Hypothermia	Measure temperature Use passive and active warming techniques
Fluid therapy	Use a syringe pump, fluid pump, or Buretrol to accurately measure fluids
Duration of anesthesia	Plan appropriately Be efficient
Airway obstruction and tracheal rupture	Use care when inserting endotracheal tubes and inflating the cuff Consider oxygen masks for short procedures Use supraglottic airway devices
Cardiovascular collapse	Monitor pulse Use a pulse oximeter
Oxygen desaturation	Use a pulse oximeter
Post-anesthetic blindness	Avoid using spring-loaded mouth gags

guidelines, improved specialty training, teamwork, and communication.[5,48] When surgical-crisis checklists were available, only 6% of lifesaving steps were missed during a crisis such as cardiac arrest compared to 23% when checklists were unavailable.[48] Incident reporting is also important for improving patient safety.[49] When an adverse event occurs in a practice, there are lessons to be learned; the incident should be documented in detail and carefully analyzed so that protocols can be adjusted to prevent the same incident in the future.

References

1. Brodbelt DC, Pfeiffer DU, Young LE, et al: Risk factors for anaesthetic-related death in cats: results from the confidential enquiry into perioperative small animal fatalities (CEPSAF). *Br J Anaesth* 99:617–623, 2007.
2. Brodbelt DC, Pfeiffer DU, Young LE, et al: Results of the Confidential Enquiry into Perioperative Small Animal Fatalities regarding risk factors for anaesthetic-related death in dogs. *J Am Vet Med Assoc* 233:1096–1104, 2008.
3. Brodbelt DC, Hammond R, Tuminaro D, et al: Risk factors for anaesthetic-related death in referred dogs. *Vet Rec* 158:563–564, 2006.
4. Brodbelt DC, Blissitt KJ, Hammond RA, et al: The risk of death: the Confidential Enquiry into Perioperative Small Animal Fatalities. *Vet Anaesth Analg* 35:365–373, 2008.
5. Haller G, Laroche T, Clergue F: Morbidity in anaesthesia: today and tomorrow. *Best Pract Res Clin Anaesthesiol* 25:123–132, 2011.
6. Brodbelt D: Perioperative mortality in small animal anaesthesia. *Vet J* 182:152–161, 2009.
7. Clarke KM, Hall L: A survey of anaesthesia in small animal practice. AVA/BSAVA report. *J Ass Vet Anaesth* 17:4–10, 1990.
8. American Society of Anesthesiologists: *ASA Physical Status Classification System*. <http://www.asahq.org>, 2014 (Accessed June 4, 2015).
9. Bille C, Auvigne V, Libermann S, et al: Risk of anaesthetic mortality in dogs and cats: an observational cohort study of 3546 cases. *Vet Anaesth Analg* 39:59–68, 2012.
10. Bainbridge D, Martin J, Arango M, et al: Perioperative and anaesthetic-related mortality in developed and developing countries: a systematic review and meta-analysis. *Lancet* 380:1075–1081, 2012.
11. Dyson DH, Maxie MG, Schnurr D: Morbidity and mortality associated with anesthetic management in small animal veterinary practice. *J Am Anim Hosp Assoc* 34:325–335, 1998.
12. Cote E, Manning AM, Emerson D, et al: Assessment of the prevalence of heart murmurs in overtly healthy cats. *J Am Vet Med Assoc* 225:384–388, 2004.
13. Paige CF, Abbott JA, Elvinger F, et al: Prevalence of cardiomyopathy in apparently healthy cats. *J Am Vet Med Assoc* 234:1398–1403, 2009.
14. Nakamura RK, Rishniw M, King MK, et al: Prevalence of echocardiographic evidence of cardiac disease in apparently healthy cats with murmurs. *J Feline Med Surg* 13:266–271, 2011.
15. Chetboul V, Petit A, Gouni V, et al: Prospective echocardiographic and tissue Doppler screening of a large Sphynx cat population: reference ranges, heart disease prevalence and genetic aspects. *J Vet Cardiol* 14:497–509, 2012.
16. Quimby JM, Smith ML, Lunn KF: Evaluation of the effects of hospital visit stress on physiologic parameters in the cat. *J Feline Med Surg* 13:733–737, 2011.
17. Rodan I, Sundahl E, Carney H, et al: AAFP and ISFM feline-friendly handling guidelines. *J Feline Med Surg* 13:364–375, 2011.
18. Carney HC, Little S, Brownlee-Tomasso D, et al: AAFP and ISFM feline-friendly nursing care guidelines. *J Feline Med Surg* 14:337–349, 2012.
19. Vasan RS: Cardiac function and obesity. *Heart* 89:1127–1129, 2003.
20. Waterman A: Accidental hypothermia during anaesthesia in dogs and cats. *Vet Rec* 96:308–313, 1975.
21. Evans AT, Sawyer DC, Krahwinkel DJ: Effect of a warm-water blanket on development of hypothermia during small animal surgery. *J Am Vet Med Assoc* 163:147–148, 1973.
22. Nickalls RW, Mapleson WW: Age-related iso-MAC charts for isoflurane, sevoflurane and desflurane in man. *Br J Anaesth* 91:170–174, 2003.
23. Yamashita K, Iwasaki Y, Umar MA, et al: Effect of age on minimum alveolar concentration (MAC) of sevoflurane in dogs. *J Vet Med Sci* 71:1509–1512, 2009.
24. Gunn-Moore DA, McVee J, Bradshaw JM, et al: Ageing changes in cat brains demonstrated by beta-amyloid and AT8-immunoreactive phosphorylated tau deposits. *J Feline Med Surg* 8:234–242, 2006.
25. Paepe D, Verjans G, Duchateau L, et al: Routine health screening: findings in apparently healthy middle-aged and old cats. *J Feline Med Surg* 15:8–19, 2013.
26. Pittari J, Rodan I, Beekman G, et al: American association of feline practitioners. Senior care guidelines. *J Feline Med Surg* 11:763–778, 2009.

27. Armstrong SR, Roberts BK, Aronsohn M: Perioperative hypothermia. *J Vet Emerg Crit Care* 15:32–37, 2005.

28. Pottie RG, Dart CM, Perkins NR, et al: Effect of hypothermia on recovery from general anaesthesia in the dog. *Aust Vet J* 85:158–162, 2007.

29. Redondo JI, Suesta P, Gil L, et al: Retrospective study of the prevalence of postanaesthetic hypothermia in cats. *Vet Rec* 170:206, 2012.

30. Bornkamp J, Robertson S: The "big chill": hypothermia in small animal patients. *Canadian Vet* 1:6, 2013.

31. Machon RG, Raffe MR, Robinson EP: Warming with a forced air warming blanket minimizes anesthetic-induced hypothermia in cats. *Vet Surg* 28:301–310, 1999.

32. Raskin RE: Hematologic disorders. In Schaer M, editor: *Clinical medicine of the dog and cat*, ed 2, London, 2009, Manson Publishing, pp 227–253.

33. Davis H, Jensen T, Johnson A, et al: 2013 AAHA/AAFP fluid therapy guidelines for dogs and cats. *J Am Anim Hosp Assoc* 49:149–159, 2013.

34. Tranquilli WJ, Thurmon JC, Benson GJ, et al: Alteration in the arrhythmogenic dose of epinephrine (ADE) following xylazine administration to halothane-anesthetized dogs. *J Vet Pharmacol Ther* 9:198–203, 1986.

35. Matthews NS, Hartke S, Allen JC, Jr: An evaluation of pulse oximeters in dogs, cats and horses. *Vet Anaesth Analg* 30:3–14, 2003.

36. Hardie EM, Spodnick GJ, Gilson SD, et al: Tracheal rupture in cats: 16 cases (1983-1998). *J Am Vet Med Assoc* 214:508–512, 1999.

37. Mitchell SL, McCarthy R, Rudloff E, et al: Tracheal rupture associated with intubation in cats: 20 cases (1996-1998). *J Am Vet Med Assoc* 216:1592–1595, 2000.

38. Bhandal J, Kuzma A: Tracheal rupture in a cat: diagnosis by computed tomography. *Can Vet J* 49:595–597, 2008.

39. Bauer MD, Clark-Price SC, McFadden MS: Anesthesia case of the month. *J Am Vet Med Assoc* 234:1539–1541, 2009.

40. Hofmeister EH, Trim CM, Kley S, et al: Traumatic endotracheal intubation in the cat. *Vet Anaesth Analg* 34:213–216, 2007.

41. Rex MA, Sutton RH, Reilly JS: The effects of lignocaine spray on the laryngeal mucosa of the cat. *Anaesth Intensive Care* 11:47–51, 1983.

42. Blunt MC, Young PJ, Patil A, et al: Gel lubrication of the tracheal tube cuff reduces pulmonary aspiration. *Anesthesiology* 95:377–381, 2001.

43. Crotaz IR: An observational clinical study in cats and rabbits of an anatomically designed supraglottic airway device for use in companion animal veterinary anaesthesia. *Vet Rec* 172:606, 2013.

44. van Oostrom H, Krauss MW, Sap R: A comparison between the v-gel supraglottic airway device and the cuffed endotracheal tube for airway management in spontaneously breathing cats during isoflurane anaesthesia. *Vet Anaesth Analg* 40:265–271, 2013.

45. Jurk IR, Thibodeau MS, Whitney K, et al: Acute vision loss after general anesthesia in a cat. *Vet Ophthalmol* 4:155–158, 2001.

46. Stiles J, Weil AB, Packer RA, et al: Postanesthetic cortical blindness in cats: twenty cases. *Vet J* 193:367–373, 2012.

47. Barton-Lamb AL, Martin-Flores M, Scrivani PV, et al: Evaluation of maxillary arterial blood flow in anesthetized cats with the mouth closed and open. *Vet J* 196:325–331, 2013.

48. Arriaga AF, Bader AM, Wong JM, et al: Simulation-based trial of surgical-crisis checklists. *N Engl J Med* 368:246–253, 2013.

49. Mahajan RP: Critical incident reporting and learning. *Br J Anaesth* 105:69–75, 2010.

Emergency Approach to Respiratory Distress: Heart Versus Lung

Elisa Mazzaferro

Cats that present for respiratory distress often are a diagnostic and therapeutic challenge. In some cases, clinical signs of open-mouthed breathing and a rapid, shallow pattern may simply be from the stress of catching a cat, placing it in a carrier, and transporting it to the hospital for a routine visit. In one study of cats with rapid, shallow respirations and respiratory difficulty, administration of a sedative alone improved respiratory rate and ease of breathing, suggesting that rapid, shallow respiration in some cats may partially be due to stress.[1] In many other cases, however, the client transports the cat for the chief complaint of increased respiratory rate or effort, or for other nonspecific signs, such as lethargy, inappetence, or vomiting. The challenge is to first anatomically localize the lesion to the upper or lower respiratory system without causing or worsening patient stress. Once the problem has been localized, diagnostic testing can ensue in an attempt to determine the cause of the lesion. The diagnostic challenge is that respiratory difficulty is not isolated to respiratory causes, and determining whether the patient has concurrent cardiac disease is important. In one study of 90 cats that presented to a referral hospital on an emergency basis with clinical signs of respiratory distress, 38% had cardiac disease, 32% had respiratory disease, and 20% had neoplastic disease.[2] In another study, use of radiographs and physical examination parameters alone were not enough to allow general practitioners to confidently make a diagnosis of cardiac versus noncardiac causes of respiratory distress in cats.[3]

TRIAGE AND INITIAL THERAPIES

Any cat that presents with signs of respiratory difficulty should be placed in a cage with supplemental oxygen (fraction of inspired oxygen 40%) and allowed to rest while the clinician is observing the patient's respiratory pattern and simultaneously obtaining a medical history from the client. If an oxygen cage is not available, flow-by oxygen with an oxygen extension line can be attached to a loose-fitting face mask and placed near the patient's nose, if tolerated. Other forms of oxygen supplementation, such as nasal or hood oxygen, are generally not well tolerated in the emergent cat with respiratory distress. While the animal is receiving oxygen, handling should be kept to a minimum to avoid stress. When possible, observation of the patient's breathing pattern, along with a physical examination, can direct the clinician toward performing appropriate diagnostic tests and therapeutic interventions.

CLINICAL SIGNS AND PHYSICAL EXAMINATION FINDINGS

Diseases of the upper airway include nasopharyngeal disease and laryngeal disease (Box 76-1). Sneezing and nasal congestion with or without nasal discharge or epistaxis can be present with bacterial, viral or fungal rhinitis, neoplasia, nasopharyngeal polyps, or nasopharyngeal foreign bodies. Cats can demonstrate signs of severe nasal congestion with stertor or a high-pitched wheeze or inspiratory stridor with nasopharyngeal polyps or laryngeal paralysis that result in upper airway obstruction. In cases of upper airway obstruction, the patient is likely to demonstrate slow, deep respirations. Cyanosis may be present. In some instances, the client may describe a change in the patient's ability to purr, vocalize, or swallow food or water or may describe gagging or coughing episodes.

Clinical signs associated with diseases of the lower airways, alveoli, or pleural space are usually associated with a shallow, rapid respiratory pattern. Cats may adopt an orthopneic stance that helps improve the work of breathing, in which the head and neck are extended, and the elbows are abducted away from the lateral thorax. Rapid, shallow respirations have commonly been called a *restrictive respiratory pattern*. More recently, attempts have been made to be more descriptive when visualizing an animal in respiratory distress.

BOX 76-1 Causes of Respiratory Difficulty in Cats

Stenotic nares
Rhinitis
- Bacterial
- Viral
- Fungal

Nasopharyngeal polyp
Neoplasia
- Lymphoma
- Adenocarcinoma
- Other

Laryngeal paralysis
Congenital anatomic laryngeal abnormality
Laryngeal masses
- Laryngeal cysts
- Neoplasia
  - Squamous cell carcinoma
  - Lymphoma
  - Round cell tumor
  - Adenocarcinoma

Oropharyngeal masses
- Neoplasia
- Foreign body
- Granuloma

Tracheal
- Neoplasia
- Foreign body
- Cuterebra
- Other parasitic
- Extraluminal masses

Lower airway diseases
  Chronic bronchitis/asthma
  Smoke inhalation
Pleural space
  Pleural effusion
  - Chylous
  - Neoplasia
  - Hemorrhage
  - Pyothorax
  - Feline infectious peritonitis
  - Modified transudate

  Diaphragmatic hernia
  Rib fracture
  Pneumothorax
Pulmonary parenchymal disease
  Pneumonia
  Pulmonary edema—cardiogenic
  Pulmonary edema—noncardiogenic
  Hemorrhage
  Pulmonary thromboembolism
  Pulmonary parasites
  Lung lobe torsion
Mediastinal
  Hemorrhage
  Neoplasia
  - Lymphoma
  - Thymoma
Cysts

Adapted from: Swift et al, 2009, Zekas et al 2002, Bordelon et al 2009, Fijuta et al, 2004; Burgu et al 2004, Brown et al 2010; Rudorf H et al, 1999 Taylor et al 2009, Hambrook et al 2012.

Synchronous respiration is associated with outward movement and expansion of the lungs, thorax, and abdomen during inspiration, and inward movement of the thorax and abdomen during exhalation.[1] Conversely, dysynchronous or inverse respiration is described as outward movement of the thorax and inward movement of the abdomen during inhalation.[1] In another study, this pattern is described as paradoxical breathing.[4] In that study, the sensitivity and specificity of paradoxical breathing in cats with pleural space disease were 90% and 58%, respectively, suggesting that the presence of paradoxical breathing should make a clinician strongly suspect a disease of the pleural space and choose diagnostic testing such as a thoracic-focused assessment with sonography for trauma (TFAST)[5], thoracic radiographs, or diagnostic thoracocentesis. In another study of 103 cats with respiratory distress, the presence of paradoxical breathing combined with decreased lung sounds on thoracic auscultation was more than 99% sensitive in detecting pleural space disease.[1] The same study confirmed that expiratory respiratory difficulty was associated with lower airway disease; however, dynamic upper airway obstruction secondary to severe asthma has also been documented to cause this

pattern.[6] Moist lung sounds, or pulmonary crackles, are commonly associated with pulmonary parenchymal disease such as pulmonary edema, pulmonary contusions, or less commonly, pneumonia. The presence or absence of a murmur can suggest the presence of cardiac disease with resultant left-sided congestive heart failure. However, the presence of pleural effusion or the severity of pulmonary crackles can make auscultation of a murmur difficult or impossible to hear. It is important to note that on physical examination, cats with heart disease may not have murmurs, and cats with murmurs may not necessarily have cardiac disease. In one study of echocardiograms performed in 103 privately owned apparently healthy cats, heart murmurs were detected in 16 (15.5%) of cats, and only five of the 16 had cardiomyopathy.[7] The same study identified cardiomyopathy in 16 other cats without a detectable murmur on auscultation. Other studies that assessed the frequency of murmurs in healthy cats demonstrated that if a murmur is detected in an otherwise healthy cat on physical examination, structural heart disease was found 53% to 88% of the time on echocardiogram.[8,9,10] Therefore, it is recommended that the presence of a murmur warrants further investigation in all healthy cats at this time.

DIAGNOSTIC TESTING

TFAST and VetBLUE

When an ultrasound machine is available, TFAST and veterinary bedside lung ultrasound examination (VetBLUE) scans can be used to diagnose pneumothorax, pleural effusion, and pericardial effusion in the emergent cat with respiratory distress.[11] Ultrasonographic images can often be obtained without the stress of restraint required for thoracic radiographs. With the patient in lateral or sternal recumbency, the lateral chest wall can be evaluated using ultrasound to determine whether air, fluid, or lung consolidation is present prior to thoracocentesis.

Radiographs

Thoracic radiographs are one of the most important first-line diagnostic tools that clinicians have available when a cat presents with respiratory distress. Radiographs should only be performed after a careful and thorough physical examination, and often after implementation of appropriate therapies to stabilize the patient's respiratory distress. For example, muffled lung sounds with respiratory difficulty in the absence of trauma are most commonly associated with pleural effusion. Performing a thoracocentesis before taking radiographs can be both diagnostic as well as therapeutic in many cats and can alleviate signs of respiratory difficulty. Administration of furosemide to a cat with suspected pulmonary edema, or a short-acting corticosteroid and bronchodilator to a cat with suspected lower airway disease can help to stabilize the patient prior to obtaining radiographs.

Standard views for thoracic radiography in cats are right and left lateral and ventrodorsal or dorsoventral views. In many cases, dorsoventral views may be less stressful for the animal than ventrodorsal views; however, it may be more challenging to obtain a perfectly straight image. Horizontal beam dorsoventral and ventrodorsal views have been shown to be more sensitive than standard dorsoventral or ventrodorsal radiographs at detecting the degree of pleural effusion and pneumothorax in cats.[12] Hanging lateral horizontal beam radiography is helpful when a mediastinal mass lesion is suspected but where pleural effusion prevents its visualization, even after thoracocentesis.[13] Characteristic radiographic findings of pleural effusion, pulmonary edema, pneumothorax, diaphragmatic hernia, and lower airway diseases are demonstrated in Figures 76-1 through 76-6. In the absence of an obvious cause of respiratory difficulty localized to the lower airways and lungs, the vertebral heart scale (VHS) can be useful in differentiating cardiac from noncardiac causes of respiratory distress in cats.[14] To assess VHS, measurements of the long and the short axis of the heart are obtained on a lateral thoracic radiograph (Figure 76-7). The long and short axis measurements are then placed against the thoracic vertebrae, starting at the cranial edge of T4. The number of vertebral bodies that are included in the cranial to caudal edge of each measurement are recorded, and the two mea-

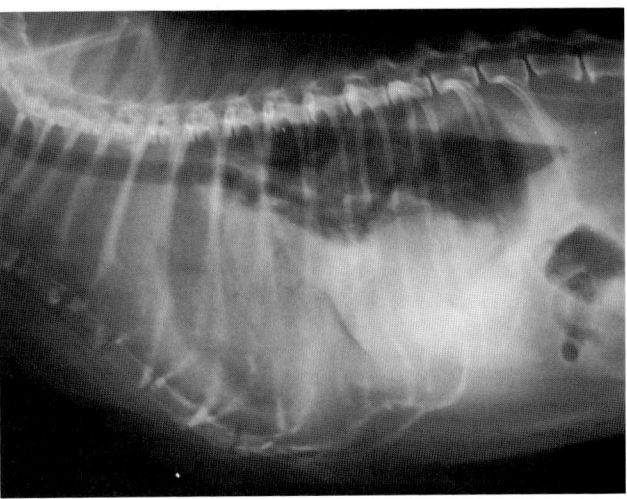

Figure 76-1: Lateral thoracic radiograph of a cat with pleural effusion. Note the soft tissue/fluid density obscuring the cranial mediastinum and cardiac silhouette, and leafing of lung lobes in the dorsocaudal thorax.

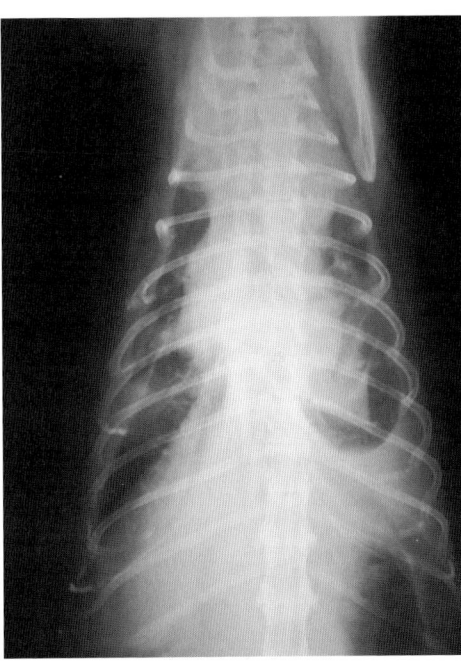

Figure 76-2: Ventrodorsal thoracic radiograph of a cat with pleural effusion. Notice the soft tissue/fluid opacity lateral to the lungs on both sides, causing retraction of the lungs away from the lateral body wall.

surements added together to sum the vertebral heart scale. Normal VHS in cats with no evidence of cardiac disease is less than 8.0.[15] A VHS greater than 8.0 vertebrae supports further investigation with echocardiogram and serum biomarkers for cardiac disease, and a VHS greater than 9.3 has been shown to be very sensitive and specific for the presence of heart disease.[14]

Pulmonary edema can be manifested secondary to cardiac and noncardiac causes, and is seen as a heavy interstitial to

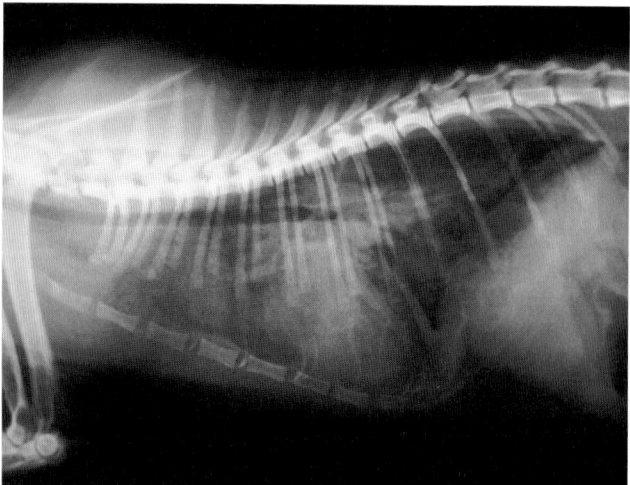

Figure 76-3: Lateral thoracic radiograph of a cat with congestive heart failure. Note the cardiomegaly with increased pulmonary infiltrates perihilar and caudal to the heart.

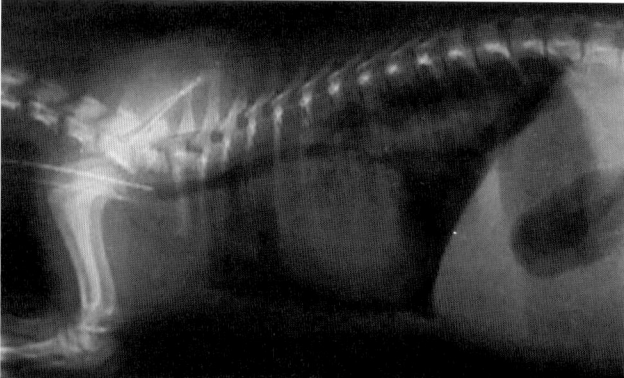

Figure 76-4: Lateral thoracic radiograph of a cat with pneumothorax. Note the elevation of the cardiac silhouette away from the sternum and retraction of the lung lobes from the diaphragm and ventral vertebral bodies.

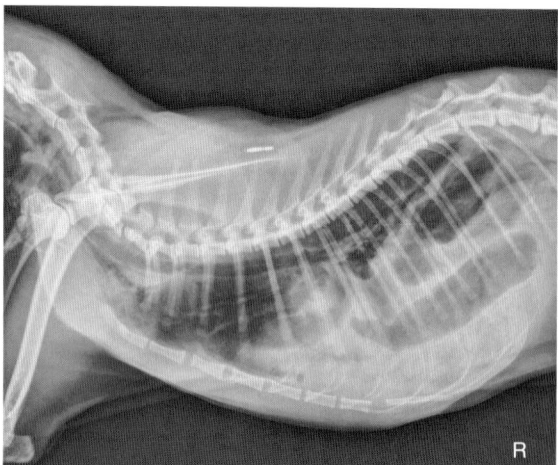

Figure 76-5: Lateral thoracic radiograph of a cat with a diaphragmatic hernia. Note the lack of diaphragmatic delineation ventrally, with a soft tissue density (liver) and air (within small intestine) within the caudoventral thorax.

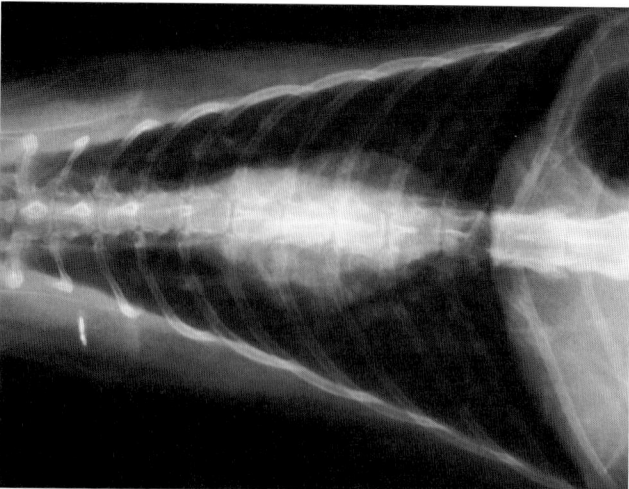

Figure 76-6: Lateral thoracic radiograph of a cat with cardiomegaly. To perform a vertebral heart score (VHS), first draw a line at the heart base in the widest spot. Next, draw a line from the carina to the apex of the heart. Superimpose both lines, starting at the cranial edge of the fourth thoracic vertebra. In this case, each line is equal to the length of 5.5 thoracic vertebrae, with a combined total VHS of 11, consistent with severe cardiomegaly.

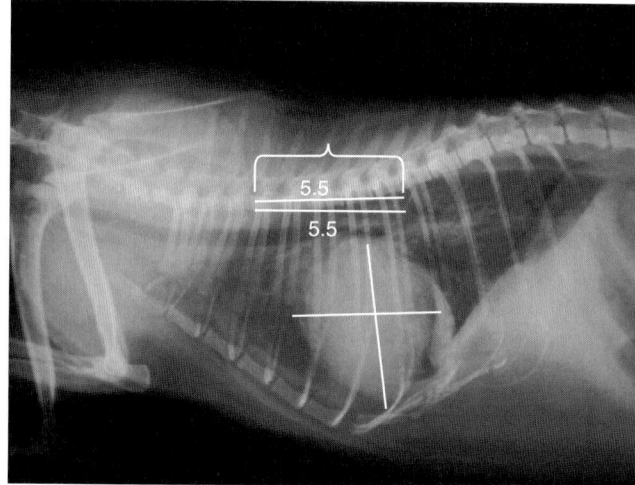

Figure 76-7: Ventrodorsal thoracic radiograph of a cat with lower airway disease/bronchitis. Note the numerous "donuts"—thickened bronchi and bronchiolar pattern consistent with airway thickening and inflammation.

alveolar radiographic pattern. With cardiac disease, perihilar edema with prominent lobar vessels may be observed, with the patchy interstitial pattern expanding as edema worsens. It is important to remember that these findings may not be present in cats, and the pulmonary edema observed with heart disease can be anywhere in the lungs. In cases of noncardiogenic pulmonary edema, however, such as that observed with electrical cord injury or airway obstruction, the edema will be present in the dorsocaudal lung fields. The location of the edema, along with VHS measurements, and careful evaluation of the patient's oral cavity for burns can help distinguish cardiac from noncardiac causes of pulmonary edema.

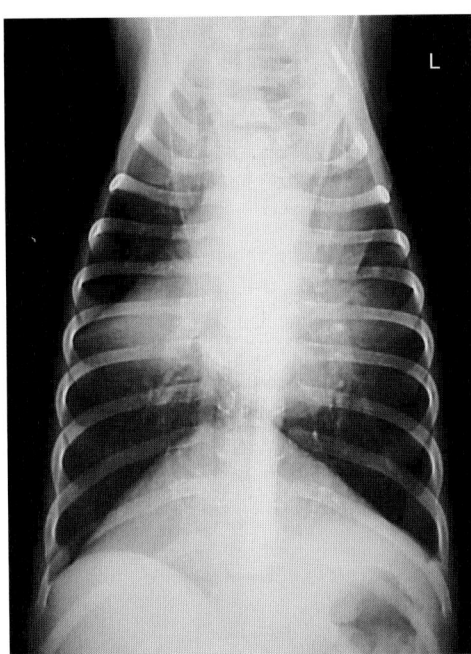

Figure 76-8: Ventrodorsal thoracic radiograph from a cat with lower airway disease and consolidation of the right middle lung lobe. Unlike aspiration pneumonia, clogging of the mainstem bronchus that supplies the right middle lung lobe with mucus causes consolidation and a lack of an alveolar pattern.

Interstitial to alveolar lung patterns can also be observed in animals with pneumonia.

The radiographic appearance of lower airway diseases such as asthma may be very classic, with caudal displacement of the diaphragm on the lateral view, tenting of the diaphragm on the dorsoventral or ventrodorsal view, and bronchiolar markings of "donuts" or "tram-lines" associated with bronchiolar thickening. Other signs, such as unstructured interstitial lung patterns and soft tissue opacities in lung fields, may also be observed.[16] In a small percentage of cats with lower airway disease, the right middle lung lobe may be atelectatic secondary to mucus plugging of the bronchus, which could be mistaken for aspiration pneumonia in some cases. (Figure 76-8).

LARYNGEAL DISEASE

In general, laryngeal disease in cats is less common than in dogs. Clinical signs of laryngeal disease include change in voice or purr, dysphagia, cough, gagging, or inspiratory stridor.[17] Causes of laryngeal disease (see Box 76-1) can include neoplasia, laryngeal paralysis, trauma, granuloma, inflammation, foreign bodies, and laryngeal cysts.[17] Cats with upper airway disease often have inspiratory stridor and a slow, deep respiratory pattern, coupled with cyanosis. At the time of presentation, once respiratory distress has been localized to the upper respiratory system, short-acting sedatives (e.g., butorphanol 0.2 to 0.4 mg/kg intravenously (IV),

subcutaneously (SC), or intramuscularly (IM) with or without midazolam 0.2 mg/kg IV, IM, SC) can be administered while the cat is given oxygen supplementation. If sedation alone is insufficient to improve the cat's respiratory status, an IV catheter should be placed, and a rapid-acting anesthetic (e.g., propofol 4 to 6 mg/kg IV to effect) should be administered to allow intubation. At the time of intubation, use of a laryngoscope or echolaryngoscopy may allow visualization of the arytenoid cartilages and larynx, and confirm the presence of laryngeal paralysis versus an oral or laryngeal mass lesion or foreign body.[17] If the sedation is too deep, and it is not possible to determine whether laryngeal paralysis is due to the effects of the sedatives versus true laryngeal paralysis, doxapram sodium (2.2 mg/kg IV given once) can be administered to counter the effects of sedation. If arytenoid abduction occurs following the administration of doxapram, the cause of inspiratory distress or stridor is not due to laryngeal paralysis. Laryngeal paralysis may be unilateral or bilateral. In cats with bilateral laryngeal paralysis, unilateral arytenoid lateralization can be performed, and has a median survival time of 157 days.[17] In cases of unilateral laryngeal paralysis, conservative medical management with exercise restriction and weight loss is favorable and has been associated with a range of survival from 300 to 2520 days.[17]

The presence of a mass lesion or vocal fold asymmetry may be characteristic of neoplasia, granulomatous disease, or cysts.[17] Fine-needle aspirates may not be sufficient to obtain a diagnostic sample;[17] therefore, biopsies of the affected tissue should be performed to obtain an accurate diagnosis. Following laryngoscopy and sample collection, the following questions should be considered:

- Is extubation possible and likely to be successful?
- Will a short-acting glucocorticoid alleviate laryngeal swelling and edema (if present)?
- Should a temporary tracheostomy be performed?

Depending on the etiology, mass lesions may respond to chemotherapy, antibiotics, glucocorticosteroids, or possible radiation therapy. If a cyst is present, aspiration of the cyst or surgical removal may be curative.[17] If extubation is chosen, the cat should receive careful observation and monitoring with oxygen supplementation as necessary until it has been determined that there are no residual signs of respiratory distress. If inspiratory stridor recurs and a definitive treatment such as arytenoid lateralization or surgical removal of a mass lesion cannot be performed, the patient should be reintubated until the time of emergent surgical intervention or a temporary tracheostomy. Heliox therapy, a mixture of helium and oxygen, could potentially be beneficial at providing oxygen to patients with upper airway obstruction.[18] For more information on feline laryngeal disease, see chapter 37.

PNEUMONIA

In general, pneumonia in cats is less common than in dogs. Aspiration pneumonia is most commonly observed as an interstitial to alveolar pattern in the right middle lung lobe.

Infectious causes of pneumonia are also possible. Unlike dogs, cats with infectious causes of pneumonia rarely cough.[19,20] Ideally, airway samples obtained from bronchoalveolar lavage or sterile transoral or endotracheal wash should be obtained for cytology, bacterial culture, and susceptibility testing prior to instituting broad spectrum antibiotics. There has been one report of a diagnosis of toxoplasmosis in a cat that presented with respiratory distress and fever using bronchoalveolar lavage.[21] If bronchoscopy is not available, transoral or transtracheal wash can be performed. The patient is placed under a light plane of anesthesia with a combination of midazolam (0.2 mg/kg IV) and propofol (4 to 6 mg/kg IV to effect) and a sterile endotracheal tube is placed. Sterile samples can then be obtained for cytology and culture as described elsewhere.[22] The clinician must weigh the potential risks of acute bronchoconstriction, oxygen desaturation, hypoxia, and cardiac arrest with the potential benefits and diagnostic yield before performing any invasive procedure that can cause further patient deterioration. In many cases of pneumonia, more than one bacterial organism is present, including *Mycoplasma* spp.[19,23,24]

PLEURAL SPACE DISEASE

Thoracic radiographs are usually sufficient to make a diagnosis of pneumothorax, diaphragmatic hernia, rib fractures, or pleural effusion. Pleural space disease should be considered in any patient that presents with a restrictive or dysynchronous respiratory pattern along with muffled heart and lung sounds. In such instances, thoracocentesis can be both diagnostic and therapeutic.

To perform a thoracocentesis, a large square of fur should be shaved on both sides of the lateral thorax. If one envisions the cat's ribcage as a box, a square in the center of the box is shaved (Figure 76-9). Following an aseptic scrub, a needle, butterfly catheter, or over-the-needle catheter can be introduced into the pleural space in the center of the shaved area to remove air or fluid. In most cases, air will be more dorsal (in the dorsal one-third of the thorax), and fluid will be more ventral (in the ventral one-third of the thorax) in location, unless pocketing occurs. Both sides of the thorax should be aspirated until no more air or fluid is obtained, and the cat is no longer demonstrating signs of respiratory distress. Although some cats may tolerate thoracocentesis without sedation, the combined stress of respiratory difficulty and thoracocentesis may worsen respiratory difficulty; therefore, sedation as described previously may be warranted. Respiratory distress will be alleviated significantly in many cats when a portion of the fluid has been removed. It is often not necessary, nor is it possible, to remove all fluid at once before the cat becomes intolerant of the procedure. Once the patient's clinical status has stabilized, additional thoracocentesis attempts can be performed as necessary. In cases of pneumothorax, if negative pressure cannot be obtained, or if free air reaccumulates frequently or rapidly, placement of a thoracic drainage catheter should be considered. Complications from thoracocentesis are rare, but include pneumothorax (increased risk if a long-standing effusion and fibrosing pleuritis is present [see chapter 84]), hemorrhage, and infection.

Whenever possible, thoracic drainage catheters should be placed while the cat is under general anesthesia and intubated. The entire lateral thorax should be clipped from the thoracic inlet caudally to the last rib, and dorsally and ventrally to midline. Following an aseptic scrub, the skin on the lateral thorax should be pulled cranioventrally to the elbow. Next, a small nick incision is made over the dorsal aspect of the tenth intercostal space. A hemostat can be used to bluntly dissect through fascia and intercostal muscles, then into the pleural cavity, where the thoracic drain is inserted. The thoracic drainage catheter should be directed cranially to the level of the fourth to fifth intercostal space. Finally, the skin is released, and the tube secured in place with suture (Figure 76-10 through 76-17).

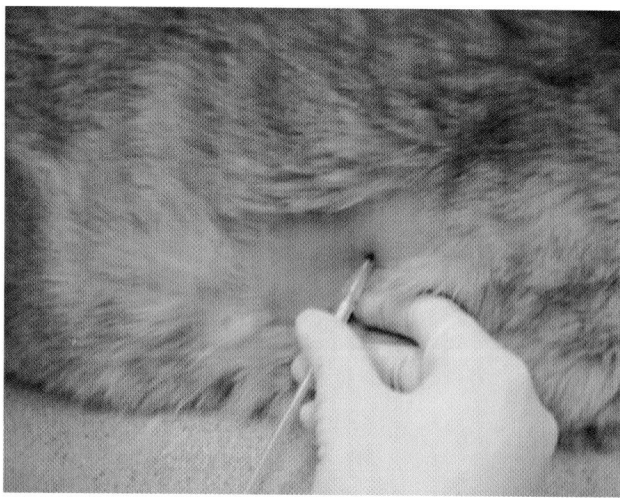

Figure 76-9: Photograph of a clinician performing thoracocentesis on a cat. Note the square of fur shaved in the center of the thorax and the needle inserted into the middle of the square.

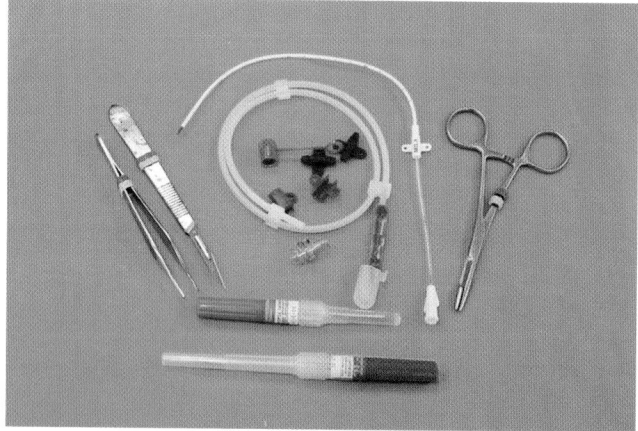

Figure 76-10: Photograph of components of an over-the-wire thoracic drainage catheter. Components of the catheter kit include a J wire, long thoracic drainage catheter, over-the-needle introducer catheter, and equipment required for suturing the catheter in place. (Photo courtesy of Vetvine® and MILA International, Inc.)

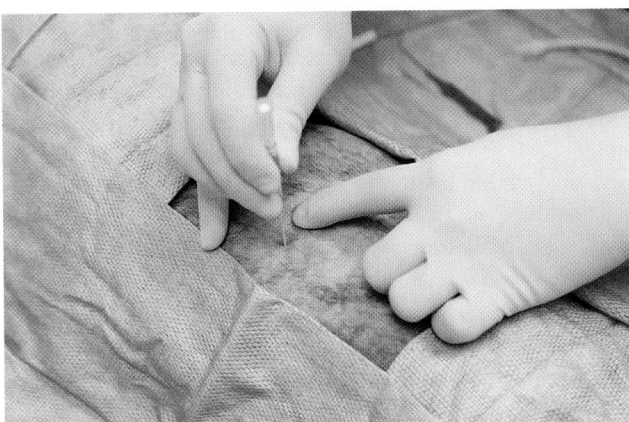

Figure 76-11: An-over-the needle catheter is inserted into the lateral thorax at the ninth to eleventh intercostal space. The needle is removed prior to introduction of the J wire through the catheter hub, into the thorax. (Photo courtesy of Vetvine® and MILA International, Inc.)

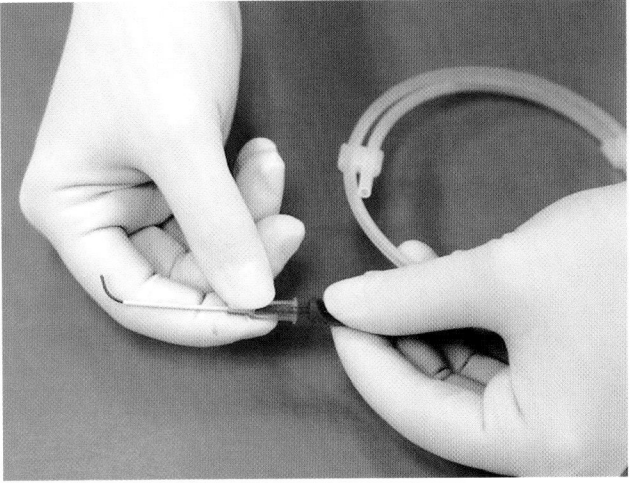

Figure 76-12: Photo of the J wire, which is curved at the end to prevent iatrogenic penetration into the lung or heart once inserted into the thorax. The J wire is pulled into the blue hub for ease of introduction into the over-the-wire-catheter hub. (Photo courtesy of Vetvine® and MILA International, Inc.)

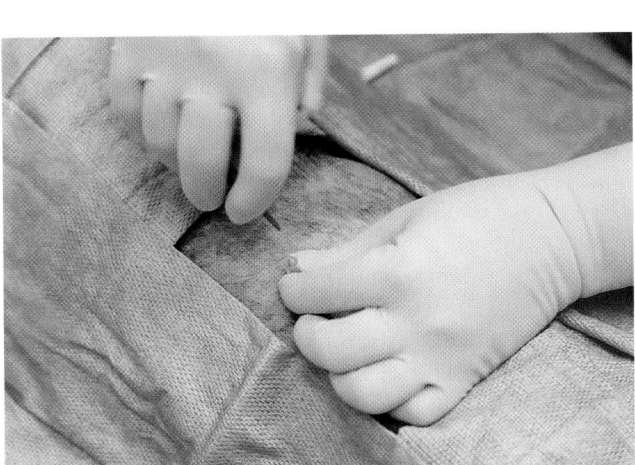

Figure 76-13: The J wire is inserted into the catheter. (Photo courtesy of Vetvine® and MILA International, Inc.)

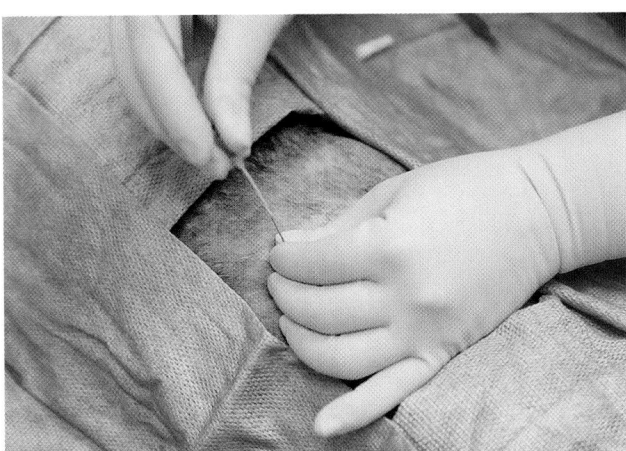

Figure 76-14: The catheter is removed from the thorax over the J wire, leaving the J wire in place. (Photo courtesy of Vetvine® and MILA International, Inc.)

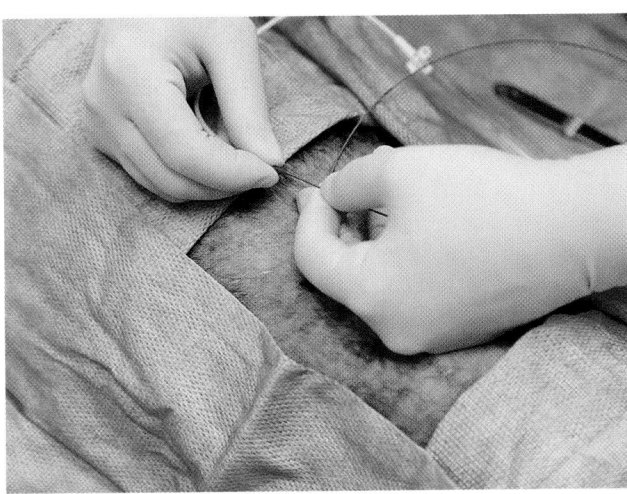

Figure 76-15: The long catheter is placed over the J wire. (Photo courtesy of Vetvine® and MILA International, Inc.)

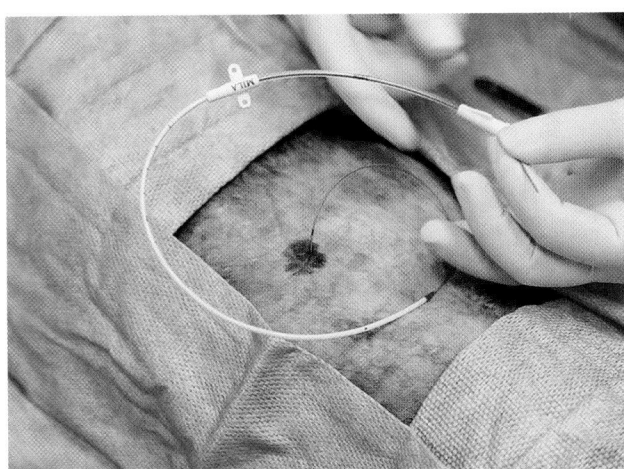

Figure 76-16: The J wire is pulled through the top catheter port, then the long catheter is pushed into the thorax. The J wire is then pulled from the thorax, leaving the long catheter in place. (Photo courtesy of Vetvine® and MILA International, Inc.)

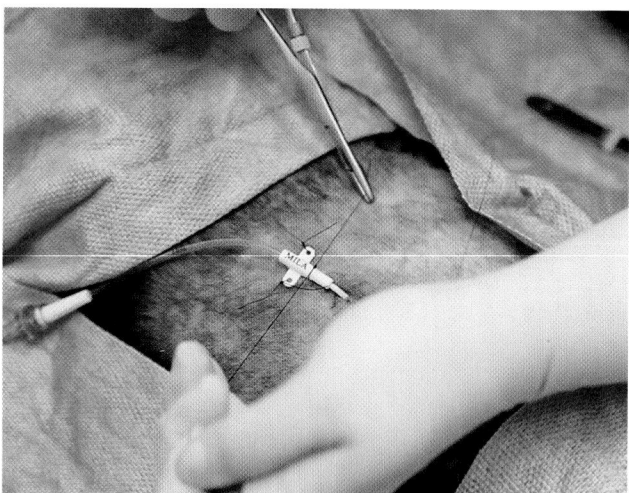

Figure 76-17: The catheter is secured in place with suture. (Photo courtesy of Vetvine® and MILA International, Inc.)

Table 76-1	Characteristics of Pleural Effusion in the Cat		
Class	**Total Protein (g/dL)**	**Nucleated Cell Count (cells/μL)**	**Differential Diagnoses**
Transudate	<2.5	<1,000	Congestive heart failure Hypooncotic state Intravascular fluid volume overload
Modified transudate	2.5 to 3.5	500-10,000	Congestive heart failure Neoplasia Chylothorax
Exudate	>3.5	>5,000	Feline infectious peritonitis Neoplasia Chylothorax Pyothorax

Many cases of pleural effusion are treated with intermittent thoracocentesis and therapy for the primary underlying disease. In some cases of chronic pleural effusion in which an underlying etiology cannot be definitively treated (e.g., idiopathic chylous effusion), pleural cavity access systems (e.g., PleuralPort, Norfolk Vet Products, Skokie, IL) have been used for recurrent thoracic drainage.[25] Following collection, the sample should be submitted for red blood cell count, cytology analysis, and culture for aerobic and anaerobic bacteria. Characteristics of the various types of pleural effusion are listed in Table 76-1. In some instances (e.g., chylous effusions, congestive heart failure, and neoplasia), nucleated cell count and protein content are insufficient to make a diagnosis

of transudate versus exudate[26,27] Measurement of triglyceride content, cholesterol, and newer biomarkers such as lactate dehydrogenase (LDH) and pleural fluid total protein : serum total protein ratio can be useful in making a more accurate diagnosis when distinguishing transudates from exudates.[27] The triglyceride content of chylous effusion is significantly higher than peripheral triglyceride concentration, and the pleural fluid cholesterol : triglyceride ratio is much lower in chylous versus nonchylous effusions.[28] In cats, pleural fluid total protein greater than 3.5 g/dL (35 g/L) and LDH greater than 226 International Unit/L are used to characterize an exudate.[27] Measurement of serum albumin concentration or colloid osmotic pressure can help to distinguish a hypooncotic state from heart disease if an echocardiogram is not immediately available. In the absence of vasculitis, pleural effusions do not usually form for purely oncotic reasons until the serum albumin level falls below 1.5g/dL (15 g/L).[29]

Malodorous pleural effusions in cats are characteristic of pyothorax until proven otherwise. Odors may be absent, however, in protozoal, fungal, and bacterial pleuritis.[26,30] The most common bacteria isolated from cats with pyothorax are anaerobic pathogens (*Peptostreptococcus anaerobius*, *Bacteroides* spp., *Fusobacterium* spp., *Porphyromonas* spp., *Prevotella* spp., less commonly *E. coli*), nonenteric pathogens (*Pasteurella* spp., *Actinobacillus ureae*, *Actinomyces* spp., *Staphylococcus intermedius*), and *Enterococcus faecalis*[31]; however, the potential for atypical bacterial isolates warrants aerobic and anaerobic culture with susceptibility testing for all samples.[32]

In-house cytologic analysis of pleural effusions can be very rewarding if degenerative neutrophils, intra- and extracellular bacteria are present with pyothorax, or if lymphoblasts are present in cases of lymphoma. Chylous effusions often appear milky white to pinkish-white in appearance, although they can be translucent if the patient has been inappetent. Without advanced training and experience in cytologic interpretation, however, differentiation of reactive mesothelial cells from carcinoma or mesothelioma can potentially be misinterpreted and thus not allow the clinician to provide an accurate treatment protocol or potential prognosis for therapy. For this reason, all pleural effusions should be investigated in-house and submitted to an outside reference laboratory for confirmatory interpretation.

TRAUMA

Trauma is a common cause of respiratory distress in cats, particularly in those that are allowed to roam outdoors. Indoor cats, too, are susceptible to trauma from other pets in the household or by falling from a height. In addition, cats are notorious for masking clinical signs until they are no longer capable of hiding distress; therefore, an acute onset of clinical signs of respiratory distress is not pathognomonic for trauma. Cats with trauma can have signs localized to the upper airways and head trauma, with open-mouth breathing, blood in the oral cavity, epistaxis, anisocoria, corneal abrasions, scleral hemorrhage, and/or dermal wounds.

Trauma to the thorax can lead to rib fractures, diaphragmatic hernia, pulmonary contusions, and pneumothorax. If pleural space disease is suspected, thoracocentesis should be performed prior to taking thoracic radiographs, whenever possible, in order to alleviate signs of respiratory distress. If rib fractures are present, systemic analgesia (e.g., fentanyl constant rate infusion at 2-4 mcg/kg/hour, or buprenorphine 0.01 mg/kg IV every 6 to 8 hours) and local rib blocks can be performed (with 0.25 mg/kg lidocaine, or 0.25 mg/kg bupivacaine administered at the dorsocaudal portion of each fractured rib, every 8 hours, with a maximum dose of 1 mg/kg). While opioids and local anesthetic agents are safe to use in cats with thoracic trauma, the use of nonsteroidal anti-inflammatory drugs and corticosteroids are contraindicated, as renal and gastrointestinal (GI) perfusion may be impaired in any traumatized animal with hypotension, and GI ulceration, decreased renal oxygen delivery and renal failure could result. In rare instances, days to weeks following a traumatic event, cats can present with clinical signs of respiratory distress and pneumothorax secondary to tracheal avulsion.[33]

CARDIAC DISEASE

Cats with cardiac disease can present with respiratory distress secondary to pleural effusion, pulmonary edema, or both. As stated previously, it may be difficult to confidently make a diagnosis of cardiac versus noncardiac causes of respiratory distress. In the acute setting, a cat with clinical signs of pulmonary crackles, orthopnea, and a rapid, shallow and restrictive respiratory pattern with a heart murmur can be considered to have cardiac disease and congestive heart failure until proven otherwise.[2] Furosemide (2 to 4 mg/kg IV, IM) should be administered, along with supplemental oxygen. Some cats will also require butorphanol (0.2 to 0.4 mg/kg IV or IM) to relieve anxiety associated with respiratory distress. Furosemide can be repeated several times, however, repeat administration can be associated with significant hypokalemia in cats. In addition, overzealous administration of furosemide can result in such a tremendous decrease in circulating intravascular fluid volume that ventricular filling pressure and stroke volume are diminished, and cardiac output is reduced to such an extent that systemic hypotension is worsened. Once clinical signs of respiratory difficulty have improved, thoracic radiographs and blood tests (complete blood count, serum chemistry panel, serum total thyroxine, and samples for cardiac biomarkers) can be obtained. It is important to recognize that elevations in blood urea nitrogen and creatinine are commonly found in cats with heart disease, even in the absence of diuretic therapy. Decreased cardiac output with systemic hypotension results in decreased renal perfusion, and thus prerenal azotemia. Fluid therapy and diuretics should be carefully balanced along with inotropic drugs, when possible, to maximize intravascular fluid volume and cardiac output, to augment systemic blood pressure, and to maintain vital organ perfusion. If possible, an echocardiogram should be performed to help determine the exact cause of the heart failure and to help gauge drug choice and the patient's response to therapy. In addition, placement of a central venous catheter into the jugular vein and monitoring central venous pressures can help guide fluid therapy. As a general guide, central venous pressure should not rise by more than 5 cm of water in any 24-hour period to avoid worsening pulmonary edema in affected patients.

Cardiac biomarkers are gaining promise as tools for helping to distinguish cardiac from noncardiac causes of respiratory distress in cats. In one study, cardiac troponin I levels were significantly higher in cats with congestive heart failure more than 50% of the time, compared with cats with primary respiratory disease as a cause of respiratory difficulty.[34] More commonly, N-terminal pro-brain natriuretic peptide (NT-proBNP) and N-terminal pro-atrial natriuretic peptide were found to be higher in cats with cardiac disease versus noncardiac causes of respiratory distress[35], and they can also be helpful in distinguishing cardiac from noncardiac causes of pleural effusion.[36] In one study, NT-proBNP greater than or equal to 49 pmol/L was 100% sensitive and 89.3% specific at predicting cardiac disease.[35] Using an optimum cut-off value, NT-proBNP greater than or equal to 258 pmol/L is very sensitive at discriminating pleural effusion secondary to congestive heart failure from pleural effusion due to noncardiac causes.[36] For more on cardiac biomarkers, see Chapter 34.

LOWER AIRWAY DISEASE

Cats with lower airway disease, more commonly referred to as asthma, may also present with clinical signs of respiratory difficulty. In such instances, the patient will have a rapid, shallow, and dysynchronous respiratory pattern and pulmonary wheezes, and in many cases they will be normo- or hyperthermic, while cats with congestive heart failure are often hypothermic.[37] In some instances, lung sounds may be normal. Careful palpation of the trachea may elicit a cough, which can open previously constricted airways and then allow turbulent flow across mucus within constricted bronchi that will be ausculted as wheezes. In the emergent setting, administration of rapidly acting glucocorticosteroids (e.g., dexamethasone or dexamethasone-sodium phosphate 0.25 mg/kg IV or IM) along with a bronchodilator (e.g., terbutaline 0.01 mg/kg IM or SC or aminophylline 4 to 8 mg/kg SC or albuterol by metered-dose inhaler) can be administered to alleviate signs of respiratory distress. In the most severe cases of status asthmaticus, a patient may require emergency intubation until the glucocorticosteroids and bronchodilators take effect.

SUMMARY

All cats with respiratory distress should be placed in supplemental oxygen and observed from a distance while gathering a history. Physical examination, along with noninvasive diagnostic techniques such as ultrasound, can be used to differentiate extrathoracic from intrathoracic causes of respiratory difficulty. Thoracocentesis may need to be performed prior to taking radiographs in the emergent patient with pleural effusion or pneumothorax. Following careful stabilization, in some cases making an educated decision to treat for congestive heart failure or lower airway disease, other diagnostic tests including blood tests, fluid or airway cytology or culture, and novel peptides can be used to make a definitive diagnosis of cardiac versus primary lung causes of respiratory difficulty. A stepwise approach, with time to allow the cat to rest in between diagnostics, is prudent in any patient with respiratory distress.

References

1. Sigrist NE, Adamik KN, Doherr MG, et al: Evaluation of respiratory parameters at presentation as clinical indicators of the respiratory localization in dogs and cats with respiratory disease. *J Vet Emerg Crit Care* 21:13–23, 2011.
2. Swift S, Dukes-McEwan J, Fonfara S, et al: Aetiology and outcome in 90 cats presenting with dyspnea in a referral population. *J Small Anim Pract* 50:466–473, 2009.
3. Singletary GE, Rush JE, Fox PR, et al: Effect of NT-pro-BPN assay on accuracy and confidence of general practitioners in diagnosing heart failure or respiratory disease in cats with respiratory signs. *J Vet Int Med* 26:542–546, 2012.
4. Le Boedec K, Arnaud C, Chetboul V, et al: Relationship between paradoxical breathing and pleural diseases in dyspneic dogs and cats: 389 cases (2001-2009). *J Am Vet Med Assoc* 240:1095–1099, 2012.
5. Lisciandro GR: Abdominal and thoracic focused assessment with sonography for trauma, triage, and monitoring in small animals. *J Vet Emerg Crit Care* 21:104–122, 2011.
6. Davis A, Khorzad R, Whelan M: Dynamic upper airway obstruction secondary to severe feline asthma. *J Am Anim Hosp Assoc* 49:142–147, 2013.
7. Paige CF, Abbott JA, Elvinger F, et al: Prevalence of cardiomyopathy in apparently healthy cats. *J Am Vet Med Assoc* 234:1398–1403, 2009.
8. Cote E, Manning AM, Emerson D, et al: Assessment of the prevalence of heart murmurs in overtly healthy cats. *J Am Vet Med Assoc* 225:384–388, 2004.
9. Nakamura RK, Rishniw M, King MK, et al: Prevalence of echocardiographic evidence of cardiac disease in apparently healthy cats with murmurs. *J Feline Med Surg* 13:266–271, 2011.
10. Dirven MJ, Cornelissen JM, Barendse MA, et al: Cause of heart murmurs in 57 apparently healthy cats. *Tijdschr Diergeneeskd* 135:840–847, 2010.
11. Boysen S, Lisciandro GR: The use of ultrasound for dogs and cats in the emergency room: AFAST & TFAST. *Vet Clin North Am Small Anim Pract* 43:773–797, 2013.
12. Lynch KC, Oliveira CR, Matheson JS, et al: Detection of pneumothorax and pleural effusion with horizontal beam radiography. *Vet Radiol Ultrasound* 53:38–43, 2012.
13. Kealy JK: The thorax. In Kealy JK, editor: *Diagnostic radiology of the dog and cat*, ed 2, Philadelphia, 1987, Saunders, p 233.
14. Sleeper MM, Roland R, Drobatz KJ: Use of the vertebral heart scale for differentiation of cardiac and noncardiac causes of respiratory distress in cats: 67 cases (2002-2003). *J Am Vet Med Assoc* 242:366–371, 2013.
15. Lister AL, Buchanan JW: Vertebral scale system to measure heart size in radiographs of cats. *J Am Vet Med Assoc* 216:210–214, 2000.
16. Gadbois J, d'Anjou M-A, Dunn M, et al: Radiographic abnormalities in cats with feline bronchial disease and intra- and interobserver variability in radiographic interpretation: 40 cases (1999-2006). *J Am Vet Med Assoc* 234(3):367–375, 2009.
17. Taylor SS, Harvey AM, Barr FJ, et al: Laryngeal disease in cats: a retrospective study of 35 cases. *J Feline Med Surg* 11:954–962, 2009.
18. Byers CG, Romeo K, Johnson TS, et al: Helium-oxygen gas-carrier mixture (heliox): a review of physics and potential applications in veterinary medicine. *J Vet Emerg Crit Care* 18:586–593, 2008.
19. MacDonald ES, Norris CR, Berghaus RB, et al: Clinicopathologic and radiographic features and etiologic agents in cats with histologically confirmed pneumonia: 39 cases (1991-2000). *J Am Vet Med Assoc* 223(1142):2003.
20. Cote E: CH 22: Pneumonia. In Silverstein DC, Hopper K, editors: *Small animal critical care medicine*, ed 2, St Louis, 2015, Elsevier/Saunders, pp 120–126.
21. Brownee L, Sellon RK: Diagnosis of naturally occurring toxoplasmosis by bronchoalveolar lavage in a cat. *J Am Anim Hosp Assoc* 37:251–255, 2001.
22. Finke MD: Transtracheal wash and bronchoalveolar lavage. *Top Companion Anim Med* 28:97–102, 2013.
23. Brady CA: Bacterial pneumonia in dogs and cats. In King LG, editor: *Textbook of respiratory disease in dogs and cats*, St Louis, 2004, Elsevier, pp 412–421.
24. Sauve V, Drobatz KJ, Shokek AB, et al: Clinical course, diagnostic findings and necropsy diagnosis in dyspneic cats with primary pulmonary parenchymal disease: 15 cats (1996-2002). *J Vet Emerg Crit Care* 15:38, 2005.
25. Brooks AC: Hardie Ruse of the PleuralPort Device for management of pleural effusion in six dogs and four cats. *Vet Surg* 40:935–941, 2011.
26. Beatty J, Barrs V: Pleural effusion in the cat, a practical approach to determining aetiology. *J Feline Med Surg* 12:693–707, 2010.
27. Zoia A, Slater LA, Heller J, et al: A new approach to pleural effusion in cats: markers for distinguishing transudates from exudates. *J Feline Med Surg* 11:847–855, 2009.
28. Fossum TW, Jacobs RM, Birchard SJ: Evaluation of cholesterol and triglyceride concentrations in differentiating chylous from nonchylous pleural effusions in dogs and cats. *J Am Vet Med Assoc* 188:49–51, 1986.
29. Guyton AC, Hall JE: The body fluid compartments: extracellular fluids, interstitial fluid and edema. In Guyton AC, Hall JE, editors: *Textbook of medical physiology*, ed 11, Philadelphia, 2006, Saunders, pp 291–305.
30. Barrs VR, Beatty JA: Feline pyothorax- new insights into an old problem part I, aetiopathologenesis and diagnostic investigation. *Vet J* 179:163–170, 2009.
31. Walker AL, Jang SS, Hirsh DC: Bacteria isolated with pyothorax in dogs and cats: 98 cases (1989-1998). *J Am Vet Med Assoc* 216:359–363, 2000.
32. Barrs VR, Allan GS, Martin P, et al: Feline pyothorax: a retrospective study of 27 cases in Australia. *J Feline Med Surg* 7:211–222, 2005.
33. Worth AJ, Row WD, Machon RG: Radiographic appearance of acute tracheal avulsion in two cats. *Aust Vet Pract* 32:160–166, 2002.
34. Herndon WE, Rishniw M, Schrope D, et al: Assessment of plasma cardiac troponin I concentration as a means to differentiate cardiac and noncardiac causes of dyspnea in cats. *J Am Vet Med Assoc* 233:1261–1264, 2008.
35. Connolly DJ, Soares Magalhaes RJ, Syme HM, et al: Circulating natriuretic peptides in cats with heart disease. *J Vet Int Med* 22:96–105, 2008.
36. Hassdenteufel E, Henrich E, Hildebrandt N, et al: Assessment of circulating N-terminal pro-B type natriuretic peptide concentration to differentiate between cardiac from noncardiac causes of pleural effusion in cats. *J Vet Emerg Crit Care* 23:416–422, 2013.
37. Goutal CM, Keir I, Kenney S, et al: Evaluation of acute congestive heart failure in dogs and cats: 145 cases (2007-2008). *J Vet Emerg Crit Care* 20:330–337, 2010.

Current Diagnostics and Therapeutics in Feline Hypercoagulability

Selena Lane and Benjamin Brainard

Hemostasis under normal conditions depends on a balance between procoagulant and anticoagulant factors in the blood, as well as contributions from cellular components, such as the vascular endothelium and platelets. Alterations in normal hemostasis may occur through changes in the function of any one (or multiple) component(s) and may lead to clinical hypocoagulability and hemorrhage or hypercoagulability and thrombotic or thromboembolic disease.

*Hypo*coagulable bleeding disorders are less commonly reported in the feline patient when compared to dogs. Inherited coagulopathies in the cat include hemophilia A,[1] hemophilia B,[2] factor X deficiency,[3] factor XII (Hageman factor) deficiency,[4,5] von Willebrand disease,[6] vitamin K-dependent coagulopathy of Devon Rex cats,[7] and platelet storage pool deficiency as part of Chediak-Higashi syndrome in blue smoke Persian cats.[8] Additionally, suspected congenital platelet function defects have been described in two unrelated domestic shorthair cats.[9] Acquired thrombocytopathia in cats has been associated with uremia, hepatic disease, and nonsteroidal anti-inflammatory drug administration, whereas thrombocytopenia has been reported to occur secondary to disseminated intravascular coagulation (DIC), neoplasia, and immune-mediated thrombocytopenia. Bleeding due to thrombocytopenia may be observed in feline patients either because of lack of platelet production from the bone marrow or secondary to consumption or destruction of the platelets. Primary immune-mediated thrombocytopenia is relatively rare in cats, with most immune-mediated destructive processes occurring secondary to infection (such as feline leukemia virus) or neoplasia. Acquired clotting factor deficiencies are commonly recognized in the clinical setting and may be associated with DIC, ingestion of vitamin K antagonists, hepatic disease,[10,11] gastrointestinal (GI) disease,[11,12] or neoplasia.[13]

In contrast to feline patients with bleeding disorders, there is little information in the veterinary literature investigating the incidence, etiology, and treatment of *hyper*coagulability in cats. However, hypercoagulability and thromboembolic disease are recognized as complicating sequelae of cardiac, endocrine, inflammatory, and neoplastic disorders. Understanding the pathophysiology of thrombus formation and the ability to diagnose and treat affected cats is limited. Further investigations into the origins of hypercoagulable conditions, diagnostic techniques for hypercoagulability and thrombosis, and the utility of thromboprophylactic and antithrombotic drugs are needed. In addition, research into invasive and alternative thrombectomy approaches may help to improve the outcome for cats affected by thrombosis or thromboembolism.

THROMBUS FORMATION

During normal hemostasis, uninterrupted blood flow is maintained throughout the vasculature while controlled coagulation and thrombus formation occur at sites of vessel trauma or injury. After the vessel heals, the thrombus is broken down by endogenous mechanisms. Abnormal thrombus formation can occur as a result of numerous underlying disease processes, all of which alter hemostatic balance by influencing one or more components of Virchow's triad. In 1856, Rudolph Virchow described these three conditions associated with the formation of thrombosis in human patients: (1) systemic hypercoagulability, (2) endothelial damage, and (3) alterations in blood flow (such as stasis or high shear).[14] Thrombi can form in the arterial or venous circulation, and the thrombus may remain *in situ* or travel to another site in the body as a thromboembolus. Arterial thrombosis occurs under conditions of high shear stress, typically after damage to the vessel wall, which exposes subendothelial collagen and activates passing platelets. This type of platelet-rich thrombus is referred to as a *white thrombus*, because it is primarily composed of a mixture of platelet aggregates and fibrin.[15,16] Venous thrombus formation is associated with low shear conditions and blood stasis, with an intact endothelium, resulting primarily from activation of soluble coagulation factors. Venous thrombi (red thrombi) are composed mostly of fibrin and red blood cells.[16,17] Arterial thromboembolism (ATE) in cats with underlying cardiac disease is a unique situation, with thrombus formation occurring in the heart (likely in areas of altered or low blood flow in the left atrium) and then becoming an ATE as the thrombus leaves the left side of the heart. Venous thrombosis and subsequent thromboembolism are associated with considerable morbidity and mortality in humans; however, venous thrombi are less commonly observed in the clinical veterinary population, which is thought to be due to species differences in platelet structure, vascular anatomy, nonbipedal circulation, and genetics.[18]

ETIOLOGIES AND PREDISPOSING CONDITIONS LEADING TO HYPERCOAGULABILITY

Hypercoagulability, or thrombophilia, can be inherited or acquired in small animals. Inherited disorders associated with hypercoagulability in cats are not completely understood, and breed predispositions are not well described. Cat breeds prone to developing hypertrophic cardiomyopathy (HCM), such as Ragdoll and Maine Coon cats, may have an increased risk of thromboembolism, although this may be secondary to the changes in cardiac blood flow that occur with HCM and not systemic hypercoagulability.[19] A family of domestic shorthair cats, all diagnosed with inherited, asymptomatic HCM, were shown to have a 75% occurrence rate of ATE;[20] however, a predisposition for ATE was not found in another study of inbred Maine Coon cats with hereditary HCM[21] (see Chapter 35 for more information on ATE in cats with cardiac disease).

Indwelling venous or arterial catheters may result in endothelial injury, and hemodialysis catheter-associated thrombosis or pulmonary thromboembolism (PTE) has been reported in cats.[22,23] Indwelling venous catheters have also been used experimentally to induce thrombosis in cats and may provide a surface for activation of the intrinsic coagulation cascade.[24] The true incidence and clinical risk for thrombosis associated with intravenous (IV) catheters in clinical treatment scenarios are unknown, but limiting the time a catheter is in place is prudent. Vascular neoplasia may directly damage or infiltrate vessels, and vasculitis associated with other systemic diseases (such as sepsis, pancreatitis, infection, or immune-mediated disease) may also predispose cats to thrombus formation secondary to endothelial damage and hypercoagulability. Occasionally, tumor thrombi may occlude blood flow in vessels or break free and result in a thromboembolus.

Acquired hypercoagulability in cats has been described to occur secondary to systemic diseases, including cardiac disease, hyperthyroidism, infectious and inflammatory diseases, protein-losing disorders, and neoplasia.[25,26] Cats affected by cardiac disease may have abnormal platelet aggregation,[27,28] which could lead to increased risk of thrombus formation in this patient population. Numerous human studies have indicated an association of hypercoagulability and hypofibrinolysis with hyperthyroidism, which is a common endocrine disease of older cats.[29-32] Increased adrenergic tone and the hypermetabolic state induced by hyperthyroidism increase the likelihood of hypercoagulability in these patients. Human studies have shown an increase in factor VIII, IX, and XI activity in hyperthyroid patients who have experienced thromboembolic events.[29-31] Abnormal clotting factor activity resolves after appropriate therapy and return to the euthyroid state, further supporting the notion

that hyperthyroidism may result in hypercoagulability.[29,31,32] Coagulation factor activity in hyperthyroid cats has not been examined, but cats with hyperthyroidism-related cardiac disease ("thyrotoxic cardiomyopathy") are predisposed to thromboembolic events, as well as abnormalities in platelet aggregation and fibrinolysis.[27,33] In another study describing ATE in cats, several cats with hyperthyroidism had echocardiographically normal hearts, suggesting that thyroid disease poses a risk factor for ATE that is independent of the cardiac effects of hyperthyroidism.[26] Further studies evaluating the effect of hyperthyroidism on feline coagulation are needed.

In humans, hypercoagulability associated with pregnancy is considered protective against the possibility of significant hemorrhage during labor and delivery. Pregnancy in queens has also been shown to result in a hypercoagulable state as assessed by thromboelastography (TEG);[34] however, further studies are needed to characterize the relationship of these changes to complications associated with pregnancy and to compare these findings with other measures of coagulation.

Protein-losing disease, such as protein-losing nephropathy (PLN) or protein-losing enteropathy (PLE), may lead to hypercoagulability and thrombus formation. Proteinuria leads to hypoalbuminemia and polycythemia, which decrease plasma volume, generating increased platelet contact and aggregation. Additionally, there is ongoing loss of endogenous anticoagulant factors, such as antithrombin (AT), protein C, and protein S. In a retrospective study of 29 cats with PTE, almost 30% of those cats had underlying PLN or PLE.[23] The true prevalence and morbidity associated with thromboembolic disease in cats affected by protein-losing disorders are unknown, and further study in this area is indicated.

Pulmonary thromboembolism, which is relatively rare in cats, has been associated with many diseases, including cardiac disease, heartworm infection, neoplasia, DIC, PLE or PLN, immune-mediated hemolytic anemia, pancreatitis, and sepsis.[23,35-36] Corticosteroid administration may also predispose to a hypercoagulable state. There are few reports of PTE in the cat; however, the disorder appears to have a similar pathophysiology and relationship to predisposing conditions in cats as compared to dogs and humans.

Thrombus formation is a complication of neoplasia and is a frequent cause of morbidity or mortality in human patients with cancer.[37-38] Tumor cells can produce and secrete procoagulant/fibrinolytic substances and inflammatory cytokines, which can lead to a prothrombotic state in affected patients. Other neoplasia-associated mechanisms that encourage thrombus formation include promotion of inflammation, abnormal protein metabolism, endothelial damage through vascular invasion, and blood stasis in large vascular tumors. Furthermore, chemotherapy, surgery, or other anticancer treatments may increase the risk of thromboembolic complications.[37] One TEG-based study of dogs with various types of neoplasia proposed that 50% of dogs with malignant neoplasia were hypercoagulable, which was significantly higher than dogs with benign epithelial neoplasia.[39] Although platelet aggregation studies have revealed increased platelet function in dogs with malignancies,[40] comparable studies of cats have not been published. A paraneoplastic thrombocytosis thought to result in aortic thromboembolism has been reported in a cat with bronchoalveolar carcinoma.[41] Thrombocytosis has been associated with paraneoplastic thromboembolic disease in humans with neoplasia of the pancreas, lung, and GI tract.[42] However, this is the only report published of this paraneoplastic phenomenon in cats.

ASSESSMENT OF COAGULATION STATUS

Traditional plasma-based coagulation testing is most useful for detecting *hypo*coagulable states. The prothrombin time (PT) assesses the integrity of the extrinsic and common pathways (Figure 77-1) and is performed by the addition of tissue factor and phospholipid to a sample of recalcified citrated plasma. The activated partial thromboplastin time (aPTT) assesses the intrinsic pathway and is initiated by the addition of a strong contact activator (e.g., kaolin) and phospholipid to the recalcified citrated plasma.[43] Depending on the methodology, the endpoint of both of these tests (fibrin formation) can be assessed by optical or mechanical means. Abnormalities in these tests may be associated with a single factor deficiency (e.g., hemophilia A) or may be associated with factor depletion due to disease, toxin, or lack of factor production. Specific coagulation factor activities may also be measured at specialty laboratories. The plasma fibrinogen concentration may also be measured in citrated plasma by a number of different assays and may be a useful parameter to test in patients at risk of hypercoagulability.[43]

Platelet function in cats may be assessed using a number of different assays. Platelet function assays are indicated to assess the effects of pharmacotherapy or to describe platelet function defects. The most specific way to assess platelet function is using platelet aggregometry. The gold standard for platelet aggregometry is light-transmission (or optical) aggregometry (LTA), which is a spectrophotometric method that uses platelet-rich plasma (PRP) to observe platelet responses to specific agonists, such as adenosine diphosphate (ADP) and collagen. Due to the tendency of feline platelets to become activated with sample handling, it is difficult to prepare PRP suitable for LTA. For this reason, the study of feline platelets has focused on whole-blood (or impedance) aggregometry, which uses citrated whole blood and a resistance circuit to evaluate the reaction of platelets to agonists. Although this method is convenient because it does not require large amounts of blood and can be performed with minimal sample processing, the interactions of red and white blood cells with platelets can result in variable outcomes. Other tests that specifically evaluate platelet function have not been extensively evaluated in cats. These methods include the platelet function analyzer (PFA-100) and the IMPACT cone and plate(let) analyzer.[44]

Coagulation also initiates fibrinolysis, the endogenous dissolution of fibrin clots through the action of plasminogen. The products of fibrinolysis are released into circulation and can be measured as fibrin(ogen) degradation products (FDPs) or D-dimers. Elevation of these products can be indicative of ongoing coagulation and fibrinolysis. D-dimers are more specific for identification of clot formation and breakdown because they are generated by the cleavage of cross-linked fibrin, whereas FDPs may be generated by breakdown of either circulating fibrinogen or cross-linked fibrin.

Although evaluation of the individual aspects of coagulation (e.g., the soluble factor and platelet contributions) can

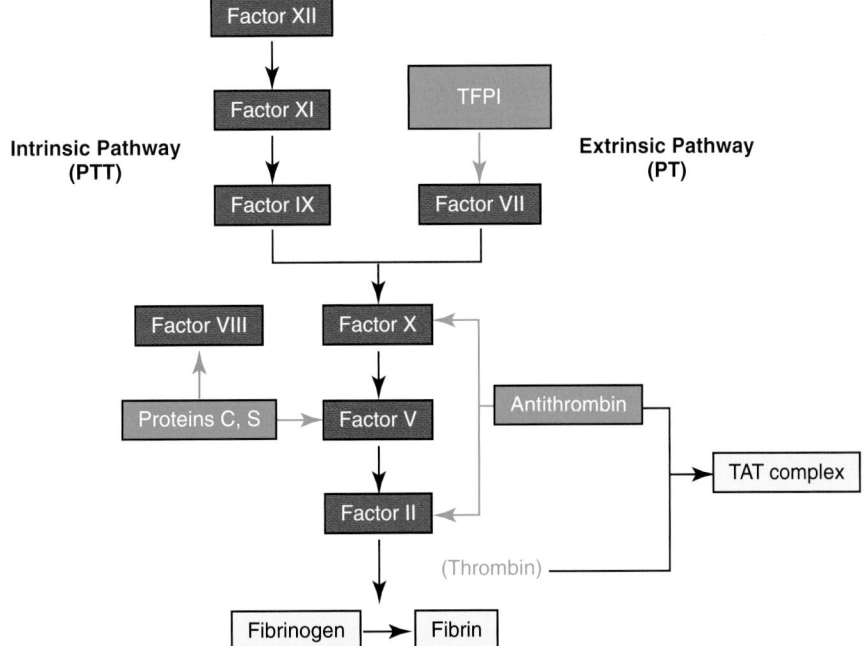

Figure 77-1: Intrinsic and extrinsic pathways of secondary hemostasis. *PT,* Prothrombin time; *PTT,* partial thromboplastin time; *TAT,* thrombin-antithrombin; *TFPI,* tissue factor pathway inhibitor.

help to identify abnormalities, coagulation *in vivo* is a process that integrates the cellular and soluble components toward the formation of a clot. For this reason, there has been a revival of interest in methodologies that evaluate coagulation, because it occurs in whole blood. Viscoelastic coagulation testing displays the change in viscosity as liquid blood transforms to a gelled clot and methodologies include TEG (Haemonetics, Braintree, MA) and the Sonoclot (Sienco, Inc., Arvada, CO). Although these assays have been studied in dogs, horses, and other veterinary species, they have not been extensively evaluated for describing feline coagulation. Part of the problem with the use of TEG in cats is difficulty in reproducibility of tracings and, in particular, the occasional appearance of tracings that seem to indicate significant fibrinolysis. Possibilities for the variability seen in feline TEG include platelet or factor activation during sample collection or a robust platelet retraction response that causes pseudofibrinolytic tracings. The use of different activators for the analysis has not reliably improved the variability in the test, but further study in this direction may make these tests useful for evaluation of feline whole blood coagulation.

DIAGNOSIS OF HYPERCOAGULABILITY

Definitive diagnosis of a hypercoagulable state is difficult in veterinary patients. Routine hemostatic evaluations (such as analysis of platelet count, PT, and aPTT) are insensitive indicators of thromboembolic risk. Most routine coagulation tests are generally unremarkable in cats that present with thromboembolic disease. In a study of cats with ATE, the majority of cats had PT and aPTT values within the reference interval.[45] In veterinary patients, factors that have been shown to reflect hypercoagulable states include decreased plasma AT, protein C, and protein S.[46] In addition, decreased plasminogen and tissue plasminogen activator with increased plasminogen activator inhibitor type 1 can predispose a cat toward a procoagulant state. Increases in thrombin-antithrombin complexes indicate that thrombin formation is ongoing and can serve as an indicator of a hypercoagulable state.[46,47] Elevations in circulating D-dimers have been attributed to consumptive coagulopathies in cats with hepatic disease[47-49] and other conditions, although elevated D-dimers were not found in cardiomyopathic cats with other markers of hypercoagulability or in another cohort of cats with DIC.[50]

ANTITHROMBOTIC THERAPIES

Indications for Use

Small animal patients may develop macrovascular or microvascular thrombosis in association with a variety of disease conditions, including cardiac disease, neoplasia, and inflammatory or infectious disease. In humans, there is a large body of evidence regarding the use of heparin, aspirin, and vitamin K antagonists for many conditions associated with

thrombosis or thromboembolism. Antithrombotic therapies that have been described in clinical feline patients consist primarily of heparins, aspirin, and clopidogrel, but outcome-based evidence is limited for the use of these medications as thromboprophylaxis. Due to undesirable side effects and frequent monitoring requirements for these drugs with relatively narrow therapeutic windows, attention has focused on development of effective and safer antithrombotic drugs. The drugs discussed in the following sections have widespread clinical use in humans, but the clinical efficacy and pharmacokinetics of these drugs in experimental and clinical cat populations remain to be seen (Table 77-1). Clinical guidelines for the management of acute thromboembolic disease in cats, as well as maintenance therapy for cats with ATE or at risk of ATE are summarized in Boxes 77-1 and 77-2.

BOX 77-1 Arterial Thromboembolism: General Guidelines for Treatment

- Rule out heart failure: Treat with oxygen, diuretics, and other cardiac medications as indicated for underlying heart disease or arrhythmias
- Analgesia: Systemic opioids (intermittent IV bolus or CRI)
- Anticoagulants: Acute therapeutic options
  - UFH: 75-200 IU/kg IV once, then 250 to 300 IU/kg SC every 8 hours[52]
  - UFH: 30 IU/kg IV once, then 20 to 40 IU/kg/hour via CRI, titrated to aPTT or anti-FXa levels (reserved for cats with acute thrombosis)
  - LMWH:
    - Dalteparin (Fragmin): 100 IU/kg SC every 4 to 12 hours[67,72]
    - Enoxaparin (Lovenox): 0.75 mg/kg SC every 6 hours[74]
  - Clopidogrel (Plavix): 18.75 mg/cat PO every 24 hours[86]
- Anticoagulants: Maintenance therapy
  - Continue clopidogrel at same dose indefinitely
  - Can consider continued LMWH for first month if finances and dosing schedule allow

aPTT, Activated partial thromboplastin time; *CRI,* constant rate infusion; *FXa,* factor Xa; *IV,* intravenous; *IU,* international unit; *LMWH,* low-molecular-weight heparin; *PO, per os* (orally); *SC,* subcutaneous; *UFH,* unfractionated heparin.

BOX 77-2 Thromboprophylaxis for Cats at Risk of Arterial Thromboembolism

- Clopidogrel (Plavix): 18.75 mg/cat PO every 24 hours[86]
- Dalteparin (Fragmin): 100 IU/kg SC every 4 to 12 hours[67,72]
- Consider oral FXa inhibitors (pending further clinical studies) such as rivaroxaban (Xarelto),[79] apixaban (Eliquis)[83]

FXa, Factor Xa; *IU,* international unit; *PO, per os* (orally); *SC,* subcutaneously.

Table 77-1	Summary of Current and Novel Antithrombotic and Thromboprophylactic Drugs for Cats		
Drug	**Mechanism of Action**	**Dosage**	**Comments**
Warfarin	Inhibits synthesis of vitamin K–dependent clotting factors	Thromboprophylaxis: 0.06 to 0.09 mg/kg/day PO[51] Antithrombotic: 0.5 mg/cat/day PO[52]	Inexpensive Requires frequent monitoring High bleeding risk Not generally recommended for thromboprophylaxis
UFH	Binds AT, inactivates thrombin and FXa	For treatment of ATE: 75 to 500 IU/kg IV once, then 250 to 300 IU/kg SC every 8 hours[52]	Inexpensive Variable dose-response relationship Requires frequent monitoring and dose adjustments
LMWHs • Dalteparin • Enoxaparin	Inhibits FXa	Dalteparin: 100 IU/kg SC every 4 to 12 hours[67,72] Enoxaparin: 1 mg/kg SC every 6 to 12 hours[63,67]	Moderately priced Cats have shorter duration of anti-FXa activity with LMWHs, so they require more frequent dosing[63] Monitor via anti-FXa activity assay[63-64]
Fondaparinux	Inhibits FXa	Thromboprophylaxis: 0.06 mg/kg SC every 12 hours[76] Antithrombotic: 0.2 mg/kg SC every 12 hours[76]	Expensive Clinical efficacy studies needed
Rivaroxaban Apixaban	Inhibits FXa	Rivaroxaban: 0.5 to 1 mg/kg PO every 12 to 24 hours[79] Apixaban: Not determined	Oral administration Clinical efficacy studies needed Clinical dosing protocols not established at this time
Aspirin	Cyclooxygenase inhibitor	Thromboprophylaxis: 81 mg/cat every 72 hours[69] 5 mg/cat PO every 72 hours[26]	No studies support use as effective thromboprophylactic drug May cause GI side effects
Clopidogrel and Ticlopidine	Binds platelet P2Y$_{12}$ ADP receptor	Clopidogrel: 18.75 mg/cat PO every 24 hours[86] Ticlopidine: 500 mg/cat/day PO[90]	Clopidogrel: Safe, inexpensive Clinical efficacy studies needed Ticlopidine: Dose-dependent anorexia and vomiting[90]
Abciximab and Tirofiban	Platelet GPIIb/IIIa receptor antagonists	Abciximab: 0.25 mg/kg IV bolus, then CRI of 0.125 µg/kg/min[93] Tirofiban: 100 µg/kg IV bolus, then CRI of 5 µg/kg/min[96]	Expensive IV injection only via CRI Not readily available Abciximab: Further safety and clinical efficacy studies needed Tirofiban: Use not recommended

ADP, Adenosine diphosphate; *AT,* antithrombin; *ATE,* arterial thromboembolism; *CRI,* constant rate infusion; *FXa,* factor Xa; *GI,* gastrointestinal; *GPIIb/IIIa,* glycoprotein IIb/IIIa; *IV,* intravenous; *LMWH,* low-molecular-weight heparin; *PO, per os* (orally); *SC,* subcutaneous; *UFH,* unfractionated heparin.

ANTICOAGULANTS

Anticoagulant therapies are used primarily in patients at risk for development of venous thrombosis and thromboembolism. Anticoagulants inhibit the generation of fibrin by interfering with the plasma coagulation cascade and are indicated for prophylaxis or therapy in clinical patients that have documented thrombosis or thromboembolism or those at risk for thrombus formation.

Vitamin K Antagonists (Warfarin)

Warfarin is one of the oldest antithrombotic medications used in human medicine, and a large body of evidence identifying dosing and monitoring regimens in various human disease states supports its use.

Mechanism of Action

Warfarin interferes with the cyclic conversion of vitamin K epoxide to vitamin K. Vitamin K-dependent coagulation proteins (factors II, VII, IX, and X) and glycoproteins (protein C and protein S) are inactive when initially synthesized. During activation, the reduced form of vitamin K, vitamin KH_2 or hydroquinone, is oxidized to vitamin K epoxide and then recycled to vitamin K by vitamin K epoxide reductase. Warfarin blocks the activity of vitamin K epoxide reductase, causing depletion of the body's vitamin K stores and eventually inhibiting the synthesis of all factors in this pathway.[51]

Pharmacokinetics and Pharmacodynamics

Healthy cats have a narrow therapeutic window of steady-state concentration of warfarin, and there is marked interindividual variation in response to warfarin in cats, much like humans. Recommended initial doses in healthy cats have ranged from 0.06 to 0.09 mg/kg/day.[51] However, a dose as high as 0.5 mg/cat/day has been used for treatment of hypercoagulable disease states and prevention of ATE in cats.[52] Warfarin tablets should not be compounded to achieve dosing in cats, as active enantiomers are not evenly distributed within the tablets and there is a risk of significant overdosing or underdosing of medication.[53]

Monitoring

Dose adjustments of warfarin therapy require frequent monitoring of PT. The optimal dose for each patient and the amount of drug to achieve a given prolongation of PT are highly individualized. In general, a therapeutic target is a prolongation of PT to 1.5 times the baseline PT; however, there is marked variability in PT reagent sensitivity, and this value may differ among machines. Due to this variability, in human medicine, PT is recorded in seconds and reported as a ratio of the PT of the patient to the mean normal PT of the laboratory (patient PT/control PT), which is the international normalized ratio (INR).[54] An INR of 2.0 to 3.0, or prolongation of PT at 1.5 to 2 times normal, has been recommended as the target therapeutic range for warfarin therapy in cats, based on extrapolation from recommendations for warfarin monitoring in human thrombotic syndromes[55] and pharmacokinetic and pharmacodynamics studies of warfarin use in healthy cats. Monitoring of INR or PT should be performed daily for the first week of therapy, or until therapeutic range has been achieved and maintained for at least 2 consecutive days, then it is monitored two to three times per week for 2 weeks, and then progressively less often depending on the stability of PT results.[54]

Adverse Effects and Client Considerations

Adverse effects of warfarin include severe, possibly fatal, hemorrhage. Hemorrhage can manifest as hemoperitoneum, hemarthrosis, GI bleeding, subcutaneous (SC) bruising, epistaxis, and excessive bleeding from traumatic or surgical wounds. This bleeding may be reversible through administration of enteral or parenteral vitamin K1 (phytonadione) or through transfusion of fresh-frozen or stored plasma. Recurrence of thromboembolism was reported in 10 out of

23 cats (43%) with cardiogenic thromboembolism that were treated with warfarin prophylaxis, and it was associated with sudden death in three out of 23 cats (12%) and bleeding episodes in five out of 23 cats (20%).[56] Warfarin is highly protein bound (greater than 96.5%) in cats, so concurrent use of other protein-bound drugs or use in hypoalbuminemic patients may result in alterations of the expected anticoagulant effects.[53] Warfarin kinetics may also be affected by diet changes, and it is important that cats receiving warfarin are kept on a strict regimen. Frequent monitoring of warfarin therapy may be costly for clients, although the drug itself is inexpensive. Given the lack of evidence of effective thromboprophylaxis and improved long-term survival in cats at risk for thromboembolic disease, in addition to the narrow therapeutic window, warfarin is not a recommended thromboprophylactic drug.

Heparins

Heparin is one of the primary anticoagulant medications used in clinical veterinary medicine. Heparin is efficacious and relatively safe in many disease states, and a large body of experimental and clinical research provides appropriate dosing and monitoring protocols in humans. Further research is needed in veterinary patients to elucidate the most appropriate use of heparin in cats and dogs, including which type of heparin is indicated and which dose is most efficacious for various disease processes.

Mechanisms of Action

Heparin produces its major anticoagulant effect by increasing AT-mediated inhibition of synthesis and activity of factors Xa (FXa) and IIa (FIIa, thrombin). Heparins also cause release of tissue factor pathway inhibitor (TFPI) from the endothelial cell surface into the blood, which further enhances the rate of inactivation of FXa.[57] Heparin binds to AT through a high-affinity pentasaccharide, which is present on one-third of heparin molecules. This results in a conformation change that leads to activation of AT, which then inactivates thrombin and FXa. By inactivating thrombin, heparin not only prevents fibrin formation but also decreases thrombin-induced activation of platelets and of factors V and VIII.[58]

Depending on the size, structure, and charge of the heparin molecules, including the length of the saccharide residues, heparins vary in their enhancement of activity of AT against target enzymes. Short molecules (i.e., the low-molecular-weight heparins [LMWHs]) retain the ability to bind to FXa but are not long enough to reach the heparin-binding site on thrombin, which is why LMWHs have relatively greater activity against FXa than they do against thrombin. Unfractionated heparin (UFH) is a mixture of heparins with a large variation in the length of the polysaccharide tails. Depolymerization of UFH into lower molecular weight fragments results in several changes in its properties, including decreased ability to bind effectively to thrombin, improved predictability of dose responses, and reduced binding to endothelial cells.[59]

Monitoring

Heparin therapy should be closely monitored to avoid adverse effects associated with over-anticoagulation and to ensure that the patient is reaching therapeutic plasma concentrations. Monitoring tests include measurement of aPTT, activated clotting time (ACT), and anti-FXa activity. The aPTT is the most commonly used diagnostic test for monitoring heparin therapy. Early studies in human medicine suggested that aPTT measurements equal to 1.5 to 2.5 times the mean control aPTT reduced the risk of recurrent thromboembolism.[60] Additionally, elevated aPTT values greater than 2.5 times the control have been correlated with a higher incidence of bleeding in humans.[61] In experimental canine studies, there is evidence that monitoring heparin therapy in dogs by aPTT should be reagent specific, due to variations in prolongation of aPTT as measured by different reagents.[62] However, comparable studies do not exist in cats and no clinical veterinary studies are available at this time. Veterinary medicine is lacking in outcome-based studies validating the target aPTT prolongation times in cats and dogs receiving heparin therapy. Prolongation of ACT measurements by 15 to 20 seconds has also been used for monitoring of UFH therapy; however, these therapeutic targets again are extrapolated from human medical literature[59] and are variably predictive of plasma heparin concentrations. Analysis of TEG parameters in cats receiving either UFH or LMWH therapy showed that anti-Xa activity significantly correlated with TEG parameters only in those receiving UFH, suggesting that TEG is not a reliable means by which to monitor cats receiving LMWH therapy.[63]

Due to unreliable aPTT prolongation by LMWHs and synthetic heparins, as well as the availability of novel oral FXa inhibitors, other methods of assessing heparin activity *in vivo* are needed, primarily by direct measurement of FXa inhibition. The use of anti-FXa activity assays, rather than coagulation screening tests, provides a more consistent basis for comparisons between species and treatment regimens. Studies exist in humans and dogs to develop target therapeutic ranges of UFH anti-FXa activity.[64-65] However, target anti-FXa activity for thromboprophylaxis has not been evaluated in cats, and further studies are needed in this patient population. A modified chromogenic assay for anti-FXa activity has been described in cats and dogs.[63-64] The anti-FXa activity range of 0.5 to 0.75 IU (International Unit)/mL caused prolongation of aPTT time to 1.5 to 2.5 times the assay mean in samples treated with UFH.[64] These results were comparable with human target therapeutic targets of 0.3 to 0.7 IU/mL. In humans, analysis of anti-FXa activity 4 hours after drug administration is recommended to monitor peak LMWH activity.[66] However, peak anti-FXa activity in cats has been reported to occur at 2 hours after administration.[63,67] Further studies based on specific outcome measures are indicated to confirm the ideal therapeutic range and dosing interval for anti-FXa activity in cats.

Unfractionated Heparin

Unfractionated heparin is rapidly absorbed from SC tissues and onset of action is immediate following IV injection. Binding of UFH to plasma proteins and cells contributes to variable pharmacokinetics of the drug in different species, and the bioavailability of SC heparin can fluctuate with changes in acute phase and inflammatory proteins during illness.[68]

Unfractionated heparin therapy requires close monitoring and dose adjustments to ensure that appropriate therapeutic levels are reached and adverse effects of inappropriate dosing are avoided. There are no studies available that indicate the most appropriate dose of heparin for cats at risk for or affected by thromboembolic disease. One retrospective study of cats with ATE presenting in acute crisis reported single IV UFH doses ranging from 75 to 500 IU/kg.[26] Following IV dosing, most of the cats in the study continued to receive SC UFH at doses between 10 to 300 IU/kg every 6 to 12 hours. The majority of cats received UFH using a low-dose or high-dose protocol, either 50 to 100 IU/kg or 200 to 250 IU/kg every 6 to 8 hours, respectively. A 2004 review of therapy for feline ATE recommended an initial SC UFH treatment protocol at dosages of 250 to 300 IU/kg every 8 hours in hospitalized cats.[69]

Bleeding is the most common adverse effect associated with heparin therapy. However, in the retrospective study of cats affected by ATE, bleeding was not observed in any cat that received heparin.[26] Heparin-induced thrombocytopenia is recognized as a serious adverse effect in people receiving UFH therapy but has not been reported in companion animals. Unfractionated heparin is widely available and inexpensive for clients, but its variability in dose-response relationship and potential for inappropriate levels of anticoagulation make it a less attractive option compared to other anticoagulant therapies.

Low-Molecular-Weight Heparins

Low-molecular-weight heparins vary in their potency, bioavailability, and cumulative effects in veterinary species. Low-molecular-weight heparins selectively inhibit FXa while minimally affecting clotting times. Low-molecular-weight heparins also exhibit decreased binding to platelets, more predictable pharmacokinetics, and greater bioavailability compared to UFH.[70] In humans, LMWHs have longer half-lives than UFH, which results in less frequent dosing, although this may not be the case with cats, due to more rapid excretion of the compounds. Low-molecular-weight heparin is moderately priced but may ultimately become expensive for clients, depending on how often the drug must be administered to achieve clinical efficacy as well as the duration of treatment.

Preliminary pharmacokinetic studies in a small number of cats receiving two different doses of LMWH (dalteparin [Fragmin; Pfizer, New York, NY]) indicated achievement of therapeutic concentrations of anti-FXa activity at a dose of 100 IU/kg SC once daily, using target therapeutic range of anti-FXa activity of 0.35 IU/mL to 0.70 IU/mL, extrapolated from human medicine.[71] Another study evaluating the effect of dalteparin on coagulation parameters in a small number of healthy cats indicated that a dosage of 100 IU/kg SC every 12 hours did not achieve therapeutic (by human standards) anti-FXa activity in 50% of the cats and failed to maintain target anti-FXa activity beyond 4 hours in the other 50% of the cats.[72] More recent evaluation of the pharmacokinetic profile of dalteparin in healthy cats revealed that the drug (administered SC) had high bioavailability and the activity was predictable, requiring little routine monitoring, similar to other species.[67] The half-life of dalteparin after SC administration was short (approximately 2 hours) compared to humans and was not dose-dependent, suggesting that multiple daily injections would be required in cats to achieve comparable pharmacokinetics to humans.[63,67] This study did not evaluate the pharmacodynamic effects of LMWHs in cats in relation to the anti-FXa levels obtained, so no conclusions can be made regarding the dose and dose frequency required to achieve antithrombotic effect in a clinical population of cats. Further research is needed to evaluate the pharmacodynamics and clinical efficacy of various dosing schemes for LMWHs used for thromboprophylaxis.

Enoxaparin (Lovenox; Sanofi, Bridgewater, NJ) is another LMWH preparation that has been evaluated in one study of healthy cats to determine pharmacokinetics of the drug[63] and in healthy cats using a venous stasis model.[73] In the pharmacokinetic evaluation of enoxaparin in healthy cats, a dosage of 1 mg/kg SC every 12 hours failed to induce sustained anti-FXa activity that was measurably different from baseline, placebo, or UFH.[63] Results of another study demonstrated that an antithrombotic effect could be achieved in this experimental setting when enoxaparin was administered at a dosage of 1 mg/kg SC every 12 hours.[73] However, the plasma anti-FXa activity was not significantly correlated with thrombus formation and supported the fact that plasma anti-FXa activity may be a poor predictor of antithrombotic effect.[73] A more recent study described the pharmacokinetics of enoxaparin in healthy cats and advocated a dosage of 0.75 mg/kg SC every 6 hours to achieve and maintain anti-FXa values between 0.5 to 1.0 IU/mL.[74] These studies had small sample sizes but do indicate that further clinical trials are needed to determine efficacy of thromboprophylaxis and antithrombotic effect of LMWHs and that conventional monitoring methods may not be appropriate to evaluate actual clinical efficacy in cats with thromboembolic disease.

Bleeding complications have been reported in cats receiving LMWHs, including bruising, bleeding around the IV catheter, and epistaxis.[63]

Fondaparinux (Synthetic Heparin Derivative)

Fondaparinux sodium (Arixtra; GlaxoSmithKline, Research Triangle Park, NC) is a synthetic pentasaccharide molecule

that is a highly specific inhibitor of FXa with no effect on thrombin or platelet function.[75] In humans, fondaparinux has 100% bioavailability and is recommended for once-daily adminstration.[75] A dose determination study of fondaparinux in healthy cats revealed that a dosage of 0.06 or 0.2 mg/kg SC every 12 hours maintained plasma anti-FXa activity within the human prophylactic or therapeutic range, respectively.[76] Clinical efficacy studies are needed before recommendations can be made for veterinary clinical patients. This relatively new drug is expensive compared to some of the other available anticoagulant options, so it may be cost prohibitive for long-term use.

ORAL FACTOR Xa INHIBITORS

Rivaroxaban (Xarelto; Janssen Pharmaceuticals, Titusville, NJ) and apixaban (Eliquis; Bristol-Myers Squibb, New York, NY) are oral FXa inhibitors that have been evaluated in experimental animal models.[77-81] These novel inhibitors of FXa are an attractive alternative to heparin therapy for anticoagulation in cats, because they can be administered orally and do not require clients to give injections at home. *In vitro* evaluation of the effect of rivaroxaban on feline coagulation indices (TEG, PT, dilute PT, aPTT, and anti-FXa activity) has shown dose-dependent prolongations in all coagulation parameters,[80] similar to coagulation effects noted in other species.[78] Kaolin-activated TEG was not sensitive to low concentrations of rivaroxaban.[80] When evaluating the pharmacodynamics of rivaroxaban in a small population of healthy adult cats using anti-FXa activity, dilute PT, and aPTT for coagulation monitoring, a single 2.5 mg dose of rivaroxaban resulted in persistent FXa inhibition at 24 hours[79] and a peak plasma drug concentration within the human therapeutic range.[82] A dose of 1 mg/kg did not result in a high anti-FXa peak but did not show sustained activity, making it likely that twice-daily dosing might be necessary for cats at this dosage. There is a need for further evaluation of oral anti-FXa inhibitors in clinical feline populations to determine appropriate dosing schemes and to identify whether these drugs can be used safely and effectively for prevention of thromboembolic disease. Additionally, anti-FXa activity reference values are extrapolated from the reference intervals used in humans, so further study to identify accurate, outcome-based reference parameters for anti-FXa activity in the cat is also warranted. Finally, initial investigation of apixaban administration in cats has been presented in abstract form and shows promise for future studies in cats.[83]

NONSTEROIDAL ANTI-INFLAMMATORY DRUGS

Aspirin, or acetylsalicylic acid, inhibits cyclooxygenase, which reduces the synthesis of thromboxane A_2 (TXA_2) in platelets, decreasing the level of activation. Low-dose aspirin therapy has been the preferred method of antiplatelet therapy and thromboprophylaxis in humans due to low risk of GI side effects and selective inhibition of TXA_2 production. Thromboprophylaxis with aspirin in cats has been suggested at doses of 81 mg/cat PO every 72 hours, but this dose can result in unwanted side effects and may not be efficacious for prevention of thromboembolism.[69] Retrospective evaluation of a large number of cats with ATE revealed that no significant differences were found in survival or recurrence of ATE between cats receiving high-dosage ($\geq$40 mg/cat PO every 72 hours) or low-dosage (5 mg/cat PO every 72 hours) aspirin therapy, although cats receiving high-dosage aspirin therapy were more likely to suffer from GI side effects.[26] One prospective study that evaluated the effects of aspirin (5 mg/kg PO every 48 hours) and meloxicam (0.05 mg/kg PO every 24 hours) on platelet aggregation in healthy cats revealed that at these dosages, neither meloxicam nor aspirin had an inhibitory effect on whole blood platelet aggregation.[84] Thromboxane (measured as the stable metabolite TXB_2) concentrations were significantly decreased in the aspirin treatment group, but this did not correlate to an antiplatelet effect.[84] There are currently no studies that support the use of low-dosage aspirin therapy as an effective thromboprophylactic in cats at risk for thromboembolism.

ADENOSINE DIPHOSPHATE RECEPTOR ANTAGONISTS

Clopidogrel and ticlopidine are thienopyridine drugs that are specific antagonists of the platelet $P2Y_{12}$ ADP receptor. The drugs themselves have no antiplatelet activity, but their metabolites bind irreversibly to the $P2Y_{12}$ receptor and inhibit platelet aggregation.[85] They are used widely in humans to prevent thrombus formation in at-risk patients, such as those with coronary artery disease.[85]

Clopidogrel (Plavix; Bristol-Myers Squibb, New York, NY) is rapidly absorbed after oral administration in humans and has good bioavailability. Clopidogrel is a prodrug and must be transformed by hepatic biotransformation into the active metabolite through the cytochrome P450 enzyme system. If this enzyme system is impaired by concurrent administration of medications (such as omeprazole), activation of clopidogrel to the active metabolite can be decreased and treatment failures may result. Investigation of the possibility for drug interactions should be assessed when using clopidogrel in cats, and appropriate substitutions should be made when indicated. When clopidogrel was administered to healthy cats at a dosage of 18.75 mg PO every 24 hours, platelet function was significantly reduced, suggesting that this dose may be useful in cats as a thromboprophylactic.[86] This effect was seen after 3 days of daily drug administration, and effects were no longer present within 1 week of stopping the medication.[86] A lower dose may be effective as well, but further studies are needed to identify the minimum effective dose for cats at risk of thromboembolic disease. No adverse effects were noted in this population of normal cats.[86] However, side effects observed in humans

include GI upset, bleeding, aplastic anemia, and thrombotic thrombocytopenic purpura.[85] The inhibitory effects of clopidogrel on human platelet function have high interindividual and intraindividual variability,[85,87] which is likely due to variation in conversion to the active metabolite. Efficacy of clopidogrel therapy can be monitored using previously referenced methods of platelet function analysis. The use of a human screening assay, Plateletworks, has been evaluated in healthy cats receiving clopidogrel.[88] Platelet aggregation after clopidogrel therapy was significantly lower than baseline aggregation measurements.[88] This monitoring tool is practical and affordable, requires a small blood sample, and may be a promising method to monitor clopidogrel therapy in cats, although it has not been validated in clinical cases. Clopidogrel is used widely for prevention of ATE in cats at risk for thromboembolism, but there continues to be a paucity of evidence regarding the clinical efficacy in this population. Further studies are needed to support its routine use and to identify optimal dose and frequency of administration.

Ticlopidine (Ticlid; Riche Pharmaceuticals, Nutley, NJ) has good bioavailability that is increased by administration with food and is decreased by antacids.[89] Ticlopidine has been evaluated in healthy cats at 100 mg/cat/day PO, which failed to consistently alter platelet function, and 500 mg/cat/day PO, which resulted in consistent reduction of ADP-induced platelet aggregation.[90] Although there were consistent antiplatelet effects at the higher dosage, there was dose-dependent anorexia and vomiting observed that cautions against the clinical usage of this drug.[90]

Novel $P2Y_{12}$ inhibitors, such as prasugrel (Effient; Eli Lilly, Indianapolis, IN) and ticagrelor (Brilinta; AstraZeneca, London, UK), are being used more frequently in humans than clopidogrel and ticlopidine, because these drugs have a more rapid onset of action and achieve more consistent platelet inhibition with less intraindividual variability.[85,91] Despite the more predictable and effective action of these drugs, widespread use continues to be limited by the expense of these novel antiplatelet drugs, and their use has not been evaluated in cats at this time.

GLYCOPROTEIN IIb/IIIa RECEPTOR ANTAGONISTS

The platelet glycoprotein IIb/IIIa (GPIIb/IIIa) receptor plays an important role in platelet-fibrinogen binding and is the therapeutic target of this class of drugs, which includes abciximab, eptifibatide, and tirofiban. These drugs are approved in humans for treatment of acute coronary syndromes and for thromboprophylaxis during percutaneous coronary interventions.[92] These drugs are for IV injection only and have relatively short half-lives, so they must be delivered as a constant rate infusion (CRI). However, there are oral GPIIb/IIIa antagonists currently undergoing clinical trials in human medicine that may become available in the future.[92] Abciximab (ReoPro; Eli Lilly, Indianapolis, IN) has been evaluated in a model of arterial injury in cats that received either aspirin alone or aspirin plus abciximab.[93] Cats that were treated with aspirin (25 mg/kg PO) plus abciximab (0.25 mg/kg IV bolus, then CRI of 0.125 µg/kg/min) had significantly less thrombus formation and significantly greater inhibition of platelet function than the control group (aspirin plus placebo).[93] Eptifibatide (Integrilin; COR Therapeutics, San Francisco, CA) has been shown to inhibit feline platelet aggregation *in vitro* but has been associated with unpredictable circulatory failure and sudden death in some cats when administered at doses necessary to maintain platelet inhibition in healthy cats.[94-95] Tirofiban (Aggrastat; Medicure Pharma, Somerset, NJ) has also been evaluated in a model of cardiac ischemia in adult, healthy cats.[96] In this study, cats receiving a loading IV dose of 100 µg/kg followed by 5 µg/kg/min via CRI showed reduction of ischemia-induced activation of feline platelets.[96] These drugs have not been evaluated in clinical veterinary patients, and their use cannot be recommended at this time without further study supporting their safe and efficacious use in cats.

SUMMARY

The understanding of hypercoagulability and thromboembolic complications in veterinary patients continues to evolve as new diagnostic testing methods are developed. Unfortunately, at this time, no one therapy has emerged as the gold standard when faced with cats that have either developed ATE or have a tendency for hypercoagulability and clot formation. Prospective, clinical studies are needed to assess the safety and efficacy of novel therapies, as well as continued evaluation of appropriate dosing and monitoring protocols in veterinary patients at risk for or affected by thromboembolic disease.

References

1. Cotter S, Brenner R, Dodds WJ: Hemophilia A in three unrelated cats. *J Am Vet Med Assoc* 172:166–168, 1978.
2. Maggio-Price L, Dodds WJ: Factor IX deficiency (haemophilia B) in a family of British shorthair cats. *J Am Vet Med Assoc* 203:1702–1704, 1993.
3. Gookin J, Brooks MB, Catalfamo JL, et al: Factor X deficiency in a cat. *J Am Vet Med Assoc* 211:576–579, 1997.
4. Dillon A, Boudreaux MK: Combined factors IX and XII deficiencies in a family of British shorthair cats. *J Am Vet Med Assoc* 193:833–834, 1988.
5. Green R, White F: Feline factor XII (Hageman) deficiency. *Am J Vet Res* 38(6):893–895, 1977.
6. French T, Fox L, Randolph JF, et al: A bleeding disorder (von Willebrand's disease) in a Himalayan cat. *J Am Vet Med Assoc* 190:437–439, 1987.
7. Maddison J, Watson A, Eade IG, et al: Vitamin K-dependent multifactor coagulopathy in Devon rex cats. *J Am Vet Med Assoc* 197:1495–1497, 1990.
8. Meyers K, Seachord C, Holmsen H, et al: Evaluation of the platelet storage pool deficiency in the feline counterpart of the Chediak-Higashi syndrome. *Am J Hematol* 11:241, 1981.
9. Callan MB, Griot-Wenk M, Hackner SG, et al: Persistent thrombopathy causing bleeding in 2 domestic shorthaired cats. *J Vet Intern Med* 14:217–220, 2000.
10. Center S, Crawford M, Guida L, et al: A retrospective study of 77 cats with severe hepatic lipidosis: 1975-1990. *J Vet Int Med* 7:349–359, 1993.
11. Center S, Warner K, Corbett J, et al: Proteins invoked by vitamin K absence and clotting times in clinically ill cats. *J Vet Int Med* 14:292–297, 2000.
12. Perry L, Williams D, Pidgeon G, et al: Exocrine pancreatic insufficiency with associated coagulopathy in a cat. *J Am Anim Hosp Assoc* 27:109–114, 1991.
13. Rogers KS: Coagulation disorders associated with neoplasia in the dog. *Vet Med* 87:55–61, 1992.
14. Kumar D, Hanlin E, Glurich I, et al: Virchow's contribution to the understanding of thrombosis and cellular biology. *Clin Med Res* 8(3–4):168–172, 2010.
15. Lippi G, Franchini M, Targher G: Arterial thrombus formation in cardiovascular disease. *Nat Rev Cardiol* 8(9):502–512, 2011.
16. Furie B, Furie B: Mechanisms of thrombus formation. *N Engl J Med* 359(9):938–949, 2008.
17. Wakefield T, Myers D, Henke PK, et al: Mechanisms of venous thrombosis and resolution. *Arterioscler Thromb Vasc Biol* 28(3):387–391, 2008.
18. Konecny F: Thromboembolic conditions, aetiology, diagnosis, and treatment in dogs and cats. *Acta Vet Brno* 79(3):497–508, 2010.
19. Payne J, Luis Fuentes V, Boswood A, et al: Population characteristics and survival in 127 referred cats with hypertrophic cardiomyopathy (1997 to 2005). *J Small Anim Pract* 51(10):540–547, 2010.
20. Baty C, Malarkey D, Atkins CE, et al: Natural history of hypertrophic cardiomyopathy and aortic thromboembolism in a family of domestic shorthair cats. *J Vet Intern Med* 15:595–599, 2001.
21. Kittleson M, Meurs K, Munro MJ, et al: Familial hypertrophic cardiomyopathy in Maine Coon cats: an animal model of human disease. *Circulation* 99:3172–3180, 1999.
22. Langston C, Cowgill L, Spano J: Applications and outcome of hemodialysis in cats: a review of 29 cases. *J Vet Intern Med* 11:348–355, 1997.
23. Norris C, Griffey S, Samii VF: Pulmonary thromboembolism in cats: 29 cases (1987-1997). *J Am Vet Med Assoc* 215(11):1650–1654, 1999.
24. Kricheff I, Zucker M, Tschopp TB, et al: Inhibition of thrombosis on vascular catheters in cats. *Radiology* 106(1):49–51, 1973.
25. Laste NJ, Harpster NK: A retrospective study of 100 cases of feline distal aortic thromboembolism: 1977-1993. *J Am Anim Hosp Assoc* 31:492–500, 1995.
26. Smith S, Tobias A, Jacob KA, et al: Arterial thromboembolism in cats: acute crisis in 127 cases (1992-2001) and long-term management with low-dose aspirin in 24 cases. *J Vet Intern Med* 17:73–83, 2003.
27. Welles E, Boudreaux M, Crager CS, et al: Platelet function and antithrombin, plasminogen, and fibrinolytic activities in cats with heart disease. *Am J Vet Res* 55(5):619–627, 1994.
28. Helenski C, Ross J, Jr: Platelet aggregation in feline cardiomyopathy. *J Vet Intern Med* 1:24–28, 1987.
29. Farid N, Griffiths B, Collins JR, et al: Blood coagulation and fibrinolysis in thyroid disease. *Thromb Haemost* 35(2):415–422, 1976.
30. Meijers J, Tekelenburg W, Bouma BN, et al: High levels of coagulation factor XI as a risk factor for venous thrombosis. *N Engl J Med* 342(10):696–701, 2000.
31. Rogers J, Shane S, Jencks FS, et al: Factor VIII activity and thyroid function. *Ann Intern Med* 97(5):713–716, 1982.
32. Hwang JU, Kwon KY, Hur JW, et al: The role of hyperthyroidism as the predisposing factor for superior sagittal sinus thrombosis. *J Cerebrovasc Endovasc Neurosurg* 14(3):251–254, 2012.
33. Bond BR, Fox PR, Peterson ME, et al: Echocardiographic findings in 103 cats with hyperthyroidism. *J Am Vet Med Assoc* 192(11):1546–1549, 1988.

34. Bille A, deLaforcade A, et al: Pregnancy is a hypercoagulable state in queens. *J Vet Intern Med* 27(3):710, 2013. (Abstract).

35. Schermerhorn T, Pembleton-Corbett JR, Kornreich B, et al: Pulmonary thromboembolism in cats. *J Vet Int Med* 18(4):533–535, 2004.

36. Davidson BL, Rozanski EA, Tidwell AS, et al: Pulmonary thromboembolism in a heartworm-positive cat. *J Vet Intern Med* 20:1037–1041, 2006.

37. Caine GJ, Stonelake PS, Lip GY, et al: The hypercoagulable state of malignancy: pathogenesis and current debate. *Neoplasia* 4(6):465–473, 2002.

38. Park H, Ranganathan P: Neoplastic and paraneoplastic vasculitis, vasculopathy, and hypercoagulability. *Rheum Dis Clin North Am* 37(4):593–606, 2011.

39. Kristensen AT, Wiinberg B, Jessen LR, et al: Evaluation of human recombinant tissue factor activated thromboelastography in 49 dogs with neoplasia. *J Vet Intern Med* 22:140–147, 2008.

40. McNiel EA, Ogilvie GK, Fettman MJ, et al: Platelet hyperfunction in dogs with malignancies. *J Vet Intern Med* 11(3):178–182, 1997.

41. Hogan DF, Dhaliwal RS, Sisson DD, et al: Paraneoplastic thrombocytosis-induced systemic thromboembolism in a cat. *J Am Anim Hosp Assoc* 35:483, 1999.

42. Bick R, Strauss J, Frenkel EP, et al: Thrombosis and hemorrhage in oncology patients. *Heme Onc Clin N Am* 10(4):875–907, 1996.

43. Lubas G, Caldin M, Wiinberg B, et al: Laboratory testing of coagulation disorders. In Weiss DJ, Wardrop KJ, editors: *Schalm's veterinary hematology*, ed 6, Ames, IA, 2010, Wiley-Blackwell, pp 1082–1089.

44. Jandrey KE: Assessment of platelet function. *J Vet Emerg Crit Care* 22(1):81–98, 2012.

45. Moore KE, Morris N, Dhupa N, et al: Retrospective study of streptokinase administration in 46 cats with arterial thromboembolism. *J Vet Emerg Crit Care* 10:245–257, 2000.

46. Bedard C, Lanevschi-Pietersma A, Dunn M, et al: Evaluation of coagulation markers in the plasma of healthy cats and cats with asymptomatic hypertrophic cardiomyopathy. *Vet Clin Pathol* 36(2):167–172, 2007.

47. Stokol T, Brooks M, Rush JE, et al: Hypercoagulability in cats with cardiomyopathy. *J Vet Int Med* 22(3):546–552, 2008.

48. Dircks B, Nolte I, Mischke R: Haemostatic abnormalities in cats with naturally occurring liver diseases. *Vet J* 193(1):103–108, 2012.

49. Tholen I, Weingart C, Kohn B: Concentration of D-dimers in healthy cats and sick cats with and without disseminated intravascular coagulation (DIC). *J Feline Med Surg* 11(10):842–846, 2009.

50. Brazzell JL, Borjesson DL: Evaluation of plasma antithrombin activity and D-dimer concentration in populations of healthy cats, clinically ill cats, and cats with cardiomyopathy. *Vet Clin Pathol* 36(1):79–84, 2007.

51. Smith SA, Kraft SL, Lewis DC, et al: Pharmacodynamics of warfarin in cats. *J Vet Pharmacol Therap* 23:339–344, 2000.

52. Smith CE, Rozanski EA, Freeman LM, et al: Use of low molecular weight heparin in cats: 57 cases (1999-2003). *J Am Vet Med Assoc* 225(8):1237–1241, 2004.

53. Smith SA, Kraft SL, Lewis DC, et al: Plasma pharmacokinetics of warfarin enantiomers in cats. *J Vet Pharmacol Ther* 23(6):329–337, 2000.

54. Ansell J, Hirsh J, Hylek E, et al: Pharmacology and management of the vitamin K antagonists: American College of Chest Physicians evidence-based clinical practice guidelines (8th edition). *Chest* 133(6 Suppl):160S–198S, 2008.

55. Dunn M, Brooks MB: Antiplatelet and anticoagulant therapy. In Bonagura JD, editor: *Kirk's current veterinary therapy XIV*, Philadelphia, 2009, Saunders, pp 24–28.

56. Harpster NK, Baty CJ: Warfarin therapy of the cat at risk of thromboembolism. In Bonagura JD, editor: *Kirk's current veterinary therapy XII*, Philadelphia, 1995, Saunders, pp 868–873.

57. Abildgaard U: Heparin/low molecular weight heparin and tissue factor pathway inhibitor. *Haemostasis* 23(Suppl 1):103–106, 1993.

58. Hirsh J, Anand SS, Halperin JL, et al: Mechanism of action and pharmacology of unfractionated heparin. *Arter Thromb Vasc Biol* 21:1094–1096, 2001.

59. Hirsh J, Warkentin TE, Raschke R, et al: Heparin and low-molecular-weight heparin: mechanisms of action, pharmacokinetics, dosing considerations, monitoring, efficacy, and safety. *Chest* 114(5 Suppl):489S–510S, 1998.

60. Basu D, Gallus A, Hirsh J, et al: A prospective study of the value of monitoring heparin treatment with the activated partial thromboplastin time. *N Eng J Med* 287:324–327, 1972.

61. Eikelboom J, Hirsh J: Monitoring unfractionated heparin with the aPTT. *Thromb Haemost* 96:547–552, 2006.

62. Mischke R: Heparin *in vitro* sensitivity of the activated partial thromboplastin time in canine plasma depends on reagent. *J Vet Diag Invest* 15:588–591, 2003.

63. Alwood AJ, Downend AB, Brooks MB, et al: Anticoagulant effects of low-molecular weight heparins in healthy cats. *J Vet Intern Med* 21:378–387, 2007.

64. Brooks M: Evaluation of a chromogenic assay to measure the factor Xa inhibitory activity of unfractionated heparin in canine plasma. *Vet Clin Path* 33(4):208–214, 2004.

65. Levine M, Hirsh J, Gent M, et al: A randomized trial comparing activated thromboplastin time with heparin assay in patients with acute venous thromboembolism requiring large daily doses of heparin. *Arch Intern Med* 154:49–56, 1994.

66. Hirsh J, Raschke R: Heparin and low molecular weight heparin: The Seventh ACCP Conference on Antithrombotic and Thrombolytic Therapy. *Chest* 126(3 Suppl):188S–203S, 2004.

67. Mischke R, Schmitt J, Wolken S, et al: Pharmacokinetics of the low molecular weight heparin dalteparin in cats. *Vet J* 192:299–303, 2012.

68. Young E, Podor TJ, Venner T, et al: Induction of the acute-phase reaction increases heparin binding proteins in plasma. *Arter Thromb Vasc Biol* 17:1568–1574, 1997.

69. Smith S, Tobias A: Feline arterial thromboembolism: an update. *Vet Clin North Am Small Anim Pract* 34(5):1245–1271, 2004.

70. Weitz JI: Low-molecular-weight heparins. *N Engl J Med* 337:688–698, 1997.

71. Goodman JS, Rozanski EA, Brown D, et al: The effects of low-molecular weight heparin on hematologic and coagulation parameters in normal cats (abstract). *J Vet Intern Med* 13:268, 1999.

72. Vargo CL, Taylor SM, Carr A, et al: The effect of a low molecular weight heparin on coagulation parameters in healthy cats. *Can J Vet Res* 73:132–136, 2009.

73. Van De Wiele CM, Hogan DF, Green HW, 3rd, et al: Antithrombotic effect of enoxaparin in clinically healthy cats: a venous stasis model. *J Vet Int Med* 24(1):185–191, 2010.

74. Mischke R, Schönig J, Döderlein E, et al: Enoxaparin: pharmacokinetics and treatment schedule for cats. *Vet J* 200(3):375–381, 2014.

75. Bauer KA, Hawkins DW, Peters PC, et al: Fondaparinux, a synthetic pentasaccharide: the first in a new class of antithrombotic agents—the selective factor Xa inhibitors. *Cardiovasc Drug Rev* 20(1):37–52, 2002.

76. Fiakpui NN, Hogan DF, Whittem T, et al: Dose determination of fondaparinux in healthy cats. *Am J Vet Res* 73(4):556–561, 2012.

77. Weinz C, Schwarz T, Kubitza D, et al: Metabolism and excretion of rivaroxaban, an oral, direct factor Xa inhibitor, in rats, dogs, and humans. *Drug Metab Dispos* 37:1056–1064, 2009.

78. Conversy B, Blais MC, Dunn M, et al: Rivaroxaban is an efficient anticoagulant in healthy dogs: time course of haemostatic parameters. *J Vet Intern Med* 27(3):709, 2013. (Abstract).

79. Dixon-Jimenez A, Rapoport G, Brainard B, et al: Pharmacodynamic evaluation of single oral dose rivaroxaban in healthy adult cats. In *International Veterinary Emergency and Critical Care Symposium*, San Diego, California, 2013. (Abstract).

80. Brainard B, Cathcart C, Dixon AC, et al: In vitro effects of rivaroxaban on feline coagulation indices. *J Vet Intern Med* 25(3):697, 2011. (Abstract).

81. He K, Luettgen J, Zhang D, et al: Preclinical pharmacokinetics and pharmacodynamics of apixaban, a potent and selective factor Xa inhibitor. *Eur J Drug Metab Pharmacokinet* 36(3):129–139, 2011.

82. Dixon-Jimenez AC, Brainard BM, Brooks MB, et al: Pharmacokinetic and pharmacodynamic evaluation of oral rivaroxaban in healthy adult cats. *J Vet Emerg Crit Care* 2015. in press.

83. Myers JA, Wittenburg LA, Olver CS, et al: Pharmacokinetics and pharmacodynamics of the factor Xa inhibitor apixaban in cats: a pilot study. *J Vet Intern Med* 28(3):1006, 2014. (Abstract).

84. Cathcart CJ, Brainard BM, Reynolds LR, et al: Lack of inhibitory effect of acetylsalicylic acid and meloxicam on whole blood platelet

aggregation in cats. *J Vet Emerg Crit Care* 22(1):99–106, 2012.

85. Wijeyeratne YD, Heptinstall S: Anti-platelet therapy: ADP receptor antagonists. *Brit J Clin Pharmacol* 72(4):647–657, 2011.

86. Hogan D, Andrews D, Green HW, et al: Antiplatelet effects and pharmacodynamics of clopidogrel in cats. *J Am Vet Med Assoc* 225:1406–1411, 2004.

87. Armero S, Camoin J, Omar Aït Mokhtar O, et al: Intra-individual variability in clopidogrel responsiveness in coronary artery disease patients under long term therapy. *Platelets* 21:503–507, 2010.

88. Hamel-Jolette A, Dunn M, Bedard C: Plateletworks: a screening assay for clopidogrel therapy monitoring in healthy cats. *Can J Vet Res* 73:73–76, 2009.

89. Farid NA, Kurihara A, Wrighton SA, et al: Metabolism and disposition of the thienopyridine antiplatelet drugs Ticlopidine, Clopidogrel, and Prasugrel in humans. *J Clin Pharmacol* 50(2):126–142, 2010.

90. Hogan D, Andrews D, Talbott KK, et al: Evaluation of antiplatelet effects of ticlopidine in cats. *Am J Vet Res* 65:327–332, 2004.

91. Ferri N, Corsini A, Bellosta S, et al: Pharmacology of the new P2Y12 receptor inhibitors: insights on pharmacokinetic and pharmacodynamics properties. *Drugs* 73(15):1681–1709, 2013.

92. Huang F, Hong E: Platelet glycoprotein IIb/IIIa inhibition and its clinical use. *Curr Med Chem Cardiovasc Hematol Agents* 2:187–196, 2004.

93. Bright J, Dowers K, Powers B: Effects of the glycoprotein IIb/IIIa antagonist abciximab on thrombus formation and platelet function in cats with arterial injury. *Vet Ther* 4(1):35–46, 2003.

94. Bright J: *In vitro* anti-aggregatory effects of the GPIIb/IIIa antagonist eptifibatide on feline platelets (correspondence). *J Vet Intern Med* 16(6):v, 2002.

95. Dowers K, Bright J: Anti-aggregatory effects of a GPIIb/IIIa antagonist on feline platelet function. *J Vet Intern Med* 14(3):335, 2000. (Abstract).

96. Fu L, Longhurst J: Activated platelets contribute to stimulation of cardiac afferents during ischaemia in cats: role of 5-HT$_3$ receptors. *J Physiol* 544(3):897–912, 2001.

Selection and Use of Blood Products in the Feline Patient

Elizabeth Thomovsky

Cats may require transfusions of blood and/or plasma as part of their treatment in the critical care unit. In the case of blood transfusions, cats most often require red blood cells (RBCs) to replace those lost through hemorrhage or via immune-mediated destruction.[1,2] Administration of blood for blood-loss anemia is the most common situation in cats (40 of 91 cats [44%] in one study[1] and 66 of 126 cats [52%] in another study[2]). This is in contrast to reports of 10% to 14%[1,2] of cats requiring transfusions to replace blood lost as a result of hemolysis and 38% to 39%[1,2] of cats requiring RBC transfusion due to a lack of production of RBCs in the bone marrow. In the relatively uncommon situations where cats require plasma transfusions, they are most typically administered to either replace clotting factors or other proteins such as albumin found naturally in plasma (2% each of total number of feline transfusions[1]).

In most situations, cats requiring blood transfusions receive fresh whole feline blood. The first reason for this is that cats can only donate a maximum of 55 to 60 mL of whole blood. Such small initial starting volumes are difficult to further separate into components such as plasma and packed RBCs.[1] Second, feline blood is collected via an "open technique" in most situations.[1,3] This means that the blood is drawn from the vein into a syringe before being placed into a collection bag, rather than being drawn directly into the collection bag. This is considered an "open" blood draw because each individual component of the blood-drawing system is packaged separately and needs to be assembled; this is in contrast to a "closed system" where the needle, tubing, and blood-collection bag are connected and packaged sterilely together. The danger of an "open technique' is that it introduces an extra step that increases the bacterial contamination risk for the blood. It is therefore not safe to separate and store or bank blood components collected via the "open technique." Third, if the blood is collected via an "open technique," it is safest to collect and then administer the blood immediately—before bacterial proliferation occurs—making whole blood the most commonly administered product.

COLLECTION OF FELINE BLOOD

Because the majority of cat blood is drawn and then administered immediately to a patient, this section details one method of collecting blood from donor cats. Donor cats should ideally be selected from a limited population that has undergone screening (see Boxes 78-1 to 78-3 for lists of preferred characteristics for donor cats). However, in an emergency setting, at times the old adage of "nearly any cat will do" may need to be followed to provide lifesaving blood to a severely anemic patient or to a patient that is hemorrhaging and cannot be stabilized without the administration of blood. Even in those emergency settings, the author suggests that the donor cats be minimally screened (see bolded items in Boxes 78-1 and 78-2) and blood-typed before transfusion.

Cats that are donating blood uniformly require sedation (in rare cases, general anesthesia) because even the best-behaved cat will rarely lie still for the entire blood draw with only manual restraint. The author typically uses a combination of butorphanol tartrate (0.2 mg/kg intravenously [IV]) and ketamine (maximum 5 to 10 mg/kg IV, given to effect) in a 1:1 combination with diazepam (maximum 0.25 to 0.5 mg/kg IV, given to effect).[3] Once the cat is sedated enough to allow for easy handling, the cervical region should be clipped around the jugular vein and aseptically prepared with 0.05% chlorhexidine solution or a mixture of betadine and water. After the skin is aseptically prepared, any individual drawing the blood, touching the region, and handling the blood collection materials should wear sterile gloves.

Open Technique for Blood Collection

Two to three 20 mL syringes are each filled with 3 mL of acid citrate dextrose or citrate phosphate dextrose anticoagulant. A needle is introduced into the jugular vein; butterfly catheters are commonly used, but hypodermic needles with attached tubing can also be used. The needle should not be less than 22 gauge to ensure that the collected RBCs are not lysed. Blood is slowly drawn into the syringe while the syringe is rotated to allow for mixing of the blood and anticoagulant. Typically 40 to 50 mL of blood is drawn from each cat (maximum 10 to 12 mL/kg).

If the only anticoagulant available is heparin, it can be combined with the blood at a ratio of 5 to 10 International Units heparin/mL of collected blood.[3] However, heparinized blood cannot be stored and should be administered

- **Clinically healthy**
- Living indoor only
- Easy to handle without sedation
- **Body weight at least 5 kg (11 lb)**
- Fully and routinely vaccinated and dewormed
- Tested negative for specific infectious diseases (Box 78-2)
- Normal complete blood count and serum chemistry panels (tested at least once a year)
- **Normal physical examination (including normal heart and lung auscultation)**
- **Packed cell volume at least 30% to 35%**

*The bolded items are recommended for ALL donors even when the cat is being used in a true emergency setting for a lifesaving blood donation.

BOX 78-2 Infectious Disease Testing Recommended in ALL Donor Cats[3],*

Nonvector-Borne Diseases
- **Feline leukemia virus**
- **Feline immunodeficiency virus**

Vector-Borne Diseases
- *Mycoplasma hemofelis/Candidatus mycoplasma haemominutum* (two species of hemotropic mycoplasmas that were formerly known as "Hemobartonella")
- *Bartonella henselae*

*The bolded items are recommended to be screened for in ALL donors even when the cat is being used in a true emergency setting for a lifesaving blood donation.

BOX 78-3 Infectious Disease Testing Recommended Contingent on Geographic Location[3]

- *Cytauxzoon felis*
- Ehrlichiosis
- Anaplasmosis
- Neorickettsiosis

immediately to a patient. Therefore, the author recommends that heparin only be used in emergency situations where blood is being drawn from a donor with the intent to administer it immediately to a patient.

Closed Technique for Blood Collection

For closed blood collection techniques, a prepackaged, commercially prepared system consisting of a collection bag (typically a 100 mL bag for cats) that is filled with anticoagulant and attached to tubing with a needle is used. This bag is opened in a sterile manner and used to collect the blood. As detailed earlier, the collection bag is agitated gently while the blood is being collected into it to allow for mixing of the blood and anticoagulant. However, at the time of this writing, no commercially prepared collection system exists that is small enough for cats. The only commercially available systems contain bags without anticoagulant. Thus, 3 mL of anticoagulant per 20 mL of collection bag capacity has to be added to the bag before the blood draw; this *opens* the system.

FELINE BLOOD TYPES

Before the administration of blood or plasma to a cat, both the donor and recipient cats must be at a minimum *blood-typed*. This is important because cats have naturally occurring alloantibodies; in short, cats are born with antibodies against blood types other than their own. Therefore, cats can react at the time of the first transfusion to blood that is not their type (see more detail in Transfusion Reactions).

Cats have traditionally been divided into three blood types: A, B, and AB. Type A cats have antibodies against type B blood and vice versa. Type AB cats are considered to be the universal recipients because they do not have any alloantibodies. Unfortunately, AB cats are extremely rare. Type A is dominant to type B, and the alleles coding for these blood types are inherited in a simple mendelian manner. The genetic mutation and inheritance pattern for blood type AB in cats has not yet been determined.

Type A cats have a low titer of naturally occurring antibodies against type B blood. However, type B cats have a high antibody titer against type A blood, making their transfusion reactions more dramatic. Antibodies against type A are largely immunoglobulin (Ig) M and cause both agglutination and lysis.[4] Antibodies against type B are both IgM (causing agglutination and lysis) and IgG (causing primarily lysis).[4] To further complicate things, an individual cat will vary seasonally in its exact antibody titer to the other blood type, making the prediction of transfusion reactions difficult.[5]

These traditional A, B, and AB blood types are distributed throughout the cat population. In general, type A predominates; the vast majority (94.5%[1]) of nonpedigreed cats in the United States are type A. Worldwide, whereas type A is always predominant among nonpurebred cats, the exact percentages have regional variances. For example, in Ireland, only 84.7% of nonpedigreed cats are type A, with 14.6% being type B and 0.7% type AB.[4] In a study of nonpedigreed cats from Turkey, 72.7% were type A, 25% were type B, and 2.2% were type AB.[6] In the United Kingdom, 68% of nonpedigreed cats were type A, 30% were type B, and 2% were type AB.[7]

Additionally, in certain breeds of cats, there is a higher percentage of type B or AB blood types. For example, a group of 61 Ragdoll cats in northern Italy showed 77% type A, 4.9% type B, and 18% type AB.[5] Conversely, 100% of Siamese cats are reported to be type A; among the Devon Rex breed, there are more type B than type A cats.[1]

As a general rule in the United States, a domestic shorthair cat is type A until proven otherwise. A Siamese cat is type A. The more exotic breeds (Persians, British Fold, Devon Rex, etc.) have a higher chance of being type B.

It is important to also realize that there are other blood types in cats that may not be described or may be incompletely described. One example is the *Mik* RBC antigen, named after incompatibility reactions were noted between a blood donor called "Mike" and cats with his same blood type.[8] It seems that cats have naturally occurring antibodies against *Mik* similar to those against the A-B RBC antigens; that is, a *Mik*-negative cat has anti-*Mik* antibodies present in its serum.[8]

Blood-Typing in Cats

There are several commercially available blood-typing kits in the United States that can differentiate the subtypes. These tests are typically done patient-side and completed within a few minutes. The tests rely on seeing a visible agglutination reaction between the test subject's blood and known antitype antibodies. For example, a type A cat will react to anti-A antibodies in the test system causing agglutination (a positive test). Even in a crisis, at the very least the donor and recipient cats must be blood-typed and given the correct type of blood to avoid the most devastating transfusion reactions.

Unfortunately, these commercially available kits do not provide a way to detect the "other" blood types in cats such as the *Mik* blood type.[8] Thus many practitioners believe that doing a crossmatch between the recipient and donor cats is the only way to be sure not to administer incompatible blood to a patient. (Always ensure that cats being crossmatched have compatible A-B blood types first!). Due to the complexity of performing crossmatches, most clinics will send all crossmatches to a commercial laboratory to receive the most reliable results. Crossmatching generally involves separating the RBCs from the plasma in both the donor and the recipient and then mixing donor plasma with recipient RBCs (minor crossmatch) and donor RBCs with recipient plasma (major crossmatch). A positive result with agglutination or lysis of the RBCs means that the samples are not compatible.

Crossmatching relies greatly on the appropriate interpretation of outcomes when donor and recipient blood components are mixed together. Bedside crossmatch kits are commercially available, but there is no published literature describing the ease of interpretation of results nor how closely the results of these test kits correlate with the gold standard (commercial laboratory testing). Crossmatching can be performed in a clinical setting as long as the practice has a centrifuge available to allow for separation of a blood sample into its constituent parts (Box 78-4). However, the author recommends performing crossmatches at a commercial laboratory if possible, for several reasons. First, because some

---

BOX 78-4 In-house Crossmatch Technique

Collect 1 mL of blood from donor and recipient in a red top tube.

1. Allow blood in red top tube to clot so that plasma is separated from the red cells.
2. Spin red top tubes in centrifuge (3000 rpm) for 5 to 10 minutes.
3. Separate serum from the red blood cells (RBCs) by decanting it. Place in a new red top tube.
4. Add 2 to 3 mL of 0.9% saline to RBCs and mix gently to resuspend RBCs.
5. Centrifuge the saline-suspended RBCs at 3400 rpm for 1 minute.
6. Decant the supernatant and add another 2 to 3 mL of 0.9% saline to the red cells.
7. Repeat steps 4 to 6 a total of 3 times to fully wash the RBCs.
8. Suspend the saline-washed RBCs in 0.9% saline in a ratio of 0.2 mL of red cells to 4.8 mL of saline (4% solution).
9. Mix the donor and recipient blood samples together in new red top tubes (be sure to label them) in the following combinations:
   - One drop of DONOR RBC suspension + 1 drop of RECIPIENT serum (major crossmatch)
   - One drop of DONOR serum + 1 drop of RECIPIENT RBC suspension (minor crossmatch)
   - One drop DONOR RBC suspension + 1 drop DONOR serum (donor control)
   - One drop RECIPIENT RBC suspension + 1 drop RECIPIENT serium (recipient control)
10. Incubate all tubes for 15 minutes at room temperature. Then spin the tubes at 3400 rpm for 15 seconds.
11. Interpret the tubes:
    - Observe for macroscopic clumping or agglutination in the tubes (visible to the naked eye). RBCs should float away from the centrifuged pellet readily and singly when the tube is moved. The supernatant should NOT be hemolyzed.
    - Place a drop of the tube contents onto a slide with a coverslip. RBCs should NOT show clumping or attachment to other cells. Rouleaux formation (RBCs lined up in a stack similar to coins) is not an indication of reaction.

Adapted from the International Society of Feline Medicine.[14]

---

samples have microscopic rather than macroscopic interactions that require further training to definitively recognize, to ensure the most reliable results it is safer to use a commercial laboratory when interpreting crossmatch results. In addition, incomplete preparation of samples by not completely separating the red cells from the plasma and/or not properly washing the separated RBCs before testing can lead to confusing or incorrect results; this is minimized by use of a commercial laboratory.

AVAILABLE FELINE BLOOD PRODUCTS

Feline blood products can be more difficult to procure than canine blood products. There are several commercial blood banks in the United States that can ship blood products regionally or nationwide. These blood banks typically have whole blood, packed RBCs, and plasma (fresh-frozen or frozen) available for purchase. However, in many cases, practitioners will use a local blood donor cat to provide the blood for a patient. These donations are almost always whole blood.

Whole blood is simply blood collected directly from a patient and mixed with anticoagulant as detailed earlier (see Collection of Feline Blood). Usually, a unit of whole blood is 50 mL of blood mixed with 9 mL of anticoagulant (a total of approximately 60 mL). If this anticoagulated whole blood is centrifuged within 6 hours of being collected, it will create packed RBCs (the RBC component of the whole blood) and fresh plasma. If not administered immediately, this fresh plasma is ideally frozen to −18°C (0°F) within 1 hour of collection. As long as the plasma is safely frozen within 6 hours from its time of collection, it is termed fresh-frozen plasma. If the plasma is frozen more than 6 hours after collection OR remains frozen for more than 1 year, it becomes frozen plasma. See Table 78-1 for indications and uses of each blood product.

Other Blood Products Used in Cats

Human Serum Albumin (5%)

There is a report about administration of human serum albumin to cats.[9] The goal was to increase oncotic support in hypoalbuminemic patients. In that study, the cats received 2 mL/kg per hour of albumin until their serum albumin levels were greater than 2.0 g/dL.[9] A total of 170 cats with low serum albumin secondary to peritonitis (decreased albumin production), liver disease (decreased albumin production), or nephropathy (albumin loss) received human serum albumin.[9] The major side effects were diarrhea, tremors, hyperthermia, or perivascular inflammation at the catheter site, but no anaphylactic or fatal reactions were recorded.[9] The author is wary of administering human serum albumin in the majority of cases because it is a xenoprotein and only shares a partial homology with cat albumin, placing patients at high risk for immune reactions to this product.

Canine Whole Blood

A 2008 report summarizing a total of 62 cats in the veterinary literature (from 1962 to 2008) described the use of canine whole blood in cats when no compatible feline blood product was available.[10] In this study, cats did not seem to have naturally occurring alloantibodies against canine red cell antigens; at most there appeared to be minor crossmatch incompatibilities between canine donor serum and feline RBCs.[10]

Table 78-1	Indications, Components, and Dosages of Commonly Used Blood Products in Cats			
	Whole Blood	**Packed Red Blood Cells**	**Fresh-Frozen Plasma**	**Frozen Plasma**
Components	RBCs, plasma	RBCs	Proteins (albumin), coagulation factors, immunoglobulin, procoagulant and anticoagulant proteins	Protein (albumin), clotting factors I, II, VII, IX, and X
Indications for use	Anemia (blood loss, hemolysis, decreased RBC production)	Anemia (blood loss, hemolysis, decreased RBC production)	Any coagulopathy secondary to dysfunction or depletion of clotting factors, liver failure	Vitamin K-dependent coagulopathy (rodenticide), inherited coagulation disorder affecting factors II, VII, IX, or X, liver failure
Storage and shelf life	28 days at refrigeration temperatures (4°C [39°F])	28 days at refrigeration temperatures (4°C [39°F])	1 year at −25°C (−13°F) or below	5 additional years[13] at −25°C (−13°F) or below (after first year as fresh-frozen plasma)
Dosage	2 mL/kg will increase the PCV by 1%	1 mL/kg will increase the PCV by 1%	5-20 mL/kg	5-20 mL/kg
Alternative dosage calculation	mL of blood = 60 mL/kg × patient's body weight (kg) × (desired PCV − patient's PCV)/(PCV of donor)		None	None

PCV, packed cell volume; RBC, red blood cell.

Therefore, using canine packed RBCs might largely eliminate these reported minor crossmatch incompatibilities.[10]

No acute major transfusion reactions were noted among the 62 cats receiving canine whole blood.[10] The only reported complications were pyrexia, tachypnea, and icterus in the week post-transfusion.[10] Due to production of anticanine RBC antibodies in the transfused cats at days 4 to 7 post-transfusion, the lifespan of a canine transfusion is approximately 4 days in all cats; any subsequent transfusions of canine RBCs will lead to anaphylactic reactions that are often fatal in cats.[10] In the event that feline blood of the correct blood type is not available and a transfusion is needed acutely to save a cat's life, this author believes that using canine blood (ideally that is crossmatched to the cat) is an acceptable substitute.

Oxyglobin

Oxyglobin is a commercially prepared bovine hemoglobin solution that is currently not available for use. When available, it was used as a hemoglobin supplement in anemic patients and to provide oncotic and vasopressor support. Because of the lack of RBCs in the product, it does not require crossmatching or blood-typing before administration and can be stored at room temperature for up to 3 years. Dosages in cats range from 2.5 to 10 mL/kg, and the calculated dosage is usually administered slowly over the course of 6 to 24 hours. Because it has a very high oncotic pressure, Oxyglobin can cause fluid overload; hence slower administration rates are typically favored in cats.

One report indicated that 53 cats safely received Oxyglobin for anemia (due to blood loss, hemolysis, and decreased red cell production).[11] A total of seven cats in this report displayed either pulmonary edema or pleural effusion, but each of these cats was believed to have pre-existing heart disease.[11] Six of these seven cats died after the Oxyglobin administration because of causes attributed to the product. The remaining 46 cats had discolored serum and urine, as expected secondary to use of this product, but did not have other significant complications attributed to the transfusion.[11] The cats in the study received 6.7 to 19.8 mL/kg Oxyglobin per 24 hours.

TRANSFUSION REACTIONS

Transfusion reactions in cats range in severity and depend on whether the cat has a high or low titer of antibodies against the other blood type. In general, type B cats have a consistently high titer of anti-A antibodies. Therefore, if they are given a transfusion from a type A cat, this will cause a dramatic lysis of the RBCs that is typically fatal. This reaction will occur after only a small amount of type A blood (even as little as 1 mL) is given to these cats. Type A cats always have a lower anti-B antibody titer than the type B cats have against type A. Therefore, transfusion reactions are much less dramatic; giving type B blood to a type A cat typically leads to shortening of the RBC lifespan rather than complete lysis

of all transfused cells. These cats will often have a fever secondary to the red cell destruction and possibly transient icterus and/or hemoglobinuria and hemoglobinemia secondary to hemolysis of the donated RBCs. Because type A cats have a wide variance in the concentration of anti-B RBCs seasonally, the intensity of the reactions is variable.[5]

Reactions against *Mik* are less well characterized. In the initial report of this blood group, the authors reported hemolysis indicated by hemoglobinemia and hyperbilirubinemia 1 to 2 days post-transfusion without an appreciable increase in the recipient cat's packed cell volume immediately post-transfusion suggesting hemolysis of the transfused cells.[8] The authors also found visible agglutination in crossmatch reactions performed involving the *Mik*-positive cats.[8] Many clinicians suspect that there are many other blood groups that, like *Mik*, are separate from the A-B system and thus can lead to incompatible crossmatches in cats given blood that is appropriately matched by A or B blood types.

In the event of immune-mediated hemolytic transfusion reactions (e.g., antitype reactions), treatment involves stopping the transfusion and administering diphenhydramine (2 to 4 mg/kg intramuscularly [IM], a maximum of two doses within a 1-hour period) to stop the reaction. Diphenhydramine stops degranulation of mast cells, the primary mediator of the immunologic allergic reaction. It is important to always give diphenhydramine to halt the ongoing immunologic reaction. In some cases when there is also significant inflammation noted in the patient, a single anti-inflammatory dose of dexamethasone sodium phosphate (0.07 to 0.14 mg/kg IM or IV) can also be administered.

Cats can also display nonhemolytic transfusion reactions induced by the transfusion of incompatible blood. These reactions (7.9%) are more common than hemolytic transfusion reactions (0.8%).[2] Nonhemolytic reactions are often self-limiting and typically involve transient increases in rectal temperature (greater than 1°C [1.8°F]), facial rubbing, angioedema, vomiting, and salivation.[2] Treatment for nonhemolytic transfusion reactions involves stopping the transfusion and administering an anti-inflammatory dosage of dexamethasone sodium phosphate (0.07 to 0.14 mg/kg IM; one to two doses total per 24 hours) to reduce proinflammatory cytokine release and reduce the severity of clinical signs.

It has also been reported that cats can have pulmonary crackles secondary to pulmonary edema.[2] Pulmonary edema can be cardiogenic or noncardiogenic in origin. Noncardiogenic pulmonary edema is caused by the leakage of fluid out of the pulmonary vessels secondary to increased vascular permeability. By contrast, cardiogenic pulmonary edema is induced by the blood volume that is administered. In the author's experience, cats with chronic anemia that have compensated for their anemia are more at risk for the induction of cardiogenic pulmonary edema. This is likely related to increases in blood viscosity secondary to the blood administration; increased viscosity can increase hydrostatic pressure in the vascular system and lead to fluid extravasation in the lung parenchyma. Cats with diagnosed or undiagnosed heart disease with pre-existing increases in hydrostatic pressure in their vascular system also seem to be at risk for the formation of cardiogenic pulmonary edema during a transfusion.

Clinical signs associated with pulmonary edema include tachypnea, dyspnea, and/or hypoxia. Treatment involves stopping the transfusion and administering 2 mg/kg furosemide IV or IM every 30 minutes as needed until the patient's clinical signs resolve. Many cats also benefit from oxygen therapy and cautious sedation while awaiting improvement of their clinical signs. There are many options for sedation, but typically an opioid such as butorphanol (0.2 mg/kg IV or IM) or oxymorphone (0.1 mg/kg IV or IM) is the safest choice for a dyspneic cat and will reduce anxiety without suppressing ventilation. If the pulmonary edema is due to fluid overload, there should be at least some improvement in the cat's clinical signs by the time 4 mg/kg of furosemide has been administered. However, because it is also possible that the pulmonary edema was induced by increased vascular permeability, furosemide may have little to no effect, and clinicians are left to provide supportive care (e.g., oxygen therapy) while awaiting resolution of the pulmonary edema over the course of 12 to 48 hours.

Much like humans, cats that give birth to kittens with a blood type differing from the queen are at risk for neonatal isoerythrolysis. Specifically, type A or AB kittens born to type B queens may have neonatal isoerythrolysis.[6] Type B queens have naturally occurring alloantibodies against type A and AB RBCs in their colostrum that, when ingested by the type A or AB neonate, lead to acute destruction of the kitten's RBCs.[6] Kittens are born healthy, but clinical signs appear within the first few hours to days of life and may range in severity from sudden death, to kittens that develop tail-tip necrosis from vessel obstruction by agglutinating erythrocytes. Some kittens develop dark-colored urine. These kittens may also stop nursing, fail to thrive or gain weight, develop anemia and icterus, and usually die within the first week after birth. The diagnosis is confirmed by blood-typing the queen and affected kittens.

There is no good treatment for neonatal isoerythrolysis, although an attempt can be made to support the kittens by administering type B blood.[12] Specifically, the type B blood should be drawn from a donor and washed with saline. The red cells can be suspended in saline and given as a transfusion to the kittens. The theory is that the maternal colostral-derived anti-A antibodies will not react to the type B red cells and the kitten will not yet have any of its own anti-B antibodies to react to the transfused cells.[12]

These kittens suffering from neonatal isoerythrolysis are usually considered "fading kittens," but not always identified as having neonatal isoerythrolysis by breeders because there are multiple causes of "fading kittens." This can be detrimental in the long term as the best recommendation to prevent neonatal isoerythrolysis is that type B queens should not be bred to type A or AB males (e.g., that breeding pair should not be bred again). However, some breeders who are aware of the high risk of neonatal isoerythrolysis will plan breedings between type B queens and type A males and be ready to (1) immediately remove the kittens from the queen prior to colostrum ingestion or (2) blood-type all of the neonates at birth (using blood from the umbilical cord) to determine which ones need to be removed from the queen and which can safely nurse.

ADMINISTRATION TIPS

Blood products can be given as fast as required for the patient's condition. Therefore, in cases where a cat is facing lethal hemorrhage or has severe clinical signs attributed to its anemia (e.g., weakness, extreme lethargy, tachycardia, hypotension), blood or plasma can be given in a bolus or over the course of 1 to 2 hours. Conversely, in cases where cats are more chronically anemic and are not showing overt clinical signs despite low packed cell volumes, blood can be given over the course of 4 to 6 hours.[3]

It is important not to keep a blood product at room temperature for more than 6 hours because of the risk of bacterial colonization.[3] If refrigerated (at 4°C [39°F]), a unit of RBCs (whole blood or packed RBCs) should be discarded within 24 hours of being opened. If an unopened bag of fresh-frozen plasma is thawed, it can be held at refrigeration temperature for 1 hour before either being given over 4 to 6 hours, discarded, or refrozen.[13]

In the event that a cat is given a portion of a unit of packed RBCs, plasma, or whole blood at time point A (with the remainder of the unit of blood refrigerated at 4°C [39°F]), a second transfusion can be given over a period of 4 to 6 hours from the refrigerated portion of the unit. However, the blood product *must* be discarded or administered by 24 hours after the bag was first opened. In short, a unit of refrigerated blood or plasma must be discarded by 24 hours after it is opened.

The author recommends calculating a blood administration rate over 4 hours (rather than 6 hours) if the blood is not being administered as a bolus (see Table 78-2 for a sample calculation). The rationale is that because of catheter issues, diagnostic testing, and other mechanical complications in the hospital, it is rare that the blood will ever be completely administered within 4 hours. The remaining 2 hours of the 6-hour window can be considered a buffer to ensure that the transfusion is completed without risk to the patient.

In all blood transfusions that are not being administered for life-threatening hemorrhage, it is best to start giving a transfusion slowly for the first 15 to 30 minutes (e.g., at 25% to 50% of the maximal calculated rate) and then gradually increase the rate to that calculated to give the dosage over 4 hours (Box 78-5). During the initial slow period of administration, the patient should be closely monitored for any indications of transfusion reaction. Clinically, increases in the patient's heart rate, respiratory rate, or temperature; signs of facial swelling, pruritus, vomiting, salivation; or—in rare cases—death, all signal a transfusion reaction.

If any of these things are noted, the transfusion should be stopped and the patient should be treated for a transfusion

Table 78-2 Administration of Blood Products

Tips/reminders	Give all products through a blood filter to remove fibrin, clots, or other large particulate matter before it is given to the patient. Discard blood and plasma after 6 h at room temperature. A unit of whole blood or packed RBCs can be refrigerated for a total of 24 h from the point of opening to the point of discard. Monitor all patients closely for the first 30 min for a transfusion reaction. Recheck PCV 1-2 h after transfusion is completed.
Example whole blood transfusion calculation	8 kg cat being administered whole blood for anemia of 1-week duration (PCV = 15%). Goal PCV is 25% post-transfusion. Weight (kg) × 2 mL whole blood/kg/1% increase PCV × (goal PCV − patient PCV) = mL of whole blood. 8 kg × 2 mL/kg/1% increase PCV × 10% = 160 mL of whole blood. Because most feline whole blood units are 60 mL, one would typically administer one unit and then recheck the cat's clinical status and PCV before determining if it requires more blood. Give 60 mL over 4 h → rate = 15 mL/h. Start at 5 mL/h for the first 15 min, then 10 mL/h for the second 15 min. At 30 min after the start of transfusion, increase to 15 mL/h. Record a temperature, pulse, and respiratory rate every 5-15 min for the first 30-60 min. Evaluate the patient every 5-15 min for the first 30-60 min for other clinical signs of a transfusion reaction (vomiting, salivation, collapse, etc.). Recheck PCV approximately 1-2 h after transfusion completed.
Treatment of a transfusion reaction	Immune-mediated transfusion reaction: • Diphenhydramine 2-4 mg/kg IM • ± Dexamethasone 0.07-0.14 mg/kg IM or IV Nonimmune-mediated transfusion reaction: • Dexamethasone 0.07-0.14 mg/kg IM or IV • Furosemide 2 mg/kg IM or IV every 30 min as needed to treat fluid overload-induced pulmonary edema (cardiogenic pulmonary edema) • Oxygen therapy with any pulmonary edema

IM, intramuscularly; *IV*, intravenously; *PCV*, packed cell volume; *RBC*, red blood cell.

BOX 78-5 Abbreviated Crossmatching Technique for Emergency Situations

1. Draw 0.5 to 1 mL of blood from the donor and recipient cats in two red top tubes. Label the tubes appropriately.
2. Allow the red top tubes to clot.
3. Spin red top tubes in centrifuge (3000 rpm) for 5 to 10 minutes.
4. Decant and collect the serum into new red top tubes.
5. Apply two drops of recipient serum and one drop of donor red blood cells (RBCs) on a glass slide (major crossmatch).
6. Apply two drops of recipient serum and one drop of recipient RBCs on a glass slide (patient control).
7. Apply two drops of donor serum and one drop of donor RBCs on a glass slide (donor control).
6. Wait 1 to 5 minutes.
7. Examine the slides for microscopic clumping of RBCs (not Rouleaux formation where RBCs stacked in a row like coins)

Adapted from the International Society of Feline Medicine.[14]

reaction as described earlier. It is then a clinician's prerogative to determine if the inciting blood product should be discarded and the cat does not receive any further transfusions, if the cat should receive a different unit of blood or plasma, or if the cat can continue to receive the original blood product.

Cats can benefit greatly from the administration of blood products. Although feline transfusion medicine has its share of challenges, with careful selection of appropriate blood products, veterinarians can safely provide cats with this potentially lifesaving intervention.

References

1. Weingart C, Giger U, Kohn B: Whole blood transfusions in 91 cats: a clinical evaluation. *J Feline Med Surg* 6:139–148, 2004.

2. Klaser DA, Reine NJ, Hohenhaus AE: Red blood cell transfusions in cats: 126 cats (1999). *J Am Vet Med Assoc* 226:920–923, 2005.

3. Barfield D, Adamantos S: Feline blood transfusion: a pinker shade of pale. *J Feline Med Surg* 13:11–23, 2011.

4. Juvet F, Brennan S, Mooney CT: Assessment of feline blood for transfusion purposes in the Dublin area of Ireland. *Vet Rec* 168:24–26, 2011.

5. Forcada Y, Guitian J, Gibson G: Frequencies of feline blood types at a referral hospital in the south east of England. *J Small Anim Pract* 48:570–573, 2007.

6. Proverbio D, Spada E, Perego R, et al: Assessment of blood types of Ragdoll cats for transfusion purposes. *Vet Clin Path* 42:157–162, 2013.

7. Gurkan M, Arikan S, Ozaytekin E, et al: Titres of alloantibodies against A and B blood types in non-pedigree domestic cats in Turkey: assessing the transfusion reaction risk. *J Feline Med Surg* 7:301–305, 2005.

8. Weinstein N, Blais M, Harris K, et al: A newly recognized blood group in domestic short hair cats: the *Mik* red cell antigen. *J Vet Intern Med* 21:287–292, 2007.

9. Bovens C, Gruffydd-Jones T: Xenotransfusion with canine blood in the feline species: review of the literature. *J Feline Med Surg* 15:62–67, 2012.

10. Weingart C, Kohn B: Clinical use of a hemoglobin-based oxygen carrying solution (Oxyglobin®) in 48 cats (2002-2006). *J Feline Med Surg* 10:431–438, 2008.

11. Yaxley P, Beal M, Jutkowitz A, et al: Comparative study of canine and feline hemostatic proteins in freeze-thaw-cycled fresh frozen plasma. *J Vet Emerg Crit Care* 20:472–478, 2010.

12. Macintire DK: Pediatric fluid therapy. *Vet Clin North Am Small Anim Pract* 38:621–627, 2008.

13. Hackner SJ: Plasma and albumin transfusions: indications and controversies. <www.cuvs.org/pdf/article-plasma-and-albumin-transfusions.pdf>, (Accessed October 8, 2013.)

14. International Society of Feline Medicine: Feline blood transfusions: practical guidelines for vets. <http://www.icatcare.org/sites/default/files/PDF/vet_0.pdf>, (Accessed October 16, 2014.)

Feline Toxins: Recognition, Diagnosis, Treatment

Tina Wismer

Many factors come into play when assessing cat exposures to various toxins. Cats have more selective eating habits than dogs; however, their fastidious grooming habits turn almost all dermal exposures quickly into oral exposures. Cats are chewers (not gulpers), which helps to decrease their exposure to ingested toxins, but they are attracted to plants.

Metabolic processes have evolved over time to allow individual species to handle various components of their diets. Animals that are true carnivores (e.g., cats) have a more restricted diet and have evolved fewer biotransformation pathways than those with more diverse diets (e.g., herbivores, omnivores).[1] This can be problematic when cats encounter a xenobiotic (foreign chemical) that requires detoxification via a biotransformation pathway they do not possess. Cats are defective in glucuronidation. They have a nonfunctional pseudogene that encodes uridine 5′-diphospho-glucuronosyltransferase, a phenol detoxification enzyme, so they are unable to glucuronidate.[1] This makes cats highly susceptible to xenobiotics that require glucuronidation for metabolism (e.g., acetaminophen, aspirin, nonsteroidal anti-inflammatory drugs [NSAIDs], phenol, or serotonin).[1] In other cases, if the metabolite is the toxin, this lack of metabolism is protective.

Cats are more sensitive to red blood cell oxidative damage than are humans or dogs. Cats have eight sulfhydryl groups on their hemoglobin (compared to four for dogs and two for humans).[2] This makes them more susceptible to developing Heinz bodies and methemoglobinemia when exposed to oxidative agents such as acetaminophen, aniline dyes, onions, garlic, and benzocaine (local anesthetic). Finally, cats have acidic urine, which can influence the rate of elimination of xenobiotics.[1] Toxins that are excreted in alkaline urine may be trapped within the body.

SELECTED TOXICITIES

Lilies

Members of the true lily family (*Lilium* and *Hemerocallis*) have been shown to cause acute kidney injury in the cat. Easter lilies (*Lilium longiflorum*), tiger lilies (*Lilium tigrinum*), rubrum or Japanese showy lilies (*Lilium speciosum*), and orange daylilies (*Hemerocallis fulva*) are all examples of true lilies.[3] All parts of the plant, including the pollen, can cause acute kidney injury if ingested. Even minor exposures may result in life-threatening toxicosis. The toxic principle is unknown, but is known to be water soluble.[4]

After ingestion, affected cats often begin to vomit within a few hours. The vomiting usually subsides, during which time the cats may appear normal or may be mildly depressed and anorexic. Blood urea nitrogen (BUN), creatinine, phosphorus, and potassium begin to rise as early as 12 hours postingestion. Around 24 hours postingestion, casts, proteinuria, glucosuria, and isosthenuria are usually detectable on urinalysis. This is due to damage to the proximal renal tubular cells. Beginning 24 to 72 hours after ingestion, oliguric to anuric renal failure develops, accompanied by depression, anorexia, dehydration, and hypothermia.[3] Disorientation, ataxia, facial and paw edema, dyspnea, and seizures have been less commonly reported.[3] Death or euthanasia due to acute anuric kidney injury generally occurs within 3 to 6 days of ingestion.

All feline exposures to true lilies should be considered potentially life threatening, and treatment should be pursued immediately. If the ingestion is recent, decontamination with emesis, oral activated charcoal, and cathartic should be performed. Early decontamination is most beneficial, but emesis induction in cats is usually unrewarding. Apomorphine is a poor inducer of emesis in the cat as it works on dopamine receptors. The feline vomiting center, the chemoreceptor trigger zone, is regulated by alpha receptors. Emesis induction can be attempted with xylazine (0.44 mg/kg intramuscularly [IM])[5] or dexmedetomidine (40 μg/kg IM) (Étienne Cote, personal correspondence). Both of these agents will cause sedation and can be reversed with either yohimbine (0.11 mg/kg intravenously [IV] slowly)[5] or atipamezole (0.2 mg/kg IV or IM).[5] See Table 79-1 for more antidotal information.

Fluid diuresis using a balanced replacement fluid at two times maintenance rate for 48 hours has been effective in preventing lily-induced acute kidney injury. When initiated within 18 hours of ingestion, prognosis is good, with most cats recovering without residual renal problems.[3] Conversely, delaying treatment beyond 18 hours postingestion frequently results in death or euthanasia due to severe acute kidney injury. Baseline renal values should be obtained upon presentation and then repeated at 24 and 48 hours. In most cases, tubular injury from lily ingestion spares the renal tubular

Table 79-1   Selected Antidote Use in the Cat

Drug	Dose	Comments
Acepromazine	0.05–0.1 mg/kg IV, IM, SC	Sedation for agitation caused by serotonergic medications (e.g., amphetamines, SSRIs)
Atipamezole	0.05–0.2 mg/kg IM, IV	Reversal of bradycardia, hypotension, and sedation from alpha agonists (e.g., amitraz, xylazine)
Cyproheptadine	2–4 mg/cat, PO or rectally every 12-24 hours (crushed in water)	Sedation for agitation caused by serotonergic medications (e.g., amphetamines, SSRIs)
Ethanol	Bolus: 20% solution, 5.5 mL/kg IV every 6 hours for 5 treatments then every 8 hours for 4 treatments CRI: 7% solution, 8.6 mL/kg (600 mg/kg) bolus, then maintain at 1.43 mL/kg per hour (100 mg/kg per hour) as a constant rate infusion	Management of ethylene glycol toxicosis
Fomepizole (4-methylpyrazole)	125 mg/kg slow IV, then 31.25 mg/kg IV at 12, 24, and 36 hours	Management of ethylene glycol toxicosis
Intravenous lipid solutions 20%	1.5 mL/kg IV over 10-20 minutes, followed by 0.25 mL/kg per min IV for 1 hour; repeat CRI every 4 hours if no longer lipemic	Management of highly lipid soluble toxicants (e.g., avermectins, baclofen, calcium channel blockers)
Methocarbamol	50–150 mg/kg slow IV, titrate up as needed	Management of muscle tremors secondary to permethrin
N-acetylcysteine	140 mg/kg, diluted to 5%, loading dose (slow IV or PO), then 70 mg/kg every 6 hours for 7+ treatments (continue if methemoglobinemia or liver enzyme elevation continues) A 280 mg/kg loading dose may be used if methemoglobinemia is already apparent	Management of acetaminophen toxicosis
Naloxone	0.05–0.1 mg/kg IV	Reversal of opioid toxicosis
Vitamin K₁ (phytonadione)	3–5 mg/kg per day PO divided, continue for 21–30 days depending on rodenticide ingested	Treatment of anticoagulant rodenticide coagulopathy
Yohimbine	0.1 mg/kg IV	Reversal of bradycardia, hypotension and sedation from alpha agonists (e.g., amitraz, xylazine)

CRI, constant rate infusion; *IM*, intramuscular; *IV*, intravenous; *PO*, per os (orally); *SC*, subcutaneous; *SSRI*, selective serotonin reuptake inhibitor.

basement membrane; thus regeneration of damaged tubules may be possible, but it takes 10 to 14 days or longer for this to occur. Treatment should be continued as long as urine is being produced and may need adjustment, based on hydration status and urine output. In severe cases, peritoneal dialysis may aid in managing acute kidney injury.[3]

Insoluble Calcium Oxalate Plants

Plants containing insoluble calcium oxalate crystals are commonly kept as houseplants. These crystals are common in thick, shiny-leaved plants. Many of these plants are members of the Araceae family, including *Aglaonema modestrum* (Chinese evergreen), *Alocasia antiquorum* (Elephant's ear), *Anthurium* spp. (Flamingo plant), *Caladium* spp., *Dieffenbachia* spp. (Dumb cane), *Monstera* spp. (split-leaf or lacy-leafed philodendron, Swiss cheese plant), *Philodendron* spp., and

Spathiphyllum spp. (Peace lily). All of these plants cause a similar clinical syndrome and contain variable amounts of oxalates.[6]

The calcium oxalate crystals are shaped like needles and are packaged in bundles called raphides. The raphides are encased in a gelatinous substance within a thick-walled structure (idioblast).[6] When the plant is damaged, these crystals are released under pressure and embed themselves in the oral cavity.[6] Hypersalivation, oral pain, vomiting, and possible swelling of the pharynx can occur, although obstruction is rare.[6] Calcium-containing products may precipitate soluble oxalates in the oral cavity, reducing pain. The mouth should be rinsed with milk or water. Sucralfate slurries can be used to reduce oral irritation. In rare cases, a tracheostomy can be lifesaving.[6] Prognosis in most cases is good, and clinical signs usually resolve within 24 hours with no lasting effects.

Acetaminophen

Acetaminophen (paracetamol) is a synthetic nonopiate derivative of N-acetyl-p-aminophenol (APAP) that has a unique mechanism of action. It inhibits prostaglandin H2 production by indirectly reducing a heme on the peroxidase portion of prostaglandin H2 synthase and indirectly inhibits cyclooxygenase activation.[7]

Acetaminophen is rapidly absorbed from the gastrointestinal (GI) tract. In humans, peak plasma levels are seen at 30 to 45 minutes (60 to 120 minutes for extended release formulations).[7] Two major conjugation pathways, glucuronidation and sulfation, are used by most species to metabolize acetaminophen. Cats are deficient in glucuronyl transferase and cannot metabolize acetaminophen to its nontoxic metabolites. Cats use the cytochrome P450 enzyme system to metabolize acetaminophen, resulting in the N-acetyl-p-benzoquinoneimine (NAPQI) metabolite. N-acetyl-p-benzoquinoneimine causes liver damage by binding to sulfhydryl groups on the hepatic cell membrane and damaging the lipid bilayer. Glutathione normally conjugates and neutralizes NAPQI, but when glutathione stores are depleted, NAPQI is able to cause liver damage. Another metabolite, para-aminophenol, appears to be responsible for methemoglobinemia and Heinz body formation.[2] Cats also have a relative deficiency of methemoglobin reductase in their red blood cells, which make it more difficult for them to reverse the hemoglobin damage.[2]

Clinical signs of acetaminophen toxicity include depression, dyspnea, tachycardia, and brown discoloration of the mucous membranes and blood due to methemoglobinemia. Swelling of the face and paws can be seen, but the mechanism is unknown. Hepatic necrosis is less common in cats than in dogs.[8]

Because of the rapid absorption from the GI tract, emesis is rarely performed. Activated charcoal adsorbs APAP and can be used before methemoglobinemia develops. A cathartic, such as sorbitol, should also be given unless the animal is dehydrated or has diarrhea. If the cat already has methemoglobinemia, do not stress the animal by administering charcoal.

Cats are very sensitive to acetaminophen, and there is a very narrow margin of safety. Almost any exposure can lead to problems, with cats developing clinical signs at doses around 10 mg/kg.[8] Affected cats should be monitored for methemoglobinemia formation over a period of 6 to 8 hours. Methemoglobin values increase within 2 to 4 hours and should be grossly visible by 6 to 8 hours. This is followed by Heinz body formation.[9] Alanine transferase, aspartate transferase, and bilirubin may rise within 24 hours after ingestion and peak within 48 to 72 hours.

If methemoglobinemia and dyspnea are present, the cat should be put in oxygen, and N-acetylcysteine (NAC; Mucomyst) therapy should be started.[10] N-acetylcysteine provides a precursor in the synthesis of glutathione, can be oxidized to organic sulfate for the sulfation pathway, and provides an alternative substrate for conjugation. N-acetylcysteine solution must be diluted to a 5% concentration with 5% dextrose or sterile water because higher concentrations can cause oral and esophageal erosions. An initial oral or IV loading dose of 140 mg/kg is given, followed by 70 mg/kg every 6 hours for seven treatments, or longer if the patient is still symptomatic.[8] If the cat already has methemoglobinemia, a loading dose of 280 mg/kg should be given. If using the IV route, give slowly over a period of 15 to 20 minutes. N-acetylcysteine should be given before activated charcoal if possible. Otherwise, a 2 to 3 hour wait after activated charcoal is needed before oral administration of NAC, because activated charcoal will adsorb NAC. Adverse effects of the oral route include nausea and vomiting. Some brands of NAC are not labeled for IV use. Fluid therapy should be used to correct dehydration and for maintenance needs.

Ascorbic acid is thought to aid in the reduction of methemoglobin back to hemoglobin. The efficacy is questionable, and vomiting is common after oral administration. Cimetidine had been historically recommended because it inhibits cytochrome P450. It is now thought to be contraindicated in cats because it has been shown that cimetidine blocks one of the only pathways that cats have to convert methemoglobin back to hemoglobin. S-adenosylmethionine (SAMe, Denosyl-SD4) at 20 mg/kg per day shows a positive effect for treatment of liver disease secondary to APAP toxicosis.[11] In severely dyspneic animals, a blood transfusion can be given to increase oxygen-carrying capacity. The cat must be monitored for volume overload. This newly formed hemoglobin can also be affected if there is still circulating free acetaminophen.

Prognosis can be good if the cat is treated promptly. Cats with severe methemoglobinemia or hepatic damage have a poorer prognosis. Methemoglobinemia can last for 3 to 4 days, and hepatic injury may be permanent.

Nonsteroidal Anti-inflammatory Drugs

Cats are sometimes inadvertently given inappropriate NSAID doses by their owners, or the cat may be attracted to chewable formulations. Chewable formulations ease administration, but have the risk for potential overdosing. Cats may also develop problems when given therapeutic doses of NSAIDs, especially during surgery (secondary to anesthesia-induced hypotension).[12]

Nonsteroidal anti-inflammatory drugs inhibit prostaglandin (PG) synthesis, which reduces pain, but also decreases the beneficial effects of PGs (e.g., decreases gastric acid secretion, increases gastric mucus secretion, opposes renal vasoconstriction). Therapeutic doses of NSAIDs can cause vomiting and diarrhea in some animals. Overdoses can cause GI upset plus gastric ulceration. The decrease in secretion of the protective mucus layer of the stomach increases the risk of GI ulcers.[12] At higher doses, acute kidney injury can occur. Renal effects of NSAIDs are from decreased synthesis of renal PGs and are associated with afferent arteriolar constriction, which leads to decreased renal blood flow and acute kidney injury.[13] Some NSAIDs, such as ibuprofen, have been associated with central nervous system (CNS) signs such as seizures or coma at very high doses. This mechanism is unknown.

Table 79-2	Acute Toxic Doses of Nonsteroidal Anti-inflammatory Drugs in Cats (Doses Are Guidelines for Healthy Cats Only)	
Drug		**Acute Kidney Injury Dose (mg/kg)**
Carprofen		8
Diclofenac		9.9
Etodolac		32.4
Ibuprofen		20
Indomethacin		5.2
Ketorolac		0.7

Source: ASPCA Animal Poison Control Center. Unpublished data 2001-2013.

Cats, due to their deficiency in glucuronidation, have a low tolerance for inappropriate use of NSAIDs. Vomiting usually starts in the first 2 to 6 hours postingestion, with GI ulcers forming after 12 hours.[12] The onset of acute kidney injury occurs usually within 12 hours, but may be delayed 3 to 5 days depending on the NSAID. Because of their relatively small size, most toxic exposures to NSAIDs in cats require treatment.

Decontamination can be attempted if the ingestion is recent (less than 1 hour) and the animal is asymptomatic. NSAIDs are quickly absorbed, and often emesis is not warranted. Activated charcoal should be administered if the dose is renal toxic (Table 79-2). Because many NSAIDs undergo enterohepatic recirculation, repeating a dose of activated charcoal in 6 hours may be considered.

Drugs to prevent or decrease GI ulceration should be started. These can include an acid reducer such as an H$_2$ blocker or proton-pump inhibitor such as omeprazole, sucralfate, or misoprostol.[12] These medications should be administered for 7 to 10 days. Patients should be monitored for signs of GI hemorrhage (e.g., melena or decreasing packed cell volume). If the dose is high enough to cause acute kidney injury (or if the cat has pre-existing renal disease), fluid diuresis at two times maintenance rate for at least 48 hours should be started and the renal profile monitored.[12] Treatment may need to be adjusted for optimal hydration and urinary output. Fluid therapy is needed to maintain adequate renal blood flow and glomerular filtration rate.[12] Prognosis for NSAID ingestion is good with early, aggressive management.

Venlafaxine

Cats are not known for inadvertently ingesting pills, but for some unknown reason they readily eat venlafaxine capsules. Venlafaxine (Effexor, Pfizer) is a bicyclic antidepressant. It is a potent serotonin and noradrenaline reuptake inhibitor as well as a weak dopamine reuptake inhibitor. Venlafaxine is available in both an immediate-release and extended-release formulation. Cats can develop signs at doses as low as 2 to 3 mg/kg. Mydriasis, vomiting, tachypnea, tachycardia, ataxia, and agitation are the most common signs. Many cats will vocalize and stare into space.[14]

In asymptomatic animals, emesis can be considered, and activated charcoal can be administered. Heart rate and blood pressure should be monitored. With agitated animals, acepromazine (0.05-0.1 mg/kg IV, IM, or subcutaneously [SC], titrate upward as needed) may be used. Cyproheptadine (2 to 4 mg per cat, PO or rectally [crushed in water] every 12 to 24 hours) may be useful in antagonizing the serotonin effects. Prognosis is good, but affected cats can be symptomatic for 24 to 72 hours (with extended-release medication). As an aside, venlafaxine will cause a false-positive reaction for phencyclidine (PCP) on over-the-counter urine drug tests.[15]

Venlafaxine is lipid-soluble, and in human medicine intravenous lipid emulsions have been used to decrease clinical signs and treatment time.[16] Lipid emulsions have been used recently to treat toxicoses in both human and veterinary medicine. The exact mechanism of action is unknown, but the prevailing theory is that the lipids act as a "lipid sink." It is thought that lipophilic drugs are redistributed (bound) in the expanded plasma lipid volume, reducing free (active) drug levels.[16] Veterinary dosing guidelines are taken from the human literature and are considered extra-label. A 20% lipid solution can be given through a peripheral catheter. A bolus of 1.5 mL/kg is given, followed by 0.25 mL/kg per minute for 30 to 60 minutes. This is repeated in 4 hours if the serum is clear.

In theory, lipids will work best on more lipid-soluble toxins, but the use of lipids unfortunately has not been shown to be effective in all cases of lipophilic drug toxicosis.[17] Adverse effects of lipids are rare but have been reported.[18] Bacterial contamination of the product can occur because the emulsion is nutrient-rich. Sterile technique must be followed. A bag should only be used for 24 hours and then discarded. The unused portion between doses should be stored in the refrigerator and discarded after 24 hours. Adverse effects reported in other species include allergic reactions to the egg or soybean oil content, lipemia, hypertriglyceridemia, immunosuppression (immune cell dysfunction), hemolysis (oxidative damage), phlebitis, thrombosis, and hepatic lipidosis.[18] Fat overload syndrome is a delayed reaction caused by excessive volumes or high administration rates overwhelming the endogenous lipid-clearance mechanisms. It is associated with hyperlipidemia, fat embolism, hepatomegaly, splenomegaly, thrombocytopenia, jaundice, increased clotting times, and hemolysis.[18] Lipids can also bind antidotes or other therapies that are being used to treat the patient and thereby may worsen the clinical condition. The use of lipids to treat intoxications can be considered if other traditional therapies are not available or successful and all adverse effects are considered.

Alpha Lipoic Acid

Alpha lipoic acid (lipoic acid, thioctic acid, acetate replacing factor, biletan, lipoicin, thioctacid, thioctan) is a fat-soluble, sulfur-containing, vitamin-like antioxidant.[19] Alpha lipoic acid increases intracellular glutathione and regenerates ascorbic acid, vitamin E, coenzyme Q10, and nicotinamide adenine dinucleotide phosphate. It acts synergistically with insulin, lowering blood glucose, increasing liver glycogenesis, and facilitating glucose uptake into cells.[19] It is primarily used to treat type II diabetes in people.

Alpha lipoic acid is available over the counter as 100 or 300 mg capsules. It is readily absorbed; peak plasma levels occur within 2 to 4 hours. The therapeutic dose for cats is 1 to 5 mg/kg, with a maximum dose of 25 mg/day.[20] It has been used in veterinary medicine to treat diabetic polyneuropathy, cataracts, glaucoma, and ischemia-reperfusion injury.[20] Alpha lipoic acid has been reported to be 10 times more toxic in cats than in humans, dogs, or rats.[21] The minimum toxic dose was calculated to be 13 mg/kg for cats. At 30 mg/kg, neurological signs and mild hepatocellular damage can occur.[21] Higher doses of 60 mg/kg were associated with ataxia, vomiting, and elevated liver enzymes.[21]

Hypoglycemia and seizures can occur, and cats showing signs should also be monitored for acute kidney injury. Signs can occur 30 minutes to several hours postingestion. For decontamination to be helpful, it must be performed immediately after ingestion. Emesis and activated charcoal with cathartic can be used as necessary. Baseline laboratory values for blood glucose, liver enzymes, BUN, creatinine, and electrolytes should be obtained. Treatment is symptomatic and supportive. Hyperglycemia, tremors, and seizures should be controlled and dehydration corrected if present. Cats without liver and kidney involvement have a better prognosis.

Ethylene Glycol

Ethylene glycol is most commonly encountered as automotive radiator antifreeze, but ethylene glycol is also present in condensers, heat exchangers, home solar units, and aircraft deicers. In addition, ethylene glycol is often used to winterize swimming pools, toilets in recreational vehicles, and summer homes in colder latitudes, and it is used in portable basketball goalpost bases. Ethylene glycol is also found in household paints, inks, ink pads, and printer cartridges, but volumes and/or concentrations are low.

Cats, rabbits, and humans are the most sensitive species to ethylene glycol. The lethal dose for cats is 1.65 g/kg,[22] but these data are based on doses that cause early deaths from acidosis and intoxication and do not take into account the fact that many animals may survive the initial stages of toxicosis only to succumb to acute kidney injury days later. Any suspected oral exposure of a cat to ethylene glycol should be considered potentially life threatening.

Ethylene glycol is a very potent alcohol, and early signs will relate to severe alcohol intoxication. As ethylene glycol is broken down into its metabolites (e.g., oxalic acid), acidosis and acute kidney injury can occur. Because of this metabolism, clinical signs frequently change throughout the course of the toxicosis.[23] The early neurological signs begin within 30 minutes of exposure and can last up to 12 hours. With large ingestions, cats can die in this stage. In other cases, these signs may pass quickly or may not be noted by the cat owner. During this time period, cats may be initially ataxic, disoriented, "drunk," and stuporous. They may be hypothermic, polyuric, and polydipsic. Coma and death can occur during this stage.[23]

As metabolism of ethylene glycol progresses, cardiopulmonary signs begin, generally 6 to 24 hours following exposure. Tachypnea, tachycardia, and depression occur. Seizures, pulmonary edema, and death may occur. Clinical pathology changes include high anion gap, increased osmol gap, and severe metabolic acidosis.[23]

Oliguric acute kidney injury can be seen as early as 12 hours in cats, but generally occurs within 24 to 72 hours following exposure. Oxalic acid binds with calcium to form calcium oxalate crystals in the renal tubules. Cats are depressed, anorexic, and vomiting and may have oliguria progressing to anuria. Seizures can occur. Urinalysis abnormalities include low urine specific gravity, glucosuria, and calcium oxalate crystalluria. Importantly, absence of crystalluria does NOT rule out the possibility of ethylene glycol toxicosis.[23] Clinical pathology changes include hyperglycemia, hyperkalemia, and hypocalcemia. Blood urea nitrogen and creatinine will elevate, but usually not before 12 hours postexposure.

Diagnosis of ethylene glycol poisoning is based on history, clinical signs, and confirmatory laboratory testing. The most reliable means of diagnosing exposure is to have blood ethylene glycol levels determined at a human hospital on an emergency basis. In cats, any ethylene glycol concentration above 20 mg/dL should be considered significant. There are two available patient-side ethylene glycol tests: the VetSpec Catachem ethylene glycol test (Catachem Inc., Oxford, Connecticut) and the Kacey ethylene glycol test (Kacey Inc, Asheville, North Carolina). The Catachem test is a colorimetric qualitative test performed on serum or plasma. It is positive for any *cis*-1-diol alcohol (ethylene glycol, propylene glycol, glycerol, sorbitol, etc.). It has both canine and feline reference levels. The Kacey strip test uses plasma and will be positive for any alcohol, including ethanol and methanol. It has both canine and feline tests on the same strip. Note that both activated charcoal and injectable diazepam will make either ethylene glycol test positive due to propylene glycol and/or glycerol in the ingredients. An increased anion gap (greater than 25 mEq/L) or serum osmol gap (greater than 20 mOsm/kg) may assist in diagnosing ethylene glycol toxicosis. A Wood's lamp can be used to fluoresce urine, stomach contents, or the paws or muzzle to look for exposure, as fluorescein dye is added to automotive antifreeze to help in detecting radiator leaks. Blood urea nitrogen and creatinine are of minimal benefit in diagnosing early exposures because they do not increase until 12 hours after ingestion.[23]

Decontamination via emesis and activated charcoal is somewhat controversial. Aliphatic alcohols are not thought to be well adsorbed by charcoal, and most cats are not presented until a later time frame.[24] Decontamination should only be tried in an asymptomatic patient. Stabilization of symptomatic cats is very important. Seizure control can be attempted with diazepam or barbiturates. Intravenous fluid therapy with high infusion rates of crystalloids is necessary to correct dehydration and hypoperfusion. Fluid intake and output should be closely monitored to avoid fluid overload and possibly pulmonary edema. Sodium bicarbonate can be used to correct acidosis. Peritoneal dialysis, hemodialysis, or charcoal hemoperfusion can be attempted on oliguric or anuric cats.[24]

Treatment of ethylene glycol toxicosis must be timely and aggressive. Failure to institute appropriate therapy within the first few hours may result in irreversible renal damage or death. Intravenous ethanol and fomepizole (4-MP, 4-methylpyrazole) have both been used to manage ethylene glycol toxicosis in cats. With both of these compounds, the goal is to delay the breakdown of ethylene glycol to its more toxic metabolites and allow the parent compound to be excreted in the urine unchanged. Ethanol competes with ethylene glycol for the alcohol dehydrogenase enzyme.[25] Fomepizole works by inhibiting the alcohol dehydrogenase enzyme so it is not available to break down the ethylene glycol.[25] Ethanol is inexpensive and readily available, but it can worsen metabolic acidosis and CNS depression. Ethanol can be administered as boluses or a constant rate infusion (CRI). Any clear liquor can be used, but vodka or grain alcohol (Everclear) are preferred. An in-line filter is recommended for ethanol infusions using nonpharmaceutical grade ethanol. The CRI method is preferred because it is less depressive of the CNS. A bolus of 8.6 mL/kg (600 mg/kg) of a 7% (70 mg/mL) ethanol solution (Box 79-1) is administered and then maintained at 1.43 mL/kg per hour (100 mg/kg per hour) as a CRI. The bolus treatment method is to make a 20% ethanol solution that is administered at 5.0 mL/kg every 6 hours for five treatments, then every 8 hours for four additional treatments. Fomepizole has been approved for use in dogs only, but has been used off-label in cats.[25] Unlike ethanol, fomepizole will not cause hyperosmolality or metabolic acidosis. Cats require much higher doses of fomepizole compared with dogs to treat ethylene glycol toxicosis (125 mg/kg, then 31.24 mg/kg at 12, 24, and 36 hours). Cats will become depressed and ataxic at these doses, but this does not affect its efficacy.

If a lethal dose of ethylene glycol is ingested, treatment must be started within 3 hours of ethylene glycol exposure. At 4 hours postexposure, fomepizole and ethanol were both unsuccessful in preventing death.[25] Treatment should be continued until cats are clinically normal and have had at least 24 hours with normal renal function and acid-base parameters. The prognosis for recovery depends on degree of exposure, length of time between exposure and treatment, and aggressiveness of treatment. Surviving cats may fully recover or may have residual chronic kidney disease. The presence of oliguria, anuria, or seizures indicates a grave prognosis.

Liquid Potpourri

Liquid simmering potpourri can contain essential oils and cationic detergents. Most significant exposures to liquid potpourri in cats occur when the product is spilled and cats groom the product off their fur.[26] The essential oils in liquid potpourri can cause mucous membrane and GI irritation, dermal hypersensitivity and irritation, and CNS depression.[26] Cationic detergents are locally corrosive and can cause dermal and oral lesions, along with hypersalivation, anorexia, oral inflammation or ulceration, dysphagia, vomiting (with or without blood), pain, and melena. Significant hyperthermia higher than 104°F (40°C) may accompany oral inflammation.[26]

Clinical signs may not develop immediately, and it may take up to 12 hours for the full extent of tissue damage to become apparent. Esophageal and/or gastric ulceration may occur.[26] Emesis should not be induced with corrosive substance exposures, nor should activated charcoal be given. Treatment of mucosal burns should include pain medication (e.g., opioids) as needed, GI protectants (e.g., sucralfate slurries), and general supportive care.[26] A gastrostomy tube may be needed in cases with severe oral or esophageal burns.

Glo-Jewelry

Cats are attracted to "glo-jewelry." These glow-in-the-dark items are popular novelties sold at fairs, carnivals, and concerts. They include both glo-sticks and glow-in-the-dark jewelry (e.g., necklaces and bracelets). The primary luminescent agent is dibutyl phthalate (n-butyl phthalate).[26] Dibutyl phthalate is a low-toxicity compound (median lethal dose greater than 8000 mg/kg in rats).[27] Cats like to bite into the glo-sticks or jewelry. The extremely bitter taste of dibutyl phthalate causes profuse salivation and occasionally retching or vomiting.[26] Signs occur within seconds of the cat biting into the item. Fortunately, signs are generally self-limiting and should resolve once the cat gets the bitter taste of the product out of its mouth. Milk or highly palatable food (e.g., canned tuna) can stop the taste reaction.[26] The cat should be placed in a dark room to visualize and remove any chemical

---

BOX 79-1   How to Make a 7% Ethanol Solution

"Proof" is double the % of alcohol (e.g., 80-proof vodka is 40% ethanol)

$$\frac{\% \text{ ETOH desired (7\%)}}{\% \text{ ETOH stock solution}} = \frac{\text{mL required of available ETOH solution}}{1 \text{L of fluids}}$$

Example:

$$\frac{7\% \text{ desired solution}}{40\% \text{ (80-proof) vodka}} = \frac{? \text{ mL of available stock solution}}{1 \text{L of fluids}}$$

Therefore, 175 mL of 40% vodka is required.

Remove 175 mL from 1 L of fluids and replace with 175 mL 40% vodka to get a 7% ETOH solution

ETOH, ethanol.

that has contaminated the hair coat and prevent re-exposure from grooming. All cats recover with minimal treatment.

Permethrin

Permethrin is a synthetic pyrethrin. Pyrethrins and pyrethroids bind to sodium channels on nerves, causing them to remain open and repetitively fire.[28] In insects, this causes paralysis and death. Permethrin exposure is commonly encountered by cats. It is used in low concentrations in many flea and tick shampoos, foggers, and sprays as well as many household and yard insecticide formulations. Spot-ons (labeled for dogs only) contain a more concentrated (45% to 65% permethrin) formulation. Concentration is the most important factor in determining toxicosis. Cats tolerate low concentrations of pyrethroids, but not high concentrations.[28]

Cats that lick low-concentration permethrin products will often have a reaction to the bitter taste, characterized by hypersalivation, gagging, and occasionally vomiting. Rinsing the mouth or offering the cat milk, canned food, or liquid from a can of tuna fish will often help the signs resolve quickly. A more severe toxicosis is seen when the concentrated dog product is applied topically to cats. Cats may also be exposed from actively grooming or engaging in close physical contact with recently treated (within 48 hours) dogs.[28]

Clinical signs of permethrin toxicosis include hypersalivation, depression, ear and facial twitching, generalized muscle tremors, hyperthermia, seizures, and possibly death. Onset of clinical signs can range from few hours after exposure up to 24 hours. The severity of clinical signs varies among individual cats.

Permethrin and its metabolites are not stored in the body nor excreted in the milk. Permethrin is also quickly broken down by the body, so activated charcoal does not need to be given. Treatment of permethrin toxicosis centers around tremor control. Methocarbamol (50 to 150 mg/kg slow IV; titrate upward as needed) is preferred to control the tremors. The maximum 24 hour dose of 330 mg/kg per day is extrapolated from the human literature. Cats do not seem to develop the respiratory and CNS depression seen in people at high doses of methocarbamol. If no injectable methocarbamol is available, the oral form may be crushed in water and administered rectally. If the cat is actively seizing, diazepam, barbiturates, or inhalant anesthesia may be needed. Once the tremors are under control, cats should be bathed. Liquid hand dishwashing soap (e.g., Dawn) should be used to bathe the entire cat. Thermoregulation is very important in these cases. Tremoring cats often present with hyperthermia, only to develop hypothermia following tremor control and bathing. Hypothermic cats will have increased tremors as well as decreased metabolism of permethrin due to decreased metabolic rate.[29] Permethrins have no direct toxic action on the liver or kidneys, but IV fluids should be used to protect the kidneys from myoglobinuria secondary to rhabdomyolysis. The prognosis for mildly tremoring cats is usually good, but treatment may be required for up to 24 to 48 hours. Some veterinarians have used intravenous lipid emulsion infusions to good effect.[30]

References

1. Toutain PL, Ferran A, Bousquet-Mélou A: Species differences in pharmacokinetics and pharmacodynamics. *Handb Exp Pharmacol* 199:19–48, 2010.
2. McConkey SE, Grant DM, Cribb AE: The role of para-aminophenol in acetaminophen-induced methemoglobinemia in dogs and cats. *J Vet Pharmacol Ther* 32:585–595, 2009.
3. Hall JO: Lilies. In Petersen ME, Talcott PA, editors: *Small animal toxicology*, St Louis, 2006, Elsevier/Saunders, pp 806–811.
4. Rumbeiha WK, Francis JA, Fitzgerald SD, et al: A comprehensive study of Easter lily poisoning in cats. *J Vet Diagn Invest* 16:527–541, 2004.
5. Plumb DC: *Plumb's veterinary drug handbook*, ed 7, Ames, 2011, Wiley-Blackwell.
6. Means C: Insoluble calcium oxalates. In Plumlee KH, editor: *Clinical veterinary toxicology*, St Louis, 2004, Mosby, pp 340–341.
7. Hendrickson RG: Acetaminophen. In Nelson LS, Howland MA, Lewin NA, et al, editors: *Goldfrank's toxicologic emergencies*, ed 9, New York, 2011, McGraw-Hill, pp 483–499.
8. Aaronson LR, Drobatz K: Acetaminophen toxicosis in 17 cats. *J Vet Emerg Crit Care* 6:65–69, 1996.
9. Fisher DJ: Disorders of red blood cells. In Morgan RV, editor: *Handbook of small animal practice*, ed 3, Philadelphia, 1997, Saunders, pp 656–673.
10. Avizeh R, Najafzadeh H, Razijalali M, et al: Evaluation of prophylactic and therapeutic effects of silymarin and N-acetylcysteine in acetaminophen-induced hepatotoxicity in cats. *J Vet Pharmacol Ther* 33:95–99, 2010.
11. Wallace KP, Center SA, Hickford FH, et al: S-adenosyl-L-methionine (SAMe) for the treatment of acetaminophen toxicity in a dog. *J Am Hosp Assoc* 38:246–254, 2002.
12. Kore AM: Toxicology of nonsteroidal anti-inflammatory drugs. *Vet Clin North Am Sm Anim Pract* 20:419–428, 1990.
13. Clive DM, Stoff JS: Renal syndromes associated with non-steroidal anti-inflammatory drugs. *N Engl J Med* 310:563–572, 1984.
14. Merola V, Dunayer E: The 10 most common toxicoses in cats. *Vet Med* 101:339–342, 2006.
15. Sena SF, Kazimi S, Wu AHB: False-positive phencyclidine immunoassay results caused by venlafaxine and O-desmethylvenlafaxine. *Clin Chem* 48:676–677, 2002.
16. Hillyard SG, Barrera-Groba C, Tighe R: Intralipid reverses coma associated with zopiclone and venlafaxine overdose. *Eur J Anaesth* 27:582–583, 2010.
17. Wright HM, Chen AV, Talcott PA, et al: Intravenous fat emulsion as treatment for ivermectin toxicosis in three dogs homozygous for the ABCB1–1Δ gene mutation. *J Vet Emerg Crit Care* 21:666–672, 2011.
18. Fernandez AL, Lee JA, Rahilly L, et al: The use of intravenous lipid emulsion as an antidote in veterinary toxicology. *J Vet Emerg Crit Care* 21:309–320, 2011.
19. Moini H, Packer L, Saris NL: Antioxidant and prooxidant activities of α-lipoic acid and dihydrolipoic acid. *Toxicol Appl Pharmacol* 182:84–90, 2002.
20. Wynn SG, Marsden S: *Manual of natural veterinary medicine: science and tradition*, St Louis, 2002, Mosby, p 236.
21. Hill AS, Werner JA, Rogers QR, et al: Lipoic acid is 10 times more toxic in cats than reported in humans, dogs, or rats. *J Anim Physiol A Anim Nutr* 88:150–156, 2004.
22. Ethylene glycol (HAZARD TEXT® Hazard Management). In Klasco RK, editor: *TOMES System*, Greenwood Village, Colorado, Thomson Micromedex.

23. Thrall MA, Grauer GF, Mero KN: Clinico-pathologic finding in dogs and cats with ethylene glycol intoxication. *J Am Vet Med Assoc* 184:37–41, 1984.

24. Thrall MA, Connally HE, Grauer GF, et al: Ethylene glycol. In Petersen ME, Talcott PA, editors: *Small animal toxicology*, ed 3, St Louis, 2013, Elsevier Saunders, pp 551–567.

25. Connally HE, Thrall MA, Hamar DW: Safety and efficacy of high-dose fomepizole compared with ethanol as therapy for ethylene glycol intoxication in cats. *J Vet Emerg Crit Care* 20:191–206, 2010.

26. Gwaltney-Brant SM: Miscellaneous indoor toxicants. In Petersen ME, Talcott PA, editors: *Small animal toxicology*, ed 3, St Louis, 2013, Elsevier Saunders, pp 291–308.

27. Rosendale ME: Glow jewelry (dibutyl phthalate) ingestion in cats. *Vet Med* 94:703, 1999.

28. Richardson JA: Permethrin spot on toxicoses in cats. *J Vet Emerg Crit Care* 10:103–106, 2000.

29. Meyer EK: Toxicosis in cats erroneously treated with 45 to 65% permethrin products. *J Am Vet Med Assoc* 215:198–203, 1999.

30. Haworth MD, Smart L: Use of intravenous lipid therapy in three cases of feline permethrin toxicosis. *J Vet Emerg Crit Care* 22:697–702, 2012.

Traumatic Brain Injury

Adesola Odunayo

DEFINITON AND ETIOLOGY

Traumatic brain injury (TBI) occurs when an external force causes injury to the brain. There is a paucity of case-controlled studies evaluating TBI in veterinary patients, and most recommendations are extrapolated from human medicine. It is thought that TBI occurs in cats secondary to crush injuries, but other types of trauma including vehicular accidents, high-rise injuries, and missiles can lead to TBI.

PATHOPHYSIOLOGY

Injuries resulting from TBI can be separated into primary and secondary injury.[1] Primary injury occurs immediately due to direct mechanical damage. Examples of primary injuries include contusions, lacerations, hematomas, and diffuse axonal injuries. Primary injury is beyond the control of the clinician but interventions can be made to prevent and treat secondary injury. Secondary injury occurs following primary injury as a result of increased activity of inflammatory cytokines, reactive oxygen species, and excitatory neurotransmitters. This can lead to cell damage and neuronal cell death. Consequences of secondary injury include increased intracranial pressure (ICP) and alterations to the blood-brain barrier.[1] Systemic derangements that can propagate and potentiate secondary injury include hypotension, hypoxia, hyperglycemia, hypoglycemia, hypercapnia, hypocapnia, and hyperthermia.

Cerebral Perfusion Pressure

Cerebral perfusion pressure (CPP) is the force driving blood into the brain, providing oxygen and nutrients. Cerebral perfusion pressure is the primary determinant of cerebral blood flow (CBF). Cerebral perfusion pressure is defined as the difference between the mean arterial pressure (MAP) and ICP (CPP = MAP − ICP). Elevated ICP is a common and life-threatening complication of TBI. The Monro-Kellie doctrine states that the skull is a rigid compartment and contains three components: brain, blood, and cerebrospinal fluid. If an increase occurs in the volume of one component, the volume of one or more other components must decrease, or ICP will be elevated. If ICP increases beyond the limit of compensatory mechanisms, cerebral perfusion can be compromised and ischemia of the brain tissue may occur.[1] Severe increases in ICP trigger the cerebral ischemic response, also known as the *Cushing reflex.* Elevation in ICP results in decreased CPP and thus CBF, which ultimately leads to an increase in carbon dioxide (CO_2). This causes a sympathetic nervous system response leading to elevated MAP in order to increase CPP. Reflex bradycardia occurs independently as a result of the elevated MAP. The Cushing reflex is characterized by a significantly increased blood pressure and concurrent bradycardia. This indicates possible life-threatening elevation in ICP and necessitates aggressive therapy.[1] Intracranial pressure can be measured using fiberoptic monitoring systems, although this is rarely used in veterinary patients.

INITIAL EVALUATION

Any patient that presents with TBI must have an initial evaluation of life-threatening abnormalities. This involves evaluation of the "ABCs" (airway, breathing, and circulation), known as the *primary survey.* Airway obstruction may be present in cases of trauma where oral or laryngeal hematomas or hemorrhage may develop. Intubation should be performed if there is concern about airway integrity. Tracheostomy should be considered in patients where a patent airway cannot be maintained with an orotracheal tube. Breathing abnormalities are not uncommon in cats with TBI. This is usually associated with concurrent injuries, such as pneumothorax, rib fracture, pulmonary contusions, or anemia. Oxygen should be provided, and the primary cause of the breathing difficulty should be addressed if possible (e.g., with thoracocentesis, analgesia, and/or blood transfusion). Mechanical ventilation may be indicated in cats with progressive hypoxemia despite oxygen supplementation.[2] Cats with cardiovascular instability may present with bradycardia, hypothermia, hypotension, weak peripheral pulses, and obtundation. A peripheral catheter should be placed and fluid or blood product therapy should be initiated to correct hypovolemic shock once it is recognized.

Neurologic Exam

A neurologic exam should be performed as soon as the animal is deemed stable. This includes assessment of the level of consciousness, respiratory pattern, pupil size and responsiveness, ocular position and movements, and the presence of motor response.[1] The modified Glasgow coma scale (MGCS) has been proposed for use in dogs with TBI and is anecdotally used in cats (Table 80-1).[3] The MGCS is thought to be best used as an objective assessment of progression of neurologic disease rather than as an initial prognostic indicator.[3] The MGCS is usually evaluated often (every 4 to 8 hours) in the hospitalized cat to monitor progression or resolution of disease.

Cats can present with varying levels of consciousness. Comatose cats will likely have global cerebral injury and a guarded prognosis, based on what is reported in human patients.[1] Pupil size should be evaluated, as well as response to light. It is important to evaluate the eyes for concurrent ocular injury (e.g., corneal ulcerations) that may interfere with interpretation of the pupillary light reflex. Miotic pupils indicate diffuse forebrain injury, whereas mydriasis may indicate brain herniation. Fixed unresponsive midrange pupils are usually seen with cerebellar herniation and are associated with a poor-to-grave prognosis in human patients.

DIAGNOSIS

Diagnosis is based on the history and physical examination findings. Skull radiographs may reveal fractures, although they provide little information regarding the severity of the brain injury. Computed tomography (CT) is considered the standard of care in human patients and can be used in cats to evaluate for fractures and peracute hemorrhage.[1] Magnetic resonance imaging (MRI) is more expensive and more time-consuming but may provide more information relevant to prognosis.[1] Cats requiring CT or MRI should be hemodynamically stable before undergoing general anesthesia. In some cases, cats that are obtunded or comatose may be able to undergo CT of the skull (a rapid procedure), yielding important information.

TREATMENT RECOMMENDATIONS

Therapeutic recommendations are generally divided into extracranial and intracranial therapy. Initial extracranial therapy is performed to ensure patient stability, and intracranial therapy follows closely afterward (or concurrently in some cases).[1]

Extracranial Therapy

Extracranial recommendations include maintenance of adequate intravascular volume, maintenance of adequate oxygenation and ventilation, and analgesia.

Maximizing MAP maximizes CPP in cats, reducing the risk of cerebral ischemia (CPP = MAP − ICP). The patient's blood pressure should be obtained shortly after presentation and monitored closely to identify hypotension. Hypotension has been identified as a primary cause of mortality in human patients with TBI.[4] Once identified, hypotension should be

Table 80-1	Modified Glasgow Coma Scale Score and Suggested Prognosis

Description	MGCS Score
Motor Activity	
Normal gait, normal spinal reflexes	6
Hemiparesis, tetraparesis, or decerebrate activity	5
Recumbent, intermittent extensor rigidity	4
Recumbent, constant extensor rigidity	3
Recumbent, constant extensor rigidity with opisthotonus	2
Recumbent, hypotonia of muscles, depressed or absent spinal reflexes	1
Brainstem Reflexes	
Normal pupillary light reflexes and oculocephalic reflexes	6
Slow pupillary light reflexes and normal-to-reduced oculocephalic reflexes	5
Bilateral unresponsive miosis with normal-to-reduced oculocephalic reflexes	4
Pinpoint pupils with reduced-to-absent oculocephalic reflexes	3
Unilateral, unresponsive mydriasis with reduced-to-absent oculocephalic reflexes	2
Bilateral, unresponsive mydriasis with reduced to absent oculocephalic reflexes	1
Level of Consciousness	
Occasional periods of alertness and responsive to environment	6
Depression or delirium, capable of responding but response may be inappropriate	5
Semicomatose, responsive to visual stimuli	4
Semicomatose, responsive to auditory stimuli	3
Semicomatose, responsive only to repeated noxious stimuli	2
Comatose, unresponsive to repeated noxious stimuli	1
Suggested Prognosis	
Grave	3 to 8
Guarded	9 to 14
Good	15 to 18

MGCS, Modified Glasgow coma scale.

corrected with fluid therapy (e.g., crystalloids, natural and artificial colloids, or blood products). Isotonic crystalloids should be administered at 10 to 15 mL/kg and given rapidly over 10 to 15 minutes using a large-bore peripheral catheter (18- to 20-gauge). This dose can be repeated up to the shock dose (45 to 60 mL/kg) if there is no evidence of improved tissue perfusion (e.g., normalization of heart rate, pulse quality, mucous membrane color, and blood pressure) after the bolus dose. Blood products (e.g., packed red blood cells and whole blood) may be considered for cats that have significant clinical signs associated with hemorrhage and blood loss. Hypertonic saline, a crystalloid that promotes movement of fluid from the interstitial and intracellular space into the intravascular space, is often recommended for resuscitation of patients with TBI.[5] Hypertonic saline works rapidly, and its effects are immediate but transient (lasting only 30 to 60 minutes). It also causes the movement of fluid out of brain tissue, thereby helping to reduce ICP. In human patients, hypertonic saline is thought to be as effective as mannitol in the treatment of elevated ICP.[6] Hypertonic saline (4 to 6 mL/kg of 7.5% sodium chloride over 10 minutes) should be given concurrently with an isotonic crystalloid when used for resuscitation.

As previously mentioned, hypoxemia contributes to the development of secondary injury in TBI. Hypoxemia may be evaluated via arterial blood gas analysis (partial arterial pressure of oxygen [PaO_2] should be greater than 80 mm Hg) or more conveniently through pulse oximetry. Pulse oximetry readings (saturation of peripheral oxygen [SpO_2]) greater than 95% are considered normal and correlate with a PaO_2 of 80 mm Hg. Oxygen therapy should be indicated with an SpO_2 value less than 95% (or PaO_2 less than 80 mm Hg). Oxygen can be provided via flow-by face mask, oxygen tent, or oxygen chamber. It is recommended that nasal oxygen tubes, oxygen cannulas, or transtracheal oxygen catheters be avoided, because these may cause sneezing or coughing that may lead to elevation of the ICP.

Ventilation should also be closely monitored in cats with TBI. Partial arterial pressure of carbon dioxide ($PaCO_2$) is the major determinant of CBF, because it regulates cerebral blood vessel diameter. Hypercapnia leads to vasodilation of the cerebral vessel in order to increase blood flow. This may ultimately lead to an increase in ICP. Hypocapnia (caused by hyperventilation) leads to vasoconstriction, which lowers ICP. However, excessive vasoconstriction may cause cerebral ischemia. An arterial blood gas measurement is the most effective way to monitor $PaCO_2$ levels, but venous blood gases may be used in its place. The end-tidal carbon dioxide ($EtCO_2$) can be used in intubated patients and is generally 5 mm Hg lower than the $PaCO_2$. Patients with TBI should ideally maintain CO_2 levels between 35 and 45 mm Hg. Aggressive hyperventilation may be considered in patients with acute decompensation of their neurologic status.

Analgesia should be provided for cats with TBI, because untreated pain may lead to significant consequences.[7] Opioids are the mainstay of analgesia in TBI due to their lack of adverse cardiovascular effects and reversibility. Fentanyl may be administered as a continuous rate infusion at 3 to 5 μg/kg/hour after an initial bolus is given (3 to 5 μg/kg). Other pure mu agonists may also be administered (e.g., morphine, hydromorphone, oxymorphone, and methadone). The partial mu agonist buprenorphine may be administered (0.01 to 0.03 mg/kg every 8 hours, intravenously [IV]), although it is more difficult to reverse with naloxone if rapid changes in neurologic status or cardiac arrest occur.[1] Body temperature should be monitored often (as long as it is not stressful to the cat) to prevent or treat hyperthermia that may develop, especially in cats managed in incubators or oxygen cages.

Intracranial Therapy

The goals of intracranial therapy include minimizing increases in ICP and maximizing CPP. Increases in ICP can be minimized by minimizing obstruction to venous drainage. This is accomplished by placing the patient's head and thorax at an elevated angle relative to horizontal (15° to 30°), usually on a backboard. The entire thorax should be included on the board to prevent bending of the neck and venous occlusion. Jugular catheters and jugular venipuncture should be avoided for the same reason.

When elevated ICP is suspected based on the presence of Cushing reflex or acute deterioration of the patient's status, hyperosmolar therapy should be initiated. The options for hyperosmolar therapy include mannitol and hypertonic saline. Mannitol works by decreasing blood viscosity immediately and providing osmotic effects about 15 to 30 minutes after administration.[1] Mannitol should be provided at a dose of 0.5 to 1.5 g/kg IV over 15 to 20 minutes. The routine use of furosemide after mannitol administration is no longer recommended for human patients with TBI.[8] Furosemide may lead to or worsen hypovolemia due to its diuretic effects, which may decrease CPP. Hypertonic saline (4 to 6 mL/kg of 7.5% sodium chloride over 10 minutes) can also be used in place of mannitol as a hyperosmolar agent for patients with suspicion for elevated ICP.

Other Supportive Therapy

Anticonvulsant therapy should be initiated as soon as a patient with TBI has a seizure. This is because seizure activity leads to hyperthermia, hypoxemia, and cerebral edema, all of which exacerbate elevated ICP.[1] Diazepam or midazolam should be used to stop any ongoing seizures. Phenobarbital should be administered for prevention of further seizures at a loading dose of 16 to 20 mg/kg divided over 1 to 24 hours, IV or orally (PO). A maintenance dose of 2 mg/kg every 12 hours IV or PO should be continued. Levetiracetam may also be used in cats at a dose of 16 mg/kg every 8 hours IV or PO.

Nutritional support should be considered early to promote healing, maintain gastrointestinal (GI) mucosal integrity, and reduce the risks of GI bacterial translocation. Esophagostomy tubes placed under general anesthesia once the animal is stable may be used with minimal compression applied around the neck. Naso-esophageal or nasogastric tubes should be avoided until the patient is stable, because nasal stimulation may lead to sneezing, which may increase ICP. Partial or total parenteral nutrition can also be initiated in cats where enteral nutrition is difficult to provide.

Electrolytes should be monitored often and supplemented as required. Special attention should be paid to serum glucose concentration, because hyperglycemia has been associated with a poor outcome in human patients.[9] Hyperglycemia has also been associated with severity of head trauma in cats.[10] Hyperglycemia can potentiate neurologic injury, and iatrogenic hyperglycemia (secondary to glucocorticoid administration or dextrose solutions) should be avoided in cats with TBI.[10] Hypoglycemia should be treated by providing dextrose supplementation in IV fluids, and serum glucose concentrations should be monitored closely to prevent hyperglycemia.

The routine use of corticosteroids is not recommended in cats with TBI. Use of corticosteroids has been shown to increase mortality in human patients with TBI because they are associated with hyperglycemia, immunosuppression, delayed wound healing, and gastric ulceration.[4,11]

Additional patient care should include bladder management via expression or indwelling urinary catheter placement. Frequent turning of the patient should be done to prevent urine scalding, atelectasis, and pressure sores. Intravenous catheter sites should be monitored daily, and catheters should be removed when not in use in order to eliminate a nidus for infection.

SURGICAL INTERVENTION

Surgery is rarely performed in cats with TBI, because many of them respond to supportive therapy. Indications for surgical intervention include the presence of an open or depressed skull fracture, ongoing hemorrhage, presence of a foreign body, or declining neurologic status despite adequate medical therapy.[1]

PROGNOSIS

There are no data regarding prognosis of cats with TBI in the veterinary literature. However many cats have a tremendous ability to compensate for loss of functional cerebral tissue. Providing an accurate prognosis is important to avoid overly negative interpretations of the cat's initial appearance, because many of them recover and regain acceptable neurologic function.[1]

References

1. Sande A, West C: Traumatic brain injury: a review of pathophysiology and management. *J Vet Emerg Crit Care* 20(2):177–190, 2010.
2. Vassilev E, McMichael ML: An overview of positive pressure ventilation. *J Vet Emerg Crit Care* 14(1):15–21, 2004.
3. Platt SR, Radaelli ST, McDonnell JJ: The prognostic value of the modified Glasgow coma scale in head trauma in dogs. *J Vet Intern Med* 15(6):581–584, 2001.
4. Ghajar J: Traumatic brain injury. *Lancet* 356(9233):923–929, 2000.
5. Rickard AC, Smith JE, Newell P, et al: Salt or sugar for your injured brain? A meta-analysis of randomised controlled trials of mannitol versus hypertonic sodium solutions to manage raised intracranial pressure in traumatic brain injury. *Emerg Med J* 8:679–683, 2014.
6. Junger WG, Rhind SG, Rizoli SB, et al: Pre-hospital hypertonic saline resuscitation attenuates the activation and promotes apoptosis of neutrophils in patients with severe traumatic brain injury. *Shock* 40:366–374, 2013.
7. Vainionpää MH, Raekallio MR, Junnila JJ, et al: A comparison of thermographic imaging, physical examination and modified questionnaire as an instrument to assess painful conditions in cats. *J Feline Med Surg* 15(2):124–131, 2013.
8. Bratton SL, Chestnut RM, Ghajar J, et al: Guidelines for the management of severe traumatic brain injury. II. Hyperosmolar therapy. *J Neurotrauma* 24(Suppl 1):S14–S20, 2007.
9. Salim A, Hadjizacharia P, Dubose J, et al: Persistent hyperglycemia in severe traumatic brain injury: an independent predictor of outcome. *Am Surg* 75(1):25–29, 2009.
10. Syring RS, Otto CM, Drobatz KJ: Hyperglycemia in dogs and cats with head trauma: 122 cases (1997-1999). *J Am Vet Med Assoc* 218(7):1124–1129, 2001.
11. Alderson P, Roberts I: Corticosteroids for acute traumatic brain injury. *Cochrane Database Syst Rev* (1):CD000196, 2005.

Pyothorax

Adesola Odunayo

DEFINITION AND ETIOLOGY

Pyothorax is defined as the accumulation of a septic, purulent effusion within the pleural space. The pleural space is a potential space between the lungs, mediastinum, diaphragm, and thoracic wall. Risk factors associated with the development of pyothorax in cats include living in a multicat household and age (i.e., younger cats are at higher risk).[1] The average age for cats with pyothorax is 4 to 6 years, although cats of any age may be affected. Breed or sex predispositions have not been identified in cats.[2]

The etiology of pyothorax is often difficult to identify due to the chronic course of the disease. By the time most cats develop clinical signs, the primary cause of the disease is often difficult to detect. Proposed bacterial sources include bite wounds to the thorax; migrating foreign bodies (e.g., grass awns); perforated esophagus, trachea, or bronchi; bacterial pneumonia; aberrant migration of *Cuterebra* larvae; or iatrogenic from thoracocentesis or thoracotomy. It has been suggested that the most likely source of bacteria associated with feline pyothorax is the aspiration of oropharyngeal flora into the lungs.[3] Development of pneumonia and extension of the infection to the pleural space subsequently result in pyothorax.[3]

Bacteria isolates in cases of feline pyothorax are usually polymicrobial and are typically similar to normal feline oropharyngeal flora. Examples of common isolates include *Bacteroides* spp., *Clostridium* spp., *Streptococcus* spp., *Mycoplasma* spp., and *Pasteurella* spp. Less than 20% of cats have infections caused by bacteria not associated with the oropharynx (including *Escherichia coli*, *Salmonella* spp., *Klebsiella* spp., *Pseudomonas* spp., and *Nocardia* spp.). Fungal causes of pyothorax are rare.[3]

CLINICAL SIGNS

The progression of pyothorax in cats can be very subtle, and it may take weeks to months before clinical signs are recognized by owners.[2] This is supported by the presence of granulation tissue and adhesions on the pleura. Many cats compensate for the gradual development of respiratory disease by reduced activity, and such signs may not be noticed by the owners. One study reports that less than 40% of owners noticed signs of respiratory compromise in their cats at home.[3] By the time clinical signs of respiratory disease are seen, it is thought that minimal respiratory reserves remain.[2]

Cats with pyothorax may have a recent history of a bite wound or external wound, although only 14.5% of cats in one study had a wound or a history of a wound.[1] The most common clinical signs associated with pyothorax in cats in order of frequency include anorexia or hyporexia, lethargy, and respiratory distress.[1,3] Cats with pleural effusion usually have a restrictive breathing pattern characterized by an increased respiratory rate and effort, as well as rapid and shallow chest excursions.[2] Auscultation of the thorax will reveal quiet lung sounds along the ventral aspect of the thorax. Heart sounds may also be muffled. Cats may present with a fever, although cats that have received antibiotics prior to presentation may be afebrile.[4] Hypothermia has been reported in cats with pyothorax and was associated with a poorer prognosis due to the possibility of severe sepsis and septic shock.[1,2] Other clinical signs include hypersalivation, dehydration, weight loss, signs of pain, and ocular and nasal discharge.[1,3,4]

DIAGNOSIS

Definitive diagnosis of feline pyothorax usually involves a combination of thoracic imaging, thoracocentesis, cytology, and aerobic and anaerobic culture and sensitivity (C&S) testing.

Thoracocentesis

Needle thoracocentesis should be performed in any cat with suspect pleural effusion based on physical examination (short and shallow respiratory pattern, quiet lung sounds ventrally) or the presence of pleural effusion on thoracic radiographs or ultrasound. If thoracocentesis is performed before radiography, it will reduce the likelihood that the patient will decompensate while radiographs are being taken. Removal of fluid will also allow better radiographic visualization of the lung fields to identify pneumonia, abscesses, or fungal/neoplastic nodules. Thoracocentesis will also facilitate the diagnosis of pyothorax through microscopic evaluation of the fluid, as well as C&S testing.

Thoracocentesis should be performed via ultrasound guidance, although it can be successfully performed blind if ultrasound is unavailable. An intravenous (IV) catheter should be placed if the cat is stable. This will allow immediate venous access if complications arise during the centesis or if the animal requires sedation. Many cats will tolerate thoracocentesis without sedation, although butorphanol (0.2 to 0.4 mg/kg IV, intramuscularly [IM], or subcutaneously [SC]) may be administered to anxious or fractious cats. Midazolam (0.1 to 0.3 mg/kg IV, IM, or SC) may also be used in addition to the butorphanol, although it may cause excitement in some cats. Eutectic mixture of local anesthetic (EMLA) cream (lidocaine/prilocaine) may also be applied to the site of thoracocentesis to provide topical anesthesia. Thoracocentesis is usually performed in sternal recumbency, although it can be successfully accomplished in lateral recumbency in animals unable to sit in sternal recumbency. The middle third (dorsoventral) of the thoracic cavity should be shaved and aseptically prepared along the sixth to ninth intercostal space. A butterfly catheter (19- or 21-gauge), three-way stopcock, and syringe are used to facilitate drainage. Due to the exudative nature of most pyothorax effusions, larger-gauge needles are usually more effective. The needle should be inserted cranial to the rib or along the intercostal space. Laceration of the intercostal vessels and nerves located along the caudal rib margins should be avoided.

The fluid associated with most cases of pyothorax is usually loculated (located in small pockets) within the pleural space and may not flow freely. In addition, fibrin plugs may obstruct the needle and prevent easy drainage of the pleural cavity. The use of ultrasound facilitates identification of the fluid pockets and drainage of the thoracic cavity.[4] However, the thorax may not be completely drained via needle thoracocentesis. In many cases, removal of only a small amount of the existing fluid can greatly improve patient respiratory status. Samples of the fluid collected should be saved for cytology, as well as aerobic and anaerobic culture. The use of glucose and lactate differentials have been described in cats with septic abdominal effusion, although their use with thoracic effusion is currently unknown at this time.[5] In animals with septic abdominal effusion, a glucose differential of 20 mg/dL (1.1 mmol/L), with the abdominal effusion having a lower concentration than the peripheral glucose concentration, is very suggestive of a septic effusion. Lactate concentration in abdominal septic effusions is generally higher than peripheral lactate concentration.[5]

Fluid Analysis, Cytology, and Culture

The fluid obtained is usually turbid and often associated with an unpleasant odor (usually indicative of an anaerobic infection). The fluid type associated with feline pyothorax is typically an exudate (protein greater than 3 g/dL and total nucleated cell count greater than 7000/µL). Neutrophils (often degenerate) are the most common cell type present. Cytology and Gram stain (if available) should be performed on all pleural fluid samples to identify the presence and morphology of bacteria or other infectious agents. Polymicrobial infection is usually present, and there should be evidence

of phagocytized infectious agents by inflammatory cells. It is important to keep in mind that infectious agents may not be seen in cases where antibiotics have been initiated prior to fluid evaluation. Bacteria that do not take up stain (e.g., *Mycoplasma* spp.) may also be difficult to identify microscopically.[2]

Acid-fast stain can be used to differentiate *Nocardia* spp. from *Actinomyces* spp. and *Filifactor* spp., because *Nocardia* spp. are partially acid-fast.[2] Modified Wright-Giemsa stains (e.g., the Diff-Quik stain) are readily available in clinical practice and can be used quickly. Any combination of filamentous bacteria, cocci, and rods may be present.[2]

Samples should also be submitted in a sterile container to a referral laboratory for both aerobic and anaerobic C&S testing. Special anaerobic containers should be used to eliminate oxygen from the specimen, because failure to do this will result in a false-negative anaerobic culture.[2,6] Special care should be taken to ensure proper handling of the fluid sample for anaerobic culture, because anaerobes make up a large percentage of bacteria identified in feline pyothorax cases.[6,7]

Thoracic Imaging

Thoracic radiographs help confirm the presence of pleural effusion; however, radiographs should be performed (or repeated) after thoracocentesis to evaluate the pleural space and pulmonary parenchyma for primary (or secondary) diseases. These may include abscesses, granuloma, pneumonia, or pulmonary nodules. Thoracic ultrasound is used to identify the presence of pleural effusion and may also be used to identify pulmonary abscesses. Thoracic cross-sectional imaging, such as computed tomography, may also be used (ideally after thoracocentesis) to identify abscesses and masses.

Blood Work

A complete blood count (CBC), serum biochemistry analysis, feline leukemia virus and feline immunodeficiency virus testing, and urinalysis should be performed in all cats presenting with pyothorax. These diagnostic tests are helpful in the therapeutic management of pyothorax. The CBC usually reveals a leukocytosis with a regenerative left shift.[1] In more severe cases, a degenerative left shift or leukopenia may be present. Cats may also be anemic—typically anemia of inflammatory disease.[8] The serum biochemistry results may reveal hypoalbuminemia, hypocalcemia, hyponatremia, hypochloremia, or hyperbilirubinemia.[1] Urinalysis may reveal proteinuria (prerenal) and low urine specific gravity, presumably from nephrogenic diabetes insipidus.

TREATMENT

Therapy for cats with pyothorax usually consists of thoracic drainage via thoracostomy tubes, antibiotics, fluid therapy, analgesia, and oxygen supplementation. In some circumstances, surgical exploration of the thorax with lavage of the chest may be performed.

Cardiovascular and Respiratory Stabilization

Cats with pyothorax may show signs of hemodynamic compromise as a result of septic shock or hypovolemia. In one study evaluating cats with pyothorax, 32 of the 80 cats with pyothorax fit the criteria for sepsis or systemic inflammatory response syndrome.[1] Signs associated with cardiovascular instability in cats may include bradycardia, hypothermia, hypotension, poor peripheral pulses, cold extremities, and/or obtundation. Serum lactate concentration may also be elevated. Cats suspected to be hypovolemic should be actively resuscitated. This should include concurrent active warming in hypothermic cats. A large-bore peripheral catheter should be placed for fluid resuscitation. Cats should be resuscitated with isotonic crystalloids, such as 0.9% sodium chloride, lactated Ringer's solution, or Normosol-R (10 to 15 mL/kg IV). This volume should be given over 10 to 15 minutes. The cat should be re-evaluated to assess response to fluid therapy, and the fluid bolus can be repeated up to a maximum of 45 to 60 mL/kg IV if response is poor or insufficient.

Cats that present in overt respiratory distress should have thoracocentesis performed immediately as both a therapeutic and diagnostic step. Thoracocentesis is usually recommended before thoracic radiographs are performed.

Antibiotic Therapy

Antibiotic therapy should be initiated as soon as pyothorax is suspected (based on historical and clinical signs, as well as purulent material from thoracocentesis) or diagnosed. Studies in people suggest that early intervention with antibiotics decreases morbidity and mortality, and recommendations are to provide broad spectrum antibiotic therapy within 1 hour of diagnosis of sepsis.[9] Initial therapy is usually empirical and should be based on cytology of the effusion. The initial antimicrobials empirically selected should be effective against obligate and facultative anaerobes and bacteria generally associated with the oropharyngeal flora. Therapy should then be adjusted after C&S testing results are finalized. Antibiotics should be administered IV at the early stages of treatment to ensure therapeutic serum concentrations. Oral antibiotics can be initiated after the patient is stable, has begun to show signs of response to therapy, and is ideally eating and drinking well. Table 81-1 provides recommended IV antibiotic therapy for cats with pyothorax.[10] The use of intrapleural antibiotics is controversial and is thought to offer no additional benefit to IV antibiotics.[11] Oral antibiotics should be initiated when appropriate, and antibiotic therapy should be maintained for at least 4 to 6 weeks.[10]

Thoracic Drainage

Placement of indwelling thoracostomy tubes is considered a standard therapy of pyothorax in cats. These tubes are usually easy to place, are well tolerated, and provide superior drainage of the pleural space compared to intermittent needle thoracocentesis.[10] Bilateral chest tubes are recommended when bilateral effusion is present. Bilateral effusion is most common in cats with pyothorax.[3,4] Needle thoracocentesis should be performed before thoracostomy tube placement to reduce the risks of complications associated with oxygenation and ventilation. The cat should be placed under general anesthesia,

Drug	Dosage	Notes
Ampicillin/sulbactam	15 to 30 mg/kg IV every 6 to 8 hours	May be used as a monotherapy drug
Clindamycin	10 to 15 mg/kg IV every 12 hours	Ineffective against *Pasteurella* spp. May be combined with penicillin G or an aminopenicillin, although antagonism may occur
Ampicillin	20 to 40 mg/kg IV every 6 to 8 hours	May be used as a monotherapy drug May also be used in combination with metronidazole
Metronidazole	10 to 15 mg/kg IV every 12 hours	Usually used in combination with other antibiotics
Amikacin	10 to 15 mg/kg IV every 24 hours	Use with caution, may cause renal toxicity Poor penetration of pleural space Infrequently used as a monotherapy drug
Enrofloxacin	5 mg/kg IM every 24 hours	May be combined with an aminopenicillin May cause retinal toxicity in cats, especially if used IV in doses exceeding 5 mg/kg/day
Penicillin G potassium/sodium	20,000 to 40,000 International Unit/kg IV every 6 hours	May be used as a monotherapy drug May also be used in combination with metronidazole

Table 81-1 Intravenous Antibiotics Recommended for the Management of Pyothorax in Cats

IM, Intramuscularly; *IV,* intravenously.

BOX 81-1 Thoracostomy Tube Placement in Cats

1. Most thoracostomy tubes are placed under general anesthesia. However, small diameter tubes can be placed using the Seldinger technique and may not require general anesthesia in calm cats.
2. The entire lateral thoracic wall should be clipped and aseptically scrubbed.
3. Have an assistant pull the skin of the lateral thoracic wall cranially and ventrally. This will help create the subcutaneous tunnel for the chest tube. The subcutaneous tunnel helps prevent iatrogenic pneumothorax from developing if the tube is inadvertently removed.
4. Consider using a local block at the tube insertion site, or consider using a paravertebral block.
5. Select an available chest tube either using silicone tubing, a trocar tube, or a red rubber catheter.
6. Measure the tube from the entrance site to the fifth intercostal space.

If using a trocar tube, follow steps 7 through 11. If using a red rubber catheter or silicone tube, begin at step 12.

7. Tent the skin at the dorsal aspect of the tenth intercostal space and make a small stab incision for the tube to pass.
8. Inset the trocar tube through the skin incision and tunnel the tube cranially.
9. When the tip of the trocar tube is over the seventh intercostal space, direct the trocar tube perpendicular to the thoracic wall and push firmly until the tube penetrates the pleural space. Use your nondominant hand to grab the tube at the level of the skin so that you can control the entry of the tube into the pleural space.
10. Once the trocar has entered the thorax, push the tube off the trocar in a cranial and ventral direction while your assistant releases the skin.
11. Have your assistant release the skin, seal the end of the tube immediately, and proceed to evacuate the thorax while securing the tube.

If using a red rubber catheter or silicon tube, follow steps 12 through 15.

12. Make an incision through the skin at the seventh to ninth intercostal space.
13. Bluntly dissect through the subcutaneous fascia and intercostal muscles with a hemostat until you have entered the pleural space.
14. Insert the red rubber catheter through the open tips of the hemostat into the pleural cavity and direct it cranioventrally so that the tip is at the fifth intercostal space.
15. Have your assistant release the skin, seal the end of the tube immediately, and proceed to evacuate the thorax while securing the tube.

Adapted from Hackett TB, Mazzaferro EM: *Veterinary emergency and critical care procedures*, ed 2, Oxford, 2012, Wiley-Blackwell.

intubated, and standard techniques should be followed for tube placement (Box 81-1).[10] Radiographs should be obtained after tube placement to assess tube position and evaluate for complications. Complications associated with thoracostomy tube placement include pneumothorax, incorrect placement leading to failure to drain, kinking, and abscess at site of drain insertion.[10] Indwelling thoracostomy tubes can be managed with continuous water seal suction or intermittent suction. Either method is effective to provide adequate thoracic drainage. Lavage of the thoracostomy tubes may be performed to facilitate drainage, prevent obstruction of the tube, and débride the pleura. It may also help identify failure of thoracostomy tube to drain the thorax if less than 75% of instilled fluid volume is recovered.[10] Lavage may be carried out with 0.9% sodium chloride at body temperature every 4 hours for the first 24 to 48 hours, after which it may be performed every 8 to 12 hours. A recommended volume of 10 to 25 mL/kg per lavage may be used.[3,10] It is important to record the volume of fluid instilled and aspirated, and the procedure should be repeated on the other tube if two thoracostomy tubes are present. Hypokalemia has been reported as a potential complication of thoracic cavity lavage.[3] The thoracostomy tube(s) should be removed when the volume of the pleural effusion has reduced to 2 mL/kg/day or less, there is cytological resolution of infection, and the fluid appears to be more serosanguineous than purulent. The median duration of thoracic drainage is 5 to 6 days.[10] The use of intrapleural fibrinolytics has been described in veterinary patients, but their efficacy is currently unknown.[10]

Intermittent needle thoracocentesis can be used to manage cats with pyothorax when owners decline thoracostomy tube placement and management. This should, however, be reserved as a last resort option, because it is uncomfortable for the patient and may not provide adequate drainage of the pleural space.

Supportive Care

Cats with pyothorax need aggressive monitoring and supportive care based on the systemic nature of their disease. Fluid therapy should be initiated as early as possible to correct intravascular deficits, prevent dehydration, and provide maintenance needs. Serum electrolytes should be evaluated often and supplementation made as soon as abnormalities are detected.

Oxygen therapy should be provided to cats with increased respiratory rate and effort or evidence of continued hypoxemia after thoracocentesis. This may be determined by a pulse oximetry reading of less than 95% obtained on room air. Nasal cannulas may be placed to provide humidified oxygen, or an oxygen chamber or cage may be used if available. The cat may be weaned from oxygen once it has a comfortable respiratory rate and effort or has evidence of increased arterial oxygenation.

Thoracostomy tubes can be painful, and a proactive analgesia plan is important. Regional analgesia can be provided by infiltration of bupivacaine (1 mg/kg every 6 to 8 hours) before tube placement or intrapleural analgesia after tube placement. Intrapleural analgesia should be administered after evacuation (and/or lavage) of thoracostomy tube(s) to ensure maximal absorption. Special caution should be taken when using bupivacaine in cats because of potential cardiac and neurologic toxicity. Systemic analgesia should also be provided using opioids. Buprenorphine (0.01 to 0.03 mg/kg every 8 hours IV) or fentanyl (3 to 5 µg/kg/hour IV) is generally well tolerated in cats. Other pure mu opioids (e.g., hydromorphone or oxymorphone) can also be used in cats. Butorphanol does not provide sufficient analgesia to be of clinical utility in this condition.

Nutritional support should be considered early, and a feeding tube should be placed in cats that remain anorexic after 24 to 48 hours of appropriate therapy. Naso-esophageal or nasogastric tubes can be placed easily without general anesthesia and can provide the resting energy requirement for that patient. Nutritional support can be initiated immediately after the patient is admitted, using a naso-esophageal tube or nasogastric tube. Esophagostomy tubes may be considered in cats that remain anorexic for an extended period of time or could be pre-emptively placed during chest tube placement if the cat is doing well under anesthesia.

Surgical Exploration, Débridement, and Lavage

Unlike dogs, surgical intervention is required infrequently for the management of pyothorax in cats, because most cases respond well to medical therapy.[10] The goals of surgery are to identify and remove any inciting cause (e.g., foreign body), remove areas of necrotic tissue, break down adhesions, and ensure proper bilateral thoracostomy tube placement. Indications for surgery in cats may include the detection of pulmonary or mediastinal abscesses, ineffective thoracostomy tube drainage, or failure of medical management that has gone on for a week or longer.[10]

PROGNOSIS AND PROPHYLAXIS

The reported prognosis of cats with pyothorax varies depending on the study evaluated, but survival rates range from 49% to 78% with almost all cases managed via medical therapy.[1,3,4] Recurrence rates have been reported to be as low as 4.5% in cats with follow-up information.[1] Because the majority of cases involve oropharyngeal flora, routine prophylactic antibiotics should be considered when cats are thought to be at risk (e.g., cats with significant dental disease undergoing dental procedures under general anesthesia).[10]

References

1. Waddell LS, Brady CA, Drobatz KJ: Risk factors, prognostic indicators, and outcome of pyothorax in cats: 80 cases (1986-1999). *J Am Vet Med Assoc* 221(6):819–824, 2002.
2. Barrs VR, Beatty JA: Feline pyothorax—new insights into an old problem: Part 1. Aetiopathogenesis and diagnostic investigation. *Vet J* 179(2):163–170, 2009.
3. Barrs VR, Allan GS, Martin P, et al: Feline pyothorax: a retrospective study of 27 cases in Australia. *J Feline Med Surg* 7(4):211–222, 2005.
4. Demetriou JL, Foale RD, Ladlow J, et al: Canine and feline pyothorax: a retrospective study of 50 cases in the UK and Ireland. *J Small Anim Pract* 43(9):388–394, 2002.
5. Bonczynski JJ, Ludwig LL, Barton LJ, et al: Comparison of peritoneal fluid and peripheral blood pH, bicarbonate, glucose, and lactate concentration as a diagnostic tool for septic peritonitis in dogs and cats. *Vet Surg* 32(2):161–166, 2003.
6. Love DN, Jones RF, Bailey M, et al: Isolation and characterisation of bacteria from pyothorax (empyaemia) in cats. *Vet Microbiol* 7(5):455–461, 1982.
7. Walker AL, Jang SS, Hirsh DC: Bacteria associated with pyothorax of dogs and cats: 98 cases (1989-1998). *J Am Vet Med Assoc* 216(3):359–363, 2000.
8. Ottenjann M, Weingart C, Arndt G, et al: Characterization of the anemia of inflammatory disease in cats with abscesses, pyothorax, or fat necrosis. *J Vet Intern Med* 20(5):1143–1150, 2006.
9. Dellinger RP, Levy M, Rhodes A, et al: Surviving sepsis campaign: international guidelines for management of severe sepsis and septic shock, 2012. *Intensive Care Med* 39(2):165–228, 2013.
10. Barrs VR, Beatty JA: Feline pyothorax—new insights into an old problem: Part 2. Treatment recommendations and prophylaxis. *Vet J* 179(2):171–178, 2009.
11. Falagas ME, Vergidis PI: Irrigation with antibiotic-containing solutions for the prevention and treatment of infections. *Clin Microbiol Infect* 11(11):862–867, 2005.

Feline Cardiopulmonary Resuscitation: Current Evidence-Based Guidelines

April E. Blong, Daniel J. Fletcher, and Manuel Boller

Cardiopulmonary resuscitation (CPR) is arguably one of the most important urgent therapeutic procedures that a veterinarian can provide to a patient; if unsuccessful, the patient will die. Although the immediate goal of CPR is the return of spontaneous circulation (ROSC), there are often more variables that ultimately determine whether or not a patient survives to discharge following a cardiopulmonary arrest (CPA) event, such as how quickly the underlying cause of the arrest can be corrected and the ability to provide adequate postcardiac arrest (PCA) care.

ETIOLOGY AND OUTCOME OF CARDIOPULMONARY ARREST

Humans who experience in-hospital CPA have a survival rate of approximately 20%, whereas cats and dogs have a survival rate of less than 6%.[1] Although many possible etiologies for CPA exist, for the purposes of discussing outcome, two categories are described here: anesthesia-related and intensive care unit (ICU) arrests. An observational study by Hofmeister and colleagues[2] demonstrated a 44% rate of ROSC but only a 7% rate of survival to discharge in all cats undergoing CPR, regardless of etiology. Among cats that were under anesthesia at the time of CPA, 71% achieved ROSC, and 43% survived to discharge. Cats that arrested in the ICU had a much lower ROSC rate (38%), and none survived to discharge. This not only demonstrates that cats with anesthesia-related CPA are more likely to survive to discharge (43%) than cats that experience CPA in the ICU (0%), but also that many cats will die in the PCA period. This phenomenon, also seen in human medicine, highlights the importance of PCA care. Among cats that obtained ROSC but did not survive to discharge, the most common reason was euthanasia, followed by recurrence of CPA. For animals that experienced a second CPA event, the median time to recurrence was 15 minutes after ROSC. Other studies have reported relatively similar numbers with 35% to 45% of cats that experience anesthesia-related CPA surviving to discharge, and none of the cats experiencing CPA in the ICU surviving to discharge.[3,4] Despite the abysmal published odds of survival for ICU patients that experience CPA, the authors have personally had ICU cases with CPA survive to discharge. Ultimately, it is likely that the severity and reversibility of the underlying disease process leading to CPA determine the chance of survival, and large veterinary data sets are needed to better understand the epidemiology of CPA in cats.

THE REASSESSMENT CAMPAIGN ON VETERINARY RESUSCITATION INITIATIVE

The Reassessment Campaign on Veterinary Resuscitation (RECOVER) initiative was intended to provide evidence-based guidelines for the care of cats and dogs experiencing CPA and to identify knowledge gaps in the literature as a foundation for future research to further strengthen and improve those guidelines.[1] In the United States, evidenced-based guidelines for human CPR have been published by the American Heart Association (AHA) since 1966, and since 1992 those guidelines have been based on a large-scale evidence evaluation process by the International Liaison Committee on Resuscitation (ILCOR).[5] Following procedures based on those used by ILCOR and the AHA to generate human CPR guidelines, the RECOVER initiative developed a list of 101 guidelines—each with an associated level and grade based on the weight of the evidence available. The majority of the recommendations discussed herein are derived from the RECOVER guidelines. The RECOVER guidelines are available in their entirety for free at http://www.acvecc-recover.org/ and in a supplemental issue of the *Journal of Veterinary Emergency and Critical Care* published in June 2012.

EARLY RECOGNITION AND PREVENTION

The adage "an ounce of prevention is worth a pound of cure" is particularly true with respect to CPA. The first step in the chain of survival involves early recognition of patients at risk for CPA, intervention to reduce this risk, and early recognition of CPA once it has occurred.[6] Given the low survival rates of patients that experience CPA, especially those in an intensive care setting,[1-4,6,7] every effort should be taken to

BOX 82-1 The Five Hs and Five Ts That May Be Useful for Identifying Patients at Risk for Cardiopulmonary Arrest

Five Hs	Five Ts
Hypovolemia or hemorrhage	Toxins
Hypoxia or hypoventilation	Tension pneumothorax
Hydrogen ions (acidosis)	Thromboembolism or
Hyperkalemia or	thrombosis
hypokalemia	Tamponade (cardiac)
Hypoglycemia	Trauma

Adapted from Boller M, Boller EM, Oodegard S, et al: Small animal cardiopulmonary resuscitation requires a continuum of care: proposal for a chain of survival for veterinary patients. *J Am Vet Med Assoc* 240:540-554, 2012.

prevent CPA. Although there is no single criterion for identification of at-risk patients, the use of a mnemonic such as the "five Hs" and the "five Ts" (Box 82-1) may help identify some of these patients. Once an at-risk patient has been identified, steps should be taken to immediately correct the detected abnormalities, and appropriate monitoring should be instituted so that further decline is rapidly recognized. Adequate education of staff, including technicians and assistants, improves the likelihood of identifying at-risk patients and intervening in time. Communication among all levels of staff, particularly at shift changes (e.g., patient rounds or written case transfers), is also important to maintain continuity of care and aid identification of at-risk patients.

Identification of Cardiopulmonary Arrest

The rapid identification of CPA is essential, because delaying the start of basic life support (BLS) results in reduced survival and worse neurologic outcome.[7-11] Unfortunately, there is little evidence to form specific guidelines for the reliable detection of CPA in humans or animals. Cardiopulmonary arrest is likely in any patient that is unresponsive, apneic (being careful not to mistake agonal breaths for breathing), and does not have obvious circulation. Rescuers are often unable to quickly and accurately assess whether or not a palpable pulse is present, and the absence of a pulse alone does not guarantee CPA; therefore, time should not be spent searching for a palpable pulse before starting CPR. In general, no more than 10 to 15 seconds should be spent diagnosing an unresponsive patient with CPA. Based on studies in humans, less than 2% of patients in whom BLS is performed experience significant injury due to chest compressions.[12,13] Given the profound potential benefit and probable lack of harm, immediate initiation of BLS is recommended in any patient in which CPA is suspected or cannot be quickly ruled out. In other words, rather than proving a patient is in CPA before starting BLS, it should be *assumed* that an unresponsive and apneic patient is experiencing CPA, and BLS should be initiated immediately.

The use of diagnostic equipment to diagnose CPA, including a stethoscope, is not recommended, except when monitoring anesthetized patients. Doppler pulse evaluation has the same potential pitfalls as digital pulse palpation. Electrocardiography (ECG) detects only the electrical activity of the heart and, therefore, is not useful for determining the presence of CPA. However, an ECG is highly valuable during the provision of CPR to guide advanced life support (ALS), which is discussed later. Capnography is potentially useful in identifying CPA in the anesthetized patient. In a patient with a constant minute ventilation, it is well known that cardiac output correlates with end-tidal carbon dioxide ($EtCO_2$) levels.[14] Cardiopulmonary arrest should be suspected in anesthetized, intubated patients undergoing constant ventilation that experience a sudden decrease in $EtCO_2$ to near zero.

Environmental Factors

A successful CPR attempt requires ready access to the appropriate equipment.[8,15] Broken or missing equipment, inadequately stocked supplies, and untrained personnel significantly delay the initiation of CPR. A crash cart or station should be maintained, regularly audited, and available at all times. All crash carts should be standardized to ensure that staff throughout the hospital are comfortable with their use. Carts should be regularly audited for completeness, equipment function, and to be sure that drugs are not expired, and ideally the carts should be sealed after auditing to ensure completeness in an emergent situation. Cognitive aids, such as charts that list emergency drug doses by body weight (Table 82-1), checklists, and CPR algorithm charts (Figure 82-1), can improve adherence to CPR protocols and should be easily visible in areas where CPA may occur. This may include the ICU, anesthesia and surgery areas, and procedure rooms. Personnel should be trained in the use of these aids.

Personnel Factors

Although no optimum team size for performing CPR has been established, one study documented that successfully resuscitated cats were treated by larger teams (for each additional team member, the odds ratio of survival was 1.68).[2] Rescuer fatigue often occurs after performing 1 to 3 minutes of continuous chest compressions.[7] Not only is a single rescuer likely to fatigue quickly, but a single person will only be able to perform BLS. Therefore, help should be called for immediately. It is important that high-quality BLS be initiated immediately; several studies have shown that the earlier high-quality BLS is initiated, the greater the survival rate—independent of other factors. When initiating CPR, seconds count.

Poor quality BLS and/or ALS due to lack of adherence to guidelines is associated with reduced survival. Staff training is a key element in the provision of high-quality CPR and achieving improved outcomes. Standardized training, incorporating both didactic and practical elements, of all staff

Table 82-1	Emergency Drugs and Doses for Cardiopulmonary Resuscitation as Published by the RECOVER Initiative											
	Weight (kg)	**2.5**	**5**	**10**	**15**	**20**	**25**	**30**	**35**	**40**	**45**	**50**
	Weight (lb)	**5**	**10**	**20**	**30**	**40**	**50**	**60**	**70**	**80**	**90**	**100**
Drug	**Dose***	**mL**	**mL**	**mL**	**mL**	**mL**	**mL**	**mL**	**mL**	**mL**	**mL**	**mL**
Arrest												
Epinephrine Low (1:1000; 1mg/mL) every other BLS cycle ×3	0.01 mg/kg	0.03	0.05	0.1	0.15	0.2	0.25	0.3	0.35	0.4	0.45	0.5
Epinephrine High (1:1000; 1 mg/mL) for prolonged CPR	0.1 mg/kg	0.25	0.5	1	1.5	2	2.5	3	3.5	4	4.5	5
Vasopressin (20 IU/mL)	0.8 IU/kg	0.1	0.2	0.4	0.6	0.8	1	1.2	1.4	1.6	1.8	2
Atropine (0.54 mg/mL)	0.04 mg/kg	0.2	0.4	0.8	1.1	1.5	1.9	2.2	2.6	3	3.3	3.7
AntiArrhythmia												
Amiodarone (50 mg/mL)	5 mg/kg	0.25	0.5	1	1.5	2	2.5	3	3.5	4	4.5	5
Lidocaine (20 mg/mL)	2 mg/kg	0.25	0.5	1	1.5	2	2.5	3	3.5	4	4.5	5
Reversal												
Naloxone (0.4 mg/mL)	0.04 mg/kg	0.25	0.5	1	1.5	2	2.5	3	3.5	4	4.5	5
Flumazenil (0.1 mg/mL)	0.01 mg/kg	0.25	0.5	1	1.5	2	2.5	3	3.5	4	4.5	5
Atipamezole (5 mg/mL)	100 μg/kg	0.06	0.1	0.2	0.3	0.4	0.5	0.5	0.7	0.8	0.9	1
Defibrillation (Monophasic)												
External defibrillation (J)	4-6 J/kg	10	20	40	60	80	100	120	140	160	180	200
Internal defibrillation (J)	0.5-1 J/kg	2	3	5	8	10	15	15	20	20	20	25

Reprinted with permission from Fletcher DJ, Boller M, Brainard BM, et al: RECOVER evidence and knowledge gap analysis on veterinary CPR. Part 7: clinical guidelines. *J Vet Emerg Crit Care* 22:S102-S131, 2012.
BLS, Basic life support; *CPR*, cardiopulmonary resuscitation; *RECOVER*, Reassessment Campaign on Veterinary Resuscitation.
*All doses are given in mL so that no calculations are required during CPR.

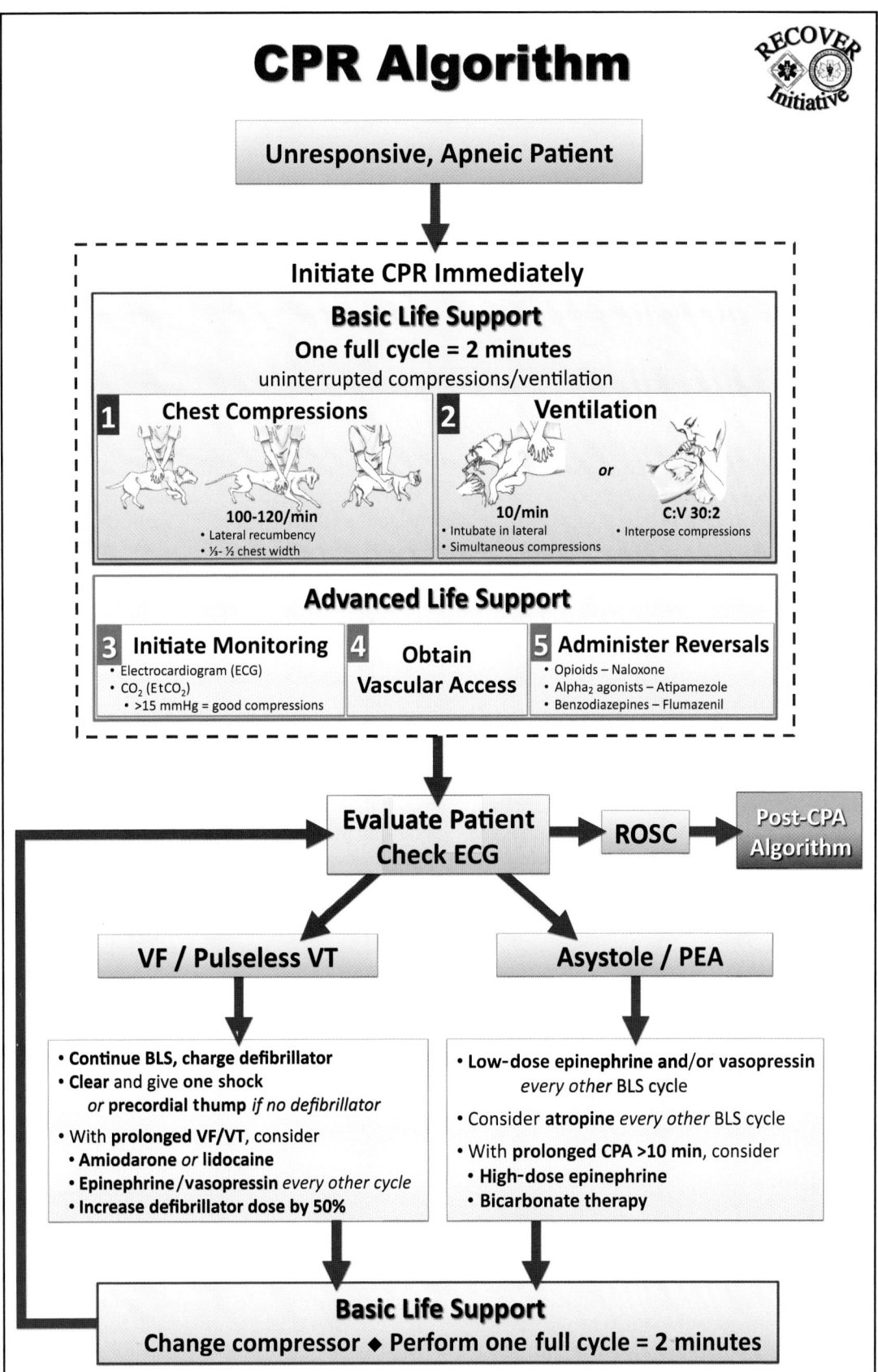

Figure 82-1: The overall basic life support *(BLS)* and advanced life support cardiopulmonary resuscitation *(CPR)* algorithm published by the Reassessment Campaign on Veterinary Resuscitation (RECOVER) initiative. *CPA,* Cardiopulmonary arrest; *C:V,* compression:ventilation ratio; *PEA,* pulseless electrical activity; *ROSC,* return of spontaneous circulation; *VF,* ventricular fibrillation; *VT,* ventricular tachycardia. (Reprinted with permission from Fletcher DJ, Boller M, Brainard BM, et al: RECOVER evidence and knowledge gap analysis on veterinary CPR. Part 7: clinical guidelines. *J Vet Emerg Crit Care* 22:S102-S131, 2012.)

members who may be involved with administration of CPR is recommended. Unfortunately, regardless of the training methods used, CPR skills begin to deteriorate within weeks, necessitating refresher training at a minimum of every 6 months. A structured debriefing session following simulated or real CPR efforts is a low-cost, safe, and readily available method to improve performance. During these sessions, participants share information about the event, discuss their performance, and identify any problems within the practice that need to be addressed.

Effective communication among team members during a CPR event is crucial to ensure that orders are followed quickly and correctly. Leadership training for individuals who head CPR efforts is recommended; in human studies, it has been shown to improve CPR performance. Using tools, such as closed loop communication, can also improve performance. Closed loop communication involves an order being given directly from one team member to another, followed by the receiving team member repeating the order back to the first team member to ensure accuracy.

BASIC LIFE SUPPORT

The remainder of this chapter reviews the RECOVER CPR algorithm (see Figure 82-1). The algorithm begins with the second link in the chain of survival, the provision of BLS.[6] Early, high-quality BLS is an independent predictor of survival following CPA.[15] Basic life support should be administered following the CAB model—first address **C**irculation, then **A**irway, then **B**reathing. This change in approach from airway-breathing-circulation to CAB is reflective of recent evidence that delays and interruptions in chest compressions are associated with worse outcomes in CPR.[7,8] Moreover, chest compressions generate some ventilation due to lung compression, whereas the reverse is not true; ventilation is unlikely to be beneficial in the absence of circulation. Despite this emphasis on the importance of early initiation of high-quality chest compressions, the recommendation for earliest possible initiation of ventilation persists. Thus, the clinical CAB recommendation has to be interpreted as starting chest compressions immediately and initiating ventilation as early as possible.

Chest Compressions

Two theories exist to account for generation of blood flow during CPR: the cardiac pump theory and the thoracic pump theory.[6,16,17] The *cardiac pump theory* posits that blood flow is created when the ventricles of the heart are directly compressed by the ribs when pressure is placed on the thoracic wall over the heart. The *thoracic pump theory* states that blood flow is generated by compressing the thorax, which increases the intrathoracic pressure, collapses the vena cava preventing backward flow of blood, and compresses the lungs and aorta, resulting in blood flow into the left side of the heart and out of the thorax. This is followed by chest wall recoil, which

creates subatmospheric pressure in the thorax, promoting venous return of blood to the right side of the heart and into the lungs. In most patients, both methods contribute to blood flow to some extent.

At best, external chest compressions during CPR achieve 25% to 30% of normal cardiac output. Numerous studies have emphasized the importance of uninterrupted chest compressions to improve the chances of achieving ROSC.[7,8] Given that the same has not been shown for ventilation, the CAB approach to BLS should be followed. Chest compressions should begin immediately after the identification of known or suspected CPA, and the frequency and duration of interruptions should be minimized.

Chest compressions should be performed with the patient in lateral recumbency. An observational study in both cats and dogs found that patients in lateral, rather than dorsal, recumbency were more likely to achieve ROSC.[2]

Cats usually have narrow and highly compliant chests, and the cardiac pump theory is thought to predominate. To maximize the effectiveness of the cardiac pump, compressions in cats should be centered over the heart, which is located between the fourth and sixth intercostal spaces. This position can be quickly located by pulling the elbow caudally until it lies approximately over the costochondral junction, which is one-third of the distance from the sternum to the spine (Figure 82-2A). In most cats, chest compressions can be performed using a one-hand technique. The nondominant hand is placed behind the spine to stabilize the cat, and the dominant hand is wrapped around the sternum at the level of the heart with the thumb on one side and the fingers on the other (see Figure 82-2B). Compressions are achieved by moving the base of the thumb toward the fingers to maximize compression of the ventricles from the apex to the base, facilitating blood flow out of the ventricles. If the tip of the thumb is pressed against the chest, the heart is compressed only at the base, resulting in poor ejection of blood from the ventricles. In obese cats, or in cases when the rescuer is fatiguing using the one-hand approach, a two-hand technique can be used instead. The hands are placed one on top of the other, and the heel of the hand in contact with the chest is placed directly over the heart (see Figure 82-2C). Care should be taken to use correct posture, with the elbows locked, shoulders centered over the hands, and the core muscles used to achieve the compressions and reduce fatigue.

Compression rates of 100 to 120 per minute are recommended, rather than higher rates approaching normal feline resting heart rates, based on neonatal human and animal studies. More rapid compressions lead to lower cardiac output due to inadequate filling times. A compression depth between one-third to one-half of the width of the thorax is likely ideal, and care should be taken to avoid overcompressing the highly compliant cat thorax. Allowing full chest wall recoil between compressions has been shown to improve hemodynamic performance during CPR. "Leaning" on the patient (which does not allow full chest wall recoil) occurs commonly during human CPR and may increase with rescuer fatigue.

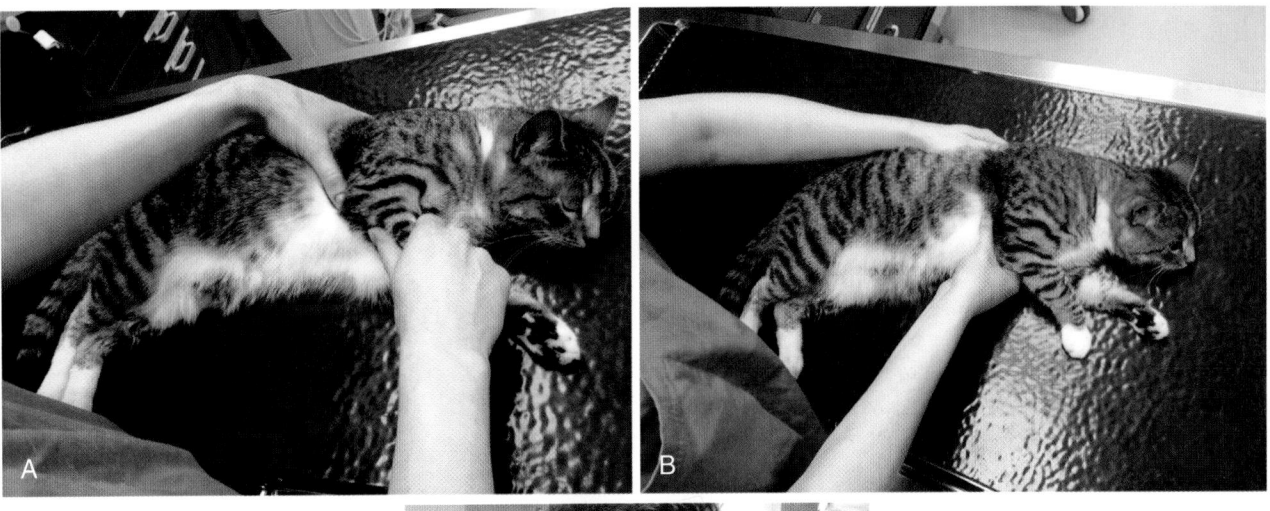

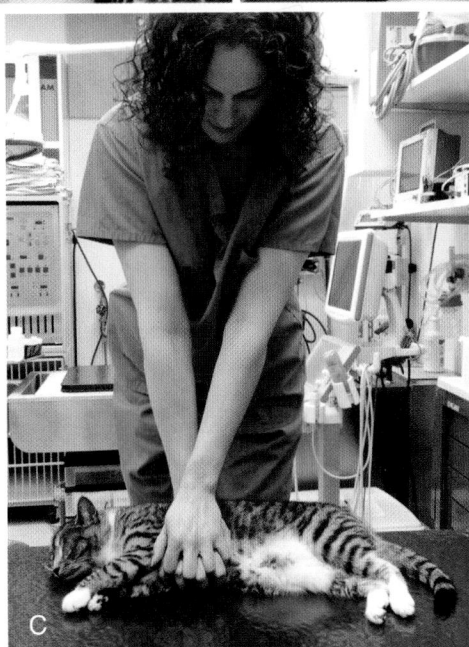

Figure 82-2: **A,** To find the optimal location for chest compressions in the cat, pull the elbow caudally until it rests over the costochondral junction, approximately one-third of the ventral-dorsal distance from the sternum to the spine. This will lie over the fourth to sixth intercostal space, approximately over the cardiac ventricles. **B,** Wrap the dominant hand around the sternum with the thumb over the heart to perform the one-hand compression technique. Compressions are achieved by pressing the entire thumb, not just the tip of the thumb, against the rest of the hand, achieving a compression of the heart from the apex to the base. The nondominant hand is placed against the spine to hold the cat in place. The compressor should convert to the two-hand technique if fatigued. **C,** Two-hand compressions are performed by placing one hand over the other with the palms aligned and the fingers interlaced. The palm of the hand in contact with the chest is placed over the location of the heart, the elbows are locked, the shoulders are located directly above the hands, and compressions are achieved by bending at the waist, engaging the core muscles.

Ventilation

The presence of either hypoxia or hypercapnia reduces the rate of ROSC; therefore, ventilation should be provided as soon as possible following the commencement of chest compressions. There is a single veterinary case report documenting successful mouth-to-snout ventilation in a dog.[18] If using this technique, ventilation should be provided using a 30:2 compression:ventilation ratio, with 30 chest compressions delivered, followed by a brief pause during which two quick mouth-to-snout breaths are delivered, and an immediate return to chest compressions.

Positive pressure ventilation with a cuffed endotracheal tube (ET) is more effective than mouth-to-snout ventilation and results in fewer pauses in chest compressions. Because cats are relatively easy to intubate, mouth-to-snout ventilation is recommended only in cases of single rescuer CPR or when intubation supplies are not available. An ET allows for delivery of 100% oxygen, enables more controlled ventilation, reduces the likelihood of aspiration, and prevents gastric distention during forced breaths.[19] Endotracheal placement should occur in lateral recumbency to avoid interruptions in chest compressions. Once in place, the cuff on the tube should be inflated and the tube secured to avoid dislodgement. Confirmation of ET placement should be achieved via direct visualization of the tube between the arytenoid cartilages, auscultation of air movement in both sides of the thorax, observation of chest wall motion, and/or by the presence of condensation in the tube. Capnography alone *cannot* be used to reliably confirm ET placement. In patients with CPA, EtCO$_2$ levels may be extremely low due to poor or absent blood flow and not due to incorrect ET placement.

Based on the evidence evaluated by the RECOVER initiative, the current recommendation is to give 10 breaths per minute, with a tidal volume of 10 mL/kg and an inspiratory time of 1 second. Studies suggest that higher rates, tidal volumes, and inspiratory times lead to decreased venous return because of a higher mean intrathoracic pressure and arterial hypocapnia due to the reduced delivery of CO$_2$ to the lungs during CPR. Hypocapnia causes vasoconstriction, resulting in decreased coronary and cerebral perfusion, which can lead to poorer outcomes.

Cycles of Cardiopulmonary Resuscitation

Occasional interruptions in chest compressions are needed for ECG rhythm assessment to guide ALS and to alternate rescuers so as to avoid fatigue. Two-minute cycles of compressions are recommended, because more frequent interruptions result in worsened outcomes. The average rescuer exhibits fatigue resulting in a deterioration of the quality of compressions within 1 to 3 minutes, and this fatigue may be more pronounced with one-hand compressions. It is not possible to interpret an ECG rhythm during chest compressions due to artifact. However, while changing which rescuer is performing compressions, the ECG can be assessed and pulses palpated to determine if a shockable rhythm is present or if ROSC has been achieved. This delay should be limited to no more than a few seconds.

ADVANCED LIFE SUPPORT

Advanced life support—including drug therapy, defibrillation, as well as correction of intravascular volume deficits, electrolyte abnormalities, and acid-base disturbances—is the third link in the chain of survival and is the next step in the RECOVER CPR algorithm (see Figure 82-1).[6,8,20] It is important that BLS not be compromised for the sake of ALS, but rather that ALS be instituted after BLS commencement. With immediate and high-quality BLS and ALS, ROSC rates may approach 50% in some subpopulations of CPA patients, such as those with perianesthetic CPA.

Routes of Drug Delivery

Intravenous Route

Venous access should be gained as rapidly as possible during ALS and ideally without interruptions of chest compressions. The use of an existing patent intravenous (IV) catheter is ideal. In the absence of an existing catheter, attempts can be made to gain peripheral or central venous access. Although either route is acceptable, drug administration via a peripheral vein results in a longer delay in the time of drug onset. The cephalic vein is preferred, because it is superior to the saphenous vein for rapidity of onset. Central or jugular venous drug administration results in the shortest time to onset of action. Following drug administration, flushing with at least 0.5 mL/kg of isotonic crystalloid can minimize the delay in drug onset when given through a peripheral vein.[21] Cut-down techniques should be employed early if a vein is not readily visible to minimize delays in achieving vascular access.

Intraosseous Route

Intraosseous (IO) catheters should be considered in cats and can be quickly placed. The use of a spinal needle with stylet is recommended to prevent plugging of the needle with cortical bone. Potential sites of access include the proximal femur and proximal humerus, with placement of the catheter perpendicular to the long axis of the bone. Specialized equipment is available to provide rapid placement of IO catheters in the tibia or humerus. These commercially available devices (EZ-IO catheter; Vidacare, Shavano Park, Texas) use single-use needle catheters placed with a reusable drill, allowing IO catheters to be placed within a few seconds.

Endotracheal Route

Many drugs can also be administered endotracheally, but absorption and onset of action are highly variable, and survival rates are lower than with IV or IO administration.

Endotracheal drug administration should only be used as a last resort when IV or IO access cannot be gained. For most drugs, the dosage should be increased at least twofold to threefold for endotracheal administration. When administering epinephrine endotracheally, a dose of 0.1 mg/kg (equivalent to high-dose epinephrine or 10 times the standard dose) should be used. All drugs should be diluted in sterile water or 0.9% saline and given via a catheter longer than the ET. Not all drugs can be given by this route, and some (such as sodium bicarbonate) may be dangerous. The use of the mnemonic NAVEL (Box 82-2) can be used as a reminder of which drugs can be administered by the endotracheal route during CPR.

Monitoring During Cardiopulmonary Resuscitation

Electrocardiogram Interpretation

An accurate rhythm diagnosis is essential for determining which ALS interventions are most likely to be of benefit. Chest compressions cause significant interference and preclude rhythm diagnosis. However, during the brief pause that occurs during exchange of the rescuer performing compressions at the end of each 2-minute cycle of BLS, a brief rhythm interpretation (lasting only a few seconds) should be done, after which chest compressions should be promptly resumed. During rhythm check, the femoral pulse or apex beat should be palpated to determine if spontaneous circulation has commenced. In cats, the apex beat is likely the more reliable sign. The goal of the rhythm analysis is to diagnose one of three types of rhythms: (1) shockable rhythms requiring defibrillation, (2) nonshockable rhythms, and (3) perfusing rhythms associated with a palpable apex beat.

The shockable arrest rhythms are ventricular fibrillation (VF) and pulseless ventricular tachycardia (VT). Ventricular fibrillation is caused by uncoordinated depolarization of many individual groups of ventricular myocardial cells, resulting in ineffective contraction. Pulseless VT is a rapid ventricular rhythm, generally occurring at greater than 200 beats per minute, which is too rapid to allow ventricular filling. Although both mechanical and electrical activity are present, no significant blood flow is generated and the patients are in CPA. Ventricular fibrillation may be diagnosed based on

small amplitude random ECG activity that does not result in repeating complexes. Pulseless VT may be diagnosed based on a repeated ECG rhythm that generally consists of wide QRS complexes at a rate of greater than 200 per minute that is not associated with a palpable pulse or apex beat, or auscultable heartbeat.

The nonshockable arrest rhythms are asystole and pulseless electrical activity (PEA). For both rhythms, there is no mechanical activity in the heart, but in PEA the electrical conduction system is conducting electrical impulses and an ECG shows waveform activity. Asystole is easily diagnosed as a flat-line ECG, whereas PEA can take on a wide variety of appearances but generally consists of repeating QRS complexes that are narrower than pulseless VT and occur at a rate of less than 200 per minute. These complexes can look like normal sinus complexes and may or may not have associated P waves, but they are not associated with a palpable apex beat or pulse.

If a pulse is palpable during the intercycle pause in chest compressions, then ROSC has likely occurred and a perfusing rhythm has been restored. Cardiopulmonary resuscitation can be discontinued and PCA care should be initiated.

End-Tidal Carbon Dioxide Monitoring

End-tidal CO_2 monitoring can be useful during CPR in several ways. First, $EtCO_2$ strongly correlates with cardiac output when minute ventilation is held constant and, therefore, can reflect the quality of BLS being provided during CPR. Several animal and human studies have demonstrated that patients with higher $EtCO_2$ levels during CPR are more likely to achieve ROSC. If capnography is available, rescuers should adjust their chest compression technique to maintain $EtCO_2$ levels of 15 mm Hg or higher. Second, because ROSC is associated with larger increases in cardiac output compared to those achievable during CPR, $EtCO_2$ will often dramatically increase when ROSC is obtained. Monitoring $EtCO_2$ may allow for early identification of ROSC without the need to interrupt cycles of CPR. Third, persistently low $EtCO_2$ levels may indicate esophageal intubation. Although it should not be used as the only criterion, persistently low $EtCO_2$ should prompt verification of correct ET placement by direct visualization.

Other Monitoring

Pulse oximetry, indirect blood pressure monitoring, and blood gases are of limited use early in CPR. Pulse oximetry and indirect blood pressure monitoring technologies require a regular, measurable pulse and are highly susceptible to motion artifact, making them unreliable during CPR. Arterial blood gas monitoring is of little value during CPR, but venous blood gas monitoring may give information about the quality of CPR. Early in CPA, blood gas values are remarkably normal, but as more time passes, low central venous CO_2, low pH, and elevated lactate are associated with poor cardiac output and, therefore, may reflect poor CPR technique. Venous blood gas sampling may also allow the identification and possible treatment of severe electrolyte disturbances, such as hyperkalemia.

Reversal Agents

Some analgesic and sedative drugs have specific reversal agents. In the case of an accidental overdose or toxicity, a specific reversal agent should be used if available. Naloxone (0.04 mg/kg IV or IO) can be used for opioid reversal, flumazenil (0.01 mg/kg IV or IO) can be given to reverse benzodiazepines, and atipamezole (0.1 mg/kg IV or IO) can be used to reverse alpha-2 agonists. In the absence of an overdose, there is no evidence documenting improved outcome with the use of reversal agents, but they are unlikely to do harm and may carry some benefit long after administration because of reduced hepatic drug metabolism in cats with CPA.

Treatment of Nonshockable Rhythms

Vasopressors should be administered as early as possible in patients with nonshockable rhythms, usually after the first cycle of BLS and as soon as an ECG rhythm diagnosis is made. In patients with shockable rhythms, vasopressors are generally reserved for patients that remain in VF or pulseless VT for more than 10 minutes and do not respond to defibrillation therapy.

Epinephrine is a nonspecific adrenergic agonist traditionally used in CPR. Benefits of epinephrine during CPR are achieved through its vasopressor activity (alpha-1 mediated). Epinephrine's beta-1 activity, and the associated increase in inotropy and chronotropy, may actually be harmful during CPR, heightening myocardial oxygen demand in a patient already experiencing hypoxia. Current guidelines recommend epinephrine at the standard dose of 0.01 mg/kg IV or IO given every 3 to 5 minutes or every other 2-minute BLS cycle when a nonshockable rhythm is present until cessation of CPR. The use of high-dose epinephrine (0.1 mg/kg) has been associated with a higher rate of ROSC in experimental studies, but both experimental and clinical studies have shown no improvement or even decreases in survival to discharge. In light of these findings, high-dose epinephrine should only be used (if at all) during a prolonged CPR attempt if standard-dose epinephrine has been unsuccessful, and it should be used with the knowledge that it may lead to poorer long-term survival. The RECOVER guidelines suggest that high-dose epinephrine may be considered after 10 minutes of CPR, but given the data on survival to discharge, it may be wise to continue longer with standard-dose epinephrine in patients with better odds of survival, such as those with perianesthetic CPA.

Vasopressin is a noncatecholamine vasopressor. It exerts its effects via the peripheral V1 receptors on vascular smooth muscle cells. In contrast to catecholamine receptors, the V1 receptor remains active in the presence of acidosis, which is common in patients with CPA. Vasopressin also lacks potentially harmful beta-1 effects. Although it has not yet been

shown to be superior to epinephrine, vasopressin seems to have efficacy equal to epinephrine. Vasopressin can be used in lieu of or in combination with epinephrine at a dose of 0.8 IU/kg IV given every 3 to 5 minutes or every other 2-minute BLS cycle when a nonshockable rhythm is present until cessation of CPR.

Atropine, a parasympatholytic agent, has been extensively used in CPR. When used at the standard dose of 0.04 mg/kg IV, there is no evidence demonstrating a clear benefit or detriment to the use of atropine, so it may be considered during CPR. Although direct evidence is lacking, cats experiencing bradycardic arrests due to high vagal tone from severe respiratory disease, asphyxia, gastrointestinal disease, or ocular disease may benefit from early administration of atropine. Higher doses of atropine are clearly associated with a worse outcome and are *not* recommended. Atropine is also not recommended in cats with shockable arrest rhythms.

Treatment of Shockable Rhythms

Shockable rhythms occur less commonly in cats with CPA than in humans,[22] but VF and pulseless VT can occur in cats and should be promptly treated with electrical defibrillation. The goal of electrical defibrillation is to depolarize as many cardiomyocytes as possible so that they then enter a refractory period, stopping the uncoordinated or rapid ventricular activity. The normal pacemaker cells of the sinoatrial node can then resume rhythm control and restore coordinated, effective ventricular contraction. Two types of electrical defibrillators are currently available: monophasic and biphasic. Monophasic defibrillators send current in one direction between the paddles, whereas biphasic defibrillators send current in one direction and then back in the opposite direction. Biphasic defibrillators can successfully terminate VF using lower energy than monophasic defibrillators, thereby causing less cardiomyocyte injury. For this reason, biphasic defibrillators are preferred over monophasic defibrillators. The recommended starting dose is 2 to 4 J/kg when using a biphasic defibrillator or 4 to 6 J/kg with a monophasic defibrillator. In cats, the use of pediatric paddle inserts is recommended, because standard adult hand paddles are likely too large and will result in current passing through an area that is too extensive. If pediatric paddle inserts are not available, internal defibrillation paddles may be used externally on cats.

To defibrillate, the cat should be placed in dorsal recumbency and paddles placed on opposite sides of the chest over the heart (Figure 82-3A). Copious amounts of an electrically conductive gel should be used to allow good contact with the patient and avoid burns. Care must be taken to ensure that the person defibrillating the cat and all other members of the team are not touching the cat during the defibrillation, because serious injury can occur. A loud, verbal "clear" should be announced before defibrillating, and the person defibrillating should visually confirm that no one is touching the cat or table. Some defibrillators are supplied with a posterior paddle assembly that can be placed under the patient, allowing defibrillation to be done by placing the single hand paddle

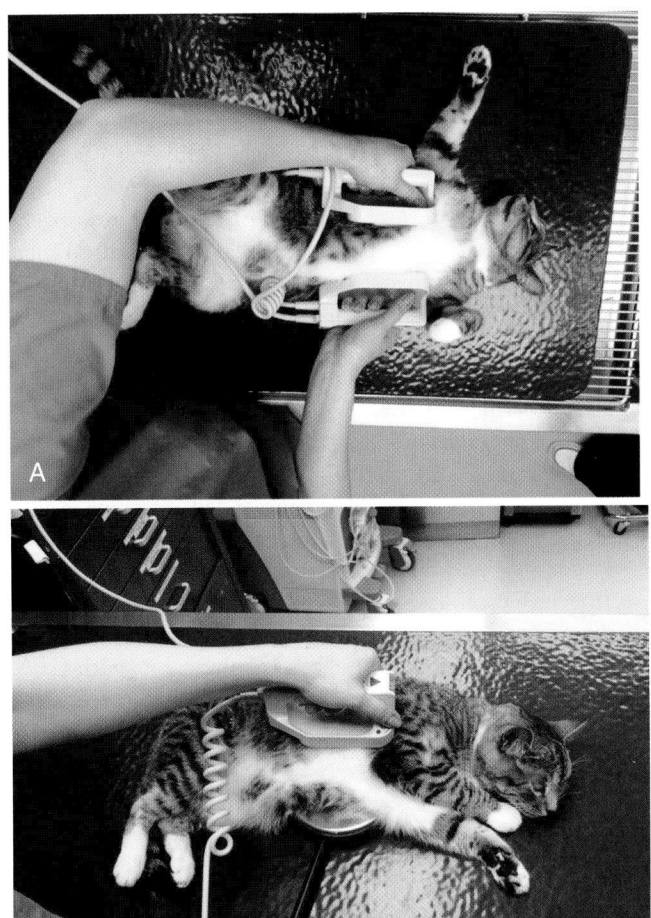

Figure 82-3: A, To defibrillate, the cat is placed in dorsal recumbency, and pediatric or internal paddles are pushed firmly against opposite sides of the chest. Nonflammable coupling gel is used to improve contact with the skin. To prevent serious injury, care must be taken to ensure that no one, including the person defibrillating, is in contact with the cat or the table before the defibrillator is discharged. **B,** A posterior paddle assembly can be used as an alternative to two hand paddles. The posterior paddle is placed below the cat in lateral recumbency. To defibrillate, the hand paddle is placed on the upper chest wall. The cat can be defibrillated in lateral recumbency using this device, making the procedure safer for the rescuers and reducing pauses in chest compressions necessitated by rolling the cat into dorsal recumbency to defibrillate.

on the upward facing chest wall, affording defibrillation in lateral recumbency (see Figure 82-3B). The posterior paddle can be left in place during chest compressions. After a single defibrillation attempt, BLS should be immediately reinitiated for a full 2-minute cycle before the next rhythm assessment and defibrillation if necessary. If more than one defibrillation attempt is needed, the energy dose may be escalated by 50% each cycle up to a maximum dose of 10 J/kg for a monophasic defibrillator or to the machine maximum dose on a biphasic defibrillator. Two-minute cycles of BLS, followed by a single defibrillation should be repeated until a nonshockable or perfusing rhythm develops.

Vasopressor administration can also be considered in the presence of a shockable rhythm, if CPR has been prolonged (i.e., more than 10 minutes), because the associated increase in myocardial blood flow and oxygenation may facilitate successful electrical defibrillation.

If an electrical defibrillator is not available, mechanical defibrillation may be attempted using a precordial thump when VF or pulseless VT is present. This is performed by striking the patient with the heel of hand, directly over the heart. In cats, this should be done carefully so as not to cause trauma to the myocardium. The efficacy of mechanical defibrillation is minimal and should never be used as a substitute if an electrical defibrillator is available.

Intravenous Fluid Therapy

Coronary perfusion pressure is determined by the difference between the aortic and right atrial pressures during diastole. The administration of high rates of IV fluids during CPR to euvolemic animals (other than following drug administration) will increase right atrial pressure, resulting in decreased coronary perfusion. Therefore, the routine use of resuscitative fluid therapy and large volume boluses in euvolemic patients during CPR is *not* recommended. The exception is patients with pre-existing hypovolemia. In these patients, the administration of fluids during CPR may improve circulating volume and perfusion.

Other Drug Therapy

Corticosteroids have historically been used for the treatment of many conditions, including shock, and as a routine part of CPR. Given that no studies show a clear benefit associated with the use of corticosteroids during CPR and their potential for deleterious side effects, the routine use of corticosteroids during CPR is *not* recommended.

The most effective therapy for VF and pulseless VT is electrical defibrillation. For this reason, the routine use of antiarrhythmic drugs during CPR is *not* recommended. However, in cases that are resistant to electrical defibrillation, drug therapy may be a useful adjunct. Amiodarone (5 mg/kg IV) is the only antiarrhythmic agent shown to have consistent benefit in treating resistant VF or pulseless VT; however, hypotension and anaphylaxis have been described in dogs, and there is no data on the use of this drug in cats in CPA. Lidocaine (0.25-0.5 mg/kg IV slowly to effect) could also be used for resistant arrhythmias, but when using a monophasic defibrillator, a higher energy dose may be required to terminate shockable rhythms after lidocaine administration based on experimental studies in dogs and other animals for reasons that are not known.[23] In the specific case of torsades de pointes, magnesium sulfate may useful.

Severe metabolic acidosis commonly occurs during CPA. The use of sodium bicarbonate during CPR is somewhat controversial, and therefore its routine use is *not* recommended. Sodium bicarbonate increases serum osmolarity, can cause alkalemia, and may cause paradoxical cerebral and metabolic acidosis. When given early in the course of CPR (in the first 10 minutes), it may actually worsen metabolic derangements and outcome. However, after prolonged CPA (greater than 10 to 15 minutes), it may improve outcome and a dose of 1 mEq/kg IV or IO may be considered.

Calcium is necessary for many processes in the body, including muscle contraction. Although the routine administration of calcium is *not* recommended, administration to patients with a documented severe ionized hypocalcemia theoretically may be beneficial. The treatment of hypokalemia during CPR has not been evaluated but may be of use. Moderate-to-severe hyperkalemia directly affects cardiac myocyte function and should be treated if present. Standard treatments for hyperkalemia (such as the administration of calcium gluconate, dextrose, and bicarbonate) could all be considered.

Open-Chest Cardiopulmonary Resuscitation

Open-chest cardiopulmonary resuscitation (OC-CPR) requires minimal equipment and training, but if ROSC is achieved, staff and facilities to handle a nonsterile thoracotomy must be available, as well as the ability to provide advanced PCA care. In canine models of VF, OC-CPR results in higher rates of ROSC and survival, as well as improved neurologic outcome. In cases where there is preexisting thoracic disease, such as tension pneumothorax or pericardial effusion, prompt OC-CPR is reasonable. Severe thoracic wall injury, diaphragmatic hernia, and pleural space disease (such as effusion and pneumothorax) are other indications for OC-CPR. If CPA develops intraoperatively when the chest or abdomen is already open, easy access to the heart (through the diaphragm in the case of abdominal surgery) is available for direct cardiac compression and, therefore, OC-CPR should be considered in these situations. However, given the high thoracic compliance and the keel-chested conformation of most cats, which lends itself to highly efficacious chest compressions, OC-CPR is rarely indicated in most cats with CPA.

POSTCARDIAC ARREST CARE

The fourth, and final, link in the chain of survival is PCA care.[24] Postcardiac arrest syndrome is a combination of anoxic brain injury, systemic ischemia, and reperfusion injury, resulting in multiorgan failure, cardiogenic shock due to postischemic myocardial dysfunction, and preexisting or precipitating diseases. Given the large number of patients that will die during this time, significant attention, monitoring, and patient care need to be devoted to the PCA patient.

Hemodynamic and ventilatory support are essential aspects of PCA care. Although not specifically validated in this patient population, using goal-directed therapy is likely of benefit in the PCA patient. This includes optimizing hemodynamic variables, such as central venous oxygen

saturation, lactate, arterial blood pressure, central venous pressure, hematocrit, and arterial oxygen saturation. Significant hypocapnia results in arteriolar vasoconstriction and can lead to brain hypoxia; alternatively, hypercapnia results in vasodilation and increased intracranial pressure.[25] To avoid both of these scenarios, it is prudent to strive for a normal partial arterial pressure of carbon dioxide of approximately 32 mm Hg. Although it is clear that hypoxemia should be avoided, hyperoxemia is also potentially harmful, because it can result in increased levels of reactive oxygen species, resulting in further cell injury. Oxygen supplementation should be provided as needed to maintain a normal oxygen tension (partial arterial pressure of oxygen of 80 to 100 mm Hg, saturation of peripheral oxygen of 94% to 98%). Assisted ventilation may be required for some patients. The RECOVER PCA algorithm (Figure 82-4) provides an overview of the concepts of goal-directed therapy for these patients.

Postcardiac arrest patients should be closely monitored in an intensive care setting on a 24-hour basis for changes in condition and additional impending episodes of CPA. Studies in humans demonstrate improved outcomes in patients treated at facilities with more PCA care experience. Referral facilities and specialty centers are more likely to have advanced monitoring and therapeutic techniques available, 24-hour care, and PCA care experience. For these reasons, referral to such an institution should be strongly considered, once the patient is stable for transport.

SUMMARY

The AHA recommends that lay-rescuers "push hard and fast" when someone experiences collapse or is found collapsed. The evidence-based guidelines recently provided by the RECOVER initiative support that statement with regard to veterinary CPR as well but suggest that in cats, one should strive to push fast and hard, but not "too hard."

Chest compressions should be immediately started in all cats suspected of experiencing CPA rather than delaying the provision of CPR in an attempt to confirm or exclude the presence of CPA. Basic life support is arguably the most important link in the chain of survival and, thus, every effort should be made to ensure adequate staff training so that high-quality BLS can be achieved as quickly as possible. Once quality BLS has been implemented, ALS interventions (such as drug therapy and defibrillation) should be added. Unfortunately, despite one's best efforts, the veterinary literature suggests that feline survival rates are very low. However, in cats with reversible, acute diseases (such as anesthetic drug reactions, witnessed asphyxiation, vagal arrest, some types of trauma, or acute hypovolemia) the odds of survival are likely much greater if high-quality CPR is initiated promptly. Ensuring that all members of the veterinary healthcare team are trained in the new evidence-based CPR guidelines and are prepared for an acute crisis has the potential to dramatically increase the odds of survival for these patients.

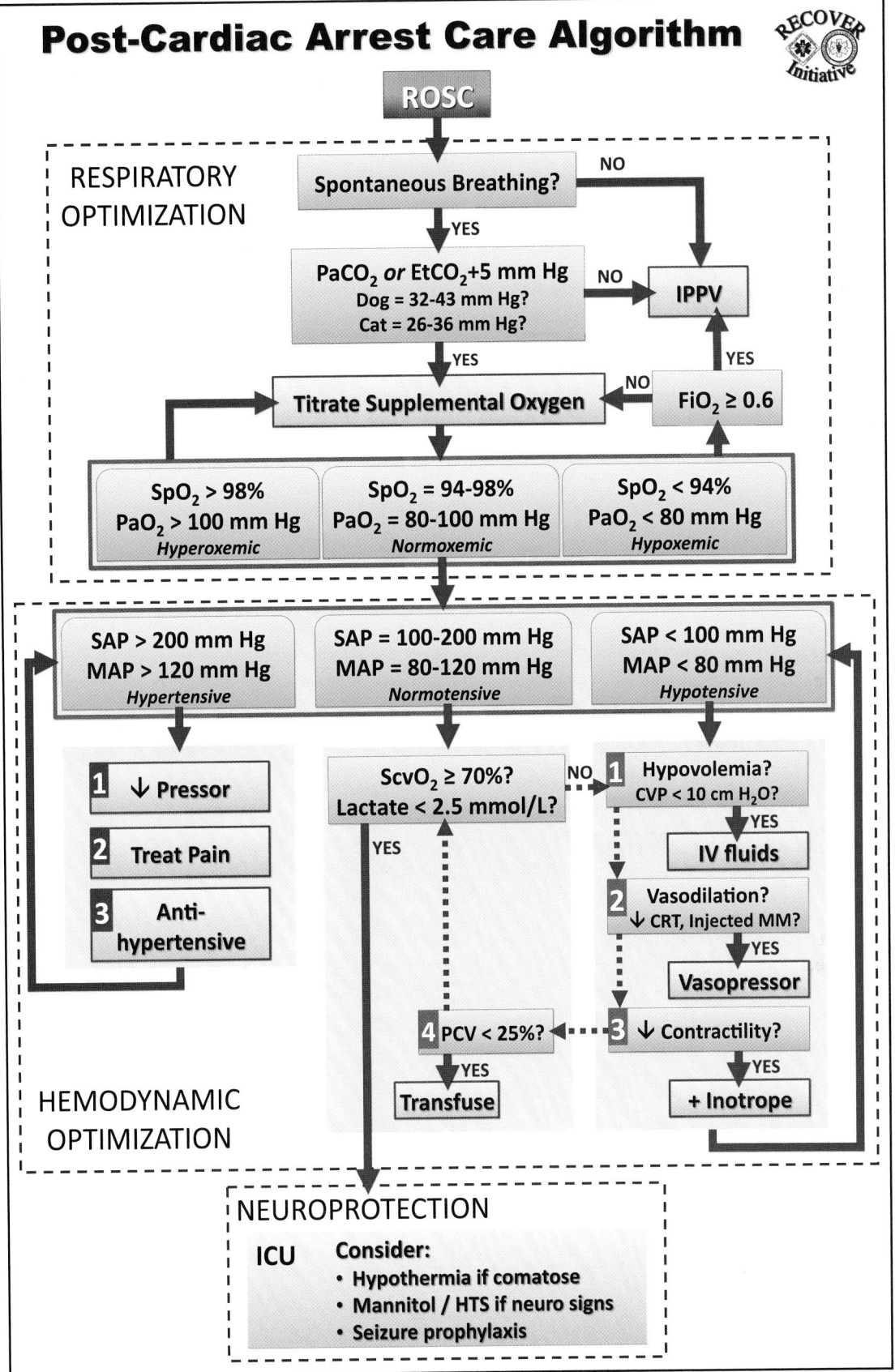

Figure 82-4: The postcardiac arrest (PCA) algorithm published by the Reassessment Campaign on Veterinary Resuscitation (RECOVER) initiative. *BLS,* Basic life support; *CPA,* cardiopulmonary arrest; *CPR,* cardiopulmonary resuscitation; *C:V,* compression:ventilation ratio; *PEA,* pulseless electrical activity; *ROSC,* return of spontaneous circulation; *VF,* ventricular fibrillation; *VT,* ventricular tachycardia. (Reprinted with permission from Fletcher DJ, Boller M, Brainard BM, et al: RECOVER evidence and knowledge gap analysis on veterinary CPR. Part 7: clinical guidelines. *J Vet Emerg Crit Care* 22:S102-S131, 2012.)

CRT, capillary refill time; *CVP,* central venous pressure; *FiO₂,* fraction of inspired oxygen; *HTS,* hypertonic saline; *ICU,* intensive care unit; *IPPV,* intermittent positive pressure ventilation; *MAP,* mean arterial pressure; *MM,* mucous membranes; *PaO₂,* partial pressure arterial oxygen; *PCV,* packed cell volume; *SAP,* systolic arterial pressure; *ScvO₂,* central venous oxygen saturation; *SpO₂,* peripheral capillary oxygen saturation.

References

1. Boller M, Fletcher DJ: RECOVER evidence and knowledge gap analysis on veterinary CPR. Part 1: evidence analysis and consensus process: collaborative path toward small animal CPR guidelines. *J Vet Emerg Crit Care* 22:S4–S12, 2012.

2. Hofmeister EH, Brainard BM, Egger CM, et al: Prognostic indicators for dogs and cats with cardiopulmonary arrest treated by cardiopulmonary cerebral resuscitation at a university teaching hospital. *J Am Vet Med Assoc* 235:50–57, 2009.

3. Kass PH, Haskins SC: Survival following cardiopulmonary resuscitation in dogs and cats. *J Vet Emerg Crit Care* 2:57–65, 1992.

4. Waldrop JE, Rozanski EA, Swanke ED, et al: Causes of cardiopulmonary arrest, resuscitation management, and functional outcome in dogs and cats surviving cardiopulmonary arrest. *J Vet Emerg Crit Care* 14:22–29, 2004.

5. Field JM, Hazinski MF, Sayre MR, et al: Part 1: executive summary: 2010 American Heart Association Guidelines for Cardiopulmonary Resuscitation and Emergency Cardiovascular Care. *Circulation* 122:S640–S656, 2010.

6. Boller M, Boller EM, Oodegard S, et al: Small animal cardiopulmonary resuscitation requires a continuum of care: proposal for a chain of survival for veterinary patients. *J Am Vet Med Assoc* 240:540–554, 2012.

7. Hopper K, Epstein SE, Fletcher DJ, et al: RECOVER evidence and knowledge gap analysis on veterinary CPR. Part 3: basic life support. *J Vet Emerg Crit Care* 22:S26–S43, 2012.

8. Fletcher DJ, Boller M, Brainard BM, et al: RECOVER evidence and knowledge gap analysis on veterinary CPR. Part 7: clinical guidelines. *J Vet Emerg Crit Care* 22:S102–S131, 2012.

9. Brainard BM, Boller M, Fletcher DJ: RECOVER evidence and knowledge gap analysis on veterinary CPR. Part 5: monitoring. *J Vet Emerg Crit Care* 22:S65–S84, 2012.

10. Deasy C, Bray JE, Smith K, et al: Cardiac arrest outcomes before and after the 2005 resuscitation guidelines implementation: Evidence of improvement? *Resuscitation* 82:984–988, 2011.

11. Hinchey PR, Myers JB, Lewis R, et al: Improved out-of-hospital cardiac arrest survival after the sequential implementation of 2005 AHA guidelines for compressions, ventilations, and induced hypothermia: the Wake County experience. *Ann Emerg Med* 56:348–357, 2010.

12. White L, Rogers J, Bloomingdale M, et al: Dispatcher-assisted cardiopulmonary resuscitation: risks for patients not in cardiac arrest. *Circulation* 121:91–97, 2010.

13. Haley KB, Lerner EB, Pirrallo RG, et al: The frequency and consequences of cardiopulmonary resuscitation performed by bystanders on patients who are not in cardiac arrest. *Prehosp Emerg Care* 15:282–287, 2010.

14. Ornato JP, Garnett AR, Glauser FL: Relationship between cardiac output and the end-tidal carbon dioxide tension. *Ann Emerg Med* 19:1104–1106, 1990.

15. McMichael M, Herring J, Fletcher DJ, et al: RECOVER evidence and knowledge gap analysis on veterinary CPR. Part 2: preparedness and prevention. *J Vet Emerg Crit Care* 22:S13–S25, 2012.

16. Tucker KJ, Savitt MA, Idris A, et al: Cardiopulmonary resuscitation: historical perspectives, physiology, and future directions. *Arch Intern Med* 154:2141–2150, 1994.

17. Cole SG, Otto CM, Hughes D: Cardiopulmonary cerebral resuscitation in small animals—a clinical practice review. Part I. *J Vet Emerg Crit Care* 12:261–267, 2002.

18. Smarick SD, Rylander H, Burkitt JM, et al: Treatment of traumatic cervical myelopathy with surgery, prolonged positive-pressure ventilation, and physical therapy in a dog. *J Am Vet Med Assoc* 230:370–374, 2007.

19. Neumar RW, Otto CW, Link MS, et al: Part 8: adult advanced cardiovascular life support: 2010 American Heart Association Guidelines for Cardiopulmonary Resuscitation and Emergency Cardiovascular Care. *Circulation* 122:S729–S767, 2010.

20. Rozanski EA, Rush JE, Buckley GJ, et al: RECOVER evidence and knowledge gap analysis on veterinary CPR. Part 4: advanced life support. *J Vet Emerg Crit Care* 22:S44–S64, 2012.

21. Gaddis GM, Dolister M, Gaddis ML: Mock drug delivery to the proximal aorta during cardiopulmonary resuscitation: central vs peripheral intravenous infusion with varying flush volumes. *Acad Emerg Med* 2:1027–1033, 1995.

22. Cole SG, Otto CM, Hughes D: Cardiopulmonary cerebral resuscitation in small animals—a clinical practice review. Part II. *J Vet Emerg Crit Care* 12:13–23, 2002.

23. Ujhelyi M, Schur M, Frede T, et al: Differential effects of lidocaine on defibrillation threshold with monophasic versus biphasic shock waveforms. *Circulation* 92:1644–1650, 1995.

24. Smarick SD, Haskins SC, Boller M, et al: RECOVER evidence and knowledge gap analysis on veterinary CPR. Part 6: post-cardiac arrest care. *J Vet Emerg Crit Care* 22:S85–S101, 2012.

25. Peberdy MA, Callaway CW, Neumar RW, et al: Part 9: post-cardiac arrest care: 2010 American Heart Association Guidelines for Cardiopulmonary Resuscitation and Emergency Cardiovascular Care. *Circulation* 122:S768–S786, 2010.

Acute Hemolytic Disorders in Cats

Christopher G. Byers

The feline body has a mechanism for responding to sudden red blood cell (RBC) loss from hemolysis and/or hemorrhage. Erythroid regeneration begins in the bone marrow and culminates in formation of reticulocytes after metarubricytes express their nuclei. Reticulocytes remain in the bone marrow for 1 to 2 days and are ultimately released as aggregate reticulocytes that have clusters of endoplasmic reticulum when stained with new methylene blue.[1] With continued maturation, aggregate reticulocytes mature to a punctate form in which the endoplasmic reticulum appears as smaller clusters. Punctate reticulocytes mature to normal erythrocytes over several weeks.[2] Peripheral blood smear analysis is always recommended in patients with hemolytic disorders, because most patients with regenerative hemolytic anemia have polychromasia, anisocytosis, macrocytosis, and increased numbers of nucleated RBCs.[1,2] Spherocytes are erythrocytes that appear spherical, and moderate spherocytosis is diagnostic of immune-mediated disease. Feline spherocytes may be challenging to identify, because they are normally smaller in diameter and have little central pallor.

Myriad causes of hemolytic anemia exist that may be classified as hereditary, immune-mediated, infectious, and toxic. Although each disease may manifest uniquely, each patient may be approached similarly by obtaining a thorough history and performing a complete physical examination. Clinical manifestations of anemia are dependent on severity and duration of tissue hypoxia. Cats with acute hemolysis may present in various stages of shock[3]: *compensatory* (normal vital signs or mild tachycardia, injected mucous membranes, rapid capillary refill time [CRT], and normal blood pressure), *early decompensatory* (with or without tachycardia, pale mucous membranes, prolonged CRT, depressed mentation, hypothermia, and hypotension), or *late decompensatory* (bradycardia, severe hypotension, absent CRT, weak or absent peripheral pulses, hypothermia, obtundation, and oliguria). In addition to the general clinical signs of anemia, evidence of hemolysis should also be observed, typically as icterus that manifests at the soft palate, gingiva, and sclera when serum bilirubin concentrations exceed 34.2 mmol/L (2 mg/dL).[4] Pigmenturia does not appear to be a consistent feature of a hemolytic crisis in cats. Patients may also have splenomegaly and/or hepatomegaly due to erythrophagocytosis. Evaluation of serum protein concentration may be helpful for differentiating a hemolytic crisis from a hemorrhagic process as a cause of regenerative anemia; serum protein concentration is usually normal-to-high-normal in hemolytic processes but is commonly low-normal-to-low with hemorrhage.

HEREDITARY CAUSES

Pyruvate Kinase Deficiency

Pyruvate kinase (PK) facilitates adenosine triphosphatase (ATP) production via the conversion of phosphoenolpyruvate to pyruvate in the Embden-Meyerhof pathway. Two genes encode PK: *pyruvate kinase, liver and RBC (PKLR)* and *pyruvate kinase, muscle*.[5] Erythrocyte PK deficiency is due to a mutation in PKLR, specifically an intron 5 single nucleotide polymorphism at position 304.[6] Clinical signs may include lethargy, diarrhea, poor hair coat quality, icterus, pica, weakness, hyporexia, weight loss, mucous membrane pallor, and occasionally splenomegaly.[7] Some cats may not manifest any clinical signs of illness. Clinical signs may be observed as early as 6 months and as late as 5 years of age. Complete blood count (CBC) typically shows a regenerative anemia with aggregate reticulocytosis. A serum biochemical profile may reveal hyperbilirubinemia, hyperglobulinemia, and liver enzyme derangements.[8,9] Pyruvate kinase deficiency has an autosomal recessive mode of inheritance.[10] The PKLR mutation has been found in significant frequency in the Abyssinian, Bengal, Egyptian Mau, La Perm, Maine Coon, Norwegian Forest Cat, Savannah, Siberian, Singapura, and Somali breeds as well as domestic shorthair and longhair cats. Genetic screening is recommended for these pedigreed breeds at risk, because a single nucleotide polymorphism has been documented in 6.31% to 9.35% of these cats.[6] As PK-deficient cats may have no clinical signs, testing for PK deficiency before breeding is strongly recommended. Exotic Shorthair, Oriental Shorthair, and Persian pedigrees have a very low frequency of the mutation. Treatment for affected patients is simply aimed at maintaining a stable oxygen-carrying capacity through provision of typed and cross-matched packed red blood cell (pRBC) transfusion(s) to alleviate clinical signs of anemia, particularly tachycardia, tachypnea, and lethargy.

Increased Osmotic Fragility

Increased osmotic fragility (OF) has been infrequently described in Somali, Abyssinian, Siamese, and domestic shorthair cats between 6 months and 5 years of age.[11,12] Increased OF is suspected to be due to a hereditary erythrocyte membrane defect and has an autosomal recessive mode of inheritance.[11] Possible clinical findings include lethargy, mucous membrane pallor, pyrexia, lymphadenomegaly, tremors, icterus, and splenomegaly. The CBC may identify a regenerative anemia with macrocytosis and occasional stomatocytosis.[12] However, macrocytosis may persist without regeneration, agglutination, or reticulocytosis. Serum biochemical profile may show hyperbilirubinemia, but this is a not a consistent finding, because some patients are thought to have low-grade hemolysis with adequate clearance of heme metabolites.

Increased OF is confirmed by exposing erythrocytes to hypotonic saline solutions ranging from 0% to 0.85%.[13] Definitive treatment has not been established, but stress avoidance is recommended to minimize possible stress-induced hemolytic events. Prednisolone therapy and splenectomy in an attempt to reduce erythrophagocytosis have been beneficial for some affected patients.[11]

Porphyrias

Porphyrias are inborn errors of metabolism that result from decreased activity of a specific enzyme in the heme biosynthetic pathway. They are commonly classified as *hepatic* or *erythroid*, depending on the predominant site of accumulation of porphyrins or porphyrin precursors. In humans, erythropoietic porphyrias include congenital erythropoietic porphyria (CEP) and erythropoietic protoporphyria (EPP), whereas the hepatic porphyrias are acute intermittent porphyria (AIP), hereditary coproporphyria (HCP) and variegate porphyria (VP). The porphyrias CEP and AIP have been rarely reported in domestic shorthair and Siamese cats.[14-19] To the author's knowledge, EPP, HCP, and VP have not been documented in cats.

Congenital erythropoietic porphyria manifests due to a severe deficiency of uroporphyrinogen-III-synthase (URO-synthase) and appears to have an autosomal dominant mode of inheritance.[16,20,21] When URO-synthase activity is deficient, hydroxymethylbilane accumulates and is converted to uroporphyrinogen I and subsequently coproporphyrinogen I. These two isomers are ultimately oxidized to form uroporphyrin I (URO I) and coproporphyrin I (COPRO I), respectively. In affected animals, URO I and COPRO I accumulate in erythroid precursors and erythrocytes, eventually causing cell rupture. These porphyrins circulate to skin, tissues, and bones and are also excreted in urine and feces. Levels of urinary 5-aminolevulinic acid (ALA) and porphobilinogen (PBG), as well as hydroxymethylbilane synthase (HMB-synthase) are normal (Table 83-1). Clinical signs include brownish colored teeth (Figure 83-1), skin that fluoresces pink with ultraviolet light, brownish urine, and hepatosplenomegaly.[22] Episodes of nasal and ocular discharge have been reported during summer months presumably due to photosensitivity. The CBC may show macrocytic hypochromic

| Table 83-1 | Similarities and Differences Between Congenital Erythropoietic Porphyria and Acute Intermittent Porphyria |

Characteristic	Congenital Erythropoietic Porphyria	Acute Intermittent Porphyria
HMB-synthase	Normal	Half normal
URO-synthase	Decreased	Normal
Erythrodontia	Present	Present
Brownish urine	Present	Present
Fluorescent bones	Present	Present
Urinary ALA	Normal	Elevated
Urinary PBG	Normal	Elevated
URO I	Elevated	Elevated
COPRO I	Elevated	Elevated

ALA, 5-aminolevulinic acid; *COPRO I*, coproporphyrin I; *HMB-synthase*, hydroxymethylbilane synthase; *PBG*, porphobilinogen; *URO-synthase*, uroporphyrinogen-III-synthase; *URO I*, uroporphyrin I.

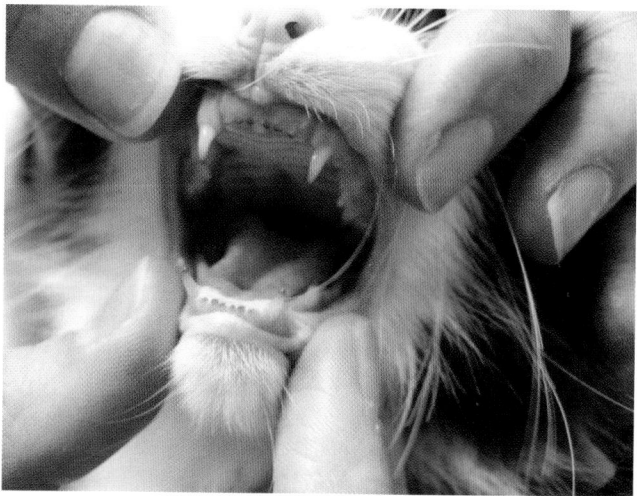

Figure 83-1: Brown discoloration of the teeth due to porphyrin deposition (erythrodontia) in a kitten with congenital porphyria. (Courtesy of Dr. Emma Thom.)

regenerative anemia with anisocytosis, poikilocytosis, target cells, and Howell-Jolly bodies.[14,16,22]

Acute intermittent porphyria was recently documented in cats as an inborn error of heme biosynthesis due to half-normal HMB-synthase.[18] As a result of this inborn error, elevated urinary levels of ALA and PBG were documented. In these cats, all had clinical signs consistent with CEP, including erythrodontia, brownish urine, and fluorescent bones when exposed to ultraviolet light. However URO-synthase activity was normal to slightly increased, and urine levels of URO I and COPRO I were markedly elevated.[17]

IMMUNE-MEDIATED HEMOLYTIC ANEMIA

Immune-mediated hemolytic anemia (IMHA) is an antibody-mediated cytotoxic destruction of circulating erythrocytes. The disease is termed *primary* or *autoimmune* when no cause of antibody production is identified and is called *secondary* when triggered by infectious diseases, inflammatory disease, drugs, and/or neoplasia. Secondary IMHA in cats has also been attributed to amyloidosis, neonatal isoerythrolysis, myelodysplasia, and systemic lupus erythematosis.[23-30]

Immunoglobulin G (IgG) is most commonly implicated in primary IMHA, but IgM, IgA, and complement may also be involved. When antibody and/or complement attaches to an erythrocyte cell membrane, cell destruction may be triggered by several mechanisms. Complement and extensive antibody attachment damages the erythrocyte membrane, causing extracellular water influx, erythrocyte swelling, and eventual rupture within the intravascular space; this process is rare in cats compared to dogs.[24,31,32] Antibody attachment without direct lysis labels erythrocytes for removal from circulation and eventual destruction by the reticuloendothelial system. A single antibody may bind two erythrocytes to cause agglutination. Antibodies may also target erythroid precursors within the bone marrow. If antibodies target membrane components shared by both mature RBCs and precursors, the patient will have a poorly regenerative hemolytic anemia. If antibodies target membrane components only found on erythroid precursors in the bone marrow, the patient will have a nonregenerative nonhemolytic anemia. Pure red cell aplasia results from a severe immune-mediated reduction of all stages of erythroid precursors.[33]

The diagnostic investigation to confirm IMHA should proceed in a manner to satisfy all components of the name of the disease: immune-mediated, hemolytic, and anemia. Clearly, anemia is usually the easiest part to confirm. There are a variety of ways to determine if an anemia is immune-mediated. Autoagglutination is definitive but must be differentiated from rouleaux formation using a saline agglutination test; if gross agglutination is not seen, microscopic evaluation to screen for microscopic agglutination is recommended. If the saline agglutination test is negative, a Coombs test can be performed. A positive Coombs test identifies bound immunoglobulins or complement on erythrocytes.[34] Spherocytosis is a strong indicator of immune mediation but is difficult to identify in feline patients, because their normal RBCs are of small size and lack central pallor. Hemolysis may also be present to help confirm IMHA. Icterus may indicate hemolysis but appears to be less common in cats compared to dogs.[23] Hemoglobinuria is a strong indicator of hemolysis in the absence of urinary disease. Measurement of OF at a reference veterinary laboratory is recommended in cats with IMHA and has been reported to be increased in all cats with primary IMHA.[23,35] Unfortunately, all pieces of the puzzle will not always fit together, and the diagnosis may merely be presumptive. If a definitive diagnosis is not attainable, frequent reassessment and further diagnostic testing (e.g., thoracic radiography or abdominal ultrasonography) are indicated to make sure another disease process has not been overlooked.

Signs typically associated with IMHA reflect the presence of both anemia (e.g., lethargy, weakness, pale mucous membranes, and systolic heart murmur) and compensatory responses caused by tissue hypoxia and stimulation of the sympathetic nervous system (e.g., tachypnea, tachycardia, and hyperkinetic peripheral pulses).[31,32] Some patients may also show clinical signs of an ongoing immunological or inflammatory process, including pyrexia, anorexia, splenomegaly, and rarely lymphadenomegaly.[22,32,36,37] Patients with acute-onset IMHA are frequently severely affected, manifesting depression, weakness, and/or collapse. Hyperbilirubinemia, bilirubinuria, and icterus are often seen during acute severe episodes of IMHA.[23,31] Whereas intravascular hemolysis is uncommon, hemoglobinemia and hemoglobinuria are observed infrequently. Patients with extravascular hemolysis due to subacute or chronic IMHA may compensate to some extent for their lack of erythrocytes and may be remarkably bright and alert despite the presence of severe anemia.

The cornerstone of IMHA treatment is corticosteroid therapy given at immunosuppressive doses. Many practitioners treat IMHA with corticosteroids alone and reserve other immunomodulatory agents for severe cases and for patients that fail to respond to initial corticosteroid therapy. However immunosuppressive agents may take weeks to be effective, so if such medications are started only after corticosteroids alone have failed, a dangerous delay of up to 1 month may ensue. Prolonged therapy appears to be the best way of minimizing relapses. Because long-term corticosteroids often cause unacceptable side effects, "steroid-sparing" combination therapy is usually needed eventually to enable reductions in corticosteroid doses. Currently, there are no meaningful studies that have documented the most effective combination therapy. The author prefers prednisolone (2 to 4 mg/kg every 24 hours orally [PO]) with an adjuvant immunosuppressive agent, such as cyclosporine (5 to 10 mg/kg every 12 hours PO), leflunomide (10 mg every 24 hours PO), cyclophosphamide (6.25 to 12.5 mg/cat every 24 hours, 4 days per week, PO), mycophenolate mofetil (10 mg/kg every 12 hours PO), or chlorambucil (0.1 to 0.2 mg/kg every 24 to 48 hours PO).[31,38,39] Azathioprine is not recommended due to the propensity to cause rapid, lethal bone marrow suppression.

Intravenous immunoglobulin G (IVIgG) has been anecdotally used successfully in dogs, but a recent blinded randomized trial evaluating the addition of IVIgG versus placebo to treatment with corticosteroids had no impact on initial response or hospitalization time.[40] To date, only anecdotal reports of IVIgG use in cats unresponsive to other immunosuppressive medications are available. As this is a human product, reactions are likely with repeated doses. Splenectomy is often performed in people with IMHA who do not respond to corticosteroids.[41] Successful use of splenectomy in dogs has been documented, and positive anecdotal reports exist for cats.[42] Splenectomy is only expected to be useful in cases where extravascular hemolysis predominates and conventional therapies have failed.

Thromboembolic events are the most common cause of mortality in dogs with IMHA but are uncommonly reported in cats. The antithrombotic medication aspirin (81 mg every 72 hours PO) reduces thromboxane A production, and its use has been advocated for patients with feline aortic thromboembolism. However, use of aspirin at standard doses is relatively contraindicated due to the concurrent administration of immunomodulatory doses of corticosteroids.[43] Newer antiplatelet medications, including clopidogrel and abciximab, may be efficacious, but further investigation is needed before routine use of anticoagulants and/or antithrombotic agents may be recommended in cats. Because a possible cause of secondary IMHA is vector-borne diseases, appropriate antimicrobial therapy should be considered in the initial treatment protocol in areas where these diseases are prevalent.

Patients should be provided a blood type–specific pRBC transfusion (10 to 15 mL/kg over 2 to 4 hours intravenously [IV]) to maintain appropriate tissue oxygen delivery if clinical signs of anemia (lethargy, tachypnea, and/or tachycardia) are present. The goal of transfusion therapy is not to normalize the RBC count or hematocrit, but rather to improve or normalize endpoints of resuscitation, particularly heart rate, respiratory rate, level of consciousness, and indicators of tissue perfusion (i.e., lactate). A bovine-derived hemoglobin-based oxygen carrier (i.e., Oxyglobin) may be an alternative to pRBCs, but current availability is limited due to discontinued production; these solutions should be administered with caution due to the possibility of pulmonary edema formation. More information on use of blood products in cats is found in Chapter 78. A balanced isotonic crystalloid should be provided IV if indicated to correct dehydration and provide daily fluid requirements. Enteral nutrition is essential, and a temporary supplemental feeding tube should be strongly considered if a patient is unwilling to eat for more than 24 hours; force-feeding is not recommended due to the potential for the development of food aversion.

Secondary IMHA is more common in cats than primary IMHA, and thus a thorough diagnostic investigation for an underlying cause is strongly recommended. Primary IMHA carries a more favorable prognosis in cats than in dogs; the reported mortality rate is 24%, and cats are more resistant to serious and potentially fatal complications, such as thromboembolic events and disseminated intravascular coagulopathy.[24,31] A recurrence rate of 31% for primary IMHA has been reported.[23] Some cats with primary IMHA may require prolonged treatment, possibly lifelong.

INFECTIOUS CAUSES

Hemotropic Mycoplasmosis

Hemotropic *Mycoplasma* species are bacteria that parasitize erythrocytes (Figure 83-2) and are the most common cause

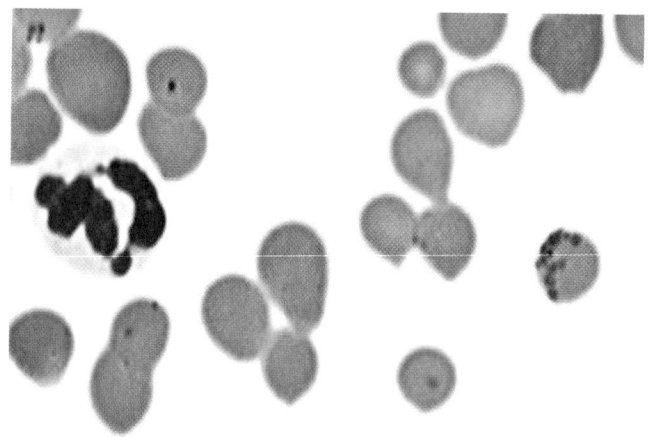

Figure 83-2: *Mycoplasma haemofelis* in a blood film from an infected cat with regenerative anemia. Ring, rod, and coccoid forms can be seen.

of infectious immune-mediated anemia in cats worldwide.[44] Three species have been documented: *Mycoplasma haemofelis*, *Candidatus Mycoplasma haemominutum*, and *Candidatus Mycoplasma turicensis*.[45-49] The former is the largest and most pathogenic of the three and may rapidly disappear and cyclically reappear from erythrocytes *in vivo*.[50-52] Cats do not need to be immunocompromised or splenectomized to be affected by clinical disease.[53] However, most studies have found an association between retrovirus infection and hemoplasmosis. Other risk factors for infection include male sex, access to the outdoors, and nonpedigreed breed status.[54] The natural route of infection has not been determined. The cat flea, *Ctenocephalides felis* (*C. felis*), is a potential vector based on experimental infections. Direct cat-to-cat transmission may occur through aggressive interactions (e.g., bite wounds, scratches).[55] Transmission can also occur through IV transfusion of infected blood; organisms can survive up to 1 week in stored blood products.[56] *M. haemofelis* is characterized by massive erythrocyte parasitemia that induces hemolytic anemia; severity of anemia is dependent on stage of infection. Clinical signs commonly include mucous membrane pallor, weight loss, cyclical pyrexia, lethargy, anorexia, icterus, splenomegaly, tachycardia, and tachypnea.[57] The CBC typically shows regenerative anemia with anisocytosis and polychromasia. Autoagglutination may be present, and Coombs test may be positive, indicating the presence of erythrocyte-bound antibodies.[57] Retroviral testing (feline leukemia virus [FeLV] and feline immunodeficiency virus [FIV]) is strongly recommended, because many clinically affected patients are concurrently infected.

Candidatus M. haemominutum may be found in some anemic cats but does not seem to produce meaningful clinical disease without concurrent retroviral infection.[51,52,58] *Candidatus M. turicensis* has been associated with intravascular hemolysis during experimental infection, but prevalence studies suggest singular infection is likely of minimal clinical importance. Risk factors for clinical disease include concurrent immunosuppression, retroviral infection, and/or infection with additional hemotropic *Mycoplasma* species.[49]

The preferred diagnostic test is detection via polymerase chain reaction (PCR) based on analysis of the 16S ribosomal RNA gene. Serology may be used to help differentiate acute from chronic *M. haemofelis* infection.[59,60] Additionally, a flow cytometry technique has been described that is rapid and capable of quantifying the level of parasitemia.[61] Peripheral blood film evaluation is not a sensitive diagnostic test, because *M. haemofelis* may rapidly and synchronously disappear from the feline RBCs and cyclically reappear *in vivo*. Treatment of choice is doxycycline (5 mg/kg every 12 hours PO; liquid form only to avoid esophageal damage), enrofloxacin (5 mg/kg every 24 hours PO), or pradofloxacin (5 to 10 mg/kg every 24 hours PO) for 14 to 21 days.[57,62-65] Pradofloxacin appears to be more effective in clearing the organism than doxycycline.[63] Concurrent immunosuppressive therapy with prednisolone (2 to 4 mg/kg every 24 hours PO) may be appropriate given the immune-mediated nature of this disease.[57] However, many Coombs-positive cats respond to antimicrobial therapy and supportive care without corticosteroid therapy, so routine use is not recommended at this time. Complete clearance of infection is difficult to confirm, because organisms may be sequestered in the liver, spleen, or lung in patients with PCR-negative blood tests. Chronically infected patients may experience recurrence of clinical signs and may serve as reservoirs of infection. Repeated PCR testing may not be clinically useful because affected patients may have persistently positive results. Certainly a negative PCR result is ideal, but cats that remain PCR-positive without clinical signs do not necessarily require continued treatment.

Viral Infections

Anemia induced by FeLV or FIV may be secondary to immune-mediated destruction, suppression of erythropoiesis in the bone marrow, chronic inflammation, and/or infiltrative neoplasia.[66] Infection may be confirmed with patient-side enzyme-linked immunosorbent assay (ELISA) tests, PCR, immunofluorescence antibody assay (IFA) and/or Western blot assays. Immunosuppressive therapy should be employed for viral-associated IMHA.

Bartonellosis

Feline erythrocytes are the main reservoirs for *Bartonella henselae* and *Bartonella clarridgeiae*; cats are also likely the reservoir for *Bartonella koehlerae*. *B. henselae* is the cause of cat-scratch disease in humans, as well as other potentially fatal disorders in immunocompromised people. *C. felis* and its feces are the known vectors for transmission, so prevention of infection focuses on flea control.[67] Infection may also be transmitted through transfusion of infected blood; all feline blood donors should therefore be screened. Most cats naturally infected with *B. henselae* are clinically normal. Clinical disease is most commonly associated with other *Bartonella* species where the cat is an accidental host; coinfection with a retrovirus may potentiate infection.[68]

Common clinical signs include lethargy, intermittent pyrexia, lymphadenomegaly, tremors, gingivitis, and uveitis.[64] Endocarditis, myocarditis, and reproductive failure have also been reported.[69-72] The CBC shows regenerative anemia, and serum biochemical profile commonly identifies hyperbilirubinemia and alanine aminotransferase (ALT) elevation.[67] Blood culture, PCR assay, and serologic testing may all be used to diagnose bartonellosis, but documentation of infection does not always correlate with clinical illness due to the high prevalence of infection in healthy cats in endemic areas.[67] Serology (IFA or ELISA) is most useful to rule out infection because of the low positive predictive value and high negative predictive value.[68] False-negative culture and PCR results, as well as false-positive PCR results, have been reported. Testing should be reserved for patients with clinical signs consistent with bartonellosis. Diagnosis should be based on a combination of the presence of clinical signs known to be associated with *Bartonella* species infection, a positive *Bartonella* species test, exclusion of other causes of clinical signs and hematologic/biochemical derangements, and a positive response to a prescribed anti-*Bartonella* medication.[68] In rare cases where clinical disease occurs, treatment may be attempted with doxycycline (10 mg/kg every 24 hours PO; liquid form only) for 2 to 4 weeks.[68] Other drug choices include marbofloxacin and azithromycin. Anti-inflammatory therapy is appropriate with anterior uveitis.[73] However, no controlled studies on efficacy have been published, and clearance of bacteremia cannot be guaranteed. Treatment of healthy carriers is not recommended as a means of eliminating zoonotic risk.[68]

Cytauxzoonosis

The protozoal organism *Cytauxzoon felis* is transmitted through the bite of *Dermacentor variabilis*, but other tick species, including *Amblyomma americanum*, may be involved.[74] Disease is geographically limited to the south central, southeastern, and mid-Atlantic United States. *Cytauxzoon* spp. infection associated with clinical disease has also been documented in cats in Italy.[75] *Cytauxzoon* spp. have been isolated and infections confirmed in bobcats, Florida panthers, and Texas cougars; domestic cats are terminal hosts.[75,76] There is no evidence that the parasite can infect humans. There are no age or sex predispositions, although younger cats seem be overrepresented. Most cases are identified in the early spring to early fall when ticks are most active. Prevention of infection is based on prevention of tick infestation. There are two distinct forms of *Cytauxzoon* spp.: sporozoite and erythrocyte form or piroplasm.[77] Ticks transmit the sporozoite to the host, which then invade reticuloendothelial cells throughout the body. Sporozoites undergo asexual reproduction within macrophages, so the cells become large enough to cause venous occlusion in multiple organs, contributing to congestion, multiple organ dysfunction syndrome, and death. The merozoites formed from asexual reproduction subsequently infect other mononuclear cells and erythrocytes. The erythrocyte form, called a *piroplasm*, may be visualized as early as

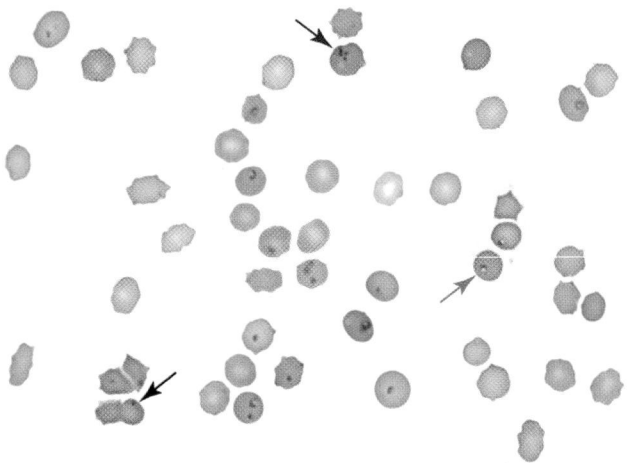

Figure 83-3: Piroplasms of *Cytauxzoon felis* within erythrocytes on a peripheral blood smear from an acutely ill infected cat. *Mycoplasma haemofelis* organisms, stain precipitate, and Howell-Jolly bodies *(black arrow)* may be confused with *C. felis* organisms. Round "signet ring" forms are commonly found *(orange arrow)*, but other forms, such as tetrads *(purple arrow)* are possible.

10 days postexperimental infection and appears as a round-to-oval signet ring (Figure 83-3). Piroplasms may undergo asexual reproduction and ultimately induce erythrocyte destruction and hemolytic anemia. The erythrocyte form develops late in the course of disease and may not occur in some patients; thus, the piroplasm form of replication is markedly less pathogenic than the sporozoite form.[77]

Clinical signs include anorexia, altered level of consciousness, seizures, lethargy, icterus, mucous membrane pallor, pyrexia, dyspnea, splenomegaly, and hepatomegaly.[74] Disease course is rapid, and patients may succumb within 1 week of clinical illness. The CBC shows acute normocytic normochromic nonregenerative anemia.[78,79] Thrombocytopenia has been documented and is thought to be secondary to a consumptive process.[79] Neutropenia is an inconsistent finding but may be due to bone marrow infiltration with infected macrophages; alternatively, neutrophilia may be documented secondary to a marked inflammatory response to infection.[74,78,80] Serum biochemical profile commonly reveals electrolyte derangements, hyperglycemia, hyperbilirubinemia, elevated liver enzymes, and occasionally azotemia.[74] Bilirubinuria is a common urinalysis abnormality. Definitive diagnosis is based on visualization of erythrocyte piroplasms, but infected macrophages may be aspirated from lymph nodes, spleen, and/or liver.[78] Testing by PCR is available and recommended.[81]

Standard treatment has not yet been determined. A recent prospective study compared the efficacy of imidocarb dipropionate (3.5 mg/kg intramuscularly [IM]; repeated 7 days after initial injection) with atovaquone (15 mg/kg every 8 hours PO for 10 days) and azithromycin (10 mg/kg every 24 hours PO for 10 days) in naturally infected cats confirmed with PCR testing. All cats received heparin (200 IU/kg every 8 hours subcutaneously [SC]) for the duration of hospitaliza-

tion), fluid therapy, and supportive care; and all cats that received imidocarb dipropionate were pretreated with atropine (0.05 mg/kg IM 15 minutes prior to treatment).[82] Although mortality remained high, cats that received atovaquone and azithromycin had improved survival to hospital discharge compared with those treated with imidocarb dipropionate (60% compared to 26%).[77] Without treatment, survival rate is reportedly 3%.

CHEMICAL AND TOXIN-INDUCED HEMOLYTIC ANEMIA

Various drugs and foodstuffs induce sufficient erythrocyte oxidative damage to cause hemolytic anemia. The agent may disrupt tissue oxygen delivery through Heinz body formation, methemoglobin production, and/or red cell membrane damage. Feline erythrocytes are uniquely susceptible to oxidant damage, because they have eight sulfhydryl groups per hemoglobin molecule as opposed to four in dogs and two in humans.[83,84] Heinz bodies form with oxidation of exposed sulfhydryl groups on hemoglobin. They are rigid and interfere with erythrocyte flexibility. When erythrocytes with Heinz bodies pass through sinusoids, intravascular hemolysis may occur when the portion of the cell containing the Heinz bodies becomes trapped. Alternatively, extravascular hemolysis occurs when sinusoidal macrophages phagocytize erythrocytes containing Heinz bodies. Diagnosis of Heinz body hemolytic anemia is based on documentation of a strongly regenerative anemia and the presence of Heinz bodies. Upon confirmation of hemolytic anemia induced by Heinz bodies, efforts should be made to identify the underlying cause. Several oxidant agents have been implicated as causes of Heinz body hemolytic anemia in the cat, including aspirin, *Allium* spp. (onion), acetaminophen, and urine acidifiers, such as D-L methionine.

Specific Agents

Acetaminophen

Acetaminophen is frequently reported to veterinary poison control centers as an intoxicant in cats, primarily associated with methemoglobinemia and hemolytic anemia.[85] In most species, acetaminophen is predominantly metabolized by sulfate and glucuronyl transferases in the liver with subsequent excretion of the conjugates by the kidneys.[86,87] A small percentage of acetaminophen is oxidized by cytochrome P450 enzymes to *N*-acetyl-*p*-benzoquinoneimine (NAPQI) that binds glutathione and is excreted via the kidneys as cysteine and mercapturic acid metabolites.[88] At toxic doses, sulfation and glucuronidation pathways are saturated, and NAPQI production increases.[89] When glutathione is depleted to less than 20% of its normal concentration, NAPQI binds to cysteine groups on other hepatocellular proteins to induce cell death.[90]

Cats also form para-aminophenol (PAP) after acetaminophen intoxication. *In vitro* investigation suggests this metabolite is the most likely causative agent for methemoglobin formation in acetaminophen intoxication in cats.[91] Para-aminophenol is removed by biliary excretion of glutathione and N-acetylation by N-acetyltransferases (NATs). Most species have two or three NATs, but cats have only one: N-acetyltransferase 1.[92,93] Subsequently cats are exposed to more PAP due to their limited ability to remove it. Para-aminophenol co-oxidizes and participates in reduction-oxidation cycling with oxyhemoglobin, culminating as prolonged methemoglobin formation.[91]

Common clinical signs include altered level of consciousness, cyanosis, generalized weakness, tachypnea, tachycardia, vomiting, hypothermia, chocolate brown mucous membranes, and facial and/or paw edema.[94] Abdominal pain and icterus may also be noted. Fulminant hepatocellular necrosis is less common in cats compared to dogs, and hepatic injury may take several weeks to resolve after appropriate medical intervention.[85,94] Clinical signs of methemoglobinemia may persist for 3 to 4 days. There is no known safe dose of acetaminophen in cats. Clinical signs of toxicity are commonly seen with dosages of 50 to 100 mg/kg, but fatalities have been documented with dosages as low as 10 mg/kg.[94-96]

A CBC, serum biochemical profile, and urinalysis should be obtained from any patient with suspected acetaminophen intoxication. Blood may appear brown-tinged due to methemoglobinemia or hemolyzed due to oxidative damage. Common abnormalities include anemia, hemoglobinemia, and hemoglobinuria.[97] Methemoglobinemia is detectable via co-oximetry within 2 to 4 hours postacetaminophen ingestion, and Heinz body formation subsequently occurs.[98] Elevation of ALT is common due to both hypoxic hepatocellular injury and direct hepatotoxicity. Liver enzymes typically increase 3 to 6 days postintoxication. Hyperbilirubinemia secondary to hemolysis occurs within 48 hours.[94] Progressive decreases in blood urea nitrogen, cholesterol, and albumin with increases in total bilirubin provide indirect evidence of hepatic dysfunction.[94,97,98] Urinalysis may identify hemoglobinuria or hematuria.[94] Urine acetaminophen concentration may be measured to confirm acetaminophen intoxication, but these assays are not yet widely available. Diagnosis is most commonly made based on correlation of clinical signs and biochemical abnormalities with documentation of exposure to the drug.

Patients should be immediately provided supplemental oxygen via the least stressful method. Induction of emesis is usually unrewarding, but administration of activated charcoal (2 g/kg PO) is recommended within the first 4 to 6 hours; repeated dosing may be required due to enterohepatic recirculation of the intoxicant. A cathartic (such as sorbitol) is also recommended unless the patient is dehydrated and/or has diarrhea. Isotonic crystalloid IV fluid therapy with appropriate vitamin and electrolyte supplementation should be administered to correct dehydration and provide daily requirements. Diuresis is not indicated, and patients should be closely monitored for signs of fluid overload. The ideal crystalloid to use has not been established, but a murine model reported improved hepatic recovery with administra-

tion of lactated Ringer's solution compared to 0.9% sodium chloride.[99] Patients may require transfusion with type-specific pRBCs; whole blood is typically not indicated, because acetaminophen does not induce hypoproteinemia. Bovine-derived hemoglobin-based oxygen carriers may also be considered but should be used cautiously due to the potential for pulmonary edema formation.

Medications to replenish glutathione stores and to promote conversion of methemoglobin to hemoglobin are essential.[100-108] N-acetylcysteine (NAC) is a glutathione precursor that replenishes glutathione stores. The initial oral loading dose (140 mg/kg, PO or IV) is followed by subsequent lower doses (70 mg/kg every 6 hours PO or IV for five to seven treatments).[102,104] If a cat already has clinical signs of intoxication, the loading dose should be increased to 280 mg/kg. Common adverse effects of oral dosing are nausea and vomiting. N-acetylcysteine may be administered IV with a micropore filter, either undiluted or diluted in a 5% dextrose solution. S-adenosylmethionine should be provided to protect erythrocytes from oxidative damage by limiting Heinz body formation and erythrocyte destruction. No optimum dosages for cats have been established, but protective benefits were confirmed in an experimental model (180 mg every 12 hours PO for 3 days; then 90 mg every 12 hours PO for 14 days).[109] Silymarin might also be beneficial as a hepatoprotective agent for stable patients that are able to tolerate oral medications.[102,104,105]

Ascorbic acid (vitamin C; 30 mg/kg every 6 hours PO for six treatments) and new methylene blue (1 mg/kg every 2 to 3 hours IV for two to three treatments) may help reduce methemoglobin to hemoglobin. Ascorbic acid has questionable efficacy and may induce nausea and gastric irritation. In a model of experimentally acetaminophen-intoxicated cats, new methylene blue with NAC provided no significant benefit compared to single agent NAC therapy.[106] New methylene blue is not toxic in cats when used at therapeutic doses for a limited number of treatments and may be superior to ascorbic acid given its more rapid onset of action.[106] Prognosis appears to be dependent upon dose received and time passed before initiation of decontamination efforts and supportive care. In a study of acetaminophen-intoxicated cats, survivors were generally treated within 14 hours, whereas nonsurvivors were not treated until 17 hours or more after intoxication.[94]

Zinc

Zinc intoxication is less common in cats compared to dogs given their more discriminating dietary nature. Potential sources of zinc include galvanized nuts, nails, or staples, as well as jewelry and zippers.[110-112] Kennels made of zinc-containing metals and/or adorned with zinc-laden paint are also potential sources. Zinc oxide ointment, calamine lotion, and various fertilizers, fungicides, antiseptics, and shampoos may be toxic sources, because cats may lick these substances from a human family member's skin and/or from their own hair coats while grooming. Pennies minted in the United States after 1982 are composed of 97.5% zinc.[113,114]

Upon ingestion, soluble zinc salts form in the stomach and are absorbed in the duodenum. Upon absorption, these salts are distributed systemically to cause direct irritant and corrosive damage to tissues and inhibit erythrocyte production and function. The mechanism of erythrocyte toxicity is currently unknown but may be associated with zinc-induced copper deficiency. Clinical signs are variable and depend on dose ingested.[115-120] Commonly reported signs are acute vomiting and anorexia with subsequent lethargy, icterus, dysrhythmias, diarrhea, and possible generalized seizure activity. The CBC typically documents a regenerative anemia, hemoglobinemia, and neutrophilic leukocytosis.[115,120] Peripheral blood smear evaluation identifies spherocytes and Heinz bodies. Biochemical profile frequently shows elevations of hepatic transaminases, alkaline phosphatase, and total bilirubin.[119] Pancreatic zinc accumulation may cause hyperamylasemia and hyperlipasemia, and glomerular and renal tubular injury may be associated with azotemia.[121] Urinalysis may manifest hemoglobinuria, bilirubinuria, cylindruria, and proteinuria.[119] Zinc levels should be measured from blood or tissue to confirm diagnosis.

Treatment must include removal of the possible source of zinc via surgery or endoscopy. Induction of emesis is typically unrewarding, because zinc-containing objects frequently adhere to gastric mucosa.[122] Patients should be provided IV isotonic crystalloid fluid therapy to correct dehydration; it is also important to provide daily fluid requirements and help reduce potential development of hemoglobinuric nephrosis. Patients may require pRBC and/or bovine-derived hemoglobin-based oxygen carrier transfusions to improve and maintain tissue oxygen delivery, and patients should be monitored closely for fluid overload. The majority of animals with zinc intoxication recover with aggressive supportive care following removal of the toxic source. Chelation therapy may be appropriate with severe intoxications that fail to respond to removal of the zinc source alone. Calcium disodium ethylenediaminetetraacetate is the most common chelator (27.5 mg/kg in 15 mL of 5% dextrose every 6 hours SC for 5 days). D-penicillamine (10 to 15 mg/kg every 12 hours PO for 7 to 14 days) and dimercaprol (3 to 6 mg/kg every 4 hours IM for 3 to 5 days) are alternative chelators.[123] Zinc levels should be monitored closely during chelation therapy to help determine duration of therapy. Prognosis is generally good when zinc intoxication is diagnosed early and treated appropriately.

Allium Species (Onion, Garlic, Leek, and Chive)

Allium cepa (onion), *Allium porrum* (leek), *Allium sativum* (garlic), and *Allium schoenoprasum* (chive) contain organic sulfur compounds that are absorbed through the gastrointestinal (GI) tract and converted to highly reactive oxidants.[124,125] Cooking does not reduce potential toxicity, and onion powder at 1% to 3% of dry matter intake may induce clinical signs.[124] Direct oxidative damage to the erythrocyte cell membrane causes cell lysis. Oxidation of exposed beta-93 cysteine residues present in hemoglobin results in the formation of sulfhemoglobin that is less soluble than hemoglobin.[126]

Sulfhemoglobin ultimately binds to erythrocyte cell membranes to form Heinz bodies and cross-links hemoglobin to form eccentrocytes.[127] The formation of Heinz bodies and eccentrocytosis increases erythrocyte fragility to cause extravascular hemolysis that impairs oxygen delivery to tissues.

Clinical signs may be observed within 1 day of ingestion, but more commonly, there is a lag period of several days between ingestion and onset of clinical signs. Clinical signs commonly include altered level of consciousness, tachypnea, tachycardia, hyporexia, weakness, lethargy, diarrhea, and abdominal discomfort.[124] The CBC typically shows anemia and hemoglobinemia, and Heinz bodies and eccentrocytes are observed during peripheral blood smear evaluation.[124] Co-oximetry may identify methemoglobinemia. Serum biochemical analysis may show hyperbilirubinemia, and urinalysis may identify bilirubinuria and cylindruria.[124]

Intoxication is commonly diagnosed through a combination of history, clinical signs, and confirmation of Heinz body hemolytic anemia. There is no specific antidote for intoxication. Early GI decontamination through induction of emesis (if within 2 hours of ingestion) and administration of activated charcoal are recommended. Supplemental oxygen should be provided via the least stressful method, and oxygen carrying capacity should be supported via pRBCs or a bovine-derived hemoglobin-based oxygen carrier to restore and maintain adequate tissue oxygen delivery. Isotonic crystalloids should be provided to correct dehydration and provide daily fluid requirements; diuresis is not indicated and patients should be monitored closely for volume overload. Prognosis depends on the species of plant involved, severity of anemia, and time to provision of appropriate medical therapy.

MISCELLANEOUS CAUSES

Fragmentation or microangiopathic hemolytic anemia (MHA) occurs when erythrocytes are lysed during circulation through abnormal vasculature. Various neoplasias, most notably hemangiosarcoma, and disseminated intravascular coagulopathy are frequently accompanied by MHA.[128,129] Cardiac valvular disease and renal disease may induce shearing injury due to turbulent blood flow.[130,131] Peripheral blood smear examination from affected patients shows schistocytes, irregularly-shaped poikilocytes that are remnants of traumatically disrupted erythrocytes. Fresh water submersion induces erythrocyte lysis secondary to hypotonic hypervolemia.[132] Thermal injury and severe hyperthermia may readily damage erythrocyte membranes.[133] Hemolytic-uremic syndrome associated with immunosuppression and allograft rejection has been documented in dogs and humans and may occur in cats.[134,135]

Phosphate is essential for ATP production, DNA, and RNA synthesis, and is also required for erythrocyte production of 2,3-diphosphoglycerate. Hypophosphatemia results in depletion of erythrocyte phosphorus and ATP. Depletion of ATP leads to erythrocyte membrane abnormalities, reducing deformability and increasing OF. Erythrocyte rheology is altered to form rigid spherocytes or echinocytes that are destroyed in the microvasculature. Hypophosphatemia has been documented in a variety of illnesses, most notably diabetes mellitus, hepatic lipidosis, refeeding syndrome, and as a result of insulin therapy.[136,137] Clinical evidence of acute hemolytic anemia may occur when serum phosphorus levels decline to values less than 25.65 mmol/L (1.5 mg/dL).[138] Treatment should focus on both oral or parenteral phosphate supplementation. Oral supplementation with a normal balanced diet, skim milk, or commercial phosphate products is preferred in cases of mild hypophosphatemia, but IV therapy is needed with severe hypophosphatemia, especially those patients that cannot tolerate enteral nutrition. An initial IV dosage of 0.01 to 0.03 mmol/kg/hour of sodium or potassium phosphate is effective, and serum phosphorus and calcium concentrations should be measured at least every 6 hours. Potential complications of IV supplementation are hypocalcemia, acute kidney injury, and dystrophic mineralization of soft tissues.

SUMMARY

Acute hemolytic anemia in cats may be triggered by a myriad of causes, including infectious organisms, genetic and hereditary disorders, toxins, and immune dysfunction. Invaluable information gleaned from obtaining a thorough history and performing a complete physical examination will guide the astute clinician in the development of an appropriate diagnostic plan. A patient's treatment(s) and prognosis are dependent on attaining a definitive diagnosis, initiating appropriate therapies, and a family's compliance with recommended treatments.

References

1. Alsaker RD, Laber J, Stevens JB, et al: A comparison of polychromasia and reticulocyte counts in assessing erythrocyte regenerative response in the cat. *J Am Vet Med Assoc* 170:39–41, 1977.

2. Fan LC, Dorner JL, Hoffman WE: Reticulocyte response and maturation in experimental acute blood loss anemia in the cat. *J Am Anim Hosp Assoc* 14:219–224, 1978.

3. Rudloff E, Kirby R: Hypovolemic shock and resuscitation. *Vet Clin North Am Small Anim Pract* 24:1015–1039, 1994.

4. Anderson JG, Washabau RJ: Icterus. *Compend Contin Educ Pract Vet* 14:1045–1059, 1992.

5. Saheki S, Saheki K, Tanaka T: Peptide structures of pyruvate kinase enzymes. I. Comparison of the four pyruvate kinase isoenzymes of the rate. *Biochim Biophys Acta* 704:484–493, 1982.

6. Grahn RA, Grahn JC, Penedo MC, et al: Erythrocyte pyruvate kinase deficiency mutation identified in multiple breeds of domestic cats. *BMC Vet Res* 30:207–217, 2012.

7. Kohn B, Fumi C: Clinical course of pyruvate kinase deficiency in Abyssinian and Somali cats. *J Feline Med Surg* 10:145–153, 2008.

8. Harvey JW: Pathogenesis, laboratory diagnosis, and clinical implications of erythrocyte enzyme deficiencies in dogs, cats, and horses. *Vet Clin Pathol* 35:144–156, 2006.

9. Owen JL, Harvey JW: Hemolytic anemia in dogs and cats due to erythrocyte enzyme deficiencies. *Vet Clin North Am Small Anim Pract* 42:73–84, 2012.

10. Giger U: Hereditary erythrocyte disorders. In August JR, editor: *Consultations in feline medicine*, ed 4, Philadelphia, 2001, Saunders/Elsevier, pp 484–489.

11. Giger U: Hemolytic anemias: is it autoimmune? In *Proceedings. American Association of Feline Practitioners Fall Meeting*, Philadelphia, PA, 2001.

12. Kohn B, Goldschmidt MH, Hohenhaus AE, et al: Anemia, splenomegaly, and increased osmotic fragility of erythrocytes in Abyssinian and Somali cat. *J Am Vet Med Assoc* 217:1483–1491, 2000.

13. Merten N, Lotz F, Kohn B: Red blood cell osmotic fragility in cats with anemia. In *Proceedings 21st European College of Veterinary Internal Medicine-Companion Animal Congress*, Sevilla, Spain, 2011.

14. Giddens WE, Labbe RE, Swango LJ, et al: Feline congenital erythropoietic porphyria associated with severe anemia and renal disease. *Am J Pathol* 80:367–386, 1975.

15. Tobias G: Congenital porphyria in a cat. *J Am Vet Med Assoc* 145:462–463, 1964.

16. Clavero S, Bishop DF, Giger U, et al: Feline congenital erythropoietic porphyria: two homozygous UROS missense mutations cause the enzyme deficiency and porphyrin accumulation. *Mol Med* 16:381–388, 2010.

17. Clavero S, Bishop DF, Haskins ME, et al: Feline acute intermittent porphyria: a phenocopy masquerading as an erythropoietic porphyria due to dominant and recessive hydroxymethylbilane synthase mutations. *Hum Mol Genet* 19:584–596, 2010.

18. Schnier JJ, Hanna P: Feline porphyria associated with anemia, severe hepatic disease, and renal calculi. *Can Vet J* 51:1146–1151, 2010.

19. Aeffner F, O'Brien M, Birkhold A, et al: Pathology in practice [congenital porphyria in a kitten]. *J Am Vet Med Assoc* 243:217–219, 2013.

20. Lyons LA: Genetic testing in domestic cats. *Mol Cell Probes* 26:224–230, 2012.

21. Glenn BL, Gleen HG, Omtvedt IT: Congenital porphyria in a domestic cat (*Felis catus*): preliminary investigations on inheritance pattern. *Am J Vet Res* 29:1653–1657, 1968.

22. Giger U, Clavero S, Bishop DF, et al: Clinical, biochemical, and molecular genetic characterization of porphyria in cats. In *Proceedings 28th American College of Veterinary Internal Medicine Forum*, Anaheim, CA, 2010.

23. Kohn B: *Erythrozytenstudien bei gesunden und anamischen katzen.* PhD thesis, FU Berlin, 2001.

24. Kohn B, Weingart C, Eckmann V, et al: Primary immune-mediated hemolytic anemia in 19 cats: diagnosis, therapy and outcome (1998-2004). *J Vet Intern Med* 20:159–166, 2006.

25. Maede Y, Hata R: Studies of feline haemobartonellosis. II. The mechanism of anemia produced by infection with *Haemobartonella felis. Jap J Vet Sci* 37:49–54, 1975.

26. Peterson ME, Hutwitz AI, Leib MS, et al: Propylthiouracil-associated hemolytic anemia, thrombocytopenia, and antinuclear antibodies in cats with hyperthyroidism. *J Am Vet Med Assoc* 184:806–808, 1984.

27. Piek CJ, Dekker A, Junius G, et al: Idiopathic immune-mediated haemolytic anaemia (IMHA) in cats: differentiation from secondary IMHA and outcome of treatment. In *Proceedings 13th European College of Veterinary Internal Medicine-Companion Animal*, Uppsala, Sweden, 2003, p 162.

28. Scott DW, Schultz RD, Post JE, et al: Autoimmune hemolytic anemia in the cat. *J Am Anim Hosp Assoc* 9:530–539, 1973.

29. Weiss DJ, McClay CB: Studies on the pathogenesis of erythrocyte destruction associated with the anemia of inflammatory diseases. *Vet Clin Pathol* 17:90–93, 1988.

30. Werner LL, Gorman NT: Immune-mediated disorders of cats. *Vet Clin North Am Small Anim Pract* 14:1039–1064, 1984.

31. Husbands BD, Smith SA, Weiss DJ: Idiopathic immune-mediated hemolytic anemia

(IMHA) in 25 cats. *J Vet Intern Med* 10:350, 2002. (Abstract).

32. Person JM, Sicard M, Pellerin JL: Les anemies hemolytiques auto-immunes chez le chat: etude Clinique et immunopathologique de cinq cas. *Revue Med Vet* 148:107–144, 1997.

33. Stokol T, Blue JT: Pure red cell aplasia in cats: 9 cases (1989-1997). *J Am Vet Med Assoc* 214:75–79, 1999.

34. Dunn JK, Searcy GP, Hirsch VM: The diagnostic significance of a positive direct antiglobulin test in anemic cats. *Can J Comp Med* 48:349–353, 1984.

35. Jain NC: Osmotic fragility of erythrocytes in dogs and cats in health and in certain hematologic disorders. *Cornell Vet* 63:411–423, 1973.

36. Engelbrecht R, Kohn B, Leibold W, et al: Klinische befunde, diagnostic und behandlungserfolge bei der primaren und sekundaren immunhamolytischen anamie beim hund. *Kleintierpraxis* 47:265–278, 2002.

37. Cuoto CG: A diagnostic approach to splenomegaly in cats and dogs. *Vet Med* 3:220–238, 1990.

38. Bacek LM, Macintire DK: Treatment of primary immune-mediated hemolytic anemia with mycophenolate mofetil in two cats. *J Vet Emerg Crit Care* 21:45–49, 2011.

39. Hanna FY: Disease modifying treatment for feline rheumatoid arthritis. *Vet Comp Orthop Traumatol* 18:94–99, 2005.

40. Whelan MF, O'Toole TE, Chan DL, et al: Use of human immunoglobulin in addition to glucocorticoids for the initial treatment of dogs with immune-mediated hemolytic anemia. *J Vet Emerg Crit Care* 19:158–164, 2009.

41. Coon WW: Splenectomy in the treatment of hemolytic anemia. *Arch Surg* 120:625–628, 1985.

42. Horgan JE, Roberts BK, Schermerhorn T: Splenectomy as an adjunctive treatment for dogs with immune-mediated hemolytic anemia: 10 cases (2003-2006). *J Vet Emerg Crit Care* 19:254–261, 2009.

43. Smith SA, Tobias AH, Jacob KA, et al: Arterial thromboembolism in cats: acute crisis in 127 cases (1992-2001) and long-term management with low-dose aspirin in 24 cases. *J Vet Intern Med* 17:73–83, 2003.

44. Maede Y, Hata R: Studies on feline haemobartonellosis. II. The mechanism of anemia produced by infection with *Haemobartonellosis felis*. *Jpn J Vet Sci* 37:49–54, 1975.

45. Foley JE, Pedersen NC: *Candidatus* Mycoplasma haemoninutum, a low-virulence epierythrocytic parasite of cats. *Int J Syst Evol Microbiol* 51:815–817, 2001.

46. Neimark H, Johansson KE, Rikihisa Y, et al: Proposal to transfer some members of the genera *Haemobartonella* and *Eperythrozoon* to the genus *Mycoplasma* with descriptions of *Candidatus Mycoplasma haemofelis, Candidatus Mycoplasma haemomuris, Candidatus Mycoplasma haemosuis* and *Candidatus Mycoplasma wenyonii*. *Int J Syst Evol Microbiol* 51:891–899, 2001.

47. Neimark H, Johansson KE, Rikihisa Y, et al: Revision of haemotrophic *Mycoplasma* species names. *Int J Syst Evol Microbiol* 52:683, 2002.

48. Willi B, Boretti FS, Baumgartner C, et al: Prevalence, risk factor analysis, and follow-up infections caused by three feline hemoplasma species in cats in Switzerland. *J Clin Microbiol* 44:961–969, 2006.

49. Willi B, Boretti FS, Cattori V, et al: Identification, molecular characterization and experimental transmission of a new hemoplasma isolate from a cat with hemolytic anemia in Switzerland. *J Clin Microbiol* 43:2581–2585, 2005.

50. Berent LM, Messick JB, Cooper SK: Detection of *Haemobartonella felis* in cats with experimentally induced acute and chronic infections, using a polymerase chain reaction assay. *Am J Vet Res* 59:1215–1220, 1998.

51. Foley JE, Harrus S, Poland A, et al: Molecular, clinical and pathologic comparison of two distinct strains of *Haemobartonella felis* in domestic cats. *Am J Vet Res* 59:1581–1588, 1998.

52. Westfall DS, Jensen WA, Reagan WJ, et al: Inoculation of two genotypes of *Haemobartonella felis* (California and Ohio variants) to induce infection in cats and the response to treatment with azithromycin. *Am J Vet Res* 62:687–691, 2001.

53. George JW, Rideout BA, Griffey SM, et al: Effect of preexisting FeLV infection or FeLV and feline immunodeficiency virus coinfection on pathogenicity of the small variant of *Haemobartonella felis* in cats. *Am J Vet Res* 63:1172–1178, 2002.

54. Sykes JE: Feline Hemotropic Mycoplasmas. *Vet Clin North Am Small Anim Pract* 40:1157–1170, 2010.

55. Woods JE, Brewer MM, Hawley JR, et al: Evaluation of experimental transmission of *Candidatus Mycoplasma haemominutum* and *Mycoplasma haemofelis* by *Ctenocephalides felis*. *Am J Vet Res* 66:1008–1012, 2005.

56. Gary AT, Richmond HL, Tasker S, et al: Survival of *Mycoplasma haemofelis* and "*Candidatus Mycoplasma haemominutum*" in blood of cats for transfusions. *J Feline Med Surg* 8:321–326, 2006.

57. Sykes JA: Feline hemotropic mycoplasmas. *J Vet Emerg Crit Care* 20:62–69, 2010.

58. Tasker S: Haemotropic mycoplasmas. *J Feline Med Surg* 12:369–381, 2010.

59. Jensen WA, Lappin MR, Kamkar S, et al: Use of a polymerase chain reaction to detect and differentiate two strains of *Haemobartonella felis* in naturally infected cats. *Am J Vet Res* 62:604–608, 2001.

60. Barker EN, Helps CR, Heesom KJ, et al: Detection of humoral response using a recombinant heat shock protein 70, DnaK, of *Mycoplasma haemofelis* in experimentally and naturally hemoplasma-infected cats. *Clin Vaccine Immunol* 17:1926–1932, 2010.

61. Sanchez-Perez A, Brown G, Malik R, et al: Rapid detection of haemotropic mycoplasma infection of feline erythrocytes using a novel cytometric approach. *Parasit Vectors* 6:158, 2013.

62. Nibblett BMD, Snead EC, Waldner C, et al: Anemia in cats with hemotropic mycoplasma infection: retrospective evaluation of 23 cases (1996-2005). *Can Vet J* 50:1181–1185, 2009.

63. Dowers KL, Tasker S, Radecki SV, et al: Use of pradofloxacin to treat experimentally induced *Mycoplasma haemofelis* infection in cats. *Am J Vet Res* 70:105–111, 2009.

64. Dowers KL, Olver C, Radecki SV, et al: Use of enrofloxacin for treatment of large-form Haemobartonella felis in experimentally infected cats. *J Am Vet Med Assoc* 221:250–253, 2002.

65. Tasker S, Caney SM, Day MJ, et al: Effect of chronic FIV infection, and efficacy of marbofloxacin treatment on *Mycoplasma haemofelis* infection. *Vet Microbiol* 117:169–179, 2006.

66. Katrin H: Clinical aspects of feline immunodeficiency and feline leukemia virus infection. *Vet Immunol Immunopathol* 143:190–201, 2001.

67. Guptill L: Bartonellosis. *Vet Microbiol* 140:347–359, 2010.

68. Pennisi MG, Marsilio F, Hartmann K, et al: Bartonella species infection in cats: ABCD guidelines on prevention and management. *J Feline Med Surg* 15:563–569, 2013.

69. Guptill L: Feline bartonellosis. *Vet Clin North Am Small Anim Pract* 40:1073–1090, 2010.

70. Chomel BB, Wey AC, Kasten RW, et al: Fatal case of endocarditis associated with *Bartonella henselae* type I infection in a domestic cat. *J Clin Microbiol* 41:5337–5339, 2003.

71. Varanat M, Broadhurst J, Linder KE, et al: Identification of *Bartonella henselae* in 2 cats with pyogranulomatous myocarditis and diaphragmatic myositis. *Vet Pathol* 49:608–611, 2012.

72. Guptill L, Slater LN, Wu CC, et al: Evidence of reproductive failure and lack of perinatal transmission of *Bartonella henselae* in experimentally infected cats. *Vet Immunol Immunopathol* 23:177–189, 1998.

73. Lappin MR, Black JC: *Bartonella* spp. associated with uveitis in a cat. *J Am Vet Med Assoc* 214:1205–1207, 1999.

74. Cohn LA, Birkenheuer AJ: Cytauxzoonosis. In Green CE, editor: *Infectious diseases of the dog and cat*, ed 4, Philadelphia, 2012, Elsevier, pp 764–771.

75. Meier HT, Moore LE: Feline cytauxzoonosis: a case report and literature review. *J Am Vet Med Assoc* 36:493–496, 2000.

76. Rotstein DS, Taylor SK, Harvey JW, et al: Hematologic effects of cytauxzoonosis in Florida panthers and Texas Cougars in Florida. *J Wildlife Dis* 35:613–617, 1999.

77. Meinkoth J, Kocan AA, Whitworth L, et al: Cats surviving natural infection with *Cytauxzoon felis*: 18 cases (1997-1998). *J Vet Intern Med* 14:521–525, 2000.

78. Cowell RL, Panciera RJ, Fox JC, et al: Feline cytauxzoonosis. *Comp Cont Edu Pract Vet* 10:731–736, 1988.

79. Franks PT, Harvey JW, Shields RP, et al: Hematological findings in experimental feline cytauxzoonosis. *J Am Vet Med Assoc* 24:395–401, 1987.

80. Hoover JP, Walker DB, Hedges JD: Cytaux-zoonosis in cats: eight cases (1985-1992). *J Am Vet Med Assoc* 205:455–460, 1994.

81. Birkenheuer AJ, Marr H, Alleman AR, et al: Development and evaluation of a PCR assay for the detection of *Cytauxzoon felis* DNA in feline blood samples. *Vet Parasitol* 137:144–149, 2006.

82. Cohn LA, Birkenheuer AJ, Brunker JD, et al: Efficacy of atovaquone and azithromycin or imidocarb dipropionate in cats with acute cytauxzoonosis. *J Vet Intern Med* 25:55–60, 2011.

83. Snow NS: Some observations on the reactive sulphydryl groups in haemoglobin. *Biochem J* 84:360–364, 1962.

84. Riggs AF, Wolbach RA: Sulfhydryl groups and the structure of hemoglobin. *J Gen Physiol* 39:585–605, 1956.

85. Allen AJ: The diagnosis of acetaminophen toxicosis in a cat. *Can Vet J* 44:509–510, 2003.

86. Prescott LF, Roscoe P, Wright N, et al: Plasma-paracetamol half-life and hepatic necrosis in patients with paracetamol over-dosage. *Lancet* 1:519–522, 1971.

87. Savides MC, Oehme FW, Nash SL, et al: The toxicity and biotransformation of single doses of acetaminophen in dogs and cats. *Toxicol Appl Pharmacol* 74:26–34, 1984.

88. Davis M, Simmons CJ, Harrison NG, et al: Paracetamol overdose in man: relationship between pattern of urinary metabolites and severity of liver damage. *Q J Med* 45:181–191, 1976.

89. Davis DC, Potter WZ, Jollow DJ, et al: Species differences in hepatic glutathione depletion, covalent binding and hepatic necrosis after acetaminophen. *Life Sci* 14:2099–2109, 1974.

90. Pumford NR, Roberts DW, Benson RW, et al: Immunochemical quantification of 3-(cysteine-S-yl) acetaminophen protein adducts in subcellular liver fractions following a hepatotoxic dose of acetaminophen. *Biochem Pharmacol* 40:573–579, 1990.

91. McConkey SE, Grant DM, Cribb AE: The role of para-aminophenol in acetaminophen-induced methemoglobinemia in dogs and cats. *J Vet Pharmacol Ther* 32:585–595, 2009.

92. Trepanier LA, Cribb AE, Spielberg SP, et al: Deficiency of cytosolic arylamine N-acetylation in the domestic cat and wild felids caused by the presence of a single NAT1-like gene. *Pharmacogenetics* 8:169–179, 1998.

93. Trepanier LA, Ray K, Winand NJ, et al: Cytosolic arylamine N-acetyltransferase (NAT) deficiency in the dog and other canids due to an absence of NAT genes. *Biochem Pharmacol* 54:73–80, 1997.

94. Aronson LR, Drobatz KJ: Acetaminophen toxicosis in 17 cats. *J Vet Emerg Crit Care* 6:65–69, 1996.

95. Sellon RK: Acetaminophen. In Peterson ME, Talcott PA, editors: *Small animal toxicology*, ed 1, Toronto, 2001, Saunders/Elsevier, pp 388–395.

96. Jones RD, Baynes RE, Nimitz CT: Nonsteroidal anti-inflammatory drug toxicosis in dogs and cats: 240 cases (1989-1990). *J Am Vet Emerg Crit Care* 201:475–477, 1992.

97. Finco DC, Duncan JR, Schall WD, et al: Acetaminophen toxicosis in the cat. *J Am Vet Med Assoc* 166:469–472, 1975.

98. Richardson JA: Management of acetaminophen and ibuprofen toxicosis in dogs and cats. *J Vet Emerg Crit Care* 10:285–291, 2000.

99. Yang R, Zhang S, Kajander H, et al: Ringer's lactate improves liver recovery in a murine model of acetaminophen toxicity. *BMC Gastroenterol* 11:125–135, 2011.

100. Oliveira CP, Lopassa FP, Laurindo FR, et al: Protection against liver ischemia-reperfusion injury in rats by silymarin or verapamil. *Transplant Proc* 33:3010–3014, 2001.

101. Gaunt SD, Baker DC, Green RA: Clinico-pathologic evaluation of *N*-acetylcysteine therapy in acetaminophen toxicosis in the cat. *Am J Vet Res* 42:1982–1984, 1981.

102. Paulova J, Dvorak M, Kolouch F, et al: Evaluation of the hepatoprotective and therapeutic effects of silymarin in an experimental carbon tetrachloride intoxication of liver in dogs. *Vet Med* 35:629–635, 1990.

103. St. Omer VV, McKnight ED: Acetylcysteine for treatment of acetaminophen toxicosis in the cat. *J Am Vet Med Assoc* 176:911–913, 1980.

104. Valenzuela A, Garrido A: Biochemical basis of the pharmacological action of the flavonoid silymarin and of its structural isomer silibinin. *Biological Res* 27:105–112, 1994.

105. Mira L, Silva M, Manso CF, et al: Scavenging of reactive oxygen species by silibinin dihemisuccinate. *Biochem Pharmacol* 48:753–759, 1994.

106. Rumbeiha WK, Lin YS, Oehme FW: Comparison of *N*-acetylcysteine and methylene blue, alone or in combination, for treatment of acetaminophen toxicosis in cats. *Am J Vet Res* 56:1529–1533, 1995.

107. Olaleye MT, Rocha BT: Acetaminophen-induced liver damage in mice: effects of some medicinal plants on the oxidative defense system. *Exp Tox Pathol* 59:319–327, 2008.

108. Avizeh R, Najafzadeh H, Razijalali M, et al: Evaluation of prophylactic and therapeutic effects of silymarin and *N*-acetylcysteine in acetaminophen-induced hepatotoxicity in cats. *J Vet Pharmaco Ther* 33:95–99, 2010.

109. Webb CB, Twedt DC, Fettman MJ, et al: S-adenosylmethionine (SAMe) in a feline acetaminophen model of oxidative injury. *J Feline Med Surg* 5:69–75, 2003.

110. Richardson JA, Gwaltney-Brant SM, Villar D, et al: Zinc toxicosis from penny ingestion in dogs. *Vet Med* 97:96–99, 2002.

111. Adam F, Elliot J, Dandrieux J, et al: Zinc toxicity in two dogs associated with the ingestion of identification tags. *Vet Rec* 168:84–85, 2011.

112. Bexfield N, Archer J, Herrtage M: Heinz body haemolytic anaemia in a dog secondary to ingestion of a zinc toy: a case report. *Vet J* 174:414–417, 2007.

113. Meerdink GL, Reed RE, Perry D, et al: Poisoning from the ingestion of pennies. *Proc Am Assoc Vet Lab Diagn* 29:141–150, 1986.

114. Latimer KS, Jain AV, Inglesby HB, et al: Zinc-induced hemolytic anemia caused by ingestion of pennies by a pup. *J Am Vet Med Assoc* 195:77–80, 1989.

115. Gandini G, Bettini G, Pietra M, et al: Clinical and pathological findings of acute zinc intoxication in a puppy. *J Small Anim Pract* 43:549–554, 2002.

116. Mikszewski JS, Saunders HM, Hess RS: Zinc-associated acute pancreatitis in a dog. *J Small Anim Pract* 44:177–180, 2003.

117. Torrance AG, Fulton RB: Zinc-induced hemolytic anemia in a dog. *J Am Vet Med Assoc* 191:443–444, 1987.

118. Luttgen PH, Whitnet MS, Wolf AM, et al: Heinz body hemolytic anemia associated with high plasma zinc concentration in a dog. *J Am Vet Med Assoc* 197:1347–1350, 1990.

119. Gurnee CM, Drobatz KJ: Zinc intoxication in dogs: 19 cases (1991-2003). *J Am Vet Med Assoc* 230:1174–1179, 2007.

120. Breitschwerdt ER, Armstrong PJ, Robinette CL, et al: Three cases of acute zinc toxicosis in dogs. *Vet Hum Toxicol* 28:109–117, 1986.

121. Volmer PA, Roberts J, Meerdink GL: Anuric renal failure associated with zinc toxicosis by dogs. *Vet Hum Toxicol* 46:276–278, 2004.

122. Talcott P, Peterson ME: Zinc poisoning. In Peterson ME, Talcott PA, editors: *Small animal toxicology*, ed 1, Toronto, 2001, WB Saunders, pp 756–761.

123. Domingo JL, Llobet JM, Patenan JL, et al: Acute zinc intoxication: comparison of the antidotal efficacy of several chelating agents. *Vet Hum Toxicol* 30:224–228, 1988.

124. Burrows GE, Tyrl RJ: Liliaceae Juss. In Burrows GE, Tyrl RJ, editors: *Toxic plants of North America*, ed 2, Ames, IA, 2001, Iowa State Press, pp 751–805.

125. Amagase H, Petesch BL, Matsuura H, et al: Intake of garlic and its bioactive components. *J Nutr* 131:955S–962S, 2001.

126. Bloom JC, Brandt JT: Toxic responses of the blood. In Klaassen CD, editor: *Casarett & Doull's toxicology: the basic science of poisons*, ed 1, New York, NY, 2001, McGraw-Hill, pp 389–411.

127. Lee KW, Yamato O, Tajima M, et al: Hematologic changes associated with the appearance of eccentrocytes after intragastric administration of garlic extract to dogs. *Am J Vet Res* 61:1446–1450, 2000.

128. Rebar AH, Hahn FF, Halliwell WH, et al: Microangiopathic hemolytic anemia associated with radiation-induced hemangiosarcoma. *Vet Pathol* 17:443–454, 1980.

129. Bull BS, Brain MC: Disseminated intravascular coagulation. Experimental models of microangiopathic haemolytic anemia. *Proc R Soc Med* 61:1134–1137, 1968.

130. Forshaw J, Harwood L: Red cell abnormalities in cardiac valvular disease. *J Clin Pathol* 20:848–853, 1967.

131. Levine H: Microangiopathic hemolytic anemia: the pathogenesis of red blood cell fragmentation, a review of the literature. *Aerospace Med* 41:331–336, 1970.

132. Powell LL: Near drowning. In *Proceedings International Veterinary Emergency and Critical Care Symposium*, San Antonio, TX, 2010.
133. Frantz K, Byers CG: Thermal injury. *Compend Contin Educ Vet* 33:2011.
134. Neild GH: Hemolytic-uraemic syndrome in practice. *Lancet* 343:398–401, 1994.
135. Holloway S, Senior D, Roth L, et al: Hemolytic uremic syndrome in dogs. *J Vet Intern Med* 7:220–227, 1993.

136. Adams LG, Hardy RM, Weiss DJ, et al: Hypophosphatemia and hemolytic anemia associated with diabetes mellitus and hepatic lipidosis in cats. *J Vet Intern Med* 7:266–271, 1993.
137. Armitage-Chan EA, O'Toole T, Chan D, et al: Management of prolonged food deprivation, hypothermia, and refeeding syndrome in a cat. *J Vet Emerg Crit Care* 16:S34–S41, 2006.

138. eClinpath: Bilirubin, Cornell University College of Veterinary Medicine: eClinpath. <http://www.eclinpath.com/chemistry/liver/cholestasis/bilirubin/>, (Accessed June 8, 2015).

Fibrosing Pleuritis

Tony Johnson

> *I was out of school a little while with pleurosis. When I came back you asked me what was the matter. I said I had pleurosis and you thought I said Blue Roses. So that's what you always called me after that!*
>
> Tennessee Williams, "The Glass Menagerie"

Fibrosing pleuritis (FP) is a disastrous complication of long-standing pleural fluid accumulation and pleural inflammation that carries a high degree of mortality. Because of the relatively little-known nature of FP and its poor prognosis, the aim of this chapter is to increase awareness and aid clinicians in recognizing FP and the clinical conditions that cause it. To date, few case reports exist in the veterinary literature, and there are no scientific studies. In humans, FP reduces total lung capacity (TLC) and residual volume (RV) and is a significant contributor to respiratory morbidity, mortality, and failure to wean from mechanical ventilation.[1]

Fibrosing pleuritis is also known as pleural fibrosis, restrictive pleuritis, and fibrotic pleurisy. Key points are summarized in Box 84-1.

PATHOPHYSIOLOGY AND RELEVANT ANATOMY

The pleural space is a potential space formed by the gap between the parietal (i.e., adherent to the body wall) and visceral (i.e., adherent to the lung) pleural surfaces. In health, only a scant amount of fluid, secreted by the serous membranes of the pleura, is present in this space. This fluid aids in lubricating the lung surface as it glides along the body wall during respiration. In disease states, this potential space can expand dramatically to accommodate large volumes of fluid.[1] In dogs and cats, the mediastinal pleura is thin but completely isolates each hemithorax. Despite this, in some disease states, pleural pathology can lead to communication between the right and left sides of the thoracic cavity.[2] Normally, pleural fluid is absorbed by the lymphatics under the parietal pleural. Fibrosing pleuritis decreases the absorptive capacity, which further promotes fluid buildup.[3]

Fibrosing pleuritis is secondary to pleural effusion and inflammation of the pleura. Pleural fluid buildup can have several causes in cats and dogs; the most common causes are listed in Box 84-2. Chyle is particularly irritating to the pleura, and patients with this condition are at high risk for FP if the disease becomes chronic.[4] Due to their nature,

it can be difficult to determine whether pleural effusion in feline patients is chronic or acute in many cases. Effusions that have been present subclinically for many weeks may suddenly cause the patient to decompensate and develop clinical signs, mimicking an acute condition. If an effusion is known to be chronic, the risk of FP increases. In the author's experience, FP occurs more frequently in cats than dogs.

The irritation caused by pleural effusion induces an inflammatory response by mesothelial cells and the formation of a fibrinous matrix. This matrix is the result of dysregulated fibrin production and degradation, wherein fibrin formation is upregulated and fibrin degradation impaired. Inflammatory cytokines, such as tumor necrosis factor-α, facilitate fibrin formation. It is largely unknown why some patients with long-standing pleural effusion will develop FP and others will not.[5]

As the fibrin matrix matures, contraction occurs,[1] which decreases the volume of the affected lung lobes and leads to the characteristic rounded appearance of the lung lobes on thoracic radiography and at surgery or necropsy. The formation of a stiff layer of scar tissue contributes to the lack of improvement after thoracocentesis and risk of pneumothorax, which may be spontaneous or seen after thoracocentesis. The lack of expansion of lung lobes following removal of pleural fluid (due to the presence of a thick "peel" of scar tissue) has been referred to as "trapped lung."[5]

CLINICAL SIGNS

Recognition of FP as a clinical entity as well as knowledge of the prognosis, underlying conditions, and radiographic signs are important points in making the diagnosis and counseling the owners of pets with this condition.

In one case study of five patients with FP (three feline, two canine), dyspnea on presentation that persisted after thoracocentesis was identified as a clinical sign.[3] Fibrosing pleuritis should also be suspected in any patient having

- Any condition that causes long-standing pleural effusion can lead to fibrosing pleuritis, but chylothorax has been described most commonly.
- Rounding of lung lobes on radiographs or computed tomography should prompt suspicion of fibrosing pleuritis.
- Dyspnea that persists after thoracocentesis may indicate failure of re-expansion of the lungs or pneumothorax.
- The prognosis for survival is poor: mortality in a published study was 86% at 72 hours.[4]

BOX 84-2 Causes of Pleural Effusion

- Chylothorax
- Pyothorax
- Decreased oncotic pressure, hypoalbuminemia
- Congestive heart failure
- Neoplasia
- Hemorrhage

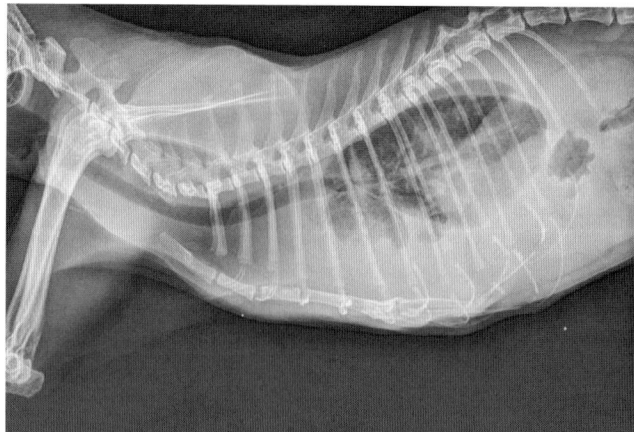

Figure 84-1: Chronic severe pleural effusion (chylothorax) has caused fibrosing pleuritis in this cat. Note the rounded margins of the lung lobes, a feature of fibrosing pleuritis.

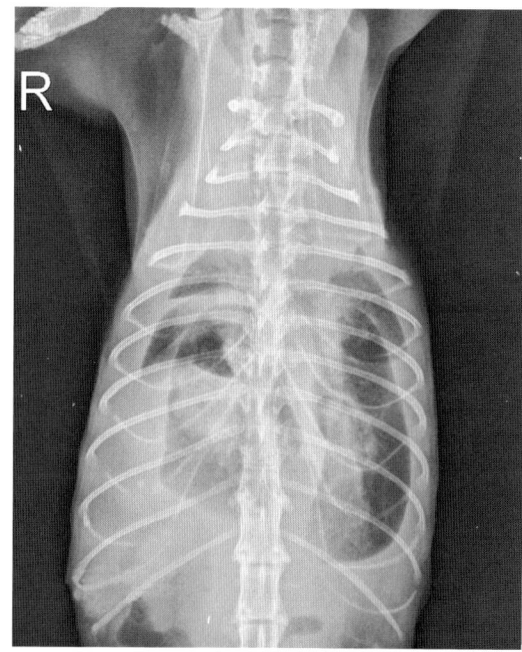

Figure 84-2: Ventrodorsal View of the Cat in Figure 84-1

suggestive radiographic changes (see Diagnostic Tests). Tachypnea and increased respiratory effort after thoracocentesis should prompt consideration of "trapped lung" or pneumothorax. If radiographs or thoracic auscultation raises suspicions of pneumothorax, repeated thoracocentesis should be considered; however, if a large leak has formed it may be difficult to achieve negative pressure. Thoracostomy tube placement or thoracotomy may be required, but the poor prognosis associated with FP (if present) should be communicated to pet owners. In addition to FP and pneumothorax, re-expansion pulmonary edema is a differential diagnosis for respiratory distress that persists after thoracocentesis.

DIAGNOSTIC TESTS

Radiographs and computed tomography may show rounded lung lobes in patients with FP, rather than the usual leaf-shaped lobes seen with acute effusions (Figures 84-1 and 84-2). Pleural fluid analysis and cytopathology may help differentiate the cause for the effusion; the interested reader is directed to other resources for a discussion of fluid analysis.

THERAPY AND PROGNOSIS

The most important therapy for FP is prevention. Addressing and treating the condition underlying the pleural effusion are necessary to prevent progression to FP. This may mean a combination of medical or surgical therapies and is of particular importance in patients with chylothorax. Once FP has progressed to the point where thoracocentesis does not relieve respiratory signs (or leads to complications such as pneumothorax), the prognosis for satisfactory quality of life is poor, in the author's opinion. The reported mortality rate in the literature (in a study of five cats and two dogs with FP) is 86% within 72 hours of diagnosis.[4] Decortication (surgical removal of the pleural layer of fibrinous scar tissue) has been described as an option for surgical management of FP,[3] but in the one extant case report re-expansion pulmonary edema led to patient death within hours of the procedure.[4]

References

1. Tortora GJ, Grabowski SR: *Principles of anatomy and physiology*, ed 13, Menlo Park, 1996, Biological Sciences Textbooks.
2. Orton EC: Pleura and pleural space. In Slatter D, editor: *Textbook of small animal surgery*, ed 2, Philadelphia, 1993, Saunders, pp 381–399.
3. Fossum TW: Surgery of the lower respiratory system: pleural cavity and diaphragm. In Fossum TW, editor: *Small animal surgery*, St Louis, 1997, Mosby, pp 675–681.
4. Fossum TW, Evering WN, Miller MW, et al: Severe bilateral fibrosing pleuritis associated with chronic chylothorax in five cats and two dogs. *J Am Vet Med Assoc* 201:317–324, 1992.
5. Huggins JT, Sahn SA: Causes and management of pleural fibrosis. *Respirology* 9:441–447, 2004.

Feline Diabetic Ketoacidosis

Gretchen Statz

Diabetes mellitus (DM) develops as a result of a relative or absolute decrease in insulin, resulting in fasting hyperglycemia and glucosuria.[1] In normal animals, insulin is necessary to transport glucose, amino acids, free fatty acids, and electrolytes into the cell for energy.[1] Insulin also serves to slow the release of free fatty acids into circulation from the adipose cells (i.e., inhibits lipolysis). In the diabetic state, lack of insulin or insulin resistance results in a buildup of these substances (glucose, free fatty acids, and electrolytes) in the bloodstream while the cells themselves are in a state of starvation.[1] The perceived starvation triggers an increase in stress hormones (e.g., epinephrine, growth hormone, and cortisol) and an increase in glucagon.[1] Glucagon stimulates gluconeogenesis (glucose production) and glycogenolysis in the liver (breakdown of glycogen to glucose), resulting in further hyperglycemia. It also promotes hepatic production of ketones from free fatty acids to provide the cells with an alternate energy source. The excess glucose, electrolytes, and gluconeogenic substrates overwhelm the proximal renal tubular resorptive capacity and are lost into the glomerular filtrate, resulting in free water loss via osmotic diuresis. The ketoacids formed in the liver include acetoacetate and beta hydroxybutyrate. Some of the acetoacetate is converted to acetone, which is then excreted in the lungs, resulting in "ketone breath."[1] If ketone production is in excess of what the tissues can use, a metabolic acidosis ensues. The result is termed *diabetic ketoacidosis (DKA)*. If left untreated, DM can progress to a ketotic state, but other disease processes can predispose a previously regulated diabetic animal to a ketotic condition by causing insulin resistance and a relative insulin deficiency. Reintroduction of insulin and a shift back to carbohydrate metabolism are needed to divert metabolism away from ketone production.

Cats with DKA are typically middle-aged to older and may have signs typical of DM (e.g., polyuria and polydipsia, polyphagia, and weight loss) or signs of generalized illness (e.g., vomiting, diarrhea, anorexia, or lethargy). Severely affected cats may be obtunded or comatose.

On physical examination, cats with DKA may have poor body condition due to unregulated DM or due to a separate underlying disease process. They are often dehydrated and may have varying degrees of shock depending on the severity of dehydration and hypovolemia. Some cats may present with ketone breath.[1]

LABORATORY FINDINGS

The hallmark laboratory findings include marked hyperglycemia, glucosuria, a metabolic acidosis (low serum pH, low serum bicarbonate—less than 12 mmol/L [less than 12 mEq/L]), and ketones in the urine or serum. Other common findings on initial presentation may include azotemia depending on the level of dehydration, elevated liver enzymes and total bilirubin due to primary hepatic disease, decreased hepatocellular perfusion and/or hepatic lipidosis, and electrolyte abnormalities. Hyperglycemia typically results in a decline in sodium levels in an effort by the body to keep serum osmolality stable.[2] Potassium and phosphorous levels may be normal initially due to the metabolic acidosis shifting potassium from the intracellular space to the extracellular space. As the metabolic acidosis is corrected and once insulin is available to move potassium into the cells, the serum potassium and phosphorous levels are likely to drop significantly.

Beta hydroxybutyrate production predominates in DKA patients and is typically found at a ratio of 3:1 to acetoacetate.[3] In states of decreased perfusion and hypoxia, the ratio of beta hydroxybutyrate to acetoacetate can reach 15:1.[3] Beta hydroxybutyrate is eventually metabolized to acetoacetate in the liver before being eliminated.[3] This concept is important to understand, because urine dipsticks measure acetoacetate and acetone but not beta hydroxybutyrate. Therefore, cats with a predominance of beta hydroxybutyrate may have negative urine ketone results despite having ketoacidosis. Despite this, the urine dipstick method is the standard method for detecting ketone bodies. Serum or plasma can be used on the urine dipstick in place of urine to measure ketones and may be a more sensitive measure of ketosis.[3] Blood may also be easier to obtain in dehydrated patients or for repeat monitoring. Benchtop and handheld meters are available that measure serum beta hydroxybutyrate (Precision Xtra; Abbott Diabetes Care Inc., Alameda, California). Serum beta hydroxybutyrate levels greater than 0.6 mmol/L are considered abnormal.[4] Beta hydroxybutyrate is not specific to diabetes or DKA and can be elevated in other disease processes, specifically hepatic lipidosis.[5]

The anion gap can be calculated and should be high in patients with DKA. The anion gap represents anions in the blood that are not routinely measured. In the case of DKA, the anions are a result of ketoacidosis and in some cases lactic acidosis from decreased tissue perfusion.[6]

$$\text{Anion gap} = (\text{Sodium [mEq/L]} + \text{Potassium [mEq/L]}) \\ - (\text{Chloride [mEq/L]} + HCO_3^- \text{ [mEq/L]})$$

A normal anion gap is between 12 and 20, whereas a typical anion gap in DKA is between 20 and 35.

Serum osmolality is typically increased in cats with DKA and can be calculated using the following equation:

$$\text{Calculated osmolality} = 2(\text{Sodium [mEq/L]} \\ + \text{Potassium [mEq/L]} + \text{BUN [mg/dL]}) \\ \div 2.8 + \text{Glucose (mg/dL)} \div 18$$

_____

BUN, Blood urea nitrogen.

Normal osmolality is between 290 and 310 mOsm/kg.

As glucose and osmolality rise, sodium levels decrease to keep the osmolality stable. Corrected sodium can be calculated using the following equation:

$$\text{Corrected Sodium} = \text{Sodium} + (1.6 \times (\text{Glucose [mg/dL]} \\ - 100) \div 100)$$

A normal measured sodium level in the face of marked hyperglycemia is inappropriate and represents some degree of free water loss.[1]

In addition to basic diagnostics (e.g., complete blood count, chemistry profile, and urinalysis), further diagnostics are often warranted to look for other disease processes. This may include urine culture, imaging (radiographs and/or abdominal ultrasound), and feline pancreatic lipase immunoreactivity.

TREATMENT AND MONITORING

The main goals of treatment include the following:
- Addressing fluid needs
- Insulin therapy to stop ketone formation
- Electrolyte replacement
- Treatment of the underlying disease process

Patients with DKA require aggressive treatment and monitoring and ideally should be managed in a 24-hour facility with the ability to place central intravenous (IV) lines, to perform laboratory tests in-house, and to provide multiple fluid pumps for the various constant rate infusions (CRIs) that may be necessary. Blood glucose and electrolytes need to be monitored frequently to adjust the insulin dose and electrolyte solutions.

Ideally, DKA patients should have a central IV line placed to easily draw blood for frequent monitoring. A second peripheral catheter can be placed to provide fluid therapy. Dextrose supplementation, if required, can be administered through the peripheral catheter to avoid effects on the glucose readings. Glucose monitoring and the insulin CRI should be administered through the central line.

Fluid Therapy

The fluid type of choice in DKA patients depends on the individual, but typically a crystalloid solution such as 0.9% sodium chloride (NaCl), Normosol-R (Abbott Laboratories, Chicago, Illinois), Plasma-Lyte 148 (Baxter Healthcare Corporation, Deerfield, IL), or lactated Ringer's solution is used. In theory, lactated Ringer's solution may be a poor choice because of the lactate that is metabolized in the liver via a similar mechanism as ketones. The metabolism of ketones could slow the lactate metabolism resulting in a buildup of lactate. As the kidneys remove the excessive negatively charged lactate, sodium and potassium may be lost in an attempt to maintain electroneutrality,[6,7] resulting in worsening hyponatremia and hypokalemia. Although this may be true in theory, it is not likely relevant in practice,[6] and any balanced electrolyte solution will suffice for the vast majority of cases. Sodium chloride is often the recommended fluid of choice due to overall body sodium depletion, but this is controversial.[6,7] Initial fluid rates should be based on the hydration status of the patient, degree of hypovolemia, maintenance needs, and ongoing losses. Fluid needs are often underestimated in cats with DKA, and fluid rates should be based on calculated needs rather than ballpark estimates or arbitrary multiples of *maintenance* fluid rates. Hypovolemia and at least some correction of the dehydration should be addressed by several hours of fluid therapy prior to insulin therapy. Rapid volume expansion can lead to hypervolemia and potentially pulmonary edema and should be approached with care[7] especially if underlying cardiac disease is suspected. Rehydration and reperfusion alone often drops the glucose by 100 mg/dL or more even without insulin therapy. Fluid therapy will also begin to correct the lactic acidosis caused by decreased perfusion. See Box 85-1 for information on calculating fluid rates.

Insulin Therapy

Once fluid therapy has been initiated for several hours and dehydration partially corrected, insulin therapy should be started. There are several insulin protocols that are designed to bring the glucose down gradually. Glucose concentrations should not drop faster than 50 to 70 mg/dL/hour

---

BOX 85-1 Calculating Intravenous Fluid Rates

Correct hypovolemia – 45 mL/kg total dose for shock, divided in $\frac{1}{4}$ dose increments given in slow boluses until hypovolemia resolved

Correct dehydration over 12 to 24 hours – % dehydration × body weight (kg) × 1000 = mL of fluids needed

Maintenance needs – 50 mL/kg/day

Estimate ongoing losses (e.g., vomit, ascites, polyuria) and add to daily fluid needs.

(3.9 mmol/L/hour) and should remain above 250 mg/dL (13.9 mmol/L) for the first 4 to 6 hours of treatment to avoid rapid osmolar shifts, which may result in cerebral edema.[6,7] Typical protocols use regular insulin (Humulin R; Eli Lilly and Co., Indianapolis, Indiana), which has a rapid onset but short duration of action, so it must be given frequently. Most protocols involve either intermittent intramuscular (IM) injections or an insulin CRI. The author finds that the blood glucose is easier to control using the CRI protocol; however, this protocol does require 24-hour hospital care. The short acting insulin protocol should be continued until the keto-acidosis is resolving and the cat is eating on its own (see Transitioning to Long-Term Care).

Constant Rate Infusion Protocol

A commonly recommended starting dose for a cat is 1.1 IU/kg/day as a CRI, which is lower than the recommended canine dose of 2.2 IU/kg/day.[6,7] In the author's experience, a starting dose of 1.5 IU/kg/day is well tolerated in both dogs and cats. Higher starting doses (2.2 IU/kg/day) were not associated with any clinically apparent detrimental effects in a study of feline patients; however, most cats in the study had their insulin CRI rate decreased over time despite the initial starting rate.[8] To make an insulin CRI, the insulin (1.1 to 1.5 IU/kg) can be added to 250 mL of 0.9% saline starting with a rate of 10 mL/**cat**/hour. (Note: *Not* 10 mL/kg/hour.) With very small cats, it may be easier to use 5 mL/**cat**/hour initially. Lower initial starting rates increase the concentration of insulin per milliliter of fluids, and adjustments in the rate make a more significant impact on glucose (i.e., smaller changes in the rate should be made). The electrolytes and dextrose will be administered from a separate bag of fluids. The fluids from both bags should be included in the total hourly fluid rate. When an insulin CRI is started, 50 mL of the solution should be discarded through the IV line after adding the insulin to saturate the plastic tubing, because insulin will adhere to the plastic. Due to the potential degradation of insulin, it is commonly recommended that the solution be replaced every 24 hours. The insulin CRI can be adjusted by 1 to 3 mL/hour as needed to decrease the glucose at the desired rate. Glucose should not drop faster than 50 mg/dL/hour (2.8 mmol/L/hour) with the initial goal of achieving a blood glucose between 200 and 250 mg/dL (i.e., between 11 and 14 mmol/L).[6,7] Dextrose supplementation (2.5% to 5%) should be added when the blood glucose drops below 250 mg/dL (14 mmol/L). Dextrose is added to avoid hypoglycemia rather than stopping the insulin to allow for continued insulin therapy, because insulin is necessary to prevent ketogenesis. Box 85-2 shows an example of how to perform the calculations for an insulin CRI. Typical insulin and dextrose CRI rates are shown in Table 85-1.

Intramuscular Intermittent Insulin Injection Technique

If an insulin CRI is not an option, an alternative technique is to give IM injections of regular insulin every 1 to 2 hours. The starting dose of insulin is 0.2 IU/kg followed by 0.1 IU/kg every 1 to 2 hours thereafter. Blood glucose should be

---

BOX 85-2 Sample Calculations for an Insulin Constant Rate Infusion

5 kg feline patient using a fluid rate of 10 mL/hour:

1.1 IU insulin/kg/hour × 5 kg = 5.5 IU insulin/hour

At an IV fluid rate of 10 mL/hour, there will be 25 hours of insulin therapy in 250 mL NaCl:

25 hours/250 mL × 5.5 IU insulin/hour = 137.5 IU insulin/250 mL of NaCl

Remove 50 mL through the IV line to saturate the plastic tubing after mixture is made.

IV, intravenous; *NaCl,* Sodium chloride.

Table 85-1 Typical Insulin and Dextrose Constant Rate Infusions*

Blood Glucose Concentration	Dextrose Supplementation	Insulin Constant Rate Infusion
>250 mg/dL (>13.8 mmol/L)	0	10 mL/hour
201-250 mg/dL (11.1-13.8 mmol/L)	2.5%	7 mL/hour
151-200 mg/dL (8.4-11.1 mmol/L)	5%	5 mL/hour
101-150 mg/dL (5.6-8.3 mmol/L)	5%	5 mL/hour
≤100 mg/dL (≤5.5 mmol/L)	5%	Stop infusion

*This chart provides general guidelines for dextrose supplementation and insulin constant rate infusion (CRI). The insulin rate can be adjusted by 1 to 3 mL/hour to achieve the desired change in glucose. If the insulin is adjusted carefully, it is often unnecessary to add more than 2.5% dextrose to the fluids. In smaller cats where the insulin CRI is calculated to start at 5 mL/hour, the rate should be adjusted by 1 mL/hour to avoid large swings in the glucose levels.

---

monitored hourly, and the insulin dose should be adjusted based on the blood glucose concentration. As with the CRI method, the goal is to slowly bring the glucose concentration down by less than 50 mg/dL/hour (2.8 mmol/L/hour) to a level between 200 and 250 mg/dL (11 to 14 mmol/L). Once the glucose dips below 250 mg/dL (14 mmol/L), the insulin can be given IM every 4 to 6 hours or switched to subcutaneous (SC) injections every 6 to 8 hours. Subcutaneous injections should only be used in cats that are well hydrated for proper absorption to occur. The SC insulin dose is 0.1 to 0.3 IU/kg and can be adjusted based on the blood glucose levels. Similar to the CRI protocol, dextrose should be added (2.5% to 5%) when the blood glucose is below 250 mg/dL (14 mmol/L) to keep blood glucose high enough to continue giving insulin. The overall goal is to keep the blood glucose concentration between 150 and 300 mg/dL (8.3 to 16.7 mmol/L), adjusting the insulin dose as needed.

Alternative Insulin Therapy Approaches

Some studies have looked at alternative approaches to treating DKA patients. One study showed success using lispro insulin (Humalog, Eli Lilly and Co.; a fast acting insulin analog) in dogs with DKA.[9] In this study, the median time to resolution of severe hyperglycemia, ketosis, and acidosis was significantly shorter in the lispro insulin group (26 hours with a range of 26 to 50 hours) compared to the regular insulin–treated group (61 hours with a range of 38 to 80 hours).[9] The time to administration of SC insulin and the time to discharge were not different between the groups. The authors concluded that lispro insulin is safe and appears to be as effective as CRI regular insulin for treatment of dogs with DKA.

A recent study in cats looked at the use of IM glargine insulin (Lantus, 100 IU/mL glargine; Aventis Pharmaceuticals, Germany) with or without concurrent SC administration in cats with DKA.[4] Cats were treated with an initial IM dose of 1 to 2 IU followed by glargine insulin at 0.5 to 1 IU IM every 2 to 22 hours as needed to bring the blood glucose down slowly (36 to 54 mg/dL/hour [2 to 3 mmol/L/hour]) until the blood glucose was below 252 mg/dL (14 mmol/L). Subcutaneous injections of insulin glargine (1 to 3 IU/cat) were given every 12 hours. The goal was to maintain the blood glucose between 180 and 252 mg/dL (10 to 14 mmol/L). Protocols varied for each case and depended somewhat on whether overnight monitoring was an option. If the blood glucose dropped below 180 mg/dL (10 mmol/L), dextrose therapy was initiated. Only two of 15 cats developed hypoglycemia (blood glucose concentration less than 54 mg/dL [3 mmol/L]), however, neither cat had associated clinical signs. All cats survived to discharge with a median hospital stay of 4 days (range of 2 to 5 days). One-third (five out of 15) of the cats in the study achieved diabetic remission. The median time to remission was 20 days (range of 15 to 29 days). Two of the cats achieving remission had received corticosteroids prior to development of the diabetes. None of the cats achieving remission relapsed during the course of the study.

The author of the study recommends the following for the majority of cats: Administer glargine insulin SC (1 to 2 IU/cat every 12 hours) starting immediately and concurrent IM glargine (0.5 to 1 IU/cat) starting several hours after fluid resuscitation. Intramuscular injections of glargine (0.5 to 1 IU/cat) are repeated as often as every 4 hours to achieve a blood glucose concentration of 180 to 252 mg/dL (10 to 14 mmol/L). The treatment is changed to SC injections alone when the cat's appetite returns and dehydration resolves.

This protocol may be more cost effective than CRI insulin (although the cost of glargine insulin has been variable) and might be easier in cases where overnight care is not available. In the study, if overnight care was not available, the evening insulin dose was conservative or withheld and IV fluids were changed to a 2.5% glucose containing solution.

Electrolyte Therapy

Once hydration is corrected and insulin is started, serum electrolytes need to be monitored closely. Insulin moves potassium and phosphorous into the cells and drops serum levels significantly. Correcting the acidosis also causes a shift in the electrolytes, which will contribute to their decrease.

Potassium

Serum potassium concentrations should be monitored every 6 to 8 hours and supplemented accordingly. The typical rates of potassium supplementation are noted in Table 85-2. This table is a guideline only, and more aggressive supplementation is often necessary in animals with DKA to achieve normal potassium levels. Table 85-3 provides guidelines for a more precise approach to potassium supplementation and takes into account fluid rates.[10] Potassium supplementation is typically provided in the form of potassium chloride, but potassium phosphate can also be used to supplement some of the potassium if phosphorous supplementation is necessary (see later).

If the potassium is severely decreased (less than 2.9 mEq/L), a potassium CRI could be considered. A potassium CRI can be administered by giving the maximum safe potassium dose over 4 to 6 hours (i.e., 0.5 mEq/kg/hour for

Table 85-2	General Guide to Potassium Supplementation for Intravenous Fluid Therapy	
Serum Potassium Concentration (mEq/L)	**Potassium Supplementation (mEq/L)**
<2.0	80
2.1-2.5	60
2.6-3.0	40
3.1-3.5	28
3.6-5.0	20

Table 85-3	A Precise Approach to Supplementing Potassium in Intravenous Fluids	
Serum Potassium Concentration (mEq/L)	**Potassium Chloride Dosage**
>3.5 (maintenance)	0.05-0.1 mEq/kg/hour
3-3.5	0.1-0.2 mEq/kg/hour
2.5-3	0.2-0.3 mEq/kg/hour
2-2.5	0.3-0.4 mEq/kg/hour
<2	0.4-0.5 mEq/kg/hour (maximum dose: 0.5 mEq/kg/hour)

4 to 6 hours). Any potassium contained in the IV fluid solution should also be considered when calculating the CRI rate. The CRI volume of potassium chloride can be diluted with an equal volume of saline for easier administration. A potassium CRI must be given via a syringe pump by qualified staff, and CRI lines must not be flushed inappropriately nor should potassium be given by bolus dosing. Rapid administration of potassium can be fatal, because it stops the ability of heart muscle cells to repolarize, resulting in bradycardia and eventually asystole. This can be detected on an electrocardiogram as peaked T waves, prolonged PR interval, widened QRS complexes, and eventually asystole. The serum potassium level should be rechecked after the CRI to determine ongoing potassium supplementation needs. Potassium can also be supplemented with ongoing IV fluid therapy instead of or after a CRI.

Phosphorous

Serum phosphorous should be monitored every 8 to 12 hours. Phosphorous can become critically low in these patients and should be supplemented if it drops below 1.5 mg/dL (0.48 mmol/L). Phosphorous is necessary for energy production and to stabilize red blood cell membranes. Because of the membrane stabilizing effects, low serum phosphorous concentration can result in hemolytic anemia if left untreated. Phosphorous can be supplemented using potassium phosphate as one-third to one-half of the potassium supplementation, or administered more precisely at a rate of 0.03 to 0.06 mmol phosphate/kg/hour, with some patients requiring doses as high as 0.2 mmol/kg/hour. Table 85-4 provides guidelines for phosphorous supplementation.[10] In the author's experience, 0.1 mmol/kg/hour will increase the phosphorous reliably, but the phosphorus must be monitored closely (4 hours after starting supplementation) to avoid overcorrection. The potassium chloride dosage should be adjusted to account for the potassium in the potassium phosphate. Potassium phosphate is incompatible with fluids that contain calcium, so lactated Ringer's solution should not be used for phosphate administration.

Magnesium

Patients with DKA can develop magnesium deficiency as a result of decreased intake, renal loss, or changes in distribu-

tion.[1] Ionized magnesium is the ideal way to measure total body magnesium. In one study of cats with DKA, ionized magnesium was found to be low in 80% of cats with DKA on presentation, whereas total magnesium levels were only decreased in 20%.[11] Hypomagnesemia can cause weakness, seizures, cardiac arrhythmias, and hypertension and can exacerbate hypokalemia and hypocalcemia.[11] Treatment is not routinely administered but could be considered if the total magnesium drops below 1 mg/dL (0.4 mml/L) or the ionized magnesium drops below 0.5 mg/dL (0.2 mmol/L), especially in cases of hypokalemia or hypocalcemia that are refractory to treatment.[6] Magnesium can be supplemented using magnesium sulfate at a rate of 0.75 to 1 mEq/kg/day IV for the first 24 hours and decreased to half that dose if continued treatment is necessary.[6]

Treating Metabolic Acidosis

Bicarbonate (HCO_3^-) therapy is rarely necessary and is somewhat controversial in treatment of DKA. The metabolic acidosis in these cases often corrects relatively quickly once fluid therapy and insulin therapy are initiated. Bicarbonate therapy is generally reserved for cases with severe, persistent metabolic acidosis (pH less than 7, HCO_3^- less than 8 mmol/L) after 24 hours of fluid therapy. Bicarbonate administration has been associated with risk for development of cerebral edema in children with DKA[12] and can cause a rebound alkalemia and paradoxical intracellular or central nervous system acidosis.[6] An example of how to calculate the bicarbonate deficit is found in Box 85-3.

Nutritional Support

It is important to provide nutritional support to cats that are anorexic or hyporexic. A feeding tube is ideal if the patient has been anorexic for more than 48 hours or hyporexic for more than 3 to 5 days. A naso-esophageal tube is easy to place without anesthesia in most patients for temporary nutritional support. For cases where prolonged anorexia is anticipated or where hepatic lipidosis is suspected or confirmed, an

---

Table 85-4	Guidelines for Phosphorus Supplementation
Serum Phosphorous Concentration	**Potassium Phosphorous Dosage**
2-2.5 mg/dL (0.64-0.81 mmol/L)	0.03 mmol/kg/hour
1.5-2 mg/dL (0.48-0.64 mmol/L)	0.06 mmol/kg/hour
1-1.5 mg/dL (0.32-0.48 mmol/L)	0.09 mmol/kg/hour
<1 mg/dL	0.12 mmol/kg/hour

BOX 85-3 Calculating the Bicarbonate Deficit

mEq bicarbonate = 0.4 × body weight (kg)
× (12 − patient's serum bicarbonate)

Give ¼ to ½ the deficit using sodium bicarbonate over 4 to 6 hours, and then reassess the blood gases.

Example:
For a 5 kg cat with a serum bicarbonate of 8 mmol/L:

0.4 × 5 kg × (12 − 8) = 8 mEq bicarbonate

Give ⅓ to ½ the deficit (2.7 to 4 mEq bicarbonate) over 4 to 6 hours, and reassess.

BOX 85-4 Calculating Resting Energy Requirements

RER in kcal/day = Body weight (kg) × 30 + 70

Example:
For a 5 kg cat:

RER = 5 × 30 + 70 = 220 kcal/day

Depending on duration of anorexia, start at ⅓ to ½ the calculated requirement (73 kcal/day to 110 kcal/day), and gradually increase.

RER, Resting energy requirement.

BOX 85-5 Concurrent Illness and Medications that Can Complicate Recovery from Diabetic Ketoacidosis

Hyperthyroidism
Inflammatory bowel disease
Eosinophilic granuloma complex
Hepatic lipidosis
Cholangiohepatitis
Chronic kidney disease
Pancreatitis
Corticosteroid use

esophagostomy tube can be placed under general anesthesia once the cat is cardiovascularly and metabolically stable. If a naso-esophageal tube is in place, a liquid diet designed for tube feeding veterinary patients must be used. If an esophagostomy tube is placed, any diet can be fed due to the large diameter of the tube, including convalescent diets. Nutritional support should be started once the cat is cardiovascularly stable and normothermic. Depending on the length of time without food, the nutritional support can be started at one-third to one-half the calculated daily maintenance calorie requirement and gradually increased over 2 to 3 days. Calculations for the daily maintenance caloric requirement can be found in Box 85-4.

Miscellaneous Therapy

Antibiotics should be given if a bacterial infection is suspected or (ideally) confirmed. Urinary tract infections are common in diabetic animals and can contribute to insulin resistance. Lower urinary tract infections can lead to pyelonephritis in some cases. Pancreatitis in cats can be bacterial in origin in some cases, resulting from ascending infection from the gastrointestinal tract.[13] Antibiotic choice should ideally be based on culture and sensitivity testing. If culture is not available, an antibiotic that targets common urinary tract isolates (*Escherichia coli, Proteus* spp., *Pseudomonas* spp., *Staphylococcus* spp., etc.) should be chosen. A good parenteral option might be potentiated penicillin, such as ampicillin/sulbactam, or enrofloxacin.

Transitioning to Long-Term Care

Once the cat is eating well or tolerating tube feeding at the maintenance requirements and the serum ketones are negative (or significantly decreased), a longer-acting insulin can be initiated. The most widely used long-acting insulin in cats is currently glargine. When preparing to switch to long-acting insulin, the first injection should be given in the morning or evening to try to mimic the insulin schedule that will be used long term by the owner. The insulin CRI should be stopped 1 or 2 hours before the first dose of long-acting insulin is administered. The blood glucose should continue to be monitored while the cat is in the hospital, but the insulin dose should not be adjusted based on the initial readings unless hypoglycemia occurs. Discharge from the hospital can take place when the cat is stable, no longer needs fluid and electrolyte supplementation, is eating well on its own or tolerating assisted tube feeding well, and is stable on the long-acting insulin. The goal of initial insulin therapy is not perfect diabetic regulation, as it takes days or weeks for the patient to adjust to the new insulin dose. A blood glucose curve should be evaluated 1 week after discharge from the hospital.

PROGNOSIS

The prognosis in cats with DKA can be considered guarded. Survival rates vary among studies with a 76% survival in one study[14] and a 100% survival rate in another.[4] Remission rates in cats with DKA have been found to be as high as 30% in one study[4] and 58% in another.[15] Death is often a result of severe concurrent illness (Box 85-5), severe metabolic acidosis, or development of complications.[6]

References

1. Kerl M: Diabetic ketoacidosis: pathophysiology and clinical and laboratory presentation. *Compendium* 23:220–227, 2001.
2. Schermerhorn T, Barr SC: Relationships between glucose, sodium and effective osmo-
lality in diabetic dogs and cats. *J Vet Emerg Crit Care* 16:19–24, 2006.
3. Brady MA, Dennis JS, Wagner-Mann C: Evaluating the use of plasma hematocrit samples to detect ketones utilizing urine dipstick colorimetric methodology in diabetic dogs and cats. *J Vet Emerg Crit Care* 13:1–6, 2003.
4. Marshall RD, Rand JS, Gunew MN, et al: Intramuscular glargine with or without

concurrent subcutaneous administration for treatment of feline diabetic ketoacidosis. *J Vet Emerg Crit Care* 23:286–290, 2013.

5. Aroch I, Shechter-Polak M, Segev G: A retrospective study of serum β-hydroxybutyric acid in 215 ill cats: clinical signs, laboratory findings and diagnoses. *Vet J* 191:240–245, 2012.

6. Feldman EC, Nelson RW: Diabetic ketoacidosis. In Feldman ED, Nelson RW, editors: *Canine and feline endocrinology and reproduction*, ed 3, Philadelphia, 2004, Saunders, pp 580–615.

7. Kerl ME: Diabetic ketoacidosis: treatment recommendations. *Compendium* 23:330–339, 2001.

8. Claus MA, Silverstein DC, Shofer FS, et al: Comparison of regular insulin infusion doses in critically ill diabetic cats: 29 cases. *J Vet Emerg Crit Care* 20:509–517, 2010.

9. Sears KW, Drobatz KJ, Hess RS: Use of lispro insulin for treatment of diabetic ketoacidosis in dogs. *J Vet Emerg Crit Care* 22:211–218, 2012.

10. Huang A, Scott-Moncrieff JC: Canine diabetic ketoacidosis. *NAVC Clinician's Brief* 9:68–70, 2011.

11. Norris CR, Nelson RW, Christopher MM: Serum total and ionized magnesium concentrations and urinary fractional excretion of magnesium in cats with diabetes mellitus and diabetic ketoacidosis. *J Am Vet Med Assoc* 215:1455–1459, 1999.

12. Dunger DB, Sperling MA, Acerin CL, et al: European Society for Paediatric Endocrinology/ Lawson Wilkins Pediatric Endocrine Society consensus statement on diabetic ketoacidosis in children and adolescents. *Pediatrics* 113:e133–e140, 2004.

13. Widdison AL, Alvarez C, Chang YB, et al: Sources of pancreatic pathogens in acute pancreatitis in cats. *Pancreas* 9:536–541, 1994.

14. Bruskiewicz DA, Nelson RW, Feldman EC, et al: Diabetic ketosis and ketoacidosis in cats: 42 cases (1980-1995). *J Am Vet Med Assoc* 211:188–192, 1997.

15. Sieber-Ruckstuhl NS, Kley S, Tschuor F, et al: Remission of diabetes mellitus in cats with diabetic ketoacidosis. *J Vet Intern Med* 22:1326–1332, 2008.

Feline Circulatory Shock

Elke Rudloff and Rebecca Kirby

The cat is not simply a small dog. The folklore that cats have nine lives illustrates their durability and acknowledges their ability to survive events that would be fatal to other species. The distinctive feline cardiovascular responses to shock may play an important role in their ability to survive.

Circulatory shock represents a critical condition where rapid and effective treatment can make the difference between life and death. The authors have recognized a triad of clinical signs specific to the cat in circulatory shock (Figure 86-1): hypotension, hypothermia, and bradycardia (i.e., an unexpectedly low heart rate given the hemodynamic status). Differences in the inciting causes, degree of physiologic response, and underlying pathology make each cat unique, warranting a goal-directed resuscitation plan individualized for that patient. An understanding of the pathophysiology of feline circulatory shock and the potential causes is essential for optimizing outcome.

PATHOPHYSIOLOGY

Circulatory shock can be defined as a condition in which oxygenation of the tissues is inadequate to meet the metabolic demands of the cells. Energy is required for all metabolic functions of the cells and is stored in the high energy bonds of adenosine triphosphate (ATP). When oxygen and glucose are available, aerobic energy production within the mitochondria results in the production of 38 ATP molecules per glucose molecule. Tissues are unable to store oxygen, making optimal ATP production dependent upon both oxygen delivery (DO_2) to the tissues and oxygen utilization (VO_2) by the mitochondria. As DO_2 declines, anaerobic energy production produces only two ATP per substrate molecule and lactic acid, which will be inadequate for anything other than a short period of inadequate DO_2.

Oxygen is transported bound to hemoglobin and, to a minor extent, dissolved in the plasma of the blood. Delivery of oxygen to the tissues depends upon a bellows capable of supplying oxygen to the capillaries (respiratory system), a functional pump (heart), sufficient intravascular volume and oxygen-carrying capacity (blood), and a patent and dynamic conduit (blood vessels). The volume of blood ejected from the heart per minute (cardiac output) is the product of stroke volume (preload, afterload, and contractility) and heart rate. Should any of these parameters function inadequately, cardiovascular and neuroendocrine compensatory mechanisms

modify one or more components with the end goal of improving tissue perfusion.

The heart and specific blood vessels are equipped with mechanoreceptors that identify the pressure within their walls. Physiologic adjustments are mediated through the stretch-detecting baroreceptors that lie within the aortic arch and carotid sinuses. Afferent signals travel from these baroreceptors through the vagus (cranial nerve X) and glossopharyngeal (cranial nerve IX) nerves to the vasomotor center in the brainstem. When adequate pressure is detected, central excitatory, sympathetic efferent nerves are suppressed and inhibitory, parasympathetic efferent nerves are enhanced, resulting in a normal heart rate and vascular tone.

Sympathetic and parasympathetic receptors are stimulated by the neurotransmitters, norepinephrine and acetylcholine, respectively. Additional receptors located in the atria and ventricles of the heart are sensitive to pressure and chemical changes. These receptors appear to play a key role in the distinctive triad of clinical signs seen in feline circulatory shock.

The cardiovascular response to shock is initiated when a significant decline in cardiac output causes a decrease in stretch of the vascular baroreceptors and cardiac mechanoreceptors. Afferent neurons stimulate the brainstem vasomotor center causing a sympathetic excitatory response and inhibition of the parasympathetic tone. This results in tachycardia, increased inotropy, and mild vasoconstriction that can be sufficient in some patients to support tissue perfusion until the cause of the shock has been rectified. This phase is recognized clinically by tachycardia, bounding peripheral pulses, a rapid capillary refill time (CRT), and bright pink or red mucous membrane (MM) color and is called the *compensatory stage of shock* (Table 86-1). This compensation is transient and requires large quantities of energy. Although this stage is commonly recognized in dogs and humans, it may be very brief (minutes) in the cat[1] and is rarely seen clinically.

After the brief compensatory stage, the cat in circulatory shock will demonstrate at least bradycardia and hypotension in the early stages, with hypothermia developing as shock progresses. The order of occurrence and the precise mechanism of the distinctive responses in cats with circulatory shock require further definition and investigation. Although no single study explains the combination of events, information exists demonstrating their interrelationships.

Within the wall of the ventricle, the cat has both mechanical and chemical volume receptors that respond to disten-

Table 86-1   Comparison of Clinical Signs Associated with the Different Stages of Hypovolemic Shock in the Cat and Dog

Stage of Hypovolemic Shock	Cat	Dog
Compensatory		
Heart rate	Rarely recognized, seconds to minutes in duration.	Increased
CRT	Rarely recognized, seconds to minutes in duration.	Less than 2 seconds
MM color	Rarely recognized, seconds to minutes in duration.	Red
Peripheral pulses	Rarely recognized, seconds to minutes in duration.	Bounding
Peripheral blood pressure	Rarely recognized, seconds to minutes in duration.	Increased, normal, or decreased
Early Decompensatory		
Heart rate	Normal or decreased	Increased
CRT	Greater than 2 seconds	Greater than 2 seconds
MM color	Pale	Pale
Peripheral pulses	Weak	Weak
Peripheral blood pressure	Decreased	Normal or decreased
Late Decompensatory		
Heart rate	Decreased	Normal or decreased
CRT	Greater than 2 seconds or absent	Greater than 2 seconds or absent
MM color	White	White
Peripheral pulses	Absent	Absent
Peripheral blood pressure (indirect)	Low or not registrable	Low or not registrable

CRT, Capillary refill time; *MM,* mucous membrane.

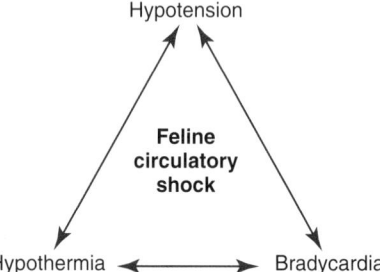

Figure 86-1: Triad of Circulatory Shock in the Cat. Typically, cats that present with circulatory shock due to hypovolemia, heart failure, or severe sepsis will be hypotensive, bradycardic, and hypothermic.

sion.[2] Small changes in blood volume appear to be primarily detected by feline-specific type-B atrial volume receptors before the carotid sinus and aortic baroreceptors are triggered.[3] The resultant increased sympathetic discharge may not have the same effect on stimulating and sustaining an increase in the heart rate in the cat as in other species.[1] It has been proposed that the activation of left ventricular mechanoreceptors and inhibition of the vascular responses may augment the bradycardia and vasodilation seen in cats with circulatory shock.[4] A pronounced bradycardia can be induced following acute rapid hemorrhage in the cat.[5] A rapid loss of

intravascular volume, extremely poor diastolic filling of the heart, and strong sympathetic excitation of the myocardium stimulate a protective cardio-cardiac inhibitory reflex. This reflex adjusts the cardiac dynamics and the efficiency of the pump to match the extent of the diastolic filling, decreasing the heart rate to allow for an increased time for the ventricles to fill. A variety of humoral substances (i.e., vasopressin, renin, and catecholamines) that are important regulators of cardiovascular and fluid volume homeostasis can also alter ventricular receptor discharge.[6] Catecholamines also play a role in inducing hypothermia as discussed later.

The release of norepinephrine from sympathetic nerve endings during the initial baroreceptor response to reduced stretch may play a role in the initiation of hypothermia. Both alpha 1- and alpha 2-noradrenergic sympathetic receptors seem to be involved in the hypothalamic mediation of the heat loss system for the control of body temperature.[7] The processes of heat loss may also include vasodilation, the inhibition of vasoconstriction, and the attenuation of metabolic heat production and shivering. In the cat, moderate hypothermia may then reduce the release of norepinephrine centrally[8] and locally in the heart,[9] which can further suppress adrenergic responses. Impaired thermoregulation will result in a cascade of events that perpetuate the triad of clinical signs associated with feline circulatory shock (Figure 86-2). Finally, an increase in parasympathetic outflow through a

Bezold-Jarisch reflex (BJR) in hypothermic cats may perpetuate a relative or true bradycardia. The BJR is a process evoked with stimulation of cardiopulmonary receptors by specific chemical and mechanical stimuli resulting in increased parasympathetic output and sympathetic inhibition.[10,11]

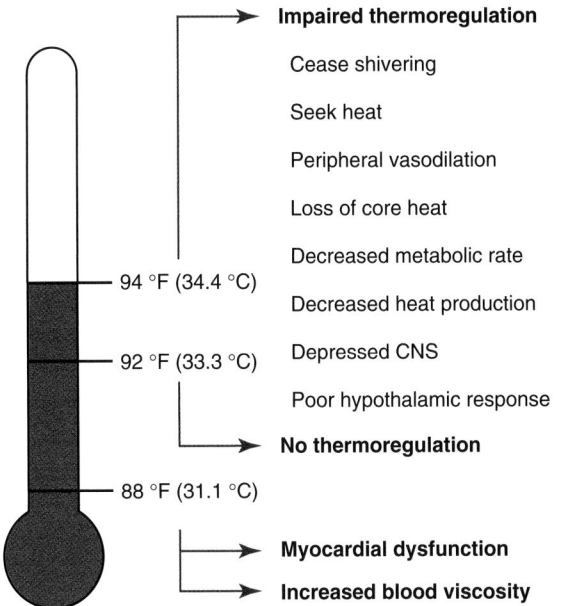

Figure 86-2: Consequences of impaired thermoregulation and hypothermia. *CNS,* Central nervous system.

In summary, it appears that reduced cardiac output in the cat causes hypotension and reduced stretch of the mechanoreceptors. There is a sympathetic response, similar to the compensatory stage of shock in other species, but it is very short (seconds to minutes) in duration. The norepinephrine released during this phase may then contribute to a centrally mediated hypothermia. Bradycardia may be a consequence of a vasovagal response elicited by mechanoreceptors in the heart and/or impaired norepinephrine release when hypothermia is present. Reduced norepinephrine release from sympathetic nerve endings and a vasovagal type response may contribute to vasodilation in the peripheral tissues, potentiating hypotension. This stage of shock is termed the *decompensatory stage.* Differentiating between early and late stages of decompensatory shock is difficult in the cat. However, the cat in late decompensatory shock is typically obtunded with no palpable peripheral pulses and significant hypothermia.

As shock progresses, prolonged tissue hypoxia leads to a cascade of events (Figure 86-3) culminating in cellular death, organ failure, and eventually the animal's death. Rapid and effective resuscitation is required to halt the decompensatory stages. However, the cardiovascular dynamics of feline shock make successful fluid resuscitation without vascular volume overload a significant challenge. The highly divergent initiating causes of feline circulatory shock are outlined in Table 86-2. Identification of the underlying cause may not be possible until the cardiovascular responses have been stabilized.

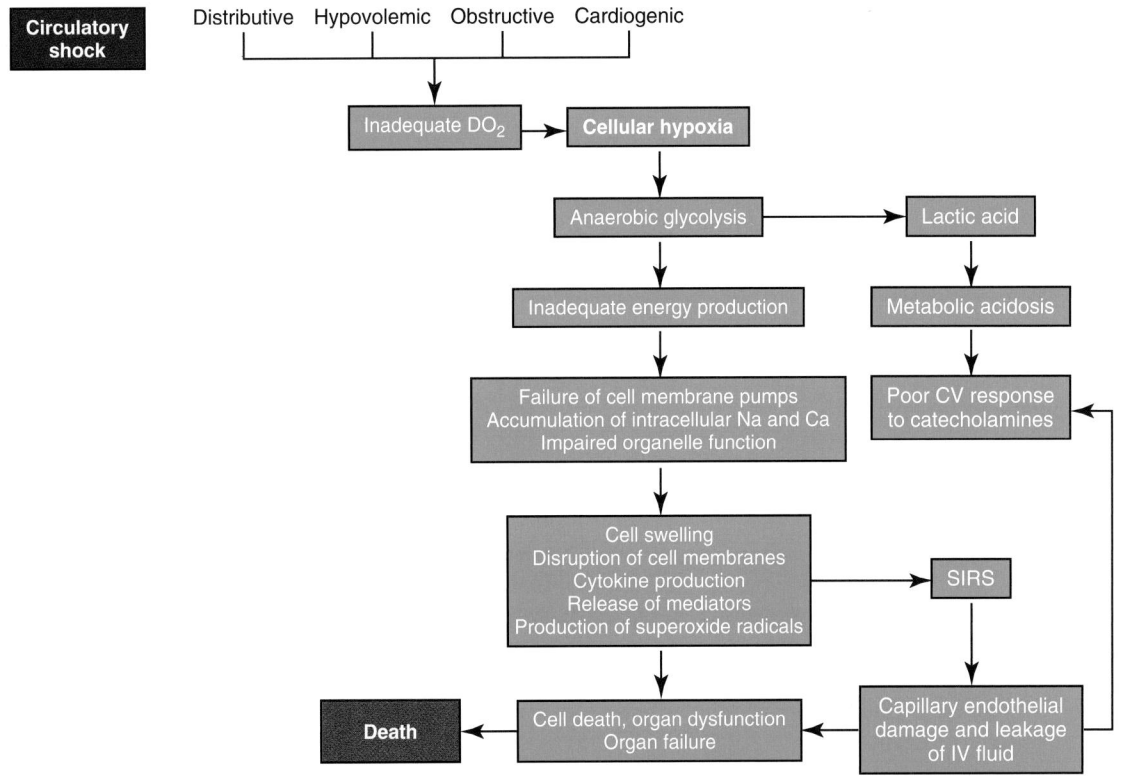

Figure 86-3: Consequences of Circulatory Shock Leading to Death. Regardless of the instigating cause and type of circulatory shock, the consequences of inadequate delivery of oxygen *(DO₂)* and cellular hypoxia culminate in a systemic inflammatory response syndrome *(SIRS),* cellular dysfunction and death, and eventually death of the animal if compensatory mechanisms or therapy is inadequate. *Ca,* Calcium; *CV,* cardiovascular; *IV,* intravenous; *Na,* sodium.

Table 86-2	Characteristics, Diagnostic Testing, Resuscitation Goals, Treatment, and Monitoring of the Different Types of Feline Circulatory Shock				
Hypovolemic	**Cardiogenic**	**Distributive**	**Obstructive**	**Common to All Forms**	
Pathophysiology					
Decreased intravascular volume, decreased cardiac output, increased peripheral SVR	Decreased pump activity, increased peripheral SVR, increased pulmonary vascular resistance, decreased cardiac output, variable intravascular volume	Decreased peripheral SVR, increased capillary permeability, decreased effective circulating volume, altered cardiac output (high early, low late)	Mechanical obstruction to venous return, reduced preload, decreased cardiac output, increased SVR	Decreased oxygen delivery Tissue hypoxia Hypotension	
Common Causes					
GI losses, third-space body fluids, lack of oral intake, hemorrhage, trauma, systemic inflammation	Cardiomyopathy Dysrhythmia Myocardial ischemia Intoxications Mitral insufficiency	SIRS diseases, spinal cord injury, anaphylaxis, severe liver disease Causes of hypoxemia	Tension pneumothorax, venous thrombosis, mechanical ventilation, severe gastric tympany Cardiac tamponade Neoplasia causing obstruction or compression, vena caval syndrome, heartworms		
Clinical Signs (Specific to Type)					
Dependent upon cause: Decreased jugular vein distensibility, with/without dehydration, evidence of systemic disease or trauma	MM: Pale CRT: Prolonged HR: Variable Pulse quality: Weak to absent With/without heart murmur and/or dysrhythmia With/without increased or decreased lung sounds With/without moist lung sounds	Dependent upon cause: With/without fever, possible evidence of systemic disease or spinal cord injury, rapid or labored breathing if hypoxemia	Dependent upon cause: Possible ascites or abdominal distension; jugular vein distension or pulse, with/without muffled heart sounds	MM: Pale CRT: Greater than 2 seconds HR: Relative or true bradycardia Pulse quality: Weak to absent Temperature: With/without hypothermia Mental depression	
Diagnostics (Specific to Type)					
Chest/abdominal radiographs, ultrasound Advanced imaging as needed	Thoracic radiographs ECG Echocardiogram Pulse oximetry Arterial blood gas analysis if respiratory distress	Diagnostic imaging Feline-specific infectious disease panel Arterial blood gas Reticulocyte count, immune panel, CBC with clinical pathology review if anemia Thoracic radiographs if hypoxia	Diagnostic imaging Echocardiogram if tamponade suspected CT if thrombosis or thromboembolism suspected Heartworm test	Immediately: PCV/TS, glucose, electrolytes, venous blood gas, blood lactate Submit: CBC, serum biochemical profile, urinalysis Coagulation profile	

Table 86-2	Characteristics, Diagnostic Testing, Resuscitation Goals, Treatment, and Monitoring of the Different Types of Feline Circulatory Shock—cont'd			
Hypovolemic	**Cardiogenic**	**Distributive**	**Obstructive**	**Common to All Forms**
Specific Resuscitation Goals (high or low end resuscitation endpoints)				

Low end if:
  Hemorrhage,
    history of trauma,
    oliguric acute
    kidney injury,
    brain or lung
    edema
High normal: Other
  causes
	Low end	High end unless oliguric
		  acute kidney injury,
		  brain or lung edema
		  or internal
		  hemorrhage
			Low end	Bring HR, BP, T, and
				  lactate to within
				  normal range

Treatment (Specific to Type)				

RBC transfusion if
  required
Treat underlying
  disease
	Inotropic support if
	  required
	Afterload and preload
	  reduction if required
	Specific dysrhythmia
	  treatment
		Antimicrobials as
		  indicated
		Positive inotrope if
		  cardiogenic
		  component
		Mechanical ventilation
		  if severe hypoxemia
		RBC transfusion if
		  severe anemia
			Relieve obstruction
			  when possible:
			  Pericardiocentesis,
			  gastric
			  decompression,
			  thoracentesis,
			  remove obstructing
			  adult heartworms
			Support collateral
			  blood flow
			Anticoagulants if
			  required
				Oxygen support
				IV fluid infusion
				Heat support

Monitoring (Specific to Type)				

PCV and TS
Rule of 20
	ECG
	Pulse oximetry
		Rule of 20	Rule of 20	Physical perfusion
				  parameters, blood
				  pressure, CVP, urine
				  output, blood lactate,
				  T, body weight

BP, Blood pressure; *CBC*, complete blood count; *CRT*, capillary refill time; *CT*, computed tomography; *CVP*, central venous pressure; *ECG*, electrocardiogram; *GI*, gastrointestinal; *HR*, heart rate; *IV*, intravenous; *MM*, mucous membrane; *PCV*, packed cell volume; *RBC*, red blood cell; *SIRS*, systemic inflammatory response syndrome; *SVR*, systemic vascular resistance; *T*, temperature; *TS*, total solids.

RESUSCITATION

The goal of resuscitation is to restore and support circulation sufficient to provide oxygen and substrate for repair and return of normal cell function. Most forms of circulatory shock require oxygen supplementation, analgesia, anxiolytic medication, and volume resuscitation. Supplemental oxygen can augment arterial oxygen concentration. Mask or hood oxygen is provided during initial resuscitation and allows continuous monitoring and treatment without interruption of oxygen therapy.

The cardiovascular response to pain stimulates the release of the same neurotransmitters as those released during circulatory shock. Pain control not only provides comfort for the cat but can also reduce the negative effects of pain-induced sympathetic stimulation. It is important to titrate analgesics and sedatives to effect after the initial infusion of fluids and target individual patient needs while reducing side effects. Reactions to the medications can be variable and their metabolism affected by underlying renal and hepatic dysfunction. For mild pain control and/or sedation, butorphanol (0.4 mg/kg intravenously [IV]) can be given. Full agonist opioids provide excellent analgesia; however, they may induce a dysphoric response. Cats have good analgesic response to the partial agonist buprenorphine (0.01 to 0.03 mg/kg IV or transmucosal) or a full agonist, such as morphine (0.2 to 0.5 mg/kg IV or intramuscularly [IM][12], lower doses may not be effective in cats due to lack of active metabolites). However, it can take 45 minutes to realize the full analgesic effects

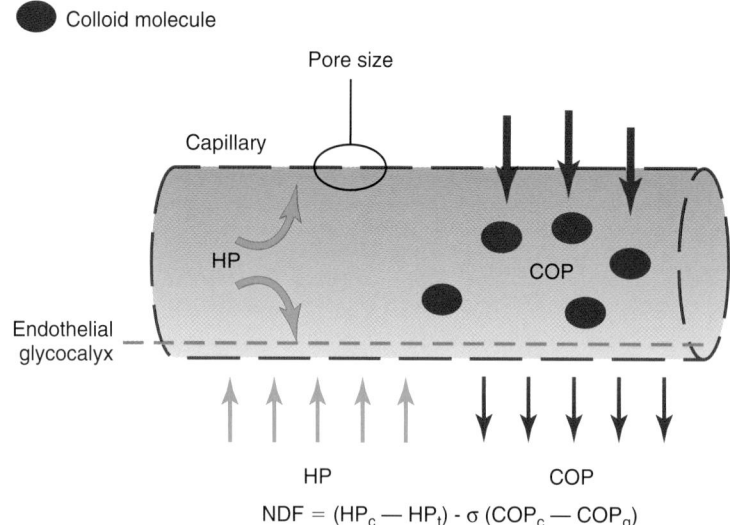

Figure 86-4: Modified Starling-Landis equation defining the driving forces for fluid movement across the normal continuous capillary membrane. Hydrostatic pressure *(HP)* within the capillary and colloid osmotic pressure *(COP)* within the subendothelial glycocalyx *(g)* compartments favor movement of fluid out of the capillary. Hydrostatic pressure within the interstitial tissue *(t)* and COP within the capillary oppose the outflow of fluid from the capillary. The difference in these forces is the net driving force *(NDF)* of fluid across the endothelial membrane. The σ is the reflection coefficient that represents the permeability of the capillary.

of buprenorphine. Methadone (0.1 to 0.2 mg/kg IV) is a rapidly acting, effective opioid analgesic, and cats have less dissociative effects with this drug compared to other pure agonists (e.g., fentanyl, hydromorphone, morphine, and oxymorphone). Methadone also antagonizes *N*-methyl-D-aspartate receptors, modulating the wind-up response. Fentanyl (1 to 5 mcg/kg/hour after 3 mcg/kg bolus infusion) can be administered as a continuous infusion and titrated to effect to maximize analgesia and minimize dysphoria.

In hypovolemic conditions, careful manipulation of Starling's forces (see later) by administering fluids is required to optimize cardiac output while avoiding harmful fluid extravasation into vital organs (i.e., lungs, brain, and heart). Cats with circulatory shock can have a blunted adrenergic response, which results in vasodilation. If large volumes of fluids are used prior to normalization of vasomotor tone, there is a high risk for fluid overload. The pulmonary vascular bed has been shown to be the main target conduit in endotoxic cats.[13-15] It has been the authors' experience that aggressive volume administration without active warming of the hypothermic cat can result in pulmonary edema and/or pleural effusion as a result of imbalances with Starling's forces irrespective of ongoing hypotension.

The amount of fluid that moves across the capillary membrane into the interstitium depends on the revised *Starling's forces:* the balance of hydrostatic pressure (HP) of the plasma and interstitium, colloid osmotic pressure (COP) of the plasma and subendothelial glycocalyx, and permeability of

the capillary (Figure 86-4). The natural particles that create COP in the blood are proteins (i.e., globulins, fibrinogen, and albumin). Albumin has a small molecular weight and is the most abundant plasma protein, so it has the most influence on plasma COP. The HP within the capillary is generated by systemic vascular resistance and cardiac output. Fluid moves into the interstitial space when intravascular HP is increased over plasma COP and interstitial HP, when endothelial membrane pore size increases, or when subendothelial glycocalyx COP increases.

Establishing a successful plan for fluid resuscitation requires four important steps that incorporate active rewarming of the hypothermic cat at the appropriate time. The primary goal is to rapidly re-establish DO_2 to core tissue beds without causing complications associated with fluid extravasation into the interstitium and third-space body fluid compartments.

Four-Step Fluid Resuscitation Plan

Step 1: Patient Assessment—Is There a Problem with Perfusion, Hydration, or Both?

The first step is to rapidly assess the patient's history and physical parameters indicative of the cat's cardiovascular status and potential mechanisms of circulatory shock. Of immediate concern is the determination of perfusion status. Circulatory shock by definition manifests with perfusion deficits. Table 86-3 provides guidelines for assessing perfusion parameters. Instrumentation and testing may be required

| Table 86-3 | Clinical Parameters and Resuscitation Endpoints during Resuscitation from Circulatory Shock |

Parameter	Normal	Poor Perfusion	High-End Resuscitation Goal	Low-End Resuscitation Goal
Mentation	Alert	Normal to decreased	Alert	Quiet but aware
Heart rate (beats per minute)	160-200	Variable Relative bradycardia	160-200	160-200
MM color	Pink	Pale	Pink	Pale pink/pink
CRT	1-2	Greater than 2	1-2	1-2
Pulse Intensity	Strong	Weak to absent	Strong	Palpable
SABP (mm Hg)	120-140	Low	90-120	80-90
MABP (mm Hg)	80-100	Low	80-100	60-80
CVP (cm H_2O)	0-2	<5	8-10	3-5
Urine output (mL/kg/hour)	1.67	<0.27	>1	>1
SpO_2	>97%	Variable	>97%	>97%
$ScvO_2$	>70%	<70%	>70%	>70%
PCV (%)	30%-45%	Variable	25%-30%	25%-30%
Hemoglobin (g/dL)	13.8-21.4	Variable	7-10	7-10
Lactate (mmol/L)	<2	Normal to increased	<2	<2
Rectal temperature	100-102.5 °F (37.8-39.2 °C)	Variable	>98 °F (36.7 °C)	>98 °F (36.7 °C)

CRT, capillary refill time; *CVP,* central venous pressure; *MABP,* mean arterial blood pressure; *MM,* mucous membrane; *PCV,* packed cell volume; *SABP,* systolic arterial blood pressure; *ScvO₂,* jugular venous oxygen saturation; *SpO₂,* saturation of peripheral oxygen.

for definitive assessment but may not be possible until perfusion has improved.

A focused physical examination can identify perfusion deficits within peripheral tissue beds (e.g. skin, MMs). Physical parameters that reflect peripheral perfusion include heart rate, MM color, CRT, pulse intensity, and body temperature (see Table 86-3). Rectal temperatures represent peripheral body temperatures and are an indirect indication of the status of peripheral blood flow. Redistribution of blood flow from the periphery to the core with vasoconstriction can give a differential core-to-peripheral temperature.

Venous volume may also be reflected through jugular vein distensibility, radiographic or ultrasonographic evaluation of central pulmonary vessel and vena cava filling, and central venous pressure (CVP). Definitive identification of an obstruction to venous return may require advanced imaging using ultrasonography or computed tomography scan to evaluate the pericardium, cardiac chambers, and major blood conduits. Trends of change identified by indirect or direct arterial blood pressure (ABP), urine output, electrocardiography, echocardiography, blood lactate, and CVP are commonly available and can provide an indirect reflection of perfusion status and the success or deficiency of resuscitation efforts within the core. Mixed venous oxygen saturation

(SvO_2) can provide more specific data regarding global DO_2 and utilization, but sampling requires placement of a pulmonary artery catheter. Jugular venous oxygen saturation ($ScvO_2$) is not as reliable an indicator as SvO_2 in people,[16] and neither one has been evaluated in feline circulatory shock. Cardiac output and pulmonary capillary wedge pressure measurement provide more specific and precise data regarding the amount of blood ejected by the heart, but they require special expertise in addition to expensive and/or invasive instrumentation.

Perfusion deficits resulting from hypovolemia typically result in concurrent hydration deficits. Hydration is a reflection of interstitial water content and is clinically assessed primarily by the following physical parameters: MM and corneal moisture, skin turgor, and eye position within the skull (Table 86-4). Dehydration will also result in fluid extravasation from the vasculature into the interstitium, which will manifest in an elevation in packed cell volume (PCV) and total solids (hemoconcentration), as well as changes in skin turgor and MM moisture. However, acute fluid movement into and out of the interstitium may not manifest with changes in skin turgor and MM moisture at the time of the initial physical examination. In addition, cats with significant fat loss or gain, and very young and very old cats can have reduced or increased skin elasticity and eye position that may not accurately reflect hydration status.

Careful patient assessment can also provide clues to the underlying mechanism of circulatory shock, which will influence fluid selection, resuscitation endpoints, and infusion technique during fluid resuscitation. Signs of potential cardiac dysfunction (e.g., heart murmur, gallop, or other dysrhythmia) should prompt evaluation of heart function (i.e., electrocardiogram, echocardiogram) early in the treatment plan. Historical and visual evidence of trauma can suggest hypo-

volemia associated with traumatic, distributive or hemorrhagic shock. True or relative hypovolemia is suspected if there is evidence of fluid loss (e.g., vomiting, diarrhea, and/or cavitary effusion), lack of fluid intake, and/or evidence of hemoconcentration.

Hemorrhage may be obvious (e.g., wounds on the external body surface or blood in vomitus, urine, or stool) or suspected with a history of trauma, evidence of cavitary fluid, or an acute decrease in PCV and total solids. The presence of significant anemia necessitates the need for a red blood cell–containing transfusion. It is ideal to type and crossmatch the donor and recipient prior to administration and to administer the transfusion over 4 to 6 hours. However, in situations where a patient is acutely decompensating, the transfusion may need to be rapidly administered with limited or no preparation. See Chapter 78 for more on use of blood products.

A history suggestive of systemic illness with compatible signs of systemic inflammation can indicate systemic inflammatory response syndrome (SIRS). Signs of circulatory shock related to a septic or SIRS condition can manifest due to a combination of hypovolemic, distributive, and cardiogenic shock (Figure 86-5). Diagnostic characteristics for SIRS and sepsis are listed in Table 86-5. Because the criteria for SIRS can be found in healthy cats, a diagnosis of SIRS is made when the criteria are found in critically ill or injured cats. The cat with sepsis-related shock may not have a significant fever response until shock has been eliminated. With sepsis and SIRS pathology, use of synthetic colloids during volume resuscitation and fluid maintenance is typically necessary, and larger volumes are usually needed compared to hypovolemic conditions not associated with SIRS.

Step 2: Fluid Selection—Crystalloid, Colloid, or Both?

The choice of fluid(s) to infuse depends on the mode of delivery, which compartment has a deficit, duration of action desired, and initiating mechanism of circulatory shock. Intravenous or intraosseous fluid administration is recommended when treating circulatory shock. Placement of a short, large-diameter catheter in a peripheral vein during the initial stages of resuscitation optimizes laminar flow and infusion rates. Fluids must be administered that will expand and remain in the body fluid compartment where the volume deficit lies.

Table 86-4	Physical Exam Findings Used to Evaluate Interstitial Dehydration
Estimated Percentage of Dehydration	**Physical Exam Findings**
4%-6%	Tacky MMs
6%-8%	Loss of skin turgor Dry MMs Slight hemoconcentration
8%-10%	Loss of skin turgor Dry MMs Retracted globes within orbits Moderate hemoconcentration
10%-12%	Persistent skin tent due to complete loss of skin elasticity Dry MMs Retracted globes Dull corneas Severe hemoconcentration
>12%	Persistent skin tent Dry MMs Retracted globes Dull corneas Signs of perfusion deficits Extreme hemoconcentration

MM, Mucous membrane.

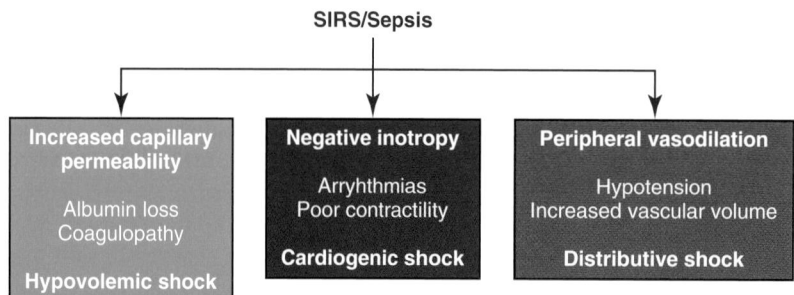

Figure 86-5: Mechanisms of shock possible with systemic inflammatory response syndrome *(SIRS)* and sepsis.

Table 86-5 Criteria for Diagnosing Systemic Inflammatory Response Syndrome, Severe Sepsis, and Septic Shock in the Cat

Term	Definition	
SIRS* Two or more of the metabolic alterations	Generalized hyperinflammatory response to inciting cause	
	Clinical Parameter	**Cat**
	Heart rate (beats per minute)	<140 or >225
	Respiratory rate (breaths per minute)	>40
	Rectal temperature	<37.8 °C (100 °F) or >39.7 °C (103.5 °F)
	Leukogram (cells/mm³)	>19,000 or <5000 or band neutrophil fraction >5%
Sepsis	SIRS caused by documented or suspected infection	
Septic shock	Sepsis associated with arterial hypotension†	
Severe sepsis	Sepsis with sepsis-induced organ dysfunction Hypotension due to sepsis Lactate above reference range Urine output <0.5 mL/kg/hour for more than 2 hours with adequate fluid support Acute lung injury PaO_2:FiO_2 ratio <250 without primary lung pathology or <200 with lung pathology Creatinine >2.0 mg/dL (176.8 mmol/L) Bilirubin >2 mg/dL (34.2 mmol/L) Platelet count <100,000/μL Coagulopathy INR >1.5	

Modified from Dellinger RP, Levy MM, Rhodes A, et al: Surviving sepsis campaign: international guidelines for management of severe sepsis and septic shock: 2012. *Crit Care Med* 41:580-637, 2013; Brady CA, Otto CM, Van Winkle TJ, et al: Severe sepsis in cats: 29 cases (1986-1998), *J Am Vet Med Assoc* 217:531, 2000.
FiO_2, Fraction of inspired oxygen; *INR*, international normalized ratio; *PaO_2*, partial arterial pressure of oxygen; *SIRS*, systemic inflammatory response syndrome.
*In the ill or injured cat
†Systolic blood pressure <90 mm Hg, mean arterial pressure <70 mm Hg, or a systolic blood pressure decrease >40 mm Hg in adults or less than two standard deviations below normal for the patient's age.

Crystalloids are water-based solutions with small molecular weight particles (e.g., electrolytes, buffers), which are freely permeable to the capillary membrane. Replacement isotonic crystalloids contain similar sodium and chloride concentration to extracellular fluid and, therefore, do not generate osmotic pressure. Over 75% of IV administered isotonic crystalloids will extravasate into the extravascular space within 1 hour, as determined by the normal distribution of replacement isotonic solutions in the extracellular compartment. More will extravasate when increased capillary permeability exists. Hypertonic saline is a crystalloid that has a higher osmolality than extracellular fluid and, when infused IV, will cause the movement of water from the interstitium into the intravascular compartment and from the intracellular into the interstitial compartment. However, this fluid will rapidly redistribute to the interstitial space during the resultant increase in intravascular HP and extracellular redistribution of serum sodium.

Colloids are isotonic crystalloid solutions that also contain large molecular weight molecules (i.e., proteins, starch) with the majority of molecules unable to freely pass across the capillary membrane. They generate COP and hold water within the intravascular compartment. Colloids are used primarily as intravascular volume replacement fluids, and isotonic crystalloids are used primarily as interstitial replacement

solutions. Intravascular retention of crystalloids depends upon intravascular HP and COP changes.

The contents of the common commercially available replacement isotonic crystalloids and synthetic colloids used during resuscitation from hypovolemic shock are listed in Table 86-6. By administering a synthetic colloid, such as hydroxyethyl starches (HESs), in conjunction with crystalloids, both intravascular and interstitial volume deficits can be corrected simultaneously. Using both HESs and replacement isotonic crystalloids may result in a reduction in the total fluid volume required to reach desired resuscitation endpoints compared to resuscitation with crystalloids alone. Therefore, shorter resuscitation times and less fluid overload may be the result.

Although HES administration can provide important and lasting benefits, it is important to recognize potential limitations. The literature has reported evidence for an increased risk for acute kidney injury (AKI) in critically ill people and people with severe sepsis when treated with HESs.[17-19] This complication has not been identified in dogs or cats. Hydroxyethyl starches have been shown to increase coagulation times, particularly when high doses are administered.

The authors have used HESs in critically ill cats for over 30 years and have not observed detrimental changes in monitored renal parameters or seen clinical evidence of bleeding

Table 86-6 Characteristics of Replacement Isotonic Crystalloids and Synthetic Colloids Used for Resuscitation from Hypovolemic Shock

Name	Fluid Compartment	Osmolarity (mOsm/L)	pH	Na⁺ (mEq/L)	Cl⁻ (mEq/L)	K⁺ (mEq/L)	Mg⁺⁺ (mEq/L)	Ca⁺⁺ (mEq/L)	Dextrose (g/L)	Buffer	COP (mm Hg)
Crystalloids											
0.9% saline	Extracellular	308 (isotonic)	5.0	154	154	0	0	0	0	None	0
Lactated Ringer's solution	Extracellular	275 (isotonic)	6.5	130	109	4	0	3	0	Lactate	0
Plasmalyte-A pH 7.4	Extracellular	294 (isotonic)	7.4	140	98	5	3	0	0	Acetate, gluconate	0
Normosol-R	Extracellular	295 (isotonic)	5.5-7	140	98	5	3	0	0	Acetate, gluconate	0
Sterofundin-ISO	Extracellular	309 (isotonic)		145	127	4	1	2.5	0	Acetate, malate	0
7.0% saline	Extracellular	2396 (hypertonic)		1197	1197	0	0	0	0	None	0
Colloids											
Synthetic											
6% HES 450/0.7 (hetastarch) Hespan	Extracellular	310 (isotonic)	5.5	154	154	0	0	0	0	None	36
6% HES 670/0.75 (hetastarch) Hextend	Extracellular	307 (isotonic)	5.9	143	124	3	0.9	5	0.99	Lactate (28 mEq/L)	36
6% HES 130/0.4 (tertrastarch) VetStarch, Voluven	Extracellular	308 (isotonic)	4-5.5	154	154	0	0	0	0	None	
6% HES 130/0.42 (tetrastarch) Tetraspan	Extracellular	296 (isotonic)		140	118	4	1	2.5	0	Acetate, malate	
10% HES 260/0.45 (pentastarch) Pentaspan	Extracellular	326 (isotonic)	5.0	154	154	0	0	0	0	None	25

COP, Colloid osmotic pressure; *HES*, hydroxyethyl starch.

at the doses recommended in this chapter. Until additional studies are done, the selection and dosing of HESs in cats with renal dysfunction or a pre-existing coagulopathy should be conservative. When cardiogenic shock is the most likely cause of hypotension, bradycardia, and hypothermia, it may be necessary to limit infusion of any fluid until treatment for the failing heart has been effective. Fluid therapy in these patients will primarily consist of careful titration of crystalloids.

Step 3: Determine Resuscitation Endpoints— High Normal or Low Normal

A goal-directed rate and volume of fluid infusion are used to reach a specific set of endpoints of resuscitation (see Table 86-3). Hypotension and hypothermia in the cat have been shown to be associated with a decreased survival and a predictor of mortality.[20,21] Efforts are made to normalize ABP and body temperature in addition to other perfusion parameters, including heart rate, MM color, CRT, and pulse intensity. If a central jugular venous catheter is in place, CVP is also maximized. Variables (e.g., renal function, presence of a third-space body fluid compartment, brain injury, lung injury, heart disease or failure, and/or closed cavity hemorrhage) require that fluid resuscitation rate and volumes be individualized for the particular patient.

When a patient is suspected of having a SIRS-related disease process (with associated vasodilation, increased capillary permeability, and depressed cardiac output), resuscitation endpoints are chosen that are at the high-normal end for blood pressure (i.e., systolic blood pressure 90 to 120 mm Hg) and cardiac output (see Table 86-3). The goal is to deliver oxygen and glucose to the cells in concentrations that promote sufficient energy production for repair and maintenance of damaged cells.

However, lung edema or hemorrhage can be worsened by aggressive and sudden increases in HP. Targeting endpoints at the low end of normal blood pressure range (i.e., systolic blood pressure 70 to 90 mm Hg) and cardiac output, also termed *permissive hypotension*,[22] provides endpoints that are at the lower than average normal values (see Table 86-3) and allows for a more gradual increase in intravascular HP. Low-normal endpoints are selected when there is a potential of closed cavity hemorrhage (e.g. trauma, coagulopathy), pulmonary contusions or edema, cardiogenic shock, or oliguric renal failure.

In people with severe sepsis or septic shock, goal-directed therapy to specific endpoint parameters within the first 6 hours of admission to an intensive care unit has been found to reduce mortality.[23,24] The targeted resuscitation goals in this study were CVP of 8 to 12 mm Hg, mean arterial pressure of 65 mm Hg, urine output of greater than 0.5 mL/kg/hour, and $ScvO_2$ greater than or equal to 70% by using fluid resuscitation. This included blood transfusion if anemic and vasopressors if unresponsive to fluid therapy. Similar endpoints have been used by the authors successfully in the cat with severe sepsis and SIRS.

Step 4: Initiation of Small Volume Infusion and Rewarming Techniques

Small volume resuscitation techniques for fluid infusion (Table 86-7; Figure 86-6) are used in the cat with circulatory shock to reach either high-end or low-end resuscitation goals. The immediate goal is to administer only the volume of fluids necessary to successfully resuscitate the intravascular compartment (Box 86-1 and Box 86-2). This technique is employed to minimize extravasation of fluids into the interstitium, titrate the amount of preload stretching a potentially disabled heart, and reduce the probability of disturbing a

Table 86-7	Resuscitation and Maintenance Fluid Types and Dosages and Endpoint Fluid Doses		
Fluid Type	**Fluid Dosage during Resuscitation**	**Fluid Endpoint Dosage for Resuscitation***	**Maintenance Fluid Dosage**
Isotonic crystalloid	10-15 mL/kg increment boluses	60 mL/kg	(30 × body weight in kg) + 70 for 24 hours
HES[†]	3-5 mL/kg increment boluses	20-30 mL/kg	0.8-2 mL/kg/hour
Hypertonic saline 7%	4-6 mL/kg single bolus	4-6 mL/kg	Not applicable
Oxyglobin	1-3 mL/kg increment boluses	15 mL/kg	0.8 mL/kg/hour
Blood transfusion	20 mL/kg single bolus	Based on PCV	Not applicable

HES, Hydroxyethyl starch; *PCV*, packed cell volume.
*When an endpoint dosage for a fluid type has been reached without successful resuscitation, then causes of nonresponsive shock are investigated.
[†]In general, the lower end of the dosage range applies to higher molecular weight HES (e.g., 6% HES 450/0.7, hetastarch), and the higher end of the dosage range applies to lower molecular weight HES (e.g., 6% HES 130/0.4, Vetstarch). Note that the published dosages for HES are anecdotal; dosages listed here are based on the authors' experience.

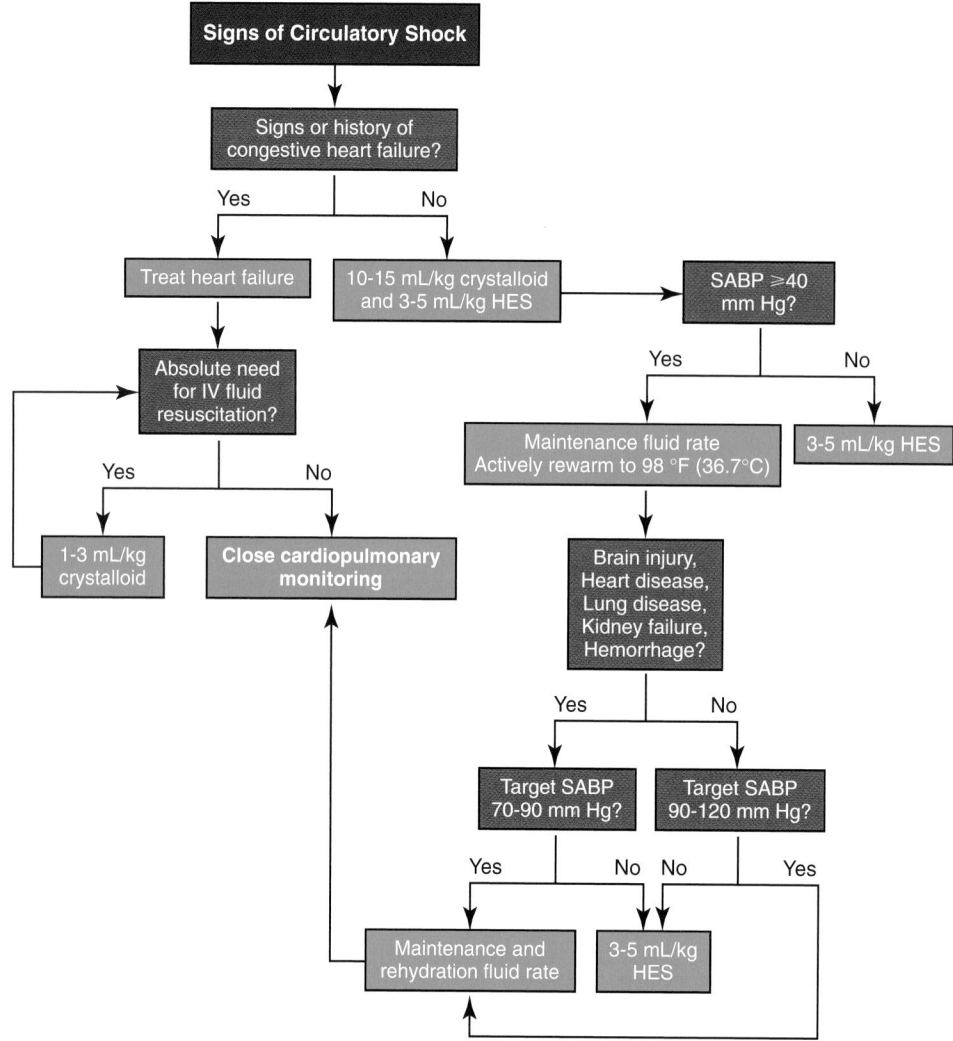

Figure 86-6: **Algorithm for Fluid Resuscitation in Cats with Circulatory Shock.** When circulatory shock is identified, it must first be determined if there is a history or clinical signs of heart failure. If there is, evaluation and treatment for heart failure is initiated. If there is a need for fluid resuscitation, replacement isotonic crystalloids are used to correct hypovolemia. If there does not appear to be the potential for heart disease, crystalloids are infused in conjunction with hydroxyethyl starch *(HES)* until a systolic arterial blood pressure *(SABP)* is detected. Active rewarming is instituted once the SABP is 40 mm Hg or greater and the cat is administered a maintenance rate of fluids. Once the rectal temperature reaches 98 °F (36.7 °C), the SABP is reassessed. If the cat has the potential for brain injury, heart disease, lung disease, oliguric renal failure, or hemorrhage, then the target SABP is 80 to 90 mm Hg. If not, the target SABP is 90 to 120 mm Hg. If the target SABP has not been achieved, HES bolus infusions are continued. Once the target SABP is reached, the cat is closely monitored for changes, and a maintenance and rehydration plan is instituted. *IV,* Intravenous.

pre-existing clot or clot formation. Fluid boluses are repeated as necessary, and rewarming techniques are employed to reach the goal resuscitation endpoints (see Table 86-3).

The presence of AKI and significant coagulopathies warrants careful fluid selection and potentially more conservative administration techniques. Crystalloids may be used as the sole resuscitation fluid when treating these patients to remove any potential for complications from colloid administration. However, when this subset of patients has SIRS or sepsis, there can be substantial benefits from HES administration. In these patients, crystalloids can be infused at 10 to 15 mL/kg and HES infused at 3- to 5-mL increments,

repeating the HES dose until reaching the desired effect. These guidelines can result in the lowest volume of HES possible to reach the targeted endpoint while supporting intravascular fluid retention.

Rewarming

Hypothermia can significantly limit the cardiovascular response to fluid resuscitation. This can lead to the administration of large cumulative volumes of fluid and extravasation of fluid into the interstitium and third-space body fluid compartments. Active external warming of the hypothermic cat

BOX 86-1 Case Example

A 4 kg (8.8 lb) cat presents with clinical signs compatible with the late decompensatory stage of shock (i.e., hypothermia, bradycardia, and hypotension). The cat is estimated to be 10% dehydrated. Thoracic auscultation finds normal heart and lung sounds. It is suspected that the cat has acute pancreatitis.

Step 1: Both perfusion and hydration deficits are found.
Step 2: A combination of isotonic balanced crystalloid (e.g., Normosol-R, Plasmalyte-A) and HES (e.g., Vetstarch) are selected. A SIRS disease process is anticipated.
Step 3: High-normal resuscitation endpoints are selected due to anticipation of SIRS disease process and normal cardiopulmonary status.
Step 4: Small volume resuscitation techniques are used. A baseline indirect ABP is not detectable. Initially, 15 mL/kg of crystalloid and 5 mL/kg of HES are given IV over 3 to 5 minutes. Systolic ABP is 30 mm Hg. A 5 mL/kg IV dose of HES over 3 to 5 minutes is repeated until the systolic ABP is 40 mm Hg or higher. Active rewarming is initiated along with maintenance fluid administration ([4 kg × 30 mL/kg] + 70 = 190 mL maintenance fluids per 24 hours) while the cat is warmed to greater than 98 °F (36.7 °C) within 30 minutes. When the temperature is greater than 98 °F (36.7 °C), the systolic ABP is 60 mm Hg. A 10 mL/kg crystalloid bolus and 5 mL/kg HES bolus is administered IV over 3 to 5 minutes. The systolic ABP is 90 mm Hg, so the rehydration and maintenance needs of crystalloids and HES are administered.

ABP, arterial blood pressure; *HES,* hydroxyethyl starch; *IV,* intravenously; *SIRS,* systemic inflammatory response syndrome.

BOX 86-2 Case Example

A 5 kg (11 lb) cat presents for persistent vomiting and hyporexia. It has clinical signs compatible with the late decompensatory stage of shock (i.e., hypothermia, bradycardia, and hypotension) with severe mental depression. The cat is estimated to be 8% dehydrated and has a string foreign body under the tongue with plication of the small intestine. Thoracic auscultation finds an intermittent gallop heart rhythm with normal lung and airway sounds. There is no increase in respiratory effort or rate.

Step 1: Both perfusion and hydration deficits are identified. The clear lung sounds support the probability that heart failure is not a significant contributor to circulatory shock at this time.
Step 2: A combination of isotonic balanced replacement crystalloids (e.g., Normosol-R, Plasmalyte-A) and HES (e.g., Vetstarch) are chosen, because the cat most likely has a SIRS process and third-spacing of fluid.
Step 3: Due to the gallop rhythm, low normal resuscitation endpoints are selected.
Step 4: Small volume infusion techniques are used to titrate the least amount of fluid necessary to reach desired endpoints. A baseline indirect ABP is found to be 30 mm Hg. Initially, 10 mL/kg of crystalloid and 3 mL/kg of HES are given IV over 3 to 5 minutes. The systolic ABP is 45 mm Hg. A 3 mL/kg HES dose IV is repeated over 3 to 5 minutes, and two additional doses are required before the systolic ABP is 40 mm Hg. The crystalloid infusion is reduced to a maintenance level ([5 kg × 30 mL/kg] + 70 = 220 mL maintenance fluids per 24 hours) while the cat is actively warmed to greater than 98 °F (36.7 °C) within 30 minutes. The heart and lungs are repeatedly auscultated and respiratory rate monitored after each fluid infusion for early detection of pulmonary edema. If the lungs start to sound congested or a significant increase in respiratory rate occurs, fluid infusion is stopped until an assessment of cardiac function can be made. When the rectal temperature is greater than 98 °F (36.7 °C), recheck systolic ABP is found to be 80 mm Hg. The hydration status is reassessed, and the rehydration and maintenance needs for crystalloids and HES are administered.

ABP, arterial blood pressure; *HES,* hydroxyethyl starch; *IV,* intravenously; *SIRS,* systemic inflammatory response syndrome.

with circulating warm air or water blankets is an essential part of the fluid resuscitation plan. It is critical to initiate rewarming procedures at the appropriate time during fluid resuscitation, beginning *after* fluid infusion has resulted in a measurable blood pressure and a palpable peripheral pulse (see Figure 86-6). The rectal temperature should be returned to 98 °F (36.7 °C) or higher within 30 minutes while giving fluids during rewarming at a daily maintenance rate and volume (30 × body weight [kg] + 70 = mL maintenance fluids per 24 hours). Commonly, hypotension present at the beginning of the rewarming period will resolve once the cat's body temperature is greater than 98 °F (36.7 °C) with little or no additional fluids. Once the body temperature is normalized, additional increments of fluids can be titrated if needed to reach the targeted endpoints with warming techniques continued to maintain core temperature.

MONITORING

Visible changes in perfusion status occur immediately after each IV fluid administration. Therefore, assessment of the patient's perfusion status is required after each titrated fluid

infusion. The first line of monitoring incorporates assessment of the trend of change in the physical peripheral perfusion parameters (heart rate, pulse intensity, MM color, and CRT) and indirect blood pressure before, during, and after resuscitation. The indirect method of measuring blood pressure is the most efficient and least expensive means. However, studies correlating indirect to direct methods of ABP measurement in normal cats have provided inconsistent results.[25-28] Indirect ABP does not accurately reflect venous return or regional blood flow,[29] so the trend of change in indirect ABP in conjunction with improved physical perfusion will imply a positive response to therapy.

Assessment of changes in body weight, urine output, CVP, and plethysmography can be indicators of changes in intravascular volume and DO_2. In general, an acute increase or decrease in body weight by 1 kg will represent an increase or decrease in total body fluid by 1 L. When clinical signs of circulatory shock occur in conjunction with an acute decrease in body weight, hypovolemia may be a component of shock.

Techniques for monitoring urine output can include the following:

1. Catching and measuring urine voided voluntarily
2. Placement of a urinary catheter and a closed collection system
3. Collecting urine from a litter box with no litter
4. Measuring the weight of absorbent urine pads before and after voiding has occurred (the pads can be placed inside a litter box)

An increase in weight of the urine pad by 1 gram is approximately equivalent to 1 mL urine. Reduced urine output (less than 1 mL/kg/hour) necessitates immediate evaluation for a urinary tract obstruction, hypotension, and/or dehydration. When those complications have been ruled out, oliguric AKI is likely. A cat with urine output that exceeds the amount of fluids infused or voluntarily taken in may be at risk for developing hypovolemia or dehydration, and the clinician should assess and possibly adjust the fluid infusion rate.

Central venous pressure can provide an indirect assessment of jugular venous volume. In the absence of increased intrathoracic pressure, right heart failure, and obstruction to pulmonary blood flow, an increasing CVP during volume resuscitation supports a volume-responsive condition. However, CVP may misrepresent venous volume when coexisting disease results in concurrent changes in heart rate, ventricular function, and venous capacitance.[30,31] To further assess venous return, additional monitoring may be required.

Dynamic changes in caudal thoracic vena cava diameter during respiration identified using M-mode ultrasonography can support a hypovolemic condition. In people, a significant diameter reduction during inspiration is characteristic for hypovolemia. Similarly, plethysmography variability index (PVI) is a monitoring variable that identifies pulse variability and measures dynamic changes in perfusion index over respiratory cycles. In mechanically ventilated hypotensive small animals, changes in the PVI to greater than 20 are reported to suggest that hypovolemia is a factor in the hypotension.[32] These particular monitoring tools have not been validated in the cat.

PERSISTENT CIRCULATORY SHOCK

Failure to reach reasonable resuscitation endpoints (see Table 86-3) with fluid therapy warrants rapid patient evaluation for complicating conditions. The more common etiologies of persistent circulatory shock (Box 86-3) are investigated and

BOX 86-3 Causes of Persistent Circulatory Shock

Inadequate intravascular volume
Ongoing fluid losses (blood or plasma)
Severe pain
Cardiac arrhythmias
Cardiac tamponade
Myocardial depression or failure
Electrolyte imbalances
Acidemia or alkalemia
Hypoglycemia
Hypocortisolemia
Neurological failure
Organ ischemia
Hypoxemia
Inadequate oxygen-carrying ability
Inadequate colloid osmotic pressure
Excessive peripheral vasoconstriction
Excessive peripheral vasodilation
Decreased venous return

specific treatment rapidly initiated as indicated. Cardiac disease should be ruled out early because treatment for the underlying heart pathology is likely required to re-establish perfusion. However, persistent hypovolemia is the most common cause of persistent or reoccurring hypotension. When a jugular venous catheter is in place, CVP is measured to determine whether the CVP endpoint has been attained (see Table 86-3). Alternatively, a fluid challenge can be given. This typically consists of a 10 to 15 mL/kg bolus of crystalloids and one or two infusions of 3 to 5 mL/kg HES (see Table 86-7). If the perfusion parameters and blood pressure improve with this challenge, then the likely cause of the nonresponsive shock is inadequate intravascular volume, and volume restoration is continued. When there is a lack of a response to the fluid challenge or the CVP is within or above the targeted range, vasopressors can be administered to support the blood pressure. If available, hemoglobin-based oxygen carriers (HBOCs; 1 to 3 mL/kg increments up to 15 mL/kg total volume) can be used to increase ABP in the cat when fluid challenges fail.[33] Although HBOCs are potent colloid fluids, it is thought that their effect on increasing blood pressure is due to the ability of hemoglobin to bind nitric oxide and increase vasomotor tone. If the HBOC has failed to increase the blood pressure or is unavailable, then dopamine (5 to 15 µg/kg/minute) or norepinephrine (1 to 20 µg/kg/minute) can be administered as a constant rate infusion (CRI). The dose is slowly reduced once the cat is able to maintain a systolic ABP greater than 70 mm Hg for 2 to 4 hours and there is evidence of improved tissue oxygenation (e.g., decreasing plasma lactate, improving acidemia, adequate production of urine, etc.).

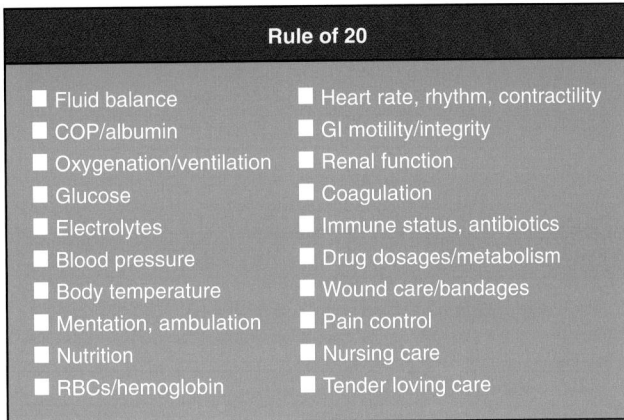

Figure 86-7: The Rule of 20. This is a list of clinical parameters that should be monitored at least twice daily in critically ill and injured cats. *COP,* Colloid osmotic pressure; *GI,* gastrointestinal; *RBC,* red blood cell.

CONTINUED CARE

Maintaining intravascular fluid volume after resuscitating patients with increased capillary permeability (e.g., SIRS) is a challenge. Hydroxyethyl starch can be administered as a CRI of 20 to 30 mL/kg/day (see Table 86-7) in the cat to promote intravascular COP and water-holding capabilities. The dose is adjusted to maintain adequate systolic arterial and CVPs. Maintenance crystalloids are administered with the CRI of colloids with the crystalloid dose reduced by 40% to 60% from what would be administered if crystalloids were used alone.

Complications associated with circulatory shock depend on the duration and extent of tissue hypoxia, magnitude of cell damage, and efficacy of treatment. Organ dysfunction or failure, electrolyte abnormalities, pain, coagulopathies, and a number of other complications can occur following circulatory shock. Assessing the parameters outlined in the "Rule of 20" (Figure 86-7) at least once daily enables the identification of organ dysfunction early and potentially prevents complications through early detection and treatment of problems. The overall prognosis depends on the success of shock resuscitation and early identification and treatment of the underlying cause.

References

1. Halinen MO, Hakumaki OK, Sarajas HSS: Circulatory reflex responses during the initial stage of feline endotoxin shock. *Acta Physiol Scand* 101:264–269, 1977.
2. Thoren PN: Characteristics of left ventricular receptors with non-medullated vagal afferents in cats. *Cir Res* 40:415–421, 1977.
3. Tomomatsu E, Gilmore JP: Blood volume changes and high and low pressoreceptor activity in cats. *Am J Phsyiol* 247:R833–R837, 1984.
4. Thoren PN: Evidence for a depressor reflex elicited from left ventricular receptors during occlusion of one coronary artery in the cat. *Acta Physiol Scand* 88:23–34, 1972.
5. Oberg B, White S: Circulatory effects of interruption and stimulation of cardiac vagal afferents. *Acta Physiol Scand* 80:395–403, 1970.
6. Zucker IH: Left ventricular receptors: physiological controllers or pathological curiosities? *Basic Res Cardiol* 81:539–557, 1986.
7. Myers RD, Beleslin DB, Rezvani AH: Hypothermia: role of alpha 1- and alpha 2-noradrenergic receptors in the hypothalamus of the cat. *Pharmacol Biochem Behav* 26:373–379, 1987.

8. Kitagawa H, Akiyama T, Yamakazi T: Effects of moderate hypothermia on *in situ* cardia sympathetic nerve endings. *Neurochem Int* 40:235–242, 2002.
9. Kawada T, Kitagawa H, Yamazaki T, et al: Hypothermia reduces ischemia- and stimulation-induced myocardial interstitial norepinephrine and acetylcholine releases. *J Appl Physiol* 102:622–627, 2007.
10. von Bezold A, Hirt L: Uber die physiologischen Wirkungen des essigsauren veratrins. Untersuchungen aus dem physiologischen laboratorium. *Wurzburg* 1:75–156, 1867.
11. Mark AL: The Bezold-Jarisch reflex revisited: clinical implications of inhibitory reflexes originating in the heart. *J Am Coll Cardiol* 1:90–102, 1983.
12. Robertson SA: Assessment and management of acute pain in cats. *J Vet Emerg Crit Care* 15:261–272, 2005.
13. Gilbert RP: Mechanisms of the hemodynamic effects of endotoxin. *Physiol Rev* 40:245–279, 1960.
14. Kuida AH, Gilbert RP, Hinshaw B, et al: Species differences in effect of gram-negative endotoxin on circulation. *Amer J Physiol* 200:1197–1202, 1961.

15. Lillehei RC, Longerbea MH, Bloch WG, et al: The nature of irreversible shock: experimental and clinical observations. *Ann Surg* 160:682–710, 1964.
16. Rivers AP, Ander DS, Powell D: Central venous oxygen saturation monitoring in the critically ill patient. *Curr Opin Crit Care* 7:204–211, 2001.
17. Myburgh JA, Finfer S, Bellomo R, et al: Hydroxyethyl starch or saline for fluid resuscitation in intensive care. *N Engl J Med* 367:1901–1911, 2012.
18. Perner A, Haase N, Guttormsen AB, et al: Hydroxyethyl starch 130/0.42 versus Ringer's acetate in severe sepsis. *N Engl J Med* 367:124–134, 2012.
19. Haase N, Perner A, Hennings LI, et al: Hydroxyethyl starch 130/0.38-0.45 versus crystalloid or albumin in patients with sepsis: systematic review with meta-analysis and trial sequential analysis. *BMJ* 346:f839, 2013.
20. Simpson KE, McCann TM, Commer NX, et al: Retrospective analysis of selected predictors of mortality within a veterinary intensive care unit. *J Fel Med Surg* 9:364–368, 2007.
21. Silverstein DC, Wininger FA, Shofer FS, et al: Relationship between Doppler blood pressure

and survival or response to treatment in critically ill cats: 83 cases (2003-2004). *J Am Vet Med Assoc* 232:893–897, 2008.

22. Duenser MW, Takala J, Brunauer A, et al: Re-thinking resuscitations: leaving blood pressure cosmetics behind and moving forward to permissive hypotension and a tissue perfusion-based approach. *Crit Care* 17:326–333, 2013.

23. Rivers E, Nguyen B, Havistad S, et al: Early goal directed therapy in the treatment of severe sepsis and septic shock. *N Engl J Med* 345:1368–1377, 2001.

24. Rhodes A, Bennett ED: Early goal-directed therapy: An evidence-based review. *Crit Care Med* 32:S448–S450, 2004.

25. Grandy JL, Dunlop CI, Hodgson DS, et al: Evaluation of the Doppler ultrasonic method of measuring systolic arterial blood pressure in cats. *Am J Vet Res* 53:1166–1169, 1992.

26. Branson KR, Wagner-Mann CC, Mann FA: Evaluation of an oscillometric blood pressure monitor on anesthetized cats and the effect of cuff placement and fur on accuracy. *Vet Surg* 26:347–353, 1997.

27. Pedersen KM, Butler MA, Ersbøll AK, et al: Evaluation of an oscillometric blood pressure monitor for use in anesthetized cats. *J Am Vet Med Assoc* 221:646–650, 2002.

28. Haberman CE, Morgan JD, Kang CW, et al: Evaluation of Doppler ultrasonic and oscillometric methods of indirect blood pressure measurement in cats. *Intern J Appl Res Vet Med* 2:279–289, 2004.

29. Greenway CV, Lawson AS: The effect of haemorrhage on venous return and regional blood flow in the anaesthetized cat. *J Physiol* 184:856–871, 1966.

30. Marik PE, Baram M, Vahid B: Does central venous pressure predict fluid responsiveness? A systematic review of the literature and the Tale of the Seven Mares. *Chest* 134:172–178, 2008.

31. Gelman S: Venous function and central venous pressure: a physiologic story. *Anesthesiology* 108:735–748, 2008.

32. Muir WW: A new way to monitor and individualize your fluid therapy plan. *Vet Med* 2:76–82, 2013.

33. Wehausen C, Kirby R, Rudloff E: Evaluation of the effects of bovine hemoglobin glutamer-200 on systolic arterial blood pressure in hypotensive cats: 44 cases (1997-2008). *J Am Vet Med Assoc* 238:909–914, 2011.

Recognition and Treatment of Hypertensive Crises

Nancy A. Sanders

Veterinary knowledge of systemic hypertension (SH) has considerably evolved for the better over the past few decades for numerous reasons. The exponential growth of the human and pet population,[1] coupled with benefits of computerized record data collection has led to an abundance of information regarding feline hypertension. Improved accuracy and availability of blood pressure (BP) measurement devices for companion animals have facilitated the ability to better diagnose feline SH. Finally, advances in the understanding of hypertension and antihypertensive pharmaceuticals in human medicine have aided the progress in effective treatment of feline SH.

Despite the many advances in the recognition and treatment of feline hypertension, cats still present in hypertensive crises without warning of pre-existing disease. This is in part due to the fact that SH is difficult to diagnose in general, let alone in aloof feline patients.

INCIDENCE OF FELINE HYPERTENSION

The estimated incidence of SH in the general feline pet population is 2.5% based upon population statistics used to determine normal ranges.[2-4] The incidence of SH dramatically increases when cats with specific illnesses or clinical signs are considered. For example, chronic kidney disease (CKD) and hyperthyroidism are among two of the most common feline diseases, and they are also significantly positively correlated with SH. Retrospective studies show the incidence of hypertension ranges from 19% to 100% in cats with CKD and from 5% to 87% in cats with hyperthyroidism.[5-22] Other less common diseases also have a high incidence of concurrent hypertension compared to the general feline population. Retrospective studies of cats with hyperaldosteronism reveal incidences of hypertension as high as 100%.[23-29] Hyperadrenocorticism is recognized with increased frequency in cats, and severe concurrent hypertension was documented in a recent case report.[30] Pheochromocytoma, although rare in cats, is also highly associated with hypertension.[31] Diabetes mellitus (DM) and obesity are common in feline patients, but they are not correlated with hypertension as they are in people and dogs. In one prospective study of 14 diabetic cats, no cats were hypertensive,[32] whereas other studies of hyper-

tensive cats revealed only a small number were diabetic.[15,18,19,24] Systemic hypertension is positively correlated with increased age in most, but not all, retrospective case studies; there is a higher prevalence of hypertension in cats over 11 years of age.* See Box 87-1 for a list of feline diseases and conditions associated with hypertension.

Cats with SH have a higher incidence of specific physical examination and diagnostic abnormalities. For example, hypertensive retinopathy is reported in up to 100% of hypertensive cats in some studies, and up to 88.4% of cats with SH have acute blindness.† Neurological abnormalities are also quite common; retrospective studies reveal 27.5% to 46% of hypertensive cats exhibit neurological signs.[9,14,18,19,37,38] Finally, cardiac changes are reported in 54% to 85% of hypertensive cases depending upon mode of detection (e.g., physical examination, thoracic radiographs, and/or echocardiography).‡

Husbandry and other conditions may also play a role in the incidence of feline hypertension. Diets high in salt are questionably associated with hypertension; studies in normal cats with high-salt diets do not show significant difference in BP from cats on normal diets.[40] However, one case report describes a cat with hypertension and hypertensive retinopathy on a high-salt diet; no underlying medical problem was found, and hypertension resolved with diet modification.[35] Female cats have a higher incidence of hypertension than males.[12]

DEFINITIONS

Systemic Hypertension

Systemic hypertension is defined as a sustained increase in blood pressure. Although the definition may be simple, determination of normal feline BP is not. Defining hypertension is even more difficult. Patient individuality, concurrent conditions, variability in response to stress, and white coat syndrome may be among the many reasons for the ambiguity.[9,10,19,41,42] Also, the studies used to determine normal feline

---

*2-4, 6, 12, 14, 15, 17, 19.
†4, 7-9, 12, 14, 16, 18-20, 25, 27, 33-36.
‡5, 6, 8, 9, 13-15, 18, 19, 21, 39.

BOX 87-1 Diseases and Conditions Associated with Feline Hypertension

Endocrinopathies
Acromegaly
Diabetes mellitus
Hyperaldosteronism
Hyperestrogenism
Hyperadrenocorticism
Hyperparathyroidism
Hyperthyroidism
Pheochromocytoma

Hyperviscosity Syndrome
Polycythemia
Hyperglobulinemia

Central Nervous System
Increased intracranial
   pressure
Vascular events

Drugs
Corticosteroids
Mineralocorticoids
Phenylpropanolamine
Estrogens
Methylxanthines
Erythropoietin

Hematological
Chronic anemia
Polycythemia

**Primary/Essential/
Idiopathic**
Renal
   Acute or chronic kidney
      disease
   Renal transplantation
Cardiovascular (cause vs
   effect)
Obesity
Paraneoplastic syndrome

Table 87-1 American College of Veterinary Internal Medicine Classification of Risk of Target Organ Damage Based on Systemic Blood Pressure

Risk Category	Systolic Blood Pressure	Diastolic Blood Pressure	Risk of Target Organ Damage
I	<150	<95	Minimal
II	150-159	95-99	Mild
III	160-179	100-119	Moderate
IV	≥180	≥120	Severe

Brown S, Atkins R, Bagley A, et al: Guidelines for the identification, evaluation, and management of systemic hypertension in dogs and cats. *J Vet Intern Med* 21:542-58, 2007.

Hypertensive Crisis

A hypertensive crisis is a serious complication of SH that warrants emergency intervention. When SH and TOD are left untreated, a hypertensive crisis can ensue. Hypertensive crises are generally confined to three of the four target organs. Neurologic and cardiovascular emergencies can cause sudden death, and ocular emergencies can cause permanent eye damage. Systemic hypertension rarely causes acute renal injury.

DISEASES AND CONDITIONS RELATED TO SYSTEMIC HYPERTENSION

Diseases and conditions associated with SH can be categorized in several ways. Systematic classification provides the following broad categories: renal, endocrine, hyperviscosity syndrome, hematologic, central nervous system (CNS), cardiovascular, paraneoplastic, iatrogenic, and idiopathic hypertension (also called *primary* or *essential hypertension*). Note that there are some areas of overlap in this classification (e.g., renal hypertension can also be classified as an endocrinopathy, and polycythemia can be included in hyperviscosity or hematological categories). Also, categories derived by this method of classification can be the cause or effect of SH. A comprehensive list of conditions associated with SH in cats is listed in Box 87-1.

PATHOPHYSIOLOGY

No single pathophysiologic mechanism can explain the cause of SH. The cause also depends upon the underlying disease. For example, increased adrenergic hormone production and/or receptor sensitivity are likely in part responsible for hypertension associated with hyperthyroidism and pheochromocytoma. The renin-angiotensin-aldosterone system (RAAS)

BP are not uniform. Interstudy differences include the use of laboratory-raised and client-owned cats, awake and anesthetized cats, and different BP–measuring instruments. Lastly, intra- and interoperator variability and interdevice differences all affect BP measurements.

Published normal values range from 105 to 181 mm Hg for systolic blood pressure (SBP), 63 to 102 mm Hg for diastolic blood pressure (DBP), and 72 to 126 mm Hg for mean arterial pressure (MAP).[2-4,9,10,43] Hypertension in cats has generally been defined as a SBP greater than 170 to 180 mm Hg. This value is based on various studies of small populations of apparently normal cats in both experimental and clinic settings, as well as on BPs of cats with signs consistent with SH. References for the definition of hypertension by DBP and MAP are even more obscure and generally not used.

Target Organ Damage

The target organs of SH are the eyes, kidneys, and cardiovascular and central nervous systems. Left untreated, sustained hypertension leads to target organ damage (TOD). Target organ damage depends upon individual variability, degree and duration of hypertension, and likely many other factors. An estimate of risk of TOD based on SBP has been previously outlined by Brown and colleagues[9] in an American College of Veterinary Internal Medicine (ACVIM) consensus statement regarding hypertension in dogs and cats (Table 87-1).

plays a part in the pathology in the hypertension associated with renal and cardiac diseases and some of the endocrinopathies. Studies show elevated renin, aldosterone, and dysregulation of the RAAS in various disease processes.[5,6,17,43-45]

In general, the heart, eyes, kidneys, and brain are targets of SH because of the insults sustained from SH (kidneys, eyes, and brain) or as a result of adaptations necessary to handle SH (heart). Strict oxygen requirements, unique vascular configuration, and susceptibility to high vascular pressure are among the reasons why target organs succumb to insult from SH. Cardiac muscle must hypertrophy to maintain cardiac output against high systemic vascular resistance. Although the hypertrophied cardiac muscle improves systolic function, it is at the expense of diastolic function. It is during diastole that coronary arterial blood flow provides oxygen delivery directly to the heart. Decreased diastolic function reduces coronary blood flow and results in ischemic insult to the heart. The heart's responses to ischemia, activated RAAS, and increased alpha- and beta-adrenergic hormones include tachycardia, arrhythmias, and additional muscle hypertrophy. This scenario results in a complex vicious cycle (Figure 87-1). Ocular and brain lesions occur as a result of compromised autoregulatory properties that arise when SBP is sustained above 160 mm Hg. In the eye, failure of the autoregulatory system causes constriction and disruption of retinal and choroidal vessels, hemorrhage and leakage of fluid and proteins into the interstitium, and subsequent damage to the choroid, retina, and optic nerve. Consequences of BP dysregulation in the brain include cerebral edema, hypoxia, ischemia, and hemorrhage. The last target organ, the kidney, suffers glomerular capillary hypertension as a result of sustained increased hydrostatic pressure. Glomerular hypertension leads to renal hyperperfusion, proteinuria, arteriosclerosis, glomerulosclerosis, and decreased tubular function.[10]

EMERGENCY PRESENTATION

Patients in hypertensive crises present with a variety of clinical signs. Signs vary based upon underlying cause and affected TOD. Signs are not specific to hypertension however; and thus, one must have a level of suspicion of hypertension to identify and treat it.

History and Presenting Complaints

Hypertensive crises are most commonly manifest by acute onset of ocular, cardiovascular, or neurologic signs. Ocular signs include hyphema, mydriasis, and acute loss of vision. Neurological signs include seizures, vestibular abnormalities, disorientation, weakness, and stroke-like events. Cardiovascular-related manifestations include respiratory distress, exercise intolerance, generalized weakness, and syncope. Pet owners may note vague signs that are more insidious in onset, such as restlessness, pacing, vocalization, inappetence or polyphagia, weight loss, polyuria, and polydipsia. Clinical signs vary depending upon the underlying disease. For a more comprehensive list of historical symptoms categorized by underlying cause, refer to Box 87-1.

Physical Examination

Similar to historical complaints, abnormal physical examination findings are confined to the target organs. Ocular defects include blindness, bullous retinal detachment (Figures 87-2 and 87-3), tortuous retinal vessels and hemorrhage (Figure 87-4), and intraretinal serous exudates. Neurological examination may reveal generalized weakness, shifting limb lameness (thromboembolic event or CNS), disorientation, mental dullness or inappropriate mentation, and central blindness. Neurological signs are common in immediately postoperative renal transplant cats, which is likely due to acute spikes in BP.[46-48] Physical examination findings consistent with cardiovascular insult include gallop rhythm, heart murmur,

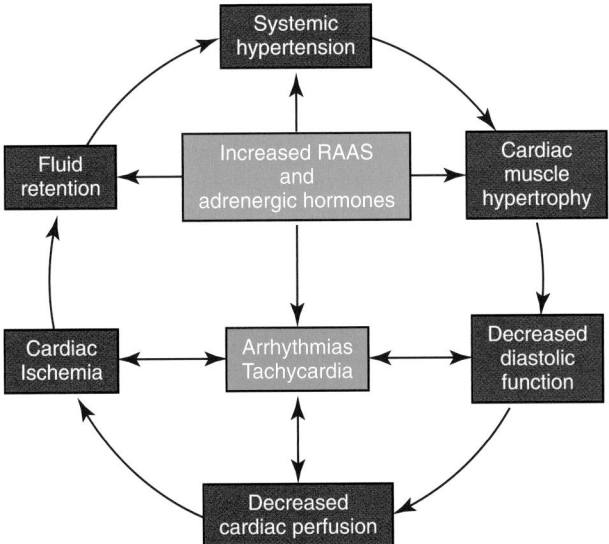

Figure 87-1: Vicious cycle of cardiac changes in hypertensive feline patient. *RAAS*, Renin-angiotensin-aldosterone system.

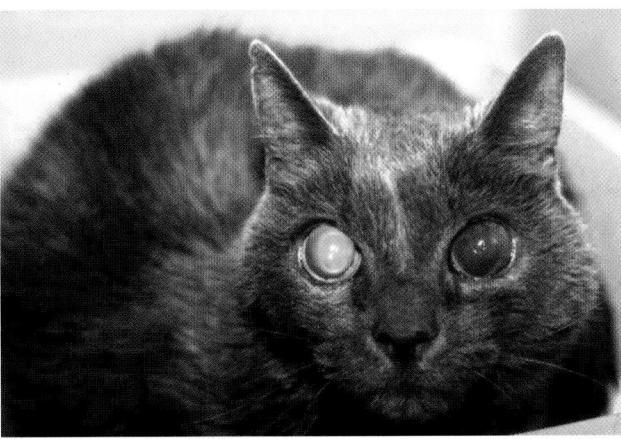

Figure 87-2: Cat with retinal detachment. Note the dilated pupils and hyphema in the left eye.

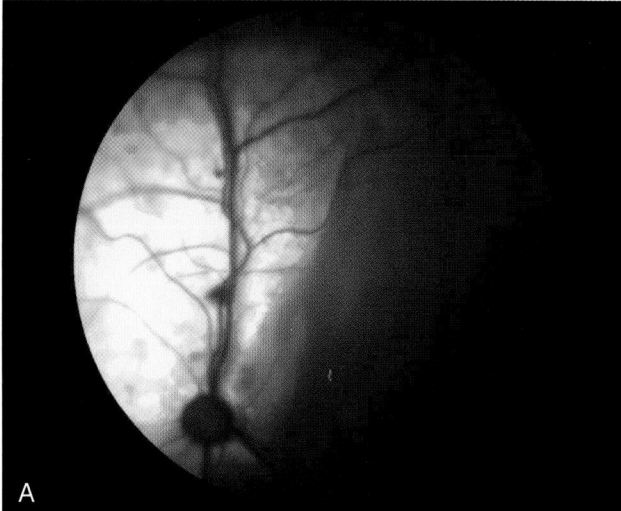

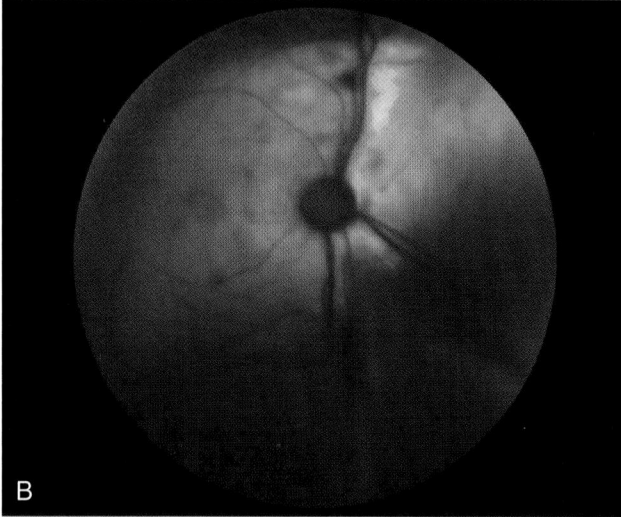

Figure 87-3: **A,** Retinal image of cat with partial retinal detachment. **B,** Retinal image of cat with near complete retinal detachment. (**A,** Courtesy of Dr. Catherine Nunnery.)

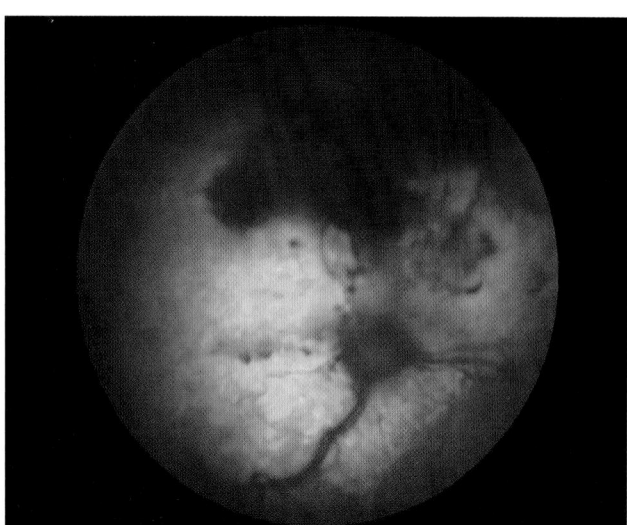

Figure 87-4: Retinal image of cat with retinal hemorrhages. (Courtesy of Dr. Catherine Nunnery.)

BOX 87-2 Clinical Signs and Physical Examination Abnormalities Associated with Hypertensive Target Organ Damage

Ocular
Acute blindness
Hyphema
Mydriasis
Retinal detachment
Retinal hemorrhages
Tortuous retinal vessels

Cardiovascular
Syncope, collapse
Exercise intolerance
Heart murmur
Gallop rhythm
"Bounding" heart sounds
Strong or weak pulses
Respiratory distress
Stroke-like events

Central Nervous System
Depression, lethargy
Behavioral changes (vocalization, pacing, disorientation, personality changes, dull or inappropriate mentation)
Syncope
Seizures
Vestibular signs
Head pressing
Central blindness
Stroke-like events

Renal
Polyuria, polydipsia
Dilute urine
Proteinuria
Hematuria
Small, irregular, and/or asymmetric kidneys

tachycardia, and weak or bounding pulses. If congestive heart failure is present, dull or harsh lung sounds and tachypnea may be present. Physical examination abnormalities indicative of renal disease include small irregular, and/or asymmetrical kidneys. A more complete list of clinical signs and abnormal physical examinations findings associated with specific diseases are listed in Box 87-2.

DIAGNOSIS

Suspicion for hypertension must exist to diagnose it. If missed, the opportunity to prevent irreversible TOD or even death is lost. Hypertension may go undiagnosed for a number of reasons, particularly in emergency situations. Reasons for lack of diagnosis of hypertension include presenting clinical signs and physical examination findings that are not specific for SH, elevated BP that is dismissed as stress or white coat syndrome, and hypertensive crisis that is not recognized and thus BP is not measured. In short, BP must be measured to diagnose hypertension.

Blood Pressure Measurement

There are a number of BP measurement devices available for use in veterinary medicine. The ideal instrument would be easy to operate, validated for use in cats, efficient, accurate, and produce repeatable results. Such a device would also be affordable and portable for cage-side use. Direct arterial blood pressure (DABP) measurement is considered the gold standard of BP measurement. However, DABP is not practical or available in most practices; it requires invasive measures, expensive equipment, advanced training, and an immobilized patient. Indirect BP devices fit many of the desirable criteria listed earlier. They use Doppler, oscillometric, high-definition oscillometric, or pressure plethysmographic methods of measurement. Oscillometric devices are particularly attractive, because in theory they can be used to take repeated measurements without operator presence and they also determine diastolic and mean arterial pressures, unlike the Doppler. The largest (and most important) issue with indirect devices, however, is accuracy. Studies have repeatedly shown that BP measurements are inconsistent and often inaccurate in feline patients. Comparison of the many studies is beyond the scope of this chapter, and the reader is encouraged to review the studies. In summary, most agree that Doppler devices are superior for use in cats, although they tend to underestimate BP and cannot be used to reliably provide DBP or MAP. There are a few studies that show oscillometric devices are the superior indirect device for BP measurement in cats.[3,10,49-55] Although hypertension may only be recognized via elevated MAP or diastolic pressure in a few select cases, the majority of cases will be identified by consistently elevated systolic pressures.[9,21]

A protocol for measuring BP should be designed for the practice and should be followed consistently to prevent erroneous measurement. Guidelines for example protocols are available in the 2007 ACVIM consensus statement regarding hypertension in dogs and cats,[9] as well as in *Kirk's Current Veterinary Therapy XIII*.[56] Protocols can and should be individualized for one's practice. Conflicting recommendations exist whether acclimatization of patients provides more or less accurate results.[3,44]

In the ideal situation, BP should be measured several times on different days before hypertension is diagnosed. In the face of a hypertensive crisis, diagnosis must be made in a short period of time and not over several days. The author recommends at least three sessions of a series of three BP measurements over a few hours. Given the accuracy of a single elevated BP measurement can be questionable, diagnosis of SH should ideally be based upon demonstration of persistently elevated BP and either evidence of TOD or proof of at least one associated disease.

Ancillary Diagnostics

Once SH is diagnosed, screening for underlying causes, associated diseases, and complications of SH should ensue. The balance between treating the patient's crisis, addressing the pet owner's concerns, and determining the underlying cause can be delicate and frustrating. Hypertension is rarely a stand-alone disease; it is more commonly a symptom of another problem. The best way to treat a symptom always includes treating the primary disease. In the emergency situation however, the underlying disease (if present) may not be

---

BOX 87-3 Initial Minimum Database for Hypertensive Feline Patients

Temperature, pulse, and respiration
Weight
Complete blood count, serum chemistry profile, and urinalysis
Total serum thyroxine
Retinal examination
Three-view thoracic radiographs
Serial blood pressure measurements

---

determined initially, and priority should be placed upon treatment of hypertension and prevention of further TOD.

Initial screening database should include complete blood count, serum biochemistry panel, total thyroxine (TT4), and urine analysis. Laboratory abnormalities that are commonly associated with, but not specific for, hypertension include dilute urine, azotemia, proteinuria, and elevated TT4. Because ocular and neurological problems are commonly associated with SH, full funduscopic and neurological examinations should be performed. Thoracic radiographs should be obtained, because cardiac abnormalities are common. See Box 87-3 for a list of initial tests for the minimum database.

Additional diagnostics should be based upon the results in combination with overall clinical picture. They may include abdominal radiographs and/or ultrasound and additional cardiac evaluation (e.g., electrocardiogram, measurement of cardiac biomarkers, and echocardiography). Radiographic and echocardiographic abnormalities associated with hypertension include aortic undulation ("lazy" or "redundant" aorta), increased cardiac sternal contact, cardiomegaly, and ventricular and interventricular septal hypertrophy.[7,13-15,21,32,57] Adrenal hormonal abnormalities are more commonly recognized in cats. If refractory hypokalemia exists, aldosterone measurement should be performed. If signs consistent with hyperadrenocorticism are present (e.g., thin and fragile skin, uncontrolled DM), adrenal function testing should be included in the medical workup.

EMERGENCY MANAGEMENT

Treatment of hypertension should never be instituted based upon a single BP measurement. The decision to institute emergency antihypertensive medications should depend upon several factors, including the patient's current BP, risk of TOD, evidence of current TOD, and any history of previously diagnosed hypertension or diseases associated with hypertension. Knowledge, detailed case history, thorough physical examination, clinical experience, and common sense must all be integrated when interpreting BP results. If BP results do not fit the case, then repeated measurements are warranted. Cats that present with historical or physical evidence of TOD are much more likely to truly be hypertensive. On occasion, cats presenting in hypertensive crises may have only moderately elevated BP. This can happen for a number of reasons. For example, patients with an acute increase in BP may be more symptomatic than patients with a slow, chronic rise.[9,37] Systolic BPs as low as 168 mm Hg have been reported in cats presenting with acute blindness and retinal detachment from hypertension. Similarly, a cat with acute hemorrhage with enough bleeding to cause hypovolemia may present with a significantly lower BP than that which incited the incident. Both examples show that constant re-evaluation of BP is important if physical examination or history suggests hypertensive disease. See Figure 87-5 for a schematic regarding decisions for emergency treatment of SH.

The ideal emergency treatment for SH should be quick in onset of action, effective, safe, free of side effects, and titratable. Availability and affordable cost are also important. Lastly, BP response to the medication should be measurable. No existent medication fits all of the criteria, so risks and

benefits of each must be carefully weighed. Intravenous (IV) medications are optimal but not practical or appropriate in all situations. Each case should be individually evaluated in light of clinical circumstances. Treatment should be chosen based on underlying or pre-existing conditions, current medications, severity of hypertension and clinical signs, if the patient is to be hospitalized or treated as an outpatient, availability of 24-hour nursing care, and availability of equipment.

Treatment

Intravenous medications that can be given as continuous rate infusions (CRIs) should be considered in dire cases. Such medications are quick, short acting, and allow quick responses to adjustments in medications. In the event of critically elevated BP from any cause (SBP higher than 220 to 250 mm Hg), sodium nitroprusside and beta-blockers are

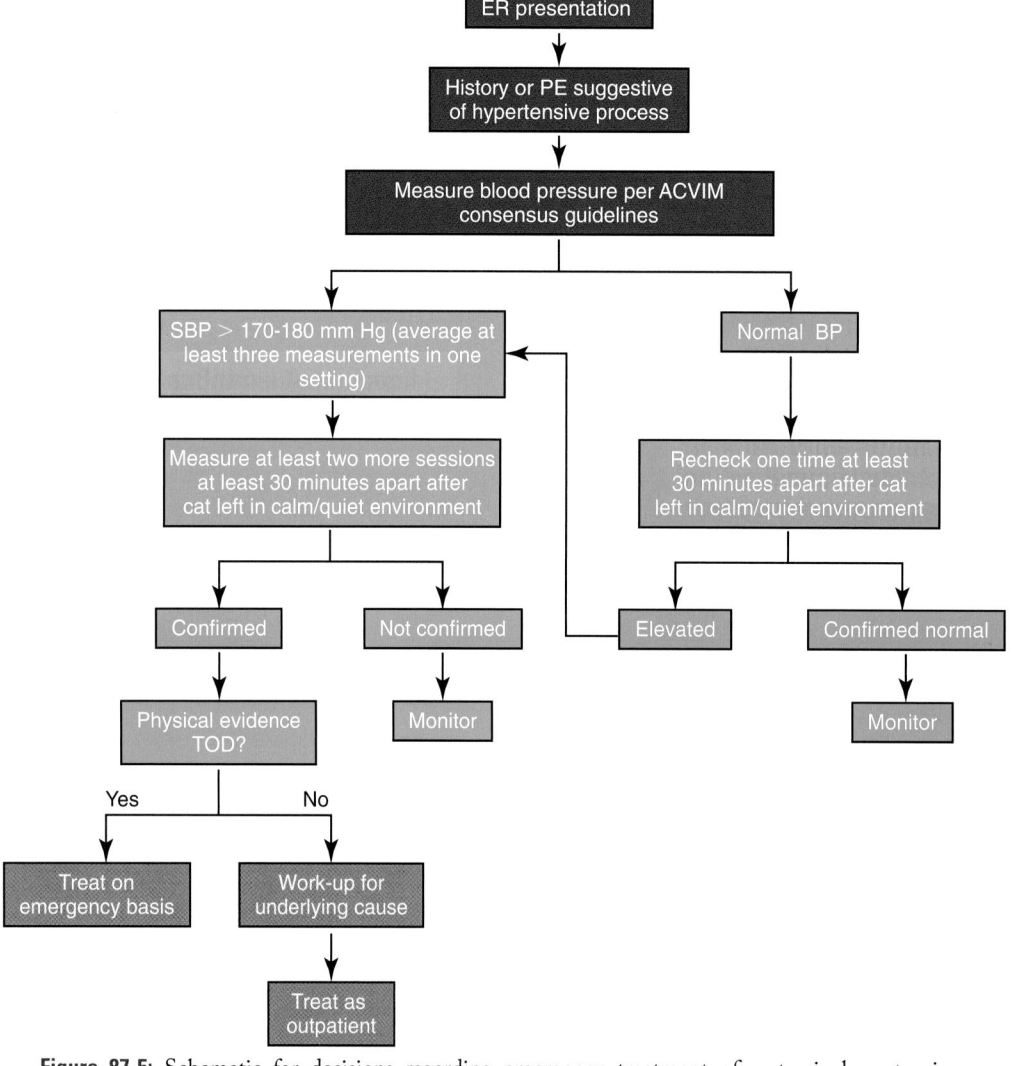

Figure 87-5: Schematic for decisions regarding emergency treatment of systemic hypertension. *ACVIM*, American College of Veterinary Internal Medicine; *BP*, blood pressure; *ER*, emergency room; *PE*, physical examination; *SBP*, systolic blood pressure; *TOD*, target organ damage.

two such medications ideal for most hypertensive crises in cats. If IV access cannot be secured, medications quickly effective by other routes must be considered. Hydralazine is effective subcutaneously; however, it is longer acting and has a narrower margin of safety, so caution and close monitoring must be used. Amlodipine is an oral medication with relatively quick onset of action (several hours) and thus is often used in emergency situations, particularly when renal azotemia exists and/or the cause of hypertension is not evident. In the author's experience, an oral loading dose of amlodipine is effective if rapid BP reduction is indicated (see Table 87-2). Amlodipine may be administered transdermally or per rectum in the event venous access is not available or oral administration is not an option; however, speed of absorption has not been determined.[58-59] Other topical medications, such as nitroglycerin ointment, can also be used until the patient is stable enough for IV catheter placement. See Table 87-2 for drugs and doses.

Table 87-2   Medications, Mode of Action, Suggested Use, and Dosages for Hypertensive Crises in Cats

Generic Drug	Brand Names	Dosage	Mode of Action/Effect	Use	Monitoring Frequency on Emergency Basis
Amlodipine	Norvasc	0.1 to 0.5 mg/kg PO every 24 hours; loading dose 0.1 to 0.2 mg/kg PO every 2 hours until SBP is <170 mm Hg *or* up to cumulative dose of 1 mg/kg (maximum of five to 10 doses)	Calcium channel blocker Arterial dilator	Emergency hypertensive crisis Renal disease Undetermined cause hypertension	At least three to four times daily every 1 to 2 hours if using loading dose protocol, including a few times after last dose
Atenolol	Tenormin	6.25 to 12.5 mg/cat PO every 12 hours	Beta-adrenergic blocker	Hyperthyroidism Cardiac disease Tachycardia	Not for emergency use
Benazepril	Lotensin, Fortekor	0.25 to 0.5 mg/kg PO every 12 to 24 hours	ACE-I	Proteinuric renal disease Cardiac disease	Not for emergency use
Enalapril	Vasotec, Enacard	0.25 to 0.5 mg/kg PO every 12 to 24 hours	ACE-I	Proteinuric renal disease Cardiac disease	Not for emergency use
Esmolol	Brevibloc	Loading dose 250 to 500 µg/kg, then 25 to 200 µg/kg/min	Beta-adrenergic blocker	Emergency hypertensive crisis, tachycardia, ventricular arrhythmias	Every 5 to 10 minutes until effective dose is determined, then hourly; wean slowly
Hydralazine	Apresoline	2.5 mg/cat PO every 12 to 24 hours *or* 0.25 to 2 mg/kg SC or IM every 8 to 12 hours	Direct arterial vasodilator	Emergency hypertensive crisis	Hourly until discontinued
Nicardipine	Cardene	Undetermined (canine dose 0.5 to 5 mcg/kg/min CRI)	Calcium channel blocker	Emergency hypertensive crisis	Suggest hourly on emergency basis
Nitroglycerin ointment	Nitrobid, Minitran	$\frac{1}{8}$ to $\frac{1}{4}$ inch applied to shaved area (e.g., inguinal area or axilla) every 4 to 8 hours as indicated, up to 24 to 48 hours maximum	Venous dilator	Emergency left-sided congestive heart failure when venous access cannot be obtained	Every 2 to 3 hours

Continued

Table 87-2		**Medications, Mode of Action, Suggested Use, and Dosages for Hypertensive Crises in Cats—cont'd**			
Generic Drug	**Brand Names**	**Dosage**	**Mode of Action/Effect**	**Use**	**Monitoring Frequency on Emergency Basis**
Nitroprusside	Nitropress	1 to 3 mcg/kg/min CRI; start at low dose and titrate up as needed	Nonspecific vasodilator	Emergency hypertensive crisis	Every 5 to 10 minutes until effective dose is determined, then hourly; wean slowly
Phenoxybenzamine	Dibenzyline	0.25 to 1.5 mg/kg PO every 8 to 12 hours, or 2.5 mg/cat every 8 to 12 hours or 0.5 mg/cat every 24 hours	Alpha-1 blocker	Pheochromocytoma	Not for emergency use
Propranolol	Inderal	2.5 to 5 mg/cat every 8 hours or 0.02 to 0.06 mg/kg IV every 8 to 12 hours	Beta-blocker	Emergency hypertensive crisis Cardiac disease Hyperthyroidism	Measure BP hourly until in reasonable range, then every 4 to 6 hours until discontinued
Spironolactone	Aldactone	1 to 2 mg/kg every 12 hours	Aldosterone antagonist	Renal disease Proteinuric renal disease	Not for emergency use

ACE-I, Angiotensin-converting enzyme inhibitor; *BP,* blood pressure; *CRI,* constant rate infusion; *IM,* intramuscularly; *IV,* intravenously; *PO,* orally; *SBP,* systolic blood pressure; *SC,* subcutaneously.

In addition to antihypertensive medications, other emergency needs should be addressed.

Treatment Goals

Specific objectives for abnormalities identified should be outlined during initiation of hypertensive treatment. In general, SBP should be decreased to 110 to 150 mm Hg over a few hours.[59] Goals should be adjusted for each individual situation. For instance, decrease to a BP higher than 150 mm Hg may be appropriate initially for cats with azotemia or severe hypertension (e.g., SBP greater than 220 mm Hg) to prevent too rapid a drop in BP that could cause further kidney damage. Other emergency conditions should not be ignored. Abnormalities of heart rate, mentation, respiratory rate, hematologic and biochemistry panels (particularly electrolytes and acid-base derangements), ophthalmologic aberrations, and hydration and neurological statuses should all be addressed.

Monitoring

Blood pressure, vital signs (heart rate, respiratory rate, and temperature), mentation, and overall patient status should be monitored as frequently as every few minutes to hourly in some situations, depending upon the drug used and initial parameters. Continuous rate infusions require minute to hourly re-evaluation; any change in dose requires appropriate re-evaluation. See Table 87-2 for monitoring suggestions associated with specific medications. Monitoring should be tailored to each individual patient.

PROGNOSIS

Prognosis depends upon the underlying cause, degree of TOD, and whether or not damage is reversible or life threatening, among other factors. Proteinuria,[7,11] age, and azotemia may be negatively related to prognosis. There are conflicting reports regarding the impact of treating SH on survival or other outcome statistics. A clinical study showed that cats with CKD and corrected hypertension had as good a prognosis as nonhypertensive cats.[11] Conflicting results from a separate study showed that control of SBP in hypertensive cats did not improve survival.[8]

PREVENTION

Prevention of hypertensive crises depends upon early detection and effective control of SH. Owner observations, veterinarian awareness, and presence of physical examination and laboratory findings commonly associated with hypertension should prompt BP monitoring. Regular screening of geriatric patients and monitoring of patients being treated for hypertension are important in the prevention of hypertensive crises.

SUMMARY

The incidence of SH in cats is likely more common than realized. Clinical signs of SH may be vague and insidious in onset, and thus signs are often missed or ignored. Unrecognized SH can lead to life-threatening hypertensive crises and severe consequences. Common laboratory abnormalities found in hypertensive cats include proteinuria, dilute urine, azotemia, and elevated thyroid values. Diseases most commonly associated with hypertension are CKD, hyperthyroidism, primary hyperaldosteronism, and hyperadrenocorticism. There is also a positive correlation between hypertension and age. The target organs of SH are the eyes, central nervous, cardiovascular, and renal systems. Signs of hypertensive crises are most commonly manifest by ocular, cardiovascular, and neurological signs.

Blood pressure should be monitored regularly in cats that are older than 11 years of age, have diseases and/or laboratory abnormalities associated with hypertension, have evidence of TOD, and/or have already been identified as hypertensive. Funduscopic examination should also be part of wellness examination in these patients. Blood pressure should be interpreted in conjunction with evaluation of the entire case, because indirect measurement devices as well as feline demeanor in general can lead to inaccurate BP measurements. Cats presenting in hypertensive crises should be treated immediately, ideally with a fast-acting, IV, titratable medication. The general goal is to lower BP to between 110 and 150 mm Hg within several hours to prevent further TOD and life-threatening complications. Treatment goals should be amended to fit individual cases. For more on the diagnosis and treatment of feline hypertension, see Chapter 38.

References

1. American Veterinary Medical Association: *U.S. pet ownership statistics* (2012 & 2007 statistics). <https://www.avma.org/KB/Resources/Statistics/Pages/Market-research-statistics-US-pet-ownership.aspx>. (Accessed July 24, 2015).

2. Lin C, Yan C, Lien Y, et al: Systemic blood pressure of clinically normal and conscious cats determined by an indirect Doppler method in clinical setting. *J Vet Med Sci* 68:827–832, 2006.

3. Sparkes AH, Caney SM, King MC, et al: Inter- and intraindividual variation in Doppler ultrasonic indirect blood pressure measurements in healthy cats. *J Vet Intern Med* 13:314–318, 1999.

4. Bodey AR, Sansom J: Epidemiological study of blood pressure in domestic cats. *J Small Anim Pract* 39:567–573, 1998.

5. Williams TL, Elliot J, Syme HM: Renin-angiotensin-aldosterone system activity in hyperthyroid cats with and without concurrent hypertension. *J Vet Intern Med* 27:522–529, 2013.

6. Syme H: Hypertension in small animal kidney disease. *Vet Clin North Am Small Anim Prac* 41:63–89, 2011.

7. Jepson RE, Brodbelt D, Vallance C, et al: Evaluation of predictors of the development of azotemia in cats. *J Vet Intern Med* 23:806–813, 2009.

8. Jepson RE, Elliot JE, Brodbelt D, et al: Effect of control of systolic blood pressure on survival in cats with systemic hypertension. *J Vet Intern Med* 21:402–409, 2007.

9. Brown S, Atkins R, Bagley A, et al: Guidelines for the identification, evaluation, and management of systemic hypertension in dogs and cats. *J Vet Intern Med* 21:542–558, 2007.

10. Egner B, Carr A, Brown S: *Essential facts of blood pressure in dogs and cats*, ed 4, Germany Babenhausen, 2007, Beate Egner Vet Verlag.

11. Syme HM, Markwell PJ, Pfeiffer D, et al: Survival of cats with naturally occurring chronic renal failure is related to severity of proteinuria. *J Vet Intern Med* 20:528–535, 2006.

12. Sansom J, Rogers K, Wood JL: Blood pressure assessment in healthy cats and cats with hypertensive retinopathy. *Am J Vet Res* 65:245–252, 2004.

13. Henik RA, Stepien RL, Bortnowski HB: Spectrum of M-mode echocardiographic abnormalities in 75 cats with systemic hypertension. *J Am Anim Hosp Assoc* 40:359–363, 2004.

14. Chetboul V, Lefebvre HP, Pinhas C, et al: Spontaneous feline hypertension: clinical and echocardiographic abnormalities, and survival rate. *J Vet Intern Med* 17:89–95, 2003.

15. Nelson OL, Reidesel E, Ware W, et al: Echocardiographic and radiographic changes associated with systemic hypertension in cats. *J Vet Intern Med* 16:418–425, 2002.

16. Elliot J, Barber PJ, Syme HM, et al: Feline hypertension: clinical findings and response to antihypertensive treatment in 30 cases. *J Small Anim Pract* 19:1981–1989, 2001.

17. Mishina M, Watanabe T, Fujii K, et al: Non-invasive blood pressure measurements in cats: clinical significance of hypertension associated with chronic renal failure. *J Vet Med Sci* 60:805–808, 1998.

18. Maggio F, DeFrancesco TC, Atkins CE, et al: Ocular lesions associated with systemic hypertension in cats: 69 cases (1985-1998). *J Am Vet Med Assoc* 217:695–702, 2000.

19. Littman MP: Spontaneous hypertension in 24 cats. *J Vet Intern Med* 8:79–86, 1994.

20. Stiles J, Polzin D, Bistner S: The prevalence of retinopathy in cats with systemic hypertension and chronic renal failure or hyperthyroidism. *J Am Anim Hosp Assoc* 26:647–651, 1994.

21. Lesser M, Fox PR, Bond BR: Assessment of hypertension in 40 cats with left ventricular hypertrophy by Doppler-shift sphygmomanometry. *J Small Anim Pract* 33:55–58, 1992.

22. Kobayashi DL, Peterson ME, Graves TK, et al: Hypertension in cats with chronic renal failure or hyperthyroidism. *J Vet Intern Med* 4:58–62, 1990.

23. Schulman RL: Feline primary hyperaldosteronism. *Vet Clin North Am Small Anim Prac* 40:353–359, 2010.

24. Reusch CE, Schellenberg S, Wenger M: Endocrine hypertension in small animals. *Vet Clin North Am Small Anim Prac* 40:335–352, 2010.

25. Ash RA, Harvey AM, Tasker S: Primary hyperaldosteronism in the cat: a series of 13 cases. *J Feline Med Surg* 7:173–182, 2005.

26. DeClue AE, Breshars LA, Pardo ID, et al: Hyperaldosteronism and hyperestrogenism in a cat with an adrenal cortical carcinoma. *J Vet Intern Med* 9:355–358, 2005.

27. Javadi S, Djajadiningrat-Laanen SC, Koistra HS, et al: Primary hyperaldosteronism, a mediator of progressive renal disease in cats. *Domest Anim Endocrinol* 28:85–104, 2005.

28. Flood SM, Randolph JF, Gelzer AR, et al: Primary hyperaldosteronism in two cats. *J Am Anim Hosp Assoc* 35:411–416, 1999.

29. Haldane S, Graves TK, Bateman S, et al: Profound hypokalemia causing respiratory failure in a cat with hyperaldosteronism. *J Vet Emerg Crit Care* 17:202–207, 2007.

30. Brown AL, Beatty JA, Lindsay SA, et al: Severe systemic hypertension in a cat with pituitary-dependent hyperadrenocorticism. *J Small Anim Pract* 53:132–135, 2012.

31. Henry CJ, Brewer WG, Montgomery RD, et al: Adrenal pheochromocytoma in a cat. *J Vet Intern Med* 7:199–203, 1993.

32. Sennello KA, Schulman RL, Prosek R, et al: Systolic blood pressure in cats with diabetes mellitus. *J Am Vet Med Assoc* 223:198–201, 2003.

33. Norsworthy GD, de Faria VP: Retrobulbar thrombus in a cat with systemic hypertension. *J Feline Med Surg* 13:144–148, 2011.

34. Komáromy AM, Andrew SE, Dennis HM, et al: Hypertensive retinopathy and choroidopathy in a cat. *Vet Ophthalmol* 7:3–9, 2004.

35. Turner JL, Brogdon JD, Lees GE, et al: Idiopathic hypertension in a cat with secondary hypertensive retinopathy associated with high salt diet. *J Am Anim Hosp Assoc* 26:647–651, 1990.

36. Morgan RV: Systemic hypertension in four cats: ocular and medical findings. *J Am Anim Hosp Assoc* 22:615–621, 1986.

37. Brown CA, Munday JS, Mathur S, et al: Hypertensive encephalopathy in cats with reduced renal function. *Vet Pathol* 42:642–649, 2005.

38. Kent M: The cat with neurological manifestations of systemic disease. Key conditions impacting the CNS. *J Feline Med Surg* 11:395–407, 2009.

39. Sampedrano CC, Chetboul V, Gouni V, et al: Systolic and diastolic myocardial dysfunction in cats with hypertrophic cardiomyopathy or systemic hypertension. *J Vet Intern Med* 20:1106–1115, 2006.

40. Reynolds BS, Chetboul V, Nguyen P: Effects of dietary sodium salt intake on renal function: a 2-year study in healthy aged cats. *J Vet Intern Med* 27:507–515, 2013.

41. Belew AM, Barlett T, Brown SA: Evaluation of the white-coat effect in cats. *J Vet Intern Med* 13:134–142, 1999.

42. Brown SA, Langford K, Tarver S: Effects of certain vasoactive agents on the long-term pattern of blood pressure, heart rate, and motor activity in cats. *Am J Vet Res* 58:647–652, 1997.

43. Klevans LR, Hirkaler G, Kovacs JL: Indirect blood pressure determination by Doppler technique in renal hypertensive cats. *Am J Physiol* 237:H720–H723, 1979.

44. Jensen J, Henik RA, Brownfield M, et al: Plasma renin activity and angiotensin I and aldosterone concentrations in cats with hypertension associated with chronic renal disease. *Am J Vet Res* 58:535–540, 1997.

45. Taugner F, Baatz G, Nobiling R: The renin-angiotensin system in cats with chronic renal failure. *J Comp Path* 115:239–252, 1996.

46. Kyles AE, Gregory CR, Wooldridge JD, et al: Management of hypertension controls postoperative neurological disorders after renal transplantation in cats. *Vet Surg* 28:436–441, 1999.

47. Mathews KG, Gregory CR: Renal transplants in cats: 66 cases (1987-1996). *J Am Vet Med Assoc* 211:1432–1436, 1997.

48. Gregory CR, Mathews KG, Aronson LR, et al: Central nervous system disorders after renal transplantation in cats. *Vet Surg* 26:386–392, 1997.

49. Ancierno MJ, Seaton D, Mitchell MA, et al: Agreement between directly measured blood pressure and pressures obtained with three veterinary-specific oscillometric units in cats. *J Am Vet Med Assoc* 237:402–406, 2010.

50. Jepson RE, Hartley V, Mendl M, et al: A comparison of CAT Doppler and oscillometric Memoprint machines for non-invasive blood pressure measurement in conscious cats. *J Feline Med Surg* 7:147–152, 2005.

51. Pederson KM, Butler MA, Esboll AK, et al: Evaluation of an oscillometric blood pressure monitor for use in anesthetized cats. *J Am Vet Med Assoc* 221:646–650, 2002.

52. Caulkett NA, Cantwell SL, Houston DM: A comparison of indirect blood pressure monitoring techniques in the anesthetized cat. *Vet Surg* 27:370–377, 1998.

53. Branson KR, Wagner-Mann CC, Mann FA: Evaluation of an oscillometric blood pressure monitor on anesthetized cats and the effect of cuff placement and fur on accuracy. *Vet Surg* 26:347–353, 1997.

54. Binns SH, Sisson DD, Buoscio DA, et al: Doppler ultrasonographic, oscillometric sphygmomanometric, and photoplethysmographic techniques for noninvasive blood pressure measurement in anesthetized cats. *J Vet Intern Med* 9:405–414, 1995.

55. Grandy JL, Dunlop CI, Hodson DS, et al: Evaluation of the Doppler ultrasonic method of measuring systolic arterial blood pressure in cats. *Am J Vet Res* 53:1166–1169, 1992.

56. Brown SA, Henik RA, Finco DR: Diagnosis of systemic hypertension in dogs and cats. In Bonagura JD, editor: *Kirk's current veterinary therapy XIII*, Philadelphia, 2000, Saunders, pp 835–838.

57. Moon MO, Keene BW, Lessard P, et al: age related changes in feline cardiac silhouette. *Vet Radiol Ultrasound* 34:315–320, 1993.

58. Helms SR: Treatment of feline hypertension with transdermal amlodipine: a pilot study. *J Am Anim Hosp Assoc* 43:149–156, 2007.

59. Labato MA: Antihypertensives. In Silverstein DC, Hopper K, editors: *Small animal critical care medicine*, St Louis, 2009, Saunders/Elsevier, pp 763–767.

Endourology in the Feline Patient: Urinary Diversion Techniques

Allyson Berent

The use of novel image-guided techniques in feline medicine is now being undertaken, particularly pertaining to upper and lower urinary tract obstructions. The relatively common incidence of urinary obstructions, combined with the invasiveness and morbidity associated with traditional surgical procedures, has made the use of minimally invasive procedures using interventional radiology (IR) and endoscopy techniques appealing. This modality is termed *endourology*. Such interventional methods have been considered the standard of care in human medicine for decades, and the same trend is following in the subspecialty of feline medicine.

Urinary outflow tract obstructions most often occur in feline patients when there is a blockage of the ureter, urethra, or bladder trigone. Various urinary diversion surgeries, along with numerous types of catheters and/or stents, can be used to accomplish decompression. Temporary drainage of the renal pelvis, ureter, or urinary bladder can be achieved with externalized tubes (e.g., nephrostomy, cystostomy, or urethral catheters), but these treatments subsequently require a more definitive approach to permanently relieve the obstruction for an indwelling alternative. Urinary "stents" are typically indwelling and can be used to divert urine internally. These types of diversion techniques are particularly useful when traditional options are considered inappropriate, difficult, or contraindicated. The most common indications for permanent urinary bypass devices are for the treatment of an unresectable malignant urethral or ureteral obstruction(s), a ureteral or urethral stricture, or obstructive ureteral stones (i.e., ureterolithiasis). Stents are available for veterinary use in different materials (e.g., metallic, silicone, polyurethane), shapes (e.g., straight, pigtail, Malecot), and sizes (0.8 mm to more than 14 mm). This chapter focuses on the use of various types of endourological procedures to treat urinary tract obstructions in feline patients, with an emphasis on catheters, stents, and implants. This chapter summarizes the current data available over the last 8 to 10 years and expands upon the author's experience in endourology. Traditional surgical procedures for the treatment of urinary tract obstructions will not be discussed in great detail in this chapter.

INTERVENTIONS IN HUMAN UROLOGY

In human urology the development and improvements in ureteroscopy, ureteral stenting, lithotripsy, laparoscopy, and percutaneous nephroureterolithotomy (PCNUL) have almost eradicated the need for open urinary surgery for stone disease, strictures, trauma, or neoplasia. Ureteroscopy is usually the firstline evaluation of ureteral neoplasia, upper tract essential hematuria, and the treatment of ureteral calculi greater than 5 mm in diameter. In addition, cystoscopy is considered a standard diagnostic tool for dysuria, providing both a diagnostic and therapeutic modality. Ureterolithiasis is routinely treated medically (stones less than 5 mm) or as an intervention in humans (stones greater than 5 mm).[1-8] Shock wave lithotripsy is effective in 50% to 81% of cases,[1,2] whereas ureteroscopy and laser lithotripsy have a near 100% success rate.[3-7] Because the human ureter is more than 4 mm in diameter, ureteroscopy is a more viable option for human patients than it is for their veterinary counterparts (canine ureteral diameter 1 to 2 mm; feline 0.3 to 0.5 mm).[9,10] Ureteral stenting was first introduced in 1967 for evaluation of human patients with malignant ureteral obstructions,[11] and it is used widely to treat both benign and malignant obstructive disease.[11-17] In children, ureteral stenting is performed routinely to encourage passive ureteral dilation in anticipation of future ureteroscopy. In addition, ureteral stents allow for immediate ureteral decompression, encourage spontaneous stone passage, and improve the outcome of large stone burden passage during extracorporeal shock wave lithotripsy.[11-17]

In children with large bladder stone burdens, transurethral lithotripsy can be traumatic and lengthy. A procedure called percutaneous cystolithotomy (PCCL) is often the treatment of choice in these patients, to avoid repetitive urethral trauma, as seen with transurethral therapy such as laser lithotripsy.[18] Percutaneous cystolithotomy has been found to be very effective in small feline patients as well in the author's practice.[19]

EQUIPMENT FOR FELINE PATIENTS

Various flexible and rigid endoscopes are used for traditional endourological procedures. Rigid cystoscopy is performed commonly in female cats for urethral, bladder, and ureteral access. The recommended equipment is the 1.9 mm rigid 30°-angle endoscope.[a] Semirigid cystoscopes[b] are available for male cats in size 3.0 to 4.5 Fr in diameter. Unfortunately, these endoscopes are only useful for diagnostic retrograde cystoscopy. Flexible ureteroscopes (2.7 mm, 0° lens)[c] can also be used for retrograde cystoscopy in female cats. For male cats, the use of percutaneous antegrade cystoureterothroscopy allows for excellent visibility of the urinary bladder, ureterovesicular junction (UVJ), and intrapelvic urethra. Rigid nephroscopes can be used (1.9- to 7.3-mm diameter) for percutaneous nephroureteroscopy when nephroliths or proximal ureteroliths must be removed. Different types of intracorporeal lithotrites and lasers are available for various procedures, including ultrasonic, pneumatic, electrohydraulic, and holmium:YAG lasers.[d] A diode laser is most often used for tissue coagulation or resection (i.e., lasering intramural ureteral ectopia, or coagulation for bleeding lesions).

For many of the more commonly performed IR procedures, a traditional fluoroscopy unit is sufficient (Figure 88-1). The C-arm fluoroscopy unit has the advantage of mobility of the image intensifier, permitting various tangential views without moving the patient. Ultrasonography is useful for percutaneous needle access into the renal pelvis or urinary bladder when needed. Guide wires of various sizes, shapes, and stiffness are needed for most procedures (Figure 88-2). Urinary catheters and stents can be used to divert urine throughout the entire urinary collection system (see Figures 88-2 and 88-3). Most catheters in the urinary system are used for temporary drainage of the renal pelvis (nephrostomy tubes), ureter, or urinary bladder (cystostomy tubes). Urinary catheters are classically soft, comfortable polyurethane tubes that have an open lumen, permitting temporary drainage, and a locking mechanism to prevent dislodgement. Stents are small tubes that are inserted across a blocked lumen to restore patency. Urinary stents are typically used for permanent or long-term diversion in the kidney, ureter, bladder, or urethra and are most often indwelling. Stents are most commonly used to bypass an obstruction secondary to either a tumor, stricture, or embedded stone(s) (i.e., ureterolithiasis).[e,f] Stents come in different materials (e.g., metal, polyurethane, plastic, rubber), shapes, and sizes (see Figures 88-2 and 88-3). The

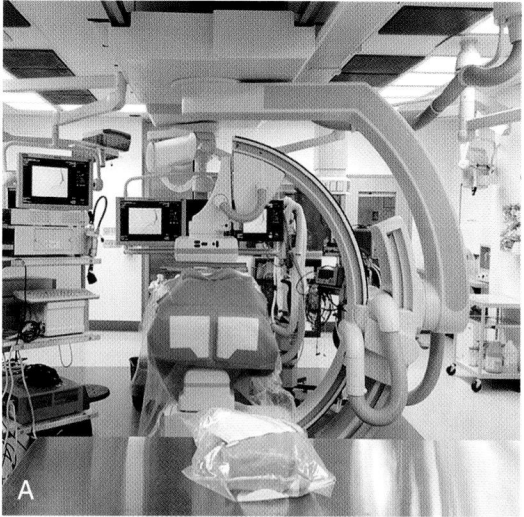
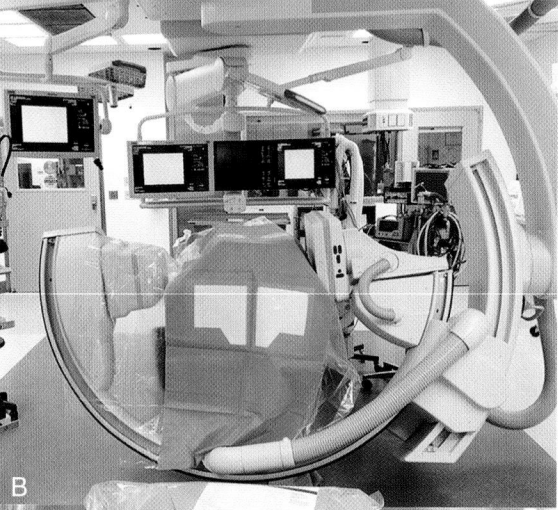

Figure 88-1: **Fluoroscopy Unit in a Minimally Invasive Operating Room.** Notice the multiple tangential views shown as the C-arm is rotated around the table.

subcutaneous ureteral bypass (SUB) device (Figure 88-4)[g] is an artificial ureter that is composed of both a nephrostomy and a cystostomy tube that are connected subcutaneously to a shunting port, allowing for urinary diversion from the renal pelvis to the urinary bladder.

Diseases of the Upper Urinary Collection System: Kidney and Ureter

Ureteral disease creates a significant dilemma in feline patients. It is the most common disease in the upper urinary tract collection system. The relatively common incidence of feline ureteral obstructions, combined with the invasiveness and morbidity associated with traditional surgical techniques,[20-22] makes the use of endourological alternatives appealing (Tables 88-1 and 88-2).

[a]Rigid endoscope, 1.9-mm 30° lens, Karl Storz Endoscopy, Culver City, CA.
[b]Semirigid male cat scope, Karl Storz Endoscopy, Culver City, CA.
[c]Flex X² Flexible ureteroscope, Karl Storz Endoscopy, Culver City, CA.
[d]200 or 400-μm Holmium:YAG laser fiber and 30-W Hol:YAG Lithotrite, Odyssey, Convergent Inc, Alameda, CA.
[e]Vet Stent ureter 2.5 Fr double pigtail ureteral stent, Infiniti Medical LLC, Menlo Park, CA.
[f]VetStent Urethra, Infiniti Medical LLC, Menlo Park, CA.

[g]Subcutaneous ureteral bypass device (SUB), Norfolk Vet, Skokie, IL.

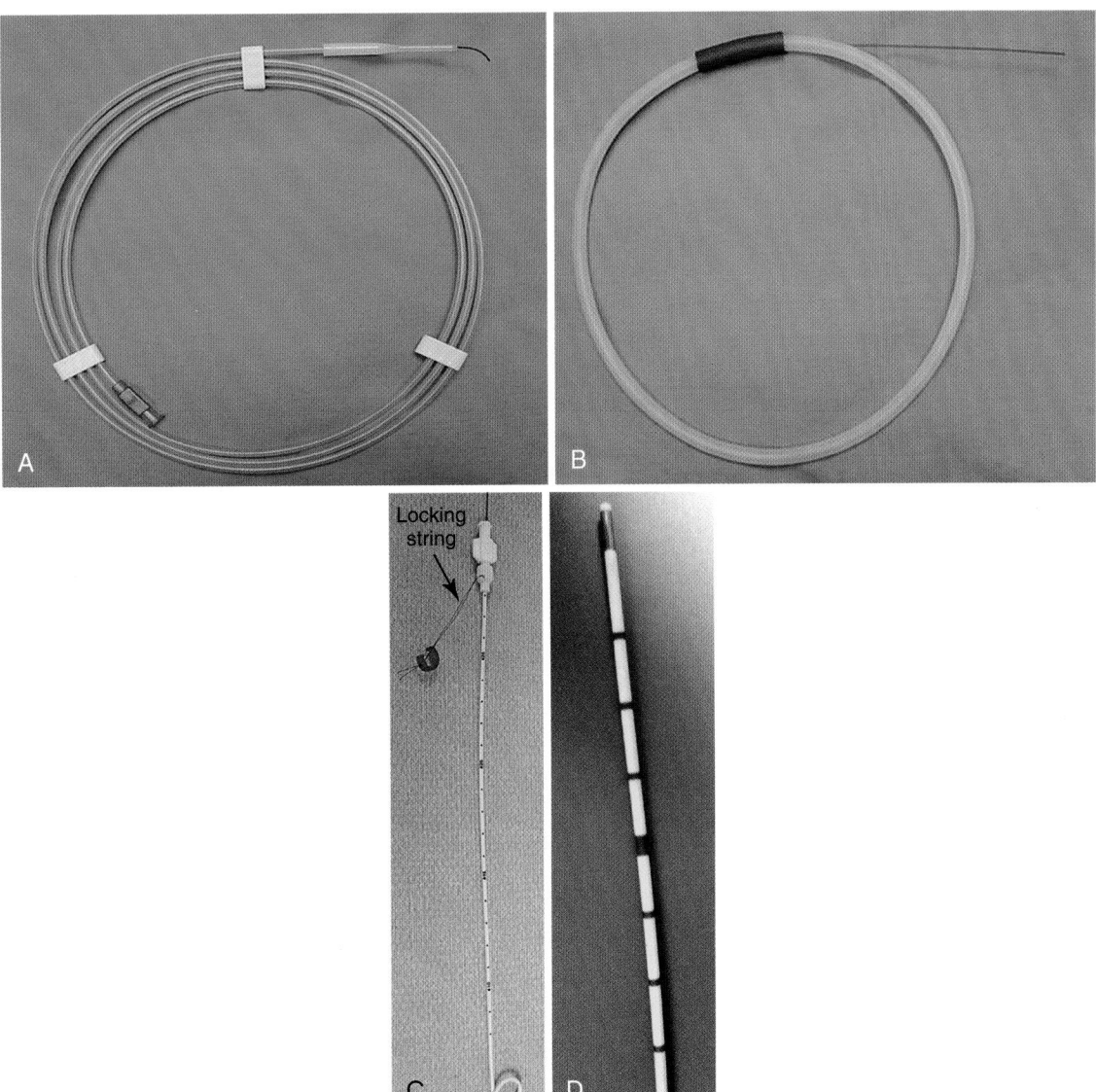

Figure 88-2: Supplies. A, Hydrophilic angle-tipped guide wire used to cannulate the lumen of an organ. This is the wire typically used for urethral and ureteral stent placement. **B,** Teflon guide wire that is needed for stiffness when a ureteral stent is placed under fluoroscopic guidance alone. **C,** Locking-loop pigtail catheter typically used for nephrostomy or cystostomy tubes; notice the locking string. **D,** Open-ended ureteral catheter; this is used when a ureteral stent is placed endoscopically to measure the ureteral lumen length to aid in choosing stent length.

Table 88-1	Treatment Options for Feline Patients Using Endourological Techniques Based on Sex							
	SUB Placement	PCNL/SENL	Cystoscopy	Urethral Stenting	Laser Lithotripsy	PCCL	CLA-EU	Polypectomy
Male cat	Yes	Yes—rarely required	Via PCCU or semirigid cystoscopy (1.9 mm)	Via antegrade urethral access	No	Yes	No	Yes (via PCCU)
Female cat	Yes	Yes—rarely required	Retrograde rigid cystoscopy (1.9 mm)	Via retrograde urethral access	Yes	Yes	Yes	Yes (via retrograde cystoscopy or PCCU)

CLA-EU, Cystoscopic guided laser ablation of ectopic ureters; *PCNL,* percutaneous nephroureterolithotomy; *PCCU,* percutaneous antegrade cystourethroscopy; *PCCL,* percutaneous cystolithotomy; *SENL,* surgically assisted endoscopic nephroureterolithotomy; *SUB,* subcutaneous ureteral bypass.

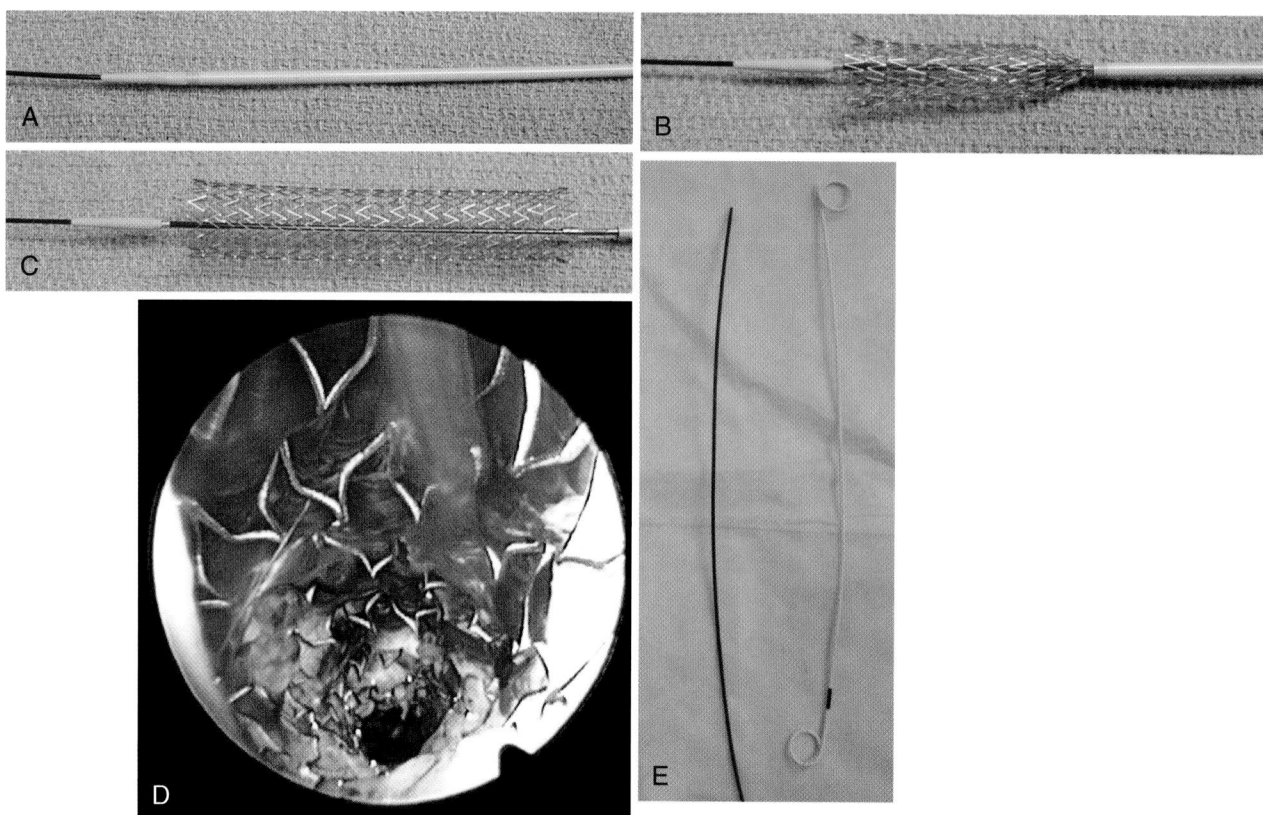

Figure 88-3: Various Types of Stents Used in the Urinary Tract. A-C, Self-expanding metallic stent typically used for urethral stenting. **D,** Endoscopic image after a urethral stent is in place showing the metallic stent material displacing the tumor to the wall of the urethra creating a patent lumen for urine flow. **E,** A double-pigtail ureteral stent used in feline patients; notice the straight ureteral dilation catheter to the left of the stent that is needed to predilate the ureter. The stent has a black mark on the distal end that is used when placing the stent endoscopically to prevent the distal loop from being pushed up the ureter.

Table 88-2	Medical Management of Ureteral Obstructions
Medications	**Dosage**
Intravenous fluid therapy	90-120 mL/kg per day Monitoring body weight, hydration status with/without central venous pressure monitoring The author will often use 0.45% NaCl at 60 mL/kg per day and replacement fluids (i.e., Plasma-Lyte) at 30-60 mL/kg per day to prevent fluid overload
Alpha-adrenergic blockage	Prazosin 0.25 mg/cat every 12 h or tamsulosin 0.01 mg/kg every 24 h Monitoring blood pressure
Diuretic therapy	Mannitol 0.25 g/kg bolus over 30 to 60 minutes, then 60 mg/kg per hour constant rate infusion for 24 hours Monitor renal pelvis size, renal biochemical parameters, and hydration status The author is cautious if there is evidence of heart disease
Amitriptyline	1 mg/kg every 24 h There is minimal evidence to support this use, and maximal effect can take a few weeks

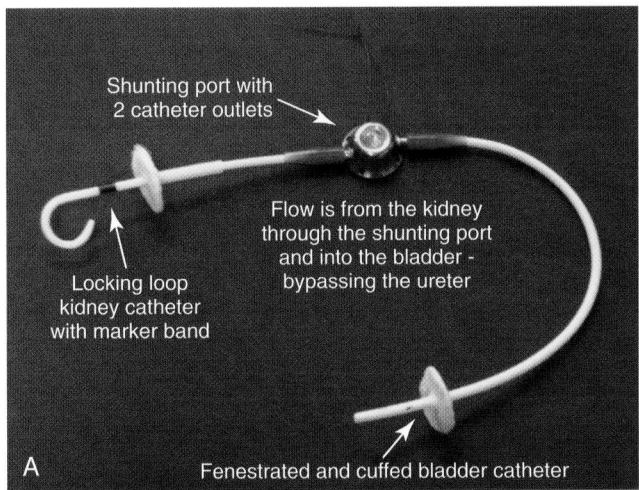

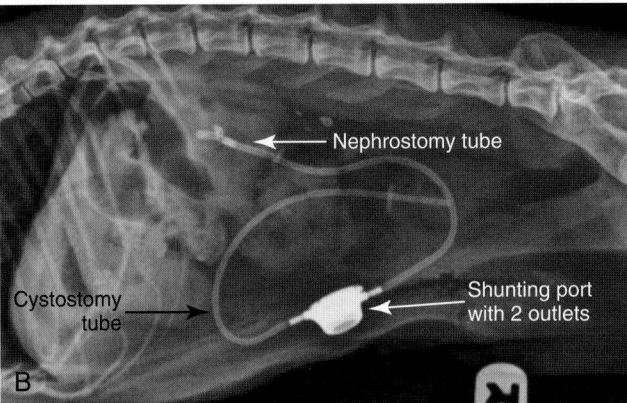

Figure 88-4: Subcutaneous Ureteral Bypass (SUB) Device. A, The device showing the locking-loop pigtail catheter with a radiopaque marker band after the distal hole to prevent leakage outside the renal pelvis; a Dacron cuff is then secured to the renal capsule to prevent leakage. This is then hooked up to a shunting port that can be flushed and sampled. Finally, the shunting port is hooked up to the cystostomy tube that enters the apex of the urinary bladder to drain urine from the renal pelvis to the urinary bladder directly. **B,** A lateral radiograph of the SUB device implanted into a cat.

Feline ureteral obstructions occur most commonly secondary to ureterolithiasis (approximately 80% of cases), ureteral stenosis (approximately 20% of cases), and trigonal neoplasia (less than 3% of cases).[23,24] Additional causes include accidental ureteral ligation during surgery, ureteral trauma, ureteral edema following ureteral surgery, and obstructions secondary to purulent material associated with pyelonephritis or pyonephrosis. Obstruction can result in life-threatening azotemia, particularly when presenting bilaterally (approximately 15% of cases)[24] or in cats with concurrent pre-existing chronic kidney disease (more than 75% to 90% of cases).[21,23,24] Greater than 98% of feline ureteroliths were documented to be composed of calcium oxalate material,[21] making medical dissolution impossible. These stones need to pass spontaneously, remain in place, be bypassed with an intervention, or be removed. Once medical management fails (see Table 88-2), intervention that is more aggressive should be considered (Table 88-3). The physiological response the body has to a ureteral obstruction is very complex. If there is

a complete ureteral obstruction, decompression of the renal pelvis becomes imperative to preserve function in the ipsilateral kidney. Studies in dogs have shown that after a complete ureteral obstruction, the renal blood flow diminishes to 40% of normal over 24 hours, and to 20% of normal by 2 weeks.[29,30] This increase in pressure generated by the ureteral obstruction is transmitted to the entire nephron, resulting in a precipitous decrease in the glomerular filtration rate (GFR).[29,31-34] After 7, 14, and 40 days, the GFR was found to permanently decline by 35%, 54%, and 100%, respectively.[29,31-34] These numbers were in a dog model with no evidence of pre-existing azotemia, chronic interstitial nephritis, chronic obstruction, or nephroureterolithiasis, and therefore a worse outcome might be expected in feline patients. Interestingly, in contrast with the irreversibility of a complete obstruction, partial obstructions result in destruction that is less severe or dramatic, as well as more frequent return to function after the obstruction is relieved. In one dog model, it was found that the GFR returned to normal after a partial obstruction was present for 4 weeks.[35] Knowing that many of feline patients are partially obstructed for weeks to months with concurrent chronic kidney disease (CKD), aggressive management and obstruction relief are recommended. Discouraging relief of a ureteral obstruction because of chronicity is not recommended, because improvement in renal function is documented routinely after fixation, regardless of chronicity.

In cases of ureteral obstruction secondary to a ureterolith, some patients can be managed medically with supportive care until the ureterolith passes (see Table 88-1). However, it is important to realize that more than 20% of feline ureteral obstructions are reported to be associated with strictures (and/or stones),[24,36,26] where medical management and traditional surgery would not be expected to be highly effective. Medical management (24 to 48 hours of intravenous [IV] fluid therapy, prazosin, and an IV mannitol constant rate infusion) has been reported to be successful in approximately 10% to 15% of cases with ureterolith-induced obstructions.[20,21,23] If medical management fails, emergency intervention should be considered to avoid permanent damage. For cats that are oliguric, anuric, hyperkalemic, or overhydrated, immediate intervention or intermittent hemodialysis therapy should be considered for stabilization. The first interventional option considered in the author's practice is the placement of a SUB device in cats. Other options include the placement of a nephrostomy tube, or a double pigtail ureteral stent. Decompression of the renal pelvis will decrease the hydrostatic pressure, allowing for immediate renal recovery and preventing permanent damage to the renal parenchyma.

Nephrostomy Tube Placement
A nephrostomy tube(s) can be placed percutaneously, or with surgical assistance, to quickly relieve the excessive hydrostatic pressure and improve renal function. Nephrostomy tubes can also be a temporary bridge to determine whether adequate renal function remains before prolonged anesthesia for a

Table 88-3 **Potential Complications of Various Ureteral Interventions**

Procedure	Operative	After Surgery (Less Than 1 wk)	Short Term (1 Week to 1 mo)	Long Term (More Than 1 mo)	Follow-up Time
Traditional feline ureteral surgery ($n = 153$, [20,21] 47[22]): Ureterotomy, reimplantation, ureteronephrectomy, renal transplantation;[20,21] ureterotomy, reimplantation.[22] Data on stones only.	• Uroabdomen (6%[22] to 15%[21]) • Presence of abdominal effusion after surgery (34%)[22]	• Persistent ureteral obstruction (7%) because of stricture, edema, persistent stones[21] • Failure of renal function to improve (17%)[21] • Second surgery required during hospitalization (13%)[21,22] • Other[21]: CHF (3%), septic peritonitis (2%), pancreatitis (1%), pyelonephritis (1%) • **Mortality (to discharge) 21%**[21,22] (25% with ureterotomy/ reimplantation; 18% if transplantation and ureteronephrectomy are included)[21]	• Failure of renal function to improve (17%)[21] • **Mortality (within 1 month) 25%**[21]	• Reobstruction (40%)[21] occurring about 1 year later, 50% mortality	From 1 to >2000 days. Major issue is postoperative complications: leakage, reobstruction, stricture formation, long-term obstruction recurrence. There were few cases followed-up long-term (approx. 50%).[21] **21% peri-operative mortality**

Feline ureteral stent[25-27,23] (n = 79,[25] 92[27]); data on 71% to 79% with stones, 21% to 28% with strictures, and 1% with obstructive pyelonephritis.	• Ureteral penetration with guide wire (17%; of little clinical consequence; no uroabdomen) • Leakage if concurrent ureterotomy is needed (6.7%) • Eversion of ureteral mucosa during stent passage • Ureteral tear during stent passage (3.8%)	• Fluid overload during postobstructive diuresis (17%) • Concurrent pancreatitis (6%) • Failure of creatinine to improve (5%) • **Mortality (to discharge) 7.5%**[25] because of nonurinary causes (pancreatitis or CHF)	• Inappetence (temporary; 25%) • Dysuria (self-limiting, 7 to 14 days, <10%)[25] • Stent migration (3%)[27]	• Dysuria (38%);[25] nearly all respond to prednisolone and/or prazosin (1.6% persist after steroid therapy) • UTI (30%, versus 34% before surgery)[25] • Reobstruction (19%, over 3.5 years)[25,27] due to stricture (58% of strictures occluded the stent), adhesions around ureter from ureterotomy, obstructive pyelonephritis, or proliferative ureteritis • Chronic hematuria (18%)[25] • Stent migration (6%)[25] • Ureteral reflux (<2%)[25]	From 2 to 1278 days. MST: 498 days. MST for renal cause of death: >1250 days; 21% of cats died of renal-related causes, the only predictor of long-term survival was creatinine concentration at 3 months.[26] Major issue is need for stent exchange in 27% of cases due to migration or occlusion of ureter and dysuria due to ureteral stent location in urinary bladder. **7.5% perioperative mortality (none related to surgical complications)**
Feline SUB device[26,27,28,23] (n = 61,[28] 71[27]); data on 20% with strictures (with/ without stones), 76% with stones, and 4% with obstructive ureteritis.	• Kinking of catheters (<5%) • Inability to place SUB (<1%)	• Leakage (5%),[28] resolved with new device • Fluid overload (<5%)[27,28] • Blockage of system (5%)[27,28] due to blood clot, purulent material, or device failure • Failure of creatinine to improve (4%)[27,28] • **Mortality (to discharge) 5.6%**[27]	• Dysuria (<2%)[27,28] • Inappetence (temporary, approx. 25%) • Seroma (1%)[28]	• UTI (15%, versus 35% before surgery)[28] • Reobstruction (9.8% total; 0% in strictures, 12% in stone cases)[27] • Dysuria (<2%)[27,28]	From 2 days to 4.5 years. Median: 571 days. Major issues: • Device occlusion (10%) which requires serial flushing or exchange, usually due to stone accumulation • Kinking • Leakage, less common with proper training **5.6% perioperative mortality (none related to surgical complications)**

CHF, Congestive heart failure; *MST,* median survival time; *SUB,* subcutaneous ureteral bypass; *UTI,* urinary tract infection.

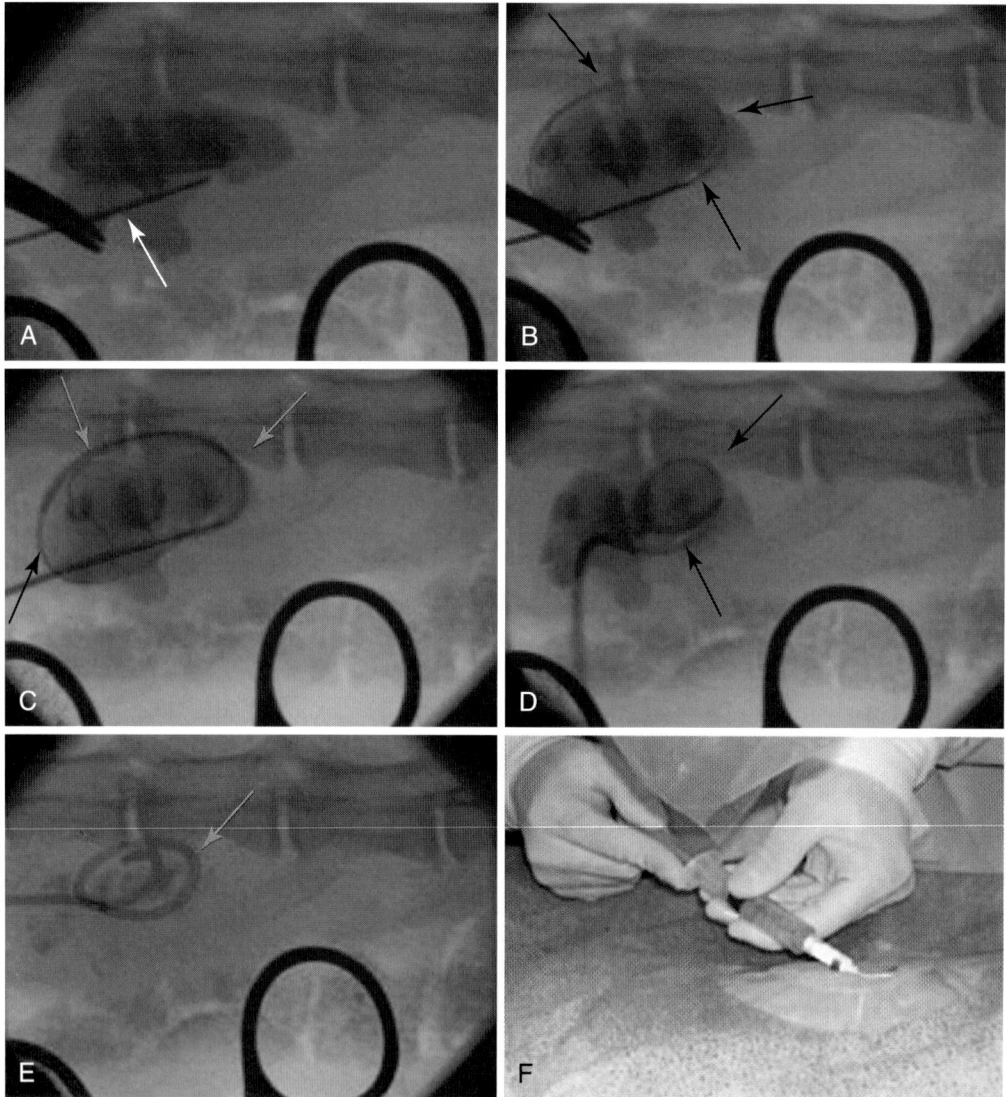

Figure 88-5: Nephrostomy Tube Placement. A, Renal access needle (*white arrow*) during pyelo-centesis and antegrade pyelogram. **B,** Guide wire advanced through the needle (*black arrows*) and coiled within the renal pelvis. **C,** Locking-loop pigtail catheter (*orange arrows*) advanced over the guide wire (*black arrow*) into the renal pelvis. **D,** Locking-loop catheter coiled within the renal pelvis (*black arrows*). **E,** Renal pelvis drained of contrast through the catheter (*orange arrow*). **F,** The neph-rostomy catheter exiting the body wall being drained of urine.

more definitive ureteral intervention. In addition, nephros-tomy tubes can be a stabilizing mechanism so a patient can be transported to a facility where a permanent ureteral inter-vention can be performed.[37] In the author's practice, external-ized nephrostomy tubes are used uncommonly because interventions that are more permanent (particularly a SUB device) have become nearly as fast to place, and are more effective in the longterm.

A locking-loop pigtail catheter is recommended (5 or 6 Fr)[h,i] to decrease the risk of inadvertent tube removal or urine leakage. Historically, nephrostomy tubes have been met with much resistance because of the high risk of complica-tions after placement (more than 50%)[21,38] that are associated with premature removal, dislodgement, urine leakage, infec-tion, or poor drainage. With the advent of sturdy, multifenes-trated tubes that form a loop that will lock the catheter within the renal pelvis, these complications have declined dramatically (see Figures 88-2 and 88-5).[23]

This procedure is typically done under ultrasound and fluoroscopic guidance if being performed percutaneously (when the renal pelvis is more than 15 mm in diameter on transverse measurement), or with surgical assistance and fluo-roscopic guidance (when the renal pelvis is under 15 mm in diameter), using the modified Seldinger technique (Figure 88-5). The author prefers to perform this procedure with surgical assistance in feline patients because of the mobile nature of the kidney and the security of performing a

[h]5 Fr Dawson Mueller Locking-loop catheter, Cook Medical, Bloomington, IN.

[i]6 Fr Locking loop catheter, Infiniti Medical, LLC, Menlo Park, CA.

nephropexy during placement to prevent urine leakage. If done *percutaneously*, a renal access needle (18 gauge) under ultrasound guidance is used for pyelocentesis and a ureteropyelogram. Then, under fluoroscopic guidance, a guide wire[j] (0.018 inch for 5 Fr and 0.035 inch for 6 Fr catheters[h,i]) is passed through the needle and coiled into the contrast-enhanced dilated renal pelvis. The appropriately sized locking-loop pigtail catheter is then advanced over the guide wire into the renal pelvis, and the curl is formed (see Figure 88-5). Once the curl in the renal pelvis is made, the pigtail is locked and the catheter is secured to the body wall for tract formation. The catheter is securely sutured to the skin by a Chinese finger trap suture pattern. The catheter should remain in place for 2 to 4 weeks for tract formation, or the hole can be closed surgically once the obstruction is relieved. *Surgically assisted nephrostomy tube placement* is performed in a similar fashion, only a smaller renal pelvis can be more safely cannulated and a nephropexy can be simultaneous performed, so that the risk of leakage decreases. During surgical nephrostomy tube placement, it may be possible to advance the guide wire down the ureter, and if it bypasses the obstruction, a ureteral stent can be attempted, allowing for a treatment that is more definitive.

Percutaneous or Surgically Assisted Endoscopic Nephroureterolithotomy

Nephroureteroscopy can be performed in an antegrade manner via renal access for proximal ureteroliths or nephroliths that are problematic or obstructive. In contrast with ureteroliths, nephroliths in cats are rarely a clinically significant problem. If nephroliths are causing chronic infections, obstructions, or worsening azotemia, then removal is recommended. This approach is considered the most renal-sparing approach in human adults and children.[39-41]

Percutaneous or surgically assisted endoscopic nephroureterolithotomy (PCNUL/SENL) is performed more commonly in dogs, but can be used in cats if the ureter and pelvis can be significantly dilated to accommodate the rigid and flexible endoscope. A renal access needle is advanced into the renal pelvis through the renal parenchyma for pyelocentesis and a pyeloureterogram, as described previously. A guide wire is advanced through the needle, down the ureter, into the urinary bladder, and out the urethra. A balloon dilator, or serial vascular dilators, is advanced over the wire, and then the access sheath (10 to 14 Fr) is placed within the renal pelvis. This procedure stretches the renal parenchyma apart rather than creating an incision through the nephrons, protecting the nephrons. The endoscope is then advanced through the sheath toward the stone. Once the stone is identified, a stone basket is used to remove the stone (Figure

88-6). If the stone is larger than the sheath, it can be fragmented with a lithotrite. If the stone is easily visualized fluoroscopically, it can be removed through a sheath without the need for endoscopy (see Figure 88-6).

Ureteral Stents

Ureteral stents are used in human patients to divert urine from the renal pelvis into the urinary bladder for obstructions secondary to ureterolithiasis, ureteral stenosis or strictures, malignant neoplasia, or trauma.[11,13-17] The main type of ureteral stent used in both human and veterinary patients is an indwelling double-pigtail ureteral stent[e] (Figure 88-3). The double-pigtail stent is completely intracorporeal and is 2.5 Fr in diameter in feline patients. In human medicine, it is recommended that the stents be removed or exchanged after 3 to 6 months,[12,13,16] but this does not seem to be necessary in feline patients because they have remained patent and in place for more than 6 years in some patients. Stent placement may be considered a long-term treatment option for various causes of ureteral obstructions; however, potential side effects and long-term complications have been documented[23,24,36,26,42-44] (see Table 88-3).

Ureteral stents have been placed for ureteral obstructions in more than 100 feline patients in the author's practice.[23,24,36,26,42-44] The benefits of ureteral stenting in feline patients are threefold: (1) to improve azotemia and ureteral decompression, (2) to create passive ureteral dilation,[17] and (3) to decrease surgical tension on the ureter after or during surgery (i.e., resection and anastomosis) and prevent leakage and reobstruction after surgery. In the author's experience, success rates in feline ureteral stent placement are more than 95% (97% when placed surgically, and only 20% when attempted endoscopically).[24]

With the *antegrade technique*, renal access is obtained with surgical renal exposure. Using a 22-gauge over-the-needle catheter from the lateral aspect of the greater curvature of the kidney, the renal pelvis is cannulated. Then, using fluoroscopic guidance, an antegrade ureteropyelogram is performed, and the location of the obstruction is documented. A 0.018-inch angle-tipped hydrophilic guide wire is passed down the ureter, around the stones, out the UVJ, and into the urinary bladder (Figure 88-7). A small cystotomy incision is then performed to externalize the wire so that through-and-through access ("flossed") is obtained. A 0.034-inch ureteral-dilation catheter[k] is then advanced antegrade over the guide wire from the kidney and into the urinary bladder, dilating the lumen for the ureteral stent. Finally, the stent is advanced over the guide wire and advanced antegrade from the kidney to the bladder. Once the stent traverses the ureter and enters the bladder, the pigtail is formed within the renal pelvis. The guide wire is then removed, and the distal end of the stent is coiled and pushed into the urinary bladder.

---

[h]5 Fr Dawson Mueller Locking-loop catheter, Cook Medical, Bloomington, IN.
[i]6 Fr Locking loop catheter, Infiniti Medical, LLC, Menlo Park, CA.
[j]0.018"-0.035" hydrophilic angle-tipped guide wires, Weasel wire, Infiniti Medical, LLC, Menlo Park, CA.

[e]Vet Stent ureter 2.5 Fr double pigtail ureteral stent, Infiniti Medical LLC, Menlo Park, CA.
[k]0.034" ureteral dilator, Infiniti Medical LLC, Menlo Park, CA.

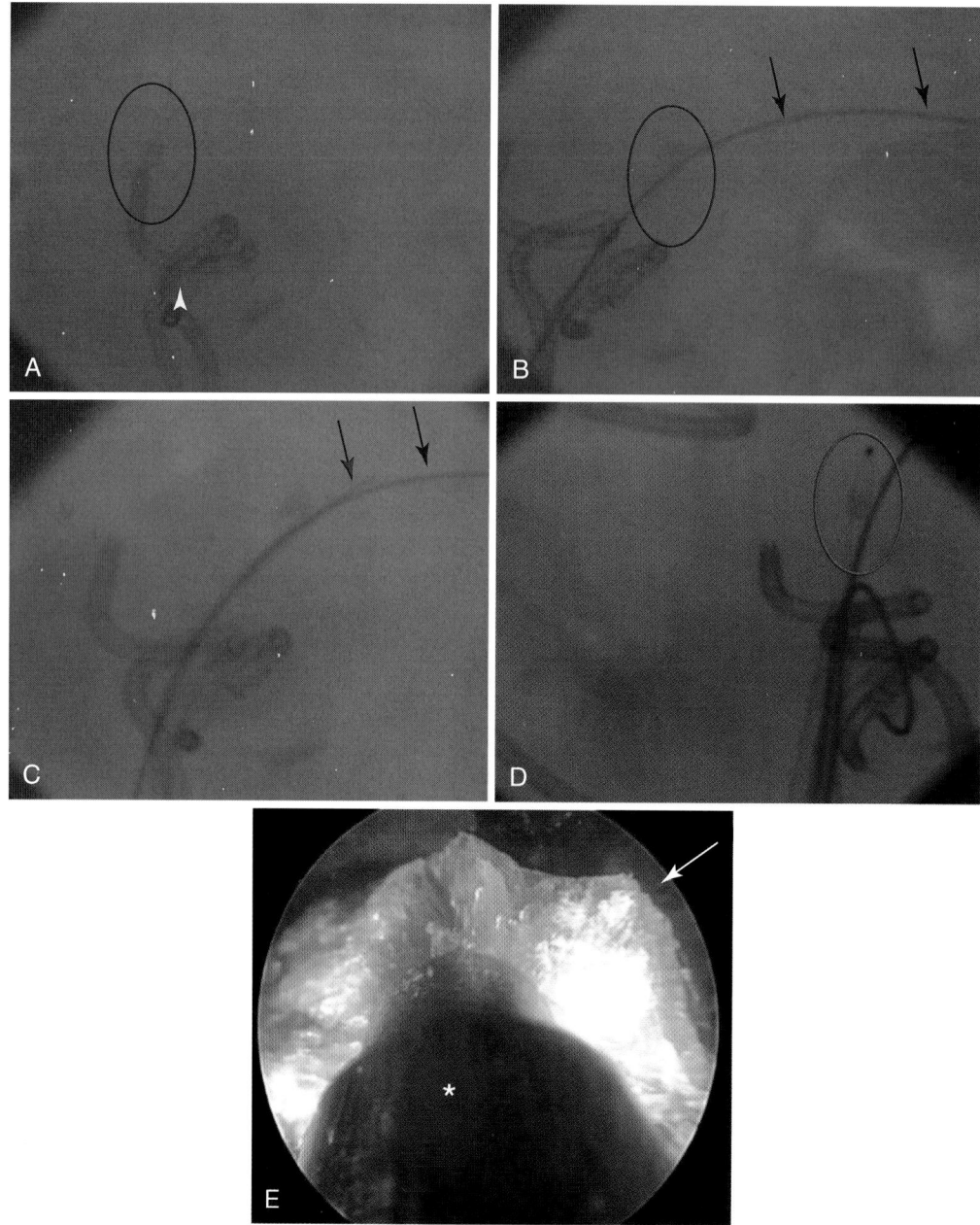

Figure 88-6: Nephrolithotomy Procedure: Images of a Cat with a Proximal Ureteral Stone during Retrieval by Fluoroscopic-Guided Nephrolithotomy. A, This cat has a locking-loop nephrostomy tube (*yellow arrow head*) within the renal pelvis. The proximal ureteral stone (*blue oval*) is identified. **B,** A guide wire (*black arrow*) is advanced down the ureter beyond the stone. **C,** A stone basket (*red arrow*) is advanced through the renal access sheath, beyond the stone. **D,** The basket is opened (*red oval*), and the stone is entrapped for removal. **E,** Endoscopic image during nephrolithotripsy (*white asterisk*) for a nephrolith (*white arrow*) that was too large to retrieve with a basket alone.

The procedure-associated complication rate for stent placement is lower[24,36] than that reported for traditional surgery,[21,22] with uroabdomen being the most common (30% with ureterotomy and reimplantation versus 6.7% with stent placement). Uroabdomen can occur if a concurrent ureterotomy is performed during stent placement and is typically self-limiting within 24 to 48 hours if a closed suction drain is left in place (see Table 88-3).

Detailed management after surgery is necessary in the treatment of feline patients after obstruction removal. Feline patients are at high risk of developing a postobstructive diuresis and potentially fluid overload. Care is taken to maintain an appropriate fluid balance using enteral hydration when possible (feeding tubes), and careful monitoring of body weight, urine production, and biochemical parameters is required. Serial urinary tract ultrasounds focusing on the renal pelvis diameter, stent location, and ureteral diameter are performed to assure that there is no evidence of stent migration, occlusion, or encrustation. The author recommends a urine culture every 3 to 6 months for proper long-term

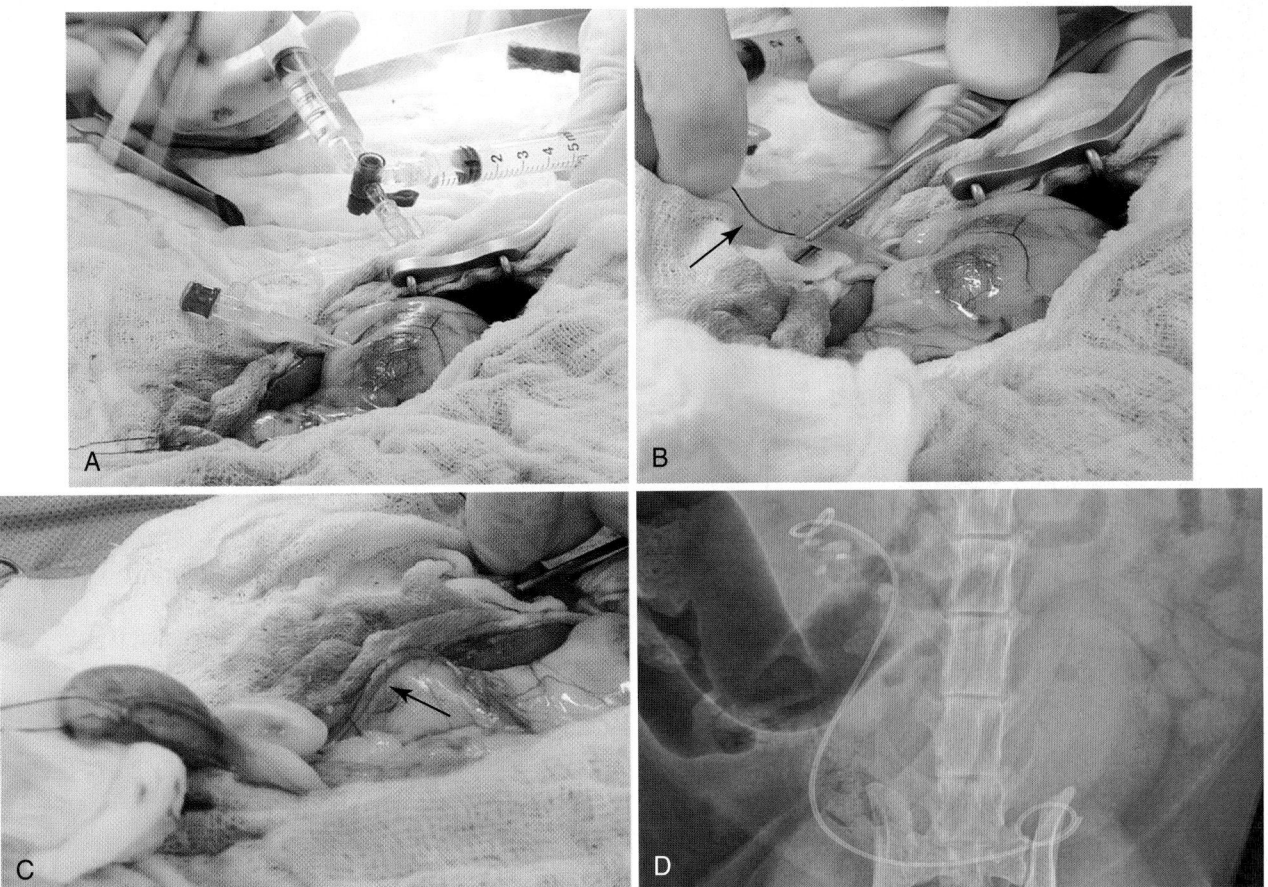

Figure 88-7: Surgical Placement of a Feline Ureteral Stent. The top of each image is cranial. **A,** Antegrade ureteropyelogram being performed using a 22-gauge over-the-needle catheter. **B,** A 0.018-inch guide wire (*black arrow*) is being advanced through the catheter and down the ureter using fluoroscopic guidance. **C,** The guide wire (*black arrow*) is in the ureteral lumen as it passes from the renal pelvis to the urinary bladder. **D,** Ventrodorsal radiograph after stent placement showing the pigtail in the renal pelvis next to a large amount of nephroliths and the shaft of the stent traveling down the ureter with the distal pigtail in the urinary bladder.

management. Traditionally, in human medicine, ureteral stents are temporary and meant to be removed, but in veterinary medicine, this is not routinely necessary. Most stents are suspected to be occluded by debris within 3 months, but with appropriate passive ureteral dilation, the ureter does not reobstruct, unless there is a concurrent ureteral stricture. Strictured tissue does not dilate passively, and this could result in ureteral reocclusion (58% of strictured cases).[24,36]

It should be emphasized that stents should be placed by those experienced with the technique and equipment because these cases are technically challenging and can become very complicated. The success rates are high, particularly when using the specific 2.5 Fr feline ureteral stent, but the procedure can be very challenging and is not recommended routinely unless the operator is trained. A study evaluating 69 feline patients (79 ureters) with ureteral obstructions treated with a ureteral stent had a 96% placement success.[24] In that study, 14% were bilaterally obstructed, 28% were associated with strictures (some with concurrent ureteroliths), and 85% of cases had concurrent nephroliths. The median number of stones in the obstructed ureter was four. Approximately one-third of cats had documentation of a urinary tract infection

before stent placement, and 30% of cats had at least one positive urine culture in their lifetime after stent placement. The median creatinine was 5.3 mg/dL (468.5 μmol/L) before surgery, and it was 2.1 mg/dL (185.6 μmol/L) after stent placement. The perioperative mortality rate after surgery was 7.5%, with no death associated with a ureteral obstruction or the procedure. This compares with an 18% to 38% mortality rate with traditional surgery.[20-22] The most common long-term (greater than 1 month) complications after ureteral stent placement were dysuria (38%, but only persistent in 2%), chronic hematuria (18%), stent occlusion (19%), stent migration (6%), and ureteritis or mucosal proliferation (4%). The dysuria typically resolved with short-term corticosteroid therapy. A ureteral stent exchange with either a bigger stent or a SUB device was needed in 27% of cats because of either occlusion or migration. This complication was most commonly associated with ureteral strictures (more than 50% of strictures reoccluded),[24,36] or an occlusion at a previous ureterotomy site. Ureters remained patent long-term in most cats, with the longest stent in place and functional for over 5 years. The median survival time was 498 days. The median survival time for only a renal cause of death was more than

1250 days, with only 21% of cats dying of suspected CKD. Another study evaluating prognostic factors for short- and long-term survivals and renal recovery before surgery did not identify any clinical, biochemical, or imaging findings that affected overall survival in patients[26] (see Table 88-3).

Subcutaneous Ureteral Bypass Device

The SUB device[g] was initially created for feline patients as an alternative to ureteral stents when either a stricture was present (higher rate of stent occlusion [greater than 50%]) or a stent was unable to be successfully placed because of excessive stones, very narrow lumen, or patient stability. The long-term outcomes documented with the SUB device found that patient comfort and reobstruction rates were superior to that of ureteral stents (see Table 88-3).[45,28] Because of these findings, the trend has moved toward using the SUB device as a primary option for treating feline ureteral obstructions in the author's practice. It is very important to understand the risks and benefits of traditional surgery, ureteral stenting, and SUB device placement to determine the best treatment option for each patient. In human medicine, a device similar to the SUB has been used for patients with extensive urinary tract malignancies, ureteral strictures secondary to renal transplantation, or when ureteral stenting or reconstructive surgery fails or is contraindicated.[46-48]

The placement of nephrostomy catheters in veterinary medicine (described earlier) has been met with excellent success when the appropriate device is used.[37] The biggest limitation is the externalized drainage, requiring careful management and hospitalization to prevent infection and dislodgement. The development of an indwelling SUB device[g] (see Figures 88-4 and 88-8), using a combination locking-loop nephrostomy catheter and cystostomy catheter connected to a subcutaneous shunting port, has been highly successful for the treatment of all causes of feline ureteral obstructions (e.g., stones, stricture, tumors, and obstructive pyelonephritis). In human patients, a similar device has been shown to reduce complications associated with externalized nephrostomy tubes and ureteral stents, and improve quality of life.[47,48]

The SUB device is placed with surgical assistance using fluoroscopic guidance. The nephrostomy catheter is 6.5 Fr in diameter, and it is placed over a 0.035-inch J-shaped guide wire using the modified Seldinger technique, as described earlier (see Figure 88-8). Then a multifenestrated catheter[g] is placed into the urinary bladder at the apex. Each catheter is secured to the renal capsule and serosal surface of the bladder, respectively, using a Dacron cuff to prevent leakage and migration (see Figure 88-8). Once the catheters are in place, they are passed through the ventral body wall, just lateral to the abdominal incision, and connected to the shunting port securely (Figure 88-9). Contrast material is infused through the shunting port before closure, to ensure patency and to check for any leakage (see Figures 88-8 and 88-9).

The management of the SUB device after surgery is similar to that described previously for ureteral stenting. Care should be taken with fluid therapy as a postobstructive diuresis is common and can lead to overzealous fluid therapy, resulting in fluid overload. Abdominal palpation is discouraged for the first 2 weeks to prevent manipulation of the device. Following discharge, patients are monitored similarly to all feline ureteral obstruction patients, including serial ultrasound examinations and urine cultures. Urine is generally sampled from the SUB device access port using a special noncoring Huber needle,[1] during which time the device can be flushed using sterile saline under ultrasound guidance. This is recommended every 3 to 6 months to help ensure and maintain patency. Cystocentesis should be discouraged in these patients.

The use of the feline SUB device has been described.[23,36,26,44,45,28] To date, more than 180 of these devices have been placed over a 6-year period with good short- and long-term success (see Table 88-3). The median creatinine before surgery was 6.8 mg/dL (601 μmol/L), and it was 2.4 mg/dL (212.2 μmol/L) after SUB device placement. The perioperative mortality rate after surgery was 5.6%, with no death associated with a procedure-related complication,[36,26,28] compared with traditional surgery (18% to 38% mortality) and ureteral stenting (7.5% mortality) (see Table 88-3). Futhermore, the median follow-up time for these patients was more than 19 months. Perioperative complications are typically rare and include leakage (at the port or nephrostomy tube insertion site in less than 5% of patients), kinking of the catheters (or failure of renal function to recover, less than 5%), and blockage of the system with either blood clots, debris, or purulent material (less than 5%). Dysuria is rarely seen in cats with a SUB device (less than 2% of patients) compared to those with a stent (38% of patients), and long-term occlusion of the device with stone debris has been seen in approximately 15% of cases (18% with stone disease and 0% with strictures), requiring either serial flushing or device exchange.

The SUB device is considered a functional option. It is currently the author's treatment of choice in cats with ureteral obstructions.

Diseases of the Lower Urinary Collection System: Urinary Bladder and Urethra

Percutaneous Cystostomy Tube Placement

Cystostomy tubes are often placed to bypass a urethral obstruction or buy time while a urethral, trigonal, or bladder lesion is healing. This can be secondary to malignant neoplasia, aggressive bladder surgeries, severe urethritis, urethral strictures, urethral tears, or urethral stones that are difficult to remove surgically. With the advent of urethral stents, the use of cystostomy tubes has declined in the author's practice, but the ease and success of placement of these tubes make them a viable option when necessary. Cystostomy tubes can be placed either percutaneously or surgically. With the locking-loop pigtail catheter (see Figure 88-2), percutaneous cystostomy tube placement has become a fast, safe, and highly effective technique. This can be done using either ultrasound

---

[g]Subcutaneous ureteral bypass device (SUB), Norfolk Vet, Skokie, IL.

[1]22 gauge Huber needle, Norfolk Vet, Skokie, IL.

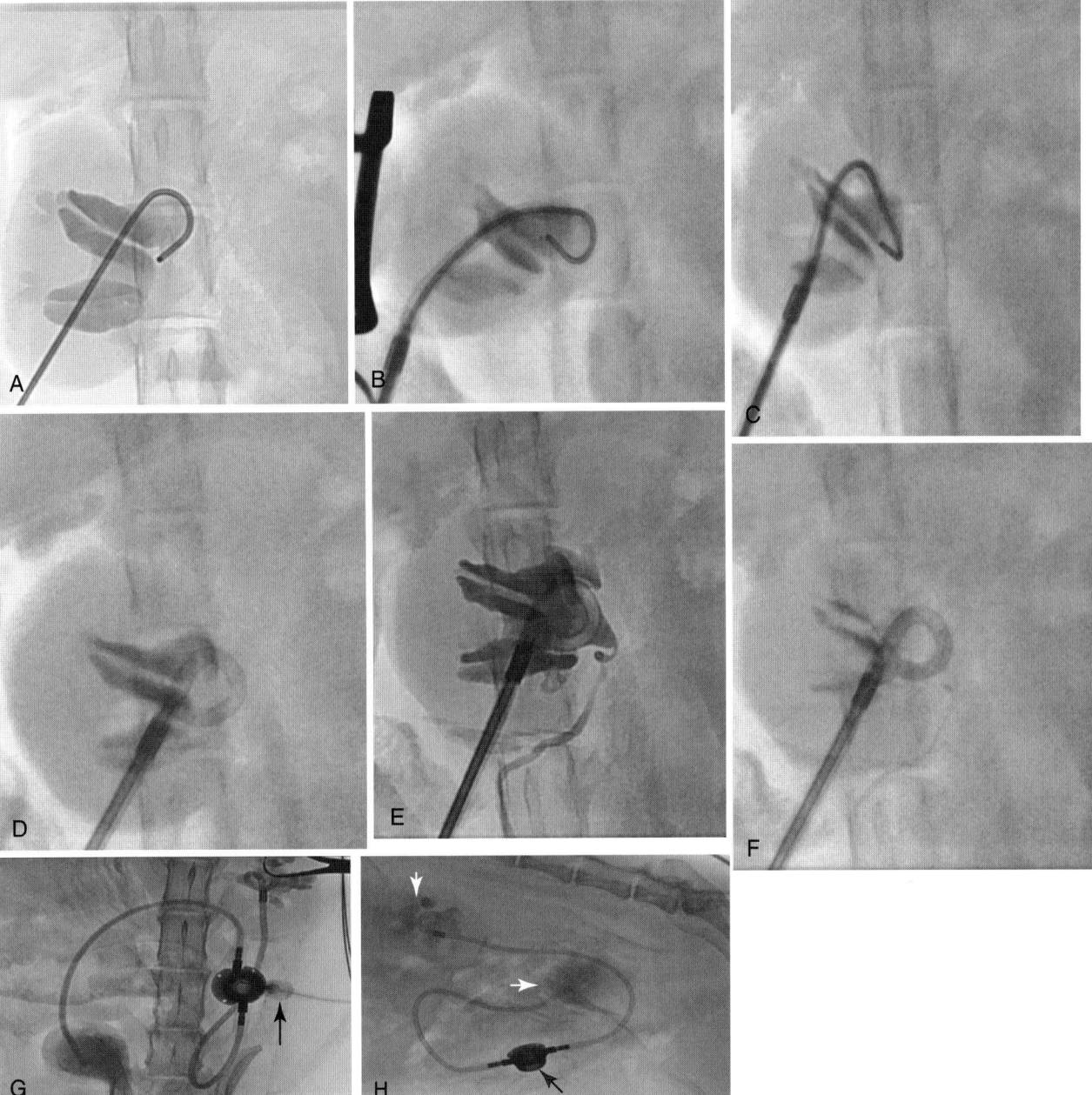

Figure 88-8: Fluoroscopic Images during Right Subcutaneous Ureteral Bypass (SUB) Device Placement. The top of each image (**A-G**) is cranial, and the left of image (**H**) is cranial. **A,** The "J-tipped" guide wire is advanced into the renal pelvis after a pyelogram is performed. This is done from the caudal pole of the kidney. **B,** A nephrostomy catheter is advanced over the wire into the renal pelvis. **C,** The nephrostomy catheter is coiled within the renal pelvis over the wire. **D,** The wire is removed, and the locking-loop pigtail catheter is locked. **E,** Ureteropyelogram through the locking-loop pigtail catheter, confirming appropriate location; this obstruction was in the distal ureter so the proximal ureterogram is visible. **F,** Renal pelvic drainage through the catheter to remove all the contrast. **G,** Image of the entire SUB device system after placement showing the pyelogram and cystogram with injection of contrast medium via a Huber needle (*black arrow*) through the port. **H,** Lateral image confirming appropriate SUB placement, in which the white arrow is the nephrostomy and cystostomy catheters, and the red arrow is the shunting port.

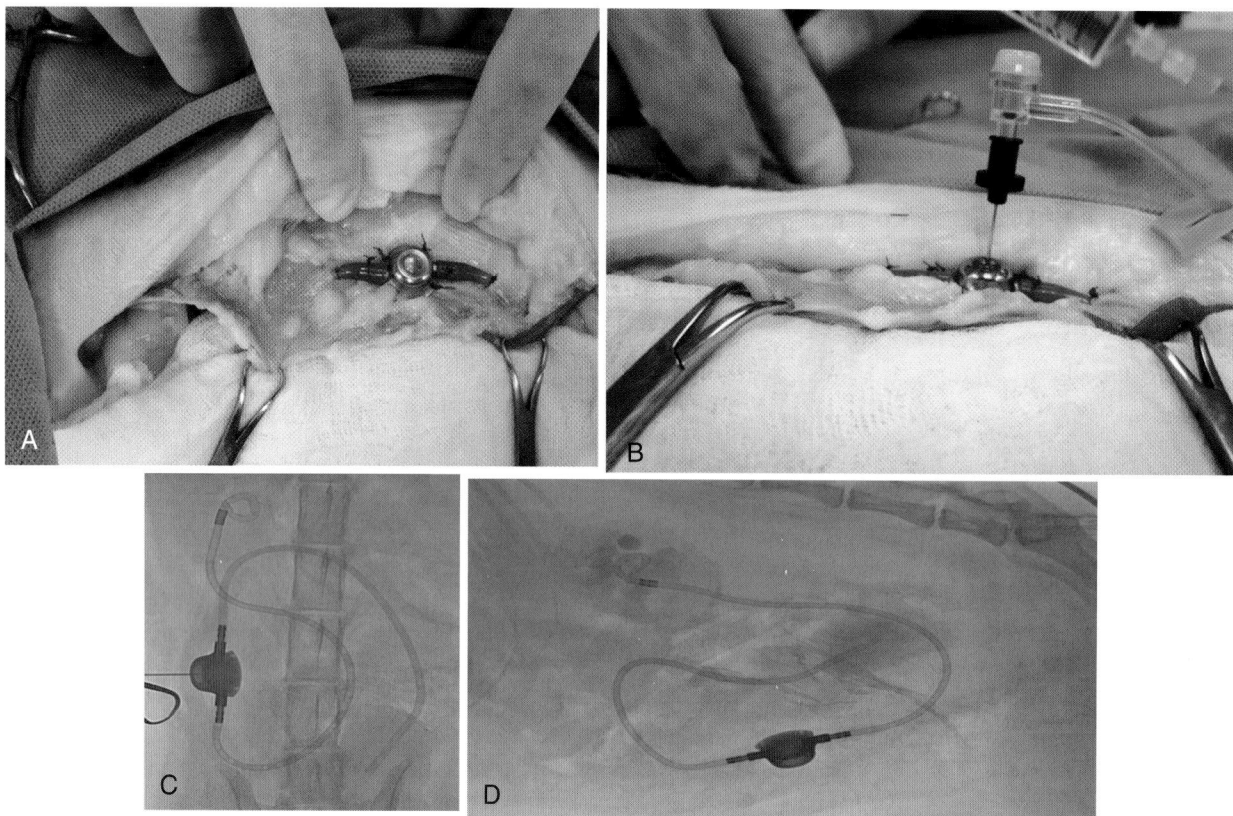

Figure 88-9: Subcutaneous ureteral bypass (SUB) device placement. A and **B** are surgical images showing the shunting port in the subcutaneous space after placement. The Huber needle is inserted into the port to ensure device patency and check for leakage before abdominal closure. **C,** Ventrodorsal fluoroscopic image of a right SUB device after placement, confirming appropriate positioning. **D,** Lateral fluoroscopic image of the SUB device.

and/or fluoroscopic guidance. The author prefers fluoroscopic guidance using the modified Seldinger technique. As described earlier for nephrostomy tubes, a stab incision is made through the skin and abdominal musculature over the area of puncture. Then, an 18-gauge over-the-needle catheter is advanced into the urinary bladder via cystocentesis (paramedian approach at the bladder body), until urine is draining. The stylet is removed, and a sterile urine sample is obtained for culture and analysis. Then a cystogram is performed using a 50% mixture of contrast medium and sterile saline to fill the bladder (approximate total bladder volume is 5 to 15 mL/kg). Next, a 0.035-inch hydrophilic angle-tipped guide wire[j] is advanced through the catheter and coiled within the urinary bladder. The guide wire can be advanced down the urethra using fluoroscopic guidance if antegrade catheterization is desired (see the next section), using this same technique.

For placement of the cystostomy tube (Figure 88-10), the locking-loop catheter is cannulated with the stiff hollow trocar and is advanced over the wire. This catheter is then punctured through the body and urinary bladder wall. Once it is well within the urinary bladder, the hollow trocar is withdrawn as the catheter is advanced over the guide wire to

ensure that the entire distal end of the catheter is within the bladder lumen. Then the locking string is engaged as the trocar and guide wire are removed, creating a loop of the pigtail catheter. The bladder is then drained and filled to ensure the entire pigtail is appropriately positioned in the bladder lumen and is functioning well. The loop of the catheter should be within the lumen of the bladder, extending approximately 1 to 2 cm from the wall, so that it is not too snug against the bladder wall. This allows movement when the bladder is both full and empty to prevent dislodgement. The catheter is then carefully secured to the body wall using a purse-string suture and Chinese finger trap suture pattern. Because there is no surgical cystopexy, this tube should remain in place for at least 2 to 4 weeks before removal. Other tubes, such as latex mushroom-tipped catheters, Foley catheters, or low-profile tubes can be placed either surgically or with laparoscopic assistance.[49-51] These tubes are placed with a surgical cystopexy. Catheter care and cleanliness should be emphasized, as cystostomy tubes are commonly associated with secondary infections (86% in one study) because of the external nature of the tube. Additional complications with cystostomy tubes have been reported in as high as 49% of patients, involving inadvertent tube removal, ingestion of the tube by the patient, fistulous tract formation, and mushroom-tip breakage during removal.[51] Cystostomy tube placement is not ideal in circumstances where chemotherapy (for

---

[j]0.018"-0.035" hydrophilic angle-tipped guide wires, Weasel wire, Infiniti Medical, LLC, Menlo Park, CA.

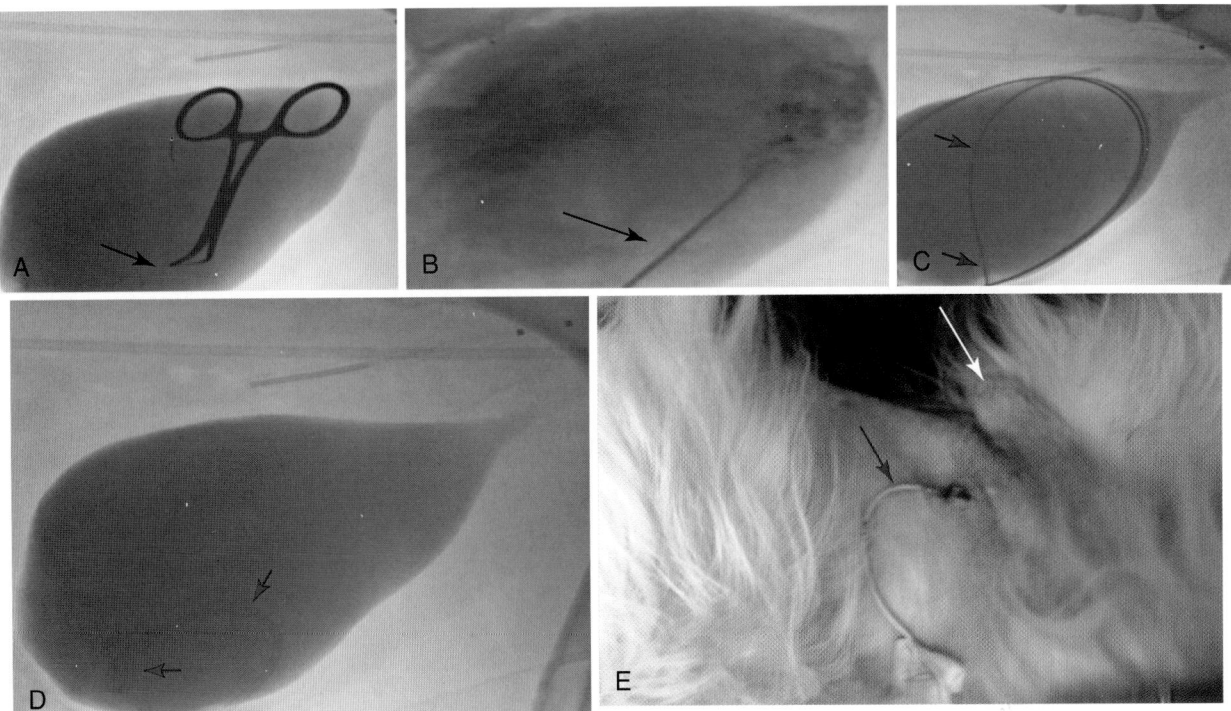

Figure 88-10: Percutaneous Cystostomy Tube Placement. A, 18-gauge over-the-needle catheter (*black arrow*) placed within the urinary bladder for cystocentesis. **B,** Cystogram performed through the catheter. **C,** Guide wire (*red arrow*) advanced into the urinary bladder through the catheter. Over the wire is a locking-loop pigtail catheter. **D,** Locking-loop pigtail catheter (*red arrows*) within the urinary bladder. **E,** Image of a male dog showing the paramedian cystostomy tube (*red arrow*) exiting the body wall; notice its location next to the prepuce (*white arrow*).

malignant obstructions) or immunosuppressive therapy (for immune-mediated proliferative urethritis) is being used as secondary infections and poor wound healing may occur. In addition, if a tube is removed prematurely and no cystopexy has been created, the risk of uroabdomen is possible.

Urethral Catheterization

Obstructions of the urethra can cause severe discomfort, dysuria, and life-threatening azotemia, requiring fast and effective relief. Urinary diversion is commonly accomplished via standard urethral catheterization techniques. This is a simple and routinely performed procedure in veterinary patients, primarily used to monitor urine output and establish urine drainage in patients that are recumbent, have mechanical or functional urethral obstructions, are healing after a urethral tear, or to provide urethral patency following urethral or urinary bladder surgery. The most common urethral catheters used in male cats are 3.5 Fr or 5 Fr red rubber catheters, as they are relatively atraumatic. In the author's opinion, rigid catheters should not be used to relieve urethral obstructions. These catheters can be a leading cause of urethral trauma and tears because of their inflexible nature. In addition, the urethral obstruction should never be physically, forcefully removed with the catheter itself, as this is how urethral tears occur. Instead, retrograde flushing should be used to dislodge the occluding object (e.g., stone, mucous plug). For this procedure, the patient should be anesthetized or heavily sedated, so that there is very little urethral spasm or reaction occurring

during manipulation. If a soft atraumatic catheter cannot be easily advanced in a retrograde manner and the bladder is turgid, the urinary bladder should be emptied by decompressive cystocentesis using a 22-gauge needle, or over-the-needle catheter, attached to an extension set (or T-port) and a three-way stopcock. The bladder should then be drained until it is soft, allowing for infusion of sterile saline (retrograde hydropropulsion) during retrograde catheter placement. All catheters in the urinary system should be placed with sterile technique. In female cats, this can be more difficult because blind catheterization of the urethral meatus is necessary. If this is not possible, the use of a speculum, cystoscope, or vaginoscope to aid papilla canalization may be needed. Once the distal end of the urethra is catheterized, 10 mL of sterile saline should be used to flush the urethra as the catheter is gently advanced. The end of the penile urethra, or the vulva, should be compressed digitally to allow pressure to build up within the urethra, ultimately distending the urethral lumen around the obstructive lesion. As the saline infusion is occurring, an assistant should advance the catheter, ensuring that no resistance is encountered. Again, it is not advisable to use the catheter tip to remove the obstruction because that can result in a urethral tear; instead, sterile flush should be used to dislodge the obstruction. It is helpful to have another assistant palpate the urinary bladder during flushing to assess size and prevent bladder overdistension or bladder rupture and urine leakage. Once the urethral catheter is in place, it should be carefully secured to the prepuce or vulva with

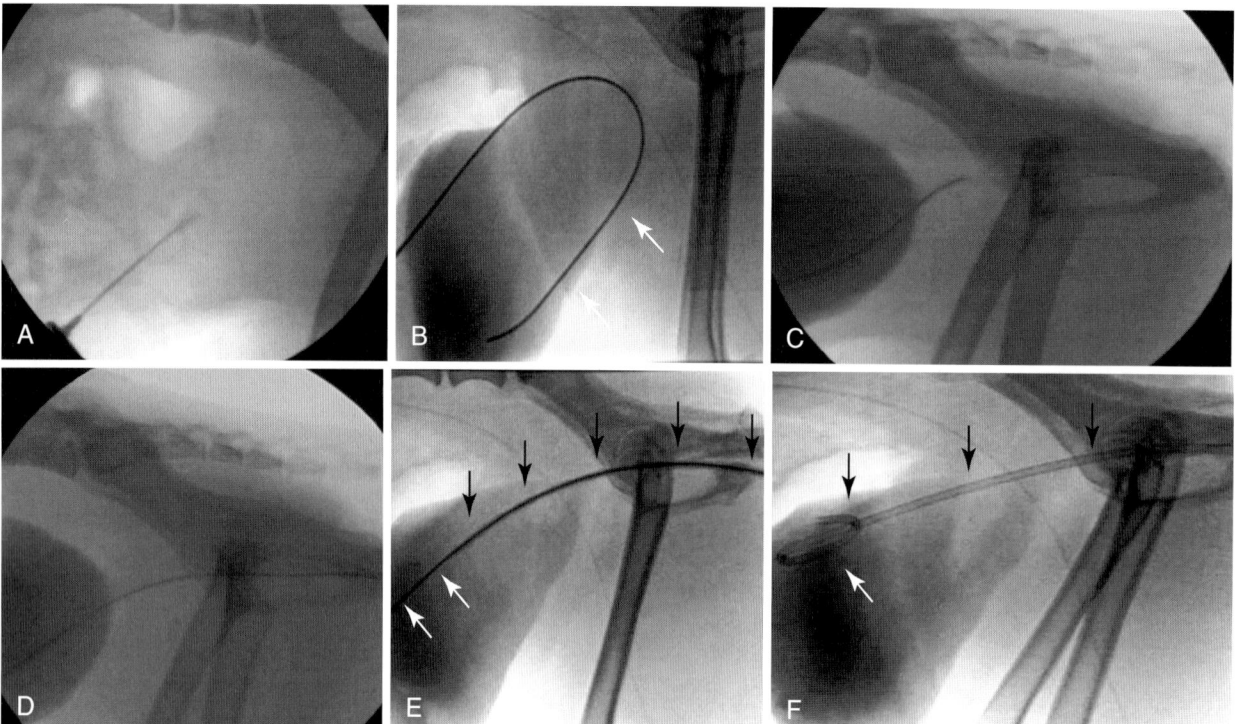

Figure 88-11: Percutaneous Antegrade Urethral Catheterization in a Male Cat with a Urethral Tear. Fluoroscopic images are showing a cat in lateral recumbency. Cranial is to the left of each image. **A,** Cystocentesis with an 18-gauge over-the-needle catheter; a cystogram is performed. **B,** A 0.035-inch guide wire (*white arrows*) advanced through the catheter. **C,** The guide wire is advanced down the urethra from the bladder. **D,** The guide wire is advanced out of the urethra for through-and-through access. **E,** Over the wire (*white arrows*) an open-ended catheter (*black arrows*) is advanced into the bladder. **F,** The wire is removed, and the catheter (pigtail [*white arrow*]) is secured in place.

suture material and then taped to the tail to prevent dislodgement. A closed sterile urinary collection system should be attached to allow constant urine drainage, and the catheter should remain clean. If this technique is not effective, a 0.018-inch hydrophilic angle-tipped guide wire[j] could be passed around the obstruction in a retrograde manner and into the bladder. This is best done under fluoroscopic guidance if possible. If this is successful, the tip of the 3.5-French red rubber catheter can be cut so that it can then be advanced over the wire and into the urinary bladder.

Urethral tears occur most commonly in male cats during procedures to relieve urethral obstruction with an excessively stiff catheter, from vehicular trauma, or during stone manipulation. The management of urethral trauma by the use of urethral catheterization alone has been reported,[52] and the patient will typically heal over a 5- to 14-day period. When retrograde catheterization is not possible, a percutaneous antegrade urethral catheterization approach can be attempted.[53]

Percutaneous Antegrade Urethral Catheterization

For animals that are difficult or too small to catheterize, have a urethral tear, or have a distal urethral obstruction, antegrade

urethral catheterization can be performed (Figure 88-11). This technique can be performed surgically or interventionally, and should be done under general anesthesia or heavy sedation.[53] When performed surgically, a ventral abdominal approach is used. In addition to normal patient preparation, the vulva or prepuce should be clipped and aseptically prepared. When performing the technique percutaneously, the patient is placed in lateral recumbency and an area in the caudal lateral abdomen over the bladder is clipped and the area, as well as the vulva or prepuce, is prepared aseptically. A cystocentesis is performed using an 18-gauge over-the-needle catheter directed toward the trigone of the bladder, as discussed in the section about percutaneous cystostomy tube placement. Urine (5 to 15 mL) is drained from the bladder and replaced with an equal amount of contrast material diluted 50% with sterile saline until the proximal urethra is identified. A hydrophilic guide wire (0.018 inch for male cats and 0.035 inch for female cats) is advanced into the bladder and aimed toward the bladder trigone and urethra, using fluoroscopic guidance. Once the urethra is cannulated with the guide wire, it is advanced down the urethra antegrade, around the obstructive lesion or tear, and out of the distal urethra, prepuce or vulva. When performed surgically, contrast enhancement and the use of fluoroscopy are not necessary. This allows for "through-and-through" guide wire access. Once the guide wire is outside the urethra, a urinary catheter

---

[j]0.018"-0.035" hydrophilic angle-tipped guide wires, Weasel wire, Infiniti Medical, LLC, Menlo Park, CA.

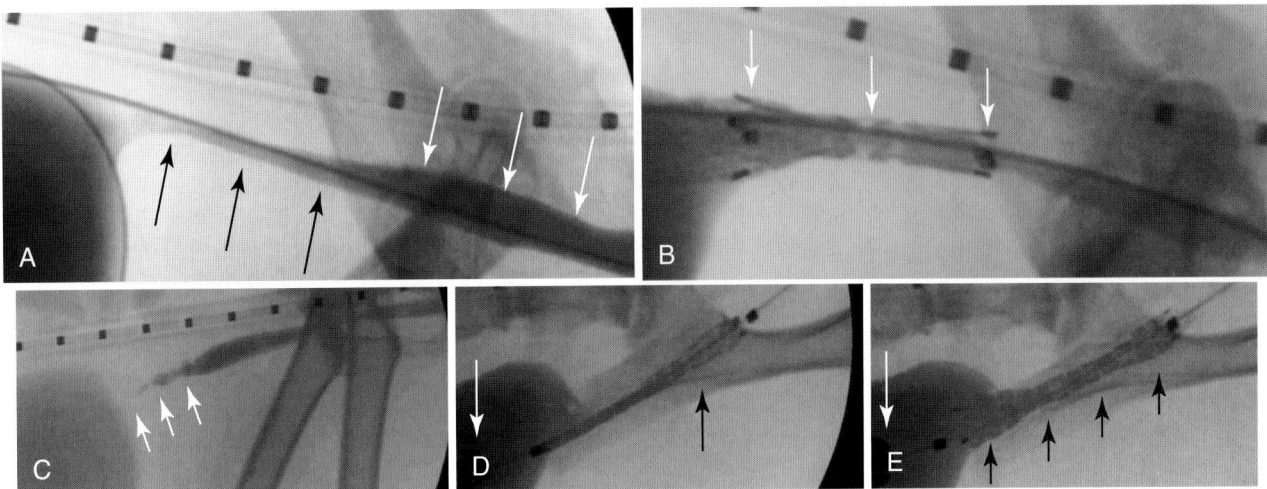

Figure 88-12: Fluoroscopic Images of Two Cats during Urethral Stent Placement. A and **B,** The cat is in lateral recumbency. This is a female cat; therefore, the stent is placed in a retrograde manner through the urethra. **A,** The obstructive lesion (*black arrows*) and normal urethra (*white arrows*) are documented during a cystourethrogram. **B,** The urethral stent (*white arrows*) is deployed over the guide wire. **C,** This is a cystourethrogram in a male cat done in lateral recumbency, documenting the urethral obstruction (*white arrows*). **D** and **E,** The urethral stent (*black arrow*) is being placed in an antegrade manner through a cystostomy sheath (*white arrow*) across the obstruction. **E,** The stent (*black arrows*) after it is deployed showing the patent urethral lumen.

(open-ended; red rubber [3.5 to 5.0 Fr for male cats and 5.0 to 8 Fr for female cats], a locking-loop pigtail catheter [5 Fr for male cats; 6 to 8 Fr for female cats], or a nonlocking pigtail catheter) is advanced over the wire in a retrograde manner, within the urethral lumen and into the urinary bladder. This is highly effective for male cats with urethral tears because the tear is typically made in a longitudinal retrograde direction, making antegrade passage easy. Longitudinal urethral tears will usually heal within 5 to 10 days without surgical intervention, and the catheter should be maintained for that length of time, using clean or sterile technique.[52]

Metallic Stenting for Benign or Malignant Urethral Obstructions

Urethral stents are used most commonly for the relief of benign or malignant obstructions in the trigone or urethra of cats.[54] The most common cause of benign obstructions in cats are strictures from urethral tears, vehicular trauma, or chronic obstructive stone disease. Transitional cell carcinoma (TCC) is less common in cats than it is in dogs, but it is the most common reason for urethral stent placement in cats to date.[55-57] Chemotherapy and nonsteroidal anti-inflammatory therapy has been successful in slowing tumor growth, but complete cure is uncommon.[56,57] When signs of obstruction occur, more aggressive therapy is indicated, with euthanasia commonly ensuing because of a lack of good alternative options. Placement of cystostomy tubes,[49-51] debulking resections,[58] and surgical diversionary procedures[59,60] have been described in dogs, but such treatments are invasive and often associated with undesirable outcomes. Urethral strictures are another obstructive lesion encountered uncommonly in cats that leave similar treatment options to that of malignant obstruction.

Placement of self-expanding metallic stents under fluoroscopic guidance via a transurethral approach can be a fast, reliable, and safe alternative to establish urethral patency regardless of the benign or malignant nature of the underlying condition.[54] This technique has been performed in more than 100 canine patients in the author's practice, but in only a small number of feline patients (Figure 88-12). Benign urethral strictures may resolve with urethral stents or balloon dilation alone. Balloon dilation has been performed in a small number of cats to date.

To place a urethral stent, the patient is positioned in lateral recumbency, and a marker catheter is placed inside the colon to allow for urethral measurement and determination of stent size. The bladder is maximally distended with contrast material, and a pull-out urethrogram is performed by injecting contrast into the catheter while pulling the catheter back caudally to allow for maximal distension of the urethra. Measurements of the normal urethral diameter and the length of the associated obstruction are obtained, and an appropriately sized self-expanding metallic urethral stent[f] is chosen (approximately 10% to 15% greater than the normal urethral diameter and 3 to 5 mm longer than the obstruction on both the cranial and caudal ends). In cats, this is usually a 5- to 6-mm-diameter and a 20- to 30-mm-length stent. The stent is deployed under fluoroscopic guidance, and a repeat contrast cystourethrogram is performed to document restored urethral patency (see Figure 88-12). For female cats, the entire procedure is done through the urethra in a retrograde manner, as previously described for dogs,[61] but in male cats, the delivery system of the stent (6 to 7 Fr) is generally too large

---

[f]VetStent Urethra, Infiniti Medical LLC, Menlo Park, CA.

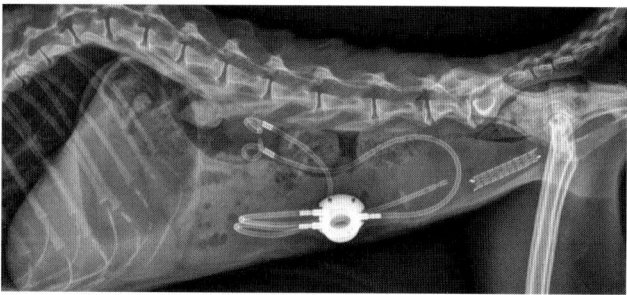

Figure 88-13: A Lateral Radiograph of a Cat that Had Bilateral Ureteral and a Urethral Obstruction from a Transitional Cell Carcinoma. This cat had bilateral subcutaneous ureteral bypass devices placed (attached to a three-way port) and a urethral stent placed to ensure patency of both ureters and the urethra.

to fit through the penile urethra, unless a perineal urethrostomy is present. Because of this, a PCCL approach, allowing antegrade cystoscopy, is used to pass the stent and delivery system through the apex of the bladder and down the diseased urethra, over a guide wire (see Figure 88-12). Once the stent is deployed and patency is confirmed, the delivery system and wire are removed and the bladder apex is repaired with a few interrupted sutures. Regardless of the approach, it is considered an outpatient procedure, and patients are typically discharged the same day. In some cases with trigonal TCC, the cat may have bilateral concurrent ureteral obstructions. When this is encountered, it is typically recommended to place bilateral SUB devices in addition to a urethral stent (Figure 88-13). This procedure can be highly successful when necessary.

For urethral strictures, balloon dilation alone can be performed using fluoroscopic guidance. After balloon dilation is complete (using a balloon size similar to that measured for stent placement), topical mitomycin C (MMC) can be applied to decrease the risk of stricture reformation. Mitomycin C is an antibiotic produced by *Streptomyces caespitosus*. Aside from being an antibiotic, it is an antineoplastic-like alkylating agent, causing single-band breakage and cross-linking of DNA at the adenosine and guanine molecules. It inhibits RNA and protein synthesis.[62,63] As an antiproliferative agent, MMC inhibits fibroblast proliferation and decreases scar tissue formation. Its antiproliferative properties on fibroblasts have been shown, in rats, dogs, and humans, to be effective in reducing stricture recurrence in the urinary tract, respiratory tract, and gastrointestinal tract.[62,63]

One study evaluated nine cats after urethral stent placement.[54] In the study the obstruction was effectively relieved in all cats, but 25% of cats were considered significantly incontinent following stenting. Long-term outcome was good to excellent in 75% of cats and fair to poor in 25%, with some cats surviving over 2.5 years after stent placement regardless of obstruction cause (benign and malignant).[54] Palliative stenting for urethral obstructions in cats can provide a rapid, effective, and safe alternative to more traditional and invasive options, and long-term survival times in cats with TCC seem to be longer than that seen in dogs.[55]

Laser Lithotripsy

Laser lithotripsy is a technique involving the intracorporeal fragmentation of uroliths during rigid or flexible cystourethroscopy. The first report of holmium laser lithotripsy was in 1995 in human medicine.[7] The holmium:YAG (yttrium, aluminum, and garnet) laser[d] is a pulsed laser that emits light at an infrared wavelength of 2100 nm.[5] The energy is absorbed in less than 0.5 mm of fluid, making it safe to fragment uroliths in tight locations, as within the urethra or urinary bladder, with limited risk to the urothelial tissue.[5] It combines both tissue cutting and coagulation properties, as well as the ability to fragment stones upon contact.[5] This technology has been used for stone fragmentation and tissue ablation in dogs, pigs, humans, horses, goats, and steers.[63-69] The procedure has become widespread for use in both dogs and cats in many veterinary facilities around the world for the treatment of bladder and urethral stones.

Small-diameter fibers (200, 365, and 550 µm) are guided through the working channel of small-diameter flexible or rigid cystoscopes or ureteroscopes. Although the various commercial models of lithotrites vary slightly, the pulse duration of the holmium laser ranges from 250 to 750 µsec, the pulse energy from 0.2 to 4.0 J/pulse, and the frequency from 5 to 45 Hz, with an average power from 3.0 to 100 W. The power that one chooses is based on the intended application. This procedure is typically only performed in female cats because of the need for cystourethroscopy and a working channel for laser fiber delivery and fluid irrigation.

For stone fragmentation, laser energy is focused on the urolith surface, directed via cystoscopy. Pulsed laser energy is absorbed by water inside the urolith, resulting in a photothermal effect, which causes urolith fragmentation. The holmium laser effect on the calculus is by a vapor bubble. The vapor bubble is created when the pulse of laser energy traveling through water from the tip of the fiber is trapped within a bubble (Moses effect). If the fiber tip is 0.5 mm or more away from the target (e.g., calculus or tissue), the vapor bubble collapses, the water absorbs the energy, and no impact is made on the target. As the fiber tip is advanced less than 0.5 mm from the target, there will be an impact. The closer the fiber tip is to the target, the larger the effect.[6] The stone is typically touched with the laser fiber and fragmented until the pieces are small enough to be removed normograde through the urethral orifice, either via voiding urohydropropulsion (for 2- to 3-mm-diameter fragments) or with the assistance of a stone basket (for 3- to 4-mm-diameter fragments). This process is useful for cystic and urethral calculi in cats. All stone types can be fragmented using laser lithotripsy. Because of the repeated need for endoscopic urethral passage, this procedure can be irritating to the urethra when a large stone burden is present, in which case the PCCL approach (described in the next section) is preferred by some operators.

Other urologic applications for laser lithotripsy (particularly a diode laser 980 nm) include incision of urethral and

---

[d]200 or 400-µm Holmium:YAG laser fiber and 30-W Hol:YAG Lithotrite, Odyssey, Convergent Inc, Alameda, CA.

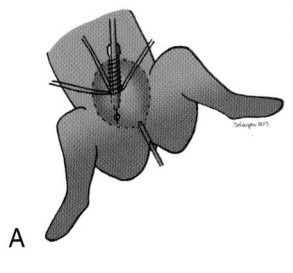
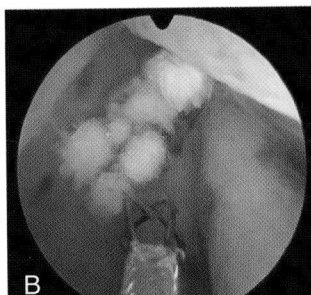
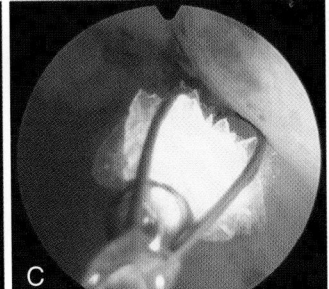
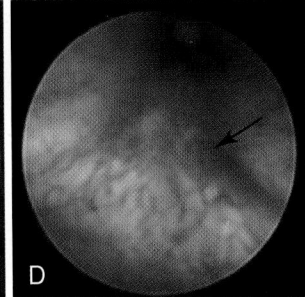

Figure 88-14: Percutaneous Cystourethroscopy. A, Schematic image showing how the trocar is advanced into the bladder using a small surgical approach so that the endoscope can be placed into the bladder and the bladder and urethra can be imaged thoroughly. **B,** Endoscopic images during the percutaneous cystolithotomy for calcium oxalate bladder stone removal. **C,** The stone basket is entrapping a stone for removal. **D,** Antegrade cystoscopy in a cat for evaluation of severe hematuria; notice the hematuria coming from the right ureteral opening (*black arrow*). A red rubber catheter is in the urethral lumen. This is likely a condition of idiopathic essential renal hematuria.

ureteral strictures, ablation of superficial TCC within the urethral lumen, and laser ablation of urinary polyps or intramural ectopic ureters.

Percutaneous Cystolithotomy and Percutaneous Cystourethroscopy

Surgical cystotomy is the most commonly used procedure to date for the retrieval of cystic and urethral calculi in small animal patients. For urethral stones, when retrograde urohydropropulsion is not possible, urethrotomy or perineal urethrostomy may be considered. Newer, minimally invasive procedures, including laparoscopic-assisted cystotomy[68] and laser lithotripsy, have shown success in stone removal.[64-67] The use of lithotripsy is limited by patient size, sex, species, stone size, and stone number. Laparoscopic-assisted cystotomy requires two incisions, a pneumoperitoneum, and additional expensive equipment. When stone retrieval is needed, urethral visualization is poor because of the large diameter, lack of flexibility, and short length of the laparoscope. The new minimally invasive technique, PCCL, combines cystic and urethral stone retrieval using cystoscopic and urethroscopic guidance in patients of any size, sex, or species; it is easy and highly effective in cats (Figure 88-14).[19] Percutaneous antegrade cystourethroscopy is a particularly useful endoscopic technique to assist in UVJ evaluation (for upper urinary tract essential hematuria) (see Figure 88-14), for urethral stent placement in male cats (see Figure 88-12), and to retrieve embedded urethral stones in the urethra of male cats.

In children, the treatment of choice for a large bladder stone burden is a similar procedure also called a PCCL.[18] After the procedure, a suprapubic cystostomy catheter is left in place for 24 hours, and a urethral catheter is left in place for 48 hours, for a seal to form in the bladder without primary closure. This was the model used for this technique in animals.

This procedure is performed under general anesthesia with the patient positioned in dorsal recumbency, with the caudal abdomen, and prepuce or vulva clipped and prepared aseptically. The apex of the urinary bladder is accessed using an atraumatic rigid trocar,[m] maintaining a seal in the bladder for fluid distension during rigid antegrade cystourethroscopy (see Figure 88-14). A rigid (1.9-mm, 30° lens) cystoscope is advanced through the trocar into the urinary bladder (see Figure 88-14). The entire mucosal surface of the bladder and proximal urethra are visualized, and the location and number of uroliths are identified. This technique can be used for evaluation of bladder polyps, ureteral bleeding, or stone retrieval. Slow saline irrigation is used to maintain bladder distension and visibility. A stone retrieval basket is advanced through the working channel of the cystoscope and guided to remove the uroliths. For any small remaining fragments that do not fit in the basket, suction is applied through the trocar as saline is irrigated through the urethral catheter. The proximal urethra is then visualized using a rigid or semirigid cystoscope in an antegrade manner. If more stones are identified, they can be removed using a stone basket or saline flush until the entire urethra is deemed to be patent, and catheter passage is smooth and easy. These patients are typically discharged on the day of their procedure, once adequate micturition is appreciated.

SUMMARY

Endourology has become one of the most progressive areas in feline medicine, following the trend seen in human medicine. Urinary diversion techniques, particularly those used for feline ureteral obstructions, are becoming the standard of care in feline medicine, and more training opportunities are available around the world. The morbidity and mortality rates with most of the interventional techniques discussed in this chapter have been shown to be superior to those previously reported for traditional surgical techniques (see Table 88-3). For the best possible outcomes, proper training is important, and operator experience is necessary.

---

[m]Endotip Trocar, Karl Storz Endoscopy, Culver City, CA.

References

1. Al-Awadi KA: Steinstrasse: a comparison of incidence with and without J stenting and the effect of J stenting on subsequent management. *BJU Int* 84:618, 1999.

2. Coe FL, Evan A, Worcester E: Kidney stone disease. *J Clin Invest* 115:2598, 2005.

3. Matsuoka K, Iida S, Nakanami M, et al: Holmium:yttrium-aluminum-garnet laser for endoscopic lithotripsy. *Urology* 45:947, 1995.

4. Bagley DH: Expanding role of ureteroscopy and laser lithotripsy for treatment of proximal ureteral and intrarenal calculi. *Curr Opin Urol* 12:277, 2002.

5. Wollin TA, Denstedt JD: The holmium laser in urology. *J Clin Laser Med Surg* 16:13, 1998.

6. Bagley DH, Das A: *Endourologic use of the holmium laser*, Jackson, 2001, Teton NewMedia.

7. Denstedt JD, Razvi HA, Sales JL, et al: Preliminary experience with holmium:YAG laser lithotripsy. *J Endourol* 9:255, 1995.

8. Al-Shammari AM, Al-Otaibi K, Leonard MP, et al: Percutaneous nephrolithotomy in the pediatric population. *J Urol* 162:1721, 1999.

9. Kochin EJ, Gregory CR, Wisner E, et al: Evaluation of a method of ureteroneocystostomy in cats. *J Am Vet Med Assoc* 202:257–260, 1993.

10. Rozear L, Tidwell AS: Evaluation of the ureter and ureterovesicular junction using helical computed tomographic excretory urography in healthy dogs. *Vet Radiol Ultrasound* 44:155–164, 2003.

11. Zimskind PD: Clinical use of long-term indwelling silicone rubber ureteral splints inserted cystoscopically. *J Urol* 97:840, 1967.

12. Yossepowitch O: Predicting the success of retrograde stenting for managing ureteral obstruction. *J Urol* 166:1746, 2001.

13. Uthappa MC: Retrograde or antegrade double-pigtail stent placement for malignant ureteric obstruction? *Clin Radiol* 60:608, 2005.

14. Goldin AR: Percutaneous ureteral splinting. *Urology* 10:165, 1977.

15. Lennon GM: Double pigtail ureteric stent versus percutaneous nephrostomy: effects on stone transit and ureteric motility. *Eur Urol* 31:24, 1997.

16. Mustafa M: The role of stenting in relieving loin pain following ureteroscopic stone therapy for persisting renal colic with hydronephrosis. *Int Urol Nephrol* 39:91, 2007.

17. Hubert KC: Passive dilation by ureteral stenting before ureteroscopy: eliminating the need for active dilation. *J Urol* 174:1079, 2005.

18. Salah MA, Holman E, Munim Khan A, et al: Percutaneous cystolithotomy for pediatric endemic bladder stone: experience with 155 cases from 2 developing countries. *J Pediatr Surg* 40:1628, 2005.

19. Runge J, Berent A, Weisse C, et al: Transvesicular percutaneous cystolithotomy for the retrieval of cystic and urethral calculi in dogs and cats: 27 cases (2006-2008). *J Am Vet Med Assoc* 239:344–349, 2011.

20. Kyles A, Hardie EM, Wooden BG, et al: Clinical, clinicopathologic, radiographic, and ultrasonographic abnormalities in cats with ureteral calculi: 163 cases (1984-2002). *J Am Vet Med Assoc* 226:932–936, 2005.

21. Kyles A, Hardie E, Wooden E, et al: Management and outcome of cats with ureteral calculi: 153 cases (1984-2002). *J Am Vet Med Assoc* 226:937–944, 2005.

22. Roberts S, Aronson L, Brown D: Postoperative mortality in cats after ureterolithotomy. *Vet Surg* 40:438–443, 2011.

23. Berent A: Ureteral obstructions in dogs and cats: a review of traditional and new interventional diagnostic and therapeutic options. *J Vet Emerg Crit Care (San Antonio)* 21:86–103, 2011.

24. Berent AC, Weisse CW, Todd K, et al: Technical and clinical outcomes of ureteral stenting in cats with benign ureteral obstruction: 69 cases (2006-2010). *J Am Vet Med Assoc* 244:559–576, 2014.

25. Berent A, Weisse C, Bagley D, et al: Ureteral stenting for benign feline ureteral obstructions in 79 ureters. *J Am Vet Med Assoc* 244:559–576, 2014.

26. Horowitz C, Berent A, Weisse C, et al: Predictors of outcome for cats with ureteral obstructions after interventional management using ureteral stents or a subcutaneous ureteral bypass device. *J Feline Med Surg* 15:1052–1062, 2013.

27. Steinhaus J, Berent A, Weisse C, et al: Circumcaval ureters in cats with and without ureteral obstructions. A comparative study. *J Vet Intern Med* 27:731–732, 2013. [Abstract].

28. Berent A, Weisse C, Bade H, et al: The use of a subcutaneous ureteral bypass device for ureteral obstructions in cats. *J Vet Intern Med* 25:1506, 2011. [Abstract].

29. Coroneos E, Assouad M, Krishnan B, et al: Urinary obstruction causes irreversible renal failure by inducing chronic tubulointerstiital nephritis. *Clin Nephrol* 48:125, 1997.

30. Wilson DR: Renal function during and following obstruction. *Annu Rev Med* 28:329, 1977.

31. Fink RW, Caradis DT, Chmiel R, et al: Renal impairment and its reversibility following variable periods of complete ureteric obstruction. *Aust N Z J Surg* 50:77, 1980.

32. Kerr WS: Effect of complete ureteral obstruction for one week on kidney function. *J Appl Physiol* 6:762, 1954.

33. Vaughan DE, Sweet RE, Gillenwater JY: Unilateral ureteral occlusion: pattern of nephron repair and compensatory response. *J Urol* 109:979, 1973.

34. Coroneos E, Assouad M, Krishnan B, et al: Urinary obstruction causes irreversible renal failure by inducing chronic tubulointerstitial nephritis. *Clin Nephrol* 48:125, 1997.

35. Wen JG, Frokiaer J, Jorgensen TM, et al: Obstructive nephropathy: an update of the experimental research. *Urol Res* 27:29, 1999.

36. Steinhaus J, Berent A, Weisse C, et al: Clinical presentation and outcome of cats with circumcaval ureters associated with a ureteral obstruction. *J Vet Intern Med* 29:63–70, 2015. [Abstract].

37. Berent A, Weisse C, Todd K, et al: The use of locking-loop nephrostomy tubes in dogs and cats: 20 cases (2004-2009). *J Am Vet Med Assoc* 241:348–357, 2012.

38. Hardie EM, Kyles AE: Management of ureteral obstruction. *Vet Clin North Am Small Anim Pract* 34:989, 2004.

39. Gupta R, Kumar A, Kapoor R, et al: Prospective evaluation of the safety and efficacy of the supracostal approach for percutaneous nephrolithotomy. *BJU Int* 90:809–813, 2002.

40. Elbahnasy AM, Clayman RV, Shalhav AL, et al: Lower-pole caliceal stone clearance after shockwave lithotripsy. Percutaneous nephrolithotomy, and flexible ureteroscopy: impact of radiographic spatial anatomy. *J Endourol* 12:113–119, 1998.

41. Meretyk S, Gofrit ON, Gafni O, et al: Complete staghorn calculi: random prospective comparison between extracorporeal shock wave lithotripsy monotherapy and combined with percutaneous nephrostolithotomy. *J Urol* 157:780–786, 1997.

42. Berent A, Weisse C, Bagley D, et al: Ureteral stenting for benign and malignant disease in dogs and cats. Abstract presented at American College of Veterinary Surgery, 18-21 October, Chicago. *Vet Surg* 36:E1–E29, 2007.

43. Berent A, Weisse C, Bagley D, et al: Ureteral stenting for obstructive ureterolithiasis. American College of Veterinary Internal Medicine. *J Vet Intern Med* 23:673–786, 2009. [Abstract].

44. Zaid M: Feline ureteral strictures: 10 cases (2007-2009). *J Vet Intern Med* 25:222–229, 2011.

45. Berent A, Weisse C, Wright M, et al: The use of a subcutaneous ureteral bypass (SUB) device for ureteral obstructions in cats. *J Vet Intern Med* 25:754, 2011. [Abstract].

46. Azhar RA: Successful salvage of kidney allografts threatened by ureteral stricture using pyelovesical bypass. *Am J Transplant* 10:1414–1419, 2010.

47. Schmidbauer J: Nephrovesical subcutaneous ureteral bypass: long-term results in patient with advanced metastatic disease-improvement in renal function and quality of life. *Eur Urol* 50:1073–1078, 2006.

48. Jurczok A, Loertzer H, Wagner S, et al: Subcutaneous nephrovesical and nephrocutaneous bypass. *Gynecol Obstet Invest* 59:144–148, 2005.

49. Smith JD, Stone EA, Gilson SD: Placement of a permanent cystostomy catheter to relieve urine outflow obstruction in dogs with transitional cell carcinoma. *J Am Vet Med Assoc* 206:496, 1995.

50. Stiffler KS, McCrackin Stevenson MA, Cornell KK, et al: Clinical use of low-profile

cystostomy tubes in four dogs and a cat. *J Am Vet Med Assoc* 223:325, 2003.

51. Beck AL, Grierson JM, Ogden DM, et al: Outcome of and complications associated with tube cystostomy in dogs and cats: 76 cases (1995-2006). *J Am Vet Med Assoc* 230:1184, 2007.

52. Meige F, Sarrau S, Autefage A: Management of traumatic urethral rupture in 11 cats using primary alignment with a urethral catheter. *Vet Comp Orthop Traumatol* 21:76–84, 2008.

53. Holmes ES, Weisse C, Berent A: Use of fluoroscopically guided percutaneous antegrade urethral catheterization for the treatment of urethral obstruction in male cats: 9 cases (2000-2009). *J Am Vet Med Assoc* 241:603–607, 2012.

54. Brace M, Weisse C, Berent A, et al: Evaluation of palliative stenting for management of urethral obstruction in cats. *Vet Surg* 3:199–208, 2014.

55. Wilson HM, Chun R, Larson VS, et al: Clinical signs, treatments, and outcome in cats with transitional cell carcinoma of the urinary bladder: 20 cases. *J Am Vet Med Assoc* 231:101, 2007.

56. Knapp DW, Glickman NW, Widmer WR, et al: Cisplatin versus cisplatin with piroxicam in a canine model of human invasive urinary bladder cancer. *Cancer Chemother Pharmacol* 46:221, 2000.

57. Norris AM, Laing EJ, Valli VEO, et al: Canine bladder and urethral tumors: a retrospective study of 115 cases (1980-1985). *J Vet Intern Med* 16:145, 1992.

58. Liptak JM, Brutscher SP, Monnet E, et al: Transurethral resection in the management of urethral and prostatic neoplasia in 6 dogs. *Vet Surg* 33:505, 2004.

59. Fries CL, Binnington AG, Valli VE, et al: Enterocystoplasty with cystectomy and subtotal intracapsular prostatectomy in the male dogs. *Vet Surg* 20:104, 1991.

60. Stone EA, Withrow SJ, Page RL, et al: Ureterocolonic anastomosis in ten dogs with transitional cell carcinoma. *Vet Surg* 17:147, 1988.

61. Blackburn A, Berent A, Weisse C, et al: Urethral stenting for malignant urethral obstructions: 42 cases. *J Am Vet Med Assoc* 242:59–68, 2013.

62. Ayyildiz A, Nuhoglu B, Gulerkaya B, et al: Effect of intraurethral mitomycin-C on healing and fibrosis in rats with experimentally induced urethral stricture. *J Urol* 11:1122, 2004.

63. Mazdak H, Meshki I, Ghassami F: Effect of mitomycin C on anterior urethral stricture recurrence after internal urethrotomy. *Eur Urol* 51:1089, 2006.

64. Streeter RN, Washburn KE, Higbee RG, et al: Laser lithotripsy of a urethral calculus via ischial urethrotomy in a steer. *J Am Vet Med Assoc* 219:640, 2001.

65. Davidson EB, Ritchey JW, Higbee RD, et al: Laser lithotripsy for treatment of canine uroliths. *Vet Surg* 33:56, 2004.

66. Halland SK, House JK, George LW: Urethroscopy and laser lithotripsy for the diagnosis and treatment of obstructive urolithiasis in goats and pot-bellied pigs. *J Am Vet Med Assoc* 220:1831, 2002.

67. Adams LG, Berent AC, Moore GE, et al: Use of laser lithotripsy for fragmentation of uroliths in dogs: 73 cases (2005-2006). *J Am Vet Med Assoc* 323:1680, 2008.

68. Rawlings CA, Mahaffey MB, Barsanti JA, et al: Use of laparoscopic-assisted cystoscopy for removal of urinary calculi in dogs. *J Am Vet Med Assoc* 222:759, 2003.

69. Grant DC, Were SR, Gevedon ML: Holmium:YAG lithotripsy for urolithiasis in dogs. *J Vet Intern Med* 22:534, 2008.

Debra F. Horwitz, DVM

Update on Feline Housesoiling and Urine Marking

Melissa Bain

Despite the fact that cats are known for their fastidious eliminative behavior, elimination outside of the litter box is the most frequent category of behavioral problems in feline practice. Additionally, it is a primary behavioral reason that cats are relinquished to shelters in the United Kingdom and the United States.[1-3] One study demonstrated that approximately 10% of cats entering a shelter were relinquished for housesoiling,[4] and another study cited housesoiling as the reason that up to 30% of cats were abandoned.[5] The problem also occurs in kittens, with approximately one-fourth of kittens adopted from a shelter demonstrating housesoiling within 30 days of adoption (decreasing to 8% approximately 1 year later).[6] Although this is a significant decrease for kittens that eliminate inappropriately, close to one in 10 cats still demonstrate this problem.

Housesoiling is also a very common reason that cats are presented to a veterinary behaviorist.[7-9] General practice veterinarians should be aware of these problems, especially urine marking, because nearly three-fourths of owners of urine-marking cats approached their veterinarian for help.[10] Even if an owner does not relinquish or euthanize a cat for these problems, they may be more likely to make the problem cat into an outdoor cat, creating many other medical problems ranging from infectious diseases to trauma.

It is important to understand that urine marking and housesoiling are two separate problems. Housesoiling (sometimes known as *toileting, periuria and perichezia,* or *inappropriate elimination*) is elimination of urine or feces in unwanted locations by emptying the bladder or bowel. Urine marking (also known as *urine spraying*) is the deposition of urine to mark a cat's territory in response to an underlying stressor and as a form of social communication.

GATHERING INFORMATION

For the general practice veterinarian, asking behavior questions at each appointment leads owners to believe that behavior problems are important and are understood by the practitioner, which in turn leads owners to ask for veterinary help when a problem behavior occurs. Owner needs for behavior information were demonstrated by one study in Brazil in which most veterinarians said that they have been consulted about pet behavior problems.[5] Unfortunately, most veterinarians do not ask the questions that would allow them to identify owner concerns about pet behaviors.[11] In a study on urine marking in cats, owners reported that their veterinarian did not provide advice about the problem behavior, thereby missing the opportunity to provide enhanced care. However, veterinarians who were able to gather a complete history of the problem and properly diagnose urine marking reported a higher success rate than those veterinarians who did not.[10]

Location of the Consultation

Information can be obtained through either a house call or an in-clinic visit. A house call allows the practitioner to observe the placement and cleanliness of the litter boxes and to directly appreciate the amount of odor present. This information may allow for a more directed treatment plan. Although some owners may want the practitioner to observe the problem behavior in person, from a safety standpoint this is not advisable if aggression is involved. Additionally, it is unlikely that the practitioner will see the cat performing the problem elimination behavior during a house call. In fact, in many cases the practitioner may not be able to observe a cat that hides from visitors and is unfriendly. House calls may decrease the ability to safely draw blood and/or urine samples, if deemed necessary. An in-clinic visit allows for more control over visit logistics; however, many cats are stressed by a visit to the veterinary clinic. Therefore, a case-by-case decision should be made in consultation with the owner and taking into account the practitioner's ability and comfort level with conducting veterinary medicine outside of the clinic. Regardless of the type of consultation chosen, practitioners should discuss appropriate fees with the client beforehand and should be sure to set aside enough time to fully evaluate the case.

Basic Information

As with all veterinary patients, it is important to gather detailed information about the cat's physical health, diet, current and past medical conditions, current and past medications, travel history, and human and animal household members. It is also important to perform a complete physical examination and any laboratory tests that are indicated based on the medical history.

Interactions with People

Before gathering information about the problem behaviors, it is necessary to know about interactions with people in the home. The age, sex, and relationships of people living in the household are important. However, it is imperative to ascertain each person's individual relationship with the cat, as well as to measure their bond and their willingness and ability to implement the treatment recommendations. Even though the presenting complaint is housesoiling, it is important to collect information on other possible behavior problems, including aggression (see Chapters 91 and 92 for more information on feline aggression).

Obtaining the Relevant Details

It is essential that practitioners gather all relevant information regarding the cat in question, other pets, and human family members—as well as to inquire about the environment, the problem in question, and the owner's relationship with the cat. Unlike physiological information gathering, which relies primarily on the practitioner's skills, behavior information gathering relies on history and behavioral observations provided by the owner. The use of a preprinted history form that the owner can fill out and submit before the appointment is efficient and allows the practitioner to review the information before the consultation. The *2014 AAFP and ISFM Guidelines for Diagnosing and Solving House-Soiling Behavior in Cats* include a downloadable cat owner questionnaire (http://www.catvets.com/guidelines/practice-guidelines/house-soiling).

Video recording the cat in its own environment is another useful tool. Even if an owner does not think casual videos of the cat are important, often there are subtle behavioral signs that reveal underlying motivations, potential anxiety, and relationships between other cats within the home. Additionally, the video can give a very accurate display of the environment and may help determine which cat is the problem cat in a multiple cat household.

Identifying the Culprits

In multiple cat households, it can be difficult to identify all the culprits for periuria and urine marking. The administration of sodium fluorescein dye *may* help identify the problem cat when urine is involved. This dye is absorbed and excreted

rapidly and can be identified in urine with a black light. Fluorescein dye can be administered in a range of dosages. For example, it can be given orally (50 mg/cat by placing fluorescein ophthalmic strips in a gelatin capsule) or subcutaneously (0.3 mL/cat of 10% solution), first to the suspected problem cat, and then to each other potential cat consecutively.[12] Because all urine will fluoresce to some degree under a black light, owners must be educated that urine from non-treated cats glows green, but not to the extent of urine from treated cats. Owners should also be advised that urine containing fluorescein could stain materials such as carpeting. Unfortunately, the amount of fluorescence may not be correlated to the dosage administered to the cat, and treated urine does not always fluoresce. The intensity of the fluorescence is influenced by the acidity of the urine, because it fluoresces more readily in alkaline solutions.

If a cat is defecating inappropriately, owners can add different brightly-colored crayon shavings to canned food. This can be administered to all cats in the home at the same time as long as the owner records the color administered to each cat (Figure 89-1).

Environmental Information

Causes of housesoiling and urine marking are often multifactorial, making it important to gather information about underlying stressors. Environmental information includes type and size of house; resting, feeding, and watering locations; time spent indoors and outdoors; and litter and litter box types, locations, and hygiene schedule. Drawings of the layout of the house, a video tour of the house, and/or photos of applicable areas are convenient ways for the owner to present this information if the practitioner is unable to do a house call.

Information on Feline Household Members

A log of the daily activities of the cat can give important information. Although cats spend what seems the majority of their day sleeping or resting, *where* they spend their time can be important as well as whether the litter box is easily accessible from this location. The percentage of time the cat spends indoors versus outdoors, whether there are interactions with other outside cats, and whether that affects the frequency of housesoiling is information that can help devise a treatment plan. In one study, one-fourth of owners stated that limiting their cats' access to outdoors was a trigger for urine marking.[13]

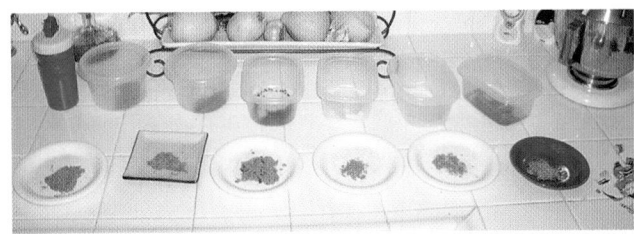

Figure 89-1: An example of a client mixing different colored crayons into canned cat food.

Information on Other Household Pets

Although it may not be directly relevant to the primary complaint, it is imperative to gather information on other pets in the household, their interactions with the problem cat, and the owner's relationships with each of them. Underlying agonistic interactions between cats (whether inside or outside of the house) can be a primary trigger for urine marking.[13] Additionally, another cat or dog can cause stress by blocking access to the litter box or, in the case of a dog in the house, pre-emptively cleaning the litter box before the cat is done eliminating.

Incident Information

Once the background information is collected, information should be collected on specific problem incidents. The "ABC" mnemonic can be used to help owners through this process:

- **A**ntecedent: What happened before the incident
- **B**ehavior: What happened during
- **C**onsequence: What did the person and cat do afterward

Owners often do not recognize early signs of anxiety, fear, and aggression; providing pictures or videos that demonstrate these behaviors may be very helpful. Regardless of whether the problem is housesoiling or urine marking, it is essential to gather data on how often the cat eliminates outside of the litter box. This information will be vital for determining treatment response; once treatment is applied, the frequency of unwanted elimination should diminish. It is noteworthy that in one study, cat owners often overestimated the number of urine marks they thought the cat deposited.[13]

The Role of the Owner

Behavioral counseling involves treating both the owner and the cat, so it is imperative to fully evaluate the owner's relationship with the cat. By the time an owner seeks help from a veterinarian, the situation is often at crisis level, leading to a break in the human-animal bond, which may have dire consequences for the pet.[14]

Practitioners may be reluctant to ask owners about their goals in seeking help in case this raises expectations that may not be met. Practitioners may also be reluctant to ask owners if they have considered euthanizing or rehoming the pet or if it has been recommended. However, once a relationship has been established with the client, it is important to ask these questions. It is important that the practitioner not appear judgmental but rather to create an environment where the client will be willing to share information necessary to resolve the problem.

It is also necessary to assess the owner's ability and willingness to implement the recommended treatment plan. Owners may unrealistically expect a quick and easy resolution to the problem, and it may take discussion and negotiation to devise a treatment plan that they will follow. This should involve a multimodal approach to delivering the information, including handouts, written treatment protocols, and how follow-up information will be obtained, because owners often do not have a clear recollection of the treatment plan after they leave the veterinary clinic.[10]

Minimum Database

As with other branches of veterinary practice, it is important to perform a full physical examination. Medical conditions should be ruled out by performing a complete blood count, serum biochemistry panel, and urinalysis. Further diagnostic testing, such as imaging, may necessary if the initial findings indicate possible medical issues. If defecation outside of the litter box is a primary complaint, the frequency, consistency, and quantity of stool on a daily basis should be determined.

Two studies have demonstrated disparate results regarding outcomes of urinalyses in cats with marking behavior. In one study, urinalysis results in cats diagnosed with urine-marking behavior were no different from those of control cats.[15] In another study that lacked controls, nine of 24 cats diagnosed with urine marking had crystalluria.[16]

DIFFERENTIATING PROBLEM ELIMINATION

There are two main classifications of inappropriate elimination: housesoiling or toileting in unwanted locations by emptying the bladder or bowel, and urine marking as a form of social communication. In this chapter, inappropriate defecation is classified as housesoiling. It is important to understand that inappropriate urination and defecation can occur together and that a complete history on all aspects of litter box use is crucial for diagnosis.

Urine marking may be readily distinguished from housesoiling (Table 89-1). Urine marking is usually performed to establish a social odor, not for the purpose of emptying the bladder. Urine marking typically is performed in a standing posture, with the hind legs straight, hind paws treading, and with the tail held straight up and quivering. The cat often sniffs the target object first. Anecdotally, the owner's odor sometimes seems to attract marking, or marking may occur on visitor's clothing. Typically a small amount of urine is sprayed on vertical surfaces (although that alone may not be diagnostic). Urine marks can also be deposited on horizontal surfaces. Common targets include doors and windows, especially if there are cats outside of the home, as well as drapes, walls, stereo speakers, heat duct openings, and kitchen appliances.

Urine may also be sprayed onto a horizontal surface, such as the owner's clothes, bedding, or new objects brought into the house (e.g., plastic shopping bags, gym bags, or strollers). Often the targets are those of social significance, such as an area frequented by another household pet causing stress in the problem cat or an object belonging to a new visitor (e.g., a suitcase or dirty laundry). Provocative stimuli including agonistic interactions with other cats are often mentioned as correlated with urine marking.[13] It is possible that volatile chemicals from the electrical insulation of speakers and

Table 89-1	Differentiating Inappropriate Urination From Urine Marking	
Trait/Characteristic	**Inappropriate Urination**	**Urine Marking**
Deposition of urine	Horizontal	Vertical
Posture	Squatting posture	Standing Treading with back legs Tail elevated
Urine amount	Generally large because bladder is emptied	Generally smaller, but not always, because bladder is not always emptied
Litter box usage	Decreased use of litter box for urination and/or defecation	Continued litter box use for normal urination and defecation; defecation is generally not used for marking
Target areas	Identifiable substrates, such as carpet, hardwood floor, soil, potted plants, and/or furniture	Target areas may have social significance, such as entryways, clothing, bedding, etc.
Preliminary signs or precipitating factors	Signs of aversion to litter, such as straddling box, shaking paws, and/or no digging or covering	Identifiable stimuli, such as agonistic interactions with housemates or outdoor cats

appliances attract marking, because these objects are frequent targets. Cats diagnosed with urine marking still use the litter box for urination and defecation, unless there is a concurrent housesoiling problem.

In housesoiling, the cat changes its toilet area to another part (or parts) of the house. The litter box may be avoided entirely, used some of the time, or used for selected elimination of either urine or stool. Unless there is an underlying medical condition causing a cat to deposit reduced amounts of urine, the amount of urine deposited is generally large. The housesoiling cat uses a typical squatting posture that is different from the standing posture of the urine-marking cat. The cat will sometimes dig at the area, sniff, and then squat to urinate or defecate. Often the cat attempts to cover the urine or feces.

However, exceptions to these general characteristics are possible. Some cats urinate while standing up, and other cats will spray larger than expected quantities of urine for marking purposes. In addition, some urine-marking cats attempt to cover the voided urine.

There are many aspects of treatment that are similar for both housesoiling and urine marking. In many cases, treatment includes reducing household stressors, eliminating aversive aspects surrounding the litter box, using appropriate cleaners, and changing the significance of the soiled areas. These are covered in more depth later.

HOUSESOILING

History and Causes

Although it is important to rule out an underlying medical condition for behavior problems, it is also important to understand that patients can have concurrent medical and behavioral causes for housesoiling. Treatment for a medical condition must be combined with the understanding of and treatment for potential behavioral causes of housesoiling. Feline lower urinary tract disease is one condition that may have both medical and behavioral underpinnings.[17] For example, patients with feline idiopathic (interstitial) cystitis will have clinical signs of the disease when they are stressed. It has also been noted that cats with housesoiling were more likely to have a history of urinary tract disorders.[18]

Other medical conditions can lead to housesoiling and must be ruled out, including causes of polydipsia and polyuria (e.g., diabetes mellitus, chronic kidney disease, hyperthyroidism), pollakiuria (e.g., urinary tract infection), dysuria (e.g., crystalluria), tenesmus (e.g., inflammatory bowel disease), and obstipation or constipation. Furthermore, in elderly cats with inappropriate elimination, practitioners must consider pain associated with osteoarthritis that may limit the cat's ability to climb or descend the stairs to access the litter box or to step into a high-sided litter box.[19] Additionally, cats should be examined for diseases of the bladder, rectal and anal area, neurological problems, cognitive changes, and sensory challenges, all of which can limit a cat's ability to find or access the litter box.

Substrate and Litter Box or Location Aversions

Elimination behavior problems may be associated with aversion to the litter box itself or its location, or a preference to eliminate elsewhere. One study comparing cats with and without behavior problems presented to the Barcelona School of Veterinary Medicine demonstrated that almost two-thirds of cats with behavior problems were diagnosed with a litter box aversion.[7] For cats that generally eliminate outdoors, inclement weather, harassing dogs, or other cats can prevent the patient from going outdoors to eliminate. The problem could also result from attraction to preferred but inappropriate places or substrates, such as a carpet. The cat may use a

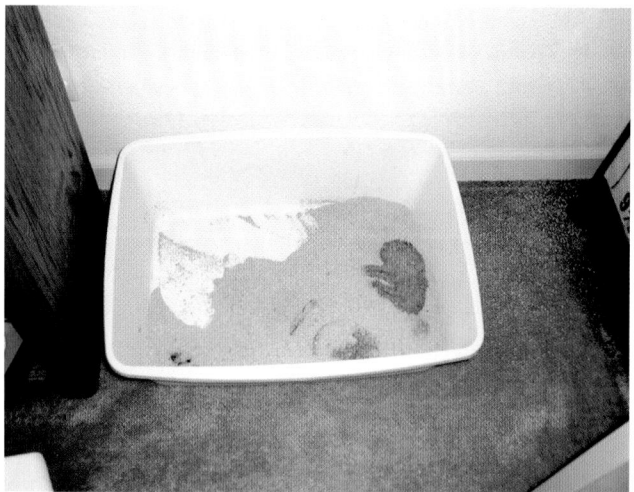

Figure 89-2: An example of an unclean litter box.

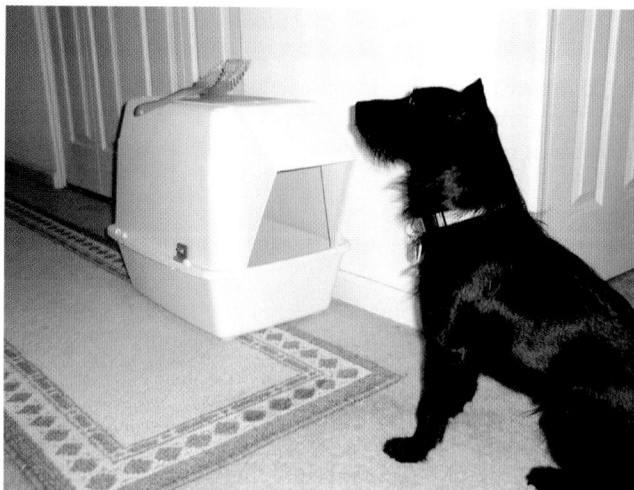

Figure 89-3: A dog sitting by a litter box can be aversive to many cats.

litter box for defecation but urinate in other places, or vice versa, or both urinate and defecate outside of the litter box.

Another underlying reason for a litter box or location aversion can stem from issues with other household cats or dogs. Inadequate numbers of litter boxes and/or placement can result in housesoiling. For example, if all litter boxes are placed in one room or one end of the house accessed by a single hallway, this can create problems. If one cat sits at the entrance to the room or hallway, another cat may not feel comfortable passing, leading to housesoiling in another part of the house when the cat needs to eliminate. Even when litter boxes are accessible, one cat (or dog) may ambush another while it is in the litter box, making elimination stressful.

Aversion to the litter or litter box may be indicated by the cat not covering feces, straddling the box to avoid touching the litter, shaking the paws after touching litter, digging outside the box on the floor, and/or running from the box after elimination.[20] Such aversion-related behavior may be a predictor that a cat that currently uses the litter box may later eliminate outside it, but this has not been substantiated with research. Aversions can be related to infrequent cleaning, cleaning with harsh cleansers, dislike of the litter (e.g., dusty, odiferous litters), introduction of new litter, use of a plastic litter box liner, or dislike of the litter depth (Figure 89-2).

A cat may display an aversion to the litter box itself. Often litter boxes are too small, not allowing enough room to turn around. Covered litter boxes, although preferred by some cats, hold odor inside. Additionally, the owner may be less likely to clean covered litter boxes (out of sight, out of mind).

A cat may refuse to use the litter box due to a location aversion. The owner's preferred location for a litter box may not be the cat's preferred location. Locations that have high traffic and noise levels can be aversive to some cats (Figure 89-3).

Substrate or Location Preferences
Cats that develop an aversion to the litter box or location often develop an alternate preferred location and/or substrate.

When the preferred substrate or litter is not offered, the cat may select a new substrate, or when a quiet, safe location for elimination is discovered, the cat may use that place to eliminate instead. Once that becomes a pattern, a concerted effort must be taken to address all of the factors that keep the cat at that location to rectify the situation.

As previously discussed, a cat may have any or all of the aforementioned reasons for eliminating outside of the litter box (i.e., aversion to the litter and/or location, preference for a substrate and/or location), and all aspects must be addressed to have a successful outcome. Stressors are often additive; and although an owner may believe they can identify the primary reason for the problem, other underlying reasons, such as intercat aggression or another cat blocking access to the litter boxes, must always be considered especially because intercat conflicts are often covert and unnoticed by cat owners.

Treatment
Eliminate Aversive Aspects of the Litter Box
Litter boxes must be kept clean. Feces and urine clumps should be removed daily, if not several times daily, and the litter should be completely changed weekly. The litter box should be cleaned with a mild, unscented detergent; the owner should be counseled to avoid bleach, ammonia, pine oil cleaners, and other strong smelling cleaning agents.

Owners should have litter boxes that are of suitable size for the cat. Under-the-bed plastic storage containers (without wheels) are a good option, because they are large, relatively shallow, and inexpensive. For cats that dig in the litter vigorously but do not prefer a covered litter box, a tall plastic storage box makes a good substitute. One side of the box can be cut to make an entrance, and the box should be kept uncovered.

Owners should provide a sufficient number of litter boxes for the household and understand that, in a multiple cat household, different cats may prefer different types of litter. A common rule of thumb is one more litter box than the number of cats (within reason). The litter boxes should be positioned to provide easy access for all cats and placed in such a way that they are not all clustered together. Owners should consider the individual cat's ability to navigate the house. Aggressive social interactions among cats may preclude access to litter boxes. Multiple litter boxes in one location are considered to be one toileting area that may not be accessible to all the cats within the home. Homes with multiple floors may require a litter box on each floor, even in single cat households.

If a cat is given the opportunity to eliminate outdoors, the owners should increase the appeal of outdoor areas by eliminating aversive elements, such as harassing dogs and the effects of inclement weather. Shelter can be provided over the toileting area for weather protection. Providing commercial sand in a sheltered area that is cleaned frequently will help encourage cats to use that area instead of a freshly planted garden bed.

Litter and Litter Box Trials

If the reason for the housesoiling is related to the litter material itself, it is essential to discover which litter material the cat prefers. This can be accomplished by creating a litter preference test using three or four litter boxes each with different litter materials. For example, one box should contain the current litter material, another should contain the cat's preferred substrate (i.e., a piece of carpet), and the remaining boxes can contain other litter options. Current research indicates that most cats prefer finely granulated clumping litters and that sand is the next most preferred substrate. Wood chips and recycled newspaper are rarely preferred materials.[21] Although one study found that scented litter was associated with a diagnosis of inappropriate elimination,[18] not all cats have a preference for whether the litter is scented or not.[22] Inherent in any litter trial is keeping the boxes clean; owners should be instructed to remove waste from the boxes frequently and to clean the boxes and refresh the litter regularly. Some cats may have a preference for the depth of the litter material. The owner can offer boxes with different depths of litter or slant the litter in one box to determine the preferred depth.

Additionally, the type of preferred litter box should be determined. Not all cats have a preference for the type of litter box, but some cats have specific preferences (e.g., larger boxes, covered or uncovered boxes).[23]

Decreasing Chance of Resoiling the Area

Soiled areas can be identified with the aid of a black light, keeping in mind that many other things beside urine will fluoresce. These areas can be cleaned with enzymatic cleaners that eliminate the problem odor by breaking down proteins in urine, perhaps decreasing the cat's desire to return and resoil the area.[24]

Owners often focus only on making the previously soiled areas aversive without addressing the precipitating cause. If the reason the cat has chosen a new toileting area is that the litter box is too dirty or the location is objectionable or unreachable, cleaning the soiled area may not keep the cat

away or prevent the cat from finding another location other than the litter box for elimination. However, the significance of the soiled areas can be changed with one of four options:
1. Block off the soiled area (e.g., behind a closed door).
2. Place a litter box on or near the soiled area.
3. Place something aversive in the soiled area.
4. Place something pleasurable in the soiled area.

Owners may need to use more than one of these tactics to address different soiled areas in the home.

Creating aversion in soiled areas can be accomplished with strong odors, such as a plug-in fragrance diffuser. Other options include aluminum foil, plastic, upside-down plastic carpet runner, or double-sided sticky tape. In some cases, more intensive aversion must be created (e.g., with motion-activated air spray canisters or alarms), but these are not recommended for cats that are already anxious.

The significance of the soiled area can be changed to something pleasant, either by making the area a feeding location or placing the cat's bed on the area. Another option is to play with the cat in that location.

Disrupting the Behavior

If an owner observes the cat beginning to approach a previously soiled area, the cat can be interrupted to stop its approach, perhaps by distracting the cat with toys. Another option is to gently toss something soft (e.g., a towel, potholder, etc.) in the cat's direction to interrupt it. It is important that the owner never yells at or physically reprimands the cat, because this can cause fear and anxiety and perhaps damage the human-animal bond. Once the cat has been disrupted, it may be useful to bring the cat to the litter box and reward the cat with a tasty tidbit for eliminating in the box. These options are only useful if issues causing aversion to the litter box or location have been addressed.

Confinement

As a last resort, it may be necessary to confine the cat in a small space where there is a high probability that it will use the litter box. Options include a small room or a large dog crate. Once the cat is regularly using the litter box, it should be gradually allowed access to the rest of the house when it can be supervised. Confinement can be aversive to both cats and owners, causing stress and anxiety, so this procedure should be instituted as a last resort. Furthermore, there is no scientific evidence that confinement will prevent the cat from resoiling previous areas again once released from confinement. If the reasons for housesoiling described earlier are not addressed, the housesoiling is likely to return.

A summary of the causes and treatment recommendations for inappropriate elimination can be found in Table 89-2.

URINE MARKING

History and Causes

Urine marking is usually a symptom of an underlying stressor. Although it is considered normal for intact male cats and

Table 89-2	Summary of the Causes and Treatments for Housesoiling
Causes	**Treatment**
Litter aversion Substrate preference	Eliminate aversive elements of the litter and litter box Provide the most attractive litter box (e.g., proper hygiene, appropriate size and location, preferred litter) Add additional litter boxes in appropriate areas Enzymatic cleaner for soiled areas Change significance of soiled areas
Location aversion Location preference	Eliminate aversive elements of the preferred location Provide an attractive location (e.g., quiet, easily accessible, unable to be blocked by other animals) Add additional litter boxes in appropriate areas Enzymatic cleaner for soiled areas Change significance of soiled areas

Table 89-3	Summary of the Causes and Treatments for Urine Marking
Causes	**Treatment**
Agonistic interactions with household cats	Surgical sterilization Improve litter box hygiene Enzymatic cleaner for soiled areas Change significance of marked areas Desensitization and counter conditioning to other cat(s) in household Arrange house to reduce intercat aggression Synthetic feline facial pheromones Anxiolytic drug therapy
Agonistic interactions with outside cats	Surgical sterilization Improve litter box hygiene Enzymatic cleaner for soiled areas Change significance of marked areas Block visual stimuli from outdoor cats Anxiolytic drug therapy and synthetic feline facial pheromones
Emotional disturbance; anxiety	Surgical sterilization Improve litter box hygiene Enzymatic cleaner for soiled areas Change significance of marked areas Desensitization and counter conditioning of cat to triggers (e.g., visitors, change in schedule) Arrange house to provide hiding places Synthetic feline facial pheromones Anxiolytic drug therapy

possibly females in estrus, this problem occurs in about 10% of castrated male cats and 5% of spayed female cats.[25] Castration is very effective in decreasing urine marking, and the age of the cat at time of castration does not affect a cat's predisposition to urine mark.[26]

Targets selected for marking usually have some form of social significance, such as windows, doorways, a dog's bed, or the owner's clothes. Target areas are marked repeatedly. Urine marking may also be performed on a horizontal surface (e.g., the owner's bed) using the squatting position. As with housesoiling, determination of the culprit in a multiple cat household is key, bearing in mind that more than one cat may be urine marking.

Male cats and cats from multiple cat households are more likely to display urine-marking behavior than female cats or those in single cat homes. Additionally, it has been documented that agonistic interactions with other cats are a significant trigger for urine marking. These could be interactions with cats in the same household or outdoor cats.[13] The urine marks from an outdoor visiting cat can trigger the household cat to begin marking its indoor territory.

Additional triggers that cannot be overlooked include: a new cat introduced into the home, moving to a new house, visitors, new family members, and/or vacations by the owner. There is conflicting evidence as to whether urine-marking cats are likely to have abnormalities on urinalysis that contribute to marking behavior.[15,16]

A summary of diagnostic criteria for urine marking can be found in Table 89-3.

Treatment

Castration

Intact cats should be spayed or castrated, because hormones can play a significant role in modulating urine-marking behavior. Castration has been shown to decrease urine marking in almost 90% of male cats.[27] Age at castration does not have an effect on the outcome.[28]

Environmental Management

Providing an appropriate environment that is as stress-free as possible is important. Alleviating household stress that originates from fighting with other household cats is especially important. For specifics on managing and treating intercat aggression, refer to Chapter 92.

Studies have shown that increasing activity levels and providing environmental enrichment for indoor cats can decrease stress.[17,29] Fortunately, there are a variety of simple ways to enrich a cat's indoor environment, including creating separate areas for each cat to decrease household tension.

Toys are an obvious method of providing enrichment, both those that do not require owner involvement (self-play toys) and those that require interaction between cat and owner (interactive toys). Any positive interaction with a cat is a form of enrichment, of course; but although owners often prefer petting the cat, the cat may prefer play.

Many self-play toys are designed to dispense food, which motivates the cat to play with the toy and may serve to distract the cat from another cat in the house or another stressor. These toys are generally filled with dry kibble, and the cat learns to manipulate the toy to release the food. Self-play toys that do not dispense food may not be as engaging for most cats. Because one of the recommendations for treatment is to change the significance of a soiled area, the food could be distributed by providing food-dispending toys. Cats are not inclined to eliminate where they eat.

Interactive toys help strengthen the bond between owner and cat. Wand-type toys with attached objects (e.g., feathers) are safe for owners to use, because they keep the cat's claws and teeth away from the owner while encouraging interactive, aerobic play.

Window perches allow cats to "virtually" spend time outside and also provide a safe place to escape from another cat. For example, the back of a sofa by a window can expand the amount of vertical space in the house. Owners need to be aware of roaming cats in the yard outside because the sight of those cats can trigger stress, and possibly urine marking and redirected aggression, in the indoor cat. If that is the case, owners should avoid placing perches near windows and/or cover the windows with opaque film to allow in light, but decrease the cat's ability to see outside. Providing places for cats to escape from one another can also decrease tension between household cats.

Eliminate Aversive Aspects

Having enough litter boxes that are properly cleaned is important in decreasing overall stress and anxiety in cats. One study demonstrated that proper litter box management (e.g., appropriate numbers of litter boxes, removing waste daily, and cleaning weekly with mild dish soap) and cleaning of urine marks with an enzymatic cleaner significantly decreased urine-marking behavior.[13] This effect was more evident in female cats than male cats but is still recommended for all urine-marking cats.

Decreasing the Chance of Remarking the Area and Disrupting the Behavior

The same recommendations as earlier for inappropriate elimination apply for cats that are displaying urine-marking behavior. It is crucial that the treatment should not increase anxiety in the cat. A summary of the treatment recommendations for urine marking can be found in Table 89-3.

Anxiolytic Medications and Pheromones

Depending upon the situation, it may be appropriate to attempt behavioral approaches first, and if not successful, augment treatment for urine marking with drug therapy (see Table 89-4 for dosages). In urine-marking situations, most owners feel that the problem is urgent and may wish to

Table 89-4	Commonly Used Medications to Treat Urine Marking		
Drug Name	**Drug Class**	**Oral Dosage**	**Published Study?**
Fluoxetine	SSRI	0.5 to 1 mg/kg once daily	Yes[32-33]
Clomipramine	TCA	0.25 to 1 mg/kg once daily or divided twice daily	Yes[32-35]
Buspirone	Azapirone	0.5 to 1 mg/kg twice daily	Yes[37]
Paroxetine	SSRI	0.5 to 1 mg/kg twice daily	No
Amitryptilline	TCA	5 to 10 mg/cat once daily	No

SSRI, Selective serotonin reuptake inhibitor; *TCA*, tricyclic antidepressant.

combine behavioral approaches and medication. Research has indicated that this approach can be successful.[30-34]

Selective Serotonin Reuptake Inhibitors. Fluoxetine has been shown to be effective in decreasing urine-marking behavior.[30] One study found a marked reduction in urine marking for cats treated with fluoxetine over placebo, with positive results usually evident within 2 weeks of initiating therapy. By 8 weeks, marking in all fluoxetine-treated cats had been reduced to less than 10% of baseline levels.[31]

Other studies of fluoxetine suggest that achieving 90% reduction in urine marking in some cats may take up to 32 weeks of treatment. Eventually most cats seem to respond. However, urine marking will resume once the medication is stopped if no environmental or behavioral recommendations are implemented. One study demonstrated that recurrence of marking to 50% or more of baseline levels occurred in most cats after cessation of drug therapy, even after as long as 32 weeks of treatment.[32] This return of marking once medication is withdrawn remains an important challenge, especially for cats that require long-term control or live in environments that continually create stress and anxiety that provoke urine marking. Cats receiving long-term medication should have regular laboratory monitoring (e.g., complete blood count and serum chemistry panel).

Cats weaned off fluoxetine that resume marking behavior seem to respond to repeat treatment as successfully as after the initial treatment.[32] Studies have not been performed on the effects of other drugs in this class on urine-marking behavior, although it is speculated that other medications in the same class may also be effective.

Tricyclic Antidepressants. Clomipramine has equal effectiveness as fluoxetine in treating urine-marking cats.[32-34] However, it has more reported side effects than fluoxetine—the most common being sedation. Practitioners must also be aware that clomipramine has been associated with decreased serum thyroid concentrations, which may affect a potential diagnosis of hyperthyroidism.[35]

Amitriptyline historically has been used to treat urine marking in cats but has fallen out of favor as newer drugs with fewer side effects have become affordable. Additionally, amitriptyline is quite bitter, which makes administration difficult.

Azapirone Medications. Buspirone is the only medication in this drug family. One study demonstrated its effectiveness in reducing urine marking; however, it appears to be less effective than fluoxetine and clomipramine. One side effect that is observed is an increase in aggression toward other cats but occasionally toward people, which is obviously not a desired outcome.[36] In addition, for best efficacy, buspirone is administered twice daily, which is often a difficult task for most owners to accomplish and hence this medication has fallen out of favor. However, one could consider this medication for a urine-marking cat whose behavior is triggered by offensively aggressive behavior by another cat within the household. There are anecdotal reports of victim cats becoming more assertive when treated with buspirone, thereby diminishing the frequency of offensive attacks by other cats.

Pheromones. A commercially available synthetic feline facial pheromone product (Feliway, Lenexa, Kansas) is promoted to prevent or reduce stress and decrease urine marking. The product should be used near the areas previously targeted for marking. Although some reduction in marking behavior has been reported, there are few controlled, blinded trials. Some papers have suggested pheromones show promise for reducing urine marking, whereas systematic reviews of pheromones for the treatment of problem behaviors in cats and dogs have provided variable evidence for efficacy.[30,37]

Other Medications. Other medications that have been studied for the treatment of urine marking in cats include diazepam and progestins. These currently are not recommended treatments due to the potential for serious side effects.[38-42]

Transdermal formulations of psychotropic medications have been evaluated in cats, because this route of administration may increase owner compliance. However, two studies have demonstrated a lack of comparable blood levels for fluoxetine, buspirone, and amitriptyline when transdermal formulations were evaluated against oral dosing.[43,44]

SUMMARY

Housesoiling and urine marking are common problems in pet cats that, once properly diagnosed and treated by a veterinarian, have a good prognosis. One study on the long-term outcome on housesoiling noted a 75% improvement, and most owners were pleased with the results.[45] A different study utilizing pheromones for the treatment of urine marking showed a long-term improvement in marking behavior in 77% of cats.[46] Veterinarians must be able to properly differentiate between marking and inappropriate elimination by asking a few key questions. With a concerted effort to address these common behavior problems, veterinarians can help curtail the rate of unnecessary relinquishment and euthanasia of cats.

References

1. Salman MD, Hutchison J, Ruch-Gallie R, et al: Behavioral reasons for relinquishment of dogs and cats to 12 shelters. *J Appl Anim Welf Sci* 3:93–106, 2000.
2. Patronek GJ, Glickman LT, Beck AM, et al: Risk factors for relinquishment of cats to an animal shelter. *J Am Vet Med Assoc* 209:582–588, 1996.
3. New JC, Salman MD, King M, et al: Characteristics of shelter-relinquished animals and their owners compared with animals and their owners in U.S. pet-owning households. *J Appl Anim Welf Sci* 3:179–201, 2000.
4. Casey RA, Vandenbussche S, Bradshaw JWS, et al: Reasons for relinquishment and return of domestic cats *(Felis silvestris catus)* to rescue shelters in the UK. *Anthrozoös* 22:347–358, 2009.
5. Souza-Dantas LMd, Soares GM, D'Almeida JM, et al: Epidemiology of domestic cat behavioral and welfare issues: a survey of Brazilian referral animal hospitals in 2009. *Int J Appl Res Vet Med* 7:130–137, 2009.
6. Wright JC, Amoss RT: Prevalence of house soiling and aggression in kittens during the first year after adoption from a humane society. *J Am Vet Med Assoc* 224:1790–1795, 2004.
7. Amat M, de la Torre JLR, Fatjó J, et al: Potential risk factors associated with feline behaviour problems. *Appl Anim Beh Sci* 121:134–139, 2009.
8. Bamberger M, Houpt KA: Signalment factors, comorbidity, and trends in behavior diagnoses in cats: 736 cases (1991–2001). *J Am Vet Med Assoc* 229:1602–1606, 2006.
9. Halip JW, Vaillancourt JP, Luescher UA: A descriptive study of 189 cats engaging in inappropriate elimination behaviors. *Feline Pract* 26:18–21, 1998.
10. Bergman L, Hart BL, Bain M, et al: Evaluation of urine marking by cats as a model for understanding veterinary diagnostic and treatment approaches and client attitudes. *J Am Vet Med Assoc* 221:1282–1286, 2002.
11. Patronek GJ, Dodman NH: Attitudes, procedures, and delivery of behavior services by veterinarians in small animal practice. *J Am Vet Med Assoc* 215:1606–1611, 1999.
12. Hart BL, Leedy M: Identification of source of urine stains in multi-cat households. *J Am Vet Med Assoc* 180:77–78, 1982.
13. Pryor PA, Hart BL, Bain MJ, et al: Causes of urine marking in cats and effects of environmental management on frequency of marking. *J Am Vet Med Assoc* 219:1709–1713, 2001.
14. Houpt KA, Honig SU, Reisner IR: Breaking the human-companion animal bond. *J Am Vet Med Assoc* 208:1653–1659, 1996.
15. Tynes VV, Hart BL, Pryor PA, et al: Evaluation of the role of lower urinary tract disease in cats with urine-marking behavior. *J Am Vet Med Assoc* 223:457–461, 2003.
16. Frank DF, Erb HN, Houpt KA: Urine spraying in cats: presence of concurrent disease and effects of a pheromone treatment. *Appl Anim Behav Sci* 61:263–272, 1999.
17. Buffington CAT, Westropp JL, Chew DJ, et al: Clinical evaluation of multimodal environmental modification (MEMO) in the management of cats with idiopathic cystitis. *J Feline Med Surg* 8:261–268, 2006.
18. Horwitz DF: Behavioral and environmental factors associated with elimination behavior problems in cats: a retrospective study. *Appl Anim Behav Sci* 52:129–137, 1997.
19. Slingerland LI, Hazewinkel HAW, Meij BP, et al: Cross-sectional study of the prevalence and clinical features of osteoarthritis in 100 cats. *Vet J* 187:304–309, 2011.

20. Sung W, Crowell-Davis SL: Elimination behavior patterns of domestic cats (*Felis catus*) with and without elimination behavior problems. *Am J Vet Res* 67:1500–1504, 2006.

21. Borchelt PL: Cat elimination behavior problems. *Vet Clin North Am Small Anim Pract* 21:257–264, 1991.

22. Neilson J: Litter preference in cats: scented vs. unscented. In *Proceedings of American College of Veterinary Behavior/American Veterinary Society of Animal Behavior Symposium*, 2011, pp 6–8.

23. Grigg EK, Pick L, Nibblett B: Litter box preference in domestic cats: covered versus uncovered. *J Feline Med Surg* 15:280–284, 2013.

24. Melese P: Detecting and neutralizing odor sources in dog and cat elimination problems. *Appl Anim Behav Sci* 39:188–189, 1994.

25. Hart BL, Cooper L: Factors relating to urine spraying and fighting in prepubertally gonadectomized cats. *J Am Vet Med Assoc* 184:1255–1258, 1984.

26. Hart BL, Eckstein RA: The role of gonadal hormones in the occurrence of objectionable behaviours in dogs and cats. *Appl Anim Behav Sci* 52:331–344, 1997.

27. Hart BL, Barrett RE: Effects of castration on fighting, roaming, and urine spraying in adult male cats. *J Am Vet Med Assoc* 163:290–292, 1973.

28. Hart BL: Effects of neutering and spaying on the behavior of dogs and cats: questions and answers about practical concerns. *J Am Vet Med Assoc* 198:1204–1205, 1991.

29. Stella JL, Lord LK, Buffington CAT: Sickness behaviors in response to unusual external events in healthy cats and cats with feline interstitial cystitis. *J Am Vet Med Assoc* 238:67–73, 2011.

30. Mills DS, Redgate SE, Landsberg GM: A meta-analysis of studies of treatments for feline urine spraying. *PLoS ONE* 6:e18448, 2011.

31. Pryor PA, Hart BL, Cliff KD, et al: Effects of a selective serotonin reuptake inhibitor on urine spraying behavior in cats. *J Am Vet Med Assoc* 219:1557–1561, 2001.

32. Hart BL, Cliff KD, Tynes VV, et al: Control of urine marking by use of long-term treatment with fluoxetine or clomipramine in cats. *J Am Vet Med Assoc* 226:378–382, 2005.

33. Landsberg GM, Wilson AL: Effects of clomipramine on cats presented for urine marking. *J Am Anim Hosp Assoc* 41:3–11, 2005.

34. King JN, Steffan J, Heath SE, et al: Determination of the dosage of clomipramine for the treatment of urine spraying in cats. *J Am Vet Med Assoc* 225:881–887, 2004.

35. Martin KM: Effect of clomipramine on the electrocardiogram and serum thyroid concentrations of healthy cats. *J Vet Behav* 5:123–129, 2010.

36. Hart BL, Eckstein RA, Powell KL, et al: Effectiveness of buspirone on urine spraying and inappropriate urination in cats. *J Am Vet Med Assoc* 203:254–258, 1993.

37. Frank D, Beauchamp G, Palestrini C: Systematic review of the use of pheromones for treatment of undesirable behavior in cats and dogs. *J Am Vet Med Assoc* 236:1308–1316, 2010.

38. Hart BL: Objectionable urine spraying and urine marking in cats—evaluation of progestin treatment in gonadectomized males and females. *J Am Vet Med Assoc* 177:529–533, 1980.

39. Cooper L, Hart BL: Comparison of diazepam with progestin for effectiveness in suppression of urine spraying behavior in cats. *J Am Vet Med Assoc* 200:797–801, 1992.

40. Hughes D, Moreau RE, Overall KL, et al: Acute hepatic necrosis and liver failure associated with benzodiazepine therapy in six cats, 1986–1995. *J Vet Emerg Crit Care* 6:13–20, 1996.

41. Center SA, Elston TH, Rowland PH, et al: Fulminant hepatic failure associated with oral administration of diazepam in 11 cats. *J Am Vet Med Assoc* 209:618–625, 1996.

42. Jacobs TM, Hoppe BR, Poehlmann CE, et al: Mammary adenocarcinomas in three male cats exposed to medroxyprogesterone acetate (1990–2006). *J Feline Med Surg* 12:169–174, 2010.

43. Mealey KL, Peck KE, Bennett BS, et al: Systemic absorption of amitriptyline and buspirone after oral and transdermal administration to healthy cats. *J Vet Int Med* 18:43–46, 2004.

44. Ciribassi J, Luescher A, Pasloske KS, et al: Comparative bioavailability of fluoxetine after transdermal and oral administration to healthy cats. *Am J Vet Res* 64:994–998, 2003.

45. Marder AR, Engel JM: Long-term outcome after treatment of feline elimination. *J Appl Anim Welfare Sci* 5:299–308, 2002.

46. Mills DS, White J: Long-term follow up of the effect of a pheromone therapy on feline spraying behaviour. *Vet Rec* 147:746–747, 2000.

Feline Anxiety and Fear-Related Disorders

Meredith E. Stepita

DEFINITION OF ANXIETY AND FEAR

Anxiety and fear are overlapping, aversive emotions, which are poorly differentiated in the literature.[1-3] The Diagnostic and Statistical Manual of Mental Disorders (DSM) defines anxiety as "apprehensive anticipation of future danger or misfortune accompanied by a feeling of dysphoria or somatic symptoms of tension."[3] Anxiety is often anticipatory to a threatening stimulus.[2] Fear differs from anxiety in that fear involves an identifiable eliciting stimulus.[2] The DSM states that "... fear is more often associated with surges of autonomic arousal necessary for fight or flight, thoughts of immediate danger, and escape behavior, and anxiety [is] more often associated with muscle tension and vigilance in preparation for future danger and cautious or avoidant behaviors."[3] According to Epstein,[4] fear turns into anxiety when coping fails.

THE ANATOMY AND PHYSIOLOGY OF ANXIETY AND FEAR

The amygdala (Figure 90-1), an almond-shaped conglomeration of nuclei found in the temporal lobe, has long been implicated in the fear response with the lateral nucleus implicated in fear acquisition and the central nucleus implicated in the acquisition and expression of fear-conditioned responses.[5-7] Other studies have shown that the hippocampus, a structure medial to the lateral ventricle in the temporal lobe and bed nucleus of the stria terminalis (see Figure 90-1) both play a role in anxiety.[8,9]

There has been extensive research into the physiology of anxiety and fear. Fear and anxiety trigger a complex set of events known as the *stress response* whose main components are endocrine and autonomic. The endocrine portion starts when sensory information enters and activates the amygdala, which in turn, activates the stress response with release of corticotropin-releasing hormone (CRH) from the hypothalamus. This response activates release of adrenocorticotropic hormone from the anterior pituitary gland, which at high levels causes cortisol to be released from the adrenal gland. Corticotropin-releasing hormone neurons in the hypothalamus are regulated by the amygdala and hippocampus. The

neurons in the bed nucleus of the stria terminalis also activate this hypothalamic-pituitary-adrenal axis and stress response.[10] Hippocampal activation is different in that it suppresses CRH release. The hippocampus contains glucocorticoid receptors that respond by inhibiting CRH when high levels of cortisol are detected. When the autonomic system is activated, stimulation of the sympathetic nervous system causes release of epinephrine and norepinephrine from the adrenal medulla, leading to an increased heart rate and blood pressure, as well as breakdown of glucose for energy.[11,12]

EFFECTS OF CHRONIC STRESS

Stress is an adaptive response necessary for self-preservation. However, chronic stressors can have detrimental effects on numerous body systems. For example, chronic exposure to cortisol kills hippocampal neurons, which play a key role in memory.[13,14] Stress suppresses the immune system and increases the chance of infectious disease primarily by way of glucocorticoids that inhibit cell growth, leukocyte activity, cytokine production, and antibody formation.[11,12] Chronic behavioral stress has resulted in increased tumor growth (weight and number of nodules), metastasis, and markedly increased tumor vascularization.[15]

BODY POSTURES

The stress response starts with physiologic changes; therefore, in the early stages, these internal changes may not be associated with external behavioral signs. When external behavioral signs are evident, it is likely that the cat has already been stressed for some amount of time.

When reading feline body postures, all components of the posture (e.g., ears, tail, etc.) must be taken into account. Body postures associated with defensive fear include ears laid back, body in a crouched position, tail tucked under the body, and the body leaning away from the fear-eliciting stimulus. The more offensively fearful cat, dubbed the *Halloween cat* has ears flattened against the head, a dorsally arched back, a tail held straight up, and piloerected hair in an attempt to appear larger. This cat has been compared to the fear-biting dog. Piloerection is not necessarily a sign of fear but does indicate

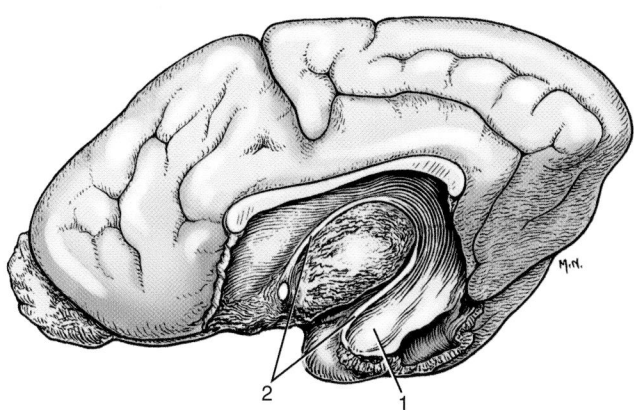

Figure 90-1: Right cerebral hemisphere (medial view) showing the amygdala *(1)* and stria terminalis *(2)*. (From de Lahunta A, Evans H: *Guide to the dissection of the dog,* ed 7, St Louis, 2010, Saunders/Elsevier.)

negative emotional arousal. It can be helpful to provide clients with a picture chart of feline body postures that they can choose from if they have difficulty describing the postures their cat displays (Figure 90-2).

Another phenomenon presumably due to stress is "feigned sleep." This posture, which mimics sleeping, is exhibited by cats subjected to chronic stress, such as in an animal shelter. In the feigned sleep posture, the body is taut rather than relaxed as in true sleep. Unfortunately at the time of this writing, feigned sleep has not been confirmed as a stress-related phenomenon with physiologic stress markers.[16]

GENETIC AND ENVIRONMENTAL CONTRIBUTIONS TO ANXIETY AND FEAR

Prevention of behavior problems, including anxiety and fear, starts with selection of an appropriate pet. This is a service veterinarians can and should offer to their clients. Factors to consider when choosing a new cat to bring into a family include owner factors (e.g., lifestyle, expectations, ability, and experience) and cat factors (e.g., behavioral and physical characteristics of particular individuals, breeds, lineages, and ages).[17]

Behavior of an individual cat is dependent on previous experiences and genetic influences; therefore, both factors should be taken into consideration with regard to prevention of fear and anxiety. When tested at 1 year of age, cats from a friendly sire or those handled between 2 and 12 weeks of age were quicker to approach, touch, and rub a test person, and spent a greater total time within 1 meter (3.3 feet) of a person or novel object compared to cats from an unfriendly sire and those not handled at a young age.[18] Other studies have also found that paternity plays some role in sociability of cats toward people, even when kittens are not exposed to their sire.[19,20]

The primary socialization period of the cat to people is from approximately 2 to 9 weeks of age, and unfortunately most kittens do not receive adequate amounts of socialization

during this time. Kitten socialization classes are becoming increasingly recognized as a way to facilitate obtaining sufficient socialization and help prevent behavior problems. These classes may include play time with people and other kittens, teaching commands using food rewards, and educating owners with regard to normal feline behavior, proper handling, grooming, appropriate play with their kittens, giving their kitten a pill, and preventing behavior problems (e.g., elimination outside of the litter box, scratching, biting, etc.). The American Association of Feline Practitioners and the American Animal Hospital Association recommend that kittens be acclimated as early as possible to any stimuli that they may encounter during their lifetime (e.g., children, dogs, nail trims, and car transport).[21] Socialization should occur at the pace of the individual cat. Care should be taken to ensure that experiences are positive (e.g., the cat is calm and relaxed and the experience is paired with a high-value food reward, play, or petting), because the quality of the experiences is just as important as the quantity. For a further discussion of socialization, see Chapter 94.

RULING OUT MEDICAL PROBLEMS

Virtually any medical problem can lead to anxiety. Therefore, the first step in assessing a patient's behavior problem should include a physical examination and diagnostic workup for underlying medical problems as warranted. A medical cause should be strongly suspected in a patient presenting with an acute onset of anxiety in which an eliciting trigger cannot be identified. If medical problems are not treated or factors prevent the necessary medical workup, complete resolution of the behavior problem is unlikely to occur until the medical problem is adequately controlled and/or treated. In one study, 76% of cats presenting to a veterinary behaviorist for presumptive psychogenic alopecia were found to have a medical cause of pruritus.[22] Medical problems causing anxiety can range from infection, inflammation, neoplasia, metabolic abnormalities, and endocrine disturbances to ocular disease, pain (including dental and orthopedic), neurologic abnormalities, and urinary tract disease. Cognitive dysfunction syndrome is another important differential diagnosis for cats over the age of 10 years with anxiety, disorientation, altered interaction with family members, changes in sleep-wake cycles, inappropriate elimination (e.g., urination, defecation), changes in activity, and excessive vocalization (see Chapter 98).

DIAGNOSIS, PROGNOSIS, AND TREATMENT OF ANXIETY AND FEAR-RELATED DISORDERS

Diagnosis

Fear is diagnosed by examining the body postures of the cat (see Figure 90-2) in response to repeated exposure to a specific and identifiable stimulus (e.g., familiar people, unfamiliar people, other animals, noises, etc.). Often the patient shows

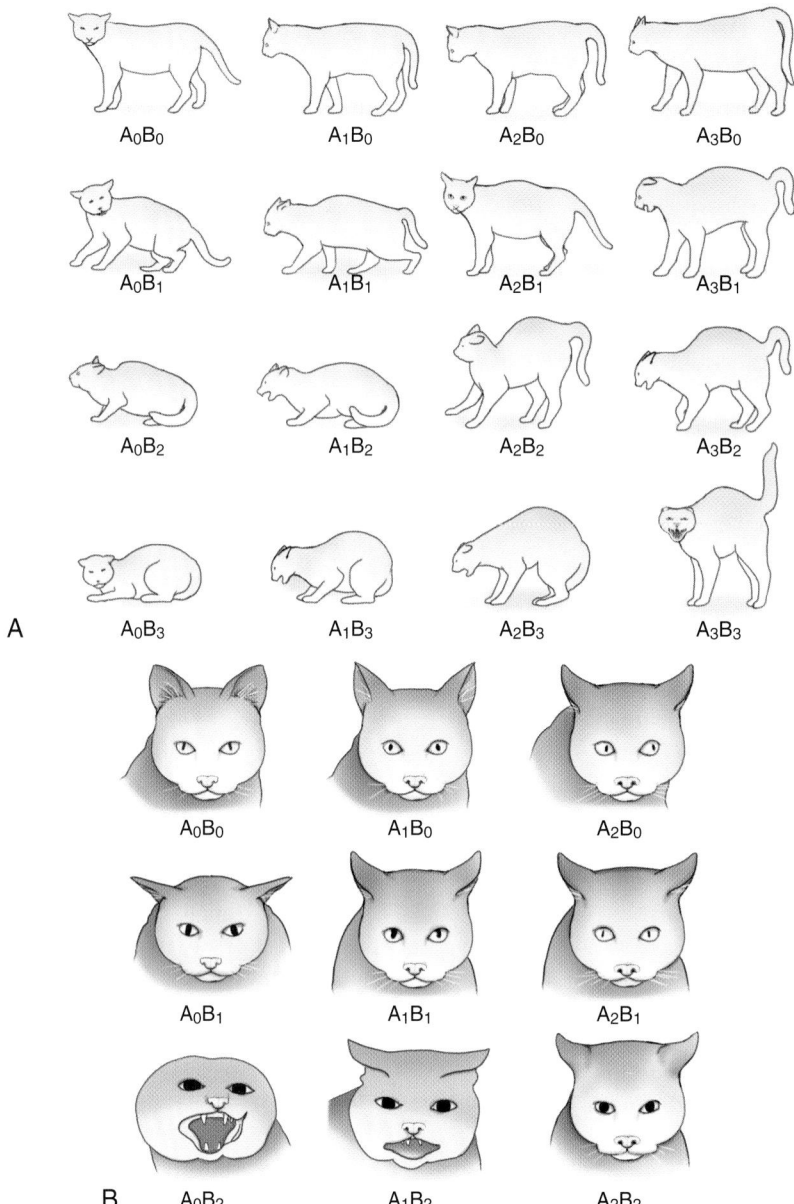

Figure 90-2: A, Feline profile body postures. A_0B_0 depicts a cat with relaxed body postures. In the first row, moving from left to right $(A_0B_0$ to $A_3B_0)$, the body postures of the cat become more confident and offensively aggressive. Note the ears slightly laid back but not laid flat back, rump elevated, and fully extended pelvic limbs. In the first column, moving from top to bottom $(A_0B_0$ to $A_0B_3)$, the body postures of the cat become more fearful and defensively aggressive. Note the ears become more laid flat back, body is crouched and leaning away, back is arched, and tail is tucked under the body. **B,** Feline facial expressions. A_0B_0 depicts a cat with a relaxed facial expression. A_2B_2 depicts an offensively and confidently aggressive cat. Note the slightly lowered head, ears slightly laid back but not laid flat back, clamping and tenseness of the mouth, and pupils in mid-dilation with a direct stare. A_2B_0 depicts a defensively fearful cat. Note the ears rotating back, neck and head are more withdrawn, and eyes in a nondirect gaze. A_0B_2 depicts an offensively fearful cat. Note the ears laid flat back against the head, teeth exposed, and pupils dilated. (From Overall KL: *Manual of clinical behavioral medicine for dogs and cats,* ed 1, St Louis, 2013, Mosby.)

other signs of fear and anxiety, including trembling, cowering, freezing, escape, hiding, hypervigilance, anorexia, pacing, anal gland expression, vomiting, diarrhea, urination and/or defecation at inappropriate times, and autonomic signs (e.g., tachycardia, mydriasis, hyperthermia, and hypertension).

Fear and anxiety may be associated with hyperarousal (e.g., piloerection, mydriasis, and tail lashing), which can last for days and increases the chance of aggression. See Chapter 91 on feline aggression toward people and Chapter 92 on intercat aggression for more information.

Prognosis

No studies are currently available that have examined the prognosis for fear and anxiety disorders in cats. Fear in response to any stimulus can be influenced by socialization, genetics, and previous experience, all of which also influence prognosis. Anecdotally, however, prognosis may be linked to many factors, including:

- Severity and duration of the problem behavior
- Predictability, consistency, number of, and ability to avoid stimuli
- How long it takes the cat to calm once the stimulus is removed
- Whether or not a genetic component exists
- Owner's ability to implement the behavior modification plan
- Patient's response to treatment

Management

For most behavior problems, including anxiety and fear, the first step is to make a list of triggers for the behavior and then avoid them. The primary reason for avoidance is safety; secondarily it can help decrease emotional arousal and therefore help decrease stress and the stress response. Some cats that are fearful will become aggressive and may bite or scratch trying to escape from the threatening stimulus. Avoidance also ensures that the cat does not continue to practice the behavior and learn that it is effective (e.g., fearful behavioral responses cause the fear-eliciting stimulus to go away); avoidance also allows the pet to relax and calm and perhaps increase receptivity to learning new things. This allows for the stimuli(us) to be successfully reintroduced in a controlled setting at a later time to change the cat's emotional response from fearful or anxious to calm and relaxed. Avoidance strategies may include:

- Placing the cat in a separate room behind a closed door with food, water, a litter box, resting areas, and hiding places prior to visitors coming to the house and for the duration of their visit
- Separating the cat from other household pets
- Playing white noise or calming music to cover up noises that cause anxiety or fear
- Not leaving a cat with separation anxiety home alone
- Putting away items that a cat with pica may ingest

Behavior Modification

The next step is behavior modification, usually systematic desensitization and counterconditioning (SD/CC). *Systematic desensitization* involves gradual exposure to a stimulus in order to raise the threshold at which the animal shows the undesirable behavior. *Counterconditioning* is teaching the animal to perform a behavior that is incompatible with the undesirable response, for example, sitting quietly and relaxed when presented with the stimulus in question. Classical counterconditioning uses an unconditioned response, such

as eating treats, to achieve the desired positive emotional response. Operant counterconditioning uses a conditioned response, such as a command, to competitively interfere with the performance of the unwanted behavior.[23] Cats are generally more amenable to classical counterconditioning, but in some cases, they can be very motivated to learn commands, and a combination of operant and classical counterconditioning can be employed. Clicker training in which the clicking noise acts as a secondary reinforcer can be highly successful. The click can be used to mark and therefore teach behaviors or commands, or otherwise reward a desirable behavior and/or emotional response. It is helpful for the cat to only receive the special reward in the presence of the anxiety-producing trigger. Physical punishment is contraindicated when using SD/CC, because it can increase fear and defensive aggression, the opposite of the desired response. These sessions are most effective when performed for short periods of time (e.g., 5 minutes or less) and frequently (e.g., daily or multiple times per day) as long as the pet is able to remain calm and relaxed.

Pharmaceutical and Ancillary Treatments

Although pheromones, supplements, and antianxiety medications can be useful in facilitating behavior modification in fearful and anxious cats, these products should never be a sole treatment for anxiety. See Table 90-1 for doses.

Feliway is a synthetic analogue of the feline facial pheromone that is available in several forms (i.e., spray, room diffuser). Some studies have demonstrated the success of pheromones in improving behaviors associated with anxiety, such as urine marking.[24-26]

A supplement containing the amino acid L-theanine (Anxitane; Virbac Corporation, Fort Worth, TX) has also been shown to significantly reduce behavioral and autonomic manifestations associated with anxiety (e.g., inappropriate elimination, aggressiveness, hypervigilance/tenseness, and physical signs, such as digestive problems and hypersalivation).[27] A diet containing alpha-casozepine, L-tryptophan, and nicotinamide (vitamin B₃) (Calm, Royal Canin Veterinary Diet; Royal Canin USA, Inc., St. Charles, MO) may help to alleviate anxiety. A study by Beata and colleagues[28] found that global scores as well as specific fears were significantly improved by the use of the milk protein hydrolysate alpha-casozepine (Zylkene; Vétoquinol USA, Fort Worth, TX).

Psychotropic Medications

In patients refractory to behavior modification or patients in which behavior modification is not possible due to extreme anxiety, antianxiety medications may be warranted in conjunction with behavior modification. Commonly used medications include selective serotonin reuptake inhibitors (SSRIs) and tricyclic antidepressants (TCAs). Multiple studies have demonstrated the success of these serotonin-enhancing medications, specifically fluoxetine and clomipramine, in improving behaviors associated with anxiety.[29-35] These are long-term anxiolytics that take 4 to 6 weeks to take effect. When using

Table 90-1	Pharmaceutical and Nonpharmaceutical Products Used to Treat Anxiety and Fear-Related Disorders in Cats	
Drug or Product	**Dosage**	**Comments**
L-theanine (Anxitane; Virbac Corporation, Fort Worth, TX)	25 mg/cat PO every 12 hours	May increase GABA, serotonin, and dopamine Reduction in behavioral and autonomic manifestations associated with anxiety
Alpha-casozepine (Zylkene; Vétoquinol USA, Fort Worth, TX)	Cats up to 5 kg: 75 mg/cat PO every 24 hours Cats 5 to 10 kg: 150 mg/cat PO every 24 hours	Similar in structure to GABA, has an affinity for benzodiazepine receptors May help alleviate anxiety Improvement in fearful behavior and autonomic signs
Fluoxetine	0.5 to 1.0 mg/kg PO every 24 hours	SSRI Side effects include sedation and GI effects
Clomipramine	0.5 to 1.0 mg/kg PO every 24 hours	Tricyclic antidepressant Side effects include sedation, anticholinergic effects, GI effects, and bone marrow suppression
Alprazolam	0.125 to 0.25 mg/cat PO up to every 8 to 12 hours	Benzodiazepine Useful for short-term treatment of an unavoidable fearful stimulus Side effects include sedation, ataxia, paradoxical excitation, increased appetite, and increased anxiety or aggression Tolerance and dependence can develop with long-term use Fatal hepatic necrosis has been reported with oral diazepam
Trazodone	50 to 100 mg/cat PO 2 hours before stressful event	Serotonin 2A receptor antagonist reuptake inhibitor Useful for short-term treatment of an unavoidable fearful stimulus, but can also be used daily Side effects include sedation, ataxia, cardiac conduction disturbances, increased anxiety, and aggression

GABA, Gamma aminobutyric acid; *GI*, gastrointestinal; *PO, per os* (orally); *SSRI*, selective serotonin reuptake inhibitor.

antianxiety medications, caution should be taken to avoid situations in which the cat may become anxious or fearful because disinhibition and worsening of aggression may occur, although this is uncommon with SSRIs and TCAs as compared to benzodiazepines.

Since fluoxetine is selective for serotonin, side effects are generally limited to sedation and gastrointestinal (GI) effects (e.g., anorexia). Side effects of clomipramine include sedation, anticholinergic effects (cardiac arrhythmias, dry mouth, urine retention, constipation, mydriasis), GI effects (anorexia, diarrhea, and vomiting), and hematological effects (bone marrow suppression). Cats have been reported to be more susceptible to adverse effects from fluoxetine and clomipramine than dogs; therefore, starting at the low end of the dosage range is advisable.

Short-acting medications, such as benzodiazepines (e.g., alprazolam) or trazodone, may be used for unavoidable fears and anxieties (e.g., leaving a cat with separation anxiety home alone or fireworks for a noise phobic cat). Regular long-term use of benzodiazepines is not recommended. Side effects of benzodiazepines include sedation, ataxia, paradoxical excitation, increased appetite, and increased anxiety or aggression. Another risk of oral diazepam administration is fatal fulmi-

nant hepatic necrosis, which appears idiosyncratic.[36] If benzodiazepines are used on a daily basis for 2 to 3 weeks, the cat will develop tolerance and dependence and will need to be weaned from the drug slowly (e.g., decreasing the dose by 25% or less per week).[37] Trazodone is a serotonin 2A receptor antagonist reuptake inhibitor for short-term or long-term use. Side effects include sedation, ataxia, cardiac conduction disturbances, increased anxiety, and aggression.

SPECIFIC ANXIETY AND FEAR-RELATED DISORDERS

Cats can be fearful of anything including specific objects (e.g., a hair dryer, broom, water bottle, etc.) and smells (e.g., other animals, people, perfumes, etc.). The more common feline fears and anxieties are discussed in this section.

Fear of Animate Stimuli
Familiar and Unfamiliar People
As is true of most species, cats are more likely to be fearful of unfamiliar people than they are of familiar people. The

fear-eliciting trigger may simply be the presence of the person, especially unfamiliar people, but for some cats, the trigger may be more specific, such as approaching, reaching for, petting, and picking up the cat or people carrying objects or moving quickly.

Systematic desensitization and counterconditioning therapy is begun by having the cat on the opposite side of the room from a person that it fears. The cat is rewarded with a favorite treat, play, or petting in the presence of this person. As long as the cat is calm and relaxed, the person can move closer to the cat over many sessions. The owner must watch the cat carefully, and if the cat becomes anxious or disinterested, the gradient should be made easier or less threatening (e.g., the distance between the cat and the person should be increased). The session can be ended on a positive note by rewarding the cat for calm, relaxed behavior.

Other Animals

Although they can be fearful of any animal, the most common animals that cats are fearful of are other cats and dogs. When a cat is fearful of another cat in the same home, environmental enrichment that increases resources and spacing and includes food-dispensing toys and more resting, hiding, feeding, climbing, and perching areas can help decrease competition for resources and therefore alleviate overall stress.[38] It is important to provide vertical space, which allows cats to increase the dimensions of their living space in multiple cat households and can help cats separate themselves in places dogs cannot access. The Indoor Pet Initiative (https://indoorpet.osu.edu) is an excellent resource for information about decreasing stress in cats. For more information on intercat aggression, see Chapter 92.

A specific SD/CC plan similar to that described for fear of familiar and unfamiliar people should be made to the dog, cat, or other animal triggering the fearful response. It is important that the other animal be under control (e.g., keeping a dog on a leash) during the sessions.

Fear of Inanimate Stimuli

Noises

Dogs are more likely to present for noise anxiety or noise phobia (an extreme fear) than cats. This is likely the case because cats often respond by running away and hiding, which is usually not a problem for the owner. Fear-eliciting noises may include fireworks, gunshots, machinery or construction noises, beeping sounds (e.g., cell phone, smoke detector), thunderstorms, wind, and other loud, acute noises.

It may be difficult to cover up noises as part of avoidance, but white noise or calming classical music can be played at times the offensive noise is likely to occur. Electronic applications and websites that play white noise are available (e.g., http://simplynoise.com). These tools may be recommended over radio or television noise, because they are continuous and do not have periods of silence that may allow the feared sound to be heard. Television or radio may also play noises the cat is fearful of. Systematic desensitization and

counterconditioning can be accomplished using a recording of the noise that causes the fearful response and adjusting the volume to stay below the threshold that elicits anxious behavior. However, not all pets will respond to recordings of noises. In that case, the actual sound (e.g., using a drill or electric saw at a distance), if possible, must be used. It can sometimes be difficult when using the actual sound to stay below the threshold that elicits anxious behavior, because the volume is not as controllable as when a recorded noise is used.

Places and Situations

Many cats are fearful of unfamiliar places. This includes the boarding kennel, veterinary hospital, other homes, etc. This can be exacerbated by situational anxiety, such as car rides, or situational anxiety can stand alone. Fear of car rides may arise due to many factors:

- The cat is placed in a small, often dark box and vision is obscured by the confines of the box.
- The ride is bumpy.
- Unusual sights, sounds, and smells are encountered.
- Motion sickness may also be a factor.
- Often the cat is only taken on these trips when absolutely necessary, which amounts to the once or twice yearly veterinary visit or boarding kennel stay.
- The conclusion of the car ride may involve fear-eliciting situations, such as handling by unfamiliar people or unfamiliar surroundings.

Fear of Veterinary Visits

Fear of the veterinary hospital has a huge impact on feline health and welfare and is a specific situational fear. The 2011 Bayer/National Commission on Veterinary Economic Issues Veterinary Care Usage Study found that 52.8% of cat owners reported that their cat hates going to the veterinarian.[39] Additionally, 37.6% of respondents reported that just thinking about veterinary visits is stressful. In another study, clients cited their stress and their pet's stress, including difficulty getting the cat into the carrier at home, driving to the hospital, and dealing with their fearful cat in the veterinary hospital, as reasons for fewer veterinary visits.[21]

Veterinarians must establish good communication with clients and help them manage and treat their pet's anxiety regarding veterinary visits, which will in turn help with their own anxiety surrounding this event. Once a good line of communication has been established between the veterinarian and client, management and treatment options can be offered.

A program for SD/CC to the veterinary hospital may take time, and the client should be apprised of the challenges. For SD/CC to be effective, the client must start where the cat is calm and relaxed.

Anxiety at the veterinary hospital usually starts at home when the owner takes out the cat carrier, so to be most effective, intervention must begin with this step. Owners can implement several steps to begin to minimize the stress associated with the carrier and hence transport to the veterinary hospital.

The first step is to leave the carrier out in a high traffic area of the house, rather than tucking it away in a closet. Spraying the interior of the carrier with feline pheromones (e.g., Feliway) can make the carrier more attractive to the cat. The pheromone product should be applied daily throughout the desensitization process. After a few days, the owner can engage the cat in a favorite activity (e.g., giving favorite treats, playing with wand-type toys, etc.) at a distance from the carrier. The cat should be calm and relaxed during these sessions. Over many sessions, the cat can be moved closer to the carrier during play or feeding until it is willing to enter the carrier on its own for treats or play. The next step is to close the carrier, first only for a second, then increasing the amount of time the carrier is closed. To make closing the carrier a positive experience, treats that the cat enjoys can be placed in the carrier. After the cat is calm and relaxed in a closed carrier, the owner can start picking the carrier up with the cat inside, and then start moving it to the car. Motion sickness should be prevented medically (e.g., maropitant 1 mg/kg, orally [PO], 2 hours before travel), and after the cat is comfortable in the parked car, SD/CC to car rides can be implemented. This should consist of short trips (e.g., backing out of the garage) and over many sessions, increasing time in the car as long as the cat is calm and relaxed. If at any time the cat shows even subtle signs of distress (e.g., freezing, not taking treats), the owner should revert back to the step the cat was last comfortable with and proceed more slowly. In severe cases, short-term anxiolytics (e.g., alprazolam, trazodone) may be warranted to facilitate behavior modification.[40-42] Owners should be encouraged to use these techniques from the very beginning, starting with their new kitten.

In the best-case scenario, the client brings the cat to the veterinary clinic for nonmedical visits once car ride anxiety is under control. These visits should provide the cat with a positive experience at the veterinary hospital (e.g., petting, play, favorite treats) without negative experiences occurring (e.g., venipuncture, vaccine administration, etc.). These visits should occur on a regular basis to maintain a positive emotional response. Systematic desensitization and counterconditioning must be performed to each fear-eliciting stimulus; therefore, fear of unfamiliar people and handling should be conducted separately and then in conjunction with veterinary visits if needed.

Another important component of management of situational anxiety of the veterinary hospital is the implementation of hospital practices aimed at reducing patient stress. The hospital waiting area can be made less stressful by providing "feline-only" zones with elevated areas so carriers can be placed above floor level. Also consider having one afternoon per week limited to appointments for feline patients. Noisy patients should be moved into an exam room quickly to minimize stress for the other patients. Calming classical music can be played throughout the hospital. Although not studied in cats, exposure to classical music resulted in shelter dogs spending significantly more time resting and less time standing, whereas heavy metal music encouraged dogs to spend significantly more time barking.[43] Feline-only exam

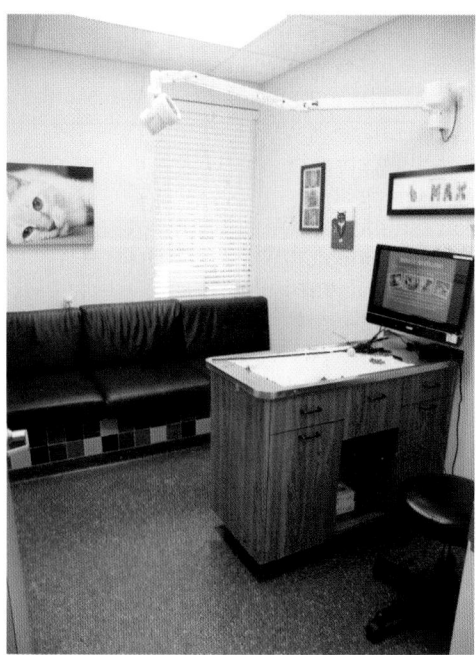

Figure 90-3: Example of a feline-friendly exam room. Note the nonslip mat on the exam table, treats, wand-type and other toys, and pheromone diffuser.

rooms will be less likely to have predator (e.g., dog) smells, thereby decreasing stress (Figure 90-3). These rooms can be stocked with cat toys, treats, and nonslip mats for the exam table and should contain pheromone diffusers. Veterinary staff should use a soft voice and slow approaches from the side rather than straight on when interacting with the patient. The least amount of restraint should be used while maintaining safety. The top of the carrier can be removed when possible and the cat examined within the carrier to decrease stress. Procedures, such as venipuncture, should be performed where the patient is most comfortable, such as in the carrier and in the exam room, as opposed to in the treatment room when possible. Chemical restraint (e.g., Dexdomitor) should be used and muzzles placed early for staff safety—before significant stress has already occurred.[40,41] Cats known to be aggressive can be counterconditioned to a muzzle prior to veterinary visits by placing treats in the muzzle and allowing the cat to approach and put its face into the muzzle. Over time, the muzzle can be buckled onto the cat, and the amount of time that the cat wears the muzzle can be increased as long as the cat remains calm and relaxed.

Other Anxieties

Generalized Anxiety

Generalized anxiety is uncommon in cats. This condition is diagnosed when the patient displays continual signs of anxiety nearly every waking moment. When awake, the cat's body posture primarily consists of ears laid back and body in a crouched position with the tail tucked underneath the body. The cat may tremble, cower, freeze, escape, hide, be hypervigilant, have a poor appetite, pace, vomit, have diarrhea, urinate or defecate at inappropriate times, and display autonomic signs (e.g., tachycardia, mydriasis, hyperthermia, and hypertension). There may be specific stimuli that elicit the anxious response and the condition may have generalized from an inciting stimulus, but anxiety is present even when anxiety-provoking stimuli are apparently absent.

The owner should allow the cat to remain where it is feels most comfortable. Forcing the cat into uncomfortable situations is called *flooding* and will likely serve to worsen the behavior and make treatment more difficult. There should be plenty of places for the cat to hide, including in boxes, cat furniture, behind or underneath furniture, etc. Behavior modification (e.g., SD/CC) will likely be very difficult before antianxiety medications have taken effect. A long-term anxiolytic, such as clomipramine or fluoxetine, can be started. Because these medications will take 4 to 6 weeks to take effect, a shorter-term medication, such as a benzodiazepine (e.g., alprazolam), can be considered for immediate relief.

Separation Anxiety
Cats were once considered an asocial species but have been found to be social. Although feline social behavior is different from that of canines and humans, cats do form groups with an internal structure in which members recognize each other and engage in social behaviors (e.g., allogrooming, cooperative rearing of kittens, nose-touch greeting behavior, etc.).[44]

Feline separation anxiety is not well understood and poorly characterized, but cats do form social bonds and are capable of becoming distressed when an attachment figure is absent. In the only published study on the topic, Schwartz[45] found that out of 716 cats evaluated over a 10-year period, 136 (19%) had clinical signs typical of dogs with separation anxiety (e.g., inappropriate elimination, excessive vocalization, destructiveness, and/or self-mutilation) only when separated from a favorite person or housemate. This is similar to the prevalence of separation anxiety in dogs diagnosed by a behaviorist (10% to 20%).[46,47] The key to a diagnosis of separation anxiety is that the behaviors occur in the absence of the favorite person or housemate; therefore, if the history does not meet this criteria, another cause of the behavior should be investigated. Because the owner is not present when this condition occurs and there are many different differential diagnoses for the behaviors associated with separation anxiety (e.g., fear of other animals and people, noise phobia, litter box aversion, boredom, medical problems, etc.), video recording when the owner is not home is usually essential to make an accurate diagnosis.

Treatment for separation anxiety should include behavior modification, as well as addressing any other contributing problems, medical and otherwise. Self-mutilation may have started in response to anxiety, but it is essential to also treat any underlying infection that has developed for resolution of the problem behavior. Likewise, if inappropriate elimination started in response to anxiety, there may be other compounding factors, such as a dirty or strong-smelling litter box or

problematic social interactions among household cats. These issues may result in the problem continuing, even if separation anxiety is successfully treated.

The time the cat is left alone should be minimized when at all possible until the cat is comfortable being left home alone. Environmental enrichment is important, especially in the absence of the owner. Cats can be taught to use food-dispensing toys by first using toys that make food retrieval easy and working up to more challenging toys. Initially the cat should be supervised to ensure that it does not destroy and consume the toy or injure itself. Although not reported, SD/CC to the owner's absence should help to change the cat's emotional response to being alone. This can be accomplished by leaving the cat with a long-lasting treat and favorite toys for gradually longer periods of time. Initially, the owner should only walk out the door, wait 5 seconds, and come back inside. If the cat is engaged in the food or toys, then the time can be lengthened. If the cat has left the food or toys or otherwise is not engaged in the same activity as when the owner left, the time should be shortened. The time the owner is away can be increased by 15 to 30 seconds, but should be varied rather than incrementally increased (e.g., 15 seconds, 30 seconds, 10 seconds, 45 seconds, etc.). Once the 15- to 20-minute mark has been reached, the owner can increase the time away by 15 to 20 minutes at a time, but care should be taken to go at the cat's pace. If the cat is not calm and relaxed, the time away should be shortened at the next session.

Treatment of cats with separation anxiety may be more dependent on antianxiety medication than is typical for dogs with a similar condition.[48] Long-term treatment with SSRIs and TCAs can help to facilitate behavior modification. If the problem is severe, benzodiazepines (e.g., alprazolam) can be used for short-term relief concurrently with either an SSRI or TCA at times when the owner has no choice but to leave the cat home alone.

COMPULSIVE DISORDERS

Definition
Compulsive disorders have been defined as repetitive behaviors in excess of that required for normal function, the execution of which interferes with normal, daily activities and functioning. The behavior is exaggerated in form and duration.[34]

Pathophysiology
The etiology of compulsive disorders is not well characterized but likely involves stress, genetics, and/or central nervous system mechanisms. These problem behaviors may be triggered or exacerbated by physical trauma and/or environmental and social stressors (e.g., moving to a new home, separation from the owner, introduction of a new pet to the household, death of an animal companion, etc.), although owners of cats with compulsive disorders are not always able to link a stressor to the onset of the behavior.[31,34,35,49] Genetic predispositions for compulsive disorders may also exist. Studies

have found that a large portion of cats ingesting fabric are Oriental breeds (e.g., Siamese, Burmese).[34,49] It has been suggested that these same breeds are predisposed to psychogenic alopecia and that early weaning might also contribute to the development of this problem.[35] Even less is known about brain mechanisms involved in feline compulsive disorders. It has been documented that in other mammalian species, opioid systems are involved in grooming, and it is theorized that there is an endogenous endorphin-mediated reward of the grooming behavior.[50-52] Naloxone, an opioid antagonist, has been shown to be effective in decreasing excessive grooming in cats.[53] Opioids are known modulators of dopaminergic activity, and haloperidol, a dopamine antagonist, has been shown to dramatically decrease time spent grooming within 24 hours of injection.[53]

Psychogenic Alopecia

Cats spend up to 50% of their awake time grooming themselves, which functions to keep them clean, control body temperature, and remove ectoparasites.[54,55] When this behavior becomes excessive so that hair loss or lesions are noted, medical problems are the most likely culprit. In one study, 76% of cats presenting to a veterinary behaviorist for presumptive psychogenic alopecia were found to have a medical cause for pruritus, with only 10% of cats having a primary diagnosis of psychogenic alopecia without an associated medical cause. In the same study, 14% of cats were diagnosed with a combination of psychogenic alopecia and a medical etiology for pruritus. Adverse food reaction was the most common medical cause of clinical signs with other causes including atopy, flea allergy dermatitis, parasitic dermatosis, bacterial dermatosis, and hyperthyroidism.[22] Other medical problems that should be excluded are anal gland disease, GI parasites, metabolic disease, and viral disease. Behavioral "rule outs" include boredom, attention-seeking behavior, displacement behavior (a normal behavior performed out of context), and compulsive disorder.

Grooming has been shown to activate an area of the brain associated with compulsive disorders.[56] In one study, owners identified environmental stresses that initiated or exacerbated psychogenic alopecia in their cats,[35] but in another study, most owners were not able to associate the onset of overgrooming with a specific triggering event.[31]

In a study investigating compulsive disorders, the most common category for cats was excessive grooming or self-mutilation, with 16 of 23 cats presenting with these symptoms.[34] Nine of 736 (1.2%) cats visiting the Animal Behavior Clinic at Cornell University from 1991 to 2001 were diagnosed with excessive grooming behavior.[46] The most common location for overgrooming is the caudal half of the body, especially the medial thigh and ventral abdomen.[35,48]

The first step in treating cats with excessive grooming is to identify and treat all contributing medical problems. Even when the cause is behavioral, a mechanical barrier (such as an Elizabethan collar) may be necessary to prevent excessive grooming if the animal is causing self-trauma while environ-

mental and behavioral modification is implemented. Environmental enrichment and mental stimulation are also important. Ways to enrich the environment and avoid boredom include food-dispensing toys, puzzle boxes, bird feeders outside of windows, crickets for the cat to hunt, scheduled play sessions with the owner, clicker training, playing with wand-type toys, fetch games, and walks outside on a harness or in a pet stroller. Toys can be rotated to keep them interesting. Any contributing anxieties should be treated with appropriate behavior modification.

Long-term antianxiety medications, specifically those that enhance serotonin (e.g., fluoxetine and clomipramine), are an integral part of treating compulsive disorders. The most studied medication for treatment of psychogenic alopecia is clomipramine. Retrospective studies and a case report have found clomipramine to be an effective treatment for psychogenic alopecia.[32,35,54,57] However, a prospective study failed to show significant changes in the number of grooming bouts, hair regrowth, and degree of alopecia in cats receiving clomipramine compared to those receiving placebo.[31] In one of the retrospective studies, three owners of cats receiving clomipramine reduced stresses in the environment. When clomipramine was discontinued, excessive grooming did not return in these cats.[35] This demonstrates that rather than relying solely on antianxiety medications, environmental modification may be the most important intervention for many patients. Amitriptyline, naloxone, and haloperidol have also been shown to be effective, but amitriptyline has more side effects than clomipramine, and naloxone and haloperidol are only available by injection, making delivery of these medications difficult.[35,53]

Pica and Wool Sucking

Pica is the ingestion of nonfood items with wool sucking being a form of pica, in which the cat sucks on the material but may not ingest it. Medical problems including nutritional deficiencies, diseases of the GI, oral, metabolic, and central nervous systems as well as restrictive diets, electrolyte imbalances, toxins, and conditions leading to polyphagia should be ruled out but are uncommon. Behavioral differential diagnoses include boredom, play or exploratory behavior, attention-seeking behavior, displacement behavior, and compulsive disorder. Cats with compulsive pica will seek out the item(s) whenever possible. Pets with other causes of pica may consume the items on a less frequent basis and may not consume the item every time they have access.

One small study of 23 cats with compulsive disorders found that 26% were diagnosed with pica of a nonfood item.[34] Wool sucking is the most common form of pica. A survey of pet owners found that wool was the fabric of choice with 93% of cats that sucked, chewed, and/or consumed items choosing this material. Other reported fabrics included cotton (64%) and synthetics (54%). Rubber or plastic materials were involved in 22% of cases (e.g., electrical insulation, rubber bands, and baby pacifiers) and paper or cardboard in 8% of cases. Most cases involved two or more types of materials. When all forms of pica were analyzed together, the researchers found that pica was most likely to appear during the first year of life and over 80% of the cats were Burmese, Siamese, or crosses of those breeds.[49] In a study by Overall and Dunham, Siamese cats were commonly diagnosed with pica involving sucking, chewing, or ingestion of fabrics. All cats that ingested fabric were Siamese.[34]

Treatment for pica is important to prevent repeated foreign body surgeries and damage to expensive household items. Although all medical problems should be treated, behavior and environmental modification should also be implemented concurrently. Items that the cat consumes should diligently be put away, out of the cat's reach. If specific items are preferred, they can be made undesirable by using an aversive taste (e.g., bitter apple or hot sauce). The owner should be counseled that aversions are specific to each individual cat and that if the taste is not aversive to their cat, ingestion of the material may still occur. Enrichment is also important, especially those types that focus on oral activities, such as food-dispensing toys. Some cats can be clicker trained to drop and leave items on command. Other items that are safer for the cat to consume can be provided (e.g., compressed rawhide, cat grass). Adding roughage and fiber to the diet has been suggested as a possible treatment. Any contributing anxieties should be treated with appropriate behavior modification techniques. Long-term antianxiety medications, specifically those that enhance serotonin (e.g., fluoxetine and clomipramine), are an integral part of treating compulsive disorders. In many cases, if the medication is effective, the cat must remain on it for years, even lifelong, for control of the problem. One study looking at all compulsive disorders together found that when medications were withdrawn, all cats relapsed and drug treatment was restarted.[34]

SUMMARY

Anxiety and fear-related disorders are underdiagnosed in our feline patients. Diagnosis is made based on examining the behavior and body postures of the cat in response to fear- and anxiety-eliciting stimuli. Treatment consists of environmental management, behavior modification including SD/CC, and antianxiety medications when appropriate. Identifying and offering treatment options for fearful and anxious patients helps to improve the human-animal bond and decrease behavior-related relinquishment and euthanasia.

References

1. Sylvers P, Lilienfeld SO, LaPrairie JL: Differences between trait fear and trait anxiety: Implications for psychopathology. *Clin Psych Rev* 31:122–137, 2011.
2. Öhman A: Fear and anxiety: overlaps and dissociations. In Lewis M, Haviland-Jones JM, Barrett LF, editors: *Handbook of emotions*, New York, 2010, The Guilford Press, pp 709–729.
3. American Psychiatric Association: *Diagnostic and statistical manual of mental disorders*, ed 5, Washington DC, 2013, American Psychiatric Association.
4. Epstein S: The nature of anxiety with an emphasis upon its relationship to expectancy. In Spielberger CD, editor: *Anxiety: current trends in theory and research*, vol 2, New York, 1972, Academic Press, pp 291–337.
5. Blanchard DC, Blanchard RJ: Innate and conditioned reactions to threat in rats with amygdaloid lesions. *J Comp Physiol Psychol* 81:281–290, 1972.
6. LeDoux JE, Cicchetti P, Xagoraris A, et al: The lateral amygdaloid nucleus: sensory interface of the amygdala in fear conditioning. *J Neurosci* 10:1062–1069, 1990.
7. LeDoux JE, Iwata J, Cicchetti P, et al: Differences projections of the central amygdaloid nucleus mediate autonomic and behavioral correlates of conditioned fear. *J Neurosci* 8:2517–2529, 1988.
8. Edinger KL, Frye CA: Intrahippocampal administration of androgen receptor agonist, flutamide, can increase anxiety-like behavior in intact and DHT-replaced mail rats. *Horm Behav* 50:216–222, 2006.
9. Walker DL, Davis M: Anxiogenic effects of high illumination levels assessed with the acoustic startle paradigm. *Biol Psychiatry* 42:461–471, 1997.
10. Bear MF, Connors BW, Paradiso MA: *Neuroscience exploring the brain*, ed 3, Baltimore, MD, 2007, Lippincott Williams & Wilkins.
11. Notari L: Stress in veterinary behavioural medicine. In Horwitz DF, Mills DS, editors: *BSAVA manual of canine and feline behavioural medicine*, ed 2, Gloucester, 2009, British Small Animal Veterinary Association, pp 136–145.
12. Carlson NR: *Physiology of behavior*, ed 10, Boston, 2010, Allyn & Bacon.
13. Uno H, Tarara R, Else JG, et al: Hippocampal damage associated with prolonged and fatal stress in primates. *J Neurosci* 9:1705–1711, 1989.
14. Sapolsky RM: *Stress, the aging brain and the mechanisms of neuron death*, Cambridge, MA, 1992, MIT Press.
15. Thaker PH, Han LY, Kamat AA, et al: Chronic stress promotes tumor growth and angiogenesis in a mouse model of ovarian carcinoma. *Nat Med* 12:939–944, 2006.
16. Dybdall K, Strasser R, Katz T: Behavioral differences between owner surrender and stray domestic cats after entering an animal shelter. *Appl Anim Behav Sci* 104:84–94, 2007.
17. Seksel K: Preventing behavior problems in puppies and kittens. *Vet Clin North Am Small Anim Pract* 38:971–982, 2008.
18. McCune S: The impact of paternity and early socialization on the development of cat's behaviour to people and novel objects. *Appl Anim Behav Sci* 45:109–124, 1995.
19. Turner DC, Feaver J, Mendl M, et al: Variation in domestic cat behaviour towards humans: a paternal effect. *Anim Behav* 34: 1890–1892, 1986.
20. Reisner IL, Houpt KA, Erb HN, et al: Friendliness to humans and defensive aggression in cats: The influence of handling and paternity. *Physiol Behav* 55:1119–1124, 1994.
21. Hoyumpa A, Rhodan I, Brown M, et al: AAFP-AAHA feline life stage guidelines. *J Feline Med Surg* 12:43–54, 2010.
22. Waisglass SE, Landsberg GM, Yager JA, et al: Underlying medical conditions in cats with presumptive psychogenic alopecia. *J Am Vet Med Assoc* 228:1705–1709, 2006.
23. Mills MS: Training and learning protocols. In Horwitz DF, Mills DS, editors: *BSAVA manual of canine and feline behavioural medicine*, ed 2, Gloucester, 2009, British Small Animal Veterinary Association, pp 49–64.
24. Frank DF, Erb HN, Houpt KA: Urine spraying in cats: presence of concurrent disease and effects of a pheromone treatment. *Appl Anim Behav Sci* 61:263–272, 1999.
25. Mills DS, Mills CB: Evaluation of a novel method for delivering a synthetic analogue of feline facial pheromone to control urine spraying by cats. *Vet Rec* 149:197–199, 2001.
26. Ogata N, Takeuchi Y: Clinical trial of a feline pheromone analogue for feline urine marking. *J Vet Med Sci* 63:157–161, 2001.
27. Dramard V, Kern L, Hofmans J, et al: Clinical efficacy of L-theanine tablets to reduce anxiety-related emotional disorders in cats: a pilot open-label clinical trial. In *Proceedings of the 6th International Veterinary Behaviour*

Meeting & European College of Veterinary Behavioural Medicine-Companion Animals European Society of Veterinary Clinical Ethology, 2007, pp 114–115.

28. Beata C, Beaumont-Graff E, Coll V, et al: Effect of alpha-casozepine (Zylkene) on anxiety in cats. *J Vet Behav* 2:40–46, 2007.

29. Hart BL, Kelly C, Tynes T, et al: Control of urine marking by use of long-term treatment with fluoxetine or clomipramine in cats. *J Am Vet Med Assoc* 226:378–382, 2005.

30. Pryor PA, Hart BL, Cliff KD, et al: Effects of a selective serotonin reuptake inhibitor on urine spraying behavior in cats. *J Am Vet Med Assoc* 219:1557–1561, 2001.

31. Mertens PA, Torres S, Jessen C: The effects of clomipramine hydrochloride in cats with psychogenic alopecia: a prospective study. *J Am Anim Hosp Assoc* 42(5):336–343, 2006.

32. Seksel K, Lindeman MJ: Use of clomipramine in the treatment of anxiety-related and obsessive-compulsive disorders in cats. *Aust Vet J* 76(5):317–321, 1998.

33. King JN, Steffan J, Heath SE: Determination of the dosage of clomipramine for the treatment of urine spraying in cats. *J Am Vet Med Assoc* 225(6):881–887, 2004.

34. Overall KL, Dunham AE: Clinical features and outcome in dogs and cats with obsessive-compulsive disorder: 126 cases (1989-2000). *J Am Vet Med Assoc* 221:1028–1033, 2002.

35. Sawyer LS, Moon-Fanelli AA, Dodman NH: Psychogenic alopecia in cats: 11 cases (1993-1996). *J Am Vet Med Assoc* 214:71–74, 1999.

36. Center SA, Elston TH, Rowland PH, et al: Fulminant hepatic failure associated with oral administration of diazepam in 12 cats. *J Am Vet Med Assoc* 209:618–625, 1996.

37. Crowell-Davis SL, Murray T: *Veterinary psychopharmacology*, ed 1, Ames, IA, 2006, Blackwell.

38. Buffington T, Westropp J, Chew D, et al: Clinical evaluation of multimodal environmental modification (MEMO) in the management of cats with idiopathic cystitis. *J Feline Med Surg* 8:261–268, 2006.

39. Spinks I: *Bayer Veterinary care usage study III: feline findings*: <http://www.bayerdvm.com/show.aspx/news-release-bvcus-iii-feline-findings>. (Accessed June 10, 2015.)

40. Rodan I, Sundahl E, Carney H, et al: AAFP and ISFM feline-friendly handling guidelines. *J Feline Med Surg* 11:364–375, 2011.

41. Yin S: *Low stress handling, restraint, and behavior modification of dogs and cats*, Davis, CA, 2009, CattleDog.

42. Catalyst Council: *Cats and carriers: friends not foes*: <http://www.catalystcouncil.org/resources/health_welfare/cat_carrier_video/>. (Accessed June 10, 2015.)

43. Wells DL, Graham L, Hepper PG: The influence of auditory stimulation on the behaviour of dogs housed in a rescue shelter. *Anim Welfare* 11:385–393, 2002.

44. Crowell-Davis SL, Curtis TM, Knowles RJ: Social organization in the cat: a modern understanding. *J Feline Med Surg* 6:19–28, 2004.

45. Schwartz S: Separation anxiety syndrome in cats: 136 cases (1991-2000). *J Am Vet Med Assoc* 220:1445–1452, 2002.

46. Denenberg S, Landsberg GM, et al: A comparison of cases referred to behaviorists in three different countries. In Mills D, Levine E, Landsberg GM, et al, editors: *Current issues and research in veterinary behavioral medicine*, West Lafayette, IN, 2005, Purdue University Press, pp 56–62.

47. Bamberger M, Houpt KA: Signalment factors, comorbidity, and trends in behavior diagnoses in dogs: 1,644 cases (1991-2001). *J Am Vet Med Assoc* 229:1591–1601, 2006.

48. Beaver BV: *Feline behavior: a guide for veterinarians*, ed 2, St Louis, 2003, Saunders.

49. Bradshaw JWS, Neville PF, Sawyer D: Factors affecting pica in the domestic cat. *Appl Anim Behav Sci* 52:373–379, 1997.

50. Gispen WH, Wiegant VM: Opiate antagonists suppress ACTH(1-24)-induced excessive grooming in the rat. *Neurosci Lett* 2:159–164, 1976.

51. Aloyo VJ, Spruijt B, Zwiers H: Peptide-induced excessive grooming in the rat: the role of opiate receptors. *Peptides* 4:833–836, 1983.

52. Zwiers H, Aloyo VJ, Gispen WH: Behavioral and neurochemical effects of the new opioid peptide dynorphin-(1-13): comparison with other neuropeptides. *Life Sci* 28:2545–2551, 1981.

53. Willemse T, Mudde M, Josephy M, et al: The effect of haloperidol and naloxone on excessive grooming behavior of cats. *Eur Neuropsychopharmacol* 4:39–45, 1994.

54. Eckstein RA, Hart BL: The organization and control of grooming in cats. *Appl Anim Behav Sci* 68:131–140, 2000.

55. Landsberg G, Hunthausen W, Ackerman L: *Behavior problems of the dog and cat*, ed 3, London, 2013, Saunders/Elsevier.

56. Fornal CA, Metzler CW, Marrosu F, et al: A subgroup of dorsal raphe serotonergic neurons in the cat is strongly activated during oral-buccal movements. *Brain Res* 716:123–133, 1996.

57. Swanepoel N, Lee E, Stein DJ: Psychogenic alopecia in a cat: response to clomipramine: clinical communication. *J S Afr Vet Assoc* 69:22, 1998.

Feline Aggression Toward People

Jeannine M. Berger

Aggression toward people is a common feline behavior problem, and broad categories include fear-related, play-related, petting-induced, redirected, and pain-related aggression. Choosing the right personality in a feline companion, proper socialization of kittens, as well as understanding feline-specific needs are crucial to prevent or treat human-directed aggression. Treatment of human-directed aggression should combine management strategies, behavior modification, and in some cases medication.

EPIDEMIOLOGY

Understanding Aggression: Physiology of Aggression

Aggression is not an antisocial behavior but one that serves multiple social and ethological functions. For example, territorial or defensive aggression is a natural defense against an intruder into one's territory; it provides defense of resources, the animal itself, or its offspring. Another form of aggression is predatory behavior, which is considered to be different from other forms of aggression and is often not classified as an aggressive behavior. The distinction between defense and predation has been confirmed by neuroanatomical and pharmacological findings and discussed by other authors.[1,2] Stalking of a prey object followed by biting the target often precedes the quiet predatory attack in natural settings. On the other hand, defensive aggression was originally described in 1943 by Hess and Brugger[3] as "affective *Abwehr*" and includes changes in body language, such as arching the back, retraction of the ears, piloerection, opening the mouth, and baring the teeth in addition to marked pupillary dilation and vocalization—all signs of high emotional arousal.

Although stress has been recognized as a major element in aggression in humans, exactly how stress mechanisms interact during feline aggression is poorly understood. In rats, plasma corticosteroids rise quickly and even before aggressive behavior can be observed.[4,5] Additional studies have shown that injections of corticosteroids into the hypothalamus of a hamster facilitate aggression. The hypothalamic-pituitary-adrenal axis is activated by behavioral responses and is strongly dependent on the behavior of the "opponent."[6] Sudden stressors often precede aggressive behaviors and can lead to escalation of violent behavior under stressful conditions.[7] It is important to keep this in mind when addressing human-directed aggression by cats. A cat might view the human as the "opponent," or threat, and therefore a stressful environment or the presence of a person will activate the physiological stress response and lead to aggression toward humans.

Differential Diagnoses: Medical or Psychological?

Pathological reasons for aggression are more common in cats than in dogs.[8] Underlying medical problems can exacerbate aggression and need to be ruled out first. Medical problems can lead to irritable, pain-induced, or truly pathological aggression; a detailed medical workup based on clinical signs is of utmost importance when diagnosing and treating any form of aggression. The minimum medical database for behavior-related problems includes a complete blood count, chemistry profile, total serum thyroxine, and a urinalysis with urine culture. Further diagnostics might be needed and depend on the problem list. For a list of medical differential diagnoses for aggression,[9] refer to Table 91-1. External triggers (e.g., people, animals, inanimate objects, noises, smells) can psychologically influence the aggression.

HISTORY AND CLINICAL SIGNS

History Taking

Taking a complete history from the owner is crucial in veterinary medicine in general, but it is especially important with regard to behavior problems. There are no laboratory tests to help determine trigger(s), threshold, and/or motivation for aggression problems, and to aid in arriving at the diagnosis. Therefore, a detailed history coupled with skilled observation techniques is required. Home videos and/or pictures and the veterinarian's observations during the examination will allow a narrowing of the differential diagnoses. To aid in this process, owners should be encouraged to fill out a specifically designed behavior questionnaire prior to the appointment. A questionnaire should ask about the pet's environment, including all other pets in the home, lifestyle, family members, visitors, a daily schedule, and detailed information about the presenting complaint and any other behavioral issues, including litter box habits. Reactions to multiple aggression and anxiety-eliciting stimuli (e.g., people, animals, noises, objects, and handling) should be detailed. Information

Table 91-1 — Medical Differential Diagnoses for Aggression

Origin	Disease
Infectious diseases	Viral: Rabies, pseudorabies, feline immunodeficiency virus, feline infectious peritonitis Bacterial: Brain abscess Protozoal: *Toxoplasma gondii* Parasites: Feline ischemic encephalopathy caused by *Cuterebra* spp.
Nutritional deficiencies	Thiamine Tryptophan
Masses	Granulomatous meningoencephalitis (rare in cats) Neoplasia (primary central nervous system or metastatic disease)
Toxins	Lead, zinc phosphate, organophosphates, marijuana, and illegal drugs
Encephalopathies	Hepatic, feline ischemic encephalopathy
Congenital	Lissencephaly, hydrocephalus
Hormonal	Hyperthyroidism, corticosteroid administration, and sex hormones
Trauma	Cranial injury or pain
Other	Seizures, changes in sensory input (vision and auditory), dermatological conditions (e.g., allergic skin disease), hyperesthesia, hypersensitivity to touch, and allodynia

Horwitz DF, Neilson JC: Aggression: medical differentials. In *Canine & feline behavior*, Ames, IA, 2007, Blackwell, pp 179-185.

should include what the cat and owner were doing before the episode, during the episode, and afterward. If they can be safely obtained, video of the aggressive episodes or feline body postures can be very useful to arrive at a diagnosis. Even video taken when the owner believes the cat is calm can be elucidating. Additionally, video of the environment may help determine if the environment is providing for the cat's needs. Because owners of problem pets are in crisis, learning the owner's point of view and understanding how the owner feels about the situation and the problem behavior is also important. History taking should also include a discussion of the owner's expectations for change, success, and tolerance for possible ongoing aggressive behavior even if greatly reduced. Guidelines for behavior history collection are available elsewhere,[10,11] and examples of detailed history forms are accessible on the websites of most diplomates of the American College of Veterinary Behaviorists (http://www.dacvb.org).

Clinical Signs

The ethogram of feline aggression directed toward humans can look very similar regardless of the motivation; hence, the importance of detail in the history and observations. As a veterinarian, one does not need to see the behavior in action to successfully address and treat the behavior problem. However, one needs to understand when the aggression occurs (threshold) and what actions (triggers) precede the aggression. The question of motivation and triggers can be answered by the circumstances in which the behavior occurs (Table 91-2), and changes in body language can help practitioners to make a diagnosis.[12] Practitioners should compare the patient's behaviors with stress-induced behaviors and scores, as well as pain-induced behaviors and scores as part of the diagnostic plan.[13,14]

DIAGNOSTIC CATEGORIES

Fear-Based Aggression

Fear responses are a combination of physiological and psychological aspects. Cats with fear-based aggression toward humans view humans as a threat. The triggers can include tactile, visual, auditory, and olfactory stimuli from humans. This form of aggression can be seen in the home environment with familiar as well as unfamiliar people and is frequently seen in the shelter or at a veterinarian's office. Fear behaviors are triggered by the "flight or fight" response of the nervous system and are not under voluntary control. Any cat that feels threatened can become fearful and consequently display anxiety that increases aggressive behavior, often with overt warning signs but not always. Due to the physiological aspect, these cats can show signs of high arousal, such as tense body language, lowered body position, withdrawal, dilated pupils, ears flattened sideways, open mouth with hissing (Figures 91-1 and 91-2), and piloerection (Figure 91-3). When not given an opportunity to flee, the cat might attack in a defensive or even offensive manner. Most cats with this form of aggression display avoidance or freeze responses first, and overt attacks are their last resort or are the consequence of learned behavior. There is no age or breed predilection for this form of aggression.

Fear-based aggression can be within the range of normal cat behavior and is mostly determined by genetics and environmental factors. The subject of sociability toward humans is the topic of multiple studies, and results suggest that it is a multifactorial process. Some authors have found the importance of a "sensitive" period (2 to 7 weeks of age) for handling kittens[15] and later found that 40 minutes of handling per day during this period had a positive effect on how fast kittens approached humans and how long they could be held by a human.[16] However, others report a relationship to human handling continues to evolve throughout the first 4 months of life, and positive effects were detectable even at 1 year of age.[17,18] Most authors agree, however, that although handling does alter sociability of cats, the results are affected by the "personality" of the kitten. Other study results indicated that being part of a certain litter or having a certain sire influenced tractability but that handling or individual caging of kittens did not.[19] A summary of different cat

Table 91-2	Clinical Signs of Fear vs Predatory Aggression	
Clinical Signs	**Fear Aggression**	**Predatory Aggression**
Posture of head and body	Flat ears, pupils dilated, mouth can be open, hissing, or growling	Head low, prepared to pounce, legs under the body in jumping position, ears forward, pupils narrow
Posture of body	Body leaning away, standing laterally, back arched	Stepping forward with body low to ground, quickly jumping and pouncing during attack
Tail position	Tail bristled or tucked under the body	Tail moving slowly back and forth, held horizontal during attack
Stalking with attack	No	Yes
Hissing, spitting	Yes	No
Growling	Yes	No
Swatting—scratching, no contact	Yes	Yes
Scratching with front paw	Yes	Yes
Scratching and kicking with hind paws	No	Yes
Biting, no breaking of skin	Yes	Yes
Biting, breaking of skin	Yes	Yes
Multiple bites, no breaking of skin	Rare	Yes
Multiple bites, breaking of skin	Rare	Yes
Circumstances		
Directed toward family members	Yes	Yes
Directed toward strangers	Yes	Rare
Location of cat	Away from action	Close to the action or behind a visual barrier

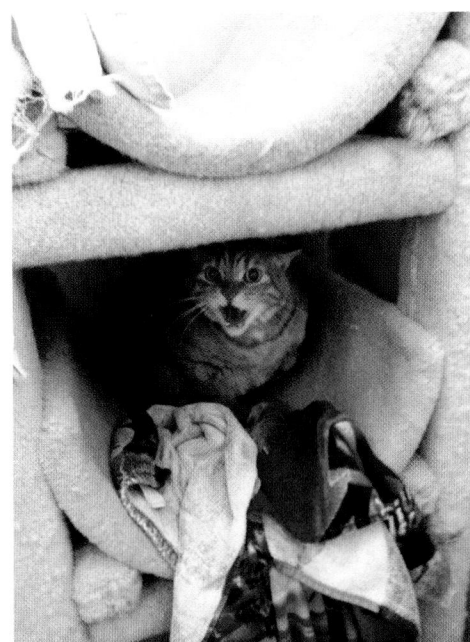

Figure 91-1: A cat with high fear arousal has a lowered tense body, slightly forward head position, dilated pupils, and open mouth with hissing.

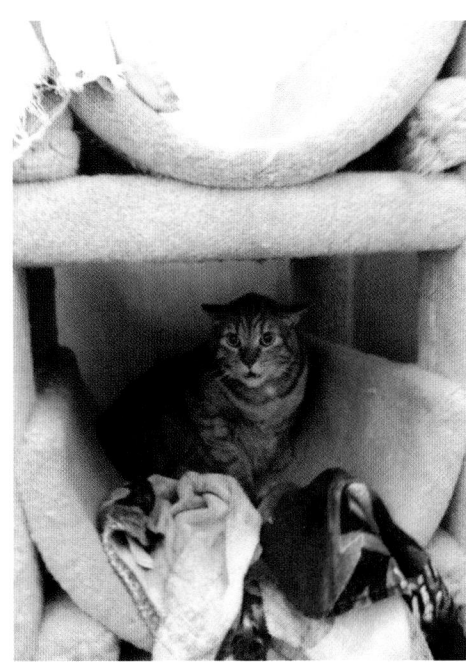

Figure 91-2: A fearful cat's body language displays withdrawal, tenseness, dilated pupils, and sideways flatting of the ears.

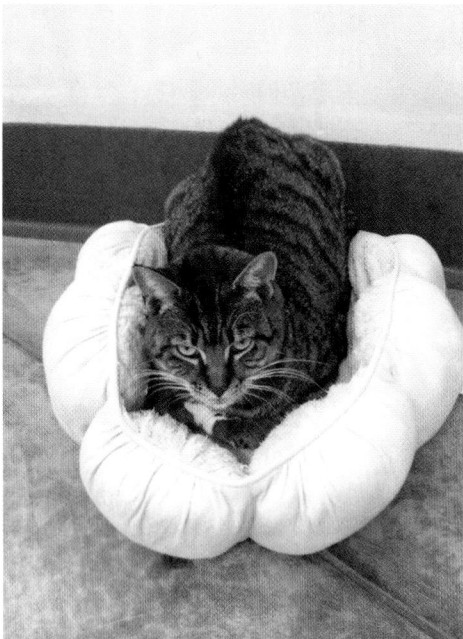

Figure 91-3: Piloerection displayed by raising of the hair over the back of the cat.

Table 91-3	Commonly Used Drugs and Dosages for Cats
Drug	**Dosage**
Class: Selective Serotonin Reuptake Inhibitors	
Fluoxetine	0.5 to 1 mg/kg PO every 24 hours
Paroxetine	0.25 to 0.5 mg/kg PO every 24 hours
Class: Tricyclic Antidepressants	
Clomipramine	0.25 to 0.5 mg/kg PO every 24 hours
Amitriptyline	2.5 to 5.0 mg/**cat** PO every 12 to 24 hours
Class: Azapirone Medications	
Buspirone	0.5 to 1 mg/kg PO every 12 hours
Class: Benzodiazepines	
Alprazolam	0.125 to 0.25 mg/kg PO every 8 to 24 hours
Lorazepam	0.03 to 0.08 mg/kg PO every 12 hours

PO, orally.

personality types was published by Bradshaw and colleagues;[20] also see Chapter 94.

The causes of fear-based aggression include a fearful personality, lack of early socialization and proper handling, lack of hiding opportunities to avoid the threatening stimulus, and medical causes (see Table 91-1).

Treatment Plan

The treatment plan for fear-based aggression must include recommendations for management, because bites can result in serious injuries. Owners should be taught how to implement safety and avoidance strategies, including watching for and avoiding triggers that elicit fearful body postures, and to never handle a fearful, aggressively aroused cat. If a fearful, aggressive cat needs to be moved, a crate can be placed close by to provide the only hiding place in the room. The owner(s) can then leave the room. When they come back later, the cat may have moved into the crate. In addition, external stressors (e.g., human interactions, noise, movement, novelties) need to be decreased as much as possible. Offering multiple hiding places and perches, providing forms of environmental enrichment that encourage play, and food-dispensing toys will also help a fearful cat. The food, water, and litter box should be close to hiding places, as a fearful cat might not want to leave a hiding place readily. However, it has been reported if the litter box, food, and resting place are less than 2 feet from each other, it can negatively affect eating behavior.[21]

Behavior modification includes desensitization and counter conditioning (DS/CC) with rewards (e.g., food) for relaxation while a person approaches and eventually handles the cat. Corrections or punishment are never appropriate for

a cat with fear aggression. Medications can prove helpful for some cases (Table 91-3).

Play-Related Aggression

Play-related aggression is the most commonly reported form of aggression toward owners in young indoor cats and involves unsolicited aggressive encounters varying from light scratches to hard, uninhibited skin-breaking bites. This form of aggression does not include overt warning signs as seen in fear or defensive aggression, likely because the underlying goal is to serve as predatory practice. This behavior usually occurs in animals less than 2 years of age, and there is no sex or breed predilection. Predatory play usually begins around 5 weeks of age and can last into adulthood.[13] Because aggression might also increase due to previous rough play experiences with humans, owners should be discouraged from play using hands or feet, but rather, should use appropriate wand or safe string toys.

Play-related aggression may arise when cats are left alone all day or when they lack outlets for appropriate play, exploratory behavior, and environmental enrichment options. Play postures include low body position, hiding, stalking, chasing, and pouncing. Owners frequently relate that play-related aggression occurs during early morning and evening hours, corresponding to natural hunting rhythms. Play-related aggression is probably a normal, but unwanted, behavior of cats.

Play-related aggression can be associated with a singly housed young cat, lack of appropriate play, lack of appropriate mental and physical stimulation, and physical restraint and confrontation during play attacks.

Treatment Plan

The treatment plan for play-based aggression must include recommendations for management, because even play-related bites can result in serious injuries. Owners should be educated on implementing environmental enrichment and how to play appropriately with their cat. For example, it is never appropriate to use hands and feet to play with the cat; wand-type toys should be used instead. Identifying body postures and triggers that lead to escalation of playful and hunting type behaviors is key to redirecting those behaviors before an attack happens. In addition, problem times can be easily managed with appropriate alternative active play options for the cat. However, a compatible feline or even canine companion can provide sufficient social or play interactions. In some cases, safe access to the outdoors with an appropriate enclosure or harness and leash can be considered.

Enriching the environment and offering multiple climbing options can serve as effective entertainment. Perches and window hammocks, toy rotation, access to a fish bowl or even a television, and bird feeders outside of the window can all enhance the environment. Foraging opportunities can increase desired activity and can be accomplished by hiding food, using food-dispensing toys or food puzzles, and using other interactive toys to keep the cat occupied. Interactive play with the owner should be scheduled using appropriate toys, such as wand and feather toys that bounce, flutter, or fly. Additional mental enrichment by teaching the cat tricks with clicker training can serve to direct the normal exploratory behaviors in a more appropriate manner.

Behavior modification includes counseling the owner never to actively escalate play behavior by rough play. All play should be ended before it escalates to aggressive behavior, and calm and relaxed behavior should be rewarded with attention and praise. Inappropriate play behavior exhibited by bites or scratches should result in all play ending. Inappropriate play behavior can be interrupted with a mild startling stimulus (e.g., a sudden noise) but it should never frighten the cat. Physical restraint or punishment is never appropriate. Playful cats need plenty of scheduled play interactions. Several 10-minute scheduled play sessions per day, especially in the morning and evening hours, are recommended.

Medication is rarely needed for play-related aggression, because this is a normal behavior and should be addressed with management.

Petting-Induced Aggression

Feline social behaviors include scent marking, allogrooming, and allorubbing, and these types of behaviors can be displayed toward humans as well.[22] Some cats use allogrooming or allorubbing to decrease stress and reduce conflict. Such cats may not enjoy petting and may respond with biting. It is important to understand that not all allogrooming or allorubbing behaviors directed toward humans are solicitations for affection. Prolonged petting or stroking a cat may also lead to overstimulation and thus consequent biting of the hands. There is no age or breed predilection for petting-induced aggression.

Petting-induced aggressive behavior can be within the normal range of cat behavior, but it can also be a defense mechanism to communicate that the cat had enough of the physical contact. Petting-induced aggression may be caused by extended or inappropriate petting and handling, lack of early socialization and proper handling, and medical reasons. Underlying pain and discomfort in response to touch in certain body areas must be ruled out.

Treatment Plan

Management, safety, and avoidance are essential to keep people safe from injuries in petting-induced aggression. It is important to keep the physical interactions below the threshold that triggers agitation and aggressive responses. Owners should stop petting and physical interaction when the cat displays a moving tail, twitching skin, ears held back, pupils dilated, or even gentle bites, because these are early warning signs of overstimulation. Some owners may be unable to read these signals and should avoid physical contact with their hands and use toys and brushes to interact with the cat instead to avoid injury. Owners should understand that individual differences and tolerances for physical interaction can vary for cats and adjust expectations to what is most comfortable for the cat.

Behavior modification includes determining alternative rewards for the cat (e.g., tasty treats, favorite toys), and then identifying the threshold for the aggressive behavior. Gradually, the cat is encouraged to accept longer periods of handling by delivering rewards for tolerance (DS/CC). Physical corrections are never appropriate for any form of aggression as they may only increase anxiety and worsen the aggression.

Medication may be needed if the problem is concurrent with other forms of aggression or anxiety but is not needed if merely decreasing physical interactions solves the problem.

Redirected Aggression

Redirected aggression occurs when the aggression is elicited by something that is not accessible, and the cat then directs aggressive intent toward a seemingly irrelevant but close-by target. Humans and other household cats are common victims of this form of aggression.[23] For example, redirected aggression may be triggered by smells that linger on the clothing of an owner who returns home after having petted a strange cat or dog. The new odor may create an aggressive response that is then redirected toward the owner. One author has described a fear-based response as the most common motivation for redirected aggression.[23] There is no age, breed, or sex predilection.

Redirected aggression is aggressive arousal elicited by any trigger other than the target and can include the sound, sight, or smell of other animals or people, as well as underlying pain and discomfort. Causes may include loud noises or interactions with other cats, other forms of aggression or fear, lack of socialization, and medical reasons.

Treatment Plan

Management, safety, and avoidance for redirected aggression include reading the cat's body language and being aware of potential triggers. Once a primary reason for the aggression has been identified, that trigger should then be avoided and the primary form of aggression addressed. Avoiding interactions, keeping physical interactions to a minimum, and giving the aggressively aroused cat some distance and time to calm are crucial steps to avoid injuries.

Behavior modification includes determining the primary form of aggression or underlying medical reasons and to treat those accordingly. Once a primary trigger has been identified, DS/CC can be applied; this technique is described later.

Medication may be needed depending on the level of anxiety and the primary form of aggression (see Table 91-3).

Territorial Aggression

Territorial aggression is a form of aggression in cats where valuable resources (e.g., territories, resting spots, food, mates, or litter boxes) are defended. This aggression occurs more commonly in sexually mature intact cats, and the motivation for this form of aggression can include fear, status or hierarchy conflicts, or sexual behavior. Territorial and status aggression can occasionally be directed toward humans but most likely will be directed toward other cats.[2] See Chapter 92 for more information about intercat aggression.

BASIC TREATMENT RECOMMENDATIONS FOR ALL TYPES OF AGGRESSION

To treat any form of aggressive behavior, a multifaceted treatment plan must be designed. The treatment plan for cats includes providing information on environmental enrichment, understanding the species-specific needs of cats, and providing specific instructions for each individual case based on a diagnosis. A complete and comprehensive treatment plan for most cases includes the design of a five-step program.[24] Specific recommendations must be discussed during the appointment and given to the client in writing.

Management: Safety and Avoidance

The first step includes a management program that is based on safety and avoidance of all triggers. Triggers that reliably cause the cat to behave aggressively should be identified during the appointment and avoided for a period of 4 to 6 weeks. This allows the pet to calm and cope with the situation. Reintroduction to the trigger(s) can occur at a later time in a step-by-step process called *desensitization*. It is important to understand and educate the client that if the aggressive behavior continues to take place, the cat cannot change its

behavior, because it is too emotionally aroused to learn anything new. If aggression results in the removal of the trigger, the cat is likely to repeat the behavior, creating an ongoing cycle that is destructive to the human-animal bond.

Improving the Pet-Owner Relationship

The second step of the plan provides direction to help build a better relationship between the owner and the cat. This can include recommendations and instructions on how to interact, play with, and train the cat. Indoor cats especially might need an active enrichment program provided by the owners. Training cats to perform certain behaviors can be fun for owners and cats alike if positive reinforcement techniques are used. Clicker training can provide mental and physical enrichment for any cat and improves the relationship with the owner by providing the cat with clear outcomes for desired behaviors.[25] When a cat consistently receives a reward for the proper response, such as getting attention for sitting on command, the cat is less likely to use less desired behaviors to get the owner's attention.

Environmental Changes and Tools

The third step involves demonstrating tools, such as play and environmental enrichment, which can help implement the designed behavior modification program.

Play can include active play with wand-like feather or string toys or fetch games with little balls or toy mice. Often, owners have to be shown creative ways to interact with their cat by providing information about what kind of toys to use, how to play with the cat properly, and which time of the day is best for play. Toys should be rotated frequently, and play should also include scheduled, regular active play between the owner and the cat.

Environment enrichment includes mental and physical stimulation for the indoor cat using interactive toys, food-dispensing toys, and creating an interesting and engaging environment. Many owners need assistance with designing an interesting and interactive home environment that includes vertical and horizontal space, access to windows and perches to rest, as well as hiding places. Owners can be taught how to create a safe place for the cat that avoids exposure to potential triggers and poisonous plants or toxins. Safe places allow the cat to escape threatening situations and create calmness. For more information on household enrichment, see Chapter 93.

Other tools that may be helpful to alleviate fear and aggression in some cases include the use of nutraceuticals, aromatherapy, pheromone therapy, regular nail trims, and the application of plastic nail caps.[26]

Psychopharmacology

The fourth step includes the use of psychopharmacology (see Table 91-3), which can help decrease overall anxiety. Medication should never be used without a diagnosis and without a comprehensive behavior modification plan in place.[27] The decision to use medications depends on many factors, such as diagnosis, availability and cost of the medication, ease of administration, and the owner's level of commitment and comfort with the medication. Medications are often prescribed for fear-related types of aggression to decrease anxiety and improve the cat's welfare. Because no medications are approved for use in cats for behavioral disorders in the United States, age-appropriate premedication laboratory testing (e.g., complete blood count, chemistry panel, urine analysis [with urine culture where appropriate], and total serum thyroxine) is prudent and when medication is used long term, yearly re-evaluations with a thorough physical examination and laboratory screening are advised.

Appropriate counseling of owners is essential and must include the extra-label usage, expectations, potential side effects, and the prolonged commitment that is required in most cases with the use of psychotropic medications. Additionally, owners may need help learning how to appropriately and safely administer medication to cats without injury to themselves.

Behavior Modification

The fifth step of behavior modification will be implemented after a period of safety and avoidance that allows the pet to become calm and more relaxed. By using steps one to four, anxiety should be reduced, enhancing the pet's ability to learn new tasks. Through the process of desensitization, the cat will be gradually reintroduced to the trigger(s) in a step-by-step fashion designed to make sure that the unwanted behavior does not recur. To change the emotional response of the animal and therefore lead to the change in motivation and behavior, highly rewarding stimuli, such as food or play, are used. This step is referred to as *counter conditioning*. Rewards are critical in activating the dopamine pathways to encourage the formation of new neuronal pathways and memories. Punishment techniques are never appropriate during DS/CC or at any time during treatment, because they can increase rather than decrease fear and anxiety.

Desensitization and counter conditioning are the major components in a behavior modification plan designed to associate a previously perceived negative stimulus with a more relaxed and calm emotional state and hopefully a new behavioral response.

A program for a cat with fear-based aggression includes the following steps:
- Determine the favored and desirable rewards for the cat (e.g., tasty treats, favorite toy).
- Establish the "safe" distance where the fearful cat can accept human presence and is comfortable eating the treats that are placed in front of it. At the beginning, this can be several feet away for some cats.
- The distance is then gradually decreased over a period of two to five brief sessions. The sessions should be repeated daily, and progress should be tracked. It is important that each session ends on a positive note.

- When an approach toward the cat does not elicit any signs of fear or aggression, it may be possible to directly give the cat rewards, such as food or treats, for calm and relaxed behavior.
- Eventually the process can include reaching toward and touching the cat.

Once handling can be tolerated and rewards are readily taken, multiple short (5 to 10 minute) positive interactions per day are recommended. Once the cat is no longer fearful and anticipates a positive outcome with the human and expects a food reward, training of certain behaviors can be implemented, such as sitting for a food reward or placement behaviors, such as going to a mat for a reward.

PROGNOSIS

The prognosis for each case has to be carefully evaluated and depends on the owner's compliance and adherence as well as patient response to the treatment plan. A prognosis may not be fully established until a few weeks into the treatment process. Owners might ask for recommendations for rehoming the patient, and this requires careful counseling. A shelter may deem cats with aggression directed toward humans as unadoptable, and owners will find it challenging to find a new home for an aggressive cat. To avoid liability issues, full disclosure of the behavior to the new owner is needed. Therefore, it might be necessary for the veterinarian to discuss the option of euthanasia for some severe cases of aggression or aggression in households where safety for people cannot be maintained. This might include homes with the elderly, immune-compromised individuals, or children who may not follow treatment plans or are at increased risk of injury or infections from cat bites and scratches. Veterinarians should discuss all treatment options with the client after having carefully evaluated and diagnosed the condition of the animal. It is crucial for the client to base such a difficult decision on the animal's welfare and human safety considerations. In cases where aggression is dangerous and severe, referral to a veterinary behavior specialist should be recommended. Euthanasia for behavioral reasons is the most difficult decision that an owner will have to make and can lead to feelings of self-blame or guilt. Counseling and comforting of the client before and after the euthanasia are needed. A good client-doctor relationship based on mutual respect and trust is necessary.

PROPHYLAXIS

Behavior problems are still the number one reason why animals are being surrendered to shelters, and aggression is the second most common behavior complaint seen at behavior specialty clinics. Prevention of aggression is therefore of utmost important. Early positive handling, proper socialization, and clear expectations and understanding of feline-specific behaviors are of great significance. Veterinarians are crucial in educating clients and providing new cat owners with information and guidance.

SUMMARY

Aggression toward people is a common behavior complaint, and the most common diagnoses are fear-related, play-related, petting-induced, redirected, and pain-related aggression. To address any form of aggressive behavior, a complete history is needed to reach a diagnosis, which is followed by

a multifaceted treatment plan. The treatment plan for aggression toward humans includes information on environmental enrichment and understanding the species-specific needs of cats. It should also include specific instructions for each individual and management recommendations based on the specific diagnosis. A complete and comprehensive treatment plan includes:

1. Management
2. Improving the human-animal interactions
3. Tools and enrichment for the home environment
4. Behavior modification
5. Medication (in some cases)

References

1. Siegel A, Roeling TA, Gregg TR, et al: Neuropharmacology of brain-stimulation-evoked aggression. *Neurosci Biobehav Rev* 23:359–389, 1999.
2. Overall KL: Undesirable, problematic, and abnormal feline behavior and behavioral pathologies. In Overall KL, editor: *Manual of clinical behavioral medicine for dogs and cats*, St Louis, 2013, Elsevier, pp 360–456.
3. Hess WR, Brugger M: Das subkortikale Zentrum der affectiven Abwehrreaktion [The subcortical center of the affective defense reaction]. *Helv Physiol Pharmacol Acta* 1:33–52, 1943.
4. Schuurman T: Hormonal correlates of agonistic behavior in adult male rats. *Prog Brain Res* 53:415–420, 1980.
5. Haller J, Barna I, Baranyi M: Hormonal and metabolic responses during psychosocial stimulation in aggressive and nonaggressive rats. *Psychoneuroendocrinology* 20:65–74, 1995.
6. Haller J, Kiem DT, Makara GB: The physiology of social conflict in rats: what is particularly stressful? *Behav Neurosci* 110:353–359, 1996.
7. Kruk MR, Halász J, Meelis W, et al: Fast positive feedback between the adrenocortical stress response and a brain mechanism involved in aggressive behavior. *Behav Neurosci* 118(5):1062–1070, 2004.
8. Reisner I: The pathophysiologic basis of behavior problems. *Vet Clin North Am Small Anim Pract* 21:207–224, 1991.
9. Horwitz DF, Neilson JC: Aggression: medical differentials. In *Canine & feline behavior*, Ames, IA, 2007, Blackwell, pp 179–185.
10. Landsberg G, Hunthausen W, Ackerman L: Behavior counseling and behavior diagnostics. In *Behavior problems of the dog and cat*, ed 3, St Louis, 2013, Elsevier, pp 65–73.
11. Overall KL: Basic history questionnaire—cats. In Overall KL, editor: *Manual of clinical behavioral medicine for dogs and cats*, St Louis, 2013, Elsevier, pp 547–557.
12. Bradshaw JWS, Casey RA, Brown SL: Communication. In *The behaviour of the domestic cat*, ed 2, Boston, 2012, CABI, pp 91–112.
13. Overall KL: Normal feline behavior and ontogeny. In Overall KL, editor: *Manual of clinical behavioral medicine for dogs and cats*, St Louis, 2013, Elsevier, pp 312–359.
14. Brondani JT, Luna SP, Padovani CR: Refinement and initial validation of a multidimensional composite scale for use in assessing acute postoperative pain in cats. *Am J Vet Res* 72:174–183, 2011.
15. Karsh EB, Turner DC: The human-cat relationship. In Turner DC, Bateson P, editors: *The domestic cat: the biology of its behavior*, Cambridge, MA, 1988, Cambridge University Press, pp 159–177.
16. Turner DC: The human-cat relationship. In Turner D, Batson P, editors: *The domestic cat: the biology of its behaviour*, ed 2, Cambridge, MA, 2000, Cambridge University Press, pp 193–206.
17. Lowe S, Bradshaw JWS: Responses of cats to being held by an unfamiliar person. *Anthrozoos* 15:69–79, 2002.
18. Casey RA, Bradshaw JWS: The effects of additional socialisation for kittens in a rescue centre on their behavior and suitability as a pet. *Appl Anim Behav Sci* 114:196–205, 2008.
19. Reisner IR, Houpt KA, Erb HN, et al: Friendliness to humans and defensive aggression in cats: the influence of handling and paternity. *Physiol Behav* 55(6):1119–1124, 1994.
20. Bradshaw JWS, Casey RA, Brown SL: The cat-human relationship. In *The behaviour of the domestic cat*, ed 2, Boston, 2012, CABI, pp 161–174.
21. Bourgeois H, Elliot D, Marniquet P, et al: *Dietary preferences of dogs and cats. Focus Special Edition Royal Canin*, Paris, 2004, Aniwa Publishing.
22. Bradshaw JWS, Casey RA, Brown SL: Social behaviour. In *The behaviour of the domestic cat*, ed 2, Boston, 2012, CABI, pp 142–160.
23. Amat M, Manteca X, Le Brech S, et al: Evaluation of inciting causes, alternative targets, and risk factors associated with redirected aggression in cats. *J Am Vet Med Assoc* 233(4):586–589, 2008.
24. Bergman L, Gaskins L: Addressing any behavior problem. *Clinician's Brief* 11(5):79–82, 2013.
25. Karen Pryor Clicker Training *(website)*: <http://www.clickertraining.com/cat-training>. (Accessed June 10, 2015).
26. Beata C, Beaumont-Graff E, Coll V, et al: Effect of alpha-casozepine (Zylkene) on anxiety in cats. *J Vet Behav* 2:40–46, 2007.
27. Crowell-Davis SL, Murray T: *Veterinary psychopharmacology*, Oxford, 2006, Blackwell.

Intercat Aggression

Diane Frank

AGGRESSIVE AND AFFILIATIVE BEHAVIORS

Aggression

Borchelt and Voith described overt aggression directed to another cat as biting and scratching, as well as threats such as hissing, spitting, and growling.[1] Most aggressive events in cats involve a combination or alternation of offensive and defensive behaviors. Changes in offensive and defensive signals occur more precisely and rapidly in facial expressions than in body postures.[1] Laboratory studies carried out by Leyhausen led to the description of offensive behavior seen during tom cat duels.[2] The first sign of an attack is a threat in which the aggressor draws itself up high on all four limbs. The back is straight and slightly elevated caudally. Piloerection along the middle of the back accentuates this slope and the base of the tail continues along this line briefly. Then, the tail is held stiffly and almost perpendicular to the ground. The distal end may twitch back and forth. The head is stretched forward, the pupils are not particularly dilated, and the ears are raised upward and outward (swiveled). The cat stares at its opponent, approaches slowly, vocalizes, and swallowes intermittently. Then, wrestling, biting, rolling, scratching, and clawing (active aggression[3]) may alternate with the previously described threat behaviors (passive aggression;[3] Figure 92-1). Although castration can decrease fighting between toms, in one study, a small percentage of castrated males (four out of 33 cats or 12%) had no behavioral change following castration and still engaged in fights.[4] Similar threats (e.g., posture, facial expression, and staring) can also be observed in housecats. They are often silent, without piloerection and thus are generally missed by owners. The threatened cat can respond defensively (hissing) to this silent aggression, leading the owners to blame the wrong cat as the aggressor.

Leyhausen also described defensive behavior in cats.[2] The cat will press itself close to the ground, shrink, and draw its head in as far as possible. Its ears are pulled down sideways, sometimes completely flat, thus becoming invisible when the cat is viewed from the front. The pupils are dilated. If the attacker continues to approach, the defensive cat rolls over on its back. The main component of defense is a paw blow. The defensive cat may also spit or wail.[5] If a forepaw blow is insufficient to stop the attacker's advance, the defensive cat grabbs the opponent with the forepaws. The attacked cat bites and vigorously scratches at the opponent's underside with the hindlimbs. The defensive posture, therefore, is not a submissive gesture, because it does not inhibit the attacker and the attacked animal does not remain passive in the face of additional threats. In fact, the attacked cat defends itself and in some cases counterattacks.[2] Figure 92-2 shows sequential changes in body language and facial expression seen within one encounter between two neutered males. Passive aggression alternates with active aggression.

Diagnostic Classification of Aggression

Aggression in the household setting has been categorized within various diagnostic classification schemes. With regard to intercat aggression, the types described, depending on authors, have included play behavior,[6] play aggression,[7,8] fear or defensive aggression,[6,7,9] social or dominance aggression,[8] territorial aggression,[7-9] intermale aggression,[9,10] and redirected aggression.[6,7,9] Diagnostic classification is based on interpretation and is not always necessary for treatment.[1] In fact, a treatment plan can be recommended based on appropriateness of the behavior and the severity and frequency of the aggressive events. Aggression can be categorized as appropriate or inappropriate and as mild, moderate, or severe, which is the author's personal preference (see Clinical Evaluation of Aggression).

Play behavior may be interpreted as aggressive behavior by another household cat if it is intense.[6] *Play aggression* or play-related aggression occurs if play is excessively rough or persistent. It may cause a problem if a very active cat pounces regularly on a less playful or even fearful cat, resulting in aggressive responses by the recipient.[7] Mild aggression may be seen during play and can be normal as long as this aggression leads to play cessation that the cats initiate themselves.[8] Intervention is required if one of the cats is being injured or is continuously attempting to escape.

Fear or defensive aggression can occur when two cats in the household that previously got along well accidently become aggressive toward each other. This problem may initially be triggered by a frightening event, such as a bookshelf falling. Both cats become startled, present piloerection, and assume defensive postures. When they see each other, they react as if the other is about to attack. Each cat acts aggressively and a fight ensues. Neither of the cats will seek the other one out, but if they encounter each other, both will act startled and attack. Thereafter, they exhibit aggressive behaviors when they see each other.[11]

In *social or dominance aggression*,[8,12] the behaviors, posture, and facial expression of the dominant cat correspond to the

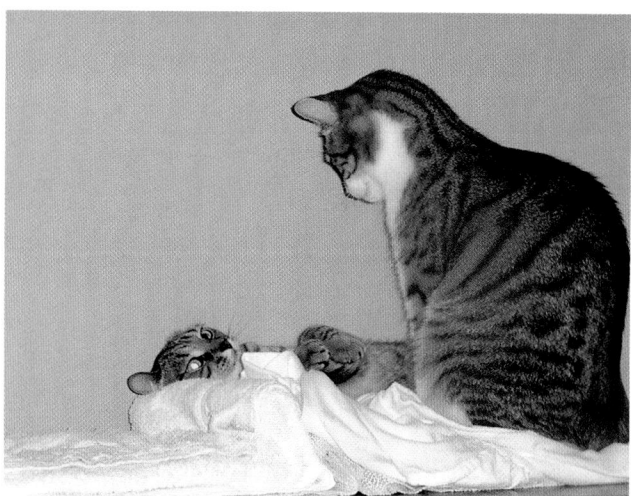

Figure 92-1: Passive aggression. The cat sitting upright is staring directly and thus silently threatening the other cat.

description of offensive aggression in toms by Leyhausen.[2] The behaviors, posture, and facial expression of the submissive cat correspond to Leyhausen's description of the defensive cat.[2] Not all veterinary behaviorists agree that the terms *dominant* and *submissive* apply to cats.

Territorial aggression has been defined by some authors as hissing and growling that progresses to swatting, chasing, relentless pursuit, and eventually results in attacks and fights.[11] Leyhausen described territorial aggression as a direct and rapid run toward the other cat along with a flurry of paw blows at the intruder.[2] His interpretation was that chases occurred only in purely territorial fights. He used as an example a queen protecting her young. However, it may be difficult in this example and others to determine the cat's true motivation (i.e., keep another cat at a safe or tolerable distance as opposed to being truly territorial). Attack and chase can in fact be the best form of self-defense. Other authors identify territorial aggression as a cat defending a specific site against another cat.[8] The same question remains: Is one cat trying to keep another cat at a safe (self-defense) or tolerable distance from itself (personal space), or is it being truly territorial of the location? Therefore, the diagnosis of territorial aggression is truly a matter of our interpretation of the cat's motivation. Borchelt and Voith report that the victim in those cases may become progressively afraid of the aggressor (possibly as a result of the severity of the attacks) and may hide, coming out only when the aggressive cat is not around.[11] Elimination problems may occur because the fearful cat is too afraid to leave the vicinity of its hiding place and find the litter box.

Intermale aggression was initially described by Leyhausen in the case of intact toms.[2] His descriptions of offensive and defensive behaviors apply to neutered cats as well.

Redirected aggression is reported when a cat cannot direct its aggression to the appropriate target and will redirect the aggression to an alternative target in the vicinity.[1] For example, if an indoor cat is threatening an outdoor cat through the

window, the threatening cat may attack a nearby inside cat. Redirected aggression can induce long-lasting social conflicts between household cats as described in one case report.[13] It can occur regardless of the type of aggression (intermale, territorial, fear-induced, or defensive).[11] In a retrospective study, *redirected aggression* was defined as aggression in which bites were uninhibited, attacks were difficult to stop, and aggressors typically stayed highly aroused long after the triggering event was over.[14] Presumptive redirected aggression was established whenever a primary inciting stimulus and an alternative target were clearly identified. Twenty-two episodes were studied. Body language description was recalled for 18 events. In 14 events, owners remembered the cat's posture with an arched lateral display, flattened ears, an inverted U-shaped tail, and piloerection, as well as hissing and high-pitched vocalization. These behaviors are compatible with high arousal. The other four owners described direct eye contact, constricted pupils, a direct gaze, and tail lashing. Chapman described the aggressive cat's behavior varying from hissing, spitting, growling, and pursuing without inflicting injury to serious attacks.[15] This publication focused on redirected aggression toward people, but cats exhibit the same range of behaviors when redirecting to another cat. The author noted that the cat's behavior was normal at all other times. Redirected aggression is not considered an abnormal behavior, but the severity may be excessive (causing injury) in some contexts.[15] The most commonly identified stimulus was the sight of or interaction with other cats, even if just visible through a window. Other stimuli included being in a strange environment (e.g., indoor cat being outdoors), high-pitched noises, visitors in the home, a dog in the house, and a peculiar odor. Some cats seemed to be aroused by more than one trigger or a combination of stimuli. Six of the 14 cats remained aroused for 30 minutes to several hours after a redirected attack,[15] indicating "increased reactivity" or arousal.

Prevalence of Aggression in Free-Roaming Cats

In one study conducted at a dairy farm over a period of more than 1 year with 10 to 11 mostly related free-roaming male and female cats, Laundré reported 202 aggressive encounters defined as striking at, or growling, of which 197 out of 202 (97.5%) occurred during milking sessions when the cats were being fed.[16] The sharp increase in aggression at those times was most likely a result of crowding close to the milk dish. These cats otherwise preyed on small rodents and birds. Up until 10 minutes prior to feeding, the cats spent most of their resting time in a communal area with very little contact of any type. Each cat seemed to maintain a personal space of approximately 0.5 meters (1.6 feet). In another study of approximately 300 dockyard cats in Portsmouth, United Kingdom, behavior of adult males over a 4-year span was recorded. Male aggression toward females was rare. A female in estrus could attract several toms, with up to six seen in attendance on one female. No fighting was observed among these waiting males. Females were frequently observed to behave aggressively toward males, but it was generally associated with a tom approaching an unreceptive early estrus

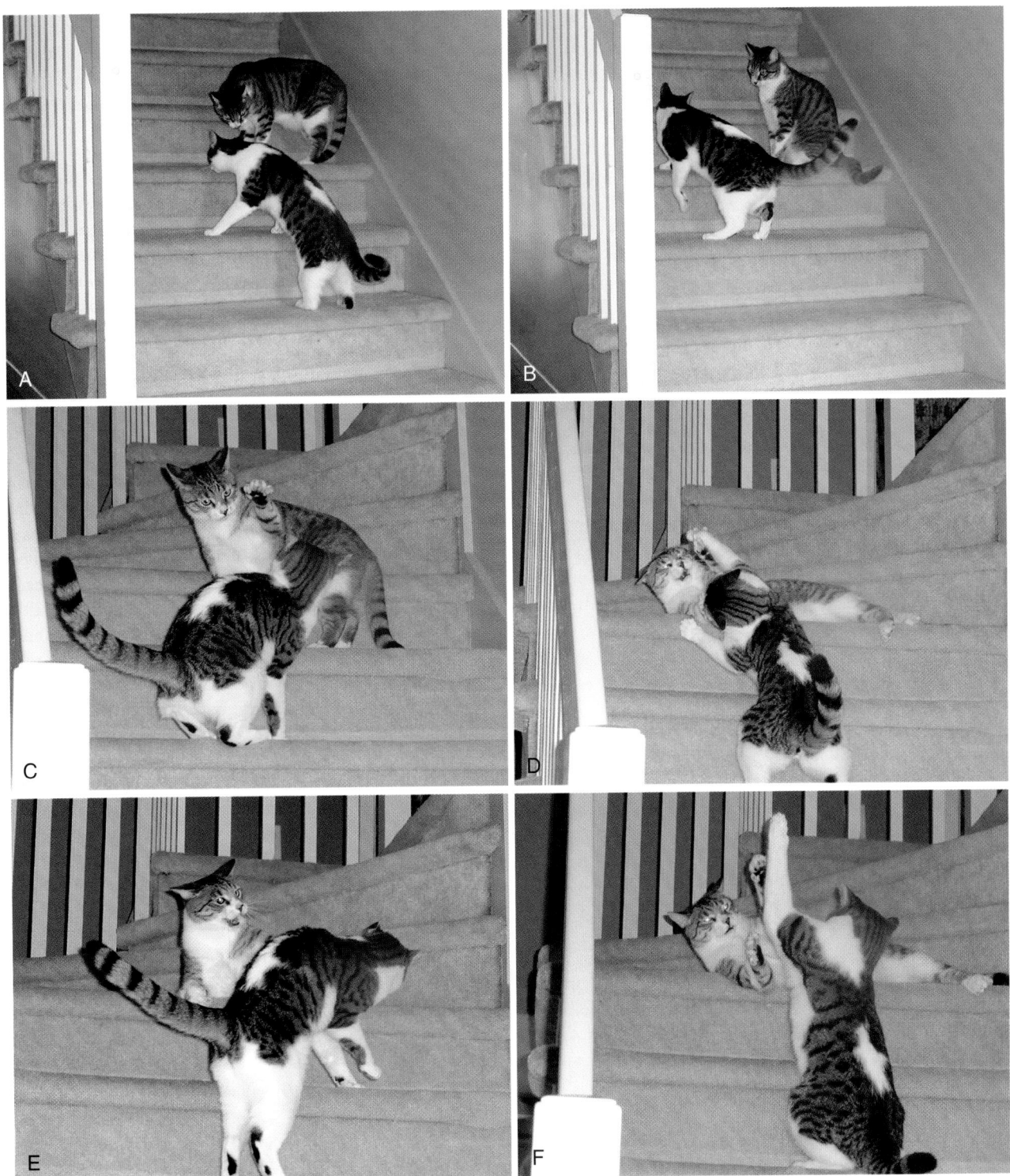

Figures 92-2: **A** to **F,** Sequential changes in body language and facial expression seen during one encounter between two neutered males. Passive aggression alternates with active aggression.

female. Agonistic interactions between adult males were generally ritualized threat postures and vocalizations. The author's description[5] of the body language is similar to Leyhausen's description[2] of offensive and defensive behaviors. Few fights between toms were observed, although some cats had wounds. An interaction resulting in one cat striking another cat occurred in only five of the 88 recorded agonistic events. In the dockyards, avoidance was the method used by toms to minimize aggression.

Natoli and De Vito studied 81 cats in a colony in Rome for a total of 315 hours.[17] They often observed a pair of animals copulating with other males calmly waiting their turn around the pair. Males that were waiting sometimes threatened each other (e.g., striking with a paw, assuming a "threatening position," hissing, or flattening ears), but they did not attack or chase one another. Threats given by the occasional male were so few that they could not be analyzed statistically. Nineteen male cats were observed mounting one female of the group. These males were subdivided into eleven "regular" males that invested a lot of time in courting behavior and eight "occasional" males that did not. For the "regular" males, urine spraying was positively correlated with threats received, amount of interference with copulation received (i.e., one male trying to push between the male and female that were copulating or even to mount the male mounting the female), and vocal duels. In another study of farm cats, Macdonald and colleagues reported aggression from one male of the group toward the three core group females.[18] The females never initiated those aggressive events. Females were aggressive to each other as well. Aggression usually consisted of mild rebuff as a consequence of an overly persistent approach. Aggression was thus mild and rare between the adult members of the core group (4.9% of 2358 observed interactions). The authors also reported that play was never observed between the male and the three females. In contrast, aggression toward out-of-group cats (both male and female) was more severe and represented a little more than half of the observed interactions (53.7% of 227) with these outsider cats. Sight of an out-of-group cat was sufficient to trigger aggression. Frequently, an attack by one of the core group female cats would result in the others joining in the aggressive event. The male always urine sprayed after these attacks.

Prevalence of Aggression in Owned Cats

Aggressive behavior in cats was the second most common behavioral complaint reported by cat owners 30 years ago.[1] In one study, 887 questionnaires were either completely or partially filled out by owners and generated data on incidence of aggressive behavior in pet cats.[11] Results showed that 80% hissed, 85% swatted, and 70% of cats fought with each other at least occasionally. When evaluated more closely, 34.4% of cats hissed, 43.1% swatted, and 28.5% fought once weekly or more. Aggression is a complex behavioral system that can be exhibited in a variety of situations and affected by multiple factors.[11] The context in which these behaviors occurred as well as the severity of the fights were not described. Some aggressive behaviors are part of normal communication between nonverbal individuals and therefore can be appropriate given the context.

A retrospective study by Blackshaw looked at 39 cats referred for behavioral inquiries over a 6-month period.[19] The most common complaint was aggression in 13 cats (33%), five of which were aggressive to cats in the same household, and one was aggressive to unfamiliar cats. Mugford also compiled information on behavioral problems seen in 100 cats.[20] Inappropriate urination and defecation were the most common complaint (31%), followed by fighting (26%), and spraying (23%). Another retrospective study showed that 64

of 179 cases (35.75%) did not have housesoiling as the primary complaint and that 23 of those cats (36%) had aggression as the presenting complaint.[10] The report did not specify if the target of aggression was another cat or a person for some of the diagnoses (e.g., fear-induced, play, or redirected) listed.

In 2006, a retrospective study on trends in behavior diagnoses in cats in the United States reported that 736 cats were presented for behavioral complaints between January 1991 and December 2001.[21] Of those, 185 (25%) were presented for intercat aggression. Cats could have up to three behavioral diagnoses, and the first three listed in the record were compiled for the purpose of the study.

Hart and Cooper did a survey to determine factors relating to urine spraying and fighting in prepubertally gonadectomized cats.[22] The authors reported that of 134 male cats, 44% engaged in fighting occasionally (once a month or less) or frequently (more than once a month) and of the 152 female cats, 30% fought occasionally or frequently. It is unclear how many of these cats were fighting with other household pets as opposed to outdoor cats or both. Context and severity of aggression were not detailed, and aggressive behaviors were not described (e.g., swatting versus biting). One factor examined was the presence of feline housemates and whether the housemates were of the same sex, opposite sex, or both. Males with female housemates fought significantly more than males with male housemates. Overall, male cats tended to fight more than female cats, although the difference was not significant. The authors also concluded that fighting was of the same order of magnitude in cats castrated between 6 and 10 months of age as those castrated after 12 months of age.

In an earlier survey conducted by Hart and Barrett, the effects of castration on fighting, roaming, and urine spraying were studied.[4] Of the 33 males cats presented for castration in adulthood because of behavioral issues, 10 were due to fighting, nine were due to fighting and roaming, nine were due to fighting and urine spraying, and five were due to fighting, roaming, and urine spraying. Over half of the males (53%) showed a pronounced and rapid decline (within 2 weeks of surgery) in fighting and 12 (35%) showed a gradual decline (significant reduction over a 2- to 6-month period). In five of the 14 cats with fighting and urine spraying, the rate of decline in fighting corresponded with the rate of decline in urine spraying.

Intercat aggression within households was examined retrospectively in a study to determine types of aggression, sex of the fighting pairs, and effectiveness of treatment.[23] Forty-eight cases of intercat aggression were studied. In 43 cases (28 males and 15 females), an aggressor and a victim were clearly identified. No additional information was given with regard to the other five cases. Anecdotally, some were unable to identify the aggressor, and in some cases, the wrong cat was accused of being the aggressor. The accused cat is seen hissing and considered the instigator, when in fact it is responding to a silent threat from the true aggressor. Information on the context of aggression, severity, and description of the behaviors was not reported. The 28 male aggressors victimized another male in 15 homes and a female in 13 homes. The 15 female aggressors fought with another female in 10 homes and with a male in five homes. Aggression was therefore equally likely to be directed toward a same sex or an opposite sex victim, unlike Hart and Cooper's finding.

Aggression in 60 households of strictly indoor cats was observed in seven of the female/female households (seven out of 20 [35%]), nine of the male/male households (nine out of 20 [45%]), and nine of the male/female households (nine out of 20 [45%]).[24] In 39 of 68 aggressive events, the approaching cat was the aggressor; and in 29 events, the approaching cat was the recipient. Some of these aggressive behaviors directed at the approaching recipient cat may have been normal communication. The initiator of the aggression was identified if it displayed any of the following behaviors first: piloerection, turning the ears toward the back of the head, flattening the ears, hissing, growling, noninhibited swat, and noninhibited bite and/or chase that resulted in the other cat hiding. Neither initiators nor recipients of aggression were more likely to spend time off the ground. There also was no difference noted in time spent by cats off the ground in households with or without aggression. There was a significant negative correlation between time spent living together and frequency of aggression in the household.

Prevalence of housesoiling and aggression (toward people or other cats) in kittens during the first year after adoption from a humane society has been studied.[25] Owners of the kittens were contacted by telephone approximately four, 18, and 52 weeks postadoption. One hundred and twenty-six kittens aged six to 13 weeks when adopted were included. The behavioral questionnaire addressed the frequency of the behavior within the preceding 30 days. For aggression between cats, information from multicat households was available for 61 kittens at the first evaluation, 55 for the second evaluation, and 42 for the last evaluation. Owners were asked how many times the kitten had attacked another cat as well as how many times the kitten had been attacked. The kitten was considered to exhibit the behavior if the owner had seen it at least once in the previous month. At the first evaluation, 15 out of 61 kittens (25%) were reported to have had an aggressive event with another cat. The proportion of kittens that attacked other cats was significantly higher for kittens that were attacked by others than for those not attacked. Of the 15 cats, seven were attackers and had been attacked (five males, two females), five were only attackers (three males, two females), and three had been attacked (all females). At the second evaluation, seven out of 55 kittens (13%) had been involved in aggressive events, five were both attacked and had attacked and two only attacked. At the last evaluation, 10 out of 42 kittens (24%) had been reported to have had an aggressive event; five were attackers and had been attacked, three were only attackers, and two were only attacked. The percentage of aggression toward other cats therefore decreased from the first to second assessment but increased again at the last evaluation. However, a description of the aggressive behaviors and the severity of the aggression

were not detailed in the publication. Some of the aggressive encounters may have been normal communication between cats.

Another survey identified the incidence of intercat aggression in households following the introduction of a new cat.[26] For this particular survey, fighting was defined as scratching and/or biting. One hundred and twenty-four multicat households were surveyed. Of these, 61 out of 123 households (49.6%) reported initial fighting between the newly adopted cat and the resident cat. In those 61 households, 59% of the owners reported that fights occurred once or several times weekly, and 41% reported fights less than once weekly. Forty-four multicat households (35%) stated that fighting still occurred 2 to 12 months postadoption. Of those 44 households, 39% indicated that fighting occurred once or several times weekly, and 61% reported fighting less than once weekly. Initial fighting was not significantly associated with number of resident cats in the household, age or sex of the adopted cat, age or sex of the original resident cats, outdoor access, or size of the residence. Current fighting was significantly associated with outdoor access in that households offering outdoor access were 3.4 times more likely to have current fighting than those with strictly indoor cats. If the adopted cat bit at least one of the resident cats when first introduced or if one of the resident cats scratched the newly adopted cat, current fighting was more likely. Initial fighting was strongly associated with current fighting. Current fighting was not associated with number of resident cats in the household, age or sex of the adopted cat, age or sex of the original resident cats, or size of residence. The original resident cats were more likely to hiss, scratch, flee, hide, ignore, and stare at the new cat. The new cat was more likely to play with the resident cat.

Amat and colleagues reported that of 336 cats seen for behavioral problems from 1998 through 2006, 171 cats (47%) were aggressive.[14] Of these, 64% were aggressive toward other cats. Nineteen cats (11 males and eight females) had displayed at least one redirected aggression, for a total of 22 episodes (16 had one reported episode, and three had two reported episodes). Seventeen of these cats lived indoors, two had access to outdoors. Eleven cats lived with other cats in the household. The authors selected 64 cats as a control group (35 males and 29 females) with 24 living indoors and 40 having access to outdoors. The reported target of redirected aggression in seven of the 22 episodes (32%) was the other household cat. Identified triggers included loud noises (e.g., falling objects, television, cellular phones, or electric drill) in 50% of cats and interaction with other cats in the other 45%. Cats with redirected aggression were significantly more likely to have a sound phobia (eight of the 11 cats reacting to loud noises had noise phobia).

Affiliative Behaviors

Leyhausen categorized friendly behaviors into six groups: sleeping together, grooming, rubbing against each other, friendly greeting (not defined specifically), running beside

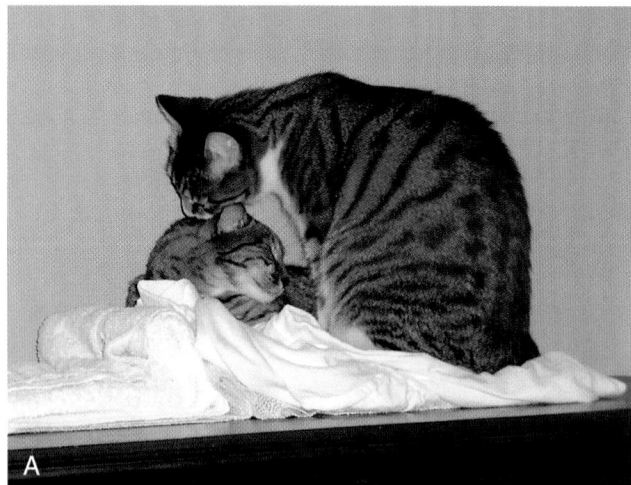

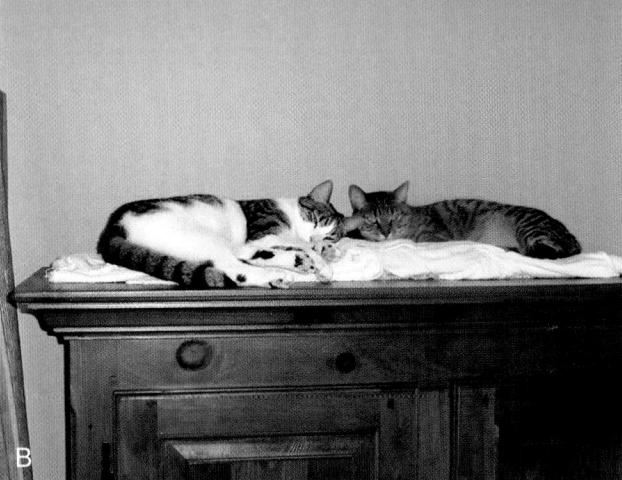

Figure 92-3: Affiliative behaviors. **A,** Grooming. **B,** Sleeping in close proximity.

each other, and purring while rubbing with the tail held up and play behavior (Figure 92-3).[2]

Prevalence of Affiliative Behaviors in Free-Roaming Cats

Affiliative behaviors described in free-roaming cats have included sleeping or sitting together. Half the observations of a group of four cats showed that when a cat was sleeping or sitting motionless, it was touching another cat.[27] Allogrooming and greeting behavior have been described as "tail up," "sniff noses," and "head rub" (either cheek-to-cheek or forehead-to-forehead); and if presented all together, they occur in that sequence.[5] "Tail-up" was the lowest intensity and the most commonly observed greeting component. The most extreme greeting behavior was head-rubbing, which could extend along the length of the body.[5] Macdonald and colleagues reported licking as the most interactive behavior (53.4% of all interactions), and rubbing was much less common (15.7% of interactions) in a group of four adult entire cats.[18] In a colony of neutered cats (four males and five females), the authors also found that the "tail up" behavior was shown more often alone rather than in association with other affiliative behaviors, such as rubbing or sniffing.[28] Most affiliative (81.75%) interactions were observed between adult females and adult males. They concluded that "tail up" was associated with other behaviors signaling amicable intentions but that it could also have an independent and different role from affiliative behaviors.

Prevalence of Affiliative Behaviors in Owned Cats

Barry and Crowell-Davis looked at 60 households of strictly indoor cats, 20 with two male cats, 20 with two female cats, and 20 with one female and one male.[24] All the affiliative behaviors (amicable approach, allogroom, and social sniff) were observed in both sexes with the exception of allorubbing, which was never seen between females during the total 10-hour observation period (2 hours per day over 5 different days). There were no significant differences in amicable approach, allogroom, or sniff by sex, household, or recipient. Male/male housemates spent significantly more time in proximity than female/female or female/male housemates. Information on the relatedness of each pair of cats was not given. No correlation between time spent living together and frequency of affiliative behaviors (allorubbing, allogrooming, sniffing, or time in close proximity) was noted, but there was a significant negative correlation between time spent together and number of affiliative approaches recorded. This study showed that sex had little effect on social behavior of the indoor neutered domestic cat.

A preliminary report on affiliative behavior in related and unrelated pairs of cats included 25 pairs, with 14 littermate pairs and 11 pairs of unrelated cats.[29] All of the littermate pairs were observed as being in physical contact (e.g., sleeping curled around one another or minimal contact with a paw or tail touching), whereas six of the unrelated pairs were never observed in physical contact. All of the related cats (except one pair) ate from the same bowl or from adjacent bowls, whereas unrelated cats tended to eat either alone (if only one bowl) or from well-spaced bowls. Almost half the littermate pairs groomed one another, but none of the unrelated pairs did.

Another study evaluated associations between relatedness and familiarity with the behaviors of allogrooming and maintaining proximity.[30] Twenty-eight privately owned, neutered cats in one colony were observed. Relatedness (only matrilineal relationships were known) and familiarity (how long the cats had lived together) was significantly associated with the number of times a cat was within 1 meter (3.3 feet) of another cat and how often a cat was groomed. The number of times a cat was within 1 meter (3.3 feet) of a studied or focal cat and allogroomed by a given cat was significantly associated with the cat being a relative and familiarity between the cats. There was a significant association between relationship and familiarity. A relative was more likely to be within 1 meter (3.3 feet) of a focal cat than a relative equivalent (i.e., a nonrelated cat that had lived with the studied cat as long as the relative). Likewise, relatives were groomed significantly more than relative equivalents.

CLINICAL EVALUATION OF AGGRESSION

The body and facial postures as well as the history and the context in which aggression occurs provide the information to make a diagnosis. It is often difficult to make a definitive diagnosis,[1] and in many cases, a tentative diagnosis must suffice. Several types of aggression require similar treatment techniques, so it is not always necessary to arrive at a definitive diagnosis (e.g., intermale, territorial, fear-induced aggression, or redirected aggression) in order to treat a problem successfully.[1]

Normal or Problematic Behavior

The context in which the aggressive events occur allows for differentiation between appropriate and inappropriate behaviors. Aggression can be an appropriate response in some contexts.[3] Defense in response to a threat would be considered appropriate aggressive behavior. Additionally, one must also remember that cats are nonverbal. To signal a desire for end of interaction for example, a cat may communicate by exhibiting aggressive behaviors, such as hissing, swatting, or biting. In the context of communication, these behaviors are generally controlled (a raised paw or an open mouth) or inhibited (a bite without teeth marks or injury). The aggression would be mild. Therefore, context is an important question to ask for each aggressive event reported by owners. In the case of severe redirected aggression, the behavior would not be appropriate given the context and from the victim's perspective.

Behavior can be thought of as a sequence of events. As an example, a normal behavioral sequence of aggression may start as an initial warning (e.g., a growl, raised paw, or open mouth [initiation]) followed by a pause. The cat is communicating and waiting for a response. The cat may end the interaction at the warning stage or in some cases may proceed to either swat or bite (action). Both the swat and the bite may be single or multiple events. The cat would then stop or release (end of sequence; volitional). Behavior becomes problematic if some of the steps in the sequence are omitted or altered. A cat growling and biting simultaneously without any other prior form of warning has an altered sequence, because there is no clear initiation phase or pause. Such a sequence could not be considered normal communication.

When considering frequency of aggressive behavior, it becomes clear that one needs to distinguish between normal communication (mild aggression) and problematic aggression. Mild aggression rarely requires intervention. The recipient may distance itself from the aggressive cat, or it may stop interacting. The recipient cat will otherwise behave normally (e.g., it does not hide, avoid, or try to escape from the aggressor).

When considering severity of the aggression, one can arbitrarily label the problematic aggression between cats as moderate in cases where the victim avoids the aggressor. The victim may have inappropriate elimination either because it is too fearful to go to the litter box or because the aggressor is preventing access (active and/or passive aggression). The aggressor and/or the victim may be urine spraying as a consequence of the fights and social stress.[31] The victim is able to avoid interactions, because it still has areas to withdraw where it can remain undisturbed. There are no physical injuries but the victim's welfare is seriously affected. This cat will increase vigilance, always trying to locate the aggressor, and may even pace in the home, if anxious. The victim may also startle more easily, indicating increased reactivity. If the aggression is strictly passive (silent threats), the owner may only notice the victimized cat behaving aggressively (usually hissing). Along those same lines, one could label the aggression between cats as severe in cases where the victim never has the option of withdrawing and being undisturbed. The aggressor appears to be obsessed with its victim, with increased duration and/or frequency of stalking and staring. The aggressor follows the victim everywhere—sometimes no longer resting or sleeping as would be normally expected. In some of these severe cases, the fights also lead to injuries. The victim is generally terrified and will exhibit behaviors compatible with fear and anxiety (e.g., hiding, avoidance, flight, defensive aggression, and so on). The aggressive behaviors of the aggressor are not appropriate given the constant nature and given that regardless of the victim's response, the threats and attacks continue. The aggression can be active and/or passive. Intervention is necessary in moderate and severe aggression cases.

Reactivity of the aggressor should also be assessed during the clinical evaluation with specific questions such as:

- How easy it is to interrupt an aggressive event (i.e., is a verbal command sufficient)?
- Does the aggressor appear unresponsive to sounds or the owner's attempts to verbally interrupt?
- How long after an aggressive event before the cat no longer exhibits aggressive behaviors (i.e., recovery time)?

A cat with redirected aggression that requires 30 minutes or more to return to unaggressive behavior (as reported by Chapman[7]) is likely exhibiting excessive reactivity. A cat that seems unresponsive to sound or that inflicts bite wounds is also most likely exhibiting excessive reactivity. All cats with excessive reactivity benefit from medication.

Active Aggression and/or Passive Aggression

Questions on the presence of passive aggression (silent threats) are essential to ask during the clinical evaluation for intercat aggression. Most owners are unaware of the importance of these threats. In a descriptive study of the use of space and patterns of interaction of 14 unrelated (seven males and seven females) neutered indoor cats in one home, a cat named Lily was the most restricted in use of space, spending almost all its time on top of the refrigerator.[32] Lily came down from the refrigerator after the death of a cat named Julius. Little overt aggression was reported in the home, but Lily was most likely a victim of passive covert aggression, unbeknownst to the owners. Recognizing passive aggression allows one to identify the true aggressor and treat accordingly.

Housesoiling or Urine Marking

Intercat aggression and urination outside the litter box occur together less often than chance would predict. In a study of 736 cats, 185 (25.1%) presented for intercat aggression and 170 (23.1%) with urination outside the litter box.[21] Therefore, the probability of having both diagnoses would be 5.8%. Of 185 cats presented for intercat aggression, 2.7% also urinated outside of the litter box. Out of 170 cats presented for urination outside the litter box, 2.9% had intercat aggression. On the other hand, aggressive interactions with other household or outdoor cats were the two factors most commonly associated with the initiation or the continuation of spraying.[31] Case reports also highlight the coexistence of urine spraying, house soiling, and intercat aggression.[33,34] In inappropriate elimination and urine cases, the owners may be aware of coexisting aggression but may not always realize that aggression is directly linked to the other problems. Treating the intercat aggression (active and passive aggression) becomes essential in order to resolve the housesoiling or urine problems.

Absence or Presence of Appropriate Affiliative Behaviors

Play is considered an affiliative behavior, but occasionally play may escalate into aggression.[8] However, aggression may be underestimated, because it may be mistaken for play. In play, one would expect an alternation of pursuit and flight. In other words, if the owner reports that it is always the same cat chasing in every play sequence, it may be worthwhile asking for videos of several cat interactions within the home. In the author's experience, there have been cases of passive aggression (silent stares missed by the owner) occurring along with mistaken "play sessions" (one cat was always chasing the other without role reversal). Therefore, it is just as important to record whether the cats show other affiliative behaviors (e.g., proximity, physical contact when sleeping or sitting, grooming, and rubbing) aside from play as it is to determine aggression severity. Together, this information will guide treatment recommendations.

Physical Environment

Important questions with regard to the multicat environment include inquiring about number of feeding and elimination areas, perches and hiding places, feeding devices, and so on. It is important for cats to have the choice of distancing themselves from one another as well as to be able to avoid certain individuals, if desired. See Chapter 93 for information on enrichment and multicat homes.

TREATMENT

Behavior Modification

As mentioned earlier, there are general treatment recommendations that apply regardless of the label that one attri-

butes to the intercat aggression. First and foremost, the fighting cats should be separated at all times when treatment techniques are not in effect[1,6] and supervision is not possible. Even low levels or infrequent aggression can perpetuate the aggression and prolong the treatment process. Initially there should be no visual contact[1] particularly because of silent threats such as stares. Prior to reintroduction exercises, both the victim and aggressor cats can be trained individually to look at the owner and come when called. Special food treats are given whenever a cat that is called and responds by looking at and running to its owner. Other rewards can be used if the cat enjoys specific activities or interactions with the owner. If a cat likes physical contact, petting, interactive play, or training sessions, these activities can also serve as a reward for looking and coming. Owners should train cats to look and come reliably prior to reintroducing them. This exercise will subsequently allow owners to interrupt undesirable behavior, such as silent threats by the aggressor, as well as assess reactivity levels when both cats are in each other's presence. If one or both cats are too aroused, they will not look at the owner when called. When the cats are initially allowed to interact, the owner must be present and must be paying attention to both cats.[6] Short intervals for interaction to set the cats up for success are more beneficial than long sessions.

Desensitization and Counter Conditioning

The reintroduction is conducted slowly and is based on desensitization and counter conditioning (DS/CC).[1,8] Cages for one or both cats may be used for the initial steps of the behavior modification, ensuring that no overt aggression takes place (the aggressor cat is placed in the cage). A harness and leash may be used on the aggressor but only if the cat does not redirect aggression to the owner during attempts to interrupt fights. The distance between cats during initial reintroduction is meant to decrease the victim's perceived level of threat associated with the presence of the aggressor. This distance must be sufficient so that the victim is relatively comfortable (i.e., exhibiting as little anxiety or fear as possible). The necessary distance varies from pair to pair. Counter conditioning involves gradually associating the sight, movement, or proximity of the cat with a behavioral response that is incompatible with fear, anxiety, or aggression, such as eating, grooming, or playing.[1] Most often counter conditioning is achieved by pairing the sight of the other cat with mealtimes or tasty treats. The aggressor must be interrupted at the first sign of threat (particularly staring at the victim) and rewarded with food or treats for complying. Interruption may be achieved by calling the aggressor by its name and rewarding it for looking at its owner. The goal of counter conditioning is to replace aggression and/or fear with relaxation, because they are incompatible emotional states. If the cats are unable to eat in each other's presence or the aggressor cannot be interrupted when it is staring, the distance between the cats must be increased. The first objective is that the cats are comfortable eating in each other's presence. Next, if both cats are capable of looking away from each other either volitionally or upon request, they are becoming more relaxed. The distance between the two cats can then be decreased very slowly as long as the cats remain relaxed. This gradual decrease in distance achieves desensitization. Figure 92-4 shows DS/CC using a cage.

Exchanging odors between cats has also been recommended,[1,6] although no studies have shown that this strategy is any more effective than other approaches. If cats are maintained in separate areas of the home, they can alternate periodically between locations,[1] or a towel may be used to rub each cat's perioral and buccal areas gently and then left in the area of residence of the other cat.[6]

Environmental Enrichment

The purpose of environmental enrichment is to provide alternative activities for the aggressor (e.g., spending more time feeding, finding other outlets for physical activity, learning new behaviors, and so on). While the aggressor is busy with

other activities, it cannot threaten or attack the victim. Offering several feeding stations and elimination areas for the victim close to where this cat spends its time, as well as perches and hiding places, reduces the need for the victim to be near the aggressor.

Medication

Prior to prescribing medication, the cat should have a thorough physical examination, and age-appropriate laboratory testing (e.g., biochemistry panel, complete blood count, urinalysis, and total thyroxine) should be performed. Currently, there are no approved drugs for the treatment of intercat aggression. One additional challenge may also be determining which cat to medicate—the aggressor, the victim, or both. Medicating the aggressor would be indicated in cases of increased reactivity. Examples include when interrupting undesirable aggressive behavior is impossible without physically placing an item between the cats (i.e., calling the cat by

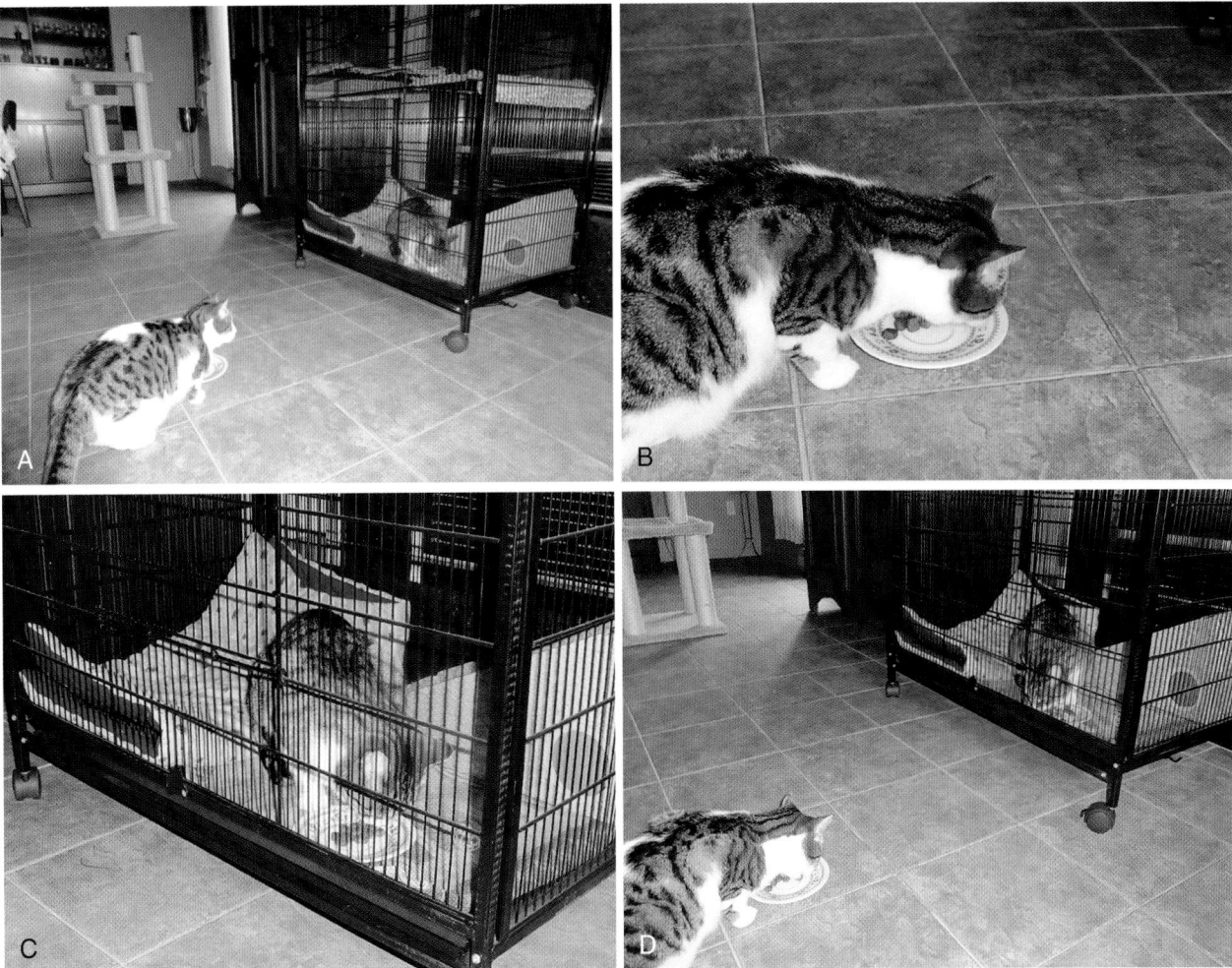

Figures 92-4: Desensitization and counter-conditioning. **A,** The aggressor is in the cage and the victim is free. Distance between the two cats is determined by the behavior of both cats. The victim should be able to eat and show only minimal signs of anxiety, if any. The aggressor should eat and not threaten (stare, vocalize, or growl) the other cat. **B,** Victim eating in the presence of the aggressor. **C,** Aggressor eating in the presence of the victim. **D,** Both cats are eating in each other's presence. *Continued*

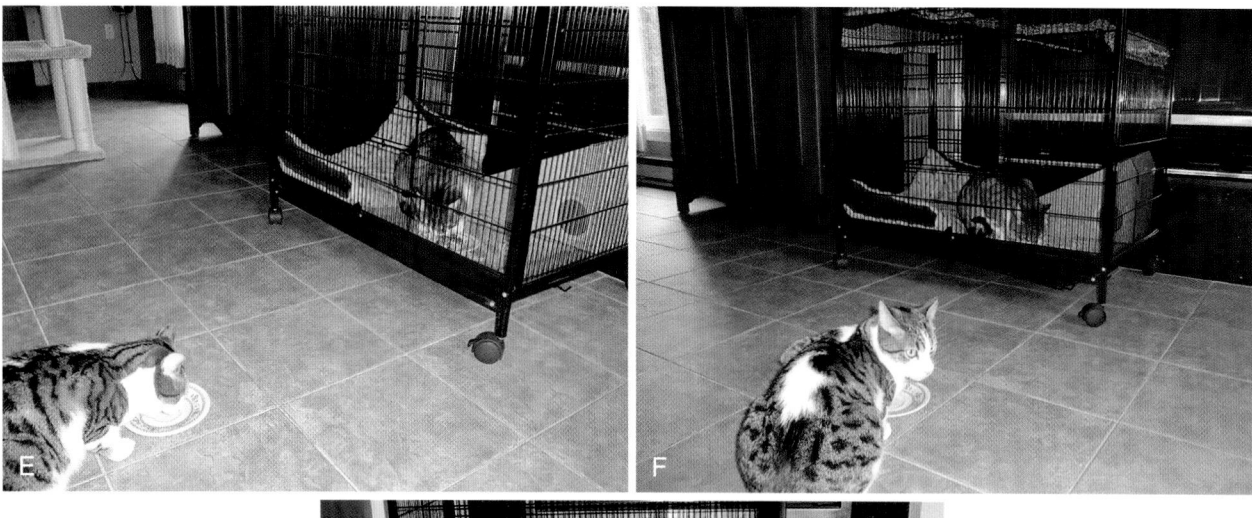

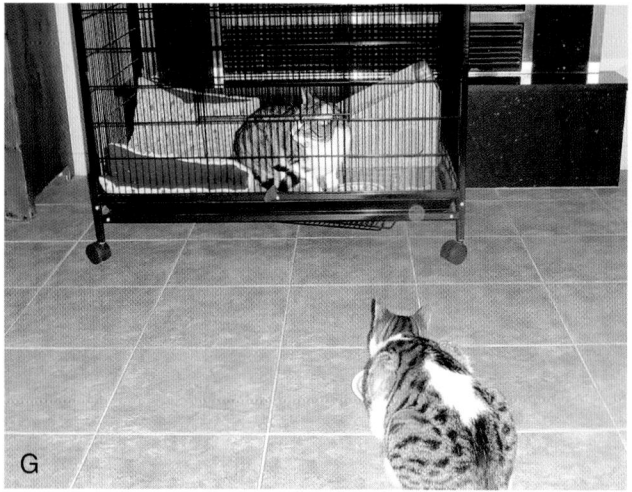

Figures 92-4, cont'd: E, Victim has eaten its entire meal. **F,** Victim feels safe enough to look away from the aggressor. **G,** Aggressor is not threatening the victim even after the end of the meal.

Table 92-1	Drugs Commonly Prescribed to Treat Intercat Aggression	
Drug Class	**Drug and Dosage**	**Comments**
Selective serotonin reuptake inhibitor	Fluoxetine: 0.5 to 1.0 mg/kg PO every 24 hours	Side effects include constipation, urinary retention, decreased appetite, and sedation
Tricyclic antidepressant	Clomipramine: 0.25 to 0.5 mg/kg PO every 24 hours	Side effects include constipation, urinary retention, decreased appetite, and sedation
Serotonin 1A partial agonist	Buspirone: 0.5 to 1.0 mg/kg PO every 12 hours	Reported to increase assertiveness in some cats and may be recommended for the victimized cat

PO, Orally.

its name or making a mild sound as distraction does not work), in cases of physical injury to the victim, or in cases where the cat remains reactive for hours after an aggressive event (as in some cases of redirected aggression). Medicating the victim would be indicated if the cat's fearful behaviors are perpetuating the cycle of violence. Unfortunately, there are no prospective studies evaluating success rates based on the severity of the aggression and whether medicating the aggressor or the victim results in better outcomes. Prospective studies on efficacy of one drug over another for either the

aggressor or the victim are also lacking. Medication is usually prescribed for several months to years; therefore, yearly or biannual (for older cats) re-evaluations are recommended. Care should be taken to verify that no contraindications exist with any concurrent medications. The commonly prescribed medications are listed in Table 92-1.

Certain medications are no longer recommended. Diazepam use was reported in one case for treatment of intercat aggression[35] but is no longer recommended because of reports of death from hepatic necrosis in cats following oral administration of the drug.[36,37] Other side effects include sedation, increased appetite, and weight gain. Medroxyprogesterone acetate has been associated with adrenocortical suppression, polydipsia, polyphagia, diabetes mellitus, and mammary adenocarcinoma. In one case report, three unrelated male housemate cats were treated repeatedly with injections of this drug over a span of many years for intercat aggression and urine marking.[38] All three cats subsequently developed multiple recurrent mammary adenocarcinomas. The delay between the last injection and the diagnosis of mammary neoplasia ranged from 2 months to 6 years.

Other products are marketed for behavior modification, but there are no published studies on efficacy for treatment of intercat aggression. These products include nutraceuticals, such as L-theanine, alpha-casozepine, tryptophan, vitamin B_3, and synthetic feline pheromones.

PROGNOSIS

Data on outcome and prognosis for treatment of intercat aggression are still lacking. One report in which two strictly indoor 2-year-old cats initially had a good relationship (e.g., allogrooming, allorubbing, mutual play, and common resting location) and then started fighting following a redirected aggression event reported that affiliative behaviors reappeared progressively during the first 6 weeks of treatment.[13] One year later, aggressive episodes were no longer observed. In the author's experience, treatment for intercat aggression requiring gradual exposure of the cats to each other may take weeks to months (as long as 6 to 12 months) and still may not be successful. The importance of previously observed affiliative behaviors prior to the onset of aggression is unknown. That is, is there a better outcome if the cats showed previous affiliative behaviors?

SUMMARY

Aggression between household cats is common. Some aggression, usually mild, may be normal and serve to communicate or preserve personal space. In other cases, aggression becomes problematic and requires intervention when the welfare of one or both cats is at risk.

References

1. Borchelt PL, Voith VL: Diagnosis and treatment of aggression problems in cats. *Vet Clin North Am Small Anim Pract* 12:665–671, 1982.
2. Leyhausen P: *Cat behavior: the predatory and social behavior of domestic and wild cats*, New York, 1979, Garland STPM Press, pp 170, 183, 189.
3. Overall KL: *Clinical behavioral medicine for small animals*, St Louis, 1997, CV Mosby, p 461.
4. Hart BL, Barrett RE: Effects of castration on fighting, roaming, and urine spraying in adult male cats. *J Am Vet Med Assoc* 163:290–292, 1973.
5. Dards JL: The behaviour of dockyard cats: interaction of adult males. *Appl Anim Ethol* 10:133–153, 1983.
6. Moesta A, Crowell-Davis SL: Intercat aggression—general considerations, prevention and treatment. *Tierärtzl Praxis* 39:97–104, 2011.
7. Chapman BL: Feline aggression: classification diagnosis and treatment. *Vet Clin North Am Small Anim Pract* 21:315–327, 1991.
8. Crowell-Davis SL, Barry K, Wolfe R: Social behavior and aggressive problems of cats. *Vet ClinNorth Am Small Anim Pract* 27:549–569, 1997.
9. Borchelt PL, Voith VL: Aggressive behavior in dogs and cats. *Comp Cont Educ* 7:949–957, 1985.
10. Beaver BV: Feline behavioral problems other than house soiling. *J Am Anim Hosp Assoc* 25:465–469, 1989.
11. Borchelt PL, Voith VL: Aggressive behavior in cats. *Comp Cont Educ* 9:49–56, 1987.
12. Crowell-Davis SL, Curtis TM, Knowles RJ: Social organization in the cat: a modern understanding. *J Feline Med Surg* 6:19–28, 2004.
13. Amat M, Manteca X, Fatjo J: Animal behavior case of the month. *J Am Vet Med Assoc* 231:710–712, 2007.
14. Amat M, Manteca X, Le Brech S, et al: Evaluation of inciting causes, alternative targets and risk factors associated with redirected aggression in cats. *J Am Vet Med Assoc* 233:586–589, 2008.
15. Chapman BL, Voith VL: Cat aggression redirected to people: 14 cases (1981-1987). *J Am Vet Med Assoc* 196:947–950, 1990.
16. Laundré J: The daytime behaviour of domestic cats in a free-roaming population. *Anim Behav* 25:990–998, 1977.
17. Natoli E, De Vito E: Agonistic behaviour, dominance rank and copulatory success in a large multi-male feral cat *Felis catus L.*, colony in central Rome. *Anim Behav* 42:227–241, 1991.
18. Macdonald DW, Apps PJ, Carr GM, et al: Social dynamics, nursing coalitions and infanticide among farm cats *Felis catus*. *Adv Ethol* 28:9–66, 1987.
19. Blackshaw JK: Abnormal behaviour in cats. *Aust Vet J* 65:395–396, 1988.
20. Mugford RA: Behavioural problems. In Chandler EA, Hilbery DR, Gaskell CJ, editors: *Feline medicine and therapeutics*, London, 1985, Blackwell Scientific, p 362.
21. Bamberger M, Houpt KA: Signalment factors, comorbidity, and trends in behavior diagnoses in cats: 736 cases (1991-2001). *J Am Vet Med Assoc* 229:1602–1606, 2006.
22. Hart BL, Cooper L: Factors relating to urine spraying and fighting in prepubertally gonadectomized cats. *J Am Vet Med Assoc* 184:1255–1258, 1984.
23. Lindell EM, Erb HN, Houpt KA: Intercat aggression: a retrospective study examining types of aggression, sexes of fighting pairs, and effectiveness of treatment. *Appl Anim Behav Sci* 55:153–162, 1997.
24. Barry KJ, Crowell-Davis SL: Gender differences in the social behavior of the neutered indoor-only domestic cat. *Appl Anim Behav Sci* 64:193–211, 1999.
25. Wright JC, Amoss RT: Prevalence of house soiling and aggression in kittens during the first year after adoption from a humane society. *J Am Vet Med Assoc* 224:1790–1795, 2004.
26. Levine E, Perry P, Scarlett J, et al: Intercat aggression in households following the introduction of a new cat. *Appl Anim Behav Sci* 90:325–336, 2005.
27. Macdonald DW, Apps PJ: The social behavior of a group of semi-dependent farm cats, *Felis catus*: a progress report. *Carniv Genet Newsl* 3:256–268, 1978.
28. Cafazzo S, Natoli E: The social function of tail up in the domestic cat *(Felis silvestris catus)*. *Behav Proc* 80:60–66, 2009.
29. Bradshaw JWS, Hall SL: Affiliative behavior of related and unrelated pairs of cats in catteries: a preliminary report. *Appl Anim Behav Sci* 63:251–255, 1999.

30. Curtis TM, Knowles RJ, Crowell-Davis SL: Influence of familiarity and relatedness on proximity and allogrooming in domestic cats *(Felis catus). Am J Vet Res* 64:1151–1154, 2003.

31. Pryor PA, Hart BL, Bain MJ, et al: Causes of urine marking in cats and effects of environmental management on frequency of marking. *J Am Vet Med Assoc* 219:1709–1713, 2001.

32. Bernstein PL, Strack M: A game of cat and house: social patterns and behavior of 14 domestic cats (Felis catus) in the home. *Anthrozoös* IX:25–39, 1996.

33. Overall KL: Animal behavior case of the month. *J Am Vet Med Assoc* 205:694–696, 1994.

34. Overall KL: Animal behavior case of the month. *J Am Vet Med Assoc* 211:1376–1378, 1997.

35. Mathews S: Dealing with feline aggression: systematic desensitization through the use of a psychoactive drug. *Feline Pract* 12:23–26, 1982.

36. Center SA, Elston TH, Rowland PH, et al: Fulminant hepatic failure associated with oral administration of diazepam in 11 cats. *J Am Vet Med Assoc* 209:618–625, 1996.

37. Hughes D, Moreau RE, Overall KL, et al: Acute hepatic necrosis and liver failure associated with benzodiazepine therapy in six cats, 1986-1995. *J Vet Emerg Cri Care* 6:13–20, 1996.

38. Jacobs TM, Hoppe BR, Poehlmann CE, et al: Mammary adenocarcinomas in three male cats exposed to medroxyprogesterone acetate (1990-2006). *J Feline Med Surg* 12:169–174, 2010.

Creating Harmony in Multiple Cat Households

Carlo Siracusa

An estimated 52% of cat owners in the United States and 37% of cat owners in the United Kingdom have more than one cat.[1,2] Therefore, cats living in a multiple cat household represent a relevant portion of a veterinarian's feline patients. The aim of this chapter is to help veterinarians and cat owners understand the social dynamics and the needs of a multiple cat household to provide cats with the best enriched environment and prevent behavior problems that may be more frequent in this unique environment. See Chapter 94 for more information about feline social behavior and personality.

UNDERSTANDING INTERACTIONS IN MULTIPLE CAT HOUSEHOLDS

The social behavior of the domestic cat, *Felis silvestris catus,* is greatly influenced by the environment in which the feline lives, because cats are able to live both in groups and as solitary individuals. This adaptability derives from the relatively recent process of domestication, which occurred about 12,000 years ago[3] and has made the solitary wildcat, *Felis silvestris* spp., a domestic animal able to share its territory with other individuals when abundant resources are available.[4-6] The wildcat diet consists of small prey animals that are consumed individually, but domestication has provided many instances where large quantities of food are often concentrated in relatively small areas that can attract and sustain numerous cats.[6] Garbage disposal areas, representing a valuable and reliable source of food, are easily accessible to cats in cities and suburbs and also attract small rodents, as do grain-storage areas on farms.[6] Nevertheless, cats are not obligate social animals (unlike the domestic dog and its ancestor, the wolf); they are phylogenetically a solitary species that has adapted to share its habitat with humans and other cats under specific environmental conditions created by human intervention. Given the relatively short history as social animals, cats do not have sophisticated communicative skills and a well-defined social structure. However, domestic cats can form social groups usually referred to as "colonies" that are based on a matrilineal composition. Females live together and cooperate in rearing each other's offspring and defending the colony from intruders.[4,6,7]

In an unrestricted environment, colonies are spontaneously formed by related individuals that retain the ability to remain in or leave the group.[6] Based on this premise, household groups of domestic cats living in confinement do not represent a colony but rather a social group artificially created by humans. Cats living in a household environment have often been "forced" to live together, without the ability to choose whether they want to join or leave the social group. These constraints may make it more difficult for some cats to peacefully manage social interactions and avoid aggressive interactions. This distinction between feline colonies and household groups is relevant to understanding and treating cat behavioral problems caused by social dysfunction.

Many obligate social species, including man, the wolf, and to a lesser extent the domestic dog,[8,9] regulate their interactions within their social unit by establishing a more or less rigid hierarchical organization. Hierarchical organization allows individuals to create a position within the group based on interactions with other individuals of the same group, providing stability, structure, and cohesion to the social unit.[4-6] Although aggressive interactions among cats of the same colony have been used to study their possible hierarchical organization, a well-defined linear hierarchical structure has not been identified in the domestic cat.[6,7] With displays of affiliative behaviors (e.g., allogrooming and allorubbing), avoidance of dangerous aggressive interactions through deference and ritualization, and maintenance of a safe interindividual distance, group-living cats are able to achieve social stability.[4-6]

Spatial Organization in Multiple Cat Households

Spatial organization in feral cats is regulated by the abundance and distribution of food. Cat populations have the highest density in environments where food is abundant and widely distributed (e.g., in urban areas). In areas where food is abundant but restricted in distribution (e.g., farms and rural environments), the cat population has a lower density.[10] In the home environment, food is usually abundant, so cats can live in a relatively crowded state. However, when food or other resources are not adequately distributed in the household, cats may be unable to regulate their distance from one

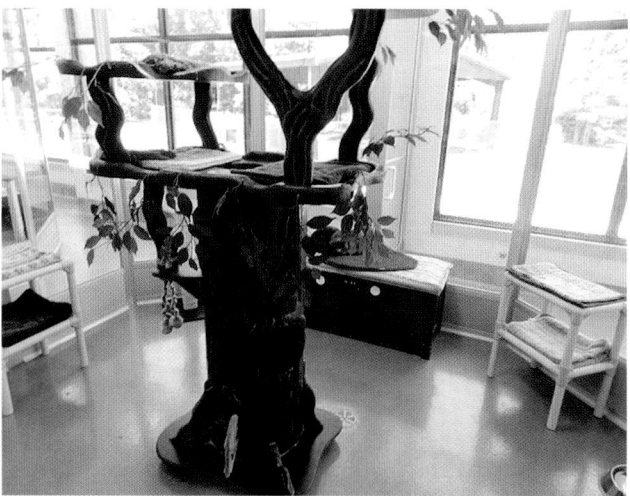

Figure 93-1: Vertical spaces and hiding places are tools to decrease hostility in a multiple cat household. Cat trees are a useful way to provide this form of environmental enrichment. (Courtesy of Monmouth County SPCA.)

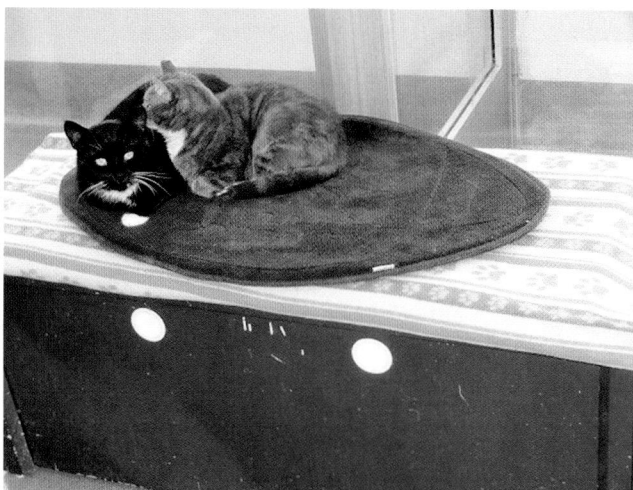

Figure 93-2: Allogrooming is an affiliative and conciliatory behavior likely to occur between preferred associates resting together. (Courtesy of Monmouth County SPCA.)

another to prevent antagonistic interactions. Cats prefer keeping an interindividual distance and may spend most of their time out of each other's sight.[11,12] If keeping safe interindividual distances is impossible or difficult, conflicts among the individuals of a group may arise. To avoid conflicts, each cat should have all the resources (e.g., food and water, resting places, litter boxes, and toys) available in the area that it uses most heavily within the home range (i.e., the core area).[12,13] To minimize social conflicts, cats should be able to avoid interactions with other cats as they access these resources. Due to the variability in sociability among individual cats, some individuals may need an exclusive core area in which they can find refuge from other cats, whereas other individuals may tolerate overlap of their core areas. However, the interindividual distance is variable for each individual and depends on the quality of the relationship and interaction between two cats in the same group. Vertical spaces can be useful to maintain individual distances and prevent aggressive interactions. Cats escaping from an aggressive interaction may prefer hiding places rather than elevated spaces (Figure 93-1).[11]

Affiliative Behaviors

Mutual affiliative behaviors are important to strengthen and confirm (after an antagonistic interaction) the social bond between two individuals and likely serve to maintain the specific common scent of the group.[5-7] Allogrooming, allorubbing, nose-touch/sniff, and prolonged proximity (e.g., lying together) are common affiliative behaviors (Figure 93-2; see Table 94-1 in Chapter 94).[4-6,11] Affiliative behaviors are more likely to be mutually displayed by *preferred associates,* which are cats in a colony or household group that spend more time together than would be expected by chance.[4] A preferred association can exist between two males, two females, or a male and a female, and it tends to persist over time even if the colony organization is disrupted.[4]

Because cats living in groups spend most of their time out of each other's sight, safe havens that allow cats to retreat and hide should be provided within the core area.[14] There are exceptions to this because preferred associates spend more time in close proximity, whereas some individuals need to consistently keep a safe distance from other cats to avoid antagonistic behaviors.[4] Littermates spend more time in close proximity and groom each other more frequently than unrelated cats, probably due to their early socialization and long-term coexistence (Figure 93-3).[15] This information can help pet owners design appropriate household environments to promote social harmony among cats.

Although adult cats play with each other, playing does not have the same relevance in strengthening social bonds between cats as it does in obligate social species. Social play is prevalent in kittens and peaks at 12 to 14 weeks, but playing with objects, which simulates predatory behavior, is prevalent is adult cats.[4,16,17] Nevertheless, providing both kittens and adult cats with objects to play with promotes correct behavioral development, helps to prevent anxiety-related behavior problems (including aggression), and facilitates safe interaction with humans.[17]

Antagonistic Behaviors

Intraspecific aggression is the most commonly reported cat behavior problem,[18] and cats living in a house with three or more cats are most likely to display intraspecific aggression (see Chapter 92).[14] When considering a sample of the general population of cats living in pairs, males are no more aggressive than females.[11] Among a sample of cats referred for evaluation of behavioral problems, males were more likely to be the aggressor than females, but the aggression was no more likely to be directed toward males than females.[19] This might mean that aggression displayed by a male cat can be more intense and more likely to be reported as a clinical problem.[11] Protection of resources does not appear to be a primary cause

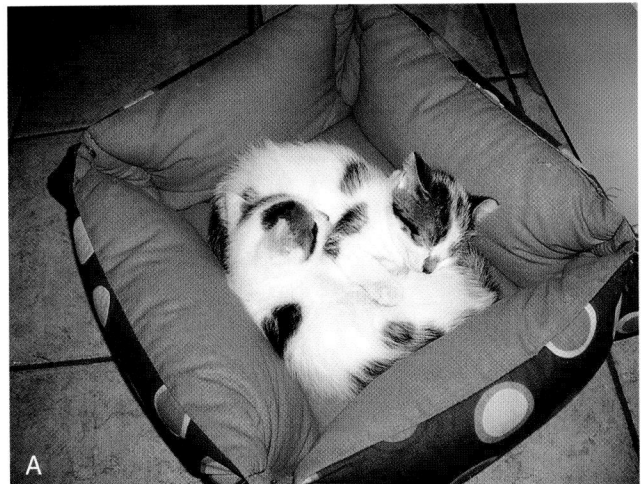

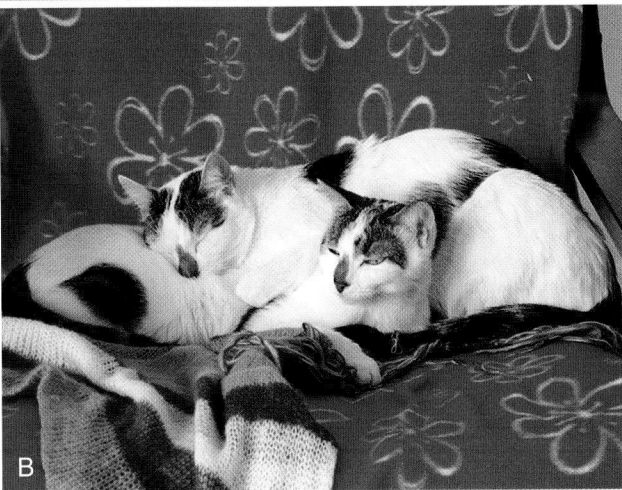

Figure 93-3: Littermates are more likely to be adult preferred associates and spend more time in close proximity. **A,** These two cats have never been separated since their birth. **B,** They continue to show strong affiliative behavior at 2 years of age. (Courtesy of S. Mariani.)

for aggression, but the lack of interindividual distance when accessing unevenly distributed resources may trigger aggression when cats are eating from a common food source.[11,13] For this reason, multiple feeding stations should be available in a multiple cat household.

There is a negative correlation between the time that cats have spent living together and the frequency of aggressive interactions; cats that have lived together longer are less likely to show aggression to each other.[11,20] Introduction of a new cat in a multiple cat household can be a trigger for aggression among cats living together, and their behavior during the first encounter may be determinant of their future relationship.[21] To keep harmony in a multiple cat household, it is extremely important to introduce a new cat following an appropriate protocol (the introduction protocol is described later in this chapter).

Aggression in a multiple cat household can be also caused by triggers different from the target of the aggressive response, such as unfamiliar cats or other animals living inside or outside the household, loud noises indoors and outdoors,

thunderstorms, etc.[14,18,22] In this case, the perception of a threatening stimulus or the frustration caused by the inability to reach a desired target (e.g., a cat that can see but not reach a bird in the yard) causes a peak of arousal that is then aggressively redirected to the nearest individual or anecdotally to an individual with whom there is a previous history of antagonistic behavior. Therefore, to keep harmony in a multiple cat household, it is also vital to control all the stimuli that may cause redirected aggression.

However, cats can also adopt a passive coping strategy in response to social and environmental stress. In this case, cats will show a reduction in their general level of activity and a lack of interaction; owners may fail to detect the suffering even though welfare can be severely compromised.

INAPPROPRIATE BEHAVIORS IN A MULTIPLE CAT HOUSEHOLDS

Some undesired feline behaviors (e.g., marking using urine, feces, and scratching) might function to deliver a social message to other cats. This may make it more likely that these behaviors are displayed in presence of other cats, and they are frequently noted in multiple cat households. In a German study, cats living in groups of two or three individuals exhibited behavior problems more often than those living alone.[23]

Scratching is used by cats to maintain the claws for predation, to increase the control over their territory,[24-26] or as a displacement behavior secondary to stress and anxiety.[17] Scratching is performed more frequently in the presence of conspecifics than when a cat is alone.[27] Therefore, cats scratch in places where other individuals can see their visual marks (scratches), usually corresponding with highly frequented areas of the house (e.g., the living room or the kitchen).[17,26] Scratching posts that are not located appropriately in highly-frequented areas may be underused.

Depositing urine or feces in places with a social significance, commonly referred to as *marking,* is also used to increase control over the territory. It can be exacerbated by anxiety and stress, and it is more frequent in multiple cat households.[5,25,26,28,29] Urine marking may serve to allow cats to control the territory and signal their own presence to conspecifics in the same space. Through social signaling, they can appropriately increase their distance from other cats and avoid confrontations. Finally, marking can communicate availability to individuals of the opposite sex for reproductive purposes.[5] Urine marking is often associated with the presence of other cats, particularly when antagonistic behaviors are shown among the cats.[30] It has been hypothesized that the frequency of urine marking is inversely proportional to the frequency of facial marking, which is also used to increase spatial organization by deposition of pheromones.[31] Therefore, providing an adequately enriched and low-stress environment to favor appropriate spatial organization and control may help reduce marking by deposition of feces and urine. The following section discusses strategies to accomplish this objective.

MANAGING THE ENVIRONMENT TO CREATE HARMONY IN A MULTIPLE CAT HOUSEHOLD

How Many Cats Are Too Many?

In a household environment, food is usually readily available, so in theory, cats could be kept at relatively high density and number. However, several limiting factors other than food availability should be considered when determining the size of a cat group. First, physical barriers preventing cats from leaving or joining the group of their own volition usually delimit the household environment. A cat may decide to leave a group because a conflict arises, because the social organization of the group is disrupted (e.g., when a cat dies), or because it reaches sexual maturity.[6,10] Moreover, some individuals may decide not to join a colony even in areas where food is not scarce or dispersed and live a solitary life.[6,10] Household cats are "prisoners" in their own environment, without the ability to choose whether to share their home with other cats. Second, as previously described, when cats live in a group, they need to keep a distance from each other. If the environment is not large enough and does not provide each cat with the horizontal or vertical individual distance needed from other cats, conflicts and other stress-related behavior problems may arise.[25,26,32,33] Third, resources (e.g., food, water, resting places, toys, and litter boxes) in the household may not be abundant enough or appropriately distributed; in these conditions, cats may not be able to safely enjoy their core area or to satisfy their behavioral needs. Ultimately, these environmental limitations may cause chronic stress to one or more cats and potentially trigger stress-related problems, including aggression or medical problems.[26,34,35] According to a recent study by Ramos and colleagues,[36] environmental factors within cat households (e.g., resource availability and distribution or interactions with the owner) may play a more important role in stress levels measured by fecal glucocorticoid metabolites than the number of cats. Cats living in groups did not have significantly higher levels of fecal glucocorticoid metabolites than cats living in single cat households. However, there was high individual variability independent from the environment in which they were living. Most of the limiting factors mentioned can be controlled to provide cats living in a group with an environment that promotes their welfare and, ultimately, their peaceful coexistence. However, in some cases, regardless of how the environment is structured, a harmonious coexistence between two or more cats might not be possible. In these cases, permanent separation of the cats may be necessary to guarantee their welfare.[14]

Environmental Enrichment: Managing Space and Resources

Environmental enrichment is defined as the addition to an impoverished environment of factors that promote animal welfare.[37] Enrichment does not always imply the introduction of new resources. Enrichment can occur by the redistribution of already existing resources in a more accessible manner. Both the addition and the redistribution of resources should be designed to favor species-typical behavior.

As previously discussed, the first essential resource to manage for harmony in a multiple cat household is space. Space should be arranged considering the individual needs of each cat, based on the quality of its relationship with each of the other individuals in the group.[11] Within the same group, there may be cats that have a preferred associate that they maintain close proximity to, other individuals that tolerate a short interindividual distance, and cats that always need to keep a safe distance from others. Therefore, subgroups of a reduced number of cats that may be kept in proximity can be identified in a multiple cat household. Individuals in the same subgroup may overlap their core areas, so they may be able to share a common space in the household. Conversely, individuals of different subgroups should have different core areas located at a distance from each other to minimize the risk of hostile behavior. Importantly, although individuals in the same subgroup can overlap their core areas, they do not necessarily share the resources present in the core areas. As discussed, cats spend most of their time out of sight of each other, even when they can spend time in close proximity.[11] Therefore, cats should be provided the ability to have their individual space within the subgroup area. This means that enough resting, sleeping, and hiding places; feeding and drinking stations; and litter boxes should be available in the area. Fortunately, cats are agile enough to use vertical spaces through the provision of available and easily accessible platforms, shelves, perches, cat trees, and hammocks. Cats housed in groups enjoy spending time on window perches to allow visual exploration of the outside environment.[38] Caution should be exercised because cats may become aggressive due to the presence of outdoor stimuli (e.g., other cats) or frustrated by their inability to reach an outdoor stimulus (e.g., a bird). Hiding places, as simple as cardboard boxes or empty space under furniture (Figure 93-4), should always be available because they are tools for a cat to stay out of sight of other individuals. To encourage cats to spend time in designated areas, a substrate that maintains a constant temperature (e.g., paper, clothes, wood, or polyester fleece) should be used on these areas.[37]

Appropriate distribution of food resources is also vital in managing the available space in the household. Generally cats do not like sharing their "small prey" (which, in the case of household cats, is represented by the portion of their daily food intake they eat in one meal), so they are unwilling to eat in close proximity to other cats.[32] Although littermates may be more likely to tolerate eating together[15] and other compatible cats might do so as well, this does not represent a species-typical behavior. Therefore, providing cats in the same household with multiple feeding stations (at least one for each core area, ideally more than one in core areas shared by multiple cats) may help to improve welfare and promote living in harmony. Feral cats spend about 30% to 40% of their daily time budget hunting,[39] so small portions of food should be made available several times during the day to approximate a species-typical feeding pattern. This may be achieved

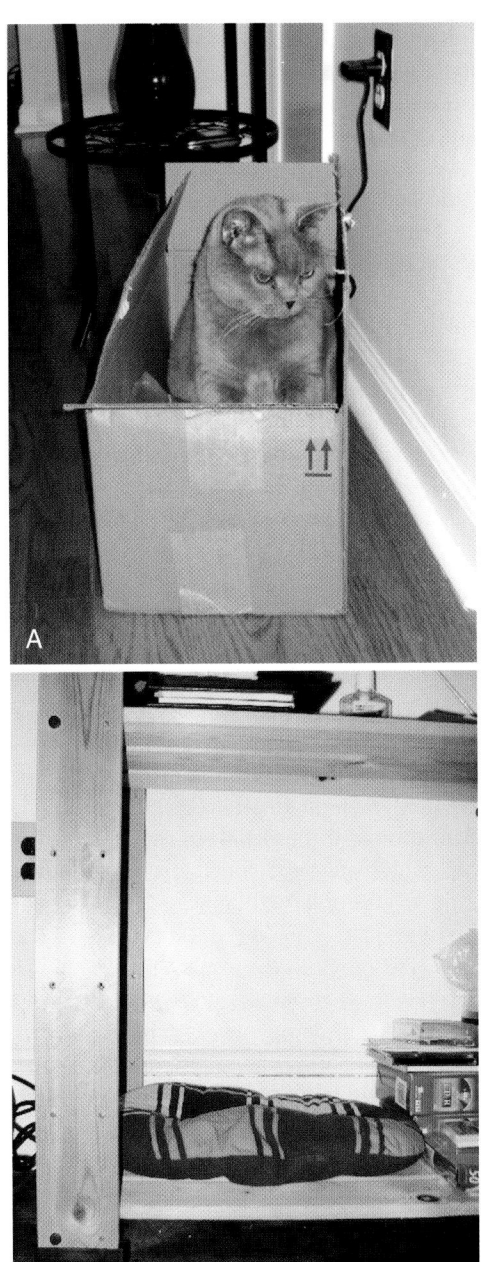

Figure 93-4: Multiple hiding and resting spots should be made available in the household. Many commonly used objects, such as cardboard boxes **(A)** and furniture **(B)**, represent hiding spots if they are large enough for the cat.

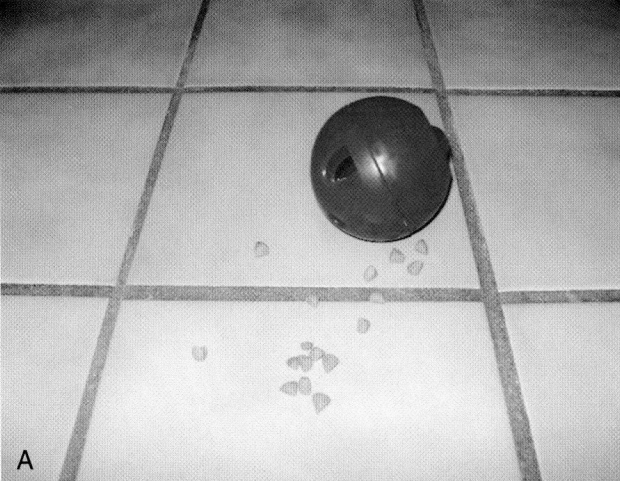

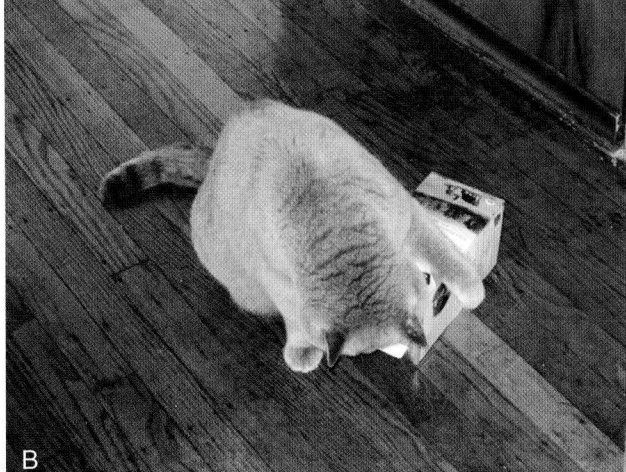

Figure 93-5: Food-dispensing toys can be used to approximate species-typical hunting and feeding behavior. Such toys are commercially available **(A)**, or can be easily made with commonly used objects such as a milk carton **(B)**.

using food-dispensing toys (Figure 93-5) or hiding small amounts of dry food in multiple locations; these strategies also promote physical activity.[37] The use of prey-like toys allows the cat to display a hunting behavior sequence, which can then be ended by the administration of a small amount of food (Box 93-1). Prey-like toys seem to be preferred by cats.[37] Robotic (i.e., automated motion) cat toys are also available. These toys can help keep the cat occupied in the absence of the owner, but they may generate frustration due to the absence of the consummation phase.

BOX 93-1 Proposed Sequence for the Use of Prey-Like Toys

A proposed sequence for the use of prey-like toys that includes a consummatory phase to prevent frustration and inappropriate play is as follows:

1. Play with a prey-like toy (see Figure 93-5) that keeps hands at a safe distance from the cat and prevents play-related aggression.
2. Before the cat may become too aroused or frustrated by the lack of a consummatory phase or before it loses interest in the toy, signal the interruption of the play session with a verbal cue (e.g., "game over"), but do not remove the toy.
3. Immediately after the verbal cue, toss a small amount of high-value food on the floor.
4. Remove the prey-like toy only after the cat has directed its attention to the high-value food.

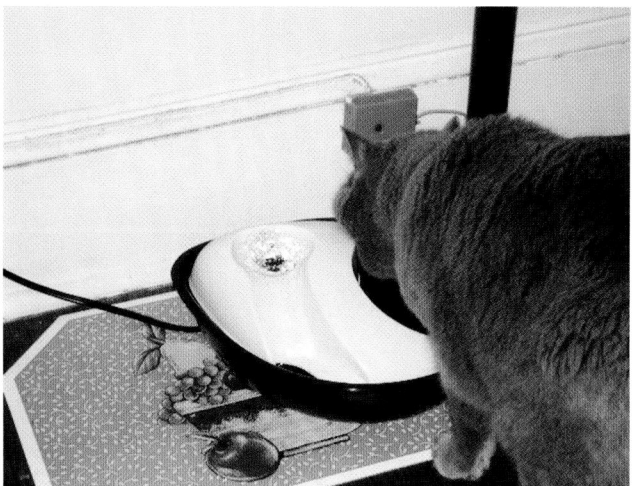

Figure 93-6: Water fountains provide a source of visual stimulation and an opportunity to play.

Multiple water sources should also be available. Water inaccessibility due to hostility between cats may affect both their mental and physical welfare, contributing to the development of pathologies, such as interstitial cystitis.[32] Although there is no scientific evidence that the use of water fountains may significantly increase water consumption,[40,41] their use might still provide a source of visual stimulation and an opportunity to play (Figure 93-6). In fact, it has been anecdotally reported by cat owners that their animals are attracted by the flowing water and spend time watching and playing with it.

Optimizing the multiple cat household territory is not only a matter of resource distribution but also of time scheduling. Cats can use common areas in the household, which usually corresponds to the shared *home range*,[14] at different times to avoid conflicts. Information about the time schedule is exchanged among cats by marking the territory, particularly by scent marking. Scent marks carry information via pheromones deposited with urine, occasionally feces, face and body rubbing, and scratching. Cats approaching the marked area can then perceive the pheromone's gradient of concentration, which will provide them with information about the cat that delivered the message, the approximate time when it was in the area, as well as the nature of its message.[24,25] Fortunately, cats other than intact males do not frequently use urine marking, although it can drastically increase in multiple cat households when hostility arises.[25,28] It is important to provide cats with plenty of opportunities to mark in ways acceptable to the owner, such as scratching in designated areas and rubbing, which will decrease hostility and increase harmony and reduce undesired urine and feces marking. Rubbing on objects and furniture is not usually perceived as a problem by cat owners, so cats are allowed to freely display this behavior. Synthetic pheromones that mimic the effect of facial pheromones deposited by rubbing are commercially available (Feliway MultiCat, Lenexa, Kansas). They can be used to increase a cat's sense of control over the environment, promote its welfare, and discourage the use of unacceptable

forms of territorial marking, such as urine spraying or scratching.[31] Scratching is often considered unacceptable by owners of non-declawed cats and therefore desirable to restrict to designated areas. To be successful in redirecting this behavior to specifically designated areas (e.g., scratching posts), the areas should be chosen taking into account the biology of scratching behavior. If this behavior is in fact performed to mark (i.e., to leave a message for other individuals), the cat wants to deposit the olfactory and visual signal in a socially relevant place, which is a place where the cat itself and the other individuals frequently spend time or transit.[26] This is the main reason why cats scratch the couch in the living room or the rug in the hall of the house, but they are unwilling to use the scratching post one has placed in the unfinished basement for them. Therefore, owners should consider installing scratching posts in socially relevant areas of the household.

Environmental Enrichment: Sharing the Households with Humans and Dogs

There is evidence that well-socialized cats benefit from regular interaction with humans. Laboratory cats tend to organize their activity pattern around the activity of human caretakers[42] and prefer human contact to toys.[38] However, early socialization with humans, the cat's temperament, and the way in which physical contact is made influence the quality of the relationship with humans.[43-45] As a general rule, interaction with cats should be established according to species-typical communicative behavior. It should be brief and limited to the body parts that are used by a cat to make physical contact in a friendly interaction: the cheeks, the chin, the temporal area, and the flanks. According to one study,[45] cats seem to respond most positively to petting by the owner on the temporal area. Consistency and predictability (i.e., repeated positive interactions with the same individual) also make the interaction less stressful for a cat.[46,47] Cats that tolerate being petted by their owner have higher fecal glucocorticoid metabolite levels than cats that run away and hide when the owner tries to make contact.[36] These results suggest that, even when cats tolerate being petted, it can still represent a stressful event for them, and paradoxically, cats that refuse contact with their owners are less likely to be actively stressed by this interaction. Therefore, physical interaction with cats should be short (to mimic a species-typical interaction between two cats meeting and rubbing), and the cat's body language should be observed to detect early signs of stress (e.g., ears back, pupils dilated, lip licking, tail twitching, and/or crouching). If, after contact is ended, the cat seeks more attention and does not display signs of anxiety, the interaction can be further extended.

Although not recommended as a first line of intervention to enrich a cat's environment, interaction with a household dog may be amicable. The gradual introduction of a dog younger than 1 year to a household where a cat younger than 6 months is already present seems to be the most successful strategy to have the two species living in harmony.[48] An introduction protocol including first an olfactory exchange through a physical barrier (but not represented by a small enclosed space, such as a crate, in which the animal may feel trapped), followed by visual contact and then by physical contact is recommended. The introduction protocol described in the Introducing a Cat to a Multiple Cat Household section can be adapted. However, it is important to keep in mind that a dog might be potentially life threatening to a cat, and so the introduction should be completed only if the dog does not show signs of aggression or predation around the cat. In some cases when owners are not present, the cat and the dog may need to be separated for safety reasons.

Environmental Enrichment: Should Outdoor Access be Provided?

Opinions on whether or not to allow outdoor access to cats greatly varies among countries. In the United Kingdom, less than 10% of cat owners do not allow outdoor access to their cats,[49] and in Germany, 55% of owners allow their cats to "run free."[23] In contrast, in the United States, the percentage of owners that never allow outdoor access to their cats is 60%.[50] The American Veterinary Medical Association, the Humane Society of the United States, and many American veterinarians encourage people that live in urban and suburban areas to keep their cats indoors.[51]

One of the main risks for outdoor cats is represented by road traffic accidents. Older, neutered females are significantly less at risk than other cats, and keeping the cat indoors at night also significantly decreases the risk that a road traffic accident may occur.[52,53] Neutered female cats, as well as older cats, may be less likely to roam than intact males that are given access to the outdoors. Households in which any cat has outdoor access have significantly more fighting than households in which the cats remained strictly indoors.[54] This finding may further support the choice to keep cats exclusively indoors.

Although it is commonly assumed that indoor cats are protected from outdoor hazards and live healthier and longer lives, it has been reported that indoor cats may be at increased risk for medical conditions (e.g., feline lower urinary tract disease, tooth resorption lesions, obesity, and hyperthyroidism) and for behavioral problems (e.g., inappropriate elimination, anxiety, and inappropriate scratching).[23,51] The indoor environment may not allow the cat to satisfy its behavioral needs, including an appropriate level of physical activity, consequently increasing its stress and decreasing its welfare. Moreover, some species-typical behaviors (e.g., urine marking and scratching) may be perceived as behavior problems for indoor cats but not for cats that are given access to the outdoors.

Concerns about the impact of cat predation on wildlife, particularly on songbirds, have also been raised, leading to restricted access to the outdoors in many areas of Australia.[49,55] Cats living outdoors frequently catch bird species that feed on the ground or on low vegetation and that live in backyards, such as robins.[56] However, it is unlikely that cat

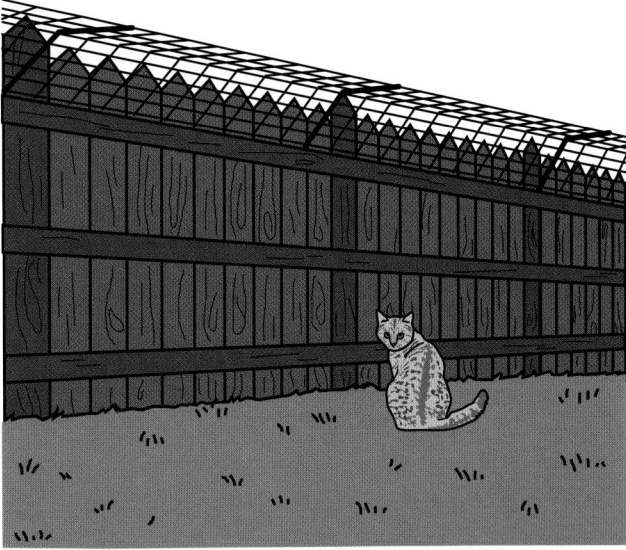

Figure 93-7: "Cat-proof" fence made by placing a soft and flexible fence, such as plastic gardening fence, on top of a solid fence. The soft fence should be angled 45 degrees.

predation would affect the overall bird population (aside from the specific case of birds living on islands, where populations are particularly vulnerable to cats). Moreover, the indirect interactions between cats and birds should also be considered. Domestic cats are in fact predators of small rodents (e.g., rats), which may in turn be predators of small birds.[55] So potentially, birds might also benefit from the presence of cats in their environment.

In conclusion, there are valid arguments to support both keeping a cat exclusively indoors or granting it access to the outdoors. However, it is imperative to provide the indoor cat with an adequate level of environmental enrichment to ensure its welfare and prevent medical and behavioral problems.[51] If an outdoor space is available, it can be secured with a fence that does not allow the household cats to leave the space and prevents unfamiliar cats from entering. A "cat-proof" fence can be easily built by placing a soft and flexible fence (e.g., plastic gardening fence) on top of a solid fence, which should not be easy for a cat to climb (e.g., solid wood). The soft fence should be angled 45 degrees toward the side where the cats are confined (Figure 93-7).

Introducing a Cat to a Multiple Cat Household

It has been reported that introducing a new cat in a multiple cat household causes initial fighting in about 50% of attempted introductions.[54] In the same study, 35% of multiple cat households reported fighting 2 to 12 months after the introduction of the new cat.[54] Unfriendly or aggressive behavior, particularly biting and scratching, during the first meeting was significantly associated with both initial and long-term fighting.[54] These data show the importance of an adequate introduction protocol.

A new cat should always be gradually introduced into an existing group of cats. The new cat should not immediately be allowed physical contact with the other cats. A safe haven should be prepared for the new cat before its arrival; this confined space should contain comfortable bedding, water and food, toys, litter box, scratching post, hiding spaces, and vertical spaces. Ideally, the safe haven should correspond to the designated core area for the new cat (although the core area may be moved to a different location in the future, based on the relationship of the newcomer with its housemates). Placing a pheromone diffuser in the safe haven may help to minimize stress for the newcomer by increasing its sense of control over the unfamiliar environment.[31,57] Physical separation of the introduced individual should be continued for some time, varying from 2 to 3 days to several weeks, depending on the cats' behavior. The safe haven should be at first completely separated from the rest of the house by means of a solid barrier, such as a closed door. In this first phase of the introduction process, only olfactory contact should be allowed between the newcomer and the other cats. The newly introduced cat and the other cats in the household should be allowed to sniff each other under the bottom of the door. High-value treats can be dispensed to the cats at opposite sides of the door to create a positive association via classical conditioning.[58] Conversely, regular meals should not be provided near either side of the door; as previously seen, cats are solitary hunters and eaters, and they may be distressed by the presence of other cats when eating. When the other cats are not present and can be confined to their respective safe havens, the new cat may be allowed to explore areas of the house that have to be shared with the other cats. Ideally, this shared space that the newcomer is allowed to explore should not include the core areas of the other cats.

Once the cats seem to be comfortable with the changes in their environment, the next step can be made in the introduction protocol. Hissing; spitting; attempting to lunge toward, bite, or scratch the other cat; stiffening of the body with prolonged staring; or active avoidance of the other cat are all signs that the cats are not comfortable with each other. If the cats seem to be comfortable with step one of the introduction protocol, a screen that allows visual contact between the cats can be used to keep the newly introduced cat in its safe haven. Only when the cats are comfortable enough with this situation can the transparent barrier be removed and the introduction completed. It is important to make sure that all cats are aware that the barrier is being removed to prevent one cat from being surprised by seeing the other (i.e., they should be allowed to see that the barrier is no longer present before they meet each other).

If any cats show signs of aggression or excessive fear, it may be necessary to confine the newcomer again in its safe haven. Punishment, even verbal, should be avoided if any cat shows aggression or fear. This may increase the undesired behavior, create a negative association with the other individuals, and delay the introduction further. Owners should

be informed that the introduction protocol might not be completed and that some degree of separation between the cats might always be necessary. When difficulties arise upon introducing new feline members, a referral to a veterinary behaviorist can be useful.

Keep It Interesting ... but Calm and Predictable!

Cats may benefit from some variability in their environment (e.g., periodically rotating toys to keep them interesting). For example, interest in catnip toys can vanish as soon as 5 days after having introduced the toy.[49] Lack of predictability and the inability to control the environment represent major sources of distress for cats.[59] As discussed, increased stress may contribute to the development of behavioral and medical problems and to increased conflicts in a multiple cat household. Therefore, it is critical to keep both the indoor and outdoor environment as calm, stable, and predictable as possible. If, for example, it is necessary to create in a household two subgroups of cats that need to be alternated in the common area of the house to avoid conflicts, this should be done on a predictable schedule. This will allow each cat to feel safer by anticipating that at a specific time of the day, no enemies are roaming free in the common area. Similarly, scheduling play sessions at specific times of the day will help a cat regulate its level of arousal throughout the day. This may also contribute to preventing undesired behaviors, such as inappropriate play.[57] Major stressors may also come from the outdoor environment, such as loud noises or the presence of cats or other animals around the house. A source of white noise, such as a radio playing classical music or a talk show, may help muffle outside noises. Similarly, putting plastic privacy film on windows and glass doors can help to decrease outdoor visual stimulation. Motion-activated citronella spray devices, compressed-air spray cans, and water sprinklers placed outdoors can keep cats and other animals away from the house.

SUMMARY

Understanding the social behavior of the domestic cat, as well as its behavioral needs, is essential to create a peaceful and harmonious environment in a multiple cat household. Cats should always be provided with the ability to keep a safe distance from their conspecifics, to hide, and to display natural behavior sequences. An inappropriate environment may cause behavior problems or undesired behaviors in a multiple cat household, which may be indicators of poor welfare.

Therefore, providing cats with an appropriate environment must first be a preventive strategy, rather than solely a treatment for behavior problems or undesired behaviors, to ensure that one's patients have an optimal quality of life and welfare.

References

1. The Humane Society of the United States: pets by the numbers, *The Humane Society of the United States* <http://www.humanesociety.org/issues/pet_overpopulation/facts/pet_ownership_statistics.html>, 2015 (Accessed June 10, 2015.).
2. Rochlitz I: A review of the housing requirements of domestic cats *(Felis silvestris catus)* kept in the home. *Appl Anim Behav Sci* 93:97–109, 2005.
3. Driscoll CA, Menotti-Raymond M, Roca AL, et al: The near eastern origin of cat domestication. *Science* 317:519–523, 2007.
4. Crowell-Davis SL, Curtis TM, Knowles RJ: Social organization in the cat: a modern understanding. *J Feline Med Surg* 6:19–28, 2004.
5. Bowen J, Heath S: An overview on feline social behavior and communication. In Bowen J, Heath S, editors: *Behavior problems in small animals*, Philadelphia, 2005, Elsevier/Saunders, pp 29–36.
6. Macdonald DW, Yamaguchi N, Kery G: Group living in the domestic cat: its sociobiology and epidemiology. In Turner B, Bateson P, editors: *The domestic cat: the biology of its behavior*, ed 2, Cambridge, 2000, Cambridge University Press, pp 95–118.
7. Natoli E, Baggio A, Pontier D: Male and female agonistic and affiliative relationships in a social group of farm cats *(Felis catus L.)*. *Behav Processes* 53:137–143, 2001.
8. Clutton-Brock J: Origin of the dog: domestication and early history. In Sepell J, editor: *The domestic dog: its evolution, behavior and interactions with people*, Cambridge, MA, 1995, Cambridge University Press, pp 7–20.
9. Boitani L, Francisci F, Cuicci P, et al: Population biology and ecology of feral dogs in central Italy. In Sepell J, editor: *The domestic dog: its evolution, behavior and interactions with people*, Cambridge, MA, 1995, Cambridge University Press, pp 217–244.
10. Liberg O, Sandell M, Pointer D, et al: Density, spatial organization and reproductive tactics in the domestic cat and other felids. In Turner B, Bateson P, editors: *The domestic cat: the biology of its behavior*, ed 2, Cambridge, MA, 2000, Cambridge University Press, pp 119–150.
11. Barry KJ, Crowell-Davis SL: Gender differences in the social behavior of the neutered indoor-only domestic cat. *Appl Anim Behav Sci* 64:193–211, 1999.
12. Broom DM, Fraser AF: *Domestic animal behavior and welfare*, ed 4, Wallingford, 2007, CABI.
13. Bernstein PL, Strack M: A game of cat and house: spatial patterns and behavior of 14 domestic cats *Felis catus* in the home. *Anthrozoos* 9:25–39, 1996.
14. Heath S: Aggression in cats. In Horwitz DF, Mills DS, editors: *BSAVA manual of canine and feline behavioral medicine*, ed 2, Gloucester, 2009, British Small Animal Veterinary Association, pp 223–235.
15. Bradshaw JWS, Hall SL: Affiliative behaviour of related and unrelated pairs of cats in catteries a preliminary report. *Appl Anim Behav Sci* 63:251–255, 1999.
16. Bateson P: Behavioral development in the cat. In Turner B, Bateson P, editors: *The domestic cat: the biology of its behavior*, ed 2, Cambridge, MA, 2000, Cambridge University Press, pp 9–22.
17. Frank D: Management problems in cats. In Horowitz D, Mills D, Heath S, editors: *BSAVA manual of canine and feline behavioral medicine*, ed 1, Gloucester, 2002, British Small Animal Veterinary Association, pp 80–89.
18. Heath S: Feline aggression. In Horwitz DF, Mills M, Heath S, editors: *BSAVA manual of canine and feline behavioral medicine*, ed 1, Gloucester, 2002, British Small Animal Veterinary Association, pp 216–228.
19. Lindell EM, Hollis NE, Houpt KA: Intercat aggression: a retrospective study examining types of aggression, sexes of fighting pairs, and effectiveness of treatment. *Appl Anim Behav Sci* 55:153–162, 1997.
20. Bradshaw JWS: *The behaviour of the domestic cat*, Wallingford, 1992, CABI.
21. Levine E, Perry J, Scarlett J, et al: Intercat aggression in households following the introduction of a new cat. *Appl Anim Behav Sci* 90:325–336, 2005.
22. Reisner I: An overview of aggression. In Horwitz DF, Mills DS, Heath S, editors: *BSAVA manual of canine and feline behavioral medicine*, ed 1, Gloucester, 2002, British Small Animal Veterinary Association, pp 173–194.
23. Heidenberger E: Housing conditions and behavioral problems of indoors cats as assessed by their owners. *Appl Anim Behav Sci* 52:345–364, 1997.
24. Bradshaw J, Cameron-Beaumont C: The signaling repertoire of the domestic cat and its undomesticated relatives. In Turner B, Bateson P, editors: *The domestic cat: the biology of its behavior*, ed 2, Cambridge, MA, 2000, Cambridge University Press, pp 67–93.
25. Overall K: Normal feline behavior and ontogeny: neurological and social development, signaling and normal feline behaviors. In Overall K, editor: *Manual of clinical behavioral medicine for dogs and cats*, St Louis, 2013, Elsevier Mosby, pp 312–359.
26. Casey R: Fear and stress. In Horwitz DF, Mills DS, editors: *BSAVA manual of canine and feline behavioral medicine*, ed 2, Gloucester, 2009, British Small Animal Veterinary Association, pp 144–153.
27. Turner DC: Cat behavior and the human/cat relationship. *Animalis Familiaris* 3:16–21, 1988.
28. Nelson J: House soiling by cats. In Horwitz DF, Mills DS, editors: *BSAVA manual of canine and feline behavioral medicine*, ed 2, Gloucester, 2009, British Small Animal Veterinary Association, pp 117–126.
29. Pryor PA, Hart BL, Bain MJ, et al: Causes of urine marking in cats and the effects of environmental management on frequency of marking. *J Am Vet Med Assoc* 219:1709–1713, 2001.
30. Horwitz D: House soiling by cats. In Horwitz DF, Mills DS, Heath S, editors: *BSAVA manual of canine and feline behavioral medicine*, ed 1, Gloucester, 2002, British Small Animal Veterinary Association, pp 97–108.
31. Pageat P, Gaultier E: Current research in canine and feline pheromones. *Vet Clin North Am Small Anim Pract* 33:187–211, 2003.
32. Heath S: Feline social behavior. In *Proceedings. Penn Vet: 111th Penn Annual Conference, Philadelphia*, 2011, pp 1–2.
33. Heath SE: Behaviour problems and welfare—multi-cat households. In Rochlitz I, editor: *Welfare of cats*, Dordrecht, 2005, Springer, pp 107–110.
34. Buffington CAT, Westropp JL, Chew DJ, et al: Clinical evaluation of multimodal environment modification (MEMO) in the management of cats with idiopathic cystitis. *J Feline Med Surg* 8:261–268, 2006.
35. Rochlitz I: Feline welfare issues. In Turner B, Bateson P, editors: *The domestic cat: the biology of its behavior*, ed 2, Cambridge, MA, 2000, Cambridge University Press, pp 207–226.
36. Ramos Dl, Reche-Junior A, Fragoso PL, et al: Are cats *(Felis catus)* from multi-cat households more stressed? Evidence from assessment of faecal glucocorticoid metabolites analysis. *Physiol Behav* 122:72–75, 2013.
37. Ellis S: Environmental enrichment—practical strategies for improving feline welfare. *J Feline Med Surg* 11:901–912, 2009.
38. De Luca AM, Kranda KC: Environmental enrichment in a large animal facility. *Lab Anim* 21:38–44, 1992.
39. Liberg O: Food habits and prey impact by feral and house-based domestic cats in a rural area in southern Sweden. *J Mammal* 65:424–432, 1984.
40. Pachel C, Neilson J: Comparison of feline water consumption between still and flowing water sources: a pilot study. *J Vet Behav* 5:130–133, 2010.
41. Grant DC: Effect of water source on intake and urine concentration in healthy cats. *J Feline Med Surg* 12:431–434, 2010.
42. Randall WR, Cunningham JT, Randall S: Sounds from an animal colony entrain a circadian rhythm in the cat. *Felis Catus L. J Interdiscipl Cycle* 21:55–64, 1990.
43. Casey RAC, Bradshaw JWS: The effects of additional socialisation for kittens in a rescue centre on their behaviour and suitability as a pet. *Appl Anim Behav Sci* 114:196–205, 2008.
44. Mendl M, Harcourt R: Individuality in the domestic cat: origins, development and stability. In Turner B, Bateson P, editors: *The domestic cat: the biology of its behavior*, ed 2, Cambridge, MA, 2000, Cambridge University Press, pp 48–64.

45. Soennichsen S, Chamove AS: Responses of cats to petting by humans. *Anthrozoos* 15:258–265, 2002.
46. Gourkow N, Fraser D: The effect of housing and handling practices on the welfare, behaviour and selection of domestic cats *(Felis sylvestris catus)* by adopters in an animal shelter. *Anim Welf* 15:371–377, 2006.
47. Kessler MR, Turner DC: Stress and adaptation of cats *(Felis silvestris catus)* housed singly, in pairs and in groups in boarding catteries. *Anim Welf* 6:243–254, 1997.
48. Feuerstein N, Terkel J: Interrelationships of dogs *(Canis familiaris)* and cats *(Felis catus L.)* living under the same roof. *Appl Anim Behav Sci* 113:150–165, 2008.
49. Rochlitz I: Housing and welfare. In Rochlitz I, editor: *The welfare of cats*, Dordrecht, 2007, Springer, pp 177–203.
50. Patronek GJ, Beck AM, Glickman LT: Dynamics of dog and cat populations in a community. *J Am Vet Med Assoc* 210:637–642, 1997.
51. Buffington CAT: External and internal influences on disease risk in cats. *J Am Vet Med Assoc* 220:994–1002, 2002.
52. Rochlitz I: Study of factors that may predispose domestic cats to road traffic accidents: Part 1. *Vet Rec* 153:549–553, 2003.
53. Rochlitz I: Study of factors that may predispose domestic cats to road traffic accidents: part 2. *Vet Rec* 153:585–588, 2003.
54. Levine E, Perry J, Scarlett J, et al: Intercat aggression in households following the introduction of a new cat. *Appl Anim Behav Sci* 90:325–336, 2005.
55. Fitzgerald BM, Turner DT: Hunting behavior of domestic cats and their impact on prey population. In Turner B, Bateson P, editors: *The domestic cat: the biology of its behavior*, ed 2, Cambridge, 2000, Cambridge University Press, pp 151–175.
56. Mead CJ: Ringed birds killed by cats. *Mammal Rev* 12:183–186, 1982.
57. Seksel K: Preventive behavioral medicine for cats. In Horwitz DF, Mills DS, editors: *BSAVA manual of canine and feline behavioral medicine*, ed 2, Gloucester, 2009, British Small Animal Veterinary Association, pp 75–82.
58. Mills D: Training and learning protocols. In Horwitz DF, Mills DS, editors: *BSAVA manual of canine and feline behavioral medicine*, ed 2, Gloucester, 2009, British Small Animal Veterinary Association, pp 49–64.
59. Casey R: Fear and stress. In Horwitz DF, Mills DS, Heath S, editors: *BSAVA manual of canine and feline behavioral medicine*, ed 1, Gloucester, 2002, British Small Animal Veterinary Association, pp 144–153.

Feline Social Behavior and Personality

Jacqui Ley

The domestic cat is an interesting and highly successful species, partly because it is capable of adapting to a wide variety of living conditions. This includes a variety of social conditions, from cats living solitary lives to multicat households and large cat colonies. The social behavior of cats has been described in some detail, but there is room for more work to capture the variability of how cats live and interact with each other and with people. The social behavior of any animal is affected, in part, by the individual's unique combination of genetics and experience. The psychological construct of personality, also known as *behavioral individual differences,* describes the effect that genetics and experience have on the way an individual tends to behave. The construct of personality has been successfully applied to several species, but only very preliminary work has been conducted on the domestic cat. This chapter summarizes feline social behavior. Personality research is reviewed briefly before discussing what a model of feline personality might look like. Lastly, how personality affects social behavior and the value of understanding feline personality are considered.

SOCIAL BEHAVIOR

Social behavior describes the behavior used by individuals to increase or decrease contact with members of their social group.[1] In some species, social behavior may be limited to defending territory, identifying a mate, and rearing offspring. This is seen in many of the solitary felid species, such as tigers and jaguars.[2,3] In other felid species, such as lions, social behavior is highly complex, building on previous interactions to forge bonds and affiliations.[2] The domestic cat defies categorization as solitary or highly social, because feral cats can be found living along a continuum from solitary cats in defended territories to large colonies of many cats in close proximity to each other.[4-6] Inspection of ethograms suggests that although social bonds do form between some cats, they are not as complex as those seen in truly social species, such as chimpanzees or elephants.[7-10] Many social species show group care of young; the domestic cat varies in social care of its young. It is well accepted that related queens will often help each other care for kittens, and there are reports of male cats interacting with and caring for kittens in colony situations.[7] This is not reported for cats living more solitary lives.

Affiliative and Agonistic Behavior

Cats vary in their social organization, but what does not vary among cats are the signals that they display to communicate their emotions and intentions to other cats. Social behaviors can increase contact among social group members or decrease contact and prevent contact with animals that are not members of the social group. Those behaviors that increase contact are considered affiliative behaviors and include such behaviors as raised tails, head rubbing, and flank rubbing. These rubbing behaviors are also known as *allorubbing.*[7] Affiliative behaviors can be organized into more complex patterns; for example, a tail up approach leads to head rubbing and mutual flank rubbing between partners.[11] What is striking among some cats is the level of affiliative behavior they may show. For example, some cats may be observed lying in groups, displaying mutual grooming and allorubbing, and can generally be found in close proximity to each other (Figure 94-1). These cats are considered to have bonded. That is, they have formed a social group and maintain the group by close contact and regular interactions. Allorubbing and lying together may help to create a group odor. This group odor appears to be important to recognition and acceptance in the group. Removing a cat from the group, for veterinary treatment for example, may affect its odor and prevent it being readmitted to the group territory.[12] Many cats show affiliative behaviors (e.g., being in close proximity, allorubbing, grooming conspecifics, and lying together) to humans and other animals such as dogs with which they have developed social bonds (Figures 94-2 and 94-3).

Agonistic behaviors are those that decrease contact among individuals. Agonistic behaviors may be displayed between members of a social group and may also be directed toward unfamiliar cats. These include behaviors such as staring, hissing, growling, and attacking. Because fighting is potentially a very costly behavior to undertake—the winner might win the battle but may sustain some fitness-reducing wounds—much agonistic behavior in cats takes the form of threats. These include controlling access to resources (e.g., sitting in doorways preventing access to food, water, litter boxes, and resting places), staring, and spraying. Table 94-1 lists some affiliative and agonistic behaviors seen in cats. See Chapters 91 and 92 for more information on agonistic behaviors and feline aggression.

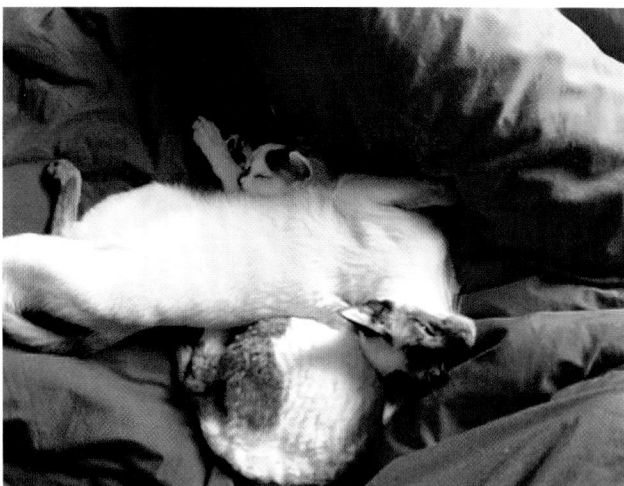

Figure 94-1: Bonded cats will lie in very close proximity to each other.

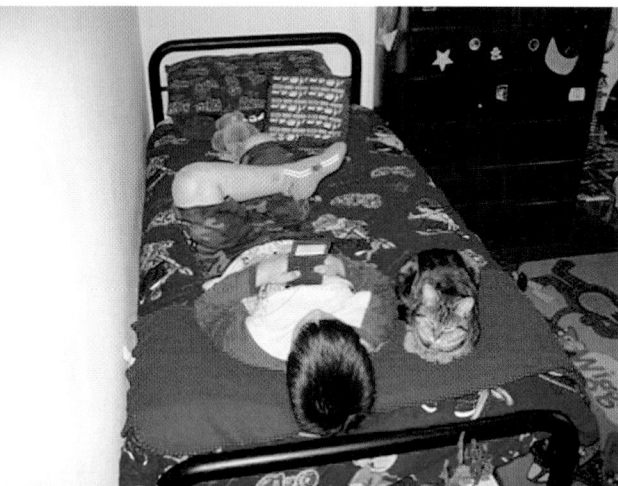

Figure 94-2: Bonded cats will spend time in close proximity with humans they have formed bonds with. (Courtesy of Mr. Damian Jeffery.)

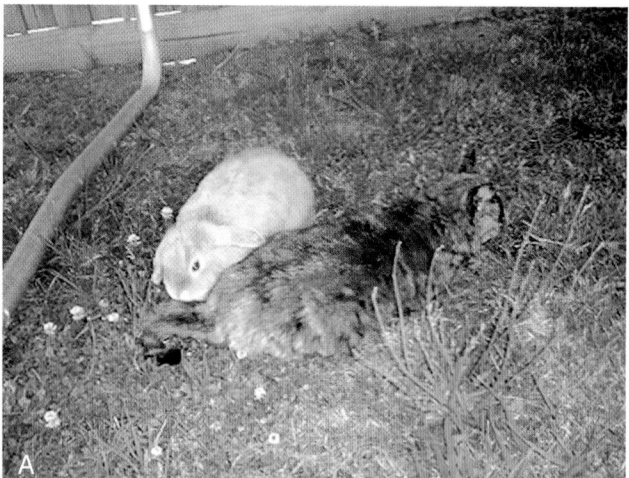

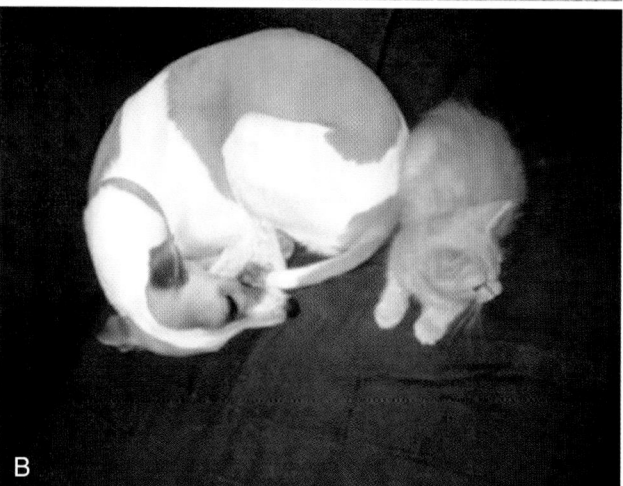

Figure 94-3: **A** and **B**, If cats spend time with animals of other species during their socialization period, they will tend to form social bonds with that species, even if they are traditionally prey species or "enemies." (Courtesy of Mr. Damian Jeffery.)

Cats that are well socialized still show a wide range of affiliative and agonistic behaviors toward others. Cats learn social behaviors as kittens through interaction with their queen, older relatives, and their littermates.

Social Behavior of Kittens

Kittens begin their lives outside the uterus as a dependent animal. They must be fed, stimulated to eliminate feces and urine, have their temperature controlled, and be defended from dangers. They gradually develop into a social animal that seeks interaction with others before maturing into a more solitary animal. Kittens learn and practice social behaviors with their littermates, their mother and related queens, and some male cats. The eyes and ears of kittens open between 5 and 14 days of age,[14] and they can send and receive information from other cats, animals, and objects in their environments. From approximately 2 weeks of age, kittens show orientation to sounds; and at about 3 weeks of age, they orientate to and show a following response to visual stimuli. By 4 weeks of age, kittens are moving and interacting with their environment, but their signals and interactions are indistinct. For example, play is restricted to just patting with the front paws at 2 weeks of age.[15] As the kittens grow and develop better muscle control and better integration of their senses, their signals become more sophisticated. The fear response, for example, is seen at about 6 weeks of age,[16] and social play develops more elements, such as "belly up" and "vertical stance" postures.[17]

The change in kittens from social animals to more solitary animals can be seen in the changes that occur in kitten play behavior. Social play involving games of chase and wrestling are seen from 4 to 16 weeks of age with a peak between 7 and 9 weeks.[15,18] A large amount of the kitten's time is spent in social play, which then wanes in favor of object-directed play. Object-directed play is generally seen at 14 days of age with a peak at about 7 weeks of age.[17,18] Whereas object-directed play involves hunting behaviors, social play involves

Table 94-1	Some Affiliative and Agonistic Behaviors Identified in Cats	
Observation	**Description**	**Type of Behavior**
Body		
Tail up	Tail raised to vertical, often as cat approaches an individual of higher status[13] Often shown by kittens toward their queen Seen between adult cats; the lower status cat keeps its tail up on approach	Affiliative
Tail horizontal	Tail is held close to level with the back Thought to indicate an interaction between two cats of similar status	Affiliative
Body: "Halloween cat"	Arched back, ears back, tail held in an inverted U shape This is a defensive posture	Agonistic
Body	Upright stance One front paw lifted ready to strike Confident, offensively aggressive cat	Agonistic
Body	Body lowered Head and front legs rolled slightly to one side ready to strike Defensive posture	Agonistic
Coat piloerection	Hair on body and tail fluffed up This makes the cat look larger and can bluff other animals, thereby avoiding fights	Agonistic
Eyes	Staring intensely	Agonistic
Eyes	Slow, exaggerated blink Signals that the cat will tolerate interaction	Affiliative
Vocalizations		
Trill/chirrup/greeting meow	Sometimes described as a chirrup or a murmur Generally made when the cat is approaching a familiar cat or person with whom it has a social bond Kittens commonly greet their queen this way Made with the mouth closed	Affiliative
Meow	Many different sounds made by altering the speed with which the mouth is closed Cats learn what sounds the people they have bonded with respond to	Affiliative
Growl, yowl, snarl	All open-mouthed sounds Used when the cat is under threat or is attacking	Agonistic
Hiss	Open-mouthed sound Used defensively	Agonistic
Behaviors		
Allorubbing	One cat approaches another and rubs the head and corner of the mouth along the approached cat's face, shoulders, and body	Affiliative
Grooming conspecific	One cat grooms by licking another cat who allows itself to be groomed	Affiliative
Sharing resting area	Two or more cats lying in a resting area touching or even intertwined (see Figure 94-1)	Affiliative
Timesharing	Two or more cats use a space sequentially—one cat leaves the area as the other approaches Avoids conflicts between the cats	Agonistic

behaviors from several different behavior patterns. For example, a game may have elements of stalking, hunting, fighting, and copulating. As kittens become older, many friendly games end in a fight, and the kittens move away from each other.[18] This behavior appears to be readying them for dispersal. Male kittens disperse between 6 and 36 months of age. They travel further away than female kittens, many of whom stay close to their mother.

Socialization

Socialization occurs as the kittens interact with their environment. Socialization describes the process by which animals become familiarized to their environment and learn what objects they can safely ignore, what things and individuals they need to be wary of, and which individuals respond positively to them. If they have contact with individuals of other species (including humans), they will become socialized to them and that species (Figures 94-2, 94-3, and 94-4). For example, kittens raised with rats in a laboratory experiment were tolerant of the strain of rat with which they were raised but would hunt rats of other strains.[19] The socialization period is the time when young animals are most receptive to learning from new experiences. This period occurs earlier in kittens than it does in puppies. The canine socialization period begins with eyes opening at approximately 21 days and ends at about 12 weeks of age. In comparison, the feline socialization period is from 14 days until 7 weeks of age, meaning most kittens are past the point of easily learning about people when they are adopted or relinquished to animal shelters. Karsh found that to become well socialized to people,

kittens should be handled from 2 weeks of age for 30 to 40 minutes a day (see Figure 94-4).[20] Cat breeders must begin to socialize their kittens to gentle handling and normal household noises and events from 2 weeks of age to maximize their chances of developing into resilient, friendly companion cats. Animal shelters have a responsibility to understand the risks and possible outcomes when rehoming older kittens that have not been socialized to humans and that do not respond positively to regular handling.

During the socialization period, kittens learn about prey species and how to hunt and dismember them; preferences for foods and prey are formed through this period. The preferences of the queen will shape her kittens' preferences for foods and prey species.[19] Kittens learn from watching their mother catch, kill, and dismember prey and are more likely to be successful with that prey species if their mother is present when they practice.[17] Substrate preferences for toileting are also formed in the socialization period. Kittens start to dig in fine soft substrates at 30 days of age, and then they progress to more adult elimination behaviors within a few days.[15] Contrary to what some owners may think, kittens that have not reached sexual maturity (between 5 and 12 months of age) that housesoil are not urine marking; they are just not properly litter trained.

Social Behavior and Being Individual

Some cats frequently display affiliative behaviors, and at the other end of the spectrum are cats that are antisocial and do not tolerate affiliative social interactions at all. These differences can be explained by the genetics and experiences of the individual cat. For example, cats are born with different genetic tolerances for close social contact and noise with genetically driven preferences for behavioral responses, including whether to be fearful and reactive or to be aggressive. These make up the cat's temperament and are purely the genetic component of how they tend to behave. As the kitten interacts with its environment and experiences other cats (including their mother and littermates), people, other animals, noises, and so on, the temperament is refined to shape how the kitten will tend to behave. The effects of learning modify the genetic tendencies. The kitten may learn that humans are good to interact with and so it will not run away from them. The way cats tend to differ in their behaviors has not been described in great depth, but the research that has been done suggests that personality is a construct that can be usefully applied to cats.[21]

PERSONALITY

The way that an individual tends to display characteristic behavior patterns, thoughts, and feelings is described as *personality*.[22] Personality is considered to be stable over time and in different situations,[23] although the exact behaviors that an individual displays vary due to the effects of affect, motivation and needs, previous learning, and the current environment.[24]

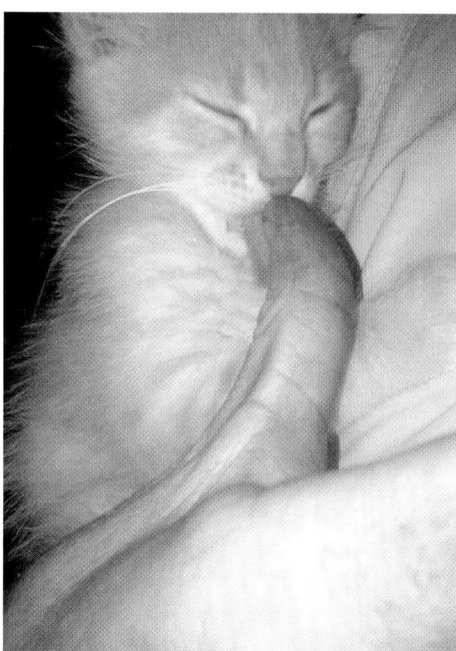

Figure 94-4: Kittens become socialized to people between the ages of 2 and 7 weeks of age. (Courtesy of Mr. Damian Jeffery.)

Personality characteristics are not static but have consequences for the individual and are the way that individuals interact with their environment, especially their social environment.[25]

There are several different theories of personality. Of these, trait theory is the system that is widely accepted in human psychology and has been most usefully applied to animals. In trait theory, the individual is described using a formal system of categorizing and measuring personality differences. Personality is considered to be made up of dimensions which are, in turn, made up of traits (Figure 94-5). Zuckerman[26] suggests that a personality trait should be:

1. Identifiable across measurement methods, sexes, ages, and cultures
2. Moderately heritable
3. Identifiable in animal species, particularly those which live in social groups or colonies
4. Identified with significant biological trait markers

These four prerequisites aim to anchor traits to the biology of the organism, and all four have empirical support.

The most widely accepted trait-based models of human personality are the Five Factor Model (FFM) and the Big Five Personality Test.[27,28] It describes human personality with five dimensions (Figure 94-6): (1) surgency (extraversion), (2) agreeableness, (3) conscientiousness, (4) intellect (openness to new ideas), and (5) emotional stability (neuroticism).

It is all well and good to recognize that cats differ from each other in how they tend to behave, but is it appropriate to apply personality theory to cats? There is a considerable body of research investigating personality in animals as diverse as chimpanzees, wolves, dogs, horses, goats, fish, and octopi (see Gosling for a complete discussion).[29-36] However, the term preferred by researchers in the fields of comparative psychology, evolutionary biology, and evolutionary ecology is *behavioral individual differences*.[37] Behavioral individual differences are considered important for individual survival and species adaptability.[38] An attempt to simply describe a model of personality that explains behavioral individual differences has been made in very few species. Figure 94-6 shows a model for canine personality. The canine five-factor model (CFFM) was developed by the author using the methodology used to define the FFM for human personality.[33]

There are not many studies that investigate feline behavioral individual differences or personality. Many studies use part of personality as a means of describing differences between cats as a fixed variable for considering physiologic or other factors. For example, Kuleshova and colleagues found significantly more interneuronal interactions in the

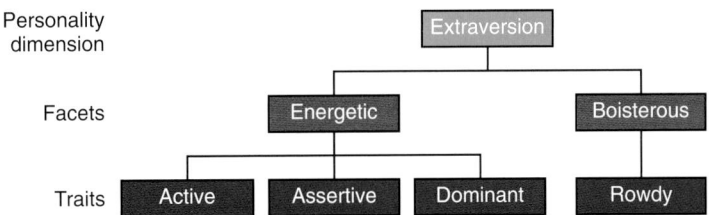

Figure 94-5: Example of hierarchical organization of traits by trait theory.

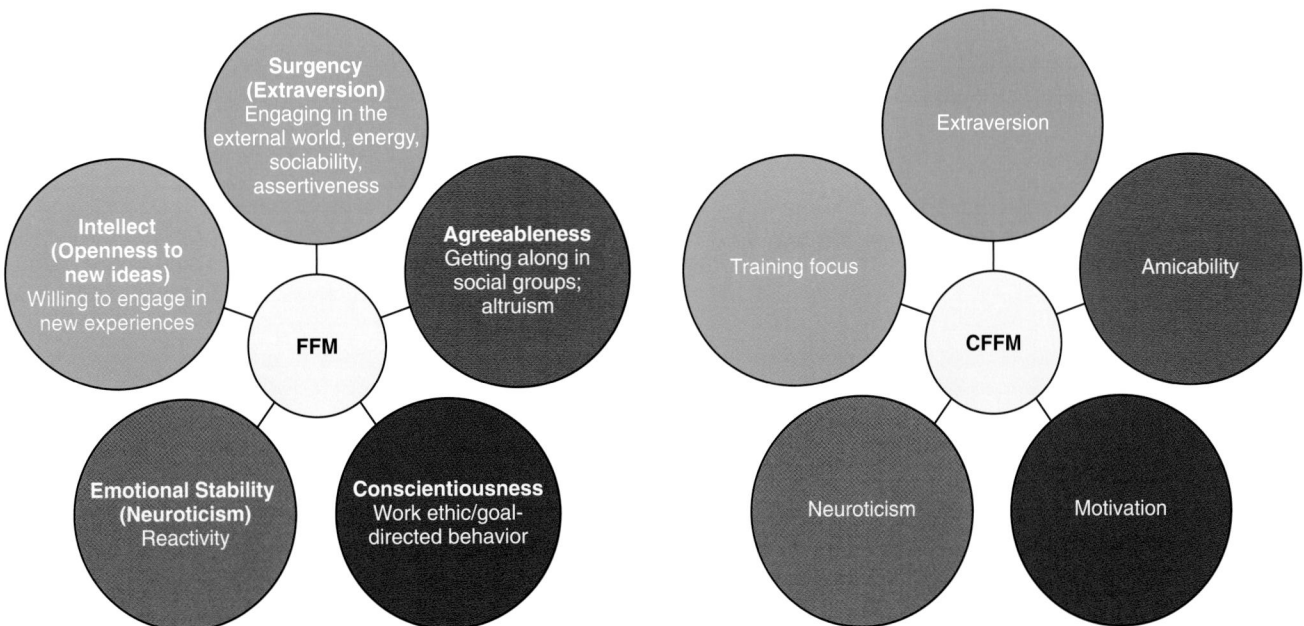

Figure 94-6: Diagrammatic representations of the Five Factor Model *(FFM)* of personality for humans and the canine five-factor model *(CFFM)* of personality.

nucleus accumbens of cats considered to have self-control compared with cats described as ambivalent or impulsive.[39] Natoli and colleagues found that feral colony cats rated as "proactive" had a greater chance of contracting feline immunodeficiency virus.[40] *Proactive cats* were described as cats that won most of their aggressive encounters, marked the most, and showed the most affiliative behaviors toward other members of their social groups. Reisner and colleagues found paternal effects for littermates and individual differences in kittens aged 8 to 20 weeks old for their sociability toward humans and objection to restraint for venipuncture regardless of the amount handling (daily or none) or the type of housing (group or solo) that the kittens experienced.[41] The Feline Temperament Profile (FTP) was developed to assess cats' affinity to humans and has been validated in one study that found a cat's preadoption scores on the FTP correlated to the postadoption scores and that preadoption FTP scores correlated with time spent sitting near an unfamiliar man in an open field test.[42]

Feaver and colleagues assessed if individual differences among cats could be reliably quantified using a rating method but did not attempt to define or describe personality in cats (see Gartner and Weiss for a review of feline personality literature).[43,44]

The research recognizes that there are differences among cats in the way that individuals behave and these differences have real effects for the cats. These differences can also be correlated with physiologic differences and have effects on what happens to the cat. However, what is missing from feline personality research is a model that describes the depth and breadth of feline personality so that it can be investigated among cats, across methodologies, and compared between species as recommended by Gosling.[36] At present, researchers have tended to use the FTP, or they have created their own questionnaire or measurements. This doesn't allow for comparison among researchers or among populations of cats or even allow the reader to be certain that the same personality dimensions are being measured. The FTP measures the cat's affinity to people, but this is likely to be the result of interactions among dimensions related to social interaction, new experiences, and timidity.

What Would a Feline Personality Model Look Like?

A model of feline personality would usefully describe behavioral tendencies of cats and allow cats to be compared along the different personality dimensions. Additionally, it would have a strong theoretical base, drawing on the fields of personality and comparative psychology.

Personality or temperament research in cats agrees that there are dimensions of personality related to shyness or timidity, energy, and sociability[44] (Figure 94-7). McCune also identifies a *bold* dimension, which is characterized as a response to novelty.[45] The author found that the cats in the study responded differently to a familiar person, an unfamiliar (novel) person, and a novel object and notes that the handling

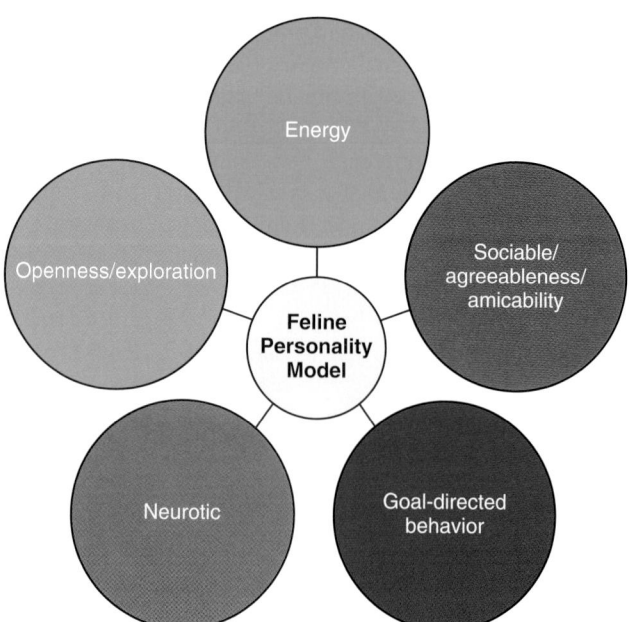

Figure 94-7: A suggested model for feline personality.

Table 94-2	List of Feline Personality Dimensions Used in Research	
Dimension	**Title/Description**	**Research Study**
Emotional stability	Nervous, timid Timid Shy and unfriendly	Feaver et al.[43] Karsh and Turner[46] Turner et al.[49]
Energy level	Active, aggressive Bold Proactive	Feaver et al.[43] Karsh and Turner[46] Natoli et al.[40]
Exploration	Bold	McCune[45]
Sociability	Sociable, confident, easygoing Confident Proactive	Feaver et al.[43] Karsh and Turner[46] Meier and Turner[48] Natoli et al.[40]
Goal-directed behavior	Impulsive, self-controlled	Kuleshova et al.[39]

effect was limited to affecting responses to humans but not novel objects.[45] In other models of personality for other species, dimensions relating to *response to novelty* (*openness* in the FFM) and interactions with others (*agreeableness* in the FFM and *amicability* in the CFFM) (see Figure 94-6) are separate dimensions. It seems likely that this would also be the case for cats.

It is possible that there are other personality dimensions in cats. Some may be unique to cats, whereas others may be analogous or limited variants of dimensions seen in other species. One possible model is a five-dimension model with dimensions relating to *energy level, sociability, response to novelty, goal-directed behavior,* and *emotional stability* (Table 94-2).

Energy Level

The *energy level* dimension typically describes the individual's tendency to be active, energetic, and outgoing. In humans, it contains traits such as talkative, assertive, and positive aspect.[47] In dogs, it is characterized more simply as the tendency to be energetic and active.[32] Research has characterized dimensions related to the activity levels of domestic cats,[43] suggesting that the feline *energy level* dimension is likely to be similar to that in dogs.

Sociability

A tendency to varying sociability has been described in cats.[43,48] In dogs, the dimension *amicability* describes the tendency to be relaxed and sociable without defining the species that is the target of the social behavior.[32] This is more limited than the human dimension of *agreeableness*, which contains traits such as affectionate, sympathetic, and unfriendly.[47] This reflects differences in the higher-order cognitive abilities between humans and animals. Thus, a dimension for sociability in cats is likely to be more similar to that for dogs than the *agreeableness* dimension for people.

Response to Novelty

In humans, *openness to experience* is the dimension of the FFM that assesses an individual's tendency to be imaginative, intelligent, and to have wide or varied interests. The CFFM lacks a dimension analogous to *openness to experience*. In cats, some studies assess the cat's response to novelty through exposure to novel objects, unfamiliar people, and open field tests. The open field test involves releasing the cat into a room or enclosure where a grid of squares has been marked on the floor. The number of squares the animal moves through is counted to generate a measure of activity. Other measures may include the total distance traveled and time spent in certain areas of the space. However, none specifically measure the tendency of the cats to be exploratory. McCune suggests that some cats may be bolder than others, but boldness is a mixture of two dimensions in personality theory, not a single dimension.[45]

A dimension related to exploration would be expected in cats, because they are a species that hunts a variety of small prey in different environments, but they are also preyed upon. Cats evolved in highly variable environments, and different strategies for exploration would have conferred different survival advantages in changing environments. The end result would be a variety of responses to novelty, from avoiding novel items and environments to reckless exploration of anything new. Research into feline personality should attempt to identify if a dimension relating to exploration can be described.

Goal-Directed Behavior

Goal-directed behavior under the heading of *conscientiousness* has only been identified in humans and chimpanzees.[30] The CFFM has a dimension labeled *motivation*, which contains the traits of assertive, determined, persevering, tenacious, and independent.[32] This dimension shares some aspects with the *conscientiousness* dimension of humans, such as continuing with a behavior to achieve a goal. Cats also show goal-directed behaviors in many parts of their lives, such as hunting and mate-seeking behaviors. Some pet cats are easily distracted from unwanted behaviors, whereas other cats persevere with behaviors, usually undesirable, until they achieve their goal. It seems likely that a personality dimension of *goal-directed behavior* exists in cats.

Emotional Stability

Turner and colleagues and Feaver and colleagues have identified differences in cats relating to *emotional stability*.[49,43] They found cats varied in shyness, timidity, and fearfulness. Traits and dimensions relating to *emotional stability* have been identified in many species, including humans, dogs, goats, and horses, suggesting that this is a personality dimension that evolved early in the evolution of behavior.[50,32,34,51]

THE INTERACTION OF SOCIAL BEHAVIOR AND PERSONALITY

Having a stable manner of responding to the environment and toward conspecifics has value for the individual and for the species. Limited work has been done in cats, but the benefits of stable *behavioral individual differences* or *personality* have been explored in species as diverse as fish, octopi, pigs, and dogs.[35,52-54] Many aspects of personality are related to surviving in variable environments and coping with interactions with other members of an individual's social group, so it is not unexpected to find similarities in personality dimensions among species even though they may exploit radically different environmental niches. Individuals of social species must balance social status in their group with the need to get along with others in the group.[55] Having a stable response to social interactions means that individuals can predict how another member of their social group will behave and alter their behavior to minimize conflict. This reduces not only actual conflict within the group but also stress, because behavioral responses become more predictable.

Diversity in ratings for personality dimensions among members of a group means that the group and the species benefit when environmental and social conditions change. For example, if some members are attracted to explore novel objects and environments, they may identify a new food source. The whole social group may benefit from this, but even if they do not, the curious animals may survive and keep the group (and the species) going. The curious individuals have an increased risk of being injured or killed by exploring new environments or eating new foods, but the rest of the group may survive. Some individuals react to novel items and environments with fear. They may attempt to avoid or escape a new enclosure or novel objects; they may be avoided or even attacked. The social group and the whole species benefit from these different strategies; in times of overcrowding or food shortages, individuals willing to explore may find new territory and more food, increasing their survival and the species survival. Being fearful of novelty can also be an effective survival strategy. By not exploring, the individual reduces its risk of dying from misadventure. In times with high food levels, the more cautious animal is less likely to die and more likely to reproduce. Depending upon environmental factors, variability in responses to novelty offers different levels of survival advantage to individuals and so variability in this trait is found throughout a population. This is also seen with cats.

Cats with a high drive to explore and a high tolerance to living close to other cats are able to exist in colonies and exploit novel food sources, such as food scraps from people. They also have increased risk of contracting diseases[40] and being injured by traffic, dogs, and people. Cats less able to tolerate social contact and that are less attracted to novelty may have a harder time finding food but will also have lower chances of contracting diseases or being injured or killed.

Within one's home, personality affects some important aspects of feline behavior. Cats with a low tolerance for change, that score low perhaps on the *response to novelty* dimension, may struggle with changes to household routines such as changes in food, litter, or litter boxes. Cats that are friendly but score high for timidity on the *emotional stability* measures may be friendly with the people they live with but may not cope with visitors. Variability in feline personality has important implications as to how well a cat will satisfy its owner's expectations for a relationship with the cat. Bold, noisy cats are not valued by everyone, and some owners find it hard to cope with a timid cat that is not friendly to people.

WHY A FELINE PERSONALITY MODEL IS NEEDED

Understanding feline personality is interesting as an intellectual pursuit, but would it result in any practical benefits for cats, their owners, breeders, veterinarians, and shelters? Research into the human-animal bond suggests that it is fragile and easily broken. Owners who are less attached to their cats report higher dissatisfaction with the level of affection their cat displays.[56] Investigation into the reasons behind an owner's decision to relinquish a pet indicates that the decision is complex involving owner, economical, and feline factors.[57] One feline risk factor is the cat not meeting the owner's expectations with regard to how it behaves.[58] Having a validated model of feline personality will allow tools to be developed that measure feline personality, allowing potential owners to quantify the personality that they would like in a cat and to identify cats that match their preferences. Breeders would have tools available to help aid selection of cats for breeding based on personality. They could also use the personality ratings to promote their cats as pets. Anecdotally, pet owners in general do not want high-maintenance pets. So the ideal cat personality for most people would be a moderately extraverted cat that has a moderate-to-high sociability rating, moderate exploratory tendencies, low-to-moderate levels of goal-directed behavior, and high levels of emotional stability. This cat would be playful some of the time, friendly most of

the time but not demanding, and be able to cope with changes in the environment and routine. But not all cats are like this.

Understanding how cats with different personalities tend to behave and cope with stressors would be invaluable for placing cats in suitable homes. Breeders and, more importantly, shelters need tools that allow them to efficiently assess many individual cats and decide what sort of homes they will best suit. Will the cat do best as a solitary cat, or could it fit in a multicat household? Does it need a regular routine, or is it emotionally stable enough to cope with an irregular routine? Shelters may also be able to identify personality patterns that make cats unsuited to be pets, allowing the shelter to identify and concentrate their often limited resources on cats that are more likely to be acceptable pets.

Identifying links between personality types and risk of developing behavioral disorders would help veterinarians give timely advice to cat owners that may help prevent clinical disorders developing and also allow closer monitoring and earlier interventions. Problem spraying (i.e., spraying inside the house and on furnishings) is a common reason for presenting cats to behavior clinics.[59] It generally occurs due to a cat feeling anxious, but not all cats with anxiety disorders show problem spraying. It may be possible to identify feline personalities at risk of developing anxiety disorders, such as problem spraying, thereby allowing early intervention.

The biggest advantage to having a feline personality model and understanding how it interacts with social behavior is that it would provide information with the potential to improve feline welfare. Cat owners who better understand their individual cat can meet its needs for social interaction and manage life-changing events, such as moving or acquiring new household members, in ways that are sensitive to the cat's personality. Having owners who understand that their cat does not enjoy a lot of social contact means that they will not expect their cat to want to be petted or to sit on their laps. Owners with highly exploratory cats may be motivated to provide toys and objects for the cat to interact with rather than becoming frustrated at their cat's destruction of household furniture. A scale for measuring personality may also help determine which cats enjoy social living and, thus, will have a better chance of being comfortable in a multicat household. Having an understanding of their cats' personalities may encourage owners of multicat households to provide the environments that each of their cats need. This could include separating cats with agonistic relationships, or providing private areas for cats with low social tolerance. It could also include instituting timesharing arrangements so that all cats have a chance to use popular resources and providing more resources, feeding stations, water, resting spots, and litter boxes for the cats.

SUMMARY

Cats are interesting and complex creatures. They can live in a variety of social systems from crowded colonies to solitary cats in large territories. Their social behavior is interesting and defies categorization into either solitary or truly social. However, cats do display agonistic and affiliative behaviors, which affect their level of social contact with other cats and also with other species to which they are socialized.

The tendency to display affiliative or agonistic behavior or exploratory or fearful behavior is described by the construct of personality. Personality trait theory has been usefully applied to many animal species. There is a small body of work looking at personality in the domestic cat, but no attempt has been made to describe the full breadth and depth of feline personality. It is likely that a feline personality model will have dimensions related to energy levels, response to novelty, and emotional stability. It is also likely that a dimension

related to being social (sociability) also exists. There are also theoretical reasons as to why a dimension related to goal-directed behavior should exist in cats. There may be further dimensions unique to cats that may be described. Any that are identified should have strong links back to personality theory in humans and nonhuman animals to increase usefulness and validity.

This work is needed because a feline personality model has potential benefits for the welfare and management of cats in homes and in shelters. The model may help in breeding decisions, in assessing cats for placement in homes, as an objective rating system for describing cats in shelters as suitable for rehoming or not, and also to help understand the needs of cats once housed.

References

1. Price EO: *Principles and applications of domestic animal behavior*, Cambridge, MA, 2008, CABI.
2. Sunquist ME: *The social organization of tigers (Panthera tigris) in Royal Chitawan National Park, Nepal*, Washington, DC, 1981, Smithsonian Institution Press.
3. Rabinowitz AR, Nottingham BG, Jr: Ecology and behavior of the jaguar *(Panthera onca)* in Belize, Central America. *J Zool (London)* 210:149–159, 1986.
4. Edwards GP, de Preu N, Shakeshaft BJ, et al: Home range and movements of male feral cats *(Felis catus)* in a semiarid woodland environment in central Australia. *Aust Ecol* 26:93–101, 2001.
5. Dickman CR: *Overview of the impacts of feral cats on Australian native fauna*, Canberra, 1996, Australian Nature Conservation Agency.
6. Natoli E: Spacing pattern in a colony of urban stray cats *(Felis catus L.)* in the historic centre of Rome. *Appl Ani Behav Sci* 14:289–304, 1985.
7. Crowell-Davis SL, Curtis TM, Knowles RJ: Social organization in the cat: a modern understanding. *J Feline Med Surg* 6:19–28, 2004.
8. Natoli E, Baggio A, Pontier D: Male and female agonistic and affiliative relationships in a social group of farm cats *(Felis catus L.)*. *Behav Proc* 53:137–143, 2001.
9. Langergraber K, Mitani J, Vigilant L: Kinship and social bonds in female chimpanzees *(Pan troglodytes)*. *Am J Primatol* 71:840–851, 2009.
10. Archie EA, Moss CJ, Alberts SC: The ties that bind: genetic relatedness predicts the fission and fusion of social groups in wild African elephants. *Proc Royal Society of Biol Sci* 273:513–522, 2006.
11. Brown SL, Bradshaw JWS: Classification of social behavior patterns in feral domestic cats. *Appl Ani Behav Sci* 35:294, 1993.
12. Horwitz D, Neilson J: *Canine and feline behavior*, Ames, IA, 2007, Blackwell.
13. Cafazzo S, Natoli E: The social function of tail up in the domestic cat *(Felis silvestris catus)*. *Behav Proc* 80:60–66, 2009.
14. Bateson P: Behavioural development in the cat. In Turner DC, Bateson P, editors: *The domestic cat: the biology of its behaviour*, ed 2, Cambridge, MA, 2000, Cambridge University Press.
15. Beaver BV: *Feline behavior: a guide for veterinarians*, ed 2, St Louis, 2003, Saunders.
16. Lowe SE, Bradshaw JWS: Ontogeny of individuality in the domestic cat in the home environment. *Anim Behav* 61:231–237, 2001.
17. Caro TM: Effects of the mother, object play, and adult experience on predation in cats. *Behav Neural Biol* 29:29–51, 1980.
18. Barrett P, Bateson P: The development of play in cats. *Behaviour* 66:106–120, 1978.
19. Kuo ZY: The genesis of the cat's response to the rat. *J Comp Psychol* 11:1–35, 1930.
20. Karsh E: Factors affecting the socialization of cats to people. In Anderson RK, Hart BL, Hart LA, editors: *The pet connection: its influence on our health and quality of life*, Minneapolis, 1984, University of Minnesota Press.
21. Morgan RS: Personality in domestic cats *(Felis catus)*: identification and description of personality structure, predictive validity, and associations with coat color characteristics. *Diss Abstr Int, B* 72(8–B):5018, 2012.
22. Phares EJ, Chaplin WF: Introduction to personality, biological influences: research and summary evaluation. In *Introduction to personality*, ed 4, Boston, 1997, Addison Wesley Longman, p 3, 9, 17, 18, 201-202.
23. Costa PT, McCrae RR: Four ways five factors are basic. *Pers Individ Diff* 13:653–665, 1992.
24. Ahadi S, Diener E: Multiple determinants and effect size. *J Pers Soc Psychol* 56:398–406, 1989.
25. Buss DM: Manipulation in close relationships: five personality factors in interactional context. *J Pers* 60:477–499, 1992.
26. Zuckerman M: What is a basic factor and which factors are basic? Turtles all the way down. *Pers Indiv Differ* 13:675–681, 1992.
27. McCrae RR, John OP: An introduction to the five-factor model and its applications. *J Pers* 60:175–215, 1992.
28. Digman JM: The curious history of the five-factor model. In Wiggins JS, editor: *The five factor model of personality: theoretical perspectives*, London, 1996, Guilford Press, pp 1–20.
29. King JE, Figueredo AJ: The five-factor model plus dominance in chimpanzee personality. *J Res Pers* 31:257–271, 1997.
30. MacDonald K: Stability of individual differences in behavior in a litter of wolf cubs *(Canis lupus)*. *J Comp Psychol* 97:99–106, 1983.
31. Ley JM, Bennett PC, Coleman GJ: A refinement and validation of the Monash Canine Personality Questionnaire (MCPQ). *Appl Anim Behav Sci* 116:220–227, 2009.
32. Le Scolan N, Hausberger M, Wolff A: Stability over situations in temperamental traits of horses as revealed by experimental and scoring approaches. *Behav Proc* 41:257–266, 1997.
33. Lyons D, Price EO, Moberg GP: Individual differences in temperament of domestic dairy goats: constancy and change. *Appl Anim Behav Sci* 36:1323–1333, 1988.
34. Kieffer JD, Colgan PW: Individual variation in learning by foraging pumpkinseed sunfish, *Lepomis gibbosus*: the influence of habitat. *Anim Behav* 41:603–611, 1991.
35. Mather JA, Anderson RC: Personalities of octopuses *(Octopus rubescens)*. *J Comp Psychol* 107:336–340, 1993.
36. Gosling SD: From mice to men: what can we learn about personality from animal research? *Psychol Bull* 127:45–86, 2001.
37. Cooper C: *Individual differences*, London, 1998, Arnold.
38. Stamps J: Behavioural processes affecting development: Tinbergen's fourth question comes of age. *Anim Behav* 66:1–13, 2003.
39. Kuleshova E, Dolbakyan E, Grigor'yan G, et al: Organization of interneuronal connections in the nucleus accumbens in "impulsive" and "self-controlled" behavior in cats. *Neurosci Behav Physiol* 39:387–394, 2009.
40. Natoli E, Say L, Cafazzo S, et al: Bold attitude makes male urban feral domestic cats more vulnerable to feline immunodeficiency virus. *Neurosci Biobehav Rev* 29:151–157, 2005.

41. Reisner IR, Houpt KA, Erb HN, et al: Friendliness to humans and defensive aggression in cats: the influence of handling and paternity. *Physiol Behav* 55:1119–1124, 1994.

42. Siegford JM, Walshaw SO, Brunner P: Validation of a temperament test for domestic cats. *Anthrozoos* 16:332–351, 2003.

43. Feaver J, Mendl M, Bateson P: A method for rating the individual distinctiveness of domestic cats. *Anim Behav* 34:1016–1025, 1986.

44. Gartner MC, Weiss A: Personality in felids: a review. *Appl Anim Behav Sci* 144:1–13, 2013.

45. McCune S: The impact of paternity and early socialisation on the development of cats' behavior to people and novel objects. *Appl Anim Behav Sci* 45:109–124, 1995.

46. Karsh E, Turner DC: The human-cat relationship. In Turner DC, Bateson PPG, editors: *The domestic cat: the biology of its behavior,* Cambridge, MA, 1988, Cambridge University Press, pp 159–177.

47. Costa PT, McCrae RR: *NEO Five Factor Inventory Test Booklet Form S (Adult),* Lutz, 2003, Psychological Assessment Resources.

48. Meier M, Turner DC: Reactions of house cats during encounters with a strange person: evidence for two personality types. *J Delta Soc* 2:45–53, 1985.

49. Turner DC, Feaver J, Mendl M, et al: Variation in domestic cat behavior towards humans: a paternal effect. *Anim Behav* 34:1890–1892, 1986.

50. McCrae RR, Costa PT: Validation of the Five-Factor Model of personality across instruments and observers. *J Pers Soc Psychol* 52:81–90, 1987.

51. Lloyd AS, Martin JE, Bornett-Gauci HLI, et al: Evaluation of a novel method of horse personality assessment: rater-agreement and links to behavior. *Appl Anim Behav Sci* 105:205–222, 2007.

52. Budaev SV: Personality" in the guppy *(Poecilia reticulata):* a correlational study of exploratory behavior and social tendency. *J Comp Psychol* 111:399–411, 1997.

53. Forkman B, Furuhaug IL, Jensen P: Personality, coping patterns, and aggression in piglets. *Appl Anim Behav Sci* 45:31–42, 1995.

54. Svartberg K, Forkman B: Personality traits in the domestic dog *(Canis familiaris). Appl Anim Behav Sci* 79:133–155, 2002.

55. Else L: Trait spotting. *New Scientist* 2451:50, 2004.

56. Serpell JA: Evidence for an association between pet behavior and owner attachment levels. *Appl Anim Behav Sci* 47:49–60, 1996.

57. Kendall K, Ley J: Cat ownership in Australia: barriers to ownership and behavior. *J Vet Behav* 1:5–16, 2006.

58. Patronek GJ, Glickman LT, Beck AM, et al: Risk factors for relinquishment of cats to an animal shelter. *J Am Vet Med Assoc* 209:582–588, 1996.

59. Mills DS, Redgate SE, Landsberg GM: A meta-analysis of studies of treatments for feline urine spraying. *PLoS ONE* 6:e18448, 2011.

Margie Scherk, DVM

Sarcopenia and Weight Loss in the Geriatric Cat

D. P. Laflamme

Weight loss is a commonly observed problem in geriatric cats. A greater proportion of geriatric cats are underweight compared to those in any other life stage.[1,2] This chapter describes what is known about the causes and consequences of weight loss and underweight conditions in aging cats, and it summarizes important management options.

WEIGHT LOSS IN AGING CATS

It is widely recognized that excess body weight is a risk factor for increased morbidity, especially from diabetes mellitus and arthritis, and earlier mortality. However, low body condition also is a significant risk factor for illness and death in cats as well as in humans.[3-6] Although obesity is common in middle-aged cats, the prevalence for underweight conditions increases with age. Underweight body condition scores (BCSs) are found in approximately 15% of cats over 12 years of age but increase dramatically beyond that.[1,2] Cats older than 14 years of age have a fifteenfold increased risk for being underweight or cachectic compared to young adults.[2] Cross-sectional epidemiological studies cannot determine if such a large proportion of geriatric cats are underweight because of weight loss associated with age, because overweight cats do not live to become geriatric due to early mortality, or both. However, longitudinal studies confirm that both of these factors play a contributory role.[3,7,8] One study that followed 90 healthy, aging non-obese cats until death from natural causes documented that nearly all cats lost weight in their senior years, with an average loss of nearly 50% of adult body weight.[8,9] The study also showed that cats losing less body weight had a longer lifespan.

Weight loss, which is commonly seen in geriatric cats, can be associated with loss of fat, loss of lean body mass (LBM), or both. Unplanned weight loss can be an early sign of disease and is a predictor of mortality in aging cats. When body weight was evaluated retrospectively in cats that had died from a variety of causes, including cancer, chronic kidney disease, and hyperthyroidism, it was found that weight loss began approximately 2 to $2\frac{1}{2}$ years before the terminal event (Figure 95-1).[7] In the previously mentioned prospective, longitudinal study of 90 aging cats, loss of body weight, body fat, and LBM were all significantly associated with increased risk for death.[8] Using the Cox proportional hazard model on the data indicated that each 100 grams of weight loss increased the risk of death by 6.4%, each 100-gram loss of LBM increased the risk of death by 20%, and each 100-gram loss of body fat increased the risk of death by 40%.[8]

These observations raise the question: If weight loss could be reduced or prevented in aging or sick cats, would it reduce morbidity or prolong survival? The research studies cited earlier as well as anecdotal reports from clinical patients suggest that the answer is "yes." Published clinical research and case studies also suggest this to be true, yet the evidence remains circumstantial. Feline cancer patients that weighed more or had a higher BCS survived up to six times longer than underweight cats.[10] Another study in lymphoma patients evaluated weight changes and correlated them with survival. Cats with large cell lymphoma that lost greater than 5% of their body weight during treatment had a significantly shorter survival time compared to those cats that maintained or gained weight.[11] In cats with heart failure, underweight cats or obese cats had shorter survival times compared to normal weight cats.[12] Although further research is required to confirm the benefit of nutrition support to prevent weight loss in sick or aged cats, it appears reasonable to expend efforts to limit weight loss in non-obese geriatric cats and cats with chronic diseases.

Sarcopenia

Sarcopenia is an age-related loss of LBM. It is a lifelong process that becomes evident later in life, and it has a complex and multifactorial etiology.[13] Sarcopenia is not caused by

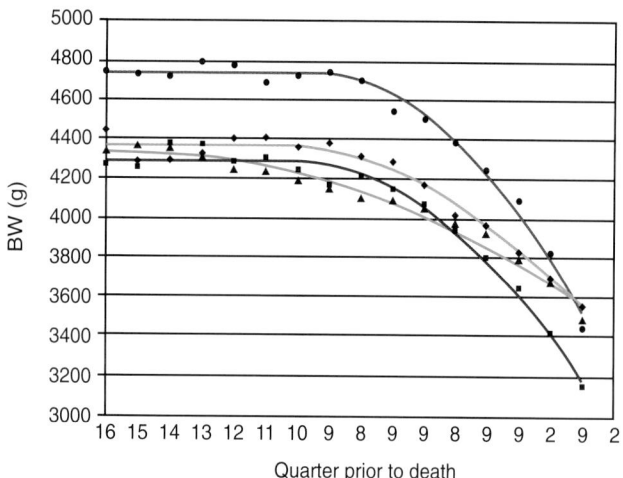

Figure 95-1: Mean body weight (BW) (in grams) during the last 4 years prior to death by quarter (3 months) in cats (*n* = 258) from a pet nutrition center. Weight loss began approximately 2 to 2½ years prior to death. Symbols/colored lines reflect primary cause of death. *Diamond/green line,* Cancer; *square/purple line,* renal; *circle/red line,* thyroid; *triangle/blue line,* other. (Figure used with permission of Nestlé Purina PetCare Research, St Louis, MO.)

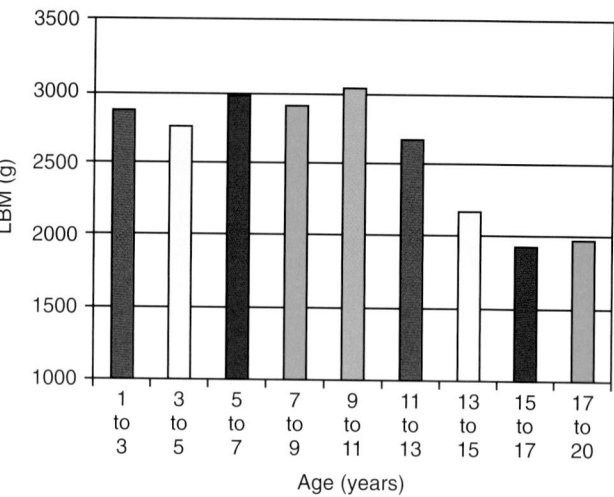

Figure 95-2: Data showing average lean body mass *(LBM)* (in grams) in cats by age (*n* = 256). Mean LBM drops dramatically after 12 years. By age 15, geriatric cats have a one-third less LBM compared to younger adult cats. (Figure used with permission of Nestlé Purina PetCare Research, St Louis, MO.)

disease, because it occurs in apparently healthy aging subjects. In most cases, the loss of LBM is offset by an increase in fat mass, resulting in little or no change in body weight. The age-related loss of LBM occurs in all species evaluated to date, including humans, dogs, and cats.[7,8,14,15]

Sarcopenia, with related loss of muscle strength and function, is associated with increased morbidity and mortality in humans. A "lean mass index," defined as LBM (in kg) divided by the square of the height in meters, was determined to be a better predictor of mortality than the traditional body mass index (weight [in kg] divided by height in m²).[16] Functional measures of muscle strength are not conducted in cats, yet significant loss of LBM, averaging 25% to 30%, has been demonstrated in geriatric cats (Figure 95-2).[7] In a longitudinal study following mature and geriatric cats over an 8-year period, mean LBM decreased by 34%.[8] As with humans, loss of LBM in cats is associated with increased mortality.[8]

In addition to aging, insufficient protein intake can contribute to loss of LBM.[17-19] Dietary protein supports both endogenous protein turnover and gluconeogenesis. When dietary protein intake is inadequate, cats and other species will gradually deplete proteins from their LBM, particularly skeletal muscle, to support these metabolic functions.[18,19] Traditional nitrogen-balance studies indicate that cats need only about 1.5 grams of protein per kilogram of body weight to maintain nitrogen (protein) balance.[18] However, when maintenance of LBM is the defining criteria, healthy adult cats require just over 5 grams of protein per kilogram of body weight or approximately 34% of calories from protein.[17,18] For cats with low energy intake, a higher percentage of calories from protein may be needed to provide sufficient protein intake. The requirement may increase further in geriatric cats due to reduced digestive function and altered metabolism.[7,20]

Gradual loss of LBM may not be readily noticeable, especially if body weight remains stable due to increasing fat mass. However, as it advances, loss of muscle mass can be detected using a simple muscle mass or muscle condition score (MCS) system (see Figure 39-1).[21,22] Both MCS and BCS systems should be used in all cats in order to evaluate both lean and fat mass independently.

Causes of Weight Loss and Sarcopenia in Apparently Healthy Cats

There are many reasons for weight loss in geriatric cats. Weight loss despite normal-to-increased appetite may indicate hyperthyroidism, diabetes mellitus, inflammatory bowel disease, neoplastic diseases, or exocrine pancreatic insufficiency. Weight loss can be associated with inappetence; and in older cats, this may result from reduced acuity in the senses of smell and taste, from pain associated with periodontal disease or arthritis, or from diseases such as chronic kidney disease. Dental disease, although common in older cats, is just one of many causes of poor appetite and weight loss.

In addition to disease, reduced calorie intake or reduced digestion and metabolic efficiency can contribute to loss of weight and LBM. Although energy requirements decrease with age in cats as in dogs and humans, this appears to be true for cats only up to about 10 to 12 years of age.[23] With advancing age, geriatric feline energy requirements actually increase despite a decrease in body size; this effect appears to accelerate after approximately 13 years of age.[7,20,24]

The increased energy requirements may be due, in part, to reduced digestive function in aging cats.[7,20,25] One study reported that older cats (approximately 10 years of age) had an average reduction in energy digestion of about 8% and in protein digestion by about 6%.[25] In another study, 20% of geriatric cats older than 12 years of age had a reduced ability to digest protein, and about 33% of geriatric cats older than 14 years of age had a significant reduction in their ability to digest dietary fat.[7] In some geriatric cats with no apparent health problems other than large stools and low body weight, fat digestibility was as low as 30%. Concurrent with the reduced fat digestion, there is reduced absorption of numerous micronutrients, including vitamin E, B vitamins, choline, sodium, phosphorus, and potassium.[26] Cobalamin deficiency occurs more commonly in older cats, although this is often associated with gastrointestinal disease. It is likely that the onset of reduced digestive function is gradual but over the long term contributes to negative protein and energy balance, weight loss, and to potential malnutrition in a large number of geriatric cats.

Additional factors contributing to weight loss in pet cats include poor intake due to stress secondary to environmental changes or due to a reduced ability to comfortably access food. Weight loss can occur secondary to low calorie intake if a low-calorie food is being fed. Some owners may be feeding a "senior" cat diet—many of these diets are formulated to be lower in calories to address the needs of mature, overweight cats. These low-calorie senior diets are generally not suitable for thin geriatric cats. A thorough dietary history should identify factors including the diet(s) fed, actual intake, and any recent changes in either (see the World Small Animal Veterinary Association Nutrition Toolkit at http://www.wsava.org/nutrition-toolkit for an example of a diet history form and other useful nutritional assessment tools). From the diet history, it can be determined if weight loss is associated with increased or decreased calorie intake.

Management of Sarcopenia and Weight Loss in Apparently Healthy Cats

Whenever possible, identification and correction of any underlying diseases or other factors contributing to reduced intake should be attempted. Reduced food intake in aging cats can be caused by oral, metabolic, and neurological diseases. Pain from arthritis, or associated inability to reach raised feeding platforms, can also contribute to reduced intake. Cats under physical or emotional stress may respond with either increased or decreased intake. For example, food refusal is a common response to perceived environmental threats.[27]

Some cats may show no evidence of disease other than weight loss. Because weight loss can be the first sign of a subclinical disease, a specific diagnosis may not be possible. In these cats, the weight loss or loss of LBM should be addressed through nutritional management.

Cats with reduced digestive efficiency may benefit from a highly digestible, high-energy diet (greater than 4 kcal metabolizable energy per gram of dry diet). Due to the recognized association between reduced vitamin and mineral absorption with reduced fat digestion, it may be reasonable to feed a diet supplemented with higher levels of these essential nutrients. Because of the tendency to lose LBM, especially when protein intake is insufficient, diets should provide increased protein content so that cats consume at least 5 to 6 grams of protein per kilogram of body weight daily. Diets providing approximately 10 to 13 grams of protein per 100 kcal of metabolizable energy will deliver sufficient protein for most geriatric cats. Relatively few "senior" diets are formulated for the "skinny old cat," because most are intended for the large numbers of overweight cats. If a high-energy, highly digestible diet formulated for geriatric cats is not available, an excellent option is to use kitten diets. These tend to be highly digestible, are fortified with increased trace nutrients, and are higher in protein compared to adult maintenance products.

Some veterinarians recommend wet or canned food for sick or aging cats to encourage water and food intake. When wet food is accepted by both cat and owner, especially if added hydration is needed, this is a reasonable approach. However, some cats and some owners prefer dry foods, and this also is completely acceptable. Due to differences in caloric density per volume fed, cats switched from dry food to canned foods may experience weight loss or have difficulty consuming adequate volumes of food. Most cats will adjust to the difference in calorie density within a month or two, but even that period can be problematic for elderly, underweight cats.

Feeding management may need to be modified to address the needs of geriatric cats. Cats, especially seniors, should be fed on a set schedule. Some cats can be stressed by unpredictable feeding times. When the owner is not able to accommodate a set schedule, automated feeders and feeding toys may be helpful. It is important that aging cats have ready access to their food. Feeding bowls should be placed in quiet areas to keep cats from being disturbed while eating. Raised locations are desirable, as long as the aging cat can easily reach the feeding perch. For arthritic cats, raising the bowl a few inches above the floor or platform (Figure 95-3) may facilitate more comfortable feeding.

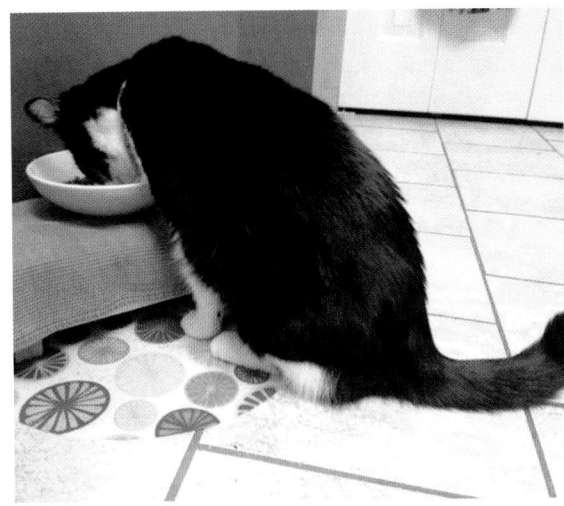

Figure 95-3: Raising the food and water bowls by a few inches can make access more comfortable for arthritic cats. (Courtesy of Dr. Margie Scherk.)

If a dietary change becomes necessary, it is best to make the change slowly. Both the old and new diets should be provided at the same time. One suggestion is to place the new food in the familiar feeding bowl and the familiar food adjacent to it in a separate bowl. Only once the cat has become accustomed to the new food should one slowly decrease the amount of the prior diet. The transition may be accomplished in as little as 1 week, but for inappetent cats or picky eaters, several weeks may be needed. More information on feeding aging cats can be found in Chapter 61.

CACHEXIA OF DISEASE

Cachexia refers to a loss of body mass and LBM, especially skeletal muscle, occurring secondary to disease and inflammation.[13] Conditions commonly associated with cachexia include heart failure, kidney disease, and cancer, among others. Unlike sarcopenia, cachexia results in more rapid depletion of LBM and is often associated with decreased body fat as well. Specific to cachexia is an inability to regulate protein degradation, resulting in catabolism of LBM, weakness, and reduced muscle function, which contribute to morbidity and mortality. Although the specific mechanisms are not yet known, ongoing research suggests that cachexia-induced loss of LBM is associated with upregulation of protein degradation via the ubiquitin-proteasome proteolytic (UPP) pathway specifically targeting myosin, actomyosin, and actin, as well as alterations in inflammatory cytokines and anabolic hormones.[13,28]

Research that is currently underway is exploring inhibition of inflammatory mediators and nuclear transcription factors as means of addressing cachexia. Oxidative stress and inflammatory mediators (e.g., tumor necrosis factor-alpha) play an important role in cachexia by stimulating upregulation of the nuclear transcription factor-kappa B (NF-κB) and activating the UPP pathway.[28] NF-κB plays a key role in protein degradation. Studies have demonstrated that inhibition of NF-κB effectively reduces muscle protein degradation, improves strength, and increases muscle regeneration in various models and species.[13,29]

In addition to inflammatory mediators and the UPP pathway, neurohormonal activation can contribute to muscle loss. Catecholamines and neurohormones (e.g., the renin-angiotensin-aldosterone system, epinephrine, and cortisol) can increase catabolism.[30] Beta-blockers and angiotensin-converting enzyme inhibitors may reduce cardiac cachexia through direct effects, as well as via decreased inflammation.[30]

Cachexia can be confounded by inappetence and made worse through malnutrition. However, the loss of LBM in cachexia differs from that in starvation in that appropriate metabolic adaptations do not occur and the effects cannot be reversed through simple nutritional supplementation. In humans with cachexia associated with human immunodeficiency virus, cancer, or sepsis, nutritional supplementation resulted in increased body weight and body fat but no increase in LBM.[28] Thus, although nutritional support is important, additional therapies are needed to manage cachexia.

Management of Cachexia

Currently there are no effective methods for reversing cachexia, so management is geared toward early recognition, addressing the underlying disease, and attempting to slow the body wasting. Early recognition is best achieved through the consistent use of BCS and MCS systems. The BCS provides an indication of body fat, whereas an MCS provides an indication of muscle and LBM. Loss of muscle can occur without loss of fat or BCS, so these must be evaluated separately.

Cachexia can be anticipated in cats with cancer, kidney disease, and heart failure. As these conditions tend to occur in older cats, age-related loss of LBM and body condition can worsen the disease-related cachexia. Although lean body condition is generally recognized to contribute to a longer, healthier lifespan, a slightly higher BCS (e.g., BCS of 6 to 7 out of 9) appears to be beneficial in the face of diseases associated with cachexia.[30] Several studies suggest that prevention of weight loss in non-obese aging cats reduces the risk for mortality.[8,10-12]

For a treatment to be effective for cachexia, it needs to provide an anticatabolic effect to decrease muscle loss, an anabolic effect to promote protein synthesis, and adequate nutritional support.[30] This requires a combination of dietary and pharmaceutical care. Unfortunately, there currently are no approved pharmaceutical treatments specific to feline cachexia, but there is considerable research underway to develop such drugs for human patients, which may ultimately lead to veterinary application. In the meantime, pharmaceutical agents should be used to control the underlying medical condition, to control pain and nausea, and to assist with appetite as needed.

Maintaining an adequate intake of calories and protein is critical for reducing cachexia. Dietary modification, assisted feeding via feeding tubes, use of appetite stimulants, or other feeding strategies that prevent or correct anorexia can be important. Appetite stimulants, such as cyproheptadine (1 to 2 mg/cat orally [PO] every 12 hours) or mirtazapine (1.88 to 3.75 mg/cat PO every 24 to 72 hours) may benefit some cats with decreased appetites.[31,32] Mirtazapine dosing frequency should be reduced for cats with liver or kidney disease, although cats with chronic kidney disease treated with mirtazapine at 1.88 mg PO every other day over 3 weeks responded well with reduced vomiting, improved appetite and bodyweight, and increased activity.[33] When relying on appetite stimulants, it is important to monitor actual food intake and body weight to confirm that intake is adequate in amount and quality. If intake is not sufficient with appetite stimulants, assisted feeding via a feeding tube should be considered (see Chapter 66).

Attention to feeding management may identify some opportunities to improve food intake. If mobility is an issue, adjustments to the environment, such as providing ramps to raised feeding platforms or raising the food bowls by a few inches, may be needed. Stress due to pain, illness, or household changes can decrease food intake in cats. Cats in multicat households may benefit from being fed in different areas, out of sight of each other.

As previously noted, any necessary dietary changes should be introduced slowly to reduce stress and increase acceptance by the cat. In addition, it is best to avoid using the same food to hide medications as the food that is given as the main meal, because this has the potential to create a food aversion. If medications need to be provided in food, one suggestion is to put it into a small amount of a different but very palatable food, separate from the main meal and given as an appetizer, before satiety is reached.

Adequate dietary protein intake is important to help reduce LBM loss. As previously noted, cats need about three times more protein to maintain LBM (about 5 g/kg body weight) compared to that needed to maintain nitrogen balance, and aging cats can require more.[17,18] It is likely that those cats with metabolic diseases require even more protein to compensate for losses, although this has not been evaluated. Some commercial diets for aging cats and some therapeutic diets may not provide sufficient protein. Although it is not possible to prevent or reverse cachexia simply by providing more protein, providing insufficient protein can make it worse.

Increased intake of long-chain omega-3 fatty acids from fish oil, specifically eicosapentaenoic acid (EPA) and docosahexaenoic acid (DHA), may be beneficial for reducing inflammatory mediators and the UPP system, helping to reduce loss of LBM.[34,35] These fatty acids also may provide various benefits for patients with cardiac, neoplastic, and kidney diseases. An optimal dosage of fish oil has not been determined, but one recommended dose is 40 mg/kg of EPA and 25 mg/kg of DHA daily for any animal with cachexia.[30]

This is approximately 1 gram of fish oil per 5 kilograms of body weight daily, some of which can be provided by the diet.

Because oxidative stress is common in cachexia, the provision of antioxidants above and beyond that needed for normally complete nutrition may be of value.[35,36] In healthy aging cats, a diet that was supplemented with vitamin E, prebiotics, and essential fatty acids contributed to an extended lifespan of approximately 1 year.[9] That diet was also associated with better preservation of body weight and LBM in those cats. However, evidence to show a benefit from antioxidants in cachectic cats is not available.

SUMMARY

Weight loss, with loss of muscle and LBM, is common among aging cats. Sarcopenia, the age-associated loss of LBM, occurs slowly over many years. Insufficient dietary protein intake can exacerbate LBM loss. Loss of body weight also tends to occur slowly in geriatric cats unless associated with disease. Loss of body fat tends to occur much later in life and is a predictor of mortality. Maintaining body weight and LBM appears to reduce the risk for morbidity and mortality in aging cats.

Cachexia is the loss of LBM and body mass that occurs secondary to disease, especially neoplasia, heart failure, and kidney failure. Although dietary management alone cannot prevent or reverse cachexia, inadequate calorie or protein intake can worsen it. Antioxidants, fish oil, and high protein diets may be beneficial in managing cachexia. Effective pharmaceutical agents to manage cachexia are not yet available, but research is underway to better understand and address the underlying mechanisms of both sarcopenia and cachexia.

References

1. Armstrong PJ, Lund EM: Changes in body composition and energy balance with aging. In *Proceedings of Health and Nutrition of Geriatric Cats and Dogs*, Topeka, KS, 1996, Hill's Pet Nutrition, Inc., pp 11–15.
2. Courcier EA, Mellor DJ, Pendlebury E, et al: An investigation into the epidemiology of feline obesity in Great Britain: results of a cross-sectional study of 47 companion animal practices. *Vet Rec* 171:560, 2012.
3. Scarlett JM, Donoghue S: Associations between body condition and disease in cats. *J Am Vet Med Assoc* 212:1725–1731, 1998.
4. Dora-Rose VP, Scarlett JM: Mortality rates and causes of death among emaciated cats. *J Am Vet Med Assoc* 216:347–351, 2000.
5. Gulsvik AK, Thelle DS, Mowe M, et al: Increased mortality in the slim elderly: a 42 years follow-up study in a general population. *Eur J Epidemiol* 24:683–690, 2009.
6. Genton L, Graf CE, Karsegard VL, et al: Low fat-free mass as a marker of mortality in

community-dwelling healthy elderly subjects. *Age Ageing* 42:33–39, 2013.
7. Perez-Camargo G: Cat nutrition: what is new in the old? *Compendium* 26(2A):5–10, 1996.
8. Cupp CJ, Kerr WW: Effect of diet and body composition on life span in aging cats. In *Proceedings of Nestlé Purina Companion Animal Nutrition Summit, Focus on Gerontology*, Clearwater Beach, 2010, pp 36–42.
9. Cupp CJ, Kerr WW, Jean-Philippe C, et al: The role of nutritional interventions in the longevity and maintenance of long-term health in aging cats. *Intern J Appl Res Vet Med* 6:69–81, 2008.
10. Baez JL, Michel KE, Sorenmo K, et al: A prospective investigation of the prevalence and prognostic significance of weight loss and changes in body condition in feline cancer patients. *J Feline Med Surg* 9:411–417, 2007.
11. Krick EL, Moore RH, Cohen RB, et al: Prognostic significance of weight changes during treatment for feline lymphoma. *J Feline Med Surg* 13:976–983, 2011.

12. Finn E, Freeman LM, Rush JE, et al: The relationship between body weight, body condition, and survival in cats with heart failure. *J Vet Intern Med* 24:1369–1374, 2010.
13. Evans WJ: Skeletal muscle loss: cachexia, sarcopenia and inactivity. *Am J Clin Nutr* 91:1123S–1127S, 2010.
14. Wolfe RR: Sarcopenia of aging: implications of the age-related loss of lean body mass. In *Proceedings of Nestlé Purina Companion Animal Nutrition Summit: Focus on Gerontology 2010*, Clearwater Beach, 2010, pp 12–17.
15. Kealy RD: Factors influencing lean body mass in aging dogs. *Comp Cont Edu Small Anim Pract* 21(11K):34–37, 1999.
16. Han SS, Kim KW, Kim LI, et al: Lean mass index: a better predictor of mortality than body mass index in elderly Asians. *J Am Geriatrics Soc* 58:312–317, 2010.
17. Laflamme DP: Loss of lean body mass in aging cats is affected by age and diet. In *Eur Society Vet Comp Nutr Annual Conference*, Ghent, Belgium, 2013 (Abstract).

18. Laflamme DP, Hannah SS: Discrepancy between use of lean body mass or nitrogen balance to determine protein requirements for adult cats. *J Feline Med Surg* 15:691–697, 2013.

19. Wolfe RR: The underappreciated role of muscle in health and disease. *Am J Clin Nutr* 84:475–482, 2006.

20. Sparkes AH: Feeding old cats—an update on new nutritional therapies. *Topics Comp Anim Med* 26:37–42, 2011.

21. Freeman L, Becvarova I, Cave N, et al: WSAVA nutritional assessment guidelines. *J Feline Med Surg* 13:516–525, 2011.

22. Michel KE, Anderson W, Cupp C, et al: Correlation of a feline muscle mass score with body composition determined by DEXA. *Brit J Nutr* 106:S57–S59, 2011.

23. Laflamme DP, Ballam JM: Effect of age on maintenance energy requirements of adult cats. *Compendium* 24(9A):82, 2002. (Abstract).

24. Cupp C, Perez-Camargo G, Patil A, et al: Long-term food consumption and body weight changes in a controlled population of geriatric cats. *Compendium* 26(2A):60, 2004. (Abstract).

25. Bermingham EN, Weidgraaf K, Hekman M, et al: Seasonal and age effects on energy requirements in domestic short-hair cats (*Felis catus*) in a temperate environment. *J Anim Physiol Anim Nutr* 97:522–530, 2012.

26. Perez-Camargo G, Young L: Nutrient digestibility in old versus young cats. *Compendium* 27(3A):84, 2005.

27. Herron M, Buffington CAT: Environmental enrichment for indoor cats. *Compend Contin Educ Vet* 32:E1–E4, 2010.

28. Tisdale MJ: Protein metabolism in cachexia. In Mantovani G, editor: *Cachexia and wasting: a modern approach*, Verlag Italia, Italy, 2006, Springer, pp 185–190.

29. Wysong A, Asher SA, Yin X, et al: Selective inhibition of NF-kappa-B with NBD peptide reduces tumor-induced wasting in a murine model of cancer cachexia in vivo. *J Cancer Sci Ther* 3:22–29, 2011.

30. Freeman LM: Cachexia and sarcopenia: emerging syndromes of importance in dogs and cats. *J Vet Intern Med* 26:3–17, 2012.

31. Caney S: Weight loss in the elderly cat. Appetite is fine, and everything looks normal. *J Feline Med Surg* 11:738–746, 2009.

32. Quimby JM, Gustafson DL, Lunn KF: The pharmacokinetics of mirtazapine in cats with chronic kidney disease and in age-matched control cats. *J Vet Intern Med* 25:985–989, 2011.

33. Quimby JM, Lunn KF: Mirtazapine as an appetite stimulant and anti-emetic in cats with chronic kidney disease: a masked placebo-controlled crossover clinical trial. *Vet J* 197:651–655, 2013.

34. Murphy RA, Yeung E, Mazurak VC, et al: Influence of eicosapentaenoic acid supplementation on lean body mass in cancer cachexia. *Brit J Cancer* 105:1469–1473, 2011.

35. Vaughan VC, Martin P, Lewandowski PA: Cancer cachexia: impact, mechanisms and emerging treatments. *J Cachexia Sarcopenia Muscle* 4:95–109, 2013.

36. Mantovani G, Madeddu C, Maccio A, et al: Cancer-related anorexia/cachexia syndrome and oxidative stress: an innovative approach beyond current treatment. *Cancer Epidemiol Biomarkers Prev* 13:1651-1659, 2004.

Osteoarthritis in the Aging Cat

David Bennett

Osteoarthritis (OA) is a very common disease in the older cat with prevalence figures for radiographic disease ranging from 6.5% to 91%,[1-5] the range reflecting the population studied and the criteria used. *Osteoarthritis* can be defined as a degenerative disorder of diarthrodial (synovial) joints characterized by the deterioration of the articular cartilage and by the formation of new bone at the joint surfaces and margins.[6] Despite many recent publications highlighting the importance of feline OA, it is still a much underdiagnosed disease in veterinary practice. Most cats show bilaterally symmetrical disease in multiple joints, with the elbow, stifle, and hip joints being most frequently affected. The term *degenerative joint disease (DJD)* is often used interchangeably with OA, but DJD is a more general term and covers other degenerative conditions besides OA, such as spondylosis and traumatic arthritis.[6] It is very common to have spondylosis coexisting with OA in the older cat.

RISK FACTORS

The main risk factor for OA is age, the prevalence increasing considerably in the older population.[7,8] Obesity is often claimed to be a risk factor, but the evidence is equivocal. Many cats lose weight and body condition with advancing age,[9,10] although they may have been overweight earlier in life. Lund and colleagues reported that the prevalence of being overweight increased in cats up to 8 to 10 years of age and decreased thereafter.[10] Obesity is certainly recognized as a risk factor in other species by causing excessive mechanical loading of joints and also by increasing levels of circulating adipokines, which can cause breakdown of articular cartilage.[11,12] Lascelles identified other possible risk factors but concluded that they were more likely to be related to age rather than directly linked to OA.[8]

ETIOPATHOGENESIS

Most cases (60% to 75%) appear to be of the primary or idiopathic type with multiple joint involvement common in an individual cat.[1,7,13,14] The systemic nature of OA in the cat does raise the possibility of genetic factors at play, although the limited studies so far have not been conclusive.[15] Other joint diseases may cause so-called *secondary OA.* Previous joint trauma, hip dysplasia, osteochondrodysplasia, muco-polysaccharidosis, patellar luxation, cranial cruciate ligament rupture, developmental elbow luxation, septic arthritis, and immune-based arthritis have all been suggested as causes of secondary OA.[1,8,13,14,16-18] A recent study has identified a flexor enthesopathy of the feline elbow joint (medial "epicondylitis"), and it is possible that this could result in altered joint loading and subsequent OA.[19] Active pronation and supination are important in feline locomotion, particularly during jumping and capture of prey. In a very active cat, the repetition of these movements could conceivably lead to joint trauma and OA. Acromegaly has also been reported as a cause of secondary OA.[20] In a recent cadaveric study of 58 aged cats by the author of this chapter and colleagues, a pituitary adenoma was found by histological examination in only one cat, and this was nonfunctional, suggesting that acromegaly is not an important underlying cause.[21] In the same study, elbow incongruity was diagnosed in six cats (nine joints) as a possible cause of elbow OA. Mineralization of the medial meniscus was identified as a possible underlying factor (decreased resilience of the meniscus resulting in increased loading of the femorotibial joint) in secondary OA of the stifle joint, although this lesion is more likely to be a consequence rather than a cause of OA. Gross degenerative changes of the cranial cruciate ligament were seen in two cats, although no complete rupture was recorded; these changes could be a consequence of OA rather than a cause.[21]

CLINICAL FEATURES

Most cats with painful OA do not show overt lameness that is perceptible to their owners; this may be one reason that cats with OA are not commonly presented to the veterinarian for evaluation. Clearly it is not easy for the owner (or veterinarian) to assess a cat's gait, because cats are seldom exercised on a lead and, due to their inquisitive nature, tend not to walk in straight lines. In the veterinary clinic, cats are often reluctant to walk and are more likely to crouch or lie down. Therefore, it is changes in the cat's normal behavior or lifestyle pattern that should alert the owner and veterinarian to the possibility of painful OA. In particular, cats with OA become less reluctant to jump and/or can only jump shorter distances, they interact and play less with their owners, hunt less, and are generally less active.[5,7,22-24] Owners feel that these are merely signs of the cat growing older and do not realize the true significance—a cat suffering from chronic arthritic pain. Affected cats can also show changes in their toilet habits, such as increased or decreased frequency, refusing to urinate outdoors, difficulty in adopting a comfortable posture to urinate and defecate, and missing the litter box when urinating and defecating. Their temperament and demeanor can also change with reduced tolerance toward their owner and other animals in the household and a change in general attitude with more aggressive behavioral responses. Grooming habits can also be affected. Their coat condition can deteriorate, because they cannot flex and extend their limb joints (or move their spine when spondylosis is present) sufficiently to allow effective grooming. As a result, the coat becomes matted, scruffy, and unkempt. Occasionally, a cat may excessively groom an area if it is painful; for example, a specific joint or the lumbar area when painful spondylosis is present. Overgrowth of the claws may result from inactivity, and this can worsen if the cat reduces its normal scratching behavior. Overgrown claws in an aged cat may indicate underlying painful OA. Although these lifestyle changes can be caused by other problems, the owner and clinician should initially conclude they are the result of painful musculoskeletal disease and assess the cat from this viewpoint.

Because it is the owner who is key in diagnosing feline OA, it is useful for the clinician to use owner assessment questionnaires similar to those reported by Bennett and Morton,[22] Lascelles and colleagues,[23] and Sul and colleagues.[24] The questionnaire used by the author of this chapter is shown in Table 96-1. The clinician (or suitably trained veterinary nurse/technician) asks the owner a series of questions relating to the cat's mobility levels, activity levels, grooming habits, and temperament. The owner is asked to compare the current behavior of the cat to when it was a young adult animal at about 2 years of age and to score any change on a scale of 0 to 10. Not only does this assessment identify the possible presence of painful OA, but it provides a baseline of severity of the disease, against which any response to therapy can be compared. Lascelles and colleagues reported the use of "client specific outcome measures" where specific activities favored by an individual cat can be interrogated.[23] For example, does the cat still jump onto the kitchen table?

The availability of personal digital devices with video capabilities makes it very easy for the veterinarian to view owner-recorded videos of their cat in the home environment to demonstrate some of the features of a cat with painful OA, which are difficult to assess in the practice environment. This includes stiffness in gait, hesitation in jumping, difficulty in urination and defecation, and difficulty in grooming.

Physical examination of the cat is often a significant challenge, particularly when trying to localize pain. Obviously the cat must be relaxed prior to the examination, and this is sometimes difficult if the cat has had to endure a car journey to the veterinary practice and then a period of waiting in an unfamiliar environment. The examination must be gentle but comprehensive. An initial quick palpation of the animal including all four limbs but without any manipulation is useful to detect any obvious thickening of, or heat associated with, individual joints and any increased sensitivity to pressure. Manipulation of joints must be methodical, and if a particular joint is suspected as being painful, this should be left until last. Elbows and hips are the most likely to be painful on manipulation. The detection of a painful joint is difficult, not least because many cats do not like their joints being manipulated through the full range of motion and may show resistance to such maneuvers even if the joint is normal. Any thickening of an OA joint is generally subtle, and any reduction in the range of motion is usually not dramatic. Synovial effusion, if present, is difficult to appreciate, and crepitus is rare. Palpation and manipulation of the vertebral column is also relevant to check for painful spondylosis but should always be left until the end of the examination.

The physical examination together with the information gleaned from the owner assessment questionnaire may be sufficient to provide a diagnosis of feline OA without any confirmatory radiographs. The latter requires sedation or general anesthesia, and because one is dealing with older cats, there may be concomitant diseases that create unacceptable risks. Even if the diagnosis is not completely certain, there may be enough evidence to justify a course of analgesia. Meloxicam is the drug of choice in most countries. A marked improvement in the cat's lifestyle and behavior is highly supportive of a correct diagnosis of painful OA (or DJD).

RADIOGRAPHY

The main feature of an OA joint is the presence of bony outgrowths or osteophytes, although in early disease they may be difficult to appreciate. Soft tissue mineralization is a common feature of feline OA and can be difficult to distinguish from osteophytes. Increased bone opacity is an important but very subjective feature and can be a result of subchondral bone thickening, osteophytes on the surface of the joint margin or areas of soft tissue mineralization superimposed on the articular bones. Soft tissue thickening and synovial effusion are less obvious features. The presence of radiographic signs of disease does not necessarily mean that the joint is painful, and conversely, a joint free of radiographic signs may still be painful due to synovial inflammation. Radiography provides information on the bony changes of OA but provides no direct information on the status of the articular cartilage or synovial membrane. The prevalence of pathological disease in the author's study of 58 feline cadavers (mean age 6.8 years, standard deviation 4.4 years), expressed as a percentage of cats affected, was 89.7% in the elbow, 87.9% in the stifle, 82.8% in the hip, 82.8% in the shoulder, 74.1% in the hock, and 50% in the carpus.[21]

Elbow Joint

Osteophytes are most often seen on the caudal aspect of the humerus and cranial aspect of the radial head on the mediolateral view (Figures 96-1 and 96-2). On the craniocaudal

Table 96-1	Examples of Behavior to Consider for Evaluation When Trying to Identify Cats Suffering from Chronic Arthritic Pain
Behavior	**Change**
Mobility	
Jumping up or down	Refusing or hesitating to jump up or down Less agile on stairs No longer attempting to reach high spots
Size/height of jump, up or down	Makes smaller jumps (e.g., takes several steps to reach high spots)
Gracefulness	Movements less graceful than before Becoming stiff and "creaky"
Changes in toileting	Changes in location (e.g., reluctant/refusing to go outside or reluctant/refusing to use litter box) Difficulties using litter box (e.g., missing litter box sometimes/often)
Activity Levels	
Sleeping habits	Sleeping or resting more Lying in the same spot for a long time, not moving location often Changes in resting place
Playing	Playing less No longer instigating play More difficult to tempt to play
Hunting	Hunting less than before
Grooming Habits	
Coat condition	Coat matted or scruffy, generally or in one particular place Observed grooming behavior less frequent or of shorter duration Overgrooming in certain areas
Scratching	Sharpens claws less frequently Change of location/height where scratching occurs Claws overgrown or catching on carpets or clicking on hard floors
Temperament (Demeanor)	
Tolerance to owner or other animals	Less keen to interact Grumpy on contact with other cats Grumpy on contact with other animals, including owner
General attitude	Quieter Spending more time alone Not seeking or avoiding contact with other cats or other animals Not seeking or avoiding contact with owner

view, osteophytes are seen on the medial aspect of the distal humerus and the medial coronoid process of the ulna. A diffuse bony reaction is sometimes seen on the medial epicondyle of the humerus and has been described as a specific entity and designated medial humeral "epicondylitis." It is a flexor enthesopathy, mainly involving the origin of the humeral head of the flexor carpi ulnaris muscle. In the author's experience, most of these cases also have typical elbow OA. The lesion may be a factor in the development of elbow OA or the result of it; in both instances, this is due to altered load bearing through the joint. Medial "epicondylitis"

can cause displacement and compression of the ulnar nerve, which might be a source of pain.[19] Increased radio-opacity beneath the ulnar semilunar notch on the mediolateral view is an important, although subjective, feature. The more consistent anatomy of the feline elbow makes this feature a little easier to assess compared to other species.

The supinator sesamoid bone (SSB) is reported as being visible in about 40% of normal elbow joints,[25] although in the author's study all elbow joints with a radiographically evident SSB had degenerative changes of the articular cartilage indicative of OA.[21] However, not all arthritic elbow

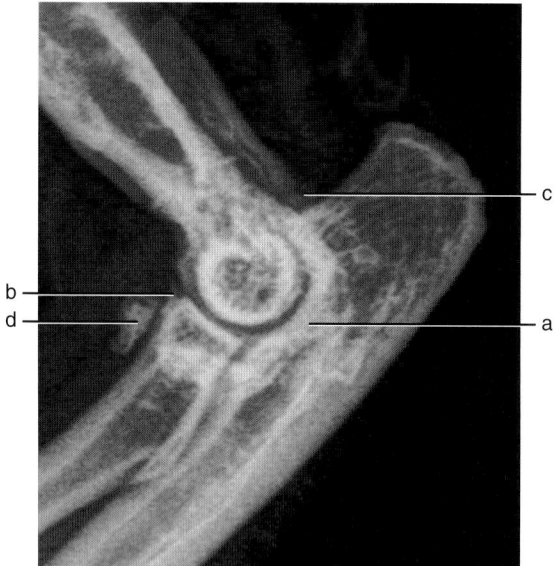

Figure 96-1: Mediolateral radiograph of an osteoarthritic right elbow joint. Increased bone opacity beneath the ulnar semilunar notch is present *(a)*. Osteophyte formation is present on the cranial aspect of the radial head *(b)* and the caudal aspect of the distal humerus *(c)*. The supinator sesamoid bone is seen on the cranial aspect of the radial head, and new bone is present on its surface *(d)*.

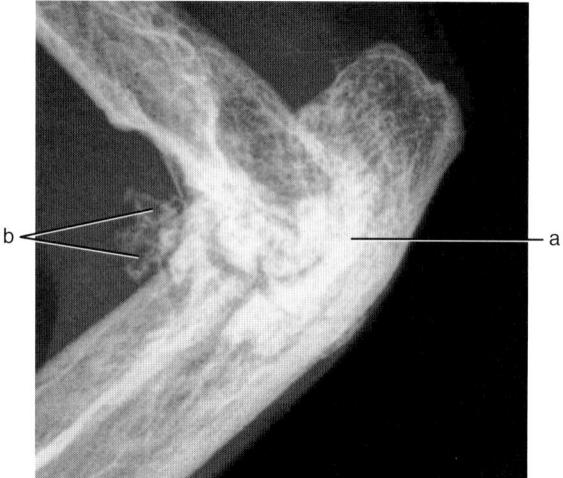

Figure 96-2: Mediolateral radiograph of a severely osteoarthritic right elbow joint. Increased bone opacity is seen affecting the proximal ulna *(a)*. There is loss of the humeroulnar joint space. There are two irregular areas of mineralization on the cranial aspect of the radial head *(b)*. These may both represent supinator sesamoid bones although one may be the result of soft tissue mineralization due to degenerative change.

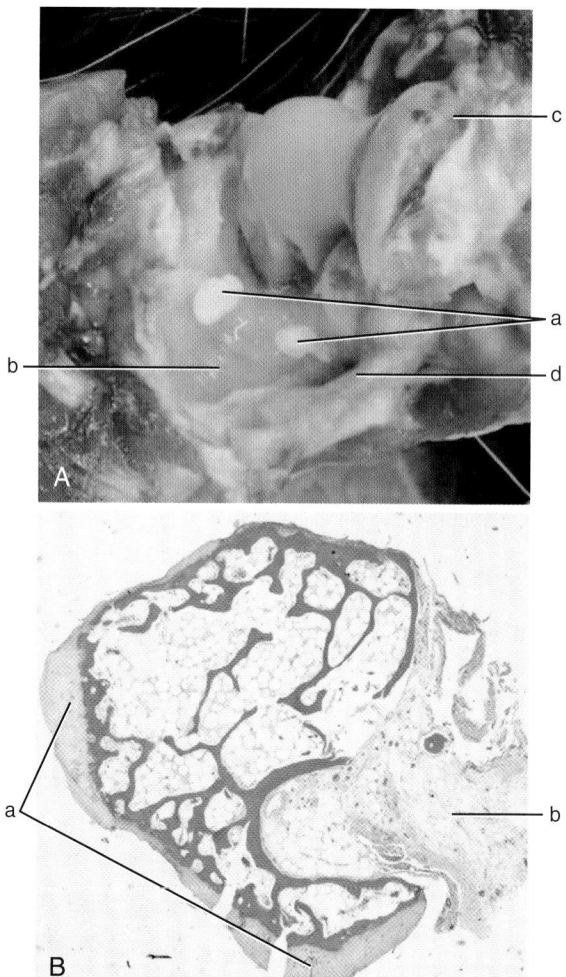

Figure 96-3: **A,** Photograph of an osteoarthritic elbow joint showing the presence of two osteochondromas ("joint mice") lying free within the articular cavity *(a)*. There are severe cartilage changes within the ulnar articular surface where marked groove formation is evident *(b)*. Osteophytes are seen at the articular margin of the humeral condyle *(c)*, and there is a large area of calcification within the joint capsule at its attachment to the ulnar semilunar notch *(d)*. **B,** Photomicrograph of an osteochondroma from an osteoarthritic elbow joint showing its typical trabecular bone structure. Cartilage covers most of its surface where it has "articulated" with the distal humerus *(a)*. This osteochondroma was firmly attached to the synovial membrane, the remnants of which can be seen *(b)*.

joints have a radiographically evident SSB. It is likely that the SSB becomes a focus of new bone formation in the arthritic joint.

Soft tissue mineralization is frequently seen in the elbow joint and may represent calcification within the elbow joint capsule, or the presence of discrete osteofibrocartilaginous bodies (osteochondromas or ossicles) either free within the articular space or adherent to the synovial surface (Figure 96-3).

In a study of 102 OA elbow joints, elbow incongruity was diagnosed in nine joints (8.8%), a relative shortening of the radius in seven joints, and a relative lengthening of the radius in two.[21] Although reported in the literature,[26] fragmentation of the medial part of the coronoid process of the ulna was not seen in any of these cadavers. The author's study also demonstrated a good correlation between the severity of the radiographic changes and the severity of the gross pathological changes of the cartilage with R values of 0.77 and 0.76 for the left and right elbow joints respectively ($p < 0.0001$).

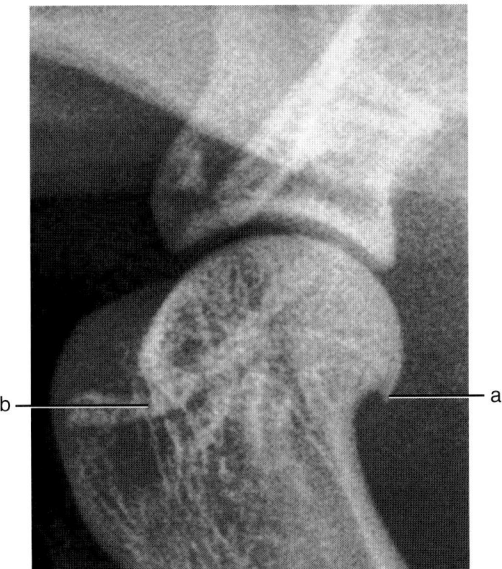

Figure 96-4: Mediolateral radiograph of an osteoarthritic shoulder joint. There is a large osteophyte on the caudal aspect of the humeral head *(a)*. The clavicle is seen superimposed on the proximal humerus *(b)*.

Shoulder Joint

Osteophyte formation is most often seen on the caudal aspects of the glenoid and humeral head on the mediolateral view (Figure 96-4). An apparent discrete mineralized body is often seen adjacent to the caudal glenoid and may represent an ossicle or a developing osteophyte (Figure 96-5). Increased radiopacity beneath the glenoid surface is sometimes appreciated, and a reduction of the caudal glenohumeral joint space may be evident. Figure 96-6 shows advanced OA of the shoulder joint with total loss of cartilage and advanced osteophyte formation.

Hip Joint

Hip dysplasia (HD) is well documented in the cat but, based on conventional radiographic diagnosis, only accounts for approximately 20% of cases of hip OA.[7,21] Feline HD has been associated with increased joint laxity,[27] but more research is required before this can become the preferred way of diagnosing HD in the cat. Clark and Bennett reported a mean Norberg angle for the dysplastic hip of 87.5 degrees compared to 100.1 degrees for the normal hip.[7] Keller and colleagues reported a 6.6% prevalence of HD in a hospital population of cats.[28] The Maine Coon breed is reported as having a higher prevalence of HD (18%), and genetic factors have certainly been implicated in this breed.[29] Subluxation of the femoral head from the acetabulum and less than 50% coverage of the femoral head by the dorsal acetabular edge are typical features of HD. In some cases of HD, an abnormally shaped femoral head is found. Osteophyte formation is seen on the cranial effective acetabular edge and on the femoral neck—where it often appears as a radiopaque line

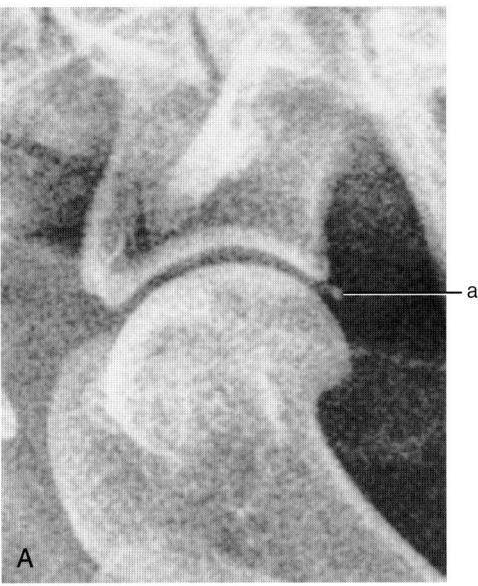

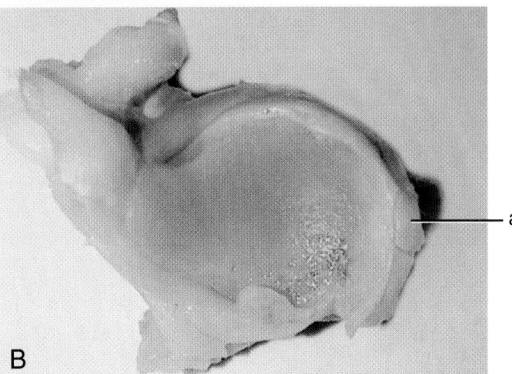

Figure 96-5: A, Mediolateral radiograph of an osteoarthritic shoulder joint. An area of mineralization is seen on the caudal aspect of the glenoid *(a)*. This may represent a developing osteophyte or mineralization within the joint capsule. **B,** Photograph of the articular surface of the glenoid, showing a discrete area of mineralization on the caudal aspect *(a)*. This specimen is from the shoulder joint whose radiograph is shown in **A.** The cartilage surface of the glenoid is discolored and fibrillated.

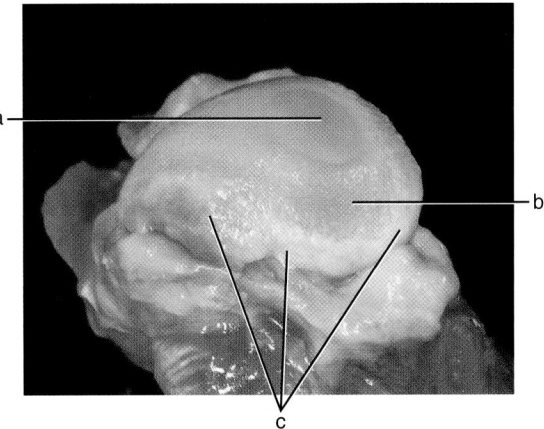

Figure 96-6: Photograph of the humeral head taken from an osteoarthritic shoulder joint. There is a large area of total articular cartilage loss with exposure of underlying subchondral bone *(a)*. The remaining cartilage is severely fibrillated *(b)*. The margin of the articular surface shows extensive osteophyte formation *(c)*.

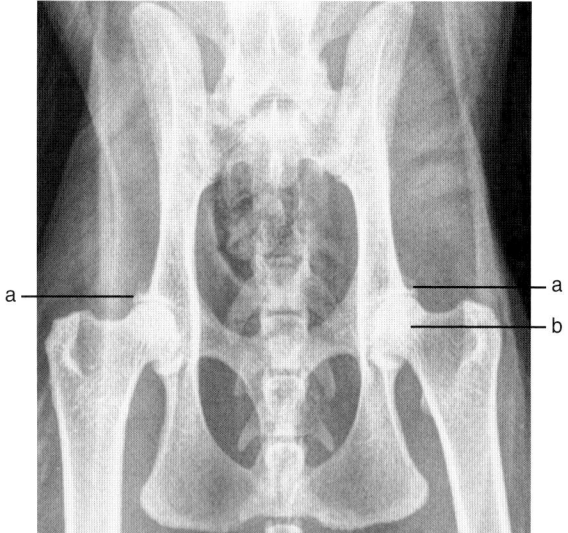

Figure 96-7: Ventrodorsal radiograph of the pelvis of a cat with hip osteoarthritis (OA). There is osteophyte formation on the cranial effective acetabular edge of both hip joints *(a)* and osteophyte formation around both femoral necks (more evident on the *left*) as shown by a linear area of increased bone opacity *(b)*. There is good coverage of the femoral head by the dorsal acetabular edge, and the Norberg angle is within the normal range. Therefore, there is no evidence of hip dysplasia. Most cases of hip OA in the cat are not associated with hip dysplasia as currently defined.

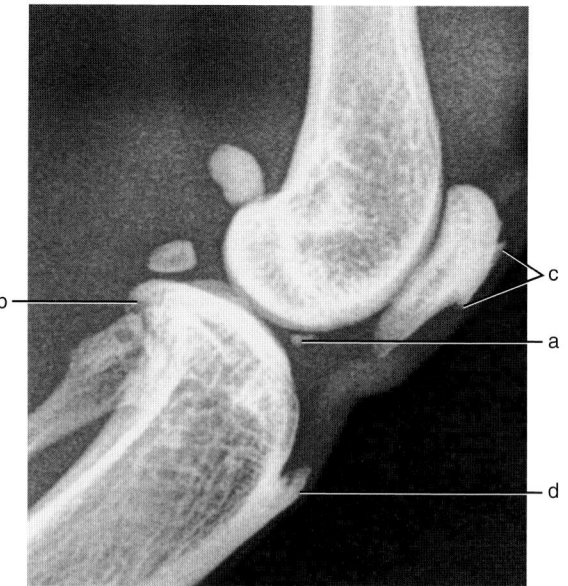

Figure 96-8: Mediolateral radiograph of the left stifle joint. An area of mineralization is seen within the joint space, which is present within the medial meniscus *(a)*. A large osteophyte is seen on the caudal edge of the proximal tibia *(b)*. There is enthesophyte formation on the cranial surface of the patella *(c)* and the tibial tuberosity *(d)*. Only one fabella is radiographically visible, which is not unusual in the feline stifle joint. The articular cartilage of both the femur and tibia of this joint showed fibrillation and erosion, which is consistent with moderately severe osteoarthritis.

(Figure 96-7). Narrowing of the joint space may also be apparent.

Stifle Joint

This joint may show quite advanced cartilaginous degeneration and loss with no evidence of osteophyte formation.[21] A common radiographic feature is mineralization within the cranial pole of the medial meniscus[13] (Figures 96-8 and 96-9), and there is an association between the presence of this mineralization and gross cartilage pathology.[30] In a recent study of 49 stifle joints with radiographic meniscal mineralization, 47 had gross pathological changes of the articular cartilage, confirming that the presence of this radiographic feature, even on its own, is most often indicative of OA. However, 52 joints without meniscal mineralization also had cartilage damage.[21] Histopathologic examination of the menisci show that in some cases this mineralization represents calcification of degenerate fibrocartilage, but in others (53.1%) it represents trabecular bone (Figure 96-10). In some of the latter cases (6.1%), the woven bone has a cartilage surface, which articulates with the femur and/or tibia. Such a structure may represent the lunula, a sesamoid bone, which is present at birth and has been described in the menisci of many different species including the cat. The exact pathogenesis of this meniscal mineralization remains unknown. Freire and colleagues were unable to show any clinical differences in cats with or without meniscal mineralization.[30]

When osteophytes occur, they appear at the poles of the patella, the supratrochlear area, along the trochlear margin

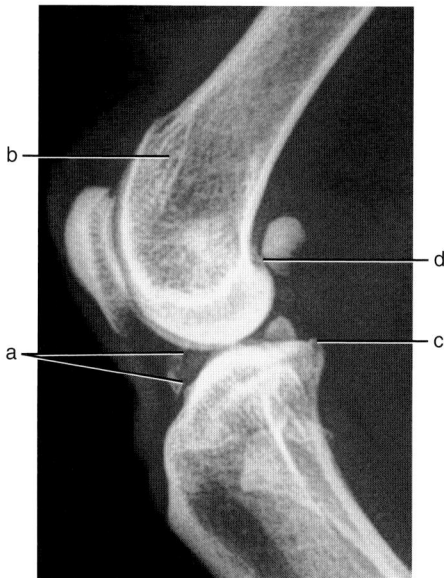

Figure 96-9: Mediolateral radiograph of the right stifle joint. There are two areas of mineralization within the medial meniscus *(a)*. Increased bone opacity is seen within the distal femur consistent with osteophyte formation along the trochlear margin *(b)*. Osteophyte formation is also seen on the caudal edge of the proximal tibia *(c)* and distal femur adjacent to the fabella *(d)*.

(where they appear as a radiopaque "line"), and on the caudal part of the tibia (see Figures 96-8 and 96-9). Increased radiopacity of the proximal tibia is another feature but is difficult to evaluate. Enthesophytosis of the tibial tuberosity at the attachment of the patellar ligament (see Figure 96-8) can be

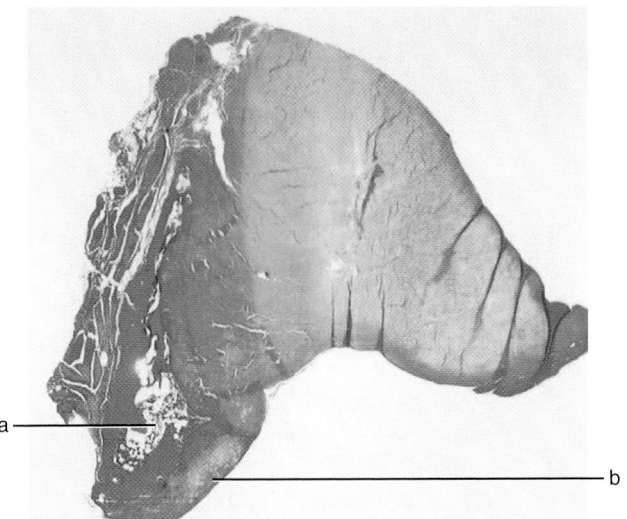

Figure 96-10: Photomicrograph of a section through the medial meniscus. Trabecular bone formation is seen within the cranial horn *(a)*. Part of the bony structure is covered with cartilage, providing an articular surface with the proximal tibia *(b)*. This structure could represent a lunula or advanced degenerative change.

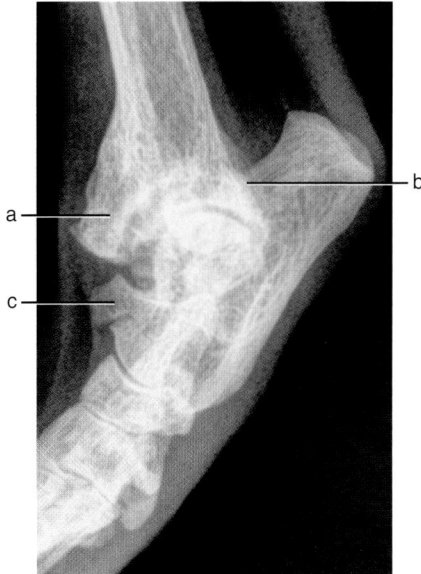

Figure 96-11: Mediolateral radiograph of an osteoarthritic hock joint. There is extensive osteophyte formation on the cranial *(a)* and caudal *(b)* aspects of the distal tibia. This has led to a marked joint remodeling (alteration in the shape of the articular surface). A large osteophyte is also seen on the cranial aspect of the tibial tarsal bone *(c)*.

a feature of stifle OA, although it is also reported as a solitary lesion, possibly traumatic in origin, which is most often not associated with pain. Gross pathology of the cruciate ligaments is seldom seen in the feline stifle joint (two cases were seen in the author's cadaveric study[21]); mineralization within the cranial cruciate ligament is sometimes radiographically visible.

It is common not to see the lateral fabella on a radiograph of a feline stifle; it may be present but not sufficiently mineralized to be visible. The absence or presence of the lateral fabella does not appear to be correlated with cartilage disease.[21]

Carpal and Tarsal Joints

The carpal and tarsal joints are the least affected. Osteophytes occur on the cranial aspect of the distal radius and the carpal and metacarpal bones. Osteophytes within the tarsal joints occur on the cranial and caudal aspects of the distal tibia and on the cranial aspects of the individual tarsal and metatarsal bones (Figure 96-11). Soft tissue mineralization may also be seen. The most severe cartilage pathology within the hock joint is seen in the lateral compartment of the tibiotarsal joint.

MANAGEMENT

Managing a cat with painful OA requires a multimodal approach. Clearly, controlling pain is important but so is adapting the environment.[14] The cat is a predatory animal with instinctive hunting behavior that enjoys freedom of movement and a high degree of independence. Chronic joint

pain can disturb the ability to perform these normal behaviors, thus becoming a significant "stressor" to the animal, possibly exacerbating other medical problems. Addressing this through modifications of the home environment is believed to help improve quality of life.

Nonsteroidal Anti-Inflammatory Drugs

There is much evidence to support the effectiveness of nonsteroidal anti-inflammatory drugs (NSAIDs) in treating feline OA,[7,22-24,31-34] but the potential toxicity of these compounds deters many clinicians from administering them to the older cat. There are several NSAIDs licensed for use in the cat (Table 96-2), but only meloxicam is licensed for long-term use in parts of the world. The liquid formulation of meloxicam makes accurate dosing relatively simple with more accurate dosing being achieved by using the provided syringe rather than counting drops from the bottle. It is highly palatable and is generally administered by mixing with food. Meloxicam is known to be metabolized by oxidative pathways, and only 21% is eliminated through the kidneys in the urine.[35] The recommended dose is 0.1 mg/kg orally (PO) on day 1 and then 0.05 mg/kg PO every 24 hours. It is always advisable to titrate to the lowest effective dose, based on the clinical response of the animal as assessed by a veterinary examination and by regular review of the owner questionnaire. In one study where this was done, the median daily maintenance oral dose was 0.03 mg/kg.[34] In cats with preexisting hepatic or renal disease, the author starts with a lower oral dose, usually 0.02 to 0.03 mg/kg/day, gradually increasing the dose if there is no initial response. If the animal is overweight or obese, the dose should be based on its ideal

Table 96-2	Nonsteroidal Anti-Inflammatory Drugs Used in Cats	
Drug	**Dosage***	**Comments**
Meloxicam (Metacam; Boehringer Ingelheim)	0.1 mg/kg PO on day 1, then 0.05 mg/kg PO every 24 hours	Easy to administer in food Cat-specific formulations should be used and administered according to the manufacturer's recommendations (e.g., dosing syringes should be used when provided) Titrate to lowest effective dose Avoid initial loading dose if CKD is present COX-2 preferential
Robenacoxib (Onsior; Novartis Animal Health)	1 to 2 mg/kg PO every 24 hours for up to 6 days	For use in acute pain and inflammation Plasma levels reduce relatively quickly, but concentrations in inflamed tissues remain high Flavored tablets—generally well accepted COX-2 specific
Ketoprofen (Ketofen; Merial)	1 mg/kg PO every 24 hours for up to 5 days	Acute pain from musculoskeletal disorders
Tolfenamic acid (Tolfedine; Vétoquinol)	4 mg/kg PO every 24 hours for 3 days	Licensed only for treatment of fever and upper respiratory tract disorders

CKD, Chronic kidney disease; *COX*, cyclooxygenase; *PO, per os* (orally).
*Dosages as given are licensed for use in the cat in the United Kingdom; licensed dosing varies in other countries.

body weight rather than its actual weight. Nonsteroidal anti-inflammatory drugs are highly protein bound in the blood, and it is suggested that the dose should be reduced by 50% if any other drug is being given or is about to be used.[36] Given that it is mainly older cats that suffer from OA, routine blood screening and urine analyses are advisable before commencing NSAID therapy, using the results to help determine what initial dose should be given. Monitoring blood pressure is also recommended, and cats receiving long-term NSAIDs should be fed moist diets. The latter is important to ensure the cat is well hydrated, particularly because many have chronic kidney disease (CKD; see later), and although cats fed dry foods drink more water than cats fed moist food, their overall fluid intake is less. Cats receiving long-term NSAIDs should be regularly monitored (every 3 to 6 months depending on their clinical status) by means of a detailed physical examination and routine hematology, serum biochemistry, and urine analysis. Owners should be made aware of possible side effects and told to report these to the veterinarian immediately when they occur. The drugs should always be stopped if the cat stops eating. Vomiting and diarrhea are common side effects and occur in approximately 4% of cats receiving meloxicam.[7,33] If they persist for more than a few days, the drug should be stopped. The NSAID can be reintroduced after 3 to 5 days at a lower dose, or an alternative drug can be selected. Gastrointestinal (GI) protectants, such as omeprazole or misoprostol, can be considered if GI side effects are a persistent problem, but these are seldom necessary.[14]

Many cats with OA also have some degree of CKD.[34] In the author's cadaveric study, 36.5% of cats with OA also had histologic evidence of CKD.[21] Gowan and colleagues

reported a group of cats with CKD that received meloxicam and showed smaller increases in blood creatinine levels over time compared with CKD cats that did not receive meloxicam.[34] This apparent beneficial effect on kidney function might be explained by the improved mobility and quality of life subsequent to pain relief, which may result in a better appetite, increased water intake, and reduced tissue catabolism. Pain relief could also reduce the animals "stress levels," because stress is known to affect other disease processes,[37] which may also be true for CKD. Meloxicam might also have a direct anti-inflammatory effect on the kidney. Inflammation and fibrosis are features of CKD, and reduction of these might slow the deterioration of renal function. In a further study by Gowan and colleagues, the long-term administration of oral meloxicam did not reduce the lifespan of cats with pre-existent CKD, even in International Renal Interest Society stages II and III.[38] The median longevity after the diagnosis of CKD was 1608 days, and the most common cause of death in these cats was neoplasia, with only 11% being attributed directly to the CKD.

Other Analgesic Therapies

There has been a recent interest in using other drugs besides NSAIDs in treating painful OA, including combinations of several different drugs, each of which acts at a different level of the pain pathway and together have a synergistic effect. This may lead to better pain control and potentially enable lower doses of individual drugs to be used.[39-41] The most frequently used drugs are shown in Table 96-3. Some authorities also advocate the use of opioids (e.g., butorphanol,

Table 96-3	Other Drugs Sometimes Used with Nonsteroidal Anti-Inflammatory Drugs for Multimodal Osteoarthritis Therapy	
Drug*	Dosage	Comments
Amantidine	3 to 5 mg/kg PO every 24 hours	No convenient size of capsules for cats Syrup available Not evaluated in the cat
Amitriptyline	0.5 to 1.0 mg/kg PO every 24 hours	Lethargy, weight gain, decreased grooming, and transient cystic calculi reported
Gabapentin	5 to 10 mg/kg PO every 12 to 24 hours	Gradually reduce dose when withdrawing drug Appears effective, especially where sensitization might be present Unpleasant taste
Tramadol	1 to 2 mg/kg PO every 12 to 24 hours	Very unpleasant taste Neurological side effects may occur May produce "opioid-like" side effects

PO, orally.
*Note: Experience is lacking with these drugs in the cat. For more information, see: Lascelles BD, Robertson S: DJD-associated pain in cats. What can we do to promote patient comfort? *J Feline Med Surg* 12:200-212, 2010.

buprenorphine, and fentanyl), but these are less frequently administered mainly due to prescribing restrictions, ease of administration, and owner safety.[14]

Glucosamine and Chondroitin Sulphate

There are numerous oral preparations available containing glucosamine and chondroitin, generally with other additives (e.g., minerals and antioxidants), and these are categorized as nutraceuticals.[6,14] The rationale for their use is based on the fact that glucosamine and chondroitin are involved in the synthesis of articular cartilage, and increasing these levels in the patient might aid in repair or slow down degradation of cartilage. There is some experimental evidence for this.[42,43] However, there is anecdotal evidence and some tissue culture studies that support an anti-inflammatory and analgesic effect. A recent prospective, double-blind, randomized, and placebo-controlled study by the author compared the efficacy of meloxicam and a glucosamine/chondroitin supplement in the management of cats with painful OA.[24] Cats with OA were divided into two groups, one group (17 cats) received meloxicam and the other group (13 cats) the glucosamine/chondroitin supplement for 70 days; both groups then

received placebo until day 98. Owner-assessed mobility was significantly improved in the meloxicam group ($P < 0.01$). There was improvement in the glucosamine/chondroitin group (58% improved their mobility scores at day 42), but this did not reach statistical significance. When the meloxicam and glucosamine chondroitin were discontinued and the placebo introduced, a significant number of cats in the meloxicam group (64.3%) showed worsening of their mobility, activity, temperament, and lifestyle scores when compared to the glucosamine/chondroitin group (27.3%). Therefore, it appeared that the potential improvement resulting from the glucosamine/chondroitin was longer lasting than that produced by the meloxicam.

These oral supplements are often used in combination with NSAIDs, although many clinicians prefer to use them as an alternative because they are regarded as being safer. There are issues with regulation and quality control of these products, and the ideal dose is not known. It is the author's belief that only those produced by reputable manufacturers should be used. Some products contain other ingredients, particularly antioxidants which may give additional benefits, such as curcumin (Seraquin, Boehringer Ingelheim) and avocado/soybean unsaponifiables and tea polyphenols (Dasuquin, Novartis Animal Health). Oxidative stress is an important aspect of joint inflammation, so the inclusion of antioxidants is relevant.

Side effects are rare, although minor GI upset has been reported. Concerns that glucosamine might precipitate diabetes mellitus have not been substantiated. Polysulfated products are used by some authorities, and these are most often given parenterally (e.g., pentosan polysulfate, Cartrophen Vet, Arthropharm [Europe] Limited), although they are not licensed for use in the cat. Polysulfated compounds must be used cautiously in combination with NSAIDs, because the former have an anticoagulant effect and may potentiate any GI bleeding caused by an NSAID.

Omega-3 Essential Fatty Acids

There are two main types of essential fatty acids (EFAs), omega-3 and omega-6, which compete for incorporation into phospholipids and can act as substrates for cyclooxygenase and lipoxygenase. A high proportion of omega-6 fatty acids within cell membranes promotes the production of inflammatory prostaglandins, leukotrienes, and thromboxanes. High levels of omega-3 fatty acids in cell membranes protect against the production of these proinflammatory prostaglandins and leukotrienes during inflammation and tissue damage.

Although there are specific omega-3 EFA preparations available for oral use, the most common way of giving these nutrients is by feeding special complete diets containing increased levels of omega-3 fatty acids. There is one published study showing that cats with DJD showed improved owner-assessed activity levels after being fed an omega-3–rich diet, although there was no improvement in activity levels as assessed by collar mounted activity monitors.[44] The main omega-3 fatty acids that appear to be important for the cat are docosahexaenoic acid and alpha-linolenic acid. These therapeutic diets contain other ingredients, which may be of benefit in reducing joint inflammation (e.g., antioxidants, glucosamine, and chondroitin). Nonsteroidal anti-inflammatory drugs can be used concurrently with the omega-3–rich diets (or other omega-3 preparations), but in these cases, the moist form of the diet should always be used to increase dietary water intake.

Contrary to common belief, there is no increased risk of weight gain in cats receiving omega-3–rich diets. These diets can be used in OA cats that also have CKD. In cats with OA and diabetes mellitus, it is preferable to use a specific metabolic diet for treatment of the diabetes rather than the omega-3 diet for the OA.

Green lipped mussel extract is popular with some clinicians in managing OA. Its mode of action is uncertain, but the extract does contain glucosamine, chondroitin, antioxidants, and omega-3 fatty acids.

Weight Reduction

Although it is unclear whether obesity is a risk factor for feline OA, it is an important factor for two reasons: first, because of the increased loading of the joints, particularly during jumping and landing; and second, because excessive fat deposits are known to produce increased amounts of adipokines, some of which cause cartilage degradation.[11,12] Only about 14% of older cats with OA are obese.[7] Therefore, weight reduction regimes are often not necessary in this population, although obviously, if the cat is overweight, weight loss through a reducing diet[45] can be very beneficial and this should be done before using any specific therapeutic diet, such as an omega-3-rich food. However, obesity in younger cats might be a risk factor for OA later in life, and these animals should be placed on a reducing diet. Weight loss in older cats is discussed at length in Chapter 95.

Environmental Modification

Because chronic arthritic pain causes many different behavioral changes in the cat, modifying the animal's environment can help to overcome some of these difficulties and improve the physical and psychological welfare of the animal.[14,38,41] Useful reviews of environmental enrichment have been published.[14,46,47] Chapters 73 and 93 address these important topics in depth. Modifications of the environment for patients with OA need not be complex (see the following information).

Improving Security
Cats are highly territorial and must feel secure in their core territory, both within the owner's home and their immediate outside territory. They need places to hide, and ideally they need more than one access route to and from their core territory. Major disturbances (e.g., introduction of other pets) can cause anxiety and stress and make it more difficult to cope with chronic pain.

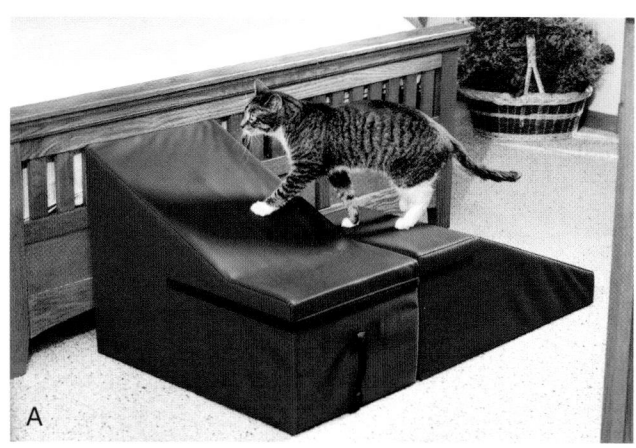

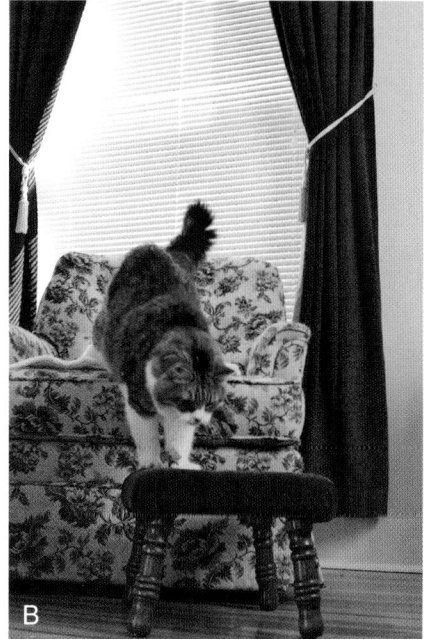

Figure 96-12: Arthritic cats have difficulty in reaching their favorite high vantage points. Providing steps/ramps **(A)** or strategically positioning furniture **(B)** can help. (Figure 96-12A, Courtesy of http://wwwDrsFosterSmith.com. B, Courtesy of Deb Given.)

Steps and Ramps
The vertical dimension is very important to cats for observation and perching. Therefore, providing steps or ramps or moving furniture (Figure 96-12) to facilitate access to beds, sofas, window ledges, and other favorite resting places is helpful. Modification of cat flaps in doors may also be required (e.g., reducing the height of the flap from the floor, increasing its size, and ensuring that the closing mechanism is not too rapid).

Access to Other Resources
The cat must have easy access to food, water, and litter boxes. There should be at least one litter box per cat in the household, and the litter should be sufficiently deep. Litter boxes must be a generous size, accessible, and easy to get into for cats with mobility problems (Figure 96-13). Several food bowls can be distributed throughout the home to encourage

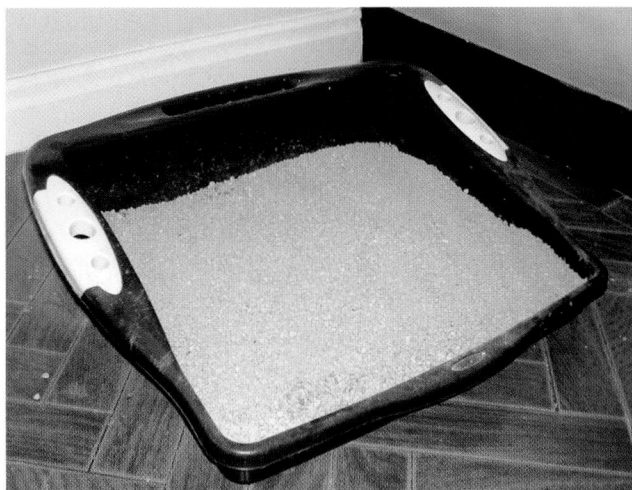

Figure 96-13: Litter boxes should be easily accessible to the arthritic cat. This litter box was made from a horticultural seedling tray. (Courtesy of Sarah Heath.)

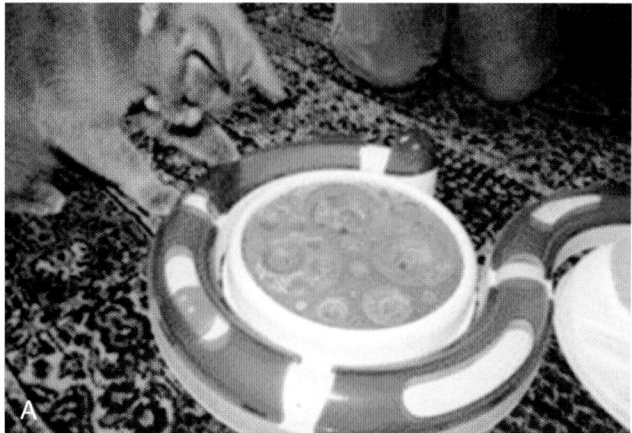

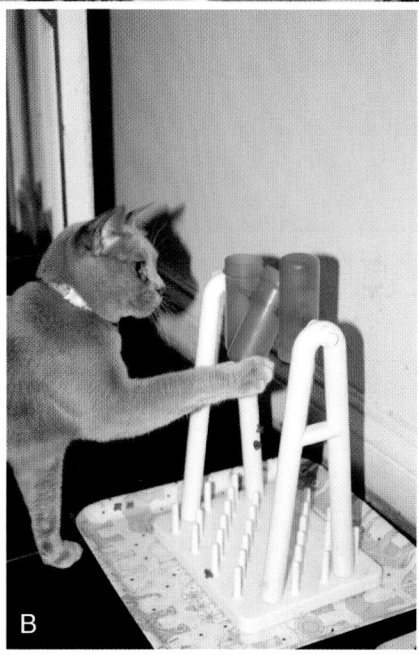

Figure 96-14: A and **B,** Playing with a selection of toys provides mental stimulation and encourages exercise, which helps to strengthen muscles and improve general fitness. (Courtesy of Sarah Ellis.)

activity and provide mental stimulation. More than one water bowl should be provided; these should not be placed adjacent to the food. Raising food and water bowls may help when there is stiffness in elbows, shoulders, or spine. Stable scratching opportunities should be provided. The provision of padded, comfortable bedding is simple but important.

Interaction and Exercise

The owner should be encouraged to actively interact with the cat and engage in play for several minutes on at least three occasions per day (or according to the wishes of the individual cat) to provide exercise and mental stimulation. Encouraging the cat to play with different toys is also useful and helps to strengthen muscle and improve general fitness (Figure 96-14). Some cats may be amenable to exercise outdoors on a leash or harness. Stroking the cat, particularly around the head, is also encouraged, because this releases neurotransmitters that can improve the cat's mood and its ability to cope with pain. Grooming the cat on several occasions during the day for several minutes will have a similar effect; grooming gloves are useful for this.

Pheromone Therapy

There are products available that contain feline facial pheromones (F3 fraction, Feliway). These are provided as a spray that can be released into the environment or as a diffuser that plugs into an electrical socket. These products can reduce stress.[48]

Physical Therapy

This type of therapy is best designed and supervised by a trained animal physiotherapist. Simple range of motion and massage techniques can be taught to owners, and these can help to alleviate the muscular pain that is often associated with OA and also improve joint mobility. This also promotes interaction between the owner and the cat. Other modalities

(e.g., shock wave therapy, laser therapy, heat and cold therapy, and even hydrotherapy) have been used in the cat but are not well evaluated.[49-51]

Surgical Treatment

Surgical therapies have been advocated but are of limited application. Total hip replacement is possible in the cat as is arthrodesis for a painful arthritic joint. Because multiple joint involvement is common in the arthritic cat, surgically targeting individual joints is of limited benefit. The age of the patient and concomitant diseases might also bring into question the value of major surgery. Joint débridement and removal of osteochondral bodies may help to relieve pain,[26,52] although these osteochondromas tend to be extensive and not necessarily mobile within the joint, making their removal challenging if not impossible.

Stem Cell Therapy and Other Therapies

Autologous, adipose-derived mesenchymal stem cell therapy is available in the United States, Australia, and some European countries. The technique requires the collection of adipose tissue under general anesthesia that is then processed at a laboratory, or even within the veterinary practice if it has the necessary equipment. After processing, the cells are injected into the affected joint. Although there are probably stem cells present, there are many other cell populations, including large numbers of adipocytes. An area of concern is that these adipose tissue cells may produce detrimental adipokines (e.g., leptin and adiponectin), which can actually promote cartilage degeneration.[11,12] Although clinical improvement has been reported in other species, the reasons for this are unclear, and such improvements are most likely due to an anti-inflammatory effect, which may be time-limited and for which the cost may not be justified. It is very unlikely that there is any regenerative effect within the joint. Although this type of therapy is generally referred to as "stem cell therapy," it is more accurate and less misleading to describe it as "cell-based therapy." Other biological therapies are being developed and/or used in feline OA (e.g., intra-articular injection of platelet-rich plasma or platelet concentrates and the use of antinerve growth factor monoclonal antibody), but clear evidence of effectiveness is awaited.

Many other therapies have been described for OA, including acupuncture;[53] however, there are no evidence-based studies to date to support efficacy in cats.

SUMMARY

Osteoarthritis is a very common disease in older cats but is still underdiagnosed in clinical practice. Many cats suffering chronic arthritic pain are not being treated, which does create important welfare concerns. Changes in the cat's behavior are an important feature of the disease, and these are best assessed by using owner questionnaires. Treatment includes the use of NSAIDs and nutraceuticals, often in combination. Recent evidence suggests that NSAIDs, if used cautiously and with proper veterinary assessment of the patient, are reasonably safe and effective in the cat. Modifications of the cat's environment are also important in helping to improve the animal's quality of life.

References

1. Clarke SP, Mellor D, Clements DN, et al: Radiographic prevalence of degenerative joint disease in a hospital population of cats. *Vet Rec* 157:793–799, 2005.
2. Hardie EM, Roe SC, Martin FR: Radiographic evidence of degenerative joint disease in geriatric cats: 100 cases (1994-1997). *J Am Vet Med Assoc* 220:628–632, 2000.
3. Godfrey DR: Osteoarthritis in cats: a retrospective radiological study. *J Small Anim Pract* 46:425–429, 2005.
4. Lascelles BDX, Henry JB, Brown J, et al: Cross-sectional study of the prevalence of radiographic degenerative joint disease in domesticated cats. *Vet Surg* 39:535–544, 2010.
5. Slingerland LT, Hazewinkel HAW, Meij BP, et al: Cross-sectional study of the prevalence and clinical features of osteoarthritis in 100 cats. *Vet J* 187:304–309, 2011.
6. Bennett D: Canine and feline osteoarthritis. In Ettinger SJ, Feldman EC, editors: *Textbook of veterinary internal medicine: diseases of the dog and cat*, ed 7, St Louis, 2010, Saunders Elsevier, pp 750–761.
7. Clarke SP, Bennett D: Feline osteoarthritis: a prospective study. *J Small Anim Pract* 47:439–445, 2006.
8. Lascelles BDX: Feline degenerative joint disease. *Vet Surg* 39:2–13, 2010.
9. Laflamme DP: Nutrition for ageing cats and dogs and the importance of body condition. *Vet Clin North Am Small Anim Pract* 35:713–742, 2005.
10. Lund GM, Armstrong PJ, Kirk CA, et al: Prevalence and risk factors for obesity in adult cats from private US veterinary practices. *Int J Appl Res Vet Med* 3:85–96, 2005.
11. Dumond H, Presle N, Terlain B, et al: Evidence for a key role of leptin in osteoarthritis. *Arthritis Rheum* 48:3118–3129, 2003.
12. German AJ, Ryan VH, German AC, et al: Obesity, its associated disorders and the role of inflammatory adipokines in companion animals. *Vet J* 195:6–9, 2010.
13. Bennett D, Zainal Ariffin SM, Johnston P: Osteoarthritis in the cat. 1. How common is it and how easy to recognize? *J Feline Med Surg* 14:65–75, 2012.
14. Bennett D, Zainal Ariffin SM, Johnston P: Osteoarthritis in the cat. 2. How should it be managed and treated? *J Feline Med Surg* 14:76–84, 2012.
15. Ryan JM, Lascelles BDX, Benito J, et al: Histological and molecular characteristics of feline humeral condylar osteoarthritis. *BMC Vet Res* 9:110, 2013.
16. Malik R, Allan GS, Howlett CR, et al: Osteochondrodysplasia in Scottish Fold cats. *Aust Vet J* 77:85–92, 1999.
17. Konde LJ, Thrall MA, Gasper P, et al: Radiographically visualized skeletal changes associated with mucopolysaccharidosis VI in cats. *Vet Radiol Ultrasound* 28:223–228, 1987.
18. Loughin CA, Kerwin SC, Hosgood G, et al: Clinical signs and results of treatment in cats with patellar luxation, 42 cases (1992-2002). *J Am Vet Med Assoc* 228:1370–1375, 2006.
19. Streubel R, Geyer H, Montavon PM: Medial humeral epicondylitis in cats. *Vet Surg* 41:795–802, 2012.
20. Petersen ME, Taylor S, Greco DS, et al: Acromegaly in 14 cats. *J Vet Intern Med* 4:192–201, 1990.
21. Zainal Ariffin SM: Radiographic and pathologic studies of feline appendicular osteoarthritis. PhD thesis, School of Veterinary Medicine, University of Glasgow, 2014.
22. Bennett D, Morton CA: A study of owner observed behavioral and lifestyle changes in cats with musculoskeletal disease before and after analgesic therapy. *J Feline Med Surg* 11:997–1004, 2009.
23. Lascelles BDX, Bernie HD, Roe S, et al: Evaluation of client-specific outcome measures and activity monitoring to measure pain relief in cats with osteoarthritis. *J Vet Intern Med* 21:410–416, 2007.
24. Sul RM, Chase D, Parkin T, et al: Comparison of meloxicam and a glucosamine-chondroitin supplement in management of feline osteoarthritis. *Vet Comp Orthop Traumatol* 27:20–26, 2014.
25. Wood AKW, McCarthy PH, Martin ICA: Anatomic and radiographic appearance of a sesamoid bone in the tendon of origin of the supinator muscle of the cat. *Am J Vet Res* 56:736–738, 1995.
26. Staiger BA, Beale BS: Use of arthroscopy for debridement of the elbow joint in cats. *J Am Vet Med Assoc* 226:401–403, 2005.
27. Langenbach A, Giger U, Green P, et al: Relationship between degenerative joint disease and hip joint laxity by use of distraction index and Norberg angle measurement in a group of cats. *J Am Vet Med Assoc* 213:1439–1443, 1998.

28. Keller GG, Reed AL, Lattimer JC, et al: Hip dysplasia: a feline population study. *Vet Radiol Ultrasound* 40:460–464, 1999.

29. Hayes HM, Wilson GP, Burt JK: Feline hip dysplasia. *J Am Anim Hosp Assoc* 15:447–448, 1979.

30. Freire M, Brown J, Robertson ID, et al: Meniscal mineralization in domestic cats. *Vet Surg* 39:545–552, 2010.

31. Lascelles BD, Henderson AJ, Hackett IJ: Evaluation of the clinical efficacy of meloxicam in cats with painful locomotor disorders. *J Small Anim Pract* 42:587–593, 2001.

32. Lascelles BD, Hardie EM, Robertson SA: Non-steroidal anti-inflammatory drugs in cats: a review. *Vet Anaesth Analg* 34:228–250, 2007.

33. Gunew MN, Menrath VH, Marshall RD: Long-term safety, efficacy and palatability of oral meloxicam at 0.01-0.03 mg/kg for treatment of osteoarthritic pain in cats. *J Feline Med Surg* 10:235–241, 2010.

34. Gowan RA, Lingard AE, Johnston L, et al: Retrospective case-control study of the effect of long-term dosing with meloxicam on renal function in aged cats with degenerative joint disease. *J Feline Med Surg* 13:752–761, 2011.

35. Thoulon F, Narbe R, Johnston L, et al: Metabolism and excretion of oral meloxicam in the cat. *J Vet Intern Med* 23:695, 2009. (Abstract).

36. Sparkes AH, Helene R, Lascelles BD, et al: ISFM and AAFP consensus guidelines: long-term use of NSAIDs in cats. *J Feline Med Surg* 13:519–538, 2010.

37. Westropp JL, Kass PH, Buffington CAT: Evaluation of the effects of stress in cats with idiopathic cystitis. *Am J Vet Res* 67:731–736, 2006.

38. Gowan RA, Baral RM, Lingard AE, et al: A retrospective analysis of the effects of meloxicam on the longevity of aged cats with and without overt chronic kidney disease. *J Feline Med Surg* 14:876–881, 2012.

39. Scherk M: Experiences in feline practice: incorporating NSAIDs in analgesic therapy. In *Proceedings of the International Society of Feline Medicine*, Amsterdam, 2010, pp 12–19.

40. Robertson S, Lascelles BD: Long term pain in cats. How much do we know about this important welfare issue? *J Feline Med Surg* 12:188–199, 2010.

41. Lascelles BD, Robertson S: DJD-associated pain in cats. What can we do to promote patient comfort. *J Feline Med Surg* 12:200–212, 2010.

42. Tiraloche G, Girard C, Chouinard L, et al: Effect of oral glucosamine on cartilage degradation in a rabbit model of osteoarthritis. *Arthritis Rheum* 52:1118–1128, 2005.

43. Naito K, Watari R, Furuhata A, et al: Evaluation of the effect of glucosamine on an experimental cat osteoarthritis model. *Life Sci* 86:538–543, 2010.

44. Lascelles BDX, De Puys V, Thomson A, et al: Evaluation of a therapeutic diet for feline degenerative joint disease. *J Vet Intern Med* 24:487–495, 2010.

45. Bissot T, Servet E, Vidal S, et al: Novel dietary strategies can improve the outcome of weight loss programs in obese client-owned cats. *J Feline Med Surg* 12:104–112, 2010.

46. Ellis S: Environmental enrichment. Practical strategies for improving feline welfare. *J Feline Med Surg* 11:901–912, 2009.

47. Ellis SLH, Rodan I, Carney HC, et al: AAFP and ISFM feline environmental needs guidelines. *J Feline Med Surg* 15:219–230, 2013.

48. Griffith CA, Steigerwald ES, Buffington T: Effects of a synthetic facial hormone on behavior of cats. *J Am Vet Med Assoc* 217:1154–1156, 2000.

49. Lindley S: Introduction to physical therapies. In Watson P, Lindley S, editors: *BSAVA manual of canine and feline rehabilitation, supportive and palliative care*, Gloucester, 2010, BSAVA, pp 85–89.

50. Sharp B: Physiotherapy and physical rehabilitation. In Watson P, Lindley S, editors: *BSAVA manual of canine and feline rehabilitation, supportive and palliative care*, Gloucester, 2010, BSAVA, pp 90–113.

51. Lindley S, Smith H: Hydrotherapy. In Watson P, Lindley S, editors: *BSAVA manual of canine and feline rehabilitation, supportive and palliative care*, Gloucester, 2010, BSAVA, pp 114–123.

52. Tan C, Allan G, Barfield D, et al: Synovial osteochondroma involving the elbow of a cat. *J Feline Med Surg* 12:412–417, 2010.

53. Lindley S: Acupuncture in palliative and rehabilitative medicine. In Watson P, Lindley S, editors: *BSAVA manual of canine and feline rehabilitation, supportive and palliative care*, Gloucester, 2010, BSAVA, pp 123–130.

Proactive Maintenance of the Aging Feline Immune System

Shila Nordone

According to veterinary demographic data published in 2013, the average lifespan for cats in the United States is 12.1 years.[1] Based on an extrapolated human-to-cat age analogy,[2] the average cat now spends 3 years as a senior patient (ages 8 to 11) and at least 1 year as a geriatric patient. These aging cats make up a substantial patient cohort; senior patients are estimated to make up 30% to 40% of veterinary general practice clientele. As such, senior care programs have been evolving for nearly two decades as veterinarians create platforms for senior-focused evaluations and protocols. Despite the clear importance of this demographic group to both veterinary practice and pet owners, there is a paucity of feline-specific data regarding age-related change in immune function. Immune function is critical to host protection against pathogens, to recognize transformed "self" cells that evolve into cancer, and control of autoreactive cells that lead to autoimmune disease. As such, the importance of immune function to the health and well-being of the aging patient is indisputable. This chapter intends to summarize what is known about the aging feline immune system and extrapolates human, canine, equine, and rodent model data to the cat when possible to enable practitioners to create senior care programs that include maintenance of the feline immune system.

THE FELINE IMMUNE SYSTEM

The immune system of cats has evolved to maintain homeostasis in an environment where the host is continually exposed to foreign, sometimes noxious, organisms that are inhaled, swallowed, or inhabit skin and mucous membranes. Whether or not these organisms cause disease is based on the integrity of the host immune system, whether it responds appropriately by ignoring or escalating, and whether the organism possesses pathogenic mechanisms to evade defense mechanisms. Therefore, host defense is a delicate balancing act between coexistence with the environment and immediate, effective removal of dangerous organisms.

The immune system can be categorized into early and delayed responders, composed of the innate and adaptive system, respectively. Cells of both systems are derived from common multipotent hematopoietic stem cells (HSCs) that differentiate into either myeloid or lymphoid progenitor cells.

Myeloid progenitors give rise to cells of the innate immune system, including basophils, neutrophils, eosinophils, dendritic cells, and monocytes. Innate immune system cells are hardwired to respond to pathogenic organisms through germline-encoded receptors that recognize molecular patterns shared by microbes and toxins that are not present in the mammalian host. Examples would be Toll-like receptors (TLRs) that recognize highly conserved pathogen-associated molecular patterns (PAMPs), such as lipopolysaccharides, lipopeptides, viral single-stranded RNA, and bacterial DNA molecules that contain a cytosine triphosphate deoxynucleotide ("C") followed by a guanine triphosphate deoxynucleotide ("G") (CpG motifs) not normally found in abundance in mammalian DNA.[3] Constitutive, broad expression of these pathogen recognition receptors on cells of the innate immune system allows immediate responsiveness to facilitate the first wave of host defense. Once triggered, TLRs induce pro-inflammatory cytokine production and upregulation of cell surface molecules necessary to start an immune response.[3] After inflammation is triggered, dendritic cells and macrophages act as professional antigen presenting cells (APCs) to cells of the adaptive immune system.[4] Professional APCs process antigen and present antigenic epitopes in the context of major histocompatibility complex (MHC) proteins to T cells, initiating the adaptive immune response. It is in the context of cytokine production and antigen presentation that the innate response facilitates activation of the adaptive response.

Lymphoid progenitors give rise to B and T cells of the adaptive immune system. Cells of the adaptive system have a high degree of plasticity in their pathogen recognition capabilities, because their antigen recognition receptors are encoded by gene elements that somatically rearrange to form infinite variations of antigen-binding molecules to enhance the likelihood of high specificity for antigenic structures. The antigen binding molecule for B cells is cell surface bound immunoglobulin (Ig) and for T cells, it is the T cell receptor (TcR). The TcR is limited to recognizing antigens in the context of MHC proteins on APCs, whereas Ig is not restricted by self-presentation and can recognize antigenic epitopes in extracellular spaces. Once engaged, cell surface Ig and TcR induce cellular proliferation and differentiation, enabling clonal expansion of antigen-specific cells and differentiation into cells with both effector and memory

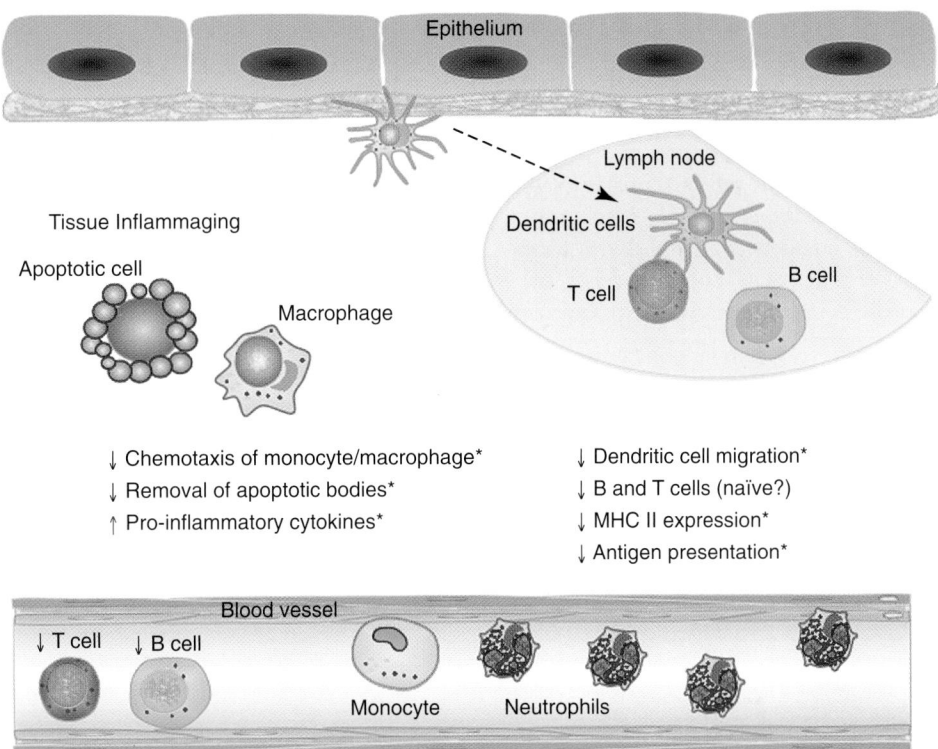

Figure 97-1: Schematic overview of age-associated decline in immune function. Asterisk *(*)* designates that experimental evidence was derived in species other than the cat. *Left side*: Age-associated decreased migration of monocytes and impaired phagocytosis by tissue macrophages leads to a delay in removal of apoptotic cellular debris, causing release of damage-associated molecular patterns and chronic, low-grade tissue inflammation known as *inflammaging*. *Right side*: Age-associated decreased dendritic cell migration, decreased antigen-presentation, and decreased naïve B and T cell numbers leads to a decline in the ability of senior animals to respond to newly encountered antigen. *MHC*, major histocompatibility complex

function. The ensuing response is highly antigen focused and capable of long-term maintenance due to persistence of memory cells. Antigen recall responses by B and T memory cells, although faster, still rely on proliferation of antigen-specific cells to mount an effective response. Estimated timelines for innate immune responses are minutes to hours, memory adaptive immune responses are within days, and *de novo* adaptive immune responses are within 1 week.

IMMUNOSENESCENCE

It is generally accepted that age-related decline in immune function, termed *immunosenescence*, occurs across all species as a result of the normal aging process.[5-9] Consensus opinion is that aging is not a disease, but rather the sum effect of time and environment on cellular and organ function. The reliance of the immune system on the highly coordinated efforts of multiple cell types described earlier, and primary and secondary lymphoid tissue makes it uniquely susceptible to generalized, age-associated tissue senescence. Vulnerabilities inflicted on the immune system as regenerative and homeostatic mechanisms fail result in a cumulative decline in immune function and, subsequently, reduced protection of the host. In simplest terms, immunosenescence can be ascribed to a reduced capacity of the host to (1) produce and mature immune cells, (2) recognize and control pathogenic organisms at the level of the innate immune system, (3) mount an adaptive immune response that will result in memory against a pathogen, and (4) control nonspecific inflammation to maintain tissue homeostasis (Figure 97-1). Ramifications of loss of immune function extend beyond pathogens to cancer[10] and autoimmune disease.[11] Although the targets of the immune response vary, the outcome remains the same—increased vulnerability of the individual due to impaired immune function with age.

IMMUNE CELL GENERATION AND MAINTENANCE

Hematopoiesis
Detailed analysis of age-related changes in HSC populations is lacking in the cat. Similar to humans, aged feline bone marrow is characterized by decreased cellularity and increased fat deposition.[12] In elderly humans, detailed phenotyping of bone marrow cells suggests that alterations in the frequency of subsets of HSC progenitor cells and function of these subsets strongly contributes to the age-associated changes in circulating cell populations.[13,14] Multipotent CD34+ HSC progenitor cells increase in frequency and are more readily

induced to proliferate in elderly patients. Elderly bone marrow consists of a higher frequency of myeloid progenitor cells and a reduced frequency of lymphoid progenitors, and it is characterized by enhanced expression of genes associated with cell cycle, myeloid lineage specification, and myeloid malignancies. These HSC changes are reflected in age-related changes in circulating populations—stable numbers of myeloid cells and reduced numbers of lymphocytes. Age-related changes in HSC are similar in rodent models,[15] suggesting that hematopoietic aging is conserved across species.

Peripheral Circulation

To date, documentation of age-related changes in feline immune cell numbers has been limited to peripheral blood analysis.[16] Differential white blood cell analysis of adult (2- to 4-year-old) and senior (10- to 14-year-old) cats revealed a significant age-related decline in total white blood cells, absolute numbers of lymphocytes and eosinophils in senior animals. Neutrophils, monocytes, and basophil numbers remain consistent across age groups. Phenotypic profiling of leukocyte populations found lower absolute counts of CD21+ B cells, CD5+ T cells (CD5 is not expressed on B cells in the cat), CD4+ T cells, CD8+ T cells, and CD56+ natural killer cells in circulation in senior cats when compared with adult cats. Most striking was the reduction in CD4+ T cells in senior cats to near half that of adults. The decline in absolute CD4 T cell numbers results in an inversion of CD4:CD8 T cell ratios from approximately 2:1 to near 1:1. These age-related changes in absolute cell numbers strongly mirror changes in other species and suggest that although relative percentages of cell populations in circulation remain somewhat consistent with age, the absolute number of immune cells declines.

IMMUNE CELL FUNCTION

Innate Immune Cells

Cells of the innate immune system, including neutrophils, monocytes/macrophages, and dendritic cells provide the first line of defense against infection. Strategically located in peripheral tissue or poised for rapid recruitment from the bloodstream, these cells recognize highly conserved PAMPs (as mentioned earlier) through cell surface and intracellular TLR.[3] Toll-like receptor activation results in initiation of inflammation and is directive of downstream adaptive immune responses involving T and B cells. Innate immune cells are also critical for removing cellular debris as cells undergo the normal process of cell death called *apoptosis*.[17,18] Prompt removal via phagocytosis of apoptotic debris is critical to prevent the release of internal damage-associated molecular patterns that can, like a pathogen, trigger and exacerbate inflammation.[19]

In cats as in humans, neutrophils and monocyte numbers in circulation remain relatively consistent throughout life.[8,16] In contrast, function of innate immune cells in humans and rodent models is significantly altered with age (reviewed in Rymkiewicz and colleagues[8]). Phagocytic clearance of foreign pathogens and autologous apoptotic debris by neutrophils, macrophages, and dendritic cells is reduced *in vitro* and *in vivo*.[20] Macrophages also exhibit reduced chemotaxis, reduced expression of MHC class II molecules, and decreased capacity for antigen presentation.[5,21-25] Collectively, impaired innate immune cell function contributes to diminished immune responses against pathogens and a failure to maintain a quiescent, noninflammatory environment.[5] As a result, chronic, mild inflammation is a common characteristic of aged tissue. Described as "inflammaging,"[5,26,27] elderly human patients have increased levels of pro-inflammatory cytokines in circulation and in tissue-resident macrophages. Similarly, senior dogs and horses have an enhanced pro-inflammatory state as evidenced by increased production of pro-inflammatory cytokines postinfection in comparison to healthy adults.[6,7] Cytokine levels increase exponentially in obese individuals and have been attributed to reservoirs of cytokines harbored by macrophages in adipose tissue.[28]

T Cells

Of all lymphocytes, T cells appear to be most dramatically affected by aging. In young individuals, bone marrow-derived lymphoid precursors seed the thymus and use the network of epithelial thymic stromal cells and dendritic cells for selection and maturation. The end result is emigration of naïve CD8 and CD4 T cells from the thymus that are capable of responding to foreign antigen in the context of MHC class I and II molecules, respectively, with minimal risk of self-recognition. The current paradigm of immunosenescence is that naive T cells are most profoundly affected by aging due to the additive effects of reduced output of lymphoid progenitors from the bone marrow and atrophy of the thymus with age.[29-31] One caveat is that dependence of naïve CD4 T cells on thymic programming and maturation is not consistent across species. In mice, thymic function is a prerequisite to maintain a naïve CD4 T cell compartment, whereas in humans, peripheral homeostatic proliferation of naïve CD4 T cells enables the maintenance of naive CD4 T cells[32], albeit at a lower level, even in the presence of thymic atrophy. The level of dependence of the cat on thymic function remains to be determined. Although it is known the feline thymus atrophies with age, it is unclear whether the cat more closely resembles the mouse or human in the mechanistic maintenance of naïve CD4 T cells.

Early murine studies suggested the reduction in T cells in the mouse was exacerbated by reduced capacity to produce interleukin-2 (IL-2),[33] a cytokine critical for T cell survival. With extensive cellular phenotyping, it is now understood that reduced IL-2 is related to the overall shift in polyfunctionality of T cells[34] rather than a loss of function. In aged human patients, memory T cells predominate,[5] and as such, they produce and use less IL-2 for survival. In place of IL-2, memory cells produce higher levels of effector cytokines, such as interferon-gamma. Finally, in humans, naïve CD8 T cells are lost more rapidly than naïve CD4 T cells with age, and the loss of naïve CD8 T cells is now known to be independent of chronic viral infections, such as cytomegalovirus.[35] Whether this is a generalized loss of production of T cell progenitors at the level of the bone marrow, a thymic loss of selection and maturation, or reduced peripheral homeostatic proliferation of naïve CD8 T cells remains to be determined.

B Cells

In cats, there is an overall reduction of circulating CD21+ B cells with age.[16] Due to phenotyping restrictions in the cat, there exists a lack of deeper understanding of whether the general decline in B cells is in memory, isotype switched memory, or naïve B cells. Serum IgG levels do not change with age in cats; however, senior cats have elevated levels of serum IgA and IgM.[16] The relationship between the change in circulating B cells and antibody levels in the cat remains to be defined. Human data suggest that the change in B cells in aged patients is both quantitative and qualitative.[36-40] B cell bone marrow precursors remain stable through life, thereby providing consistent naïve and IgM+ memory B cells in circulation. The reduction in peripheral B cells is attributed to a decline in isotype switched ("switch") memory B cell pool and B cells capable of responding to antigens independent of T cell support.

Flexibility of B cells to respond to antigen in the presence or absence of T cell help is critical, and the differential ability of B cells to perform this function is highly conserved across species. These B cell responses are termed *T dependent* or *T independent*, respectively, and are defined by the antigen itself. T-independent antigens are those containing epitopes of repetitive biochemical structures, such as bacterial capsular polysaccharides, lipopolysaccharide, or polymeric protein antigens. These antigens cross-link B cell surface Ig to stimulate clonal expansion and antibody production but do not drive differentiation of cells into memory cells. As such, T-independent antigens do not result in immunological memory. B cells capable of responding to T-independent antigen reside in the peritoneal cavity and mucosa, are maintained by self-renewal of cells, and use a limited repertoire of germline variable-region genes. In contrast, T-dependent antigens are usually proteins processed and presented by APCs. B cell responses against T-dependent antigen occur in secondary lymphoid tissue, such as lymph nodes, where B and T cells can comingle. In order for B cells to respond to T-dependent antigen, activated CD4+ T cells are required for optimal B lymphocyte proliferation, production of Ig, Ig class switching (from IgD/IgM to IgG and IgA), rescue of B lymphocytes from apoptotic death, germinal center formation, and generation of B lymphocyte memory.

In humans, the ability of B cells to respond to T-independent versus T-dependent antigens varies with age.[41,42] B cell responses to T-independent antigens develop after the age of 2 years and are reduced in senior patients. In contrast, B-cell T-dependent antigen responses appear to be intact in elderly humans. Conjugation of T-independent antigens to

T-dependent antigen enhances efficacy of the humoral immune response in neonatal and senior humans, suggesting that antigen formulation can rescue age-related limitations in antibody responses to T-independent antigen.[30]

MANAGEMENT OF IMMUNOSENESCENCE IN THE CAT

Cats have benefited extensively from improvements in routine veterinary healthcare, diet, dental care, and immunization protocols as evidenced by their prolonged lifespan. Despite these improvements, the primary ailments of aged cats are immune-mediated in nature, including diabetes mellitus, kidney disease, cancer, infectious disease, and perhaps a subset of cats with hyperthyroidism. Maintenance of a robust and balanced immune system is therefore paramount to extending not just the quantity of years for cats but the quality of those years.

Vaccination

Vaccination has profoundly changed the landscape of feline infectious disease and is arguably one of the most cost-effective interventions veterinarians perform for the health of cats. Vaccine products and protocols protect cats from the most common pathogens that cause morbidity and mortality.[43] Despite these gains, vaccination of senior cats is a work in progress. Because there exists a lack of some very basic understanding of immunologic aging in the cat, there is a simultaneous lack of understanding of whether current products and protocols are optimal for seniors. Although limited in scope, data suggest that cats, like humans, retain antigen-specific memory into old age, and thus, protective cell-mediated immunity and antibody against core vaccine viruses should remain intact if animals are routinely immunized as adults. It is well established that adult cats (between 4 months and 8 years of age) respond adequately to feline parvovirus, feline calicivirus, and feline herpesvirus vaccination.[43] As duration of immunity is 3 to 7 years on average, it is likely that protection is achieved and maintained through the life of the cat if immunization occurs on schedule during adulthood. What is less clear is the protection afforded by noncore vaccines in senior cats, including those against feline immunodeficiency virus and feline leukemia virus, or core vaccines to unimmunized, naïve senior (greater than 8 years old) animals. In one reported immunization trial performed in senior animals, cats older than 8 years had a greater chance of not reaching protective rabies titers of 0.5 International Unit/mL in comparison to adult cats.[44] Imbedded in these results was the observation that the two most important factors in achieving successful antibody titers are the number of doses of vaccine and the interval between vaccination and blood draw to evaluate titers. Therefore, in the absence of challenge studies that would define optimal vaccination protocols for senior cats, it is recommended to vaccinate naïve senior animals at least twice, in a 3- to 4-week period.

Immunization protocols should then be continued through-out the life of the cat, following label recommendations for duration of immunity and reimmunization.

The optimal choice of vaccine type (e.g., modified live, killed, or vectored) in aged cats remains to be determined. Beyond what is known in humans with respect to reduced responsiveness to T-independent antigens in aged patients, studies in horses have shown that old animals have limited antibody responses to standard inactivated vaccines.[45,46] In the horse, canarypox-vectored equine influenza virus vaccine protects naïve young horses and significantly decreased clinical disease in old horses, suggesting that vectored vaccines remain effective in aged animals.[47-49] Similar to humans, older horses display evidence of chronic inflammation, or inflammaging.[7] Beyond reduction of clinical signs, immunization of older horses with the canarypox vectored vaccine also blunted the severity of pro-inflammatory cytokines associated with infection.[49] Therefore, in the absence of feline-specific data, it may be prudent to choose modified live or vectored vaccines in senior cats until further studies determine whether differences exist in vaccine efficacy in the aged cat.

Immunonutrition

Over 65% of immune cells and 90% of antibody-producing cells reside in the gastrointestinal (GI) tract, making the GI tract the cat's largest immune system organ. Understanding the role of the GI tract in overall health and the complex interplay between commensal microbes and the host has greatly changed the view of nutrition and, more importantly, shown how the GI tract can be manipulated to improve health in the aging cat.[6,8,26,50-52] Colonization of the feline GI tract by microbes begins during vaginal delivery and is further enhanced by nursing, maternal contact, environment, and diet.[52,53] The end result is a diverse array of microbes, collectively known as the *microbiome*, with which cats have a symbiotic relationship. Microbes assist in digestion and form a barrier that protects the GI tract from harmful bacteria and viruses. They also actively maintain GI homeostasis through direct suppression of GI inflammation. The symbiotic relationship between microbe and host is evidenced by active regulation of microbe growth by the immune system, using both the innate and adaptive systems to prevent overgrowth of microbes in mucosa. As previously discussed, decline of both the innate and adaptive immune systems with age has broad impact, and the GI tract is collaterally affected. In animal models, the gut-associated lymphoid tissue has a reduced capacity to synthesize and secrete IgA, and has impaired innate immune cell production of alpha-defensins, antimicrobial peptides, and mucus (reviewed in Rymkiewicz and colleagues[8]). Collectively, the end result is overgrowth of the resident microbiota. These microbes trigger inflammaging in the GI tract and contribute to ongoing, low-grade GI inflammation. There is growing opinion that this self-sustaining pro-inflammatory loop creates an environment conducive to both autoreactivity in the form of inflammatory bowel disease (IBD), complex endocrine and metabolic dis-

eases (e.g., diabetes mellitus and obesity), and increased susceptibility to infection.[8]

The microbiome is an intense area of study because the specific species that make up the microbiome appear to influence GI homeostasis, immune responsiveness, and overall health. The few feline studies performed using the most powerful DNA-based sequencing technology available have identified the predominant microbial taxa in healthy feline GI tracts. In these animals, the microbiome consists of 97% to 99% bacteria, 0.02% to 0.4% fungi, 0.09% to 1% archaea, and 0.09% to 0.25% viruses.[54,55] Bacteroidetes (36% to 68% of sequences), Firmicutes (13% to 36% of sequences), Proteobacteria (6% to 12% of sequences), and Actinobacteria (1% to 8% of sequences) are the predominant bacterial phyla present.[54,55] Reports of microbiome changes with age in the cat have been noted but are inconsistent. Bifidobacterium, generally regarded as "good bacteria" for their ability to contribute to GI homeostasis, were noted to be lower in elderly animals in two studies but unchanged in another study (reviewed in Kerr and colleagues[56]). Authors noted that this is likely because macronutrient composition (dietary fiber, prebiotics, and protein-to-carbohydrate ratios) and dietary format (wet versus dry) in commercial cat food alter the microbiome. As such, direct administration of prebiotics and probiotics to cats remain an intense area of study. Prebiotics are specialized plant fiber that nourishes beneficial bacteria, whereas probiotics are live bacteria themselves. Both prebiotics and probiotics alter the microbiota, suggesting that manipulation of the GI landscape is possible and can be used to foster overall feline health, support immune system function with age, and potentially mitigate the severity of chronic disease, such as IBD.[57,58] Despite these comprehensive background studies, there is a lack of understanding of whether there is a causal relationship between a specific population of microbes and immune system decay that contributes to disease. Research to define the bacteria directly associated with disease signatures and/or GI health is paramount for making progress in dietary regulation of immunosenescence.

Finally, there is growing recognition that optimizing the macronutrients and micronutrients in the feline diet may have a direct effect on immune function outside of its influence on the microbiome (reviewed in Satyaraj[52]). Adequate nutrition may not be the equivalent of optimal nutrition when considering the increased need to manage tissue damaging oxidative stress, cardiovascular disease, joint degeneration, pain, cognitive function, and neurologic disease in senior feline patients. Inflammation has become pivotal in the outcome of all of these conditions, and there is growing recognition that "personalized nutrition" that tailors diet to patient need is part of the paradigm shift in the care of senior cats.

SUMMARY

In summary, there is no debate that geriatric feline patients are a substantial and growing part of veterinary practices, and they require a different level of care than healthy adult patients. Unfortunately, research into the most basic aspects of immunologic aging in the cat has yet to be performed. Given the lack of evidence-based best practices at the current time, clinicians must draw from other species when making decisions regarding how best to support optimal immune function in the senior cat. Obviously, lifelong healthcare from kitten through adulthood provides a preventative course of treatment that is easier to support as cats transition into seniors. Once they transition, continuation of immunization protocols that minimize unnecessary vaccination (i.e.,

following duration of immunity-based vaccination schedules) and judicious use of any potential inflammation-inducing drugs should be the platform of senior care. Use of diet modification, supplementation, prebiotics, and probiotics are also attractive options to manage detrimental inflammaging in the senior patient. Although substantial gaps in knowledge of optimal feeding and supplementation protocols exist, research advances are expected to close these gaps over the next few years to provide veterinarians with the evidence they need to optimize immune health in aging feline patients.

References

1. Banfield Pet Hospital: 2013 Banfield State of Pet Health. <http://www.stateofpethealth.com/Content/pdf/Banfield-State-of-Pet-Health-Report_2013.pdf>, (Accessed July 29, 2015).
2. Fortney WD: Implementing a successful senior/geriatric health care program for veterinarians, veterinary technicians, and office managers. *Vet Clin North Am Small Anim Pract* 42:823–834, viii, 2012.
3. Kawai T, Akira S: Toll-like receptors and their crosstalk with other innate receptors in infection and immunity. *Immunity* 34:637–650, 2011.
4. Medzhitov R, Janeway CA, Jr: Innate immune induction of the adaptive immune response. *Cold Spring Harb Symp Quant Biol* 64:429–435, 1999.
5. Aw D, Silva AB, Palmer DB: Immunosenescence: emerging challenges for an ageing population. *Immunology* 120:435–446, 2007.
6. Day MJ: Ageing, immunosenescence and inflammageing in the dog and cat. *J Comp Pathol* 142:S60–S69, 2010.
7. Horohov DW, Adams AA, Chambers TM: Immunosenescence of the equine immune system. *J Comp Pathol* 142:S78–S84, 2010.
8. Rymkiewicz PD, Heng YX, Vasudev A, et al: The immune system in the aging human. *Immunol Res* 53:235–250, 2012.
9. Schultz RD, Thiel B, Mukhtar E, et al: Age and long-term protective immunity in dogs and cats. *J Comp Pathol* 142:S102–S108, 2010.
10. Sidler C, Woycicki R, Ilnytskyy Y, et al: Immunosenescence is associated with altered gene expression and epigenetic regulation in primary and secondary immune organs. *Front Genet* 4:211, 2013.
11. Goronzy JJ, Weyand CM: Immune aging and autoimmunity. *Cell Mol Life Sci* 69:1615–1623, 2012.
12. Schalm OW: Interpretations in feline bone marrow cytology. *J Am Vet Med Assoc* 161:1418–1425, 1972.
13. Pang WW, Price EA, Sahoo D, et al: Human bone marrow hematopoietic stem cells are increased in frequency and myeloid-biased with age. *Proc Natl Acad Sci U S A* 108:20012–20017, 2011.
14. Wang J, Sun Q, Morita Y, et al: A differentiation checkpoint limits hematopoietic stem cell self-renewal in response to DNA damage. *Cell* 148:1001–1014, 2012.
15. Chambers SM, Shaw CA, Gatza C, et al: Aging hematopoietic stem cells decline in function and exhibit epigenetic dysregulation. *PLoS Biol* 5:e201, 2007.
16. Campbell DJ, Rawlings JM, Koelsch S, et al: Age-related differences in parameters of feline immune status. *Vet Immunol Immunopathol* 100:73–80, 2004.
17. Erwig LP, Henson PM: Immunological consequences of apoptotic cell phagocytosis. *Am J Pathol* 171:2–8, 2007.
18. Napoli I, Neumann H: Microglial clearance function in health and disease. *Neuroscience* 158:1030–1038, 2009.
19. Said-Sadier N, Ojcius DM: Alarmins, inflammasomes and immunity. *Biomed J* 35:437–449, 2012.
20. Li W: Phagocyte dysfunction, tissue aging and degeneration. *Ageing Res Rev* 12:1005–1012, 2013.
21. Butcher SK, Chahal H, Nayak L, et al: Senescence in innate immune responses: reduced neutrophil phagocytic capacity and CD16 expression in elderly humans. *J Leukoc Biol* 70:881–886, 2001.
22. Hearps AC, Martin GE, Angelovich TA, et al: Aging is associated with chronic innate immune activation and dysregulation of monocyte phenotype and function. *Aging Cell* 11:867–875, 2012.
23. Plowden J, Renshaw-Hoelscher M, Engleman C, et al: Innate immunity in aging: impact on macrophage function. *Aging Cell* 3:161–167, 2004.
24. Simell B, Vuorela A, Ekstrom N, et al: Aging reduces the functionality of anti-pneumococcal antibodies and the killing of *Streptococcus pneumoniae* by neutrophil phagocytosis. *Vaccine* 29:1929–1934, 2011.
25. Wenisch C, Patruta S, Daxbock F, et al: Effect of age on human neutrophil function. *J Leukoc Biol* 67:40–45, 2000.
26. Franceschi C: Inflammaging as a major characteristic of old people: can it be prevented or cured? *Nutr Rev* 65:S173–S176, 2007.
27. Franceschi C, Capri M, Monti D, et al: Inflammaging and anti-inflammaging: a systemic perspective on aging and longevity emerged from studies in humans. *Mech Ageing Dev* 128:92–105, 2007.
28. Han JM, Levings MK: Immune regulation in obesity-associated adipose inflammation. *J Immunol* 191:527–532, 2013.
29. Czesnikiewicz-Guzik M, Lee WW, Cui D, et al: T cell subset-specific susceptibility to aging. *Clin Immunol* 127:107–118, 2008.
30. Duraisingham SS, Rouphael N, Cavanagh MM, et al: Systems biology of vaccination in the elderly. *Curr Top Microbiol Immunol* 363:117–142, 2013.
31. Pawelec G, Larbi A, Derhovanessian E: Senescence of the human immune system. *J Comp Pathol* 142:S39–S44, 2010.
32. den Braber I, Mugwagwa T, Vrisekoop N, et al: Maintenance of peripheral naive T cells is sustained by thymus output in mice but not humans. *Immunity* 36:288–297, 2012.
33. Gillis S, Kozak R, Durante M, et al: Immunological studies of aging. Decreased production of and response to T cell growth factor by lymphocytes from aged humans. *J Clin Invest* 67:937–942, 1981.
34. Gupta S, Bi R, Su K, et al: Characterization of naive, memory and effector CD8+ T cells: effect of age. *Exp Gerontol* 39:545–550, 2004.
35. Nikolich-Zugich J, Li G, Uhrlaub JL, et al: Age-related changes in CD8 T cell homeostasis and immunity to infection. *Semin Immunol* 24:356–364, 2012.
36. Ademokun A, Wu YC, Dunn-Walters D: The ageing B cell population: composition and function. *Biogerontology* 11:125–137, 2010.
37. Dunn-Walters DK, Ademokun AA: B cell repertoire and ageing. *Curr Opin Immunol* 22:514–520, 2010.
38. Rossi MI, Yokota T, Medina KL, et al: B lymphopoiesis is active throughout human life, but there are developmental age-related changes. *Blood* 101:576–584, 2003.

39. Sanz I, Wei C, Lee FE, et al: Phenotypic and functional heterogeneity of human memory B cells. *Semin Immunol* 20:67–82, 2008.

40. Tangye SG, Tarlinton DM: Memory B cells: effectors of long-lived immune responses. *Eur J Immunol* 39:2065–2075, 2009.

41. Avci FY, Li X, Tsuji M, et al: A mechanism for glycoconjugate vaccine activation of the adaptive immune system and its implications for vaccine design. *Nat Med* 17:1602–1609, 2011.

42. Clutterbuck EA, Lazarus R, Yu LM, et al: Pneumococcal conjugate and plain polysaccharide vaccines have divergent effects on antigen-specific B cells. *J Infect Dis* 205:1408–1416, 2012.

43. Scherk MA, Ford RB, Gaskell RM, et al: 2013 AAFP Feline Vaccination Advisory Panel Report. *J Feline Med Surg* 15:785–808, 2013.

44. Mansfield KL, Burr PD, Snodgrass DR, et al: Factors affecting the serological response of dogs and cats to rabies vaccination. *Vet Rec* 154:423–426, 2004.

45. Goto H, Yamamoto Y, Ohta C, et al: Antibody responses of Japanese horses to influenza viruses in the past few years. *J Vet Med Sci* 55:33–37, 1993.

46. Horohov DW, Dimock A, Guirnalda P, et al: Effect of exercise on the immune response of young and old horses. *Am J Vet Res* 60:643–647, 1999.

47. Paillot R, Kydd JH, MacRae S, et al: New assays to measure equine influenza virus-specific type 1 immunity in horses. *Vaccine* 25:7385–7398, 2007.

48. Paillot R, Kydd JH, Sindle T, et al: Antibody and IFN-gamma responses induced by a recombinant canarypox vaccine and challenge infection with equine influenza virus. *Vet Immunol Immunopathol* 112:225–233, 2006.

49. Adams AA, Sturgill TL, Breathnach CC, et al: Humoral and cell-mediated immune responses of old horses following recombinant canarypox virus vaccination and subsequent challenge infection. *Vet Immunol Immunopathol* 139:128–140, 2011.

50. Jia J, Frantz N, Khoo C, et al: Investigation of the faecal microbiota of geriatric cats. *Lett Appl Microbiol* 53:288–293, 2011.

51. Jirillo E, Jirillo F, Magrone T: Healthy effects exerted by prebiotics, probiotics, and symbiotics with special reference to their impact on the immune system. *Int J Vitam Nutr Res* 82:200–208, 2012.

52. Satyaraj E: Emerging paradigms in immunonutrition. *Top Companion Anim Med* 26:25–32, 2011.

53. Jia J, Frantz N, Khoo C, et al: Investigation of the faecal microbiota of kittens: monitoring bacterial succession and effect of diet. *FEMS Microbiol Ecol* 78:395–404, 2011.

54. Barry KA, Middelbos IS, Vester Boler BM, et al: Effects of dietary fiber on the feline gastrointestinal metagenome. *J Proteome Res* 11:5924–5933, 2012.

55. Tun HM, Brar MS, Khin N, et al: Gene-centric metagenomics analysis of feline intestinal microbiome using 454 junior pyrosequencing. *J Microbiol Methods* 88:369–376, 2012.

56. Kerr KR, Beloshapka AN, Swanson KS: 2011 and 2012 Early Careers Achievement Awards: use of genomic biology to study companion animal intestinal microbiota. *J Anim Sci* 91:2504–2511, 2013.

57. Inness VL, McCartney AL, Khoo C, et al: Molecular characterisation of the gut microflora of healthy and inflammatory bowel disease cats using fluorescence in situ hybridisation with special reference to *Desulfovibrio* spp. *J Anim Physiol Anim Nutr (Berl)* 91:48–53, 2007.

58. Janeczko S, Atwater D, Bogel E, et al: The relationship of mucosal bacteria to duodenal histopathology, cytokine mRNA, and clinical disease activity in cats with inflammatory bowel disease. *Vet Microbiol* 128:178–193, 2008.

Cognitive Dysfunction in the Cat

Danièlle Gunn-Moore

With improvements in nutrition and veterinary medicine, the life expectancy of pet cats is increasing. In the United States over the last two decades, the percentage of pet cats older than 7 years of age has increased to over 40%,[1] there has been a 15% increase in cats older than 10 years of age,[2] and over 10% of pet cats are older than 12 years of age.[1] In Canada, it is estimated that 35% of pet cats are older than 8 years of age, including 24% older than 10 years of age.[3] In the United Kingdom, it is estimated that there are currently over 2.5 million "senior" cats,[4] and because this accounts for about 30% of the pet cat population, appropriate management of these individuals is becoming an increasingly more important consideration for small animal veterinary practitioners.

Unfortunately, accompanying this growing geriatric population are increasing numbers of pets with signs of altered behavior and apparent senility.[5] These behavioral changes may result from many different disorders (Box 98-1), including systemic illness (e.g., hyperthyroidism), organic brain disease (e.g., brain tumor), true behavioral problems (e.g., separation anxiety), or cognitive dysfunction (Figure 98-1). Diagnosis involves a full investigation for underlying illness (Box 98-2 and Box 98-3) and assessment for behavioral problems. Once these have been ruled out, cognitive dysfunction syndrome (CDS) should be considered, although, *antemortem*, this is a diagnosis of exclusion. Changes in interaction with the family occur frequently (Table 98-1). Overall, the most commonly seen changes include spatial or temporal disorientation, altered interaction with the family, changes in sleep-wake cycles, housesoiling with inappropriate urination/defecation (most typically urination), changes in activity, and/or inappropriate vocalization (often displayed as loud crying at night)[9] (Box 98-4).

PREVALENCE OF COGNITIVE DYSFUNCTION SYNDROME

Cognitive dysfunction syndrome refers to an age-related deterioration of cognitive abilities characterized by behavioral changes (as described earlier and in Table 98-1 and Box 98-4) where no medical cause can be found.[10-13] A survey of cats aged 7 to 11 years revealed that 36% of owners reported behavioral problems,[14] and this increased with age to 88% in cats aged between 16 and 19 years. A later study suggests that 28% of pet cats aged 11 to 14 years develop at least one geriatric-onset behavior problem that appears to relate to

CDS, and this increases to over 50% for cats aged 15 years or older. Excessive vocalization and aimless activity are the most common problems in this older age group.[13,15]

PATHOPHYSIOLOGY OF COGNITIVE DYSFUNCTION SYNDROME

The cause of CDS is still unknown, but compromised cerebral blood flow and chronic free radical damage are both believed to be important.[13,16] Numerous vascular changes can occur in the brain of old cats, including a decrease in cerebral blood flow, the presence of small hemorrhages around the blood vessels, and a form of arteriosclerosis.[12,13] In addition, the brain of elderly cats may also be subject to compromised blood flow and hypoxia due to heart disease, anemia, blood clotting defects, and/or underlying hypertension. A small amount of the oxygen that is used by cells in energy production is normally converted to free radicals. As cells age, they become less efficient, producing less energy and more free radicals. Normally, these free radicals are removed by the body's natural antioxidant defenses, including a number of special enzymes and free radical scavengers, such as vitamins A, C, and E. The balance between the production and removal of free radicals can be upset by disease, age, and stress. An excess of free radicals can lead to damage, and the brain is particularly susceptible because of its high fat content, a high demand for oxygen, and a limited ability to self-repair.[12,17,18] Ultimately, chronic damage can eventually lead to disease processes similar to those seen in humans suffering from Alzheimer's disease with alteration of proteins within nerve cells (e.g., tau hyperphosphorylation) and deposition of protein plaques outside the nerve cells (made from beta-amyloid protein).[16] In humans and dogs, genetics, diet, and lifestyle choices have all been found to influence the prevalence and pattern of neuropathological changes (particularly beta-amyloid plaques) and the nature of the cognitive dysfunction. Although these relationships have still to be determined in cats, it is likely that they will be similar.

MANAGEMENT OF COGNITIVE DYSFUNCTION SYNDROME

Although CDS cannot be cured, its clinical signs can be reduced with suitable intervention; treatment options are

BOX 98-1 Potential Causes of Behavioral Changes in Geriatric Cats

Cognitive dysfunction syndrome
Pain in any body system
Arthritis*
Systemic hypertension (primary, or secondary to hyperthyroidism, chronic kidney disease, diabetes mellitus, acromegaly, hyperadrenocorticism, hyperaldosteronism, chronic anemia)
Hyperthyroidism
Chronic kidney disease
Diabetes mellitus
Urinary tract infection (especially some quinolone-resistant toxin-producing strains of *Escherichia coli*—as can be found in elderly humans[6])
Gastrointestinal disease
Liver disease (hepatic encephalopathy)
Neurological defects (sensory or motor deficits)
Reduced vision or hearing
Brain tumors (e.g., meningioma, lymphoma)
Infectious disease (e.g., feline immunodeficiency virus, feline leukemia virus, toxoplasmosis, feline infectious peritonitis, etc.)
Dental or periodontal disease
Inflammatory disease in any body system
Primary behavioral problems

*The importance of arthritis is often under-recognized in elderly cats and should not be overlooked. Radiographic evidence of degenerative joint disease is present in 70% to 90% of cats over 10 years of age.[7] Associated pain and dysfunction can result in reduced activity and mobility, aggression, altered interactions with the family, loss of litter box training, and crying out loudly. Owners can help their arthritic cats by making minor modifications in their house; for example, by raising food and water bowls a few centimeters or inches off the floor to reduce stress on arthritic elbows, adding ramps to allow easier access to favored sleeping areas, providing deep comfortable bedding that will support and protect the cat's joints (heated beds can be particularly soothing), and placing low-sided litter boxes, food bowls, and water bowls all within easy reach of the cat (for more information, see Chapter 96).

BOX 98-2 Investigation of Behavioral Changes in Geriatric Cats

Initial Investigations

Full history, including the possibility of previous trauma (which may have led to arthritis), any potential exposure to toxins or drugs, and any recent environmental changes (in the household, family members, diet, etc.). Asking specific questions about alterations in the cat's behavior can help in determining how the cat has changed (see Box 98-3).

Full physical examination, including assessment of body weight, calculation of percentage weight change, body condition score, muscle condition score, and retinal examination.

Assessment of systemic blood pressure is particularly important because hypertension occurs commonly in older cats and may cause many of the same signs as CDS.

Mobility assessment, plus neurological and orthopedic examinations, although these can be challenging in some cats.

Assessment of hematology and serum biochemistry, including total thyroxin concentration.

Urine analysis, including urine protein-to-creatinine ratio and bacterial culture (even if the urine sediment appears nonreactive) to detect occult infection.[8]

Further Investigations

Where appropriate, serological testing for feline leukemia virus infection, feline immunodeficiency virus infection, toxoplasmosis, and other infectious diseases; diagnostic testing for feline infectious peritonitis.

Thoracic, abdominal or skeletal radiography, abdominal ultrasound examination, electrocardiography, echocardiography, intestinal endoscopy or exploratory laparotomy and biopsy collection, as indicated from initial findings.

Computed tomography or magnetic resonance imaging of the head.

CDS, Cognitive dysfunction syndrome.

Table 98-1	Changes in Interaction with the Family from Questionnaire Studies*	
Interaction	**1995 Data from 1134 Cat Owners**	**2010 Data from 1016 Cat Owners**
Increased affection to owner	81%	30%
Less tolerant of other animals in the house	26%	21%
More tolerant of other animals in the house	24%	12%
More vocal[†]	66%	54%
More vocal at night[†]	30%	37%

*Questionnaire studies of cats 12 years of age and older (median of 15 years) as observed in two studies from the United Kingdom performed 15 years apart; V. Halls, unpublished data, 2002; and author's unpublished data.
[†]Cries out loudly for no apparent reason and/or to try to gain attention.

BOX 98-3 Mobility and Cognitive Dysfunction Questionnaire*

My cat	Yes	Maybe	No
Is less willing to jump up or down	☐	☐	☐
Will only jump up or down from lower heights	☐	☐	☐
Shows signs of being stiff at times	☐	☐	☐
Is less agile than previously	☐	☐	☐
Shows signs of lameness or limping	☐	☐	☐
Has difficulty getting in or out of the cat flap	☐	☐	☐
Has difficulty going up or down stairs	☐	☐	☐
Cries when picked up	☐	☐	☐
Has more accidents outside the litter tray	☐	☐	☐
Spends less time grooming	☐	☐	☐
Is more reluctant to interact with me	☐	☐	☐
Plays less with other animals or toys	☐	☐	☐
Sleeps more and/or is less active	☐	☐	☐
Cries out loudly for no apparent reason/to try to gain my attention	☐	☐	☐
Appears forgetful	☐	☐	☐

It can be difficult to differentiate between many of the changes caused by cognitive dysfunction syndrome and those caused by arthritis. Indeed, the two conditions often occur concurrently in old cats and many of the treatments for one condition also help the other. For more information about arthritis, see Chapter 96.

*Ensure there have been no environmental reasons for the change(s).

BOX 98-4 Behavioral Changes That Can Be Seen in Geriatric Cats and May Be Associated with Cognitive Dysfunction Syndrome

Spatial disorientation or confusion, such as getting trapped in corners or forgetting the location of the litter box; housesoiling is the most common reason for referral of old cats to behavior specialists[11]

Altered social relationships, either with their owners or other pets in the household; for example, increased attention seeking or aggression

Inappropriate vocalization, such as loud crying at night; this may appear to be for no apparent reason and/or to try to gain the owner's attention

Altered behavioral responses, such as increased irritability or anxiety, or decreased response to stimuli

Changes in sleep/wake patterns

Altered learning and memory, such as forgetting commands or breaking housetraining

Changes in activity, such as aimless wandering or pacing, or reduced activity

Altered interest in food, either increased or, more typically, decreased

Decreased grooming

Temporal disorientation, such as forgetting that they have just been fed

usually extrapolated from studies of humans with Alzheimer's disease and/or dogs with CDS. In general, potential interventions include environmental management and modification, dietary modification, and drug therapies.[9,19] To date, there have been a small number of dietary studies that have been shown to increase activity and/or reduce the signs of CDS in cats (Hill's Pet Nutrition, data on file, 2008),[20,21] plus a single placebo-controlled study investigating the use of a dietary supplement.[22]

Environmental Management and Dietary Modification

Environmental factors can have positive or negative influences on the signs of CDS (Table 98-2). Environmental enrichment can lead to mental stimulation, increased activity, an increase in nerve growth factors, the growth and survival of nerves, and an increase in cognitive function.[13] In contrast, lack of environmental stimulation may increase the risk of CDS when older, and factors within the environment that cause frustration can exacerbate signs of CDS. These could include, for example, inconsistent feeding times or inconsistent locking of a cat flap that provides access to outdoors. Many older cats have concurrent disease, and this can lead to further frustrations. Examples include moving food bowls or litter boxes to different areas of the house when a cat with CDS is also blind, and supplying a high-sided litter box to a cat with CDS that also has severe arthritis. Environmental

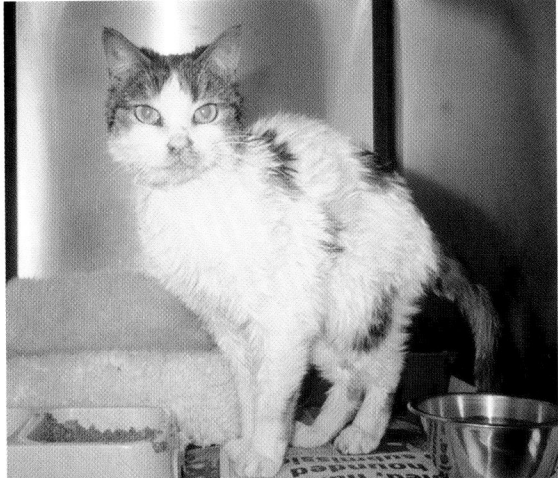

Figure 98-1: Elderly (14-year-old) domestic shorthair cat that has been showing signs of cognitive dysfunction syndrome (night crying and inappropriate elimination). The picture shows that the cat has stopped grooming, and the odd stance suggests significant osteoarthritis—particularly affecting the lower back and stifles.

Table 98-2	Environmental Adjustments for Aging Cats
Category	**Environmental Adjustments**
Key resources (i.e., food, water, resting places, litter box, a place to hide, or an escape route)	All key resources must be easily accessible. There should be at least one set of key resources for each "group" of cats in the household. A "group" of cats are those that will comfortably sleep together and groom each other. If an elderly cat has to walk too far for its food or water, it may do without, risking weight loss and dehydration. If it has to walk too far for its litter box, it may develop inappropriate elimination. Key resources should not be moved from their usual place, because this can cause significant confusion and anxiety in a cat with CDS.
Food	Raising the food bowl up by a few centimeters or inches allows arthritic cats (especially those with arthritis in their elbows) to eat more comfortably (Figure 98-2). For elderly cats that prefer not to eat at floor level, place their food bowls on a low, easily accessible surface or provide ramps for easy access. Food bowls should be placed away from water bowls and litter boxes. Feed elderly cats separately so that they do not feel stressed by their companions and can eat at their own pace. Monitor the food intake of elderly cats to ensure that they do not lose weight; they should also be regularly weighed. Elderly cats typically have a reduced ability to digest and absorb their food; to counter this and reduce the risk of weight loss, feed *ad libitum* or as a number of small meals throughout the day. If a prescription diet is needed, it should be introduced slowly over 1 to 2 weeks; place a small amount of the new food in a favorite bowl beside the old food at each meal. The cat will smell the new food while gaining the gratification of the old diet; with time, the amount of the old food can be reduced and the amount of the new food increased.
Water	Raising the water bowl up by a few centimeters or inches allows arthritic cats (especially those with arthritis in their elbows) to drink more comfortably. Water bowls should be placed away from food bowls and litter boxes. Cats typically prefer a large, wide water bowl so that they can drink without getting their whiskers wet. Elderly cats with poor vision may agitate the water with a paw as this may help them to see the water surface meniscus better—placing a few flakes of fish (or similar) on the top of the water can help them to see or sense the meniscus if they are too arthritic to use their paw in this way. Pet water fountains can be useful and may stimulate elderly cats to drink more. If an elderly cat does not drink sufficiently, it will become dehydrated; this can exacerbate constipation and also lead to inappropriate elimination.
Resting places	Ideally, provide multiple, elevated platforms and sleeping places with padded, comfortable bedding and, where needed, ramps for easy access (Figure 98-3). Warmed beds can be particularly welcome for all elderly cats, especially for arthritic cats or cats with a poor hair coat. There should be sufficient beds so that the elderly cat can always gain access to one of its choosing.
Litter boxes or access to outdoor latrine sites	Cats with CDS frequently develop inappropriate elimination, so it is essential that owners do everything they can to facilitate their cat's use of its litter box and/or outdoor latrine site(s). In a multicat household, there should be sufficient litter boxes so that each "group" of cats has its own litter box, plus one extra. Use large, low-sided boxes for easy access. Litter boxes need to be within easy reach; if the cat has access to more than one floor of the home, there should be at least one litter box on each level. Sandy-type litter is generally more comfortable for elderly cats' paws and joints. Litter box liners are not recommended because elderly cats may get their claws caught in them. Elderly cats that go outside to eliminate often become less able to cope with climbing through the cat flap and/or confronting other cats from outside the family group. If they wish to keep going outside, ensure there is enough "cover" for them to leave the house and get to the latrine site; this may entail placing large plant pots near the cat flap so that the cat can leave the house without being seen by other cats. Alternatively, the owner could "cat-proof" the outdoor space with high fencing so that other cats cannot gain entry (Figure 98-4). Cats typically have a preferred latrine site; if the ground becomes compacted or frozen, the owner needs to dig over the area to loosen the soil for the elderly cat. Adding sand to the area will help to keep it from compacting or freezing and will make it more comfortable for elderly paws.

Table 98-2	Environmental Adjustments for Aging Cats—cont'd
Category	**Environmental Adjustments**
Hiding places or exit routes	It is important to provide easily accessible hiding places. If the cat prefers an elevated site, a ramp needs to be provided (Figure 98-5). In multipet households, it is important that the cat can have time alone if it desires. If they are in their hiding place, they should not be disturbed (e.g., to be medicated). It is essential that the hiding place remains a place of safety. Do not presume an elderly cat can comfortably use the cat flap if it needs to escape.
Companionship	Elderly cats may have a decreased or increased desire for human companionship, and/or the companionship of other animals. Cats may grieve at the loss of a long-time companion and may need much reassurance to get over the loss. The introduction of a new cat or dog can be very stressful, especially for elderly cats. Do not presume that because the cat is grieving for the loss of a long-term companion that it will benefit from a new animal being introduced into the household.
Environmental enrichment	This can be achieved by ensuring that each cat has more than sufficient key resources. Using feeding balls or puzzle feeders can make feeding time more stimulating; however, they can be confusing if introduced late in a cat's life and difficult to use if the cat has significant arthritis. Even elderly cats should have regular access to toys. These should be changed regularly to create stimulation and need to be suitable for elderly cats: blind cats need toys that make a noise (e.g., with a bell inside), whereas cats with arthritis need light-weight easily moved toys (Figure 98-6). Climbing frames need to have flat steps rather than circular rope-covered ones, because the latter can be difficult for arthritic cats to use. At least one scratching post should be available. However, many older cats are unable to scratch sufficiently to keep their claws short; because of this, they will need to have their claws trimmed regularly to prevent them from catching in carpet, and leading to pain in arthritic paws and confusion in cats with CDS. Cats with CDS often become easily anxious, and this can exacerbate their confusion. The environmental application of synthetic feline facial pheromone (Feliway, Ceva Animal Health) or herbal anxiolytic (Pet Remedy, www.petremedy.co.uk) may help reduce anxiety, preferably by being applied using a plug-in diffuser. Cats with CDS may show signs suggestive of separation anxiety; leaving a radio or television on when leaving the house may help these cats to cope with being left alone.

CDS, Cognitive dysfunction syndrome.

modifications should be made to improve ease of access for the cat with CDS, just as for the poorly visual or arthritic individual.

Diets enriched with antioxidants and other supportive compounds (e.g., vitamin E, beta carotene, and essential fatty acids) are believed to reduce oxidative damage, reduce beta-amyloid production, and improve cognitive function.[9,23] In humans, studies have shown that a high intake of fruits, vegetables, vitamins E and/or C, folate, and/or B[12] may improve cognition. In addition, alpha-lipoic acid and L-carnitine enhance mitochondrial function, and omega-3 fatty acids promote cell membrane health and have, in humans, been found to be beneficial in the treatment of dementia. In general, combinations of these compounds are believed to work best; however, excessive intake of some of these compounds can be harmful.

The combination of environmental stimulation (e.g., toys, companionship, interaction, and food hunting games; see Table 98-2) and a diet enriched with antioxidants has been shown in dogs to have a synergistic action in improving cognitive function. In aged dogs, a 4-year study on the use of an antioxidant-enriched diet (Hill's Prescription Diet b/d, Hill's Pet Nutrition, containing vitamins E and C, selenium, fruit and vegetable extract [beta carotene, other carotenoids, flavonoids], mitochondrial co-factors (DL-lipoic acid and L-carnitine), and omega-3 fatty acids plus environmental enrichment (e.g., toys, kennel mate, walks, and cognitive experience testing) revealed rapid (onset of 2 to 8 weeks into treatment) and significant improvements in learning and memory that lasted throughout the 2 years of the study. Interestingly, although there was no reversal of existing pathology, the antioxidants did appear to prevent the deposition of more beta-amyloid, whereas the environmental enrichment did not.[24,25]

The clinical signs of CDS in dogs have also been reduced by feeding a diet supplemented with plant-derived medium-chain triglycerides (MCTs), which provide ketones as a more efficient energy source for the brain (Purina One Vibrant Maturity 7+, Nestlé Purina Pet Care).[26] Unfortunately, cats generally do not find diets enriched with MCTs to be

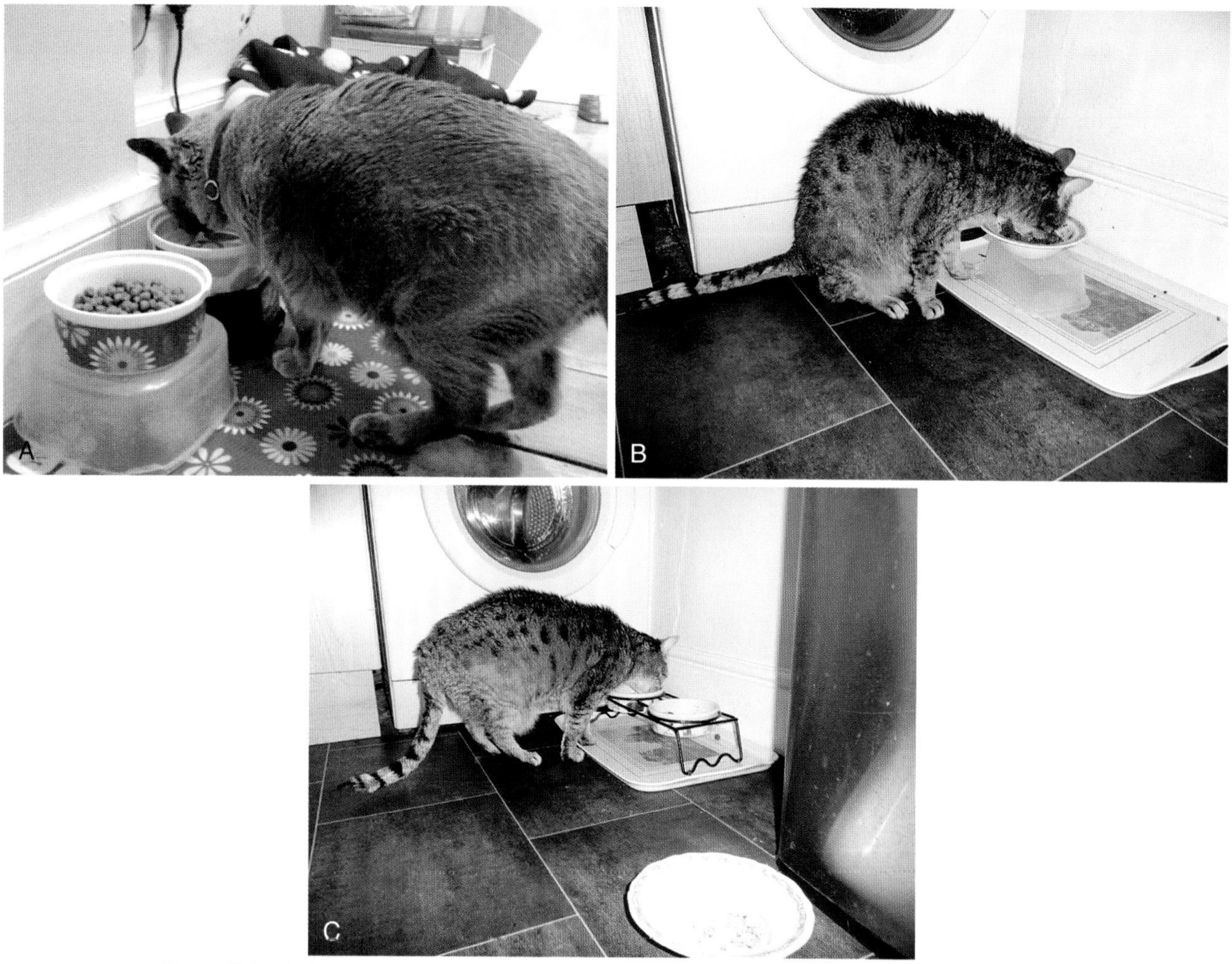

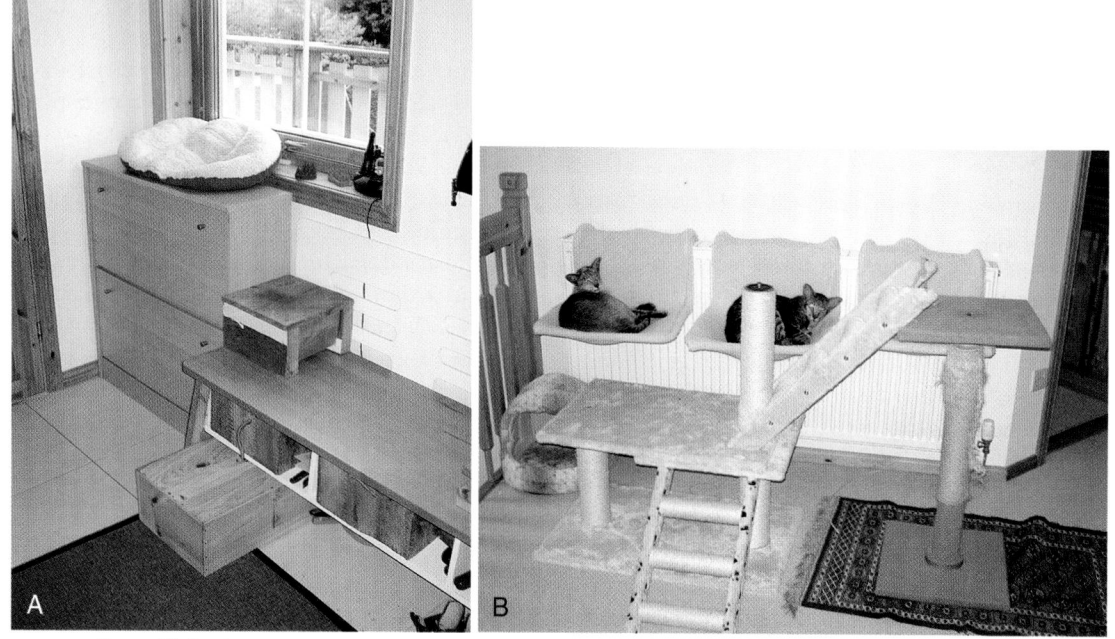

Figure 98-2: A, Raising food and water bowls can make an elderly cat more comfortable when eating and drinking. Upturned plastic tubs serve the purpose well **(B)** and commercially available food bowl stands may also be used **(C). (A,** Courtesy of Stephanie Brinkman.)

Figure 98-3: A and **B,** Ramps or steps can be added to enable cats to gain access to favored resting places. (Courtesy of John Purves.)

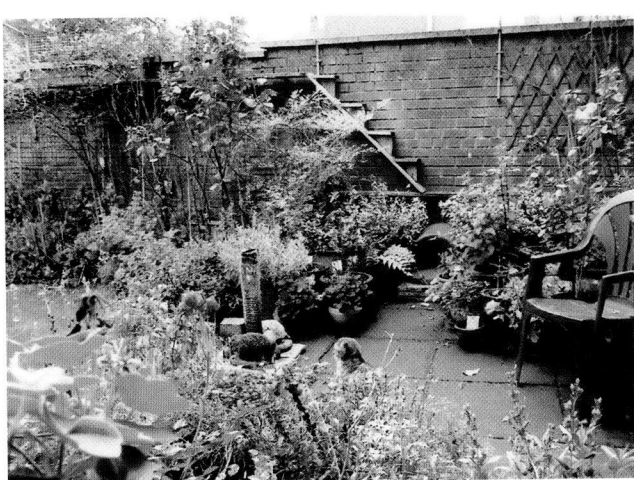

Figure 98-4: A small garden can be fenced so that elderly cats have access to raised walkways, and other cats cannot gain access to the garden. Note the mesh fencing above the walkway to the left of the picture. (Courtesy of Catherine Martin.)

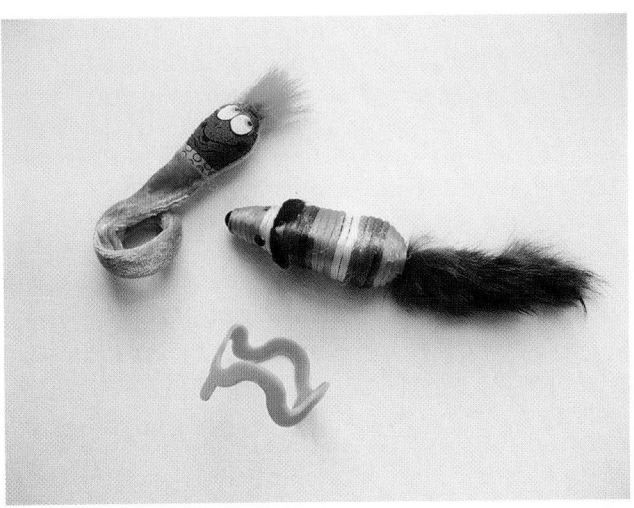

Figure 98-6: Lightweight toys that are easier for elderly cats to play with are available.

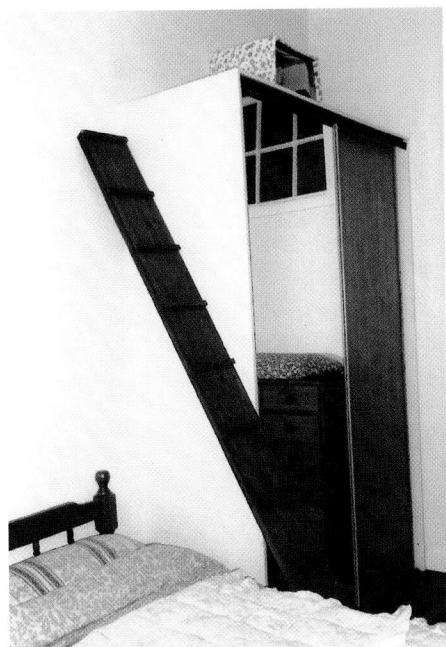

Figure 98-5: A ramp with steps added enables an elderly cat to gain access to a favorite hiding place (in this case a box on top of the wardrobe). (Courtesy of Catherine Martin.)

palatable, so it is unclear if this approach will be useful for cats with CDS.

Although a study similar to that using Hill's b/d plus environmental enrichment has not yet been performed in cats with CDS, a 5-year study feeding healthy older cats (7 to 17 years old) a diet (Nestlé Purina Pro Plan Age 7+, Nestlé Purina Pet Care) supplemented with antioxidants (vitamin E and beta-carotene), essential fatty acids (omega-3 and omega-6 fatty acids), and dried whole chicory root (which

contains the prebiotic inulin to modify intestinal flora) resulted in the supplemented cats living significantly longer (and more healthily) than the nonsupplemented ones.[27,28] The most convincing data comes from a recent study of middle-aged and older cats that were fed a diet supplemented with a combination of fish oil, antioxidants, arginine, and key B vitamins; they were found to have enhanced brain functions compared to those fed a control diet.[21] A deficiency of these nutrients, especially omega-3 fatty acids and B vitamins, are proven risk factors for brain aging, stroke, and dementia in humans. In another study, supplementing the diet of elderly cats with tocopherols, vitamin C, beta-carotene, L-carnitine, docosahexaenoic acid, and sulfur amino acids resulted in increased activity compared to controls.[20] Other similarly supplemented diets are now available (e.g., Hill's Prescription Diet Feline j/d, Hill's Pet Nutrition; Royal Canin Mobility Support, Waltham Pet Nutrition), although they are actually designed for cats with osteoarthritis. For example, Hill's Prescription Diet Feline j/d is supplemented with a mixture of antioxidants (vitamins C and E, and beta carotene), essential fatty acids, chondroprotectants (methionine, glycosaminoglycans, glucosamine, and chondroitin sulphate), L-carnitine, and lysine. In a 2-month study of 75 cats aged 12 years and older that were not selected for signs of CDS or osteoarthritis, owner questionnaires suggested that more than 70% of the cats improved in one or more signs of cognitive function (and more than 50% improved in one or more signs of mobility) (Hill's Pet Nutrition, data on file, 2008).

There have been a small number of studies investigating the potential benefit of various dietary supplements in dogs with CDS.[9,18,19,23,29] For example, a study of 11 dogs older than 8 years of age given a supplement containing omega-3 fish oils, vitamins E and C, L-carnitine, alpha-lipoic acid, coenzyme Q, phosphatidylserine, and selenium (sold in the United Kingdom as Aktivait, VetPlus) over a 2-month period showed significant improvements in signs of disorientation, social interaction, and housesoiling when compared to 11 placebo-treated controls.[30] Unfortunately, a different formula is needed for cats because alpha-lipoic acid is toxic in this species,[31] so products containing it should not be given. Although the new feline-safe version of Aktivait is on the market, trials in cats are still needed to determine its efficacy.

A number of other supplements have also been suggested for the treatment of dogs and cats with CDS. For example, a placebo-controlled crossover study showed significant improvements in nine dogs with CDS when given a supplement containing ginkgo biloba, vitamins B6 and E, and resveratrol (Senilife, Ceva Animal Health),[32] and two studies of seven and 17 dogs aged over 8 years (compared with seven and 19 placebo-treated controls, respectively), showed significant improvements in activity and awareness when S-adenosylmethionine (SAMe) was given as a supplement for up to 2 months.[22,33] A recent study gave SAMe to eight cats with signs of CDS (and compared them to eight placebo-treated cats); it appeared to show that the treated cats had improved executive function. This study, like the studies investigating the use of nutraceuticals in the management of dogs with CDS, suffered from involving a small number of animals and with assessments typically being subjective. The latter study suggests that SAMe may be worth considering in the management of feline dementia.[22] Although there is now a growing list of compounds that have been suggested to have beneficial effects on the aging feline brain,[9] there is an urgent need for more placebo-controlled studies looking at the use of dietary supplements in cats, either as single ingredients or in potentially synergistic combinations.

Management of Severe Cognitive Dysfunction Syndrome

Unfortunately, once cats develop significant clinical signs of CDS, instigating environmental or dietary change can actually have a negative effect. This is because affected cats often become stressed and cope poorly with change, whether in their environment, their daily routine, their diet, or the members of the household. The cat's response to this stress is to show more obvious signs of CDS (e.g., anorexia, hiding, and/or housesoiling).[34] For these cats, where possible, change should be kept to a minimum. When change cannot be avoided, it should be made slowly and with much reassurance. The owner should be present to comfort the cat if it appears to be confused by the change. Some cats may become so demented and cope so poorly with change that they may benefit from having their area of access reduced in size. For example, this could be a single room containing the key resources for cats: food, water, litter box, resting places, either somewhere to hide and/or some way of escaping, and companionship (as dictated by the particular needs of the individual cat). This core territory can then be kept safe and constant. Environmental application of synthetic feline facial pheromone (Feliway; Ceva Animal Health) can also help in reducing feline anxiety.[35]

Potential Drug Therapies

There are a growing number of possible drug options for Alzheimer's disease in humans and CDS in dogs. These include various cholinesterase inhibitors (to increase the availability of acetylcholine at the neuronal synapses), selegiline (to manipulate the monoaminergic system), antioxidants (e.g., vitamin E), and nonsteroidal anti-inflammatory drugs (to reduce neuronal damage). However, very few have actually been approved for the treatment of human dementia. Selegiline (Selgian, Ceva Animal Health; Anipryl, Pfizer), propentofylline (Vivitonin, MSD Animal Health), and nicergoline (Fitergol, Merial Animal Health) are the only drugs that have been approved for the treatment of canine dementia in either the United Kingdom or the United States.

Although there are no drugs licensed for the treatment of CDS in cats, a number of drugs have been used "off label."[9,12,19,36,37] These include selegiline (suggested dosage: 0.25 to 1.0 mg/kg orally [PO] every 24 hours), propentofylline (suggested dosage: 12.5 mg/cat PO every 24 hours) and, where available, nicergoline (suggested dosage: 0.25 to 0.5 mg/kg PO every 24 hours), all of which have been used in cats with varying degrees of success. For example, a small open trial using selegiline showed a positive effect.[19] Other drugs that have been used to treat particular signs of CDS in cats include anxiolytic drugs, such as a number of nutraceuticals (e.g., Zylkène, MSD Animal Health), buspirone and benzodiazepines (e.g., diazepam, although hepatotoxicity is a particular risk with this drug when given orally), or antidepressants (that lack anticholinergic effects), such as fluoxetine.

SUMMARY

Increasing numbers of cats are living to old age, and behavioral changes are common in these cats. The behavioral changes reported most frequently to veterinarians are loss of litter box training (particularly inappropriate urination) and crying loudly at night. The most typical causes of these problems are CDS, osteoarthritis, systemic hypertension (commonly secondary to chronic kidney disease or hyperthyroidism), hyperthyroidism (even without hypertension), deafness, and brain tumors. Almost one-third of pet cats aged 11 to 14 years develop at least one geriatric-onset behavior problem that appears to relate to CDS. This increases to over 50% for cats aged 15 years and older. These conditions occur frequently in older cats, and many older cats suffer from a number of concurrent interacting conditions. Unfortunately, owners and veterinarians often mistake these for "normal aging changes," so many treatable conditions are neglected and go untreated.

References

1. Laflamme DP, Abood SK, Fascetti AJ, et al: Pet feeding practices of dog and cat owners in the United States and Australia. *J Am Vet Med Assoc* 232:687–694, 2008.
2. Broussard JD, Peterson ME, Fox PR: Changes in clinical and laboratory findings in cats with hyperthyroidism from 1983 to 1993. *J Am Vet Med Assoc* 206:302–305, 1995.
3. Perrin T: The business of urban animals survey: the facts and statistics on companion animals in Canada. *Can Vet J* 50:48–52, 2009.
4. Gunn-Moore DA: Considering older cats. *Compend Contin Educ Pract Vet Suppl* 26:1–4, 2003.
5. Gunn-Moore DA: Cognitive dysfunction in cats: clinical assessment and management. *Top Companion Anim Med* 26:17–24, 2011.
6. Colodner R, Kometiani I, Chazan B, et al: Risk factors for community-acquired urinary tract infection due to quinolone-resistant *E. coli. Infection* 36:41–45, 2008.
7. Bennett D, Zainal Ariffin SM, Johnston P: Osteoarthritis in the cat: how common is it and how easy to recognise? *J Feline Med Surg* 14:65–75, 2012.
8. Mayer-Ronne B, Goldstein RE, Erb HN: Urinary tract infections in cats with hyperthyroidism, diabetes mellitus and chronic kidney disease. *J Feline Med Surg* 9:124–132, 2006.
9. Landsberg G, Denenberg S, Araujo J: Cognitive dysfunction in cats: a syndrome we used to dismiss as "old age." *J Feline Med Surg* 12:837–848, 2010.
10. Chapman BL, Voith VL: Behavioral problems in old dogs: 26 cases (1984-1987). *J Am Vet Med Assoc* 196:944–946, 1990.
11. Ruehl WW, Bruyette DS, DePaoli A, et al: Canine cognitive dysfunction as a model for human age-related cognitive decline, dementia, and Alzheimer's disease: clinical presentation, cognitive testing, pathology and response to L-deprenyl therapy. *Prog Brain Res* 106:217–225, 1995.
12. Landsberg GL, Araujo JA: Behavior problems in geriatric pets. *Vet Clin North Am Small Anim Pract* 35:675–698, 2005.
13. Gunn-Moore DA, Moffat K, Christie LA, et al: Cognitive dysfunction and the neurobiology of aging in cats. *J Small Anim Pract* 48:546–553, 2007.
14. Landsberg G: Behavior problems of older cats. In Schaumburg I, editor: *Proceedings of the 135th Annual Meeting of the American Veterinary Medical Association*, San Diego, CA, 1998, pp 317–320.
15. Moffat KS, Landsberg GM: An investigation of the prevalence of clinical signs of cognitive dysfunction syndrome (CDS) in cats. *J Am Anim Hosp Assoc* 39:512, 2003. (Abstract).
16. Gunn-Moore DA, Gunn-Moore FJ: Growing old is not for wimps. *J Feline Med Surg* 12:835–836, 2010.
17. Dimakopoulos AC, Mayer RJ: Aspects of neurodegeneration in the canine brain. *J Nutr* 132(6 Suppl 2):1579S–1582S, 2002.
18. Roudebush P, Zicker SC, Cotman CW, et al: Nutritional management of brain aging in dogs. *J Am Vet Med Assoc* 227:722–728, 2005.
19. Landsberg G: Therapeutic options for cognitive decline in senior pets. *J Am Anim Hosp Assoc* 42:407–413, 2006.
20. Houpt K, Levine E, Landsberg G, et al: Antioxidant fortified food improves owner perceived behaviour in aging the cat. In *Proceedings of the European Society for Feline Medicine Conference*, Prague, Czech Republic, 2007.
21. Pan Y, Araujo JA, Burrows J, et al: Cognitive enhancement in middle-aged and old cats with dietary supplementation with a nutrient blend containing fish oil, B vitamins, antioxidants and arginine. *Br J Nutr* 110:40–49, 2013.
22. Araujo JA, Faubert ML, Brooks ML, et al: NOVIFIT (NoviSAMe) tablets improve executive function in aged dogs and cats: implications for treatment of cognitive dysfunction syndrome. *Intern J Appl Res Vet Med* 10:90–98, 2012.
23. Head E, Zicker SC: Nutraceuticals, aging and cognitive dysfunction. *Vet Clin North Am Small Anim Pract* 34:217–228, 2004.
24. Milgram NW, Head E, Zicker SC, et al: Long-term treatment with antioxidants and a program of behavioral enrichment reduces age-dependent impairment in discrimination and reversal learning in beagle dogs. *Exp Gerontol* 39:753–765, 2004.
25. Milgram NW, Head E, Zicher SC, et al: Learning ability in aged Beagle dogs is preserved by behavioural enrichment and dietary fortification: a two year longitudinal study. *Neurobiol Aging* 26:77–90, 2005.
26. Pan Y, Larson B, Araujo JA, et al: Dietary supplementation with medium-chain TAG has long-lasting cognition-enhancing effects in aged dogs. *Br J Nutr* 103:1746–1754, 2010.
27. Cupp CJ, Jean-Philippe C, Kerr WW, et al: Effect of nutritional interventions on longevity of senior cats. *Int J Appl Res Med* 4:34–50, 2006.
28. Cupp CJ, Kerr WW, Jean-Philippe C, et al: The role of nutritional interventions in the longevity and maintenance of long-term health in aging cats. *Int J Appl Res Vet Med* 6:69–81, 2008.
29. Ikeda-Douglas CJ, Zicker SC, Estrada J, et al: Prior experience, antioxidants, and mitochondrial cofactors improve cognitive function in aged Beagles. *Vet Ther* 5:5–16, 2004.
30. Heath S, Barabas S, Craze P: Nutritional supplementation in cases of canine cognitive dysfunction. *J Appl Anim Behav Sci* 105:284–296, 2007.
31. Hill AS, Werner JA, Rogers QR, et al: Lipoic acid is 10 times more toxic in cats than reported in humans, dogs or rats. *J Anim Physiol Anim Nutr (Berl)* 88:150–156, 2004.
32. Araujo JA, Landsberg GM, Milgram NW, et al: Improvement of short-term memory performance in aged beagles by a nutraceutical supplement containing phosphatidylserine, *Ginkgo biloba*, vitamin E, and pyridoxine. *Can Vet J* 49:379–385, 2008.
33. Rème CA, Dramard V, Kern L, et al: Effect of S-adenosylmethionine tablets on the reduction of age-related mental decline in dogs: a double-blinded, placebo-controlled trial. *Vet Ther* 9:69–82, 2008.
34. Houpt KA, Beaver B: Behavioral problems of geriatric dogs and cats. *Vet Clin North Am Small Anim Pract* 11:643–652, 1981.
35. Griffith CA, Steigerwald ES, Buffington CAT: Effects of a synthetic facial pheromone on behavior of cats. *J Am Vet Med Assoc* 217:1154, 2000.
36. Landsberg GL, Hunthausen W, Ackerman L: The effects of aging on behavior in senior pets. In *Handbook of behavior problems in the dog and cat*, ed 2, London, 2003, Saunders, pp 269–304.
37. Studzinski CM, Araujo JA, Milgram NW: The canine model of human cognitive aging and dementia: pharmacological validity of the model for assessment of human cognitive-enhancing drugs. *Prog Neuropsychopharmacol Biol Psychiatry* 29:489–498, 2005.

Anesthesia for the Aging Cat

Tamara Grubb

The phrase "cats are not small dogs" is just as true in anesthesia as it is in any other discipline. Compared to healthy, young adult dogs (0.5 to 5 years of age), healthy, young adult cats are at greater risk for anesthesia-related death (0.05% versus 0.11%, respectively).[1] Although one study found no relationship between age and risk of anesthesia-related death,[2] a larger study found that cats 12 years of age or older are twice as likely as young adult cats to die from anesthesia-related causes.[3] The risk of anesthesia-related death for unhealthy cats (American Society of Anesthesiologists [ASA] status 3 to 5; Box 99-1) increases to 1.40% (compared with 1.33% for unhealthy dogs).[1] Thus, aged cats, especially those with concurrent disease, are at increased risk for anesthesia-related mortality.

RISKS OF BEING A CAT

There are several factors that put cats at higher risk of anesthesia-related adverse events. Their small body size makes them more prone to hypothermia, easier to overdose, and potentially, makes it more difficult to monitor their physiologic parameters.[4] Their temperament may make performing a comprehensive physical examination challenging and may require the use of higher dosages of sedative and induction agents. They have a greater propensity for upper airway problems during intubation.[4] Cats also have species-specific differences in metabolism (e.g., metabolism of nonsteroidal anti-inflammatory drugs [NSAIDs]) and responses to drugs (e.g., potential for opioid-mediated excitement) that must be considered when planning an anesthetic protocol. However, the most significant factor for greater anesthetic risk compared to dogs is the fact that different standards of anesthesia appear to exist for dogs and cats. In a study of 79,178 anesthetic procedures in cats, provision of intravenous (IV) fluids and/or ventilatory support was "infrequent in the anesthetized cats" and patient monitoring was "often superficial."[4] For more information about anesthesia-related morbidity and mortality in cats, see Chapter 75.

RISKS OF BEING A GERIATRIC CAT

The average lifespan of a cat in 2012 was 12.1 years, an increase of 10% over previous reports from the same database,[5] with many cats living into their late teens or early twenties. They are generally classified as "geriatric" having reached 75% of their expected lifespan.[6] Although age is not a disease in any species, compared to young and middle-aged adults, geriatric patients have an increased likelihood of comorbidities and an increased so-called "sensitivity" (see later) to anesthetic drugs that is manifested as exaggerated or prolonged effects to dosages appropriate for young adults. They also have limited organ reserve, decreasing their ability to respond to a physiologic challenge or change (Table 99-1). This makes them more prone to the "five Hs:" hypovolemia, hypothermia, hypotension, hypoxemia, and hypoglycemia. Not all of these changes occur to an equal extent in all geriatric patients, because aging is a very individual process and each patient must be treated as an individual. Most of the data regarding age-associated changes are extrapolated from aging humans,[7,8] but one can expect aging to result in similar pathologic alterations in other mammals.

In geriatric humans, comorbidities are a major risk factor for anesthesia-related complications,[9] and one can presume that the same is true for cats, because, as previously mentioned, sicker cats (ASA status 3 to 5), regardless of age, were more likely to die during anesthesia than healthy cats.[4] Comorbidities associated with aging in cats include hyperthyroidism, chronic kidney disease (CKD), diabetes mellitus (DM), cardiac disease, and neoplasia. Patients with concurrent diseases should be stabilized to the fullest extent possible prior to anesthesia.

Key Point. Geriatric patients are not actually more "sensitive" to the effects of anesthetic drugs *per se*, but age-related changes often dictate that lower doses be used to achieve the same level of sedation or anesthesia compared to younger patients (see Table 99-1).

Age-related changes that may impact the response to anesthetic drugs include (1) lower plasma albumin concentrations resulting in higher levels of the free, metabolically active portion of highly protein-bound drugs; (2) less skeletal muscle mass for initial drug redistribution, resulting in longer drug activity; (3) increased body fat resulting in greater sequestration of fat-soluble drugs, slowing their elimination and prolonging recovery; (4) decreased glomerular filtration rate (GFR) and excretory capacity of the kidney, prolonging the half-life and duration of effect of renally excreted drugs; (5) reduced hepatic mass and total hepatic blood flow, resulting in reduced hepatic clearance and prolonged effect of

The American Society of Anesthesiologists classification system is based on the physical status of the patient. Five categories are defined as follows:

- Class 1: A normal, healthy patient
- Class 2: A patient with a mild systemic disease
- Class 3: A patient with a moderate systemic disease
- Class 4: A patient with a severe systemic disease that may be a threat to life
- Class 5: A moribund patient not expected to survive without the operation

drugs metabolized by the liver; and (6) a 20% to 30% loss of total body water with subsequent decrease in blood volume, allowing a greater proportion of the drug to be delivered to highly perfused tissues, including the brain (so-called "centralized" circulation).[10] All of these factors lead to one major clinically important conclusion: The dose of anesthetic drugs in geriatric patients should be reduced or overdose is likely to occur.

In addition, there are numerous changes in the physiologic systems. In the cardiovascular system, myocardial contractility declines because of loss of contractile tissue. Maintenance of cardiac output depends on preload (cardiac filling) because maximum achievable heart rate is lower with age in humans, yet preload is reduced due to decreased vascular compliance. Whether this occurs in nonhuman animals is not known. The propensity for arrhythmias increases, which can further affect heart rate. Changes in the sympathetic nervous system lead to decreased baroreceptor response to hypotension.[10] Clinically, the end result is a patient that may need intervention with a positive inotrope (e.g., dopamine or dobutamine) to maintain cardiac output and/or may need antiarrhythmic therapy. Carefully balanced support of circulating volume must be achieved. Dehydration and hypovolemia can have a major adverse impact, and the patient should be carefully volume-loaded to the point that preload is supported but the ejection capacity of the heart is not overloaded. Appropriate fluid therapy also impacts other organ systems, as described later.

With age, the respiratory system undergoes loss of functional alveoli and lung elasticity, which can cause ventilation/perfusion mismatch and decreased partial arterial pressure of oxygen (PaO_2). There is a decrease in maximum achievable PaO_2 with subsequent decreased oxygen reserve. The ventilatory response to hypoxia and hypercarbia is reduced. Ventilatory muscle strength is decreased which, along with increased thoracic wall rigidity, makes breathing more difficult.[10] The result is a patient with minimal oxygen reserve, so hypoxemia can occur very quickly, yet the patient may not be able to respond by increasing ventilatory drive. Clinically, the end result is a patient that requires oxygen supplementation and may need mechanical or manual positive-pressure ventilation. Oxygen support should begin as soon as an older patient is even lightly sedated (i.e., "preoxygenation") and should continue well into recovery. Utilization of the pulse oximeter can help determine whether the geriatric patient needs oxygen supplementation in the postoperative period.

Changes in the urinary system include decreases in renal blood flow, kidney mass, GFR, and tubular function. These changes lead to decreased elimination of drugs and metabolites excreted in the urine[10] and to an increased likelihood of damage from drugs that have adverse renal effects. Old cats are predisposed to CKD, and anesthesia, especially if accompanied by hypoxemia and/or hypotension, can mildly to profoundly exacerbate this disease. Thus, maintaining normal oxygenation and perfusion is critical in the aged cat. Because of the decreased blood volume, decreased renal blood flow, and dependence on preload for cardiac output, the geriatric patient is fairly intolerant of hypovolemia. However, the geriatric kidney is not efficient at excreting a fluid load, and excessive fluid therapy is not well-tolerated. Clinically, the end result is a patient that requires a careful balance between fluid needs and fluid load, and the judicious use of appropriate IV fluids is important.[10]

Hypothermia has been implicated as a contributing factor to anesthesia-related death.[1] High-risk cats, which may include geriatric cats, are more likely to develop hypothermia.[11] An age-associated decrease in basal resting metabolic rate results in less body heat being produced, leading to a decreased ability to maintain core body temperature and to rewarm once hypothermic. Hypothermia increases the incidence of myocardial dysfunction, increases the incidence of surgical wound infection, adversely affects antibody- and cell-mediated immune defenses, changes the kinetics and action of various anesthetic and paralytic drugs, increases thermal discomfort, and is associated with delayed postanesthetic recovery.[12] Because shivering during recovery increases oxygen consumption by as much as 200% to 300%, perianesthetic hypothermia alone may place severe demands on the cardiopulmonary system.

ANESTHESIA

Regardless of the species or health status of the patient, anesthesia is often most efficiently and safely planned if the anesthetic period is thought of as four distinct and equally important periods: (1) preparation and premedication, (2) induction, (3) maintenance, and (4) recovery. The importance of preparation and premedication and recovery is often overlooked, and yet these phases contribute as much to successful anesthesia as induction and maintenance. Decreasing the patient's ASA status can decrease the risk of anesthesia-related death,[1] and this can often be achieved with appropriate patient preparation prior to anesthesia. Most anesthesia-related deaths occur during the recovery phase of anesthesia and "greater patient care in the postoperative period could reduce fatalities."[1]

Table 99-1   Pathophysiologic Characteristics of Geriatric Patients That May Affect Anesthesia

Physiologic Characteristic	Effect on Anesthesia
General	
Hypoalbuminemia	Exaggerated effect from standard drug dosage for young adult patients— decreased dosage required
Neuronal degeneration	
Decrease in neurons and neurotransmitters	Decreased tolerance to fluid load—do not overhydrate
Decrease in skeletal muscle	Fat may act as drug reservoir and contribute to delayed recovery
Increase in body fat	Hypothermia contributes to delayed recovery—keep warm
Impaired thermoregulatory system	
Renal/Urinary System	
Decreased RBF, GFR and tubular function	Prolonged duration of action of renally cleared drugs—may prolong recovery time
Decreased filtration rate and excretory capacity	Decreased tolerance to fluid load—do not overhydrate
Hepatic System	
Decreased hepatic mass and hepatic blood flow	Prolonged duration of action of hepatically cleared drugs—may prolong recovery time
Respiratory System	
Loss of strength of muscles of ventilation	Decreased respiratory reserve, both oxygen and ventilatory support are required for most patients
Thorax becomes rigid, lungs lose elasticity	
Increased closing volume	
Reduction in arterial oxygen	
Cardiovascular System	
Myocardial atrophy	Decreased cardiac reserve, cardiovascular system must be supported with IV fluids and some patients may need chronotropic or inotropic support
Fibrosis of the endocardium	Anticipate need for dopamine or dobutamine
Decreased myocardial contractility	
Loss of vascular distensibility	
Maximum heart rate decreases	
Cardiac output is SV dependent	
SNS less responsive to stress	
Decreased vasoconstrictor and baroreceptor responses	

Adapted from: Pettifer GR, Grubb T: Neonatal and geriatric patients. In Tranquilli WJ, Thurmon JC, Grimm KA, editors: *Lumb and Jones veterinary anesthesia and analgesia*, ed 4, London, 2007, Wiley-Blackwell, pp 985–992.
GFR, Glomerular filtration rate; *IV*, intravenous; *RBF*, renal blood flow; *SNS*, sympathetic nervous system; *SV*, stroke volume.

Key Point. With all drugs used for anesthesia and analgesia, the concurrent or sequential use of multiple drugs reduces the doses required of each drug, thereby reducing their propensity for adverse effects.

Key Point. Sedative, analgesic, and anesthetic drugs should be titrated "to effect" in all patients, and this is especially critical in geriatric patients because of the physiologic changes that result in decreased drug dosages required for clinical effect. However, decreased cardiac output with subsequent slower delivery of anesthetic drugs to the brain may cause delayed onset of anesthetic effects, which may lead the anesthetist to assume that the original dose was ineffective. The key is to administer a dose appropriate for a geriatric patient and to refrain from redosing for a time period that is 1.5 to 2 times longer than expected in a young, healthy adult patient.

Phase 1: Preparation and Premedication

A thorough physical examination is essential to preanesthetic assessment in all patients. Pre-existing abnormalities that could have an impact on the outcome of anesthesia should be corrected, if at all possible, prior to induction. Left untreated, abnormalities may be exacerbated by anesthesia. The preanesthetic assessment for geriatric cats should include arterial blood pressure measurement, a complete blood count, serum chemistry profile with electrolytes and serum total thyroxine, and urinalysis.[13] Electrocardiographic analysis is highly recommended. Specific tests might include thoracic radiographs and/or an echocardiogram, depending on concurrent disease and physical examination findings. Although the routine use of preanesthesia diagnostic tests is occasionally criticized, routine testing in geriatric patients is a critical step in anesthetic safety. In one study, routine screening in apparently healthy cats over 10 years of age revealed numerous health concerns, many of which could have had an adverse impact on anesthetic safety (e.g., increased blood pressure, heart murmur, anemia, hypoalbuminemia, and changes in renal values), that were not present, or were present to a lesser extent, in younger cats.[14]

An IV catheter should be placed in all geriatric cats prior to anesthesia. If the patient reacts to catheter placement after administration of opioids and/or sedatives, a topical local anesthetic (2.5% lidocaine and 2.5% prilocaine) cream can be placed under a bandage on the skin at the catheter site and the cat returned to its cage for 20 to 30 minutes while dermal desensitization occurs. Hydration status should be critically evaluated. Because geriatric patients adapt poorly to hypovolemia and may be prone to dehydration, preoperative fluid therapy is often necessary. However, as previously stated, fluid needs should be carefully calculated to avoid overhydration. Correction of preoperative hypotension is important because it is a risk factor for intraoperative hypotension, especially in geriatric patients.[15] Blood glucose concentrations must be evaluated in patients with DM. Because of low oxygen reserve, potential intubation-related delay in the initiation of oxygen supplementation, and the propensity of induction

agents to cause apnea, geriatric cats should be preoxygenated for 2 to 5 minutes before induction to anesthesia.

Key Point. Warming of the patient should begin *prior* to induction if the body temperature is below normal, because warmer preoperative body temperature was found to be a significant protective factor against intraoperative hypothermia.[11] Body temperature starts to drop immediately after induction and cats can develop moderate (36.5 to 34.0 °C [97.7 to 93.2 °F]) to severe (less than 34.0 °C [93.2 °F]) hypothermia within 1 hour of induction.[11]

Drugs for Premedication

Although overt sedation is not generally needed in quiet or debilitated geriatric cats, low dosages of sedatives should be strongly considered in this patient group to alleviate stress, and to decrease the dosage of drugs needed for induction and maintenance (Table 99-2). The potential adverse effects of a low dose of sedative should be weighed against the adverse effects of needing larger doses of induction and maintenance drugs (e.g., hypotension, hypoventilation). Opioids provide analgesia, are reversible, and often provide adequate sedation when used alone in geriatric dogs. In cats, with the exception of butorphanol, opioids generally require the addition of a tranquilizer. Opioids are discussed in more detail later.

Table 99-2 Dosages of Anesthetic Drugs for Geriatric Patients*

Drug	Dosage, Interval, and Route	Comments
Opioids[†]		
Buprenorphine	0.01 to 0.03 mg/kg; every 6 to 8 hours; IM, IV, SC, or transmucosal	Excellent choice for geriatric patients Moderate to long duration, moderate analgesia, minimal adverse effects, minimal to no sedation
Butorphanol	0.2 mg/kg (up to 0.4 mg/kg); every 2 to 4 hours; IM, IV, SC	Provides moderate analgesia and sedation of fairly short duration
Fentanyl	1 to 5 μg/kg (up to 20 μg/kg); every 20 minutes if needed; IV	Excellent choice for geriatric patients Potent opioid with minimal adverse effects Consider administering as a CRI
Hydromorphone	0.1 mg/kg; every 4 to 6 hours; IM, IV, SC	Excellent choice for geriatric patients Potent opioid with minimal adverse effects Consider administering as a CRI Important note: Implicated for contributing to hyperthermia in some populations of cats
Methadone	0.1 to 0.2 (up to 0.3) mg/kg; every 4 to 6 hours; IM, IV, SC	Excellent choice in cats Tends to cause less excitement than other mu-opioid agonists
Morphine	0.1 to 0.2 (up to 0.3) mg/kg; every 1 to 6 hours; IM, SC, IV (*slowly* if IV)	Also consider administering morphine in the epidural space (0.1 mg/kg) or as a CRI
Sedatives		
Acepromazine	0.02 to 0.03 mg/kg; not usually repeated; IM, IV, SC	Not commonly used in compromised geriatric cats because effects may be prolonged Can be used up to 0.05 mg/kg in healthy geriatric cats
Dexmedetomidine	5 to 15 μg/kg; repeated if more sedation needed; IM, IV, SC	Used only in patients with healthy hearts; dose can be doubled if necessary—rarely necessary in geriatric cats

Continued

Table 99-2 Dosages of Anesthetic Drugs for Geriatric Patients—cont'd

Drug	Dosage, Interval, and Route	Comments
Induction Drugs: *Titrate All Drugs to Effect*		
Alfaxalone	1 to 3 (up to 5) mg/kg; once; IV 0.5 to 1.0 mg/kg; once; IM for light sedation in geriatric or sick cats	Excellent choice for geriatric patients Effects are similar to those achieved with propofol
Etomidate	0.5 to 1.0 mg/kg; once; IV	No cardiovascular depression Good for patients with moderate to profound cardiovascular disease
Ketamine	1 to 3 (up to 5) mg/kg; once; IV 5 to 7 (up to 10) mg/kg; once; IM	May not be appropriate for patients with hepatic or renal disease Avoid large boluses of IM drugs in frail geriatric patients
Propofol	2 to 4 (up to 6) mg/kg; repeat as needed; IV	Excellent choice for geriatric patients Fast onset makes propofol easy to titrate to effect; eliminated from the body by multiple routes Causes mild to moderate respiratory and cardiovascular depression
Maintenance Drugs: *Titrate to Effect*		
Isoflurane and Sevoflurane	Keep dose as low as possible	The inhalants cause dose-dependent hypotension, hypoventilation, and hypothermia Keep dose as low as possible
Other Drugs		
Local anesthetic drugs	4 mg/kg lidocaine; once or every 2 to 4 hours; inject around nerves 1 mg/kg bupivacaine; once or every 6 to 8 hours; inject around nerves	Excellent choice for geriatric patients Profound analgesia, slow presentation of drugs for metabolism, no systemic effects when dosed appropriately Adverse effects include CNS and cardiovascular events
Drug Antagonists		
Naloxone	0.002 to 0.04 mg/kg; every 1 hour, as needed; IV (0.005 to 0.01 mg/kg is a good dose to start) Best protocol: Dilute the naloxone to a volume that is easy to titrate; administer $\frac{1}{4}$ of calculated dose every 3 to 4 minutes until desired reversal is achieved	Reversal drug for opioids Reverses all effects mediated at both the mu and kappa receptors Be sure that analgesia is provided by another drug class prior to reversing
Butorphanol	0.1 to 0.2 mg/kg; every 2 to 4 hours, as needed; IM, IV, SC IV route should be used if rapid reversal is necessary	Reversal for opioids but only reverses effects mediated by the mu receptors, leaving kappa receptor-mediated analgesia
Atipamezole	Administer the same *volume* as the volume of dexmedetomidine or medetomidine that was administered There is a sliding dose scale on the drug label If no label is available, average the dosing scale at roughly 250 µg/kg	Reversal for alpha-2 agonists Reverses both sedation and analgesia Duration is longer than the duration of the alpha-2 agonists, so redosing is generally not required
Flumazenil	0.01 to 0.02 mg/kg every 1 hour, as needed; IV only	Reversal for benzodiazepines Duration is shorter than that of the benzodiazepines so redosing may be necessary Causes tissue necrosis if administered by any route other than IV

CNS, Central nervous system; *CRI*, constant rate infusion; *IM*, intramuscular; *IV*, intravenous; *SC*, subcutaneous.
*Drug dosages for geriatric patients are generally 25% to 50% lower than dosages for young, healthy patients. The low end of the dose range should be effective in most compromised patients, and the higher end is more likely to be effective in healthy patients. Intravenous administration provides the most profound and consistent response. The SC route provides the least profound and consistent response and the slowest onset of action. Thus, SC administration should be avoided if a rapid, consistent response is required; for example, when opioids are administered to treat existing pain.
†Frequency of administration should be patient-dependent and based on response to pain assessments.

Benzodiazepines do not provide consistent or deep sedation in very active or anxious animals but can provide mild-to-moderate sedation in calm, geriatric cats, especially when combined with an opioid. The benzodiazepines are reversible and produce little to no cardiovascular and respiratory depression, making them an ideal choice in patients with pre-existing, or the potential to develop, cardiovascular and/or respiratory compromise. The judicious use of low dosages of alpha-2 adrenergic agonists may also be considered for use in healthy geriatric cats. Drugs in this class can produce profound cardiovascular side effects and should not be used in cats with cardiovascular disease. Acepromazine may also be used for sedation but may cause prolonged sedation (due to impaired metabolism), hypotension (due to vasodilation), and hypothermia (also due to vasodilation) in geriatric animals. Acepromazine is not reversible and does not provide analgesia.

There are no age limits for pain relief, and *every* patient anesthetized for a painful procedure should receive appropriate analgesic therapy. Analgesia should be started with premedication and continue throughout the anesthetic period and beyond. In fact, analgesia in geriatric patients may be even more critical than previously realized,[16] as evidenced by the fact that untreated pain leads to a more rapid decline in physical abilities, cognitive function, and quality-of-life measures in geriatric humans than in young adult humans.[17] Analgesia is also necessary if the patient has pre-existing pain, even if the procedure requiring sedation or anesthesia is not painful (e.g., anesthesia for radiographs). Pre-existing painful conditions, such as osteoarthritis, are common in geriatric cats,[18,19] and manipulation of the anesthetized patient can aggravate the pre-existing pain. Procedural pain (e.g., surgery or painful diagnostic procedures) added to the pre-existing pain can increase the likelihood of central sensitization. As with other drugs, dosages of the analgesic drugs may need to be decreased in geriatric cats and patients should be closely monitored for signs of adverse effects, but pain management should not be withheld because of age. The fact that the effects of opioids are reversible makes them an excellent choice for analgesia in any patient with reduced capacity for metabolism. Mu-opioid agonists (e.g., morphine, hydromorphone, methadone, fentanyl, and oxymorphone) provide the most profound analgesia but may be more likely to cause adverse effects, although most effects are generally clinically manageable (or even insignificant) and are reversible. Partial agonists (e.g., buprenorphine) and agonist-antagonists (e.g., butorphanol) provide only mild to moderate analgesia but also tend to have minimal adverse effects. Buprenorphine provides medium-to-long duration (6 to 8 hours) analgesia with minimal adverse effects and is an excellent choice for analgesia in geriatric cats. Butorphanol provides short duration analgesia (90 minutes). Selection of an appropriate opioid is best made based on the particular analgesic requirements, the health status of the cat, and the pain intensity and duration expected from the intended procedure. Other analgesic classes that could be used as a premedicant include the alpha-2 agonists (previously discussed) and NSAIDs (discussed in Phase 4: Recovery in this chapter). Local anesthetic drugs are among the most useful analgesic drugs in all species and patients of all ages, and they are discussed in Phase 3: Maintenance of Anesthesia. Because each of these drugs or drug classes provide analgesia by a different mechanism, the use of more than one drug or drug class (i.e., multimodal analgesia) provides analgesia that is generally more profound and of longer duration than the use of any one drug or drug class used alone.

Key Point. Multimodal analgesia is more effective than analgesia provided by one drug class used alone. This increased efficacy often allows a decreased dose of each of the drugs, thus decreasing the likelihood of dose-related adverse effects.

Routine premedication with anticholinergic drugs to decrease oral and respiratory secretions is generally not recommended and may lead to unwanted tachycardia with subsequent increased cardiac workload, which may not be sustainable by the geriatric myocardium. However, bradycardia that is contributing to hypotension should be treated with an anticholinergic. Administration of anticholinergics should also be considered for surgical procedures that are likely to stimulate a vagal reflex (e.g., many ocular procedures).

Phase 2: Induction to Anesthesia

Key Point. For all induction protocols, administration of a sedative or analgesic drug as a premedicant will reduce the dose of drug needed for induction and decrease the risk of dose-related adverse effects.

Although mask delivery of inhaled anesthetics was advocated in the past, use of inhalants alone (i.e., without sedative or induction drugs) increases the risk of anesthesia-related mortality[1] and is no longer recommended as a routine induction technique, especially in the high-risk cat. The dose of inhalant required to anesthetize the nonpremedicated cat is fairly high, and the adverse effects of inhalant anesthetics (primarily hypotension and hypoventilation) are dose dependent. Also, the prolonged excitement phase that occurs during induction in unsedated animals may be more physiologically detrimental than a judiciously dosed injectable anesthetic. However, if venous access is not possible, an inhalant could, if titrated very carefully, be used in patients that have received sedative and/or analgesic drugs. Extra caution must be exercised because induction with inhalant gases can occur very quickly in geriatric, or otherwise compromised, patients and excessive anesthetic depth may be reached very rapidly. Thus, ongoing and repeated assessment of response to the drugs is imperative. Environmental pollution and personnel exposure are also concerns during mask inductions with inhaled anesthetics.

Anesthesia can be induced with a variety of injectable anesthetic drugs (see Table 99-2). Propofol, alfaxalone, and etomidate are readily titrated to effect. Although the pharmacokinetic profile for propofol in cats is not completely elucidated, it is known that this drug is rapidly eliminated by a variety of routes in other species so that termination of activity does not depend on the function of a single organ system.[20] Propofol produces dose-related respiratory and cardiovascular depression and should be incrementally dosed to achieve the desired depth of anesthesia. There are no data for geriatric cats, but the dose of propofol required to induce anesthesia in dogs over 8½ years of age was lower, the incidence of apnea higher, and the rate of clearance slower when compared to the same criteria in young adult dogs.[21] Results are expected to be similar for cats. The clinical effect of propofol is not affected by hepatic lipidosis, even in geriatric cats (age range for the study was 3 to 15 years, median 8 years).[22] Although there are no specific data for geriatric cats, the benzyl alcohol preservative present in newer versions of propofol does not cause adverse effects when the propofol is administered at clinically appropriate dosages.[23]

Etomidate[24] and alfaxalone[25] depend on hepatic metabolism, but redistribution and clearance are rapid following administration of either drug to young adult cats. No information for geriatric cats is available for either drug. The dose-dependent cardiovascular and respiratory effects of alfaxalone are very similar to those induced by propofol,[26] and the drug should be carefully titrated to achieve the desired depth of anesthesia. Alfaxalone is more likely than propofol to cause excitement.[27] Although anecdotally supported, the intramuscular (IM) or subcutaneous (SC) routes of administration are not recommended because large volumes of drug are required and a prolonged period of hyperexcitability can occur following administration by either route in healthy, young cats.[28] Sedation of hyperthyroid cats occurred 45 minutes after SC alfaxalone injection, but tremors occurred in a number of cats, and cats reacted to the large volume of injection,[29] which is a potential problem in the geriatric patient with expected decreased muscle mass. However, in the author's experience, a low dose of alfaxalone (0.5 to 1.0 mg/kg) combined with an opioid can be administered IM for light sedation in geriatric or aged cats.

No data are available for etomidate use in geriatric cats, but etomidate causes minimal-to-no cardiovascular changes when compared to alfaxalone[30] or propofol[31] administered to young, healthy dogs. The cardiovascular effects of etomidate in geriatric humans were similar to those produced by propofol.[32] The results in cats are expected to be the same, and etomidate is used clinically in geriatric cats.[33] Etomidate does cause adrenal suppression, and whether or not this suppression might be clinically relevant in geriatric cats is unknown.

Induction to anesthesia with ketamine, in combination with a benzodiazepine, causes only mild respiratory depression and may actually improve cardiovascular function through stimulation of the sympathetic nervous system.[34] Stimulation of cardiovascular function could be detrimental in cats with hypertrophic disease or pre-existing tachycardia, but the use of low-dose ketamine with an opioid and/or benzodiazepine decreases the clinical impact of the ketamine-mediated cardiovascular effects. Ketamine is partially metabolized by hepatic microsomal enzymes to the active metabolite norketamine.[35] Both ketamine and norketamine are excreted unchanged in the urine in cats.[35] The effects of ketamine may be prolonged, and thus not the best choice, in patients with failing hepatic and renal systems.[34] Data on clearance of tiletamine/zolazepam in the cat is limited but expected to be similar to ketamine/benzodiazepine.

Barbiturates could be used in low dosages, but the response to barbiturates can be both pronounced and prolonged in geriatric patients with reduced plasma protein concentrations and/or failing hepatic or renal function.

Once the cat is induced, it should be carefully intubated. Intubation was identified as a risk factor for anesthesia-related death,[4] but the explanation for this result is not that intubation is an inherent risk but that cats are difficult to intubate and inappropriate intubation techniques can lead to increased morbidity or mortality.

Phase 3: Maintenance of Anesthesia

Inhaled anesthetics are minimally metabolized and readily cleared regardless of hepatic or renal health, making them metabolically ideal for maintenance of anesthesia. However, they cause dose-dependent hypotension, hypoventilation, and hypothermia. Because of these adverse effects, inhaled anesthetics must be very carefully titrated, and vigilant monitoring is required to avoid excessive anesthetic depth. Unfortunately, geriatric patients may be easier to overdose if the inhalant is not titrated to effect because the minimum alveolar concentration (MAC) of an inhalant required to keep a patient anesthetized decreases with age,[36] resulting in overdose if the MAC for young healthy patients is used in geriatric patients. The concurrent administration of analgesic and sedative drugs will reduce the inhaled anesthetic requirement, thus decreasing the magnitude of dose-dependent adverse effects.

Injectable anesthetics can also be used for maintenance, and protocols are generally ketamine or tiletamine based. However, injectable anesthetic protocols with these drugs should be limited to very short procedures with no repeat dosing, especially in geriatric cats with hepatic or renal insufficiency because injectable drugs, when compared to inhalant drugs, require a higher degree of metabolism for termination of activity. Short-duration propofol infusions may be an option for geriatric cats when inhalant maintenance is not possible, for instance for airway procedures, such as bronchoalveolar lavage. Analgesia should be provided regardless of whether anesthesia is maintained by inhalant or injectable drugs.

Monitoring and Support

Along with a carefully chosen anesthetic protocol and conservative drug dosing, vigilant monitoring and aggressive physiologic support are imperative for a successful anesthetic outcome. The limited physiological reserves in geriatric patients increase the possibility of anesthetic complications, and these must be prevented if at all possible or recognized early should they occur. In the studies describing anesthesia-related risk for death, monitoring was the only factor that statistically decreased the risk of death.[1] A staff member should be dedicated to careful monitoring of the geriatric patient throughout the entire procedure. Monitoring should include basic parameters (e.g., heart rate, respiratory rate, degree of thoracic excursions or reservoir bag movement [i.e., respiratory depth], mucous membrane color, capillary refill time, pulse quality, body temperature, response to surgery, jaw tone, and palpebral reflex) along with more advanced parameters, such as arterial blood pressure, electrocardiography waveforms, SpO_2 (pulse oximetry), and end-tidal carbon dioxide.

Intravenous fluids should be administered during anesthesia, and specific concerns regarding fluid therapy in geriatric cats have already been mentioned. Fluid therapy should be targeted at correcting specific deficits while maintaining adequate perfusion and oxygen delivery without delivering excessive electrolyte or fluid volumes that could result in intravascular and extravascular fluid overload, and lead to congestive heart failure and peripheral edema. Fluid therapy was identified as a risk factor for anesthetic death in cats, but the conclusion of the study was not that fluids present an inherent risk to cats but that cats are extremely easy to volume overload because of their small body size and reduced blood volume when compared to dogs.[1]

Analgesia

Analgesia should be addressed in the maintenance phase of anesthesia and boluses of opioids, constant rate infusions of opioids and/or ketamine, and local anesthetic blockade can all be useful. The addition of local anesthetic techniques to anesthetic protocols is particularly appropriate. In humans, local anesthetic techniques result in decreased anesthesia-related morbidity,[7] although the largest impact occurs when techniques are used instead of, rather than along with, general anesthesia. In animals, local anesthetics are generally used in addition to general anesthesia, but the advantages are still significant. Local anesthetic drugs provide profound analgesia, which allows reduction in the requirement for general anesthetics, thereby improving anesthetic safety. Because the local anesthetics have a fairly slow uptake from the tissues, the drugs are presented to the liver in low amounts and are unlikely to be affected by impaired metabolism. However, because geriatric patients have decreased muscle mass and require lower dosages of most drugs, the low end of the dosage range should be used, and the drug should be carefully injected into the tissue to be desensitized using a small-gauge needle and delicate injection technique. Adverse effects of local anesthetics include central nervous system effects that can range from muscle tremors to coma and cardiovascular effects that can range from decreased myocardial contractility to cardiovascular collapse. Cats appear to be more likely to suffer dose-dependent adverse effects of local anesthetics than dogs, emphasizing the need to use lower dosages.

Phase 4: Recovery

Most anesthetic deaths occur in the recovery phase of anesthesia.[1,4] Young, healthy patients recover quickly, limiting the

monitoring and support time that is required postoperatively. Aged and compromised patients, on the other hand, may recover very slowly requiring a longer monitoring and support period. During this time, support should include IV fluids, active warming, analgesic drugs, and supplemental oxygen. Those patients experiencing excitement in recovery must also be addressed. Additional opioids or micro-doses of alpha-2 agonists (if appropriate for the patient) may be beneficial for these patients. Postoperative delirium is a common problem in geriatric humans,[7,8] and control of the delirium may require sedation and environmental modulation (i.e., decreased sound and light stimuli). A risk factor for delirium is cognitive dysfunction and because geriatric cats experience cognitive dysfunction,[37,38] postanesthetic delirium might be anticipated in these patients. Treatment with sedatives (e.g., midazolam) is appropriate, but it is also important to treat pain that might be causing signs that appear to be delirium (e.g., excitement, vocalization).

The NSAIDs are among the few drugs available that actually treat the source of the pain (inflammation) as well as the pain itself. Because of this impact on the pathology, NSAIDs should be considered any time that pain due to inflammation is present. Most pain involves some degree of inflammation (e.g., surgery, trauma, osteoarthritis, or cancer). However, the adverse effects of NSAIDs, especially the negative impact on renal function, may be exacerbated in geriatric cats. Thus, NSAIDs should be used cautiously in geriatric cats and may be inappropriate in some cats. But age alone, and even the presence of CKD, does not necessarily eliminate NSAID therapy, as evidenced by the fact that painful osteoarthritic geriatric cats with CKD had slower progression of renal disease if treated with daily, long-term meloxicam when compared to untreated cohorts.[39] Patients should be well hydrated, and doses should be calculated based on lean body weight. Nonsteroidal anti-inflammatory drugs are appropriate in patients with competent hepatic and renal function and are commonly administered to geriatric patients with inflammatory disease, such as osteoarthritis or cancer.

SUMMARY

No single ideal anesthetic protocol exists for all geriatric feline patients. An understanding of the pathophysiological changes and the alterations in pharmacodynamics and pharmacokinetics that arise in conjunction with aging is necessary when choosing an anesthetic protocol for any geriatric animal. Particular attention to decreasing and titrating anesthetic dosages and using multiple drugs concurrently to achieve the central nervous system depression necessary for a specific surgical or other procedure is advocated. Appropriate anesthetic management of geriatric animals includes thorough evaluation and assessment; preoperative correction of identified abnormalities; vigilant, aggressive perianesthetic monitoring; careful titration of anesthetic drugs; provision of analgesia; and appropriate perianesthetic support.

References

1. Brodbelt DC, Blissitt KJ, Hammond RA, et al: The risk of death: the confidential enquiry into perioperative small animal fatalities. *Vet Anaesth Analg* 35:365–373, 2008.

2. Hosgood G, Scholl DT: Evaluation of age and American Society of Anesthesiologists (ASA) physical status as risk factors for perianesthetic morbidity and mortality in the cat. *J Vet Emerg Crit Care* 12:9–15, 2002.

3. Brodbelt D: Feline anesthetic deaths in veterinary practice. *Top Comp Anim Med* 25:189–194, 2010.

4. Brodbelt DC, Pfeifer DU, Young L, et al: Risk factors for anaesthetic-related death in cats: results from the confidential enquiry into perioperative small animal fatalities (CEPSAF). *Br J Anaesth* 99:617–623, 2007.

5. Banfield Applied Research & Knowledge (BARK) Team: The state of pet health report, *Banfield Pet Hospital* (website): <http://www.stateofpethealth.com/state-of-pet-health>. (Accessed June 11, 2015.).

6. Hoskins J: *Geriatrics and gerontology of the dog and cat*, ed 2, St Louis, 2004, Saunders.

7. Jin F, Chung F: Minimizing perioperative adverse events in the elderly. *Br J Anaesth* 87(4):608–624, 2001.

8. Yang R, Wolfson M, Lewis MC: Unique aspects of the elderly surgical population: an anesthesiologist's perspective. *Geriatr Orthop Surg Rehabil* 2:56–64, 2011.

9. Pelavski AD, Lacasta A, Rochera MI, et al: Observational study of nonogenarians undergoing emergency, non-trauma surgery. *Br J Anaesth* 106:189–193, 2011.

10. Pettifer GR, Grubb T: Neonatal and geriatric patients. In Tranquilli WJ, Thurmon JC, Grimm KA, editors: *Lumb and Jones veterinary anesthesia and analgesia*, ed 4, London, 2007, Wiley-Blackwell, pp 985–992.

11. Redondo JI, Suesta P, Gil L, et al: Retrospective study of the prevalence of postanaesthetic hypothermia in cats. *Vet Rec* 170:206–209, 2012.

12. Doufas AG: Consequences of inadvertent perioperative hypothermia. *Best Pract Res Clin Anaesthesiol* 17:535–549, 2003.

13. Metzger FL: Senior and geriatric care programs for veterinarians. *Vet Clin North Am Small Anim Pract* 35:743–753, 2005.

14. Paepe D, Verjans G, Duchateau L, et al: Routine health screening: findings in apparently healthy middle-aged and old cats. *J Feline Med Surg* 15:8–19, 2013.

15. Reich DL, Hossain S, Krol M, et al: Predictors of hypotension after induction of general anesthesia. *Anesth Analg* 101:622–628, 2005.

16. Halaszynski T: Influences of the aging process on acute perioperative pain management in elderly and cognitively impaired patients. *Ochsner J* 13:228–247, 2013.

17. Caltagirone C, Spoletini I, Gianni W, et al: Inadequate pain relief and consequences in oncological elderly patients. *Surg Oncol* 19:178–183, 2010.

18. Hardie EM, Roe SC, Martin FR: Radiographic evidence of degenerative joint disease in geriatric cats: 100 cases (1994–1997). *J Am Vet Med Assoc* 220:628–632, 2002.

19. Lascelles BD, Henry JB, 3rd, Brown J, et al: Cross-sectional study of the prevalence of radiographic degenerative joint disease in domesticated cats. *Vet Surg* 39:535–544, 2010.

20. Simons PJ, Cockshott ID, Glen JB, et al: Disposition and pharmacology of propofol glucuronide administered intravenously to animals. *Xenobiotica* 22:1267–1273, 1992.

21. Reid J, Nolan AM: Pharmacokinetics of propofol as an induction agent in geriatric dogs. *Res Vet Sci* 61:169–171, 1996.

22. Posner LP, Asakawa M, Erb HN: Use of propofol for anesthesia in cats with primary hepatic lipidosis: 44 cases (1995–2004). *J Am Vet Med Assoc* 232:1841–1843, 2008.

23. Taylor PM, Chengelis CP, Miller WR, et al: Evaluation of propofol containing 2% benzyl alcohol preservative in cats. *J Feline Med Surg* 14:516–526, 2012.

24. Wertz EM, Benson GJ, Thurmon JC, et al: Pharmacokinetics of etomidate in cats. *Am J Vet Res* 51:281–285, 1990.

25. Whittem T, Pasloske KS, Heit MC, et al: The pharmacokinetics and pharmacodynamics of alfaxalone in cats after single and multiple intravenous administration of Alfaxan at clinical and supraclinical doses. *J Vet Pharmacol Ther* 31:571–579, 2008.

26. Martinez Taboada F, Murison PJ: Induction of anaesthesia with alfaxalone or propofol before isoflurane maintenance in cats. *Vet Rec* 167:85–89, 2010.

27. Mathis A, Pinelas R, Brodbelt DC, et al: Comparison of quality of recovery from anaesthesia in cats induced with propofol or alfaxalone. *Vet Anaesth Analg* 39:282–290, 2012.

28. Grubb TL, Greene SA, Perez TE: Cardiovascular and respiratory effects, and quality of anesthesia produced by alfaxalone administered intramuscularly to cats sedated with dexmedetomidine and hydromorphone. *J Feline Med Surg* 15:858–865, 2013.

29. Ramoo S, Bradbury LA, Anderson GA, et al: Sedation of hyperthyroid cats with subcutaneous administration of a combination of alfaxalone and butorphanol. *Aust Vet J* 91:131–136, 2013.

30. Rodríguez JM, Muñoz-Rascón P, Navarrete-Calvo R, et al: Comparison of the cardiopulmonary parameters after induction of anaesthesia with alphaxalone or etomidate in dogs. *Vet Anaesth Analg* 39:357–365, 2012.

31. Sams L, Braun C, Allman D, et al: A comparison of the effects of propofol and etomidate on the induction of anesthesia and on cardiopulmonary parameters in dogs. *Vet Anaesth Analg* 35:488–494, 2008.

32. Larsen R, Rathgeber J, Bagdahn A, et al: Effects of propofol on cardiovascular dynamics and coronary blood flow in geriatric patients: a comparison with etomidate. *Anaesthesia* 43(Suppl):25–31, 1988.

33. Shilo Y, Pypendop BH, Barter LS, et al: Thymoma removal in a cat with acquired myasthenia gravis: a case report and literature review of anesthetic techniques. *Vet Anaesth Analg* 38:603–613, 2011.

34. Wright M: Pharmacologic effects of ketamine and its use in veterinary medicine. *J Am Vet Med Assoc* 180:1462–1471, 1982.

35. Heavner J, Bloedow D: Ketamine pharmacokinetics in domestic cats. *Vet Anesth* 6:16–19, 1979.

36. Nickalls RW, Mapleson WW: Age-related iso-MAC charts for isoflurane, sevoflurane and desflurane in man. *Br J Anaesth* 91:170–174, 2003.

37. Gunn-Moore D, Moffat K, Christie LA, et al: Cognitive dysfunction and the neurobiology of ageing in cats. *J Small Anim Pract* 48:546–553, 2007.

38. Gunn-Moore DA: Cognitive dysfunction in cats: clinical assessment and management. *Top Companion Anim Med* 26:17–24, 2011.

39. Gowan RA, Baral RM, Lingard AE, et al: A retrospective analysis of the effects of meloxicam on the longevity of aged cats with and without overt chronic kidney disease. *J Feline Med Surg* 14:876–881, 2012.

Cardiorenal Syndrome

Marie C. Bélanger

Myocardial and chronic kidney diseases (CKDs) are common disorders of the geriatric cat.[1,2] The coexistence of heart failure (HF) and CKD is often associated with an adverse outcome, because combined cardiac and renal dysfunctions amplify the progression of failure of each system through complex neurohormonal feedback mechanisms.[3]

In humans, the term *cardiorenal syndrome* (CRS) has traditionally been reserved to describe declining renal function in the face of advanced congestive heart failure (CHF). Recently, a more specific schema for CRS has been published.[4] In this classification, CRS is divided into five subtypes that reflect the pathophysiology, time frame, and nature of concomitant cardiac and renal dysfunction (Table 100-1). Patients with types 1 and 2 have cardiac disease, acute or chronic respectively, with the subsequent development of acute kidney disease or CKD. In types 3 and 4, renal dysfunction (acute exacerbation or CKD) precedes deterioration of cardiac function. Type 5 refers to systemic disease unrelated to renal or cardiac systems that results in disease of both of those organs.

Whether this negative spiral of primary CKD causing cardiac dysfunction occurs in small animals is unknown, although uremic cardiopathies have been observed in dogs.[5] Except for the consequences of hypertension, CRS types 3 and 4 are probably uncommon in cats. For the purpose of this chapter, CRS will refer to type 2 in the human classification, in which the function of relatively normal or susceptible kidneys declines secondary to HF or chronic cardiac dysfunction. A special focus on the therapeutic strategies of feline cardiorenal syndrome will be presented.

PREVALENCE

Comorbid dysfunction of the heart and kidney has been reported to be as high as 30% to 50% in hospitalized humans.[6,7] A similar prevalence of 15% to 50% has been found in dogs with mitral valve disease.[8,9] The true incidence of CRS in cats is still unknown, but a study evaluating 102 cats with hypertrophic cardiomyopathy (HCM) reported a 59% prevalence for azotemia as compared to 25% in an age-matched control population.[10]

PATHOPHYSIOLOGY

The pathophysiology of CRS is complex and not completely understood. Cardiorenal syndrome becomes relevant when therapy to relieve HF is limited by progressively worsening renal function. The etiology of CRS is multifactorial and involves bidirectional interactions between the heart and kidneys. These include activation of the renin-angiotensin-aldosterone system (RAAS) and the sympathetic nervous system, potentiation of oxidative stress, endothelial dysfunction, and defective nitric oxide metabolism (Figure 100-1). In chronic myocardial dysfunction, long-term reduction of renal perfusion is responsible for worsening renal function. However, hypoperfusion alone cannot explain progressive renal dysfunction as the cause of CKD. Numerous neurohormonal mechanisms are implicated and include vasoconstrictive (epinephrine, angiotensin II, endothelin), vasodilatory (brain natriuretic peptide, nitric oxide) and inflammatory (C-reactive protein) mediators.[11] Other contributing factors include anemia, the deleterious effects of uremia and acidemia on cardiac inotropy, and the hypotensive effects of diuresis-associated hypovolemia and RAAS blockade.[12,13] Whether all of these mechanisms are responsible for CRS in cats remains a speculation.

DIAGNOSIS

Clinicians should monitor for, and anticipate, CRS while managing any cat with chronic HF. It is suspected when progressive increases in serum creatinine level (eventually leading to azotemia) are observed in cats treated for HF or in cats with CKD that develop HF. For both medical and prognostic purposes, the glomerular filtration rate (GFR) should be estimated and included in the initial database. In a clinical setting, creatinine concentration can be used as an indirect, albeit insensitive, estimate of GFR. However, numerous nonrenal factors affect serum creatinine levels, most notably a decline in muscle mass, giving a false sense of improvement in GFR. Single injection iohexol plasma clearance can also be used to estimate GFR clinically in cats.

Table 100-1 Classification of Cardiorenal Syndrome in Humans

Type of Cardiorenal Syndrome	Definition
Type 1	Abrupt worsening of cardiac function (e.g., acute cardiogenic shock or decompensated CHF) leading to acute kidney injury
Type 2	Chronic abnormalities in cardiac function (e.g., CHF) causing progressive and permanent chronic kidney disease
Type 3	Abrupt worsening of renal function (e.g., acute kidney ischemia or glomerulonephritis) causing acute cardiac disorder (e.g., heart failure, arrhythmia, ischemia)
Type 4	State of chronic kidney disease (e.g., chronic glomerular disease) contributing to decreased cardiac function, cardiac hypertrophy, and/or increased risk of adverse cardiovascular events
Type 5	Systemic condition (e.g., diabetes mellitus, sepsis) causing both cardiac and renal dysfunction

Adapted from Ronco F, Ronco C: Cardiorenal syndrome, current understanding. *Recenti Prog Med* 100:202, 2009.
CHF, Congestive heart failure.

The diagnosis of CKD is difficult in cats already being treated for HF. The diagnostic hallmark of isosthenuric urine in the presence of azotemia cannot be used in patients receiving diuretics. Also, mild or moderate prerenal elevation of blood urea nitrogen (BUN) and creatinine are expected in animals on diuretics.[8,9,14] However, finding a progressive increase in BUN and especially creatinine, with or without a decreasing urine specific gravity (USG), in a cat with chronic HF should alert the practitioner to potential development of CRS. Longitudinal assessment of serum creatinine is important, because a progressive rise can indicate declining renal function even when values remain within the normal reference interval, such as in cats with International Renal Interest Society (IRIS) CKD stage 1 and early-to-mid stage 2. Other indices of CKD include hyperphosphatemia, hypokalemia, nonregenerative anemia, and proteinuria. Evidence of the clinical signs of CKD (e.g., increasing polyuria and polydipsia, inappetence and anorexia, vomiting, weight loss) should also increase suspicion for CRS.

Diagnosis of kidney disease requires a complete blood count, serum chemistry profile, urinalysis, and urinary protein : creatinine ratio. Abdominal ultrasound should be performed to recognize the typical architectural changes of CKD (e.g., irregular kidneys with poor corticomedullary

definition) and to suggest underlying causes such as pyelonephritis, nephrolithiasis, neoplasia, polycystic kidney disease, etc. for which there may be specific treatments. Thromboembolism resulting in renal infarction and an acute decline in renal function should be suspected when a cat with HF presents with acute renal failure. Urine culture should be performed to identify and treat possible urinary tract infection.[15] Systemic blood pressure should be evaluated in all cats with CRS because the presence of hypotension will worsen renal perfusion, whereas hypertension will negatively affect cardiac output and renal function. In calm, conscious cats, a systolic blood pressure over 150 mm Hg should be regarded as suspicious for hypertension.[16] A complete echocardiogram is warranted to enable more optimal treatment of the primary cardiomyopathy and to assess the risk for pending or potential embolic events. Thoracic radiographs should be performed to evaluate the degree of control of the HF and to adjust the medical plan accordingly. Finally, identification of reversible causes of decompensation (e.g., ingestion of sodium-rich treats, glucocorticoid administration, a recent stress-causing acute tachycardia such as a veterinary visit or chasing prey) should be identified and addressed.

A promising tool in the diagnosis of CRS is the measurement of biomarkers, such as serum N-terminal pro-brain natriuretic peptide (NT-proBNP) for cardiac disease and urinary neutrophil gelatinase-associated lipocalin or serum symmetric dimethylarginine (SDMA) for renal disease, respectively.[17-21] Neutrophil gelatinase-associated lipocalin has recently been shown to increase in dogs with kidney injury before GFR declines and is predictive of prognosis.[22-25] A recent study in geriatric cats showed that serum SDMA concentration was significantly correlated with GFR and increased before creatinine in cats with CKD.[26]

Prospective studies are needed to assess the usefulness of such biomarkers in the diagnosis and management of CRS in cats.

THERAPY

Treatment of CRS in cats is largely empiric, because no clinical trials have been performed with this species. It is important to recognize that cats with CRS are fragile and that every change in medication and hydration status may threaten equilibrium and may cause cardiac or renal decompensation. Close monitoring and follow-up evaluations are essential. Table 100-2 summarizes the general approach to the cat presented with CRS. The goals are to recognize the syndrome, reverse it as much as possible, and deal with the renal consequences of chronic HF.

The main challenge in treating comorbid HF and CKD is to balance two organs with opposing volume requirements.[27] The objective is to find a balance between "drying-out" HF and "hydrating" CKD. Prioritizing the predominant clinical disorder and decompensated organ is essential. The clinician will have to decide whether or not to implement treatments that favor intravascular volume. Unfortunately,

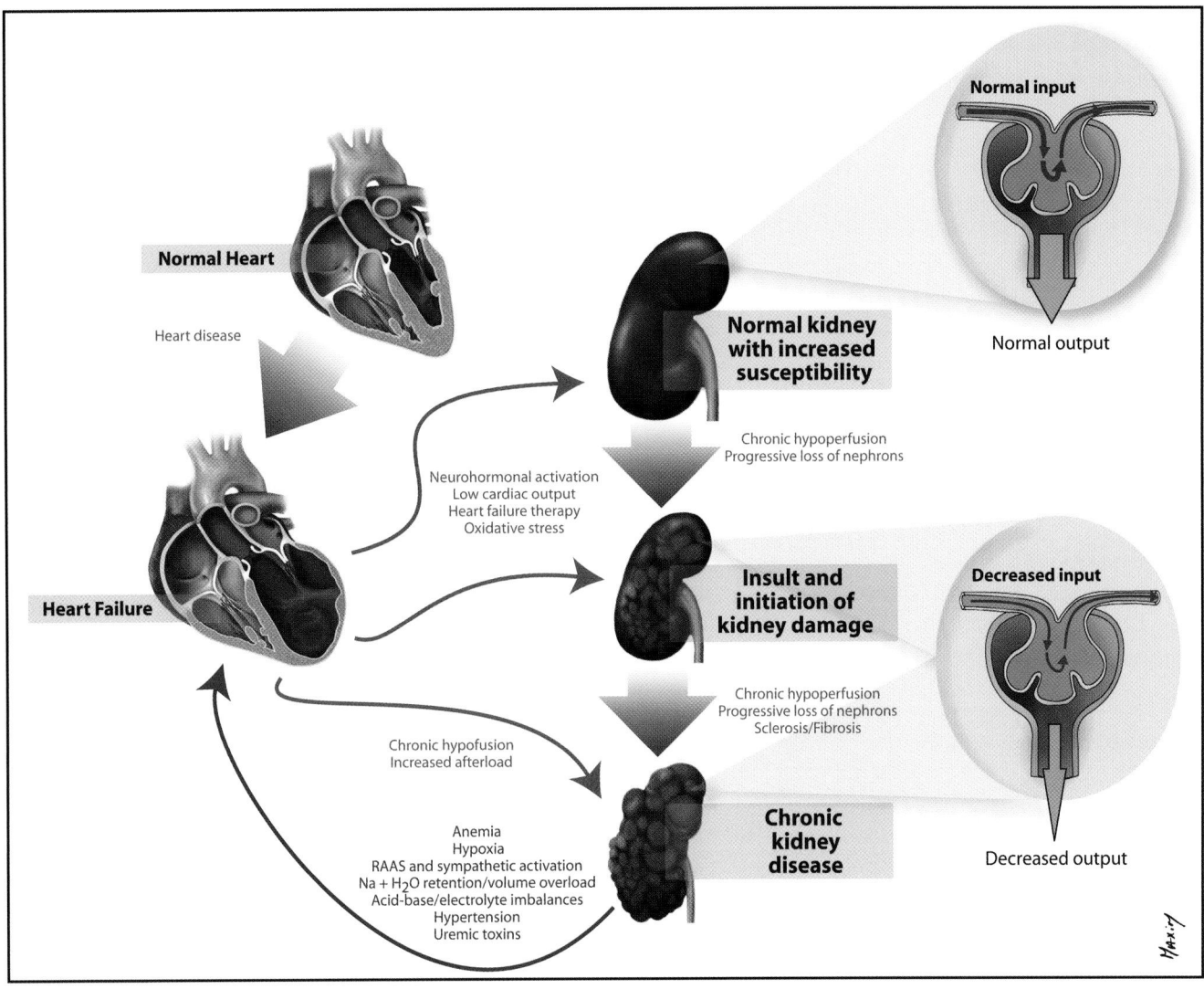

Figure 100-1: Pathophysiology of cardiorenal syndrome. *RAAS,* Renin-angiotensin-aldosterone-system.

control of HF is often favored to the detriment of optimal renal support, leading to adverse long-term consequences for the kidneys. It should not be assumed that the heart is more important than the kidneys, due to the aforementioned complex neurohormonal interactions; renal compromise is detrimental to cardiac function. Table 100-3 outlines specific treatment plans for different CRS situations.

Adjust Drug Dosages

Because cats with CRS are on many drugs, it is important to review and adjust the doses, if appropriate, on each visit. In general, a good strategy is to "start low and go slow," titrating dose increases in order to find the optimal therapeutic and dosing combination that will return the patient to a state of equilibrium. Special care should be taken to check for drug interactions and to prolong the dosing interval of renally excreted drugs such as atenolol, propranolol, and enalapril. Dose adjustments are appropriate for drugs that are administered to effect, such as amlodipine. Heart failure may

affect hepatic biotransformation of drugs (e.g., diltiazem) in some cats.

Optimize Heart Failure Therapy

Angiotensin-Converting Enzyme Inhibitors

Because of RAAS activation, angiotensin-converting enzyme (ACE) inhibitors are the mainstay of therapy for concomitant HF and CKD, especially in the presence of hypertension and/or proteinuria. Although activation of RAAS is beneficial in the early stages of renal disease, prolonged renal ischemia exacerbates renal injury and may cause fibrosis as it does in other species.[28] In small animals with CKD, ACE inhibitors limit systemic and glomerular capillary hypertension, have an antiproteinuric effect, and delay development of glomerulosclerosis and tubulointerstitial lesions.[29] In cats with uncomplicated CKD, benazepril has been shown to counteract proteinuria, improve control of hypertension, delay the onset or progression of azotemia, and potentially prolong survival.[30-33]

Table 100-2   **Approach to the Cat with Cardiorenal Syndrome**

1. Recognize and anticipate cardiorenal syndrome	• Record baseline BUN/creatinine/USG/UPC ratio • Monitor for increasing creatinine over time
2. Optimize heart failure therapy	• Use lowest effective dose of furosemide • Consider dual-diuretic therapy • Consider torsemide if diuretic resistance • Use ACE inhibitors • Consider other cardiac drugs directed at primary disease • Perform thoracentesis/abdominocentesis as needed
3. Evaluate and monitor renal function	• CBC/serum chemistry profile/urinalysis ± UPC ratio • Every 1-3 months or when changing treatment plan • Urine culture • Abdominal ultrasound
4. Control hypertension	• Assess SBP • Treat when SBP is >150 mm Hg • Use amlodipine
5. Avoid hypotension	• If SBP is <100 mm Hg • Re-evaluate use of potential hypotensive drugs • Consider positive inotropes
6. Improve renal therapy	• Supplement with omega-3 PUFAs • Feed a renal therapeutic diet • Consider phosphate binders • Potassium supplementation • H_2 blockers if gastrointestinal signs present • Consider long-term low-sodium SC fluids • Consider renal replacement therapy
7. Improve cardiac output	• Consider positive inotropes • Dobutamine unconvincing • Pimobendan promising
8. Correct anemia	• When hematocrit is less than 17% to 20% • Erythropoietin or darbepoietin administration • Iron supplementation
9. Review and modify drug dosages	• Extend dosage interval of renally excreted drugs • Check for drug interactions

ACE, Angiotensin-converting enzyme; *BUN,* blood urea nitrogen; *CBC,* complete blood count; *PUFAs,* polyunsaturated fatty acids; *SC,* subcutaneous; *SBP,* systemic blood pressure; *UPC,* urine protein/creatinine ratio; *USG,* urine specific gravity.

Cats with CRS should be volume-repleted cautiously before being started on low dose ACE inhibitors (benazepril or enalapril, 0.25 mg/kg, every 24 hours, orally [PO]). This dose can eventually be increased (0.5 to 1 mg/kg, every 24 hours, for benazepril, every 24 to 48 hours for enalapril) for better control of HF. Benazepril is only metabolized in the liver, whereas enalapril is metabolized by both the liver and kidneys. Consequently, cats with CRS might need a lower dose or prolonged dosing interval of enalapril than benazepril or a prolonged dosing interval. Initiation of ACE inhibition therapy is associated with a transient decrease in GFR and increase in BUN and creatinine concentrations. Cats showing an increased creatinine or those already on an ACE inhibitor while developing renal failure can remain on therapy. Angiotensin-converting enzyme inhibitors should not be stopped in the face of azotemia in cats with renal disease and HF; lowering the dose is generally sufficient.[34] In CRS, ACE inhibitors are beneficial in the long term and generally not responsible for worsening renal function. In general, vasodilators improve cardiac output and renal blood flow by decreasing systemic vascular resistance.

Diuretics

If progressive azotemia becomes a concern in cats with CRS, decreasing the furosemide dose should be the first approach. By lowering cardiac output and renal blood flow, diuretics tend to cause prerenal increases in BUN and creatinine. However, it is recommended not to go below the lowest effective dose of furosemide that controls signs of HF. This dose has to be continuously reassessed depending on the type

Table 100-3	Therapeutic Strategies in Different Cardiorenal Syndrome Situations	
	RENAL DYSFUNCTION	
Heart Failure	**Normal Creatinine**	**Increased Creatinine**
Resolved	Find lowest effective diuretic dose Optimize follow-up evaluations	Reduce furosemide dose Reassess ACE-I dosage Consider positive inotropes Stimulate water consumption Consider SC fluids
Unresolved, Progressive, or Severe	Increase furosemide dose Consider dual-diuretic therapy Consider furosemide CRI Consider torsemide Control arrhythmias (check for hypokalemia and/or hypomagnesemia) Increase ACE-I dosage/frequency Consider pimobendan Consider afterload reduction: arteriodilator/amlodipine therapy	Optimize positive inotrope use Consider dual diuretic therapy Control signs of uremia Maintain SC fluids Increase arteriodilator dose Control hypertension Avoid iatrogenic hypotension Consider renal replacement therapy

ACE-I, Angiotensin-converting enzyme inhibitor; *CRI*, constant rate infusion; *CRS*, cardiorenal syndrome; *HF*, heart failure; *SC*, subcutaneous.

and progression of heart disease, dietary salt intake, and renal adaptation to the diuretic. During any tapering process, the owner can monitor daily resting respiratory rate (RRR) and respiratory effort to identify signs of recurring CHF (i.e., increasing RRR and effort). Owners should be instructed to report any progressive increase of RRR or sudden increase greater than 30 to 40 breaths per minute.[35]

An important principle when determining the ideal furosemide dosage for an individual HF patient is that the threshold rate of drug excretion must be achieved for optimal efficacy.[36] In other words, the single effective dose resulting in adequate natriuresis must be found; a cat nonresponsive to 5 mg of furosemide once a day will need 10 mg (once, twice, or three times a day) rather than increasing to 5 mg twice a day. Adequate natriuresis can be grossly assessed in a clinical setting by observing increased urine volume and decreased USG. Constant rate infusion (CRI) of furosemide should also be considered in acute HF because it produces superior diuresis in dogs,[37] and likely in cats.[38] Another important principle to remember when attempting rapid fluid elimination in a cat with CRS is that furosemide is more effective in removing interstitial fluid (e.g., pulmonary edema) than body cavity effusions. Periodic centesis of significant pleural effusion or ascites is advocated to avoid excessive diuretic use.[38]

Diuretic resistance may be associated with chronic therapy for HF. It is defined as a clinical state in which diuretic response is reduced or absent before therapeutic relief from pulmonary edema is attained. Cats receiving chronic furosemide should have a USG less than 1.030.[34] Values higher than this suggest noncompliance, malabsorption, or incomplete or absent diuretic effect. Multiple factors account for

diuretic resistance, including insufficient diuretic dose, excessive sodium intake, impaired intestinal absorption of oral drugs, increased sodium reabsorption at diuretic-insensitive sites in the nephrons, decreased renal perfusion, and excessive urinary excretion of the diuretic.[39] When diuretic resistance occurs in cats, furosemide CRI (0.25 to 0.6 mg/kg per hour intravenously [IV]) can achieve natriuresis by inhibition of sodium reabsorption more consistently than oral or IV bolus therapy. Once the volume-overloaded state has resolved, most cats will once again respond to oral diuretics.

An alternate strategy for diuretic resistance is to switch to a different oral loop diuretic. Torsemide (0.1 to 0.3 mg/kg every 24 hours PO or divided every 12 hours) is useful in CRS patients because of excellent bioavailability, superior diuretic action, and a long half-life.[38] A recent study of healthy dogs showed that diuretic resistance developed after 14 days of furosemide, but not torsemide, administration.[40] Torsemide has been evaluated in cats with experimentally induced left ventricular hypertrophy; it appears to be 10 times more potent than furosemide.[41] Its effects peak at 4 hours and persist for 12 hours.

Dual-diuretic therapy is an option when diuretic resistance is suspected or when a furosemide dose needs to be decreased. Combination therapy potentiates diuretic effects by acting at multiple sites within the nephron. Spironolactone (1 to 2 mg/kg PO every 12 hours) may occasionally cause a reversible facial dermatitis in cats.[42] In the author's experience, spironolactone use in patients with renal dysfunction occasionally causes significant hyperkalemia. A thiazide diuretic (e.g., hydrochlorothiazide, 1 to 2 mg/kg PO every 12 hours) can also be used, but this is less effective than loop diuretics.

Normalize Blood Pressure: Control Hypertension and Avoid Hypotension

Systemic hypertension is common in feline CKD.[43] It complicates management of HF by increasing the afterload, consequently aggravating ventricular hypertrophy and reducing cardiac output and renal blood flow. Uncontrolled hypertension worsens renal lesions; it should be aggressively controlled in cats with CRS. Angiotensin-converting enzyme inhibitors are not effective as monotherapy for hypertension in cats with CKD.[44] Amlodipine (0.625 to 1.25 mg/cat PO every 24 hours) should be added to the therapeutic plan and can be used concurrently with ACE inhibitors. Blood pressure monitoring should be performed regularly to avoid iatrogenic hypotension, especially in a patient receiving other drugs for HF that have hypotensive effects. Systolic blood pressure should ideally be maintained between 100 and 150 mm Hg in cats with CRS.

Improve Cardiac Output

The role of positive inotropes in feline CRS is unclear. Most HF in cats is due to HCM, which is mainly a disease of diastolic dysfunction. Nevertheless, in advanced stages of HF and CKD, a positive inotrope can be helpful in improving renal blood flow and azotemia. Use of pimobendan increases cardiac output, improves renal blood flow, and may allow reduction in the diuretic dosage. However, its use is still controversial in cats with obstructive HCM (i.e., having moderate to severe systolic anterior motion of the mitral valve).[45,46] Although unapproved in this species, the author has used pimobendan (0.25 mg/kg PO every 12 hours or 1.25 mg/cat every 12 hours) on several cats with end-stage CRS, resulting in improved azotemia, demeanor, and appetite. Further study is needed in that area, because a small but significant increase in BUN has been reported in dogs with HF treated with pimobendan.[47] Dobutamine (2 µg/kg per minute IV) is another positive inotrope that can be used in hospitalized cats with CRS, but its real benefit is still unproven.

Improve Renal Therapy

Management of feline CKD is discussed in detail in Chapter 47. Specific strategies to optimize renal function in CRS follow.

Diet

Appropriate diet therapy is essential in the management of CRS, and the nutritional needs of both cardiac and renal dysfunction should be taken into consideration. In HF, high sodium intake can prevent net fluid loss even when adequate diuresis is achieved. Therefore, cats with CRS should eat a diet with sodium content of no more than 0.25% to 0.33% dry matter basis (e.g., Hill's Prescription Diet k/d Feline Renal Health). More stringent sodium restriction is sometimes needed in CRS cats with severe or progressive HF (e.g.,

Purina VD Feline NF-Formula and Royal Canin Renal LP). Distilled or low-sodium bottled water can also be offered for drinking. Owners should be advised to avoid feeding treats with high sodium content. Examples of low-sodium treats for cats include Purina Whisker Lickin's brands and Stewart Fiber Formula.

In CKD, dietary modification is recommended in cats in IRIS stages 2 to 4.[48] Besides protein and phosphorus reduction, diets designed for feline CKD usually differ from maintenance diets in several ways that are also beneficial in HF. These modifications include reduced sodium content (minimizing diuretic need), increased B vitamin content, increased caloric density, neutral effect on acid-base balance, and supplementation of potassium and omega-3 polyunsaturated fatty acids (PUFAs). Protein restriction should be tailored on an individual basis in cats with CRS. Adequate high-quality, biologically available protein is important in HF to avoid cardiac cachexia. Protein should be given at the highest level tolerated by the renal dysfunction without increasing azotemia. A home-made diet formulated with the assistance of a board-certified veterinary nutritionist and tailored to the individual patient's needs may be considered for cats with CRS.

Omega-3 Polyunsaturated Fatty Acids

Omega-3 PUFAs have many beneficial effects on both the heart and the kidney. Dietary supplementation with omega-3 PUFAs may be renoprotective early in the course of kidney disease.[49] In a study of experimentally induced kidney disease, dogs receiving omega-3 PUFA supplementation had fewer structural renal lesions, less proteinuria, and preservation of GFR when compared with dogs fed a control, low-PUFA-content diet.[50] A retrospective study on the effects of renal diets found that survival was greatest among cats with CKD that were fed the diet with the highest omega-3 PUFAs content.[51]

Omega-3 fatty acids are also beneficial in animals with cardiac disease. In one study of dogs with HF, fish oil supplementation decreased cytokine production and improved cachexia and appetite.[52] Antiarrhythmic effects of fish oil have also been reported in humans and animals.[53,54] Although these effects have not been studied in cats with CRS, omega-3 PUFAs can be given at the following suggested dosage: eicosapentaenoic acid at 40 mg/kg PO every 24 hours and docosahexaenoic acid at 25 mg/kg PO every 24 hours.

Fluid Therapy

In volume-depleted CRS patients, administration of IV fluids may be essential to reduce uremia (via improving renal flow and promoting diuresis) but may precipitate CHF. Therefore, the main focus during fluid administration is to determine when euvolemia is achieved and to avoid fluid overload. A good strategy is to use replacement-type fluids (e.g., Plasma-Lyte 148, lactated Ringer's solution) to slowly correct dehydration, and then change to low-sodium maintenance crystalloid fluids (e.g., NaCl 0.45%-dextrose 2.5%, Plasma-Lyte 56 with 5% dextrose) to further reduce azotemia. Constant-rate fluids are preferable to an IV bolus, and the rate and amount of fluids must be determined on a case-by-case basis. Monitoring patient weight is an easy tool to use in deciding how to adjust fluid rates. Auscultation of a new gallop sound or finding a progressive increase in the respiratory and/or heart rate in a cat with pre-existing heart disease warn of impending or existing CHF and the need for immediate reduction of fluid rate.

Cage-side echocardiography can also be used to assess left atrial size and guide fluid rate decisions.[55] A normal left atrial size in a severely azotemic patient suggests that cautious IV fluid therapy may be well tolerated. Conversely, if the echocardiogram shows a marked enlargement of the left atrium with dilation of the pulmonary vein, IV fluids may precipitate or worsen pulmonary edema, and reduction of azotemia may be effected by manipulating cardiac output through use of positive inotropes and vasodilators. Echocardiography is useful for assessing the accumulation of effusions. The gold standard for monitoring the risk of CHF in CRS patients remains pulmonary artery catheterization for evaluation of capillary wedge pressure. The clinical limitation of this tool in cats is the requirement of anesthesia for placement of a Swan-Ganz catheter (6 to 8 Fr) in the pulmonary artery. An alternative is the measurement of central venous pressure (CVP) from the jugular vein in a sedated cat.[56] Because CVP reflects the pressure reaching the right ventricle, it cannot replace arterial catheterization, which detects left-sided changes where the majority of feline heart diseases are located.[38] Normal CVP in cats is 4.2 ± 1.1 mm Hg.[57]

Although there are no supportive scientific studies, many cardiologists consider administration of fluids via the subcutaneous (SC) route less likely to worsen signs of CHF than by the IV route, due to slower absorption.[55] Subcutaneous fluid administration can correct dehydration and azotemia in cats with CKD. This strategy is also helpful in cats with CRS, but SC fluids, like IV fluids, ultimately increase blood volume and constitute a risk for cardiac decompensation. It is therefore essential to educate the owner regarding the risk of acute HF and how to monitor for signs of fluid overload (e.g., monitoring of the RRR). Administration of fluids and diuretics should generally not be given concurrently. Decreasing the dose of diuretics should be attempted before SC fluids are prescribed for an azotemic cat with CRS. Cats with IRIS stage 3 and 4 CKD with normal cardiac function may typically receive 75 to 100 mL/cat of a balanced electrolyte solution (e.g., lactated Ringer's solution) every 24 to 72 hours or up to 60 mL/kg per day.[58] In fragile CRS patients, it is recommended to start with a much smaller volume (30 mL/cat every 48 hours) and, if the effect on uremia is suboptimal, the volume can cautiously be increased to 50 mL/cat every 48 hours and then to every 24 hours if needed and tolerated. Serial assessment of hydration, signs of uremia, and renal function should be performed and fluid therapy adjusted accordingly.

Placing a feeding tube for administration of water is another option; this has the additional advantage of providing a means to improve the nutritional plane of an inappetant or anorectic patient.[58] Oral fluid supplementation (e.g., water

fountains or slow dripping faucets in addition to fresh water provided in bowls) is another easy, often overlooked, approach to improve hydration in cats with CKD.[38]

Electrolytes, especially potassium, should be monitored closely in animals with CRS. Hypokalemia is common in cats with CKD[59] and is aggravated by the use of furosemide in CRS management. Serum potassium is ideally measured from blood drawn into a heparinized (green top) tube because red-top tubes allow blood clotting, which releases potassium from activated platelets, thereby potentially masking hypokalemia.[60] Hypokalemia causes muscle weakness and anorexia and triggers ventricular tachyarrhythmias and refractoriness to some antiarrhythmic drugs (e.g., lidocaine). Hypokalemia can be corrected through fluid therapy supplementation (potassium chloride 0.05 to 0.5 mEq/kg per hour) or via oral supplementation (potassium citrate 40 to 75 mg/kg every 12 hours or potassium gluconate 1 to 4 mEq every 24 hours).

Magnesium, like potassium, plays an important role in the maintenance of resting membrane potential and regulation of ion shifts within cardiomyocytes. Hypomagnesemia increases the risk and severity of cardiac arrhythmias. Diuretics increase the risk for hypomagnesemia, whereas ACE inhibitors and spironolactone can induce hypermagnesemia.[61] Toll and colleagues[62] reported that critically ill cats with magnesium abnormalities had a longer period of hospitalization and were more likely to die or be euthanized than cats that remained normomagnesemic. Correction of hypomagnesemia in cats can be achieved by CRI of magnesium sulfate (0.01-0.04 mEq/kg per hour IV).

Renal replacement therapy such as hemodialysis or ultrafiltration can improve survival and quality of life in cats with end-stage CRS. Availability, feasibility, and costs of renal replacement therapy are limiting factors for many cat owners.

Manage Anemia

Correction of anemia when heart disease is present results in lower risk of cardiac arrhythmias and improved tissue delivery of oxygen.[38] Anemia is relatively common in cats with CKD. Several mechanisms may be involved: anemia of chronic disease (iron sequestration), decreased erythropoietin (EPO) production, inadequate dietary protein intake for normal hemoglobin production, or azotemia-induced destruction of red blood cells. In humans with advanced HF, anemia may be secondary to defective erythropoiesis and represents an independent risk factor for worse outcome.[63] Dogs with HF have been shown to have lower hematocrits than healthy controls.[64]

There has been a growing interest in the pathogenic link between EPO deficiency and progression of CRS. Cardiac EPO receptor activation protects the cardiomyocytes from apoptosis, inflammation, and fibrosis; EPO supplementation in anemic humans with CRS has been shown to improve cardiac function.[65] In cats with CRS, significant anemia (packed cell volume less than 17% to 20%) can be corrected with EPO or darbepoietin administration (see Chapter 47). Caution is advised when blood transfusions are given to anemic cats with CRS, because they can precipitate volume overload and CHF. Chronic gastrointestinal blood loss should also be considered and treated in anemic cats with CRS with the use of proton pump inhibitors (e.g., omeprazole), H2 antagonists (e.g., famotidine), or barrier protectants (e.g., sucralfate).

PROGNOSIS

Patients with both HF and CKD experience worse outcomes than those with either disease alone. In humans with HF,

renal dysfunction is strongly linked to increased morbidity.[66] Negative predictive indicators for development of renal failure in people with HF include old age, low cardiac output, elevated baseline creatinine concentration, progressive rise in creatinine concentration, hypertension, diuretic therapy, and calcium channel blocker therapy.[67] In a study of cats with HCM, azotemia was associated with older age, lower body weight, and higher systolic blood pressure.[10] Although renal function may remain stable for months in cats with HF, once CRS occurs, it leads to frequent hospitalization, difficulty maintaining a good quality of life, and eventually, euthanasia. The therapeutic strategies discussed are mainly directed at improving the quality of life for cats with CRS. Whether they also contribute to prolonged survival is unknown.

References

1. Paige CF, Abbott JA, Elvinger F, et al: Prevalence of cardiomyopathy in apparently healthy cats. *J Am Vet Med Assoc* 234:1398–1403, 2009.
2. Lund EM, Armstrong PJ, Kirk CA, et al: Health status and population characteristics of dogs and cats examined at private veterinary practices in the United States. *J Am Vet Med Assoc* 214:1336 1341, 1999.
3. Ronco C, Haapio M, House AA, et al: Cardiorenal syndrome. *J Am Coll Cardiol* 52:1527–1539, 2008.
4. Ronco C, House AA, Haapio M: Cardiorenal syndrome: refining the definition of a complex symbiosis gone wrong. *Intensive Care Med* 34:957–962, 2008.
5. Chetboul V: Échocardiographie des cardiopathies acquises. In de Madron É, editor: *Échocardiographie clinique du chien et du chat,* Issy-les-Moulineaux, 2012, Elsevier Masson, pp 214–215.
6. Ronco C, Cruz DN, Ronco F: Cardiorenal syndromes. *Curr Opin Crit Care* 15:384–391, 2009.
7. McClellan V, Langston R, Presley R: Medicare patients with cardiovascular disease have a high prevalence of chronic kidney disease and a high rate of progression to end-stage renal disease. *J Am Soc Nephrol* 15:1912–1919, 2004.
8. Nicolle A, Chetboul V, Allerheiligen T, et al: Azotemia and glomerular filtration rate in dogs with chronic valvular disease. *J Vet Intern Med* 21:943–949, 2007.
9. Pouchelon J, King J, Martignoni L, et al: Long-term tolerability of benazepril in dogs with congestive heart failure. *J Vet Cardiol* 6:7–13, 2004.
10. Gouni V, Chetboul V, Pouchelon JL, et al: Azotemia in cats with feline hypertrophic cardiomyopathy: prevalence and relationships with echocardiographic variables. *J Vet Cardiol* 10:117–123, 2008.
11. Arici M, Walls J: End-stage renal disease, atherosclerosis, and cardiovascular mortality: is C-reactive protein the missing link? *Kidney Int* 59:407–414, 2001.
12. Meyer TW, Hostetter TH: Uremia. *N Engl J Med* 357:1316–1325, 2007.

13. Nohria A, Hasselblad V, Stebbins A, et al: Cardiorenal interactions: insights from the ESCAPE trial. *J Am Coll Cardiol* 51:1268–1274, 2008.
14. Boswood A, Murphy A: The effect of heart disease, heart failure and diuresis on selected laboratory and electrocardiographic parameters in dogs. *J Vet Cardiol* 8:1 9, 2006.
15. White JD, Stevenson M, Malik R, et al: Urinary tract infections in cats with chronic kidney disease. *J Feline Med Surg* 15:459–465, 2013.
16. Brown S, Atkins C, Bagley R, et al: Guidelines for the identification, evaluation, and management of systemic hypertension in dogs and cats. *J Vet Intern Med* 21:542–558, 2007.
17. Kuster N, Moréna M, Bargnoux A-S, et al: Biomarkers of cardiorenal syndrome. *Ann Biol Clin (Paris)* 71:409–418, 2013.
18. Ronco C, Kaushik M, Valle R, et al: Diagnosis and management of fluid overload in heart failure and cardio-renal syndrome: the "5B" approach. *Semin Nephrol* 32:129–141, 2012.
19. Cobrin AR, Blois SL, Kruth SA: Biomarkers in the assessment of acute and chronic kidney diseases in the dog and cat. *J Small Anim Pract* 54:647–655, 2013.
20. Hall JA, Yerramilli M, Obare E, et al: Comparison of serum concentrations of symmetric dimethylarginine and creatinine as kidney function biomarkers in healthy geriatric cats fed reduced protein foods enriched with fish oil, L-carnitine, and medium-chain triglycerides. *Vet J* 202:588–596, 2014.
21. Braff J, Obare E, Yerramilli M, et al: Relationship between serum symmetric dimethylarginine concentration and glomerular filtration rate in cats. *J Vet Intern Med* 28(6):1699–1701, 2014.
22. Nabity MB, Lees GE, Cianciolo R, et al: Urinary biomarkers of renal disease in dogs with X-linked hereditary nephropathy. *J Vet Intern Med* 26:282–293, 2012.
23. Segev G, Palm C, LeRoy B, et al: Evaluation of neutrophil gelatinase-associated lipocalin as a marker of kidney injury in dogs. *J Vet Intern Med* 27:1362–1367, 2013.

24. Lee YJ, Hu YY, Lin YS, et al: Urine neutrophil gelatinase-associated lipocalin (NGAL) as a biomarker for acute canine kidney injury. *BMC Vet Res* 8:1–9, 2012.
25. Kai K, Yamaguchi T, Yoshimatsu Y, et al: Neutrophil gelatinase-associated lipocalin, a sensitive urinary biomarker of acute kidney injury in dogs receiving gentamicin. *J Toxicol Sci* 38:269–277, 2013.
26. Hall JA, Yerramilli M, Obare E, et al: Comparison of serum concentrations of symmetric dimethylarginine and creatinine as kidney function biomarkers in cats with chronic kidney disease. *J Vet Intern Med* 28(6):1676–1683, 2014.
27. Côté E: Seeking the perfect balance: management of concurrent cardiac and renal disease. In *Proceedings of the American College of Internal Medicine Medicine Forum,* Montreal, Quebec, 2009.
28. Brewster UC, Setaro JF, Perazella MA: The renin-angiotensin-aldosterone system: cardiorenal effects and implications for renal and cardiovascular disease states. *Am J Med Sci* 326:15–24, 2003.
29. Lefebvre HP, Toutain PL: Angiotensin-converting enzyme inhibitors in the therapy of renal diseases. *J Vet Pharmacol Ther* 27:265–281, 2004.
30. Watanabe T, Mishina M: Effects of benazepril hydrochloride in cats with experimentally induced or spontaneously occurring chronic renal failure. *J Vet Med Sci* 69:1015–1023, 2007.
31. Mizutani H, Koyama H, Watanabe T: Evaluation of the clinical efficacy of benazepril in the treatment of chronic renal insufficiency in cats. *J Vet Intern Med* 20:1074–1079, 2006.
32. Brown SA, Brown CA, Jacobs G, et al: Effects of the angiotensin-converting enzyme inhibitor benazepril in cats with induced renal insufficiency. *Am J Vet Res* 62:375–383, 2001.
33. King JN, Gunn-Moore DA, Tasker S, et al: Tolerability and efficacy of benazepril in cats with chronic kidney disease. *J Vet Intern Med* 20:1054–1064, 2006.
34. Côté E, MacDonald KA, Meurs KM, et al: Congestive heart failure. In *Feline Cardiology,*

West Sussex, 2011, Wiley-Blackwell, pp 257–302.

35. Ljungvall I, Rishniw M, Porciello F, et al: Sleeping and resting respiratory rates in healthy adult cats and cats with subclinical heart disease. *J Feline Med Surg* 16(4):281–290, 2014.

36. Geisberg C, Butler J: Addressing the challenges of cardiorenal syndrome. *Cleve Clin J Med* 73:485–491, 2006.

37. Adin DB, Taylor AW, Hill RC, et al: Intermittent bolus injection versus continuous infusion of furosemide in normal adult greyhound dogs. *J Vet Intern Med* 17:632–636, 2003.

38. Côté E, MacDonald KA, Meurs KM, et al: Comorbidities: managing cats that have coexistent cardiac disease and extracardiac disorders. In *Feline Cardiology*, West Sussex, 2011, Wiley-Blackwell, pp 368–373.

39. Rose BD: Diuretics. *Kidney Int* 39:336–352, 1991.

40. Hori Y, Takusagawa F, Ikadai H, et al: Effects of oral administration of furosemide and torsemide in healthy dogs. *Am J Vet Res* 68:1058–1063, 2007.

41. Uechi M, Matsuoka M, Kuwajima E, et al: The effects of the loop diuretics furosemide and torasemide on diuresis in dogs and cats. *J Vet Med Sci* 65:1057–1061, 2003.

42. MacDonald K, Kass P, Kittleson M: Effect of spironolactone on diastolic function and left ventricular mass in Maine Coon cats with familial hypertrophic cardiomyopathy. *J Vet Intern Med* 21:335–341, 2007.

43. Syme HM, Barber PJ, Markwell PJ, et al: Prevalence of systolic hypertension in cats with chronic renal failure at initial evaluation. *J Am Vet Med Assoc* 220:1799–1804, 2002.

44. Steele JL, Henik RA, Stepien RL: Effects of angiotensin-converting enzyme inhibition on plasma aldosterone concentration, plasma renin activity, and blood pressure in spontaneously hypertensive cats with chronic renal disease. *Vet Ther* 3:157–166, 2002.

45. Gordon SG, Saunders AB, Roland RM, et al: Effect of oral administration of pimobendan in cats with heart failure. *J Am Vet Med Assoc* 241:89–94, 2012.

46. MacGregor JM, Rush JE, Laste NJ, et al: Use of pimobendan in 170 cats (2006-2010). *J Vet Cardiol* 13:251–260, 2011.

47. Gordon SG, Miller MW, Saunders AB: Pimobendan in heart failure therapy—a silver bullet? *J Am Anim Hosp Assoc* 42:90–93, 2006.

48. International Renal Interest Society website. IRIS staging of CKD. Available at: <www.iris-kidney.com>. (Accessed August 24, 2015.)

49. Brown SA, Brown CA, Crowell WA, et al: Effects of dietary polyunsaturated fatty acid supplementation in early renal insufficiency in dogs. *J Lab Clin Med* 135:275–286, 2000.

50. Brown SA, Brown CA, Crowell WA, et al: Beneficial effects of chronic administration of dietary omega-3 polyunsaturated fatty acids in dogs with renal insufficiency. *J Lab Clin Med* 131:447–455, 1998.

51. Plantinga EA, Everts H, Kastelein AM, et al: Retrospective study of the survival of cats with acquired chronic renal insufficiency offered different commercial diets. *Vet Rec* 157:185–187, 2005.

52. Freeman LM, Rush JE, Kehayias JJ, et al: Nutritional alterations and the effect of fish oil supplementation in dogs with heart failure. *J Vet Intern Med* 12:440–448, 1998.

53. Smith CE, Freeman LM, Rush JE, et al: Omega-3 fatty acids in Boxer dogs with arrhythmogenic right ventricular cardiomyopathy. *J Vet Intern Med* 21:265–273, 2007.

54. Kang JX, Leaf A: Antiarrhythmic effects of polyunsaturated fatty acids. Recent studies. *Circulation* 94:1774–1780, 1996.

55. DeFrancesco TC: Maintaining fluid and electrolyte balance in heart failure. *Vet Clin North Am Small Anim Pract* 38:727–745, 2008.

56. de Laforcade AM, Rozanski EA: Central venous pressure and arterial blood pressure measurements. *Vet Clin North Am Small Anim Pract* 31:1163–1174, 2001.

57. Lamont LA, Bulmer BJ, Grimm KA: Cardiopulmonary evaluation of the use of medetomidine hydrochloride in cats. *Am J Vet Med Assoc* 62:1745–1762, 2001.

58. Polzin DJ: Chronic kidney disease. In Ettinger SJ, Feldman EC, editors: *Textbook of veterinary internal medicine*, ed 7, St Louis, 2010, Elsevier Saunders, pp 1990–2021.

59. DiBartola SP, Rutgers HC, Zack PM, et al: Clinicopathologic findings associated with chronic renal disease in cats: 74 cases (1973-1984). *J Am Vet Med Assoc* 190:1196–1202, 1987.

60. Sevastos N, Theodossiades G, Archimandritis AJ: Pseudohyperkalemia in serum: a new insight into an old phenomenon. *Clin Med Res* 6:30–32, 2008.

61. Thomason JD, Rockwell JE, Fallaw TK, et al: Influence of combined angiotensin-converting enzyme inhibitors and spironolactone on serum K^+, Mg^{2+}, and Na^+ concentrations in small dogs with degenerative mitral valve disease. *J Vet Cardiol* 9:103–108, 2007.

62. Toll J, Erb H, Bimbaum N, et al: Prevalence and incidence of serum magnesium abnormalities in hospitalized cats. *J Vet Intern Med* 16:217–221, 2002.

63. Horwich TB, Fonarow GC, Hamilton MA, et al: Anemia is associated with worse symptoms, greater impairment in functional capacity and a significant increase in mortality in patients with advanced heart failure. *J Am Coll Cardiol* 39:1780–1786, 2002.

64. Farabaugh AE, Freeman LM, Rush JE, et al: Lymphocyte subpopulations and hematologic variables in dogs with congestive heart failure. *J Vet Intern Med* 18:505–509, 2004.

65. Palazzuoli A, Silverberg DS, Iovine F, et al: Effects of beta-erythropoietin treatment on left ventricular remodeling, systolic function, and B-type natriuretic peptide levels in patients with the cardiorenal anemia syndrome. *Am Heart J* 154:645.e9–15, 2007.

66. Hillege H, Nitsch D, Pfeffer M, et al: Renal function as a predictor of outcome in a broad spectrum of patients with heart failure. *Circulation* 113:671–678, 2006.

67. Cohen N, Gorelik O, Almoznino-Sarafian D, et al: Renal dysfunction in congestive heart failure, pathophysiological and prognostic significance. *Clin Nephrol* 61:177–184, 2004.

Medicating the Very Young and the Very Old Cat

Dawn Merton Boothe

Understanding the ways in which pediatric and geriatric animals are physiologically and pathologically different from adults is essential for successful drug therapy. This chapter focuses on some of the clinically important parameters that are likely to alter response to drugs in these age extremes. Data in animals are limited, and as such, disposition pattern changes described for humans, and when appropriate, dogs, are discussed where feline-specific data is lacking. Although some of these extrapolations appear to be relevant,[1-4] limitations do exist. The impact of age-related diseases is not addressed in a comprehensive manner in this chapter. Key points for drug therapy in pediatric and geriatric cats are summarized in Boxes 101-1 and 101-2.

Drug disposition in the cat is characterized by unique differences in drug movement and responses, including predisposition to toxicities; these have been reviewed thoroughly elsewhere.[3-6] The effects of age extremes in drug disposition in cats are summarized in Tables 101-1 and 101-2. Because the impact depends, in part, on the physiochemical characteristics of the drug, particularly water versus lipid solubility, examples of commonly used drugs that fall in either category are listed in Table 101-3.

DRUG DISPOSITION IN THE PEDIATRIC CAT

For the purposes of this chapter, the term *pediatric* generally refers to the first 12 weeks of life.[7] Identifying the distinct age at which cats transition from neonate to infant to pediatric to young adult is difficult. Although no clear physiologic endpoints occur for each of these stages, changes in physiology and anatomy are profound and impact drug disposition. Changes associated with each of these stages affect drug disposition, rendering the pediatric patient more susceptible to drug-induced adverse reactions. All four determinants of drug disposition (i.e., absorption, distribution, metabolism, and excretion [ADME]) undergo dramatic changes as the neonate matures (see Table 101-1),[2,8] and the clinical significance of these sequelae varies with age and stage of development.

Absorption

Young kittens have decreased ability to digest energy, carbohydrate, and organic matter compared with kittens older than

19 weeks of age.[9] Because of the large surface area of the small intestine, even in neonates, the *extent* of absorption of orally administered drugs probably does not differ clinically between healthy pediatric and adult animals. However, the rate of absorption tends to be slower in pediatric animals probably because of decreased gastric emptying and irregular intestinal peristalsis. As a result, peak plasma drug concentrations (PDCs) may be lower in pediatric patients. The decreased rate of absorption might actually protect against toxic drug concentrations.[10,11] However, before colostrum has been absorbed, the permeability of the intestinal mucosa is increased, leading to an increased rate and extent of drug absorption, even allowing drugs not normally absorbed from the gastrointestinal (GI) tract (e.g., aminoglycosides, acid-sensitive beta-lactams, and enteric sulfonamides) to reach the systemic circulation. Intestinal permeability decreases rapidly following the ingestion of colostrum,[11,12] possibly because of the endogenous release of hydrocortisone or adrenocorticotropic hormone. Exogenous supplementation of either of these hormones to the queen during the 24 hours prepartum prevents increased permeability but also absorption of colostrum.

A number of other factors may alter small intestinal drug absorption in pediatric patients:

- Gastric pH is neutral in the newborn, and adult acidic levels are not reached until sometime after birth, depending on the species.[10,12] The neonate's higher gastric pH (achlorhydria) may decrease the absorption of many drugs that require disintegration and dissolution or that are ionized in a less acidic environment (e.g., weak acids, such as penicillins).
- Milk diets can reduce drug absorption by either decreasing gastric emptying or directly interacting with drugs (e.g., milk can impair absorption of tetracyclines).
- An "unstirred water layer" found adjacent to the surface area of the mucosal cells in animals of all ages is thicker in the neonate than in the older pediatric patient; this may limit the rate of absorption of some drugs, particularly those that are water soluble.
- Absorption of fat-soluble drugs (e.g., griseofulvin, fat-soluble vitamins) increases as biliary function matures.
- The importance of microbial colonization of the GI tract and the impact of drugs has not been evaluated but is potentially profound in the pediatric patient. In addition

Table 101-1	Projected Clinically Relevant Changes in Drug Disposition in the Pediatric Patient
Drug Disposition Determinant	**Projected Changes in Drug Disposition**
Absorption	Increased oral absorption for first 24 hours of life (during colostrum absorption)
	Decreased GI acidity leading to decreased absorption of weak acids
	Milk possibly binding to luminal contents decreases absorption of some drugs
	Reduced absorption of fat-soluble drugs
	Non-IV parenteral absorption may be slowed by hypothermia
Distribution	Increased volume of distribution, reduced plasma concentrations for most drugs leads to longer elimination half-life
	Greater proportion of extracellular fluid reduces plasma concentrations of water-soluble compounds more than lipid-soluble drugs; leads to longer elimination half-life
	Decreased distribution of compounds that accumulate in fat
	Decreased protein binding of highly protein-bound drugs, possibly increasing distribution of unbound drug; PDCs decreased, half-life prolonged
	Decreased distribution to peripheral organs in hypothermic patients
	Increased permeability of blood-brain barrier increases risk of CNS toxicity
Metabolism	Decreased phase I metabolism, being absent for first weeks and reaching adult levels at 3 to 4 months; this may be challenged by evidence that some metabolism may exceed that of adults
	Increased oral bioavailability of drugs that normally undergo first-pass metabolism; decreased response to compounds that must be metabolized to active state (prodrugs); prolonged elimination (half-life) of drugs metabolized by liver
	Decreased peripheral metabolism of compounds
Excretion	Decreased renal clearance until 2 to 3 months of age results in generally prolonged half-life for water-soluble drugs

CNS, Central nervous system; *GI,* gastrointestinal; *IV,* intravenous; *PDC,* plasma drug concentration.

BOX 101-1 Key Points for Drug Therapy in Pediatric Patients

- In general, higher doses and longer intervals should be expected for most drugs used in pediatric patients. Exceptions include CNS active drugs because of an immature blood-brain barrier.
- Predicting hepatic metabolism is difficult in pediatric patients, because evidence is emerging that they may actually metabolize drugs more rapidly than adults.
- Several antimicrobials are not recommended for pediatric patients. These include chloramphenicol, tetracyclines, doxycycline, and drugs that undergo enterohepatic circulation (e.g., clindamycin and to some degree, doxycycline), because they are more likely to disrupt the normal colonization of the alimentary tract in pediatric patients.

CNS, Central nervous system.

BOX 101-2 Key Points for Drug Therapy in Geriatric Patients

- In general, changes associated with aging predispose the geriatric patient to adverse drug reactions as organ clearance and protection decrease. "Start low and go slow" is appropriate.
- As cardiac function decreases, secondary compensatory responses redistribute blood flow to the brain and heart, increasing the risk of adverse reactions to drugs toxic to these tissues. Cardiac disease can exacerbate these changes.
- Dose water-soluble drugs in the geriatric cat based on lean body weight; dose lipid-soluble drugs based on mg/kg.
- Changes in plasma albumin can be clinically important to patients receiving highly protein-bound drugs, with the risk of adverse reactions greater for those drugs that are potentially toxic, such as nonsteroidal anti-inflammatory drugs.
- The risk of drug interactions is increased in geriatric patients because of comorbidities and the need for polypharmacy.

Table 101-2 **Projected Clinically Relevant Changes in Drug Disposition in the Geriatric Patient**

Drug Disposition Determinant	Projected Changes in Drug Disposition
Absorption	Decreased esophageal motility may increase risk of drug-induced mucosal erosion
	Decreased gastric motility prolongs time to peak effect
	Altered gastric acidity may increase risk of bacterial overgrowth or alter impact of antimicrobials on GI microbiota
	Generally decreased absorption of oral drugs
	Decreased gastroprotection
Distribution	Decreased fat mass and decreased lean body weight results in decreased distribution, higher PDCs, and shorter half-life of water-soluble drugs
	Decreased body fat and lean body mass results in higher drug concentrations and potentially a shorter half-life; if obese, decreased lean body mass also results in higher concentrations and shorter half-life of water-soluble drugs, as well as an increased distribution and prolonged half-life of lipid-soluble drugs
	Decreased protein binding may be compensated for by clearance of free compound
	Increased distribution to heart and brain as cardiac function declines
	Decreased distribution of water-soluble drugs resulting in increased drug concentrations, shorter half-life
Metabolism	Decreased hepatic mass and drug metabolizing enzymes (phases I and II) result in prolonged half-life of most drugs, decreased formation of prodrugs, and increased oral bioavailability of drugs which undergo first-pass metabolism
	Decreased hepatic blood flow, decreased clearance of flow-limited drugs, and increased absorption of drugs that undergo first-pass metabolism
	Decreased hepatoprotection increases risk of drug-induced hepatotoxicity
Excretion	Decreased GFR, decreased renal clearance results in proportional prolongation of elimination half-life
	Decreased renal protection increases risk of drug-induced nephrotoxicity

GFR, Glomerular filtration rate; *GI,* gastrointestinal; *PDC,* plasma drug concentration.

to the immune system, altered microflora may subsequently alter the response to antimicrobial drugs, extrahepatic metabolism, or enterohepatic circulation.[13,14]

Absorption of drugs administered parenterally to pediatric animals also varies from that of adults. The rate of absorption after intramuscular administration changes with age as muscle mass and its accompanying blood flow increase and as vasomotor responses mature.[13] Because muscle mass is small, subcutaneous administration is frequently preferred for pediatric patients. Again, variability in subcutaneous absorption rates can be anticipated with age. A smaller fat—but greater water—compartment may result in faster absorption compared with that in adults.[15] The newborn is more subject to the effect of environmental temperature on subcutaneous absorption until thermoregulation matures; subcutaneous drug absorption may require that the neonate be kept warm and hypothermia be corrected.

Alternative routes of administration should be considered in the neonate and pediatric patient. Absorption from the rectal mucosa is rapid. Rectal administration of drugs or fluids can be used for pediatric patients when venous catheterization is difficult, to reduce complications associated with intravenous administration (e.g., sedation, anesthesia), or when oral administration is undesirable (e.g., antiemetics). Limited data from studies of human infants indicate that peak plasma concentrations after rectal administration may be higher than those obtained by other routes.[13]

Intraperitoneal administration can be a lifesaving route of blood and fluid administration, particularly for the newborn with inaccessible central veins. Isotonic fluids are rapidly absorbed, and up to 70% of red blood cells are absorbed in 48 to 72 hours.[16] However, because this route of administration is accompanied by the risk of peritonitis or trauma, intraosseous administration of blood and fluids into the medullary cavity of large bones (e.g., trochanteric fossa of the femur in larger kittens 4 weeks of age or older) is preferred.[17,18]

Absorption of volatile anesthetics from the pediatric respiratory tract is rapid because minute ventilation is greater, making them more sensitive to the effects of gas anesthetics.[7] Although not a common route of drug administration, transdermal absorption of drugs is likely to be greater in pediatric patients because it is directly related to skin hydration, which is greatest in neonates. Topical administration of potentially toxic lipid-soluble drugs (e.g., hexachlorophene, organophosphates) is not recommended. Administration of transdermal opioids (e.g., fentanyl patch) is likewise not recommended.

Lactation

The nursing animal is an inadvertent recipient of drugs administered to the mother. Most of the pertinent information in the veterinary literature is concerned with excretion of drugs in the milk of food animals; there appears to be no

Table 101-3 Examples of Drugs Characterized as Either Lipid Soluble (Lipophilic, Hydrophobic) vs Water Soluble (Hydrophilic, Lipophobic)

Water-Soluble Drugs	Lipid-Soluble Drugs
Antimicrobials	**Antimicrobials**
Beta-lactams (*penicillins, *cephalosporins)	Fluorinated quinolones
Aminoglycosides	"Potentiated" sulfonamides (*sulfadiazine, *trimethoprim)
	Macrolides (e.g., *azithromycin)
Cardiac Drugs	Clindamycin
Atenolol	Chloramphenicol
Lisinopril	Doxycycline
*Enalapril	Metronidazole
Analgesics	**Cardiac Drugs**
*Morphine	Metoprolol
	Carvedilol
	Benazepril
	*Enalapril
	Amlodipine
	Analgesics
	Bupivacaine
	*Morphine
	Fentanyl
	Buprenorphine
	Central Nervous System Active Drugs
	Tricyclic antidepressants
	Anticonvulsants (most)
	Toxins
	Organophosphates
	Glucocorticoids

*These agents (marked with asterisks) can be either water soluble or lipid soluble.

information regarding small animals. Studies of humans indicate that drugs diffuse into the milk from maternal circulation. Low-molecular-weight (<200 Daltons), un-ionized, highly lipid-soluble drugs that are minimally protein bound diffuse into the lactating mammary gland rapidly, whereas water-soluble drugs diffuse more slowly.[19] The acid-base dissociation constant (pK_a) of a drug largely determines its concentration in milk. Animal milk tends to be acidic compared with plasma pH. Consequently, although a drug may be non-ionized in the plasma and thus more likely to diffuse into milk, it may become ionized and nondiffusible once in the milk. Such "ion trapping" can concentrate drugs in milk. The ratio of a drug in milk to plasma is predictable, being greater for weak bases and weak acids whose pK_as differ from the pH of milk by 2 pH units (+2 for acids and −2 for bases).[20]

Generally, the amount of drugs excreted in milk is less than 2% of the maternal dose.[19] However, greater concentrations can be expected if a drug is administered to the mother intravenously, as a bolus or an infusion, or in repeated doses.

Not all drugs ingested with milk during nursing will be absorbed from the GI tract of the nursing animal. For example, milk may decrease the absorption of some drugs, whereas the pharmacokinetic properties of other drugs (e.g., aminoglycosides) preclude their absorption except in the very young. However, not all drugs need to be absorbed to cause adverse effects. For example, antimicrobials can sometimes alter the developing flora of the pediatric alimentary tract.[14,21] Thus, it is prudent to refrain from administering potentially toxic drugs to the lactating queen.

Distribution

The two most important factors contributing to drug distribution in pediatric patients are differences in body fluid compartments and drug binding to serum proteins. Body fluid compartments undergo profound changes with the growth of the neonate. Both the percentage of total body water and the ratio of compartmental volumes change with maturation. The percentage of total body water decreases with age, but the decrease is more substantial in the extracellular versus the intracellular compartment (see Table 101-1; Figure 101-1).[22] Daily fluid requirements are greater in neonatal and pediatric patients, in part because a larger proportion of their body weight is represented by body water. The effects of these body compartment differences depend on the normal distribution of the drug in question. Most water-soluble drugs are distributed to extracellular fluids. In pediatric patients, the volume to which these drugs is distributed is higher than in adults. Although decreased PDCs resulting from increased distribution may protect the pediatric patient from potentially toxic drug concentrations,[23] higher (e.g., 20% to 30%) mg/kg doses may be necessary to provide therapeutic efficacy. A different pattern might be expected for lipid-soluble drugs, because they tend to be distributed to total body water (both intracellular and extracellular distribution). Such drugs should be dosed according to body weight (e.g., mg/kg). The disposition of several antimicrobials in neonatal animals has been reviewed by Baggot,[24] with differences in disposition generally found to be similar to those described for humans. Ampicillin, a water-soluble drug, is characterized by volumes that are larger in puppies and kittens (threefold to fourfold higher) compared with adults, resulting in clinically significant lower drug concentrations.[25,26] Distribution of enrofloxacin, a lipid-soluble drug, is somewhat unpredictable and age-dependent in kittens, being smaller at 2 to 4 weeks but greater at 4 to 6 weeks.[27] Those drugs that are distributed to a larger volume in pediatric patients are characterized by a longer half-life and as such, the dosing interval of the drug may need to be prolonged. In some cases, this effect may be balanced by increased clearance of a drug, as has been demonstrated for enrofloxacin in 6- week-old kittens.[27]

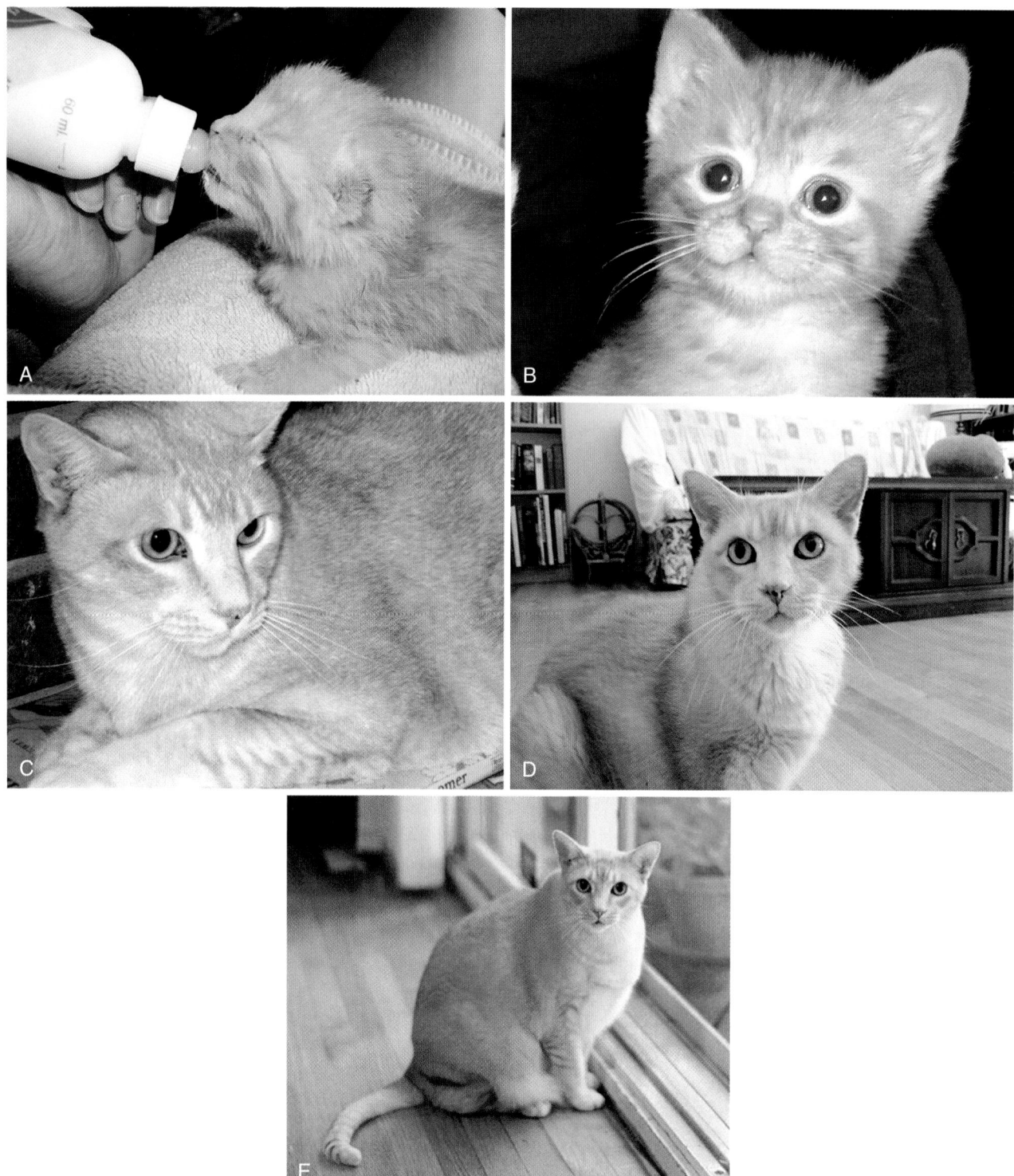

Figure 101-1: With aging, the body composition of a cat changes. The extracellular fluid compartment represents a greater proportion of total body mass in the neonate **(A)**, and this progressively decreases until adult age is reached (3 weeks **[B]**, adult **[C]**). Doses of all drugs, but particularly water-soluble drugs, may need to be increased by 25% to 10% (decreasing the percentage as the kitten ages) to achieve the same plasma drug concentration that might be obtained in the adult cat. **D,** The geriatric cat generally has a marked loss of total body weight, including both lean body weight and fat. Overdosing is easier in these patients because of the loss of all mass. **E,** Less commonly, some older cats may be obese. In these cats, overdosing with water-soluble drugs may be an issue if they are dosed on a mg/kg basis, because such drugs will not distribute to fat (e.g., meloxicam). (**A** and **B,** Courtesy of Chantal Bourdon. **C, D,** and **E,** Courtesy of Dr. Susan Little.)

Because the proportion of body fat is smaller in pediatric patients than in adults, the distribution of lipid-soluble drugs that accumulate in fat (e.g., organophosphates, chlorinated hydrocarbons, and ultrashort thiobarbiturates) may be proportionately decreased. As a result, although drug half-life decreases, PDCs may become toxic. Many lipid-soluble drugs have a high affinity for, and are bound by, plasma proteins, facilitating their movement through the body. Binding, however, limits their distribution to tissues. Predicting the distribution of highly protein-bound drugs is complicated in the pediatric patient. Serum concentrations of both albumin, the protein to which most drugs are bound, and alpha-1 glycoproteins (to which basic drugs preferentially bind) are decreased in pediatric patients.[28] Protein binding of drugs may also be reduced because of differences in albumin structure or because drugs compete with endogenous substrates (e.g., bilirubin) for binding sites.[11,29] When drugs are displaced, their concentration in plasma and the distribution of free, pharmacologically active forms into tissues increase. The risk of adverse reactions may also increase.[29] As the distribution increases, drug half-life may become longer, necessitating longer dosing intervals if the drug is potentially toxic. However, increased clearance of unbound drug may balance the impact of displaced protein binding.

Differences in regional organ blood flow might cause clinically important changes in drug disposition in pediatric animals due to differences in drug excretion.[30,31] Because blood flow to vessel-rich tissues of the body (e.g., heart, brain) is greater and faster;[7] the pediatric patient is more susceptible to drug-induced cardiac and central nervous system (CNS) toxicity. The potential for CNS toxicity is further increased because the blood-brain barrier is poorly developed immediately after birth. Accordingly, although opioids generally are the preferred sedative, premedicant, or analgesic for some clinicians,[7] one may need to be prepared to reverse them in these patients. Increased permeability protects the neonatal brain from a lack of nutritional fuels in stressful states (e.g., hypoglycemia, hypoxia, and acidosis) by allowing the movement of oxidizable substrates, such as lactate, into brain cells.[32] However, drugs normally incapable of reaching the adult brain are also able to reach susceptible brain cells, increasing the risk of CNS toxicity.[33]

Fluid therapy in pediatric patients is impacted by several characteristics of drug distribution. Pediatric patients are predisposed to dehydration because the extracellular fluid compartment is increased, their renal capacity to conserve water is decreased, the ratio of surface area to body weight is large, and fluid loss through immature skin is greater.[34] Fluids can be administered by several routes. Crystalloids administered rectally should be isotonic; rapid rectal absorption of hyperosmolar solutions can lead to life-threatening hyperosmolarity. Subcutaneous administration may be an acceptable route if small volumes of warmed isotonic fluids are administered in patients with normal hydration. Intraosseous fluid administration is an acceptable route of administration if a central vein is not accessible.[18,35] Oral rehydration is recommended

as the preferred therapy for dehydration caused by diarrhea in human pediatric patients.[36]

Differential distribution of drug to growing tissues may also predispose the pediatric patient to toxicities or side effects. For example, tetracyclines may bind to cations in the developing teeth prior to deposition of enamel, causing a brown discoloration.

Metabolism

Drug elimination, via hepatic metabolism and renal excretion, is limited in neonatal and pediatric patients. Thus, many drugs administered to the young animal are characterized by decreased clearance.[8,11] In contrast to human infants, hepatic metabolism of drugs is immature in the near-term and neonatal puppy.[37-39] Both phase I (i.e., oxidative) and phase II (i.e., glucuronidation) reactions are reduced. The various metabolic pathways mature at different rates. In puppies, phase I activity may not occur or may not be evident until 9 days of age if it does occur. Activity appears to increase progressively after day 25, potentially not reaching adult levels until 135 days postpartum.[38] Drug metabolism in pediatric patients, however, is quite complex. For example, Ecobichon and colleagues[40] found that in Beagle puppies, phase I metabolites decreased with age; and for phase II metabolism, glucuronidation predominated with sulfonation decreasing as puppies got older. The relevance to cats is not clear, but it does suggest that the traditional expectation of when drug-metabolizing enzymes mature should be challenged.

Generally, decreased hepatic drug metabolism is reflected by decreased plasma clearance, increased plasma half-life, and potentially toxic PDCs. Dose reduction, prolongation of dose intervals, or both, may be indicated for some drugs. Several antimicrobials are not recommended for pediatric patients. These include chloramphenicol, tetracyclines, doxycycline, and drugs that undergo enterohepatic circulation (e.g., clindamycin and to some degree, doxycycline) because they are more likely to disrupt the normal colonization of the alimentary tract in pediatric patients.

Oral bioavailability of drugs characterized by significant first-pass metabolism in adults (e.g., opioids) is probably greater in puppies and kittens. On the other hand, response to prodrugs (e.g., prednisone) may be reduced because of decreased formation of active drug products. This might also affect other drugs whose active metabolites contribute significantly to drug efficacy (e.g., tramadol). Pediatric hepatic drug-metabolizing enzymes do appear to be inducible by phenobarbital and other drugs. Nonhepatic drug-metabolizing enzymes also appear to be decreased in pediatric patients. For example, lower plasma cholinesterase in puppies can result in increased sensitivity to organophosphates, succinylcholine, and procaine; the same is likely to be true for kittens.[40]

Excretion

Reduced renal excretion results in decreased clearance of renally excreted parent drugs and products of phase II drug metabolism in pediatric puppies. Although the number of glomeruli remains constant throughout pediatric development, both glomerular filtration and renal tubular function progressively increase.[31,41] Adult values may not be reached until approximately 10 weeks of age. In contrast to glomerular filtration and secretion, renal tubular reabsorption in puppies appears to be similar to that in adults as long as the volume and composition of body fluids and electrolytes are maintained.[42,43] The results of developmental changes in pediatric renal function include decreased clearance and prolonged half-life of (primarily water-soluble) drugs excreted by the kidneys. Such a pattern has been shown for several drugs. Compared with current recommendations for adults, pediatric patients may require a higher dose of gentamicin due to increased volume of distribution. However, with once-daily administration, the need to prolong dosing intervals is less clear unless there is evidence of renal dysfunction in unhealthy kittens that are affected by conditions that increase the potential for gentamicin-induced nephrotoxicity (e.g., dehydration). Interestingly, in puppies, underdeveloped glomeruli may actually protect them from aminoglycoside-induced nephrotoxicity.[2] Further investigations are needed to establish safe yet effective doses of gentamicin for the neonatal kitten.

PHYSIOLOGIC CHANGES IN THE GERIATRIC PATIENT

Aging changes impact both the disposition (pharmacokinetics) of the drug (ADME) which influences plasma (and thus tissue drug concentrations), as well as the body's responses to the drug (pharmacodynamics). Selected clinically important changes are outlined in Table 101-2. Age-related changes in pharmacokinetics (gerontokinetics) and pharmacodynamics have been described in general, although most data is extrapolated from humans.[44-46] Aging in most species results in impaired adaptive and homeostatic mechanisms, resulting in increasing susceptibility to external and internal stressors.[44] Oxidative stress, mitochondrial aging, and apoptosis contribute to changes in drug disposition compared to the younger adult. Geriatric animals are at a greater risk for therapeutic failure or adverse drug events because of normal aging-related changes in physiology, an increased incidence of disease, and the likelihood of polypharmacy in response to disease. Moreover, a decrease in normal organ protective mechanisms may increase the risk of adverse events. The age at which body functions shift from a period of growth to one of decay (16 to 18 years in humans) has not been established in cats. Aging is accompanied by permanent loss of up to 30% of body cells, with a parallel loss in oxygen consumption. Body composition and regional blood flow rates change and physiologic functions generally decline steadily with increasing age. Whereas in humans and dogs, decreases in basal metabolic rates (in humans at a rate of 0.4% per year[45]) are accompanied by a corresponding decrease in caloric needs; in the cat, there is no evidence of age-related decline in energy intake, and

energy and protein requirements actually increase after 11 years of age.[47] Statistics on organ mass and function are not available in cats, but again, in humans, organ mass reduces in size and function by approximately 25%, resulting in corresponding changes in drug disposition. The combined impact of these changes among the body systems can influence all four drug movements. In human medicine, the approach of "start low and go slow" might apply to geriatric cats as well.

Age-related changes in the central and peripheral nervous systems are characterized by a decrease in brain weight and the number of peripheral fibers and peripheral connective tissue infiltration.[45] Oxygen consumption and cerebral blood flow decrease, as does the number of neurotransmitters. In dogs, changes in the blood-brain barrier have been documented.[48]

In the geriatric cardiovascular system, cardiac output decreases and circulation transit time increases. In humans, cardiac output decreases by about 1% per year for a total decline of 30% to 40% in the aged. Regional and organ blood flow rates similarly decrease.[45] The net effect of these changes depends on each drug movement. Absorption, metabolism, and excretion are likely to decrease, whereas distribution may increase or decrease depending on the state of vascular responses or fluid retention.[45,49,50] As cardiac function decreases, secondary compensatory responses redistribute blood flow to the brain and heart, increasing the risk of adverse reactions to drugs toxic to these tissues. Cardiac disease can exacerbate these changes.

In the geriatric human respiratory tract, residual lung volume decreases by 50% with accompanying decreases in vital capacity, partial pressure of oxygen, and maximum oxygen uptake. In addition, the central response to hypoxia and hypercapnia, such as that induced by opioid analgesics, decreases.[45] Anesthetic or other sedating agents must be used more cautiously.

With aging, deglutition decreases as a result of decreased salivation and pharyngeal and esophageal motility. In general, oral administration of drugs in cats presents a greater risk due to reduced esophageal motility, and the risk of esophageal erosions is probably greater in geriatric cats.[51,52] Gastric function is impacted by mucosal atrophy and reduction of hydrochloric acid secretion with a subsequent increase in gastric pH. Gastrointestinal motility is generally reduced. The intestinal macrovilli and microvilli atrophy, increasing the risk of bacterial overgrowth. These sequelae tend to reduce the absorption, and thus the PDC, of orally administered drugs. Changes in GI function (including a reduction in gastroprotective mechanisms) may also predispose the geriatric patient to GI adverse drug events, including those associated with chemotherapeutic agents and nonsteroidal anti-inflammatory drugs (NSAIDs). Digestibility of key nutrients, such as fat and protein, tends to decrease in elderly cats.[53] As with humans, the intestinal microbiota population shifts in elderly dogs and cats, with the proportions of lactobacilli decreasing and clostridia increasing (in dogs)[54] and bifidobacteria decreasing in cats.[55] In addition to their response to antimicrobials, these changes might influence the enterohepatic circulation of bile acids and thus potentially some drugs.[56]

Changes in hepatic function are important to the geriatric animal for those drugs requiring hepatic metabolism.[57] Hepatocyte numbers and function decrease, as do hepatic and splanchnic blood flow, hepatic oxidation, and cytochrome P450 content (the primary drug-metabolizing enzyme). Both flow-limited and capacity-limited drugs are affected. For example, hepatic clearance of both opioid analgesics (which are characterized by first-pass metabolism; i.e., flow limited) and nonsteroidal analgesics (eliminated principally by hepatic metabolism; i.e., capacity limited) is decreased in geriatric patients. The increased responsiveness of human geriatric patients to opioid analgesics, leading them to require 60% to 75% less drug than younger patients, has been attributed to changes in drug elimination.[58,59] Changes in hepatic function, oxygenation, and nutrition may also predispose the liver to drug-induced hepatotoxicity. Because of reduced hepatic function, the geriatric cat, even more so than other species, may be less able to generate endogenous hepatoprotective agents, increasing the risk of drug-induced hepatotoxicity.[4]

As renal blood flow decreases, the glomerular filtration rate and active secretory capacity of the nephron unit progressively decrease with age. Both result in a similar decline in renal clearance. Renal excretion is the major route of elimination of many drugs; therefore, changes in renal clearance tend to prolong the elimination and increase PDCs in the geriatric patient. Changes in renal function also render the geriatric patient more susceptible to adverse drug reactions, such as those induced by aminoglycosides, angiotensin-converting enzyme inhibitors, and NSAID analgesics.

Changes in Distribution

Drug disposition is influenced by a number of factors that change with age. These include, but are not limited to, body composition, and plasma and tissue proteins that influence drug movement from plasma and into tissues and back. Changes in body composition may be among the most complex in the geriatric animal.[60] The impact of aging on body composition in cats varies. Although middle-aged cats tend to be overweight, geriatric cats often become thin.[53] Thus, the proportion of total body water, including both extracellular and intracellular fluid is likely to decline. Plasma drug concentrations of water-soluble drugs might be expected to be higher in older animals compared with those of young adults, even if dosing on a mg/kg body weight basis, whereas for lipid-soluble drugs, dosing on a mg/kg body weight basis might compensate for potential changes in plasma concentrations (see Table 101-3). Erring on the side of underdosing (e.g., dose reduction of 25%) might be prudent for those drugs characterized by a narrow therapeutic window. It is important to note that the elimination half-life of such drugs might be shorter (rather than longer), so a change in dosing interval may not be as effective as a change in dose.

Tissue Proteins

Drugs are carried in plasma by proteins to the tissues where they are inactivated via binding to tissue proteins. Although total plasma protein content probably remains the same in the geriatric animal, the proportion represented by albumin decreases and that represented by globulins increases. Changes in plasma albumin can be clinically important to patients receiving highly protein-bound drugs, with the risk of adversity greater for those drugs that are potentially toxic, such as NSAIDs. Decreased albumin can result in a greater proportion of free drug; importantly, most NSAIDs are close to 99% protein bound. A decrease of only 1% (i.e., 99% to 98% binding) doubles the concentration of a pharmacologically active drug. The consequences of an increased PDC may be offset by a compensatory increased clearance, because only unbound drugs are generally conducive to hepatic or renal clearance. This balance might be compromised, however, if organs of clearance are negatively affected. As such, caution is recommended in simultaneously administered drugs that are highly protein bound if one of them is potentially toxic.

A number of transport proteins are responsible for binding drugs in tissues. Among the most notable are influx and efflux proteins, which move drugs into and out of cells.[4] Because such proteins tend to be located in portals of entry (sites where drugs enter the body) and sanctuaries (sites the body protects from unwanted drug influx), altered drug movement can lead to higher—or lower—than desired drug concentrations. Differences, and specifically, deficiencies noted in the cat have been demonstrated for proteins responsible for efflux of phototoxic fluoroquinolones from the retina.[61] The geriatric cat is likely to be predisposed to the consequences of deficiencies from changes in efflux protein number or function, as well as changes in elimination of the drugs (particularly enrofloxacin) as renal function declines.

Receptor Sensitivity and Pharmacodynamics

Geriatric patients respond differently to some drugs, suggesting that tissue receptor sensitivity to the drugs is altered. Changes in receptor number or responsiveness have been implicated but not documented.[45,46] Physiologic changes, such as altered neurotransmission or intracellular constituents, have also been suggested. For example, although human geriatric patients are more likely to experience pain compared with young adults, changes in neurologic function may decrease the perception of pain.[62] Thus, the need for analgesic therapy is often not detected and alternative pain assessment tools have been developed for the geriatric human patient.[62] In addition, geriatric patients are less able to respond to many analgesic drugs.

Diseased Geriatric Cat

Aged animals are more likely to be suffering from diseases that affect not only drug disposition but also tissue receptivity to drugs and organ protection.[59] Recommended changes in

BOX 101-3 How to Adjust Doses or Intervals for Drugs That Are Potentially Toxic

Creatinine clearance or serum creatinine can be used to adjust doses or intervals for drugs that are potentially toxic:

$$\text{New dose} = \text{old dose} \times \frac{\text{patient creatinine clearance}}{\text{normal creatinine clearance}}$$

or

$$\text{New dose} = \text{old dose} \times \frac{\text{normal serum creatinine}}{\text{patient serum creatinine}}$$

A more appropriate response might be a change in the interval:

$$\text{New interval} = \text{old interval} \times \frac{\text{normal creatinine clearance}}{\text{patient creatinine clearance}}$$

or

$$\text{New interval} = \text{old interval} \times \frac{\text{patient serum creatinine}}{\text{normal serum creatinine}}$$

For example, if the serum creatinine is twofold higher than normal, a drug normally given every 12 hours would be given every 24 hours, or the dose could be reduced by 50%. If only half of the drug is eliminated by the kidneys, the interval would need to be prolonged only by 50% (i.e., to 18 hours). Thus, it might be more practical to reduce the dose by 25%.

drug disposition in the presence of disease can be profound. Changes have been reviewed elsewhere and should be considered.[4] However, among the changes that have the most predictable effects on drug disposition is renal disease. In general, clearance of any drug (or any proportion of the drug) will change in concert with renal blood flow (see Box 101-3). For hepatic disease, although no clinical laboratory test accurately predicts the impact of disease on drug disposition, as a rule of thumb, if albumin is normal, drug metabolism is not likely to be substantively impacted. Drugs which undergo high first-pass metabolism, however, will be proportionately impacted in cases of portosystemic shunting.

The immune system of the geriatric patient is not as effective as that of the adult[63] (see Chapter 97). As a result, it may be prudent to use bactericidal antimicrobials and minimize the use of immunosuppressive drugs. In addition, the geriatric patient is more likely to be receiving multiple drugs, which increases the likelihood of drug interactions. Finally, diseases of selected organs may predispose these organs to drug-induced toxicity.

References

1. Dowling P: Geriatric pharmacology. *Vet Clin North Am Small Anim Pract* 35(3):557–569, 2005.
2. Boothe DM, Tannert K: Special considerations for drug and fluid therapy in the pediatric patient. *Compend Contin Educ Pract Vet* 14:313–329, 1991.
3. Jolivette LJ, Ward KW: Extrapolation of human pharmacokinetic parameters from rat, dog, and monkey data: molecular properties associated with extrapolative success or failure. *J Pharm Sci* 94:1467–1483, 2005.
4. Boothe DM: Factors affecting drug disposition. In Boothe DM, editor: *Small animal clinical pharmacology and therapeutics*, ed 2, St Louis, 2012, Elsevier, pp 34–70.
5. Shah SS, Sanda S, Regmi NL, et al: Characterization of cytochrome P450-mediated drug metabolism in cats. *J Vet Pharmacol Ther* 30:422–428, 2007.
6. Boothe DM: Drug therapy in cats. Mechanisms and avoidance of adverse drug reactions. *J Am Vet Med Assoc* 196:1297–1306, 1990.
7. Robinson EP: Anesthesia of pediatric patients. *Compend Contin Educ Pract Vet* 5(12):1004–1011, 1983.
8. Green TP, Mirkin BL: Clinical pharmacokinetics: pediatric considerations. In Benet LZ, Massoud N, Gambertoglio JG, editors: *Pharmacokinetic basis for drug treatment*, New York, 1984, Raven Press, pp 269–282.
9. Harper EJ, Turner CL: Age-related changes in apparent digestibility in growing kittens. *Reprod Nutr Dev* 40:249–260, 2000.
10. Heimann G: Enteral absorption and bioavailability in children in relation to age. *Eur J Clin Pharmacol* 18:43–50, 1980.
11. Rane A, Wilson JT: Clinical pharmacokinetics in infants and children. In Gibaldi M, Prescott L, editors: *Handbook of clinical pharmacokinetics*, New York, 1983, ADIS Health Science Press, pp 142–168.
12. Gillette DD, Filkins M: Factors affecting antibody transfer in the newborn puppy. *Am J Physiol* 210(2):419–422, 1966.
13. Morselli PL, Morselli RF, Bossi L: Clinical pharmacokinetics in newborns and infants: age-related differences and therapeutic implications. In Gibaldi M, Prescott L, editors: *Handbook of clinical pharmacokinetics*, New York, 1983, ADIS Health Science Press, pp 99–141.
14. Jones RL: Special considerations for appropriate antimicrobial therapy in neonates. *Vet Clin North Am Small Anim Pract* 17(3):577–601, 1987.
15. Shifrine M, Munn SL, Rosenblatt LS, et al: Hematologic changes to 60 days of age in clinically normal beagles. *Lab Anim* 23(6):894–898, 1973.
16. Authement JM, Wolfsheimer KJ, Catchings S, et al: Canine blood component therapy: product preparation, storage, and administration. *J Am Anim Hosp Assoc* 23:483–493, 1987.
17. Fiser DH: Intraosseous infusion. *N Engl J Med* 322(22):1579–1581, 1990.
18. Little S: Feline pediatrics: how to treat the small and the sick. *Compendium* 33:E1–E6, 2011.
19. Berlin CM: Pharmacologic considerations of drug use in the lactating mother. *Obstet Gynecol* 58(5):17S–23S, 1981.
20. Rasmussen F: Excretion of drugs by milk. In Brodie BB, Gillette JR, editors: *Handbook of experimental pharmacology, vol 28: concepts in biochemical pharmacology, part I*, New York, 1979, Springer-Verlag, p 390.
21. Smith HW: The development of the flora of the alimentary tract in young animals. *J Pathol Bacteriol* 90:495–513, 1965.
22. Sheng HP, Huggins RA: Growth of the beagle: changes in the body fluid compartments. *Proc Soc Exp Biol Med* 139:330–335, 1972.

23. Davis LE, Westfall BA, Short CR: Biotransformation and pharmacokinetics of salicylate in newborn animals. *Am J Vet Res* 34(8):1105–1108, 1973.

24. Baggot JD: Principles of antimicrobial bioavailability and disposition. In Prescott JF, Baggot JD, Walker RD, editors: *Antimicrobial therapy in veterinary medicine*, ed 3, Ames, IA, 2000, Blackwell, pp 50–87.

25. Goldstein R, Lavy E, Shem-Tov M, et al: Pharmacokinetics of ampicillin administered intravenously and intraosseously to kittens. *Res Vet Sci* 59:186–187, 1995.

26. Lavy E, Goldstein R, Shem-Tov M, et al: Disposition kinetics of ampicillin administered intravenously and intraosseously to canine puppies. *J Vet Pharmacol Ther* 18:379–381, 1995.

27. Seguin MA, Papich MG, Sigle K: Pharmacokinetics of enrofloxacin in neonatal kittens. *Am J Vet Res* 65:350–356, 2004.

28. Poffenbarger EM, Ralston SL, Chandler ML, et al: Canine neonatology, part I. Physiological differences between puppies and adults. *Compend Contin Educ Pract Vet* 12(11):1601–1609, 1990.

29. Ehrnebo M, Agurell S, Jalling B, et al: Age differences in drug binding by plasma proteins: studies on human fetuses, neonates and adults. *Eur J Clin Pharmacol* 3:189–193, 1973.

30. Horster M, Kemler BJ, Valtin H: Intracortical distribution of number and volume of glomeruli during postnatal maturation in the dog. *J Clin Invest* 50:796–800, 1971.

31. Horster M, Valtin H: Postnatal development of renal function: micropuncture and clearance studies in the dog. *J Clin Invest* 50:779–795, 1971.

32. Hellmann J, Vannucci RC, Nardis EE: Blood-brain barrier permeability to lactic acid in the newborn dog: lactate as a cerebral metabolic fuel. *Pediatr Res* 16:40–44, 1982.

33. Ginsberg G, Hattis D, Russ A, et al: Pharmacokinetic and pharmacodynamic factors that can affect sensitivity to neurotoxic sequelae in elderly individuals. *Environ Health Perspect* 113:1243–1249, 2005.

34. Kerner JA, Sunshine P: Parenteral alimentation. *Semin Perinatol* 3(4):417–434, 1979.

35. Otto CM, Kaufman GM, Crowe DT: Intraosseous infusion of fluids and therapeutics. *Compend Contin Educ Pract Vet* 11(4):421–431, 1989.

36. Hirschhorn N: Oral rehydration therapy for diarrhea in children: a basic primer. *Nutr Rev* 40(4):97–104, 1982.

37. Reiche R: Drug disposition in the newborn. In Ruckesbusch P, Toutain P, Koritz D, editors: *Veterinary pharmacology and toxicology*, Westport, CT, 1983, AVI Publishing, pp 49–55.

38. Peters EL, Farber TM, Heider A, et al: The development of drug-metabolizing enzymes in the young dog. *Fed Proc Am Soc Biol* 30:560, 1971.

39. Inman RC, Yeary RA: Sulfadimethoxine pharmacokinetics in neonatal and young dogs. *Fed Proc Am Soc Biol* 30:560, 1971.

40. Ecobichon DJ, D'Ver AS, Ehrhart W: Drug disposition and biotransformation in the developing beagle dog. *Fundam Appl Toxicol* 11:29–37, 1988.

41. Cowan RH, Jukkola AF, Arant BS: Pathophysiologic evidence of gentamicin nephrotoxicity in neonatal puppies. *Pediatr Res* 14:1204–1211, 1980.

42. Kleinman LI: Renal bicarbonate reabsorption in the newborn dog. *J Physiol* 281:487–498, 1978.

43. Bovee KC, Jezyk PF, Segal SC: Postnatal development of renal tubular amino acid reabsorption in canine pups. *Am J Vet Res* 45(4):830–832, 1984.

44. McLean AJ, Le Couteur DG: Aging biology and geriatric clinical pharmacology. *Pharmacol Rev* 56(2):163–184, 2004.

45. Ritschel WA: *Gerontokinetics: the pharmacokinetics of drugs in the elderly*, Caldwell, NJ, 1988, Telford Press, pp 1–16.

46. Feely J, Coakley D: Altered pharmacodynamics in the elderly. *Clin Pharm* 6:269–283, 1990.

47. Harper EJ: Changing perspectives on aging and energy requirements: aging and digestive function in humans, dogs and cats. *J Nutr* 128(12 Suppl):2632S–2635S, 1998.

48. Morita TY, Mizutani Y, Sawada M, et al: Immunohistochemical and ultrastructural findings related to the blood-brain barrier in the blood vessels of the cerebral white matter in aged dogs. *J Comp Pathol* 133:14–22, 2005.

49. Benowitz NL: Effects of cardiac disease on pharmacokinetics: pathophysiologic considerations. In Benet LZ, Massoud N, Gamberto-glio JG, editors: *Pharmacokinetic basis for drug treatment*, New York, 1984, Raven Press, pp 89–104.

50. Aucoin DP: Drug therapy in the geriatric animal: the effect of aging on drug disposition. *Vet Clin North Am Small Anim Pract* 19:41–48, 1989.

51. Westfall DS, Twedt DC, Steyn PF, et al: Evaluation of esophageal transit of tablets and capsules in 30 cats. *J Vet Intern Med* 15(5):467–470, 2008.

52. Carlborg B, Densert O: Esophageal lesions caused by orally administered drugs. An experimental study in the cat. *Eur Surg Res* 12(4):270–282, 1980.

53. Perez-Camargo G, Young L: Nutrient digestibility in old versus young cats. *Compendium* 27(3A):84, 2005.

54. Benno Y, Nakao H, Uchida K, et al: Impact of the advances in age on the gastrointestinal microflora of beagle dogs. *J Vet Med Sci* 54:703–706, 1992.

55. Patil AR, Czarnecki-Maulden GL, Dowling KE: Effect of advances in age on fecal microflora of cats. *FASEB J* 14(4):A488, 2000.

56. Hickman MA, Bruss ML, Morris JG, et al: Dietary-protein source (soybean vs casein) and taurine status affect kinetics of the enterohepatic circulation of taurocholic acid in cats. *J Nutr* 122:1019–1028, 1992.

57. Sheaker S, Bay M: Drug disposition and hepatotoxicity in the elderly. *J Clin Gastroenterol* 18:232–237, 1994.

58. Enck RE: Pain control in the ambulatory elderly. *Geriatrics* 46:49–60, 1991.

59. Workman BS, Ciccone V, Christophidis N: Pain management for the elderly. *Aust Fam Physician* 18:1515–1527, 1989.

60. Lawler DE, Evans RH, Larson BT, et al: Influence of lifetime food restriction on causes, time, and predictors of death in dogs. *J Am Vet Med Assoc* 226:225–231, 2005.

61. Wiebe V, Hamilton P: Fluoroquinolone-induced retinal degeneration in cats. *J Am Vet Med Assoc* 221:1508–1571, 2002.

62. Schofield PA: The assessment and management of peri-operative pain in older adults. *Anaesthesia* 69(Suppl 1):54–60, 2014.

63. Schultz RD: The effects of aging on the immune system. *Compend Contin Educ Pract Vet* 6(12):1096–1105, 1984.

Neonatal Resuscitation and Supportive Care in Cats

Michelle Kutzler

The unique anatomical and physiological characteristics of neonatal feline patients make emergency care and resuscitation efforts especially challenging. Adult parameters cannot be relied upon in these patients. For the purposes of this chapter, neonates are defined as kittens under 3 weeks of age. To provide optimal care to kittens in a neonatal intensive care situation, a veterinarian should be familiar with normal vital signs, nursing care (e.g., pain management), cardiovascular and fluid-resuscitation therapies, and probable diseases (e.g., neonatal isoerythrolysis).

PHYSICAL EXAMINATION OF CRITICAL NEONATES

When presented with a critically ill neonate or one in need of resuscitation, it is important for the practitioner to take a few moments to complete a physical examination. In human medicine, routine evaluation is performed immediately after birth to identify newborns that require prompt medical intervention. In 1952, Dr. Virginia Apgar[1] developed a simple, reliable scoring system for evaluating human babies that has also been used to evaluate the effectiveness of neonatal resuscitation efforts.[2] The Apgar scoring system has been modified for puppies and shown to correlate well with assessments of newborn viability and short-term survival prognoses (Table 102-1).[3] Although similar research has not been published for neonatal kittens, this scoring system has been used by clinicians in newborn cats.

The normal heart rate for neonatal kittens is greater than 220 beats per minute. At birth, the normal respiratory rate ranges from 10 to 18 breaths per minute, and increases to 16 to 32 breaths per minute (comparable to that of an adult animal) by 1 week of age.[4] Normal rectal temperatures in kittens during the first week of life are from 94.5 to 97.5 °F (35 to 36 °C) and then increase to 98.6 to 100 °F (37 to 38.2 °C) during the remainder of the neonatal period.[4] Mucous membrane color and capillary refill time are good indicators of hydration and perfusion in neonates.[5] Neonates normally have hyperemic mucous membranes for the first week of life.[6] Typical methods for assessing hydration in adult animals (e.g., skin tenting) are unreliable in neonates because of increased body water content and decreased fat content of the skin compared with adults. In addition, urine is not concentrated in neonates even in cases of severe dehydration.

CARDIOPULMONARY RESUSCITATION IN NEONATES

At birth, initial survival depends upon the ability of the neonate to clear the lungs of amniotic fluid, expand the lungs with air, and begin breathing. Bulb suctioning of the airways can help to clear out accumulated fluid (Figure 102-1). Aggressive suctioning of the airways with suctioning devices should be avoided because it can cause a vagal response or laryngospasm. Gentle but brisk rubbing of the neonate over the entire body will stimulate respirations. Specifically, stimulation of the neonatal genital or umbilical region induces reflex respiration during the first 3 days of life. This can be used to stimulate respiration in weak or ineffectively breathing neonates.[7]

Traditional recommendations to gently "swing" newborns (where the neonate is cradled in cupped hands and swung in a downward motion from midtorso height to knee height to remove amniotic fluid from the airways and lungs) can result in intracranial trauma. Although the head and neck are typically supported while "swinging," the rapid deceleration (linear or rotational) is sufficient to induce significant intracranial (subdural and intracerebral) hemorrhage consistent with "shaken baby syndrome."[8]

Although no clinical trials have been performed in kittens, the use of the Renzhong (JenChung, GV26) acupressure point may stimulate respiration as well.[9] A 25-gauge needle is inserted into the nasal philtrum at the base of the nostrils and rotated when bone is contacted. Doxapram has been commonly used for neonatal resuscitation, but its use in veterinary medicine is controversial.[9] Doxapram is rarely used in resuscitation of human neonates. Doxapram can be given under the tongue (sublingually) to stimulate respirations in a newborn with no respiratory drive. However, the effectiveness of doxapram is greatly decreased if the brain is hypoxic, so administration during hypoventilation is unlikely to result in a favorable response.[10]

Neonates have profoundly different responses to hypoxia than adult animals. For example, hypoxic neonates experience bradycardia that is not mediated vagally despite evidence of parasympathetic maturity.[7] In fact, administration of parasympatholytic agents (e.g., atropine) to neonates only exacerbates myocardial hypoxia by increasing oxygen demand and is therefore contraindicated.[9] The most effective treatment for

Table 102-1	Apgar Scoring Modified for Use during Resuscitation of Neonatal Puppies		
	SCORE		
Parameter	**0**	**1**	**2**
Heart rate	Less than 180 beats/min	180-220 beats/min	Greater than 220 beats/min
Respiratory effort	No crying with fewer than 6 breaths/min	Mild crying with 6-15 breaths/min	Crying with more than 15 breaths/min
Mucus membrane color	Cyanotic	Pale	Pink
Reflex irritability	No vocalization with no leg retraction	Weak vocalization with weak leg retraction	Crying with quick leg retraction
Spontaneous movement	Absence of movement	Weak movement	Strong movement

Reprinted with permission from Veronesi MC, Panzani S, Faustini M, et al: An Apgar scoring system for routine assessment of newborn puppy viability and short-term survival prognosis. *Theriogenology* 72:401-407, 2009.
Although similar research has not been published for neonatal kittens, this scoring system has been used by clinicians in newborn cats. A score of 7 to 10 is indicative of no distress; a score of 4 to 6 indicates moderate distress; a score of 0 to 3 is indicative of severe distress. Apgar scores of 6 or lower require immediate action.

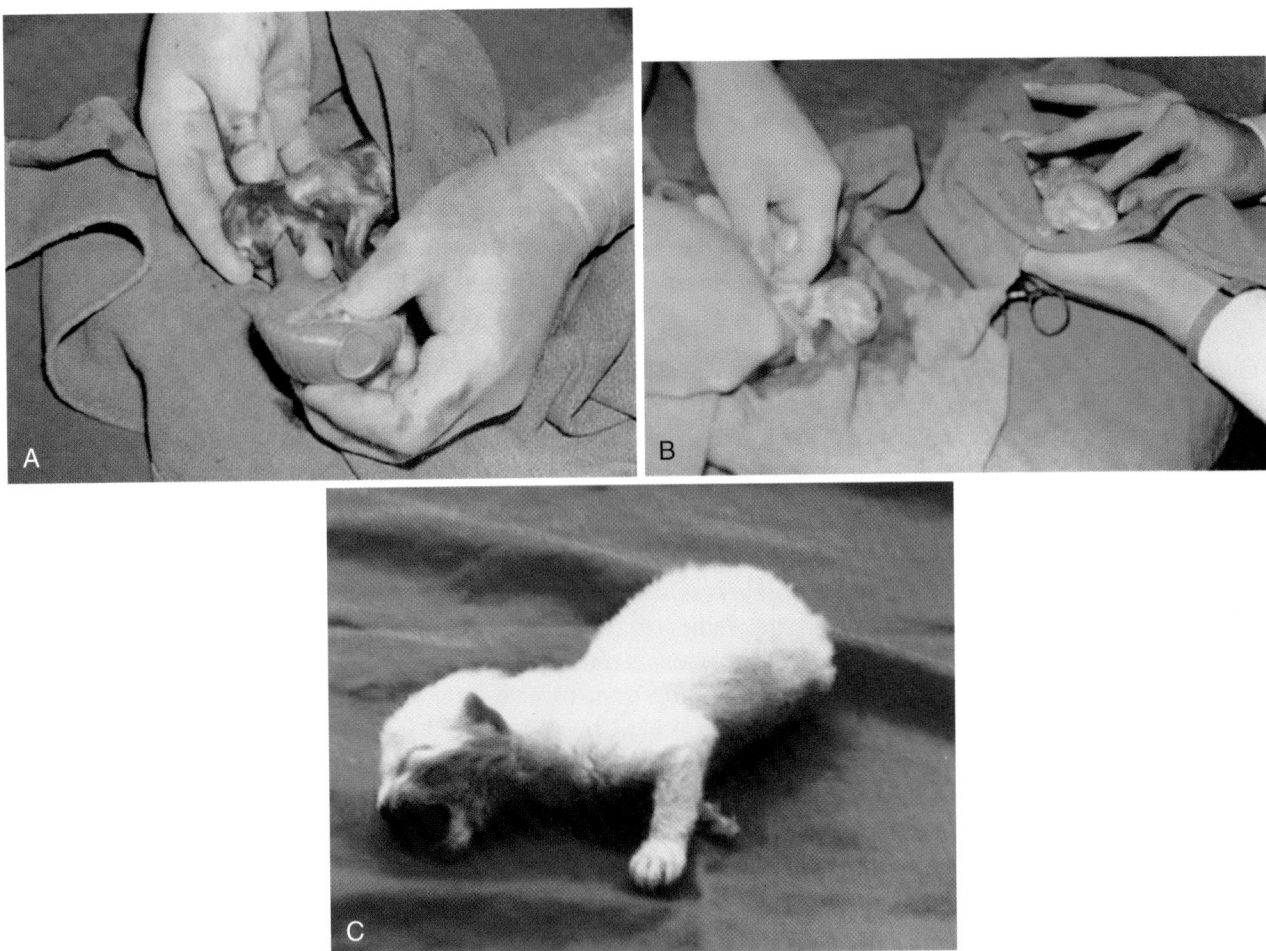

Figure 102-1: Stimulation of respiration is a critical component of neonatal resuscitation. **A,** At birth, bulb suctioning of the airways can help to clear out any accumulated fluid. **B,** Gentle but brisk rubbing of the neonate over the entire body will stimulate respirations. However, if respiration distress continues (**C**), oxygen therapy and positive pressure ventilation will be needed. (Reprinted with permission from McMichael M: Emergency and critical care issues. In Peterson ME, Kutzler MA, editors: *Small animal pediatrics: the first twelve months of life,* St Louis, 2011, Elsevier Saunders, pp 73-81.)

neonatal bradycardia is to increase partial pressure arterial oxygen through supplemental oxygen. According to human guidelines on neonatal resuscitation, "ventilation of the lungs is the single most effective step in cardiopulmonary resuscitation of the compromised infant."[11] Oxygen should be supplied via a tight-fitting facemask or endotracheal tube (size 1 and 2 standard uncuffed tubes). For very small patients, a 12- to 16-gauge intravenous (IV) catheter can be substituted for an endotracheal tube.[9] If there are no respirations, the neonate should be ventilated at 40 to 60 breaths per minute. Respiratory resuscitation should be performed for about 30 seconds before cardiac compressions are started, should they be required. If the chest is not expanding, the seal on the facemask or the endotracheal tube should be checked. The head and neck should be extended to facilitate movement of air into the trachea and limit the amount of air forced into the stomach via the esophagus.

Although lung expansion is essential for adequate ventilation, overexpansion also causes serious damage, so minimal pressure (20 to 30 cm of H_2O pressure applied for about 3 seconds) should be used for ventilation.[9] A resuscitation bag designed for human pediatric patients (e.g., Pediatric Bag Valve Mask, Galls Emergency Medical Products, Carlsbad, California) should be used. Oxygen therapy should be kept at or below a fraction of inspired oxygen of 0.4 to avoid oxygen toxicity, which is an even greater concern in neonates than in adults. Excess oxygen supplementation in neonates can cause retrolental fibroplasia, which can lead to permanent blindness.[12]

Following respiratory resuscitation, in kittens with persistently low heart rates (40 to 60 beats per minute), lateral chest compressions with the thumb and forefinger should be begun at a rate of 1 to 2 beats per second, pausing for respiratory exertions.[9] For neonates in cardiac arrest, and when respiratory support and chest compression have failed to elicit a heartbeat, epinephrine may be administered (0.1 to 0.3 mg/kg) IV or intraosseously (IO).[9] Naloxone used to be recommended for use in all apneic neonates. This was based upon findings that there was a surge of endorphins at the time of parturition (especially during a stressful birth), which was associated with respiratory depression. However, research has shown that the use of naloxone is not effective and may even be detrimental if given to a hypoxemic patient, as it may worsen the existing bradycardia. It may still be beneficial in cases where the neonate shows signs of respiratory depression and the queen received an opiate injection before or during a cesarean (C-section).

When IV or IO access is unavailable, endotracheal administration of epinephrine at two to three times the IV dose has been recommended. The drug should be diluted in an appropriate volume of saline (0.9% NaCl) solution (0.5 mL/2 kg of body weight) and injected through a catheter that extends just beyond the tip of the endotracheal tube. Endotracheal administration of the standard IV dose of epinephrine is to be avoided because it causes a decrease of arterial blood pressure mediated by beta-adrenergic receptors unopposed by alpha-adrenergic vasoconstriction. However, endotracheal

administration of vasopressin (1 International unit/kg) may be a better option for the treatment of cardiac arrest because it stimulates blood pressure instead of decreasing blood pressure and has a more rapid, vigorous, and protracted effect.[13] Vasopressin was successful as a rescue therapy for children after prolonged cardiac arrest.[14]

The use of sodium bicarbonate in neonatal resuscitation is controversial. The guidelines from the American Heart Association Manual on Neonatal Advanced Life Support in humans do not recommend bicarbonate as frontline therapy because evidence for its efficacy is lacking.[15] However, in cases in which adequate ventilation is established but there has been no response to other therapies and a prolonged resuscitation effort is unsuccessful, sodium bicarbonate may be useful.[9] If more than 15 minutes of resuscitation has failed to return spontaneous respiration and adequate circulation, some cases have anecdotally responded to the administration of 0.5 to 1.0 mL/kg sodium bicarbonate (8.4%) IV in the umbilical vein, diluted 1:2 with sterile water or normal saline.[9] Sodium bicarbonate should not be administered by the endotracheal route. Ventilation must be continued during and after administration because bicarbonate is metabolized to carbon dioxide and must be cleared via the lungs.[9]

Poor patient outcome (i.e., severe illness or death) in patients that survive the immediate resuscitation phase can be attributed to postcardiac arrest syndrome, the systemic ischemia and reperfusion response, and precipitating pathological changes.[16] Any precipitating disease may complicate further the treatment regimen, as will organ dysfunction such as ileus and renal injury. Hofmeister and colleagues reported that only 16% of dogs and cats that had a return of spontaneous circulation after in-hospital cardiac arrest and cardiopulmonary resuscitation survived to discharge from the hospital. However, there is no data published regarding outcomes after resuscitation in neonates.[17]

FLUID THERAPY IN NEONATES

Neonatal fluid requirements are higher than in adults, and dehydration can rapidly progress to hypovolemia if not adequately treated. In adults, hypovolemia is compensated for, or partially compensated for, by increasing the heart rate, concentrating the urine, and decreasing urine output. In neonates, these compensatory mechanisms do not exist.[18-20] Neonates have a greater body surface-area-to-volume ratio and increased skin permeability, which make them susceptible to rapid fluid losses. Neonates also have higher total body water content (80% of body weight compared with 60% in adult animals) and have immature renal function. Kittens are unable to concentrate urine until 8 weeks of age.

Because of rapid water turnover, dehydration and hypovolemia occur much more acutely in neonates.[21] Hypovolemia results in decreased perfusion and subsequent decreases in oxygen delivery to tissues. Aggressive fluid resuscitation is associated with decreased mortality in children with sepsis.[22] Neonates with hypovolemia may have normal skin turgor even when mucous membrane color and capillary refill time indicate shock. Because of the difficulties in adequately assessing hypovolemia in neonates, the practitioner should assume that all neonates with inadequate intake or with vomiting and diarrhea are dehydrated and potentially hypovolemic.

Treatment of hypovolemia in neonates includes fluid replacement and nutritional support. The patient should be weighed at least every 12 hours, preferably every 8 hours. On average, kittens should gain 10% of their body weight each day for the first few weeks of life. Any day a kitten fails to gain weight should alert the care-giver to dehydration. The normal birth weight of a kitten is 100 g ± 10 g. Birth weights lower than 90 g are associated with an increased risk of neonatal mortality. Methods for fluid replacement and nutritional support will vary depending upon the stage of life and severity of the underlying condition.

Oral Fluid Therapy

Oral fluid therapy can be an effective method for providing rehydration and nutrition to neonates that cannot suckle from the queen if they are not hypothermic, hypoglycemic, or hypotensive. Neonates can be fed with a syringe, dropper, or bottle (Figure 102-2). If using a syringe or dropper, care must be taken not to administer the liquid too quickly, because aspiration is a common complication. If using a bottle, the hole in the nipple may need to be enlarged with a hot needle so that a drop of milk forms easily when the bottle is turned upside down. The bottle should not be squeezed while feeding, to avoid aspiration. In a clinical setting, oral fluid therapy is often best accomplished via a 5 to 8 Fr feeding tube. The tube is measured from the tip of the nose to the last rib and marked, then lubricated. With the kitten in sternal recumbency (normal nursing position),

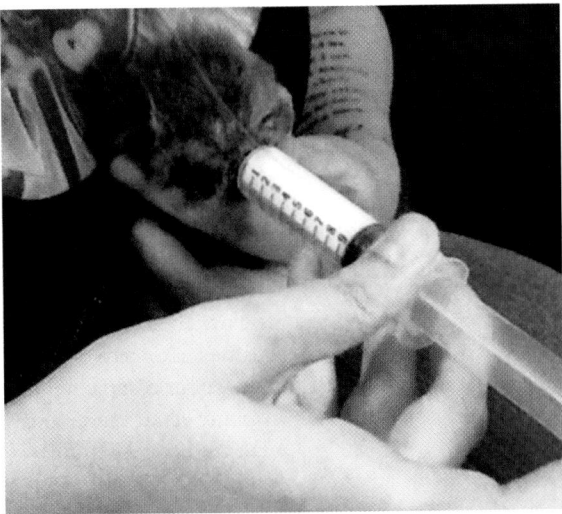

Figure 102-2: Oral fluid therapy can be an effective method for providing rehydration and nutrition to neonates that cannot suckle from the queen, if they are not hypothermic, hypoglycemic, or hypotensive. Neonates can be fed with a syringe, dropper, or bottle. (Photo courtesy of Dodi Reesman.)

the tube should be passed down the left side of the mouth. It should pass easily because neonates under 10 days of age lack a gag reflex.[23] Proper placement can be assured by instilling a small amount of sterile saline first and making sure that it does not come out of the nose. It is not recommended to fill the stomach to capacity (approximately 50 mL/kg) because of the increased risk of aspiration.[23] For newborn kittens on a commercial kitten milk replacer, a maximum of 5 mL should be given every 2 to 4 hours, increasing by 1 mL per day. Although the caloric density of commercial kitten milk replacers varies somewhat, most commercial milk replacers deliver approximately 1 kcal metabolizable energy (ME)/mL. The nutritional requirements for a kitten during first 3 days of life are 15 kcal ME/100 g of body weight, 20 kcal ME/100 g of body weight for days 4 to 6, and 20 to 25 kcal ME/100 g of body weight after day 6. The milk should be warmed to body temperature (approximately 100°F [37.7°C]) before feeding to reduce risk of chilling and aspiration. When removing the stomach tube after feeding, it is important to kink it to prevent aspiration of liquid that otherwise could drain from the tube as it is being pulled out. Opened liquid milk replacer or reconstituted powdered milk replacer should be used within 48 hours, provided the unused portion is refrigerated in a glass container. After use, the feeding tube and syringe should be disinfected and rinsed thoroughly in hot water between feedings.

Subcutaneous Fluid Therapy

Neonates with mild to moderate dehydration but normal perfusion can be treated with subcutaneous (SC) fluid therapy. Maintenance requirements are two to three times higher than for adult animals (120 to 180 mL/kg per day).[21] The best fluid to correct mild dehydration is a balanced electrolyte solution (e.g., lactated Ringer's solution or Normosol-R). If dextrose supplementation is desired, 0.45% NaCl with 2.5% dextrose can be administered SC. However, adding dextrose to isotonic fluids creates a hypertonic solution, which can draw fluid into the SC space. If hypokalemia is present, up to 30 mEq/L of KCl can be added to fluids for SC administration.

Intravenous or Intraosseous Fluid Therapy

Neonates with perfusion deficits do not absorb oral or SC administered fluids because of the peripheral vasoconstriction. In these hypovolemic patients, fluid resuscitation must be accomplished via the IV or IO route. In some patients, a 24-gauge, 3/4-inch catheter can be placed in the cephalic or femoral vein. However, these small-gauge catheters can easily burr when being driven through the skin. A small skin puncture can be made with a 20-gauge needle while keeping the skin elevated to create a pilot hole that the catheter can then be fed through to prevent burring of the catheter. More commonly, the jugular vein is used for IV catheterization. A 20- to 22-gauge, 1-inch catheter usually can be placed in the jugular vein.

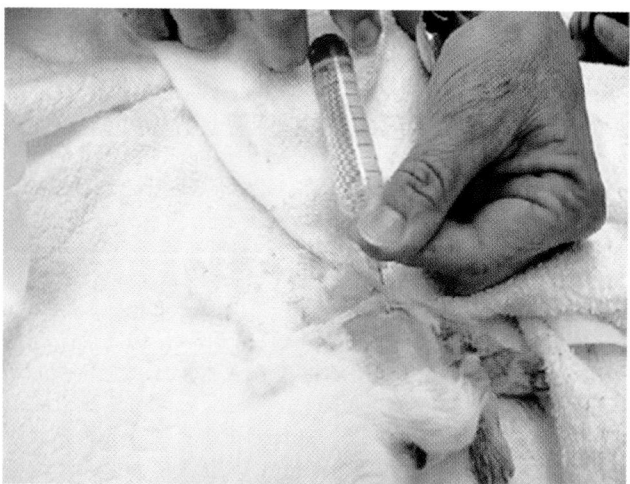

Figure 102-3: Fluid resuscitation of critically ill neonates can be accomplished by placing a spinal needle in the shaft of the femur and administering warmed fluids by the intraosseous route. (Reprinted with permission from Macintire D: Pediatric fluid therapy. *Vet Clin N Am Small Anim Pract* 38(3):621-627, 2008.)

If attempts at IV catheterization fail, an IO catheter should be placed. An IO catheter can be inserted in the proximal femur (greater trochanter) or humerus using an 18- to 22-gauge (1- or 2-inch) spinal needle or an 18- to 25-gauge, 1-inch hypodermic needle. Any fluid that can be given IV (e.g., blood, balanced electrolyte solution, or glucose) can also be given by the IO route at the same dose and rate.[24] The catheter placement area must be aseptically prepared, and the needle is inserted into the bone parallel to the long axis of the bone (Figure 102-3). The cortical bone is hard compared with the softer medullary cavity. Once the needle is firmly seated, the stylet can be removed and blood can be gently aspirated to ensure patency. Then, the catheter should be secured with a sterile bandage. However, if the patient is active or mobile, an IO catheter can be readily dislodged. Once the hypovolemia has been corrected, an IV catheter should be placed so that the IO catheter can be removed. Rarely should an IO catheter stay in place longer than 24 hours. The risk of IO catheter complications (e.g., infections) is directly correlated with the duration of use.[25]

For moderate to severe dehydration, an initial fluid bolus of 30 to 45 mL/kg (0.03 to 0.045 mL/g) of a warm crystalloid solution can be given over a period of 5 to 10 minutes.[26] Lactated Ringer's solution may be ideal because lactate is the preferred metabolic fuel in the neonate during times of hypoglycemia.[27,28] Following the initial bolus, fluid resuscitation should be continued by a constant rate infusion of 80 to 120 mL/kg per day.[26] Neonatal fluid-resuscitation efforts should be evaluated hourly by monitoring heart rate, respiration rate, mucous membrane color, pulse quality, extremity temperature, and mentation.

It is important always to administer warmed fluids to treat or prevent hypothermia. Neonates are at increased risk of hypothermia compared with adults because they have an immature thermoregulatory system, a large surface area-to-body weight ratio (which has high radiation and evaporative heat losses), an inability to shiver and vasoconstrict in response to decreasing temperatures, a small amount of SC fat, and a high water composition.[21] A fluid warmer that is placed in the line is a better option than heating a bag of fluids before use because a liter of fluids warmed to 104°F (40°C) will cool down to room temperature within about 10 minutes. Hypothermic neonates develop bradycardia and gastrointestinal ileus. Oral fluid replacement and feeding should not be attempted if neonates are hypothermic.

In addition to being prone to dehydration, neonates also are at much higher risk for hypoglycemia than adult animals are. Neonates have inefficient hepatic gluconeogenesis, have limited glycogen stores, and lose glucose in the urine.[29] The need for glucose must always be considered during rehydration and resuscitation of sick neonates. Dextrose (1.25% to 5%) can be added to IV fluids at the lowest amount that maintains normoglycemia. Some neonates may develop refractory hypoglycemia and may only respond to hourly boluses of dextrose in addition to IV fluids supplemented with dextrose.[30]

Large volumes of fluid are often needed for hypovolemic patients, but overhydration can be a serious concern because the kidneys cannot dilute the urine to rid the body of excess fluid.[31] The best way to monitor for overhydration is to frequently weigh the patient, as previously mentioned. Baseline thoracic radiographs may also be helpful; however, radiographs can be challenging to interpret in neonatal patients because of normal age-related anatomical differences. The thymus is located in the cranial thorax on the left side and can mimic a mediastinal mass or lung consolidation on thoracic radiographs. Because the heart takes up so much of the thoracic cavity in neonates, it can appear falsely enlarged. The neonatal lung parenchyma also has increased water content such that the interstitial tissue appears more radiographically opaque than in adults, which can make it difficult to diagnose fluid overload without having baseline radiographs.[32]

Response to fluid therapy can also be assessed by sequentially checking the hematocrit and total solid values. Laboratory testing in neonates is often limited because of the patient's estimated blood volume of 90 mL/kg.[7] This translates into a mere 9 milliliters for a 100-gram newborn kitten. Reference guidelines for the hematologic values of feline neonates may be found in Table 102-2. At birth, the hematocrit may be as high as 60%, causing the mucous membrane color to be dark pink to red.[33] By 3 days of age, the hematocrit has decreased dramatically and continues to decrease until reaching a nadir of about 26% at around 4 weeks.[34] This initial decrease is likely caused by a change from the relatively hypoxic prenatal environment to an oxygen-rich postnatal environment.[35] The sustained decrease in the 3 weeks after birth is likely caused by a lack of iron in the diet because the nadir occurs just before weaning to solid foods containing iron.

Table 102-2	Hematologic Reference Values for Healthy Neonatal Cats	
Hematologic Parameter	**AGE**	
	0-2 weeks	**2-4 weeks**
Hematocrit	35.3% ± 1.7%	26.5% ± 0.8%
Red blood cell concentration	$5.29 ± 0.24 × 10^6/\mu L$	$4.67 ± 0.10 × 10^6/\mu L$
Hemoglobin	12.1 ± 0.6 g/dL	8.7 ± 0.2 g/dL
Mean corpuscular volume	67.4 ± 1.9 fL	53.9 ± 1.2 fL
Mean corpuscular hemoglobin	23.0 ± 0.6 pg	18.8 ± 0.8 pg
Mean corpuscular hemoglobin concentration	34.5% ± 0.8%	33.0% ± 0.5%

Modified from Meyers-Wallen VN, Haskins ME, Patterson DF: Hematologic values in healthy neonatal, weanling and juvenile kittens. *Am J Vet Res* 45:1322-1327, 1984.

NEONATAL ISOERYTHROLYSIS

Neonatal isoerythrolysis (NI) is a life-threatening hemolytic condition of kittens. It occurs when kittens with blood type A or blood type AB are born to queens with blood type B.[36] Cats with blood type B have naturally occurring anti-A antibodies. The highest prevalence of cats with blood type B (up to 60%) is reported in certain cat breeds (e.g., British Shorthair, Birman, Devon Rex, Turkish Van, and Turkish Angora).[37-39]

It is critical to blood-type every queen regardless of ancestry because the prevalence of blood type B in nonpurebred cats has been reported as high as 11.4%[40] and 36%, depending on the country and region.[41] However, in nonpurebred cats, the prevalence of blood type B has been reported as high as 11.4%[40] and 36%, depending on the country and region.[41]

Kittens with NI are normal at birth, but when they begin to nurse, they ingest anti-A antibodies in the colostrum, which results in isoerythrolysis. Clinical signs develop within hours to days and may include lethargy, anemia, icterus, hemoglobinuria, tail-tip necrosis, and death. The majority of kittens die within the first week of life, with a smaller percentage dying between 1 and 8 weeks of age.[42]

The prognosis is poor. Kittens should be removed from the queen (if less than 18 hours old) and aggressively treated as soon as a problem is suspected.

If anemia is severe and a transfusion is required, washed red blood cells from the queen or other type B cat can be administered IO at a dose of 5 to 10 per kitten over several hours. This blood is not lysed by the colostral antibodies. The red cells should be suspended in saline rather than plasma so the kitten does not receive more anti-A antibodies.

Subsequent transfusions administered later in life to kittens that survive should consist of type A blood.

Neonatal isoerythrolysis should be prevented by blood typing breeding pairs and not breeding toms with blood type A to queens with blood type B when possible. When such a breeding is necessary, kittens can be removed from the queen for the first 18 hours of life to prevent ingestion of colostrum. Serum from a donor with the same blood type as the kittens can be administered to provide passive immunity. Subcutaneous or intraperitoneal administration of serum (15 mL per kitten; approximately 150 mL/kg) will correct immunoglobulin G deficiency in colostrum-deprived kittens.[43]

CLINICAL PATHOLOGY IN CRITICAL NEONATES

Clinical laboratory testing is restricted in neonates because of their limited blood volume. Normal hepatobiliary biochemical values for neonatal kittens include lower levels of blood urea nitrogen (BUN), creatinine (Cr), cholesterol, albumin, and total protein than in adults (Table 102-3). Alkaline phosphatase (ALP) and gamma-glutamyltransferase (GGT) liver enzyme activities are markedly elevated in neonates.[44] Elevations in ALP and GGT enzyme activity have been attributed to placental, colostral, and intestinal activity.[45] Lower Cr is thought to be caused by decreased muscle mass, and lower BUN and cholesterol are thought to be a result of immature liver function.[44] Knowledge of these values is crucial to prevent a misdiagnosis of liver disease in the neonate.

Although urine is easy to obtain from the neonate with genital stimulation, interpretation of a neonatal urinalysis can be misleading because of renal immaturity. As mentioned earlier, BUN and Cr are lower in neonates than in adults, making monitoring of azotemia challenging. Both protein and glucose may be detected in urine because of immaturity in the proximal tubules.[46] Low urine specific gravity (1.006 to 1.017) is normal in neonates,[31] and they lack the ability to concentrate urine in response to hypovolemia.[19] A diagnosis of dehydration is likely when the urine specific gravity reaches 1.020.[47] As discussed earlier, the neonatal kidney is not only unable to concentrate urine, but also less able to dilute urine because renal blood flow parallels blood pressure and there is altered sodium excretion by the proximal tubule. Appropriate concentration and dilution of urine are not seen until approximately 10 weeks of age.[30,48] A decline in urine specific gravity should be monitored as an indicator of rehydration.

PAIN MANAGEMENT FOR NEONATES

Pain sensation is present at birth, and analgesia is essential for all procedures that are anticipated to be painful.[49] Unmanaged painful experiences, especially when the nervous system is developing, may have a permanent negative effect on the individual. Studies in neonates have revealed that when anesthesia or analgesia is withheld during painful experiences,

Table 102-3	Normal Hepatobiliary Biochemical Values for Neonatal Kittens			
Biochemical Value	**AGE**			
	2 Days	**1 Week**	**2 Weeks**	**4 Weeks**
Total bilirubin	0-0.7 mg/dL	0-0.6 mg/dL	0-0.2 mg/dL	0-0.3 mg/dL
ALT	12-84 IU/L	11-76 IU/L	10-21 IU/L	14-55 IU/L
ALP	275-2021 IU/L	126-363 IU/L	116-306 IU/L	97-274 IU/L
GGT	0-5 IU/L	0-5 IU/L	0-4 IU/L	0-1 IU/L
Total protein	3.9-5.8 g/dL	3.5-4.8 g/dL	3.7-5.0 g/dL	4.5-5.6 g/dL
Albumin	1.6-2.6 g/dL	2.0-2.5 g/dL	2.1-2.6 g/dL	2.4-2.9 g/dL
Cholesterol	80-175 mg/dL	119-213 mg/dL	137-223 mg/dL	173-253 mg/dL
Glucose	75-154 mg/dL	105-145 mg/dL	107-158 mg/dL	117-152 mg/dL
BUN	24-71 mg/dL	16-36 mg/dL	11-30 mg/dL	10-22 mg/dL
Creatinine	0.5-1.1 mg/dL	0.3-0.7 mg/dL	0.4-0.6 mg/dL	0.4-0.7 mg/dL

Modified from Levy J, Crawford P, Werner L: Effect of age on reference intervals of serum biochemical values in kittens. *J Am Vet Med Assoc* 228:1033-1037, 2006.
ALP, Alkaline phosphatase; *ALT,* alanine aminotransferase; *BUN,* blood urea nitrogen; *GGT,* gamma-glutamyltransferase; *IU,* international unit.

Table 102-4	Analgesic Drug Dosages for Neonatal Kittens		
Drug	**Dose (mg/kg)**	**Route of Administration**	**Interval (h)**
Morphine	0.05-0.1	IM, SC	1-4
	0.025 (or to effect)	IV, SC (per hour)	Constant rate infusion
	0.25 (or to effect)	PO, titrate to effect	4-6
Methadone	0.1-0.5	IV, IM, SC	1-4
Fentanyl	0.002-0.01	IV loading	0.5-1
	0.001-0.005	IV (over 20-60 min)	Constant rate infusion
Meperidine	2-5	IM	0.5-1
Butorphanol	0.1-0.2 (or to effect)	IV, IM, SC	1-4
	0.05-0.1 (or to effect)	IV, SC (per hour)	Constant rate infusion
Buprenorphine	0.005-0.010	SC	Approximately 6

Modified from Mathews KA: Pain management for the pregnant, lactating, and neonatal to pediatric cat and dog. *Vet Clin North Am Small Anim Pract* 38:1291-1308, 2008.
IM, Intramuscular; *IV,* intravenous; *PO,* per os; *SC,* subcutaneous.

altered pain sensitivity and increased anxiety occurred with subsequent painful experiences later in life.[50-51]

Although neonates do feel pain, the nociceptive threshold may be higher than in adults because of a potential delay in development of the descending inhibitory mechanism. The slower development of some neurotransmitters and receptors means that certain drugs (e.g., ketamine) are not effective at this stage of development. Based upon human neonatal studies, dosing depends upon the degree of pain and the stage of maturation.[51] Immature hepatic metabolism and renal clearance contribute to differences in drug concentrations and high risk for overdose in neonates.[31,52]

Because of altered metabolism and the potential for renal toxicity, nonsteroidal anti-inflammatory drugs should not be used in neonates.

Opioids are a good choice for analgesia because of their reversibility, but neonates must be monitored closely as these drugs will depress respiratory rates.[9,53-54] Practitioners should start at lower dosages and increase to effect (Table 102-4). Intravenous routes seem to be the most predictable and are preferred over intramuscular or SC routes.[31] The blood-brain barrier is more permeable in neonates, allowing drugs that do not normally cross over to enter the central nervous system.[31] Oral drug absorption is significantly higher in the first

3 days of life because of increased permeability of the gastrointestinal tract. The presence of milk in the stomach may inhibit the absorption of some drugs. Transdermal and transmucosal routes of fentanyl administration have not been studied in neonatal cats or dogs.

Reversal of any adverse opioid effects may be titrated using one drop of naloxone (0.4 mg/mL) sublingually.[53] Repeat dosing in 30 minutes may be required if the neonate becomes depressed again.[53] Opioids are often profoundly sedating in neonates. If further sedation is required, a low dose of a sedative may be administered after the opioid has had time for full effect. In general, sedatives should be used with caution in neonates because they induce peripheral vasodilation resulting in hypotension and subsequent hypothermia.[55]

For minor superficial procedures (e.g., IV catheter placement), local anesthesia may be adequate without the risks associated with systemic administration of analgesics. Eutectic mixture of local anesthetic cream (EMLA, AstraZeneca LP, Wilmington, Delaware) is a frequently used topical local anesthetic. This is a prescription-only mixture of lidocaine (2.5%) and prilocaine (2.5%) combined with thickening agents to form an emulsion. The EMLA cream should be applied to intact skin and covered with an occlusive dressing for at least 30 minutes to provide for maximal analgesia.[53] This product is not sterile.

For more invasive procedures (e.g., IO catheter placement), local anesthesia will be necessary. However, lidocaine infiltration is extremely painful in neonates even with 27- to 30-gauge needles.[56] To reduce pain, warming the solution (100.0 to 107.6 °F [37 to 42 °C]), slow administration, and

buffering are recommended. Buffering can be accomplished by mixing a 10:1 ratio of 1% lidocaine with sodium bicarbonate before administration. The maximum dose of lidocaine recommended for use in neonatal kittens is 3 mg/kg. This dose may be diluted in 0.9% saline for more accurate dosing, ease and safety of administration, and distribution over a larger site. As an alternative to lidocaine, bupivacaine may be used at a maximum dose of 1 mg/kg in neonatal kittens.[53] A 0.5% bupivacaine solution (5 mg/mL) can also be buffered to minimize discomfort during administration, but it requires a higher ratio of sodium bicarbonate (20:1).[53]

SUMMARY

Preventing problems with neonates begins with good prenatal maternal care (e.g., nutrition, vaccination, and hygiene) and prompt identification of problems during parturition. For queens needing to undergo a C-section, risk of neonatal losses can be minimized by preoxygenating the queen before surgery and by preventing neonatal hypothermia after delivery. Hypothermia decreases neonatal responsiveness to resuscitation attempts. Bradycardia is often the result of hypothermia and hypoventilation, so correcting these underlying conditions should be the primary objective before using medication to increase heart rate. Clinicians should be able to identify these critically ill neonates readily by the presence of meconium staining, limp body tone, no body movement, persistent crying, temperature, etc., so that there is no delay in treatment implementation (Figure 102-4).

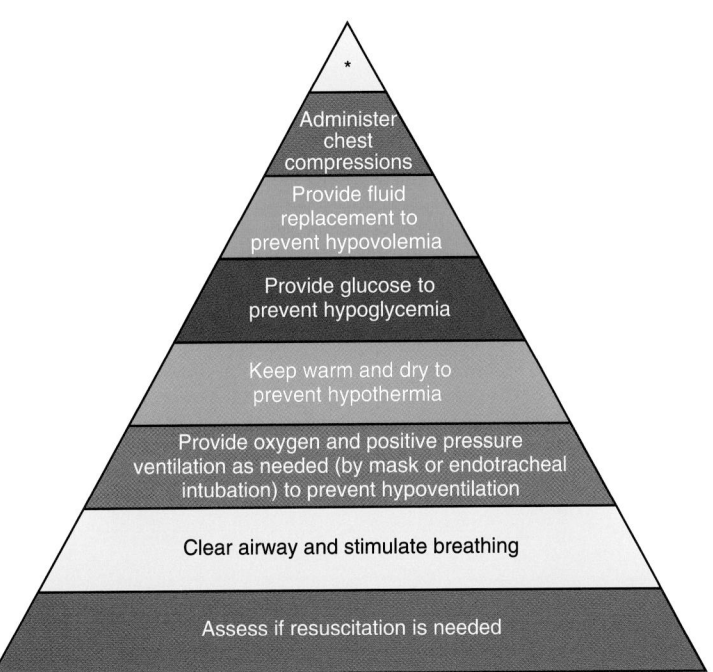

Figure 102-4: Neonatal resuscitation pyramid, where the base of the pyramid is always necessary in critically ill neonates and the apex (* = drug therapy) is rarely indicated. (Modified from: Kattwinkel J, editor: *Textbook of neonatal resuscitation*, ed 5, Elk Grove, 2006, American Academy of Pediatrics and American Heart Association, pp 1-2.)

The pyramid (from top to bottom) reads:
- *
- Administer chest compressions
- Provide fluid replacement to prevent hypovolemia
- Provide glucose to prevent hypoglycemia
- Keep warm and dry to prevent hypothermia
- Provide oxygen and positive pressure ventilation as needed (by mask or endotracheal intubation) to prevent hypoventilation
- Clear airway and stimulate breathing
- Assess if resuscitation is needed

References

1. Apgar V: A proposal for a new method of evaluation of the newborn infant. *Curr Res Anesth Analg* 32(4):260–267, 1953.
2. Finster M, Wood M: The Apgar score has survived the test of time. *Anesthesiology* 102:855–857, 2005.
3. Veronesi MC, Panzani S, Faustini M, et al: An Apgar scoring system for routine assessment of newborn puppy viability and short-term survival prognosis. *Theriogenology* 72:401–407, 2009.
4. Root Kustritz MV: History and physical examination of the neonate. In Peterson ME, Kutzler MA, editors: *Small animal pediatrics: the first twelve months of life*, St Louis, 2011, Elsevier Saunders, pp 20–27.
5. Poffenbarger EM, Ralston AL, Chandler ML, et al: Canine neonatology: part 2, disorders of the neonate. *Compend Contin Educ Pract Vet* 13:25–37, 1991.
6. Lawler DF: Care and diseases of neonatal puppies and kittens. In Kirk RW, editor: *Current veterinary therapy X: small animal practice*, Philadelphia, 1989, Saunders, pp 1325–1333.
7. Grundy SA: Clinically relevant physiology of the neonate. *Vet Clin North Am Small Anim Pract* 36:443–459, 2006.
8. Grundy SA, Liu S, Davidson A: Intracranial trauma in a dog due to being "swung" at birth. *Top Companion Anim Med* 24(2):100–103, 2009.
9. Traas AM: Resuscitation of canine and feline neonates. *Theriogenology* 70:343–348, 2008.
10. Moon PF, Erb HN, Ludders JW, et al: Perioperative risk factors for puppies delivered by cesarean section in the United States and Canada. *J Am Anim Hosp Assoc* 36:359–368, 2000.
11. Aggarwal R, Paul VK, Deorari AK: Latest guidelines on neonatal resuscitation. *Indian J Pediatr* 70(1):51–55, 2003.
12. Jenkins S: Oxygen toxicity. *J Crit Care Med* 3:137–152, 1988.
13. Efrati O, Barak A, Ben-Abraham R, et al: Should vasopressin replace adrenaline for endotracheal drug administration? *Crit Care Med* 31(2):572–576, 2003.
14. Mann K, Berg RA, Nadkarni V: Beneficial effects of vasopressin in prolonged pediatric cardiac arrest: a case series. *Resuscitation* 52(2):149–156, 2002.
15. Niermeyer S, Kattwinkel J, Van Reempts P, et al: International guidelines for neonatal resuscitation: an excerpt from the guidelines 2000 for cardiopulmonary resuscitation and emergency cardiovascular care: international consensus on science. contributors and reviewers for the neonatal resuscitation guidelines. *Pediatrics* 106(3):E29, 2000. [Abstract].
16. Neumar RW, Nolan JP, Adrie C, et al: Post-cardiac arrest syndrome: epidemiology, pathophysiology, treatment, and prognostication. *Circulation* 118:2452–2483, 2008.
17. Hofmeister EH, Brainard BM, Egger CM, et al: Prognostic indicators for dogs and cats with cardiopulmonary arrest treated by cardiopulmonary cerebral resuscitation at a university teaching hospital. *J Am Vet Med Assoc* 235:50–57, 2009.
18. Mace SE, Levy MN: Neural control of heart rate: a comparison between puppies and adult animals. *Pediatr Res* 17:491–495, 1983.
19. Kleegman LI, Lube RJ: Factors affecting maturation of the glomerular filtration rate and renal plasma flow in the newborn dog. *J Physiol* 223:395–409, 1972.
20. Margin F: Hemodynamic determinants of the arterial blood pressure rise during growth in conscious puppies. *Cardiovasc Res* 12:422–428, 1978.
21. Poffenbarger EM, Ralston AL, Chandler ML, et al: Canine neonatology: part 1, physiologic differences between puppies and adults. *Compend Contin Educ Pract Vet* 12:601–609, 1990.
22. Thomas NJ, Carcillo JA: Hypovolemic shock in pediatric patients. *New Horiz* 6(2):120–129, 1998.
23. Hoskins JD: Pediatric health care and management. *Vet Clin North Am Small Anim Pract* 29(4):837–852, 1999.
24. Otto C, Kaufman G, Crowe D: Intraosseous infusion of fluids and therapeutics. *Compend Contin Educ Pract Vet* 11(4):421–430, 1989.
25. Fiser DH: Intraosseous infusion. *N Engl J Med* 322(22):1579–1581, 1990.
26. Macintire D: Pediatric fluid therapy. *Vet Clin North Am Small Anim Pract* 38(3):621–627, 2008.
27. Levitsky LL, Fisher DE, Paton JB, et al: Fasting plasma levels of glucose, acetoacetate, D-beta-hydroxybutyrate, glycerol, and lactate in the baboon infant: correlation with cerebral uptake of substrates and oxygen. *Pediatr Res* 11(4):298–302, 1977.
28. Hellmann J, Vannucci RC, Nardis EE: Blood-brain barrier permeability to lactic acid in the newborn dog: lactate as a cerebral metabolic fuel. *Pediatr Res* 16(1):40–44, 1982.
29. Atkins C: Disorders of glucose homeostasis in neonatal and juvenile dogs: hypoglycemia—part 1. *Compend Contin Educ Pract Vet* 6(2):197–204, 1984.
30. Holster M, Keeler BJ: Intracortical distribution of number and volume of glomeruli during postnatal maturation in the dog. *J Clin Invest* 50:796–800, 1971.
31. Boothe DM, Tannert K: Special considerations for drug and fluid therapy in the pediatric patient. *Compend Contin Educ Pract Vet* 14:313–329, 1992.
32. Partington B: Diagnostic imaging techniques. In Hoskins JD, editor: *Veterinary pediatrics: dogs and cats from birth to six months*, Philadelphia, 1995, Saunders, pp 7–21.
33. Windle WF, Sweet M, Whitehead WH: Some aspects of prenatal and postnatal development of the blood in the cat. *Anat Rec* 78:321–332, 1940.
34. Meyers-Wallen V: Hematologic values in healthy neonatal, weanling and juvenile kittens. *Am J Vet Res* 45:1322–1327, 1984.
35. Earl FL, Melveger BE, Wilson RL: The hemogram and bone marrow profile of normal neonatal and weanling beagle dogs. *Lab Anim Sci* 23(5):690–695, 1973.
36. Clinkenbeard KD, Cowell RL, Meinkoth JH, et al: The hematopoietic and lymphoid systems. In Hoskins JD, editor: *Veterinary pediatrics: dogs and cats from birth to six months*, ed 3, Philadelphia, 2001, Saunders, pp 301–343.
37. Knottenbelt CM, Addie DD, Day MJ, et al: Determination of the prevalence of feline blood types in the UK. *J Small Anim Pract* 40(3):115–118, 1999.
38. Giger U, Bucheler J, Patterson DF: Frequency and inheritance of A and B blood types in feline breeds of the United States. *J Hered* 82(1):15–20, 1991.
39. Arikan S, Duru SY, Gurkan M: Blood type A and B frequencies in Turkish Van and Angora cats in Turkey. *J Vet Med A Physiol Pathol Clin Med* 50:303–306, 2003.
40. Zheng L, Zhong Y, Shi Z: Frequencies of blood types A, B, and AB in non-pedigree domestic cats in Beijing. *Vet Clin Pathol* 40(4):513–517, 2011.
41. Malik R, Griffin DL, White JD, et al: The prevalence of feline A/B blood types in the Sydney region. *Aust Vet J* 83(1–2):38–44, 2005.
42. Sparkes AH, Rogers K, Henley WE, et al: A questionnaire-based study of gestation, parturition and neonatal mortality in pedigree breeding cats in the UK. *J Feline Med Surg* 8:145–157, 2006.
43. Levy JK, Crawford PC, Collante WR, et al: Use of adult cat serum to correct failure of passive transfer in kittens. *J Am Vet Med Assoc* 219:1401–1405, 2001.
44. Center SA, Hornbuckle WE, Hoskins JD: The liver and pancreas. In Hoskins JD, editor: *Veterinary pediatrics: dogs and cats from birth to six months*, ed 2, Philadelphia, 1995, Saunders, pp 189–225.
45. Center SA, Randolph JF, ManWarren T, et al: Effect of colostrum ingestion of gamma-glutamylaminotransferase and alkaline phosphatase activity in neonatal pups. *Am J Vet Res* 52:499–504, 1991.
46. Fettman MJ, Aleen TA: Developmental aspects of fluid and electrolyte metabolism and renal function in neonates. *Compend Contin Educ Pract Vet* 13:392–397, 1991.
47. McIntire D: Pediatric intensive care. *Vet Clin North Am Small Anim Pract* 29:837–852, 1999.
48. Fetuin M, Allen T: Development aspects of fluid and electrolyte metabolism and renal function in neonates. *Compend Contin Educ Pract Vet* 13(4):392–402, 1991.
49. Averill DR, Jr: The neurologic examination. *Vet Clin North Am Small Anim Pract* 11(3):511–521, 1981.
50. Taddio A, Katz J, Ilersich AL, et al: Effect of neonatal circumcision on pain response during

subsequent routine vaccination. *Lancet* 349: 599–603, 1997.

51. Lee BH: Managing pain in human neonates-application for animals. *J Am Vet Med Assoc* 221(2):233–237, 2002.

52. Short CR: Drug disposition in neonatal animals. *J Am Vet Med Assoc* 184(9):1161–1162, 1984.

53. Mathews KA: Pain management for the pregnant, lactating, and neonatal to pediatric cat and dog. *Vet Clin North Am Small Anim Pract* 38:1291–1308, 2008.

54. Moon PF, Massat BJ, Pascoe PJ: Neonatal critical care. *Vet Clin North Am Small Anim Pract* 31:343–367, 2001.

55. Hosgood G: Surgical and anesthetic management of puppies and kittens. *Compend Contin Educ Small Anim Pract* 14(5):345–357, 1992.

56. Rodriguez E, Jordan R: Contemporary trends in pediatric sedation and analgesia. Pediatric emergency medicine: current concepts and controversies. *Emerg Med Clin North Am* 1:199–222, 2002.

Disorders and Normal Variations of the Oral Cavity of Kittens and Senior Cats

Judy Rochette

The majority of notable findings in the oral cavity of the kitten are related to its formation and development as well as development and eruption of teeth, whereas problems seen in senior cats reflect the gradual aging of the dental hard tissues and their supporting structures.

CLEFTS

The head, face, and oral cavity are some of the first structures to manifest in the developing embryo. The fetus is very susceptible to teratogenic influences during this time, and developmental failures can occur. The primary etiologies of facial and oral clefts are hereditary predilection and maternal environmental effects. The latter includes nutritional imbalances,[1,2] metabolic/systemic disease, medications,[3,4] and mechanical interference with the fetus, as well as some viral infections or vaccination with live and/or modified live vaccines.[5]

Clefts can occur in several areas of the face, but those affecting the oronasal area are the most common congenital defects found in cats.[6] Genetic studies have shown variable heritability depending on the breed.[6,7] As so many neonates with this disorder die early or are euthanized by the breeder, accurate statistics on the true incidence of this problem are difficult to obtain. Brachycephalic dogs are reported to be at increased risk,[7] but this does not seem to translate to feline breeds. Clefts have been reported in Siamese[6,8] and Abyssinians, but also in the Bengal, Manx, Persian, Ragdoll, Ocicat, Savannah, Burmese, and Norwegian Forest cat breeds, in addition to many other purebreds and nonpurebreds alike.[9,10]

Clinical Signs

Clinical signs of a cleft palate vary depending on what embryologic process failed to complete. Those involving the oronasal cavity can be primary (anterior to the incisive foramen) or secondary (caudal to the incisive foramen) with the latter potentially involving the hard and/or soft palates. Severity of each type can range from minor soft and hard tissue deformities[11,12] to severe forms in which the majority of the hard and/or soft palate is missing. For these reasons, clinical signs of an incomplete, primary cleft may be limited

to being aesthetic (Figure 103-1A), whereas severe secondary clefts can be life-threatening (see Figure 103-1B). Any oronasal communication allows fluids into the nasal cavity, where they may be seen coming from the nostrils and/or cause sneezing, snuffling, rhinitis, and coughing or gagging. If a kitten is unable to take in adequate calories due to inefficient nursing, it will fail to gain weight and growth will be stunted. Fluid flow into the lungs may result in aspiration pneumonia, a major cause of death in animals with severe cleft palate.

Clefts are often associated with congenital deformities in other areas of the head and body, including the tympanic bullae, nasal turbinates and septum, vomer bone, frontal sinuses, maxillary bones, and nasopharynx.[7,8,13] A heritable condition in Burmese cats may also manifest with encephaloceles, hydrocephalus, cranioschisis, and microphthalmia.[14] These associated cranial defects can seriously affect quality of life for the kitten in other ways not directly associated with the cleft.

Treatment

Nutritional support of the newborn kitten by hand or tube feeding may be required to ensure adequate caloric intake until the kitten is at least 3 months of age at which time surgery can be performed. Presurgical radiology, or ideally computed tomography, to assess the extent of bony defects and other possible cranial defects is necessary. Thoracic radiographs should be taken to detect aspiration pneumonia. If severe rhinitis exists, samples should be collected for culture and sensitivity testing prior to liberal flushing of the nasal cavity to remove debris before surgery. Should aspiration pneumonia be present, culture of bronchoalveolar wash samples for detection of microbes would optimize antimicrobial therapy.

Consideration should be given to placement of an esophageal feeding tube to decrease inflammatory irritation of the nasal passages and risk of pneumonia. The presence and location of deciduous and permanent teeth should be documented.

Closure of Primary Cleft Palate Defects

Supernumerary teeth are commonly found in primary clefts. Dental radiographs of the cleft, and graft source areas will

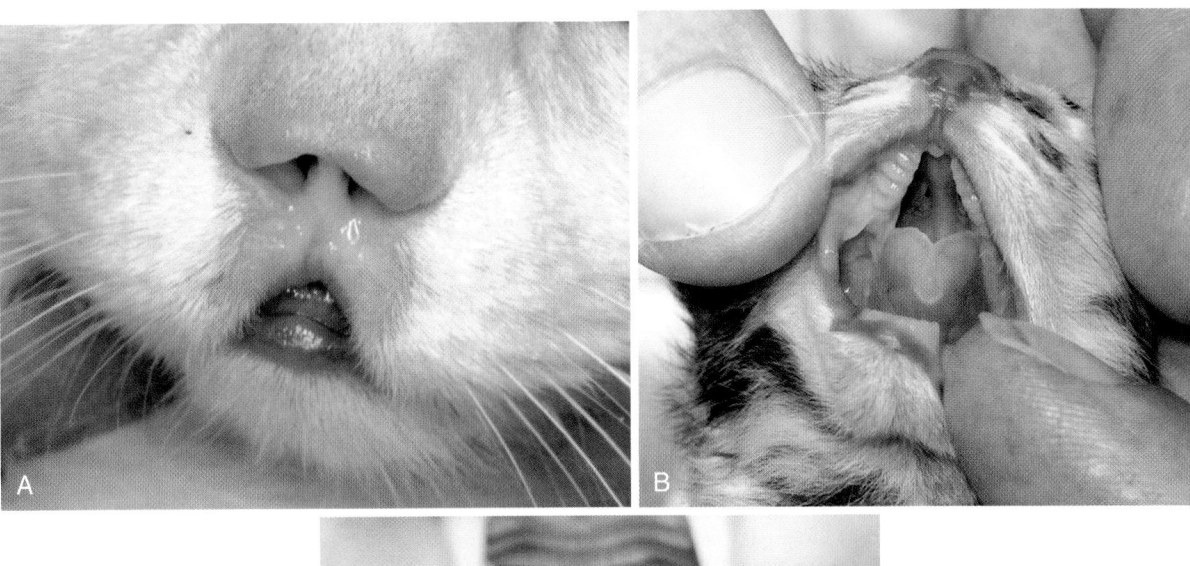

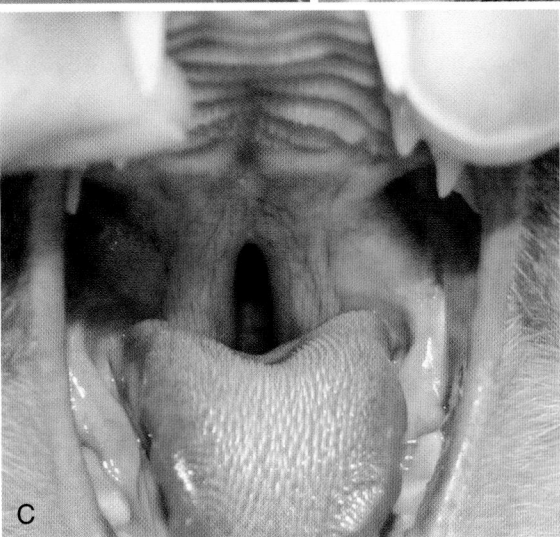

Figure 103-1: A primary cleft **(A)** may have minimal clinical significance beyond the aesthetic, whereas a large secondary cleft **(B)** may have life-threatening sequelae, such as aspiration pneumonia. **C,** A cleft soft palate can cause dysfunctional deglutition with secondary respiratory disease.

locate the deciduous and permanent incisors and canines, and any supernumerary teeth that may be present. All teeth within these areas should be extracted 6 to 8 weeks prior to cleft closure. Formation and/or rotation of one large flap that will span the full width of the defect ensures that suture lines are supported by the far edge of the defect and are not spanning a void. Overlapping of flap edges ("vest-over-pants" technique) also provides strength to the suture line. Sliding/advancement, rotational, and/or transpositional flaps can be used as appropriate to the situation. Reconstruction of the cutaneous surface of the lip requires restoration that provides symmetry of the rhinarium, a straight philtrum, a continuous lip, and, if possible, proper hair alignment.

Closure of Hard and Soft Palate Clefts

The primary goal of repair is to reconstruct the nasal floor so that integrity of separate oral and nasal cavities is achieved. As with primary clefts, preparatory procedures may be necessary before the definitive closure surgery can be performed.

Initial investigation should document the extent of the bony defect underlying the existing rugae. The flap technique should be chosen based on blood supply and the amount of soft tissue that is available compared to the size of defect. "Hinged" flaps, single and bipedicle rotational flaps, the von Langenbeck technique, and other techniques exist. However, for very large defects, a flap may need to extend onto, or beyond, the alveolar ridge to include tissues from the buccal mucosa. Detailed descriptions of surgical techniques can be found elsewhere.[15] Dehiscence may occur as a result of tension on suture lines from normal actions including tongue movements, ingestion of food, yawning, and grooming. Use of a surgical implant can provide critical support to reduce the likelihood of this complication. Use of commercially produced collagen membranes may be helpful. However, auricular cartilage is more supportive,[16,17] and commercially prepared, freeze-dried bone sheets are most likely to be associated with successful surgery. The maximum size of the auricular graft is determined by the size of ear from which the graft is being created. The bone membranes, by comparison, can be very large, can be commercially acquired before surgery, do not require surgery time to acquire the graft, and do not compromise the aesthetics of the patient's ear.

There have been a small number of case reports describing the use of a Silastic button to occlude an oronasal defect. These are often difficult to fit and maintain and should only be offered when all other options have been exhausted.[18,19]

Defects of the soft palate (see Figure 103-1C) can occur with, or in isolation from, a hard palate cleft. Coordinated muscular movements during deglutition produce periods of tension on the tissues of the soft palate. Therefore, it is critical that cleft closure involves adequate tissue to span the defect with tension-free closure.

Small and/or unilateral clefts can be closed with simple apposition and two-layer suturing so that nasal and mucosal layers are created and sutured only to their self-layers. With larger defects, when harvesting flaps from the buccal pharyngeal wall, one must avoid vital structures in close proximity to the donor sites, yet provide sufficient size and integrity to be able to avoid surgical failure. Multiple flap techniques and source sites have been documented for large defects;[20,21] however, bilateral soft palate clefts result in a shortened soft palate. Recreating a reasonable length of soft palate in these animals can be very challenging. Reconstruction may not return full function due to lack of normal innervation and muscle mass;[22] oronasal reflux may still occur with ongoing rhinitis.

A visual reassessment of the surgery site should be conducted 2 weeks postoperatively, with further evaluation conducted under sedation at 6 weeks postoperatively. Should revisional surgery be needed, it is more likely to succeed at this second (6-week) visit because healing and revascularization of tissues will be well advanced.

Postoperative care should include antibiotic therapy and fluid and nutritional support as needed. Consideration should be given to placing an esophageal feeding tube to ensure caloric intake, administer medications, avoid aspiration, and eliminate the need to handle the oral cavity during early healing. If an esophageal feeding tube is not placed, blenderized food should be fed for 2 weeks after surgery, with gradual transition to a soft diet over the next 4 weeks. All hard diets and toys should be removed for at least 6 weeks.[15]

Patients that have had reconstructive surgery that continue to experience oronasal reflux should be fed foods that maintain a bolus form, such as large kibble. Raising food and water bowls may help with swallowing.[23]

In cases in which extractions were necessary for surgical closure, the remaining teeth in the apposing arcade may accumulate calculus rapidly and develop periodontal disease more quickly than the rest of the mouth. Areas of soft tissue trauma from the cusps of the apposing teeth may arise and require extraction of the offending teeth, or crown amputation with immediate endodontics, to resolve pain. Owners should have the affected animal surgically sterilized to prevent transmission of the defect to offspring.

MALOCCLUSION

Healthy occlusion resembles that of the "wild" phenotype with interdigitating cheek teeth that create a "pinking shears" effect, a mandibular canine tooth that occludes between the maxillary third incisor and canine tooth, and mandibular incisors that rest immediately distal to the maxillary incisor teeth. This occlusal design is the most efficient and durable to cope with the diet of a predator. The skeletal architecture complements this oral arrangement by having strut reinforcement of the facial bones in the areas in which maximum forces occur. Genotypic and/or phenotypic variations from normal can be detrimental; what is considered acceptable as a breed standard may not be ideal for a pet's quality of life.

The prevalence of malocclusion in domesticated cats has been poorly documented, but one study in the United Kingdom reported the prevalence as 3.9% in all breeds of cats, with an increased prevalence (13%) in the longhaired cats.[24] It was not specified that the longhaired cats were brachycephalic breeds, but Stockard's study[25] proved that malocclusion is primarily a genetic problem and that most clinically significant malocclusions result from discrepant jaw lengths due to selection for specific breed standards.

A Class 1 malocclusion defined by the American Veterinary Dental College as a "normal rostral-caudal relationship of the maxillary and mandibular dental arches with malposition of one or more individual teeth" can include rotation, tipping, and physical displacement.[26] An example of a Class 1 malocclusion involves the maxillary canine tooth being facially tipped and has been called a *lance canine tooth* (Figure 103-2). This tipping causes loss of the diastema where the mandibular canine tooth would normally occlude. The mandibular canine is forced to tip buccally, and the tooth-on-tooth contact between the mandibular and maxillary canine

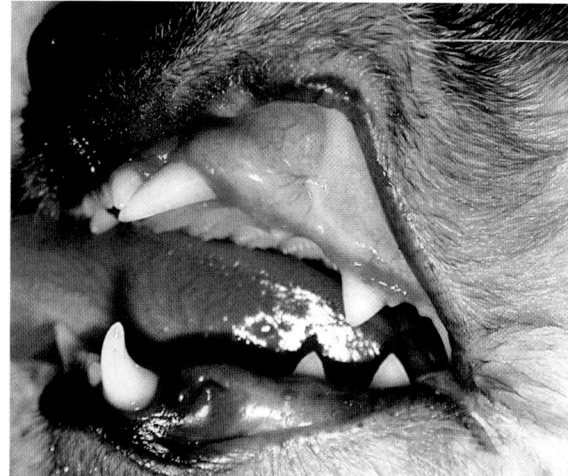

Figure 103-2: A "lance" canine is an example of a Class 1 malocclusion. The maxillary canine tooth prevents the ipsilateral mandibular canine from occluding in its correct position, causing it to tip buccally. Periodontal disease, traumatic pulpitis, and soft tissue trauma to the maxillary lip can all occur with this malocclusion.

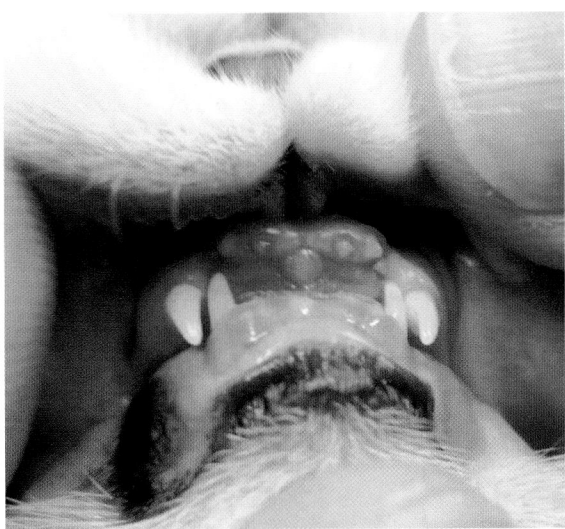

Figure 103-3: This kitten demonstrates a Class 2 malocclusion with the mandibular teeth occluding caudal to the expected position relative to the maxillary teeth. Soft tissue trauma is common with Class 2 malocclusions.

teeth can result in concussive pulpitis with subsequent tooth death. The mandibular canine tooth can also cause recurring soft tissue trauma to the maxillary lip, which is painful. Periodontal disease can also develop around the crowded maxillary incisor and "lance" canine tooth.

A Class 2 malocclusion (Figure 103-3) occurs when the mandibular arch occludes caudal to its normal position relative to the maxillary arch. This occlusal abnormality is not as common in the cat as in the dog but can occur in all species.[2] In a kitten, interlocking of the mandibular canine teeth interfering with the distal surface of the maxillary canine teeth can impede any corrective growth that may occur. Trauma to the soft tissues of the palate and maxillary alveolar ridge is common with this type of malocclusion. Periodontal disease secondary to damage to the attached gingiva of the maxillary canine tooth, oronasal fistula formation, and dysmastication are possible.

Likely the most common occlusal problem seen in cats is a Class 3 malocclusion; symptomatic cases almost always accompany brachycephalism. The mandibular arch occludes rostral to its normal position relative to the maxillary arch usually due to maxillary brachygnathia. Rotation of the maxillary cheek teeth to accommodate the smaller space results in dental crowding, which prevents maintenance of an intact collar of attached gingiva around each tooth, predisposing to periodontal disease. The maxillary incisors may damage the lingual aspects of the mandibular canine teeth or the mandibular soft tissues.

Treatment of malocclusion should be directed towards removing the source of soft tissue trauma, relieving crowding, arresting tooth-on-tooth concussion, and restoring functional occlusion. Appropriate corrective procedures include orthodontic movement, crown amputation with immediate endodontic treatment to reseal the pulp chamber, or extraction of the offending tooth/teeth. The option chosen depends

on the skills of the operator; the temperament of the patient; and the dedication, patience, and financial means of the owner.

ABNORMALITIES OF TEETH

The formation, eruption, and loss of deciduous and permanent dentition are a tightly choreographed series of events. Disruption anywhere along this sequence can result in visible oral pathology.

During eruption, the tooth moves from within the bone of the jaw to its functional occlusive position; the primary movement is coronal/axial. If the tooth is abnormal or another dental structure is in the way, eruption is impeded. If the impediment is removed before apical closure of the successional (adult) tooth, the potential for normal eruption still exists, and the tooth may take its proper position within the dental arcade. The apex of the permanent mandibular molar is usually fully formed by 7 months of age, but the maxillary canine tooth is not complete until 11 months of age. Structural interference is most often secondary to retained deciduous teeth; extraction of the deciduous precursors must occur prior to these ages to allow full eruption.[27]

Retained Deciduous Teeth

Exfoliation of deciduous teeth is the result of resorption of the tooth roots and the associated periodontal ligament. Resorption is triggered by pressure on the deciduous tooth from a successional tooth, from growth-related increases in forces of mastication that overwhelm the support structures of the deciduous tooth, and from apoptotic cell death.[28]

Missing, or impacted, successional teeth will delay shedding—as will occlusal interference that removes necessary mastication forces from a tooth.[29] Apoptotic cell death is 80% genetically controlled,[30] so familial tendencies for retained deciduous teeth have been identified. If deciduous teeth are present when the adult tooth is erupting, they must be removed to prevent displacement of the adult tooth as well as crowding-induced periodontal disease.

Odontomas and Dentigerous Cysts

When a developmental accident occurs, the resulting dental structure may not be able to erupt. An odontoma is an uncommon, but dramatic, cause for failure of eruption. These hamartomas may be composed of relatively organized dental anatomy (denticles) or the conglomerate of dental tissues may bear no resemblance to teeth. The former mass is called a *compound odontoma* and the latter, a *complex odontoma*. It is not uncommon for these masses to be mixed, making definitive labelling as either compound or complex arbitrary.[31,32]

Odontomas are not neoplastic and will not metastasize, but they can be disfiguring (Figure 103-4A-B). The radiologic appearance (see Figure 103-4C) is characteristic, exhibiting either a sharply defined mass of calcified material

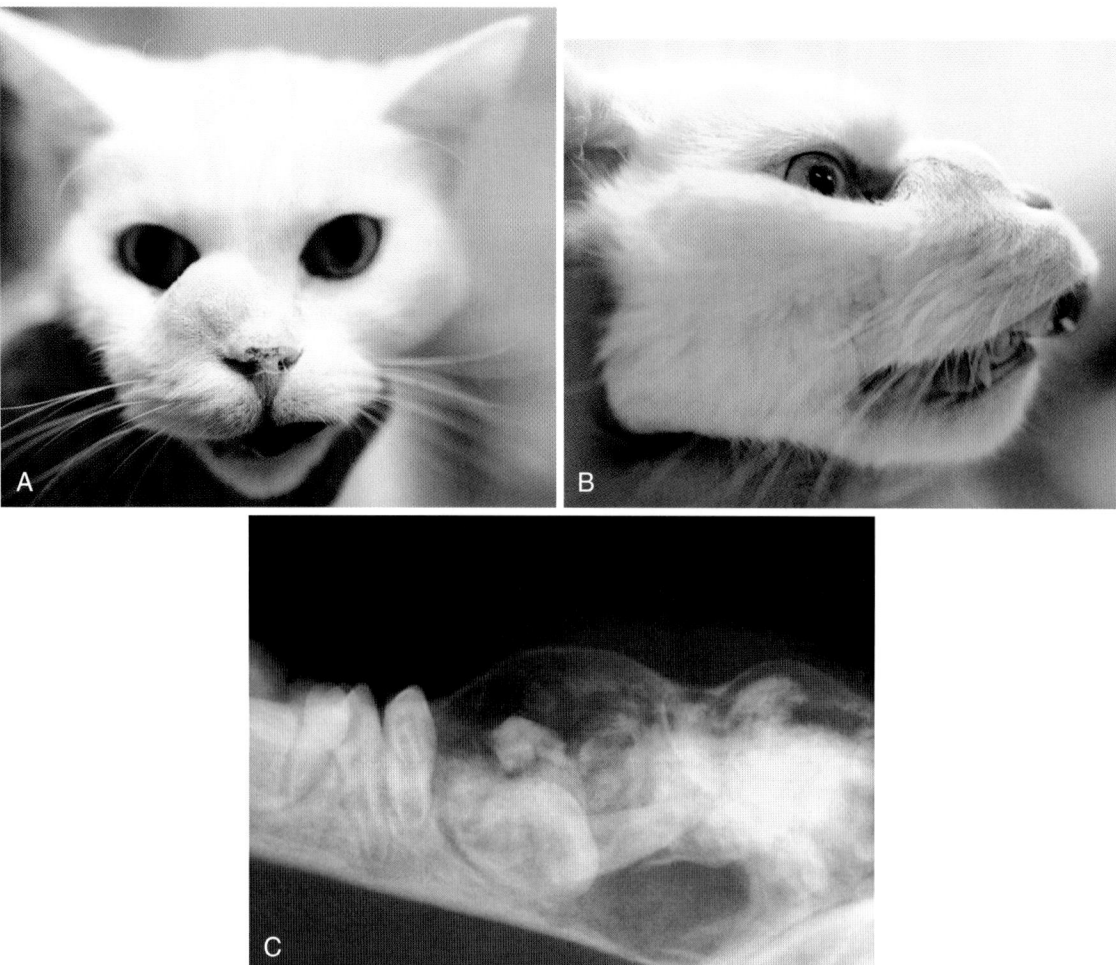

Figure 103-4: An odontoma can inhibit tooth eruption. **A** and **B** show a large maxillary odontoma in a cat. **C,** Radiographic characteristics include a radiolucent area, with the missing tooth and mineralized dental materials and/or denticles contained within. (**A** and **B,** courtesy of Dr. Susan Little.)

surrounded by a narrow radiolucent band, or an accumulation of a variable number of tooth-like structures.[33] The literature on odontomas in cats is sparse; a maxillary case has been reported.[34] Anecdotally, and in the author's own experience, odontomas can occur anywhere along the dental arcade. Surgical removal is curative. If the mass has formed around an unerupted tooth, the unerupted tooth must also be removed.

Any unerupted tooth that is not removed is at risk of forming a dentigerous cyst. These cysts develop from the dental sac (from within which teeth form) and can become quite large. Slow expansion causes thinning and eventual loss of the overlying cortical bone. The mass may be either firm, if bone is still present, or fluctuant if the bone is completely lost. Overlying soft tissues may appear normal or have a bluish tint. Aspiration usually yields a clear, poorly cellular, slightly viscous fluid, but this can change if the cyst becomes infected. Dental radiographs will demonstrate an unerupted tooth with a radiolucent area girdling the crown. Compaction of alveolar bone by cyst expansion creates a radiodense outline of the lucent area. Pressure-induced resorption of adjacent tooth roots and alveolar bone, mandibular fracture, and

respiratory compromise if expansion invades the nasal cavity are possible sequelae of ongoing enlargement.

Treatment requires removal of the cyst lining as well as the embedded tooth. If adjacent teeth are fatally compromised, they should also be surgically extracted. Cyst linings should always be submitted for histopathology to verify that the cyst is truly dentigerous and not a more aggressive tumor masquerading as a benign cyst. Follow-up radiographs should be used to monitor bone healing and that the cyst does not recur.[35-37]

Abnormalities in Tooth Number

Failure of tooth formation results in the absence of a single tooth or multiple teeth (oligodontia or partial anodontia). Global disruption of tooth formation results in absence of all teeth (anodontia). Reports of oligodontia or anodontia in cats are very sparse in the literature,[38-39] and the cause of this problem is unknown. In people and dogs, there is a strong genetic association. In some geographically restricted cat populations, oligodontia may be more common. For example, the maxillary second premolar was found to be missing in 3.4% of cats in the United Kingdom, but the prevalence was 23.6% for a group of cats in Mexico, suggesting a genetic role for cats as well.[40]

Although alopecia, or hypotrichosis, has been associated with oligodontia in dogs and people, the feline breeds with known ectodermal defect syndromes (e.g., Sphynx and Devon Rex) do not seem to have oligodontia as well, suggesting a different genetic modification for these phenotypes in the feline species.[6,41] Radiographs are required to confirm that teeth are absent rather than having failed to erupt. As mentioned earlier, embedded teeth pose a risk for the formation of a dentigerous cyst and must be removed.

Supernumerary Teeth

When the molecular signaling pathways involved in normal tooth development are overactive, single or multiple supernumerary teeth can develop. These pathways are under genetic control, but environmental factors and/or metabolic disturbances can also disrupt formation.[42-43]

Problems that can arise from supernumerary tooth formation include crowding with subsequent development of periodontal disease, concussive trauma with the apposing arcade, failure of eruption of either the extra tooth or an adjacent tooth, displacement of neighboring teeth, and pathology relating to dentigerous cyst formation.

Treatment involves extraction of any teeth that are compromised or causing pathology elsewhere in the oral cavity. Dental radiographs are required to accurately identify which tooth should be removed and to confirm that the extra tooth is not fused with the original tooth.

Abnormal Tooth Appearance

Formation of a tooth begins at the occlusal surface and progresses toward the root. A limited number of ameloblasts are available to produce enamel along the surface of the developing tooth; these are activated in sequence and decommissioned once their task is completed. Deleterious influences have their most severe effects on the activated ameloblasts, resulting in cessation of enamel production in the area of tooth that is under formation. Removal of the insult permits the ameloblasts to resume function.[44] Disturbance in the normal synthesis and secretion of enamel leads to enamel hypoplasia. If the enamel volume is normal but its mineralization is defective, the enamel is said to be *hypomineralized*. Hypoplasia is manifested by pitting, furrowing, or even total absence of the enamel, whereas hypomineralization appears as opaque or chalky areas on normally contoured enamel surfaces. The causes of such defective enamel formation can be generally classified as systemic, local, or genetic. The most common systemic influences are nutritional deficiencies,[2] endocrinopathies, fever, and certain chemical intoxications, such as excessive ingestion of fluoride (greater than 1.5 parts per million).[45] "Temporal hypoplasia" manifests as narrow bands of horizontal agenesis with normal enamel coronal and apical to the affected areas. Temporal hypoplasia is a lasting reminder of a systemic problem that disrupted enamel production for only a short duration.

Generalized enamel abnormalities require prolonged failure of amelogenesis and are usually heritable.[46] The entire enamel surface of both deciduous and permanent teeth is affected. The anomaly is transmitted as an autosomal dominant defect in people. The exact mode of transmission has not been identified in cats, but breeds with reduced hair coats often have enamel abnormalities, suggesting an association with the genes for hairlessness.

Local disturbances tend to affect a single tooth or a focal area. Infection of the periapical tissues of a nonvital deciduous tooth during enamel formation of the permanent successor, surgical manipulation of tissues in the vicinity of a developing tooth, or trauma may all produce localized pathology.

Affected teeth are prone to plaque and tartar accumulation leading to periodontal disease and are susceptible to bacterial penetration through exposed dentinal tubules with concurrent dental sensitivity and possible pulpitis. Diligent dental hygiene involving daily brushing, and possibly the use of barrier products, is critical in reducing the incidence of complications. Affected teeth should be radiographically monitored for continued vitality. Composite resin and/or glass ionomer products can be used to cover defects, thus reducing sensitivity and risk of bacterial ingress. Fluoride application may be beneficial under very specific conditions, such as when used in a single application to help strengthen enamel in newly erupted teeth or to decrease sensitivity secondary to root exposure.

Abnormal tooth appearance may also be a result of abnormal occurrences affecting dentin layers. Odontoblasts produce dentin and are susceptible to the same conditions that harm ameloblasts. Unlike the enamel-producing cells, odontoblasts can be replenished, even during their active state; therefore, negative influences are mitigated and damage tends to be less visible.

Odontodystrophies and osteodystrophies tend to be associated with genetic diseases and severely affect both enamel and dentin production.[2] Dentinogenesis imperfecta is an odontodystrophy associated with failure of dentin production. The teeth are effectively blue-hued enamel shells with very thin walls; they are extremely fragile and fracture easily. Treatment is limited to extractions as needed.

Other causes of abnormal tooth color are extrinsic staining and deposition of intrinsic pigments. Intrinsic staining (Figure 103-5) tends to occur from deposition of pigments within the enamel and/or dentin matrix as the tooth is forming, or from pigments entering hematogenously to discolor subsequently forming dentinal layers. As a result, intrinsic staining cannot be removed through polishing. For example, tetracycline (yellow/brown) staining occurs when the antibiotic is given to a pregnant queen, or directly to the kitten while the dentition is still forming. Porphyrins (pink fluorescence [see Figure 103-5A-B]), bilirubin (green), and high iron content (brown/black) in water sources are other sources of intrinsic staining. In human patients, external and

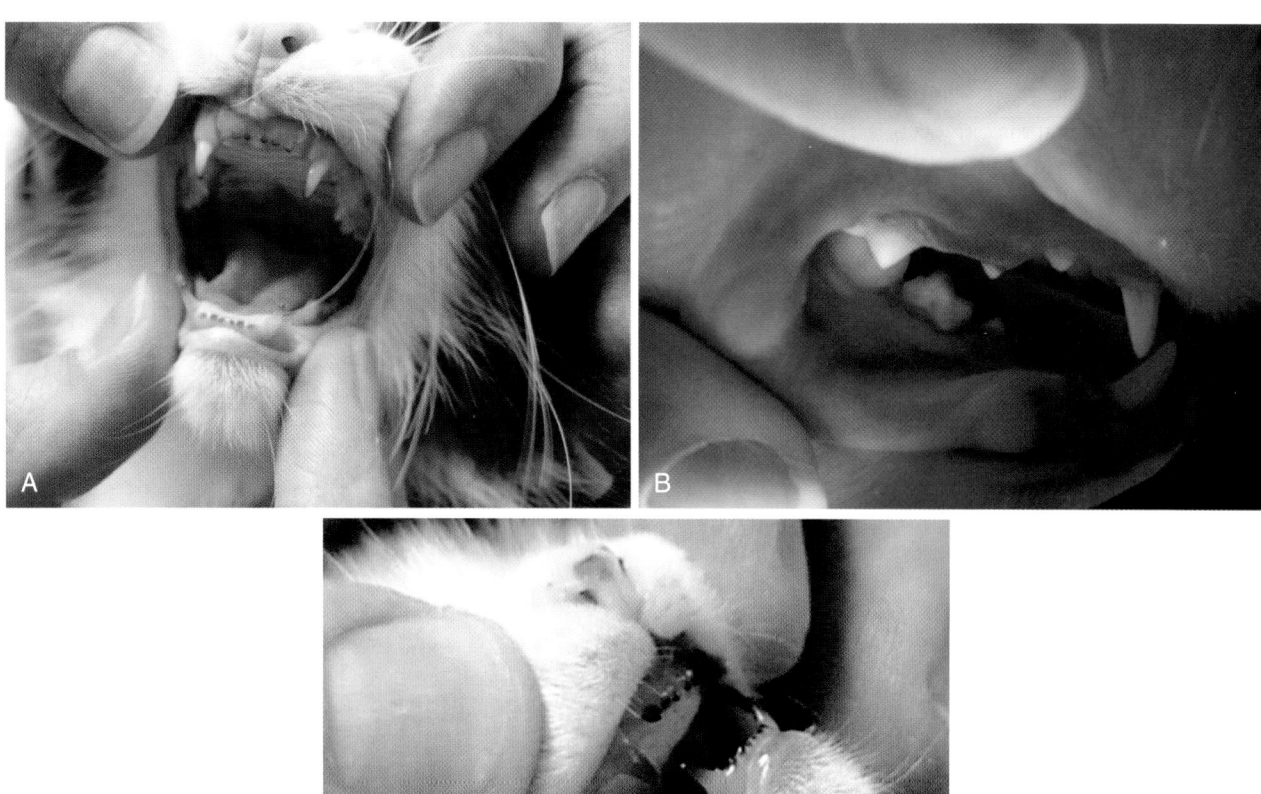

Figure 103-5: Intrinsic staining pigments the teeth as they are forming and cannot be removed by polishing the teeth. Porphyria causes a visible discoloration to the tooth crowns **(A)** that fluoresces pink under black light **(B)**. **C,** Tetracycline causes a yellow-brown discoloration. (**A** and **B,** courtesy of Dr. Emma Thom.)

internal bleaching can lighten stains, and veneers may provide further aesthetic camouflage. These measures are rarely taken in pets.

Extrinsic staining tends to be from contact with a pigmenting substance found in the kitten's environment. An example of this includes the brown discoloration Sphynx kittens are reported to acquire from accumulation of skin oils/waxes on the teeth during nursing and grooming. This extrinsic staining should not be confused with enamel hypoplasia. Chlorhexidine mouth rinses used long term can stain surface plaque brown. Food coloring and dyes from chew objects/toys can also transfer color to the oral cavity. Removal of the inciting agent may be sufficient to allow the discoloration to fade. Polishing of the teeth with a medium grit pumice or polishing paste should result in removal of the extrinsic stain in most cases.

Supereruption

Supereruption can be an age-related manifestation of the normal posteruption physiologic processes that maintain the tooth position within the alveolar bone, or it may be associated with pathology. The normal eruptive tension within the periodontal ligaments continues throughout life and is usually offset by occlusal intrusive forces. An imbalance between eruptive and intrusive forces, combined with cemental hypertrophy (see Hypercementosis) along with senile atrophy of the alveolar processes and gingival recession may increase the length of the clinical crown.[2] Close examination of these teeth will reveal a visible cementoenamel junction, because it is coronal to the alveolar ridge. Prolonged supereruption results in a tooth becoming so extruded that its anchorage is compromised, it may become loose, and the tooth may even get lost during normal mastication. Affected cats may show sensitivity from root exposure. Treatment to reduce this sensitivity may include the professional application of unfilled resins and/or fluoride products.

Pathologic extrusion can occur in association with tooth resorption.[47] Radiographic and histologic assessment of teeth affected with resorption and/or extrusion showed a statistical association between extrusion and root resorption. For this reason, any extruded tooth should be assessed for resorption.

However, because loss of the periodontal ligament space in early replacement resorption can be difficult to differentiate from hypercementosis radiographically, clinical judgment must be employed when making decisions whether or not to extract the tooth.

Hypercementosis

Hypercementosis is a normal, age-related infilling phenomenon,[48-49] which is secondary to the axial movement typically seen in older cats. Radiographs show increased density and thickening of the periapical area secondary to the benign deposition of layers of cementum and increased deposition of periapical alveolar bone. In many cases, the periodontal ligament space is no longer clearly discernible, and the tooth may appear to be fused with the bone. This condition must be distinguished from ankylosis associated with root resorption, because these roots are not undergoing pathologic change and should never be crown amputated. If the tooth requires extraction, the tooth must be extracted in total.

Chronic Alveolitis/Osteitis

Feline chronic alveolitis is a species-specific manifestation of chronic periodontal disease. Alveolitis/osteitis is characterized by inflammation and outward expansion of the bone around a canine tooth, (Figure 103-6) and in some cases, loss of supporting periodontal structures. Treatment involves therapy for periodontal disease and alveoplasty to return the

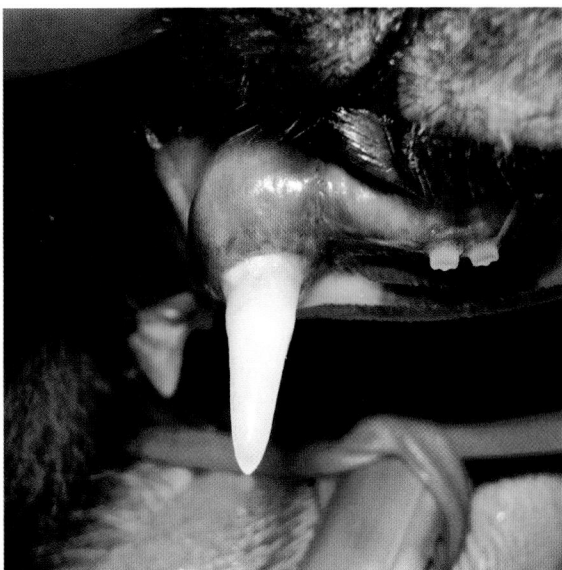

Figure 103-6: Osteitis with bony expansion around the canine tooth and supereruption, which causes the cementoenamel junction to be coronal to the gingiva, can both be signs of periodontal disease in the cat.

bone to more anatomically correct contours, which in the case of extraction, will allow for tension-free closure of the socket.[50-51]

SYMPHYSEAL BONE LOSS AND OPEN-MOUTH JAW LOCKING

In the majority of mammals, the symphysis is a fibrous union joining the two mandibles together to form the lower jaw. With aging, that joint may become lax. Radiographic examination may show a widened symphysis that may be mistaken for traumatic separation. Irregularities in density can also be seen in aging cats, often exacerbated by severe periodontal disease of the mandibular incisor or canine teeth.[52] The significance of a mobile symphysis is controversial. If the cat is asymptomatic, treatment is not needed. If mobility is affecting the ability to eat or is causing pain, dental acrylic can be used to stabilize the fibrous union. Wiring is not recommended as a long-term solution, because the wire can cause inward rotation of the mandibles, which will stress the temporomandibular joints. Additionally, the wires may contribute to gingival trauma.

A small number of cats are presented to practitioners because they are unable to close their mouth. Open-mouth jaw locking likely occurs as a result of symphyseal laxity combined with mildly deformed temporomandibular fossae, which may allow for buccal rotation of the mandibular body and interference of the coronoid process with the zygomatic process. Open-mouth jaw locking with lateral displacement of the coronoid process has been reported in several head types, including dolicocephalic and bracycephalic.[53] Patients present in acute distress, unable to close their mouths, having a palpable swelling lateral to the zygomatic arch on the affected side. Skull radiographs confirm the displacement. Analgesics combined with sedation or anesthesia may allow the mandible to be opened maximally so that the dislocation can be reduced through manipulation of the coronoid process. Recurrence is common. Some cats learn to unlock their jaws themselves. The permanent solution to this problem is to remove a portion of the zygomatic arch and/or the coronoid process,[54] but it may be controlled with intermandibular arthrodesis.[53]

SUMMARY

In the majority of cats with oral variations, early detection via thorough oral examination and dental radiographs, and treatment by astute veterinary practitioners will limit the comorbidity from the conditions described. To date, the veterinary literature has sparse information about many of the conditions listed in this chapter, but as veterinarians become more knowledgeable about genetics and more consistent at detecting and documenting these problems, they should get better data on the frequency and causes of these conditions.

References

1. Wiersig DO, Swenson MJ: Teratogenicity of vitamin A in the canine. *Fed Proc* 26:486, 1967.
2. Barker IK, Van Dreumel AA, Palmer N: The alimentary system. In Jubb KVF, Kennedy PC, Palmer N, editors: *Pathology of domestic animals* (vol 2), ed 3, San Diego, CA, 1985, Academic Press, pp 2–203.
3. McDevitt JM, Gautieri RF, Mann DE, Jr: Comparative teratogenicity of cortisone and phenytoin in mice. *J Pharm Sci* 70(6):631–634, 1981.
4. DeSesso JM: Cell death and free radicals: a mechanism for hydroxyurea teratogenesis. *Med Hypotheses* 5(9):937–951, 1979.
5. Maxwell HS, Nettleton P, Kirkland PD: Overview of congenital and inherited anomalies, *The Merck Veterinary Manual* (website): <www.merckmanuals.com/vet/generalized_conditions/congenital_and_inherited_anomalies/overview_of_congenital_and_inherited_anomalies.html>, (Accessed June 15, 2015).
6. Shelton L, Helmrich HG: Heritable diseases and abnormalities in cats, *The Cat Fanciers' Association* (PDF online): <www.catdnatest.org/pdf/heritable-diseases.pdf>, (Accessed June 15, 2015).
7. Provet: Cleft palate, *Provet Healthcare Information* (website): <www.provet.co.uk/health/diseases/cleftpalate.htm#c>, (Accessed June 15, 2015).
8. Ingwersen W: Congenital and inherited anomalies of the mouth: cleft palate or cleft lip (harelip) complex, *The Merck Veterinary Manual* (website): <http://www.merckmanuals.com/vet/digestive_system/congenital_and_inherited_anomalies_of_the_digestive_system/congenital_and_inherited_anomalies_of_the_mouth.html>, (Accessed June 15, 2015).
9. de Souza HJM, et al: Oronasal fistula repair. In Norsworthy B, Fooshee Grace S, Crystal MA, editors: *The feline patient*, ed 4, New Jersey, 2011, John Wiley & Sons.
10. Vella CM, Shelton LM, McGonagle JJ, et al: *Robinson's genetics for cat breeders and veterinarians*, ed 4, Oxford, 1999, Butterworth-Heinemann.
11. Coruh A, Gunay GK: A surgical conundrum: Tessier number 4 cleft. *Cleft Palate Craniofac J* 42(1):102–106, 2005.
12. Onizuka T, Hosaka Y, Aoyama R, et al: Operations for microforms of cleft lip. *Cleft Palate Craniofac J* 28(3):293–300, 1991.
13. Nemec A, Daniaux L, Johnson E, et al: Craniofacial defects in dogs with congenital palatal defects: CT findings in 9 cases. In *Proceedings of European Congress of Veterinary Dentistry*, Prague, Czech Republic, 2013, pp 98–100.
14. Zook BC, Sostaric BR, Draper DL, et al: Encephalocele and other congenital craniofacial anomalies in Burmese cats. *Vet Med Small Anim Clin* 83:695–701, 1983.
15. Marretta SM: Cleft palate repair techniques. In Verstraete FJM, Lommer MJ, editors: *Oral and maxillofacial surgery in dogs and cats*, Philadelphia, 2012, Saunders, pp 351–361.
16. Cox CL, Hunt GB, Cadier MM: Repair of oronasal fistulae using auricular cartilage grafts in five cats. *Vet Surg* 36(2):164–169, 2007.
17. Lorrain RP, Legendre LF: Oronasal fistula repair using auricular cartilage. *J Vet Dent* 29(3):172–175, 2012.
18. Coles BH, Underwood LC: Repair of the traumatic oronasal fistula in the cat with a prosthetic acrylic implant. *Vet Rec* 122(15):359–360, 1988.
19. de Souza HJ, Amorim FV, Corgozinho KB, et al: Management of the traumatic oronasal fistula in the cat with a conical Silastic prosthetic device. *J Feline Med Surg* 7(2):129–133, 2005.
20. Griffiths LG, Sullivan M: Bilateral overlapping mucosal single-pedicle flaps for correction of soft palate defects. *J Am Anim Hosp Assoc* 37(2):183–186, 2001.
21. Sager M, Nefen S: Use of buccal mucosal flaps for the correction of congenital soft palate defects in three dogs. *Vet Surg* 27(4):358–363, 1998.
22. Shelton GD: Swallowing disorders in the dog. *Compend Contin Educ Pract Vet* 4:607–613, 1982.
23. Sylvestre AM: Management of a congenitally shortened soft palate in a dog. *J Am Vet Med Assoc* 211(7):875–877, 1997.
24. Crossley DA: Survey of feline dental problems encountered in a small animal practice in NW England. *Brit Vet Dent Assoc J* 2:3–6, 1991.
25. Stockard CR: *The genetic and endocrine basis for differences in form and behavior as elucidated by studies of contrasted pure-line dog breeds and hybrids, Am Anat Memoirs*, Philadelphia, 1941, Wistar Institute.
26. American Veterinary Dental College (AVDC): *Classification of dental occlusion in dogs, American Veterinary Dental College* (website): <AVDC.org/nomenclature.html#occlusion>, (Accessed June 15, 2015).
27. Wilson G: Timing of apical closure of maxillary canine teeth and mandibular first molar teeth of cats. *J Vet Dent* 16(1):19–21, 1999.
28. Ten Cate AR: Tooth eruption. In Bhaskar SN, editor: *Orban's oral histology and embryology*, ed 11, St Louis, 1991, Mosby.
29. Ten Cate AR, Anderson RD: An ultrastructural study of tooth resorption in the kitten. *J Dent Res* 65:1087, 1986.
30. Ten Cate AR: *Oral histology, development, structure and Function*, St Louis, 1989, Mosby.
31. Rawlinson JE, Lewis JR: Oral masses: cystic, benign and malignant. In *Proceedings of American College of Veterinary Internal Medicine Forum*, San Antonio, 2008, pp 49–51.
32. Kramer IRH, Pindborg JJ, Shear M: *Histological typing of odontogenic tumours*, ed 2, Berlin, 1992, Springer-Verlag, pp 16–21.
33. Verstraete FJM: Odontogenic tumors. In *Proceedings of World Small Animal Veterinary Association Congress*, Jeju, Korea, 2011.
34. Papadimitriou S, Kouki M, Doukas D, et al: Compound maxillary odontoma in a young cat. In *Proceedings of European Congress of Veterinary Dentistry*, Lisbon, Portugal, 2012, pp 187–188.
35. Hoffman S: Abnormal tooth eruption in a cat. *J Vet Dent* 25(2):118–122, 2008.
36. Gioso MA, Gomes Carvalho VG: Maxillary dentigerous cyst in a cat. *J Vet Dent* 20(1):28–30, 2003.
37. D'Astous J: An overview of dentigerous cysts in dogs and cats. *Can Vet J* 52(8):905–907, 2011.
38. Vieira AL, Ocarino NM, Boeloni JN, et al: Congenital oligodontia of the deciduous teeth and anodontia of the permanent teeth in a cat. *J Feline Med Surg* 11(2):156–158, 2009.
39. Elzay RP, Hughes RD: Anodontia in a cat. *J Am Vet Med Assoc* 154(6):667–670, 1969.
40. Verstraete FJM, van Aarde RJ, Nieuwoudt BA, et al: The dental pathology of feral cats on Marion Island, part 1: congenital, developmental and traumatic abnormalities. *J Comp Path* 115(3):265–282, 1996.
41. Moriello KA: Hereditary alopecia and hypotrichosis, *The Merck Veterinary Manual* (website): <www.merckmanuals.com/vet/integumentary_system/congenital_and_inherited_anomalies_of_the_integumentary_system/hereditary_alopecia_and_hypotrichosis.html>, (Accessed June 15, 2015).
42. Fleming PS, Xavier GM, DiBiase AT, et al: Revisiting the supernumerary: the epidemiological and molecular basis of extra teeth. *Br Dent J* 208(1):25–30, 2010.
43. D'Souza RN, Klein OD: Unraveling the molecular mechanisms that lead to supernumerary teeth in mice and men: current concepts and novel approaches. *Cells Tissues Organs* 186(1):60–69, 2007.
44. Kallenbach E: Fine structure of differentiating ameloblasts in the kitten. *Am J Anat* 145:283, 1976.
45. Weinmann JP: Developmental disturbances of the enamel. *Burns* 43:20, 1943.
46. Weinmann JP, Svoboda JF, Woods RW: Hereditary disturbances of enamel formation and calcification. *J Am Dent Assoc* 32:397, 1945.
47. Harvey CE, Flax BM: Feline oral-dental radiographic examination and interpretation. *Vet Clin North Am Small Anim Pract* 22(6):1279–1295, 1992.
48. Reiter AM: Symphysiotomy, symphysiectomy, and intermandibular arthrodesis in a cat with open-mouth jaw locking—case report and literature review. *J Vet Dent* 21(3):147–158, 2004.
49. Lantz GC: Temporomandibular joint dysplasia. In Verstraete FJM, Lommer MJ, editors: *Oral and maxillofacial surgery in dogs and cats*, Philadelphia, 2012, Saunders, pp 531–537.

50. Lewis JR, Okuda A, Shofer FS, et al: Significant association between tooth extrusion and tooth resorption in domestic cats. *J Vet Dent* 25(2):86–95, 2008.

51. Grue H, Jensen B: Review of the formation of incremental lines in tooth cementum of terrestrial animals. *DRGBAH* 11(3):3–44, 1979.

52. Nakanishi N, Ichinose F, Higa G, et al: Age determination of the Iriomote cat by using cementum annuli. *J Zool* 279:338–348, 2009.

53. Southerden P: Review of feline oral disease: 2. Other common conditions. *In Pract* 32:51–56, 2010.

54. Peak M: Managing mouths in cats. In *Proceedings of North American Veterinary Conference*, Orlando, FL, 2005, p 219.

Index

Page numbers followed by "*f*" indicate figures, "*b*" indicate boxes, and "*t*" indicate tables.

1034